# SPINE SURGERY

**VOLUME TWO**

Second Edition

## Techniques, Complication Avoidance, and Management

WITHDRAWN

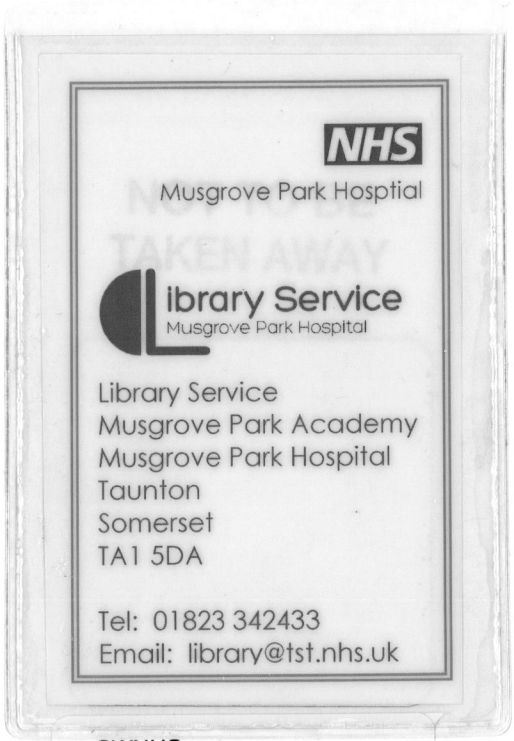

# SPINE SURGERY

**VOLUME TWO**

**Second Edition**

## Techniques, Complication Avoidance, and Management

### EDWARD C. BENZEL, MD

Chairman, Cleveland Clinic Spine Institute
Vice Chairman, Department of Neurosurgery
The Cleveland Clinic Foundation
Cleveland, Ohio

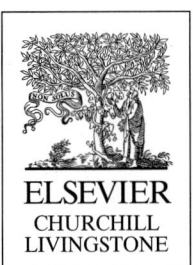

**ELSEVIER**
CHURCHILL
LIVINGSTONE

**ELSEVIER**
CHURCHILL
LIVINGSTONE

The Curtis Center
170 S Independence Mall W 300E
Philadelphia, Pennsylvania 19106

SPINE SURGERY: TECHNIQUES, COMPLICATION AVOIDANCE,
AND MANAGEMENT
**Copyright 2005, Elsevier, Inc. All rights reserved.**

ISBN 0-443-06616-7

---

**NOTICE**

Surgery is an ever-changing field. Standard safety precautions must be followed, but as new research
and clinical experience broaden our knowledge, changes in treatment and drug therapy become
necessary or appropriate. Readers are advised to check the product information currently provided by
the manufacturer of each drug to be administered to verify the recommended dose, the method and
duration of administration, and contraindications. It is the responsibility of the treating physician,
relying on experience and knowledge of the patient to determine dosages and the best treatment for
the patient. Neither the Publisher nor the editor assumes any responsibility for any injury and/or
damage to persons or property.

---

First edition 1999.

**Library of Congress Cataloging-in-Publication Data**

Spine surgery: techniques, complication avoidance, and management / [edited by] Edward
  C. Benzel.– 2nd ed.
    p. ; cm.
  Includes bibliographical references and index.
  ISBN 0-443-06616-7
    1. Spine–Surgery. I. Benzel, Edward C.
  [DNLM: 1. Spinal Diseases–surgery. 2. Spinal Diseases–complications.
  3. Spine–surgery. WE 725 S7599 2005]
  RD768.S684 2005
  617.5'6059–dc22

                                                    2004045517

Acquisitions Editor: *Rebecca Schmidt Gaertner*
Developmental Editor: *Agnes Hunt Byrne*
Publishing Services Manager: *Joan Sinclair*
Project Manager: *Daniel Clipner*

Printed in the United States of America.

Last digit is the print number:   9   8   7   6   5   4   3   2   1

*This book is dedicated to my wife, Mary; my children, Morgan, Jason, Brian, and Matthew; and my mother and father, Anna and Carl, for their past and present encouragement, tolerance, and guidance.*

*A special thanks to Christine Moore for her energy, diligence, and effort, as well as her continued and perpetual commitment to this project; to all the contributors for their masterful "works" and for the privilege of their friendships, both new and old; and to prior residents and fellows, who have provided energy, encouragement, and guidance.*

# Contributors

Mark F. Abel, MD
Professor, Department of Orthopedics, University of
Virginia School of Medicine, Charlottesville, Virginia

Kuniyoshi Abumi, MD, Dr Med Sci
Professor, Department of Orthopaedic Surgery, Health
Administration Center, Hokkaido University, Sapporo,
Japan

Mark S. Adams, MD
Saginaw Valley Neurosurgery, Saginaw, Michiga

Cary D. Alberstone, MD
Ventura County Neurosurgery Associates, Oxnard,
California

Joseph T. Alexander, MD
Assistant Professor, Department of Neurosurgery, Wake
Forest University School of Medicine, Winston-Salem,
North Carolina

John A. Anson, MD, FACS
Las Vegas, Nevada

Ronald I. Apfelbaum, MD
Professor of Neurosurgery, Department of Neurosurgery,
University of Utah Health Sciences Center, Salt Lake
City, Utah

Paul M. Arnold, MD
Professor of Neurosurgery, Department of Surgery,
University of Kansas Medical Center, Kansas City,
Kansas

L. Brett Babat, MD
Premier Orthopaedics and Sports Medicine, Nashville,
Tennessee

Julian E. Bailes, MD
Professor and Chairman, Department of Neurosurgery,
West Virginia University, Morgantown, West Virginia

Jamie Baisden, MD
Assistant Professor of Neurosurgery, Medical College
of Wisconsin, Milwaukee, Wisconsin

Nevan G. Baldwin, MD, FACS
Clinical Associate Professor, Texas Tech University,
Lubbock, Texas

Perry A. Ball, MD
Dartmouth-Hitchcock Medical Center, Lebanon,
New Hampshire

Giancarlo Barolat, MD
Thomas Jefferson University Hospital, Philadelphia,
Pennsylvania

H. Hunt Batjer, MD
Department of Neurosurgery, Northwestern University
Medical School, Chicago, Illinois

Thomas W. Bauer, MD, PhD
Departments of Orthopaedic Surgery and Pathology, The
Cleveland Clinic Foundation, Cleveland, Ohio

James R. Bean, MD
Neurosurgical Associates, Lexington, Kentucky

Brion J. Beerle, MD
Chair, Department of Anesthesiology, Alaska Regional
Hospital, Anchorage, Alaska

Gordon R. Bell, MD
The Cleveland Clinic Foundation, Cleveland, Ohio
Cleveland Clinic Spine Institute

Gregory J. Bennett, MD
Clinical Director-Neurosurgery, Erie County Medical
Center, Buffalo, New York

Edward C. Benzel, MD
Chairman, Cleveland Clinic Spine Institute,
Vice Chairman, Department of Neurosurgery,
The Cleveland Clinic Foundation, Cleveland, Ohio

Darren Bergey, MD
Loma Linda University Medical Center, Loma Linda,
California

Marc L. Bertrand, MD
Assistant Professor and Director, Neuroanesthesia,
Department of Anesthesiology, Dartmouth-Hitchcock
Medical Center, Lebanon, New Hampshire

Mark H. Bilsky, MD
Memorial Sloan Kettering Cancer Center, New York,
New York

Barry D. Birch, MD
Department of Neurosurgery, Mayo Clinic Scottsdale,
Scottsdale, Arizona

Robert S. Biscup, MS, DO, FAOAO
Cleveland Clinic Florida Spine Center, Weston, Florida

Kevin Blaylock, CPA
CFO, Neuroscience Specialists, CEO, Oklahoma Spine
Hospital, LLC, Oklahoma City, Oklahoma

Oheneba Boachie-Adjei, MD
Hospital for Special Surgery, New York, New York

Maxwell Boakye, MD
Assistant Professor of Neurosurgery,
Stanford School of Medicine, Stanford, California

**Scott D. Boden, MD**
Professor of Orthopaedics, Director, The Emory Spine
Center, Emory University School of Medicine, Atlanta,
Georgia

**Henry Bohlman, MD**
Professor, Case Western Reserve University and
University Hospitals, Cleveland, Ohio

**Michael Bolesta, MD**
Associate Professor, Department of Orthopedics,
Southwestern Medical School, Dallas, Texas

**Mary B. Bondy, MBA**
Cleveland Clinic Spine Institute, The Cleveland Clinic
Foundation, Cleveland, Ohio

**Christopher M. Boxell, MD**
Oklahoma Spine & Brain Institute, Tulsar, Oklahoma

**Keith H. Bridwell, MD**
Washington University School of Medicine, St. Louis,
Missouri

**Darrell S. Brodke, MD**
Associate Professor, Department of Orthopedics,
Director, Spine Service, University of Utah, Salt Lake
City, Utah

**James Butler, MD**
Resident, Department of Neurosurgery, The Cleveland
Clinic Foundation, Cleveland, Ohio

**David W. Cahill, MD (deceased)**
Department of Neurosurgery, College of Medicine,
University of South Florida, Tampa, Florida

**Robert C. Cantu, MA, MD, FACS, FACSM**
Chief, Neurosurgery Service and Director, Service
Sports Medicine, Emerson Hospital, Concord,
Massachusetts; Adjunct Professor, Exercise and Sport
Science, University of North Carolina, Chapel Hill,
North Carolina

**Allen L. Carl, MD**
Professor, Division of Orthopaedic Surgery, Albany
Medical College, Albany, New York

**John A. Carrino, MD, MPH**
Assistant Professor of Radiology, Harvard Medical
School, Clinical Director, Magnetic Resonance Therapy
Program, Co-Director, Spine Intervention Service,
Boston, Massachusetts

**John R. Caruso, MD**
Neurosurgical Specialists, LLC, Hagerstown, Maryland

**Andrew G. Chenelle, MD, MS**
DuPage Neurosurgery, S.C., Glen Ellyn, Illinois

**Joseph S. Cheng, MD**
Assistant Professor and Co-Director, Section of Spinal
Surgery, Department of Neurosurgery, Vanderbilt
Medical Center North, Nashville, Tennessee

**Yong-Jun Cho, MD**
Department of Neurosurgery, Stanford University,
Stanford, California

**Tanvir F. Choudhri, MD**
Assistant Professor and Director, Neurosurgery Spine
Program, Department of Neurosurgery, Mount Sinai
Medical Center, New York, New York

**Frank Conguista, MD**
Resident, Division of Orthopaedic Surgery, Albany
Medical College, Albany, New York

**Edward S. Connolly, MD**
Professor of Neurosurgery, Ochsner Clinic Foundation,
Louisiana State University School of Medicine, New
Orleans, Louisiana

**Paul R. Cooper, MD**
Professor of Neurosurgery, New York University School
of Medicine, New York, New York

**Jean-Valéry C.E. Coumans, MD**
Department of Neurosurgery, Massachusetts General
Hospital, Boston, Massachusetts

**Albert E. Cram, MD**
Professor, Department of Neurosurgery, University of
Iowa Hospitals and Clinics, Iowa City, Iowa

**H. Alan Crockard, MD**
The National Hospital for Neurology and Neurosurgery,
London, United Kingdom

**Richard Crownover, MD**
The Cleveland Clinic Foundation, Cleveland,
Ohio

**Bryan W. Cunningham, MD**
Director, Biomechanics Laboratory, Union Memorial
Hospital, Baltimore, Maryland

**William T. Curry, Jr, MD**
Department of Neurosurgery, Massachusetts General
Hospital, Boston, Massachusetts

**Joseph F. Cusick, MD**
Professor, Medical College of Wisconsin, Madison,
Wisconsin

**Scott D. Daffner, MD**
Thomas Jefferson University, Philadelphia,
Pennsylvania

**Mark D. D'Alise, MD, FACS**
Neurosurgical Associates, Complex and Reconstructive
Spinal Surgery, Lubbock, Texas

**Vinay Deshmukh, MD**
Carolina Neurosurgery and Spine, Charlotte,
North Carolina

**Denis DiAngelo, MD**
Associate Professor, School of Biomechanical
Engineering, University of Tennessee Health Science
Center, Memphis, Tennessee

**Curtis A. Dickman, MD**
Associate Chief, Spine Section, Director, Spinal
Research, Division of Neurological Surgery, Barrow
Neurosurgical Associates, Phoenix, Arizona

**Thomas B. Ducker, MD**
Maryland Neurological Institute, Annapolis, Maryland

**Scott T. Dull, MD, FACS**
Neurosurgical Network, Toledo, Ohio

**Stewart B. Dunsker, MD**
Emeritus Faculty, Mayfield Clinic and Spine Institute,
Cincinnati, Ohio

**Michael J. Ebersold, MD**
Professor of Neurosurgery, Mayo Clinic College of
Medicine, Department of Neurologic Surgery, Luther
Middlefort Clinic—Mayo Health System, Eau Claire,
Wisconsin

**Jason Eckhardt**
Spine Research Laboratory, The Cleveland Clinic
Foundation, Cleveland, Ohio

**Bruce L. Ehni, MD**
Neurosurgical Group of Texas; and Clinical Associate
Professor, Baylor College of Medicine, Houston, Texas

**Matthew Eichenbaum, MD**
Spine Research Fellow, Department of Orthopaedic
Surgery, Thomas Jefferson University and the Rothman
Institute, Philadelphia, Pennsylvania

**Kurt M. Eichholz, MD**
Resident, Department of Neurosurgery, University
of Iowa, Iowa City, Iowa

**Marc E. Eichler, MD**
Division of Spine Surgery, Department of Neurosurgery,
Brigham and Women's Hospital, Boston, Massachusetts

**Samer K. Elbabaa, MD**
Resident, Division of Neurosurgery, Department of
Surgery, University of North Carolina at Chapel Hill,
Chapel Hill, North Carolina

**Sanford E. Emery, MD, MBA**
Professor and Chairman, Department of Orthopaedics,
West Virginia University, Morgantown, West Virginia

**Nancy E. Epstein, MD**
Clinical Professor of Neurological Surgery,
The Albert Einstein College of Medicine, Bronx;
Attending in Neurosurgery, Winthrop University
Hospital, Mineola; and The North Shore-Long Island
Jewish Health System, Manhasset, New York

**Jennifer Erdos, MD**
Resident in Orthopedic Surgery, Allegheny General
Hospital, Pittsburgh, Pennsylvania

**Thomas J. Errico, MD**
Associate Professor of Orthopedic and Neurologic
Surgery, New York University School of Medicine,
Chief of the Spine Service, Department of Orthopedic
Surgery, NYU/Hospital for Joint Diseases, New York,
New York

**Tom Faciszewski, MD**
Chairman, Department of Orthopedic Spine Surgery,
Marshfield Clinic, Marshfield, Wisconsin

**Michael G. Fehlings, MD, PhD, FRCS(C)**
Professor of Neurosurgery, Krembil Chair in
Neurological Repair and Regeneration, University
of Toronto; Director Krembil Neuroscience Program,
Heed Spinal Program, Toronto Western Hospital,
University Health Network, Toronto, Ontario,
Canada

**Lisa A. Ferrara, MS, PhDc**
Spine Research Laboratory, The Cleveland Clinic
Foundation, Cleveland, Ohio

**Richard G. Fessler, MD, PhD**
Professor and Chairman, Section of Neurological
Surgery, University of Chicago Hospital, Chicago,
Illinois

**Kevin T. Foley, MD**
Associate Professor, Neurosurgery, University of
Tennessee, Memphis, Tennessee

**Robert M. Galler, DO**
Assistant Professor of Neurosurgery, Stony Brook
University Medical Center, Stony Brook,
New York

**John W. German, MD**
Albany Medical College, Department of Neurosurgery,
Albany, New York

**Alexander J. Ghanayem, MD**
Associate Professor and Chief, Division of Spine Surgery,
Department of Orthpaedic Surgery, Loyola University
Medical Center, Maywood, Illinois

**Zoher Ghogawala, MD**
Assistant Clinical Professor of Neurosurgery, Yale
University School of Medicine, New Haven,
Connecticut

**Vijay K. Goel, PhD**
Professor and Chair, Department of Bioengineering,
University of Toledo, Director, Spine Research Center,
Department of Orthopedics, Medical College of Ohio,
Toledo, Ohio

**Jan Goffin, MD, PhD**
Department of Neurosurgery, Catholic University of
Leuven, University Hospital Gasthuisberg, Leuven,
Belgium

**Ziya L. Gokaslan, MD**
Professor of Neurosurgery, Johns Hopkins University,
Baltimore, Maryland

**Sohrab Gollogly**
University of Utah, Salt Lake City, Utah

**Jorge Gonzalez-Martinez, MD**
Resident, Department of Neurosurgery, The Cleveland
Clinic Foundation, Cleveland, Ohio

**James E. Greensmith, MD, PhD**
Department of Anesthesia, Saint Elizabeth Hospital,
Appleton, Wisconsin

**Jeffrey D. Gross, MD**
Comprehensive Spine and Wellness Center, Ladera
Ranch, California

**Regis W. Haid, Jr, MD**
Atlanta Brain and Spine Care, Atlanta, Georgia

**Andrea L. Halliday MD, PA**
Center for Neurological Disorders, Fort Worth Brain
and Spine Institute, Fort Worth, Texas

**Allan J. Hamilton, MD**
Head of Surgery, University of Arizona Health Sciences
Center, Tucson, Arizona

**Fadi Hanbali, MD**
Assistant Professor of Neurosurgery, University of Texas
Medical Branch, Galveston, Texas

**Jürgen Harms, MD**
Center for Spine Surgery, Department of Orthopedics
and Traumatology, Klinikum Karlsbad-Langensteinbach,
Karlsbad-Langensteinbach, Germany

**James S. Harrop, MD**
Assistant Professor, Division of Spinal Surgery,
Department of Neurosurgery, Neurosurgical Director,
Delaware Valley Spinal Cord Injury Center, Thomas
Jefferson University, Philadelphia, Pennsylvania

**Blaine I. Hart, MD**
Professor, Department of Radiology, University of
New Mexico School of Medicine, Albuquerque,
New Mexico

**Robert A. Hart, MD, MA**
Chief, Spine Section, Assistant Professor, Department
of Orthopaedic Surgery, Oregon Health and Science
University, Portland Shriner's Hospital, Portland, Oregon

**Robert F. Heary, MD**
Associate Professor of Neurological Surgery, University
of Medicine and Dentistry-New Jersey, New Jersey
Medical School; Director, The Spine Center of New
Jersey, Neurological Institute of New Jersey, Newark,
New Jersey

**Fraser C. Henderson, MD**
Associate Professor of Neurosurgery, Director of
Neurosurgery of the Spine and Craniocervical Junction,
Georgetown University Medical Center, Washington, D.C.

**Patrick W. Hitchon, MD**
Professor, Department of Neurosurgery, University of
Iowa Hospitals and Clinics, Iowa City, Iowa

**James P. Hollowell, MD**
Integrated Spine Care, Milwaukee, Wisconsin

**Paul J. Holman, MD**
Department of Neurosurgery, Cleveland Clinic
Foundation, Cleveland, Ohio

**John K. Houten, MD**
Associate Professor, Department of Neurological Surgery,
Montefiore Hospital, Albert Einstein/Jaboni Hospital,
Bronx, New York

**Robert E. Isaacs, MD**
Head, Section of Minimally Invasive Spine Surgery,
Cleveland Clinic Florida Spine Institute, Weston, Florida

**Manabu Ito, MD, Dr Med Sci**
Assistant Professor, Department of Orthpaedic Surgery,
Hokkaido University Graduate School of Medicine,
Sapporo, Japan

**John A. Jane, Jr, MD**
Department of Neurological Surgery, University of
Virginia, Charlottesville, Virginia

**J. Patrick Johnson, MD**
Co-Director, Cedars-Sinai Institute for Spinal Disorders,
Los Angeles, California

**Christopher Kager, MD**
Lancaster Neuroscience and Spine Association,
Lancaster, Pennsylvania

**Iain H. Kalfas, MD**
Head, Section of Spinal Surgery, Department
of Neurosurgery, Cleveland Clinic Foundation,
Cleveland, Ohio

**George J. Kaptain, MD**
Loma Linda University Medical Center, Loma Linda,
California

**Saad Khairi, MD**
Spine Fellow, Cedars-Sinai Institute for Spinal Disorders,
Los Angeles, California

**Daniel H. Kim, MD**
Associate Professor and Director, Spinal and Peripheral
Nerve Surgery, Depatment of Neurosurgery, Stanford
University Medical School, Stanford, California

**David H. Kim, MD**
Attending Spinal Surgeon, The Boston Spine Group,
Boston, Massachusetts

**Thomas A. Kopitnik, Jr., MD**
University of Texas Southwestern Medical Center at
Dallas, Dallas, Texas

**Robert J. Kowalski, MD, MS, PE**
Resident, Department of Neurosurgery, The Cleveland
Clinic Foundation, Cleveland, Ohio

**Ajit A. Krishnaney, MD**
Department of Neurosurgery, Cleveland Clinic
Foundation, Cleveland, Ohio

**John A. Lancon, MD**
Associate Professor of Neurosurgery and Pediatrics,
Blair E. Batson Hospital for Children, The University
of Mississippi Medical Center, Jackson, Mississippi

**Giuseppe Lanzino, MD**
Associate Professor, Department of Neurosurgery,
University of Illinois College of Medicine at Peoria, Peoria,
Illinois

**Sanford J. Larson, MD, PhD**
Medical College of Wisconsin, Department of
Neurosurgery, Milwaukee, Wisconsin

**Jorge Lastra-Power, MD**
Assistant Professor, Neurosurgery Section, University
of Puerto Rico, San Juan, Puerto Rico

**Nathan H. Lebwohl, MD**
Voluntary Associate Professor, Clinical Orthopaedics and
Rehabilitation University of Miami School of Medicine,
Miami, Florida

**Isador H. Lieberman, MD, MBA, FRCS(C)**
Department of Orthopaedics and The Cleveland Clinic
Spine Institute, The Cleveland Clinic Foundation,
Cleveland, Ohio

**Donlin M. Long, MD**
Johns Hopkins University Medical School, Baltimore,
Maryland

**Mark G. Luciano, MD, PhD**
Head, Section of Pediatric and Congenital Neurosurgery,
Department of Neurological Surgery, The Cleveland
Clinic Foundation, Cleveland, Ohio

**Charles A. Luevano, BS**
Component Reliability Development, General Motors
Corp., Milford, Michigan

**Parley M. Madsen III, MD, PhD**
Microsurgery and Brain Research Institute, St. Louis,
Missouri

**Dennis J. Maiman, MD, PhD**
Professor of Neurosurgery, Medical College of Wisconsin
and Clement J Zablocki VA Medical Center, Milwaukee,
Wisconsin

**Jacek M. Malik, MD, PhD**
Peninsula Neurosurgical Associates, Salisbury, Maryland

**David G. Malone, MD**
Oklahoma Spine & Brain Institute, Tulsa, Oklahoma

**Joseph C. Maroon, MD**
Clinical Professor and Vice Chairman, Department of
Neurosurgery, University of Pittsburgh Medical Center,
Pittsburgh, Pennsylvania

**Eric M. Massicotte, MD, MSc, FRCS(C)**
Assistant Professor of Neurosurgery, University
of Toronto, Toronto, Ontario, Canada

**Shunji Matsunaga, MD**
Assistant Professor, Department of Orthopedic Surgery,
Kagoshima Graduate School of Medical and Dental
Sciences, Kagoshima, Japan

**Daniel J. Mazanec, MD, FACP**
Vice Chairman, Cleveland Clinic Spine Institute, The
Cleveland Clinic Foundation; and Associate Professor of
Medicine, Cleveland Clinic Lerner College of Medicine,
Cleveland, Ohio

**Paul C. McAfee, MD**
Chief of Spine Surgery, St. Joseph's Hospital, Baltimore,
Maryland

**Bruce M. McCormack, MD**
Clinical Faculty, University of California San Francisco
Medical Center, San Francisco, California

**Paul C. McCormick, MD, MPH**
Professor of Clinical Neurosurgery, Columbia University
College of Physicians and Surgeons, New York,
New York

**William E. McCormick, MD**
Schwartzapfel Novick, West Islip, New York

**Robert A. McGuire, Jr., MD**
University of Mississippi Medical Center, Jackson, Mississippi

**Robert F. McLain, MD**
The Cleveland Clinic Spine Institute, The Cleveland Clinic Foundation, Cleveland, Ohio

**Nagy Mekhail, MD, PhD**
The Cleveland Clinic Foundation, Cleveland, Ohio

**D. Mark Melton, MD**
Resident, Department of Neurosurgery, College of Medicine, University of South Florida, Tampa, Florida

**Carole A. Miller, MD**
Ohio State University, Department of Neurological Surgery, Columbus, Ohio

**Jared H. Miller, BA**
Case Western Reserve University, Cleveland, Ohio

**Sung Min, MD**
The Cleveland Clinic Foundation, Cleveland, Ohio

**William Mitchell, MD**
Attending Neurosurgeon, JFK Medical Center, Edison, New Jersey

**Junichi Mizuno, MD, PhD**
Associate Professor, Department of Neurological Surgery, Aichi Medical University School of Medicine, Aichi, Japan

**Michael T. Modic, MD**
The Cleveland Clinic Foundation, Cleveland, Ohio

**Howard W. Morgan, Jr, MD**
University of Texas, Southwestern Medical School, Dallas, Texas

**Robert J. Morlock, PhD**
Pfizer Incorporated, Worldwide Outcomes Research, Ann Arbor, Michigan

**Michael A. Morone, MD, PhD**
Deaconess Billings Clinic, Billings, Montana

**Wade M. Mueller, MD**
Assistant Professor of Neurosurgery, Medical College of Wisconsin, Madison, Wisconsin

**Praveen V. Mummaneni, MD**
Assistant Professor, Department of Neurological Surgery, Emory University School of Medicine, Atlanta, Georgia

**John S. Myseros, MD**
Assistant Professor, Division of Neurosurgery, Cincinnati College of Medicine, Staff Pediatric Neurosurgeon, Cincinnati Children's Hospital

**Sait Naderi, MD**
Associate Professor, Department of Neurosurgery, Dokuz Eylul University, Izmir, Turkey

**Dileep Nair, MD**
The Cleveland Clinic Foundation, Cleveland, Ohio

**Hiroshi Nakagawa, MD, PhD**
Professor and Chairman, Department of Neurological Surgery, Aichi Medical University School of Medicine, Aichi, Japan

**Jaime H. Nieto, MD**
Divisions of Neurosurgery and Orthopedic Surgery, Maimonides Medical Center, Brooklyn, New York

**Russ P. Nockels, MD**
Associate Professor, Neurological Surgery, Orthopaedic Surgery and Rehabilitation, Loyola University Medical Center, Maywood, Illinois

**Bruce E. Northrup, MD**
Professor Emeritus, Department of Neurosurgery, Thomas Jefferson University, Philadelphia, Pennsylvania

**Chima Ohaegbulam, MD**
Resident, Department of Neurosurgery, Brigham and Women's Hospital, Harvard Medical School, Boston, Massachusetts

**Tunc Oktenoglu, MD**
VKV Amerikan Hastanesi, Nisantasi, Istanbul, Turkey

**Bernardo Jose Ordonez, MD**
Neurosurgical Associates, Norfolk, Virginia

**Jeffrey H. Owen, PhD**
Sentient Medical Systems, Cockeysville, Maryland

**A. Fahir Özer, MD**
American Hospital, Istanbul, Turkey

**Stephen M. Papadopoulos, MD**
Director of Surgical Navigation, Barrow Neurosurgical Institute, Phoenix, Arizona

**Christopher G. Paramore, MD**
Lake Norman Neurological and Spine Surgery, Mooresville, North Carolina

**Robert S. Pashman, MD**
Director, Scoliosis and Spinal Deformity, Cedars-Sinai Institute for Spinal Disorders, Los Angeles, California

**Warwick J. Peacock, MD**
Professor Emeritus, Department of Neurosurgery, University of California, San Francisco, San Francisco, California

**Stanley Pelofsky, MD**
Neuroscience Specialists, Oklahoma City, Oklahoma

**Noel I. Perin, MD, FRCS, FACS**
Clinical Associate Professor, Department of
Neurosurgery, St. Luke's/Roosevelt Hospital Center,
New York, New York

**Christopher J. Pham, DO**
Department of Neurosurgery, Stanford University
Hospital School, Stanford, California

**Rick J. Placide, MD, PT**
West End Orthopaedic Clinic, Richmond, Virginia

**Branko Prpa, MD**
All Saints Healthcare, Racine, Wisconsin

**Gregory J. Przybylski, MD**
John F. Kennedy Medical Center, Edison, New Jersey

**Ashraf A. Ragab, MD**
University of Mississippi Medical Center, Jackson,
Mississippi

**Y. Raja Rampersaud, MD, FRCS(C)**
Assistant Professor, Division Orthopedic Surgery,
University of Toronto; Spinal Program, Krambil
Neuroscience Center, Toronto Western Hospital,
University Health Network, Toronto, Ontario, Canada

**Peter A. Rasmussen, MD**
Department of Neurosurgery, The Cleveland Clinic
Foundation, Cleveland, Ohio

**Richard B. Raynor, MD**
Clinical Professor of Neurosurgery, New York University
School of Medicine, New York, New York

**Gary L. Rea, MD, PhD**
Department of Orthopaedics, Ohio State University
Hospital East, Columbus, Ohio

**Glenn R. Rechtine, MD**
Dunspaugh-Dalton Professor of Spinal Surgery,
Department of Neurosurgery, University of Florida,
Gainesville, Florida

**John Regan, MD**
Medical Director, Institute for Spinal Disorders,
Cedars-Sinai Medical Center, Los Angeles, California

**Setti S. Rengachary, MD**
Associate Chairman and Professor, Department of
Neurological Surgery, Wayne State University, Detroit
Medical Center, Detroit, Michigan

**Daniel K. Resnick, MD**
Associate Professor, Department of Neurosurgery,
University of Wisconsin Medical School, Madison,
Wisconsin

**Laurence D. Rhines, MD**
Assistant Professor and Director, Spine Program,
Department of Neurosurgery, University of Texas MD
Anderson Cancer Center, Houston, Texas

**Albert J. Rhoton, MD**
Chairman Emeritus, Department of Neurosurgery,
University of Florida – Gainesville, Gainesville, Florida

**Donna J. Rodriguez, MS, RD, CNSD**
Former Visiting Professor/Lecturer, College of
Education, Nutrition/Dietetics Program, University of
New Mexico; Professional Healthcare Writer, Lovelace
Healthcare Innovations, Lovelace Health Systems,
Albuquerque, New Mexico

**Gerald E. Rodts, Jr, MD**
Associate Professor and Director of Neurosurgery Spine,
Department of Neurological Surgery, Emory University,
Atlanta, Georgia

**Michael J. Rosner, MD**
Department of Neurosurgery, Walter Reed Army
Medical Center, Washington, DC

**Alexander Sah, MD**
Resident, Harvard Medical School Combined
Orthopedic Residency Program, Boston, Massachusetts

**Jared P. Salinsky, DO**
Resident, Department of Orthopedic Surgery,
NSUCOM/Parkway Regional Medical Center, North
Miami Beach, Florida

**Paul Santiago, MD**
Assistant Professor, Department of Neurological Surgery,
Washington University School of Medicine, St. Louis,
Missouri

**Mehdi Sarkarati, MD**
Assistant Clinical Professor, Department of Physical
Medicine and Rehabilitation Tufts University School of
Medicine, Healthsouth N.E. Rehabilitation Hospital,
Woburn, Massachusetts

**Richard L. Saunders, MD**
Professor Emeritus of Surgery, Dartmouth-Hitchcock
Medical Center, Lebanon, New Hampshire

**Paul D. Sawin, MD**
Orlando Neurosurgery, Orlando, Florida

**Edward H. Scheid, MD**
Senior Resident, Thomas Jefferson University,
Department of Neurosurgery, Philadelphia,
Pennsylvania

**Meic H. Schmidt, MD**
Assistant Professor and Director, Spinal Oncology,
Department of Neurosurgery, University of Utah
Medical Center, Salt Lake City, Utah

**Michael Schneier, MD**
Neurological Surgery, Philadelphia, Pennsylvania

**Dilip K. Sengupta, MD, Dr Med**
Professor, Department of Orthopaedics, Dartmouth-
Hitchcock Medical Center, Lebanon, New Hampshire

**Christopher I. Shaffrey, MD**
Professor, Department of Neurological Surgery,
University of Virginia School of Medicine,
Charlottesville, Virginia

**Mark E. Shaffrey, MD**
Department of Neurosurgery, University of Virginia
Health System, Charlottesville, Virginia

**Alok D. Sharan, MD**
Albany Medical College, Albany, New York

**Ashwini D. Sharan, MD**
Assistant Professor, Department of Neurosurgery,
Thomas Jefferson University, Philadelphia, Pennsylvania

**Christopher B. Shields, MD, FRCS(C)**
Professor and Norton Hospital Chairman, Department
of Neurological Surgery, University of Louisville,
Louisville, Kentucky

**Frederick A. Simeone, MD**
Department of Neurosurgery, Thomas Jefferson
University, Philadelphia, Pennsylvania

**Kern Singh, MD**
Department of Orthopedic Surgery, Rush Presbyterian
St. Luke's Medical Center, Chicago, Illinois

**Ran Vijai P. Singh, MD**
Neurological Associates, Norfolk, Virginia

**Donald A. Smith, MD**
Associate Professor, Department of Neurosurgery,
College of Medicine, University of South Florida,
Tampa, Florida

**Maurice M. Smith, MD**
Semmes-Murphey Clinic, Germantown, Tennessee

**Volker K.H. Sonntag, MD, FACS**
Vice Chairman and Chief, Spine Section, Division of
Neurological Surgery; Barrow Neurosurgical Associates;
and Director, Residency Program, University of Arizona,
Phoenix, Arizona

**Ivan J. Sosa, MD**
Chief Resident, Neurosurgery Section, University
of Puerto Rico, San Juan, Puerto Rico

**Micheal J. Speck, MD**
The Cleveland Clinic Spine Institute, The Cleveland
Clinic Foundation, Cleveland, Ohio

**Robert F. Spetzler, MD**
Director, Department of Neurosurgery, Barrow
Neurological Institute, Phoenix, Arizona

**Sudhakar T. Sridharan, MD**
Research Director, Department of Rheumatic and
Immunologic Diseases, The Cleveland Clinic
Foundation, Cleveland, Ohio

**Loretta A. Staudt, MS, PT**
University of California Los Angeles, Los Angeles,
California

**Michael P. Steinmetz, MD**
Resident, Department of Neurosurgery, The Cleveland
Clinic Foundation, Cleveland, Ohio

**Charles B. Stillerman, MD**
Clinical Professor of Surgery, University of North Dakota
School of Medicine, Minot, North Dakota

**Kota Suda, MD, Dr Med Sci**
Spine Surgeon, Center for Spinal Injury and Disorder,
Bibai Rosai Hospital, Bibai, Japan

**Sonia Suys, MD**
General Surgeon, Virginia Beach, Virginia

**George W. Sypert, MD**
Southwest Florida Neurosurgical Association, Fort
Myers, Florida

**Charles H. Tator, MD, PhD, MA, FRCSC, FACS**
Director, Canadian Paraplegic Association Spinal Cord
Injury Research Centre, Toronto Western Hospital,
Toronto, Ontario, Hospital

**Nicholas Theodore, MD**
Director, Neurotrauma, Division of Neurological
Surgery, Barrow Neurosurgical Associates, Phoenix,
Arizona

**Ajith J. Thomas, MD**
MeritCare Neuroscience, Fargo, North Dakota

**Nicholas W.M. Thomas, MD**
Department of Neurosurgery, Kings College Hospital,
London, England

**Robert E. Tibbs, Jr., MD**
Mercy Health Center, Oklahoma City, Oklahoma

**Daisuke Togawa, MD, PhD**
Department of Orthopaedics and The Cleveland Clinic
Spine Institute, The Cleveland Clinic Foundation,
Cleveland, Ohio

**Frank J. Tomecek, MD**
Oklahoma Brain & Spine Institute, Tulsa, Oklahoma

**Richard M. Toselli, MD**
University of North Carolina at Chapel Hill, Chapel Hill,
North Carolina

**Vincent C. Traynelis, MD**
Professor, Department of Neurosurgery, The University
of Iowa, Iowa City, Iowa

**Gregory R. Trost, MD**
Assistant Professor, Departments of Neurosurgery and
Orthopaedic Surgery, University of Wisconsin Medical
School, Madison, Wisconsin

**Eeric Truumees, MD**
Staff Spine Surgeon, William Beaumont Hospital, Royal Oak, Michigan; Orthopedic Director, Gehring Biomechanics Laboratory; and Adjunct Faculty, Wayne State University Biomechanics Center, Detroit, Michigan

**Gary W. Tye, MD**
Department of Neurosurgery, Virginia Commonwealth University Health System, Richmond, Virginia

**Abm Salah Uddin, MD**
John F. Kennedy Medical Center, Edison, New Jersey

**Alexander R. Vaccaro, MD**
Professor of Orthopaedic Surgery, Co-Chief of Spine Surgery, Jefferson Medical College, Thomas Jefferson University, The Rothman Institute; and Co-Director, Delaware Valley Regional Spinal Cord Injury Center, Philadelphia, Pennsylvania

**Ceslovas Vaicys, MD**
Division of Neurosurgery, Memorial Healthcare System, Hollywood, Florida

**Alex Valadka, MD**
Baylor College of Medicine, Texas Medical Center, Houston, Texas

**Arnold B. Vardiman, MD**
Neurological Associates of San Antonio, San Antonio, Texas

**Anthony A. Virella, MD**
Chief Resident, Division of Neurosurgery, University of California Los Angeles Medical Center, Los Angeles, California

**Elizabeth Vitarbo, MD**
University of Miami, Miami, Florida

**Todd W. Vitaz, MD**
University of Louisville, Louisville, Kentucky

**Dennis G. Vollmer, MD**
Division of Neurosurgery, University of Texas Health Science Center at San Antonio, San Antonio, Texas

**Jean-Marc Voyadzis, MD**
Resident, Department of Neurosurgery, Georgetown University Hospital, Washington, D.C.

**John D. Ward, MD**
Professor and Vice Chairman, Department of Neurosurgery, Chief, Pediatric Neurosurgery, Virginia Commonwealth University Health System, Richmond, Virginia

**Joseph Watson, MD**
Assistant Professor, University of California Davis School of Medicine, Davis, California

**John K. Webb, FRCS**
Chairman, Center for Spinal Studies and Surgery, University Hospital, Nottingham, United Kingdom

**Philip R. Weinstein, MD**
University of California San Francisco School of Medicine, San Francisco, California

**Martin W. Weiser, PhD**
Technical Product Manager, Johnson Matthey Electronics, Spokane, Washington

**William C. Welch, MD, FACS**
Associate Professor, Department of Neurological Surgery, University of Pittsburgh Medical Center, Pittsburgh, Pennsylvania

**Simcha J. Weller, MD**
Director, Neurosurgery Spinal Disorders Program, Beth Israel Deaconess Medical Center, Boston, Massachusetts

**L. Erik Westerlund, MD**
CORE Orthopaedic Medical Center, P.C., Encinitas, California

**Jonathan A. White, MD**
University of Texas, Southwestern Medical Center, Dallas, Texas

**Melvin D. Whitfield, MD**
The Cleveland Clinic Spine Institute, The Cleveland Clinic Foundation, Cleveland, Ohio

**Gregory C. Wiggins, MD**
David Grant Medical Center, Travis Air Force Base, California

**Jack E. Wilberger, MD**
Acting Chairman, Department of Neurosurgery, Allegheny General Hospital, Pittsburgh, Pennsylvania

**William S. Wilke, MD**
Department of Rheumatic and Immunologic Diseases, The Cleveland Clinic Foundation, Cleveland, Ohio

**Diana Barrett Wiseman, MD**
Department of Neurosurgery, Naval Hospital, Okinawa, Japan

**W. Putnam Wolcott, MD**
Neurosurgeon, Newport News, Virginia

**Eric J. Woodard, MD**
Assistant Professor and Chief, Section of Spine Surgery, Department of Neurosurgery, Harvard Medical School, Brookline, Massachusetts

**Philip Yazback, MD**
Neuroscience Group of NE Wisconsin, Neenah, Wisconsin

**Narayan Yoganandan, PhD**
Department of Neurosurgery, Medical College of
Wisconsin, Milwaukee, Wisconsin

**Kenneth S. Yonemura, MD**
Assistant Professor, SUNY-Upstate Medical University,
Syracuse, New York

**Kazuo Yonenobu, MD**
Department of Orthopaedic Surgery, Osaka University
Medical School, Osaka, Japan

**Hansen A. Yuan, MD**
Professor, SUNY-Upstate Medical University, Syracuse,
New York

**Seth M. Zeidman, MD**
University of Rochester Medical Center, Rochester,
New York

**Barry M. Zide, MD**
Professor, Department of Surgery (Plastic), New York
University Medical Center, New York, New York

**Mehmet Zileli, MD**
Professor of Neurosurgery, Ege University Faculty of
Medicine, Department of Neurosurgery, Bornova, Izmir,
Turkey

# Preface

This, the second edition, is bigger and (I think) better than the first. This preface is as appropriate for the second edition, as I feel it was for the first. Therefore, it is presented again with minimal modification.

The purpose of this book is to assist the spine surgeon with the avoidance, identification, and management of complications. This differs little from a presentation of operative technique and medical management. Therefore, this book in many respects is a *techniques* book. To achieve its purpose, an understanding of history, decision making, medical management, differential diagnosis, ethics, and even discussions of problems associated with related disorders (such as peripheral nerve injury and metabolic bone diseases) is mandatory. This process requires an understanding of the fundamental basic science components of spine surgery (e.g., anatomy, biomechanics, and physiology).

The book's style was created by its authors, as well as their interactions with each other. In most cases, two or more senior authors were assigned to most chapters. These senior authors were not necessarily chosen on the basis of their philosophical compatibility with their coauthor(s). In fact, coauthors with opposing viewpoints were chosen in many circumstances. Authors were also selected on the basis of experience, educational adeptness, and communication and writing skills. The greater-than-usual number of expert authors contributing to each chapter achieves continuity within the text itself that would not be possible otherwise.

## Risk Taking

Surgery is a risk-taking process. The patient places himself or herself in the hands of the surgeon, and the ensuing decision-making process involves the resolution (or the attempts at such) of many technical and quality-of-life–related issues and dilemmas. A surgical procedure may be warranted if the sum of the costs (both financial and personal) and risks is less than the sum of the benefits. This risk/benefit analysis should be of paramount concern and should be emphasized by the surgeon and realized by the patient. This book is designed to help surgeons achieve their goals, by minimizing the *risk-taking* component of this "equation."

## Opinion and Dogmatism

This book is intended to be used as a textbook, to serve as a reference, and to function as a resource for information. Much information is available in the pages that follow. Perspectives, *pearls*, conventional wisdom, and objective data are presented, as is opinion. Great care has been taken to identify opinion when presented, and to avoid its extreme dogmatism.

It is important to be objective, fair, and nonjudgmental when assessing complications, particularly those of others. There are clearly many ways to effectively and safely accomplish a task. Very infrequently, if ever, does a single method *always* work. What works for one surgeon may not work for another, and vice versa.

## Nomenclature

In this book, some standardization of nomenclature was thought to be important. For example, *ventral* (according to Dorland's, pertaining to the belly or to any venter; denoting a position more toward the belly surface than some other object of reference) is used instead of *anterior* (according to Dorland's, situated in front of or in the forward part of an organ toward the head end of the body; a term used in reference to the ventral or belly surface of the body).[1] Similarly, *dorsal* is used instead of *posterior; rostral* instead of *cephalad;* and *caudal* instead of *caudad.* Exceptions to this are situations in which the term designates a structure or concept that is clearly established (e.g., *anterior* longitudinal ligament).

## Repetition

We learn most effectively by having data presented in a repetitive manner, often from different perspectives, using differing techniques (e.g., written, mathematical, or visual). Truly understanding a concept involves a *spiral*, which often involves multiple exposures to information, so that a solid data base is acquired. New data (raw data) are then added and assimilated. This "expanded" knowledge base can then be applied to, and enhanced by, additional basic science and clinical applications. This entire process is perpetually refined by new experiences, such as clinical encounters or through reading (Figure 1). Repetition is good.

## Standard of Care

Before undertaking the definition of a complication, the issue of standard of care deserves consideration. S. Haines (personal communication) illustrates the discrepancy between the legal definition (the degree of care a reasonable person would take to prevent injury to another) and the evidence-based definition (a generally accepted principle for patient management reflecting a high degree of clinical certainty) of the standard of care. Emphasis on "certainty" by clinicians and its de-emphasis by the legal system are most certainly noteworthy.

## What is a Complication?

Peter McL. Black addressed the issue of defining a complication of neurological surgery in the front matter to *Brain Surgery: Complication Avoidance and Management.*[2] Much of what Black addressed is pertinent to spine surgery. The unique nature of spine surgery, however, dictates the examination of complications from a slightly different approach. The nuances and complexities of the spine and spine surgery are associated with unique concerns.

In order to more clearly understand the nature of a spine surgery complication, each author (of the first

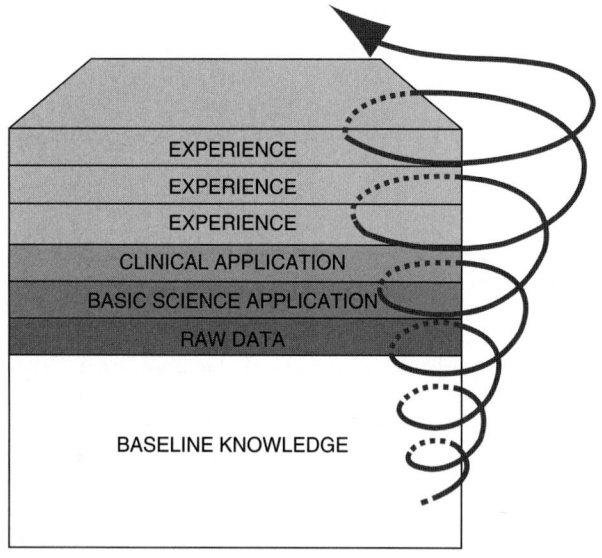

**Figure 1** The Learning Spiral.

The others, which are more routine, are listed. For instance, a urinary tract infection is merely listed, but a wound infection or meningitis is discussed.

4. Any surgical or postsurgical event that prolongs the expected hospitalization must be discussed.
5. Any failure of equipment must be discussed. This includes shunts, stimulators, and internal fixators.
6. All serious events involving non-neurosurgical organ systems are discussed.
7. All postanesthetic complications are discussed in anesthesia morbidity and mortality conference but also must be listed at the neurosurgery morbidity and mortality conference.

Excessive cost is treated as a complication. If there is an outlier, when the cost is extreme, that patient case is discussed.

D. Long reported that after the monthly meeting at his institution, chief residents who present the cases produce a written summary that goes into the minutes of the conference. This details the complication that occurred and the discussion that centered on prevention.

Question 3 shows that the majority of respondents thought that a complication was an adverse event that occurred within 1 month of surgery. This has constituted traditional thinking, but without an objective rationale. Question 4 "spreads out" this field even further.

The majority of authors who responded to Question 5 believed that the younger and healthier the patient in whom a pneumonia occurs after routine surgery, the greater the probability that the pneumonia should be considered a complication. Perhaps this should apply to selected other complications as well.

Regarding Question 6, the authors were split on whether a dural tear that was successfully repaired during surgery signifies a complication. Clinical manifestations of this "tear," however, were relatively consistently considered complications by the authors.

Question 7 revealed an interesting response by the authors. Generally, a pedicle screw fracture was not considered to be a complication if asymptomatic and associated with a solid fusion. However, if there was an associated pseudarthrosis, with or without back pain, this same fracture was generally considered to be a complication. Finally, if the back pain persisted but the fusion was solid, no complication was believed to be present. Therefore, in the authors' opinion, the acquisition of fusion was the main determinant regarding definition of a complication in this circumstance.

Similarly, the responses to Question 8 depict a relatively clear demarcation between symptomatic and asymptomatic pseudarthroses after anterior cervical discectomies. The case of a symptomatic patient with a pseudarthrosis was regarded by the majority of respondents to be a complication, whereas those cases in which a pseudarthrosis was asymptomatic, no complication was thought to be present.

Regarding Question 9, a complaint of back pain at the rostral implant insertion site was not believed to be indicative of a complication by the majority of authors, almost regardless of circumstance.

Question 10, although theoretic, elicited consistent responses. The majority of respondents thought that the quality of *our* medical practices and medical reporting

edition) completed a questionnaire that incorporates some of the concepts and questions used in Black's questionnaire. It was specifically designed to facilitate an understanding of a complication. The results of this questionnaire are reported and discussed for our enlightenment regarding the complications of our "trade." There was a 98% response rate by spine surgeon authors. Fourteen authors, who do not participate significantly in clinical decision making (i.e., engineers, nurses, anesthesiologists, and physiologists), did not complete the questionnaire. What is particularly interesting and revealing is the commentary by the majority (73%) of the respondents.

The first section (Questions 1 and 2) explores surgeon and institutional policy regarding complications. The second section (Questions 3 through 9) concerns the specifics of defining a complication and involves surgeon opinion to a significant degree. Nevertheless, this section provides a baseline for those wishing to derive an "operational definition(s)" of complications. The final question (Question 10) provides a philosophical and speculative slant.

## The Responses

Question 1 reveals that spine surgeons do not have an adequate definition of what constitutes a surgical complication. Question 2 implies that in teaching institutions, there is variability regarding what is to be presented at a morbidity and mortality conference. D. Long provides a pertinent response that is worth sharing. He outlines seven rules for morbidity and mortality conferences:

1. All mortality must be discussed. The case must be presented by the residents and the responsible faculty surgeon must be at the meeting to summarize the mortality.
2. All postoperative neurological change, expected or unexpected, must be presented. The responsible surgeon must be present to discuss the case.
3. All postoperative infections are discussed. Those with serious patient implications are discussed in detail.

would be improved by a more accurate definition of what constitutes a complication. They also believed that quality assurance would be enhanced. They, however, had mixed feelings about whether the medical-legal climate would be improved.

## Author Commentary

The majority of authors not only completed the questionnaire but added comments that were of significant relevance. Although most thought that the questionnaire was of some utility, the responses in this regard varied. They ranged from statements such as "Nice try, Ed, but I think this standardization would be difficult to do and really does not matter. . ." (anonymous) to ". . . a very thought-provoking questionnaire that illustrates well the 'gray areas' involved with the definition of complications." (M. Gallagher)

"You touch on a very important point in that standard agreement of what constitutes a complication is highly subjective. We need to develop an analogue of the Glasgow Outcome Scale for spine that can be more universally applied." (E. Woodard) It is in this vein that perhaps the most clear and concise response regarding the definition of a complication was derived. P. McCormick defined a complication as "an untoward unanticipated adverse event." Although this is clear and concise, it is made more specific by J. Lancon. He defined a complication as "any perioperative event which results in persistence or recurrence of symptoms or the development of new symptoms." B. Northrup defined a complication as "a preventable symptomatic maloccurrence that requires additional treatment. . ." This adds specificity to Lancon's definition while broadening McCormick's.

A. Hamilton defines a complication ". . . as any untoward event occurring to a patient while on the neurosurgical service. These are usually subdivided into errors in diagnosis, errors in management, or errors in technique. By this definition, therefore, the development of a urinary tract infection in a patient who had Foley catheter is considered a complication."

J. Bean provided a particularly relevant medical-legal slant to the definition. He stated, "A complication has no generally agreed meaning until it is operationally defined. A medicolegal definition will of necessity vary from a 'scientific' or clinical definition because the responses to and uses of the information will be different. One focuses on culpability, one on the modification of clinical behavior or decision making."

The most pertinent question, perhaps, is not necessarily what constitutes a complication but what constitutes an avoidable versus non-avoidable complication. More importantly, what constitutes negligence? In this vein, R. Apfelbaum responded, "Complication to me doesn't imply failure to provide adequate care—although it can mean that. Most often, it reflects the fact that we work with a biologic system with multiple variables acting concomi-

tantly. We therefore need to evaluate 'complications,' which can be anything short of a perfect result . . ."

In the future, we should perhaps focus on a further breakdown of the term "complication." Perhaps a simple discussion of the concept of "avoidable" and "nonavoidable" complications is the place to start. The use of refined outcome assessment tools will clearly facilitate this process in the future.

## The Canadian Thistle

What is a complication? We still have not answered this question. Perhaps we never will. It, indeed, has different meanings and implications, depending on both its definer and the circumstances.

Perhaps an analogy is in order. The *Canadian thistle* is considered a weed on the eastern Washington farm on which I grew up. This weed is a destroyer of wheat crops and the *enemy* of the farmer. Its mere presence in a field, in a sense, is a *complication* of farming; a manifestation, perhaps, of inadequate *control* measures and of less than optimal surveillance, early detection, and eradication techniques. If left unchecked, the Canadian thistle is associated with serious detrimental consequences.

In Albuquerque, New Mexico, where my family had made our home in years gone by, the Canadian thistle is annoying to some, unnoticed by others, and considered a flower by many. Beauty is in the eye of the beholder, and, perhaps more relevant here, *ugly* is clearly a matter of perception and perspective, as is fault and blame.

To the spine surgeon, the patient, and the attorney, a complication has different meanings, and often different consequences. Whereas postoperative pain (as subjective as it may be) may not be considered a complication by the surgeon, and occasionally may be annoying and a source of distress to the patient, it may be a source of revenue, and therefore joy, for the attorney. Beauty is clearly in the eye of the beholder, and without question, *ugly* is indeed a matter of perception and perspective.

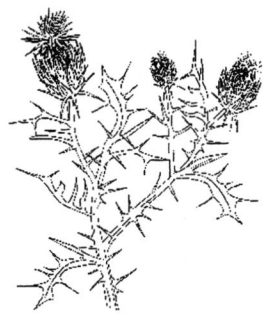

## The Components And Factors Involved With The Definition Of A Complication Of Spinal Surgery: A Survey

1. Does your service have an explicit written (or "understood") definition of what constitutes a surgical complication? If so, could you append it to this questionnaire? If not, would you briefly describe your own concept of a complication under comments below?
   *Yes 9%        No 88%        No response 3%*

2. How do you decide what will be presented at a Morbidity and Mortality conference?
   *Residents decide 31%        Faculty decides 24%*
   *Faculty/residents decide 35%   Other 10%*

3. Do you consider a complication as an adverse event occurring (check all that apply):
   a. *Within 48 hours of surgery 45%*
   b. *Within a week of surgery 46%*
   c. *Within a month of surgery 75%*
   d. *While the patient was in the hospital 43%*
   e. *With reasonable assurance as a result of the surgical manipulation 75%*
   f. *None 23%*

4. Do you consider recurrent sciatica, that is identical to the preoperative lumbar laminotomy pain pattern, to be a complication if it occurs (check all that apply):
   a. *Within 48 hours of surgery 35%*
   b. *Within a week of surgery 36%*
   c. *Within a month of surgery 41%*
   d. *Within 2 months of surgery 25%*
   e. *Within 6 months of surgery 35%*
   f. *None 1%*

5. Do you consider the occurrence of pneumonia to be a complication if it occurs (check all that apply):
   a. *In a 25-year-old postoperative ventilated cervical quadriplegic patient 57%*
   b. *In a 65-year-old postoperative lumbar fusion patient with chronic obstructive pulmonary disease 13%*
   c. *In a 25-year-old nonoperated ventilated cervical quadriplegic patient 45%*
   d. *In a 40-year-old healthy nonsmoker on day 2 following a routine lumbar discectomy 96%*

6a. Do you consider a dural tear, that is successfully repaired during surgery and that has no adverse sequelae, to be a complication of surgery?
   *Yes 43%        No 57%*

6b. Do you consider this same dural tear to be a complication of surgery if (check all that apply):
   a. *It is associated with 2 days of severe positional headaches 74%*
   b. *It is associated with CSF leakage through the wound and that requires lumbar drainage to successfully manage 96%*
   c. *It requires reoperation to manage 96%*

7. Do you consider pedicle screw fracture at 6 months following surgery to be a complication if (check all that apply):
   a. *It is asymptomatic and associated with a solid fusion 24%*
   b. *It is asymptomatic and associated with a pseudarthrosis 65%*
   c. *It is associated with persistent back pain and a solid fusion 38%*
   d. *It is associated with persistent back pain and a pseudarthrosis 86%*
   e. *None of the above 13%*

8. In a patient who has undergone an anterior cervical discectomy with fusion, do you consider a pseudarthrosis (without excessive movement on flexion/extension x-rays) to be a complication if (check all that apply):
   a. *It is asymptomatic 24%*
   b. *It is associated with neck pain 80%*
   c. *It is associated with radicular pain 80%*
   d. *None 15%*

9. One year following a fusion and the placement of a hook-rod system for an unstable L1 fracture in a patient without neurological deficit, the patient complains of back pain at the rostral implant insertion site. Do you consider this a complication if (check all that apply):
   a. *You successfully manage the pain with an exercise program 12%*
   b. *Narcotic analgesics are required to manage the pain 30%*
   c. *The pain is managed successfully by surgical removal of the spinal implant 40%*
   d. *None 52%*

10. If we as surgeons could more accurately define what constitutes a complication (check all that apply):
   a. *Would the quality of our practices be improved?*
      *Yes 63%    No 28%        No response 9%*
   b. *Would medical reporting in the literature be enhanced?*
      *Yes 92%        No 6%        No response 2%*
   c. *Would quality assurance be enhanced?*
      *Yes 76%        No 14%        No response 10%*
   d. *Would the medico-legal climate be:*
      *Worsened  Improved        No effect No*
      *29%        38%            29%        response 4%*
   e. *And if we could simultaneously standardize which complications were the result of negligence, would the medico-legal climate be:*
      *Worsened 20%  Improved 50%  No effect 23%*
      *No response 7%*

The definition of a complication is not as clear as *outsiders* (e.g., the lay public and the legal system) often believe is the case. With all this in mind, and in the best interest of our patients, we should attain and maintain objectivity. We should not be swayed by uneducated or undeserved accolades from the medically naive, or by *threats* from entrepreneurs. Complications must be defined, avoided, identified, and aggressively managed. Their avoidance, identification, and management should not be charged with emotion and anger but attacked with an armamentarium of logic, thoughtfulness, science, and objectivity.

The avoidance, identification, and management of the complications of spine surgery are addressed in the pages that follow by experts in the field. These experts themselves are not infallible. They address complications with which they have had first-hand experience. We must seize the opportunity to benefit from their wisdom and experience. A wise person can learn from the observations and mistakes of others.

Like a Canadian thistle, a complication means different things to different people. We must put complications in their appropriate perspective by clarifying their definition. Then we should actively avoid them and aggressively identify and manage them when they occur.

## Final Comments

Chapter 1 by Robert Grossman, in the sister volume to the first edition of this textbook, is worthy of careful review.[3] His "Maxims Concerning Complications" are repeated here, to emphasize their value.

MAXIMS CONCERNING COMPLICATIONS

Some aphorisms that are useful in guiding one's practice to avoid complications are as follows:

1. There is no such thing as a *simple* neurosurgical (spine surgery) operation.
2. It is easier to stay out of trouble than to get out of trouble.
3. The time expended in avoiding complications will be more than compensated by the time saved in not having to treat them.
4. The patient's well-being is paramount. A neurosurgeon (spine surgeon) should never hesitate to request consultation, or assistance, during surgery.
5. Surgeons should always operate with the meticulousness that they would wish for if they were the patient. It is a salutary exercise for surgeons to think of their own feelings and reactions if they had to undergo the procedures being carried out.

## REFERENCES

1. *Dorland's Illustrated Medical Dictionary,* ed 26. Philadelphia, WB Saunders, 1981.
2. Black P McL: What is a complication in neurological surgery? A practical approach. In Apuzzo MLJ (ed): *Brain Surgery: Complication Avoidance and Management. Supratentorial Procedures.* New York, Churchill Livingstone, 1994, pp xxv-xxviii.
3. Grossman RG: Preoperative and surgical planning for avoiding complications. In Apuzzo MLJ (ed): *Brain Surgery: Complication Avoidance and Management. Supratentorial Procedures.* Churchill Livingstone, New York, 1994, p 9.

# Contents

# Conflict of Interest

In order to minimize bias, the disclosure of potential conflicts of interest is imperative. The following contributors to this book have disclosed financial relationships with industrial partners. These relationships could bias the author's opinion and, therefore, should be considered accordingly.

| Author | Industrial Partner |
|---|---|
| Ronald I. Apfelbaum, MD | Aesculap Instrument Co, Medtronic |
| Giancarlo Barolat, MD | Advanced Neuromodulation System (ANS), Medtronic |
| Edward C. Benzel, MD | DePuy Spine, NuVasive, Orthovita, & Spinal Concepts |
| Scott D. Boden, MD | Medtronic, Centerpulse, Osteotech, & Wright Medical |
| Joseph S. Cheng, MD | Medtronic Sofamor Danek |
| Curtis A. Dickman, MD | Johnson and Johnson & Medtronic |
| Thomas J. Errico, MD | Fastenetix, Medtronic, & Synthes Spine |
| Jan Goffin, MD, PhD | Spinal Dynamics, Medtronic Sofamor Danek |
| Regis W. Haid, Jr., MD | MedTronic; Johnson & Johnson; |
| Allan J. Hamilton, MD | Biogen & Guilford Pharmaceuticals |
| Robert A. Hart, MD, MA | Stryker Howmedic, MedTronic Sofamor Danek; Depuy Spine; Kyphon; Synthes/AO; Orthovita |
| Robert F. Heary, MD | DePuy Spine |
| Patrick W. Hitchon, MD | |
| Iain H. Kalfas, MD | DePuy Spine, Medtronic Sofamor Danek, Synthes Spine, Spine Tech |
| Lawrence G. Lenke, MD | Medtronic Sofamor Danek |
| Alan D. Levi, MD | DePuy Spine & Medtronic |
| Isador H. Lieberman, MD | Kyphon, DePuy Spine, Orthovita |
| Paul C. McAfee, MD | DePuy Spine |
| Nagy Mekhail, MD, PhD | Pfizer, Merck, Medtronic |
| Hiroshi Nakagawa, MD, PhD | Ammtec (Tokyo, Japan) |
| Daniel K. Resnick, MD | NuVasiv, Orthovita |
| Gerald E. Rodts, Jr., MD | Medtronic |
| Christopher B. Shields, MD, FRCS(C) | Norton Healthcare |
| Vincent C. Traynelis, MD | Medtronic Sofamor Danek |
| Kenneth S. Yonemura, MD | Smith & Nephew – Spine |

# CHAPTER 81

# Occult Spinal Dysraphism and the Tethered Spinal Cord

**Gary W. Tye, John D. Ward, and John S. Myseros**

In this chapter the term *occult spinal dysraphism* describes a group of primary embryonic myelodysplastic syndromes that present with or without cutaneous manifestations and frequently, but not invariably, with tethering of the spinal cord. Spinal dysraphism is more common in females than in males by a ratio of at least 2:1. Although not all subtypes of occult spinal dysraphism (e.g., spina bifida associated with congenital lesions of the caudal spinal cord) present with tethering of the distal cord, many do. Their symptoms are frequently quite similar. Therefore, this chapter includes a discussion of the tethered cord syndrome. In addition to the tethered cord from a thickened filum terminale, the clinical entities covered in this chapter include the structural defects found in split cord syndrome, congenital dermal sinuses, and spinal lipomas.

This overlapping of structural pathology and clinical findings may present with few or minimal neurologic deficits, particularly if tension on the ascending spinal cord is not present. Symptoms such as isolated back or lower extremity pain in the young adult may be the first and only symptoms referable to such a congenital lesion. Regardless, the proper surgical treatment of these anomalies is paramount to preserve and improve neurologic function, prevent potential infection, and relieve pain.

Because of the nature of these dysraphic lesions (i.e., breeching of the natural protective barriers of the distal neuraxis, such as incomplete or absent closure of the dorsal elements, enteric or subcutaneous communications with the subarachnoid space, and compromised soft tissues over the spine), repair and treatment are occasionally complicated by infection, cerebrospinal fluid (CSF) leak, and breakdown of compromised tissues. Timing of surgery, meticulous surgical technique, and close postoperative examinations, as always, may aid in avoiding potentially devastating results.

Each entity is approached in the following format: (1) a brief discussion of the basic embryology and pathology, (2) the clinical presentation and appropriate work-up, (3) the indications for surgery, (4) a description of the technical aspects of the operative treatment (with empha-

sis on complication avoidance), (5) the recognition and treatment of complications, and (6) outcome.

## The Tethered Cord Syndrome

### Pathology

The term *tethered cord syndrome,* as used in this chapter, signifies a pathologic fixation of the spinal cord in an abnormally low position so that the spinal cord, with activities and growth, undergoes mechanical stretching, distortion, and ischemia.[22] Many conditions can cause tethering of the spinal cord; these include tight filum terminale, split cord malformations, lipoma, dermal sinus, and meningomyelocele. The remainder of this section addresses the care and treatment of these conditions, excluding meningomyelocele.

### Presentation

The patient with tethered cord presents in one of two groups: symptomatic or asymptomatic. Both groups frequently, but not invariably, have a midline cutaneous dorsal abnormality. These may consist of a dimple, hairy patch, hemangioma, lipoma, or a skin tag (Figure 81.1). If there is no external manifestation, the problem usually goes unrecognized until symptoms begin to develop.

Symptoms, when present, can be grouped into three general areas: sensorimotor, sphincteric, and orthopedic. Sensorimotor symptoms can include pain, delayed walking, sensory loss (usually in the dermatomes of the lumbosacral roots), and motor weakness of the distal leg or foot (the most common symptom, presenting in 76% of cases).[38] Sphincteric symptoms are usually insidious, with frequent urinary tract infections secondary to incomplete emptying, hydronephrosis with renal involvement secondary to reflux, and fecal incontinence. In addition, these patients may develop urinary incontinence or become impotent. The orthopedic problems are related to gait disturbance and abnormalities of the foot or scoliosis. Adult patients with tethered cords may also present with back pain that may radiate to the legs, urinary difficulties, and lower extremity weakness.[1] Patients may present either as asymptomatic in childhood and symptomatic in adulthood or as a progression of symptoms once they reach adulthood perhaps due to repeated microtrauma to the cord.[21] Often in adults the disease may have an insidious onset or may have a predisposing factor such as exercise, lifting heavy loads, or even birth trauma.[1,10]

### Diagnostic Aids

Any infant or child with a midline cutaneous lesion such as a dimple, hair patch, or hemangioma or symptoms mentioned earlier may be suspected as having a tethered cord[7]; the work-up is to determine the anatomy of the anomaly.

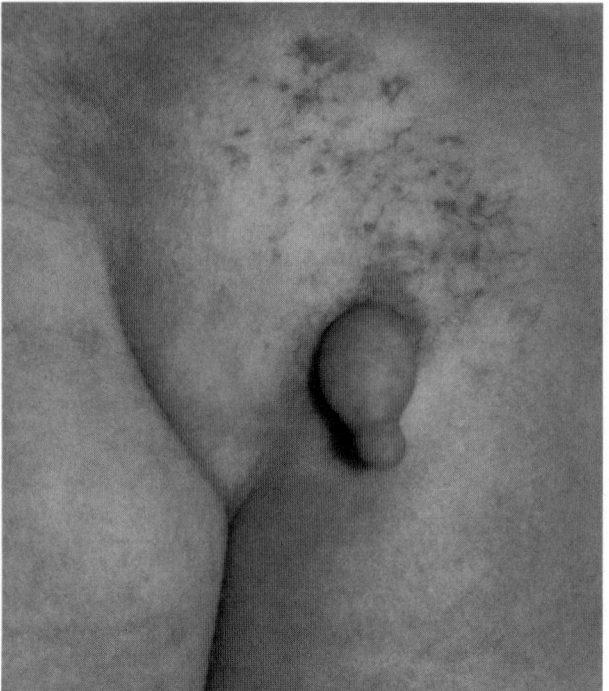

**Figure 81.1** Skin tag and angiomatous changes in a child with a tethered cord and spinal lipoma.

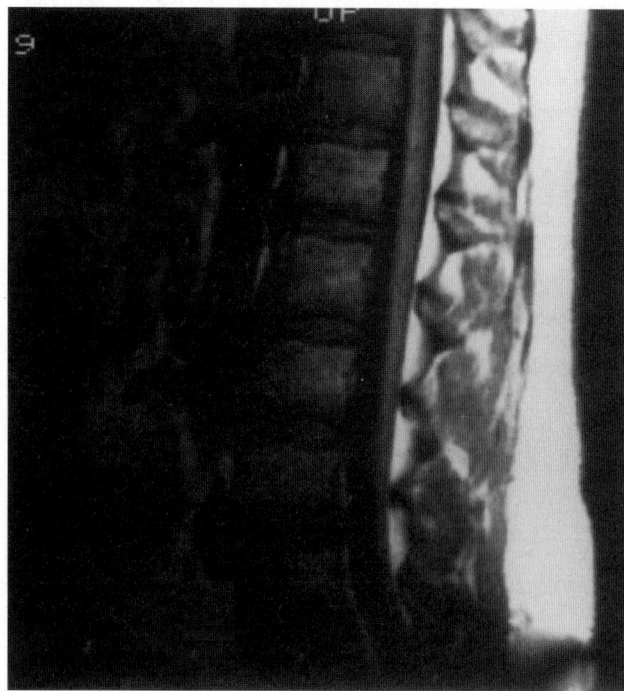

**Figure 81.2** $T_1$-weighted MRI scan demonstrating a tethered spinal cord.

A careful neurologic examination with attention paid to evaluation of motor and sensory function as well as sphincter tone is imperative. If the history indicates possible bladder involvement, a urologic evaluation is indicated. Plain films may be obtained as a screening procedure and may show a widened interpedicular distance and defects at one or more levels. The procedure of choice is magnetic resonance imaging (MRI) (Figure 81.2). Often, this is the only necessary imaging study, and treatment can be planned on the basis of MRI alone. It is generally prudent to image the entire spinal cord at least once to rule out other associated anomalies such as a syrinx or a type I Chiari malformation. If there are any remaining concerns or issues, a myelogram with subsequent computed tomography (CT) may be helpful.

## Treatment

Once the problem is identified, the treatment of the tethered cord is surgical. Although controversy existed in the past (over the concept of prophylactic surgery of asymptomatic patients), most surgeons now believe that the risk of waiting for deterioration to occur is not justified because the deficit is often not reversible. Therefore, surgery is recommended, even in the asymptomatic patient,[43] although, a recent study[11] suggests that careful follow-up and monitoring for upper motor neuron signs using urodynamic assessments, in order to time surgical intervention with the appearance of upper motor neuron signs, may be possible. In adults, those with back pain and lower extremity pain seem to benefit more than those with sphincter problems.[1]

The goal of surgery is to untether the spinal cord and to avoid incurring further neurologic deficit. It is crucial to expose areas of normal anatomy and then proceed to the abnormal area. Electrophysiologic monitoring, especially the use of intraoperative electromyography (EMG), may be helpful. This is performed by inserting needle electrodes into the appropriate muscles and the anal sphincters under anesthesia. Then during surgery the level of each root is accurately established by intradural nerve root stimulation, and before dividing any structure, it is stimulated to confirm that no neural structures are involved. The same probes that are used for a dorsal rhizotomy may be employed, although any nerve stimulator may be used. The advantage of this technique is that the response to EMG is very rapid and provides a substantial safety margin during the surgery for the tethered cord syndrome.

## Complications

Several complications may occur during surgery. The incidence of infection should be low, as with any clean neurosurgical procedure.

CSF leak is a most uncommon complication. After careful dural closure, fibrin glue is used and a Valsalva procedure usually performed to check for leakage. If postoperative cutaneous leakage occurs, reoperation is mandatory. The patient should be kept flat for 3 days after surgery, with sedation if necessary.

Another potential complication is that of urinary retention. A Foley catheter is always inserted after induction of anesthesia and removed on the third to fifth day. If the child is unable to initiate micturition after catheter removal, intermittent catheterization is used until normal voiding is reestablished. If the child does void, a postvoid residual urine volume should be checked to verify adequate emptying. No more than 10 to 30ml of urine should be left after the child has voided.

## Outcome

The shorter the duration of symptoms, the better the prognosis.[10] A study by Archibeck et al.[4] demonstrated a 50% revision rate by 5 years after initial revision and a 57% revision rate by 2 years after the second release. In addition, 50% of patients required at least one orthopedic procedure after tethered cord release.[4] In a study by Cornette et al.[11] of 12 patients operated on for tethered cord, none required a second operation. However, the series is small, although the follow-up period was reasonable (58 months). In terms of urologic outcome, improvement in symptoms as well as urologic dynamic parameters is expected in most patients, although few if any will return to normal.[5] Improvements may be noted in detrusor function, EMG recordings, and pressures.[6]

## Split Cord Malformations

### Embryology and Pathology

Split cord malformation (SCM) is a term that was introduced by Pang et al.[41] in 1992 to describe diastematomyelia based on the dural tube and the nature of the septum. Two types of SCM exist: Type I (diastematomyelia with septum) and Type II (diastematomyelia without septum). Type II is usually more common.

By the end of the second week of gestation, the human embryo normally consists of a bilaminar structure: (1) an epiblast, or layer of cells next to the amnion and (2) a hypoblast, or layer of cells next to the yolk sac. From there, the cells divide to form the primitive streak. During gastrulation the embryo becomes trilaminar as adjacent epiblastic cells migrate medially toward the primitive streak to become mesoderm. The primitive streak begins to regress by day 16,[41] and the notochordal process begins. As the notochord elongates, it canalizes, initially forming a connection through the embryo to join the amnion and yolk sac. This connection is then lost as the open notochord separates from the endoderm and again forms a blind tube.[41]

In the case of the split cord malformations, there is an adhesion between the ectoderm and endoderm. This leads to the formation of an "accessory neurenteric canal around which condenses an endomesenchymal tract that bisects the developing notochord and causes formation of two hemineural plates."[41] The formation of Type I or Type II SCM depends on what happens to the endomesenchymal tract. If it develops toward bone and cartilage, there will be two dural sacs and a Type I. If the tract regresses or leaves a fibrous septum, a Type II will develop.[48]

The spinal cord above and below the split is normal. The two hemicords themselves are usually the same size, but in 10% of patients, they are grossly asymmetric. When this occurs, the spinal cord itself, above and below the bifurcation, is asymmetric, being smaller on the side of the smaller hemicord.

The anterior spinal artery and the central canal bifurcate to accompany each hemicord,[17] so that each has its own blood supply. The two hemicords give rise to the spinal nerve roots on their respective sides. Although splitting of the spinal cord at more than one site and cases of incomplete splitting of the spinal cord with a resultant partial cleft cord have been reported, the majority of cases involve a single, complete cleft through the spinal cord and meninges. In cases in which there are two hemicords without an intervening septum, a single dural sac surrounds both. In such cases, symptoms may result from tethering of the cord by fibrous bands or a thickened filum terminale.

In cases in which the meninges themselves are also bifurcated, there is almost always an intervening septum. Its position is at the caudal end of the split; therefore, ascent of the neural elements is prohibited. The septum, or spur, is usually attached to both the dorsal elements and the dorsal aspect of the vertebral body. Because of the incidence of spina bifida, the spur may continue dorsally between unfused laminae. These spurs may present anywhere along the spine, but 70% of the time they are between L1 and L5. They are less likely in the thoracic spine and occur with only a 1% incidence in the cervical spine.[18,23] The spur is initially cartilaginous and may mature to calcified bone with time.

Other associated anomalies, such as vertebral body abnormalities, may occur. Hemivertebrae, butterfly vertebrae, blocked vertebrae, and spina bifida may contribute to a kyphoscoliosis. The scoliotic defect and segmental vertebral anomalies are commonly located near the level of the split cord malformation. In addition, many children with these anomalies have hypertrichosis over the level of the spur, clubfoot, or pes cavus. Twenty percent of cases are associated with other abnormalities of the spine, including hydromyelia, lipoma, dermal sinus, and neurenteric, epidermoid, and arachnoid cysts. Unless a preexisting myelomeningocele exists, Chiari malformations are not usually associated with split cord malformations.

### Pathophysiology

The clinical symptoms most likely evolve from traction of the spinal cord against the restricting septum or bony spur.[22,30] As with other forms of tethered spinal cord, the ascent of the cord within the dural sac and spinal canal is prohibited. The average age of presentation is 6½ years, with neurologic symptoms first becoming evident with the onset of walking.[23] With the onset of walking, however, increased traction of the distal spinal cord against the restricting septum results in new symptoms. To support this, Yamada et al.[54] have studied the oxidative metabolism of the distal spinal cord and have found a decrease when the cord is under axial tension.

### Presentation

Boxes 81.1 and 81.2 include some of the presenting symptoms and physical signs of patients with split cord malformations.[28] In general, signs and symptoms fall into three categories: (1) cutaneous abnormalities, (2) pain, and (3) neurologic deficits (from spinal cord traction).

In newborns and infants in whom neurologic deficits may not yet have developed, cutaneous lesions bring the child to the attention of the neurosurgeon. Most commonly, a patch of hair or hypertrichosis is noted in the thoracic or lumbosacral midline posteriorly. This hair, usually

**81.1**

**Split cord malformation: common presenting complaints**

**Symptoms arising from pain**
Low backache
Shooting pains down leg

**Symptoms arising from cutaneous abnormalities**
Hairy patch
Prominence in lumbar midline
Skin discoloration
Skin defect

**Symptoms arising from traction injury to spinal cord**
Limp
Deformity or smallness of leg and foot
Sensory disturbance
Bladder disorder
Impotence
Abnormal spinal curvature

**Incidental radiographic findings**

Mathern GW, Peacock WJ: Diastematomyelia. In Park TS (ed): *Spinal Dysraphism*, Boston, Blackwell Scientific, 1992, p 91.

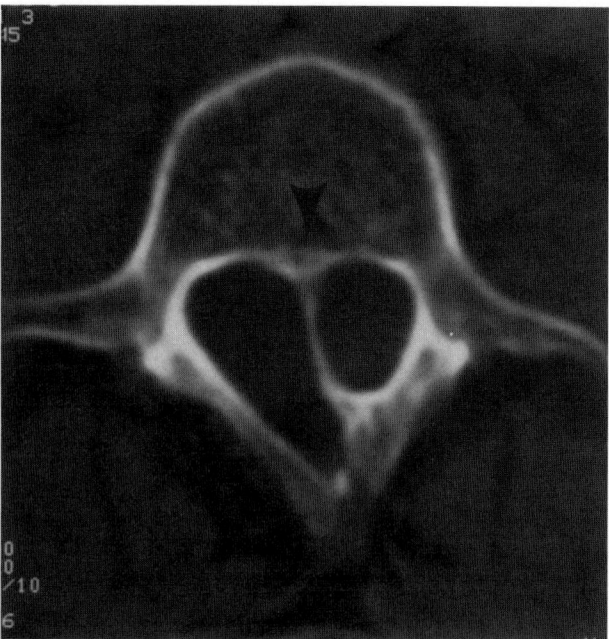

**Figure 81.3** Plain axial CT scan revealing the bony septum (*arrow*) of split cord malformation.

**81.2**

**Split cord malformation: common physical signs**

**Elicitation of pain**
Straight leg raising test
Flexion of spine

**Cutaneous abnormalities**
Faun's tail or hypertrichosis
Lipoma
Prominent spinous process
Meningocele
Angiomatous malformation
Dermal sinus or dimple

**Neurologic abnormalities**
Short leg and hypoplasia of calf and thigh
Varus or cavus deformity of foot
Adducted forefoot
Clawed toes
Muscle weakness
Depressed ankle and knee reflexes
Diminished sensation in dermatomes of leg or perianal
  area
Distended bladder
Scoliosis

Mathern GW, Peacock WJ: Diastematomyelia. In Park TS (ed): *Spinal Dysraphism*, Boston, Blackwell Scientific, 1992, p 91.

coarse and long, is sometimes referred to as *faun's tail*. The surrounding skin is associated with an intradermal angiomatous malformation, giving the skin a pinkish blue color. In addition, a dermal sinus, lipoma, abnormally protuberant spinous process, or meningocele may be associated with the spur.

As the child develops, begins to walk, and acquires bowel and bladder control, the neurologic sequelae of split cord malformations usually appear. A hypoplastic lower extremity and foot deformities are sometimes present at birth. Progressive kyphoscoliosis may also become noticeable. With the onset of walking, a limp, an ulcer secondary to areas of anesthesia, and the new onset of bowel or bladder incontinence after a period of normally developed continence all indicate tethering. Although spasticity and other long-tract signs are not common, hyperreflexia and loss of sensation in the sacral dermatomes are common.

If the patient with split cord malformation has successfully progressed through development with few or none of the aforementioned symptoms, the most common complaint, particularly in older children and adults, is back or leg pain.[42] This may be due to subtle concomitant scoliosis or to the spinal bony deformity itself.

### Diagnostic Aids

Aids that confirm the diagnosis of split cord malformation are usually radiologic. Although plain radiographs or unenhanced computed tomographs of the spine may reveal the bony spur, a widened interpedicular distance, spina bifida occulta, or other segmental vertebral anomalies, MRI in all three axes can be more revealing and is the procedure of choice (Figures 81.3 through 81.5). Associated lipomas, hydromyelia, and other intraspinal and intradural defects may also be observed incidentally, allowing for a more focused treatment approach. If there are any questions or further clarification is required, myelography and postmyelographic CT best delineate the hemicords, the dural sac, and the presence and extent of the intervening bony septum (Figure 81.6).[24] Plain and CT myelography may reveal aberrant nerve roots, intradural bands, a thickened filum terminale, or a concomitant

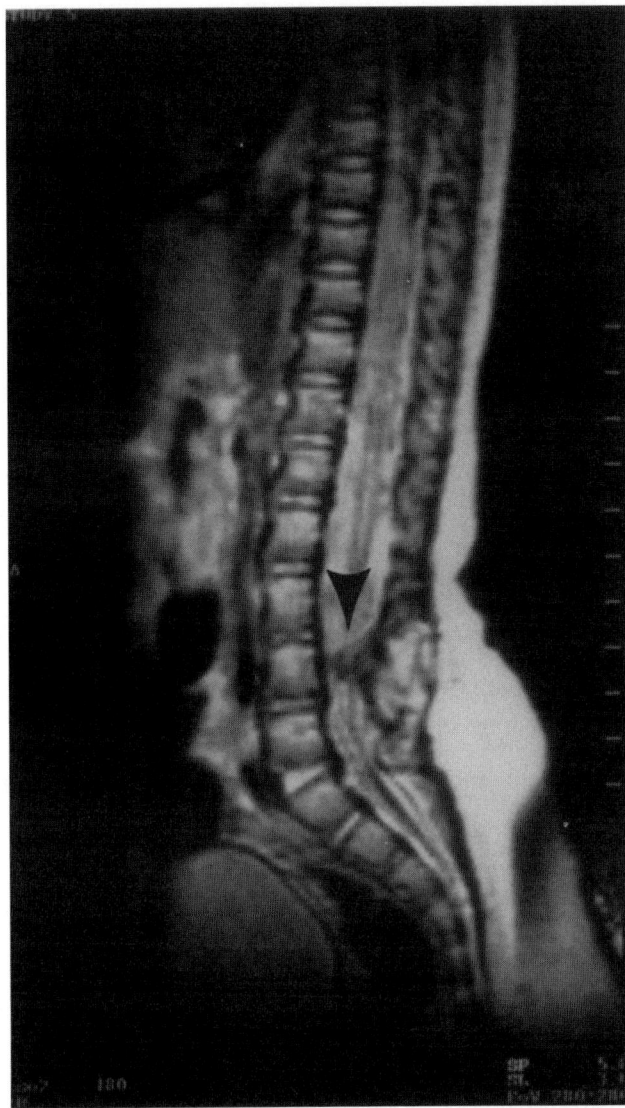

**Figure 81.4** Sagittal T$_2$-weighted MRI scan demonstrating split cord malformation, with the septum spanning from the ventral to the dorsal elements *(arrow)*.

intradural lipoma. In addition, a recent study[44] reported up to a 75% incidence of abnormal urologic dynamic studies in patients with SCM, despite a lack of symptoms. Therefore obtaining preoperative and postoperative urologic dynamic studies may be of some benefit. Again, as in the tethered cord syndrome, the entire spinal cord should be imaged.

## Treatment

Other than incidental findings of split cord malformation in newborns, any patient with signs or symptoms referable to split cord malformation should be promptly untethered to relieve symptoms, preserve function, and possibly reverse neurologic deficits. In the otherwise normal newborn, surgery should be delayed for about 3 months because the older child will be larger, will tolerate anesthesia better, and will have developed more resilient meninges and soft tissues, allowing for more secure surgical closure.

The goal of surgery is to untether the hemicords by removing the cartilaginous, fibrous, or bony septum, as well as the dural tunnel about the septum, which itself tethers the cord. In addition, any surrounding dural adhesions restricting the motion of the spinal cord should be lysed.

Under general anesthesia the patient should be positioned as for a laminectomy, in the prone position, either on chest rolls or on a flexed frame with adequate room for abdominal-wall motion. Unless an associated tethered filum terminale that requires incision is expected, there is no need for preoperative placement of sphincter and lower extremity EMG electrodes.

Before making a standard midline incision to the lumbosacral fascia, the spine should be palpated. Occasionally, a protruding spinous process or bony spur may be felt, allowing for a more localized incision. In addition, a localizing plain radiograph with a skin marker is used and correlated with the preoperative MRI. If a cutaneous lesion, such as a patch of hair, is present, it may be beneficial to create an elliptical incision circumferentially around the defect. Because the underlying bony and soft-tissue defect may not be clear, it is helpful to incise the fascia and perform a subperiosteal reflection of the paraspinous musculature at the levels above and below the level of the lesion, understanding that midline fusion defects may also exist here. The monopolar electrocautery should be used cautiously in retracting the muscles, because areas of expected protective bone may be missing. After the lamina above and below the lesion are exposed, their spinous processes are removed using a rongeur. A partial laminectomy is then performed at the caudal aspect of the lamina above the septum and the rostral aspect of the lamina below the septum. After careful curettage of the underside of both these lamina, the ligamentum flavum, if still intact, is elevated laterally with Penfield forceps and incised longitudinally through its outer layer. A blunt instrument is then gently inserted through the remaining ligament, and a small cottonoid patty is placed between the dura mater and the ligamentum flavum for protection. A small, angled Kerrison punch is then used to remove the ligamentum flavum until the dura mater is exposed completely laterally. With a Penfield no. 4 dissector, the septum is then felt over the dura from above and from below. A small-mouthed rongeur or angled Kerrison punch or high-speed drill is used to remove the lamina and overhanging bone of the involved level until only the spur is left. Because of the substantial epidural venous plexus associated in and around the bony spur and deep to the two hemicords, control of bleeding and cauterization of these vessels should be performed prior to and during the removal of the spur (Figure 81.7). After decompression, with movement of the hemicords, hemostasis may be very difficult. Any extruding segment of spur is removed using a rongeur, and a small dissector is used to probe and dissect the dural sheath away from the bony spicule down to the level of the dorsal vertebral body. A high-speed diamond-bit drill is then used to carefully thin down the spicule as far as possible.

At this point, the dura mater is opened along the midline above and below the spur and elliptically around the spur remnant. After the dural edges are tacked up, the two hemicords become evident. The ventral dural sac is

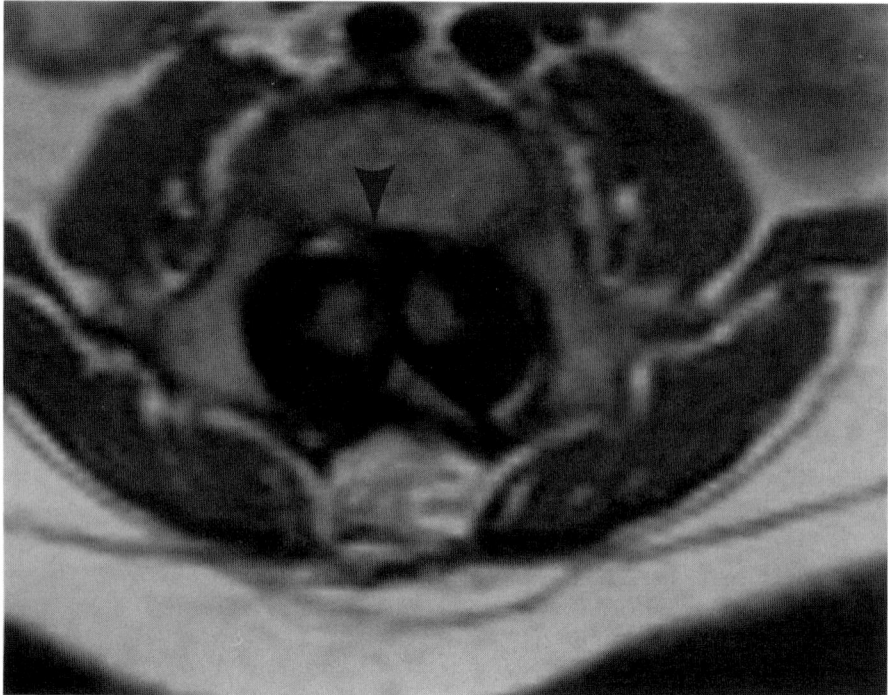

**Figure 81.5** Axial T$_1$-weighted MRI scan revealing the septum (*arrow*) and hemicords of split cord malformation.

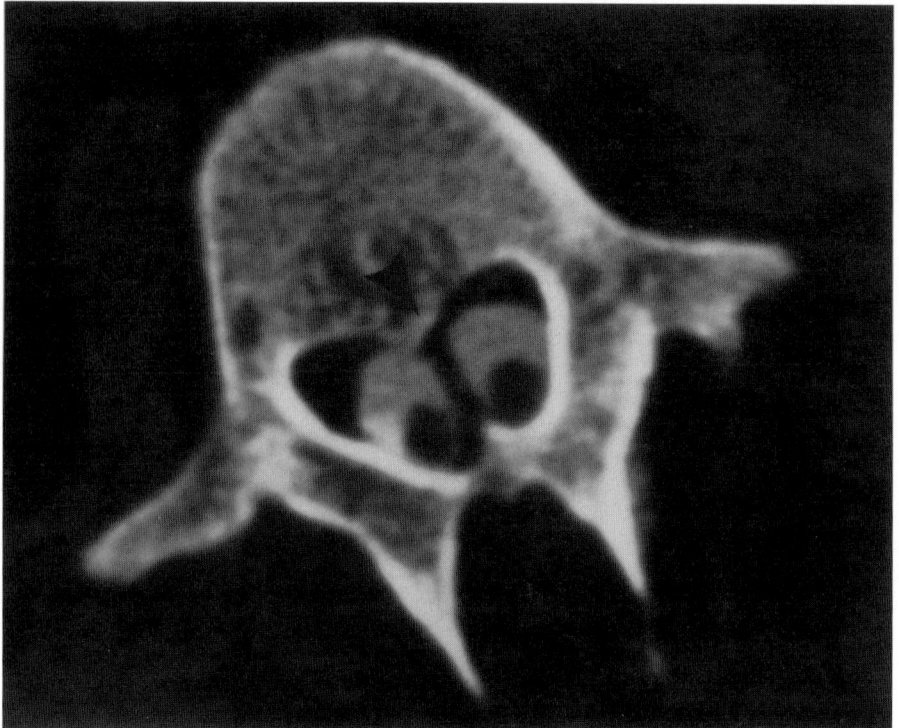

**Figure 81.6** Axial postmyelogram CT scan demonstrating split cord malformation resulting from a nonossified fibrous septum (*arrow*). Note the delineation of the hemicords.

then incised along the midline above the spicule and circumferentially around it. The dural "chimney" is removed, and the resultant dural edges are teased laterally so that the remainder of the spur may be completely drilled off, with the spinal cord being protected at all times. With the removal of the spur, the entire cord may migrate rostrally. Microinstruments should be used to break or cut any additional adhesions that may be tethering the spinal cord to the dura mater. A watertight closure of the dorsal dural opening is then performed, with

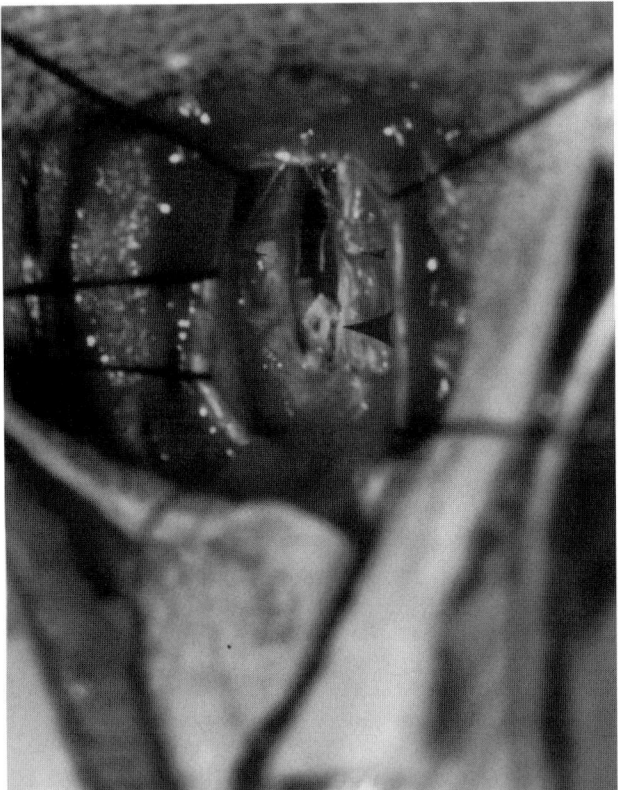

**Figure 81.7** Intraoperative photograph showing the bony spicule *(large arrow)* and two hemicords *(small arrows)* in a patient with split cord malformation.

interrupted sutures used over the elliptical incision to avoid the unraveling of a running stitch over this area of tension; again, fibrin glue is used. The ventral dura mater does not require closure. A small drain is inserted, and the soft tissues are closed in anatomic layers. The patient should then be kept flat for 3 days postoperatively to avoid CSF leak.

### Complications

If there are persistent CSF leaks from the suture line, the suture line should be oversewn or patched until the leak stops. It is not uncommon to have a small amount of CSF leakage from the suture holes of the dural closure. If it is minimal, it should not pose a problem. Although infrequent, a persistent CSF leak must be addressed to avoid incision breakdown, infection, and possibly meningitis. If a CSF leak from this source should occur, placing a lumbar subarachnoid drain above the incision and having the patient lie flat in bed for 3 days should allow for closure. If the leak is from the dorsal dural suture line, a drain may again avoid reoperation, but failure to stop the leak will necessitate reexploration and primary dural closure. If the meningeal tissues are found to be weak and nonresilient, a pericardium, fascia lata, or other dural graft may be required. Fibrin glue or DuraGen may also be of some value.

As always, postoperative epidural hemorrhage is possible. Because of the apparent increased venous drainage in the defect, hemostasis may be difficult. A delayed postop-

erative neurologic deficit should be worked up immediately, either with MRI or myelography. Both epidural hematomas and subdural extension secondary to ventral durotomy should be evacuated immediately. Normal coagulation studies and adequate hematologic status should be verified, and correction should be initiated if needed. As mentioned earlier, the placement of a drain in the epidural space for 24 hours may be considered at the time of initial repair, although this should not replace meticulous surgical technique. This may prevent the accumulation of a mass lesion, and rarely does it induce leakage of CSF from the underlying suture line.

Sterility, perioperative antibiotics, and gentle handling of tissues will all aid in preventing meningitis and wound infections. If these should occur, appropriate intravenous antibiotics should be administered. The goal is to prevent a subsequent epidural or subdural empyema.

Iatrogenic traction, contusion, or direct injury with an instrument or a drill may inadvertently occur intraoperatively. Care should be exercised continuously to prevent unnecessary manipulation and traction on the spinal cord.

### Outcome

In symptomatic patients, bowel and bladder dysfunction may improve up to 40% of the time, but stabilization of progressive urologic symptoms may also be noted.[39] Neurologic sensorimotor deficits only return to normal 5% to 10% of the time. Patients whose main complaint is pain in general improve. Also included in improvement of pain is the dysesthetic component. A higher surgical morbidity has been reported in cases in which the bony septum is present, perhaps due to removal of the bony septum.[39] It is important to remember that preserving neurologic function is as important as improving it. Recent studies[3,39] also report untethering the cord may have no effect on the neuro-orthopedic syndrome (e.g., lower limb asymmetry, foot deformities), perhaps due to irreversible changes in the ligaments.

## Congenital Dermal Sinus

### Pathology and Embryology

Dorsal congenital dermal sinus (a subtype of spinal dysraphism not associated with spina bifida or bony abnormalities) is defined as an epithelium-lined tract from the skin of the back, usually the lumbosacral midline (although they are possible in the thoracic and cervical spine),[48] that passes through the soft tissues toward the spine, the thecal sac, and even into the neural elements. These tracts, which are usually very thin, are thought to develop because of adhesion and failure of separation between the superficial cutaneous ectoderm and the neural tube.[37] This usually occurs at the fourth week of fetal development, after neurulation of the tail bud. As such, this attachment between skin and spinal cord is lengthened and thinned with the ascent of the cord and fixation of the skin. Because of its small size, the surrounding bone-forming mesoderm may produce little or no spina bifida. Also, the remainder of the vertebral body at the affected levels is usually normal. Although not usually a cause of tethering of the spinal cord, the cutaneous origin of the sinus tends to be two to three vertebral levels caudal to its adhesion to the neural elements.

Because of the epithelial lining and potential communication with the skin, the dermal sinus may result in an expanding dermoid or epidermoid tumor in the subdural or epidural space, in the same manner that such tumors arise from iatrogenic implantation of such elements with spinal needles.[49] These tumors may present as mass lesions or as a simple dermal sinus associated with a possible communication between the skin and subarachnoid space. Therefore, they are a nidus for infection, meningitis, and possibly abscess formation. Microscopically, they consist of dermal elements, such as sweat and apocrine glands and hair follicles.

Most dorsal dermal sinuses are lumbosacral, with occipital sinuses being less common. Although about 60% of dermal sinuses end in dermoid or epidermoid tumors, only 30% of these tumors are associated with dermal sinuses.[20,52] In addition, the dermal sinus may be involved in tethering of the spinal cord, not by itself, but either by a thick band of tissue attached to the spinal cord or conus medullaris or as a result of inflammatory scarring.

## Pathophysiology and Presentation

Because of the low incidence of tethering with dermal sinuses, symptoms are usually the result of infectious etiologies. Bacteria may include *Staphylococcus aureus, Staphylococcus epidermidis, Escherichia coli,* and even proteus species.[31] The tract from the bacteria-laden epidermis to the intraspinous space and even subarachnoid space provides opportunities for intermittent, chronic, and acute infections.[13,51] Although the incidence of meningitis is higher with the presence of a concomitant dermoid or epidermoid tumor, simple tracts carry this risk as well.[29] In fact, dermal sinuses may be the cause of infection in up to one quarter of cases of intramedullary spinal abscesses, with approximately 70% of patients having neurologic deficits.[9] Because of the dimple formed in the skin over the tract, infections are noticed and addressed, often before clinical symptoms have surfaced. The dimple, or the external ostium of the sinus, is usually in the midline and may be associated with a hemangioma, a nevus, or short tufts of hair protruding from the sinus. Parents, caretakers, or physicians may notice caseous discharge from this area or perhaps some erythema or inflammation. Because of the usual lumbosacral location, fecal and skin organisms may be the cause of meningitis. Frank neurologic symptoms or neurogenic pain are rarely present unless there is compression from an associated tumor or tethering of the spinal cord or conus as mentioned previously.

By examination, neurologic function is usually preserved. The dimple should not be probed in order to avoid lodging infection-forming organisms into the deeper sinus. Manipulation and pulling of the skin around the ostium in different directions often reveal further umbilication of the tract, thus confirming that the margins of the tract are fixed to the deeper tissues. Palpation of the spine itself may reveal prominent or

absent spinous processes, indicating a dorsal element malformation. It is important, however, to distinguish a low-lying dermal sinus pore from a simple pilonidal dimple, which is usually more caudal, is near the tip of the coccyx, and usually requires no further work-up. However, if the dimple is over the sacrum or higher, further evaluation is indicated.

## Diagnostic Aids

Although the index of suspicion for congenital dermal sinus is high solely on the basis of the examination, neuroimaging is helpful to discern its extent and the presence of associated tethering and tumors. Injection of contrast material is not recommended because of the risk of inducing meningitis and infection.

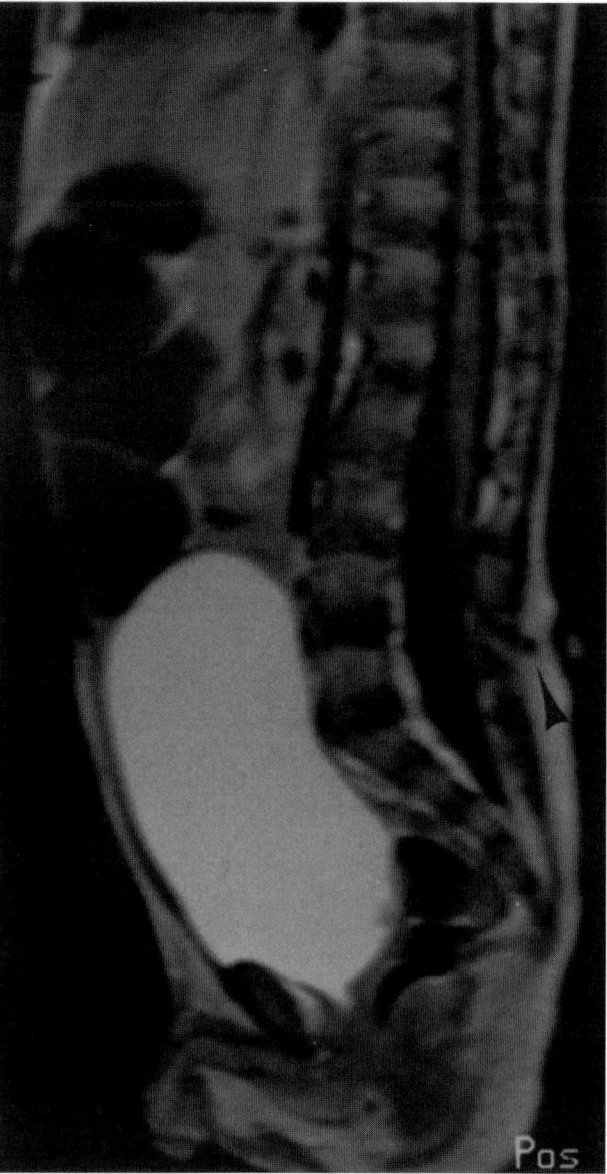

**Figure 81.8** Sagittal $T_1$-weighted MRI scan revealing a tethered spinal cord that appears to be contiguous with a dermal sinus tract *(arrow)*. Note the overdistended, previously undiagnosed, neurogenic bladder.

MRI is the initial imaging modality of choice (Figure 81.8). It is useful to follow the denser, low-signal sinus through the high-signal subcutaneous fat toward the dura mater. The intraspinal course of the tract, however, may not in all cases be well-displayed by MRI. Dermoid and epidermoid tumors have variable signal intensity on MRI. Dermoids, with increased $T_1$ and $T_2$ signals compared to water (because of the cholesterol, fat, and protein content), image well. However, if there has been chemical meningitis from leakage of the tumor, detection may be more difficult. Although containing only epithelial elements, epidermoid tumors are equally well-defined by MRI.

Axial CT imaging reveals the dense sinus tract through its course from the skin into the dura mater. Occasionally, the lumen of the tract may be visualized as a more hypo-dense line within the tract. The use of intra-arachnoid myelographic contrast before a CT is the most useful method to image the course of the sinus in the subdural space as it ascends toward the conus medullaris.[47] Water-soluble contrast or air should be used in order to avoid leaving oily droplets that could act as potential foreign bodies. A lucent mass along the tubular filling defect may represent dermoid or epidermoid tumors. However, since the advent of MRI, the use of contrast material has been reduced dramatically. Even in the presence of a normal MRI scan, if a cutaneous lesion seems to truly represent a dermal sinus in a suspicious location, surgical exploration may be warranted.

## Treatment

The treatment of a true dermal sinus is surgical. Even if the MRI is normal, the sinus tract should be excised. Technically, surgical excision of the dermal sinus may range from a very simple procedure (when it ends in the soft tissue) to a very difficult and complex operation (if it is adherent to the conus medullaris or is associated with one or more dermoid or epidermoid tumor). When a patient presents with soft-tissue infection or meningitis, the infection first should be treated adequately with intravenous antibiotics. The surgery should not be performed until the CSF is sterile. In any case, antibiotics should be used both perioperatively and postoperatively.

Loupe or microscope magnification should be used after the dura mater is exposed. As for a laminectomy, the patient is placed on chest rolls or on a frame after general anesthesia. The skin and ostium of the sinus should be sterilized, and access should be available from the spinous process of T11 to the coccyx. A midline incision is then performed from at least two spinous processes rostral to the dimple to one spinous process below it. An elliptical incision is made around the ostium itself, including any associated nevus or other cutaneous abnormality. The skin edges around the sinus may then be secured and manipulated with a heavy silk suture or a clamp with teeth.

Using traction on the elliptically incised skin and ostium allows for easier dissection along the tract. With the use of Metzenbaum-type scissors, the tract is followed as it dives into the soft tissues, until the lumbosacral fascia is reached. A blunter instrument, such as a small curved hemostat, is then used to follow the tract through the fascia, caudally to rostrally, while holding traction on the tract

in the rostral direction. Care should be taken not to incise or avulse the tract, lest the remaining stump retracts under the fascia and becomes very difficult to locate. Care should also be exercised to avoid undue traction on the sinus tract in case it is contiguous with the neural elements. When the direction and location of the subfascial tract has been determined, the fascia above and below may be incised on either side of the spinous processes above and below the tract. Again, using subperiosteal dissection, either with a gauze and periosteum elevators or with traction and a monopolar electrocautery, the laminae are exposed. This leaves the line of spinous processes, usually with the dermal sinus tract disappearing into the interspinous ligament of the involved level. In the case of dorsal element abnormalities and spina bifida, care should be taken, particularly with the electrocautery, to protect the underlying dura mater and its contents. A Penfield no. 4 dissector is then used to probe the tract as it enters the spine, to determine the tract's position and direction. The flavum ligamentum, under upward traction with forceps, can be carefully incised. Often, the sinus tract may end in the interspinous ligament, and amputation here can be followed by thorough washing of the incision and closure. If the tract indeed pierces the ligamentum flavum, a laminectomy above this should be performed, with rongeurs and an angled Kerrison punch. As with a standard laminectomy, if there is no access to the epidural space after bony removal, an incision through the ligamentum flavum, under traction with subsequent protection of the dura mater with a cottonoid, is warranted. The ligamentum flavum is then removed completely laterally and caudally to the tract. A small cottonoid should first be advanced under the ligamentum flavum and above the dura mater to avoid incision of the tract as it is neared or to avoid performing an incidental durotomy. The same is accomplished at the lamina below the tract, although only the rostral half of the spinous process, lamina, and ligamentum flavum need to be removed, because intradurally the sinus tract rarely travels caudally.

If at this time the tract appears to extend rostrally beyond the level of the laminectomy, the next lamina should be removed. Further exposure may be necessary until the tract is not visualized or until its termination at the conus medullaris can be visualized. The dura mater is then incised along the midline at the rostral end of the exposure, well away from the site of entry of the tract, and carefully extended in the direction of the tract. To approach the entry site, an elliptical incision is made circumferentially around the tract, and finally the midline incision is continued to the caudal end of the exposed dura mater. The dural ellipse that is incised around the tract should be kept as small as possible to preclude the use of graft material when closing the dura mater. Care should be taken to keep the force of suction minimal in order to avoid inadvertent aspiration of free-floating nerve roots. If the arachnoid has been preserved after the durotomy, it may be opened in the midline with a small hook or knife. The dural leaves may then be tacked to the musculature with 4-0 silk or woven nylon sutures.

With gentle traction on the tract, microinstruments are used to dissect away any adhesions between the tract, the dura mater, and the nerve roots. Some adhesions, particularly postmeningitic scars, may require incision. In this way the tract is followed to its attachment, usually dorsally above the tip of the conus. The sides of the tract at this point are completely identified by using a small blunt hook, and microscissors are used to detach it. If the stump bleeds, it is lightly coagulated with bipolar forceps. After verifying the absence of other mass lesions or areas of tethering, the subarachnoid space is copiously irrigated with warm saline, and the dura mater is closed in a watertight fashion with 4-0 silk or woven nylon suture, using a graft if necessary. Fibrin glue is then applied. A drain may be placed in the epidural space and brought through the skin for 24 hours. The soft tissues are then closed in anatomic layers, with some undermining of the subcutaneous tissue occasionally necessary to bring together the skin edges in the area of the elliptical excision. The patient should remain flat in bed for 3 days and should be administered antibiotics postoperatively for 3 days or longer if a previous infection was present.

If preoperatively or during the course of the procedure a dermoid or epidermoid tumor is encountered, it should be completely extirpated, with great care taken to avoid a rupture of its contents. If the tumor itself is at the end of the tract and situated within the substance of the spinal cord, it cannot be completely removed; it should be amputated with an adequate stump to avoid injuring the spinal cord.

### Complications

As with other intradural procedures, CSF leakage may occur postoperatively. A Valsalva maneuver (safe to 40mmHg) after closing the dura mater is helpful for finding any obvious areas of leakage. To avoid the problem of wound breakdown and postoperative meningitis, particularly with a dermal sinus and exposure to its intraluminal debris, a watertight closure (again using fibrin glue, saline irrigation before dural closure, and antibiotic irrigation after dural closure) is helpful. If meningitis should occur, the appropriate antibiotics should be administered. In the case of a superficial wound infection, the area should be opened and drained and packed and the patient should be treated with antibiotics. If, however, the fascia has been violated by the infection, reoperation is necessary to open the fascia, to verify a clean epidural and, if necessary, subdural space, and to close the fascia primarily. All efforts should be made to avoid leaving the dura mater exposed to the environment.

Iatrogenic injury to the conus medullaris, spinal cord, and nerve roots is minimized by gentle handling of the tissues, avoidance of traction, and protection of the neural elements. If preoperatively it is thought that the sinus may end in the conus medullaris or in a tumor adherent to the conus, somatosensory-evoked potentials may be monitored during the procedure. Division of a nerve root, particularly with the absence of EMG monitoring and uncertainty as to its function, should be primarily repaired with 8-0 or 9-0 absorbable monofilament sutures. Because the incidence of postoperative neurologic deficits from dermal sinus surgery is small, no evidence supports the use of perioperative or postoperative steroids for neural protection.

Emphasis should be placed on the complete excision of the sinus tract. Because of its epithelial lining, the potential for dermoid or epidermoid formation remains if part of the tract remains. If a lumen is apparent in the stump of the tract after it is incised near the spinal cord or conus medullaris, it should be trimmed until no lumen is apparent. It should then be well-cauterized.

### Outcome

Most patients with simple tracts do well, and the incidence of neurologic injury is low. Even in the case of spinal cord infection, a positive outcome may be obtained. In a report by Morandi et al.,[35] 10 of 16 patients with spinal cord abscess had complete recovery.

## Spinal Lipomas

### Pathology and Embryology

Although associated with other forms of occult spinal dysraphism, spinal lipomas are connective tissue and fat collections that are distinct, partially or completely encapsulated, and definitely attached to the spinal cord.[25] It is thought that during the process of primary neurulation improper disjunction of surface ectoderm and neuroepithelium may lead to inclusion of fat.[25] Distinct from lipomyelomeningoceles, isolated lipomas technically are fibrolipomas of the filum terminale or dural fibrolipomas, as defined by Emery and London.[14] In simple lipomas the neural elements remain within the spinal canal, whereas lipomyelomeningoceles are marked by herniation of the neural elements out of the canal into the subcutaneous portion of the lipoma.[16] Strictly intradural lipomas associated with an intact dura mater are lesions of subpial fat found in the cervical and thoracic spinal cord.[2] In a large series reported by McLone and Naidich,[33] intradural lipomas comprised 4% of the lipomas treated surgically. More common, however, are lipomas that involve the dura mater and extend from the spinal cord to the subcutaneous tissue.[2,27,46]

More than with the previously described dermal sinus, lipomas are associated with more severe bony changes, including scalloping of the dorsal vertebral body, widening of the interpedicular space, hemivertebrae, or even hypoplasia of the iliac wing.[16] These sequelae of the mass effect associated with lipomas suggest that resultant neurologic deficits occur not only by spinal cord tethering (see Pathophysiology and Presentation) but also by direct neural compression.

### Pathophysiology and Presentation

Spinal lipomas, accounting for up to 35% of skin-covered lumbosacral masses, may extend to the superficial subcutaneous tissues and present in the infant as a visible and palpable mass.[50] As with other forms of the tethered cord syndrome, children with spinal lipomas may present with several complaints. At this age, before the onset of walking and the development of bladder control, a concomitant hairy patch may accompany an otherwise unnoticed lipoma. If the condition is unnoticed or disregarded, the infant without neurologic abnormalities may, with age, develop sphincter disturbance, postural and lower extremity deformities and weakness, or even verbalized discomfort.[8]

As mentioned, lipomas may cause neurologic symptoms through a combination of neural compression and spinal cord tethering. Lipomas, therefore, may present in much the same manner as do split cord malformations, thickened filum terminale, and congenital dermal sinus. As always, failure to attain developmental landmarks, as well as progressive loss of neurologic function, particularly lumbosacral function, should alert the health care provider to investigate the spine.

### Diagnostic Aids

Lipomas constitute only 1% of primary intraspinal tumors and are almost always associated with dysraphic spines.[19] Varying from intramedullary to extradural, their histologic nature and relative position to the spinal canal make them definable by both CT and MRI.[36]

Although spina bifida occulta, widening of the interpedicular distance, hemivertebrae, and vertebral body scalloping may all be observed on plain radiographic studies in the patient with a lipoma, these films may be difficult to interpret. As with other spinal anomalies, lipomas are usually best worked up with MRI as the initial study (Figure 81.9). CT is usually reserved for better definition of bony anatomy, if needed. Although not as detailed, myelograms may help define the extent of the mass (Figure 81.10). Intradural lipomas are low density or even radiolucent on CT and have a high signal on $T_1$-weighted MRI.[15] Both techniques are useful, however, in axial section. Extradural lipomas are usually more diffuse and contiguous with the nearby epidural fat. They must be considered, even in the light of unclear CT and MRI images.

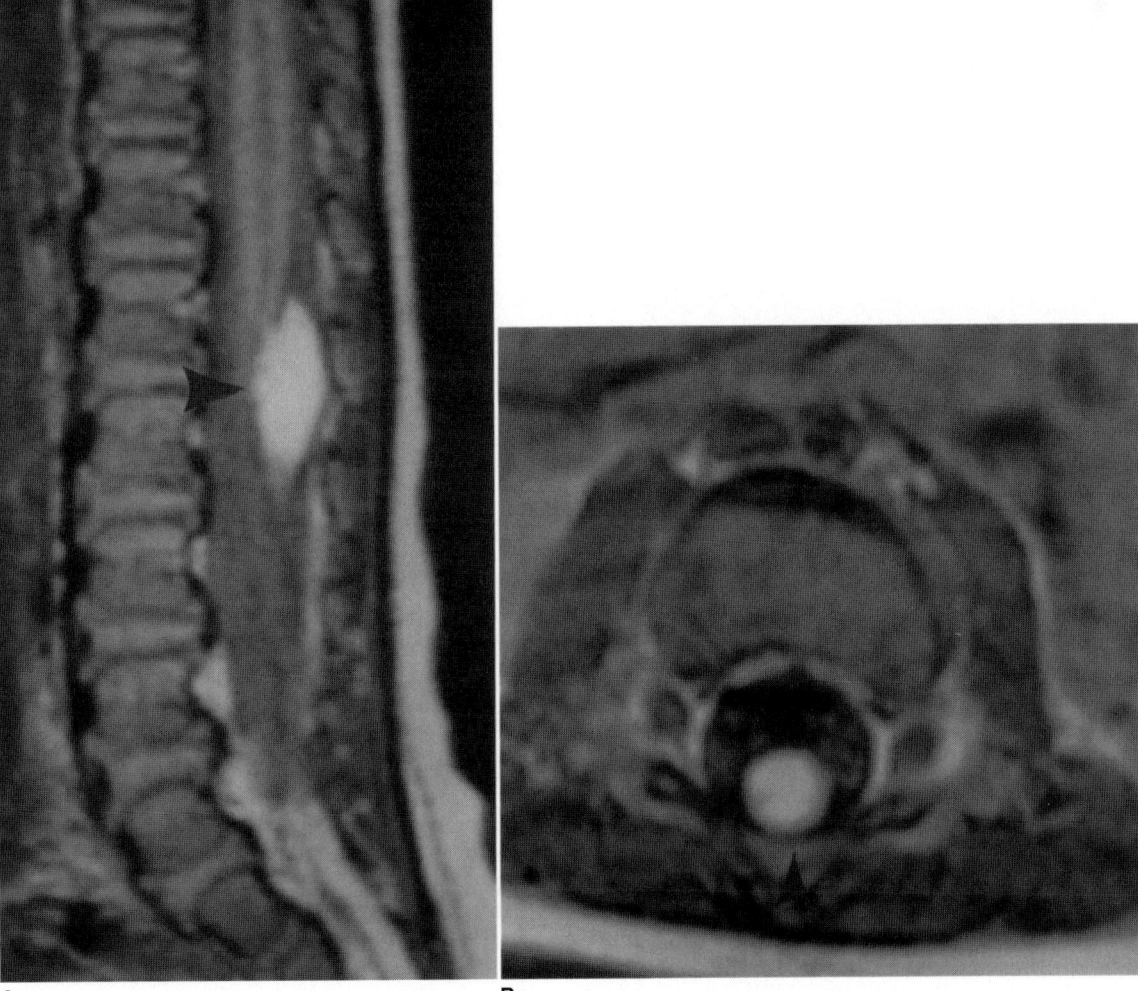

**A**  **B**

**Figure 81.9** **(A-B)** Sagittal and axial MR images of a tethered spinal cord with an intradural spinal lipoma *(arrows)*.

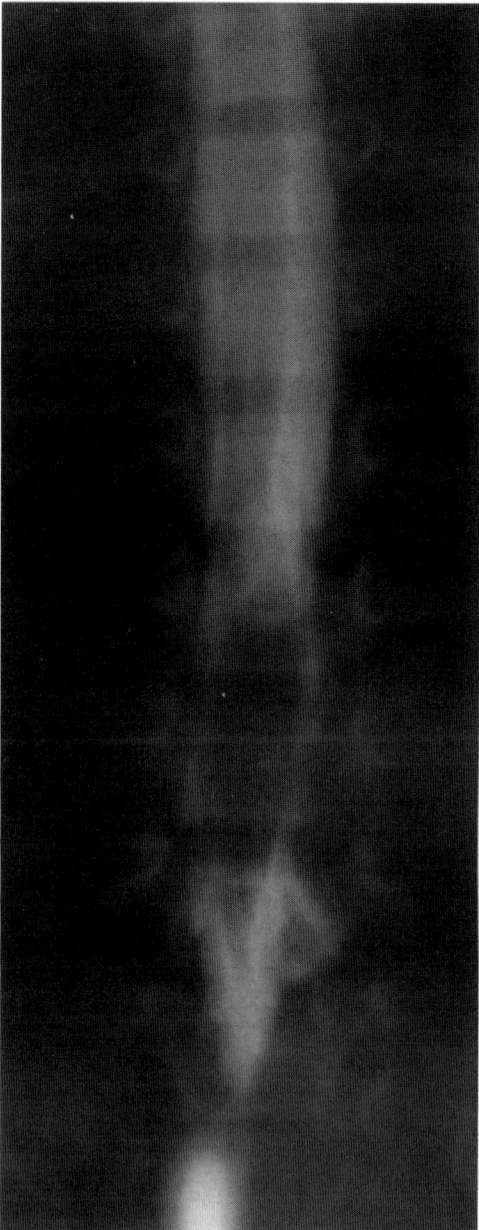

**Figure 81.10** Anteroposterior lumbar myelogram revealing the filling defect caused by an intradural lipoma, causing a tether of the cord in the lumbosacral region.

McLone and Naidich[34] also support the use of ultrasonography in managing these lesions. The lack of calcium in immature bones allows for penetration and evaluation of structural detail, often well enough to verify the lesion, determine the extent of tethering, and proceed straight to surgery without the need for additional radiographic studies.

## Treatment

Whether by tethering of the filum terminale and spinal cord, the direct neural compression, or both, surgery for spinal lipomas is warranted in the child with neurologic deficits. Operating on the asymptomatic patient has been controversial. However, today most neurosurgeons feel

that if possible, lipomas and lipomeningoceles should be operated on before neurologic sequelae occur.[8,26,45] Unlike split cord malformations, in which involvement of the neural elements in the substance of the pathology is rare, such involvement is common in spinal lipomas. Therefore, even with detailed and defining preoperative studies, intraoperative electrophysiologic studies perhaps should be considered during resection of spinal lipomas; however, not all surgeons feel this is necessary. The authors, however, find it quite useful and use intraoperative EMG monitoring and insert needle electrodes in the muscles of the lower extremities as well as in the sphincter. Stimulation is performed with the same probes that are used for dorsal root rhizotomy. With this type of monitoring, one can ascertain whether there is undue traction on the conus medullaris and if it is safe to incise tissues that are near nerves or the spinal cord.

After sterilization of the skin, a midline incision should be performed over the palpable or visible subcutaneous portion of the lipoma. If there is no evidence of such a superficial lesion, needle localization with anteroposterior and lateral radiographs is useful. After incision of the fascia and lateral exposure of the laminae, microscopic enhancement, either with loupe magnification or the operating microscope should be used. As with all occult dysraphic spines, care should be taken with both the scalpel and the electrocautery because the unformed or bifid laminae may offer no protection for the thecal sac. Before the bony structures are reached, the extradural portions of the lipoma may require resection. If so, circumferential dissection of the lipoma is important so as to allow complete resection. The actual resection of the extradural portion of the lipoma is usually fairly straightforward. However, the location of the nerve roots relative to the lipoma-cord junction vary with the type of attachment that the lipoma has with the conus medullaris.[12] If the lipoma attaches to the dorsal surface of the conus, the nerve roots are ventral to the lipoma-conus interface. If, however, the lipoma is a caudal extension of the conus medullaris, the course of the nerve roots through the lipoma can be variable and great care has to be exerted to prevent damage to neural structures (Figure 81.11).

At the time of the durotomy, all anesthetic muscle relaxants should be avoided. Extradural lipomas that traverse the thecal sac into the intradural compartment may require resection of some dura mater. At this point, although some surgeons advocate the use of the carbon dioxide laser to vaporize the fatty lesion, the authors also suggest the use of the ultrasonic aspirator. Although relief of neural compression is one principle of surgery, particularly for lipomas on the dorsal surface of the spinal cord, the primary goal is to untether the spinal cord. Therefore, the surgery should be directed at accomplishing this goal. In such cases, sectioning of the filum terminale caudal to the sacral nerve roots may be required. Electrophysiologic monitoring is particularly useful at this point, not only to determine where the filum terminale may be incised and to ensure that no neural structures are coursing within the filum, but also to take care to not excessively manipulate functional nerve roots and the spinal cord. Often it is not possible or even necessary to completely resect the lipoma (Figure 81.12). Prudence should be the rule, and one

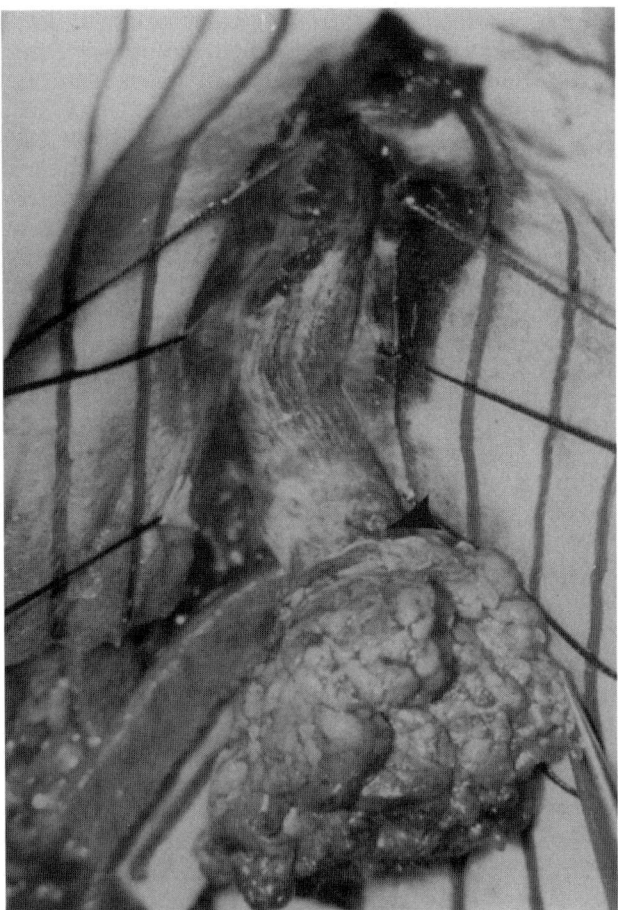

**Figure 81.11** Intraoperative photograph showing the continuity of this large subcutaneous lipoma with the spinal cord *(arrow)*. Note the caudal attachment, making dissection of the nerve roots very difficult.

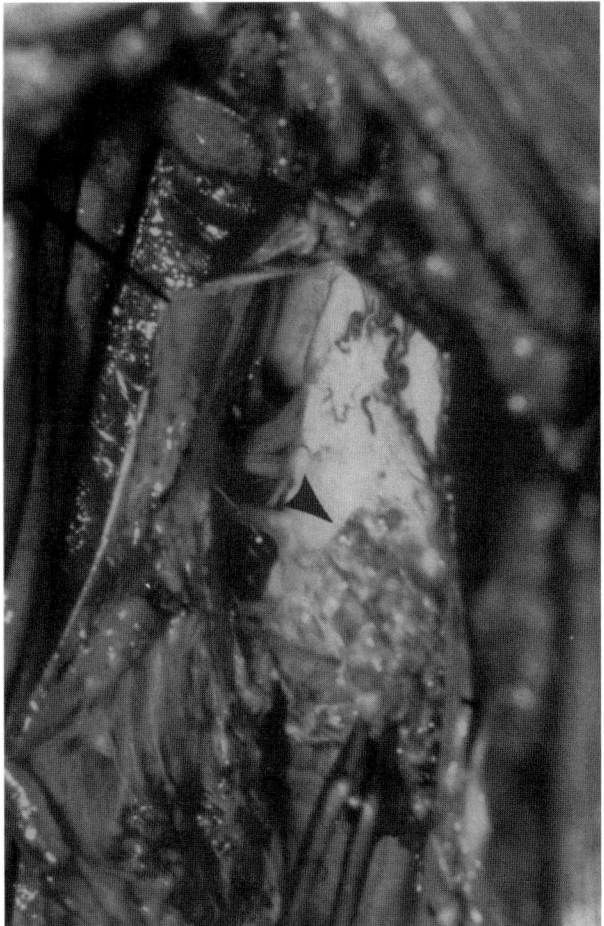

**Figure 81.12** Intraoperative photograph demonstrating residual lipoma at the lipoma-conus interface, stimulation of which verified the presence of functional neural elements *(arrow)*. Note the slack nerve roots verifying successful untethering of the cord from the dura.

should not take any chances of injuring the conus medullaris or the nerve roots. It should be remembered that the primary goal of surgery is to untether the spinal cord and at the same time cause no deficits.

After removal of the lipoma, untethering of the surrounding neural structures, and possible sectioning of the filum terminale, dural closure must be watertight. Although reapproximation of two of the three meningeal layers may decrease the change of retethering, the pia and arachnoid are often incompetent after removal of the lipoma. As such, careful closure of the dura mater, which may include a graft, is important. As with other intrathecal operations, leaving the child flat in bed for 3 days allows for tissue healing and helps avoid collection of CSF, particularly if a large "dead space" has resulted from excision of an extradural component of the lipoma. Special techniques of closure to prevent retethering have been reported, but the patients have not been followed long enough to determine whether these techniques are better than conventional methods of closure.[55]

## Complications

Infection, CSF leaks, and iatrogenic neurologic deficits are all complications that should be avoidable with metic-

ulous surgery and disciplined technique. Preoperative administration of antibiotics is paramount, although postoperative doses depend on the surgeon. Although the literature does not firmly support the use of antibiotics after elective, clean surgery, the authors prefer three postoperative doses to cover common skin flora. If postoperative infection should occur, appropriate drainage and débridement are necessary. Prolonged antibiotic treatment is indicated, and concerns about subsequent meningitis must be addressed with lumbar puncture. In the absence of obvious superficial infection, prolonged fever, or progressive worsening of neurologic function, MRI is necessary to rule out epidural abscess. In such cases, well-intentioned lumbar punctures may result in unintended meningitis.

The avoidance of CSF leaks, as previously mentioned, depends on watertight dural closure, anatomic approximation of all tissue planes, and placement of the child in the supine position postoperatively for recovery. A Valsalva maneuver at the end of the initial surgery may help expose any occult areas of leakage. Continued leaking requires decompression of the intradural pressure with a lumbar subarachnoid drain. Persistence despite these measures requires prompt reexploration, repair of obvious areas of CSF escape, and the appropriate use of dural substitutes and cryoprecipitate-based fibrin glue, with the possible addition of a lumbar subarachnoid drain. In extreme cases of dural incompetence, particularly in the face of a soft-tissue defect and a potential space for CSF collection, a rotated or free-pedicle tissue flap may be required.

Immediate postoperative neurologic deficits often resolve. Manipulation of the distal spinal cord and nerve roots may result in traction injury and edema, resolution of which should imply return of neurologic function. This is not always the case, and prudence should be used while handling neural tissue during surgery. Deficits that result from definitive sectioning of the filum terminale or nerve roots are not reversible. With time, however, motor and sensory function may improve with reorganization of cortical neurons.

## Outcome

Successful resection and untethering of these lipomas is now associated with little or no morbidity and mortality.[12,32,33] The best outcomes may be achieved with respect to pain, with most of the pain decreasing or disappearing within 3 months. Bladder dysfunction may also respond to resection of the lipoma in 20% to 30% of patients; of these patients, those with a spastic bladder respond best.[40] In a study by La Marca et al.,[26] 213 patients were operated on over a 20-year period from 1975 to 1995. In patients with filum lipomas, 28 were asymptomatic and 27 were symptomatic. None of the asymptomatic patients worsened after surgery (mean follow-up 3.4 years) and of the symptomatic group, there were no further deteriorations noted (follow-up 6 months to 9 years). Of the group with conus lipomas, 9 of the 71 children (12.7%) operated on prophylactically later deteriorated (mean follow-up 6.2 years) and required a second untethering operation. Symptoms of deterioration included urinary retention, pain, gait difficulty, urinary incontinence, and spasticity. In the symptomatic group (87 patients), 41% further deteriorated and required further surgery. At the final follow-up, however (mean 6.6 years), 51% remained at clinical baseline and 26% improved. In a study by Xenos et al.,[53] their reoperation rate was 12% for signs of recurrent spinal cord tethering.

## REFERENCES

1. Akay KM, Ershin Y, Cakir Y: Tethered cord syndrome in adults. *Acta Neurochir (Wien)* 142:1111, 2000.
2. Ammerman BJ, Henry JM, De Girolami U, et al: Intradural lipomas of the spinal cord: clinicopathological correlation. *J Neurosurg* 44:331, 1976.
3. Andar UB, Harkness WFJ, Hayward RD: Split cord malformations of the lumbar region. *Pediatr Neurosurg* 26:17, 1997.
4. Archibeck MJ, Smith JT, Carroll KL, et al: Surgical release of tethered cord: survivorship analysis and orthopedic outcome. *J Pediatr Orthop* 17:773, 1997.
5. Basar H, Aydoganli L, Yuksel M, et al: The outcome of urologic findings in operated tethered cord patients. *Int Urol Nephrol* 29:167, 1997.
6. Balkan E, Kilic N, Avsar I, et al: Urodynamic findings in the tethered spinal cord: the effect of tethered cord division on lower urinary tract functions. *Eur J Pediatr Surg* 11:116, 2001.
7. Boop FA, Russell A, Chadduck WM: Diagnosis and management of the tethered cord syndrome. *J Ark Med Soc* 89:328, 1992.
8. Bruce DA, Schut L: Spinal lipomas in infancy and childhood. *Childs Brain* 5:192, 1979.
9. Chan CT, Gold WL: Intramedullary abscess of the spinal cord in the antibiotic era: clinical features, microbial etiologies, trends in pathogenesis, and outcomes. *Clin Infect Dis* 27:619, 1998.
10. Chong C, Molet J, Oliver B, et al: The tethered cord syndrome: a review of causes. *Neurologia* 9:12,1994.
11. Cornette L, Verpoorten C, Lagae L, et al: Tethered cord syndrome in occult spinal dysraphism: timing and outcome of surgical release. *Neurology* 50:1761, 1998.
12. Chapman PH: Congenital intraspinal lipomas: anatomic considerations and surgical treatment. *Child's Brain* 9:37, 1982.
13. El-Gindi S, Fairburn B: Intramedullary spinal abscess as a complication of a congenital dermal sinus: case report. *J Neurosurg* 30:494, 1969.
14. Emery JL, London RG: Lipomas of the cauda equina and other fatty tumors related to neurospinal dysraphism. *Dev Med Child Neurol* 20:62, 1968.
15. Fitz CR: Neuroradiology of spinal dysraphism. In Park TS (ed): *Spinal Dysraphism*, Boston, Blackwell Scientific, 1992, p 161.
16. French BN: Abnormal development of the central nervous system. In McLauren RL, Schut L, Venes JL, Epstein FL (eds): *Pediatric Neurosurgery*, ed 2. Philadelphia, WB Saunders, 1989, p 9.
17. Garzo-Mercado R: Diastematomyelia and intramedullary epidermoid spinal tumor combined with extra-dural teratoma in an adult. *J Neurosurg* 58:954, 1983.
18. Geremin GK, McNeil TW: CT demonstration of cervical diastematomyelia. *J Comput Assist Tomogr* 9:592, 1985.
19. Giuffre R: Intradural spinal lipomas. *Acta Neurochir* 14:69, 1966.
20. Guidetti B, Gagliardi FM: Epidermoid and dermoid cysts: clinical evaluation and late surgical results. *J Neurosurg* 47:12, 1977.
21. Gupta SK, Kosla VK, Sharma BS, et al: Tethered cord syndrome in adults. *Surg Neurol* 52:362, 1999.
22. Guthkelch AN: Diastematomyelia with median septum. *Brain* 97:729, 1974.
23. Hamby WB: Pilonidal cyst, spina bifida occulta and bifid spinal cord: report of a case and review of the literature. *Arch Pathol* 21:831, 1936.
24. Hilal SK, Marton D, Pollack E: Diastematomyelia in children. *Radiology* 112:609, 1974.
25. Knepper DA, McLone DA: Development of the spinal cord: normal and abnormal neurulation. In Park TS (ed): *Spinal Dysraphism*, Boston, Blackwell Scientific, 1992, p 1.

26. La Marca F, Grant JA, Tomita T, McLone DG: Spinal lipomas in children: outcome of 270 procedures. *Pediatr Neurosurg* 26:8, 1997.

27. Lassman LP, James CCM: Lumbosacral lipomas: critical survey of 26 cases submitted to laminectomy. *J Neurol Neurosurg Psychiatry* 30:174, 1967.

28. Mathern GW, Peacock WJ: Diastematomyelia. In Park TS (ed): *Spinal Dysraphism.* Boston, Blackwell Scientific, 1992, p 91.

29. Matson DD, Jerva MJ: Recurrent meningitis associated with congenital lumbo-sacral dermal sinus tract, *J Neurosurg* 25:288, 1966.

30. Matson DD, Woods RP, Campbell JB et al: Diastematomyelia (congenital clefts of the spinal cord): diagnosis and surgical treatment. *Pediatrics* 6:98, 1950.

31. McComb JG: Congenital dermal sinus. In Pang D (ed): *Disorders of the Pediatric Spine,* Raven Press, 1995, p 349-360.

32. McLone DG, Hayashida SF, Caldarelli M: Surgical resection of lipomyelomeningoceles in 18 asymptomatic infants. *J Pediatr Neurosci* 1:239, 1985.

33. McLone DG, Naidich TP: Laser resection of fifty spinal lipomas. *Neurosurgery* 18:611, 1986.

34. McLone DG, Naidich TP: The tethered spinal cord. In McLauren RL, Schut L, Venes JL, Epstein FL (eds): *Pediatric neurosurgery,* ed 2, Philadelphia, WB Saunders, 1989, p 76.

35. Morandi S, Mercier P, Fournier HD, Brassier G: Dermal sinus and intramedullary spinal cord abscess: report of two cases and review of the literature. *Child Nerv Syst* 15:202, 1999.

36. Morano JU, Miller JD, Connors JJ: MR imaging of spinal epidural lipoma. *Am J Neuroradiol* 10:102, 1989.

37. Mount LA: Congenital dermal sinuses as a cause of meningitis, intraspinal abscess and intracranial abscess. *JAMA* 139:1263, 1949.

38. Muraszko K, Youholis A: Intramedullary spinal tumors of disordered embryogenesis. *J Neurooncology* 47:271, 2000.

39. Pang D: Split cord malformation: part II: clinical syndrome. *Neurosurgery* 31:481, 1992.

40. Pang D: Spinal cord lipomas. In Pang D (ed): *Disorders of the Pediatric Spine.* Raven Press, 1995, p 175-201.

41. Pang D, Dias MS, Ahab-Barmada M: Split cord malformation: part I: a unified theory of embryogenesis for double spinal cord malformations. *Neurosurgery* 31:451, 1992.

42. Pang D, Wilberger JF Jr: Tethered cord syndrome in adults. *J Neurosurg* 57:32, 1982.

43. Pierre-Kahn, Lacombe J, Pinchon J et al.: Intraspinal lipomas with spina bifida. *J Neurosurg* 65:756, 1986.

44. Proctor M, Bauer SB, Scott MR: The effect of surgery for split spinal cord malformation on neurologic and urologic function. *Pediatr Neurosurg* 32:13, 2000.

45. Reigel DH: Tethered spinal cord. In Humpreys RP (ed): *Concepts in Pediatric Neurosurgery,* vol 4. Basel, S Karger AG, 1983, p 142.

46. Rogers HM, Long DM, Chou SN, et al: Lipomas of the spinal cord and cauda equine, *J Neurosurg* 34:349, 1971.

47. Scott G, Harwood-Nash DC, Hoffman HJ: Congenital thoracic dermal sinus: diagnosis by computer-assisted metrizamide myelography. *J Comput Assist Tomogr* 4:675, 1980.

48. Tortori-Donati P, Rossi A, Cama A: Spinal dysraphism: a review of neuroradiological features with embryological correlations and proposal for a new classification. *Neuroradiology* 42:471, 2000.

49. Van Gilder JC, Schwartz HG: Growth of dermoids from skin implants to the nervous system and surrounding spaces of the newborn rat. *J Neurosurg* 26:14, 1967.

50. Villarejo FJ, Blasquez MG, Guierrez-Diaz JA: Intraspinal lipomas in children. *Child's Brain* 2:361, 1976.

51. Walker ARE, Bucy PC: Congenital dermal sinuses: source of spinal meningeal infection and subdural abscesses. *Brain* 57:401, 1936.

52. Wright RL: Congenital dermal sinuses. *Prog Neurol Surg* 4:175, 1971.

53. Xenos C, Sgouros S, Walsh R, Hockley A: Spinal lipomas in children. *Pediatr Neurosurg* 32:295, 2000.

54. Yamada S, Zinke DE, Sanders DC: Pathophysiology of "tethered cord syndrome." *J Neurosurg* 54:499, 1981.

55. Zide BM: How to reduce the morbidity of wound closure following extensive and complicated laminectomy and tethered cord surgery. *Pediatr Neurosurg* 18:157, 1995.

# CHAPTER 82

# Myelomeningocele and Associated Anomalies

**Samer K. Elbabaa and Mark G. Luciano**

Myelomeningocele, or spina bifida aperta, is defined as a dorsally protruding open spinal cord defect that is usually associated with spinal nerve paralysis and anomalies throughout the spinal axis. The goal of this chapter is to discuss and provide a description of the current management of myelomeningocele and its common associated anomalies in general, with special emphasis on associated spinal anomalies.

## History and Epidemiology

Many epidemiologic studies have combined myelomeningocele with other defects such as anencephaly under the term *neural tube defect* (NTD). This grouping has a rationale in embryology since both are open lesions that arise as a result of failure of primary neurulation and are separated in time only by one embryonic stage (2 days).

When describing NTD at birth, the term *incidence* is more clinically descriptive than is the term *prevalence*, since many NTD occurrences spontaneously abort. NTDs are known to exhibit wide geographic, ethnic, and gender variation. In the United States, NTD rates have declined from 1.3 per 1000 births in 1970 to 0.6 per 1000 births in 1989.[86] Worldwide, numbers range from 1 to 6 per 1000 births.[52] Superimposed on a general worldwide decrease in the incidence at birth of myelomeningocele, a number of influences cause both a reduction in prevalence at birth and increased prevalence in the general population. Reduction of myelomeningocele at birth may result from maternal use of folates and a higher rate of pregnancy termination due to availability of maternal serum α-fetoprotein and refined resolution of ultrasound for *in utero* fetal examination.

Improved neonatal and postoperative care in recent years has resulted in increased survival rates and, therefore, an increased prevalence in the general population. Zachary[87] felt that all affected infants should be operated on, even if it is certain that many survivors will suffer from multiple handicaps. Worldwide, there are several variables and degrees of selection for candidacy for myelomeningocele treatment. The predominant factors are the level of myelomeningocele and associated paralysis, severity of associated hydrocephalus, and gross deformities. It is well-known that the overwhelming majority of untreated infants with myelomeningocele will die early in life.[36]

The history of myelomeningocele treatment over the last few decades has also lead to a tremendous change in quality of life of myelomeningocele patients. McLone[42] estimated that more than 75% of surviving myelomeningocele infants will have normal intelligence; however, the frequency of learning disabilities is likely to be high. More than 80% will be ambulators by school age, while more than 90% will have bladder and bowel control.

## Embryogenesis and Pathophysiology

During the last 100 years, various hypotheses have been proposed concerning the embryogenesis of myelomeningocele. Multiple experimental models and autopsy specimens were studied thoroughly. Myelomeningocele was produced in animal models genetically (e.g., curly tail mouse)[1] or induced by medical or environmental factors such as vitamin A,[75] valproic acid,[53] salicylates,[80] insulin,[15] and hyperglycemic[60] and hyperthermic[22] conditions.

Current theories regarding the embryogenesis of dysraphic spinal lesions in general, and of myelomeningocele in particular, invoke a primary disorder of early neural tube development. This early defect of embryogenesis occurs in the fourth week of gestation. In normal embryos the central nervous system originates from the neural tube, which is the thickening of the dorsal ectoderm. By the gradual elevation of the lateral margins of the neural tube, which are termed *neural folds*, the neural groove is formed. The neural folds meet in the midline and then form the neural tube. This process begins at the mesencephalic level and proceeds rostrally and caudally with latest tube formation in the caudal spine at the caudal level.

Four different theories have been described: simple nonclosure theory, overgrowth and nonclosure theory, reopening (overdistention) theory, and primary mesodermal insufficiency theory.[75] Since its introduction, nonclosure theory has gained almost universal acceptance because of its consistency with observations of early human embryos in which NTDs have been studied during or shortly after neural tube closure. Additional support came from animal models of dysraphism, virtually all of which displayed a primary defect of neural tube closure.[16]

Myelomeningocele includes other consistent anomalies through the central nervous system axis; these include Chiari II malformation and hydrocephalus. After studying the initial developmental defects of the Chiari II malformation using a genetically mutated NTD mouse model, McLone and Knepper[45] proposed a unified theory that describes and emphasizes the developmental sequence of associated anomalies. This pathophysiologic sequence starts with cerebrospinal fluid (CSF) leakage from the unclosed spinal defect. As a result the usual distention and expansion of the developing ventricular system fails. The lack of distention of rhombencephalic vesicles alters the inductive effect of pressure on the surrounding mesenchyme and endochondral bone formation and results in small posterior fossa. Consequently, the development of the cerebellum and brainstem with a small posterior fossa leads to upward herniation and a dysplastic tentorium. Downward herniation results in a large foramen magnum and cerebellar vermis and brainstem displacement into the cervical segments (Chiari II malformation). Hydrocephalus is secondary to maldevelopment of the CSF pathways in the posterior fossa.

The highest percentage of myelomeningoceles occur in the distal thoracic to lumbosacral spine (85%). About 10% are detected in the higher thoracic area, and an additional 5% in the cervical area.[25] Typically, a neural placode (plaque), which is unfolded neural tissue, appears at the center with a pia mater on the ventral surface. The ventral and dorsal nerve roots arise from the central surface of the placode, with the dorsal roots originating more laterally. Rostrally, the placode is continuous with the normal spinal cord within the spinal canal. At the periphery of the defect, the placode is circumscribed by arachnoid membrane that fuses with the free margins of the skin, fascia, and dura mater (Figure 82.1). At involved levels, pedicles of vertebrae are displaced laterally, creating a widened spinal canal diameter. Vertebral bodies may be normal or wedge-shaped in the anteroposterior diameter, resulting in a kyphotic deformity.[55]

## Etiology

It has been established that the etiology of myelomeningocele is multifactorial and heterogeneous. Experimental teratology has shown that several agents can increase occurrence rates; alcohol, carbamazepine,[61] valproic acid,[64] salicylates,[80] insulin,[15] clomiphene, influenza virus,[19] and chemotherapeutic agents have all been incriminated. Population studies, however, have provided strikingly little evidence to suggest the role of a single teratogen as the sole cause of a significant number of myelomeningoceles.[9] Maternal age and birth order may also contribute to the risk of NTDs. Most studies show an excess of first-born children in the population of NTDs.[12] In addition, the majority of affected mothers are younger than 20 years of age or older than 35.[11]

Although rarely clustered in families, a mendelian pattern of inheritance is evident. The recurrence risk for siblings of an affected individual is 2% to 5%, representing a twenty-five-fold to fifty-fold increase in recurrence risk compared with the general population incidence.[20] A multicenter NTD genetic study reviewed the identification of genes predisposing to NTD through linkage analysis and candidate gene analysis along with characteristics of a large nationally ascertained cohort of families. Results from specific assessments of p53, PAX3, and MTHFR failed to suggest that these genes play a major role in NTD development in these families.[47] Frequent association was found between trisomy 13 and 18 and myelomeningocele in the fetus less than 24 weeks of age (as high as 14%) but was rare in full-term infants, suggesting fetal demise.[38]

Dietary factors related to NTDs were investigated extensively after several studies showed a progressive increase in the prevalence rate of NTDs in lower socioeconomic classes. Zinc deficiency has been considered because of known increased risk of congenital defects in the offspring of animals fed a zinc-deficient diet;[81] however, human studies have been inconclusive so far.[9]

Folic acid antagonists, such as aminopterin, were shown to cause NTDs in animal studies, and since the publication of these studies, the effect of folic acid on prevention of myelomeningocele has been studied. In one study, serum and RBC folate were decreased in mothers of children with myelomeningocele compared with controls.[65] Folic acid and multivitamin supplementation to high-risk mothers has been demonstrated to reduce the prevalence at birth of myelomeningocele in some populations.[33,65] However, adherents to the folic acid prevention philosophy acknowledge that they cannot provide a reasonable mechanism of action.[64]

## Repair of Myelomeningocele
### Evaluation of the Newborn

Prenatal diagnosis and counseling have a significant effect on the preparation and decision-making process in myelomeningocele cases.[13] Prenatal diagnosis of myelomeningocele involves the combined use of maternal serum α-fetoprotein screening and fetal ultrasonography.[3] The advances in ultrasound imaging lead to an increased rate of identification of fetuses with myelomeningocele during intrauterine life. Obstetricians then commonly refer the mother and family to a multidisciplinary team that includes a pediatric neurosurgeon, neonatologist, social worker, and spina-bifida team coordinator. This referral facilitates postnatal treatment, including surgery, to be planned in a timely fashion and informs and educates the family about the nature of myelomeningocele and its associated anomalies.[25]

Early closure of the spinal defect remains an important part of the modern management of children born with myelomeningocele. The rationale for early closure includes the prevention of ascending infection; preservation of motor, sensory, and intellectual function; establishment of a suitable environment for continued development of neural tissue; and cosmetic reconstruction.[40] Most pediatric neurosurgeons agree that closure of the open myelomeningocele within the first 24 to 48 hours after birth decreases morbidity and mortality rates. Initiating surgery after 72 hours carries a significant risk of meningitis and ventriculitis,[43] a decrease of motor function, and an increase in neurologic deficits.[25]

Postnatally, the myelomeningocele defect should be covered with a sterile dressing (wet or nonadherent dressing)

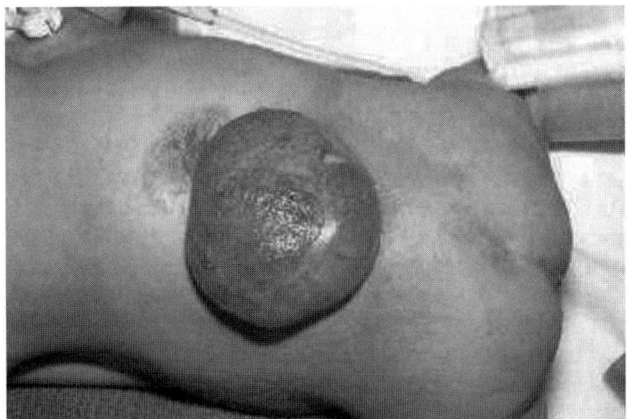

**Figure 82.1** Preoperative photograph demonstrating the typical myelomeningocele.

before the infant is transferred to the neonatal intensive care unit. The newborn is kept in a prone or lateral recumbent position to protect the neural tissue by avoiding pressure on the placode. A thorough examination of the neonate should be conducted to assess the degree of neurologic deficit, the functional level, and associated concerns such as hydrocephalus and cardiopulmonary, genitourinary, and gastrointestinal conditions that could interfere with surgery of the myelomeningocele. Early urologic consultation is obtained with intermittent catheterization until adequate bladder function is ascertained.

A segmental motor examination should be obtained for future comparison. Observation of spontaneous hip flexion (L1-3), knee extension (L2-4), knee flexion (L5-S1), foot dorsiflexion (L4-5), and foot plantar flexion (S1-S2) should be noted. If painful stimulus is required to elicit movement, it should be applied in a sensory dermatome well above those related to the lesion. Painful stimuli applied below the level of the lesion may elicit stereotypical reflex movements, which may be falsely interpreted as a functional motor segment. Gross asymmetry between the two lower extremities may indicate a more proximal lesion in the spinal cord (e.g., diastematomyelia, hemimyelocele).

More than 90% of neonates with myelomeningocele have some form of neurogenic bladder. Dribbling of urine as the neonate cries or moves is a strong indicator of future urinary incontinence, whereas periodic micturition with a good stream suggests a possibility of partial incontinence.[66] These infants should also be carefully inspected for characteristic external features that point to severe chromosomal abnormalities. Examination of the placode includes noting its shape and circumference, skin integrity, and extent of the cutaneous and epithelialized layers. The spinal column is examined for early congenital scoliosis, kyphosis, and palpable prominent laminae at the lateral margin of the lesion.

## Surgical Repair

After the identification of the neural placode and cerebrospinal fluid flowing from the central canal, dissection begins and is continued in a circumferential fashion, dividing the placode from the epithelial layer. This will allow the surgeon to see the pia-arachnoid attached at the periphery of the neural placode. It is essential to understand that, developmentally, the lateral edges of the ventral surface of the placode are the alar plate or the dorsal root entry zones. Dorsal nerve roots (sensory) are observed in this region. The medial portion of the ventral surface of the placode is the basal plate, which contains the ventral nerve roots (motor). Thus, the pia-arachnoid meets the neural placode at the lateral margin of the ventral surface of the placode.

The neural tissue is then gently freed from any ventral arachnoid adhesions, using microdissection techniques. When this has been completed, the flat neural placode should be free throughout its circumference and ready for dorsal reapproximation. Beginning rostrally, the pia-arachnoid neural junction of each lateral edge should be brought together in the dorsal midline. Care should be taken to engage only the pia with each pass of the suture, avoiding injury to the sensory roots.

The dura mater is located just beneath the skin edge laterally. Its lateral attachment is incised and the epidural space identified (often marked by the presence of epidural fat). The dura mater should be freed rostrally and caudally to the apices of the defect on each side so that the free edges come together in the midline dorsally. The dura mater is closed in a watertight fashion. The closure should be patulous to prevent spinal cord ischemia and tethering. Occasionally, a dural graft may be required. Intradural hemostasis should be meticulous to minimize late fibrosis and scarring. With all these surgical procedures, latex reactions should be considered.[6]

Reapproximation of the paraspinous muscles over the repair may require some lateral dissection for mobilization. In the presence of a kyphos, the paraspinous muscles can act as spine flexors because of their lateral position, which owing to the deformity, is ventral to the neural axis of the spine. The paraspinous muscles may then be repositioned in the normal anatomic location: dorsal and paramedian. The dorsal fascia can now be reapproximated. A continuous suture with intermittent, interrupted sutures can be used for this layer to further reinforce the watertight dural closure. It is important to note that adequate mobilization of the paraspinous muscles is crucial to prevent constriction of the underlying neural elements.[25]

Closure of the skin in the midline can be facilitated by a generous blunt subcutaneous dissection for mobilization. The proper plane for this blunt dissection is just superficial to the dorsal fascia. Continuous monofilament suture is used for skin closure, which further reinforces the layer by watertight closure. Occasionally, the defect is so large that skin closure cannot be accomplished without undue tension. Plastic surgical consultation may be obtained if adequate skin closure is difficult or even impossible. Several surgical techniques have been used in this situation, including local rotated skin flaps, tissue expansion,[70] relaxations of the lateral incisions with a skin graft,[51] and a Limberg-latissimus dorsi myocutaneous flap.[39]

A recent development in myelomeningocele closure involves the *in utero* closure of myelomeningocele defects. The rationale for fetal repair of myelomeningoceles and initial clinical outcomes have been discussed over the last few years. The development of techniques to close open neural tube malformations prior to birth has generated great interest and hope for fetal interventions and their outcomes. In most recent series of patients, intrauterine myelomeningocele repair appeared to decrease the incidence of hindbrain herniation and shunt-dependent hydrocephalus in infants with myelomeningocele, but increased the incidence of premature delivery. Long-term improvement of neurologic outcome and prevention of hindbrain herniation and hydrocephalus has yet to be proven.[8,14,69,78]

## Associated Anomalies

A multitude of associated anomalies are common in an infant with myelomeningocele. Central nervous system anomalies are more common than other systemic anomalies. Microgyria, polygyria, enlargement of the massa intermedia, agenesis or dysgenesis of the corpus callosum, and cerebellar dysgenesis along with Chiari II malformation are frequent findings that can be encountered on magnetic resonance imaging (MRI). The midbrain, especially the tectal area, can be beaked, and the aqueduct of Sylvius can be anomalous. The pons and medulla oblongata are bowed dorsally and often extend into the rostral cervical spinal canal along with the cerebellar vermis and tonsils.[25]

In a series of autopsies on infants with the myelomeningocele and Chiari malformations, cerebral and cerebellar cortical malformations were found in 92% and 72% of cases, respectively. Heterotopias (i.e., displaced, well-formed gyri and folia), heterotaxias (i.e., disordered combinations of mature neurons and germinal cells), immature germinal cell collections, microgyria, and polymicrogyria were observed. Ventricular system anomalies were present in 92% of cases in the same series, including atresia, stenosis, and forking of the cerebral aqueduct. Atresia of the third ventricle and stenosis of the fourth ventricle occurred rarely. Other infrequent findings included septum pellucidum cysts and agenesis of the olfactory tracts and bulbs.[24]

Systemic anomalies also occur and should be considered independently when assessing infants with the myelomeningocele and Chiari malformations for surgical intervention. Associated systemic anomalies appear in the gastrointestinal, pulmonary, and cardiovascular systems and in the craniofacial structures.[41] The most common anomalies in the genitourinary system include hydroureter and hydronephrosis, which usually occur after long-standing neurogenic bladder. Gastrointestinal anomalies include inguinal hernia, Meckel's diverticulum, malrotation, omphalocele, and imperforate anus. Cardiovascular anomalies include ventricular or atrial septal defects, patent ductus arteriosus, and coarctation of aorta.[7]

## Hydrocephalus

CSF shunting for hydrocephalus is required in approximately 80% of infants born with myelomeningocele.[68] Most clinical signs develop in the first 3 weeks of life, but clinical signs occasionally develop at an older age.[68] It is possible that the rapid onset of hydrocephalus after birth is due to the myelomeningocele acting as a compensatory reservoir that is terminated by defect closure.[55]

Advanced gestational age and severity of posterior fossa deformity have both been shown independently to correlate with the size of ventricles in infants born with myelomeningocele.[4] The sites of obstruction of CSF pathways are variable and include the aqueduct, outlet of the fourth ventricle, arachnoid space at the level of foramen magnum, and tentorium. Wills *et al.*[82] showed that hydrocephalus itself has a very minor effect on intellectual development; however, prior shunt infections and ventriculitis in the neonatal period are major factors limiting intelligence.

Head circumference is less than the fiftieth percentile in most infants born with myelomeningocele. However, serial measurement of head circumference and ultrasound examination of the head should be obtained after closure of the myelomeningocele defect to identify infants who will subsequently need shunting. A mean increase of 2mm per day was found to have a predictive value. Infants born

with overt hydrocephalus signs such as large head circumference, bulging fontanelle, split cranial sutures, and dilated scalp veins generally require early CSF diversion to relieve the intracranial hypertension and prevent myelomeningocele wound dehiscence. Signs of increased intracranial pressure in the newborn such as bradycardia, poor sucking, apnea, and decreased spontaneous activity indicate the need for shunting. The function of the shunt should always be considered and checked before any surgical treatment of Chiari II malformation or syringomyelia after symptoms deteriorate.[42] Although variable, a common practice is to wait 5 days or more after myelomeningocele closure before shunting. Most infants will tolerate this waiting period.[55] In one series, shunt infection and malfunction rates were comparable between infants undergoing a simultaneous myelomeningocele closure and shunting procedures and those infants with the delayed-onset hydrocephalus and shunting.

## Chiari Malformation and Syringomyelia

Virtually all children with myelomeningocele have a Chiari II malformation.[76] The hallmark of the Chiari II malformation is the caudal displacement of the cerebellar vermis, medulla, and lower brainstem below the level of foramen magnum into or below the craniocervical junction. The caudal descent of the lower brainstem into the cervical canal may create a kink or spur of medulla behind the cervical spinal cord in up to 70% of Chiari II patients.[17] The cerebellum of the Chiari II patient is smaller than normal; however, it resides in a proportionately smaller posterior fossa. The tentorium has a low insertion and is frequently hypoplastic (Figure 82.2).

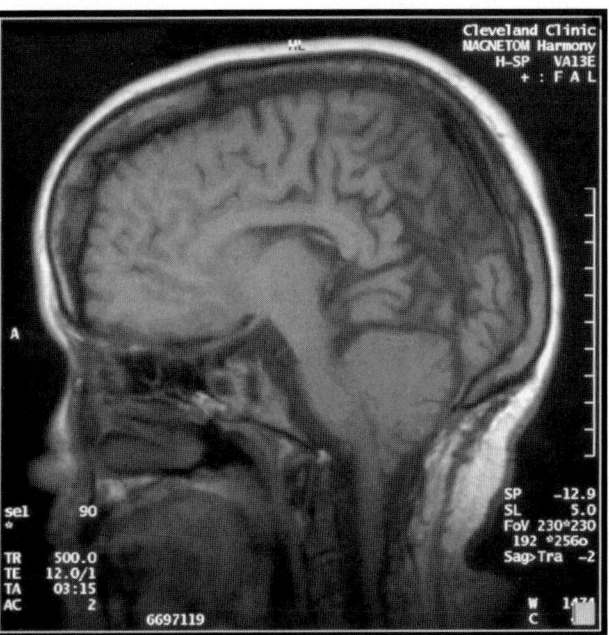

**Figure 82.2** Sagittal $T_1$-weighted magnetic resonance image of the Chiari II malformation. Note the herniation of the cerebellar vermis through the foramen magnum, low-lying tentorium, beaked appearance of the tectal plate, and enlargement of the massa intermedia.

The frequency of hydrosyringomyelia in Chiari II patients has varied in reports from 44% to 88%.[30,62] The true frequency in recent series may be underestimated secondary to collapse of the syrinx after shunting and/or Chiari's decompression[59] (Figure 82.3).

Between 20% and 33% of Chiari II patients become symptomatic from hindbrain herniation.[59] Of these symptomatic children, nearly one third do not survive beyond infancy, making the symptomatic hindbrain herniation the leading cause of mortality in treated myelomeningocele in the first 2 years of life.[42] Between 1983 and 1992, four different retrospective studies indicated that there are basically two types of presentation that are clearly

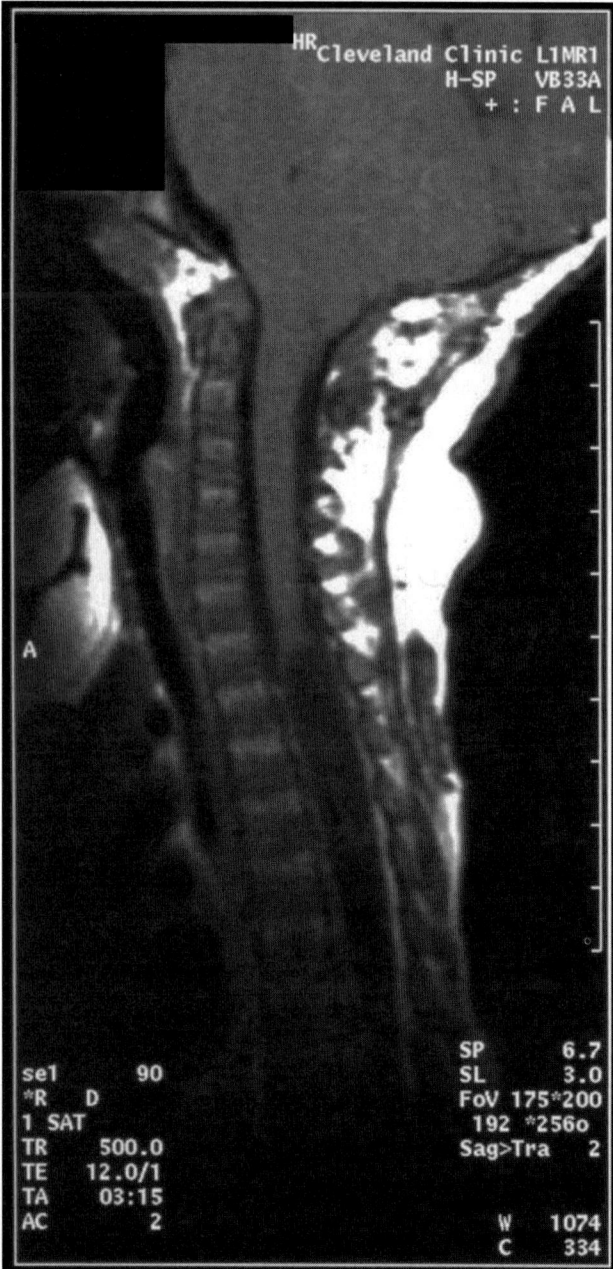

**Figure 82.3** Sagittal $T_1$-weighted magnetic resonance image of a child with Chiari II demonstrating hydrosyringomyelic cavities of the cervical and upper thoracic spinal cord.

age-dependent and may reflect different pathophysiologies[57-59,76] Neonatal patients present with symptoms referable to lower cranial nerve and brainstem dysfunction, and older children present with spasticity, cerebellar signs, and weakness.[59] Infantile symptoms include swallowing difficulty, stridor, aspiration, apnea, bradycardia, arm weakness, and opisthotonic posturing.

The surgical treatment of Chiari II malformation usually consists of decompressive laminectomy at the C1 level and lower as needed, excision of the constrictive dural band at the C1 level, and a cautious suboccipital craniectomy due to the low-lying transverse sinus. Fourth ventricular exploration may be performed to ensure that a CSF outlet and dural graft may be used in closure. The timing of surgery is controversial.[57] The surgical treatment of older children can be rewarding, with almost all patients showing stabilization or return to normal function.[59] Irreversible compressive or ischemic brainstem injury has been proposed as the cause of the high mortality and as an argument for relatively emergent surgical intervention. Two of the retrospective studies have noted no obvious evidence of brainstem dysfunction at birth.[58] In autopsy specimens from infants dying with Chiari II malformation, ischemic medullary hemorrhages confirmed that vascular compromise is a contributing cause.[50] It is likely that in one third of myelomeningocele patients that become symptomatic before 3 years of age there is greater degree of brainstem dysmorphism, creating a brainstem at risk that would have little tolerance for compression or ischemia. In these patients, rapid deterioration would be expected and the results of prompt surgical intervention with the initial symptoms may be favorable.[59]

There are more clear-cut indications for surgery in patients with syringomyelia. Between 60% and 73% improved after treating a symptomatic syrinx, and none worsened after surgery in two series.[30,56] Typically patients have an initial stable neurologic examination and then present with progressive spasticity and scoliosis. An expanding cervical hydrosyringomyelic cavity classically results in dissociative sensory loss of the upper extremities caused by interruption in the crossing spinothalamic tracts. Weakness, hyporeflexia, and atrophy of the upper musculature may result from involvement of the anterior horn cells. Motor and sensory findings can be asymmetric, and a worsening scoliosis may be the sole manifestation of an expanding cavity of the thoracic spinal cord.[57,84] Also, an expanding cervical cavity can result in a worsening lower cranial nerve dysfunction.[59] Different treatment strategies have been followed. In the presence of ventriculomegaly, ventricular shunting reduces the syrinx size when there is a communication between the syrinx and fourth ventricle (in about 10% of cases).[77,84] When a shunt is already in place, its function should be evaluated and corrected. A decompressive laminectomy and opening of the foramen of Magendie to restore normal CSF hydrodynamics is indicated when a functional shunt is confirmed.[84] Obex plugging, fourth ventricle to subarachnoid shunts, syringosubarachnoid, and syringopleural shunts have all been used but are controversial.[48,72,77,84] However, syrinx shunts have been used successfully when decompression alone fails to result in clinical improvement and as a primary treatment of thoracic lesions.[48]

## Tethered Spinal Cord

After primary repair of myelomeningocele, late progressive neurologic deterioration commonly occurs due to a tethered spinal cord at the site of previous closure secondary to scarring and adherence of the neural placode to the dorsal dura mater[29] (Figure 82.4). Tethered cord is the result of fixation of the spinal cord, which limits motion in the caudal-rostral direction. Yamada *et al.*[85] correlated the pattern of gradually developing tethered cord symptoms with impairment of oxidative metabolism and mitochondrial anoxia as a result of excessive steady traction of the spinal cord in experimental animal models.

In some series, neurologic deterioration due to tethered cord occurred in 27% of children.[42] The average onset of symptoms occurs at 10 years of age and correlates with period of accelerating growth. Presenting symptoms include gait imbalance, lower back pain, weakness in the lower extremities, bladder or bowel incontinence, scoliosis, and orthopedic deformities. MRI of the lumbar spine is the gold standard of anatomic diagnosis. However, since all spinal cords in myelomeningocele patients appear elongated and tethered, the decision to operate depends on the demonstration of clinical progression. The decision to treat may result from a deterioration seen on a urodynamic study or ascending sensory or motor neurologic loss of function.

Surgical release involves laminectomy at the vertebral level just rostral to the defect and lysis of adhesions. Additional pathology such as hydromyelia, thickened filum terminale, dermal sinus tracts, and diastematomyelia can present in 30% of patients.[29] The stretched spinal cord tissue should appear relaxed at the completion of the procedure. Duraplasty may be considered to prevent postoperative dural adhesions in the repair of the tethered spinal cord.[2]

The timing of the surgical release of the tethered spinal cord is controversial. However, early diagnosis and early treatment are essential to provide patients with the best chance of recovery. In one report, 82% of patients who were followed closely and treated early had improvement, whereas only 54% of those not followed closely had improvement.[29] Another report showed that delayed untethering, following the onset of a neurological deficit, may reverse some lost motor function but is unlikely to restore bladder and bowel function.[46]

## Scoliosis

Deformity of the spine is common in patients with myelomeningocele. The most frequently encountered spinal deformities are scoliosis and kyphosis. Scoliotic deformities typically develop over years as a result of imbalance of the spinal musculature and abnormal posture.[26] The frequency of spinal deformities is related to the neurologic level, with nearly 100% of thoracic level myelomeningocele children requiring corrective surgery.[32] Other important factors include age, and the presence of syringomyelia,[28] and tethering of the spinal cord.[44]

Scoliosis presents in two forms in these patients: congenital and developmental.[21] Congenital scoliosis arises from vertebral anomalies, particularly hemivertebrae and segmentations defects. Developmental scoliosis (majority) has a delayed onset and a progressive course producing considerable functional decline at advanced stages and is generally believed to result from muscular imbalance leading to progressive deformity during growth. Scoliotic curves usually develop between 5 and 10 years of age, but most deterioration occurs between 10 and 15 years of age.[21]

The higher the level of paralysis, the greater the incidence of spinal deformity.[10] Scoliosis develops in up to 100% of patients with thoracic lesions, but in less than 10% of patients with sacral lesions. In a large series of 465 patients, Carstens *et al.*[10] showed that the patient's neurologic level of the lesion is the most important factor determining the development of scoliosis in myelomeningocele. A 3.5-degree deterioration of the angle every year occurred in patients with levels of paralysis between T3 and T12, and a 2.5-degree deterioration in patients with levels of paralysis between L1 and L3.

The natural history of untreated scoliosis in myelomeningocele is that of deformity progression, with a rate of deterioration significantly higher than in idiopathic scoliosis. The aims of treatment are preservation of respiratory function, maintenance of sitting stability, achievement

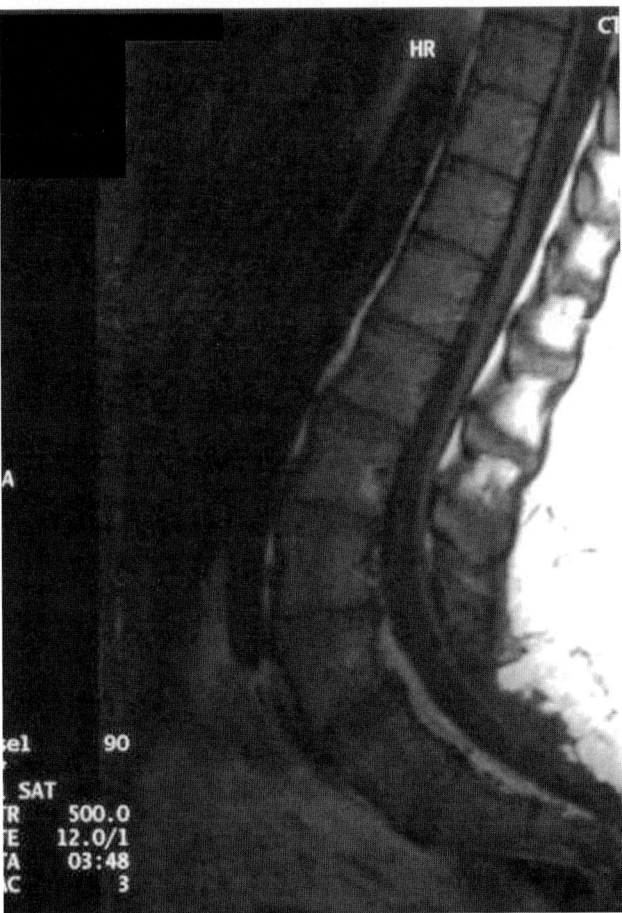

**Figure 82.4** Sagittal T$_1$-weighted magnetic resonance image showing tethering of the spinal cord 15 years after myelomeningocele closure.

of maximal trunk length, and stabilization of the trunk.[21] Corrective bracing is used as the initial management while the child matures. Children with myelomeningocele should be examined yearly for the presence or progression of scoliosis. Once spinal curvature surpasses 30 degrees, bracing usually fails and fusion surgery is required to control progression.[26] However, spinal orthoses in children with myelomeningocele may lead to deformity of the ribs, decreased pulmonary function, ischemia of the skin, and pressure ulcerations.[83] Progressive scoliosis is often the result of other correctable neurologic pathologies such as syringomyelia, hydromyelia, tethered spinal cord, or hydrocephalus shunt malfunction.[32] Stability or improvement of the scoliosis can be anticipated following untethering of the spinal cord.[44] Tomlinson et al.[73] found that syringomyelia is associated with a high incidence of developmental scoliosis and that decompression of the syrinx either leads to improvement in, or stabilization of, the majority of scoliotic curves or postpones the need for fusion surgery. If a neurosurgical cause is discovered and treated, spontaneous improvement in the scoliosis may be seen if the curve is small in magnitude. Large curves do not resolve despite neurosurgical intervention.[27]

The definitive treatment of scoliosis in the myelomeningocele patient is spinal fusion. The entire curve must be included in the fusion. Distally, the fusion should extend to include the lumbosacral joint if there is pelvic obliquity and the patient does not walk.[32] Combined ventral and dorsal spinal fusions have been recommended because dorsal fusion alone can result in a high rate of pseudoarthroses due to incomplete solid fusion at the defective laminar defects. Most arthroses occur at the lumbosacral junction. However, bilateral transpedicular fixation of L5 and S1 levels can be performed as a prophylactic procedure.[23] The role of ventral fusion is controversial and may be unnecessary for routine curves.[79] The most common complications are infection, loss of correction, and pseudoarthrosis.[54]

## Kyphosis

A kyphotic deformity of the spine, in association with a myelomeningocele, is present in approximately 10% of patients.[31] Progression of the kyphotic deformity can be seen in the sagittal plane of affected children.[49] Unrelenting progression of 8 degrees per year is seen in most of them.[63] Congenital kyphoses progress not only because of the deficiencies of the dorsal elements of the spine but also because of the effects of gravity during sitting and standing, as well as the subluxation of the extensor spinal muscles laterally and the unopposed psoas muscles anteriorly.[5] A kyphotic deformity can interfere with sitting and prevents supination. There is frequently skin ulceration over the gibbus and crowding of the thoracic and abdominal contents. Kyphosis is usually associated with pulmonary and digestive compromise, owing to the crowding of the lungs by the intraabdominal contents, which are forced upward by the flexion of the trunk.[32,35] Neurologic deterioration is usually not a concern since there is no useful neurologic function distal to the kyphosis in most children so affected.

The goal of a kyphectomy procedure is restoration of complete sagittal alignment, balance, and stability, while allowing for growth.[37] The preferred age for surgery appears to be 2 to 5 years of age, when the anteroposterior vertebral diameter reaches a 25mm minimum. McLone[42] recommended a kyphectomy procedure prior to 2 years of age for children born with a thoracolumbar kyphosis and motor function at or below L4 level. Corrective surgery may also be performed at the time of myelomeningocele closure, with resection of misaligned segments. In severe cases this may be needed to obtain adequate closure.

Optimal surgical results require resection of the vertebral bodies at the apex of the kyphos to facilitate complete correction, without which recurrence is likely.[74] Published reports of long-term follow-up of resection of the rostral portion of the kyphotic deformity demonstrate that most patients improved but a residual deformity persisted and that some degree of a loss of correction of sagittal balance was observed over time.[34,37] A number of methods of internal fixation have been described. Aggressive deformity correction procedures that achieve satisfactory results have been described. However, this was associated with significant blood loss and a significant recurrence at 1 year of age, when limited internal fixation is used.[35]

In general, a correction of 45 degrees per vertebral level can be expected, and the lumbar lordosis can be restored, along with thoracic kyphosis and comprehensive sagittal balance. Postoperative wound breakdown is a common complication and can be managed by a postoperative full-thickness flap advancement or preoperative placement of tissue expanders.[35,63]

## Other Spinal Anomalies

Other vertebral anomalies include an absence of the spinous processes and laminae, a reduction in the anteroposterior dimension of the vertebral body, an increase of the interpedicular distance, a decrease in the height of the pedicle, lateral extension of the large transverse processes, hemivertebrae, partial or complete vertebral fusion, and fusion of transverse processes.[25] Spinal cord anomalies other than open myelomeningocele include hydromyelia, diplomyelia, diastematomyelia, and defective myelinization; these were found in 88% of autopsy cases having spinal cord anomalies.[24]

## Postoperative and Chronic Care

About 15% of patients with myelomeningocele are born with clinical signs of hydrocephalus, but 80% or more develop hydrocephalus in early infancy. In most instances, the clinical features and diagnosis become obvious within a week or two.[67] Performing a CSF diversion procedure (e.g., ventriculoperitoneal shunt) will relieve the ventricular pressure and tension on the myelomeningocele closure site to permit healing without CSF leakage. Third ventriculostomy may be considered for treatment of aqueductal stenosis in myelomeningocele patients with a reported success rate that ranges between 65% and 80%. Third ventriculostomy is also a safe and effective means of treating hydrocephalus in the older myelomeningocele population even after years of shunting and offers the possibility of a long-term, shunt-independent life for selected patients.[18,71]

A thorough urologic evaluation should determine the degree of sphincter impairment, bladder dysfunction, and infection. Clean intermittent catheterization is utilized by 90% of children with myelomeningocele in the United States; 75% perform self-catheterization.[42] Bowel management programs are easily achieved by supplementing proper nutrition, using laxatives, and taking advantage of the normal physiologic response of the gastrointestinal tract.[25]

Optimal care of a patient with myelomeningocele in the long term requires a comprehensive coordinated plan of treatment usually in a myelomeningocele clinic that includes neurosurgery, urology, orthopedic surgery, neurology, and rehabilitation. Neurosurgical follow-up should include periodical evaluation of the status of hydrocephalus, tethered spinal cord, Chiari II malformation, and syringomyelia. Deterioration of function must be investigated, and this investigation should begin with ensuring proper CSF diversion. Multiple surgical procedures usually include urologic and orthopedic operations, as well as shunt revisions, Chiari decompressions, tethered cord releases, or spinal fusions.

Over the last 30 years, continual progress has been made in the outcomes of children born with myelomeningocele. Survival rates dramatically improved once hydrocephalus was controllable. Survival rates range between 80% and 85% at 15-year follow-up in treated group of patients.[42] Hindbrain dysfunction caused by Chiari II malformation remains the principal cause of mortality. With an ongoing coordinated care plan, the affected patient's level of function can be expected to be maintained.[42]

# REFERENCES

1. Adinolfi M, Beck S, Embury S, *et al*: Levels of alpha-fetoprotein in amniotic fluids of mice (curly-tail) with neural tube defects. *J Med Genet* 13:511-513, 1976.
2. Aliredjo RP, de Vries J, Menovsky T, *et al*: The use of Gore-Tex membrane for adhesion prevention in tethered spinal cord surgery: technical case reports, *Neurosurgery* 44:674-677, 1999.
3. Babcook CJ: Ultrasound evaluation of prenatal and neonatal spina bifida, *Neurosurg Clin N Am* 6:203-218, 1995.
4. Babcook CJ, Drake CM, Goldstein RB: Spinal level of fetal myelomeningocele: does it influence ventricular size? *Am J Roentgenol* 169:207-210, 1997.
5. Banta JV: The evolution of surgical treatment of spinal deformity in myelomeningocele. *Z Kinderchir* 42(suppl 1):10-12, 1987.
6. Banta JV, Bonanni C, Prebluda J: Latex anaphylaxis during spinal surgery in children with myelomeningocele. *Dev Med Child Neurol* 35:543-548, 1993.
7. Brown SF: Congenital malformations associated with myelomeningocele. *J Iowa Med Soc* 65:101-104, 1975.
8. Bruner JP, Tulipan N, Paschall RL, *et al*: Fetal surgery for myelomeningocele and the incidence of shunt-dependent hydrocephalus. *JAMA* 282:1819-1825, 1999.
9. Campbell LR, Dayton DH, Sohal GS: Neural tube defects: a review of human and animal studies on the etiology of neural tube defects. *Teratology* 34:171-187, 1986.
10. Carstens C, Vetter J, Niethard FU: Development of paralytic scoliosis in myelomeningocele. *Z Ortho Ihre Grenzgeb* 128:174-182, 1990.
11. Carter CO, Evans K. Children of adult survivors with spina bifida cystica. *Lancet* 2:924-926, 1973.
12. Carter CO, Evans KA, Campbell S. Letter: neural-tube malformations in offspring of spina-bifida patients. *Lancet* 1:685, 1975.
13. Charney EB, Weller SC, Sutton LN, *et al.*: Management of the newborn with myelomeningocele: time for a decision-making process. *Pediatrics* 75:58-64, 1985.
14. Cochrane DD, Irwin B, Chambers K: Clinical outcomes that fetal surgery for myelomeningocele needs to achieve. *Eur J Pediatr Surg* 11(suppl 1):S18-S20, 2001.
15. Cole WA, Trasler DG: Gene-teratogen interaction in insulin-induced mouse exencephaly. *Teratology* 22:125-139, 1980.
16. Dias MS, Walker ML: The embryogenesis of complex dysraphic malformations: a disorder of gastrulation? *Pediatr Neurosurg* 18:229-253, 1992.
17. el Gammal T, Mark EK, Brooks BS: MR imaging of Chiari II malformation. *Am J Roentgenol* 150:163-170, 1988.
18. Elbabaa SK, Steinmetz M, Ross J, *et al*: Endoscopic third ventriculostomy for obstructive hydrocephalus in the pediatric population: evaluation of outcome. *Eur J Pediatr Surg* 11(suppl 1):S52-S54, 2001.
19. Elwood JH: Epidemics of anencephalus and spina bifida in Ireland since 1900. *Int J Epidemiol* 2:171-175, 1973.
20. Elwood M: Folic acid prevents neural tube defects. *Med J Aust* 155:579-581, 1991.
21. Eysel P, Hopf C, Schwarz M, Voth D: Development of scoliosis in myelomeningocele: differences in the history caused by idiopathic pattern. *Neurosurg Rev* 16:301-306, 1993.
22. Finnell RH, Moon SP, Abbott LC, *et al*: Strain differences in heat-induced neural tube defects in mice. *Teratology* 33:247-252, 1986.
23. Geiger F, Parsch D, Carstens C: Complications of scoliosis surgery in children with myelomeningocele. *Eur Spine J* 8:22-26, 1999.
24. Gilbert JN, Jones KL, Rorke LB, *et al*: Central nervous system anomalies associated with meningomyelocele, hydrocephalus, and the Arnold-Chiari malformation: reappraisal of theories regarding the pathogenesis of posterior neural tube closure defects. *Neurosurgery* 18:559-564, 1986.
25. Hahn YS: Open myelomeningocele. *Neurosurg Clin North Am* 6:231-241, 1995.
26. Hall JE, Poitras B: The management of kyphosis in patients with myelomeningocele. *Clin Orthop* Oct:33-40, 1977.
27. Hall PV, Campbell RL, Kalsbeck JE: Meningomyelocele and progressive hydromyelia: progressive paresis in myelodysplasia. *J Neurosurg* 43:457-463, 1975.
28. Hall PV, Kalsbeck JE, Wellman HN: Clinical radiosotope investigations in hydrosyringomyelia and myelodysplasia. *J Neurosurg* 45:188-194, 1976.
29. Herman JM, McLone DG, Storrs BB, Dauser RC: Analysis of 153 patients with myelomeningocele or spinal lipoma reoperated upon for a tethered cord: presentation, management, and outcome. *Pediatr Neurosurg* 19:243-249, 1993.
30. Hoffman HJ, Neill J, Crone KR, *et al*: Hydrosyringomyelia and its management in childhood. *Neurosurgery* 21:347-351, 1987.

31. Hoppenfeld S: Congenital kyphosis in myelomeningocele. *J Bone Joint Surg Br* 49:276-280, 1967.

32. Karol LA: Orthopedic management in myelomeningocele. *Neurosurg Clin N Am* 6:259-268, 1995.

33. Laurence KM, James N, Miller MH et al: Double-blind randomised controlled trial of folate treatment before conception to prevent recurrence of neural-tube defects. *Br Med J (Clin Res Ed)* 282:1509-1511, 1981.

34. Leatherman KD, Dickson RA: Congenital kyphosis in myelomeningocele: vertebral body resection and posterior spine fusion. *Spine* 3:222-226, 1978.

35. Lindseth RE, Stelzer L, Jr: Vertebral excision for kyphosis in children with myelomeningocele. *J Bone Joint Surg Am* 61:699-704, 1979.

36. Lorber J: Results of treatment of myelomeningocele: an analysis of 524 unselected cases, with special reference to possible selection for treatment. *Dev Med Child Neurol* 13:279-303, 1971.

37. Lowe GP, Menelaus MB: The surgical management of kyphosis in older children with myelomeningocele. *J Bone Joint Surg Br* 60:40-45, 1978.

38. Luthy DA, Wardinsky T, Shurtleff DB, et al: Cesarean section before the onset of labor and subsequent motor function in infants with meningomyelocele diagnosed antenatally. *N Engl J Med* 324:662-666, 1991.

39. McDevitt NB, Gillespie RP, Woosley RE, et al: Closure of thoracic and lumbar dysgraphic defects using bilateral latissimus dorsi myocutaneous flap transfer with extended gluteal fasciocutaneous flaps. *Childs Brain* 9: 394-399, 1982.

40. McLone DG: Technique for closure of myelomeningocele. *Childs Brain* 6:65-73, 1980.

41. McLone DG: Treatment of myelomeningocele: arguments against selection. *Clin Neurosurg* 33:359-370, 1986.

42. McLone DG: Continuing concepts in the management of spina bifida. *Pediatr Neurosurg* 18:254-256, 1992.

43. McLone DG, Dias MS: Complications of myelomeningocele closure. *Pediatr Neurosurg* 17:267-273, 1991.

44. McLone DG, Herman JM, Gabrieli AP, Dias L: Tethered cord as a cause of scoliosis in children with a myelomeningocele. *Pediatr Neurosurg* 16:8-13, 1990.

45. McLone DG, Knepper PA: The cause of Chiari II malformation: a unified theory. *Pediatr Neurosci* 15:1-12, 1989.

46. McLone DG, La Marca F: The tethered spinal cord: diagnosis, significance, and management. *Semin Pediatr Neurol* 4:192-208, 1997.

47. Melvin EC, George TM, Worley G, et al: Genetic studies in neural tube defects: NTD Collaborative Group. *Pediatr Neurosurg* 32:1-9, 2000.

48. Milhorat TH, Johnson WD, Miller JI, et al: Surgical treatment of syringomyelia based on magnetic resonance imaging criteria. *Neurosurgery* 31:231-244, 1992.

49. Mintz LJ, Sarwark JF, Dias LS, et al: The natural history of congenital kyphosis in myelomeningocele: a review of 51 children. *Spine* 16:S348-S350, 1991.

50. Morley AR: Laryngeal stridor, Arnold-Chiari malformation, and medullary haemorrhages. *Dev Med Child Neurol* 11:471-474, 1969.

51. Munro IR, Neu BR, Humphreys RP, Lauritzen CG: Limberg-latissimus dorsi myocutaneous flap for closure of myelomeningocele. *Childs Brain* 10:381-386, 1983.

52. Myrianthopoulos NC, Melnick M: Studies in neural tube defects. I. Epidemiologic and etiologic aspects. *Am J Med Genet* 26:783-796, 1987.

53. Naruse I, Collins MD, Scott WJ Jr: Strain differences in the teratogenicity induced by sodium valproate in cultured mouse embryos. *Teratology* 38:87-96, 1988.

54. Osebold WR, Mayfield JK, Winter RB, Moe JH: Surgical treatment of paralytic scoliosis associated with myelomeningocele. *J Bone Joint Surg Am* 64:841-856, 1982.

55. Pang D: Surgical complications of open spinal dysraphism. *Neurosurg Clin N Am* 6:243-257, 1995.

56. Park TS, Cail WS, Maggio WM, Mitchell DC: Progressive spasticity and scoliosis in children with myelomeningocele: radiological investigation and surgical treatment. *J Neurosurg* 62:367-375, 1985.

57. Park TS, Hoffman HJ, Hendrick EB, Humphreys RP: Experience with surgical decompression of the Arnold-Chiari malformation in young infants with myelomeningocele. *Neurosurgery* 13:147-152, 1983.

58. Pollack IF, Pang D, Albright AL, Krieger D: Outcome following hindbrain decompression of symptomatic Chiari malformations in children previously treated with myelomeningocele closure and shunts. *J Neurosurg* 77: 881-888, 1992.

59. Rauzzino M, Oakes WJ: Chiari II malformation and syringomyelia. *Neurosurg Clin North Am* 6:293-309, 1995.

60. Reece EA, Pinter E, Leranth CZ, et al: Ultrastructural analysis of malformations of the embryonic neural axis induced by in vitro hyperglycemic conditions. *Teratology* 32:363-373, 1985.

61. Rosa FW: Spina bifida in infants of women treated with carbamazepine during pregnancy. *N Engl J Med* 324: 674-677, 1991.

62. Samuelsson L, Bergstrom K, Thuomas KA, et al: MR imaging of syringohydromyelia and Chiari malformations in myelomeningocele patients with scoliosis. *Am J Neuroradiol* 8:539-546, 1987.

63. Sarwark JF: Kyphosis deformity in myelomeningocele. *Orthop Clin North Am* 30:451-5, i-ix, 1999.

64. Shurtleff DB, Lemire RJ: Epidemiology, etiologic factors, and prenatal diagnosis of open spinal dysraphism. *Neurosurg Clin N Am* 6:183-193, 1995.

65. Smithells RW, Nevin NC, Seller MJ, et al: Further experience of vitamin supplementation for prevention of neural tube defect recurrences. *Lancet* 1:1027-1031, 1983.

66. Stark G: Prediction of urinary continence in myelomeningocele. *Dev Med Child Neurol* 13:388-389, 1971.

67. Stark GD: Neonatal assessment of the child with a myelomeningocele. *Arch Dis Child* 46:539-548, 1971.

68. Stein SC, Schut L: Hydrocephalus in myelomeningocele. *Childs Brain* 5:413-419, 1979.

69. Sutton LN, Adzick NS, Bilaniuk LT, et al: Improvement in hindbrain herniation demonstrated by serial fetal magnetic resonance imaging following fetal surgery for myelomeningocele. *JAMA* 282:1826-1831, 1999.

70. Teichgraeber JF, Riley WB, Parks DH: Primary skin closure in large myelomeningoceles. *Pediatr Neurosci* 15:18-22, 1989.

71. Teo C, Jones R: Management of hydrocephalus by endoscopic third ventriculostomy in patients with myelomeningocele. *Pediatr Neurosurg* 25:57-63, 1996.

72. Tognetti F, Calbucci F: Syringomyelia: syringo-subarachnoid shunt versus posterior fossa decompression. *Acta Neurochir (Wien.)* 123:196-197, 1993.

73. Tomlinson RJ, Jr., Wolfe MW, Nadall JM, *et al:* Syringomyelia and developmental scoliosis. *J Pediatr Orthop* 14:580-585, 1994.

74. Torode I, Godette G: Surgical correction of congenital kyphosis in myelomeningocele. *J Pediatr Orthop* 15:202-205, 1995.

75. Urui S, Oi S: Experimental study of the embryogenesis of open spinal dysraphism. *Neurosurg Clin North Am* 6:195-202, 1995.

76. Vandertop WP, Asai A, Hoffman HJ, *et al:* Surgical decompression for symptomatic Chiari II malformation in neonates with myelomeningocele. *J Neurosurg* 77:541-544, 1992.

77. Vaquero J, Martinez R, Arias A: Syringomyelia-Chiari complex: magnetic resonance imaging and clinical evaluation of surgical treatment. *J Neurosurg* 73:64-68, 1990.

78. Walsh DS, Adzick NS, Sutton LN, Johnson MP: The rationale for in utero repair of myelomeningocele. *Fetal Diagn Ther* 16:312-22, 2001.

79. Ward WT, Wenger DR, Roach JW: Surgical correction of myelomeningocele scoliosis: a critical appraisal of various spinal instrumentation systems. *J Pediatr Orthop* 9:262-268, 1989.

80. Warkany J, O'Toole BA: Experimental spina bifida and associated malformations. *Childs Brain* 8:18-30, 1981.

81. Warkany J, Petering HG: Congenital malformations of the central nervous system in rats produced by maternal zinc deficiency. *Teratology* 5:319-334, 1972.

82. Wills KE, Holmbeck GN, Dillon K, McLone DG: Intelligence and achievement in children with myelomeningocele. *J Pediatr Psychol* 15:161-176, 1990.

83. Winter RB, Carlson JM: Modern orthotics for spinal deformities. *Clin Orthop* 74-86, 1977.

84. Wisoff JH, Epstein F: Management of hydromyelia. *Neurosurgery* 25:562-271, 1989.

85. Yamada S, Iacono RP, Andrade T, *et al:* Pathophysiology of tethered cord syndrome. *Neurosurg Clin North Am* 6:311-323, 1995.

86. Yen IH, Khoury MJ, Erickson JD, *et al:* The changing epidemiology of neural tube defects: United States, 1968-1989. *Am J Dis Child* 146:857-861, 1992;.

87. Zachary RB: Moral and social problems in intensive treatment of myelomeningocele. Moral, philosophical, religious and social bases of intensive treatment of severe forms of myelomeningocele. *Ann Chir Infant* 10:7-14, 1969.

# CHAPTER 83

# Anterior Sacral Meningocele

**John A. Lancon, Edward C. Benzel, and Robert E. Tibbs, Jr.**

Sacral meningocele may be congenital or acquired. Most acquired sacral meningoceles are a consequence of dural ectasia in association with the neurofibromatoses, Marfan syndrome, and Ehlers-Danlos syndrome.[*] These meningoceles are usually single and may expand into the intrasacral, presacral, and parasacral spaces. Traumatic avulsion of sacral nerve roots may produce sacral pseudomeningoceles in conjunction with profound neurologic deficits.[6,32] These sacs are more likely to be multiple and located in the lateral presacral space.

The congenital anterior sacral meningocele (ASM) was first described by Bryant in 1837.[10] It is rare in comparison to its dorsal counterpart. Matson noted only three examples in his analysis of 1390 cases of spina bifida cystica.[31] A congenital ASM characteristically occurs as a cystic presacral mass connected to the caudal thecal sac by a pedicle of variable size. Meningocele volumes up to 1 to 2L have been described.[41,48,50] Anorectal, genitourinary, and sacral anomalies may also be present.

In addition to the reported incidence, congenital ASM and dorsal lumbosacral meningocele differ from one another with respect to their pathogenesis, presentation, prognosis for neurologic improvement, and surgical approaches. Both anomalies may be associated with significant morbidity and mortality if not managed in a logical fashion, based on an understanding of their pathogenetic origins and surgical anatomy. This chapter reviews the pathogenesis, clinical presentation, and preoperative evaluation of congenital ASM. Needle aspiration and surgical approaches, including the transabdominal-transpelvic, presacral, parasacral, and dorsal transsacral routes, are described. In addition, guidelines for the avoidance and management of perioperative complications are reviewed.

## Pathogenesis

The processes of spine and spinal cord development span the period from embryogenesis to postnatal development. Similar to more rostral vertebrae, the sacral vertebrae develop from sclerotomes. However, the sacral pattern requires additional centers of ossification. This process occurs slowly and is not completed until the third or fourth decade of life. Developmental sacral osseous anomalies (mesodermal) include sacralization of lumbar and coc-

cygeal segments; lumbarization of the first sacral segment; stenosis or dilatation of the sacral foramina; isolated defects of the dorsal, lateral, and ventral elements; and sacral agenesis.[34]

The sacrococcygeal neural elements develop after closure of the posterior neuropore. Beneath an intact surface ectoderm, the caudal cell mass enlarges and undergoes canalization. This occurs from the fourth to sixth week of life, forming spinal cord segments extending from S2 to S3 to the coccygeal terminus. Extensive cellular degeneration along the distal neural tube produces a fibrous remnant at the caudalmost tip of the developing central nervous system. This remnant becomes the filum terminale. The ventriculus terminalis lies at the level of the S5 entry zone, marking the point of transition between the conus medullaris and filum terminale.[34] Lying at the distal end of the filum terminale, the coccygeal medullary vestige may be the origin of the intrasacral meningocele.[17,20,27]

Before the ninth week of life, spinal cord and vertebral segments are aligned level for level. With the dura mater now forming a complete covering, the spinal cord and dura mater begin to ascend in relation to the growing vertebral column, albeit at different rates. The conus medullaris rises to L3 at birth and to L1-2 by 3 months. The dural sac constricts terminally, rising only to S4 at birth and to S2-3 in the adult. Developmental sacrococcygeal neuroectodermal anomalies include meningocele, myelomeningocele, lipomyelomeningocele, myelocystocele, anomalies of the conus medullaris, tethered filum terminale, intrasacral meningocele, and caudal regression syndromes.[34]

In contrast to dorsal meningoceles that arise from failure of the posterior neuropore to close or dehiscence of a formed neural tube, a congenital ASM arises after failure of one or more sacral sclerotomes to develop. The meningeal sac expands through the sacral defect driven by cerebrospinal fluid (CSF) pulsations. The sacral defect enlarges only slightly, while the developing pelvic viscera offer less resistance to the budding meningocele. The sac enlarges tremendously in the presacral space, remaining attached to the thecal sac by a smaller pedicle. Although spontaneous regression of the meningocele does not occur after birth, progressive enlargement may occur and is associated with the development of symptoms. The large volume attained by some meningoceles causes crowding of the pelvic viscera.[41] The ventral sacral defect is usually parasagittal, less commonly midline or lateral. The typical anatomic relationships of an anterior sacral meningocele are depicted in Figure 83.1.

Complex interactions between adjacent germ cell substrata in the embryonic caudal midline give rise to varying cascades of maldevelopment, which comprise a spectrum of mesectodermal dystrophies. The embryologic event that initiates these patterns of maldevelopment is distinct from the insult that causes failure of the posterior neuropore to close. Although the precise event is not clearly defined, evidence for a vascular etiology exists.[7,8,34] In addition to anomalies of the conus medullaris, sacral nerve roots, and sacral dura mater, the clinical manifestations of these patterns of maldevelopment include the development of congenital tumors (e.g., dermoid, epidermoid, hamartoma, lipoma, teratoma, and teratocarcinoma) and

---

[*]References 26,33,37,40,43,44.

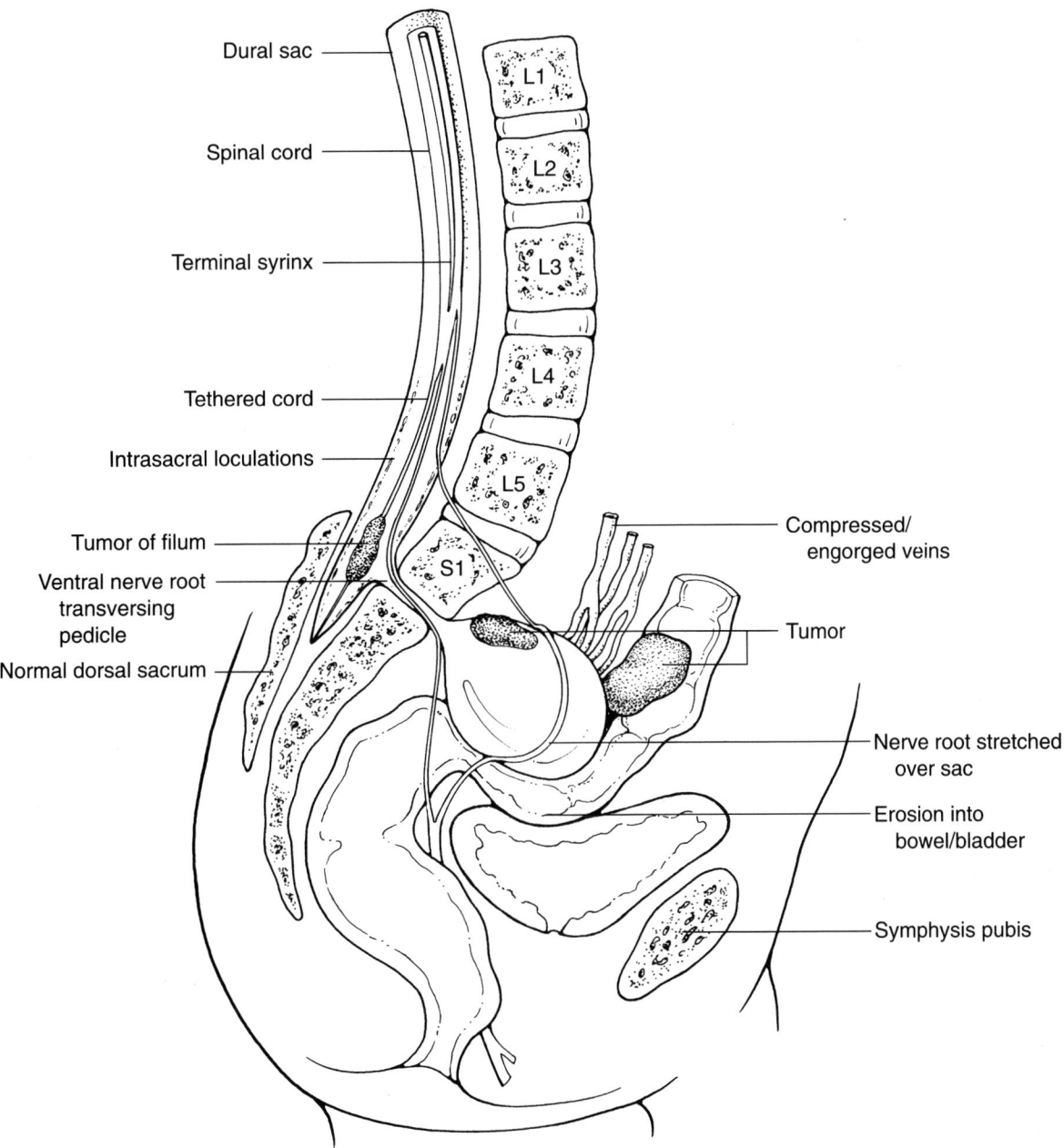

Dural sac

Spinal cord

Terminal syrinx

Tethered cord

Intrasacral loculations

Tumor of filum

Ventral nerve root
transversing
pedicle

Normal dorsal sacrum

L1
L2
L3
L4
L5
S1

Compressed/
engorged veins

Tumor

Nerve root stretched
over sac

Erosion into
bowel/bladder

Symphysis pubis

**Figure 83.1** Illustration of a typical anatomic scenario regarding a congenital anterior sacral meningocele. Intrathecal (filum terminale), intracystic, and extracystic-intrapelvic tumors may be associated.

anomalies of the colorectal, genitourinary, and reproductive systems.°

Most congenital ASMs appear to occur sporadically, although familial and X-linked dominant inheritance have been reported.[1,11,36,42] The seemingly greater incidence in females is a manifestation of the tendency toward symptomatology in the presence of sacral crowding, as well as the greater likelihood of female patients in the second and third decades of life to undergo palpation of the presacral space during routine physical examination. When cases up to 20 years of age are considered, the female-to-male ratio is approximately 1:1.[3,48]

## Clinical Presentation

Congenital ASM has a trimodal pattern of presentation.° Some ASMs are recognized at the time of birth when they are discovered in association with anorectal anomalies and sacral defects (Currarino's triad).[14] Most commonly, however, ASMs present during the first and second decades of life with progressive constipation or other symptoms referable to the colorectal, genitourinary, and reproductive systems.† Less commonly, low back pain, headache, or sacral radiculopathy may be the initial manifestation.[29,48,50]

°References 1,23,29,33,34,36,39.

°References 4,12,19,22,33,39,46,48,50.
†References 3,12,19,22,24,25,33,39,46,48,50.

A small congenital ASM may remain occult for life, particularly in the male patient.[48,50] An occasional meningocele is discovered incidentally during the initiation of routine prenatal care in a new mother. In the rare case of a pregnant woman with no prenatal care, the meningocele may present as dystocia. In this setting the characteristically benign ASM may threaten serious morbidity and even death.

### Colorectal

The most common symptom in patients with congenital ASM is chronic constipation or obstipation. This usually manifests in the first two decades of life. Fecal incontinence and soiling rarely predominate the clinical picture. Communication between congenital ASM and the rectum may be congenital or acquired and may produce fulminant meningitis. The anal canal may be duplicated or atretic.[1,48,50]

### Genitourinary

Urinary incontinence may be due to tethering of the spinal cord or direct pressure on the bladder, ureters, or S1, S2, and S3 nerve roots, or rarely may be the result of congenital deficits in the innervation of the lower urinary tract. Enuresis and recurrent infections affecting either the upper or the lower tract may occur. Coexisting anomalies include horseshoe-shaped kidneys and duplication of the kidneys, renal pelvis, or ureter.[48,50]

### Reproductive

Dysmenorrhea, dystocia, and dyspareunia occur less commonly. Dysmenorrhea may be secondary to compression of retropelvic veins resulting in pelvic venous congestion. Duplication of the uterus and vagina and vaginal atresia may be present.[23,48,50]

### Neurologic

True neurologic symptoms are rare and typically mild when present because the distal spinal cord and nerve roots develop normally. However, progressive leg or perineal weakness, numbness, and pain may develop as a result of stretching of the sacrococcygeal nerve roots by the meningocele.[3,48,50] These patients will usually have some symptoms suggestive of involvement of the pelvic visceral innervation. Chronic pelvic pain may occur resultant to involvement of the pelvic autonomic plexi. That such symptoms are typically progressive and do not develop until later in life implies the potential for reversibility after treatment if they are recognized early. Coexisting tethering of the spinal cord may actually lessen the amount of tension exerted on the nerve roots by the enlarging meningocele.[33] The presence of severe neurologic dysfunction from birth indicates a more severe myelodysraphic state and is associated with a greater tendency toward anomalous development in adjacent viscera. The patient whose clinical picture is characterized by prominent sacrococcygeal radiculopathy that worsens after a Valsalva maneuver is more likely to harbor an intrasacral meningocele or an ASM based on a

large pedicle.[17,27,33,48,50] The sacrococcygeal radiculopathies are listed in Table 83.1.

Mild to moderate headache-associated symptoms occur and are of two forms[3,9,22,33]: a high-pressure variant secondary to pressure exerted on the meningocele during pregnancy or after a Valsalva maneuver has been reported occasionally; or less commonly, a low-pressure headache may occur with a rising to the standing position and is caused by the displacement of CSF from the thecal sac into the meningocele. Pressure-related headaches are more likely in the presence of a large communication between the thecal sac and the meningocele.[48,50]

Congenital ASM may be a cause of meningitis. Bacterial meningitis resulting from erosion of the meningocele into the bowel or bladder lumina or resulting from the presence of a congenital rectothecal or vesiculothecal fistula and aseptic meningitis resulting from leakage of an intraspinal dermoid cyst have been described.[3,33,36]

## Preoperative Evaluation

The most consistent physical finding in congenital anterior sacral meningocele is a soft, cystic, retrorectal mass that appears fixed to the sacrum.[48,50] The mass is felt most commonly on rectal examination but may be felt on pelvic, abdominal, gluteal, or inguinal examination as well. With a Valsalva maneuver a transmitted pulse wave may sometimes be appreciated.[48,50] Dyck and Wilson[18] described a patient who presented with a sliding groin hernia and was found to harbor a congenital ASM. They postulated crowding of the pelvic viscera as a significant contributing factor in the development of the hernia, which contained a portion of the urinary bladder.

Although a congenital ASM can usually be felt easily on rectal or pelvic examination, the main limitation to premorbid discovery is a failure to suspect its presence. This failure is a result of both its secluded location within the deep pelvis and the great variety of typically mild, nonspecific symptoms with which it presents. The evaluation of a male or female patient presenting within the first three

**TABLE 83.1**

**Sacrococcygeal Radiculopathies**

| Level | Motor | Sensory | Autonomic |
|-------|-------|---------|-----------|
| S1 | Gluteus maximus<br>Hamstrings<br>Gastrocnemius/<br>  soleus<br>Intrinsic foot<br>  muscles<br>FDL, FHL | Lateral<br>  aspect and<br>  sole of foot | |
| S2 | Gastrocnemius/<br>  soleus<br>FDL, FHL | Dorsal thigh | Detrusor |
| S3 | | Outer perineal | Detrusor |
| S4 | | Inner perineal | Detrusor |
| S5 | | Perianal | |
| S0 | | Coccyx | |

FDL, Flexor digitorum longus; FHL, flexor hallucis longus.

decades of life with progressive constipation or obstipation should include a careful history and physical examination directed toward the gastrointestinal, genitourinary, and reproductive systems. Specific examination of the sacrococcygeal innervation should be performed.

## Imaging

Preoperative planning for surgery of congenital anterior sacral meningocele begins with the radiologic delineation of the surgical anatomy of the meningocele. Specific considerations are (1) confirmation of the cystic nature of the mass; (2) identification of the pedicle, associated mass lesions, and any other abnormalities of the neural, dural, or vertebral components of the sacrum; (3) determination of the relationship between the meningocele and the sacral nerve roots; and (4) determination of the relationship to the pelvic viscera. Bone window computed tomography and magnetic resonance imaging (MRI) are the primary diagnostic studies performed.[15,28,30,32,49] Myelography and postmyelographic computed tomography do not offer an equivalent amount of noninvasive surgically useful information.[5] Adjuvant evaluation of the pelvic viscera may provide additional useful information in selected cases.

The sacrum is difficult to evaluate with plain radiography owing to its curvilinear shape and overlying soft tissue and bowel gas patterns. The pathognomonic sickle-shaped sacral deformity, or scimitar sign, and a presacral mass may be present (Figure 83.2). Less obvious findings include widening of isolated sacral foramina, increases in interpedicular distance or flattening of the pedicles, and abnormalities of curvature.[48,50] Transforaminal sacral views may better demonstrate these changes. Calcification within an associated presacral mass may be difficult to discern.

The development of myelography allowed better visualization of the meningocele and its pedicle but contributed little to the diagnosis of associated pelvic visceral anomalies. Only masses within the meningocele could be seen, and in the presence of a very small pedicle, the fistulous communication was not always demonstrated.[48,50] Delayed imaging at 24 to 48 hours and the use of large volumes of contrast material increased the chance of identifying the pedicle. Balériaux-Waha et al.[5] described the utility of computed tomography (CT) in differentiating anterior sacral meningocele from solid masses of the presacral space. Computed tomographic bone windows are particularly helpful in delineating osseous anatomy. However, as with myelography, CT (even with intrathecal contrast) may fail to demonstrate a small pedicle.

In 1988, Lee et al.[28] reported on the use of MRI to demonstrate familial anterior sacral meningoceles in a father and daughter. The authors were able to noninvasively demonstrate a horseshoe-shaped kidney, didelphic uterus, and associated pelvic teratoma, which were not shown by other imaging studies. This is a critical advantage of MRI over other diagnostic imaging in the evaluation of congenital ASM, considering the extensive differential diagnoses of a presacral mass (Box 83.1).[38,45,47]

In cases where ASM is present, the MRI appearance of a congenital ASM is characteristic.[21,28,30,49] $T_1$-weighted images show a homogeneous low-signal cyst extending from the sacral thecal sac into the presacral space. It is usually possible to identify the communicating pedicle. The thickened filum terminale and any associated tumors may be identified. $T_2$-weighted images show high signals, although occasionally both high and low signals may be present within the meningocele as a consequence of fluid movements during imaging (Figure 83.3).

## Management

An understanding of the pathogenesis of ASM and the anatomic confines of the sacrococcygeal region allows the surgeon to devise a systematic, logical approach to deal with each anomaly. Important surgical goals are (1) visual confirmation of the anomalous anatomy depicted by MRI, (2) aspiration of the meningocele, (3) detethering of the spinal cord, (4) ligation of the pedicle or creation of a dural sleeve around exiting nerve roots, (5) excision of associated masses, and (6) dural closure.

Five surgical approaches have been described during the evolution of the surgical treatment of congenital ASM (Figure 83.4). Transrectal or transvaginal aspiration and the inferior presacral approach (e.g., Kraske approach) are associated with prohibitive risks of morbidity and mortality.[3,19,22,33,35] The oblique parasacral approach of Demel[16] and Coqui[13] was described for the rare gluteal meningocele. The ventral transabdominal-transpelvic approach was recommended by Leibowitz et al.[29] to prevent missing an occult tumor. With MRI, this is no longer necessary. However, this approach may still be useful in cases of large abdominopelvic masses or when nerve roots are known to traverse the pedicle of the meningocele. Only the dorsal transsacral approach allows the surgeon to carry out each of the aforementioned goals in a planned, logical progression, while minimizing the risks of injury to the pelvic viscera and presacral neurovascular networks.[2,41]

### Aspiration

Transrectal and transvaginal aspiration were abandoned after mortality rates of 80% to 90% were reported. However, direct aspiration of the meningocele should be a deliberate goal of any surgical exposure of an anterior sacral meningocele.

### Inferior Presacral Approach (Kraske-Pupovac Approach)

With the inferior presacral approach an incision is extended from just dorsal to the rectum to the dorsal surface of the coccyx. A plane is developed in the retrorectal space, and the coccyx is excised. The pedicle is identified and ligated, after which the sac may be aspirated via direct puncture. This approach has several disadvantages. First, the pedicle and its relationship with adjacent sacral nerve roots and the filum terminale are not fully visualized. An associated mass lesion within the meningocele or ventral to it can be difficult or impossible to expose via this approach. Inadvertent entry into the bowel or

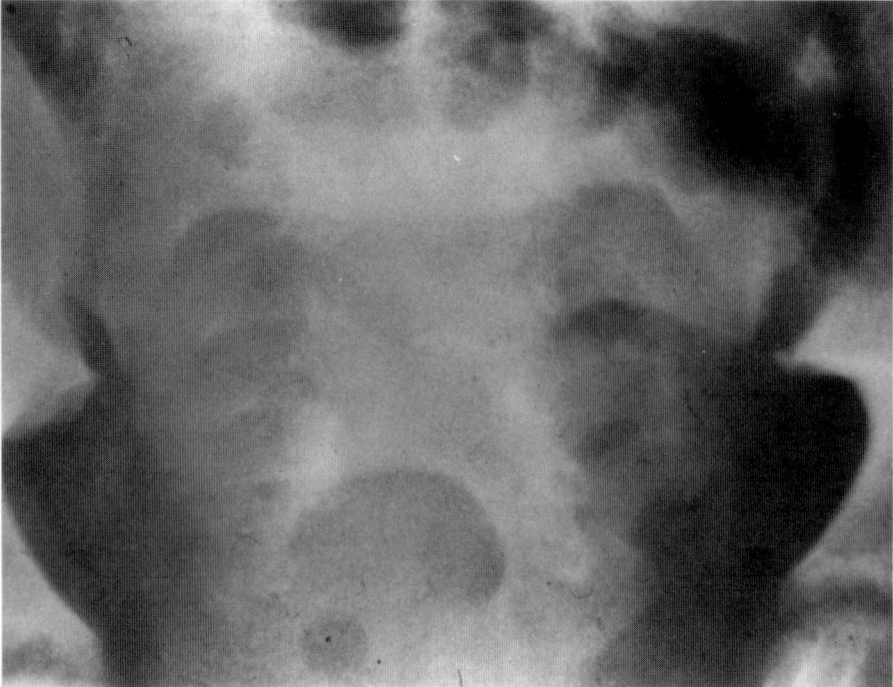

A

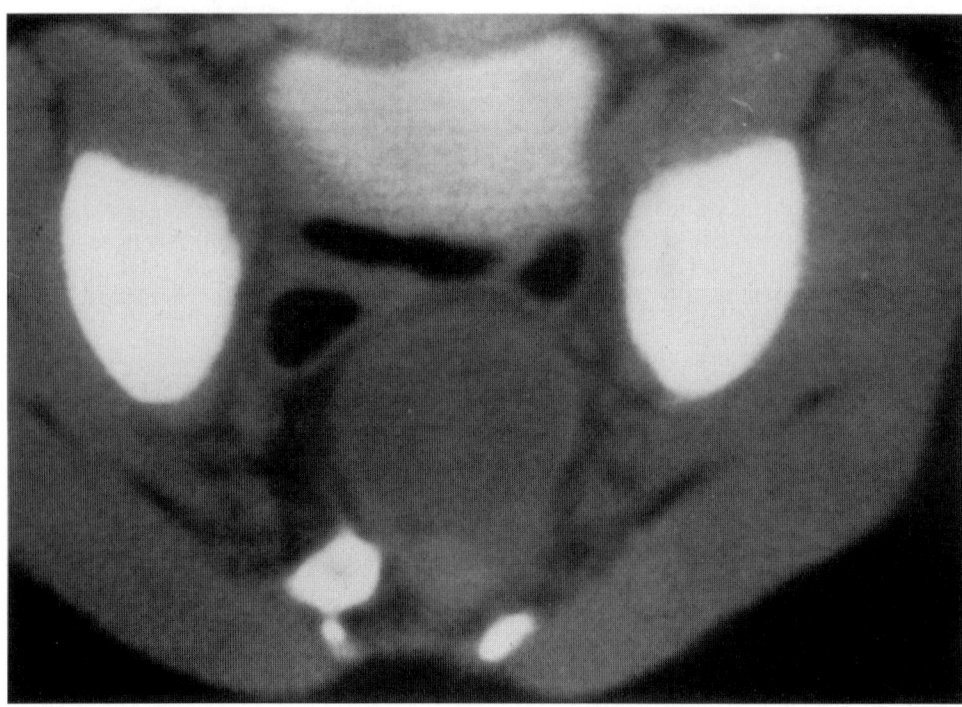

B

**Figure 83.2** **(A)** Anteroposterior radiograph of a patient with an anterior sacral meningocele. Note the classic presence of the "scimitar sign" configuration of the eroded sacrum. **(B)** Pelvic CT scan demonstrating the presacral mass associated with the meningocele.

bladder may occur. Finally, because any opening in the dural sac will occur in its most dependent portion, the incidence of a postoperative CSF fistula is increased. Proximity of the incision to the rectum may result in postoperative wound infection, pararectal abscess formation, or meningitis. This is particularly problematic in extremely young children.

## Oblique Parasacral Approach (Demel and Coqui Approach)

Originally described as an approach to the rare anterior sacral meningocele presenting as a gluteal mass, the oblique parasacral approach also does not allow surgical correction of associated tethering or mass lesions. An

83.1

BOX

**Differential diagnosis of sacral or presacral mass**

Aneurysmal bone cyst
Anterior sacral meningocele
Chondrosarcoma
Chordoma, chondroma
Dermoid cyst
Ependymoma
Epidermoid
Fibroma
Fibrosarcoma
Gastrointestinal tract tumors
Genitourinary tract tumors
Giant cell tumor
Hamartoma
Intrasacral meningocele

Lipoma
Nephroblastoma
Neuroblastoma
Osteoblastoma
Osteomyelitis
Perineurial cyst
Pheochromocytoma
Plasmacytoma
Polycystic kidney
Reproductive tract tumors
Rhabdomyosarcoma
Seminoma
Teratoma, teratocarcinoma

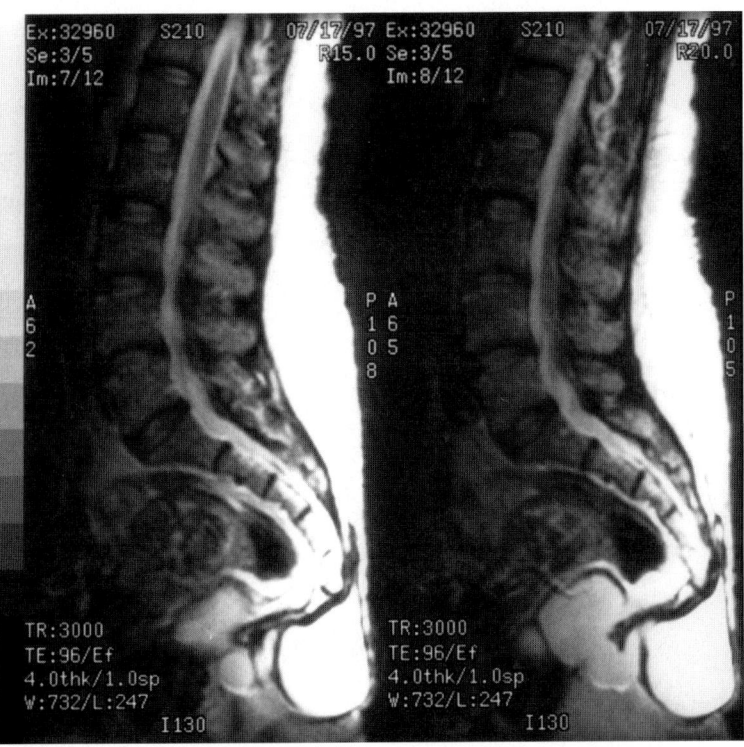

**Figure 83.3** Axial $T_2$-weighted magnetic resonance images of the sacral spine demonstrating a caudal anterior sacral meningocele extending into the presacral space.

incision on the buttocks allows identification of the gluteus maximus, which is reflected. The underlying piriformis, superior gemellus, obturator internus, inferior gemellus, and quadratus femoris muscles are identified. The superior and inferior gluteal arteries and nerves, sciatic nerve, and posterior femoral cutaneous nerves are identified in relation to the meningocele that will emerge in the space between the piriformis and quadratus femoris muscles. Although the sac may be aspirated and the protruding portion of the meningocele excised and oversewn, this approach leaves residual meningocele ventral to the sacrum and allows for further growth of the sac into the

presacral or parasacral space. Unless an associated tumor has been identified in the gluteal region by preoperative imaging, this approach should not be used.

### Transabdominal-Transpelvic Approach

During a transabdominal-transpelvic approach with the patient in the lithotomy Trendelenburg's position, a midline incision is made from the symphysis to just above the umbilicus. The small intestine is packed off. The ureters are then identified and preserved. The peritoneum is opened on the right side of the rectum, and

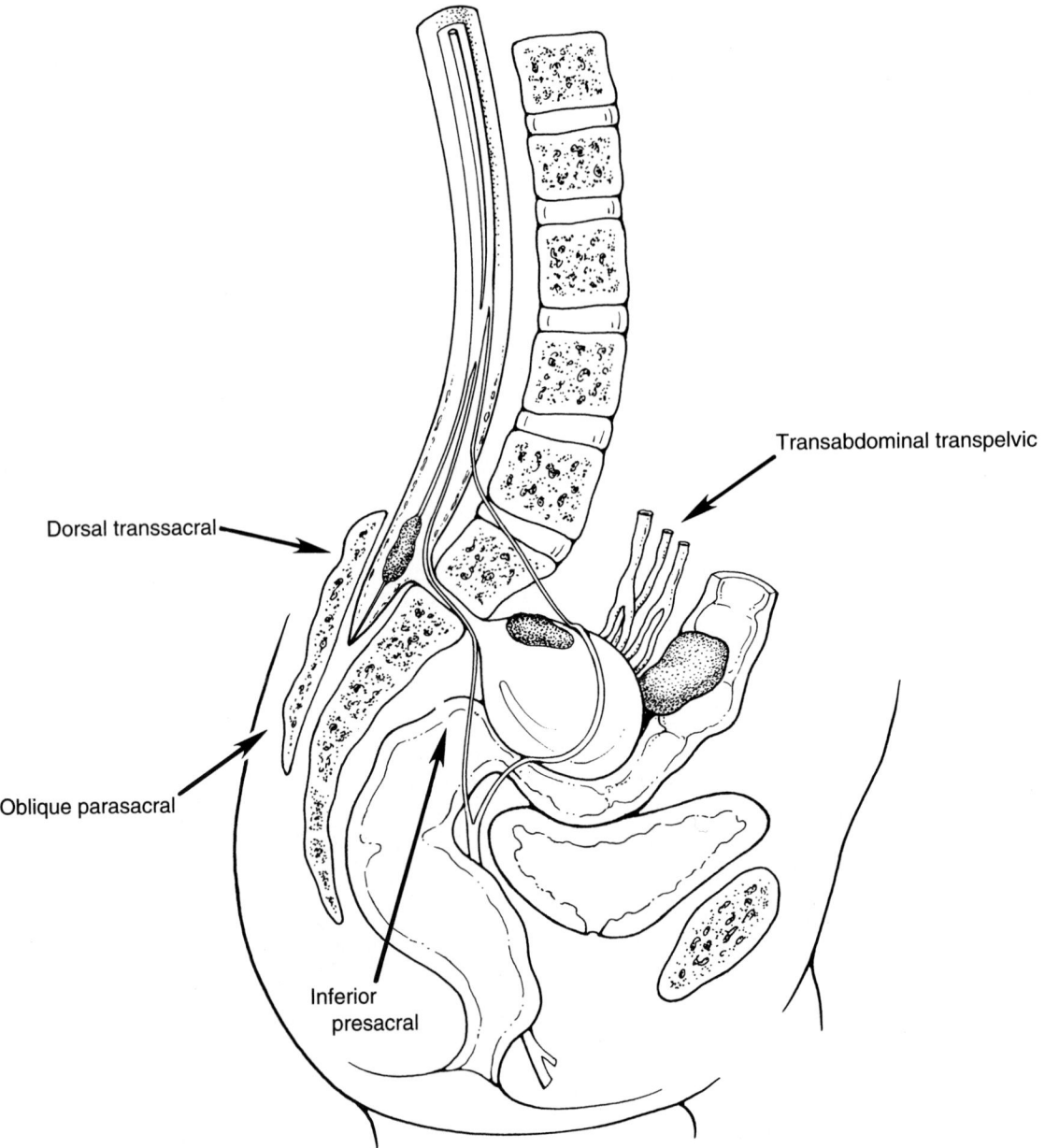

**Figure 83.4** Depiction of the orientation of the variety of surgical approaches used for the management of anterior sacral meningoceles.

the meningocele is identified. The meningocele may be aspirated and the pedicle ligated, or the meningocele may be opened and the dural sac plicated around any neural elements traversing the pedicle. The primary utility of this approach is in the management of large associated abdominopelvic masses, meningoceles arising from extremely large pedicles, and cases in which multiple sacral nerve roots traverse the ostium of the meningocele. Release of an associated tethering may be difficult by this approach, and the large retropelvic veins may hinder bloodless exposure. Preoperative consultation with general or colorectal surgery colleagues is important to adequately assess the risk-to-benefit ratio of the potential exposure gained by this approach within a small pelvis.

## Dorsal Transsacral Approach (Adson Approach)

The dorsal transsacral approach allows inspection of intrasacral anatomy, direct visualization of the sacral nerve roots, aspiration and collapse of the meningocele, detethering of the spinal cord, ligation of the pedicle, excision of associated tumors, and access to the sacral nerve roots for intraoperative stimulation. Rarely, a large abdominopelvic mass cannot be completely excised via this exposure. If sacral nerve roots traverse the pedicle, creation of a dural sleeve around the exiting roots may also be difficult by a dorsal exposure.[36] Because the meningocele is not excised, dissection in the presacral space is minimized. There have been no reported surgical deaths with this approach since 1965. A staged dorsal transsacral and transabdominal-transpelvic approach may be required in some cases.

## Surgical Technique

Care must be taken to avoid using inappropriate surgical approaches, particularly ventral approaches, that may not provide the most direct exposure of the pathology and that, in addition, may be associated with significant morbidity. For the vast majority of cases, the dorsal transsacral approach of Adson, or a variant thereof, is recommended. With this approach, the patient is positioned prone on two longitudinal chest rolls, and all pressure points are carefully padded. The bowel is prepared preoperatively. Prophylactic antibiotics are administered and continued for 48 hours postoperatively. Intraoperative monitoring, if employed, is planned in advance and is now checked. A Foley catheter, arterial line, and two large-bore peripheral intravenous lines are placed. The skin is cleansed with 0.25% triclosan (Septisol) and alcohol and prepared with povidone-iodine (Betadine).

The skin incision is placed in the midline and extends from the level of the iliac crests to the tip of the coccyx. The dorsal sacral fascia is identified and divided, allowing reflection of the erector spinae musculature to either side. The dorsal sacral foramina and sacroiliac ligaments should not be damaged. Sacral laminectomy is then performed. In cases of a small pedicle and no associated mass, a small laminotomy of the appropriate hemisacrum may be all that is required for ligation of the pedicle and aspiration of the meningocele.

The dural sac is then opened in the midline centered at the level of the pedicle of the meningocele. Inspection of the intrasacral anatomy is directed at identifying any intrasacral loculations, the anatomy of the sacral nerve roots, the ostium of the pedicle of the meningocele, and the relationship between the sacral nerve roots and the pedicle. The filum is identified and should not be divided until the meningocele has been aspirated. All visible nerve tissue must be preserved. In the absence of a more ventral mass lesion, the pedicle is ligated. The meningocele is aspirated by way of a soft angiocatheter or ventricular catheter attached to a syringe before placement of the final stitch. Alternatively, a fascial patch may be sewn over the ostium of the meningocele. At this point, tethering may be released.

If entry into the meningocele is desired for approach to an associated mass lesion or for plication of a dural sleeve around nerve roots traversing the pedicle, an opening should be made in the ventral surface of the dural sac adjacent to the pedicle. A fibrous plane is usually found between the ventral surface of the thecal sac and the dorsal surface of the meningocele, although venous bleeding from this space may occasionally be problematic. The sac is then opened, and the associated mass lesion is excised. The thecal sac is irrigated with warm antibiotic-containing solution to remove any blood that may have run down into the exposure. A watertight closure of the dural openings with 4-0 to 6-0 monofilament or braided nylon is confirmed by a Valsalva maneuver. After closure of the dorsal thecal sac, the paraspinous tissues are reapproximated. With meticulous hemostasis, a drain is not placed. Skin closure should be cosmetic. In the infant or young child, 5-0 to 4-0 Vicryl is placed in inverted fashion at the subdermal plane. The skin edges may then be held in approx-imation using Steri-Strips or 5-0 monofilament nylon in simple interrupted fashion. In the older child or adult, the subdermal closure is done with 3-0 Vicryl in a similar fashion, and the final layer consists of 4-0 monofilament nylon in a simple interrupted manner.

## Complications

Some of the operative and postoperative complications associated with the dorsal transsacral approach of Adson and the transabdominal-transpelvic approach are listed in Box 83.2. The discussion that follows addresses some of these procedures' common complications and their prevention and management.

### Dural Closure

The dura mater should be handled delicately to avoid inadvertent tears that would prevent watertight closure. Cautery of dural bleeding should be minimized or avoided entirely to prevent contraction of the dural surface. Closure with 4-0 to 6-0 braided or monofilament nylon or Prolene in watertight fashion is the most important step in preventing a postoperative CSF fistula. When a CSF leak occurs, a

**83.2**

BOX

### Perioperative complications

**Operative complications**
Positioning injuries
Prone anesthetic complications
Wound infection
Osteomyelitis
Meningitis (bacterial or aseptic)
CSF headache
CSF fistula
Failure to aspirate sac
Failure to obliterate pedicle
Failure to detether
Premature release of tethering
Direct injury to nerve root
Direct injury to ureter
Direct injury to bowel
Direct injury to bladder

**Postoperative complications**
Ileus
Malnutrition
Fluid and electrolyte abnormalities
Fecal impaction
Urinary retention
Urinary tract infection
Atelectasis
Pneumonia
Deep venous thrombosis
Pulmonary embolism
Sepsis
Decubitus
Pain

*CSF*, Cerebrospinal fluid.

lumbar subarachnoid drain may be placed percutaneously into the lumbar cistern and the patient turned to the prone position. CSF drainage should be continued for 5 days, at which point the drain is clamped for 24 hours. If the leak does not recur, the drain may be removed. Failure to resolve the leak requires reoperation for primary closure. In the extremely young child, primary reexploration may be preferable to a trial of lumbar drainage so as to avoid having to maintain the child in a prone position for an extended period of time.

### Nerve Injury

The sacral nerve roots should be assumed to be physiologically stressed by the stretch imparted by the meningocele and may be easily injured by improper handling. They should be identified at the time of initial dural opening and handled with great care. They may be injured during drilling of the dorsal sacrum, dural opening, pedicle ligation, formation of a dural sleeve, or aspiration of the sac and by premature release of tethering. The relationship between the pedicle and the adjacent nerve roots must be clearly determined before ligation of the pedicle. Any nerve roots observed to traverse the ostium of the pedicle should be preserved, and the dural sac plicated around them. Although sacral radiculopathies may worsen transiently after surgery, they almost always improve. Conversely, damage to the presacral autonomic plexus may result in debilitating chronic pelvic pain.

### Tethering

Complications related to tethering of the spinal cord result from both failure to detether and premature release of tethering. Release of a tethered spinal cord should be performed only after aspiration of the sac. This prevents sudden upward traction on the sacral nerve roots, which are already stretched tenuously by the meningocele. Failure to identify and release a tethered spinal cord may result in postoperative persistence or worsening of bowel and bladder symptoms. Because both aberrant sacral nerve roots and the filum terminale may enter the meningocele, the routine use of intraoperative electrophysiologic monitoring for identification of the filum terminale may assist with the prevention of accidental division of a sacral root.

### Meningitis

Meningitis may occur secondary to bacterial contamination of the CSF by skin flora or as a result of entry into the rectum or bladder. Preoperative bowel preparation and parenteral antibiotic coverage should be used. Aseptic meningitis may occur from leakage of an associated dermoid cyst or failure to remove blood that has run down into the thecal sac. Copious irrigation of the caudal thecal sac before final dural closure should always be performed and noted in the operative dictation.

### Pelvic Visceral Injury

Injury to the pelvic viscera is minimized by use of the dorsal transsacral approach and by limiting dissection in the presacral space. In addition to direct injury to the ureters, rectum, bladder, and their neurovascular supply, delayed hematoma formation secondary to inadequate hemostasis of retropelvic veins and venous thrombosis with central extension are potential serious risks of transabdominal-transpelvic approaches. Retropelvic hemorrhage may be life threatening.

### Postoperative Care

Urinary retention, urinary tract infection, atelectasis and pneumonia, ileus, fecal impaction, decubitus formation, sepsis, and deep venous thrombosis with pulmonary embolism may occur postoperatively. A definitive plan for bowel, bladder, pulmonary, skin, and nutritional management should be formulated for each case on an individual basis by considering preoperative and postoperative deficits. Mobilization, including physical and occupational therapy, should begin immediately after surgery.

## REFERENCES

1. Aaronson I: Anterior sacral meningocele, anal canal duplication cyst, and covered anus occurring in one family. *J Pediatr Surg* 5:559, 1970.
2. Adson AW: Spina bifida cystica of the pelvis: diagnosis and surgical treatment. *Minn Med* 21:468, 1938.
3. Amacher AI, Drake CG, McLachlin AD: Anterior sacral meningocele. *Surg Gynecol Obstet* 126:986, 1968.
4. Anderson FM, Burke BL: Anterior sacral meningocele: a presentation of three cases. *JAMA* 237:39, 1977.
5. Balériaux-Waha D, Osteaux M, Terwinghe G, et al: The management of anterior sacral meningocele with computed tomography. *Neuroradiology* 14:42, 1977.
6. Barberá J, Broseta J, Argüelles F, et al: Traumatic lumbosacral meningocele. *J Neurosurg* 46:536, 1977.
7. Bavinck JN, Weaver DD: Subclavian artery supply disruption sequence: hypothesis of a vascular etiology for Poland, Klippel-Feil, and Mobius anomalies. *Am J Med Genet* 23:903, 1986.
8. Brill CB, Peyster RG, Keller MS, et al: Isolation of the right subclavian artery with subclavian steal in a child with Klippel-Feil anomaly: an example of the subclavian artery supply disruption sequence. *Am J Med Genet* 26:933, 1987.
9. Brown MH, Powell LD: Anterior sacral meningocele. *J Neurosurg* 2:535, 1945.
10. Bryant T: Case of deficiency of the anterior part of the sacrum with a thecal sac in the pelvis, similar to the tumor of spina bifida. *Lancet* 1:358, 1837.
11. Cohn J, Bay-Nielsen E: Hereditary defect of the sacrum and coccyx with anterior sacral meningocele. *Acta Pediatr Scand* 58:268, 1969.
12. Coller FA, Jackson RG: Anterior sacral meningocele. *Surg Gynecol Obstet* 76:703, 1943.
13. Coqui: Beitrag zur Kasuistik, Diagnose und Therapie der Meningocele sacralis anterior, *Z Geburtshilfe Gynakol* 78:609, 1916.
14. Currarino G, Coln D, Votteler T: Triad of anorectal, sacral, and presacral anomalies. *Am J Radiol* 137:395, 1981.

15. Davis SW, Levy LM, LeBihan D, *et al:* Sacral meningeal cysts: evaluation with MR imaging. *Radiology* 187:445, 1993.

16. Demel R: Meningocele sacralis anterior. *Deutsch Z Chir* 209:90, 1928.

17. Doty JR, Thomason J, Sinods G, *et al:* Occult intrasacral meningocele: clinical and radiographic diagnosis. *Neurosurgery* 24:616, 1989.

18. Dyck P, Wilson CB: Anterior sacral meningocele. *J Neurosurg* 53:548, 1980.

19. Eder D: Anterior sacral meningocele: survey of literature and report of case. *Bull Los Angeles Neurol Soc* 14:104, 1949.

20. Enderle C: Meningocoele intrasacrale occulto (rivelato con la mielografia). *Riv Neurol* 5:418, 1932.

21. Enzmann DR, DeLaPaz RL, Rubin JB: *Magnetic Resonance of the Spine.* St Louis, Mosby, 1990.

22. Haddad FS: Anterior sacral meningocele: report of two cases and review of the literature. *Can J Surg* 1:230, 1958.

23. Henley RB, Lawrence LB: Pelvic meningocele: a case report. *J Neurosurg* 23:206, 1965.

24. Ivamoto HS, Wallman LJ: Anterior sacral meningocele. *Arch Neurol* 31:345, 1974.

25. Jabre A, Ball JB, Tew JM: Anterior sacral meningocele: current diagnosis. *Surg Neurol* 23:9, 1985.

26. Klenerman L, Merrick MV: Anterior sacral meningocele occurring in a family. *J Bone Joint Surg* 55B:331, 1973.

27. Lamas E, Lobato RD, Amor T: Occult intrasacral meningocele. *Surg Neurol* 8:181, 1977.

28. Lee KS, Gower DJ, McWhorter JM, *et al:* The role of MR imaging in the diagnosis and treatment of anterior sacral meningocele. *J Neurosurg* 69:628, 1988.

29. Leibowitz E, Barton W, Sadighi P, *et al:* Anterior sacral meningocele contiguous with a pelvic hamartoma: case report. *J Neurosurg* 61:188, 1984.

30. Martin B, de Latour FB: MR imaging of anterior sacral meningocele. *J Comput Tomogr* 12:166, 1988.

31. Matson DD: *Neurosurgery of Infancy and Childhood,* ed 2, Springfield, IL, Charles C Thomas, 1969.

32. McLennan JE, McLaughin WT, Skillicorn SA: Traumatic lumbar nerve root meningocele: case report. *J Neurosurg* 39:528, 1973.

33. Oren M, Laber B, Lee SH, *et al:* Anterior sacral meningocele: report of five cases and review of the literature. *Dis Colon Rectum* 20:492, 1977.

34. Pang D: Sacral agenesis and caudal spinal cord malformations. *Neurosurgery* 32:755, 1993.

35. Pupovac CD: Zur Kenntnis der pathologischen Anatomie und Genese der Hydromeningocele sacralis anterior. *Arb Geb Klin Chir* 1:533, 1903.

36. Quigley MR, Schinco F, Brown JT: Anterior sacral meningocele with an unusual presentation: case report. *J Neurosurg* 61:790, 1984.

37. Raftopoulous C, Pierard GE, Retif C, *et al:* Endoscopic cure of a giant sacral meningocele associated with Marfan's syndrome: case report, *Neurosurgery* 30:765, 1992.

38. Rengachary SS: Masses of the sacrum. In Wilkins RH, Rengachary SS (eds): *Neurosurgery.* New York, McGraw-Hill, 1985, p 1079.

39. Silvis RS, Riddle LR, Clark GG: Anterior sacral meningocele. *Am Surg* 22:554, 1956.

40. Smith MD: Large sacral dural defect in Marfan syndrome. *J Bone Joint Surg* 75A:1067, 1993

41. Smith HP, Davis CH: Anterior sacral meningocele: two case reports and discussion of surgical approach. *Neurosurgery* 7:61, 1980.

42. Solopaev AA, Mylkinokov PI, Gerber IVM, *et al:* Anterior sacral meningocele (in Russian). *Zh Vopr Neiro* 5:18, 1977

43. Stern WE: Dural ectasia and the Marfan syndrome. *J Neurosurg* 69:221, 1988.

44. Strand RD, Eisenberg HM: Anterior sacral meningocele in association with Marfan's syndrome. *Radiology* 99:653, 1971.

45. Tarlov IM: Perineurial cysts of the spinal nerve roots. *Arch Neurol Psychiatry* 40:1067, 1938.

46. Thierry A, Archimbaud JP, Ficher G, *et al:* La meningocèle sacrée antérieure: revue de la litérature et présentation d'un cas. *Neurochirurgie* 15:389, 1969.

47. Turner ML, Mulhern CB, Dalinka MK: Lesions of the sacrum: differential diagnosis and radiological evaluation. *JAMA* 245:275, 1981.

48. Villarejo F, Scavone C, Blazquez MG, *et al:* Anterior sacral meningocele: review of the literature. *Surg Neurol* 19:57, 1983.

49. Wetzel LH, Levie E: MR imaging of sacral and presacral lesions. *Am J Radiol* 154:771, 1990.

50. Wilkins RH, Odom GL: Anterior and lateral spinal meningocele. In Vinken PJ, Bruyn GW (eds): *Handbook of Clinical Neurology,* New York, Elsevier Biomedical, 1978, p 193.

# CHAPTER 84

# Chiari Malformation and Syringomyelia

## Albert L. Rhoton and Allan J. Hamilton

The term *Chiari malformation* refers to a group of anomalies involving the caudal displacement of the hindbrain; ranging from a mild form, in which only the cerebellar tonsils are displaced below the foramen magnum, to more severe forms, in which the tonsils, medulla, and fourth ventricle are caudally displaced. The terminology for this group of malformations is associated with a history of controversy. The malformation was named for Chiari,[7] although he was not the first to describe it. It later became known as Arnold-Chiari malformation.[1,26] The recent trend has been to use the original eponym, *Chiari malformation*.

The term *syringomyelia* refers to a relentlessly progressive clinical entity caused by a destructive process originating in regions adjacent to the central canal of the spinal cord and extending into the gray and white matter. Syringomyelia is associated with a chronic accumulation of fluid anywhere within the substance of the spinal cord. By contrast, the term *hydromyelia* refers to a condition in which the central canal of the spinal cord communicates with the fourth ventricle and is distended by cerebrospinal fluid (CSF) (Figure 84.1).

Hydromyelia is seldom found in the absence of Chiari malformation, but Chiari malformations often occur in the absence of hydromyelia. Hydromyelia is the most common cause of spontaneously appearing syringomyelic spinal cord syndrome. It often coexists with Chiari malformation. Therefore, the combination has been termed the *syringomyelia-Chiari complex*.[27] The frequency with which Chiari malformation and hydromyelia are discovered on magnetic resonance imaging (MRI) scans in patients who have no neurologic deficit makes it likely that these disorders are much more common than previously suspected.[6]

## Neurologic Manifestations

The clinical hallmarks of the syringomyelic spinal cord syndrome are atrophy and dissociated anesthesia beginning in the upper extremities. The first manifestation is often a loss of sensation to pain and temperature in the involved dermatomes. This is caused by destruction of the pain fibers crossing ventral to the central canal of the spinal cord. The area of destruction forms a cavity, which extends into the anterior horn and destroys the motor neurons, eventually causing atrophy and weakness in the involved segments. Extension of the cavity into the posterior horns may produce loss of touch and proprioception as well. As the disease progresses, evidence of involvement of the long motor and sensory pathways in the spinal cord often appears.

Frequently, scoliosis is present, and neurogenic arthropathies develop in the later stages of the disorder.

The dysfunction of the lower brain stem caused by Chiari malformation includes upper and lower motor neuron signs in the bulbar musculature, gait difficulties caused by involvement of cerebellar and corticospinal pathways, and variably, nystagmus. When these deficits are present, the typical syringomyelic spinal cord syndrome is said to be accompanied by syringobulbia. In most cases, however, it is Chiari malformation that compresses and distorts the brain stem. Infrequently, the hydromyelic cavity extends rostrally into the brain stem and rarely into the cerebrum (Figure 84.2).[24]

## Pathophysiology

The pathologic basis of the syringomyelic spinal cord syndrome is frequently misunderstood. Because of the initial description of the clinical syndrome in the last century,[14] syringomyelia has incorrectly become synonymous with an untreatable degenerative condition rather than with a pressurized distention of the spinal cord caused by a developmental anomaly.[14,15] The inaccuracy of this traditional concept is evident because none of the more than 60 patients who were treated for a spontaneously appearing syringomyelic spinal cord syndrome had degenerative cavitation and gliosis within the spinal cord. The most common cause of the syndrome was hydromyelia associated with Chiari malformation as reported in other large series.[3,10-12]

In response to these findings, Gardner[10] put forth the so-called hydrodynamic theory of the development of the syringomyelia. This theory attributes extension of the hydromyelia to the "water hammer" effect created by the blockage of the foramen of Magendie. The transmission of CSF from the fourth ventricle via a patent central canal results in a slowly progressive dilatation of the central canal or in the development of a ramifying diverticulum that originates in the central canal and communicates with the CSF pathways through the fourth ventricle. Communication between the fourth ventricle and the syrinx has been demonstrated both on neuroradiologic examination and on postmortem studies.[22] Recently, Oldfield *et al.*[18] proposed that the downward movement of the cerebellar tonsils with systole, as visualized on dynamic MRI, creates a piston effect in the spinal subarachnoid space that forces CSF through the perivascular and interstitial spaces into the syrinx.

The second most common cystic spinal lesion that produces a syringomyelic spinal cord syndrome is an intramedullary tumor associated with a cyst (see Figure 84.1D).[22,23] The cysts, in general, do not communicate with the central canal and are not associated with a hindbrain malformation. Such tumor-related cysts contain yellow or brown fluid with an elevated protein content.

Cysts in the spinal cord may also develop after any of a wide variety of insults, including acute or chronic spinal cord compression, trauma, meningitis, abscess, or surgery.[3,9] In most cases, there is a clear-cut history of the initial insult to the spinal cord. Posttraumatic cysts can produce a progressive deficit long after the initial injury. The expanding posttraumatic cyst most commonly causes an ascending progressive deficit because of damage to the spinal cord above the level of the initial injury, but it may also be associated with further loss at or below that level. Barnett *et al.*[3] differentiated cystic lesions in the spinal cord into noncommunicating and communicating forms, based on whether they communicate with the central canal. The noncommunicating form was associated with an intramedullary tumor and posttraumatic myelopathy. The communicating form resulted from persistent dilatation of the central canal, secondary to pressure from the developmental anomaly of the cerebellum and brain stem at the level of the foramen magnum.

## Clinical Factors

The improved understanding of pathophysiology underlying Chiari malformation and syringomyelic spinal cord syndrome has led to a more rational approach to surgical treatment. Both Chiari malformation and hydromyelia are surgically treatable. Early diagnosis and treatment, however, are essential because patients who have progressed beyond a moderate stage of disability have little likelihood of achieving a useful recovery.

Patients with Chiari malformation or hydromyelia have their initial onset of symptoms between 16 and 72 years of age. A prior history of hydrocephalus or myelomeningocele is uncommon. All patients with hydromyelia have symptoms or signs referable to it but only one-third have signs referable to Chiari malformation. Sensory loss usually precedes lower motor neuron signs. The neurologic deficits produced by hydromyelia range in severity from a subjective sensory loss or minimal motor deficit (or both) to a widespread sensory loss and quadriparesis with marked atrophy of the upper extremity musculature and atrophy or spasticity in the lower extremities. In the early stages, the sensory deficit frequently is greater on one side than on the other. Occasionally, patients present with a burning discomfort in an area of sensory loss or pain, suggesting a cervical radiculopathy. The weakness and atrophy are most commonly manifest in the hands. In the later stages, compression of the corticospinal tracts and long sensory pathways results in a spastic gait and sensory loss in the lower extremities. Most of the patients with minimal neurologic deficits at the time of diagnosis who were not treated surgically eventually worsen and undergo surgery.

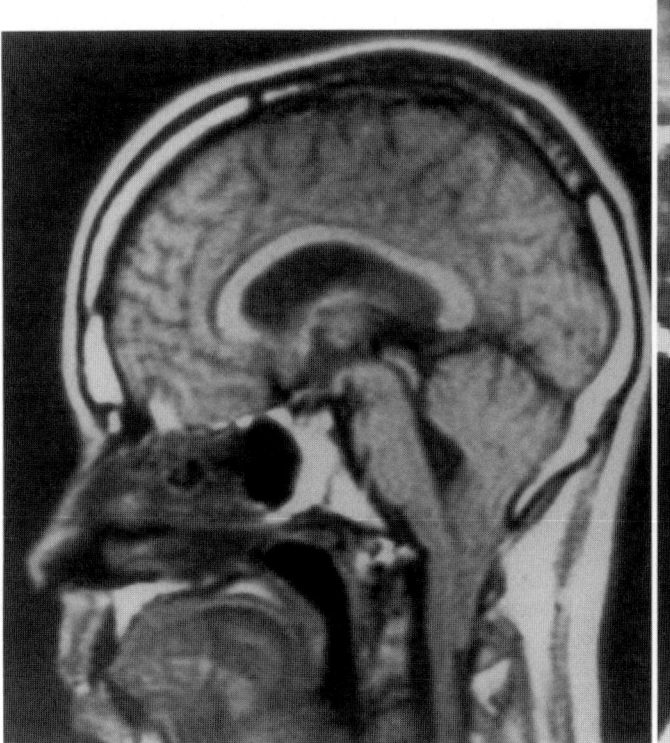

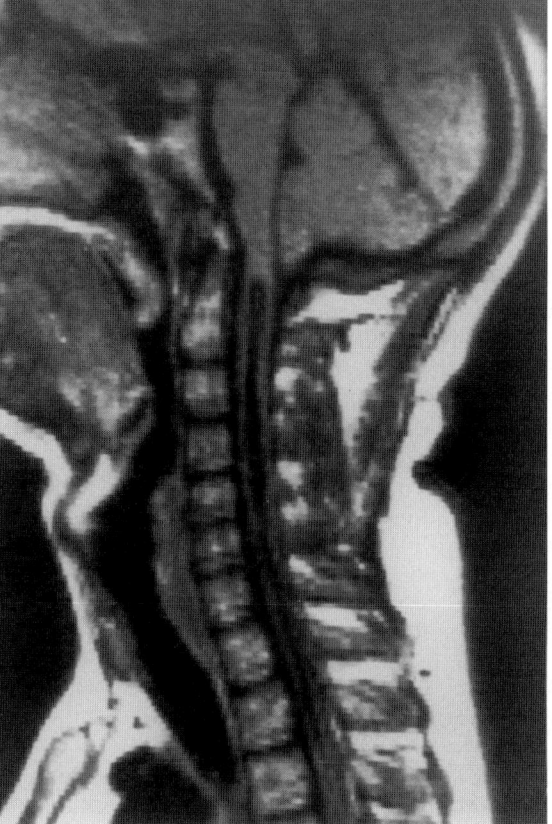

A                                                                 B

**Figure 84.1** MRI of Chiari malformations with and without hydromyelia. **(A)** Sagittal image shows Chiari malformation without hydromyelia. The cerebellar tonsils extend down to the level of C2. **(B)** Sagittal image of Chiari malformation with hydromyelia. The cavity in the spinal cord extends from the level of the foramen magnum, through the cervical region, into the upper thoracic area.

*Continued*

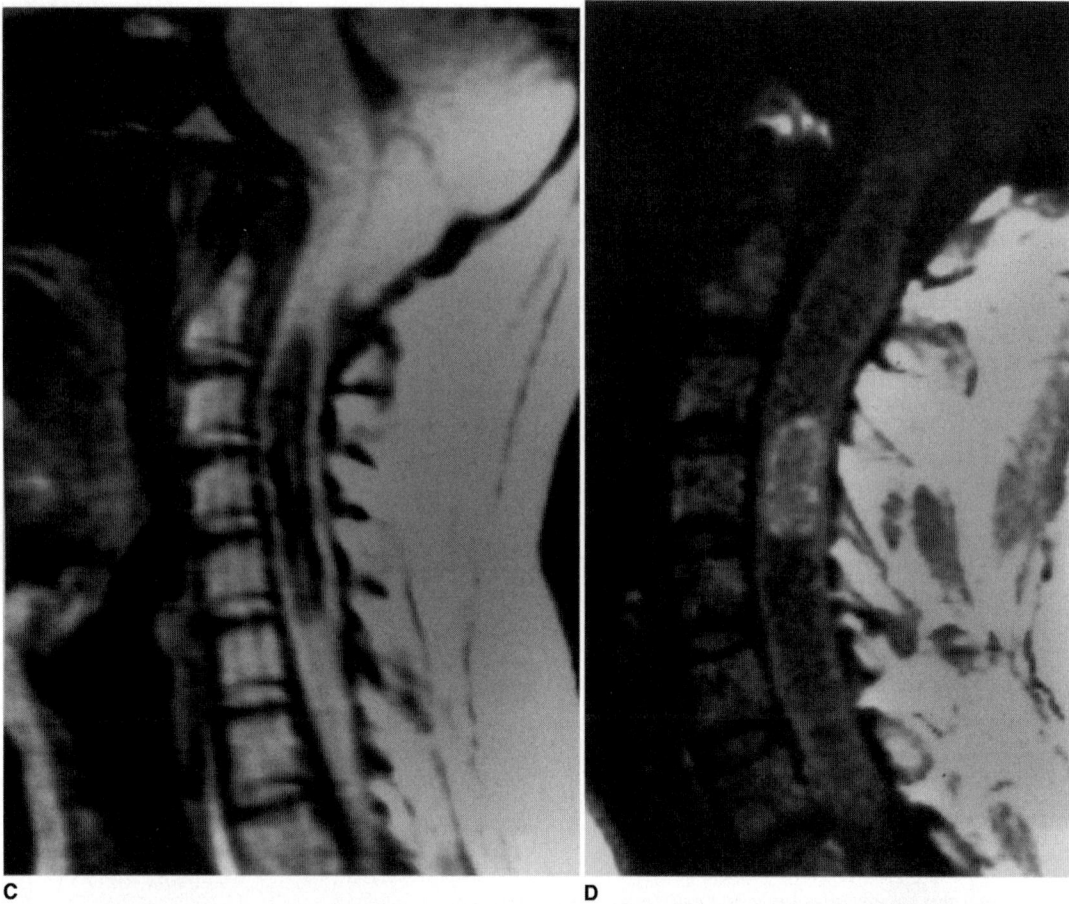

C                                                    D

**Figure 84.1 *cont'd*** (**C**) Sagittal image of a hydromyelic cavity with a septum in the central part of the cavity. (**D**) Sagittal image shows a cyst associated with an intramedullary tumor in the cervical region.

The patients with brain stem symptoms caused by Chiari malformation have a combination of upper and lower motor neuron signs in the bulbar musculature, gait difficulties caused by cerebellar and long-tract involvement, and nystagmus. Some patients with Chiari malformation can have sudden severe respiratory stridor caused by bilateral vocal cord paralysis and rapid onset or progression of other symptoms. Bertrand[5] has described the mechanism for a sudden onset or change of symptoms in cases of Chiari malformation. Although defective ventricular drainage has been implicated in the development of hydromyelia, no patient in this series had hydrocephalus or evidence of increased intracranial pressure.

## Radiographic Evaluation

Plain films of the skull and cervical spine in patients with Chiari malformation and hydromyelia frequently show no abnormalities. It was once assumed that radiologic evidence of a normal skull and cervical spine excluded the diagnosis of Chiari malformation and hydromyelia. However, anomalies of the skull, cervical spine, or craniovertebral junction, such as a basilar impression, Klippel-Feil deformity, atlanto-occipital fusion, or widening of the anteroposterior diameter of the cervical spinal canal, have

been identified on plain films. In patients with hydromyelia, the anteroposterior diameter of the spine may be enlarged, but none of the features of focal expansion associated with intramedullary tumors are present.

MRI is the method of choice to evaluate patients suspected of having Chiari malformation and hydromyelia (see Figure 84.1). MRI scans show the extent that the cerebellar tonsils and fourth ventricle have been displaced into the foramen magnum and upper spinal canal, the transverse diameter and rostrocaudal extent of the hydromyelic cavity, and the size of the lateral ventricles. MRI also demonstrates extension of the cavity into the brain stem (an infrequent finding) and tracking into the cerebrum, which is also rare (see Figure 84.2).[24] MRI usually provides all the information needed to plan the surgical approach and to demonstrate the resolution or reduction in size of the hydromyelic cavity postoperatively.

If MRI cannot be performed or does not provide the information needed for diagnosis and treatment, myelography with water-soluble contrast medium can be used in conjunction with computed tomography (CT) (Figure 84.3). Plain CT scans show caudal displacement of the fourth ventricle and cerebellar tonsils, but rarely demonstrate spinal cord enlargement or the hydromyelic cavity. CT scans obtained after an intrathecal injection of water-soluble iodinated contrast material will show tonsillar

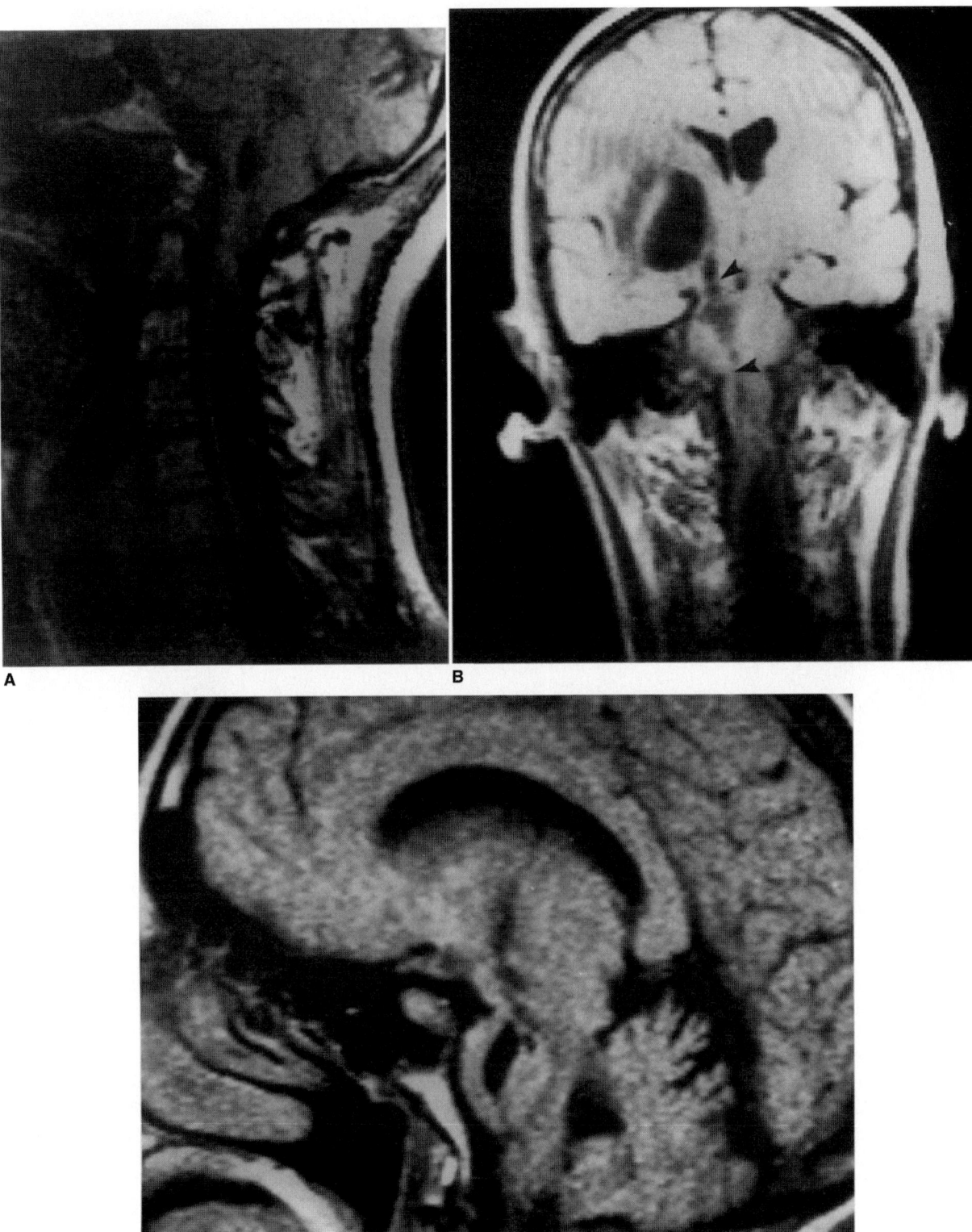

**Figure 84.2** MRI of a patient with Chiari malformation and hydromyelia extending into the brain stem and cerebrum. (**A**) Sagittal image shows Chiari malformation and hydromyelia. (**B**) Coronal image shows a tract (*arrows*) in the medulla, pons, and midbrain that connected with the large cyst in the cerebrum. (**C**) Sagittal MRI shows the tract in the pons. (*From Rhoton EL, Rhoton AL: Chiari malformation with syringocephaly.* J Neurosurg *75:791, 1991.*)

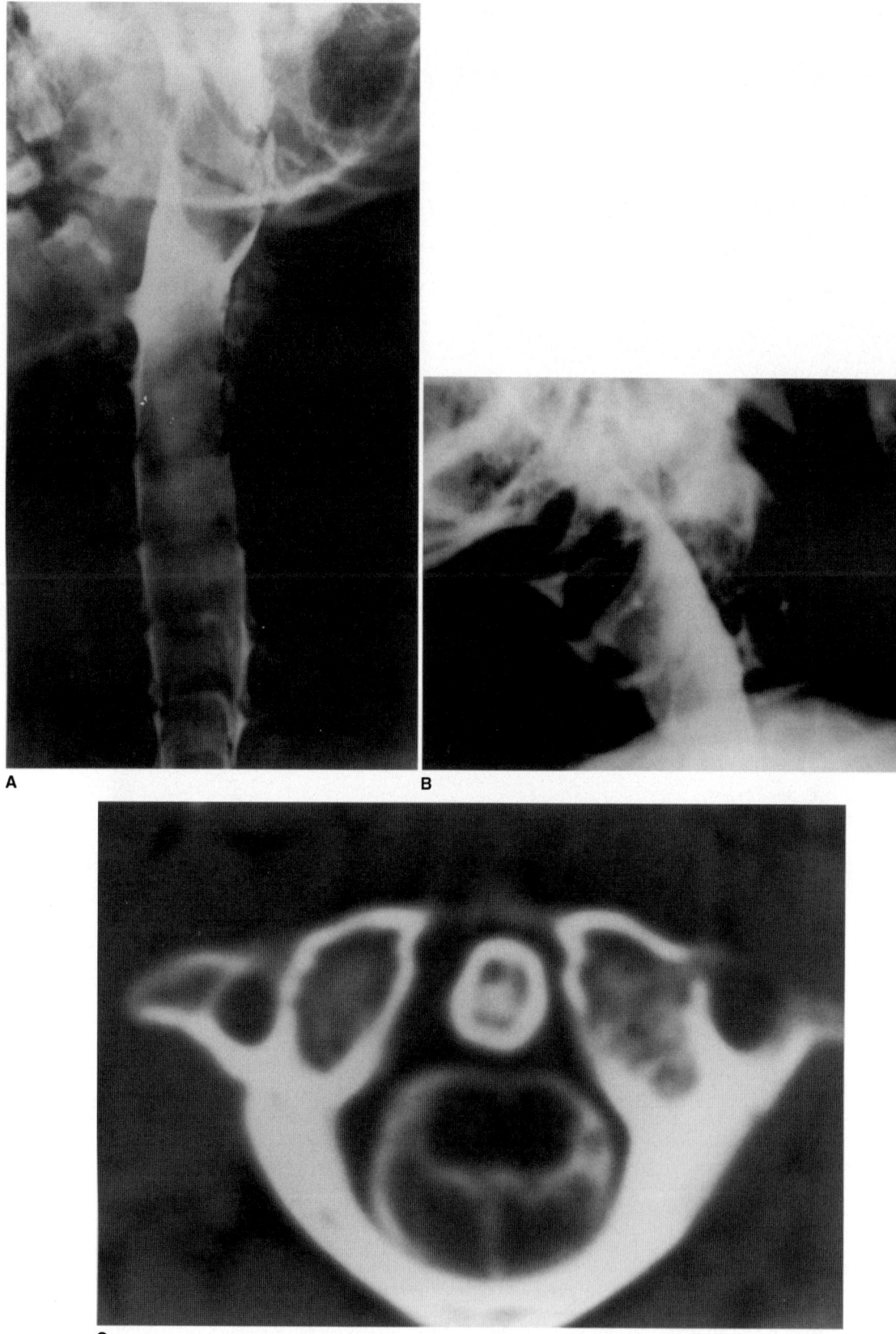

**Figure 84.3** Myelograms obtained after the injection of water-soluble contrast agent and CT scans from selected patients with Chiari malformation and hydromyelia; studies (**A**) to (**E**) are from the same patient. (**A**) Oblique view shows the herniated cerebellar tonsils and the enlarged cervical spinal cord. (**B**) Right lateral view shows the herniated cerebellar tonsils. (**C**) Axial CT at the level of the odontoid process shows the cerebellar tonsils in the upper spinal canal behind the spinal cord.

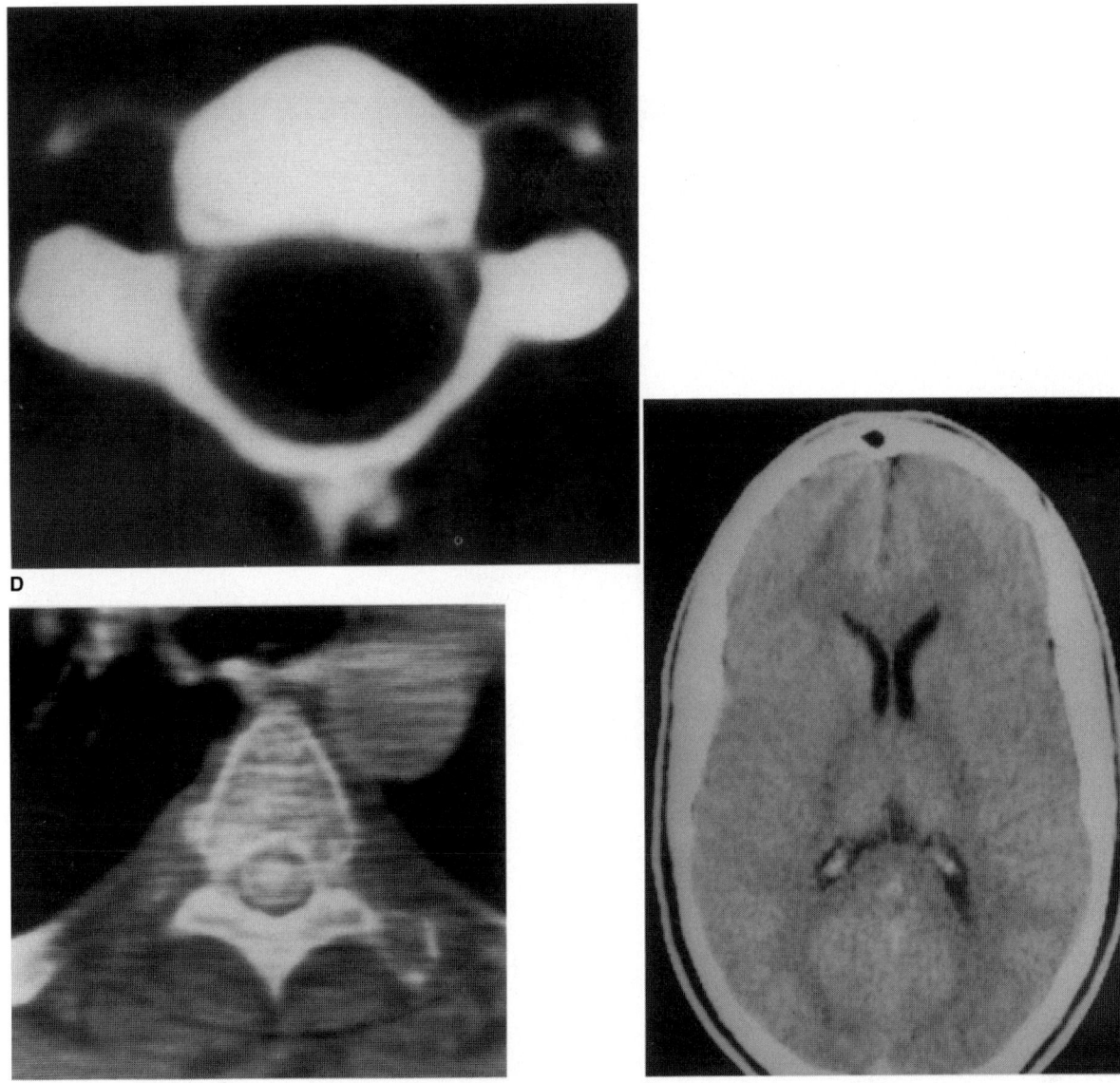

**Figure 84.3** *cont'd* (**D**) CT scan shows the enlarged spinal cord. (**E**) CT scan of the head shows lateral ventricles of normal size. (**F**) CT scan from another patient obtained 12 hours after intrathecal administration of metrizamide shows the accumulation of contrast medium within the spinal cord. Studies (**G**) to (**I**) are from another patient with Chiari malformation.

*Continued*

herniation and enlargement of the spinal cord (see Figure 84.3). CT scans obtained 8 to 24 hours after the injection may show contrast medium that has entered the hydromyelic cavity in the spinal cord. The cavity may be located centrally or asymmetrically within the cord, and its position may vary from level to level (see Figure 84.3*H-I*). Plain films rarely show contrast medium that has entered the hydromyelic cavity (see Figure 84.3*G*).

Angiograms are rarely useful. Although angiograms demonstrate the displacement of the cerebellar tonsils associated with Chiari malformation, as defined by the descent of the posterior inferior cerebellar artery and the size of the lateral ventricles, this information is better demonstrated by CT scans and MRI. Angiography may be indicated if the CT or MRI findings suggest that a vascular tumor, such as a hemangioblastoma, is the cause of the tonsillar herniation or cord enlargement.

## Surgical Treatment

The most effective treatment for Chiari malformation and hydromyelia is a suboccipital craniectomy, upper cervical laminectomy, and duraplasty to decompress the Chiari malformation, combined with drainage of the hydromyelic cavity through the dorsal root entry zone into the subarachnoid space (Figure 84.4).[20-23] Decompressing the Chiari malformation alone has been advocated, but, in the first author's (A.L. Rhoton) experience, it has not been as effective as decompression of the Chiari malformation and drainage of the syrinx. However, decompression alone has proven more effective in reducing the size of a hydromyelic cavity than drainage of the cavity alone.[4,23] Numerous patients treated with a Chiari decompression without drainage of the hydromyelia have continued to have significant fluid collection in the spinal cord, whereas in those treated with

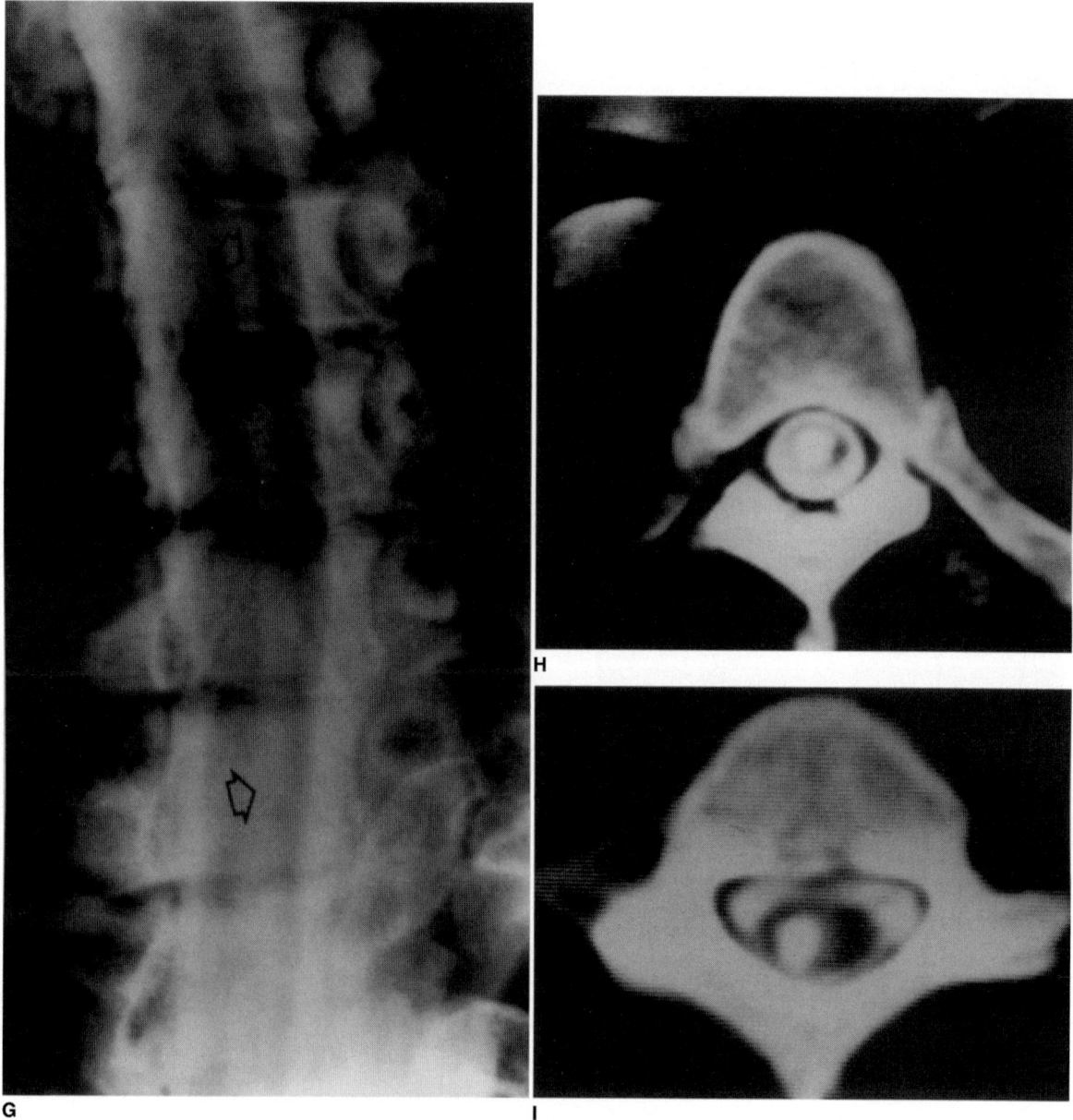

**Figure 84.3 *cont'd*** (**G**) During myelography, metrizamide entered the hydromyelic cavity in the central part of the spinal cord *(arrows)*. (**H**) Axial CT scan shows the metrizamide in the hydromyelic cavity in the central part of the spinal cord. (**I**) Axial CT at another level shows the cavity situated in one half of the cord. *(From Rhoton AL Jr: Microsurgery of syringomyelia and syringomyelic cord syndrome. In Schmidek HH, Sweet WH (eds): Operative Neurosurgical Techniques: Indications, Methods, and Results, ed 3, vol 2. Philadelphia, WB Saunders, 1998, pp 1745-1774.)*

decompression and dorsal root entry zone myelotomy, the syrinx disappeared or the residual cavity became slitlike. The first postoperative MRI scan is obtained about 4 months after surgery, and by that time most cavities have become slitlike or have disappeared after the treatment described below (Figure 84.5).

### Decompression of Chiari Malformation

In the past, this operation was performed with the patient in the semisitting position and the neck in a neutral position. In recent years, the first author has been using the three-quarter prone position, with the table tilted to place the head slightly above the trunk. Marked flexion of the neck during surgery for Chiari malformation has been reported to increase the neurologic deficit or cause respiratory problems and should be avoided.[16] A suboccipital craniectomy and upper cervical laminectomy to decompress Chiari malformation are accomplished through a midline skin incision (see Figure 84.4). If only a Chiari malformation is present, the laminectomy should include C1 and C2 and lower levels as needed to ensure that the herniated tonsils are well decompressed. If hydromyelia is also present, the laminectomy should include C3 to prepare for

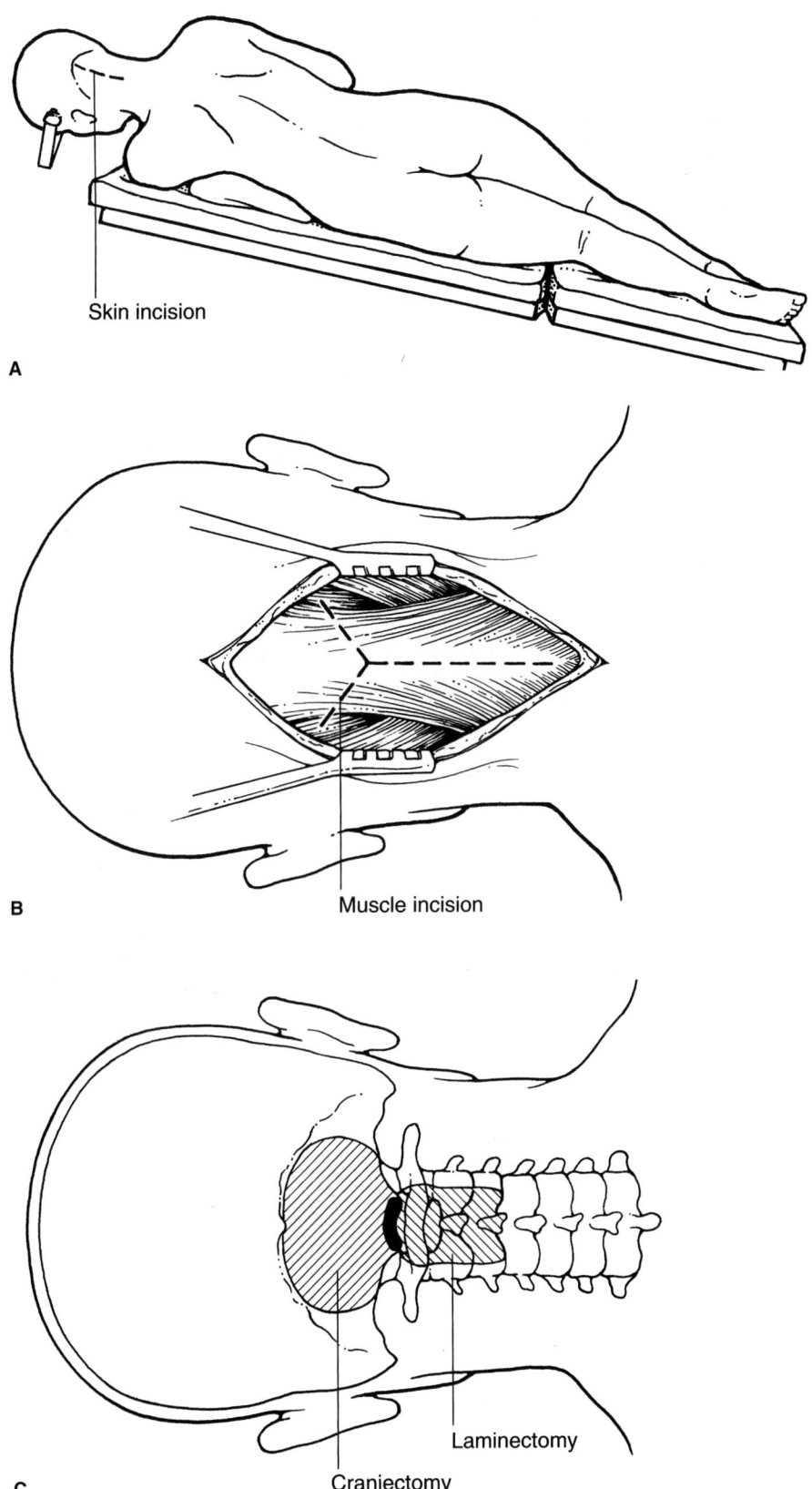

**Figure 84.4** Surgical exposure of Chiari malformation and hydromyelia. **(A)** The three-quarter prone position is used. The head is positioned higher than the feet. The face is turned 45 degrees toward the floor, and a midline skin incision is used. The side of the dorsal root entry zone to be drained is placed uppermost. **(B)** Site of muscle incision. A Y-shaped incision is made to provide a muscle flap attached to the superior nuchal line and inion, which facilitates closure. **(C)** Site of craniectomy and laminectomy. The laminectomy is extended to include C3 if a hydromyelic cavity is to be drained through the exposure.

*Continued*

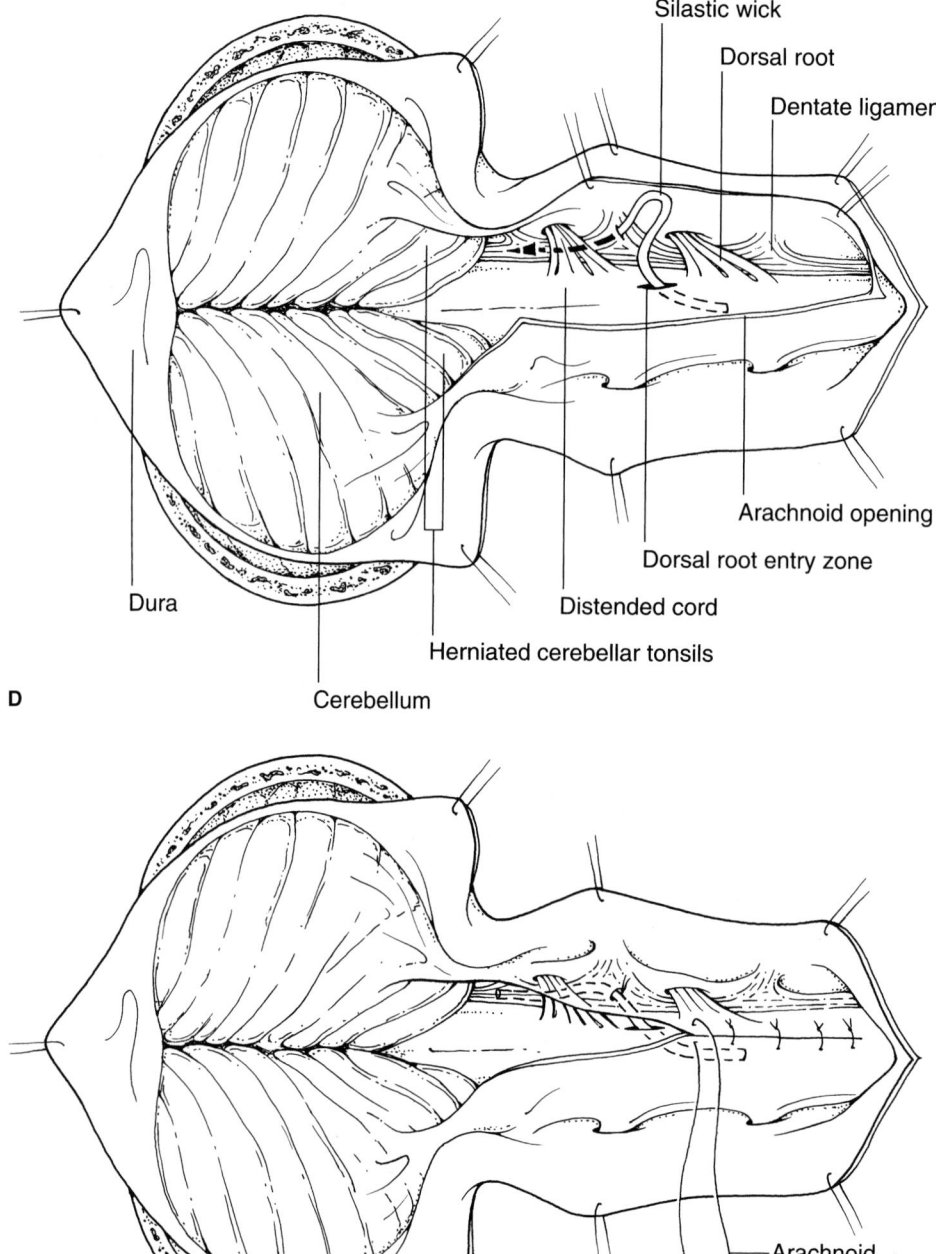

**D**

**E**

**Figure 84.4** *cont'd* (**D**) The suboccipital craniectomy and laminectomy have been completed and the dura and arachnoid have been opened. The myelotomy has been completed in the dorsal root entry zone. A 26-gauge Silastic wick is anchored to the arachnoid membrane and threaded downward into the hydromyelic cavity and upward into the subarachnoid space ventral to the nerve roots and dentate ligament. The tube is approximately one-half the diameter of the standard tubing used for a ventriculoperitoneal shunt. (**E**) The tube is anchored to the arachnoid membrane and not to the dura. The arachnoid is closed at the myelotomy site with a few 8-0 sutures in order to prevent the cord from becoming tethered to the dura at the site of the myelotomy. No attempt is made to close the arachnoid over the cerebellum or at the cervicomedullary junction and the outlet of the fourth ventricle. Closure of thickened arachnoid membrane at this site could constrict the cervicomedullary junction and block the outlet of the fourth ventricle.

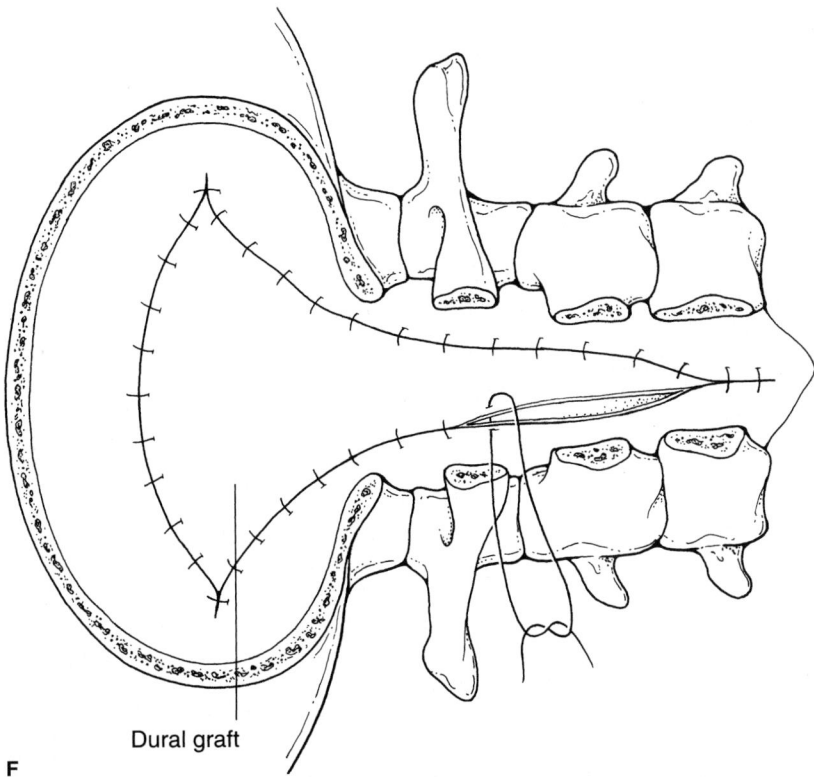

**F**

**Figure 84.4** *cont'd* **(F)** A dural graft is used to complete the closure in order to avoid constriction of the cervicomedullary junction and Chiari malformation.

drainage of the cavity at this level. The elongated cerebellar tonsils vary in appearance from those that are normal in color and consistency to those that are white and firm because of scarring and gliosis (Figures 84.6 and 84.7).[20] The caudal loop of the posterior inferior cerebellar artery often descends to the level of C2, marking the lower margin of the cerebellar tonsils (see Figure 84.6).

It is essential that the dura mater be opened and then closed with a dural graft that is tailored to relieve the constriction of the medulla and cerebellar tonsils (see Figure 84.4). The degree to which the dura mater and arachnoid adhere to the spinal cord and medulla can be predicted from neuroradiologic studies (see Figure 84.6). If CSF can be demonstrated between the dura mater and the cerebellar tonsils, the meninges can be separated easily from the tonsils. If the tonsils are pressed against the dura mater lining the cisterna magna, and no CSF is visualized between the tonsils and dura mater, the cerebellar tonsils may be adherent to the arachnoid and the dura mater. If a plaque of arachnoid and dura mater is adherent to the dorsal surface of the medulla and the spinal cord it should be left attached, because an attempt to disconnect it might injure the neural tissue (see Figures. 84.6 and 84.7).[20] If the foramen of Magendie is blocked, as occurs in a few cases, an outlet should be established by microsurgical techniques. Care should be taken to ensure that the dissection is rostral enough to enter the fluid cavity of the fourth ventricle rather than the medulla. After the fourth ventricle is opened, a Silastic wick (Dow Corning Corp., Midland, MI) is attached to the dura and passed upward into the new opening in the midline (Figure 84.8; see Figures 84.4 and 84.7). The wick serves to maintain the

patency of the outlet rather than to provide a conduit for drainage.

## Drainage of the Syrinx

After the Chiari malformation has been decompressed, the syrinx is drained into the subarachnoid space through a longitudinal incision in the dorsal root entry zone at the C2-3 level. The dorsal root entry zone between the lateral and posterior columns is selected for the myelotomy because it is consistently the thinnest area in patients with hydromyelia (see Figures 84.4, 84.7, and 84.8). The natural dissection of the cavity along the dorsal root entry zone also leads to a proprioceptive deficit in the upper extremities; hence, incision here minimizes the possibility of increasing the patient's neurologic deficit because the arm fibers course in the lateral part of the dorsal columns adjacent to the dorsal root entry zone.

The nerve root entry zone that has been most severely damaged and into which the hydromyelia has dissected the closest to the spinal cord surface is selected for the incision. The side with the greater involvement can usually be predicted from the neurologic findings, and one usually selected is the side showing increased sensory nerve deficit. MRI in the axial plane commonly shows that the cavity has dissected further into either the left or the right dorsal horn. The side with the greater damage and the side to be drained are usually placed uppermost if the operation is in the three-quarter prone position.

The dorsolateral myelotomy used to treat hydromyelia is different from the midline myelotomy between the gracile fasciculi (which carry the lower extremity fibers)

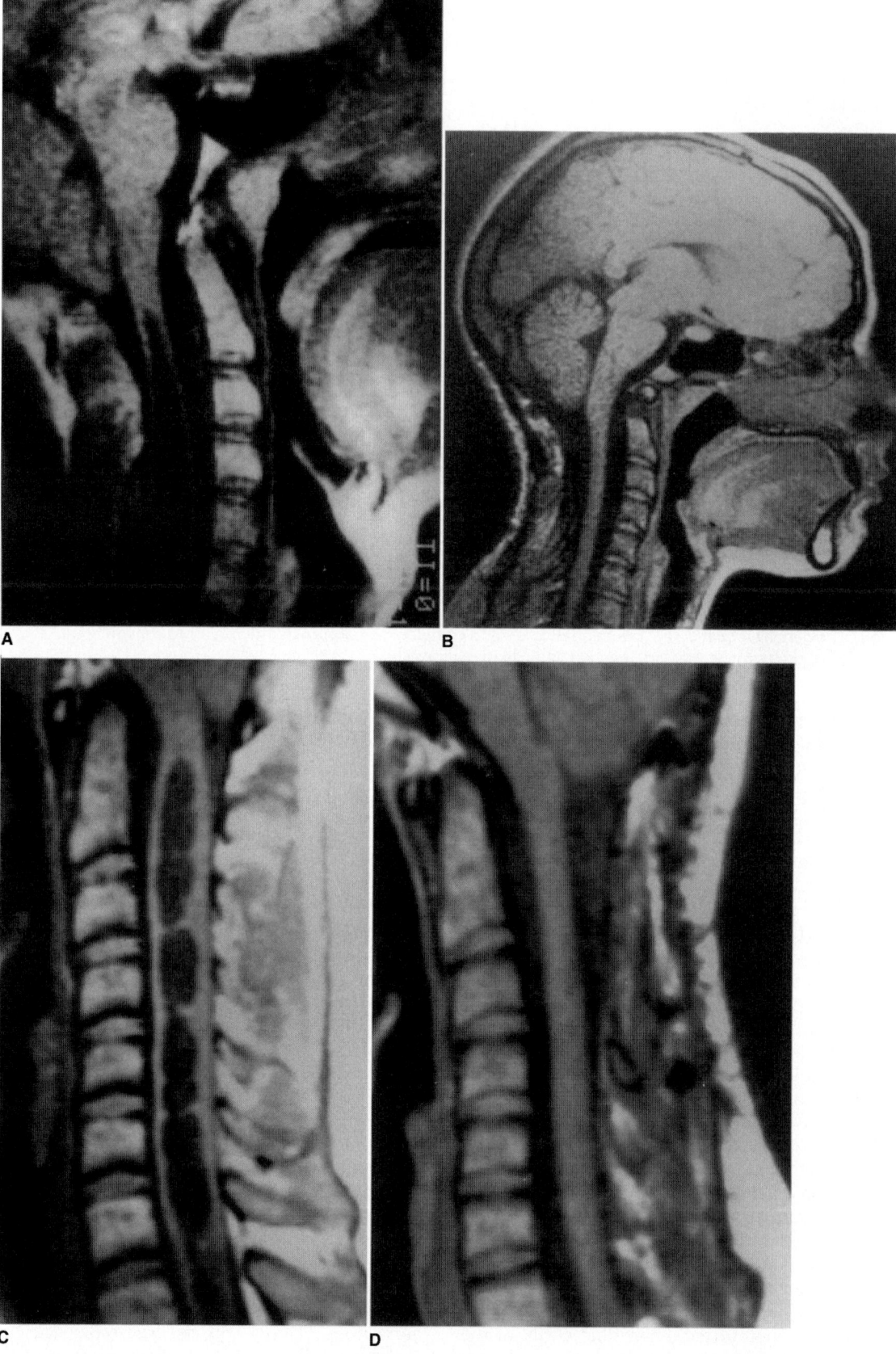

**Figure 84.5** Preoperative and postoperative MRI of Chiari malformations with hydromyelia. (**A** and **B**; **C** and **D**; **E** and **F**; **G** and **H**) Preoperative and postoperative sagittal images of individual patients before and after decompression of Chiari malformation and drainage of the hydromyelia.

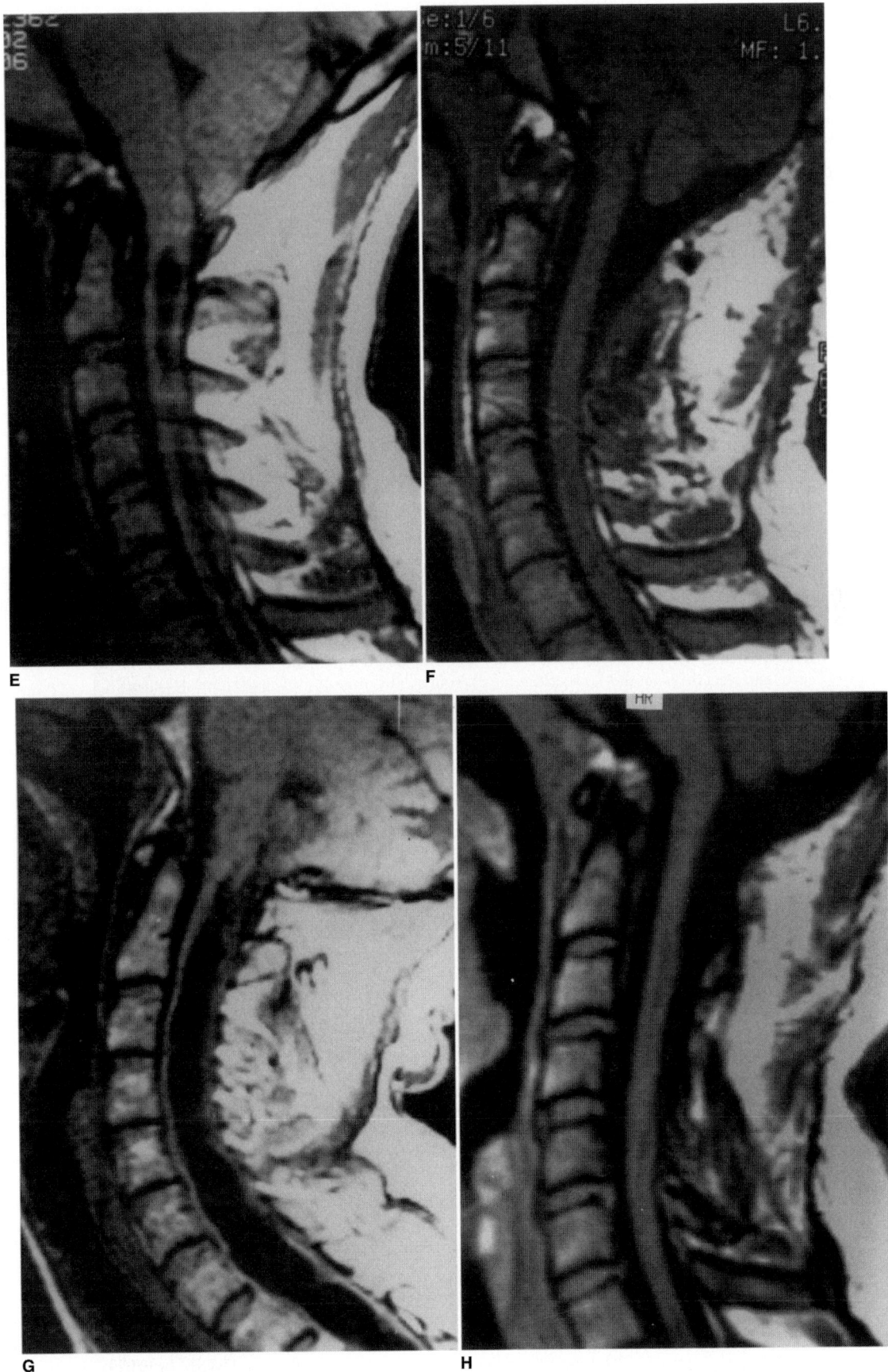

**Figure 84.5** *cont'd*

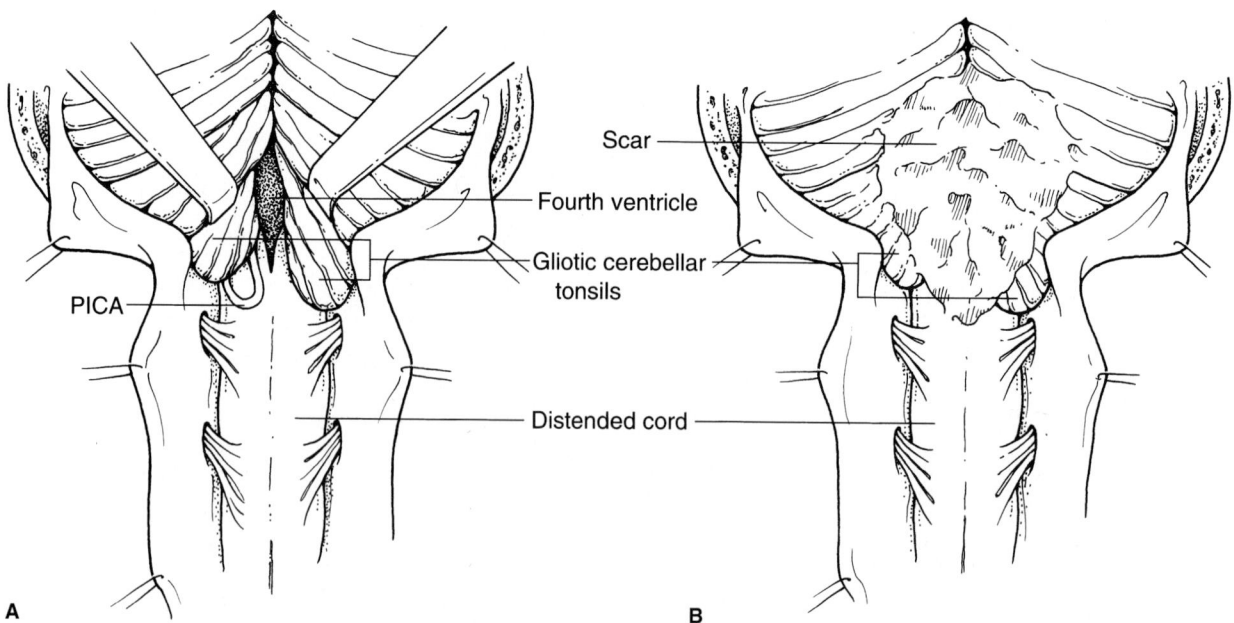

**Figure 84.6** Abnormalities at the outlet of the fourth ventricle with Chiari malformation. **(A)** A less complicated form of Chiari malformation in a patient with herniated gliotic cerebellar tonsils, ascending cervical nerve roots, abnormal caudal descent of the posterior inferior cerebellar artery, loss of normal folial patterns over the tips of the herniated cerebellar tonsils, an elongated fourth ventricle, and distended spinal cord. **(B)** A more complex malformation. The foramen of Magendie is occluded by a plaque of scar, and the pia, dura, and arachnoid are adherent to the dorsal medulla and cerebellum, occluding the outlet of the fourth ventricle. Disconnecting this mat of scar from the neural tissue could injure the medulla, cervical spinal cord, and structures on the floor of the fourth ventricle; therefore, the scar is not detached. Instead, the dura is opened by incising around the scar, which is left attached to these vital structures.

that is made to expose and remove an intramedullary tumor. In hydromyelia, usually, the dorsal root entry zone is thinnest on the side of the greater neurologic deficit. Before the spinal cord is incised, a needle may be introduced into the cavity at the thinnest area to collect fluid for cell count and protein determinations. Clear fluid with a normal protein level indicates hydromyelia, whereas colored fluid or an elevated protein level indicates an intramedullary tumor. A longitudinal incision approximately 8mm long is made into the thinnest area along the dorsal root entry zone, and a small, thin Silastic wick, approximately half the size of the standard tube used for ventricular shunting, is anchored to the arachnoid above and threaded downward into the myelotomy (see Figures 84.4, 84.7, and 84.8). The myelotomy is long enough to ensure that there is no tendency for spontaneous closure. The subarachnoid end of the tube is placed in the ventral subarachnoid space in front of the dentate ligament. An attempt is made to preserve the arachnoid at the time of opening the dura mater, so that the tube can be anchored to the arachnoid in the area lateral to the arachnoid incision rather than to the dura mater. The subarachnoid end of the tube is passed along the edge of the spinal cord ventral to the dentate ligament so that it is less likely to be adversely affected by scarring in the arachnoid and dura along the dorsally situated opening. The arachnoid is closed at the level of the myelotomy with a few 8-0 sutures in order to prevent the spinal cord from becoming tethered to the dura mater at the site of the myelotomy. No

attempt is made to close the arachnoid over the cerebellum or at the cervicomedullary junction and the outlet of the fourth ventricle. Closure over the outlet of the fourth ventricle in a patient with an extremely thick arachnoid, which is occasionally associated with Chiari malformation, could result in persistent postoperative compression at the cervicomedullary junction. Care is taken to avoid closure that could result in tethering of the spinal cord or adherence to the dura mater. The dura mater is closed with a loose-fitting triangular dural graft to ensure that the region around the Chiari malformation is not constricted and to create a generous cisterna magna.

Should every spinal cord be drained if there is a hydromyelic cavity in association with Chiari malformation? The first author has cared for a few patients in whom the decision has been made to not drain the syrinx, because the cavity was small and there was a significant thickness of the spinal cord overlying the cavity, both of which increase the risk of the myelotomy. On the other hand, a dorsal root entry zone myelotomy is done if the spinal cord is particularly thin in the region of the dorsal root entry zone, as is observed in most cases.

The first author has been referred numerous patients in whom neurologic deficits continued to progress after a decompressive suboccipital craniectomy and upper cervical laminectomy, either with or without plugging of the obex, without drainage of the hydromyelic cavity. Several of these patients, who had an MRI scan that demonstrated a poorly decompressed cisterna magna, had a repeat

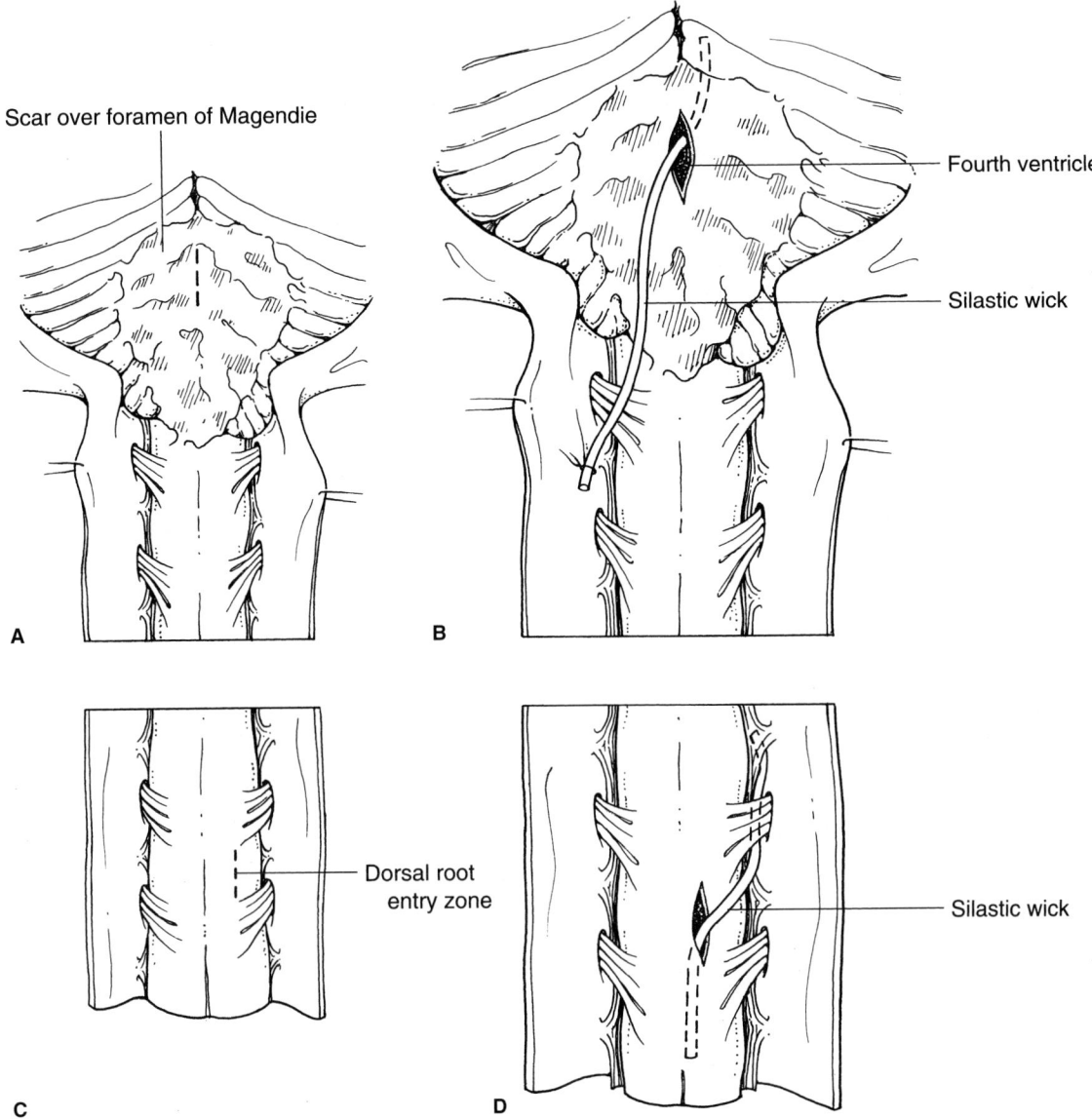

Scar over foramen of Magendie

Fourth ventricle

Silastic wick

**A**

**B**

Dorsal root entry zone

Silastic wick

**C**

**D**

**Figure 84.7** Surgical approach used by the authors to treat Chiari malformation with hydromyelia. A suboccipital craniectomy and upper cervical laminectomy are performed to expose and decompress the Chiari malformation (**A** and **B**) and to expose the hydromyelic spinal cord (**C** and **D**). If the foramen of Magendie is blocked by dense scar it is reestablished by opening through the upper part of the scar into the fourth ventricle (**A**). A Silastic wick is anchored to the dura and passed through the opening into the fourth ventricle (**B**). The hydromyelic cord is decompressed by opening the thinnest area (the dorsal root entry zone) with a longitudinal incision that follows the course of the entering dorsal nerve roots (**C**). A Silastic wick is then anchored to the arachnoid and advanced downward into the hydromyelic cavity and upward into the subarachnoid space ventral to the dentate ligament (**D**).

suboccipital craniectomy or upper cervical laminectomy, combined with duraplasty and drainage of the syrinx. If the Chiari malformation was shown to be decompressed with an open cisterna magna, a hemilaminectomy was performed in the thoracic region over the lower extent of the hydromyelic cavity, and the fluid was drained through the dorsal root entry zone into the subarachnoid space, with insertion of a Silastic wick, anchored to the arachnoid (Figure 84.9).

A myelotomy of the dorsal root entry zone was the initial surgical procedure in several patients with hydromyelia

without Chiari malformation who had progressive neurologic deficits caused by hydromyelia (see Figure 84.9). If this procedure is to be performed as the primary operation, the hemilaminectomy is performed in the upper thoracic region, below the cervical enlargement on the side of the greater deficit.

Shunting of CSF from the lateral ventricles to the peritoneum would be indicated if the ventricles are large or if there is evidence of increased intracranial pressure.[8] These findings of hydrocephalus on a scan or evidence of increased intracranial pressure, however, are uncommon.

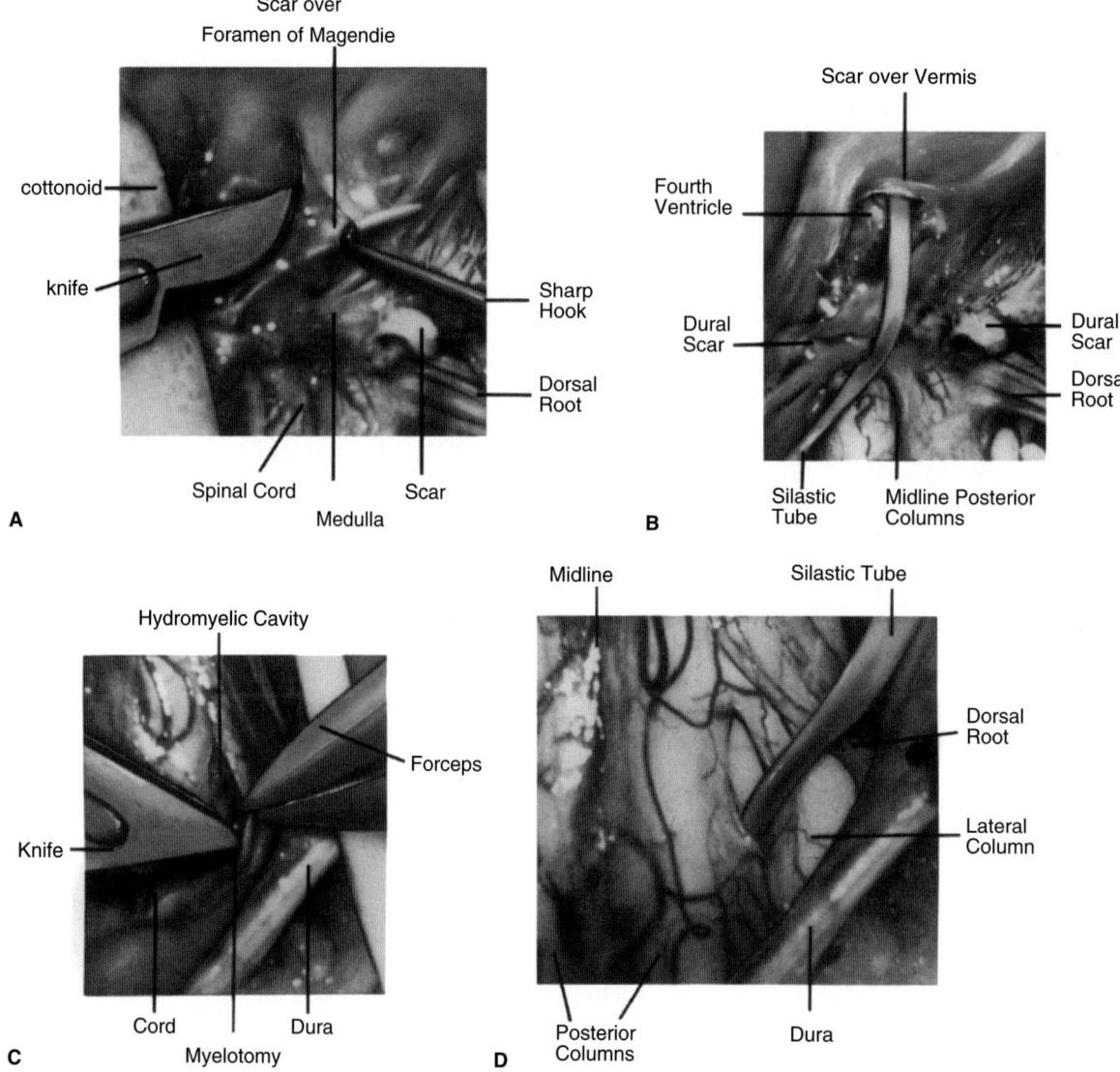

**Figure 84.8** Chiari malformation and hydromyelia as seen through a suboccipital craniectomy and a C1-4 laminectomy through the surgical microscope (x6). (**A**) Incision of the dense mat of scar over the foramen of Magendie. (**B**) Opening into the fourth ventricle is completed; a Silastic wick, anchored to the dura below, is threaded rostrally. (**C**) An incision, 8 to 10mm long, is made with a no. 11 knife blade in the dorsal root entry zone. (**D**) A Silastic wick is attached to the arachnoid above and inserted into the hydromyelic cavity. (*From Rhoton AL Jr: Microsurgery of Arnold-Chiari malformation in adults with and without hydromyelia.* J Neurosurg 45:473, 1976.)

If a deficit continues to progress after decompression alone of Chiari malformation, the hydromyelic cavity should be drained. If this proves ineffective, a syringoperitoneal shunt should be used.[2,8,28] Two patients in this series, having Chiari malformation and hydromyelia, also had marked ventral compression of the cervicomedullary junction requiring transoral odontoidectomy in addition to the posterior decompression.

## Results

In the first author's experience, there have been no deaths after surgery on more than 60 patients. Furthermore, the neurologic deficit increased in only two patients as a result of surgery. One patient developed a mild proprioceptive sensory loss in the right thumb of which he was unaware but which was demonstrable on examination. Another patient who had the Chiari malformation decompressed and two previous operations to drain the syrinx (before referral) and who was quadriparetic and bedridden had a further mild loss of strength in her only functional extremity after a third operation directed through an extensive scar to drain the syrinx.

A careful preoperative explanation of the reasonable potential benefits a patient may expect from the operation is helpful to obtain an optimal result from surgical therapy. Most patients report functional improvement after the

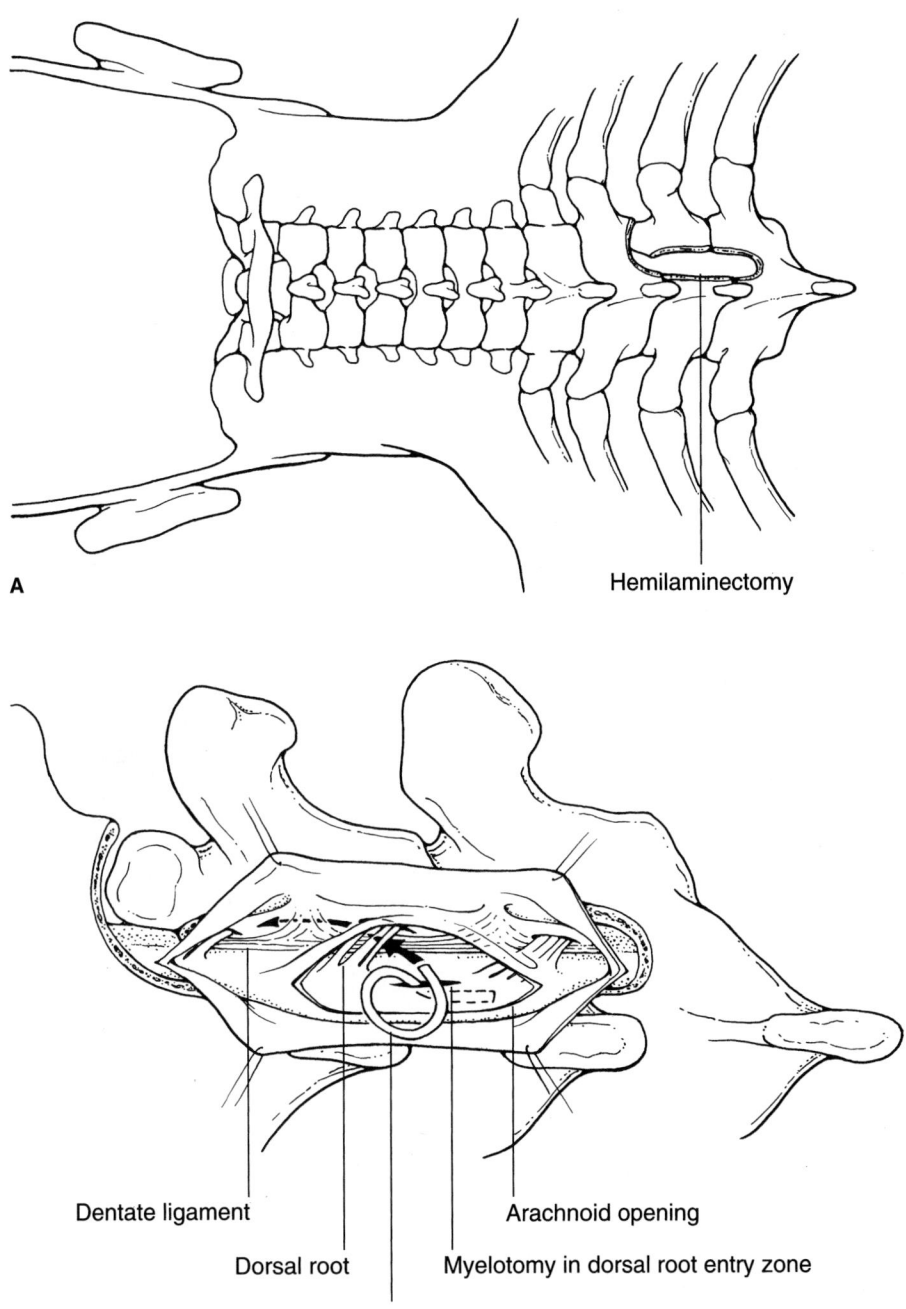

**Figure 84.9** Dorsal root entry zone myelotomy in the upper thoracic region. This approach is used if the patient with a hydromyelia has minimal Chiari malformation or if a suboccipital craniectomy and decompression of Chiari malformation has failed to arrest the progression of a spinal cord deficit. (**A**) The operation is usually done with the patient in the three-quarter prone position. The side of the dorsal root entry zone to be drained is placed uppermost if the three-quarter prone position is used. The hemilaminectomy is positioned below the cervical enlargement of the spinal cord in the upper thoracic area. (**B**) The myelotomy is located in the dorsal root entry zone.

*Continued*

operation, although the neurologic examination usually reveals little or no change in the deficit. Therefore, patients are advised that the operation usually halts the progression of their deficit but may not restore them to normal. The operation commonly arrests the progression of muscle atrophy, prevents the areas of numbness from increasing in size, and may result in some improvement of strength. In most patients who have anesthesia dolorosa postoperatively, the pain continues to be exacerbated by emotional stress, hunger, cold weather, and fatigue. This type of pain seems to recur 6 to 12 weeks postoperatively, after patients have returned to employment and resumed full-time work. Spasticity also fluctuates under the same conditions postoperatively, although motor testing shows

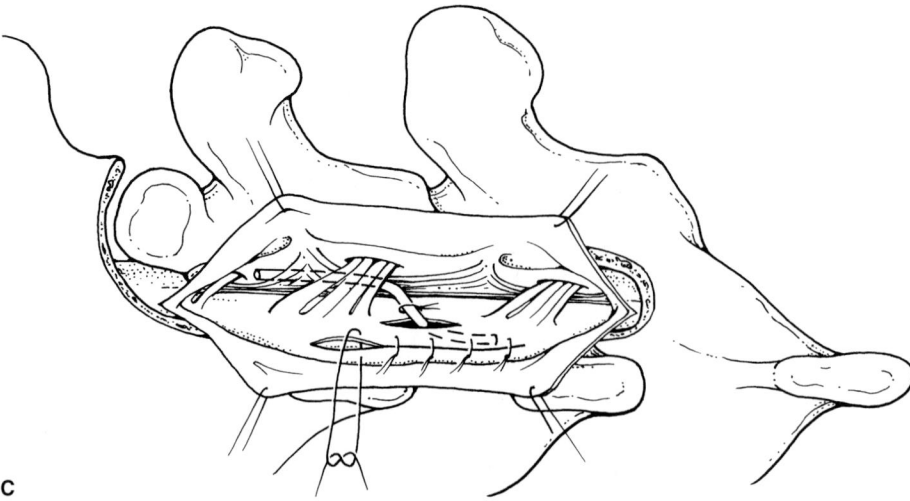

C

**Figure 84.9 *cont'd*** (**C**) A Silastic wick is anchored to the arachnoid and threaded downward into the hydromyelic cavity and upward anterior to the nerve roots and dentate ligament into the ventral subarachnoid space. The wick is anchored to the arachnoid and not the dura. The arachnoid membrane is closed with a few 8-0 sutures in order to prevent the cord from becoming tethered by scar to the dura at the site of the myelotomy.

no further loss of strength. Deformities at joints associated with muscle atrophy may increase during the years after surgery, even though there has been no further atrophy or loss of strength. MRI has provided an excellent way to follow these patients (see Figure 84.5). However, even when postoperative MRI shows the hydromyelia to be absent or markedly reduced in size, patients may continue to experience fluctuations in pain and spasticity, even though the size of analgesic areas and the extent of muscle atrophy and weakness do not progress.

## Alternative Therapies

A variety of surgical treatments have been proposed for hydromyelia associated with Chiari malformation (Figure 84.10).[21] Gardner[10-12] initially recommended a suboccipital craniectomy and cervical laminectomy to decompress the malformation and subsequent plugging of the obex with a small piece of muscle. He subsequently reported that most of the patients treated in this fashion later developed progressive neurologic deficits (personal communication). Plugging the obex increases the chance of damaging the hypoglossal and vagal nuclei that are located at the level of the obex near the rostral end of the central canal.

Gardner *et al.*[13] have also described a procedure called *terminal ventriculostomy*. The terminal ventricle is the dilated portion of the central canal that extends below the tip of the conus medullaris into the filum terminale (see Figure 84.10). A laminectomy is performed over the caudal limit of the fluid sac, and the filum is opened. This procedure does not decompress the malformation at the foramen magnum but may prove satisfactory if the patient has symptoms of hydromyelia only. The procedure is inappropriate in cases in which the hydromyelic cavity does not extend into the lumbar portion of the spinal cord or into the filum terminale.

Shunting of CSF from the lateral ventricle to the atrium or peritoneum has been considered a mode of treatment.[17] However, patients in the first author's series, even those with marked hydromyelic deficits, had no significant ventricular dilatation. Furthermore, the small ventricles make shunting difficult. Shunting is indicated if the ventricles are large or if there is increased intracranial pressure. Lumboperitoneal shunting has been advocated. It has not been used frequently because of concern that it may increase the risk of herniation at the foramen magnum.[19] Percutaneous needling of the hydromyelic cavity has been advocated as a possible mode of therapy; however, aspiration of fluid at the time of surgery is followed by rapid refilling of the hydromyelic cavity from the ventricular system, and it seems unlikely that a needle track would remain open.[25]

## Perspective

The authors have found that the most effective treatment of syringomyelia associated with Chiari malformation is a suboccipital craniectomy and upper cervical laminectomy with duraplasty to decompress the malformation in combination with drainage of the hydromyelia through the dorsal root entry zone into the subarachnoid space to decompress the syrinx. If the foramen of Magendie is blocked, it is reestablished using microsurgical techniques. If a previous adequate decompression of Chiari malformation has been performed, without drainage of the hydromyelia, a myelotomy of the dorsal root entry zone may be performed below the cervical enlargement in the thoracic region. If the neurologic deficit progresses after decompression of Chiari malformation and syringosubarachnoid shunting, a syringoperitoneal shunt should be employed. Shunting of CSF from the lateral ventricles to the peritoneum is indicated if hydrocephalus is present. This is uncommon in adult patients.

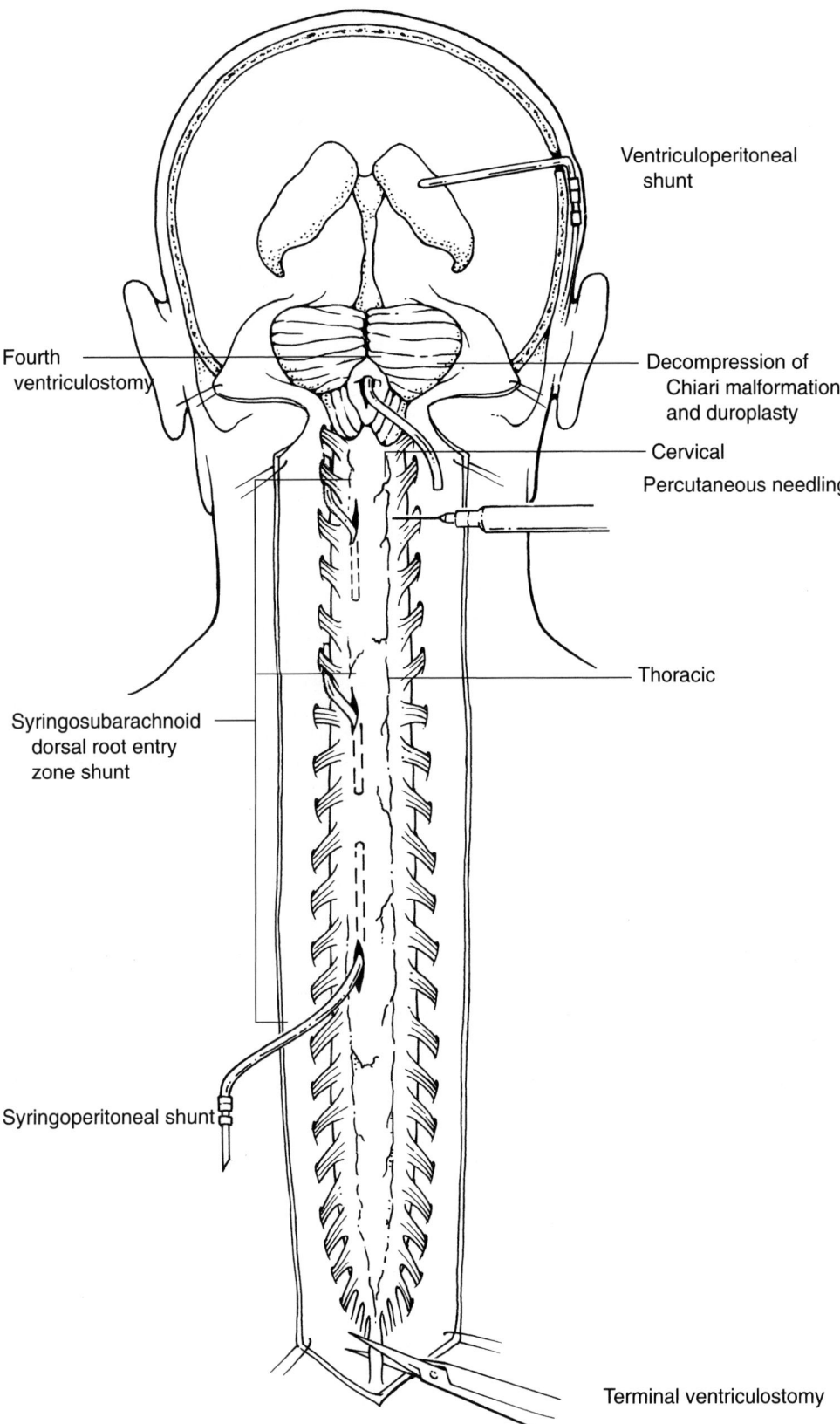

**Figure 84.10** Procedures for the treatment of syringomyelia associated with Chiari malformation.

# REFERENCES

1. Arnold J: Myelocyste: transposition von Gewebskeimen und Sympodie. *Beitr Pathol Anat Pathol* 16:1, 1894.
2. Barbaro NM, Wilson CB, Gutin PH, *et al:* Surgical treatment of syringomyelia: favorable results with syringoperitoneal shunting. *J Neurosurg* 61:531, 1984.
3. Barnett HJM, Foster JB, Hudgson P: *Syringomyelia.* Philadelphia, WB Saunders, 1973.
4. Batzdorf U: Chiari I malformation with syringomyelia: evaluation of surgical therapy by magnetic resonance imaging. *J Neurosurg* 68:726, 1988.
5. Bertrand G: Dynamic factors in the evolution of syringomyelia and syringobulbia. *Clin Neurosurg* 20:322, 1973.
6. Brewis M, Poskanzer DC, Rolland C, *et al:* Neurological disease in an English city. *Acta Neurol Scand* 42 (suppl 24):1, 1966.
7. Chiari H: Uber die pathogenese der sogenannten syringomyelie. *Heilkunde* 9:307, 1888.
8. Conway LW: Hydrodynamic studies in syringomyelia. *J Neurosurg* 27:501, 1967.
9. Ellertsson AB: Syringomyelia and other cystic spinal cord lesions. *Acta Neurol Scand* 45:403, 1969.
10. Gardner WJ: Hydrodynamic mechanism of syringomyelia: its relationship to myelocele. *J Neurol Neurosurg Psychiatry* 28:247, 1965.
11. Gardner WJ: Myelocele: rupture of the neural tube? *Clin Neurosurg* 15:57, 1968.
12. Gardner WJ, Angel J: The mechanism of syringomyelia and its surgical correction. *Clin Neurosurg* 6:131, 1959.
13. Gardner WJ, Bell H, Poolos PN, *et al:* Terminal ventriculostomy for syringomyelia. *J Neurosurg* 46:609, 1977.
14. Gowers WR: *A Manual of Disease of the Nervous System,* vol 1. London, Churchill, 1886.
15. Merritt HH: *A Textbook of Neurology,* ed 5. Philadelphia, Lea & Febiger, 1973.
16. Mullan S, Raimondi AJ: Respiratory hazards of the surgical treatment of the Arnold-Chiari malformation. *J Neurosurg* 19:675, 1962.
17. Ogilvy CS, Borges LF: Treatment of symptomatic syringomyelia with a ventriculoperitoneal shunt: a case report with magnetic resonance scan correlation. *Neurosurgery* 22:748, 1988.
18. Oldfield EH, Muraszko K, Shawker TH et al: Pathophysiology of syringomyelia associated with Chiari I malformation of the cerebellar tonsils. *J Neurosurg* 80:3, 1994.
19. Park TS, Cail WS, Broaddus WC et al: Lumboperitoneal shunt combined with myelotomy for treatment of syringohydromyelia. *J Neurosurg* 70:721, 1976.
20. Rhoton AL Jr: Microsurgery of Arnold-Chiari malformation in adults with and without hydromyelia. *J Neurosurg* 45:473, 1976.
21. Rhoton AL Jr: Syringomyelia. In Wilson CB, Hoff JT (eds): *Current Surgical Management of Neurological Disease.* New York, Churchill Livingstone, 1980, p 29.
22. Rhoton AL Jr: Microsurgery of syringomyelia and syringomyelic cord syndrome. In Schmidek HH, Sweet WH (eds): *Operative Neurosurgical Techniques: Indications, Methods, and Results,* ed 3, vol 2. Philadelphia, WB Saunders, 1998, pp 1745-1774.
23. Rhoton AL Jr, Fessler RG: Surgical treatment of Chiari malformation and hydromyelia in adults. In Wilson CB (ed): *Neurosurgical Procedures: Personal Approaches to Classic Operations.* Baltimore, Williams & Wilkins, 1992, p 170.
24. Rhoton EL, Rhoton AL: Chiari malformation with syringocephaly. *J Neurosurg* 75:791, 1991.
25. Schlesinger ER, Tenner MS, Michelsen WH: Percutaneous spinal cord puncture in the analysis and treatment of hydromyelia. Presented at the Annual Meeting of the American Association of Neurological Surgeons, Houston, Texas, April 1971.
26. Schwalbe E, Gredig M: Uber entwicklungsstorungen des kleinhirns, hirnstamms und halsmarks bei spina bifida (Arnoldshe and Chiarishe missbildung). *Beitr Path Anat* 40:132, 1907.
27. Vaquero J, Martinez R, Arias A: Syringomyelia-Chiari complex: magnetic resonance imaging and clinical evaluation of surgical treatment. *J Neurosurg* 73:64, 1990.
28. Wisoff JH, Epstein F: Management of hydromyelia. *Neurosurgery* 25:562, 1989.

# CHAPTER 85

# Chiari Malformation and Chronic Fatigue Syndrome/Fibromyalgia: A Paradigm for Care

**Sudhakar T. Sridharan and William S. Wilke**

The Chiari Malformation is an extraordinarily common problem. It is not necessarily a disease or truly a malformation. Perhaps, in the adult form (Chiari Malformation I [CMI]), it should be considered a normal variant. The diagnosis is established by observing the cerebellar tonsils to be below the foramen magnum on magnetic resonance imaging (MRI). Depending on the examiner's definition of the CMI (as assessed by the amount of descent below the foramen magnum in mm), the incidence of the diagnosis may vary considerably. The extent of descent of cerebellar tonsils does not necessarily correlate with symptoms, physical findings, or neurologic findings. The coexistence of a CMI with syringomyelia indicates that the CMI is more physiologically significant. However, this does not necessarily imply that surgery is indicated.

## Characterization of CMI

In 1891, Hans Chiari (1851-1916) first characterized and classified these alterations, and he recognized three types. Modern neuropathologists continue to accept Chiari's seminal observations and classification design. Contemporary neuroradiologic imaging facilitates the determination of the type of malformation without the need for invasive techniques. However, varying degrees of cerebellar ectopia are increasingly being recognized on midsagittal MRI in asymptomatic subjects, and in some patients with a wide variety of clinical symptoms.[1] There is continued debate regarding the significance of these incidental changes observed on MRI. Today, we face a challenge that Chiari did not consider: to determine the significance of incidental changes in the context of often vague and difficult to localize symptoms.

The CMI is a herniation of the cerebellar tonsils into the foramen magnum. This herniation creates a crowding of the craniocervical junction. Although the incidence of CMI is unknown, it is not uncommon.[19] Unlike patients with the more severe Chiari II malformation, which typically manifests in infancy, patients with Chiari I lesions may remain asymptomatic or experience symptoms in adulthood with subtle clinical findings related to brainstem compression or coexistent syringomyelia.[5]

Before the past decade, the diagnosis of CMI relied on strong clinical suspicion, coupled with a specifically tailored imaging examination that consisted of cervical myelography and/or computerized tomography (CT).[50] In the 1980s, however, newer technologies such as MRI made it possible to make an accurate, noninvasive diagnosis of this disorder for the first time.[49] MRI is now the diagnostic tool of choice.[4] The following criteria are used for diagnosis[35]:

1. Caudal descent of the cerebellar tonsil at least 3 to 5mm below the plane of the foramen magnum
2. "Pegged or pointed" appearance of the tonsillar tips
3. Crowding of the subarachnoid space in the area of the craniocervical junction

Associated abnormalities primarily occur in the spinal cord and skeletal system. A syrinx is present in 20% to 40% of all patients; however, 60% to 90% of symptomatic patients have a syrinx. A syrinx usually involves the cervical spinal cord; however, occasionally it involves the entire spinal cord. Skeletal abnormalities occur in approximately 25% of all patients with CMI that include basilar invagination, Klippel-Feil syndrome, atlantooccipital assimilation, platybasia, fused cervical vertebrae, cervical ribs, spina bifida, and aqueductal stenosis.[17] In addition, in a study of 50 patients with CMI, Dyste[15] found 57% had scoliosis, 57% had a shallow posterior fossa, and 51% had a widened spinal canal. Milhorat,[35] in a large prospective study of 364 symptomatic patients, found that 65% had an associated syrinx, 42% had scoliosis, and 12% had basilar invagination.

## Workup

To appropriately care for patients with the CMI and syringomyelia, one must first define the presence of tonsillar herniation, its extent, and its physiologic and clinical significance. The history and physical examination are extraordinarily important in this regard. These often lead to imaging studies, such as MRI. The definition of a Chiari Malformation is usually an indicator for further diagnostic workup. This usually entails an MRI of the head to demonstrate the presence or absence of hydrocephalus and other associated anomalies. MRI of the cervical and thoracic spine is also appropriate to rule in or out the presence of syringomyelia. If a syrinx is present, a contrast-enhanced MRI (MRI following the injection of a contrast and enhancing agent, gadolinium) may be indicated in some circumstances. Finally, many surgeons feel that a cervicomedullary junction cine MRI is appropriate to determine if an obstruction of cerebrospinal fluid (CSF) flow occurs in this region.

Patients who have significant symptoms and who have a physiologic explanation for these symptoms (the presence of an MRI, evidence of a syringomyelia, and/or obstruction to CSF flow in the region of the CMI) may have a clinical and physiologically significant Chiari Malformation. This constellation, in fact, may constitute an indication for surgical decompression in many patients.

These aforementioned studies, combined with the history, physical examination, and neurologic examination, define the optimal surgical candidates. One must then define a care plan for the patient. Aside from surgery, further treatment is usually indicated. This includes pain management and rehabilitation. Most importantly, it also includes the establishment of a working diagnosis of concomitant or related illnesses and a treatment plan. This is best accomplished by a multidisciplinary team.

## Fibromyalgia and Chronic Fatigue Syndrome

Symptoms of CMI vary significantly. The symptom complex may be difficult to differentiate from symptoms of syringomyelia. The determination that the Chiari Malformation is causally related to the symptom complex is often complicated by the overlap of similar symptoms caused by stress-related disorders; hence, the alleged association between the CMI and the diagnosis of fibromyalgia (FMS) and chronic fatigue syndrome (CFS). This association has perhaps been taken to an extreme by some, that is, those who consider the coexistence of FMS and CFS symptoms and the CMI as an indication for Chiari Malformation surgery. A recent, highly publicized theory attempted to link these two syndromes by suggesting that surgery for CMI may be curative for FMS/CFS,[7] leading to intense media coverage and speculation. Unfortunately, no peer-reviewed manuscripts have yet been published

that confirm this relationship, or document outcomes.[52] Regardless of the presence or absence of an association, it is evident that the complex nature of the diagnosis and treatment of the CMI and syringomyelia deserves a comprehensive and methodologic approach.

Perhaps most important in the aforementioned diagnostic and treatment algorithm (Figure 85.1) is the management of those patients who are felt to have symptoms associated with the Chiari Malformation but do not have indications for surgery, as well as for those patients who are felt to have unrelated symptoms (such as those related to the FMS or CFS).

Fibromyalgia is relatively common in the general population, occurring in 3.4% to 4.9% of women and 0.5% of 1.6% of men.[51,58] The majority of patients with FMS also have symptoms of chronic fatigue syndrome, which suggest that there is significant overlap and little difference between these two illnesses. Approximately 10% to 20% of new patients in a rheumatology practice and 2% to 6% of patients in primary care practices have FMS.[34] The concept of FMS as a distinct nosologic entity is controversial. Some authorities argue that when the diagnosis is made, a nondisease is medicalized.[24] Unfortunately, to simply tell patients that they are "out of sorts" is unlikely to benefit FMS patients.[24] In fact, recognition of this illness construct facilitates study of symptoms that may be related to distress and/or a genetic, physiologic diathesis.

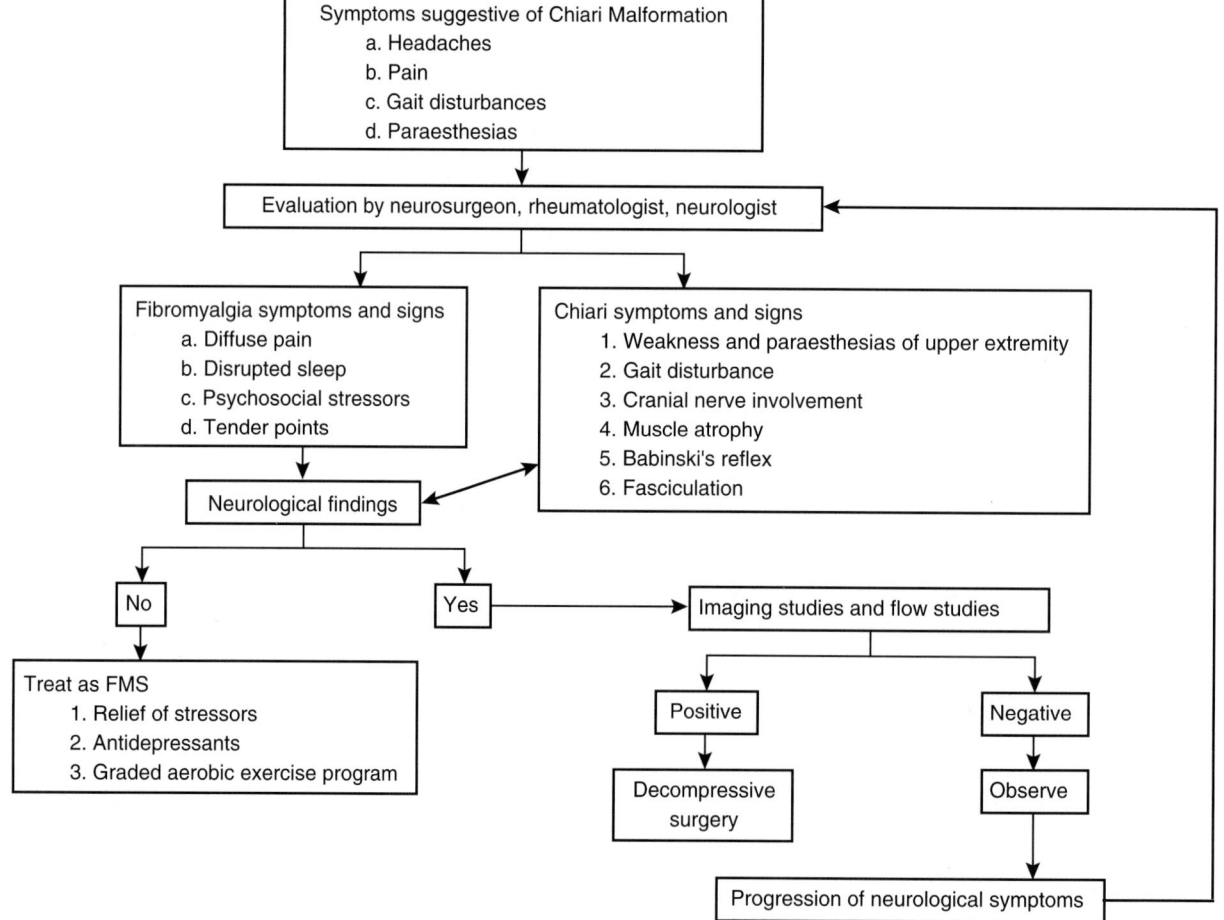

**Figure 85.1** Algorithm for the management of a patient with symptoms of Chiari Malformation.

The definition criteria for CFS require that debilitating fatigue be present for at least 6 months and result in functional impairment.[46] Minor criteria for CFS, which are also common in FMS and include sleep disturbance, headaches, and postexertional malaise, demonstrate the overlap between these two entities.[31] The American College of Rheumatology classification criteria for FMS was published in 1990.[59] The combination of widespread pain in four quadrants of at least 3 months duration, and tenderness in at least 11 out of 18 designated tender points was found to be 84.4% sensitive and 81.1% specific for the diagnosis.[59] In general, the pain of FMS worsens at rest and improves during physical activity, only to reoccur afterward. A variety of other symptoms are also associated. The most common, which occur in 75% of individuals include fatigue, nonrestorative sleep, distress, and morning stiffness; and the less common include irritable bowel syndrome, urinary frequency, headache, subjective swelling, diffuse paresthesias, psychologic distress, and marked functional disability.[12,56-58,61-63]

Unfortunately, the ACR criteria are flawed. They suggest that FMS is a homogeneous illness. In fact the two diagnostic criteria, a high number of tender points and chronic widespread pain, when studied in a large German population, appeared to have different background risk variables.[48] Those symptoms that carried a higher risk for positive tender points included low physical mobility, pain and bodily complaints; and of those for chronic widespread pain included poor health status, catastrophizing, emotional reactions, low energy level, and sleep disturbances. Furthermore, these factors appear to operate independent of each other.

A recent cluster analysis of 97 patients who met ACR criteria for FMS confirms the heterogeneous nature of this disorder and adds a cluster of patients with minimal psychological dysfunction who had the highest pain responses.[20] This information suggests that neurobiologic mechanisms may be more important than psychologic factors in some patients.

This is not to deemphasize the importance of psychologic factors. In fact, they may play a part in the genesis of a variety of pain disorders. A prospective study of 829 individuals engaged in diverse occupations demonstrated that factors such as individual psychologic distress, increasing job demands, poor support from colleagues, and dissatisfaction with work were highly associated with regional pain syndromes.[27] This observation helps one understand why FMS symptoms occur at a higher point frequency in chronic illnesses such as systemic lupus erythematosus and rheumatoid arthritis. They are probably results of distress caused by the primary disease.[21,57]

## Pathogenesis of Fibromyalgia and Chronic Fatigue Syndrome

Any hypothesis of the pathogenesis of FMS remains a work in progress. A number of statements, however, can be made with reasonable certainty:

1. Patients with FMS have diffusely lower pain threshold than healthy control patients.
2. The mechanisms responsible for lower pain thresholds are central.

3. FMS is not a discrete disorder but represents a distal point on a continuum of disorders related to distress.[53]

Furthermore, genetic factors appear to influence susceptibility to this disorder. FMS patients are more likely to have a certain genotype for the promoter region of the serotonin transporter gene.[38] Individuals with this particular genotype demonstrate increased blood flow to the amygdala in response to fearful stimuli versus controls.[26] This finding suggests that individuals with this gene polymorphism may in fact have a more cautious/fearful view of reality, which might explain increased perceived distress.

## Treatment of Fibromyalgia and Chronic Fatigue Syndrome

The cornerstone of treatment for FMS includes education, methods to increase aerobic capacity, and measures to improve mood/sleep. Tricyclic antidepressant drugs have been demonstrated to be superior to placebo in two metaanalyses.[3,39] Although, selective serotonin reuptake inhibitors alone have not been demonstrated to be beneficial,[37,55] when combined with 25mg of amitriptyline, the combination was superior to placebo or single agents.[22] Higher doses of selective serotonin reuptake inhibitors, when given alone, may in fact be efficacious.[2] Other agents such as alprazolam, bromazepam, moclobemide, 5-HT3 receptor antagonists, 5-hydroxytryptophan, S-adenosylmethionine, zolpidem, zopiclone, and tramadol are superior to placebo for control of some symptoms of FMS.[°] Importantly, prednisone, nonsteroidal anti-inflammatory drugs, and acetaminophen have not been demonstrated to be more effective than placebo.[9,54,60] None of these drugs, when tested in CFS, demonstrated efficacy. One trial of low-dose hydrocortisone showed modest improvement in the symptoms of chronic fatigue but caused hypothalamic pituitary axis suppression as a serious adverse effect, and for this reason is not recommended.[11]

Behavioral therapies and education may be of benefit in both of these conditions.[23,41,44,48] Cardiovascular fitness and the strength training exercises have been demonstrated to be superior to placebo in the above conditions,[18,30,43] and as might be expected, a combination of such interventions is more efficacious than any one intervention alone.[33] Newer agents such as milnacipran may be more effective than previous pharmacologic therapy. However, as the heterogeneous nature of these disorders is increasingly recognized, no one pharmacologic intervention or, for that matter, combination of interventions, is likely to be universally effective. Further understanding of pathogenic mechanisms in individual patients can help to identify subsets that may be better suited to one or a combination of therapies. It is unlikely that one size will ever fit all.

A great deal of excitement was generated in the mass media and on the Internet by claims of curative surgery for FMS/CFS in patients in whom the Chiari malformation was incidentally discovered.[7] However, this belies important differences between these two conditions; the weakness in FMS is subjective and objective in Chiari, and fatigue, widespread pain, and disturbed sleep are not

---

°References 6,8,14,25,28,29,36,42,45.

features of abnormal hindbrain anatomy. Other important differences also exist (see Table 85.1).

Undoubtedly, multiple factors contribute to the complexity of assessing patients with a Chiari malformation, some of whom may develop "secondary" forms of FMS. A small proportion of patients with FMS may also have anatomic abnormalities consistent with a Chiari malformation, which may or may not be itself symptomatic. Also, some patients with Chiari malformation and/or syringomyelia experience symptoms such as weakness and sensory abnormalities, much like FMS patients, underscoring the immense complexity of assessing and treating these patients.

The symptomatic Chiari neurologic syndrome appears rare: a total of 147 patients were seen over 6 years at a tertiary care center specializing in cervical cranial malformations.[17] Since chronic and regional pain syndromes are very common in the general population, with prevalence rates between 10% and 20%, one must conclude that only a very small subset of patients with CFS will also demonstrate symptomatic Chiari malformation, or this neurologic entity is grossly underreported in the general population. A pilot prevalence of MRI findings showed that 8 of 26 patients with FMS (31%) had some degree of tonsillar herniation compared to 11 of 15 healthy controls (73%).[10] This report suggests a much higher prevalence of

this asymptomatic anatomic finding in the general population. Most importantly, however, FMS patients did not have a higher prevalence of this radiographic finding, suggesting little or no relationship between the symptoms of chronic pain and fatigue and this malformation.

A review of selected series of classic symptomatic Chiari patients (Table 85.2)* demonstrates key features of the syndrome that occur in descending order of frequency to be: (1) weakness, (2) paresthesias of the upper extremities, (3) gait disturbances, (4) cranial nerve involvement, and (5) cervical pain with headaches. Corresponding findings at physical examination demonstrate (1) cranial nerve palsy, (2) upper extremity weakness and muscle atrophy with sensory abnormalities, (3) hyporeflexia in the upper extremities and hyperreflexia in the lower extremities, (4) Babinski and Hoffman signs, and (5) fasciculation. Although headaches are common in patients with FMS, the pain is diffuse, fatigue nearly universal, and the only reproducible finding is tenderness on palpation. If reflexes are brisk, they are exaggerated in all four extremities. In fact, the signs and symptoms of FMS and Chiari are largely mutually exclusive. Some patients, however, may have both syndromes. It is possible that a small subset of patients has both conditions by chance alone. Certainly, patients with a chronic progressive neurologic condition that goes undiagnosed for years will experience great stress, a key etiologic factor associated with FMS. If surgery improves the symptoms of the anatomic syndrome, it will also improve stress and, thus, the symptoms of FMS and chronic fatigue. Rosner and Heffez[52] emphasize that gainful improvement of FMS may take many months, in keeping with the hypothesis of secondary benefit.

## Diagnostic and Treatment Paradigm

All patients with a Chiari malformation who are referred to the Neurosurgery Service at The Cleveland Clinic

**TABLE 85.1**

**Differences Between CMI and FMS/CFS**

| Parameter | CMI | FMS/CFS |
|---|---|---|
| Pain | Localized | Generalized |
| Non-restorative sleep | No | Yes |
| Primary mood disorder | No | Yes |
| Weakness | Objective | Subjective |
| Sensory findings | Objective | Subjective |
| Deep tendon reflexes | Brisk, asymmetric | Brisk, symmetric |

CFS, Chronic fatigue syndrome; CMI, Chiari malformation I; FMS, fibromyalgia.

*References 10,13,15-17,32,40.

**TABLE 85.2**

**Symptoms of Chiari Malformation**

| Reference Number | Arm/Leg Weakness (%) | Numbness (%) | Pain (%) | Gait Disturbance (%) | Cranial Nerve Involvement (%) | Headache (%) |
|---|---|---|---|---|---|---|
| 1 | 43 (arms) 23 (legs) | 60 | 60 | 40 | 10 | 60 |
| 2 | 30 | 50 | 11 | 15 | 15 | 10 |
| 3 | — 57 | 74 — | — — | 62 57 | 74 66 | 88* —† |
| 4 | 33 (arms) 43 (legs) | 50 | 65‡ | 43 | 31 | 65 |
| 5 | 80 (arms) | 30 (62§) | 54‖ | 24 | 28 | 24 |
| 6 | 56 | 52 | 69¶ | 40 | 37 | 34 |

*, Chiari malformation I.
†, Chiari malformation II.
‡, Cervical.
§, Sensory.
‖, Central.
¶, Regional.

undergo a careful history and thorough neurologic examination. "Hard" neurologic findings such as nystagmus, external ophthalmoplegia, absent "gag" reflex, reproducible sensory abnormalities, lower extremity brisk reflexes and upper extremity hyporeflexia, quantifiable weakness, muscle atrophy, fasciculations, and Babinski and Hoffmann signs are noted. An MRI of the brain and the spinal cord is performed, along with cine flow studies to delineate the extent of physiologic and anatomic abnormalities. The patients are then referred to a rheumatologist. A careful history with emphasis on psychosocial factors and current levels of stress is now obtained. The cardinal symptoms of chronic fatigue and FMS are sought, and an extensive sleep history is obtained. A neurologic examination is performed and previous findings confirmed. New findings are noted. The rheumatologist is blinded to the previous neurologic examination and testing to prevent bias. A screening FMS Questionnaire, Beck Depression Inventory, and tender points are quantitated. With this information, an independent assessment is made by the rheumatologist considering the nature of the patient's complaints. The MRI findings are reviewed, and a final assessment is made.

It is usually possible to assign patients into one of three different categories:

1. Patients who have clinical features of Chiari malformation as evidenced by neurologic findings that are consistent with disruption of central pathways involving the cerebrospinal, cerebellospinal or sensory spinothalamic pathways. Corroborative findings include cerebellar tonsillar herniation, syringomyelia, and obstruction to CSF flow at these levels. Such patients are the best candidates for corrective surgery.
2. Patients who have features of FMS and CFS. These patients have sleep disturbances, psychosocial stressors, active tender points (greater than 11), and elevated FIQ-DI and BDI scores. No neurologic findings are demonstrated, although many subjective symptoms are present. They may or may not have a Chiari malformation/syringomyelia (herniation less than or equal to 8mm), which is usually mild in degree. Most importantly, there is no obstruction to spinal flow on cine flow studies. These patients will not benefit from surgery.
3. A "mixed" pattern, where (1) and (2) coexist. These patients represent a unique challenge, since there may be features of FMS in the setting of an anatomic and physiologic Chiari malformation. While a minority of these patients may actually benefit from surgery, conservative management is recommended for most. Frequently, the authors obtain a neurology consult and objectively confirm the symptoms and physical findings by electrophysiologic studies. These patients are closely followed, and progression of their neurologic findings triggers a repeat evaluation. Most importantly, these patients are educated about the nature of FMS and associated disrupted sleep and dysthymia. They are aggressively treated with appropriate medications and a graded aerobic exercise program.

The factors that favor the diagnosis of FMS are premorbid history, diffuse pain, sleep disturbances, dysthymic mood, stressors, "soft" neurologic signs, hyperreflexia in all four extremities, patchy nondermatomal sensory findings, and postural hypotension. On the other hand, the diagnosis of CMI is more likely if any of the following are present: no premorbid history, localized pain, ataxia, cerebellar symptoms, "hard" neurologic signs such as upper limb hyporeflexia, lower limb hyperreflexia, Babinski's or Hoffman's signs, atrophy, wasting, or cerebellar signs. However, the "gold" standard of evaluation remains an appropriate history and physical examination, confirmed by neuroradiologic testing. This approach often requires collaboration among interested neurosurgeons, rheumatologists, and neurologists.

# REFERENCES

1. Arnett B, Huckmann MS, Moore CM: Comparison of presenting symptoms and neurologic signs in incidental tonsillar ectopia, abstracted. *Neurology* 58(7):A116, 2002.
2. Arnold LM, Hess EV, Hudson JI, *et al*: A randomized, placebo-controlled, double-blind, flexible-dose study of fluoxetine in the treatment of women with fibromyalgia. *Am J Med* 112(3):191-197, 2002.
3. Arnold LM, Keck PE, Jr., Welge JA: Antidepressant treatment of fibromyalgia: a meta-analysis and review. *Psychosomatics* 41(2):104-113, 2000.
4. Ball W, Crone K: Chiari I malformation: from Dr. Chiari to MR imaging. *Radiology* 195:602-604, 1995.
5. Banerji NK, Millar JHD: Chiari malformation presenting in adult life. *Brain* 97:157-168, 1974.
6. Biasi G, Manca S, Manganelli S, Marcolongo R: Tramadol in the fibromyalgia syndrome: a controlled clinical trial versus placebo. *Intl J Clin Pharmacol Res* 18(1):13-19, 1998.
7. Burton TM: High hopes. Surgery on the skull for chronic fatigue? Doctors are trying it. This and related syndrome lead to operation some praise but others decry. Bit more room for the brain. *The Wall Street Journal*, November 11, 1999:A8.
8. Caruso I, Sarzi Puttini P, Cazzola M, Azzolini V: Double-blind study of 5-hydroxytryptophan versus placebo in the treatment of primary fibromyalgia syndrome. *J Int Med Res* 18(3):201-209, 1990.
9. Clark S, Tindall E, Bennett RM: A double blind crossover trial of prednisone versus placebo in the treatment of fibrositis. *J Rheumatol* 12(5):980-983, 1985.
10. Clauw DJ, Bennett RM, Petzke F, Rosner MJ: Prevalence of Chiari malformation and cervical stenosis in fibromyalgia, abstracted. *Arthritis Rheum* 43(suppl):173, 2000.
11. Cleare AJ, Heap E, Malhi GS, *et al*: Low-dose hydrocortisone in chronic fatigue syndrome: a randomised crossover trial. *Lancet* 353(9151):455-458, 1996.
12. Croft P, Schollum J, Silman A: Population study of tender point counts and pain as evidence of fibromyalgia. *BMJ* 309:696-699, 1994.
13. Curnes JT, Oakes WJ, Boyko OB: MR imaging of hindbrain deformity in Chiari II patients with and without symptoms of brainstem compression. *Am J Neuroradiol* 10:293-302, 1989.

14. Drewes AM, Andreasen A, Jennum P, Nielsen KD: Zopiclone in the treatment of sleep abnormalities in fibromyalgia. *Scand J Rheumatol* 20(4):288-293, 1991.

15. Dyste GN, Menezes AH, Van Gilder JC: Symptomatic Chiari malformations: an analysis of presentation, management, and long-term outcome. *J Neurosurg* 71: 159-168, 1989.

16. Eisenstat DDR, Bernstein M, Fleming JFR, *et al:* Chiari malformation in adults: a review of 40 cases. *Can J Neurol Sci* 13:221-228, 1986.

17. Elster AD, Chen MYM: Chiari I malformations: clinical and radiological reappraisal. *Radiology* 183:347-353, 1992.

18. Fulcher KY, White PD: Randomised controlled trial of graded exercise in patients with the chronic fatigue syndrome. *BMJ* 314(7095):1647-1652, 1997.

19. Gardner W: The cause of syringomyelia and its surgical treatment. *Cleve Clin Quart* 25: 4-8, 1958.

20. Giesecke T, Williams DA, Harris RE, *et al:* Subgrouping of fibromyalgia patients on the basis of pressure-pain thresholds and psychological factors. *Arthritis Rheum* 48:2916-2922, 2003.

21. Gladman DD, Orowitz MB, Gough J, *et al:* Fibromyalgia is a major contributor to quality of life in lupus. *J Rheumatol* 24:2145-2148, 1997.

22. Goldenberg D, Mayskiy M, Mossey C, *et al:* A randomized, double-blind crossover trial of fluoxetine and amitriptyline in the treatment of fibromyalgia. *Arthritis Rheum* 39: 1852-1859, 1996.

23. Goossens ME, Rutten-van Molken MP, Leidl RM, *et al:* Cognitive-educational treatment of fibromyalgia: a randomized clinical trial. II. Economic evaluation. *J Rheumatol* 23(7):1246-1254, 1996.

24. Hadler NM: The dangers of the diagnostic process: iatrogenic labeling as in the fibrositis paralogism. In Hadler NM (ed): *Occupational Musculoskeletal Disorders.* New York, Raven Press, 1993, pp 16-33.

25. Hannonen P, Malminiemi K, Yli-Kerttula U, *et al:* A randomized, double-blind, placebo-controlled study of moclobemide and amitriptyline in the treatment of fibromyalgia in females without psychiatric disorder. *Br J Rheumatol* 37(12):1279-1286, 1998.

26. Hariri AR, Mattay VS, Tessitore A, *et al:* Serotonin transporter genetic variation and the response of the human amygdala. *Science* 297(5580):400-403, 2002.

27. Harkness EF, Macfarlane GJ, Nahit ES, *et al:* Effects of psychosocial and individual psychological factors on the onset of musculoskeletal pain: common and site-specific effects. *Ann Rheum Dis* 62(8):755-760, 2003.

28. Haus U, Varga B, Stratz T, *et al:* Related articles, links oral treatment of fibromyalgia with tropisetron given over 28 days: influence on functional and vegetative symptoms, psychometric parameters and pain. *Scand J Rheumatol Suppl* 113:55-58, 2000.

29. Jacobsen S, Danneskiold-Samsoe B, Andersen RB: Oral S-adenosylmethionine in primary fibromyalgia. Double-blind clinical evaluation. *Scand J Rheumatol* 20(4):294-302, 1991.

30. Jones KD, Burckhardt CS, Clark SR, *et al:* A randomized controlled trial of muscle strengthening versus flexibility training in fibromyalgia. *J Rheumatol* 29(5):1041-1048, 2002.

31. Komaroff AL, Buchwald DS: Chronic fatigue syndrome: an update. *Ann Rev Med* 49:1-13, 1998.

32. Levy WJ, Mason L, Hahn JF: Chiari malformation presenting in adults: a surgical experience in 127 patients. *Neurosurgery* 12:377-380, 1983.

33. Marlin RG, Anchel H, Gibson JC, *et al:* An evaluation of multidisciplinary intervention for chronic fatigue syndrome with long-term follow-up, and a comparison with untreated controls. *Am J Med* 105(3A):110S-114S, 1998.

34. Martinez JE, Ferraz MB, Sato EI, *et al:* Fibromyalgia versus rheumatoid arthritis: a longitudinal comparison of the quality of life. *J Rheumatol* 22(2):270-274, 1995.

35. Milhorat T, Chou M, Trinidad E, *et al:* Chiari I malformation redefined: clinical and radiological findings. *Neurosurgery* 44:1005-1017, 1999.

36. Moldofsky H, Lue FA, Mously C, *et al:* The effect of zolpidem in patients with fibromyalgia: a dose-ranging, double-blind, placebo-controlled, modified crossover study. *J Rheumatol* 23(3):529-533, 1996.

37. Norregaard J, Volkmann H, Danneskiold-Samsoe B: A randomized controlled trial of citalopram in the treatment of fibromyalgia. *Pain* 61(3):445-449, 1995.

38. Offenbaecher M, Bondy B, de Jonge S, *et al:* Possible association of fibromyalgia with a polymorphism in the serotonin transporter gene regulatory region. *Arthritis Rheum* 42(11):2482-2488, 1999.

39. O'Malley PG, Balden E, Tomkins G, *et al:* Treatment of fibromyalgia with antidepressants: a meta-analysis. *J Gen Intern Med* 15(9):659-666, 2000.

40. Paul KS, Lye RH, Strang FA, Dutton J: Arnold-Chiari malformation: review of 71 cases. *J Neurosurg* 58:183-187, 1983.

41. Prins JB, Bleijenberg G, Bazelmans E, *et al:* Cognitive behaviour therapy for chronic fatigue syndrome: a multicentre randomised controlled trial. *Lancet* 357(9259):841-847, 2001.

42. Quijada-Carrera J, Valenzuela-Castano A, Povedano-Gomez J, *et al:* Comparison of tenoxicam and bromazepan in the treatment of fibromyalgia: a randomized, double-blind, placebo-controlled trial. *Pain* 65(2,3):221-225, 1996.

43. Rooks DS, Silverman CB, Kantrowitz FG: The effects of progressive strength training and aerobic exercise on muscle strength and cardiovascular fitness in women with fibromyalgia: a pilot study. *Arthritis Rheum* 47(1):22-28, 2002.

44. Rossy LA, Buckelew SP, Dorr N, *et al:* A meta-analysis of fibromyalgia treatment interventions. *Ann Behav Med* 21(2):180-191, 1999.

45. Russell IJ, Fletcher EM, Michalek JE, *et al:* Treatment of primary fibrositis/fibromyalgia syndrome with ibuprofen and alprazolam: a double-blind, placebo-controlled study. *Arthritis Rheum* 34(5):552-560, 1991.

46. Schluederberg A, Strauss SE, Peterson P, *et al:* Chronic fatigue syndrome research. Definition and medical outcome assessment. *Ann Intern Med* 117:325-331, 1992.

47. Schochat T, Raspe H: Elements of fibromyalgia in an open population. *J Rheum* 42:829-835, 2003.

48. Sim J, Adams N: Systematic review of randomized controlled trials of nonpharmacological interventions for fibromyalgia. *Clin J Pain* 18(5):324-336, 2002.

49. Spinos E, Laster DW, Moody DM, *et al:* Magnetic resonance imaging of the Chiari I malformation at 0.15 T. *Am J Neuroradiol* 6:203-208, 1985.

50. Weisberg L, Shraberg D, Meriwether RP, *et al:* Computerized tomography findings in the Arnold-Chiari type I malformation. *CT* 5:1-9, 1981.

51. White KP, Speechley M, Harth M, *et al:* The London Fibromyalgia Epidemiology Study: the prevalence of fibromyalgia syndrome in London, Ontario. *J Rheumatol* 26:1570-1576, 1999.

52. Wilke WS: Can fibromyalgia and chronic fatigue syndrome be cured by surgery? *Cleve Clin J Med* 68(4):277-279, 2001.

53. Wilke WS: The clinical utility of fibromyalgia. *J Clin Rheumatol* 5:97-102, 1999.

54. Wolfe F, Anderson J, Harkness D, *et al:* A prospective, longitudinal, multicenter study of service utilization and costs in fibromyalgia. *Arthritis Rheum* 40(9):1560-1570, 1997.

55. Wolfe F, Cathey MA, Hawley DJ: A double-blind placebo-controlled trial of fluoxetine in fibromyalgia. *Scand J Rheumatol* 23(5):255-259, 1994.

56. Wolfe F, Cathey MA, Kleinheksel SM, *et al:* Psychological status in primary fibrositis and fibrositis associated with rheumatoid arthritis. *J Rheumatol* 11:500-506, 1984.

57. Wolfe F, Cathey MA, Kleinheksel SM: Fibrositis (fibromyalgia) in rheumatoid arthritis. *J Rheumatol* 11: 814-818, 1984.

58. Wolfe F, Ross K, Anderson J, *et al:* The prevalence and characteristics of fibromyalgia in the general population. *Arthritis Rheum* 38:19-28, 1995.

59. Wolfe F, Symythe HA, Yunus MB, *et al:* The American College of Rheumatology 1990 criteria for the classification of fibromyalgia. Report of the Multicenter committee. *Arthritis Rheum* 33:160-172, 1990.

60. Wolfe F, Zhao S, Lane N: Preference for nonsteroidal antiinflammatory drugs over acetaminophen by rheumatic disease patients: a survey of 1,799 patients with osteoarthritis, rheumatoid arthritis, and fibromyalgia. *Arthritis Rheum* 43(2):378-385, 2000.

61. Wolfe F: Fibromyalgia: the clinical syndrome. *Rheum Dis Clin North Am* 15:1-18, 1989.

62. Wolfe F: The relationship between tender points and fibromyalgia symptom variables: evidence that fibromyalgia is not a discrete disorder in the clinic. *Ann Rheum Dis* 56:268-271, 1997.

63. Yunus M, Masi AT, Calabro JJ, *et al:* Primary fibromyalgia (fibrositis): clinical study of 50 patients with matched normal controls. *Semin Arthritis Rheum* 11(1):151-171, 1981.

# 3.9 ADJUNCTIVE MANAGEMENT DILEMMAS AND COMPLEX SURGICAL PROBLEMS

# CHAPTER 86

# Evaluation of the Cervical Spine after Trauma

Mark D. D'Alise, Edward C. Benzel,
Blaine I. Hart, and Arnold B. Vardiman

The absence of injury to the cervical spine after trauma is both difficult and imperative to define. Methodology for such, however, has been disputed. An algorithm for the "clearing of the cervical spine" for several clinical circumstances is presented here. It is emphasized that the schemes presented here are only a few of the many rational approaches to the clearance of the posttraumatic cervical spine.

The American College of Surgeons Committee on Trauma[1] published recommendations for the initial cervical spine radiographic evaluation in trauma victims. The committee included anteroposterior, lateral, and odontoid views of the cervical spine in this evaluation. Optimally, the lateral view images the rostral aspect of the first thoracic vertebra.

Often, conventional lateral radiographs are not sufficient, and a "swimmer's" view may be necessary (Figure 86.1). Despite aggressive attempts at radiographic clearance, failure of diagnosis may occur. McDonald et al.[15] and Chakeres et al.[5] independently demonstrated that a three-view series (including a lateral view of the rostral aspect of T1) misses approximately 3% of traumatic cervical spine lesions.[5,14]

After the recommended radiographic series is obtained, the next step is situation dependent. Thus, several algorithms are presented as alternatives to traditional management options.

## Radiographic Injury or Neurologic Deficit

Perhaps the least controversial clinical scenario is that of the patient with an obvious radiographic injury or localizing neurologic deficit. Radiographic evidence of fracture and extent of neural compression should be pursued further via magnetic resonance imaging (MRI) or myelogram-computed tomography (CT). The number and location of the injured spinal levels and extent of soft-tissue injury may be determined (Figure 86.2). These vital observations are the basis for the formulation of a sound

management plan. The author's[6] preference is to begin with an MRI evaluation, including sagittal $T_2$-weighted images with axial cuts targeted to the areas of concern, as identified by MRI. The target areas should include those that were identified by radiographs and levels adjacent to soft-tissue injuries demonstrated by the sagittal MRI (Figure 86.3).

Computed tomography provides the best view of the spine axially[3,16] and is the best test for visualizing bony anatomic detail.[16] Concomitant administration of intrathecal water-soluble contrast medium may be a useful adjunct to CT to evaluate the extent of neural compression from bone fragments. Sagittal or coronal reconstruction of the axial CT scan, in some cases, adds useful information to MRI and the targeted axial CT cuts, especially in assessing the facets and neural foramina. Kyphotic deformity and degree of vertebral body compression can be adequately assessed with plain radiographs.

Spinal canal compromise is best assessed by a combination of sagittal and axial views. Sagittal and parasagittal reconstructions, in particular, are helpful in understanding the anatomy of the pedicle at all levels and the location of the vertebral arteries in the cervical spine.

## Inadequate Initial Radiographs

A patient with inadequate radiographs and no localizing neurologic deficit who complains of neck pain or who is found to have tenderness on palpitation represents a complex clinical problem. Often, the initial radiographic survey is suboptimal because of body habitus, inadequate caudal visualization, or a concurrent therapy, such as an endotracheal or nasogastric tube (Figure 86.4; see Figure 86.3).[18]

Limited MRI (sagittal $T_1$- and $T_2$-weighted images) are used as the subsequent imaging study. This enables full visualization of the cervical spine for alignment, as well as for identification of soft-tissue injury.[2,4-6,10,12,14] The areas of abnormality on the screening MRI can be further imaged with a targeted CT scan.

Many centers use the CT as the first subsequent study. Because the best CT images are axially oriented, nearly all fractures can be identified. Many malalignments and subluxations, however, are missed by relying on axial cuts.[3,17]

Although flexion-extension lateral radiographs are considered the standard for identifying ligamentous instability, their role should be considered carefully. Perhaps their greatest utility is for the determination of the clinical significance of ligamentous disruption in the awake patient several days after the injury. Paraspinous muscle spasm and patient guarding are known factors that may lead to a false-negative interpretation.[11,13,16] In addition, when evaluating the cervical spine in flexion and extension, one must visualize T1 on both views. An inability to visualize to the rostral aspect of T1 should be considered inadequate. Dynamic studies in comatose, obtunded, or pharmacologically sedated

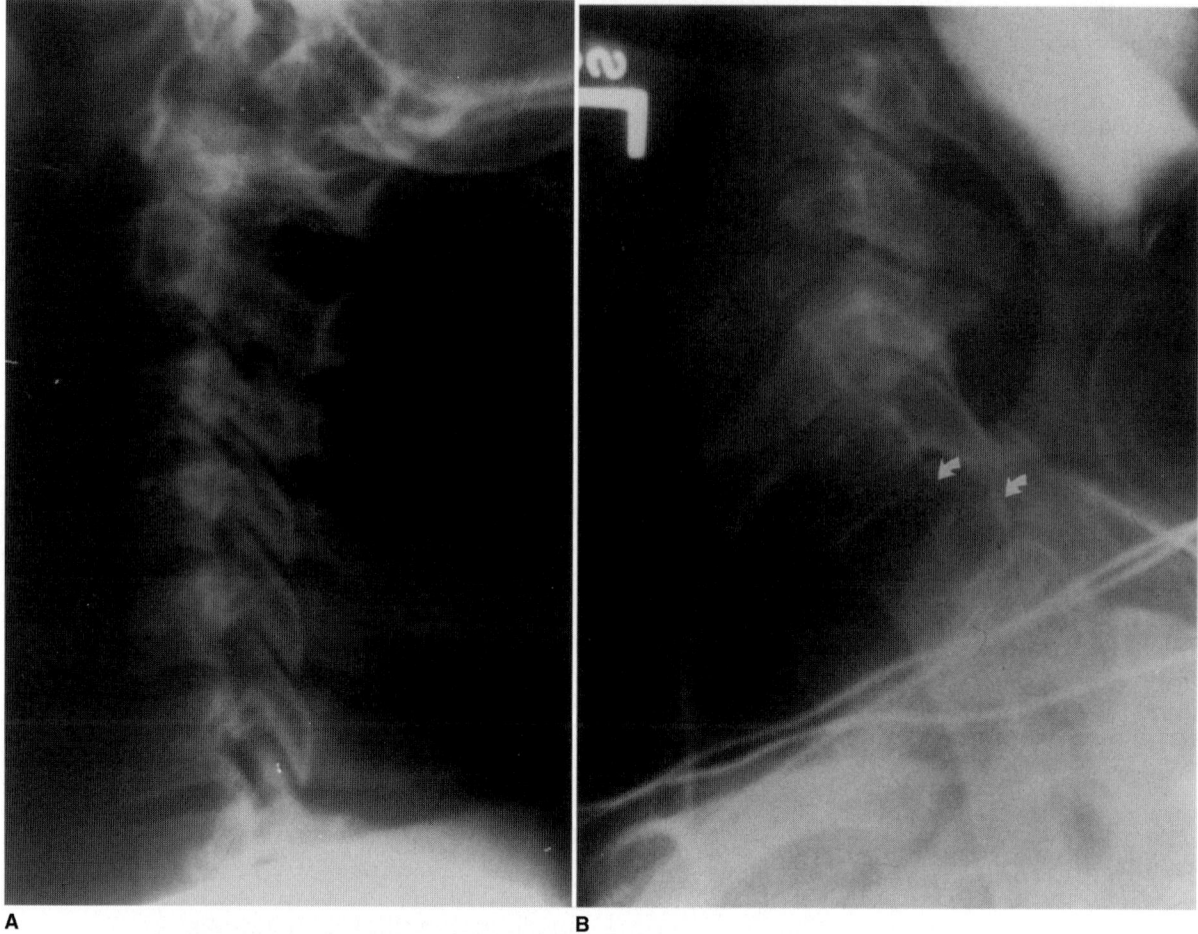

**Figure 86.1** (**A**) Initial lateral radiograph with inadequate caudal visualization. (**B**) "Swimmer's view" demonstrating distraction/subluxation injury at C7-T1 level (*white arrows*).

or paralyzed patients should be performed only with extreme caution, because the patients' intrinsic guarding mechanisms are not intact.

## Obtunded and Comatose Patients

Obtunded and comatose patients should be treated as though they have a cervical spine injury (even with a normal three-view series) until their soft tissues can be studied adequately. Many methods have been used to address this problem.[2,4-6,8,17] A common method is to simply take spinal precautions until either the patients are medically stabilized or their neurologic condition improves to a level that allows an adequate examination for pain, neurologic deficit, or radiographic abnormality. This philosophy may hinder the delivery of pulmonary care because of concerns about positioning. It may lead to preventable skin infections and pressure sores from prolonged rigid collar immobilization. Therefore, early identification of patients without bony or soft-tissue cervical spine injuries is extremely important so that unnecessary and potentially harmful precautions can be discontinued.

A series of 121 comatose or obtunded trauma patients with no obvious radiographic injury who were evaluated by limited MRI within 48 hours of admission were found to have a 26% incidence of significant soft-tissue injury that warranted further treatment. The remaining 74% of this patient population were cleared by MRI, thus facilitating nursing care and the delivery of other medical therapies.[6] The limited (sagittal $T_1$- and $T_2$-weighted) MRI is associated with an acquisition time of about 10 minutes. $T_1$-weighted images are valuable for demonstrating anatomic detail, and $T_2$-weighted images are most sensitive for soft-tissue injury. For the latter, fat suppression is also very helpful. This can be accomplished with an inversion recovery sequence or with a fast spin-echo sequence using chemical fat saturation; either sequence takes only a few minutes. Complications related to ventilator management or other complex therapies, such as central venous lines or intracranial pressure monitor devices, are minimal with modern techniques.

Some surgeons use flexion-extension radiography or fluoroscopy to evaluate these patients. As mentioned, it is important to consider the hazards of these techniques carefully in comatose patients. These procedures should

(Continued on p. 1200)

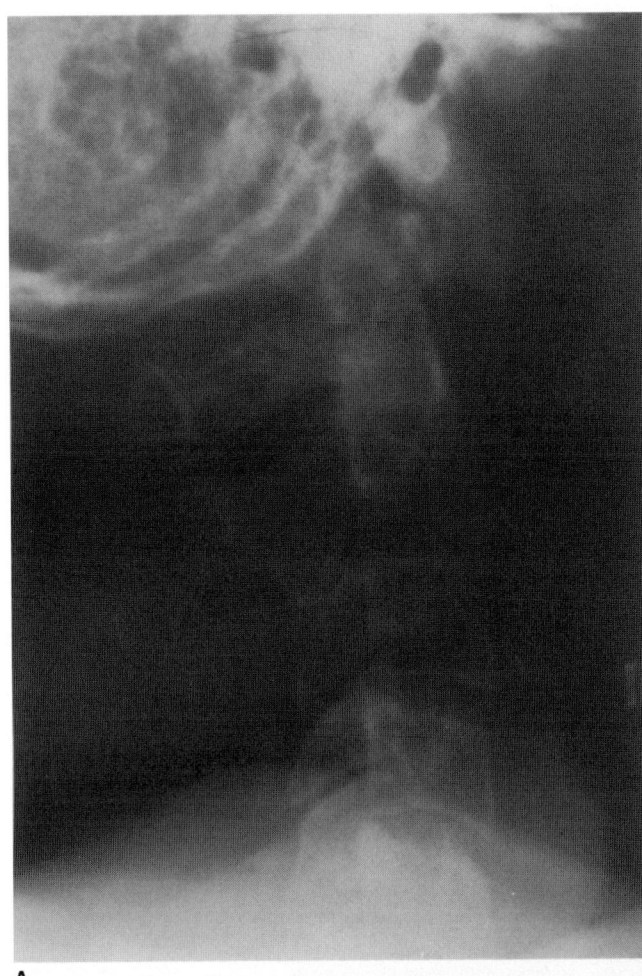

A

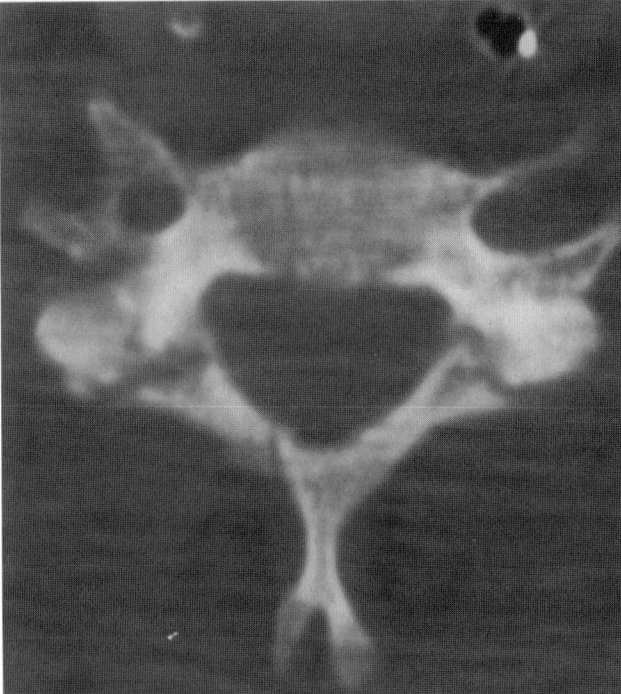

C

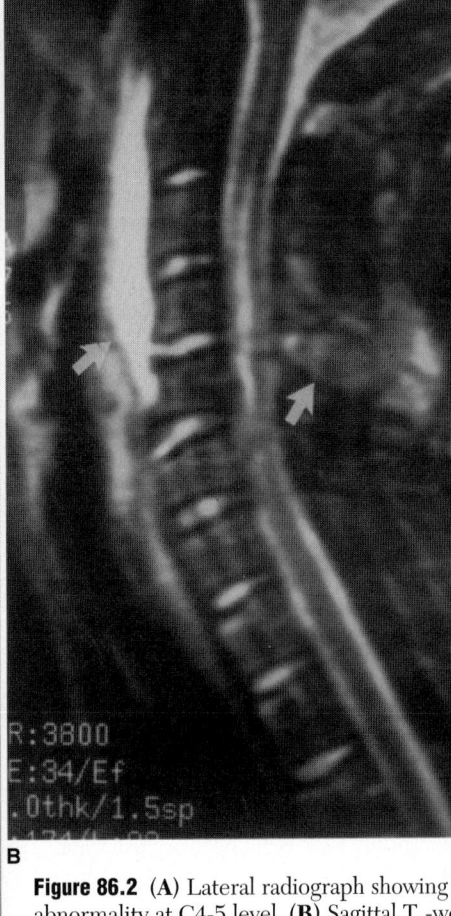

B

**Figure 86.2** (**A**) Lateral radiograph showing minor alignment abnormality at C4-5 level. (**B**) Sagittal T$_2$-weighted MRI scan demonstrating injury to the anterior longitudinal ligament and interspinous ligament *(white arrows)*. (**C**) Targeted axial CT scan showing bilateral laminar fractures with extension into the lateral masses at the level of the interspinous ligament injury.

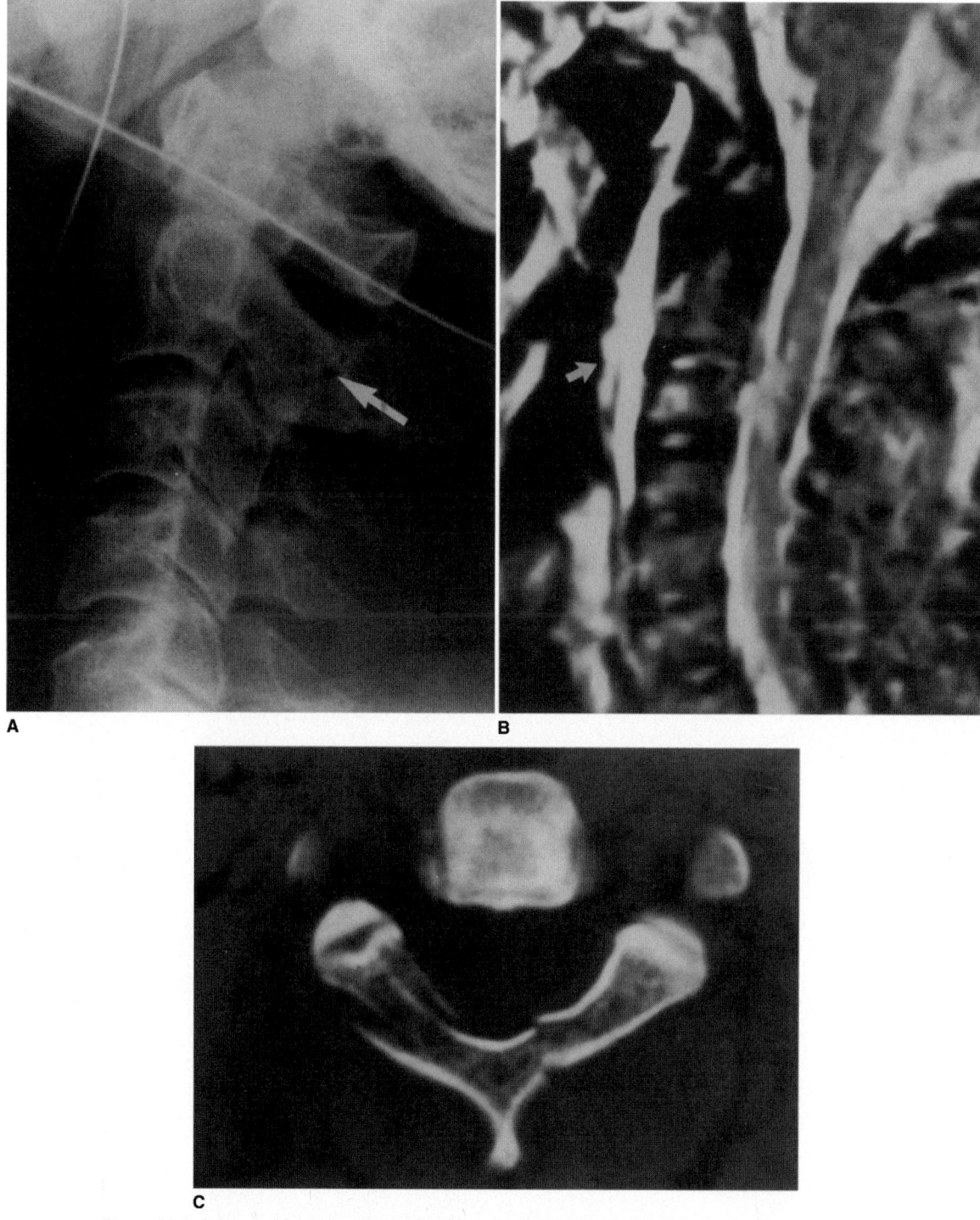

**Figure 86.3** (**A**) Initial lateral radiograph in an awake patient complaining of neck pain after a motor vehicle accident. A subtle radiographic sign of fracture was not noted on initial emergency room reading *(white arrow)*. (**B**) Sagittal $T_2$-weighted MRI scan demonstrated signal abnormality in ventral upper cervical spine, consistent with injury to anterior longitudinal ligament. (**C**) Targeted axial CT scan showing left laminar fracture of C2.

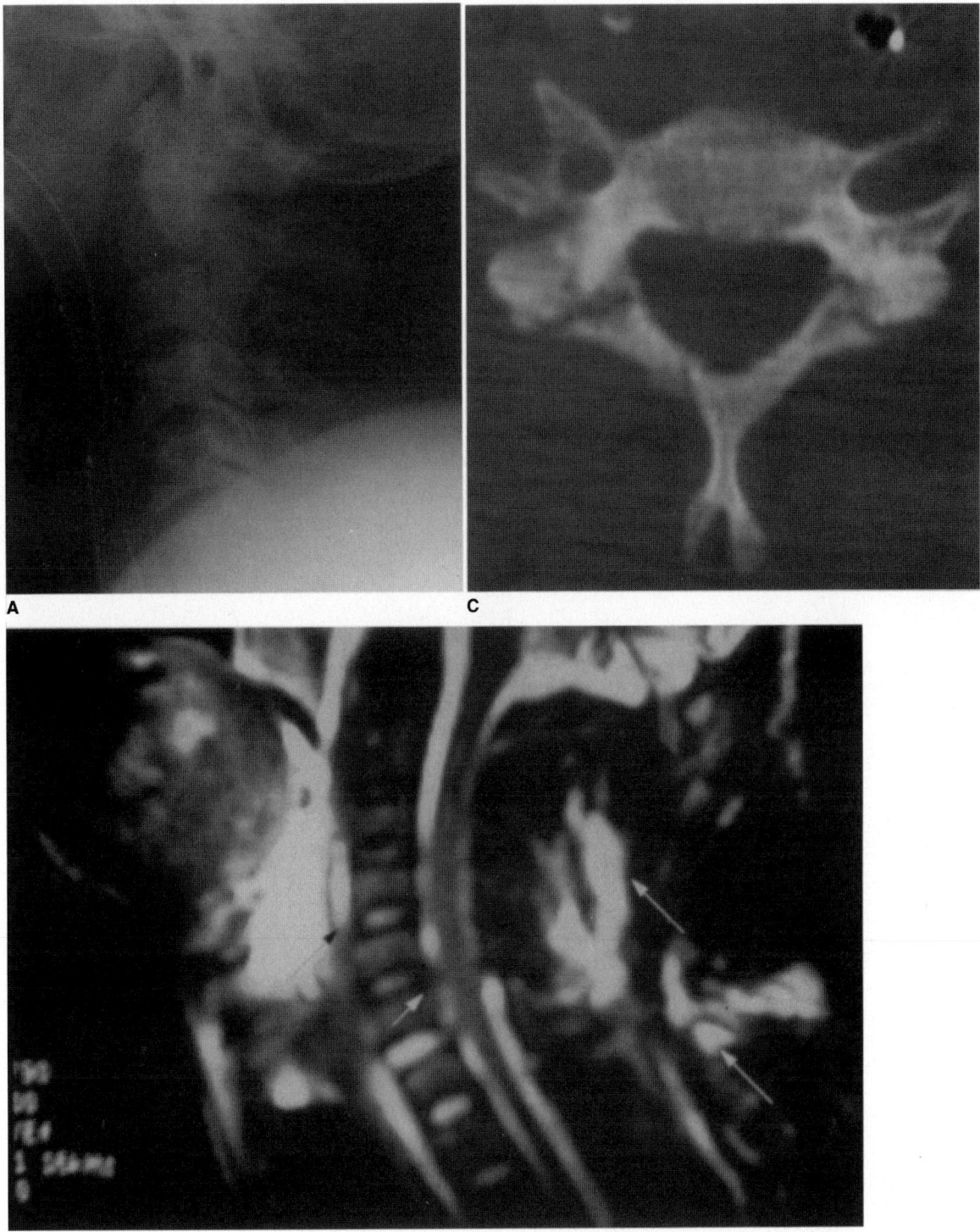

**Figure 86.4** (**A**) Initial lateral radiograph with inadequate caudal visualization (multiple attempts). (**B**) Sagittal T₂-weighted MRI scan demonstrating injury to the posterior ligamentous complex *(long arrows)*, the prevertebral region *(short black arrow)*, and the posterior longitudinal ligament *(short white arrow)*. Alignment is normal in the lower cervical levels. (**C**) Targeted CT scan demonstrating fracture of both facet joints and the lamina of C5.

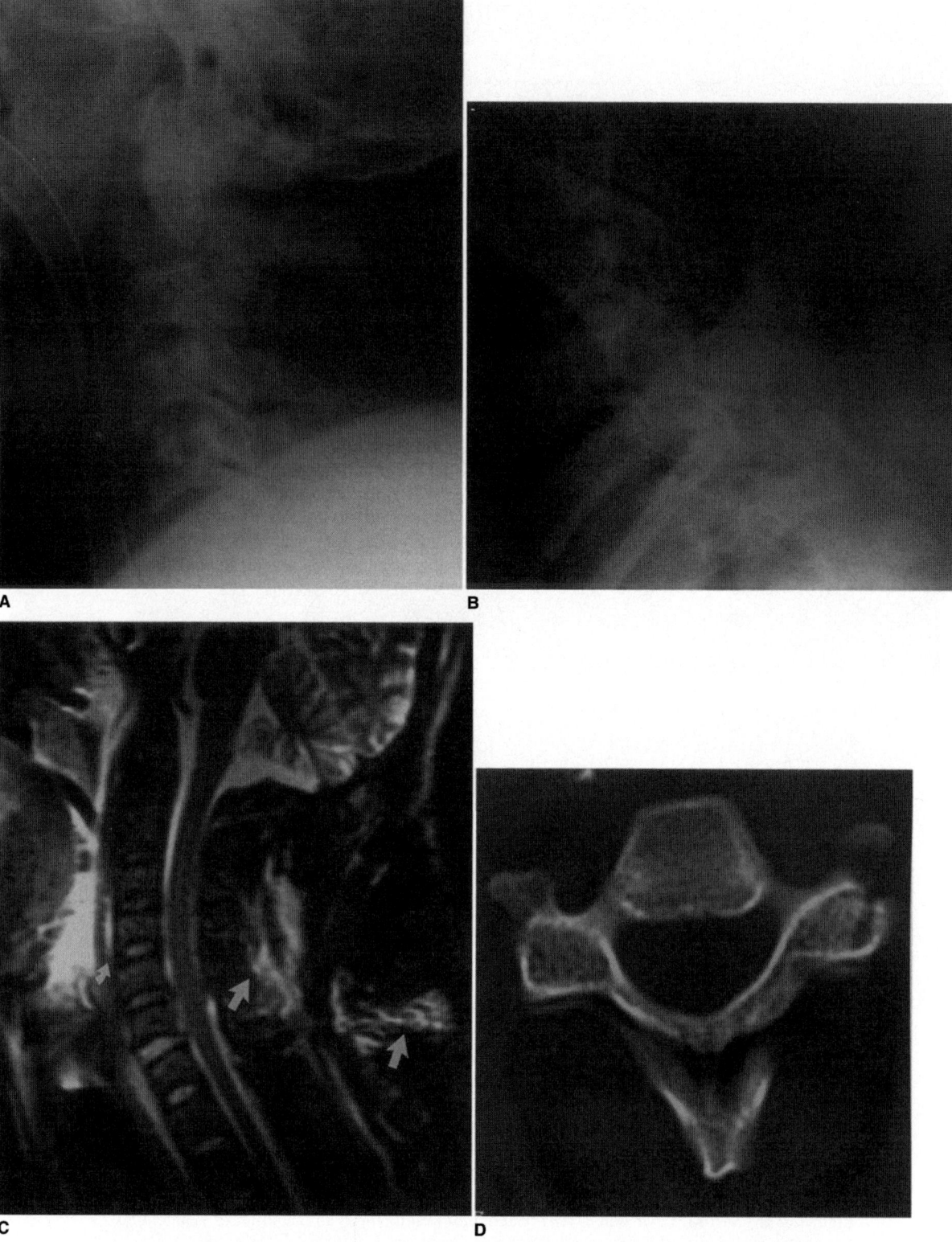

**Figure 86.5** (A) Lateral radiograph with (B) swimmer's view of a comatose trauma patient. There is no obvious radiographic injury. (C) Sagittal $T_2$-weighted MRI scan showing injury of the anterior longitudinal ligament, interspinous ligament, and supraspinous ligament (*white arrows*). (D) Targeted axial CT scan demonstrating fracture of the left lateral mass of C5.

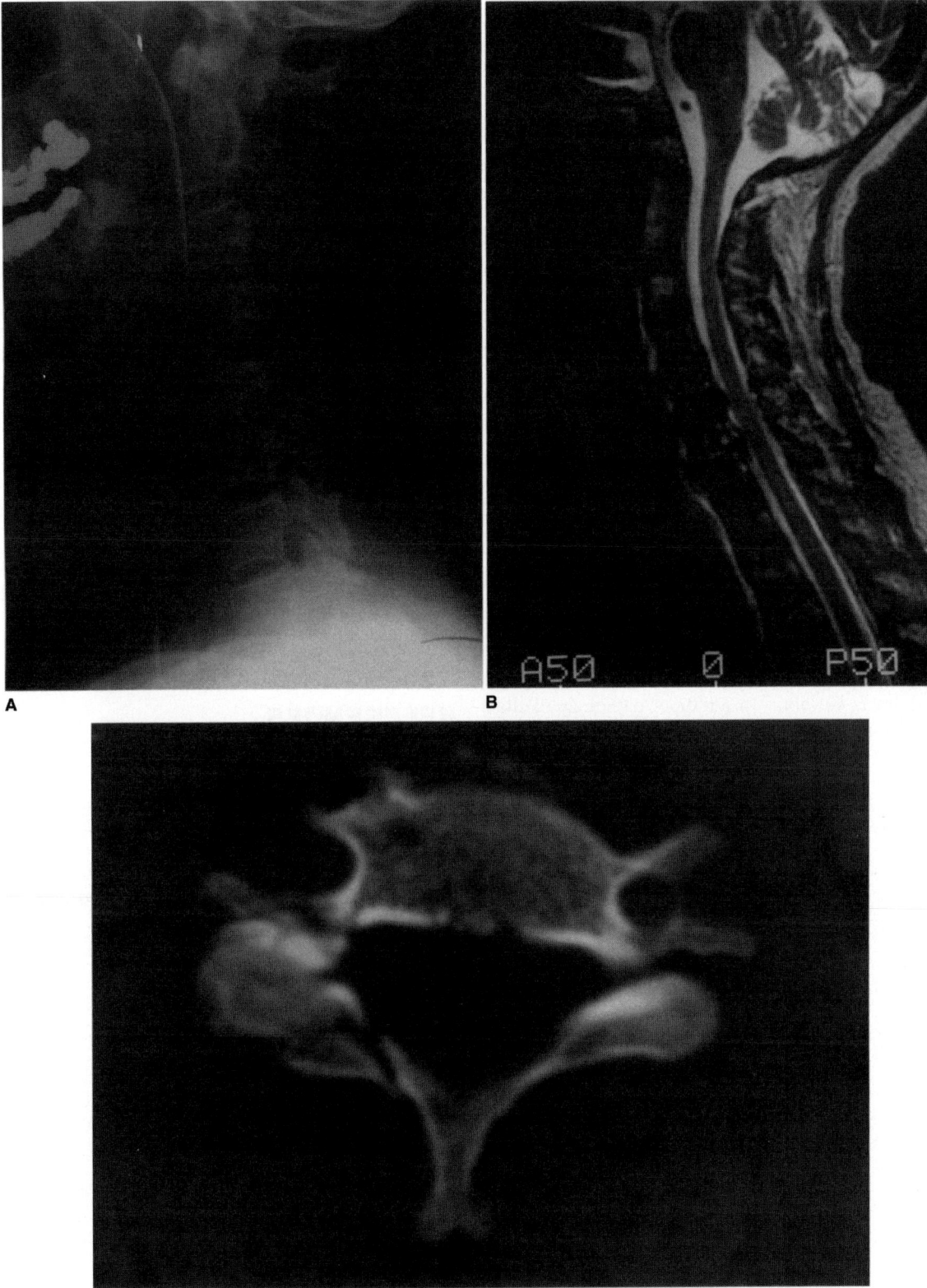

A

B

C

**Figure 86.6** (**A**) Lateral radiograph of a trauma patient, intubated for severe multisystem injuries. Straightening is probably caused by the rigid cervical collar. (**B**) Sagittal $T_2$-weighted MRI scan showing disk interspace injury at C6-7 level. (**C**) Targeted axial CT scan demonstrating associated right lamina and lateral mass fracture of C6.

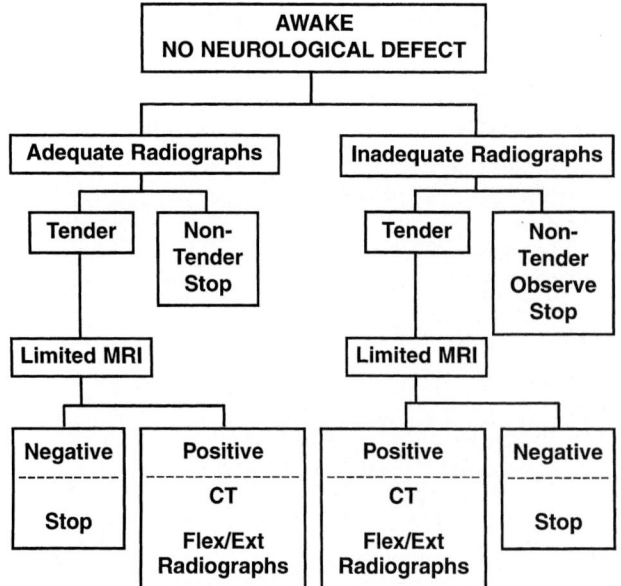

**Figure 86.7** Clearance algorithm for awake trauma patients.

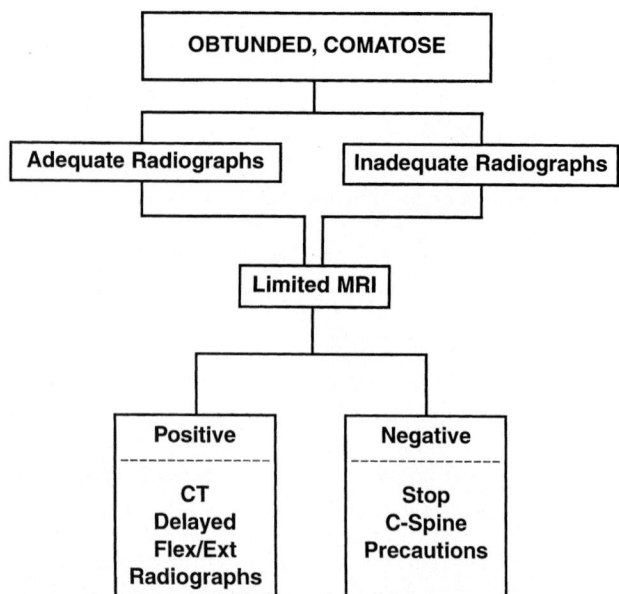

**Figure 86.8** Clearance algorithm for comatose or obtunded trauma patients.

always be performed with physician guidance and with manual axial traction to prevent subluxation of the unstable cervical spine. The false-negative rate may be high because of guarding and inadequate visualization of bony structures. This is especially true for the rostral aspect of the first thoracic vertebra. In addition, pathology of the disk interspace may be completely missed by static and dynamic radiography in the comatose, obtunded, or intubated multisystem trauma patient. In fact, worsening of a disk herniation with flexion and extension could cause spinal cord compression in the previously uncompromised spinal canal.

For these reasons, an algorithm that includes early limited MRI as a screening test for soft-tissue injury of the supporting ligaments and disk interspaces in comatose and obtunded patients is a rational alternative to dynamic radiography.[4,6,8] Dynamic radiography may then be reserved for subsequent use at follow-up to determine the stability of known injuries (Figures 86.5 and 86.6).

Any of several algorithms may be appropriate. The availability of MRI (or CT) obviously dictates, in part, the algorithm chosen. Physician philosophy and local expertise impact this as well.

## Summary

Occult cervical spine injury can have devastating sequelae if undetected. Physicians treating traumatized patients must maintain a high level of suspicion when attempting to clear the cervical spine. It cannot be overstated that the *completeness* of imaging studies is mandatory. The odontoid process and the rostral aspect of T1 must be included in each evaluation. Patients with equivocal neurologic examinations must undergo some form of soft-tissue imaging evaluation. The author's algorithms for radiographic clearance are presented in Figures 86.7 and 86.8. These reflect this philosophy but honor the mandate of visualiz-

ing the entire cervical spine and radiographically evaluating soft-tissue structures in patients with unreliable clinical examinations.

## REFERENCES

1. Alexander RH, Proctor HJ: ATLS: course for physicians, student manual, ed 5.
2. Beers GJ, Raque GH, Wagner GG, *et al:* MR imaging in acute cervical spine trauma. *J Comp Asst Tomogr* 12: 755-761, 1988.
3. Benzel EC: *Biomechanics of Spine Stabilization: Principles and Clinical Practice.* New York, McGraw-Hill, 1995, p 278.
4. Benzel EC, Hart BL, Ball PA, *et al:* Magnetic resonance imaging for the evaluation of patients with occult cervical spine injury. *J Neurosurg* 85:824-829, 1996.
5. Chakeres DW, Flickinger F, Bresnahan JC, *et al:* MR imaging of acute spinal cord trauma. *Am J Neuroradiol* 8:5-10, 1987.
6. D'Alise MD, Benzel EC, Hart BL: Identification of occult cervical spine injuries in obtunded trauma victims using early limited MRI in progress, abstracted. Presented at the 46th annual meeting of the Congress of Neurological Surgeons, Montreal, October 1996.
7. Davis JW, Phreaner DL, Hoyt DB, Mackensie RC: The etiology of missed cervical spine injuries. *J Trauma* 34: 342-346, 1993.
8. Davis JW, Parks SN, Detlefs CL, *et al:* Clearing the cervical spine in obtunded patients: the use of dynamic fluoroscopy. *J Trauma* 39:435-438, 1995.
9. Denis F: The three-column spine and its significance in the classification of acute thoracolumbar spine injuries. *Spine* 8:817-831, 1983.
10. Doran SE, Papadopoulos SM, Ducker TB, Lillehei KO: Magnetic resonance imaging documentation of coexistent traumatic locked facets of the cervical spine and disc herniation. *J Neurosurg* 79:341-345, 1993.

11. Fazi M, LaFebvre J, Willinsky RA, Gertzbein S: Posttraumatic ligamentous disruption of the cervical spine and easily overlooked diagnosis: presentation of three cases. *Neurosurgery* 26:674-678, 1990.

12. Hall AJ, Wagle VG, Raycroft J, *et al:* Magnetic resonance imaging in cervical spine trauma. *J Trauma* 34:21-26, 1993.

13. Hart BL, Orrison WW, Benzel EC: Imaging spinal trauma. In Lee RR (ed): *Spinal Imaging: State of the Art Reviews.* Philadelphia, Hanley & Belfus, 1995, pp 93-118.

14. McArdle CB, Crofford MJ, Mirfakhraee M, *et al:* Surface coil MR of spinal trauma: preliminary experience. *Am J Neuroradiol* 7:885-893, 1986.

15. McDonald RL, Schwartz ML, Mirich D, *et al:* Diagnosis of cervical spine injury in motor vehicle crash victims: how many x-rays are enough? *J Trauma* 30:392-397, 1990.

16. Webb JK, Broughton RBK, McSweeney T, Park WM: Hidden flexion injury of the cervical spine. *J Bone Joint Surg* 58:322-327, 1976.

17. Woodring JH, Lee C: The role and limitations of computed tomographic scanning in the evaluation of cervical trauma. *J Trauma* 33:698-708, 1992.

18. Woodring JH, Lee C: Limitations of cervical radiography in the evaluation of acute cervical trauma. *J Trauma* 34:32-39, 1993.

# CHAPTER 87

# Revascularization and Scar Prevention: Omental Transposition and Spine Surgery

**L. Brett Babat, Edward C. Benzel, and Stephen M. Papadopoulos**

Omental transposition to the brain and spinal cord is based, in part, on the omentum's unusual biochemical properties. Omentum contains high levels of neurotransmitters and lipid-soluble factors that induce growth of new blood vessels[9,24,35,47] as well as neurite outgrowth in cultured neurons.[45] After experimental spinal cord transection, omentum has been shown to enhance neurite outgrowth across a collagen bridge.[13] Blood flow experimentally provided to the brain by pedicled omentum is sufficient to prevent infarction after middle cerebral artery occlusion.* Angiographs of children with moyamoya disease who underwent omental transposition have shown vascular communications between the omental graft and the brain.[37] There are many reports of omental transposition to the brain of patients after stroke.[2,17,51,52]

## Omental Transposition for the Enhancement of Neural Function

### Background

Goldsmith[20] first proposed the concept of omental transposition to the brain and spinal cord. His work showed the development of vascular communications from omentum to neural tissue in animals in which pedicled omentum was subcutaneously tunneled from the abdomen and placed against the brain or spinal cord.[19,20] This was supported by MacMillan and Stauffer.[34] Based on the ability of the *in situ* omentum to remove inflammatory exudates and to revascularize regions of ischemia, they proposed that pedicled omental transposition could improve vascularity, aid in the removal of necrotic tissue from the spinal cord, and reduce scar formation. Using a dog laminectomy model, they transferred pedicled omentum either to dura mater or directly to the neural elements. After an unspecified period, the animals were re-anesthetized, and the pedicle was injected with latex. They noted vascular communication between the graft and spinal nerves, through the local segmental arteries. However, there was no direct communication with the spinal cord. They hypothesized that this was because they had produced no cord injury in the animals, so there was no ischemia or necrosis to stimulate omental adherence to the cord. However, they felt that local trauma to paraspinal tissues during the initial surgery was sufficient to allow the omentum to anastomose with the segmental vessels. Histologically, they found that the omentum prevented the formation of a "laminectomy membrane or epidural fibrosis." They speculated that the vascularized graft removes postoperative hematoma, thus decreasing fibroblast proliferation.

Eight clinical reports have described omental transposition after spinal cord injury (SCI) in more than 160 patients.* The basic surgical procedure was described by Goldsmith.[27] The omentum is pedicled by dividing its vascular supply so that the right gastroepiploic artery and vein provide the blood supply, and the omentum may be lengthened (Figure 87.1). Once pedicled, the graft is tunneled subcutaneously to the neck or lateral chest wall. Either a thoracic or a cervical laminectomy is performed, depending upon the level of the lesion. The graft is tunneled subcutaneously to the incision, the dura mater and arachnoid are opened, and the graft is applied to the spinal cord in the region of the injury, plus several centimeters above and below it. The graft is then sutured to the opened dura.

Although substantial recovery of function has been reported, actual details of neurologic outcome are scant. Widely performed throughout the world, omental transposition has been reported recently in 40 patients in the United States.[19] In this report, 40% of SCI patients who underwent omental transposition showed "varying degrees of neurologic involvement."[19] No systematic follow-up using anatomic, neurophysiologic, and neurologic measures was reported in these retrospective series.

### Prospective Studies

Clifton *et al.*[10] reported on two groups of SCI patients who underwent omental transposition with frequent multimodality follow-up measures to determine whether the procedure could offer benefit. A pilot series of four patients with tetraplegia underwent omental transposition. Two underwent long-term follow-up. Patients were given standard neurologic examinations developed by the National Acute Spinal Cord Injury Study (NASCIS)[8] on two different occasions before surgery, at 4, 8, 12, and 20 months after surgery, and again at 4½ years after surgery. Somatosensory evoked potentials were performed preoperatively and at 1 year postoperatively. Magnetic resonance imaging (MRI) scans of the cervical spine were performed before surgery, 1 year after surgery, and 4½ years after surgery.

A second, larger series of eleven patients underwent omental transposition with more outcome measures tested at more frequent intervals. These patients underwent detailed assessment twice at 2-month intervals before surgery and at 4-month intervals for 1 year after surgery. Baseline MRI scans through the area of injury were obtained within 1 month before surgery for four patients. Seven other patients had immediate postoperative MRI

---

*References 4,12,14,21,23,39,40.

*References 3,19,25,36,38,41,46,53.

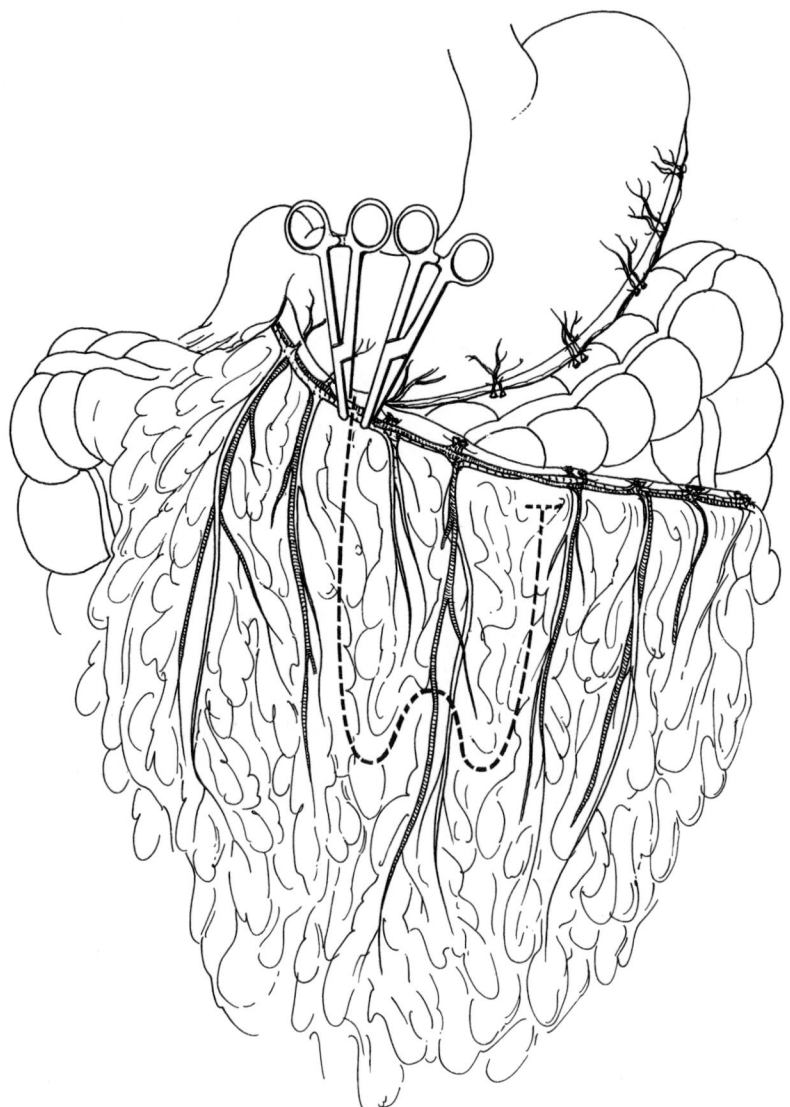

**Figure 87.1** The left gastroepiploic artery has been divided after separation from the greater curvature of the stomach. The omentum is then divided to provide length. The right gastroepiploic artery provides the blood supply to the pedicled omentum. (*Adapted from Goldsmith HS, Neil-Dwyer MS, Barsoum FFS: Omental transposition to the chronically injured human spinal cord.* Paraplegia 24:173, 1986.)

after metal fixation devices were removed at surgery. MRI, with and without contrast, was again performed at 4, 8, and 12 months after surgery. Cervical and lumbosacral somatosensory evoked potentials, motor evoked potentials, and brain motor control assessment (BMCA) for evaluation of spasticity and motor control were performed. Spasticity was assessed using BMCA of upper and lower limbs.[15,44] This technique measures electromyographic (EMG) activity in response to voluntary and passive movement. Changes in spasticity of the lower extremities were assessed by patient self-reports and by BMCA. These were then correlated. A comparable group of eight patients who met the inclusion criteria for the study but declined the operation were followed for 1 year.

In the first series, one patient had slight motor improvement for the first 12 months after injury, then plateaued neurologically. Functionally, this patient was unimproved. Somatosensory evoked potentials were unchanged from the preoperative study. MRI scan repeated 4½ years after surgery showed there was no fat overlying the spinal cord. The area dorsal to the spinal cord where fat had been seen 1 year after surgery was occupied by cerebrospinal fluid (CSF). The spinal cord was more atrophic than at 1 year after surgery.

The second patient, with C5 ASIA Impairment Scale C injury, had incomplete sensory function and was motor complete below C5 in the period immediately after injury. Before omental transposition, he had grade five biceps and deltoid flexion bilaterally, consistent trace toe flexion on the right side, and intermittent toe flexion on the left side. He had impaired touch sensation in all dermatomes below T1 bilaterally. By 18 months after surgery he had gained grade two to grade three quadriceps, iliopsoas, and toe flexion bilaterally, as well as grade two triceps function bilaterally. Sensation to light touch improved below T6. These neurologic findings were unchanged at 4½ years after surgery. He reported improved truncal control, decreased spasticity, and increased sensation beginning at 8 months after surgery, and that was maximal at 2 years. Somatosensory evoked potentials were unchanged. At 1 year after surgery, MRI showed some increase in apparent size of the spinal cord. There were no definite changes between the 1-year postoperative MRI and the scan obtained 4½ years after surgery. Fat was still observed to be abutting the spinal cord.

Based on the outcomes from the first series, 11 more SCI patients underwent omental transposition. Five reported that spasticity was not a major problem preoperatively. In three patients, it did not change postoperatively, whereas two patients reported increases in spasticity. Three of six patients in whom spasticity was a major problem preoperatively reported a significant decrease in spasticity. Six of the 11 patients also reported improved truncal control.

Slight improvement in all the sensations of touch, pain, heat, and cold below the level of injury was reported by four patients at 4 to 8 months after surgery. One patient reported a decrease in touch. There were no consistent reports of changes in bowel and bladder sensations or functions. Subjective improvement in function of specific muscle groups was reported by five patients in their arms and by three patients in their legs beginning at about 8 months after surgery. One patient, with C6 sensory incomplete tetraplegia, noted decrease in bilateral biceps and wrist extensor function 4 months after surgery.

Changes in neurologic examination scores were calculated between the baseline examination and at 1 year follow-up. The effect of surgery was evaluated by comparing the mean change between the operated and nonoperated patients. None of these comparisons showed any evidence of improved neurologic functioning in the operated patients. There was a decrease in the mean ASIA light touch score in the operated patients but not in the nonoperated patients. The comparison between these mean change scores fell just short of the statistical significance level. The arm motor, pinprick, and light touch change scores were compared between operated and nonoperated patients. None of the between-group differences were statistically significant ($p > .40$, two-tailed).

No changes in cervical somatosensory evoked potentials were noted following any surgery, nor were there any changes in lumbosacral somatosensory evoked potentials attributable to surgery. No subject in the surgery group had motor evoked potentials in lower limb muscles, either before or after surgery. No consistent changes in upper limb motor evoked potentials attributable to surgery were found. BMCA of lower limbs indicated decreased spasticity in four patients in the 4 to 8 months after surgery that extended to the twelfth month. Six patients showed change in measured spasticity of less than 15%, and one

subject demonstrated increased spasticity beginning at 8 months after surgery.

MRI was performed at 4, 8, and 12 months after surgery. The omentum enhanced with gadolinium in all patients, and there was contact with the dorsum of the cord in 9 of 11 cases. In two cases, there was evidence of compression of the cord at 4 months, which decreased at 8 months. These patients did not change neurologically. Spinal cord size increased in six patients by 4 to 8 months after surgery, but then remained stable at 12 months.

Thus, in this second series of omental transpositions there were no overall improvements in ASIA scores; rather, there was slight worsening in scores that did not reach the level of significance, both when the operated and nonoperated groups were compared collectively to themselves and to each other over time. Nonetheless, objective improvement or worsening was recorded for a select few individuals within both groups.

In 2001, Duffil et al.[16] reported a prospective series of omental transposition in 17 patients with chronic spinal injuries. Each patient underwent at least two physical and functional examinations preoperatively. Assessment included degree of spasticity, as determined by the modified Ashworth scale, motor power, and light touch. Additionally, arm and hand function was determined with a writing test and a nine-hole peg test, as well as tests of dexterity. Activities of daily living (ADL) function was documented with two separate tests, wheelchair use was recorded, as were pain levels. Furthermore, each patient underwent urodynamic, neurophysiologic, and pulmonary function testing.

At 12 months postoperatively, most patients showed no significant change in spasticity. One of the two patients who had a significant reduction in spasticity had a similar reduction in power, which prevented her from being able to transfer, though she had been able to do so preoperatively. No patient had an objective improvement in motor score, and 15 of the 17 patients had no change in sensation. One patient had a small improvement in sensation, and another had a significant loss of sensation, accompanied by increased pain and paresthesias. Function in ADLs was largely unchanged, and there was a tendency toward increased pain postoperatively. No patient showed EMG or SEP changes.

Sgouros and Williams[43] reported similar results in a retrospective review of 10 patients who underwent pedicled omentum transfer to either the cervical or the thoracic spine for deteriorating spinal cord function. One patient died of a perioperative myocardial infarct. Of the remaining nine patients, seven reported worse overall ADL performance, one was unchanged, and one was improved. No patient had improved arm or leg function, though several worsened. Two patients reported improved bladder function.

## Complications

Clifton et al.[10] reported that three patients developed persistent subcutaneous CSF accumulations requiring lumboperitoneal shunts. Two of these three patients also required a dorsal wound revision, and one developed a progressive decrease in bilateral biceps and wrist extensor function. One patient required revision of a lateral abdominal wall hernia at the site at which the graft was brought through the abdomen. Likewise, Sgouros and Williams[43] noted considerable morbidity from the procedure, including protracted ileus, wound infections, one CSF leak, and one perioperative death. Duffil et al.[16] encountered similar difficulties. Ray et al.[42] reported a case of recurrent gastric volvulus that eventually necessitated gastrojejunostomy.

## Omental Transposition for Wound Problems

The use of omental flaps, either pedicled or free, has been reported to aid coverage and closure in multiple sites, including the face,[47] chest wall,[1,30] and thoracolumbar defects.[29,33] Giordano[18] transferred the omentum to the thoracolumbar spine of a patient with a chronic postoperative infection. This patient with Pott's disease fell from a scaffold and required multiple corpectomies (T12 through L2). He developed a fistula from his graft site, which was contaminated with *Peptostreptococcus magnus*. An attempt at dorsal stabilization and "massive bone grafting" failed, along with surgical debridement. A second debridement was performed, and the defect was filled with a pedicled omental graft. At 32 months, there were no signs of recurrent infection.

In the first edition of this text, Clifton[11] reported omental transposition to prevent scarring of the dura mater to the cervical spinal cord. A 43-year-old woman underwent resection of a meningioma at C1-2. Postoperatively she developed CSF leakage through her wound, with meningitis. She recovered after a lengthy hospitalization but developed a gradually worsening myelopathy 1 year after the surgery. MRI showed tethering of the spinal cord to the dorsal dura at C2, which was confirmed at laminectomy. The portion of the dura adherent to the spinal cord was left to avoid damaging the spinal cord. The freed-up dural edges were sutured to a large cadaveric dural patch, and fibrin glue was applied. The patient's myelopathy rapidly improved. Postoperative MRI showed relief of the tethering with CSF present over the dorsum of the spinal cord.

At 1 year after this procedure, she again became progressively myelopathic. MRI showed that the spinal cord had retethered to the dural patch dorsally. At the next procedure, the spinal cord was found to be adherent to the patch. The dura mater and dural patch were completely dissected from the spinal cord, and a large omental pedicle was tunneled subcutaneously and sutured to the dural defect. The patient recovered rapidly, although with much more postoperative pain than after her previous surgeries. One week postoperatively, her MRI showed a large omental graft with obliteration of CSF spaces. Her myelopathy resolved, and her MRI scan, 6 months postoperatively, showed dissolution of the fat dorsally, with no tethering.

Recently, Heller et al.[28] reported two patients with subarachnoid-pleural fistulae that were managed with a pedicled omental flap. They noted that, in the thoracic spine, a dural tear or defect might be exposed to the negative intrathoracic pressure associated with respiration. This presents a path of least resistance to CSF flow, preventing the arachnoid mater from sealing the thecal sac. In this situation, lumbar drains may be inadequate treatment. In closing the defect, the authors performed a transdiaphragmatic pedicled omental flap, isolating the pressure gradient from the dura, with excellent results.

In another example of a wound problem, Clifton[11] performed a laminectomy and resection of a recurrent intramedullary cervical spinal cord ependymoma. The patient had received extensive radiation therapy 15 years earlier, making the cervical musculature and skin fibrous and avascular. The patient recovered well from resection of the tumor, but his wound completely dehisced 3 weeks after surgery. An omental pedicle was used to cover the defect, and the skin was closed over the omentum. There was no CSF leakage observed, and the wound healed. Lantieri[31] described similar treatment of a lumbar soft-tissue defect in the face radionecrosis. The morbidity of the graft harvest was decreased by an endoscopic technique.

In 1987, Benzel et al.[5] reported the use of a free omental flap in a complex cranial reconstruction on a 38-year-old man who, at age 9, had undergone a right frontotemporal craniotomy for removal of an astrocytoma, with postoperative irradiation. He subsequently incurred further trauma to the area, and, at age 18, the bone flap was removed due to osteomyelitis. Wound breakdown resulted in the loss of the skin flap, which was treated by a split thickness skin graft over the dura mater and bone margins. However, the patient continued to experience repeated episodes of purulent drainage. At age 30, biopsy of hyperpigmented areas of the graft demonstrated basal cell carcinoma. Plain films and CT scan (Figure 87.2) showed the 13cm × 16cm defect.

At surgery, the skin graft, dura mater, and surrounding skin and bone were removed. An autologous fascia lata graft was used to repair the dura. Autologous rib and iliac crest grafts were fashioned into a meshwork over the cranial defect. A free omental graft was harvested and placed in the cranial defect. Prior to surgery, an angiogram had demonstrated the superficial temporal artery to be an inadequate donor vessel. Therefore, the pedicle was tunneled to an incision in the neck, where the gastroepiploic vein was anastomosed with the common facial vein, and the gastroepiploic artery was attached to the lingual artery. A split thickness skin graft was then placed over the omentum. At 3 months, the wound was completely healed. However, at 1 year postoperatively, the defect was sunken. An angiogram demonstrated adequate blood supply to the flap (Figure 87.3). A partially resorbed cranioplasty was removed and replaced with a methylmethacrylate cranioplasty. The cosmetic result was excellent (Figure 87.4). The authors note that omental grafts shrinkage of 30% to 50% must be planned for at the time of the procedure. This omental free flap technique may have utility in spinal pathology when a significant volume must be filled for adequate coverage.

## Summary

By 1994, Goldsmith[19] had performed omental transposition on approximately 40 patients with chronic SCI in the United States. By 1992, at least 120 patients had undergone omental transposition in China, Japan, Mexico, Great

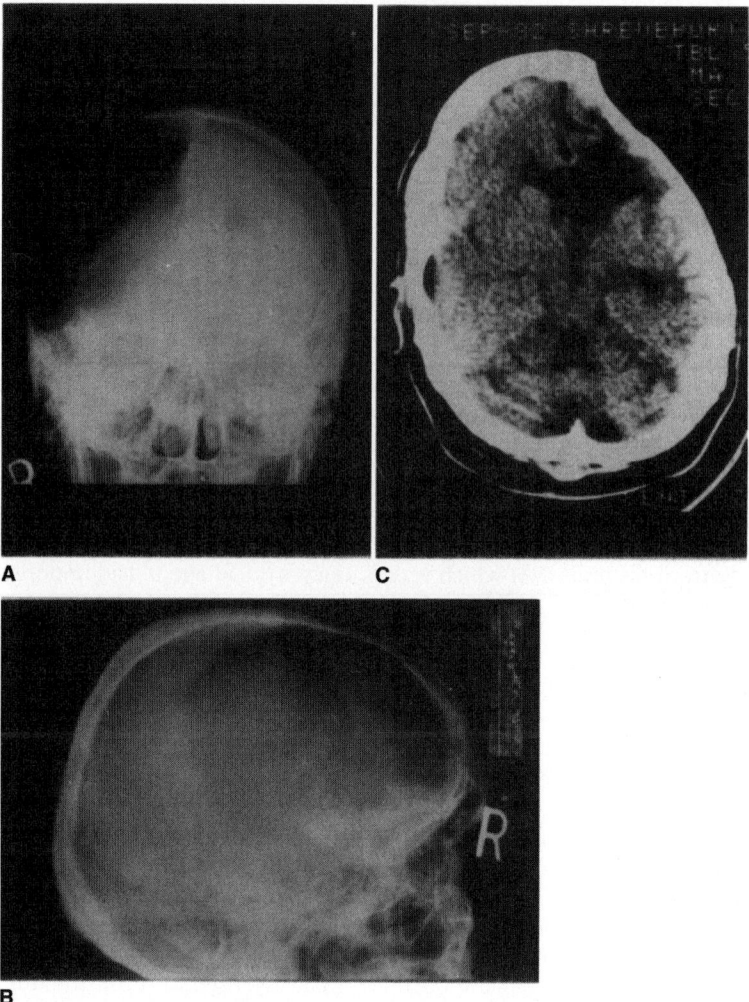

A          C

B

**Figure 87.2** (**A**) Anteroposterior, (**B**) lateral radiographs, and (**C**) CT scan demonstrating the preoperative defect. *(From Benzel EC, LeBlanc KA, Hadden TA, et al: Management of a large skull defect utilizing a vascularized free omental transfer.* Surg Neurol 27:223, 1987.)

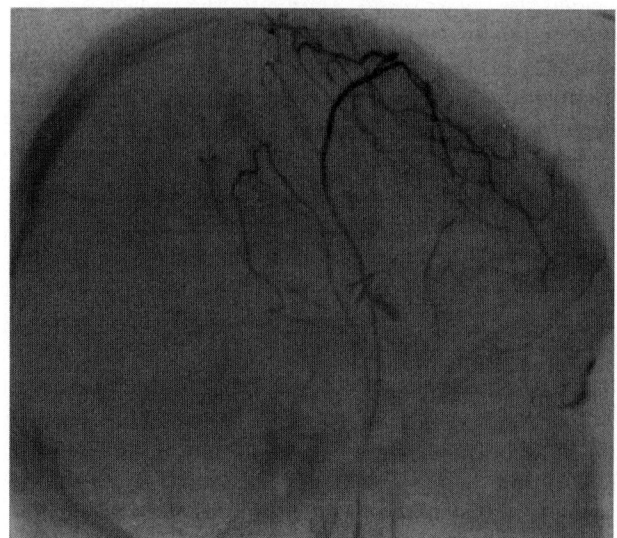

**Figure 87.3** One year postoperatively, angiogram of the external carotid artery demonstrated good flow through the free omental flap. *(From Benzel EC, LeBlanc KA, Hadden TA, et al: Management of a large skull defect utilizing a vascularized free omental transfer.* Surg Neurol 27:223, 1987.)

Britain, and India.* Except for a few detailed case reports, the published data are often in abstract or summary form, which does not provide sufficient data to allow the reader to form conclusions. Nonetheless, 40% of patients were reported to have improved after surgery.[19]

The hypothesis that omental transposition may improve conduction within existing fiber tracts in the chronically injured spinal cord is worth considering. Blight and Young[7,50] have shown that relatively few axons are needed for locomotion in cats. As many as 84% of SCI patients with complete motor injury may have only partial neurophysiologic injury,[44] and neuropathologic studies of patients with complete SCIs have shown that 78% of patients have anatomic continuity of the spinal cord.[31] Demyelination of axons is commonly found after SCI, and remyelination is associated with neurologic and neurophysiologic recovery.[7,48,50] Axonal conduction can be improved in chronically injured cat spinal cords pharmacologically.[6] Omentum contains a lipid-soluble angiogenic factor that enhances new vessel growth and contains high levels of neurotransmit-

---

*References 3,25,36,38,41,46,53.

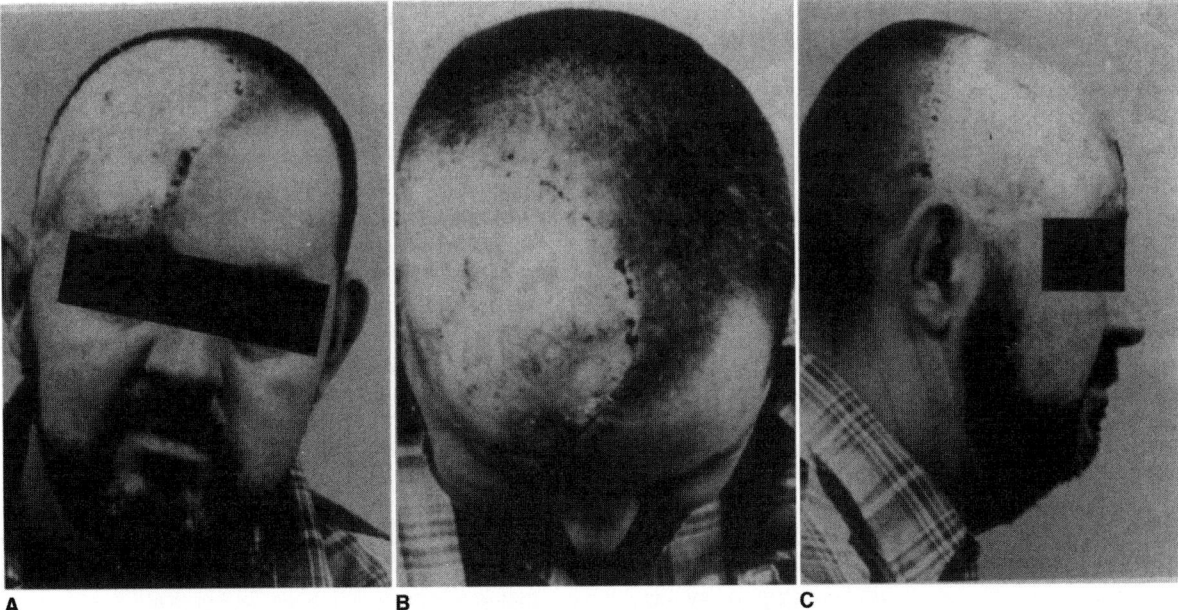

**Figure 87.4** (**A**) Anteroposterior, (**B**) vertex, and (**C**) lateral photographs after removal of the partially resorbed autogenous cranioplasty and revision with methylmethacrylate. *(From Benzel EC, LeBlanc KA, Hadden TA, et al: Management of a large skull defect utilizing a vascularized free omental transfer. Surg Neurol 27:223, 1987.)*

ters.[9,24,35] Omental transposition has been reported to enhance axonal growth across a collagen bridge and to contain a lipid-soluble factor that enhances neurite outgrowth in neuronal cell culture.[13,45] Therefore, it is conceivable that omental transposition could enhance function of existing tracts, either by remyelination, by provision of deficient neurotransmitters, or by both mechanisms.

The first attempt to use omentum to revascularize the spinal cord was in a nontraumatized dog model.[22] Studies from the same lab[26] in a traumatized cat spinal model demonstrated that omental transposition performed within 3 hours of injury improved electrical function. Transposition at 6 to 8 hours was no better than control. Sgouros and Williams[43] made note that after 3 to 6 months, established gliosis and leptomeningeal fibrosis would likely interfere with new anastomoses between neural elements, even in the face increased vascular supply. Given these time constraints, it may well be that optimal timing for an omental transposition to the spinal cord would be within days or even hours of the initial trauma. However, it is probably not advisable to perform such a significant procedure on an acutely injured patient. Furthermore, many patients who initially appear to have a complete injury make remarkable spontaneous recovery and would not be well served by such an invasive procedure as omental transposition in the acute setting.[43]

On the basis of the complications encountered, the length of the operative time, the modest nature of patient reported improvements, the lack of objectively measured neurologic improvement, and evidence of sensory deterioration, there is no apparent justification for further performance of this procedure. Pedicled omentum, however, may be useful in difficult spinal wound problems to seal thoracic dural defects, to fill soft-tissue defects, especially in previously irradiated tissue, or to prevent scarring of the dura mater to the spinal cord.

## REFERENCES

1. Abbes M, Mateu J, Giordano P, *et al:* Chest wall reconstruction after full thickness resection: an experience with 22 patients. *Eur J Surg Oncol* 17:342, 1991.
2. Abraham J: Omental transposition to the brain: experimental and human applications. In Goldsmith H (ed): *The Omentum.* New York, Springer-Verlag, 1990, p 147.
3. Abraham J, Paterson A, Bothra M, *et al:* Omentomyelo-synangiosis in the management of chronic traumatic paraplegia: case report. *Paraplegia* 25:44, 1980.
4. Azzena GB, Campus G, Mameli O, *et al:* Omental transposition or transplantation to the brain and superficial temporal artery: middle cerebral artery anastomosis in preventing experimental cerebral ischemia. *Acta Neurochir* 68:63, 1983.
5. Benzel EC, LeBlanc KA, Hadden TA, *et al:* Management of a large skull defect utilizing a vascularized free omental transfer. *Surg Neurol* 27:223, 1987.
6. Blight AR, Gruner JA: Augmentation by 4-aminopyridine of vestibulospinal free-fall responses in chronic spinal-injured cats. *J Neurol Sci* 82:145, 1989.
7. Blight AR, Young W: Central axons in injured cat spinal cord recover electrophysiological function following remyelination by Schwann cells. *J Neurol Sci* 91:15, 1989.
8. Bracken MB, Shepard MJ, Collins WF, *et al:* A randomized control trial of methylprednisolone or naloxone in treatment of acute spinal-cord injury: results of the National Acute Spinal Cord Injury Study. *N Engl J Med* 322:1405, 1990.

9. Cartier R, Brunette I, Hashimoto K, *et al:* Angiogenic factor: a possible mechanism for neurovascularization produced by omental pedicles. *J Thorac Cardiovasc Surg* 99:264, 1990.

10. Clifton GL, Donovan WH, Dimitrijevic MD, *et al:* Omental transposition in chronic spinal cord injury. *Spinal Cord* 34:193, 1996.

11. Clifton GL, Donovan WH, Dimitrijevic MD, *et al:* Revascularization and scar prevention: omental transposition and spine surgery. In Benzel E (ed): *Spine Surgery: Techniques, Complication Avoidance, and Management.* New York, Churchill Livingstone, 1999, p 825.

12. Cucca GS, Papavero L, Pau A, *et al:* Effect of omental transposition to the brain on protein synthesis in experimental cerebral ischemia. *Acta Neurochir (Wien)* 51:253-257, 1980.

13. De La Torre JC, Goldsmith HC: Collagen-omental graft in experimental spinal cord transection. *Acta Neurochir (Wien)* 102:152, 1990.

14. DeRiu PL, Rocca A, Falzoi A, *et al:* Physiological function after middle cerebral artery occlusion in rabbits with neovascularization of the brain by transposed omentum. *Neurosurgery* 7:57, 1980.

15. Dimitrijevic MM, Dimitrijevic MR, Sherwood AM, *et al:* Clinical neurophysiological techniques in the assessment of spasticity. *Phys Med Rehab* 3:64, 1989.

16. Duffil J, Buckley J, Lang D, *et al:* Prospective study of omental transposition in patients with chronic spinal injury. *J Neurol Neurosurg Psychiatry* 71:73, 2001.

17. Frackowiak R, Neil-Dwyer G: Studies on cerebral blood flow and oxygen metabolism in patients with established cerebral infarct undergoing omental transposition. *Stroke* 18:46, 1987.

18. Giordano PA, Griffet J, Argenson C: Pedicled greater omentum transferred to the spine in a case of postoperative infection. *Plast Reconstr Surg* 93:1508, 1994.

19. Goldsmith HS: Brain and spinal cord revascularization by omental transposition. *Neurol Res* 16:159, 1994.

20. Goldsmith HS, Chen WF, Duckett SW: Brain vascularization by intact omentum. *Arch Surg* 106:695, 1973.

21. Goldsmith HS, Duckett S, Chen WF: Prevention of cerebral infarction in the dog by intact omentum. *Am J Surg* 130:317, 1975.

22. Goldsmith HS, Duckett S, Chen WF: Spinal cord vascularization by intact omentum. *Am J Surg* 129:262, 1975.

23. Goldsmith HS, Duckett S, Chen WF: Prevention of cerebral infarction in the monkey by omental transposition of the brain. *Stroke* 9:224, 1978.

24. Goldsmith HS, Griffith AL, Catsimpoolas N: Increased vascular perfusion after administration of an omental lipid fraction. *Surg Gynecol Obstet* 162:579, 1986.

25. Goldsmith HS, Neil-Dwyer MS, Barsoum FFS: Omental transposition to the chronically injured human spinal cord. *Paraplegia* 24:173, 1986.

26. Goldsmith HS, Stewart E, Ducket S: Early application of pedicled omentum to the acutely traumatised spinal cord. *Paraplegia* 23:100, 1985.

27. Goldsmith HS, Saunders RL, Reeves AG, *et al:* Omental transposition to brain of stroke patients. *Stroke* 10:471, 1979.

28. Heller JG, Kim HS, Carlson GW: Subarachnoid-pleural fistulae management with a transdiaphragmatic pedicled greater omental flap: report of two cases. *Spine* 26:1809, 2001.

29. Hosono N, Yonenobu K, Ono K: Postoperative pseudomeningocele with herniation of the spinal cord. *Spine* 20:2147, 1995.

30. Jurkiewicz MJ, Arnold PG: The omentum: an account of its use in the reconstruction of the chest wall. *Ann Surg* 185:548, 1977.

31. Kakulas B: The applied neurobiology of human spinal cord injury: a review. *Paraplegia* 26:371, 1988.

32. Lantieri LA, Tantaoui B, Rimareix FA, *et al:* Lower back coverage with endoscopically harvested pedicled greater omental flap. *Plast Reconstr Surg* 103:960, 1999.

33. Lefourn B, Loirat Y, Sartre JY, *et al:* Covering of a thoraco-lumbar defect by omentoplasty. *Ann Chir Plast Esthet* 42:70, 1997.

34. Macmillan M, Stauffer ES: The effect of omental pedicle graft transfer on spinal microcirculation and laminectomy membrane formation. *Spine* 16:176, 1991.

35. McIntosh TK, Goldsmith HS: Vasoactive neurochemicals in the omentum: implications for CNS injury. In Goldsmith H (ed): *The Omentum.* New York, Springer-Verlag, 1990, p 75.

36. Min-Shu Z, Hua-Cheng J, Rong-Giu W, *et al:* Experimental and clinical use of omental transposition for spinal cord pathology. In Goldsmith H (ed): *The Omentum.* New York, Springer-Verlag, 1990, p 173.

37. Miyamoto S, Kikuchi H, Karasawa J, *et al:* Cerebral revascularization by omental graft for moya-moya disease. In Goldsmith H (ed): *The Omentum.* New York, Springer-Verlag, 1990, p 159.

38. Nagashima C, Masumori Y, Kubota S, *et al:* Omentum transplantation to the cervical cord with microangio anastomosis. *No Shinkei Geka* 19:309, 1991.

39. Pau A, Sehrbundt Viale E, Turtas S, *et al:* Cerebral water and electrolytes in experimental ischemia following omental transposition to the brain. *Acta Neurochir (Wien)* 54:213, 1982.

40. Pau A, Sehrbundt Viale E, Turtas S: Effect of omental transposition to the brain on the cortical content of norepinephrine, dopamine, 5-hydroxytryptamine, and 5-hydroxyindoleacetic acid in experimental cerebral ischemia. *Acta Neurochir (Wien)* 66:159, 1982.

41. Rafael H, Malpica A, Espinoza M, *et al:* Omental transplantation in the management of chronic traumatic paraplegia. *Acta Neurochir (Wien)* 114:145, 1992.

42. Ray A, Savich G, Gardner B: Gastric volvulus: a complication of spinal cord omental transposition. Case report. *Paraplegia* 33:536, 1995.

43. Sgouros S, Williams B: A critical appraisal of pediculated omental graft transposition in progressive spinal cord failure. *Br J Neurosurg* 10:547, 1996.

44. Sherwood AM, Dimitrijevic MR, McKay WB: Evidence of subclinical brain influence in clinically complete spinal cord injury: discomplete SCI. *J Neurol Sci* 110:90, 1992.

45. Siek GC, Marquis JK, Goldsmith HS: Experimental studies of omentum-derived neurotrophic factors. In Goldsmith H (ed): *The Omentum.* New York, Springer-Verlag, 1990, p 83.

46. Song MF: Indications and complications of omental transposition to the spinal cord. *Chung Hua Wai Ko Tsa Chih* 28:342, 1990.
47. Wallace JG, Schneider WJ, Brown RG, *et al:* Reconstruction of hemifacial atrophy with a free flap of omentum. *Br J Plast Surg* 32:15, 1979.
48. Waxman SG: Demyelination in spinal cord injury. *J Neurol Sci* 91:1, 1989.
49. Williams R: Angiogenesis and the greater omentum. In Goldsmith H (ed): *The Omentum.* New York, Springer-Verlag, 1990, p 45.
50. Young W: Recovery mechanisms in spinal cord injury: implications for regenerative therapy. In Seil F (ed): *Frontiers of Clinical Neuroscience: Neural Regeneration and Transplantation,* vol. 10. New York, Alan R. Liss, 1987, p 156.
51. Zhang C: Intracranial free omentum with microsurgical technic in the treatment of ischemic cerebrovascular disease. *Chung Hua Shen Ching Ching Shen Tsa Chin* 16:23, 1983.
52. Zhu ZC, Wu WL, Mo YZ: Omental transposition to the brain for cerebrovascular occlusive disease. *Chung Hua Wai Ko Tsa Chih* 20:11, 1982.
53. Zou XW: Omental transposition in the surgical treatment of spinal cord injuries. *Clin J Neurosurg* 1:107, 1985.

# CHAPTER 88

# Spinal Wound Closure

**Patrick W. Hitchon, James E. Greensmith, and Albert E. Cram**

## Anatomic Layers

Deep to the skin is the subcutaneous fascia of the back, a thick, fibrous layer extending from the scalp to the gluteal region. The deep fascia overlying the spine comprises the nuchal fascia from the subocciput to T6 and the thoracolumbar fascia caudally to the iliac crests. The nuchal fascia attaches caudally to the superior nuchal line of the subocciput and to the spinous processes of the seventh cervical and upper six thoracic vertebrae. It is adherent to the fascia of the deep surface of the trapezius caudally and is continuous with the thoracolumbar fascia.[3] The thoracolumbar fascia attaches medially to the spinous processes of the lumbar and sacral vertebrae and caudally to the iliac crests. Laterally, it attaches to the ribs and intercostal fascia. The dorsal layer of the thoracolumbar fascia is termed the lumbar aponeurosis and serves as the origin of the latissimus dorsi muscle.

The trapezius muscle is the most superficial of the muscles overlying the spine and arises from the external occipital protuberance and superior nuchal line rostrally, the spinous process of C7, and the spinous processes of all the thoracic vertebrae caudally.[3] The trapezius muscle inserts into the clavicle, acromion, and dorsal border of the spine of the scapula. Deep to the trapezius muscle are the splenius capitis and splenius cervicis muscles, the latter extending caudally to the spinous process of T6. The erector spinae muscles, comprising the iliocostalis laterally and the longissimus and spinalis muscles medially, constitute the deepest of the three superficial muscles of the spine. The deep muscle stratum of the spine is made up of the semispinalis capitis and cervicis rostrally and the thoracis caudally. Deep to the semispinalis muscle is the multifidus muscle that extends from the axis to the sacrum. In the lumbar spine, the superficial stratum of spinal muscles is made up of the latissimus dorsi muscle and fascia and the erector spinae muscles. The deep layer consists of the multifidus muscle. The latissimus dorsi muscle arises from the spinous processes of T6, to and including the sacral vertebrae, by way of the dorsal layer of the thoracolumbar fascia or lumbar aponeurosis and the crest of the ilium. The fibers of the latissimus dorsi muscle proceed rostrally and laterally to a 7cm quadrilateral tendon that passes ventral to the teres major muscle, inserting into the intertubercular groove of the humerus.

The trapezius muscle thus spans the entire breadth of the interscapular distance and longitudinally extends from the subocciput to T12. The latissimus dorsi muscle likewise extends from T6 caudally to the sacrum, inserting lat- erally into the humerus. These muscles belong to the superficial stratum of spinal muscles deep only to the superficial fascia. It is by virtue of their location and span that they provide a ready mechanism for the closure and repair of open spinal wounds.

## Basic Principles of Spinal Closure

Nowhere is the basic principle of a layered anatomic closure more important than with the structures overlying the spine. If the spinous processes have been removed, the erector spinae and multifidus muscles are approximated in the midline using heavy absorbable suture, such as 0 Vicryl. If the spinous processes are intact, the fascia is approximated in the midline, again with heavy absorbable sutures. In the presence of a gibbus deformity, or if the subcutaneous fat is sparse, it may be advisable to excise the rostral and caudal spinous processes to attain a lower profile. Postoperatively, these bony prominences can create a major ulceration problem, particularly in the presence of neurologic deficit or prior radiation therapy. Suction drains are often placed in extensive wounds, as in fractures with instrumentation or vascular neoplasms. Dual drains can be inserted, one in the epidural space and a second in the subcutaneous layer. These drains diminish the occurrence of hematomas and seromas that hamper wound healing.[6,33] If cerebrospinal fluid (CSF) is noted to accumulate in the suction canister, the drain must be removed immediately to prevent a persistent CSF leak and complications associated with CSF overdrainage. The superficial fascia and subcutaneous tissue are approximated to obliterate dead space. A watertight closure of the skin is accomplished with nonabsorbable nylon or staples. In the presence of wound dehiscence or infection before attempted closure, extensive debridement is necessary. In cases in which preoperative radiation therapy has been received or postoperative radiation is anticipated, closure of the fascia should be accomplished with nonabsorbable 0 or 2-0 monofilament or braided nylon. Wound closure in general is uncomplicated in the cervical and lumbar region. This is because of the thickness of the muscle layer and the lordotic curvature of the spine. A spinal incision in the upper thoracic spine is subject to horizontal tensile forces caused by shoulder movement. It is this area that is notorious for dehiscence in as much as 30% of cases with cancer or spinal implants.[3] In addition to spinous process excision, a figure-eight brace may be worn postoperatively to reduce tensile forces across the vertical incision. Drains are usually left in place for 2 days (if used) or until the drainage is less than 50ml per shift. Sutures are removed 2 or more weeks postoperatively.

When the quality of the tissue present at the wound edge or the amount of tissue damaged or missing precludes primary closure, one must consider either a skin graft or some other type of flap closure. Split thickness skin graft can be used for closure in rare instances in which the underlying soft tissue is adequate to protect underlying structures and also has adequate circulation to support survival of the skin graft. Modern electric and nitrogen gas pressure powered dermatomes make the harvest of high-quality split thickness autograft a simple and predictable procedure. Graft may be taken from any suitable donor site, usually at a thickness between 0.012 and 0.015 inches. This is applied to the wound bed. Fixation of the graft for 4 to 5 days prevents movement between the graft and the recipient bed. This usually results in graft acceptance.

## Myocutaneous Flaps

Closure of large soft-tissue defects currently relies heavily on the use of myocutaneous and fasciocutaneous flaps. In the back, the most commonly used musculocutaneous flap for defects of the upper third of the thoracic spine is the trapezius muscle. Variations of flap design can cover upper third defects over a relatively wide arc of rotation, as long as the transverse cervical artery is intact. Defects in the middle third of the back are most frequently closed by use of the latissimus muscle. This is based on its thoracodorsal blood supply or on the paraspinous perforators. Defects of the lower third of the back are often closed with gluteus muscle myocutaneous flaps, most often based on the inferior gluteal artery. In the lower third, the latissimus dorsi muscle may also be used. This must be based on a free flap using vein grafts from the thoracodorsal trunks or by anastomosis to the superior or inferior gluteal vessels, if it is to reach the caudal most portions of the lower third of the back.

### Trapezius Muscle and Myocutaneous Flaps

By virtue of its length extending from the superior nuchal line to the spinous process of T12 and its width from one acromial process to the other, the trapezius muscle is suitable for rotation, with or without overlying flaps of skin (Figure 88.1). The blood supply to the trapezius muscle is via the type II vascular pattern characterized by one dominant vascular pedicle with other minor contributing pedicles.[20,23,27] The principal pedicle consists of the dorsal scapular artery, which constitutes the descending branch of the transverse cervical artery. The latter arises from the subclavian artery or thyrocervical trunk. The dorsal scapular artery courses caudally, medial to the scapula and ventral to the rhomboid muscle, supplying these muscles as well as the latissimus dorsi and trapezius muscles and eventually anastomosing with the suprascapular, subscapular, and some of the intercostal arteries. The minor pedicle consists of branches of the occipital artery perfusing the rostral segments of the muscle.[4,6] With careful dissection, the caudal pole of the trapezius muscle can be dissected from the spinous processes and underlying latissimus and rhomboid muscles. Careful attention must be paid to preserve the integrity of its blood supply, which can be observed on the ventral aspect of the caudal and medial fibers.

Trapezius flaps, with or without attached cutaneous pedicles, can be used to repair defects overlying the kyphotic curvature of the thoracic spine. Spinal wound closure can be a challenge in patients who are being treated for thoracic spinal metastases. The apex of the thoracic kyphosis is most prone to dehiscence in patients whose wound healing capability has been compromised by chemotherapy and radiation therapy. Radiation therapy contributes to impairment of circulation by virtue of endothelial swelling and subintimal fibrosis. This results in an obstructive endarteritis with the subcutaneous tissue being replaced by dense fibrosis.[6] Shoulder movement further contributes traction on the skin edges increasing their predilection for separation and dehiscence. This is further expedited in cases of wound infection or diabetes or in the elderly. When such wound dehiscence fails to heal by secondary intention, alternative approaches must be sought. Failure of healing with superimposed infection can result in dural erosion and CSF leaks. Spinal drainage is insufficient to provide for dural closure in the depths of an open infected wound. Under those circumstances, extensive debridement of the wound in the operating room is necessary. Excision of all infected bone is undertaken until bleeding cancellous bone is encountered. Dural repairs are undertaken with free or pedicle fascial grafts attached to a trapezius flap. The trapezius flap can obliterate the dead space in the depths of the spinal wound, providing for an optimal watertight closure. The wound is further approximated in layers, usually over drains. The approximation is usually undertaken with heavy, nonabsorbable sutures such as 0 or 2-0 braided nylon and the skin closed with heavy monofilament of 0-Prolene. It is important to maintain an optimum nutritional status of the patient and use blood transfusions to enhance wound healing. The patient is usually maintained in a figure-of-eight brace for up to 4 weeks.

### Latissimus Flaps

The latissimus dorsi muscle, owing to its location and blood supply, provides muscle or myocutaneous flaps for the closure of spinal defects overlying the lower thoracic and lumbar spine (Figure 88.1). Its blood supply is type V, consisting of one dominant vascular pedicle, which in this case is the thoracodorsal artery arising from the subclavian artery and secondary midline and paramedian pedicles. This is comprised of the dorsal cutaneous branches of the intercostal and lumbar arteries.[6,20] The intercostal arteries contributing most to the secondary pedicles are those of the ninth, tenth, and eleventh intercostal arteries as confirmed on cadaveric dissections.[29] These perforators usually enter the latissimus muscle approximately 5cm from the midline. Latissimus dorsi flaps, with and without skin, are based on the thoracodorsal artery and are dissected away from the spinous process attachments. Such flaps are generally suited for repair of large thoracic wall or lateral iliac decubiti.

Reverse latissimus flaps, on the other hand, are dissected laterally or rostrally and thus maintain the blood supply of the flap from the midline paraspinal secondary vascular pedicles. The integrity of the penetrating vessels on the ventral surface of the muscle is preserved because the supply from the thoracodorsal artery is sacrificed for distal mobilization. Such latissimus dorsi flaps are referred to as reverse flaps and are suited for the repair of spinal defects of the lower thoracic and lumbar spines (Figure 88.2). The muscle flap is based medially on the ninth, tenth, and eleventh intercostal feeders.

The length of the pedicle is geared to the size of the spinal defect to be repaired. The portion of the latissimus

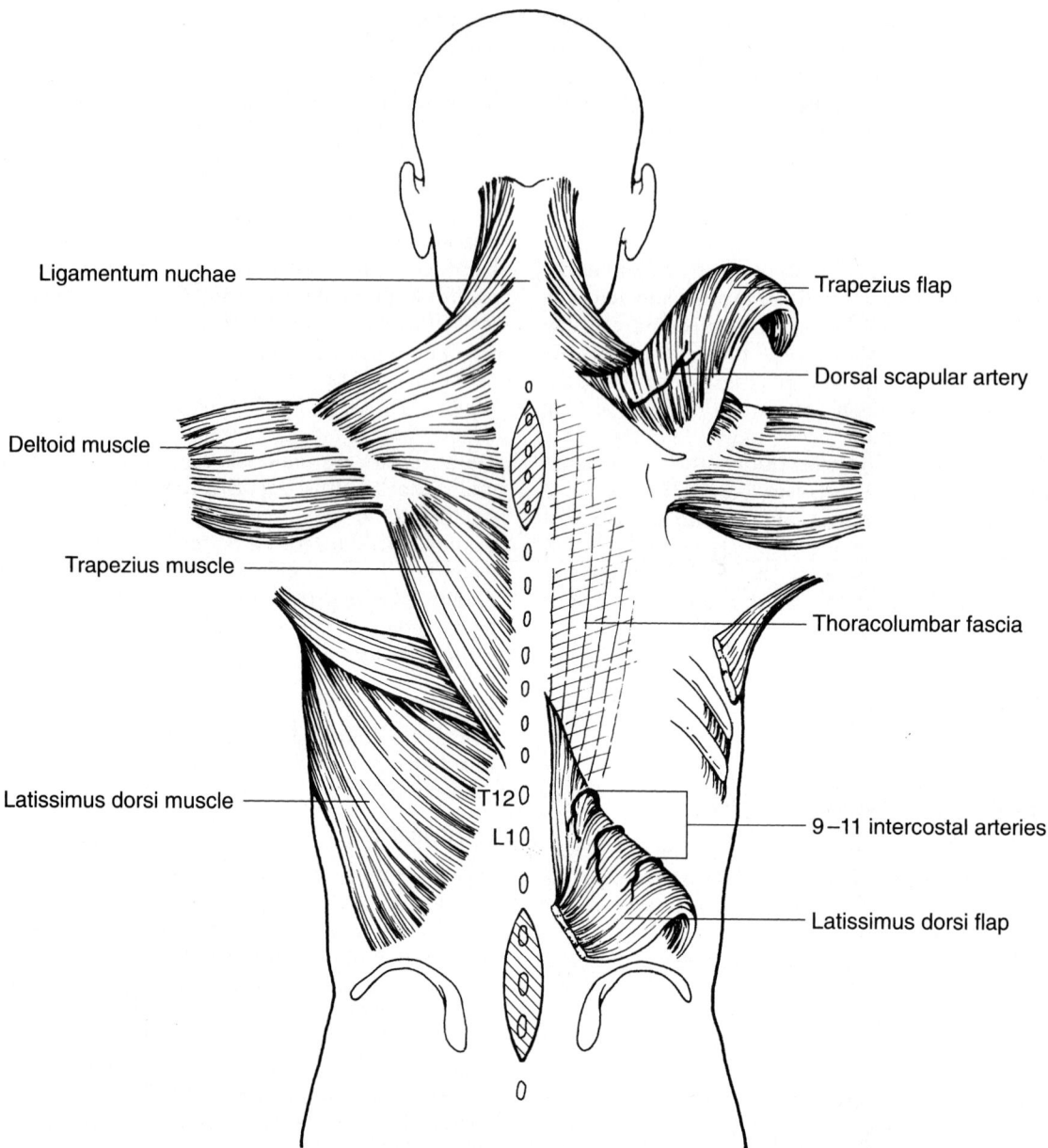

Ligamentum nuchae

Deltoid muscle

Trapezius muscle

Latissimus dorsi muscle

T12
L1

Trapezius flap

Dorsal scapular artery

Thoracolumbar fascia

9–11 intercostal arteries

Latissimus dorsi flap

**Figure 88.1** Normal anatomy of the trapezius and latissimus dorsi muscles (*left*). Trapezius and reverse latissimus dorsi flaps (*right*) are used for coverage of defects over the upper thoracic and lumbar spines, respectively. Mobilization of these flaps requires preservation of their blood supply.

dorsi muscle mobilized and its width are customized to the case at hand (Figure 88.3). The latissimus dorsi muscle provides a large muscle mass capable of filling far larger spinal defects than is possible with trapezius muscle flaps. The reverse latissimus flap, with or without its cutaneous pedicle, when necessary, is tunneled subcutaneously to the midline incision. The site of the cutaneous pedicle is then repaired with a split thickness skin graft. Reverse latissimus flaps are usually adequate when used unilaterally.

Bilateral large musculocutaneous latissimus flaps may be advanced medially to cover large midline spinal defects. In these circumstances, the flaps are based on the thoracodorsal artery with partial preservation of the sec-

ondary intercostal blood supply. Skin grafting may be necessary to cover the relaxing incisions made on either side of the torso to facilitate advancement.[3]

It is possible to create a large muscle or skin and muscle flap using the latissimus dorsi muscle based on a vein graft extension of the thoracodorsal artery.[23] This approach requires a microsurgical team and the harvest of saphenous or other suitable vein to interpose on both the arterial and venous circulation. The vein interposition can be performed below the subscapularis branch, and a large muscle advancement can be carried out. This overcomes the problems that occasionally occur when using the most medial portions of the flap with complete ligation of the paraspinous

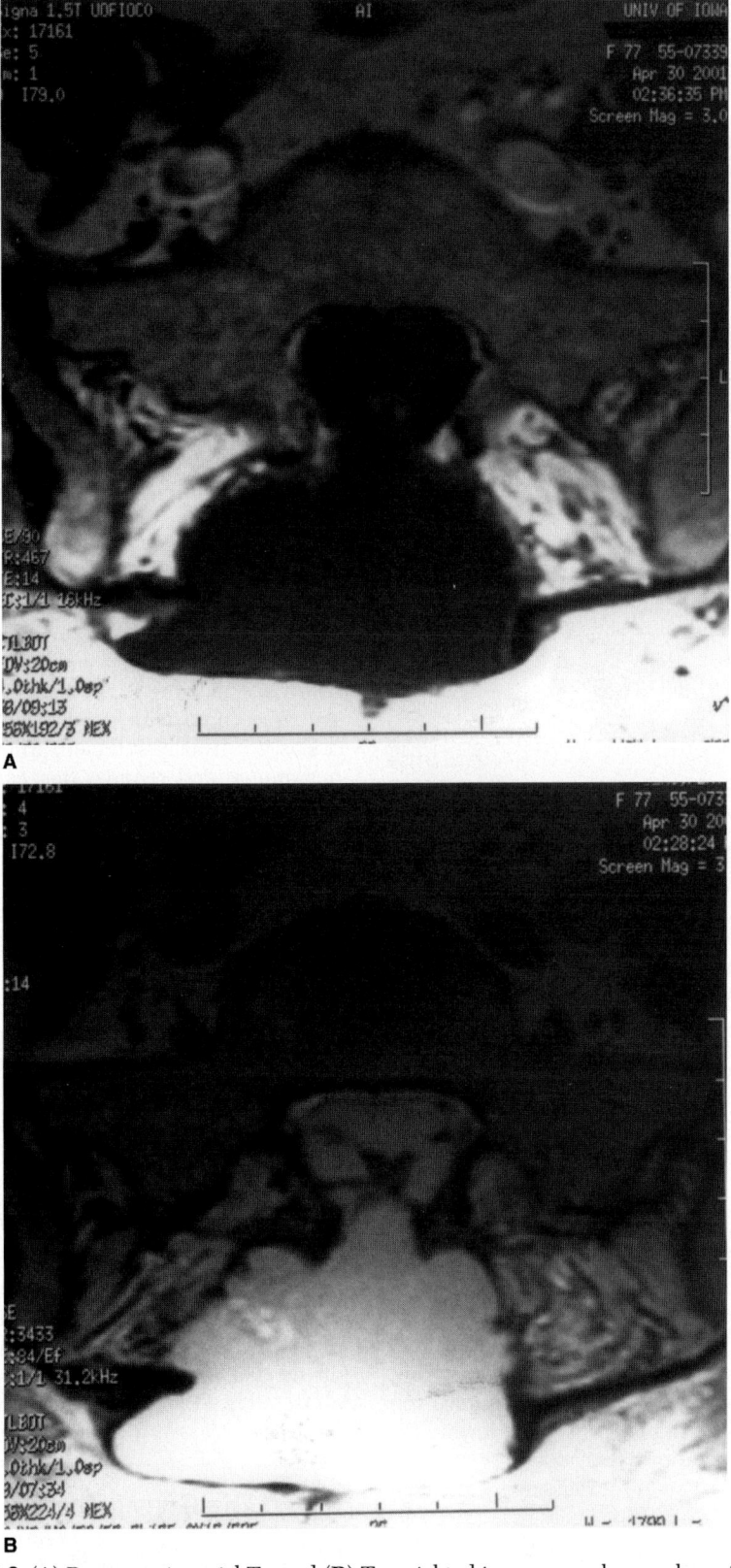

**Figure 88.2** **(A)** Postoperative axial T₁- and **(B)** T₂-weighted images reveal a sacral meningocele in a 77-year-old lady who underwent release of a tethered cord. Though no external CSF leakage was present, the patient was symptomatic with postural headaches and a large subcutaneous fluid collection.

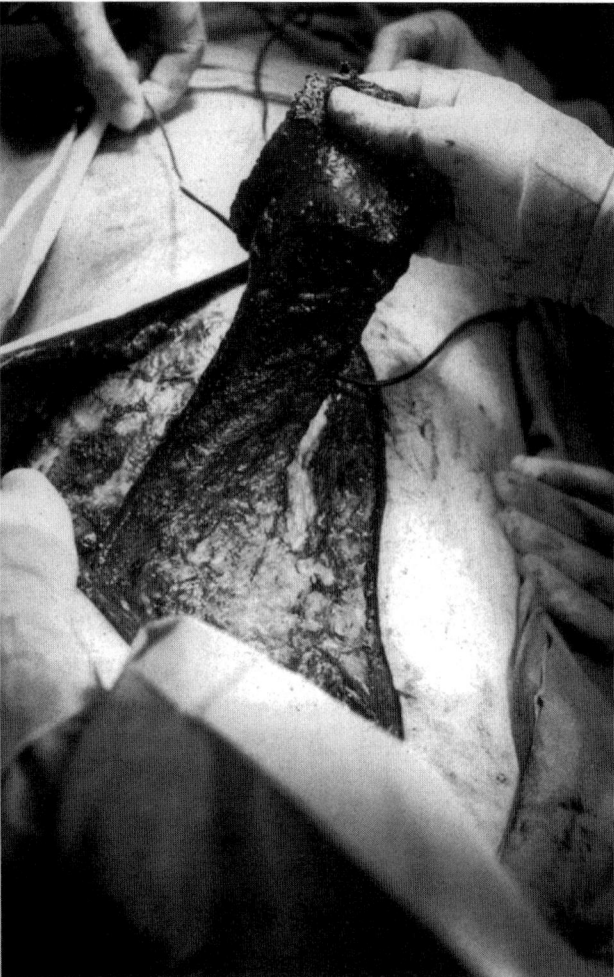

**Figure 88.3** The patient from Figure 88.2 was explored, and no frank CSF leak was identified. A reverse latissimus dorsi flap was used for obliteration of the dead space. The midline incision was extended rostrally, and the latissimus muscle sectioned below its insertion. The muscle head is held up and reflected into the lumbosacral incision while safeguarding its vascular supply. On follow-up she was asymptomatic, and her lower back was flat.

perforators. This medial most portion of the flap is primarily fascial and of marginal circulation. It depends entirely on the thoracodorsal vessel for inflow. Use of the vein graft and transection of the insertion of the muscle permits safe movement of more reliable muscle and skin medially. A "V-to-Y" technique allows movement of relatively large skin-muscle flaps, when such flaps are needed. Conversely, this technique can be used to advance only the latissimus dorsi muscle, and the epithelial coverage is provided by application of split thickness graft to the exposed portion of the latissimus muscle.

### Gluteus Maximus Flaps for the Sacral Region

The gluteus maximus is a large buttock muscle with a quadrilateral shape. It extends from the ilium, sacrum, coccyx, and sacrospinal aponeurosis to the greater trochanter of the femur and the iliotibial band of the fascia lata.[3] This large muscle has a type III vasculature, with two dominant arteries, the superior and inferior gluteal arteries, arising

from the internal iliac artery.[20,22] Owing to its location, the gluteus maximus muscle, with or without an attached skin flap, is suited for repair of sacral, ischial, trochanteric, and ilial open wounds. The muscle mass and overlying skin have sufficient size and redundancy, such that a unilateral myocutaneous flap is often sufficient to provide coverage for a midline defect. For the coverage of a sacral decubitus, the skin incision extends along the caudal margin of the iliac crest laterally from the edges of the wound that had been debrided. The incision is carried through the subcutaneous tissue, and a plane is created between the gluteus maximus and medius muscles. It is important to maintain the integrity of the superior gluteal artery as it enters the deep surface of the gluteus maximus muscle. However, if the superior gluteal artery interferes with the mobility of this muscle flap, it can be sacrificed for increased mobility. In instances in which this has been done, the blood supply provided by the inferior gluteal artery has proven sufficient.[22] The muscle and skin edges are then sutured to the contralateral debrided edge of the exposed wound after incision of all infected and devascularized bone. Depending on the size of the defect to be covered, the lateral caudal margin of the myocutaneous flap can extend inferiorly to the greater trochanter. The gluteus medius muscle provides adequate soft-tissue padding of the iliac crest. The donor site of the skin is covered with a split thickness skin graft. Vacuum drains are usually sufficient to avoid the accumulation of hematomas and seromas that can complicate and impede healing. The muscle flap is usually sutured in place with heavy-gauge absorbable suture such as 0 and 2-0 Vicryl, and the skin is sutured with monofilament nylon or Prolene. Heavy dressings are applied to prevent pressure upon the flap that may impair adequate perfusion. The patient is to be kept on the side or in the prone position for at least 2 weeks subsequent to flap rotation.

The rotational advancement of gluteus-based flaps for sacral wounds has been largely replaced by "V-to-Y" techniques. The sacral lesion is debrided, and depending on the transverse diameter of the wound, either a single or a bilateral V incision is designed. The origins of the gluteus maximus are freed up as needed and the muscle is dissected free at the lateral margin, dissecting medially as needed to free the flap. The superior or inferior gluteal artery must be kept intact. This myocutaneous flap is then advanced medially and sutured to the wound edge or to its mirror image flap from the opposite side, if the size of the wound dictates a bilateral approach. As the lateral portion of the flap is moved by this advancement, a linear closure of the defect results in the Y-shaped final appearance as observed in Figures 88.4 and 88.5.

## Hyperbaric Oxygen Therapy (HBO)

### Introduction and Rationale

Although the vast majority of primary surgical closures heal without difficulty, there are occasionally wounds that fail to heal. The sequelae of these nonhealing surgical wounds can be as minor as the need for additional home nursing care or as severe as patient demise. Risk factors for nonhealing wounds include: malnutrition, diabetes mellitus,

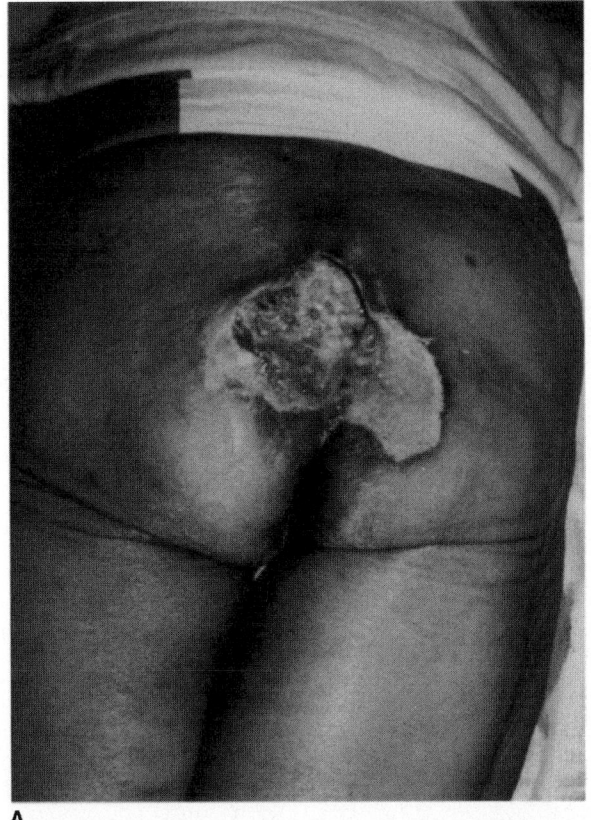

A

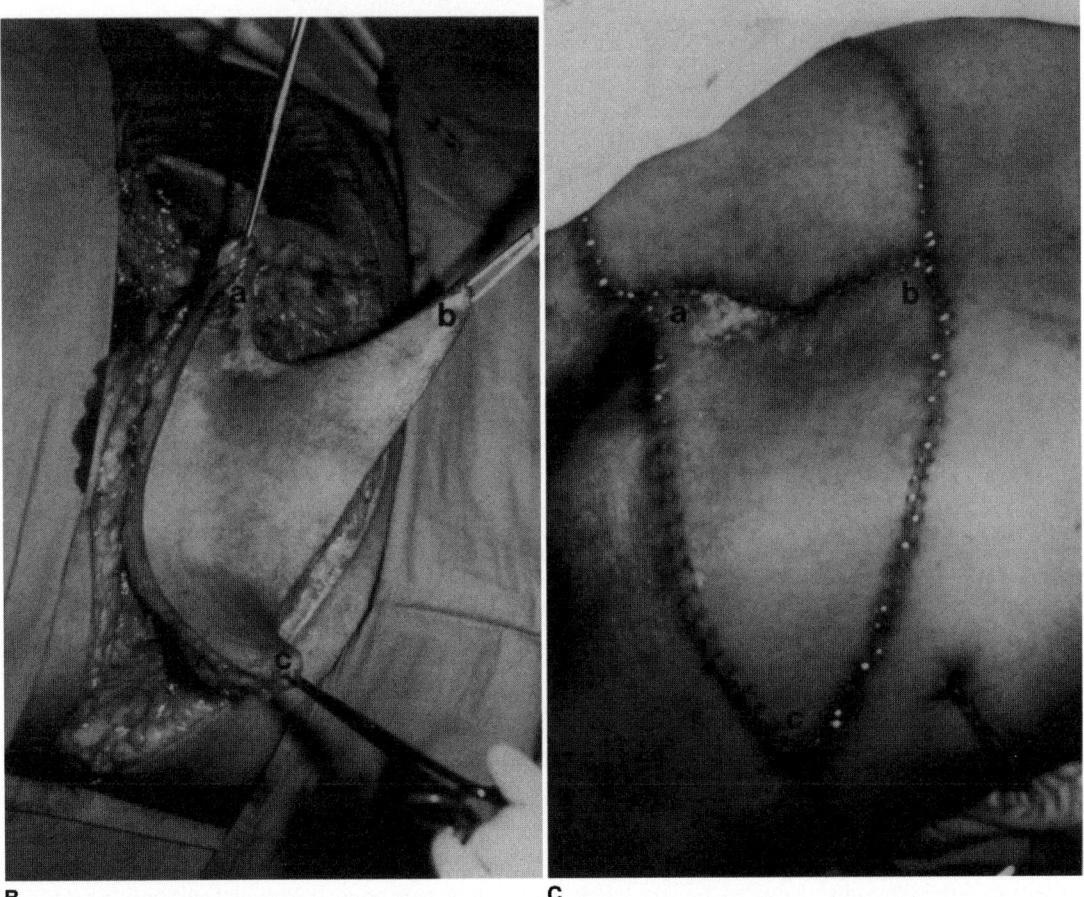

B                                    C

**Figure 88.4** (A) Sacral decubitus ulcer with exposure of sacrum. (B) V-shaped myocutaneous flap. (C) Completed bilateral gluteal myocutaneous flaps approximated in midline.

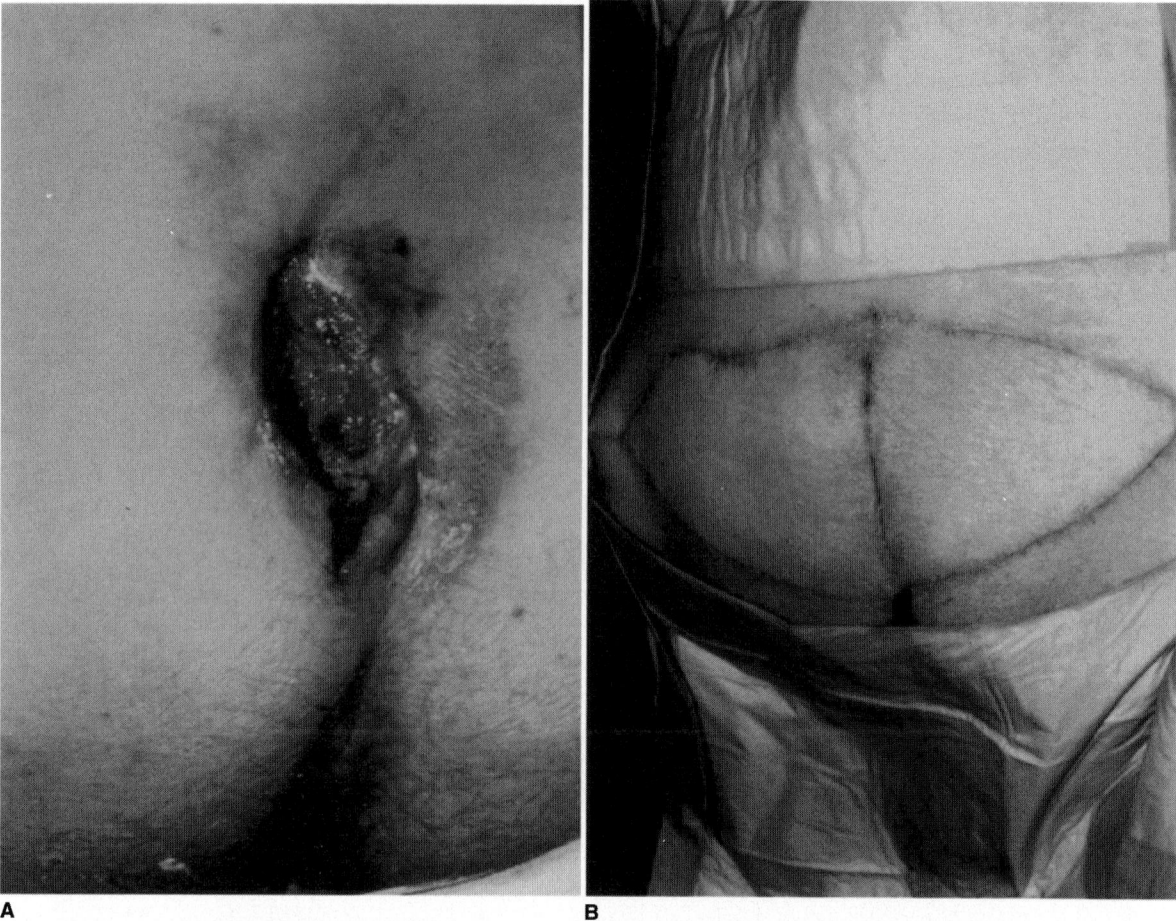

**A**                                                              **B**

**Figure 88.5** (**A**) Sacral decubitus ulcer with sacral osteomyelitis. (**B**) After closure.

peripheral vascular insufficiency, smoking, collagen vascular disorders, steroid use, immunosuppressive therapy, and a history of radiation therapy in proximity to the surgical site.

A common feature in several of these risk factors is a hypoxic state at the wound edge. T. K. Hunt[11,31] has used microelectrode studies to plot a tissue oxygen profile from an experimentally induced wound edge back to normal tissue. Several salient features emerge in this model of wound healing. First, the center of a wound can be very hypoxic (i.e., $Po_2$ = 0-10 TORR). Second, the measured oxygen tension is a balance between the oxygen supply to the microenvironment and tissue use. Regions of high leukocyte activity or rapid collagen formation (a needed step in wound closure) act as oxygen "sinks" and rapidly consume the oxygen dissolved in the interstitial fluid. In some cases, the oxygen demand outstrips the ability to supply this vital substrate. Hydroxylation of lysine and proline (rate limiting in collagen formation) slows or halts in a hypoxic setting.[14,21] Furthermore, polymorphonuclear (PMN) leukocyte activity in killing bacteria is highly dependent upon the presence of oxygen for the "oxidative burst" that is lethal to bacteria. Incapacitation of the white blood cell by tissue hypoxia may explain why hypoxic wounds not only do not heal but also tend to become infected.[10,12]

It is possible to measure oxygen levels transcutaneously and to predict which wounds will fail to heal. Transcutaneous oximetry ($T_{COM}$) is widely used in the orthopedic, peripheral vascular, and wound management communities for the quantitative assessment of oxygen balance in failing wounds.[28] A series of small wells (Figure 88.6) are sealed to skin that has been shaved and cleaned with a mild astringent cleanser. A conductive solution fills the well. Modified Clark oxygen electrodes are sealed in the wells. The electrode contains a small heating coil that heats the skin underlying the well to 43° to 45°C. The vasodilation under the heated $T_{COM}$ electrode "arterializes" the capillary and venous blood and yields the best measure of underlying tissue oxygenation. $T_{COM}$ values can be normal or low and, if they are low, they may be either responsive to oxygen administration or oxygen nonresponsive. Each of these findings provides valuable prognostic and diagnostic information.

Normal $T_{COM}$ values (30-60 TORR) predict a wound that is not hypoxic and should heal without difficulty. Should the wound still fail to heal, a vigorous search for aggravating causes of wound nonhealing should be initiated. Retained

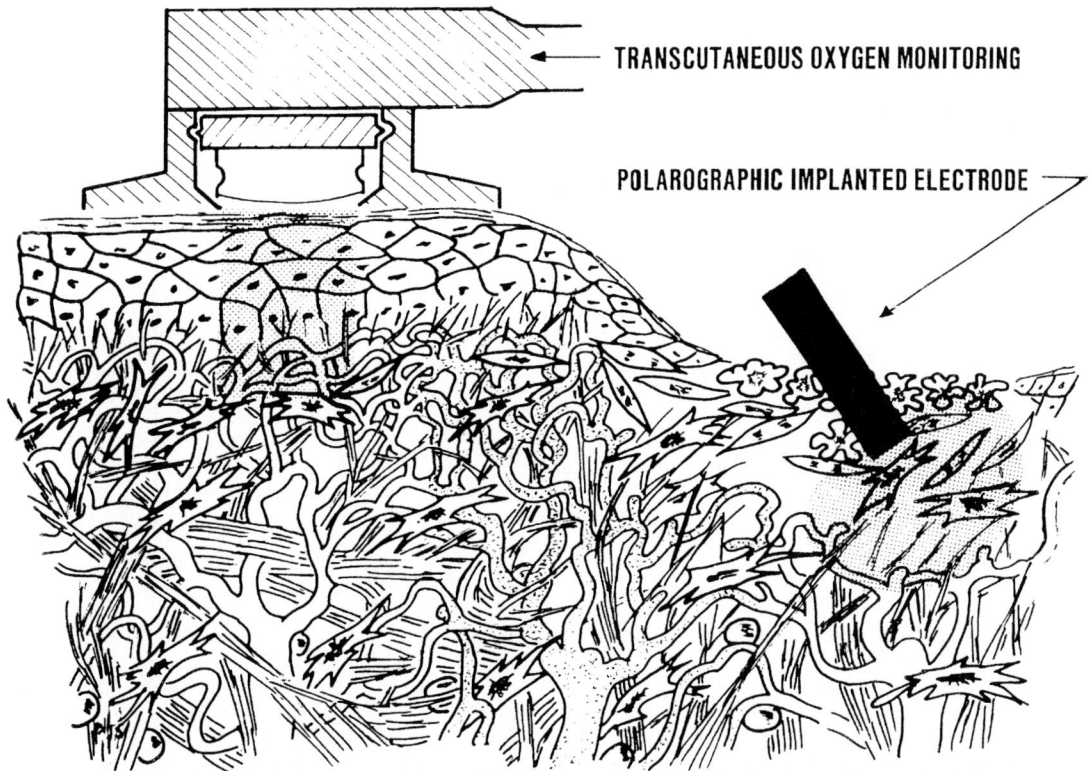

**Figure 88.6** Transcutaneous oximetry uses a polarographic (Clark) electrode to measure $Po_2$ in a fluid-filled well, sealed over an area of prepared skin. A heating element within the electrode warms the underlying skin to generate a local cutaneous vasodilation. This technique is easily replicated and less invasive than implanted platinum electrode studies that are now used only in the research setting.

foreign bodies, metabolic disarray, reaction to suture material, wound infection, nutritional factors, and Münchhausen syndrome are a few of the conditions that should be ruled out. Diabetic patients, perhaps as a result of their microvascular disease, appear to have a higher threshold for wound healing and typically require at least 40 TORR for tissue oxygen levels to ensure wound healing.

Patients with subnormal (less than 40 TORR) $T_{COM}$ values are given an "oxygen challenge" with 100% $F_{I}O_2$ administered via a hood (most "nonrebreather" masks administer only 70% to 80% $F_{I}O_2$). Those skin areas without at least a doubling in $T_{COM}$ values are both hypoxic and oxygen nonresponsive. This is the hallmark of macrovascular insufficiency and generally requires a procedure to enhance macrovascular flow to the area. The specific procedure can range from an arterial bypass graft to a vascularized flap to angioplasty of a stenosed feeding vessel. Success in any of these revascularization procedures should be heralded by substantially increased $T_{COM}$ values on a post-procedure measurement.

$T_{COM}$ values that are low (0-40 TORR) but respond briskly with a doubling of $T_{COM}$ value upon "oxygen challenge" predict wounds that will benefit from hyperbaric oxygen therapy. The best data interpretation is that there is evidence of microvascular insufficiency with a high likelihood of a favorable response to a course of hyperbaric oxygen.[29,30]

## HBO Treatment

HBO involves patients breathing 100% $F_{I}O_2$ in a chamber where the entire body is exposed to increased barometric pressure. The general public is familiar with these devices as "decompression chambers." The advantage of HBO is that tissue oxygen levels can intermittently be raised quite high (generally several 100 TORR) (Figure 88.7). These ultra high oxygen tensions inhibit anaerobic bacteria, enhance leukocyte function in killing bacteria, accelerate collagen formation, and ultimately contribute to neovascularization of the hypoxic tissue, particularly in tissues made hypovascular by wounding or prior radiation therapy.[1,20,27] HBO is relatively safe; for example, oxygen-related seizure activity occurs at a rate of approximately 1:10,000 at the most common treatment settings.[5]

HBO is not universally available; there are about 300 chambers in the entire country. Typical treatment schedules for nonhealing wounds involve a 2-hour "dive" daily for 3 weeks. HBO therapy is expensive (about $500 per session), but nonhealing wounds are expensive in general, with most refractory wounds costing thousands of dollars in addition to patient morbidity.[17] Careful patient selection and pretreatment $T_{COM}$ screening helps identify those patients most likely to benefit from hyperbaric therapy. Typical patients include those with radiation-damaged tissues (soft tissue or bone), chronic refractory osteomyelitis, documented hypoxic wounds unresponsive

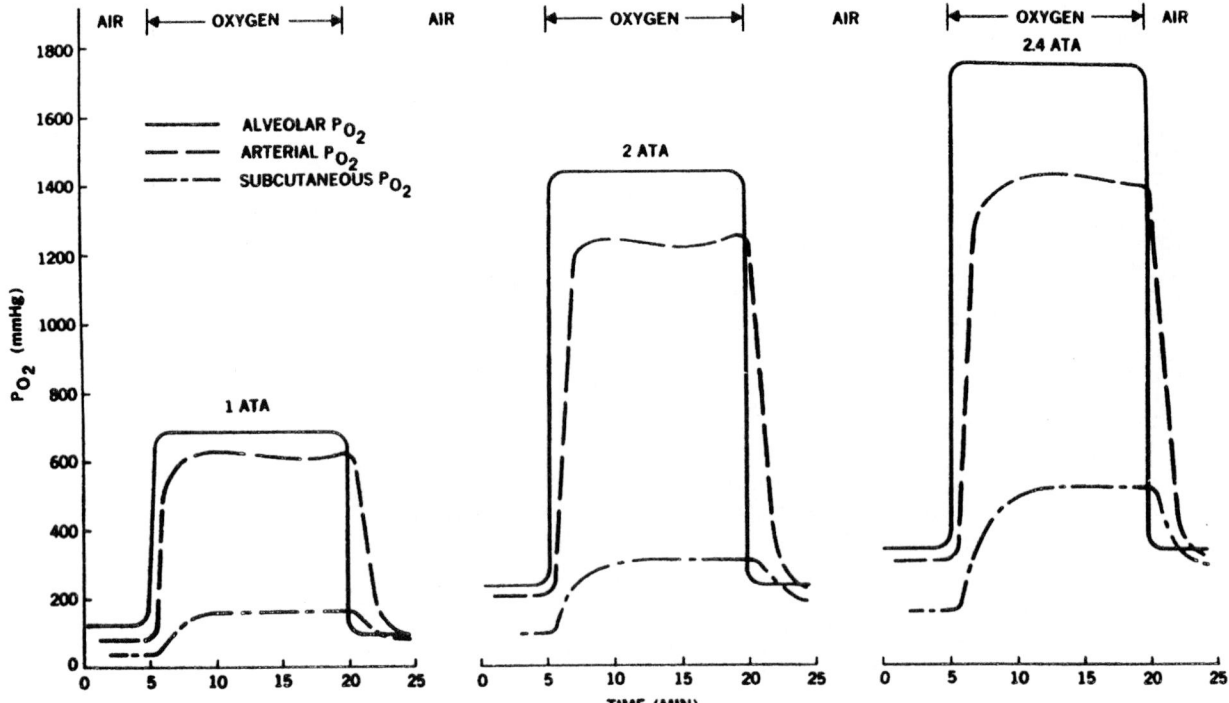

**Figure 88.7** Alveolar, arterial, and tissue oxygen tension during normobaric and hyperbaric oxygen breathing. *ATA* refers to "atmosphere's absolute." One ATA is 1 atmosphere, that is, 760mmHg of barometric pressure. A typical wound treatment depth is 2.4 ATA which corresponds to the same pressure as 45 feet of sea water. *(From Sheffield PJ: Tissue oxygen measurements. In Davis JC, Hunt TK [eds]:* Problem Wounds: The Role of Oxygen. *New York, Elsevier, 1988, 17-51.)*

to conventional therapy, and grafts and flaps at risk of failure.

If the surgery is elective and the patient has a history of radiation therapy near the proposed surgical site, it is recommended that the patient receive 20 HBO treatments *prior to the surgery,* followed by 10 treatments after the procedure. The necessity of HBO in this setting rises in proportion to the intensity of the RT treatments, the lapse of time since the RT and the proximity of the RT ports to the area of surgery. Anything more than 5000cGY of radiation therapy is considered a significant exposure and is likely to result in a progressive and linear loss in microvascular density in the path of the RT beam.[19] Tissue oxygen levels are roughly proportional to vascular density. A progressive paucity of vessels results in hypoxic tissue that is incapable of supplying the elevated oxygen demands of wound healing. The authors' HBO treatment recommendations are based on the elegant basic and clinical investigation of Marx and Johnson[18] working to find the cause and cure of osteoradionecrosis of the mandible following RT therapy for head and neck cancer. These investigators found that adding HBO to the standard treatment regimen increased their cure rate twelvefold and actually decreased overall medical expenses.[18] Although there are no specific investigations of HBO use for healing back wounds, logic suggests that the same principles should apply at other anatomic locations, particularly those without the profuse and redundant vascular supply of the head and neck.

For chronic, nonhealing wounds without prior radiation exposure, HBO was commonly used as part of the "preparation or preservation of a graft." A frequent outcome was that the wound rapidly progressed to complete healing after HBO is initiated, without the need for graft. In an unfortunate twist of events, HCFA has recently ruled that "preparation for a graft" can only take place *after* a graft has been placed and then failed. Because of this, patients must now have a graft before initiating the HBO therapy, or they may be personally liable for the costs of HBO therapy.

If there is exposed bone or other clinical or radiographic evidence of chronic osteomyelitis as part of a nonhealing wound, there is an indication for HBO therapy. Not only does HBO itself enhance WBC function against bacteria,[17] HBO greatly enhances the efficacy of certain classes of antibiotics such as aminoglycosides, vancomycin, clindamycin, sulfonamides, and quinolone.[2,7,8,15,27] HBO is one component of comprehensive therapy for chronic, refractory osteomyelitis, along with debridement, culture-driven antibiotics, smoking cessation, and adequate nutrition.

In summary, the vast majority of surgical wounds will heal without recourse to HBO therapy (although increased inspired oxygen at one atmosphere in the perioperative period has been shown to reduce the incidence of wound infections).[9,13] Those wounds that are refractory to conventional therapy frequently have hypoxia as a component of their failure to heal. Transcutaneous oxygen mapping

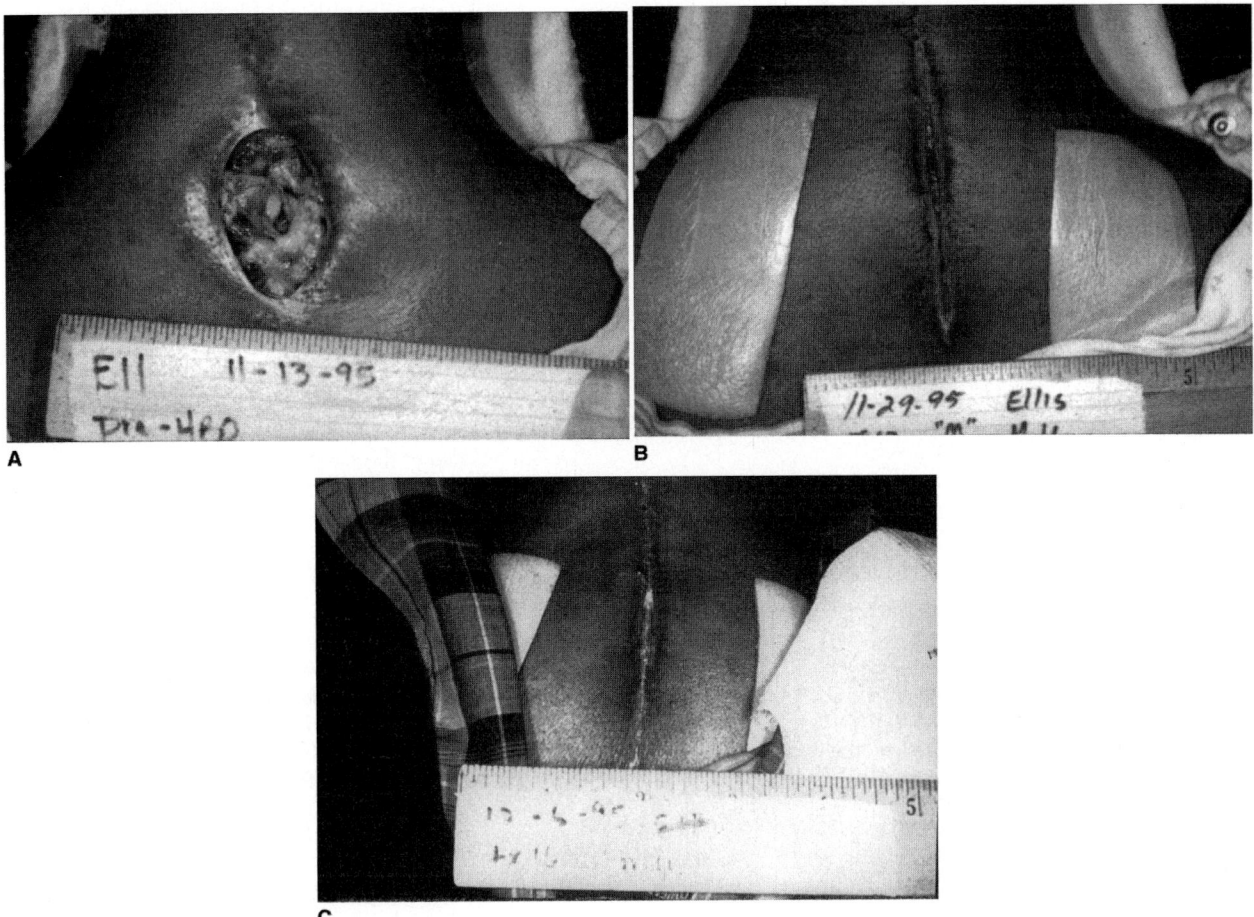

**Figure 88.8** Three views of a nonhealing wound over the cervical spine. (**A**) Initial HBO clinic visit. Rolled wound edges indicate chronicity of wound with healing "stalled." Suture material is visible at the base of the wound. (**B**) Wound closing after 10 HBO treatments at 2.4 ATA. (**C**) Full wound edge apposition after 16 HBO treatments.

around the wound edge can document tissue oxygen levels, and an "oxygen challenge" can identify those tissues that will require macrovascular intervention versus those that should respond to HBO therapy. When administered for the proper indications and with due diligence for patient safety, HBO is frequently an integral component in resolving the problem wound (Figure 88.8).

## Summary

Successful treatment of dorsal trunk defects depends on adherence to sound basic surgical principles. Debridement of necrotic tissue, elimination of dead space, elimination of pressure points, aggressive treatment of infection, and the provision of an adequate quantity of vascularized tissue should result in successful closure of most soft-tissue defects. The specific surgical option chosen depends on the anatomic location of the wound, its size, and the quality and quantity of tissue missing. Defects that do not expose underlying bone or hardware and that exhibit good blood supply may be closed with skin grafts, local flaps, or by tissue expansion techniques. Larger and deeper wounds require a combination of surgical techniques, often including pedicled myocutaneous flaps. In severe cases, it may be necessary to provide wound closure using microvascular anastomoses to import adequate tissue based on vasculature outside the zone of injury. In most cases, early debridement and closure provide the best opportunity to minimize complications and result in satisfactory wound healing.

## REFERENCES

1. Adams KR, Roberts RM, Mader JT: In vitro killing of *Clostridium perfringens* by oxygen with and without polymorphonuclear leucocytes. *Undersea Biomed Res* 17(suppl):123, 1990.

2. Bryan LE, Kwan S: Mechanisms of aminoglycoside resistance of anaerobic bacteria and facultative bacteria grown anaerobically. *J Antimicrob Chemother* 8D:1, 1981.

3. Clemante CD: Muscles and fascia. In *Gray's Anatomy*, ed 13. Philadelphia, Lea & Febiger, 1985, p 429.

4. Clemante CD: The arteries. In *Gray's Anatomy*, ed 13. Philadelphia, Lea & Febiger, 1985, p 648.

5. Davis JC: Complications. In Davis JC, Hunt TK (eds): *Problem Wounds: The Role of Oxygen*. New York, Elsevier, 1988.

6. El-Tamer MD, Chaglassian T: Wound management in spinal surgery. In Sundaresan N, Schmidek HH, Schiller AL, Rosenthal DI (eds): *Tumors of the Spine: Diagnosis and Clinical Management*. Philadelphia, WB Saunders, 1990, pp 504-519.

7. Gottlieb SF, Conley J: Interactions of increased pressures of oxygen and sulfonamides on the in vitro and in vivo growth of pathogenic bacteria. *Undersea Biomed Res* 7:95, 1980.

8. Gottlieb SF: Effect of hyperbaric oxygen on microorganisms. *Annu Rev Microbiol* 25:111, 1971.

9. Greif R, Akca O, Horn EP, *et al:* Supplemental perioperative oxygen to reduce the incidence of surgical-wound infection. *N Engl J Med* 342:161, 2000.

10. Hohn DC, MacKay RD, Halliday B, *et al:* The effect of $O_2$ tension on the microbiocidal function of leukocytes in wounds and in vitro. *Surg Forum* 27:18, 1976.

11. Hunt TK, van Winkle Jr.: Wound healing: disorders of repair. In Dunphy JE (ed): *Fundamentals of Wound Management in Surgery*. South Plainfield, NJ, Chirurgecom, 1976, p 37.

12. Klebanoff SJ: Oxygen metabolism and the toxic properties of phagocytes. *Ann Intern Med* 93:480, 1980.

13. Kotani N, Hashimoto, Sessler DI, *et al:* Supplemental intraoperative oxygen augments antimicrobial and proinflammatory responses of alveolar macrophages. *Anesthesiology* 93:15, 2000.

14. Lind F: How do tissue cells react to varying $O_2$ tensions? In Bakker DJ, Le Pechon JC, Marroni A (eds): *Hyperbaric Oxygen: Wound Healing, Safety, Cost-effectiveness*. Flagstaff, AZ, Best Publishing Company, 1998, pp 55-62.

15. Mader JT, Adams KR, Couch LA, Sutton TE: Potentiation of tobramycin by hyperbaric oxygen in experimental *Pseudomonas aeruginosa* osteomyelitis. Twenty-seventh Interscience Conference on Antimicrobial Agents and Chemotherapy, 1987, p 1331.

16. Mader JT, Brown GL, Guckian JC, *et al:* A mechanism for the amelioration by hyperbaric oxygen of experimental staphylococcal osteomyelitis in rabbits. *J Infect Dis* 142:915, 1980.

17. Marroni A, Hamilton-Farrell MR, Oriani G, Longobardi P: Cost-effectiveness of hyperbaric oxygen therapy. In Bakker DJ, Le Pechon JC, Marroni A (eds): *Hyperbaric Oxygen: Wound Healing, Safety, Cost-effectiveness*. Flagstaff, AZ, Best Publishing Company, 1998, pp 179-199.

18. Marx RE, Johnson RP: Studies in the radiobiology of osteoradionecrosis and their clinical significance. *Oral Surgery* 64:379, 1987.

19. Marx RE: Radiation injury to tissue. In Kindwall EP (ed): *Hyperbaric Medicine Practice*. Flagstaff, AZ, Best Publishing Company, 1955, pp 448-503.

20. Mathes SJ, Nahai F: Classification of the vascular anatomy of muscles—experimental and clinical correlation. *Plast Reconstr Surg* 67:177-187, 1981.

21. McGilvery RW: *Biochemistry: A Functional Approach*. Philadelphia, WB Saunders, 1970, pp 85, 93.

22. Minami RT, Mills R, Pardoe R: Gluteus maximus myocutaneous flaps for repair of pressure sores. *Plast Reconstr Surg* 60:242, 1977.

23. Nahai F, Hagerty R: One-stage microvascular transfer of latissimus flap to the sacrum using vein grafts. *Plast Reconstr Surg* 77:312, 1986.

24. Nahai F, Seheflan M, Bostwick J: Reconstruction. In Mathes SJ, Nahai F: *Clinical Applications for Muscle and Musculocutaneous Flaps*. St Louis, CV Mosby, 1982, pp 349-361.

25. Park MK, Muvich KH, Myers RAM, Marzell L: Hyperoxia prolongs the aminoglycoside-induced postantibiotic effect in *Pseudomonas aeruginosa*. *Antimicrobial Agents and Chemotherapy* 35:691, 1991.

26. Park MP, Muhvich KH, Meyers RAM, Marzella L: Effects of hyperbaric oxygen in infectious diseases: basic mechanisms. In Kindwall EP (ed): *Hyperbaric Medicine Practice*. Flagstaff, AZ, Best Publishing Company, 1955, pp 141-172.

27. Seyfer AE, Joseph AS: Use of trapezius muscle for closure of complicated upper spinal defects. *Neurosurgery* 14: 341-345, 1984.

28. Sheffield PJ: Measuring tissue oxygen tension. In Bakker DJ, Le Pechon JC, Marroni A (eds): *Hyperbaric Oxygen: Wound Healing, Safety, Cost-Effectiveness*. Flagstaff, AZ, Best Publishing Company, 1998, pp 25-41.

29. Sheffield PJ: Measuring tissue oxygen tension: a review. *Undersea Hyper Med* 25(3):179, 1998.

30. Sheffield, PJ: Tissue oxygen measurements. In Davis JC, Hunt TK (eds): *Problem Wounds: The Role of Oxygen*. New York, Elsevier, 1988.

31. Silver IA: The measurement of oxygen tension in healing tissue. Presented at the International Symposium on Oxygen Pressure Recording, Nijmegan, 1968. *Int Anesthesiol Clin* 4(1):135-153, 1966.

32. Stevenson TR, Rohrich RJ, Pollock RA, *et al:* More experience with the "reverse" latissimus dorsi musculocutaneous flap: precise location of blood supply. *Plast Reconstr Surg* 74:237, 1984.

33. Zide BM, Wisoff JH, Epstein FJ: Closure of extensive and complicated laminectomy wounds: operative technique. *J Neurosurg* 67:59, 1987.

# CHAPTER 89

# Spinal Reoperations

## Edward S. Connolly and Donlin M. Long

Often reoperations on the spinal column are more technically difficult than previous operations, and the risk of surgical complications is potentially greater. In addition to the technical problems of reoperations, the clinical and radiographic evaluation of the patient is more difficult. Because normal anatomic relationships and normal tissue planes have been altered, imaging is less accurate, and the surgical pathology is more difficult to recognize.

Magnetic resonance imaging (MRI) remains the most valuable imaging study, but it may not be adequate for examination of bony detail. Plain films are of great importance for determining exactly what was done previously, and computed tomography (CT) scanning with two- and three-dimensional reconstruction can provide bony detail that is very useful during surgery. The techniques are particularly useful for recognizing failed fusion or instability secondary to pars fracture. CT myelography is still useful when there is question about pathology definition.

When reoperating on the spine, some general principles of wound healing should be kept in mind. If the reoperation is being performed through the same approach as previous surgical interventions, the scar in the skin may be excised so that fresh skin edges are approximated. This may reduce the chance of superficial wound infection, wound dehiscence, and a poor cosmetic outcome. Also, in a reoperation, the surgical field should be exposed beyond the scar tissue and into normal surgical planes, so that the surgeon is working from normal anatomy on either side of the scar. Foreign material in the wound, which could be a source for bacterial contamination, is removed unless doing so would create excessive tissue destruction or unacceptable instability.

Usually, reoperations on the spinal column are performed for the following reasons and each requires specific experience and each involves specific consideration: (1) recurrent or persistent neural compression, (2) development of, or persistence of, instability, (3) cerebrospinal fluid (CSF) leak, and (4) infection.

## Neural Compression

The most common reason for reoperation on the spine is recurrent or persistent neural compression. Of all the indications for reoperation for neural compression, recurrent or persistent radiculopathy (radiculitis secondary to disc or scar), is by far the most common.* Other indications include persistent radiculitis with an inadequate decompression of the nerve root in patients with a large foraminal osteophyte and inadequate decompression of the spinal cord or cauda

*References 4,7,8,10,11,15,21,23,28.

equina in spinal stenosis, calcified nerve, ossification of the posterior longitudinal ligament, or in neoplasia.[20,31]

The differentiation of a recurrent disc from an epidural scar presents a dilemma. A recurrent disc has a substantially better prognosis with reoperation. However, the discovery of a focal mass of scar that is obviously compressing a nerve root may still be an indication for surgery. Diffuse epidural scar without nerve root compression, however, is not.

## Lumbar Radiculopathy or Radiculitis

Reoperation for a recurrent lumbar disc herniation requires lengthening the surgical excision to fully expose the normal laminae above and below the interspace and the freeing of the scar from the previous laminotomy using sharp dissection with a tool such as a sharp curette or a no. 15-blade knife. A high-speed drill or angled punch is used to obtain further bony decompression and to allow visualization of normal epidural tissue. Persistent ligamentum flavum remaining from less extensive laminotomies should be removed and the disc space approached rostrally to caudally, working from normal epidural tissue rostrally toward the disc space and nerve root. It is important to completely dissect out the nerve root, with good exposure of the axilla of the nerve root and its entire course in the lateral recess. If the dura mater or the nerve root is firmly attached to a recurrent disc fragment, sharp dissection and magnification should be used to free it so that no dural tear occurs during manipulation of the disc fragment. Utmost care should be taken to visualize the paramedian aspect of the disc, which is frequently the site of residual or persistent compressive disc herniations. Exploration, both above and below the disc space, should be carried out to ensure that at the conclusion of the second procedure, no extruded fragment has migrated over the body of the vertebra above or below the disc space. Using a microinstrument, the surgeon should circumferentially feel around the nerve root as it passes through the lateral recess and along its course in the neural foramen. Any dural tears that occur during the dissection should be repaired, if possible, before further dissection is performed. Repairing the dura mater prevents significant CSF fluid loss with a resultant decompression of the dural sac and increased risk of epidural venous bleeding. If the dura mater cannot be repaired using microsurgical suturing techniques, absorbable gelatin sponge and fibrin tissue adhesive are usually effective in closing the rent. Fat is an alternative seal.

## Reoperation for Thoracic Disc Herniation

Reoperation for thoracic disc is usually due to persistent or inadequately removed centrally located calcified discs. The removal of these centrally located discs requires a ventral approach, usually transthoracic, with a partial carpectomy and interbody fusion. Other indications for reoperation for thoracic disc herniation are missed level at the first operation, missed intradural herniation, and CSF leaks. The leaks are managed with fibrin glue, dura gel, or muscle followed by a lumbar subarachnoid drain for a few days.[6]

## Inadequate Decompression of the Nerve Root in Patients with a Large Foraminal Osteophyte

Reoperation for persistent cervical nerve root compression can usually be undertaken via one of several options. In a patient with a previous ventral cervical diskectomy and fusion and with a persistent large osteophyte in the neural foramen, correction may be accomplished by performing a simple cervical foraminotomy from a dorsal approach, with or without drilling off the osteophyte. This procedure is probably easier than reoperating from the ventral approach and drilling out the previous fusion and decompressing the foramen. If, however, the osteophyte is ventral and medial and cannot be decompressed adequately from a dorsal approach, a reoperation from the ventral approach should be performed. Soft-tissue problems associated with reoperating in the ventral cervical region are usually not prohibitive. The tissue planes may be slightly scarred, but the tissue plane between the carotid sheath and the esophagus and trachea is usually relatively maintained and easily dissected. If the soft-tissue scarring is due to previous infection or radiation therapy, the operation may be simplified by operating from the opposite or virgin side. An operation being performed by the ventral approach for inadequate neural decompression requires increased bone resection, at least a minicorpectomy, to obtain a 7-mm or 8-mm removal of each vertebral body rostrally and caudally to the disc space and definitive visualization of both nerve roots with magnification. This is often best accomplished by using a high-speed drill and an operating microscope. If the problem is a persistent central osteophyte or ossification of the posterior longitudinal ligament, corpectomy is the safest ventral approach, allowing complete decompression of the spinal cord. The corpectomy is followed by a ventral interbody fusion.

## Inadequate Decompression of the Cauda Equina in Spinal Stenosis

Reoperations from a dorsal approach after a laminectomy or foraminotomy require great care to prevent injury to the dura mater and the neural structures. Again, the incision is extended both rostrally and caudally. After the previous skin scar has been excised and the deep fascia exposed, the vertebrae above and below the laminectomy defect are exposed. Next, with the surgeon working from both a rostral and caudal direction, the soft tissues are removed from the remaining lateral mass and facet joints, with care taken to avoid the midline scar. The bone above and below the scar is then freed with a small, sharp curette or periosteal elevator and drilled off. This exposes normal ligamentum flavum, which is then sharply removed. Both above and below the scarred site, a dissection plane can be developed between the dura mater and the previous scar using a small dissector, and the scar can be opened and sharply removed. The widening of a previous laminectomy can often be best accomplished with a high-speed drill under magnification. After the bone is drilled down to a thin shell, the last millimeter of bone is removed with a small, sharp curette or an angled punch. A malleable retractor may be used to protect the dura from possible damage by the drill. Drilling requires substantial experi-

ence, best gained in the laboratory or in less demanding surgeries.

## Inadequate Decompression of the Spinal Cord in Neoplasia

A reoperation for persistent spinal cord compression, secondary to epidural tumor, usually results from a dorsal decompression that was performed on a ventrally or ventrolaterally situated tumor. A different surgical approach, either a lateral extracavitary or a ventral approach, is required for resection of tumor and decompression of the spinal cord, as well as for appropriate stabilization of the spinal column. Reexposure of the dorsal spine may also be necessary for performing dorsal arthrodesis and segmental instrumentation to supplement the ventral arthrodesis.

Reoperation for intradural tumors requires exposing the dura mater in the same manner as previously described. Intraoperative real-time ultrasound is extremely helpful for planning the dural opening and its extent. If a previous dural incision with retained suture material is present, the dura mater should be opened above and below the previous dural closure, and a small blunt dissector should be used to free the underlying spinal cord or arachnoid from the dura mater as the dura is opened. When the dura mater has been opened a second time, placing a dural patch graft on the closure is usually prudent, both to reduce the chances of the dura mater adhering to the spinal cord and to provide increased room for the spinal cord.

Dissection of recurrent tumor from nerve roots and the spinal cord needs to be accomplished under high magnification. Great care regarding hemostasis is necessary to allow good visualization under high magnification. Dissection is obtained best by using sharp dissection with two-point microcoagulation. If no neurologic structures are deep to the tumor, a laser may be used. The laser is particularly effective in removing ventrally based dural tumors.

## Extrusion of a Bone Graft

The development of instability, extrusion of a bone graft, failure of fusion, or failure of instrumentation is an indication for reoperation.* Extrusion of a cervical interbody bone graft may not require surgery if the spine is stable and no associated pain or swallowing difficulty is present. If, however, persistent pain, cervical deformity, or swallowing difficulty is present, reoperation is indicated. The extruded bone fragment is removed; the graft site is freshened, usually by use of a high-speed drill to accomplish good exposure of cancellous bone, and a new graft is inserted. If any question arises about the security of this graft, a ventral plate-and-screw construct provides further assurance of retention of the bone graft. A ventral plate is indicated if the graft extrusion occurs in the setting of an unstable spine. The extrusion of a strut graft associated with a corpectomy may have been caused either by a poorly fitting graft or by fracture of the vertebral body into which the graft is fixed. This allows for the caudal portion of the graft to extrude ventrally. The dislocation of the

---

*References 1,2,9,14,16-18,20,25-27,31-34.

graft may be associated with collapse of the disc spaces that, in turn, may cause nerve root irritation and pain. Furthermore, the extruded graft may result in esophageal compression. If symptoms are present, reoperation is indicated. If the vertebral body is fractured as well, a partial corpectomy of the fractured segment must be performed and the graft refitted. This necessitates a longer graft. Ventral plating with screw fixation may add to the stability of the new construct. A supplement to fixation via a dorsal approach should often be considered. Postoperatively, it is prudent for the patient to wear an orthosis.

## Failure of Fusion

The development of a pseudarthrosis of a dorsal cervical fusion is most common in rheumatoid arthritis at the C1 or C2 vertebral level.[5] Realignment should be attempted with mild traction and neck extension. At reoperation, the previous bone graft and wire constructs are removed. If acrylic was placed, it must be removed. Sometimes a high-speed burr is required to remove this material or to free the wires from the acrylic. If the arch of C1 is still intact, the fusion is carried out by using a dorsal iliac crest graft, saddled between the arch of C1 and the spinous process of C2 and secured in place with wire or cable. The cortical surfaces of C1 and C2 are scored laterally with a high-speed burr, and onlay grafts of cancellous bone are placed from C1 to C2. Halo or Minerva orthoses should be employed postoperatively. If the arch of C1 is incompetent, or as an alternative to the previously described scheme, lateral mass screw fixation or transarticular screw fixation of C1 and C2 can be performed. One should ascertain that no defect is present in the lateral mass that could cause a potential injury to the vertebral artery.[22] If screw fixation is performed, an onlay graft is still indicated, with use of cancellous bone from the dorsal ilium.

If this technique is not practical or if the bone quality is poor, a fusion of occiput to C2 or C3 should be performed. A Luque rectangle that has been bent to provide the proper occipitocervical angle may be wired to the occiput and to C2 and C3 with sublaminar wires. Cancellous bone grafts are onlayed from the occiput to C3. A recent report of a higher fusion rate with a Y-plate-and-screw fixation suggests that screw fixation may be the procedure of choice for occipitocervical fusion in rheumatoid arthritis.[13]

Instability may develop after ventral diskectomy without fusion or after a failed ventral fusion. Refusion may be performed via direct reexploration and the refashioning of the bone plug. The chance of healing of the second fusion is improved with ventral plating.

An alternative technique is to leave the ventral fusion as is and simply carry out a dorsal fusion with wired spinous processes and dorsolateral fusion. In most cases, this leads to prompt healing of the ventral pseudarthrosis.

### Development of Instability

Reoperation for the development of instability after decompressive laminectomies in the lumbar spine is best handled by intertransverse process and lateral mass onlay graft fusions, supplemented with pedicle screw fixation. Reoperation for pseudarthrosis of the lumbar spine requires reexposure of the graft site and removal of dead or nonviable bone graft, with meticulous care taken to denude the bone of all soft tissue and dead bone until good bleeding surfaces are exposed. The onlay bone grafts may be supplemented with pedicle screw-and-rod constructs. Direct current electrical stimulation appears to help in patients who have a high risk of fusion failure, such as patients who are diabetic or who have rheumatoid arthritis, those who smoke, and those with malnutrition or osteoporosis.[19] For failed interbody fusions, magnetic field stimulation is reported to improve fusion rates.[24,29] These cases are probably best handled by performing a dorsolateral onlay autogenous graft fusion with pedicle screw fixation.

## Failure of Instrumentation

Reoperation for screw backout or for poorly placed screws, in which the screw is placed in the disc space instead of in the vertebral body, simply requires removal of the screws and proper repositioning of the plate. However, a different plate length may be required. The screws are placed with use of real-time imaging. If screw backout occurs with lateral mass plates, the involved screws should be removed along with the plate or rods. An arthrodesis should then be performed, using another type of instrumentation and bone graft. Alternately, a ventral fusion with instrumentation may provide a better alternative.

Reoperation to remove instrumentation that has either failed or has eroded through the skin requires full exposure of the instrumentation and construct, with care taken to not create fracture of the bone grafts or vertebral column when removing the implant. Large metal shears and rod cutters may create enough torque to actually fracture the dorsal elements of the vertebra and should be used with great caution. A high-speed carbide burr may be used to cut the rods, but all exposed soft tissue should be covered to prevent the small metal filings from being spread throughout the wound. Otherwise, these filings cause a great deal of artifactual change on future imaging studies.

## Cerebrospinal Fluid Leak

Reoperation for CSF leak requires adequate exposure of the dural defect. This may require further bone removal. A patch of autologous fascia and fibrin tissue adhesive,[3,12,30] followed by placement of a CSF drain for 5 days may be used for dural repair if primary dural closure fails. The deep fascia is closed tightly with interrupted sutures and a continuous locking suture is then placed over the interrupted suture closure, thus providing a watertight fascial closure.

## Infection

Reoperation for wound infection is best handled by reopening the complete length of the incision to the depth of infectious involvement. After all suture material is removed, along with any dead tissue, the wound is debrided to bleeding tissue. The wound should then be irrigated thoroughly with antibiotic solution. If the infection is superficial, the wound is closed with a single layer of through-and-through monofilament mattress sutures, and for 10 days the patient is given the appropriate intravenous antibiotics to which the organism is susceptible. For deep infections and for infections in the presence of instrumentation or bone grafts, a similar procedure is carried out, but the deep fascia is closed with polyglycol absorbable sutures over multiple-holed catheters for antibiotic irrigation and drainage. Occasionally, a badly infected wound may be packed open for secondary closure when granulation is satisfactory. If osteomyelitis or diskitis is present, debridement of the involved bone and disc is performed via an extraperitoneal approach in the lumbar spine, a lateral extracavitary approach in the thoracic spine, and a ventral approach in the cervical spine. A fresh autologous cortical bone graft is inserted for ventral stabilization. The antibiotics are usually continued for 6 weeks or even longer if the C-reactive protein level has not returned to normal by that time. The patient is kept in an orthosis until fusion has occurred.

## Summary

Compared with virgin spine operations, reoperations require more extensive exposures. Therefore, the risk of spinal instability, neural damage, and infection is increased. The same techniques as used in the virgin operation are used in reoperations, but limitations created by scar tissue and the loss of bone and ligamentous structures that aid in spinal stability are present. When undertaking any reoperation on the spine, the surgeon must keep in mind that with each succeeding operation, the challenge is increased, and the chance of a good result is reduced.

Pain alone is not an indication for reoperation. Correctable anatomic abnormalities must be present to warrant repeat surgery.

It is always worthwhile to remember that the most common cause of failure of spinal surgery is not a technical error or complication, but failure of appropriate patient selection. When patients have been improperly chosen for surgery in the first place, it is not likely that repair of an unintended consequence of the first operation will be beneficial. On the other hand, it is unfair to leave patients with an uncorrected abnormality that is symptom producing. Repair of the demonstrated problem in such patients is reasonable. All patients with failed spinal surgery should, however, be carefully assessed for the presence of important comorbidities that may exaggerate the complaint of pain. These should be addressed simultaneously with reparative surgery.

## REFERENCES

1. Andrew TA, Brooks S, Piggott H: Long-term follow-up evaluation of screw-and-graft fusion of the lumbar spine. Clin Orthop 203:113-119, 1986.
2. Brodsky AE, Khalil MA, Sassard WR, Newman BP: Repair of symptomatic pseudarthrosis of anterior cervical fusion: posterior versus anterior repair. Spine 17:1137-1143, 1992.
3. Cain JE, Jr., Rosenthal HG, Broom MJ, et al: Quantification of leakage pressures after durotomy repairs in the canine. Spine 15:969-970, 1990.
4. Cauchoix J, Ficat C, Girard B: Repeat surgery after disc excision. Spine 3:256-259, 1978.
5. Clark CR, Goetz DD, Menezes AH: Arthrodesis of the cervical spine in rheumatoid arthritis. J Bone Joint Surg 71A:381-391, 1989.
6. Dickman CA, Rosenthal D, Regan JJ: Reoperation for herniated thoracic discs. J Neurosurg 91(2 suppl):157-162, 1999.
7. Ebeling U, Kalbarcyk H, Reulen HJ: Microsurgical reoperation following lumbar disc surgery: timing, surgical findings, and outcome in 92 patients. J Neurosurg 70: 397-404, 1989.
8. Echlin FA, Selverstone B, Scribner WE: Bilateral and multiple ruptured discs as one cause of persistent symptoms following operation for a herniated disc. Surg Gynecol Obstet 83:485-493, 1946.
9. Farey ID, McAfee PC, Davis RF, Long DM: Pseudarthrosis of the cervical spine after anterior arthrodesis. J Bone Joint Surg 72A:1171-1177, 1990.
10. Finnegan WJ, Fenlin JM, Marvel JP, et al: Results of surgical intervention in the symptomatic multiply-operated back patient: analysis of sixty-seven cases followed for three to seven years. J Bone Joint Surg 61A:1077-1081, 1979.
11. Frymoyer JW, Matteri RE, Hanley EN, et al: Failed lumbar disc surgery requiring second operation: long-term follow-study. Spine 3:7-11, 1978.
12. Gibble JW, Ness PM: Fibrin glue: the perfect operative sealant? Transfusion 30:741-747, 1990.
13. Grob D, Dvorak J, Panjabi MM, Antinnes JA: The role of plate and screw fixation in occipitocervical fusion in rheumatoid arthritis. Spine 19:2545-2551, 1994.
14. Grubb SA, Lipscomb HJ: Results of lumbosacral fusion for degenerative disc disease with and without instrumentation: Two- to five-year follow-up. Spine 17: 349-355, 1992.
15. Hardy RW: Repeat operation for lumbar disc. In Hardy RW (ed): Lumbar Disc Disease. New York, Raven Press, 1982, pp 193-202.
16. Hartman JT, McCarron RF, Robertson WW Jr.: A pedicle bone grafting procedure for failed lumbosacral spinal fusion. Clin Orthop 178:223-227, 1983.
17. Herkowitz HN, Kurz LT: Degenerative lumbar spondylolisthesis with spinal stenosis: a prospective study comparing decompression with decompression and intertransverse process arthrodesis. J Bone Joint Surg 73A:802-808, 1991.
18. Jackson RK, Boston DA, Edge AJ: Lateral mass fusion: a prospective study of a consecutive series with long-term follow-up. Spine 10:828-832, 1985.
19. Kane WJ: Direct current electrical bone growth stimulation for spinal fusion. Spine 13:363-365, 1988.
20. Katz JN, Lipson SJ, Larson MG, et al: The outcome of decompressive laminectomy for degenerative lumbar stenosis. J Bone Joint Surg 73A:809-816, 1991.
21. Law JD, Lehman RAW, Kirsch WM: Reoperation after lumbar intervertebral disc surgery. J Neurosurg 48: 259-263, 1978.

22. Marcotte P, Dickman CA, Sonntag VKH, et al: Posterior atlantoaxial facet screw fixation. *J Neurosurg* 79:234-237, 1993.

23. Martin G: Recurrent disc prolapse as a cause of recurrent pain after laminectomy for lumbar disc lesions. *N Z Med J* 91:206-208, 1980.

24. Mooney V: A randomized double-blind prospective study of the efficacy of pulsed electromagnetic fields for interbody lumbar fusions. *Spine* 15:708-712, 1990.

25. Mutoh N, Shinomiya K, Furuya K, et al: Pseudarthrosis and delayed union after anterior cervical fusion. *Int Orthop* 17:286-289, 1993.

26. Newman M: The outcome of pseudarthrosis after cervical anterior fusion. *Spine* 18:2380-2382, 1993.

27. Shinomiya K, Okamoto A, Kamikozuru M, et al: An analysis of failures in primary cervical anterior spinal cord decompression and fusion. *J Spinal Disord Tech* 6:277-288, 1993.

28. Silvers HR, Lewis PJ, Asch HL, Clabeaux DE: Lumbar diskectomy for recurrent disc herniation. *J Spinal Disord Tech* 7:408-419, 1994.

29. Simmons JW: Treatment of failed posterior lumbar interbody fusion (PLIF) of the spine with pulsing electromagnetic fields. *Clin Orthop* 193:127-132, 1985.

30. Stechison MT: Rapid polymerizing fibrin glue from autologous or single donor blood: preparation and indications. *J Neurosurg* 76:626-628, 1992.

31. Tuite GF, Stern JD, Doran SE, et al: Outcome after laminectomy for lumbar spinal stenosis. Part I. Clinical correlations. *J Neurosurg* 81:699-706, 1994.

32. West JL, III, Bradford DS, Ogilvie JW: Results of spinal arthrodesis with pedicle screw-plate fixation. *J Bone Joint Surg* 73A:1179-1184, 1991.

33. Wetzel FT, LaRocca H: The failed posterior lumbar interbody fusion. *Spine* 16:839-845, 1991.

34. Zindrick MR: The role of transpedicular fixation systems for stabilization of the lumbar spine. *Orthop Clin North Am* 22:333-344, 1991.

# CHAPTER 90

# Penetrating Spinal Cord Injuries

**Michael P. Steinmetz, William E. McCormick, Alex Valadka, Perry A. Ball, Philip A. Yazbak, and Edward C. Benzel**

Penetrating spine injury is a major cause of spinal cord injury (SCI) in the United States. Gunshot injuries have been reported to be the third leading cause of SCI.[46] Stab wounds and other penetrating injuries tend to occur less in the United States but are more common in some other countries. In South Africa, they account for 25% of all SCI.[25]

Avoiding complications in the management of patients with penetrating SCIs begins with meticulous attention to evaluation, resuscitation, and operative and surgical techniques.

## Military Versus Civilian Gunshot Injuries

Most experience with the management of penetrating spinal cord injuries has been gained during wartime. During Word War I survival was uncommon after a complete myelopathy (72% mortality). Treatment of these injuries consisted of laminectomy for incomplete myelopathy and debridement of the entry and exit wounds for complete myelopathy.[39] A high operative mortality (62%) added to the dismal outcome.

During World War II advances were made in trauma resuscitation and therapy. These advances decreased the mortality from penetrating SCI dramatically.[12,13,15] Some surgeons reported neurologic improvement in those that were managed surgically.[8] During the Korean war, most cases of penetrating SCI underwent surgical exploration. There were reports of significant improvement.[41] The treatment of civilian penetrating SCI, however, has generated less optimism than previous military reports.[14,19,35,36,45] This is likely related to the pathophysiology of this type of injury.

Military weapons fire high-velocity missiles, and civilian weapons (typically handguns) fire low-velocity missiles. The pathophysiology of the SCI differs based on velocity. High-velocity missiles may produce SCI by a concussive effect of the bullet passing close to, but not through, the spinal canal.[20] Most SCIs caused by high-velocity missiles may fit into this pattern. These types of injuries may have a slightly better prognosis. Low-velocity missiles are more likely to injure the spinal cord directly, without a significant concussive effect; therefore, the prognosis for recovery is worse due to the direct cord injury. This phenomenon may also explain the large percentage of civilian gunshot SCIs appearing as complete myelopathies.[3,7,14,35]

## IMPALEMENT PATHOPHYSIOLOGY

A weapon (knife) that penetrates the spinal canal may damage the spinal cord directly or indirectly. The direct injury may range from a dural tear to a total cord transection. Indirectly, there may be spinal cord contusion from the weapon impacting the cord against the bony spinal canal. The anatomy of the spinal canal may protect the spinal cord from a complete transection (Figure 90.1). The weapon usually enters the spinal canal in the gutter between the spinous process and transverse process, thus leading to an incomplete spinal cord injury. Classically, the Brown-Sequard syndrome or a variant results.[4]

## Resuscitation

The initial management of patients suffering from penetrating spinal cord injuries begins with advanced trauma life support (ATLS) measures. The airway should be evaluated and secured. If necessary, endotracheal intubation should be performed. Oral intubation using manual in-line traction has been shown to be both safe and effective in patients with suspected SCI.[11] Tracheostomy is indicated if the injury involves the trachea or larynx.[17] Chest radiographs and arterial blood gas analysis (if indicated) should be part of the initial evaluation.

The patient's early course may be complicated by hypotension. This may be as a result of blood loss (hypovolemia) or to neurogenic shock from the loss of sympathetic vasomotor tone. Determining the exact cause of the hypotension is often difficult in the acute setting. However, tachycardia and cool extremities are often observed with hypovolemia, and bradycardia is often observed with spinal shock.[4] The treatment for either condition is aggressive volume resuscitation. A central venous catheter is often helpful for monitoring the volume resuscitation. If the hypotension persists despite adequate intravascular volume replacement, vasopressor agents such as phenylephrine or dopamine should be employed. Vagolytic agents like atropine may also be used. An indwelling pulmonary artery catheter may be useful if hypotension persists despite the use of vasopressor agents.

A Foley catheter should be placed. This allows bladder decompression and assists with gauging of the effectiveness of volume resuscitation. It also decreases the likelihood of subsequent urologic complications.[4]

Once the patient is stable from a cardiopulmonary standpoint, a more thorough history and physical examination should be performed. Information about the mechanism of injury and the caliber of the weapon should be obtained. The physical examination should note if the patient has suffered a complete or incomplete myelopathy. If the injury is incomplete, the level of the SCI should be noted. The entry and exit sites should be inspected, and notation of cerebrospinal fluid or foreign material should be made.[8]

Treatment of nonneurologic injuries is of primary importance because such treatment is usually lifesaving (rather than function-preserving).[4] Because the course a penetrating object takes within the torso is unpredictable, there may be an associated visceral injury.[4] A trauma surgeon should assist with the evaluation for such potential injuries. Explorations or the neck, chest, and abdomen take precedence over spinal surgeries.[38]

Some advocate exploration for wounds that penetrate the platysma, whereas others advocate the individualization of surgical planning.[4] The two approaches appear equally effective if injuries to the great vessels, upper airway, and upper gastrointestinal tract can be ruled out via angiography, endoscopy, or swallowing studies.[21,22,27,32]

Pharyngeal perforation carries the risk of osteomyelitis.[1,17,32] There are divergent views on the appropriate management of pharyngeal perforation. Some advocate broad-spectrum antibiotics, debridement of bone and soft tissue, drainage, and immobilization.[17] Other authors[40] have reported a lower infection rate with neural decompression and debridement of the wound.

Penetrating thoracic injuries may damage the lungs or mediastinum. Chest radiography, computed tomography, and/or angiography may be used to define the extent of the injury. Tube thoracostomy or surgical exploration may be indicated.

## Radiographic Evaluation

Initial evaluation should begin with routine radiographs. Fractures and bullet fragments may be seen (Figure 90.2). A CT through the area of involvement should be performed next. This modality is generally superior to plain radiographs for the evaluation of the injury and for localizing the fracture or bullet fragments (Figure 90.3). The aforementioned will also give the surgeon a sense of spinal stability or instability. CT-myelography may be used to assess for neural compression. This modality may also aid in the evaluation of a CSF fistula. If there is a question of spinal instability, passive flexion/extension radiographs may be used.

Magnetic resonance imaging (MRI) may also be used in the evaluation. There will be artifact from the bullet fragments, but valuable information, such as the presence of extradural hematoma, disk herniation, or spinal cord

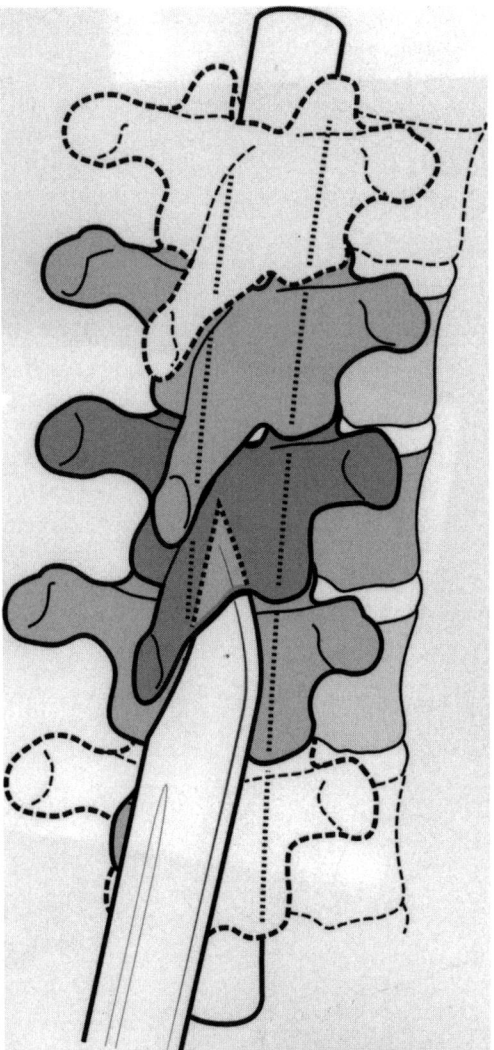

**Figure 90.1** A depiction of a stab wound to the spine. The weapon enters in the gutter between the spinous process and the transverse process. This anatomy prevents the weapon from crossing midline as it enters the spinal canal. A spinal cord hemisection, rather than a transection, often results.

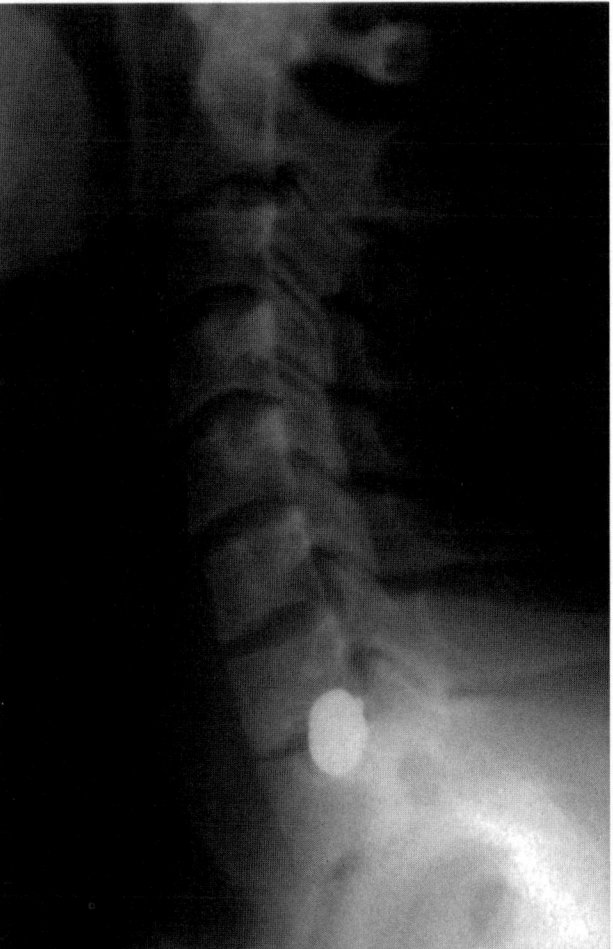

**Figure 90.2** Lateral radiograph demonstrating a bullet that has entered the spinal canal. It is in the proximity of the neural foramen.

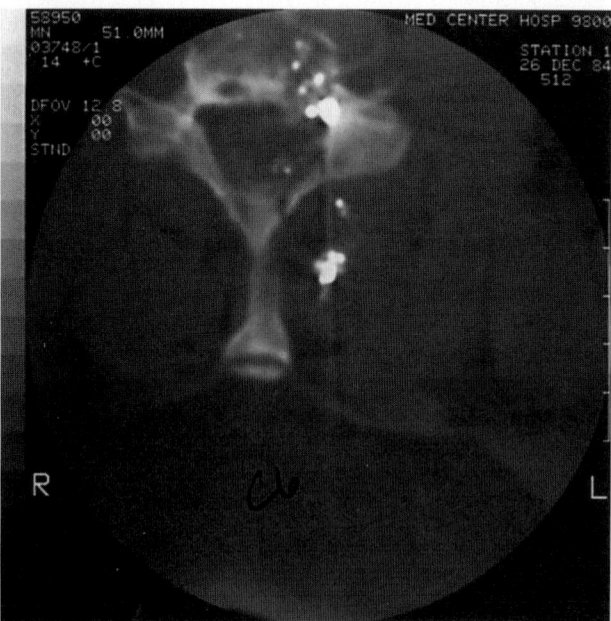

**Figure 90.3** Axial CT scan of a gunshot wound to the cervical spine demonstrating multiple fragments and a resultant fracture of the vertebral body.

contusion, may be gained. There is a risk of fragment migration in the magnetic field, so only those in whom the information gained would have been difficult to obtain with other imaging modalities should undergo MRI.[10]

## Steroids and Antibiotics

Experience with large patient populations has shown no improvement in outcome from using steroids in patients with penetrating spinal injuries.[4,6,26,34] This lack of efficacy and the potential adverse effects on wound healing and infection suggests no role for steroids in penetrating spinal injury patients.

The rate of infection in penetrating SCI during the Vietnam war was lower compared to prior conflicts. The reason for the lower incidence was predominantly the use of antibiotics.[16] Therefore, one may reasonably conclude that prophylactic antibiotics are of benefit in penetrating SCI. At least 7 days of antibiotic treatment for penetrating abdominal wounds with accompanying involvement of the spine have been shown to result in fewer infectious complications than shorter courses of antibiotic treatment.[31] The antibiotic agents should be chosen based on the region of the body injured and on local hospital bacterial sensitivities.

## Surgical Management

Protection of the integument, support of pulmonary function, and prophylaxis against deep vein thrombosis should be addressed immediately. Specialized nursing care is of the utmost importance. This should begin immediately. The patient should be turned frequently, and an aggressive pulmonary toilet program should be instituted.

## Surgical Indications
### Missile Injuries

Surgery may be indicated in the following circumstances: (1) cord compression with an incomplete injury, (2) a discrepancy between the clinical examination and the missile trajectory with a complete myelopathy, (3) a migratory missile fragment, (4) spinal instability, (5) associated infection, and (6) persistent CSF leak[3,4,7] (Figure 90.4). Consideration should be given to surgical exploration of lesions of the cauda equina regardless of neurologic status. Because such injuries involve nerve roots as opposed to the spinal cord proper, they have a better prognosis.[8] Surgery to remove a bullet fragment is not warranted except if there exists compression of the cauda equina. The composition of the bullet fragments has not been shown to adversely affect neurologic function.[24,33,36]

### Impalement Injuries

Indications for surgery include neural element compression by bone or soft-tissue fragments, retained fragments, CSF fistula, and infection. As opposed to gunshot injuries, retained foreign material should be removed after a stab wound. Because stab wounds are rarely delivered with enough force to cause spinal instability, this is an uncommon indication for surgery after these types of injuries.

## Surgical Techniques
### Dorsal Approach

The dorsal approach is used most commonly for treatment of penetrating SCIs.[4] A midline incision is made over the area of injury, and a standard subperiosteal dissection is used to gain access to the spine. Laminectomy or laminotomy is performed to expose the area of injury. Care should be taken to remove all compressive elements. Of particular importance is preservation of the facet joints to preserve spinal stability. The dura mater is often opened to expose the injured spinal cord or nerve roots. If an intramedullary mass with associated neurologic deficit is identified, it can be approached via midline myelotomy. Unnecessary injury to the posterior columns can be avoided by a strict adherence to the placement of the midline myelotomy, and liquefied clot can be removed from within the spinal cord with gentle irrigation and suction[4] (Figure 90.5).

Bullet and bone fragments that are compressing neural elements are removed. Not all fragments need be removed, especially if they are intramedullary. Foreign objects associated with an impalement injury should be removed.

Dural closure should be pursued aggressively, with care taken to not compromise intradural contents[4] (Figure 90.6). Watertight closure should be performed, either primarily, or with patching. Every effort should be made to use autologous material, such as local fascia or fascia lata. Ventral dural tears represent a challenge to repair from the dorsal approach. They may be left alone or may be loosely patched with muscle or other tissue. Fibrin-based tissue sealants are often helpful in treating such dural

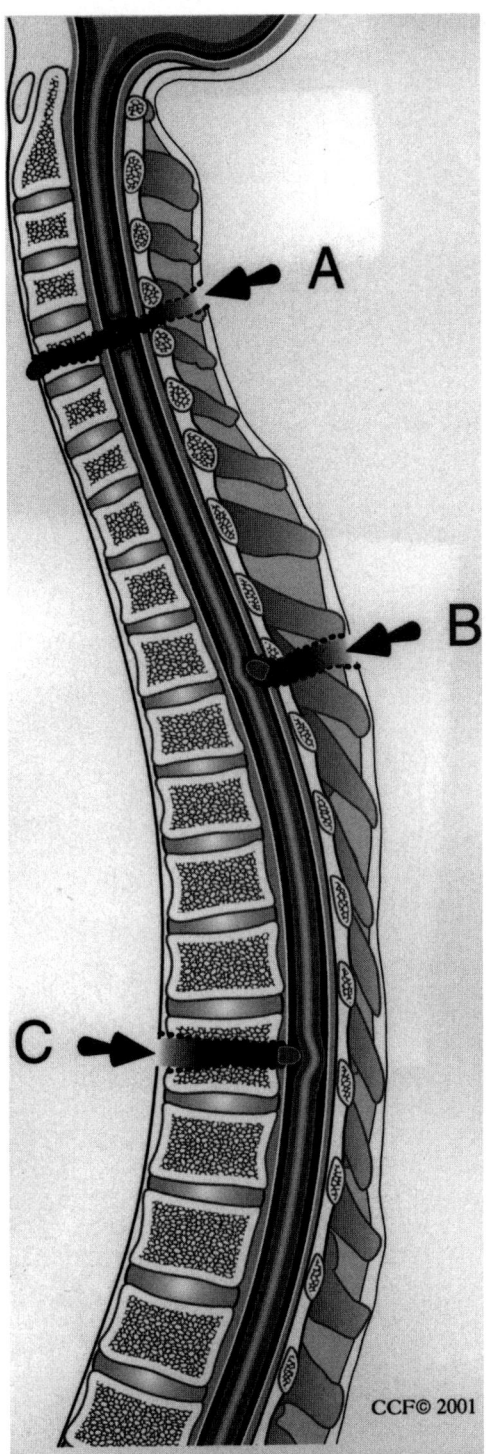

**Figure 90.4** Illustrations depicting injury types that may be treated surgically. **(A)** Through-and-through gunshot wound, which has resulted in a complete myelopathy with spinal instability or a neurologic level of injury that is significantly higher than the level of spinal injury. **(B)** A dorsal gunshot wound to the spine that has resulted in an incomplete myelopathy with spinal cord compression. Surgical decompression via laminectomy is indicated. **(C)** A gunshot wound has caused a ventral compression and an incomplete myelopathy. Surgical decompression is warranted. In the thoracic or lumbar spine, a ventral or dorsolateral strategy may be used.

lacerations. Cerebrospinal fluid diversion is another useful adjunct.

### Dorsolateral and Ventral Approaches

If a compressive lesion is lateral or ventral to the spinal cord, a dorsolateral or ventral approach may be indicated. Options include a transpedicular or costotransversectomy approach or a thoracotomy and lateral extracavitary approach for a more ventral exposure. Because these approaches do not provide wide exposure of the dura, they are rarely indicated.[3] If the spine has been judged unstable, appropriate fixation and fusion techniques should be employed.

### Closure

All closures should be accomplished in multiple layers. Drains should be avoided if at all possible.

## Prognosis

Prognosis is better after an impalement injury compared to a missile injury. Overall, 60% of patients with stab wounds are able to ambulate at follow-up, compared to 24% of those with SCI resulting from gunshot wounds.[43] Prognosis is poor with complete injury in either group.

## Complications

CSF fistula may occur at the entrance or exit site. Fistulous connections with the bowel, bladder, and pleural cavity have also been reported.[5,9,42] The initial management should be with subarachnoid drainage. If this fails, surgical exploration is warranted.

With the institution of prophylactic antibiotics, the incidence of infection after gunshot wounds has dramatically decreased.[31] The antibiotics should be given for 7 to 14 days and should be tailored to the body site violated and to local hospital sensitivities. The combination of removal of retained foreign material, debridement, and prophylactic antibiotics should achieve a low infection rate after an impalement injury.

Fever should prompt lumbar puncture to rule out meningitis. Late deterioration after penetrating SCI may indicate an infectious source, such as epidural abscess.

Metallic fragments have been reported to migrate in the CNS.[2,18,23,28] If there has been migration and the patient is asymptomatic, no treatment may be needed, and they may simply be followed. If the patient is or becomes symptomatic (e.g., radiculopathy or paresthesias), the fragment should be retrieved.

Lead intoxication after a gunshot injury is rare. Bullets become encapsulated by poorly vascularized fibrous tissue.[37] In addition, the lead from a bullet is relatively insoluble. Removal of a bullet for the purpose of decreasing lead intoxication is not warranted.

Penetrating spinal injuries often lead to deafferentation pain. This pain is problematic in that it is often refractory

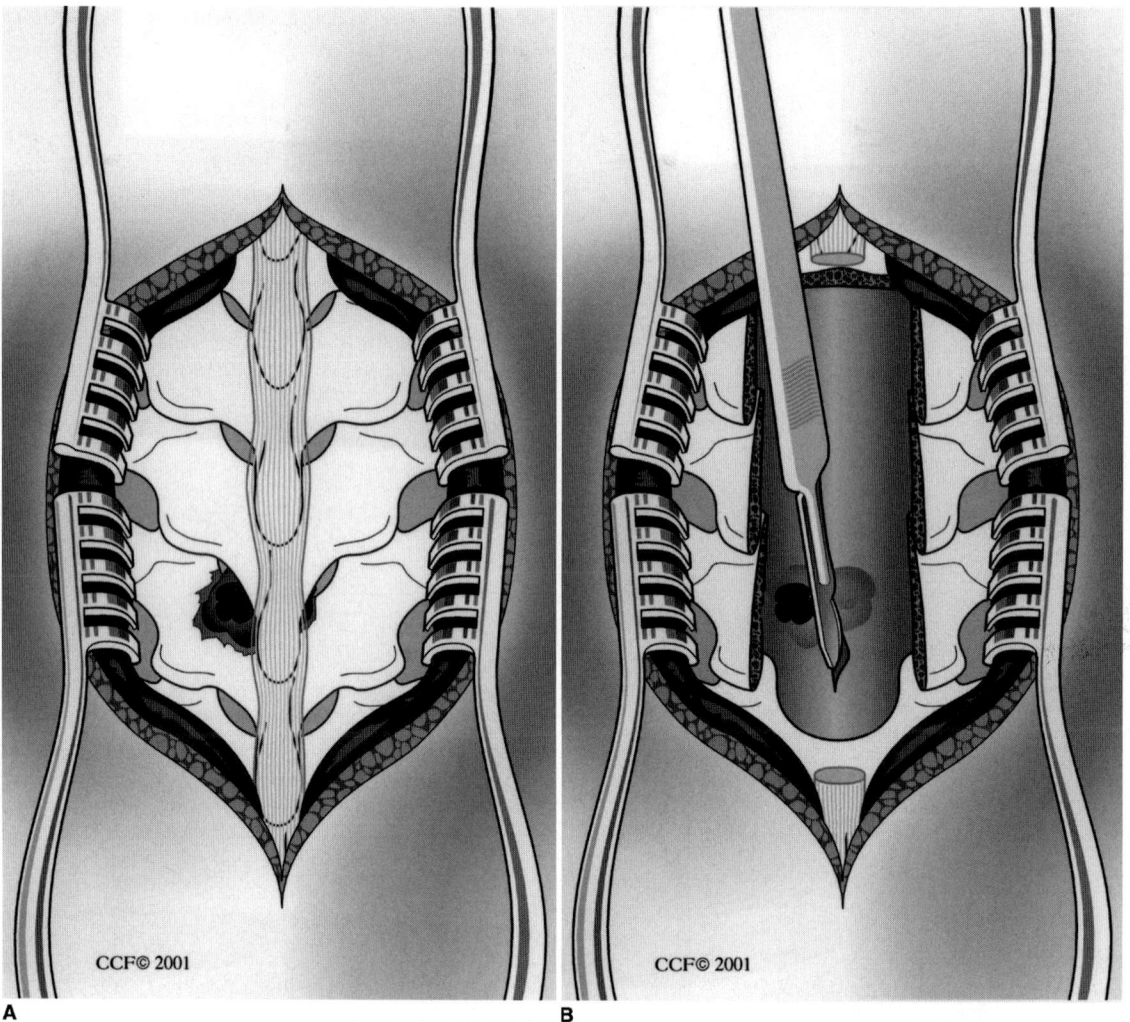

A        B

**Figure 90.5** **(A)** A wide exposure has demonstrated the bullet's entry site. **(B)** A generous laminectomy is performed, both above and below the level of entry.

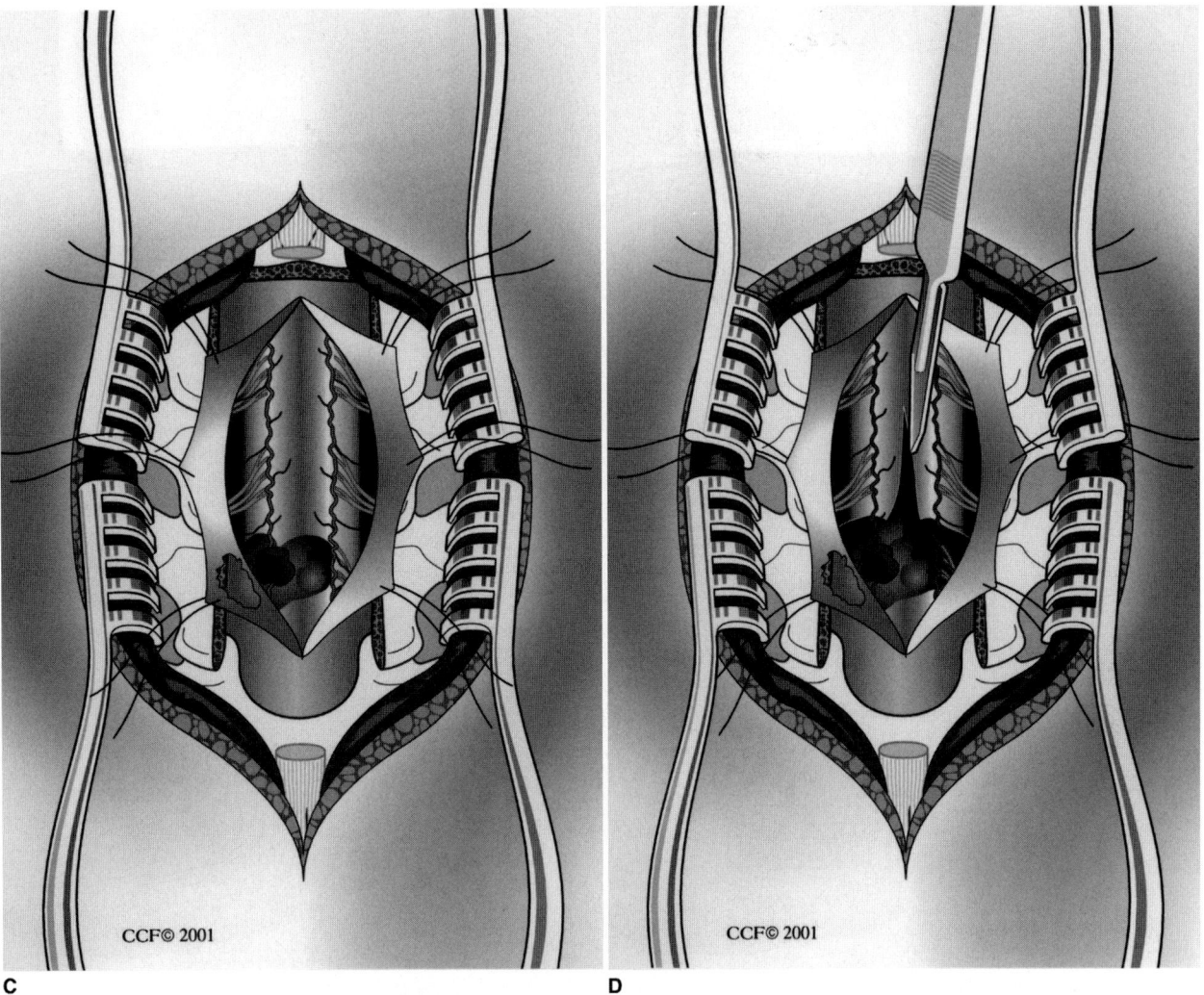

C                                                   D

**Figure 90.5 *cont'd*** (**C**) The durotomy should also be generous. (**D**) If an intramedullary hematoma has been identified, a midline myelotomy may be performed to evacuate the clot.

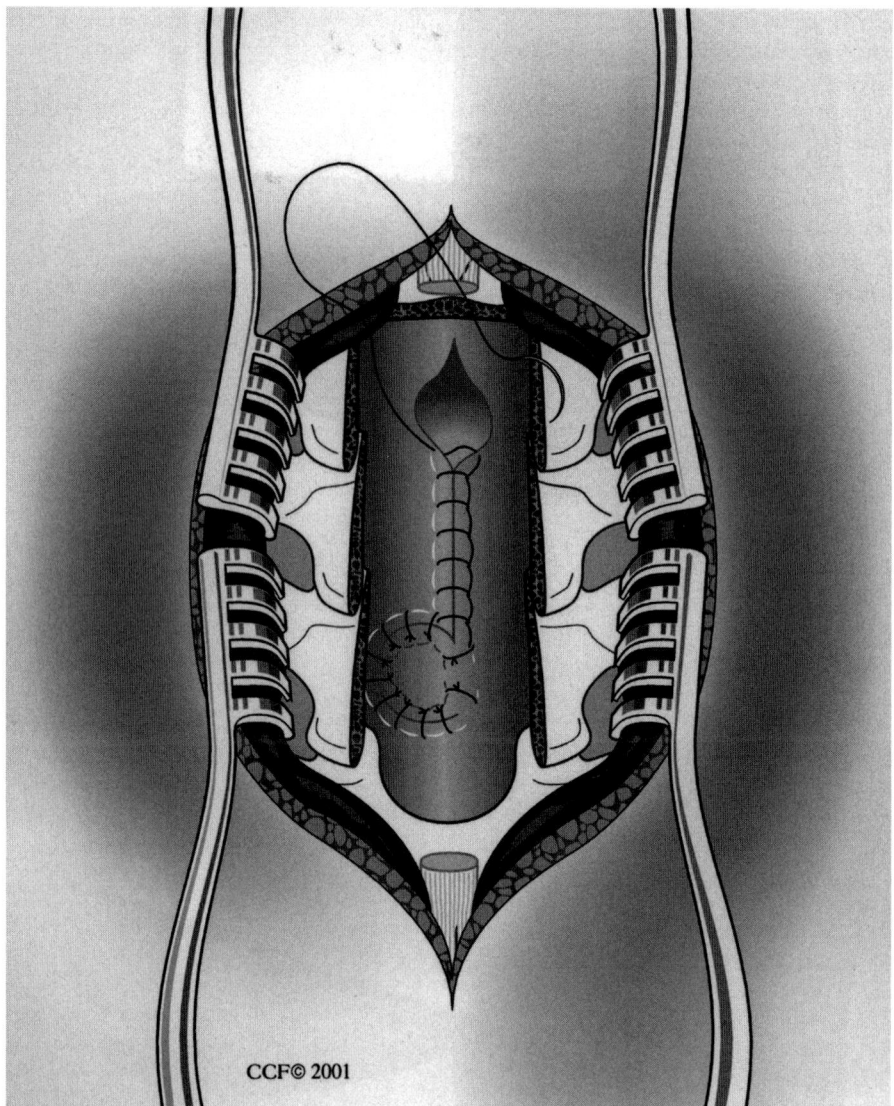

CCF© 2001

**Figure 90.6** The dura mater is closed in a watertight fashion. Any dural defect should be patched.

to treatment.[17] The problem is usually managed medically, but often with no or minimal success. Surgery to remove bullet fragments thought to be related to pain has not been shown to provide improvement.[29,30,43] Procedures such as spinal cord stimulation may be an option if medical therapy fails.

## Summary

Penetrating injuries are important causes of spinal cord injury. Despite a better understanding of the pathophysiology and improved surgical care, the prognosis is still poor. Surgery does not play a significant role in gunshot wounds unless there is an incomplete myelopathy with a surgically correctable cause. Surgery plays a larger role in impalement injuries. These types of injuries have a better prognosis then gunshot injuries. Complications such as infection and lead intoxication are rare and do not warrant removal of retained fragments, whereas in stab injuries, retained foreign objects should be removed.

## REFERENCES

1. Altman MM, Joachims HS: Osteomyelitis of the cervical spine after neck injuries. *Arch Otolaryngol* 96:72-75, 1972.
2. Arasil E, Tascioglu AO: Spontaneous migration of an intracranial bullet to the cervical spinal canal causing Lhermitte's sign: case report. *J Neurosurg* 56:158-159, 1982.
3. Benzel EC, Hadden TA, Coleman JE: Civilian gunshot wounds to the spinal cord and cauda equina. *Neurosurgery* 20:281-285, 1987.
4. Benzel EC, Ball PA: Controversies: penetrating injuries. In Garfin SR, Northrup BE (eds): *Surgery for Spinal Cord Injuries*. New York, Raven Press, 1993, pp 269-278.
5. Beutel WE, Roberts JD, Langston HT, et al: Subarachnoid-pleural fistula. *J Thorac Cardiovasc Surg* 80:21-24, 1980.
6. Bracken MB, Shepard MJ, Collins WF, et al: A randomized controlled trial of methylprednisolone or naloxone in the treatment of acute spinal-cord injury. *N Engl J Med* 332:1405-1411, 1990.

7. Cloeman JE, Benzel EC, Hadden T: Gunshot wounds to the spinal cord and cauda equina in civilians. *Surg Forum* 37:496-498, 1986.

8. David CA, Landy HJ, Green BA: Penetrating wounds of the spine. In Wilkins RH, Rengachary SS (eds): *Neurosurgery*. New York, McGraw-Hill, 1996, pp 3055-3061.

9. Djergaian RS, Roberts JD, Ditunno JF, et al: Subarachnoid-pleural fistula in traumatic paraplegia. *Arch Phys Med Rehabil* 63:488-489, 1982.

10. Finitsis SN, Falcone S, Green BA: MR of the spine in the presence of metallic bullet fragments: is the benefit worth the risk? *Am J Neuroradiol* 20:354-356, 1999.

11. Grande CM, Baron CR, Stene JK: Appropriate techniques for airway management of emergency patients with suspected spinal cord injury, letter. *Anesth Analg* 67:714-715, 1988.

12. Guttman L: *Spinal Cord Injuries: Comprehensive Management and Research*. Oxford, Blackwell Scientific Publications, 1976.

13. Haynes WG: Acute war wounds of the spinal cord: analysis of 184 cases. *Am J Surg* 72:424-433, 1946.

14. Heiden JS, Weiss MH, Rosenberg AW, et al: Penetrating gunshot wounds of the cervical spine in civilians: review of 38 cases. *J Neurosurg* 42:575-579, 1975.

15. Hopkins DA, Marshall TK: Firearm injuries. *Br J Surg* 54:344-353, 1967.

16. Jacobs GB, Berg RA: The treatment of acute spinal cord injuries in a war zone. *J Neurosurg* 34:164-167, 1971.

17. Jones RE, Bucholz RW, Schaefer SD, et al: Cervical osteomyelitis complicating transpharyngeal gunshot wounds to the neck. *J Trauma* 19:630-634, 1979.

18. Karim NO, Nabors MW, Golocovsky M, et al: Spontaneous migration of a bullet in the spinal subarachnoid space causing delayed radicular symptoms. *Neurosurgery* 18:97-100, 1986.

19. Kupcha PC, An HS, Cotler JM: Gunshot wounds to the cervical spine. *Spine* 15:1058-1063, 1990.

20. Matson DD: *The Treatment of Acute Compound Injuries of the Spinal Cord Due to Missiles*. Springfield, IL, Charles C. Thomas, 1948.

21. May M, Chadaratana P, West JW, et al: Penetrating neck wounds: selective exploration. *Laryngoscope* 85:57-75, 1975.

22. Meinke AH, Bivins BA, Sachatello CR: Selective management of gunshot wounds to the neck: report of a series and review of the literature. *Am J Surg* 138:314-319, 1979.

23. Milhorat TH, Elowitz EH, Johnson RW, et al: Spontaneous movement of bullets in the brain. *Neurosurgery* 32:140-143, 1993.

24. Ott K, Tarlov E, Crowell R, et al: Retained intracranial metallic foreign bodies: report of two cases. *J Neurosurg* 44:80-83, 1976.

25. Peacock WJ, Shrosbree RD, Key AG: A review of 450 stab wounds of the spinal cord. *S Afr Med J* 51:961-964, 1977.

26. Prendergast MR, Saxe JM, Ledgerwood AM, et al: Massive steroids do not reduce the zone of injury after penetrating spinal cord injury. *J Trauma* 37:576-580, 1994.

27. Rao PD, Bhatti FK, Gaudindo J, et al: Penetrating injuries of the neck: criteria for exploration. *J Trauma* 23:47-49, 1983.

28. Rengachary SS, Carey M, Templer J: The sinking bullet. *Neurosurgery* 30:291-294, 1992.

29. Richards JS: Pain secondary to gunshot wound during the initial rehabilitation process in spinal cord injury patients. *J Rehabil Res Dev* 25:75, 1988.

30. Richards JS, Meredith RL, Nepomuceno C, et al: Psycho-social aspects of chronic pain in spinal cord injury patients. *Pain* 8:355-366, 1980.

31. Roffi RP, Waters RL, Adkins RH: Gunshot wounds to the spine associated with a perforated viscus. *Spine* 14:808-811, 1989.

32. Schafer SD, Bulcholz RW, Jones RE, et al: The management of transpharyngeal gunshot wounds to the cervical spine. *Surg Gynecol Obstet* 152:27-29, 1981.

33. Sherman IJ: Brass foreign body in the brain stem: a case report. *J Neurosurg* 17:483-485, 1960.

34. Simpson RK, Venger BH, Narayan RK: Treatment of acute penetrating injuries of the spine. *J Trauma* 29:42-46, 1989.

35. Six E, Alexander E, Jr., Kelly DL, Jr., et al: Gunshot wounds to the spinal cord. *South Med J* 72:699-702, 1979.

36. Stauffer ES, Wood RW, Kelly EG: Gunshot wounds of the spine: the effects of laminectomy. *J Bone Joint Surg Am* 61A:389-392, 1979.

37. Switz DM, Elmorshidy ME, Deyerle WM: Bullets, joints, and lead intoxication: a remarkable and instructive case. *Arch Intern Med* 136:939-941, 1976.

38. Tanguy A, Chabannes J, Debuelle A, et al: Intraspinal migration of a bullet with subsequent meningitis. *J Bone Joint Surg* 64A:1244-1245, 1982.

39. Tinsley M: Compound injuries of the spinal cord. *J Neurosurg* 3:306-309, 1946.

40. Venger BH, Simpson RK, Narayan RK: Neurosurgical intervention in penetrating spinal trauma with associated visceral trauma. *J Neurosurg* 70:514-518, 1989.

41. Wannamaker GT: Spinal cord injuries: a review of the early treatment in 300 consecutive cases during the Korean conflict. *J Neurosurg* 11:517-524, 1954.

42. Ward WE, Maltby GL: Associated complications in war wounds of the spine. *JAMA* 129:155-157, 1945.

43. Waters RL, Adkins RH: The effects of removal of bullet fragments retained in the spinal canal: a collaborative study by the National Spinal Cord Injury Model Systems. *Spine* 16:934-939, 1991.

44. Waters RL, Adkins RH, Hu SS, et al: Penetrating injuries of the spinal cord: stab and gunshot injuries. In Frymoyer JW, Ducker JW, Hadler NM, et al (eds): *The Adult Spine*. Philadelphia, Lippincott-Raven, 1997, pp 919-930.

45. Yashon D, Jane JA, White RJ: Prognosis and management of spinal cord and cauda equina bullet injuries in sixty-five civilians. *J Neurosurg* 32:163-170, 1970.

46. Young JS, Burns PE, Bowen AM, McCtchen R: *Spinal Cord Injury Statistics: Experience of the Regional Spinal Cord Injury Systems*. Phoenix, AZ, Good Samaritan Medical Center, 1982.

# CHAPTER 91

# Vascularized Bone Grafts in Spine Surgery

**Alok D. Sharan, Frank Conguista, Ashwini D. Sharan, and Allen L. Carl**

Bone grafting has had an important role in surgery since Barth first introduced bone-grafting techniques in the late nineteenth century.[5] Typically, bone grafts are used in the treatment of nonunions, arthrodesis of joints, filling of bone cavities, replacement of bone lost due to infection, trauma, tumor, augmentation of fracture healing, and spinal fusion. The variety of bone grafts used today include autogenous cancellous, nonvascularized autogenous cortical, vascularized autogenous cortical, allogeneic cancellous, allogeneic cortical, allogeneic demineralized bone matrix, and allogeneic inductive proteins.

Bone grafts are commonly used in spine surgery to provide stability in areas where defects are created by decompressive procedures. Currently, the gold standard for bone grafts is the autograft. This type of graft has the best biologic compatibility and leads to fewer nonunions. The most common complications associated with its use include donor site pain and a suboptimal incorporation rate of the graft. The advent of the use of vascularized bone grafts has given the spine surgeon a potentially powerful tool to treat difficult spinal problems. This chapter presents a brief discussion on bone grafts and the basic biology behind their incorporation, along with causes for a nonunion. Its indications in spine surgery and a review of the results are also presented.

## Bone Grafts in Spine Surgery

Albee[1] first described the utilization of bone graft for spinal fusion in 1911 as a treatment for Pott's disease. There have been many advances since that time. Fusion is now the standard treatment for a variety of spinal disorders. All fusions involve two key components: (1) preparation of the site to be fused and (2) the stimulation of bone formation with a bone graft or bone graft substitute. In general, grafts should have a large surface area of contact with the recipient bed. This facilitates vascularization and incorporation.

Because of diminished number of osteoblasts that survive the grafting process and the slower rate of revascularization of the graft, cortical bone grafts are associated with a slow rate of incorporation, thus limiting their use.[28] However, the advantage of cortical grafts lies in the fact that they provide structural support and are available in larger sizes to fill multilevel defects. These grafts provide immediate support, but their strength decreases over time. This is due to a process termed *creeping substitution*, whereby the avascular nature of the graft causes resorption by osteoclasts (while new bone is laid down by osteogenic cells originating from the recipient bed rather than the graft). This was first observed and described by Phemister in 1914.[30] For this reason a cortical graft, such as a strut graft used in the treatment of kyphosis, may take up to 2 years to completely incorporate. Due to creeping substitution, the bone graft is found to be weakest at 6 months, thus increasing the risk of developing a fracture at the graft site.[10] By retaining its vascular supply and viability of the osteocytes, a vascularized bone graft provides a mechanically stronger support than a nonvascularized graft.

## Vascularized Bone Grafts

The use of vascularized bone grafts parallels the developments marking the history of vascular surgery. The advent of this field can be traced back to Carrel's classic paper published in 1908, "Results of the Transplantation of Blood Vessels, Organs, and Limbs,"[9] in which he describes a technique whereby blood vessels can be anastomosed. In the years following this publication, various tools and techniques used to anastomose small vessels were designed and tested: Androsov[2] designed the first vascular stapling machine, Jacobsen and Suarez[20] demonstrated the utility of using the microscope in the operating room, and Buncke and Schulz[8] improved microsurgical instrumentation and completed much of the early experimental work in this field in the 1960s. In 1971, Strauch et al.[33] used a canine model to transpose a rib to the mandible on its internal mammary pedicle, and in 1973 a free vascularized rib graft was performed in a dog by McCullough and Fredrickson.[24] The first free skin flap using microvascular anastomoses was reported by Taylor et al.[36] in 1973, and in 1975, Taylor and Daniel[35] transferred a fibula to a tibial defect, thus performing as the first free vascularized bone graft.

The vascularized bone graft has traditionally been used in refractory nonunions or in areas with a large segmental defect. The history of its use in spine surgery began out of a need to find a more mechanically supportive bone graft. Surgery for severe kyphosis secondary to infection or trauma obligates the spanning multiple spinal segments. A nonvascular rib or fibula is commonly used for this purpose, but due to the length of the graft and the slow rate of incorporation, a high nonunion rate can be expected. Bradford et al.[7] encountered fatigue fractures in 4 of 23 patients when a nonvascularized fibula was used for spinal kyphosis surgery. These results caused spine surgeons to seek out alternatives to traditional bone grafts. In two separate reports, Bradford[6] and Rose et al.[31] described the successful use of rib graft with a vascular pedicle. Since the cross-sectional area of the rib was too small and could not provide the structural support needed for certain areas of spinal fusion, surgeons began to explore the use of the fibula as a vascularized graft.[21,27] Rib, fibula, and iliac crest are used as primary donors for a vascularized grafting (Table 91.1).

**TABLE 91.1**

### Summary of Different Spinal Uses of Vascularized Bone Grafts

| Author | Indication | Graft Used |
| --- | --- | --- |
| Bradford et al.[7] | Severe kyphosis | Rib |
| Meyers et al.[25] | Salvage reconstruction in severe spondylolisthesis | Fibula |
| Nakamura et al.[28] | Anterior thoracic and lumbar fusion | Folded rib |
| Freidberg et al.[11] | Replacement of resected cervical vertebral bodies | Fibula |
| Govender et al.[13] | Tuberculosis kyphosis | Rib |
| Wright et al.[37] | Anterior decompression and fusion in the setting of radiation therapy for cervical chordoma | Fibula |
| Asazuma et al.[3] | Cervical kyphosis due to neurofibromatosis | Fibula |
| Wuisman et al.[40] | Thoracolumbar scoliotic deformity in the setting of osteogenesis imperfecta | Fibula |

## Indications and Principles

A vascularized bone graft would be indicated in the following situations:

1. When the bone graft length is greater than 5cm[18]
2. When the strut graft is to be greater than 4cm from the ventral border of the spine (and thus more prone to fracture)[18]
3. In the presence of a pseudoarthrosis after a nonvascularized bone graft[26]
4. In the setting of a malignancy[39]
5. In cases of infection where placing instrumentation or avascular bone may propagate the infection[14]
6. In cases in which the fusion is associated with a low fusion rate, such as with neurofibromatosis[3]

## Surgical Technique

The three most common locations from which a vascularized bone graft may be taken are the rib, iliac crest, and fibula. In spine surgery the rib is the easiest location from which to harvest a vascularized bone graft. Unfortunately, due to its thin cylindrical structure, the rib does not provide the necessary mechanical stability required to fill large segmental defects. The fibula is a relatively larger cylindrical structure that has robust mechanical properties. It can be used to span multiple levels. The major disadvantage of using the fibula is donor site morbidity.

### Preoperative Planning

The surgeon should be well trained in microvascular techniques. Multiple types of anastomoses may be required in vessels that could be potentially scarred or traumatized. A preoperative angiogram should be performed to elucidate the vasculature of the donor and recipient sites. Of particular note, however, is that a normal angiogram may be misleading, as scarred blood vessels may appear normal. Oftentimes the surgeon must make an intraoperative decision regarding the viability of a blood vessel.

### Fibula

The fibula is a long bone that is triangular in cross-section and has a high cortical-to-cancellous bone ratio. Up to 25cm of length can be harvested safely for long grafts. The medullary vascular supply to the fibula arises as a branch of the peroneal artery. It enters the fibula at the junction of the proximal and middle thirds of the bone. The venous system is similar to the arterial system, with drainage occurring through the venae comitantes of the peroneal artery and the medullary sinusoidal system.

The procedure described herein was initially described by Vail and Urbaniak,[38] using an extraperiosteal dissection. This procedure has also been described by Gore et al.[13] using a subperiosteal plane. As described by Vail and Urbaniak, the extraperiosteal dissection is associated with fewer pain-related complaints.

To obtain the fibula graft, the patient is placed supine on the operating table. The leg is prepped from the hip to the toes, and a tourniquet is applied to the thigh. After the tourniquet has been inflated, the limb should be exsanguinated with an elastic bandage.

A straight lateral incision should be made directly over the fibula, with further dissection performed between the posterior and lateral compartments of the calf. The peroneal muscle should be separated from the ventral aspect of the fibula to the intramuscular septum. Elevating the muscles of the anterior compartment reveals the intraosseous membrane. The muscles of the posterior compartment are also dissected extraperiosteally. The superficial peroneal nerve and a portion of the peroneal artery deep to the fibula are protected, and the fibula is divided with a Gigli saw.

The flexor hallucis longus, the posterior tibial muscle, and the remaining muscles of the anterior compartment are separated from the fibula extraperiosteally. The fibula is elevated from the wound distally to proximally, while the pedicle is left intact. Vascular branches entering the soleus muscle are clipped and divided. The peroneal vessels are dissected proximally to its bifurcation from the tibial vessels. The fibular diaphyseal segment, along with approximately 4 to 6cm of the peroneal vessels, is ligated and dissected.

The donor site is closed primarily over suction drains. Postoperative aspirin is often administered. In uncomplicated free flap procedures, dextran and heparin play a minimal role. A splint with the foot in dorsiflexion is utilized for approximately 5 to 7 days, followed by active range-of-motion exercises. A radionuclide bone scan, using technetium 99–labeled methylene diphosphonate, is the most useful study to assess the viability of the vascularized bone. This bone scan has been shown to be a reliable indicator of microvascular patency and correlates with clinical outcome if performed within the first postoperative week. Thereafter, false positives are more frequent.

### Iliac Crest

Grafting of the iliac crest is based on the fact that the most reliable pedicle is the deep circumflex iliac artery. This artery has been shown to supply the majority of the ilium.[37] The following technique has been described by Mezera and Weiland and is based on the original work by Taylor.[25]

The patient is placed supine on the operating table with a small bump under the donor hip. An incision should be made from the femoral artery to a point 10cm dorsal to the anterior superior iliac spine (ASIS). The external oblique muscle should be exposed and incised in line with its fibers to a point 3cm rostral to the iliac crest. The incision should be curved toward the ASIS and parallel to the inguinal ligament so that the inguinal canal can be entered. The spermatic cord or round ligament should be identified and retracted upward and medially. The fascia at this point should be incised, and the deep circumflex iliac artery and vein should be identified. The vessels should be traced laterally, dividing the transversalis fascia, internal oblique, and transversus abdominis muscle from the inguinal ligament. The ascending branch of the deep circumflex iliac artery is identified as the ASIS is approached. Its origin from the superficial circumflex iliac artery can be identified medially by incising the internal oblique muscle 3cm above and behind the ASIS.

Incising the transversus muscle parallel to the iliac crest at this point isolates the ilium. The transversalis fascia is incised, the extraperitoneal fat is retracted, and a line between the transversalis and the iliacus fascia is exposed. The iliacus is incised 1cm medial to this line to expose the periosteum of the iliac fossa. The iliacus muscle is dissected from the remainder of the ilium. The attachment of the tensor fasciae latae and glutei muscles is separated from the ilium. The inguinal ligament and the origin of the sartorius muscle are divided just medial to the ASIS.

The graft can now be osteotomized to isolate it with its vascular pedicle. The flap should be allowed to sit for 20 minutes to ensure its viability. Occasionally, the lateral femoral cutaneous nerve will require sectioning to remove the graft; however, every attempt should be made to preserve it. Using an oscillating saw, the graft can be cut first laterally then medially to a depth of 2.5cm. The iliac crest graft should now be present with the deep circumflex iliac artery and vein. The graft can be no longer than 10cm due to the curvature of the ilium.

During closure, careful attention must be paid to securing the layers to avoid herniation of abdominal contents. The iliacus fascia and muscle should be sutured to the transversalis fascia and muscle. Next, the internal and external oblique muscles should be sutured to the glutei, the fascia lata, and its muscle. Finally, the inguinal canal should be repaired and the inguinal ligament reattached laterally.

### Rib

Injection studies have demonstrated that the rib receives its primary blood supply from the posterior intercostal vessels. The posterior intercostal artery is a branch of the aorta that forms the dorsal and ventral ramus. The dorsal ramus provides branches to the spinal cord and the paraspinous muscles. The ventral ramus anastomoses with the anterior intercostal artery and also provides a nutrient artery to the rib. The anterior intercostal artery provides vascular supply mainly to the periosteum and therefore is not as important as its posterior counterpart.

As first described by Bradford, a vascularized rib graft should be planned so that the rib removed will be long enough to span the defect. The rib to be used should be two to three segments below the level of the rostral vertebrae.[6] The patient is placed in the lateral decubitus position. A skin incision is made over the rib to be resected. The intercostal musculature is incised 0.5 to 1cm above the rib. The rib is divided at the costochondral junction, and the intercostal musculature is then caudal to the rib from distal to proximal. A wide margin is left to avoid dividing the vascular complex. Chest retractors are placed into the wound, and the intercostal vasculature is identified. Dissection is carried out dorsally, and the rib is divided at the rib–transverse process junction. At this point the rib can be mobilized along with its vascular complex. The vessels are dissected and then mobilized to the junction of the intervertebral foramen. A pleural centimeter of rib should be dissected subperiosteally so that bone-to-bone contact can be made with the adjacent vertebra. The rib is then rotated and mobilized to span the vertebra above and below. Incising the periosteum 1cm over the rib can test circulation to the graft. If brisk bleeding is encountered, an intact vascular pedicle is confirmed. The chest can now be closed in the usual fashion.

### Results and Complications

As first reported in 1980 by Bradford, a vascularized rib graft is suitable for situations that require strong biomechanical support and in which a large defect must be spanned.[6] By avoiding the process of creeping substitution, the vascularized bone graft prevents microfracture and nonunions commonly observed when a large nonvascularized graft is used. Most of the cases reported in the literature have used the graft in areas where mechanical support is essential while awaiting bone graft incorporation.

Vascularized bone grafts are also useful in the setting of malignancy that requires radiation therapy. Often a subtherapeutic dose of radiation therapy must be applied at the site of the bone fusion to minimize the chance of nonunion of the bone graft.[16,17] Due to the greater number of viable osteocytes and osteoblasts available, along with a lesser requirement of ingrowth and neovascularization, a vascularized graft may better tolerate the deleterious effects of the radiation.[12,32]

The superior mechanical stability afforded by a vascularized graft is also useful in the setting of infection. When nonoperative therapy has failed to eradicate a spinal infection, operative intervention requires decompression of the infected bone along with fusion for stabilization. Using instrumentation or long segments of nonvascularized bone can provide a nidus for the infection. In these cases a vascularized bone graft has been successful in increasing the speed of acquisition, as well as the ultimate stability of the fusion.

## Complications

Most of the complications involving vascularized bone grafts in spine surgery are related to donor site morbidity. In 1996, Vail and Urbaniak[38] reported on complications of harvesting vascularized fibular grafts. He noted that pain and motor weakness were the most prevalent complications. Sensory deficits were also noted along with rare cases of skin breakdown secondary to loss of vascular supply. In a separate report a functional iatrogenic valgus of the ankle joint was reported when resection of the fibula extended too caudally.[19] Other morbidities include transient peroneal nerve palsy, flexor hallucis longus contracture, compartment syndrome, and fracture of the ipsilateral tibia.[15]

Persistent pain following removal of the iliac crest has been reported with chronic disability when a large graft is harvested.[4,22,34] There have also been reports of infection, hematoma, and fracture of the ASIS.[23]

## Summary

Vascularized bone grafts offer an additional tool for the spine surgeon to use when the achievement of bony union proves difficult. It is a technically demanding procedure. As with all surgical interventions, patient selection is extremely important. Removal of the graft has known associated morbidities, and the patients should be apprised of these. Overall, the vascularized bone graft provides a mechanically strong construct with a successful rate of incorporation in cases with a significant choice of pseudoarthrosis.

## REFERENCES

1. Albee FH: Transplantation of a portion of the tibia into the spine for Pott's disease. *JAMA* 57:885, 1911.
2. Androsov PI: New methods of surgical treatment of blood vessel lesions. *Arch Surg* 73:902, 1956.
3. Asazuma T, Yamagishi M, Nemoto K, *et al:* Spinal fusion using a vascularized fibular bone graft for a patient with cervical kyphosis due to neurofibromatosis. *J Spinal Disord* 10(6):537, 1997.
4. Banwart JC, Asher MA, Hassanein RS: Iliac crest bone graft harvest donor site morbidity: a statistical evaluation. *Spine* 20:1050, 1995.
5. Barth H: Histologische Untersuchchungen Uber Knochen Transplantation. *Beitr Pathol Anat Allg Pathol* 17:65, 1895.
6. Bradford DS: Anterior vascular pedicle bone grafting for the treatment of kyphosis. *Spine* 5:318, 1980.
7. Bradford DS, Winter RB, Lonstein JE, *et al:* Technique of anterior spinal surgery for the management of kyphosis. *Clin Orthop* 128:129, 1977.
8. Buncke HJ, Schulz WP: Experimental digital amputation and reimplantation. *Plast Reconstr Surg* 36:62, 1965.
9. Carrell A: Results of the transplantation of blood vessels, organs, and limbs. *JAMA* 51:1661, 1908.
10. Cervansky J, Skovring B, Moor D: Use of fibular bone grafts in reconstructive surgery. *Chir Narzadow Ruchu Ortop Pol* 27:297, 1962.
11. Freidberg SR, Gumley GJ, Pfeifer BA, *et al:* Vascularized fibular graft to replace resected cervical vertebral bodies. *J Neurosurg* 71:283, 1989
12. Goldberg V, Shaffer JW, Field G, *et al:* Biology of vascularized bone grafts. *Orthop Clin North Am* 18:197, 1987.
13. Gore DR, Gardner G, Sepic S, *et al:* Function following partial fibulectomy. *Clin Orthop* 220:206, 1987.
14. Govender S, Suresh Kumar KP, Med PC: Long-term follow-up assessment of vascularized rib pedicle graft for tuberculosis kyphosis. *J Pediatr Orthop* 21:281, 2001.
15. Han CS, Wood MB, Bishop AT, *et al:* Vascularized bone transfer. *J Bone Joint Surg* 74:1441, 1992.
16. Harrington KD: The use of methylmethacrylate for vertebral body replacement and anterior stabilization of pathological fracture-dislocation of the spine due to metastatic disease. *J Bone Joint Surg* 63:36, 1981.
17. Harrington KD: Anterior cord decompression and spinal stabilization for patients with metastatic lesions of the spine. *J Neurosurg* 61:107, 1984.
18. Honma T, Yoshizu T: Vascularized fibular bone graft in spinal surgery. *Monthly Book Orthop* 5:71, 1992.
19. Hsu LC, Yau AC, O'Brien JP, *et al:* Valgus deformity of the ankle resulting from fibular resection for a graft in subtalar fusion in children. *J Bone Joint Surg* 54:585, 1972.
20. Jacobsen JH, Suarez EL: Microsurgery in anastomosis of small vessels. *Surg Forum* 11:243, 1960.
21. Kaneda K, Kurakami C, Minami A: Free vascularized fibular strut graft in the treatment of kyphosis. *Spine* 13:1273, 1988.
22. Kreibich DN, Scott IR, Wells JM, *et al:* Donor site morbidity at the iliac crest: comparison of percutaneous and open methods. *J Bone Joint Surg* 76:847, 1994.
23. Kurz LT, Garfin SR, Booth RE Jr.: Harvesting autogenous iliac crest bone grafting: a review of complications and techniques. *Spine* 14:1324, 1989.
24. McCullough DW, Fredrickson JM: Neovascularized rib grafts to reconstruct mandibular defects. *Can J Otolaryngol* 2:96, 1973.
25. Mezera KK, Weiland AJ: Vascularized bone grafts. In Chapman MW, Szabo RM (eds): *Operative Orthopaedics.* Philadelphia, Lippincott Williams & Wilkins, 2001, pp 1209-1223.
26. Meyers AM, Noonan KJ, Mih AD, *et al:* Salvage reconstruction with vascularized fibular strut graft fusion using posterior approach in the treatment of severe spondylolisthesis. *Spine* 26(16):1820, 2001.
27. Minami A, Kaneda K, Satoh S, *et al:* Free vascularized fibular strut graft for anterior spinal fusion. *J Bone Joint Surg* 79:43, 1997.
28. Motoki DS, Mulliken JB: The healing of bone cartilage. *Clin Plast Surg* 17:527, 1990.
29. Nakamura H, Yamano Y, Seki M, *et al:* Use of folded vascularized rib graft in anterior fusion after treatment of thoracic and upper lumbar lesions. *J Neurosurg* (Spine 2) 94:323, 2001.
30. Phemister DB: The fate of transplanted bone and regenerative power of its constituents. *Surg Gynecol Obstet* 19:303, 1914.

31. Rose GK, Owen R, Sanderson JM: Transposition of rib with blood supply for stabilization of spinal kyphosis. *J Bone Joint Surg* 57:112, 1975.

32. Shaffer JW, Field GA, Goldberg VM, *et al:* Fate of vascularized and nonvascularized autografts. *Clin Orthop* 197:32, 1985.

33. Strauch B, Bloomberg AE, Lewin ML: An experimental approach to mandibular replacement: island vascular composite grafts. *Br J Plast Surg* 24:334, 1971.

34. Summers BN, Eisenstein SM: Donor site pain from the ilium: a complication of lumbar spine fusion. *J Bone Joint Surg* 71:677, 1989.

35. Taylor GI, Daniel RK: The free flap: composite tissue transfer by vascular anastomoses. *Aust N Z J Surg* 43:1, 1973.

36. Taylor GI, Miller GDH, Ham FJ: The free vascularized bone graft: a clinical extension of microvascular techniques. *Plast Reconstr Surg* 55:533, 1975.

37. Taylor GI, Townsend P, Corlett R: Superiority of the deep circumflex iliac vessels as the supply for free groin flaps: experimental work. *Plast Reconstr Surg* 64:595, 1979.

38. Vail TP, Urbaniak JR: Donor-site morbidity with use of vascularized autogenous fibular grafts. *J Bone Joint Surg Am* 78(2):204, 1996.

39. Wright NM, Kaufman BA, Haughey BH, *et al:* Complex cervical spine neoplastic disease: reconstruction after surgery by using a vascularized fibular strut graft. *J Neurosurg* (Spine 1) 90:133, 1999.

40. Wuisman PIJM, Jiya TU, Van Dijk M, *et al:* Free vascularized bone graft in spinal surgery: indications and outcome in eight cases. *Eur Spine J* 8:296, 1999.

# CHAPTER 92

# Pain and Spasticity

**Giancarlo Barolat, Warwick J. Peacock, and Loretta A. Staudt**

The surgical management of chronic pain and spasticity share many features. The goal of these procedures is not to cure the conditions but to alleviate the symptoms. Complete elimination of the symptomatology of either condition is seldom possible. Recurrences are frequent, especially with chronic pain. In general, the procedures are aimed at interrupting, either anatomically or functionally, the undesirable signals that maintain the pain or the spasticity. Often, pain and spasticity coexist in the same patient, especially the patient with spinal cord injury (SCI).

The procedures performed for these conditions fall into two major categories: ablative and neuromodulatory. Ablative procedures rely on anatomic interruption of the desired pathways by the sectioning of nerves, nerve roots, or tracts of the spinal cord. Such procedures include neurectomies, dorsal and ventral rhizotomies, dorsal root entry-zone lesioning, and various forms of cordotomies. When performed for chronic pain, a neurectomy or a dorsal rhizotomy attempts to eliminate all the sensory input from the painful area. However, a dorsal root entry-zone lesion carries more specificity and attempts to destroy the sensory neurons in the dorsal horn. Interruption of the spinothalamic tract is the objective of a ventrolateral cordotomy. These procedures usually provide relief for a few months, after which the pain usually returns. For this reason, the procedures have been successfully used mainly to treat pain arising from terminal cancer. They have seldom been found useful for management of chronic nonmalignant pain. The development of neuromodulation interventions has allowed a substantial improvement in the management of some chronic pain conditions. Neuromodulation procedures include neurostimulation using electrodes implanted on the peripheral nerves or spinal cord or in the brain and implantation of pumps that deliver drugs (e.g., morphine and other narcotic medications) into the intrathecal space. The use of intrathecal opioids has been popularized mainly for the management of cancer pain; its use in chronic noncancer pain has been more controversial and is under investigation.

For the management of spasticity, the goal is to reduce the hyperexcitability of the spinal cord, including the monosynaptic and polysynaptic reflexes that lead to uncontrollable reflex muscle contractions. This can be accomplished by sectioning the dorsal roots, making a lesion in the spinal cord at the level of the interneurons, enhancing the presynaptic inhibition locally within the spinal cord with an intrathecal baclofen infusion, or electrically stimulating the spinal cord and possibly inhibiting the hyperactive interneurons.

The management of spasticity has been revolutionized by the advent of implantable pumps that deliver baclofen to the spinal fluid cavity in the spine. The amount of intrathecal baclofen necessary to reduce spasticity is infinitesimal compared with the oral dosage. However, the use of neurostimulation procedures to treat spasticity is more limited because of the effectiveness of the intrathecal baclofen. Ablative procedures such as functional selective dorsal rhizotomy have recently regained popularity for the treatment of spastic cerebral palsy.

Many of the procedures for management of chronic pain and spasticity are similar in concept and share the same implant technology.

## Spinal Neuromodulation Procedures

### Spinal Cord Stimulation

Epidural spinal cord stimulation (SCS) has been performed since the 1970s. The main indication for the procedure is intractable chronic pain that has not responded to conservative therapeutic modalities.[47,51,62,76,84] The most commonly treated pain is the one that occurs in failed back syndrome, which occurs in persons who have undergone multiple lumbar spine operations and have developed adhesive arachnoiditis or epidural fibrosis. Pain resulting from nerve injury or from reflex sympathetic dystrophy has been shown to respond to SCS.[13] The procedure is also widely used in Europe for the treatment of pain arising from critical limb ischemia (particularly in the lower extremity) and for intractable angina pain.[7,8,20]

The basic SCS unit consists of one or more electrodes implanted in the dorsal epidural space and a pulse generator implanted in a subcutaneous pocket (Figures 92.1 through 92.3). The electrodes are of two types: percutaneous electrodes and plate electrodes. Percutaneous electrodes are inserted under fluoroscopy through a specially modified Tuohy needle and are manipulated into the epidural space until the desired location is reached. Plate electrodes must be inserted under direct vision. Their placement usually requires the removal of the ligamentum flavum and some of the spinous process. With modern technology, both types of electrodes are safe and effective means of delivering electrical stimulation to the spinal cord.

Currently, two types of power sources are available. The totally implantable pulse generators contain an internal lithium battery as the power source. They are activated and controlled by outside transcutaneous telemetry and, once activated, do not require any patient input for function. They can be turned on and off through a small magnet that patients carry. By contrast, radio-frequency B–driven systems consist of a passive receiver that is implanted under the skin and a transmitter that is worn outside the body. For the system to function, the transmitter must contain charged alkaline batteries, and the antenna must be adequately juxtaposed to be in contact with the receiver. Both systems present advantages and disadvantages; thus the implanting team should select the appropriate system on an individual patient basis.

### Neurologic Damage

The most dreaded complication of SCS is neurologic damage, either from intraoperative nerve root injury, SCI, or

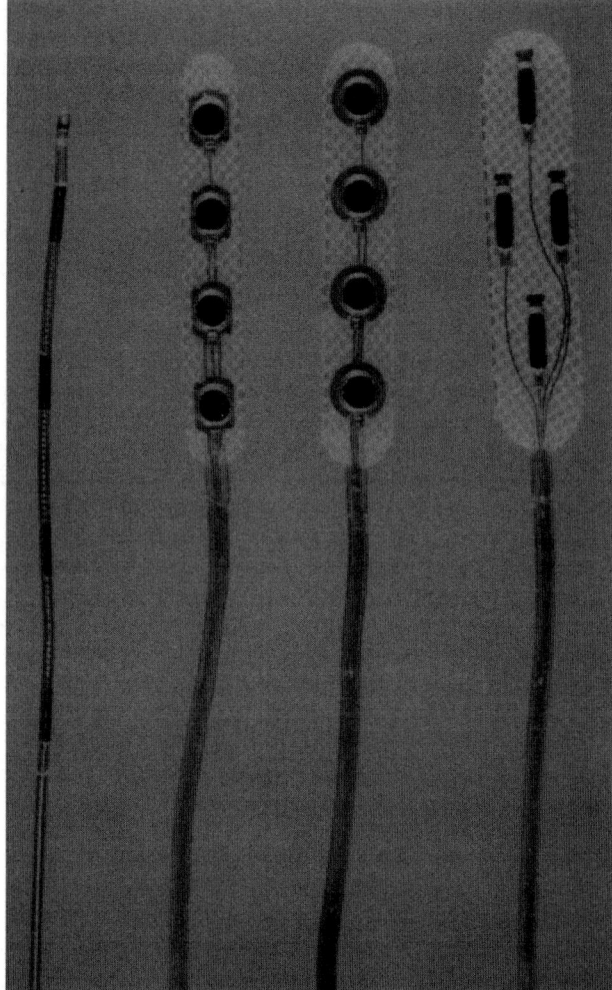

**Figure 92.1** Percutaneous and plate electrodes for spinal cord stimulation manufactured by Medtronic Inc. (*Courtesy of Medtronic Inc, Minneapolis, Minn.*)

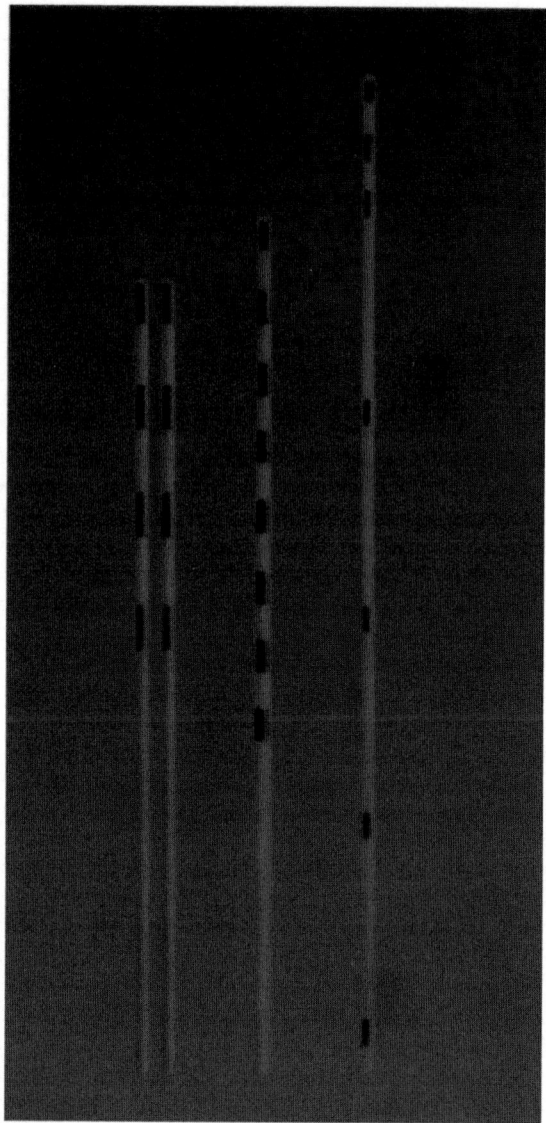

**Figure 92.2** Percutaneous electrodes manufactured by Neuromed Inc. (*Courtesy of Neuromed Inc, Ft. Lauderdale, Fla.*)

subsequent spinal cord compression from an intraspinal clot. Intraoperative injury is possible during implantation of percutaneous or plate electrodes. Percutaneous needle placement could result in direct penetration of the spinal cord. The first author (Barolat) is aware of such a case, in which the patient was rendered quadriplegic during a low cervical needle placement. Another instance of neurologic damage was a reoperative case (with dense epidural adhesions) of nerve root injury incurred during implantation of a plate electrode. During epidural dissection under inadequate intravenous sedation, the patient received a sudden jolt, and a Penfield dissector (placed under the lamina) connected with neural structures. Pain and allodynia developed immediately in the L1 nerve root distribution. The symptoms subsided after several weeks and after the patient received a series of lumbar sympathetic blocks.

Epidural hematoma can also be a cause of postoperative neurologic deficit. This can occur with both percutaneous and laminotomy electrode placement.[36,51] In a consecutive series of 700 implanted plate electrodes, one instance of postoperative paraplegia resulted from epidural hematoma at the site of electrode implantation.[11] The symptoms were not defined clearly until about

20 hours after the implant. The clot was immediately evacuated. In the subsequent months the patient experienced improvement in his neurologic function but was left with a significant neurologic deficit.

### Electrode Migration

Electrode migration most commonly occurs within the first few days after implantation. After approximately 3 weeks, substantial scar tissue forms around a plate electrode and prevents movement in any direction. This does not hold true for percutaneous electrodes, because the sleeve of scar tissue never completely prevents caudal migration. The exact incidence of electrode dislodgment is unclear. In early series the incidence of migration was 5% to 17%.[76,77,99] More recently, the development of stiffer multicontact percutaneous electrodes appears to have reduced the incidence of electrode migration. Young found the migration to occur almost exclusively with percutaneous electrodes.[99] Migration occurred in 1.5% of patients in a

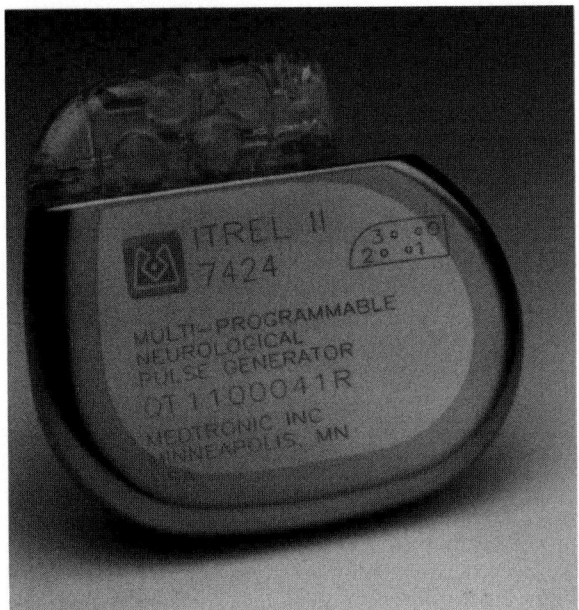

**Figure 92.3** Lithium-powered spinal cord stimulation pulse generator (Medtronic Itrel II). (*Courtesy of Medtronic Inc, Minneapolis, Minn.*)

series of 509 patients in whom plate electrodes were implanted.[11] Electrode migration most often results in loss of the appropriate stimulation-induced paresthesias. Multipolar electrodes or multiarray constructs are more forgiving because the stimulation can be reprogrammed to recapture the desired paresthesias.

### Infection

Infections of the implanted hardware have been reported with an incidence varying between 0.5% and 15%. An infection rate not in excess of 3% to 5% is considered acceptable. Infection most often affects the implanted pulse generator or radio receiver and the cabling connecting these to the electrode. Very seldom does the infection spread to the epidural space. Infections can occur from a few days to a few years after implantation. Infection usually presents with persistent tenderness over the implanted hardware. Swelling, redness, and other signs of inflammation may not be present. A rampant postoperative infection presents with purulent drainage and dehiscence of the wound to such an extent that the hardware can be seen. Other infections may take a very indolent course with moderate but persistent tenderness that occurs over the pulse generator and spreads along the subcutaneous cabling toward the electrode. These instances may create a serious differential diagnosis dilemma in patients with reflex sympathetic dystrophy (RSD) who often complain of long-lasting pain at the implant site.

The ultimate treatment for infection is complete removal of the hardware followed by a 6-week treatment with intravenous antibiotics. If the infection is confined strictly to the radio receiver or pulse generator, it may be tempting to leave the electrode in place, particularly in the case of the plate electrodes, with which successive reimplantation may be difficult, but this course may not be prudent. Occasionally, however, with the patient's full understanding of the possible risks involved, the electrode may be left in place. Infection of implanted hardware must be distinguished from a superficial wound infection, which should be treated with antibiotics and does not require removal of the hardware.

### Cerebrospinal Fluid Leakage

Persistent cerebrospinal fluid (CSF) leakage has occurred after implantation of both percutaneous electrodes and plate electrodes. The clinical presentation is usually characterized by headaches and CSF accumulation at the pulse generator site. The initial approach should be to prescribe bed rest for a few days and to place a fairly tight abdominal binder over the pulse generator. This technique usually generates enough pressure in the pocket to stop the tracking of the CSF and, eventually, the dural leakage. The binder should be worn for at least 2 to 3 weeks. If leakage persists, the options are either to inject a blood patch or to perform surgical exploration. Rarely is the problem of such magnitude as to actually threaten the integrity of the incisions and result in external fluid leakage through the wounds. However, if this does occur, prompt surgical intervention is imperative.

### Pain

Some patients experience prolonged or exaggerated postoperative pain, sometimes localizing to the incision and sometimes occurring more diffusely over the axial parts of the body. In patients with failed back syndrome or neurogenic thoracic outlet syndrome, the pain may be associated with severe, persistent muscle spasms. In subjects with RSD, this may be accompanied by allodynia and the spread of symptoms to previously unaffected body parts. These pain symptoms may last for weeks and months, and occasionally they may be permanent. In Simpson's series, prolonged postoperative pain affected about 5% to 10% of patients implanted with thoracic plate electrodes.[85] It is extremely important for this possibility to be explained to the patient preoperatively, and such an explanation is part of the operative consent. Persistent pain at the implanted pulse generator site or along the subcutaneous cabling can also be experienced by patients with RSD and may require repositioning of the implant. As mentioned previously, persistent pain at the implant site must be carefully differentiated from an indolent infection of the implanted equipment.

Persistent radicular irritation may be due to impingement on a nerve root by the electrode. This has been seen mostly in patients with RSD, moderate spinal stenosis, and plate electrodes. The irritation can be managed successfully by performing a limited decompressive laminotomy over the electrode.

### Intrathecal Drug Delivery Pumps

Implanted intrathecal pump systems consist of a catheter implanted in the subarachnoid space, usually in the lumbar area, and a fluid-containing device, the pump, connected to the catheter and implanted in a subcutaneous pocket (Figure 92.4). The pump requires refilling periodically

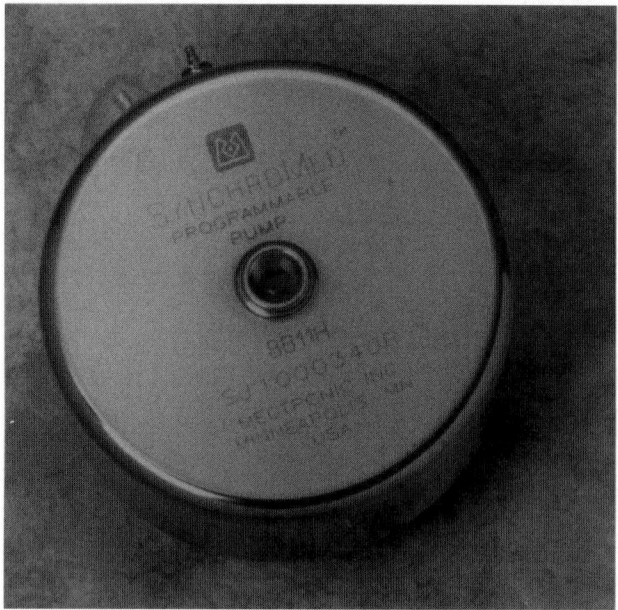

**Figure 92.4** Medtronic Synchromed pump for intrathecal drug delivery. (*Courtesy of Medtronic Inc., Minneapolis, Minn.*)

through a needle inserted into the access port through the skin. The pump is driven by a lithium-powered motor or by a gas-expansion mechanism. The motor can be programmed noninvasively through a telemetry unit, whereas the gas-expansion mechanism requires changes in the concentration of the injected medication in order to modify the dosage delivered to the subarachnoid space.

Implanted intrathecal pumps are most often used for management of intractable pain and of spasticity. Traditionally, the most common indication has been management of cancer pain with intrathecal morphine administration.[5,24,34,39,64] More recently, other chronic pain syndromes (e.g., failed back syndrome and various forms of neuropathic pain) have been successfully treated with this modality.[26,32,72] Intrathecal infusion of local anesthetics and other types of medications is also being explored to treat these pain conditions.

Another increasingly popular application of pumps is the intrathecal infusion of baclofen for the treatment of spasticity.[3,21,53,63,70] This application has been uniformly successful in the treatment of spasticity of spinal origin (e.g., SCI or multiple sclerosis) and is being investigated for treatment of spasticity of cerebral origin.

When dealing with complications from implanted drug delivery pumps, one has to distinguish among complications related to the surgical procedure, complications related to the implanted hardware, and complications related to the drug being delivered. This review does not consider the long-term implications of drug delivery because many of these are still unknown.

The incidence of complications in relatively large series has been reported recently. Levin and Sperling[50] reported a total of 20 complications arising after 33 infusion pumps were implanted for delivery of morphine or baclofen between 1986 and 1994. The most common complication was disconnection of the catheter at its connection with the pump (five instances in four patients). This occurred with the Medtronic Syndromed pump exclusively. In five

instances, the catheter migrated outside the spinal canal and had to be repositioned. Wound dehiscence occurred in three cases. Meningitis (all caused by *Pseudomonas* species) occurred in three patients. Bloomfield and Gross[16] reported their experience with 50 patients implanted with intrathecal morphine-delivery pumps for chronic pain (not caused by a malignant tumor). There were 22 catheter revisions because of catheter disconnection, migration, or obstruction. Hormonal dysfunction was found in 18% of patients, diffuse polyarthralgias in 24%, and sleep disturbances in 8%. Three patients experienced urinary retention, which limited dose escalation.

## Cerebrospinal Fluid Leakage

CSF leakage usually occurs along the catheter track and into the pump pocket. If all the incisions have healed, CSF will accumulate under the skin along the implanted hardware. Accumulation of large quantities of CSF may result in substantial distention of the pocket and potential disruption of wound integrity. The first author has treated a patient with copious external CSF drainage through a nonhealed abdominal incision.

Placement of a figure-of-eight nonabsorbable suture in the interspinous ligament and fascia around the catheter may help prevent fluid escape and catheter migration. The suture must be placed before the Tuohy needle is withdrawn but must be tied down around the catheter after removal of the needle. Meticulous watertight wound closure in multiple layers is mandatory. The first author maintains the patients flat at bed rest for 2 to 3 days after implantation of an intrathecal pump.

Mild internal leaks, manifesting only with headaches, can be handled initially with prolonged flat bed rest. If the headaches persist, an epidural blood patch can be injected, with great care taken not to shear the catheter. If there is visible accumulation of CSF along the catheter track and in the pocket, use of a tight abdominal binder for 2 weeks is usually sufficient. If wound integrity is threatened, hospitalization and placement of an external lumbar drain for 5 to 7 days may be necessary. If CSF is leaking externally through a small opening, the hole can be closed with one or two skin sutures. The patient must be administered antibiotics, because a leak poses a significant risk for infection. If there is wound dehiscence, the patient must undergo wound revision and meticulous closure. Flat bed rest, a lumbar drain, and intravenous antibiotics should also be parts of the therapeutic regimen. If wound dehiscence is such that the internal hardware is externally visible, removal of the entire implanted system should be considered.

## Infection

Infection can be of several types, with varying degrees of severity. A distinction must be made between a purely localized infection and one that affects the nervous system because, if untreated, a localized infection may lead to an infection that affects the nervous system. A superficial wound infection usually manifests with erythema, some swelling, and tenderness. A deep wound infection is often purulent and is accompanied by wound dehiscence.

Localized epidural and subdural abscesses may lead to paraplegia, if not recognized immediately. The first author has treated a patient with a subdural abscess along the catheter track that manifested clinically only with persistent low back pain and no other signs of infection. Meningitis and meningoencephalitis can be the result either of wound infection or pump refills performed without use of proper sterile technique.

Proper patient selection and meticulous sterile technique at surgery and during pump refills are the mainstays of infection prevention. Patients who are heavy smokers, who have diabetes, who are immunosuppressed, who have poor nutrition, or who are either obese or extremely thin are at great risk for healing problems and, therefore, for infection. Whether or not prophylactic antibiotics play a significant role is still debated. The first author orders administration of one dose of antibiotics before surgery and four more doses postoperatively. The regimen may vary in patients who are in a high-risk category.

Any infection related to an intrathecally implanted device must be viewed as very serious and potentially dangerous. An infection that clearly involves only the superficial tissues should be treated with intravenous antibiotics without removal of the hardware. Any other infection commands immediate removal of the implanted hardware and long-term administration of the appropriate intravenous antibiotics. In the instance of an epidural or subdural abscess, prompt surgical evacuation is mandatory.

### Catheter Migration

A catheter usually migrates in a caudal direction, with multiple causes accounting for downward catheter migration. If not enough slack is left in the back incision, continuous trunk rotation and bending will affect the intraspinal part of the catheter and will gradually pull it out. Another mechanism is related to the pump. If the pump is not securely sutured to the fascial layers, it may entangle the catheter. This may eventually result in complete migration of the catheter into the pump pocket. In one case in the first author's experience, the entire catheter, including the tip, was coiled into the pump pocket.

To prevent migration, some slack must be left in the catheter, both in the lumbar incision and in the pump pocket. At least 3 inches of catheter should be inserted in the subarachnoid space. The pump must be securely sutured to the fascial layers in at least two places in order to avoid rotation of the reservoir.

Caudal catheter migration does not have to be treated unless the catheter has migrated outside the intrathecal space, thereby preventing access of the drug to the spinal fluid compartment. However, if progressive caudal displacement can be demonstrated on successive radiographs, surgical repositioning of the catheter may be an elective consideration.

### Radicular Irradiation

Irritation of the lumbar nerve roots has been observed occasionally, especially in patients with RSD. The exquisite sensitivity of the nerves to mechanical stimulation may explain the high susceptibility of patients to this complica-tion. The patient usually complains of shooting pain along the exact distribution of the affected nerve root. The pain can be severe and incapacitating, and it may command surgical revision. The first author has been able to correct this problem successfully either by gently pulling the catheter caudally by a few centimeters or by reinserting it at a different level.

### Catheter Occlusion

Occlusion of the catheter usually occurs at the tip. The rate at which the flow slows down depends on the degree of obstruction. Catheter occlusion is much more common with epidural than with intrathecal catheters. Catheter occlusion is not symptomatic, except for the effects related to the lack of delivery of the medication to the nervous system. Because of the continuous pushing of the fluid by the pump, the pressure build-up in the catheter may cause the catheter to disconnect at the connector site. Diagnosing an obstructed catheter may be difficult if a direct access port is unavailable. The most direct diagnosis is by injection of opaque contrast through the port, with radiographic demonstration of the obstruction.

Clogging of the tip of the catheter is a function of the properties of the catheter material, the fluid, and the milieu in which the catheter tip lies. Whereas with intracranial catheters placement of the tip near the choroid plexus has been shown to lead inevitably to obstruction, no specific anatomic guidelines have emerged for spinal intrathecal placement.

When an obstruction is demonstrated, one may initially attempt to unplug the catheter by injecting fluid through the access port. If this is not successful, replacement of the catheter becomes necessary.

### Formation of a Granuloma at the Catheter Tip

The first author has observed two instances in which the tip of the intrathecal catheter became encased in a mass of granulomatous tissue. In one patient the mass had become sizable and impinged substantially on the intraspinal contents. Figures 92.5 and 92.6 show a myelogram and a magnetic resonance imaging scan, respectively, of the intrathecal mass. At surgical exploration, the nerve roots appeared to adhere tenaciously to the mass and could not be dissected free; however, substantial debulking of the mass resulted in resolution of the symptoms. A similar occurrence was reported by North et al.[61] in which the patient had developed a severe paraparesis over a 1-month period. A computed tomography (CT) myelogram showed an intrathecal mass at the T10 level. At surgery a mass measuring $6 \times 8 \times 40$ mm surrounded the catheter tip. Microscopic examination showed chronic inflammatory cells and large areas of necrosis consistent with a foreign body reaction.

### Overdose

**Morphine.** Accidental overdose can occur either as a result of a pump malfunction or as a result of accidental injection of the refill dose directly through the direct access port. The latter mechanism is, by far, the most common. Death has occurred after accidental bolus injection of large doses of morphine through the direct access port rather than through the chamber port. To avoid this potentially fatal complication, the design of the pumps has been modified either by elimination of the direct access port or by requiring two different needles to access the two ports. The best prevention, of course, is education and avoidance of human error.

Sauter *et al.*[82] reported on the treatment of massive intrathecal morphine overdose in a patient who had an intrathecal pump implanted to treat chronic pain because of failed back syndrome. During a refill, 450mg of morphine

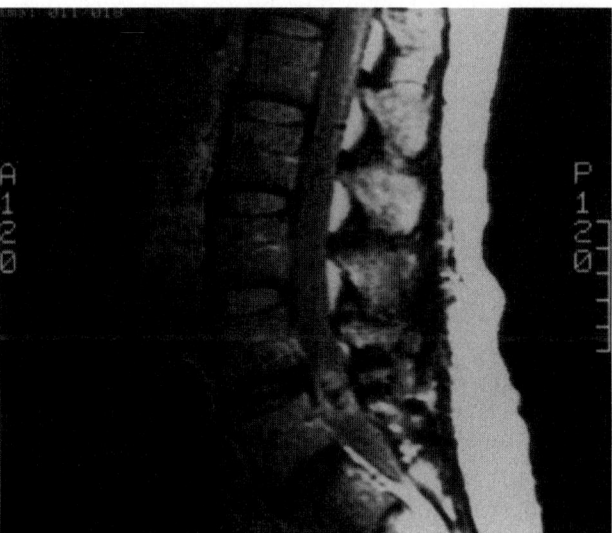

**Figure 92.5** Myelogram showing the granulomatous intrathecal mass in the lower lumbar area.

sulfate was inadvertently injected into the bolus side port. The patient became drowsy, agitated, and hypertensive (blood pressure 200/150mmHg) and developed tonic-clonic seizures. She was intubated and mechanically ventilated, and an intravenous naloxone drip was begun immediately. Because of status epilepticus, intravenous phenytoin and intravenous phenobarbital were immediately administered. Attempts to withdraw CSF through the pump were unsuccessful. A spinal intrathecal catheter was inserted, and continuous spinal fluid drainage was instituted at approximately 10ml/hr. A CT scan showed a left frontal intracerebral hemorrhage and a left sylvian subarachnoid hemorrhage, presumably secondary to the hypertensive episode. The patient continued to improve and was extubated after 4 days. She had received a total of 884mg of naloxone, and 550ml of CSF had been removed. Morphine concentrations in the spinal fluid were obtained at approximately 6-hour intervals for the first 36 hours. These levels progressively decreased in the CSF from an initial value of 404µg/ml to a final concentration of 0.38µg/ml. The calculated volume of distribution was 13.9ml/kg.

Erroneous injection of refill doses of morphine subcutaneously has been reported by Wu and Patt.[98] In this instance, 2 to 3ml of fluid was aspirated, but this may have been taken from a subcutaneous seroma, giving the erroneous impression of CSF aspiration. Upon being injected with 450mg of morphine subcutaneously, the patient became confused and lethargic but not comatose. Prompt administration of naloxone fully reversed the process, with no prolonged side effects.

As a precaution, in the case of massive overdose, naloxone should be administered cautiously to avoid severe hypertension, dysrhythmias, and pulmonary edema, which might be lethal.

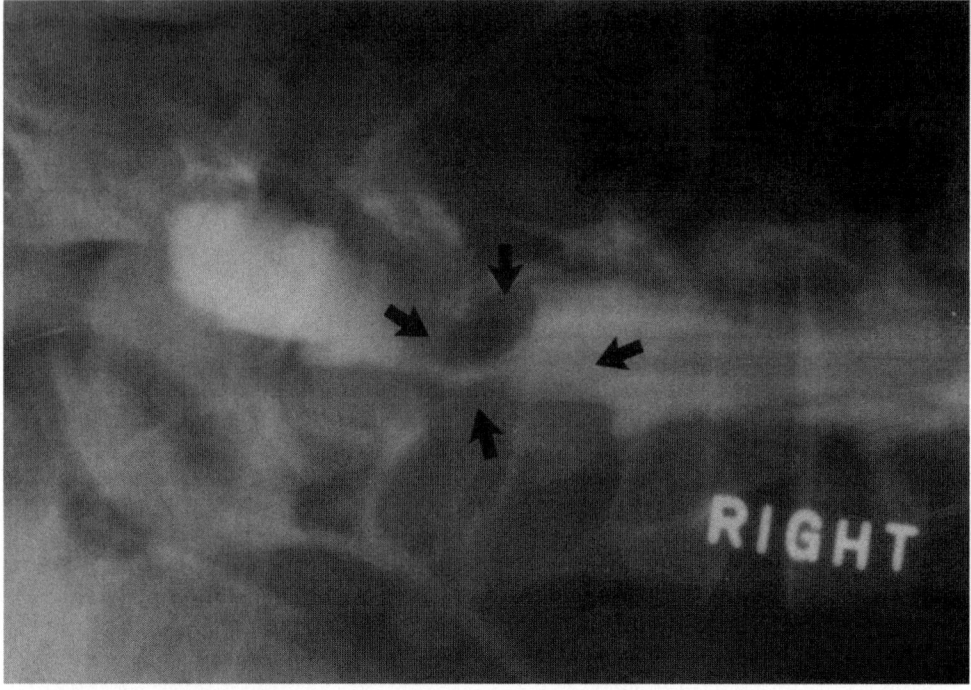

**Figure 92.6** Magnetic resonance imaging scan showing the granulomatous intraspinal mass.

**Baclofen.** Intrathecal baclofen overdose has been reported in the literature. Symptoms of overdose usually include severe sedation, followed by coma and respiratory depression. According to Kroin,[44] the initial elimination half-time ($t_{1/2}$) after a bolus dose of intrathecal baclofen is about 1.5 hours, but there may be a later, slower elimination phase with a $t_{1/2}$ of 4.6 hours during the 8- to 24-hour period postinjection. This has been confirmed, because in most reported instances the overdose clinically lasted 2 to 3 days.

Teddy et al.[92] reported two instances of serious drug overdose in a series of 46 patients implanted for intrathecal baclofen infusion. In both instances, the patients became unresponsive and required intubation and artificial ventilation. The supportive treatment could be discontinued after 2 days, and the patients did not suffer any adverse long-term effects. Kofler et al.[43] described the electrophysiologic findings in a case of serious intrathecal baclofen overdose. The patient received 10mg of baclofen intrathecally in a bolus dose and became comatose and apneic. Transcranial electrical stimulation up to 750V did not evoke any responses in the hand muscles the first day of intoxication. An improvement to normal values was observed within 3 days, paralleling the patient's neurologic improvement. Cervical electrical stimulation was largely unaffected by baclofen. Median nerve somatosensory-evoked potentials and brain stem acoustic potentials revealed few or no differences.

Delhaas and Brouwers[23] reported seven events of intrathecal baclofen overdose in five patients in a group of 43 patients suffering from previously intractable spasticity and a total treatment time of 2422 weeks. On two occasions, bolus injection doses of 50 and 280μg caused overdose symptomatology. The five events of intoxication during continuous infusion occurred only in patients receiving high doses. The overdose symptoms occurred in one patient when she was supine (baclofen dose of 800μg/24hr) and in another patient after repair of CSF leakage with an autologous epidural blood patch (baclofen dose of 1920μg/24hr). In tolerant patients, one event occurred during maximal dose adjustments (baclofen dose of 2400μg/24hr), and two events occurred 6 hours after reinitiation of the intrathecal baclofen infusion after a "drug holiday" treatment (baclofen doses of 27μg/hr and 55μg/hr).

The mainstay of therapy for severe cases of overdose is support of cardiovascular and respiratory functions in an intensive care unit. In most reported cases the symptoms and signs completely regressed in 24 to 72 hours, with no residual effects. Whether the intravenous administration of physostigmine has a significant role in the management of such an overdose remains controversial.[54,81] Patients receiving massive overdoses of baclofen may not respond to physostigmine. Penn and Kroin[71] recommend the use of intravenous physostigmine (1 to 2mg over a 5-minute period) only in cases of mild bolus overdose without any cardiac compromise. It has also been suggested, in cases of early detection of a massive bolus overdose, that drainage of spinal fluid could be beneficial. Delhaas and Brouwers[23] believe that the occasionally doubtful antidotal benefits of physostigmine must be weighed against major side effects. They believe that the classic approach of decreasing the absorption of a drug by lowering baclofen levels in the CSF by lumbar puncture drainage is indicated.

No other major complications of long-standing therapy with intrathecal baclofen have been identified in two large multicenter studies.[21,63]

Acute withdrawal can also have disastrous consequences. Siegfried et al.[83] reported one patient for whom timely refill of the implanted pump was not performed. The patient started to develop paresthesias, severe headache, and disorientation that progressed to intermittent loss of consciousness and seizures. The pump was immediately filled, and oral baclofen was promptly started. The patient's symptoms promptly cleared, and he was discharged 48 hours after admission. In their series, Meythaler et al.[53] also reported one instance in which withdrawal from baclofen because of occlusion of the catheter led to a grand mal seizure.

## Intraspinal Ablative Procedures

### Dorsal Rhizotomy

A dorsal rhizotomy consists of complete or partial sectioning of one or more dorsal nerve roots in the spinal canal. The sectioning can be performed extradurally, at the level of the dorsal root ganglion, or intradurally. The procedure has been performed for the management of intractable pain and for the treatment of spasticity or spasms in patients with conditions affecting the central nervous system. When used for chronic pain management, the procedure has been performed mostly to treat nociceptive pain arising from cancer. Foerster reported the use of dorsal rhizotomy for the treatment of spastic patients in the early 1900s.[31] There were few subsequent reports until the procedure was reintroduced by Gros et al. in 1967.[37] Fasano et al.,[29] Fasano et al.,[30] Peacock and Staudt,[68] and others[10] subsequently popularized it for the management of spasticity in subjects with cerebral palsy. Dorsal rhizotomies have also been used successfully to manage severe flexor spasms in patients with SCI or multiple sclerosis.[9] The indications for dorsal rhizotomy have substantially decreased since the advent of intrathecal delivery of morphine and baclofen for pain and spasticity management. However, selective dorsal rhizotomy to treat children with spastic cerebral palsy is used widely.

Selective dorsal rhizotomy has been successful for selected children with spastic diplegic or spastic quadriplegic cerebral palsy. Although the motor disabilities of cerebral palsy include many factors such as weakness, impaired balance, and difficulties with motor control, spasticity often has a major impact on and can interfere with function or care. Spastic diplegic patients who have relatively good strength and motor control are usually the best surgical candidates for improvement of function via rhizotomy. More severely involved patients also benefit, especially in the areas of positioning and daily care. Spasticity contributes to contracture and deformity in the growing child. Therefore, it is best to intervene in the early childhood years before growth is complete.

Reduction of spasticity is achieved after selective division of approximately 25% to 50% of lumbosacral sensory nerve rootlets. Precautions are taken to prevent interruption of lower sacral nerve rootlets involved in bowel and bladder function and to avoid excessive deafferentation. Intraoperative electromyography of the major lower extremity muscle groups and external anal sphincter muscles is performed. Postoperative physical and occupational therapy is considered important for functional recovery and improvement after surgical reduction of spasticity. Several authors report reduction of spasticity and functional improvement in children with cerebral palsy after rhizotomy.[15,25,68,87] Outcome studies have shown reduction of lower extremity muscle tone to near normal levels; increase in passive range of motion at hips, knees, and ankles; and functional benefits.[68] Increased stride length, walking speed, and range of gait-motion have been documented with instrumented analyses.[17,19,96] Positive changes in upper extremity function have been noted by several authors and appear to occur in about 50% of patients who have upper limb impairment before surgery.[6,14,30,67]

### Hypoesthesia

Sectioning of one nerve root alone (except possibly for S1) usually does not lead to any significant sensory loss. Two or three adjacent dorsal roots must be sectioned for a clinically detectable sensory loss to result. Because the nerve roots can be subdivided in a variable number of rootlets (five to six in the cervical area, 10 to 15 in the lower lumbar area), partial section of multiple adjacent roots can be accomplished safely. If one fifth of the rootlets of each root are spared, no sensory loss will occur. This strategy has been used extensively in selective dorsal rhizotomies performed for management of spasticity in patients with cerebral palsy.[29,37,69,87] With chronic pain, however, leaving some rootlets intact will inevitably lead to early recurrence of the pain. This is true particularly for rhizotomies performed for cancer pain resulting from excessive nociception. Sensory loss can be an acceptable trade-off when the pain is in the thoracic area or when the affected limb is already not functional. In Abbott's[1] and Abbott et al.'s,[2] series of children with cerebral palsy, three patients sustained loss of proprioception, and two had loss of pain or temperature sensation.

Some patients who have complete motor but incomplete sensory paraplegia are considered for a dorsal rhizotomy for treatment of severe flexor spasms (which may be responsible for pressure sores). This approach must be evaluated carefully. Partial section of the lumbar roots, in this instance, inevitably leads to early recurrence of the spasms. However, complete section of the lumbar roots eliminates all sensation from the buttocks. The patient will lose sensory feedback from the very area that is most susceptible to decubitus ulcers. This, in turn, may make the patient more prone to this complication. In these patients (as with others with severe flexor spasms), the first treatment choice should be intrathecal baclofen infusion, and a destructive procedure should be considered only if there are contraindications to dorsal rhizotomy.

### Painful Dysesthesias

Anesthesia dolorosa and painful dysesthesias can result after extensive multilevel rhizotomies, accompanied by complete sensory loss. This usually occurs when extensive rhizotomies are performed for nonmalignant pain conditions, because it takes several months for the condition to develop. The painful dysesthesias can be as troublesome as

the pain that was meant to be relieved. It is not unusual for children with spasticity, who undergo the selective dorsal rhizotomy, to complain of unpleasant dysesthesias in the distribution of the sectioned dorsal roots. Forty percent of the patients in Abbott's[1] series experienced uncomfortable dysesthesias in the lower extremities. Usually, these last only a few days and then disappear. This can also occur after selective cervical rhizotomy. The first author has never observed a situation in which painful dysesthesias resulted permanently after a partial selective rhizotomy.

### Lower Bowel or Bladder Dysfunction

Lower bowel or bladder dysfunction is encountered exclusively after rhizotomies at the low lumbar or sacral levels. Usually bilateral section of S2 and S3 is required to severely impair sphincter function. The situation may be different in persons who already have weakened bladder function because of a preexisting condition. In this situation the individual must be informed of the high risk for complications. Children with spastic cerebral palsy are at risk for developing a symptomatic neurogenic bladder. McNeal et al.[52] found an 8% incidence of bladder dysfunction from cystometrograms and a 36% incidence from suggestive symptoms. In Abbott et al.'s[2] series of 250 rhizotomies in patients with spastic cerebral palsy, 5% reported urinary retention. This problem was transient (5 to 21 days) in 12 patients and permanent in one. Whereas 11 of these patients had both the left and right S2 roots cut, two of them had only one S2 root cut. None of the patients in whom the rhizotomy only extended to the S1 nerve root experienced any bladder dysfunction, but 20% experienced constipation. Park Gaffney et al.[65] did not report any bladder problems in their series of 66 children who underwent the selective dorsal rhizotomy. Deleits et al.[22] showed that intraoperative monitoring of the dorsal sacral roots may minimize the risk of iatrogenic micturition disorders.

### Impaired Motor Function

Impaired motor function is observed in patients with various forms of hypertonic spasticity who undergo dorsal rhizotomy to improve their function.

Two mechanisms can negatively affect motor function. First, unmasked excessive weakness after reduction of tone when associated with reduced preexistent trunk balance can lead to an inability to sit or stand, even with support. A similar situation can occur in patients with substantial motor weakness of the lower extremities but who are able to use the extensor spasticity to ambulate. In this situation, removing the spasticity significantly would be disastrous for ambulation. Second, in patients who have severe athetotic or chreic movements, reducing the spasticity may result in marked worsening of the involuntary movements, a condition for which no treatment has been uniformly successful.

### Progressive Spinal Deformity and Hip Subluxation

Progressive spinal deformity and hip subluxation have been reported in children with spastic cerebral palsy who undergo dorsal selective rhizotomy. The exact role of surgery, if any, is unknown because children with spastic cerebral palsy are predisposed to these deformities. Several factors play a role in the potential development of this complication: (1) the number of levels in laminectomy, (2) the compromise of the articular facets, (3) the performance of a laminoplasty, and (4) the condition of the spine before surgery. Theoretically, either a short laminectomy or a laminoplasty in a child with a preoperatively normal spine should minimize the risk for deformity.

In 1990, Peter et al.[73] reported on 55 children with cerebral palsy who underwent multilevel laminectomies for selective dorsal rhizotomies to relieve spasticity. They were followed up clinically and radiologically to assess spinal stability and the possible development of a post-laminectomy deformity of the spine. The majority of deformities found were related to cerebral palsy and did not appear to be due to the laminectomy: 16% of the patients had scoliosis; 5%, kyphosis; 7%, lordosis; and 9%, spondylolysis or spondylolisthesis.

Progression of hip subluxation has been reported after dorsal rhizotomy in patients with cerebral palsy who had preexisting hip dysplasia. The exact mechanism is unknown, although the reduction in tone itself may lead to subluxation in predisposed individuals. The exact incidence of this complication is unknown. Greene et al.[35] observed rapid progression of hip subluxation in the year after selective dorsal rhizotomy in seven instances of hip dysplasia (six patients). The hips that subluxed progressed from a lateral extrusion index averaging 25% preoperatively to an average extrusion index of 50% after rhizotomy. Although preexistent hip dysplasia was a predisposing factor, hips with an intermediate degree of preoperative lateral extrusion (12% to 25%) had variable results. In contrast, Park et al.[66] found that lateral migration of the femoral head was unchanged in 75% of hips studied in 67 children (134 hips) 6 to 10 months after selective dorsal rhizotomy. Decreased migration occurred in 17% of the children, and increased migration was observed in only 7%. This larger series suggests that hips tend to remain stable or improve after rhizotomy. In Abbott et al.'s[2] series, six of the patients underwent osteotomy of the hip for progressive hip dislocation after the rhizotomy. All of these children were crawling before the surgery. After the rhizotomy, they advanced to walking as their main mode of locomotion. Regular periodic evaluation of hip stability is necessary after dorsal rhizotomy.

## Ventral Rhizotomy

Currently, section of the ventral roots is seldom performed. Ventral rhizotomy was used in selected situations to control severe flexor spasms in patients with spastic paraplegia resulting from SCIs or multiple sclerosis.[12,55] Since the advent of the intrathecal baclofen delivery pumps, the already limited indication for this procedure has been even further reduced. However, in cases of severe flexor spasms that have been refractory to all other treatment modalities, including intrathecal baclofen infusion, ventral rhizotomy is used either alone or in combination with a dorsal rhizotomy.

### Paralysis

Complete loss of voluntary and reflex motor function in the distribution of the sectioned nerve root is an expected effect of the section. It is extremely important that patients fully understand that this is an irreversible procedure that will make them ineligible for possible future advances in the field of neurorehabilitation (such as functional electrical stimulation or spinal cord implants or transplants).

### Muscle Atrophy

This complication may negate the potentially positive effects of the root section, even in patients with complete paraplegia. Muscle atrophy will inevitably follow section of the ventral roots, an effect that is also shared with peripheral neurectomies. The severity and distribution of the atrophy is directly related to the topography and number of sectioned nerve roots. In a paraplegic patient, atrophy of the quadriceps and hip flexor muscles is usually of no great consequence. However, atrophy of the glutei and hamstring muscles may have disastrous consequences for the patient. Decubitus ulcers may occur and, because of the complete lack of underlying viable muscle, may become unmanageable. Because this procedure is almost always performed to prevent or treat pressure sores in paraplegic patients, the complication completely defeats the purpose of the procedure. For this reason, one should always avoid sectioning L5 and S1 when a ventral rhizotomy is performed.

### Other Atrophic Complications

Because the ventral roots carry trophic factors besides motor impulses, other structures will undergo variable degrees of atrophic change. The bones in the affected limbs will demineralize rapidly, although the exact extent of demineralization is unclear. The skin will become delicate and will be prone to breakdown, therefore compromising pressure sore healing.

In summary, ventral rhizotomy for management of severe spasticity in paraplegic patients is a very effective but irreversible procedure. When indicated, the section should be limited to the L1-4 nerve roots and should never involve L5 and S1. Usually, this is not a vital issue because the most severe spasms in paraplegics affect the hip flexors and adductors and can be abolished by sectioning L1 to L3.

## Cordotomy

Currently, cordotomy is performed infrequently because it is usually confined to cancer pain that has not responded to intrathecal narcotic administration. Usually, a laminectomy is performed in the thoracic area and, percutaneously, at C1-2 in the cervical area. The purpose is to destroy the contralateral spinothalamic tract in order to abolish pain resulting from excessive nociception.

### Thoracic Cordotomy

The most common complication of unilateral thoracic cordotomy is damage to the corticospinal tract. Classically, the landmarks for the spinothalamic and corticospinal tracts are well known, and if the section is limited to the spinal cord quadrant that is dorsal to the dentate ligament, there should be no damage to the pyramidal tract. If the section is carried dorsal to the attachment of the dentate ligament, weakness or paralysis will inevitably occur. It has been shown that each lower limb runs a greater risk for paralysis from a bilateral cordotomy than does a single limb from a unilateral cordotomy. Temporary weakness of the ipsilateral lower extremity after unilateral cordotomy has been reported, with rates as high as 14%.[38,88] Young reported a 27% incidence of transient ipsilateral leg weakness after unilateral cordotomy and an 8% incidence of significant permanent weakness.[101] After bilateral cordotomy, new bilateral leg weakness was observed in his series in 26% of patients, and inability to walk was observed in 16% of patients. Tasker[89] reported significant paresis in 15% of patients after unilateral cordotomy and in 39% of patients after bilateral cordotomy.

During the sectioning, attention must also be directed to not damaging the anterior spinal artery, which may result in infarction of the spinal cord. The pathways for micturition are situated in a narrow band extending from the periphery to the lateral horn of the gray matter, just medial to the spinothalamic tract. Bilateral sectioning of the spinothalamic tract dorsally to interrupt sacral fibers will inevitably impair micturition and defecation significantly. Unilateral thoracic cordotomy does not lead to permanent impairment of bladder or bowel function. Young[101] reported temporary urinary retention in 21% of patients after unilateral cervical or thoracic cordotomy and in 65% after bilateral thoracic cordotomy. Twenty-seven percent of the patients who underwent bilateral thoracic cordotomy developed permanent urinary retention. To minimize these side effects of the bilateral procedure, the levels of the spinothalamic tract sections should be at least one or two levels apart.

The level of analgesia invariably drops with time, usually by 4 to 5 spinal cord segments. Pain recurrence inevitably occurs, unless the cordotomy is performed at a substantially higher level than the painful area. This usually implies a cordotomy at T2-3 for pain in the lower extremities.

Unpleasant or frankly painful dysesthesias have been reported after spinothalamic tractotomy performed for nonmalignant pain, and these have been known to be long lasting or even permanent. They were reported by Nathan and Smith[60] in 3 cases in a series of 114 cordotomies and by White and Sweet[97] in 12 cases in a series of 276 cordotomies. The painful sensations appear in areas that are rendered analgesic by the cordotomy. The dysesthesias usually appear only when analgesia has given way to hypoesthesia and, therefore, are more likely to affect patients who live longer. Occurrence of a new pain or a mirror-image pain shortly after a cordotomy has also been described.[56,57]

Bowsher[18] hypothesized that the occurrence of mirror-image pain after pain relief by ventrolateral cordotomy may depend on some nociceptive neurons in the deep spinal gray matter that have bilaterally symmetric receptive fields; one half of the neurons are normally subject to tonic descending inhibitory control. He suggested that

some cordotomy lesions may damage this descending inhibitory pathway and that this inhibitory mechanism may normally involve enkephalinergic interneurons.

## Cervical Cordotomy

Cervical cordotomy is most commonly performed for malignant pain through a percutaneous approach at C1-2.* Most commonly, the lesion is made with a radiofrequency probe inserted within the spinothalamic tract. The procedure is performed with the patient awake and with an intrathecal contrast injection. The procedure has been performed successfully either with fluoroscopic imaging or, more recently, with CT guidance.[42,45]

Physical trauma to the spinal cord could cause an intraparenchymal hemorrhage. Correct placement of the probe in the spinothalamic tract is confirmed by eliciting warmth paresthesias in the appropriate topographic distribution at a low voltage. During the lesioning, ipsilateral motor function is continuously monitored. Should any weakness occur, the lesioning should be stopped immediately.

## Paralysis

Paralysis can occur several hours after cervical cordotomy because of progressive damage to the spinal cord. Tasker[90] reported a 1.6% incidence of significant persistent paresis after bilateral cordotomy and a 1% incidence after unilateral cervical cordotomy. Ischia et al.[41] reported 36% incidence of transient paresis and 1.8% incidence of permanent paralysis after bilateral cervical cordotomy. Rosomoff[78] reported a 5% incidence of temporary hemiparesis and a 3% incidence of permanent motor deficit in his series. He found transient ataxia to be the most common motor complication, occurring in 20% of the cases.

## Respiratory Depression

Respiratory depression is the most serious complication of cervical cordotomy when it is performed bilaterally. Two descending respiratory pathways separately control voluntary and automatic breathing. Voluntary breathing is controlled by the spinothalamic tract, which is seldom damaged significantly by percutaneous cordotomy. The pathways for automatic breathing have been postulated to run in the lateral column of the spinal cord, possibly in conjunction with the reticulospinal tract. Nathan,[59] in a careful postmortem study, localized the descending pathways for respiration in the reticulospinal fibers lying on the surface of the ventral horn, medial to the spinothalamic tract. Strictly ipsilaterally distributed, its unilateral interruption eliminates automatic breathing, but only on the side of the lesion. These tracts are very closely related to the spinothalamic tract and are at high risk for damage during percutaneous cordotomy. Damage to the descending reticulospinal tracts results in ipsilateral loss of automatic respiration. If the contralateral lung is well functioning, it can satisfactorily support respiration. On the other hand, a lesion in the reticulospinal tract ipsilateral to a solitary, adequately functioning lung will have dis-

---

*References 4,38,48,78,79,90,91.

astrous consequences. Therefore, unilateral cervical cordotomy is unlikely to cause any respiratory impairment, unless the contralateral lung is hypofunctional. Bilateral high cervical cordotomy, on the other hand, carries a very high probability of apnea. The apnea may not occur immediately but can occur during sleep several days later.

In Tasker's[90] series, transient respiratory failure requiring ventilation occurred in 0.3% of unilateral cordotomies and 3.2% of bilateral cordotomies. Awareness of the pathophysiologic factors of the cordotomy-related respiratory depression enabled him to avoid any respiratory complications in his more recent series. Kühner[46] reported a 2.6% respiratory failure rate after unilateral cordotomy and a 20% failure rate after bilateral cordotomy. Rosomoff[78] reported a 2% incidence of major temporary respiratory depression and a 1% incidence of major permanent respiratory depression in his series of 1279 percutaneous cervical cordotomies.

Lahuerta et al.[49] studied the spinal cord of 12 patients who died during sleep at postoperative intervals of 1 to 8 days after high cervical percutaneous cordotomy for pain in malignant disease. Nine died after a first cordotomy and three after a second (contralateral) procedure. All patients who died of presumed respiratory dysfunction syndrome had lesions involving the region of the anterolateral funiculus in the C2 segment containing "pain" fibers activated from the second to the fifth thoracic dermatomes. The fibers whose destruction appeared to be responsible for respiratory dysfunction syndrome were completely intermingled with ascending pain fibers.

Rosomoff et al.[80] studied the predictive value of several preoperative respiratory parameters but could not find any significant predictors.

Tranmer et al.[95] reported six patients who died of sleep apnea after cervical cordotomy procedure. Five patients (16%) died following bilateral cordotomy and one (1%) patient with pulmonary disease died after unilateral cordotomy.

Polatty and Cooper[74] reported the case of a 33-year-old woman who developed Ondine's curse after high cervical cordotomy for relief of chronic pain. The patient maintained adequate ventilation while awake but became apneic as she progressed from light sleep toward stages of deep sleep. She died suddenly after 14 months of successful nocturnal ventilatory support.

### Dorsal Root Entry Zone Lesioning

Dorsal root entry zone lesioning has been popularized by Nashold et al.[58] via RF coagulation for the treatment of intractable pain and by Sindou and Jeanmonod[86] via microsurgical bipolar coagulation for the treatment of painful spasticity.* The procedure has been performed successfully for the treatment of brachial plexus avulsion pain, segmentary SCI pain, and severe spasticity, in both the upper and the lower extremities. The procedure entails a laminectomy extending over the spinal cord segments to be lesioned. Several lesions at the dorsal root entry zone levels are then made in the dorsal horn. The various techniques are described elsewhere.[33,86,94]

*References 27,28,33,40,93,94.

Inevitably, some sensory loss accompanies the procedure. If the lesion is limited to the lateral aspect of the dorsal root entry zone, as popularized by Sindou and Jeanmonod, one can selectively interrupt only the small myelinated contingent, sparing the large lemniscal contingent. If the lesion is limited to the dorsal root entry zone or the dorsal horn, any sensory loss is limited to the lesioned segments. If the lesion extends into the dorsal column(s), the sensory loss affects the entire hemibody below the lesion. If the lesion extends into the pyramidal tract, various degrees of motor loss will occur.

Young[100] reported his experience with dorsal root entry zone lesioning to treat intractable pain resulting from deafferentation in 78 patients managed between 1981 and 1988. Three different lesioning techniques were employed: a radiofrequency method using a $0.5 \times 2mm$ stainless steel electrode with control of electric current and duration (group 1: 21 patients); a carbon dioxide laser (group 2: 20 patients); and a radiofrequency method, using a $0.25 \times 2mm$ stainless steel electrode with control of electrode temperature and duration (group 3: 37 patients). Neurologic complications including mainly ipsilateral leg weakness or loss of proprioception occurred in 52.3% of the group 1 patients, 15% of the group 2 patients, and 8.1% of the group 3 patients. The first author concluded that dorsal root entry zone lesions may be made most effectively and safely with the radiofrequency lesioning technique associated with control of electrode temperature and duration.

Thomas and Kitchen[94] reported the long-term results of 44 patients who underwent dorsal route entry zone lesioning for pain secondary to brachial plexus avulsion with a mean clinical follow-up of 63 months. Eight cases (18%) had persisting neurologic deficits, although these were generally mild. In Nashold et al's,[58] series, up to 50% of the patients suffered from at least transient weakness of the ipsilateral lower extremity, with the early lesions treated with a non-temperature–controlled cordotomy electrode. Subsequent to the use of smaller thermo-controlled electrodes, the incidence was reduced to less than 5%.

## REFERENCES

1. Abbott R: Complications with selective posterior rhizotomy. *Pediatr Neurosurg* 18:43-47, 1992.
2. Abbott R, Johann-Murphy J, Shiminski-Maher T, *et al*: Selective dorsal rhizotomy: outcome and complications in treating spastic cerebral palsy. *Neurosurgery* 33:851-857, 1993.
3. Albright AL: Neurosurgical treatment of spasticity: selective posterior rhizotomy and intrathecal baclofen. *Stereotact Funct Neurosurg* 58:3-13, 1992.
4. Amano K, Kawamura H, Tanikawa T, *et al*: Bilateral versus unilateral percutaneous high cervical cordotomy as a surgical method of pain relief. *Acta Neurochir Suppl (Wien)* 52:143-145, 1991.
5. Andersen PE, Cohen JL, Everts EC, *et al*: Intrathecal narcotics for relief of pain from head and neck cancer. *Arch Otolaryngol Head Neck Surg* 117:1277-1288, 1991.
6. Arens LJ, Peacock WJ, Peter J: Selective posterior rhizotomy: a long-term follow-up study. *Childs Nerv Syst* 5:148-152, 1989.

7. Augustinsson LE: Spinal cord electrical stimulation in severe angina pectoris: surgical technique, intraoperative physiology, complications, and side effects. *Pacing Clin Electrophysiol* 12:693-694, 1989.

8. Augustinsson L, Holm J, Jivegard L: Epidural electrical stimulation in severe limb ischemia: evidence of pain relief, increased blood flow and a possible limb-saving effect. *Ann Surg* 202:104-111, 1985.

9. Barolat G: The surgical management of spasticity and spasms in spinal cord injury: an overview. *J Am Paraplegia Soc* 11:9-13, 1988.

10. Barolat G: Dorsal selective rhizotomy through a limited exposure of the cauda equina at L-1: technical note. *J Neurosurg* 75:804-807, 1991.

11. Barolat G: Experience with 509 plate-electrodes implanted epidurally from C1 to L1. *Stereotact Funct Neurosurg* 61:60-79, 1993.

12. Barolat G: Surgical management of spasticity in spinal cord injury. In Northrup B, Garfield R (eds): *Surgery for Spinal Injuries.* Philadelphia, Lippincott-Raven, 1993, pp 297-304.

13. Barolat G, Schwartzman RJ, Woo R: Epidural spinal cord stimulation in the management of reflex sympathetic dystrophy. *Stereotact Funct Neurosurg* 53:29-39, 1989.

14. Beck AJ, Gaskill SJ, Marlin AE: Improvement in upper extremity function and trunk control after selective posterior rhizotomy. *Am J Occup Ther* 47:704-707, 1993.

15. Bloom KK, Nazar GB: Functional assessment following selective posterior rhizotomy in spastic cerebral palsy. *Childs Nerv Syst* 10:84-86, 1994.

16. Bloomfield S, Gross R: Intrathecal morphine infusion for chronic intractable benign pain: experience with 50 patients. In *Proceedings of the 1995 Quadrennial Meeting of the American Society for Functional and Stereotactic Neurosurgery,* 1995

17. Boscarino LF, Ounpuu S, Davis RB III, *et al:* Effects of selective dorsal rhizotomy on gait in children with cerebral palsy. *J Pediatr Orthop* 13:174-179, 1993.

18. Bowsher D: Contralateral mirror-image pain following anterolateral cordotomy. *Pain* 33:63-65, 1988.

19. Cahan LD, Adams JM, Perry J, Beeler LM: Instrumented gait analysis after selective dorsal rhizotomy. *Dev Med Child Neurol* 32:1037-1043, 1990.

20. Claeys L, Horsch S: Epidural spinal cord stimulation in treatment of refractory Fontaine stages III and IV arterial occlusive disease: indications, use and clinical results. *Vasa Suppl* 32:406-410, 1991.

21. Coffey RJ, Cahill D, Steers W, *et al:* Intrathecal baclofen for intractable spasticity of spinal origin: results of a long-term multicenter study. *J Neurosurg* 78:226-232, 1993.

22. Deletis V, Vodusek DB, Abbott R, *et al:* Intraoperative monitoring of the dorsal sacral roots: minimizing the risk of iatrogenic micturition disorders. *Neurosurgery* 30:72-75, 1992.

23. Delhaas EM, Brouwers JR: Intrathecal baclofen overdose: report of 7 events in 5 patients and review of the literature. *Int J Clin Pharmacol Ther Toxicol* 29:274-280, 1991.

24. Dennis GC, DeWitty RL: Long-term intraventricular infusion of morphine for intractable pain in cancer of the head and neck. *Neurosurgery* 26:404-407, 1990.

25. Dudgeon BJ, Libby AK, McLaughlin JF, *et al:* Prospective measurement of functional changes after selective dorsal rhizotomy. *Arch Phys Med Rehabil* 75:46-53, 1994.

26. Ebel H, Buschmann D, Conzen M, Oppel F: Initial experiences with implantable pump systems for intrathecal therapy of chronic pain conditions. *Nervenarzt* 64:468-473, 1993.

27. Edgar RE, Best LG, Quail PA, Obert AD: Computer-assisted DREZ microcoagulation: posttraumatic spinal deafferentation pain. *J Spinal Disord* 6:48-56, 1993.

28. Esposito S, Delitala A, Nardi PV: Microsurgical DREZ-lesion in the treatment of deafferentation pain. *J Neurosurg Sci* 32:113-115, 1988.

29. Fasano V, Barolat G, Broggi G: La radicotomie posterieure fonctionnelle dans le traitment de la spasticite cerebrale. *Neurochirurgie* 22:23-24, 1976.

30. Fasano VA, Broggi G, Barolat-Romana G, Sguazzi A: Surgical treatment of spasticity in cerebral palsy. *Childs Brain* 4:289-305, 1978.

31. Foerster O: On the indications and results of the excision of posterior spinal nerve roots in men. *Surg Gynecol Obstet* 16:463-464, 1913.

32. Follett KA, Hitchon PW, Piper J, *et al:* Response of intractable pain to continuous intrathecal morphine: a retrospective study. *Pain* 49:21-25, 1992.

33. Friedman AH, Nashold BS Jr: DREZ lesions for relief of pain related to spinal cord injury. *J Neurosurg* 6:465-469, 1986.

34. Goucke R: Continuous intrathecal analgesia with opioid/local anaesthetic mixture for cancer pain. *Anaesth Intensive Care* 21:222-223, 1993.

35. Greene WB, Dietz FR, Goldberg MJ, *et al:* Rapid progression of hip subluxation in cerebral palsy after selective posterior rhizotomy. *J Ped Orthop* 11:494-497, 1991.

36. Grillo PJ, Yu HC, Patterson RH: Delayed intraspinal hemorrhage after dorsal column stimulation for pain. *Arch Neurol* 30:105-106, 1974.

37. Gros C, Ouakine G, Vlahovitch B, Frerebeau P: La radicotomie selective posterieure dans le traitment neurochirurgicale de l'hypertonie pyramidal. *Neurochirurgie* 13:505-515, 1967.

38. Gybel JM, Sweet WH: *Neurosurgical Treatment of Persistent Pain,* Basel, S Karger AG, 1989.

39. Hassenbusch SJ, Pillay PK, Magdinec M, *et al:* Constant infusion of morphine for intractable cancer pain using an implanted pump. *J Neurosurg* 73:405-409, 1990.

40. Iacono RP, Guthkelch AN, Boswell MV: Dorsal root entry zone stimulation for deafferentation pain. *Stereotact Funct Neurosurg* 59:56-61, 1992.

41. Ischia S, Luzzani A, Maffezzoli G: Bilateral percutaneous cordotomy: immediate and long-term results in 36 patients with neoplastic disease. *J Neurol Neurosurg Psychiatry* 47:141-147, 1984.

42. Kanpolat Y, Akyar S, Caglar S, *et al:* CT-guided percutaneous selective cordotomy. *Acta Neurochir* (Wien) 123:92-96, 1993.

43. Kofler M, Saltuari L, Schmutzhard E, *et al:* Electrophysiological findings in a case of severe intrathecal baclofen overdose. *Electroencephalog Clin Neurophysiol* 83:83-86, 1992.

44. Kroin SJ: Intrathecal drug administration. *Clin Pharmacokinet* 22:319-326, 1992.

45. Krol G, Arbit E: Percutaneous lateral cervical cordotomy: target localization with water-soluble contrast medium. *J Neurosurg* 79:390-392, 1993.

46. Kühner A: La cordotomie percutanee: sa place actuelle dans la chirurgie de la douleur. *Anesth Analg* (Paris) 38:357-359, 1981.

47. Kumar K, Nath R, Wyant GM: Treatment of chronic pain by epidural spinal cord stimulation: a 10-year experience. *J Neurosurg* 75:402-407, 1991.

48. Lahuerta J, Bowsher D, Lipton S, Buxton PH: Percutaneous cervical cordotomy: a review of 181 operations on 146 patients with a study on the location of "pain fibers" in the C-2 spinal cord segment of 29 cases. *J Neurosurg* 80:975-985, 1994.

49. Lahuerta J, Buxton P, Lipton S, Bowsher D: The location and function of respiratory fibers in the second cervical spinal cord segment: respiratory dysfunction syndrome after cervical cordotomy. *J Neurol Neurosurg Psychiatry* 55:1142-1145, 1992.

50. Levin AB, Sperling KB: Complications associated with implanted infusion pumps. In *Proceedings of the 1995 Quadrennial Meeting of the American Society for Functional and Stereotactic Neurosurgery*, 1995, p 95.

51. Long DN, Erickson DE: Stimulation of the posterior columns of the spinal cord for relief of intractable pain. *Surg Neurol* 4:134-141, 1975.

52. McNeal DM, Hawtrey CE, Wolraich ML, Mapel JR: Symptomatic neurogenic bladder in a cerebral palsy population. *Dev Med Child Neurol* 25:612-616, 1983.

53. Meythaler JM, Steers WD, Tuel SM, *et al:* Continuous intrathecal baclofen in spinal cord spasticity. *Am J Phys Med Rehabil* 71:321-327, 1992.

54. Muller-Schwefe G, Penn RD: Physostigmine in the treatment of intrathecal baclofen overdose. *J Neurosurg* 71:273-275, 1989.

55. Munro D: The rehabilitation of patients totally paralyzed below the waist: anterior rhizotomy for spastic paraplegia. *N Engl J Med* 233:456-461, 1945.

56. Nagaro T, Amakawa K, Arai T, Ochi G: Ipsilateral referral of pain following cordotomy. *Pain* 5:275-276, 1993.

57. Nagaro T, Kimura S, Arai T: A mechanism of new pain following cordotomy: reference of sensation. *Pain* 30: 89-91, 1987.

58. Nashold BS Jr, Vieira J, el-Naggar AO: Pain and spinal cysts in paraplegia: treatment by drainage and DREZ operation. *Br J Neurosurg* 4:327-335, 1990,

59. Nathan PW: The descending respiratory pathways in man. *J Neurol Neurosurg Psychiatry* 26:487-499, 1963.

60. Nathan PW, Smith PC: Dysesthesie apres cordotomie. *Med Hyg* 42:1788-1790, 1984.

61. North RB, Cutchis PN, Epstein JA, Long DM: Spinal cord compression complicating subarachnoid infusion of morphine: case report and laboratory experience. *Neurosurgery* 29:778-784, 1991.

62. North RB, Kidd DH, Zahurak M, *et al:* Spinal cord stimulation for chronic, intractable pain: experience over two decades. *Neurosurgery* 32:384-394, 1993.

63. Ochs G, Struppler A, Meyerson BA, *et al:* Intrathecal baclofen for long-term treatment of spasticity:

64. Onofrio BM, Yaksh TL: Long-term pain relief produced by intrathecal morphine infusion in 53 patients. *J Neurosurg* 72:200-209, 1990.

65. Park TS, Gaffney P, Kaufman B, Molleston M: Selective lumbosacral dorsal rhizotomy immediately caudal to the conus medullaris for cerebral palsy spasticity. *Neurosurgery* 33:929-934, 1993.

66. Park TS, Vogler GP, Phillips LA II, *et al:* Effects of selective dorsal rhizotomy for spastic diplegia on hip migration in cerebral palsy. *Pediatr Neurosurg* 20:43-49, 1994.

67. Peacock WJ, Arens LJ, Berman B: Cerebral palsy spasticity, selective posterior rhizotomy. *Pediatr Neurosci* 13:61-66, 1987.

68. Peacock WJ, Staudt LA: Functional outcomes following selective posterior rhizotomy in children with cerebral palsy. *J Neurosurg* 74:380-385, 1991.

69. Peacock WJ, Staudt LA: Selective posterior rhizotomy: evolution of theory and practice. *Pediatr Neurosurg* 17:128-134, 1991.

70. Penn RD: Intrathecal baclofen for spasticity of spinal origin: seven years of experience. *J Neurosurg* 77:236-240, 1992.

71. Penn RD, Kroin JS: Failure of physostigmine in treatment of acute severe intrathecal baclofen intoxication: answer to a letter to the editor. *N Engl J Med* 322:1533-1534, 1990.

72. Penn RD, Paice JA: Chronic intrathecal morphine for intractable pain. *J Neurosurg* 67:182-186, 1987.

73. Peter JC, Hoffman EB, Arens LJ, Peacock WJ: Incidence of spinal deformity in children after multiple level laminectomy for selective posterior rhizotomy. *Childs Nerv Syst* 6:30-32, 1990

74. Polatty RC, Cooper KR: Respiratory failure after percutaneous cordotomy. *South Med J* 79:897-899, 1986.

75. Privat JM, Benezech J, Frerebeau P, Gros C: Sectorial posterior rhizotomy: a new technique of surgical treatment of spasticity. *Acta Neurochir* 35:181-195, 1976.

76. Racz GB, McCarron RF, Talboys P: Percutaneous dorsal column stimulator for chronic pain control. *Spine* 14:1-4, 1989.

77. Robaina FJ, Dominguez M, Diaz M, *et al.:* Spinal cord stimulation for relief of chronic pain in vasospastic disorders of the upper limbs. *Neurosurgery* 24:63-67, 1989.

78. Rosomoff HL: Stereotaxic cordotomy. In Youmans J (ed): *Neurological Surgery*, ed 2. Philadelphia, WB Saunders, 1982, pp 3672-3685.

79. Rosomoff HL, Carroll E, Brown J, Sheptak P: Percutaneous radiofrequency cervical cordotomy: technique. *J Neurosurg* 23:639-644, 1965.

80. Rosomoff HL, Kreiger AJ, Kuperman AS: Effects of percutaneous cervical cordotomy on pulmonary function. *J Neurosurg* 31:620-627, 1969.

81. Saltuari L, Baumgartner H, Kofler M, *et al:* Failure of physostigmine in treatment of acute severe intrathecal baclofen intoxication: letter to the editor. *N Engl J Med* 322:1533, 1990.

82. Sauter K, Kaufman H, Bloomfield S, *et al:* Treatment of high dose intrathecal morphine overdose. *J Neurosurg* 81:143-146, 1994.

83. Siegfried R, Jacobson L, Chabal C: Development of an acute withdrawal syndrome following the cessation of

intrathecal baclofen in a patient with spasticity. *Anesthesiology* 77:1048-1050, 1992.

84. Simpson BA: Spinal cord stimulation in 60 cases of intractable pain. *J Neurol Neurosurg Psychiatry* 54: 196-199, 1991.

85. Simpson BA: Spinal cord stimulation. *Pain Rev* 1:199-230, 1994.

86. Sindou M, Jeanmonod D: Microsurgical DREZ-otomy for the treatment of spasticity and pain in the lower limbs. *Neurosurgery* 24:655-670, 1989.

87. Steinbok P, Reiner A, Beauchamp RD, *et al:* Selective functional posterior rhizotomy for treatment of spastic cerebral palsy in children. *Pediatr Neurosurg* 18:34-42, 1992.

88. Sweet WH: Recent observations pertinent to improving antero-lateral cordotomy, *Clin Neurosurg* 23:80-95, 1976.

89. Tasker RR: Open cordotomy. *Progr Neurol Surg* 8:1-14, 1977.

90. Tasker RR: Percutaneous cordotomy. In Youmans J (ed): *Neurological Surgery*, ed 3. Philadelphia, WB Saunders, 1990, pp 4045-4058.

91. Tasker RR, Evans RJ: Experience with percutaneous cordotomy. *Can J Surg* 16:1-3, 1973.

92. Teddy P, Jamous A, Gardner B, *et al:* Complications of intrathecal baclofen therapy. *Br J Neurosurg* 6:115-118, 1992.

93. Thomas DG: Brachial plexus injury: deafferentation pain and dorsal root entry zone (DREZ) coagulation. *Clin Neurol Neurosurg* 95(suppl):S48-S49, 1993.

94. Thomas DG, Kitchen ND: Long-term follow up of dorsal root entry zone lesions in brachial plexus avulsion. *J Neurol Neurosurg Psychiatry* 57:737-738, 1994.

95. Tranmer BI, Tucker WS, Bilbao JM: Sleep apnea following percutaneous cervical cordotomy. *Can J Neurol Sci* 14:262-267, 1987.

96. Vaughan CL, Berman B, Peacock WJ: Cerebral palsy and rhizotomy: a 3-year follow-up evaluation with gait analysis. *J Neurosurg* 74:178-184, 1991.

97. White JC, Sweet WH: *Pain and the Neurosurgeon: a Forty-Year Experience*, Springfield, Ill, Charles C Thomas, 1969.

98. Wu CL, Patt RB: Accidental overdose of systemic morphine during intended refill of intrathecal infusion device. *Anesth Analg* 75:130-132, 1992.

99. Young RF: Evaluation of dorsal column stimulation in the treatment of chronic pain. *Neurosurgery* 3:373-379, 1978.

100. Young RF: Clinical experience with radiofrequency and laser DREZ lesions. *J Neurosurg* 72:715-720, 1990.

101. Young RF: Cordotomy by open operative techniques. In Youmans J (ed): *Neurological Surgery*, ed 3. Philadelphia, WB Saunders, 1990, pp 4059-4069.

# CHAPTER 93

# Bone Graft Harvesting

**Mehmet Zileli, Edward C. Benzel, and
Gordon R. Bell**

Spinal operations frequently attempt to provide stability after it has been adversely affected by a variety of pathologies such as trauma, tumor, or spondylosis. The operations themselves may also cause significant instability. In these cases, fusion, with or without instrumentation, is often used. Because instrumentation provides only a temporary support, solid bony union must be achieved in order to provide permanent stability.

## The Bone Graft

An ideal bone graft would be (1) able to incorporate rapidly, (2) structurally sound, (3) antigenically compatible, (4) readily available and easily shaped, (5) associated with a low incidence of graft site complications, and (6) cost-effective. Regrettably, none of the grafts available today have all of these features.

Cortical bone is primarily advantageous for structural support, whereas cancellous bone is advantageous for osteogenesis.[50] Cancellous grafts have the highest fusion rates. All cellular elements in grafts die and are slowly replaced by "creeping substitution." The graft itself acts as a scaffold for the new bone formation. With hard cortical bone, this process is slower than with cancellous bone. Conversely, cancellous bone is not as strong as the cortical bone. The harvesting technique for cancellous bone is easier and carries a lower complication rate than full-thickness graft harvesting.

Cancellous grafts are primarily used during dorsal spinal fusions because they do not need to bear compressive forces. Cortical grafts, however, are predominantly used for ventral fusions. It is clearly more advantageous to use corticocancellous bone grafts for ventral fusions because in this situation both load-bearing capacity and osteogenesis are necessary.

## Autografts

Autografts are the most frequently used bone grafts in spinal surgery. They are considered the "gold standard" since they provide the most predictable results. Key features of autografts included (1) osteoinduction (i.e., biologically mediated recruitment and differentiation of cell types essential for bone formation), (2) osteoconduction (i.e., the opposition of growing bone to the three-dimensional surface of a suitable scaffold provided by the graft), and (3) osteogenesis (i.e., the process of bone formation through cellular osteoblastic activity properties). The capacity for rapid regeneration comes mostly from fresh cancellous bone, which contains bone matrix proteins and mineral collagens.

An ideal autograft includes strong cortical bone to provide structural support when needed and cancellous bone for augmented incorporation and fusion characteristics.[11,41]

Revascularization of cancellous bone is completed within 2 weeks, whereas the same process takes 2 months for corticated bone.[24] An additional advantage of autogenous bone graft is that it does not carry transmissible diseases to the host. It is not immunogenic.

Cortical and cancellous graft material is generally obtained from the iliac crest. Purely cortical bone is usually obtained from the fibula or tibia.

## Allografts

Allografts are tissues obtained from human cadavers or living donors. They are associated with delayed vascularization and delayed incorporation, perhaps because of antigenic recognition.

Allografts have osteoinductive and osteoconductive properties. However, they have lost their osteogenic property.

Allografts are appropriate in several clinical circumstances.[8,31,45] One is ventral cervical interbody fusion, in which single-level allografts can achieve a solid arthrodesis, with a fusion rate similar to that of the autograft.[32] However, allografts incorporate relatively slowly, and when they are used for multilevel ventral cervical fusions, pseudoarthrosis rates range from 63% to 70%.[49] In general, fibular allografts are preferred for cervical corpectomy, because harvesting autogenous fibula grafts is associated with significant morbidity.[31] Autogenous bone should be used for dorsal onlay fusions because allografts are associated with a low fusion rate. Fibula, iliac crest, femoral neck, patella, and bone chip allografts are chosen for ventral cervical fusion.

One of the disadvantages of allografts is the potential risk of viral disease transmission, such as human immunodeficiency virus (HIV) infection. Gamma radiation and freezing techniques seem to be inadequate in decontaminating the HIV virus from allografts.[9]

## Xenografts

Xenografts are tissues transplanted from one species to another. Xenografts provide less satisfactory results than do autografts and allografts due to histocompatibility differences. Kiel bone grafts have also been used in spinal surgery.

## Osteoinductive Growth Factors

Autologous bone marrow or demineralized bone matrix (DBM) may be added to autogenous and homogenous bone grafts to stimulate osteogenesis. Another experimental material is bone morphogenic protein (BMP). Its inherent advantage lies in its ability to stimulate bone growth and incorporation. Addition of this material to ceramics may improve the fusion capacity of these substitutes.[9]

### Ceramics and Bone Graft Substitutes

Some of the substitutes that have been suggested in lieu of bone grafts are nonbiologic materials, such as hydroxyapatite (HA)[10,23,37] and tricalcium phosphate (TCP).[27] Polymethylmethacrylate has even been suggested as a bone graft substitute[21]; however, it does not incorporate. Although their biologic properties vary and are generally poor, these three nonbiological materials can be manufactured or formed in different sizes and quantities. Their combination with other materials, such as autografts, may be useful. Ceramic substances have osteoconductive properties. Ceramics present with a specific porosity and act as scaffold for further osteoblastic ingrowth.[27] Calcium sulfate pellets (plaster of Paris) have been used in place of morselized cancellous bone graft to fill bone defects.[22] Calcium phosphate ceramics have been helpful in lumbar posterolateral fusion.[15,16]

## Autogenous Bone Graft And Harvesting Techniques

There are five fundamental types of grafts: (1) dual onlay and strut grafts (e.g., fibula or rib graft), (2) tricortical graft (e.g., full-thickness iliac crest graft), (3) bicortical graft (e.g., iliac grafts obtained below the crest), (4) unicortical graft (e.g., grafts obtained from one cortex of the bone), and (5) cancellous bone chip grafts.

In general, it is advantageous to suture the periosteum over a bone graft harvest defect. The periosteum thus serves as a structurally solid membrane that prevents irregular callus formation. Bone cells under the periosteum may help to form new bone to fill the defect.

Although most surgeons prefer to harvest the graft before primary surgery, this may cause the material to dry and lose some proteins, which are valuable for a good fusion. Therefore, the graft should be soaked in blood and covered with moist gauze.[4]

### Iliac Crest

The most commonly used donor site for spinal surgery is the iliac crest.[46] Its advantages are rapid incorporation and ease of harvesting. Its disadvantages are donor site pain and limited length.

#### *Ventral Iliac Crest Grafts*

Ventral iliac crest graft harvesting is usually chosen for ventral cervical fusions (Figure 93.1). The incision should be just inferior to the crest and 3 to 4cm lateral to the anterior superior iliac spine. This protects the inguinal ligament, lateral femoral cutaneous nerve, and attachments of the sartorius muscle. In 10% of cases the lateral femoral cutaneous nerve may be located 2cm lateral to the anterior superior iliac spine, so dissection should be lateral to this point to prevent injury to this nerve (Figure 93.2). A 6 to 8cm incision is made with a subperiosteal dissection using monopolar cautery and a Cobb periosteal elevator. Medially, the iliohypogastric and ilioinguinal nerves can be injured over the iliacus muscles if careful subperiosteal dissection is not performed. To prevent a herniation of

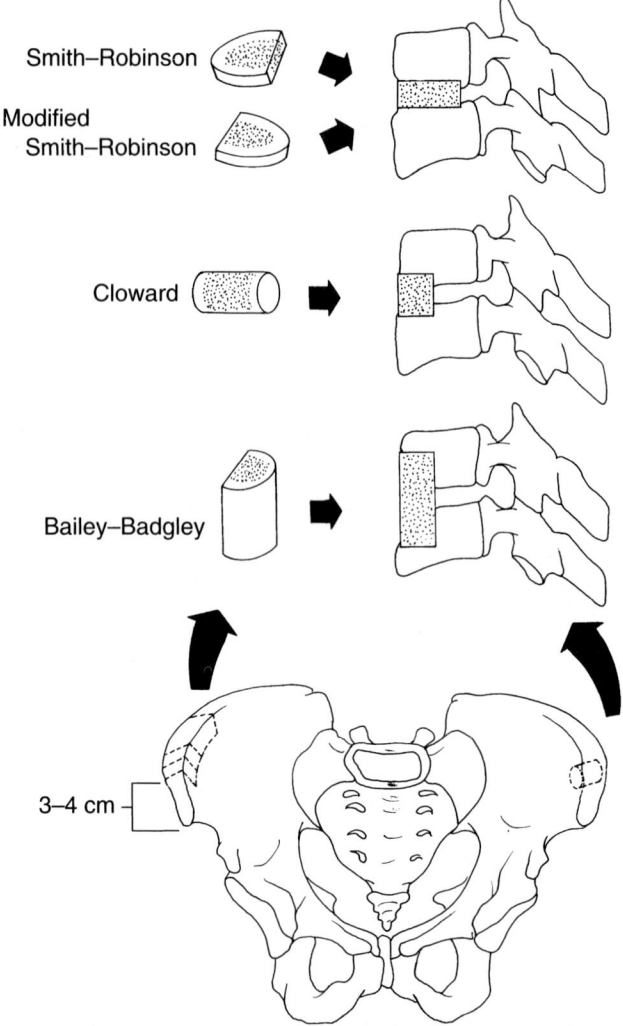

**Figure 93.1** Ventral iliac crest graft harvesting and ventral cervical fusion techniques. *(Redrawn with permission from White AA, Hirsch C: An experimental study of the immediate load bearing capacity of some commonly used iliac bone grafts.* Acta Orthop Scand 42:482-490, 1971.)

pelvic contents, the fascia should be closed securely (see Figure 93.1).

After obtaining the graft, the bone surfaces may be sparingly covered with bone wax or thrombin-soaked Gelfoam. A drain is not usually necessary. Care should be taken during graft harvest to avoid proximity to the anterior superior iliac spine in order to minimize risk of avulsion fracture, which can lead to significant persistent pain.

A vascularized ventral iliac crest graft with the attached deep circumflex iliac artery and vein was proposed for spinal reconstruction to promote rapid fusion and higher resistance to infection.[47] Such grafts, however, have not become popular. Vascularized grafts in general can overcome the problems of strut allografts, such as fatigue fracture and nonunion.

#### *Dorsal Iliac Crest Grafts*

The dorsal iliac crest is an excellent source for large quantities of cancellous graft. If the operation is in the

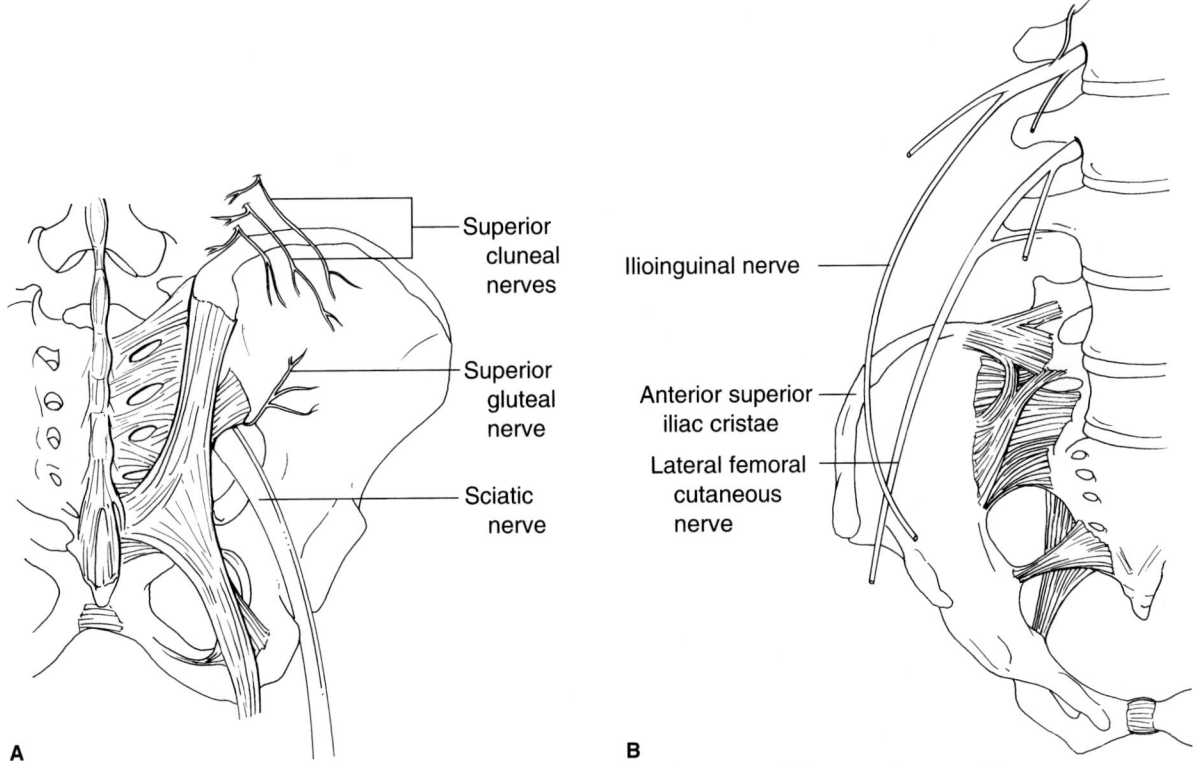

**Figure 93.2** Possible nerve injury sites during (**A**) dorsal and (**B**) ventral iliac crest bone graft harvesting.

lumbosacral region, the midline incision is often sufficient to obtain dorsal iliac grafts through the same midline but separate fascial incision. The disadvantage of taking bone graft from the same deep incision as the laminectomy and fusion incision is that an infection at the bone graft site can cross-contaminate the laminectomy and fusion site.

For cervical or thoracic operations a second incision that is parallel to the lateral iliac crest is used (Figure 93.3). The dorsal portion of the iliac crest is palpated, and a curvilinear incision is made over the iliac crest. An incision approximately 6 to 8cm long is necessary. The medial border of the facial incision should be 6 to 8cm lateral to the midline in order to avoid injury to the cluneal nerves, which may cause sensory loss or pain over the buttocks. This is more likely if a large amount of graft is required. Medially, the sacroiliac ligaments and joints must be avoided. If the dissection is performed subperiosteally, the superior gluteal artery and nerve will not be injured. The junction of the thoracodorsal fascia and the gluteal fascia is incised over the iliac crest, and muscles are dissected subperiosteally from both sides of the crest.

The sciatic nerve or the ureter (just ventral to the sciatic notch) can be injured if the dissection is taken very deep and inside the muscles. If an osteotomy cut is made lateral to the posterior superior iliac spine, then entry into the sciatic notch and injury to superior gluteal artery and sciatic nerve is unlikely.

A gouge is helpful for removing strips of cancellous bone. An osteotome or an oscillating saw may be used to resect the cortical portion of the crest (Figure 93.4). A gouge or curette is used to remove cancellous bone.

Some surgeons prefer to open a cortical bone window on the superior aspect of the crest, remove cancellous bone, and replace this piece to prevent a large defect. However, if a bicortical graft is needed, this method is not applicable.[5]

For unicortical and cancellous bone graft harvesting, a subcrestal exposure is also described.[48] With this technique, only gluteal muscles are retracted from the dorsal surface of the iliac crest. Without disturbing the entire thickness of the crest, unicortical and cancellous bone graft is harvested with the aid of osteotomes, and a portion from the outer table of the ilium is resected. Cancellous bone is usually removed with gouges. However, entering the inner table of the ileum can damage the sacroiliac joint. If only cancellous bone graft is needed, it can be harvested by trephine curettage by entering the ventral or dorsal iliac spine with minimal exposure.[36]

In general, it is better to irrigate the wound generously and to use Gelfoam packing instead of bone wax because bone wax does not permit bony regeneration.

## Fibula

Fibular grafts have the advantages of strength, length, and relative ease of harvest. The disadvantages are slow incorporation and harvest site complications. Fibula struts should be removed from the middle third of the fibular shaft through the lateral intermuscular septum, preserving the periosteum.

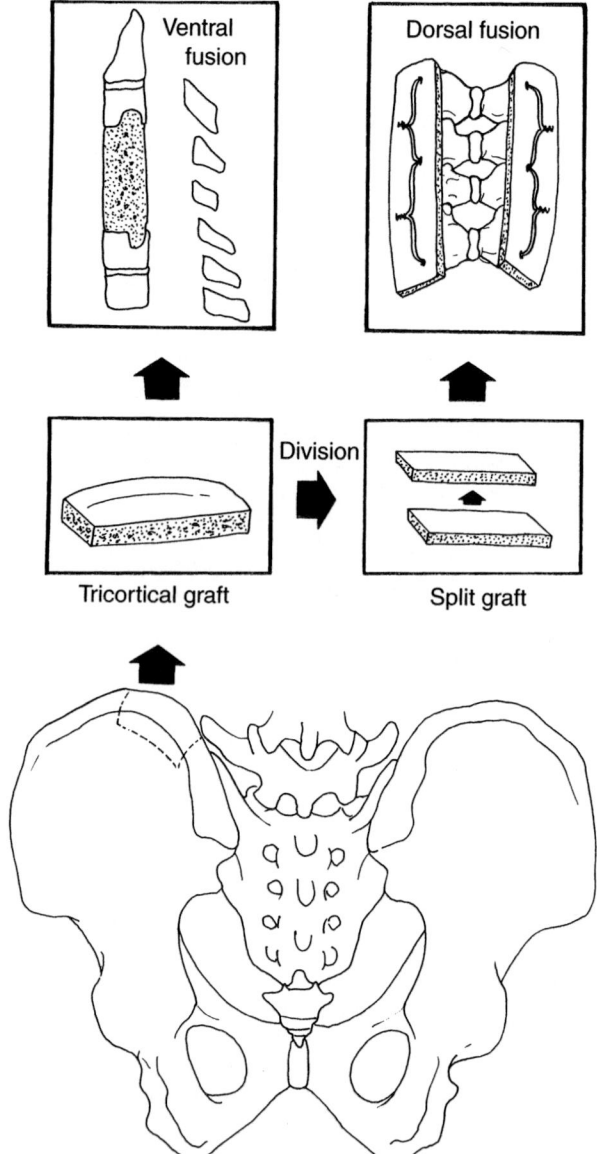

**Figure 93.3** Dorsal iliac crest graft harvesting. Both tricortical and split techniques are depicted.

The rostral two thirds of the fibula may also be removed to use as a graft. However, such a procedure may cause excessive pain and weakness.[19] This technique also involves a significant risk of peroneal nerve injury, as well as intolerability.

The use of a vascularized fibula with the peroneal artery and vein may result in a more rapid incorporation of the graft. However, the muscle sleeve interferes with lateral incorporation and causes an impairment of foot function, secondary to muscle harvest with the fibula.

### Tibia

The main advantages of tibia grafts are their strength, compact cortical bone, and their length. The subcutaneous proximal ventromedial aspect of the tibia is suitable for graft harvest. Donor site fracture is a disadvantage. The tibia must be protected for 6 to 12 months to prevent fractures.[11] It should be understood that this technique is infrequently employed because of the significant chance of morbidity.

To harvest a graft from the tibia, a longitudinal incision is made over the proximal ventromedial surface of the tibia. The periosteum is incised and retracted. Because the proximal portion of the tibia is larger than its distal counterpart, the graft shape is asymmetrical. Because the cortex is thinner in the proximal tibia, it is better to harvest grafts from the distal part of the tibia. An oscillating saw can be used to remove a square-shaped graft easily. Fractures of the tibia occur most commonly in the distal portion. Care should be taken to not remove excessive bone, particularly in the distal portion (see Figure 93.5).

### Rib

Rib bone is easily harvested, especially during ventral thoracic spine operations. However, it is a weak graft material that is poorly vascularized. Some surgeons prefer to use a rib graft for its unique curvature that conforms to normal cervical lordosis.[35] Although it may cause more serious donor-site complications, including pneumothorax and intercostal neuralgia, a study comparing rib grafts with posterior iliac crest grafts in posterior cervical fusions showed that donor site morbidity with rib grafts (3.7%) occurred with much less frequency than it did with iliac crest grafts (25.3%).[35]

A vascular pedicle rib graft has been proposed for ventral thoracic fusion operations.[12]

### Skull

Skull is a strong graft material. Its curvature facilitates incorporation for selected applications, particularly upper cervical and occipitocervical applications. However, the donor site usually requires some form of a reconstruction procedure. The skull's thickness is variable, and it is limited by cranial sutures.

Cranial bone is used predominantly for craniofacial surgery and for plastic surgery. Most unicortical grafts are taken from the outer surface of the parietal bone (so-called in situ grafts) that do not require the aid of a spine surgeon[26]; their complication rate is low.

After fibula harvest, a few days of compressive leg wrapping with leg elevation minimizes swelling and discomfort.

During fibula graft harvesting, the peroneal nerve must be protected. The distal portion of the fibula must be left (i.e., to avoid injury to the tibia-fibular syndesmosis) in order to preserve the ankle joint. The peroneal muscles should also be preserved.

A long skin incision is made on the lateral side of the leg. Dissection is carried out between the peroneus longus and triceps surae muscles. Peroneal muscles are retracted ventrally after subperiosteal dissection. Because the peroneal muscles attach to the fibula in an oblique fashion (at both the proximal and distal ends of the fibula), they tend to resist the retraction. The middle third of the fibula may be osteotomized, using an oscillating saw. An osteotome may be harmful because it can cause a fracture on the graft or of the remainder of the fibula (Figure 93.5).

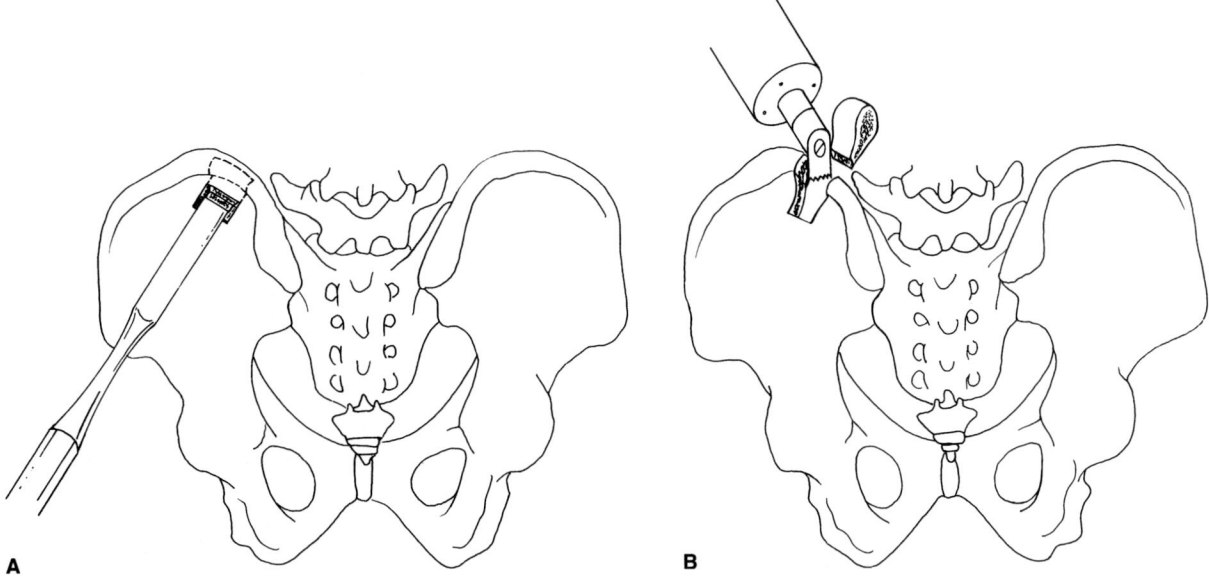

**Figure 93.4** **(A)** Unicortical graft harvesting from the dorsal iliac crest using an osteotome. **(B)** Tricortical graft harvesting from dorsal iliac crest using an oscillating saw.

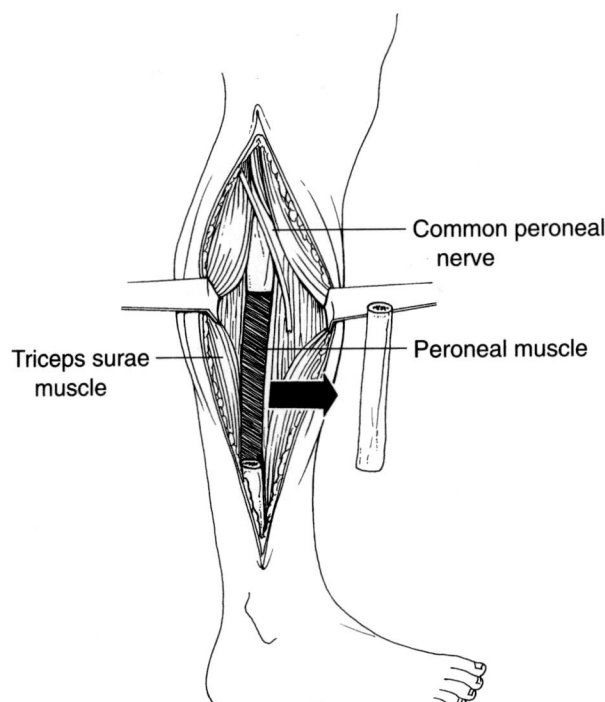

Common peroneal nerve

Peroneal muscle

Triceps surae muscle

**Figure 93.5** Fibula graft harvesting. The midportion of the fibula is removed with a saw or osteotome.

## Complications of Graft Harvesting

Graft harvesting complications are common.[3,26] Although they are generally minor in nature, a review of 1244 cases from multiple series demonstrated that their occurrence is about 20%.[44]

### Chronic Persistent Pain

Graft donor site pain is a complaint of nearly all patients, particularly in the early postoperative period. Pain may persist throughout the first 3 months in up to 15% of the patients.[26] Chronic persistent pain for up to 10 years, however, has been observed in up to one third of the patients.[13,15] The reason for this chronic pain is not well understood but is frequently associated with an overall pain syndrome. There are other uncommon specific reasons for chronic donor site pain. These include injury to the sacroiliac joints, hernia through the graft site, pelvic fracture through the graft donor site (predominantly on the ventral ilium), and heterotopic bone formation.[3]

The extent of the acute pain depends in part on the size of the graft and the breadth and depth of the wound. Therefore, one should attempt to minimize soft tissue injury. If the gluteal fascia is not approximated to the periosteum properly, gait disturbance may arise from gluteus maximus muscle weakness.

In a prospective study, dorsal iliac crest bone graft harvest was found to result in morbidity in 35% of the patients.[33] The major component was donor site pain. Pain scores tended to be higher at 6 months, but significantly decreased at 12 months. The pain was more significant in lumbar spinal surgery than other primary surgeries.

Preserving the outer and inner tables of the ilium and harvesting cancellous bone by an intracortical method did not reduce the donor site pain and postoperative bleeding.[28] By contrast, less bone is harvested and longer operation duration is required in the intraosseous method.

### Nerve Injury and Pain

Incisions for bone grafts may injure nerves or may cause entrapment of nerves because of scar formation. The lateral femoral cutaneous nerve can be injured during ventral iliac crest harvest procedures. This complication has been reported in up to 10% of cases. It may cause either sensory loss on the lateral side of the thigh or meralgia paresthetica.[42] The nerve usually crosses the iliac fossa and passes under the inguinal ligament, 1cm medial to the anterior superior iliac spine. However, in 10% of cases, it may pass above the inguinal ligament and just lateral to the anterior superior iliac spine.[17] Meralgia paresthetica was observed in 1% to 14% of the patients.[43]

The cluneal nerves arise from the superficial fascia, 6 to 8cm lateral to the posterior superior iliac spine. Injury to these nerves during dorsal iliac crest graft harvesting may cause analgesia over the buttock or painful neuromas. A hockey-stick or longitudinal incision may help to avoid this problem.

Other cutaneous nerves, such as the ilioinguinal, iliohypogastric, genitofemoral, superior gluteal, and femoral nerves, may be injured, though this rarely happens. Ilioinguinal, iliohypogastric, and genitofemoral nerves can be injured during iliac muscle splitting for ventral iliac crest harvesting. The superior gluteal and sciatic nerve may be injured during gluteal muscle splitting for dorsal iliac crest harvesting.

### Vascular Injury

Vascular injury during dorsal iliac crest graft harvesting includes damage to the superior gluteal artery. This can cause severe hemorrhaging. The superior gluteal artery lies between the gluteus medius and minimus muscles and is preserved with careful subperisoteal dissection.

### Hematoma Formation

Hematoma formation has been reported in 9% of cases.[13] The bleeding arises from the adjacent muscles and bone surfaces. Meticulous hemostasis is, therefore, mandatory. Hematoma formation can result in excessive blood loss (i.e., into the retroperitoneum) and an increased chance of infection.

### Pelvic Fracture or Instability

Fortunately, pelvic fracture or instability is a rare complication. Pelvic fractures may arise from ventral iliac graft harvests performed too close to the anterior superior iliac spine. This type of fracture is usually an avulsion fracture of the ventral wing of the ilium. It causes severe pain with ambulation. Symptomatic treatment (e.g., decreased activity) usually suffices. A vertical fracture through the pelvis may occur during dorsal iliac harvest. If this fracture is complete, the whole hemipelvis may "drop" due to additional instability through the symphysis pubis.

Disruption of the sacroiliac joint and its ligaments during dorsal operations is also to be avoided. Painful instability can result. In a retrospective study examining the computed tomography findings of 22 patients with pain persisting more than 24 months after posterior iliac bone graft harvesting, Ebraheim et al.[14] found a high prevalance of inner table disruption of sacroiliac joint.

### Local Infection

Local infections occur in less than 1% of cases.[26] As mentioned earlier, meticulous hemostasis and technique should minimize this complication.

### Herniation Through Graft Site

Herniation, including bowel contents, is rare and may occur after both ventral[29] and dorsal[7,40] iliac crest harvesting procedures. A common cause for herniation is excessive iliacus muscle dissection, which, therefore, should be minimized.

### Cosmetic Deformity

Cosmetic deformity may occur after ventral iliac crest full-thickness tricortical graft harvest procedures. Several techniques, such as longitudinal iliac crest splitting,[46] have been used to minimize the incidence of this complication. The use of the subcrestal window technique[4,26] and reconstruction with synthetic material[21] may diminish its incidence. If this material is made of bioactive ceramic, new bone formation may be obtained in addition to the cosmetic result.[1]

## Grafts for Ventral Cervical Spine Operation

### Interbody Strut Grafts

The Smith-Robinson graft is a tricortical horseshoe strut graft. Smith and Robinson described the harvesting of the graft from the ventral iliac crest at a depth of approximately 1cm and a width of 5 to 6mm.[39] This graft is inserted into the intervertebral space, so that its cancellous portion is directed dorsally. To prevent collapse, extrusion, or nonunion, Bloom and Raney have modified the graft position, with the cortical portion directed dorsally (see Figure 93.1).[6]

The Bailey-Badgley graft is a strut graft. A trough is prepared in the ventral aspect of the vertebral body at a limited depth (0.5cm).[2] The trough is then deepened to the full vertical height of the vertebra, and the discs are cleaned with a rongeur to a depth of approximately 1.2 cm.[2,44] A cortical-cancellous graft is placed into the trough (see Figure 93.1).

### Cloward Graft

The Cloward graft is a dowel graft (see Figure 93.1). After harvesting from the iliac crest with a cylindric saw, the iliac crest is impacted in the place prepared with a 1mm narrower burr. A special instrument set is used for graft harvesting, graft bed preparation, and graft impaction.

If a Cloward graft is used in multilevel fusions, avasacular necrosis of the vertebra may occur.[30] Using Cloward grafting at two adjacent vertebrae can cause this complication. For this, Cloward has advocated an alteration of his technique. If multilevel fusions are required, a Smith-Robinson graft may be inserted with a dowel of bone at an adjacent space.

Sutures placed through the prevertebral fascia are tied over the graft in order to hold it in position.

## Graft Preparation Considerations

The strongest constructs are provided by the Smith-Robinson type grafts.[43] Tricortical grafts are stronger than the split grafts.[45] The more extensive the cancellous portion of the graft junction, the greater the bony ingrowth, but the greater the graft subsidence. The optimal autologous graft has a substantial cancellous surface.

After central corpectomy, either an iliac crest graft or a fibula graft is inserted into the corpectomy space (similar to a Smith-Robinson graft). Iliac crest graft can be used in shorter segments but may not withstand the axial stresses associated with multilevel corpectomies.[23] A fibular allograft may be considered for three or more vertebrectomies. Others have found iliac crest to be satisfactory, even for long grafts.

Some surgeons advise preparation of a hole (mortise), at both the rostral and caudal ends of the fusion bed in the middle of the vertebral body (keystone method).[31,38] In the dovetail method, however, the mortises are in the ventral cortex of the vertebral body (see Figure 93.6).[18] The graft is first inserted into the rostral mortise and then gently tapped into the caudal end. In this instance, manual or skeletal traction may be helpful.[34] In both instances, the iliac crest graft is tailored in a T-shaped form, and the cortical portion of the graft is positioned dorsally.

## Grafts for Ventral Thoracolumbar Operations

With anterior thoracic and lumbar operations, dorsal iliac crest grafts can also be used because the patient is usually positioned laterally. The shape and size of the thoracic and lumbar vertebral bodies are relatively large, and therefore, a more generous graft harvest is necessary. If the donor site is the iliac crest, a tricortical graft is preferred for ventral interbody struts.

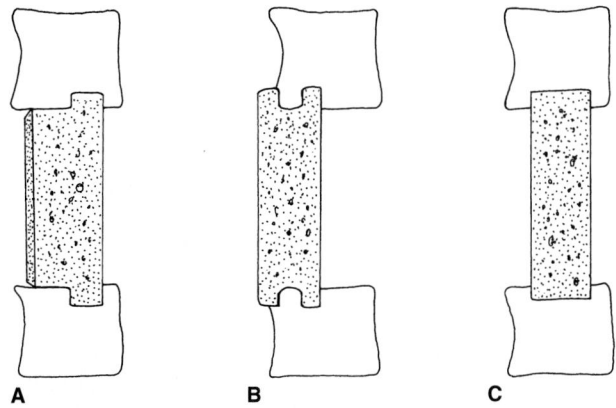

**Figure 93.6** Cervical graft insertion after central corpectomy. **(A)** T-shaped iliac crest graft; **(B)** notched fibula graft (dovetail method); **(C)** straight fibula graft (keystone method). *(Redrawn with permission from Whitecloud TS: Cervical spondylosis: the anterior approach. In Frymoyer JW (ed): The Adult Spine: Principles and Practice, New York, Raven Press, 1991, pp 1165-1185.)*

## Grafts for Dorsal Cervical, Thoracic, and Lumbar Spine Operations

Dorsal cervical, thoracic, and lumbar grafts do not need to be bicortical or tricortical in nature. Usually, cancellous bone is harvested from the dorsal iliac crest, using an osteotome gauge or curette. If the operation includes the removal of spinous processes or lamina, the grafts can also be prepared by removing attached ligaments and muscles and can be used as onlay autografts. The use of allograft as an onlay bone graft material is not recommended.

For wiring and fusion of the dorsal cervical spine, unicortical grafts can be used after decortication of the dorsal elements. These are bone graft plates that can be prepared by splitting the full-thickness bicortical iliac crest graft horizontally. The convex cancellous side of the graft can be placed against the cervical spine to help maintain stability. Wires or cables help fasten unicortical grafts onto the laminar facet surfaces. It is also possible to use a strip graft from the proximal metaphysis of the tibia or to use a split rib graft for this purpose. Cancellous graft chips are then placed laterally between the strut grafts and the lateral musculature.

Local bone, such as lamina and spinous processes, may provide bone graft material for dorsal onlay or interbody fusions. The incorporation potential of such bone is not as high as that of an autogenous iliac crest graft. Therefore, its use is usually as a bone graft extender, rather than as the sole source of bone graft.

## Factors that Facilitate Graft Fusion

Incorporation of a bone graft is dependent on multiple processes related to both the graft and the perigraft environment. One of these factors is the histocompatibility antigen incompatibility.[41] Another important issue is the biologic activity of the surrounding tissue. If the tissue is irradiated, badly vascularized (scar tissue), or osteoporotic, its fusion rate will be lower and slower. Cigarette smoking has an inhibitory effect on fusion, with diminished vascularization of graft bed. Electrical stimulation, some endocrine hormones (e.g., estrogen, testosterone, growth hormone, thyroxine, insulin), vitamin D, and calcitonin all have positive effects an bone graft fusion.

## REFERENCES

1. Asano S, Kaneda K, Satoh S, *et al*: Reconstruction of an iliac crest defect with a bioactive ceramic prosthesis. *Eur Spine J* 3:39-44, 1994.
2. Bailey RW, Badgley CE: Stabilization of the cervical spine by anterior fusion. *J Bone Joint Surg (Am)* 42:565-594, 1960.
3. Banwart JC, Asher MA, Hassanein RS: Iliac crest bone graft harvest donor site morbidity: a statistical evaluation. *Spine* 20:1055-1060, 1995.
4. Behairy YM, Al-Sebai W: A modified technique for harvesting full-thickness iliac crest bone graft. *Spine* 26:695-697, 2001.
5. Bernardi R, Mueller W: Thoracic fusion techniques using bone. In Menezes AH, Sonntag VKH (eds): *Principles*

*of Spinal Surgery.* New York, McGraw-Hill, 1996, pp 1173-1183.

6. Bloom MH, Raney FL: Anterior intervertebral fusion of the cervical spine: a technical note. *J Bone Joint Surg (Am)* 63:842, 1982.

7. Bosworth DM: Repair of herniae through iliac-crest defects. *J Bone Joint Surg (Am)* 37:1069-1073, 1955.

8. Cloward RB: Gas-sterilized cadaver bone grafts for spinal fusion operations: a simplified bone bank. *Spine* 5:4-10, 1980.

9. Cook SD, Salheld SL, Prewett AB: Simian immunodeficiency virus (Human HIV II) transmission in allograft bone procedures. *Spine* 20:1338-1342, 1995.

10. Cook SD, Whitecloud TS, Reynolds MC, et al: Hydroxylapatite graft materials for cervical spine fusions. In Kehr P, Weidner A (eds): *Cervical Spine I.* Strasbourg, Springer Wien NewYork, 1987, pp 257-262.

11. Crenshaw AH: *Campbell's operative orthopaedics,* vol 1, St Louis, Mosby Year Book, 1992.

12. Deen HG, Zimmerman RS, Lanza LA: Vascular pedicle rib graft in anterior transthoracic fusion procedures: technical note. *J Neurosurg* 90:155-158, 1999.

13. DePalma AF, Rothman RH, Lewinnek GE, et al: Anterior interbody fusion for severe cervical disc degeneration. *Surg Gyn Obst* 134:755-758, 1972.

14. Ebraheim NA, Elgafy H, Semaan HB: Computed tomographic findings in patients with persistent sacroiliac pain after posterior iliac graft harvesting. *Spine* 25:2047-2051, 2000.

15. Frymoyer JW, Howe J, Kuhlmann D: The long-term effects of spinal fusion on the sacroiliac joints and ilium. *Clin Orthop* 134:196-201, 1978.

16. Fujibayashi S, Shikata J, Tanaka C, et al: Lumbar posterolateral fusion with biphasic calcium phosphate ceramic. *J Spinal Disorders* 14:214-221, 2001.

17. Ghent WR: Further studies on meralgia paresthetica. *Can MAJ* 85:871-875, 1961.

18. Gore DR: Technique of cervical interbody fusion. *Clin Orthop* 188:191-195, 1984.

19. Gore DR, Gardner GM, Sepic SB, et al: Function following partial fibulectomy. *Clin Orthop* 220:206, 1987.

20. Hamby WB, Glaser HT: Replacement of spinal intervertebral discs with locally polymerizing methylmethacrylate: experimental study of effects upon tissue and report of a small clinical series. *J Neurosurg* 16:311-313, 1959.

21. Hochshuler SH, Guyer RD, Stith WJ, et al: Proplast reconstruction on iliac crest defects. *Spine* 13:378-379, 1988.

22. Kelly CM, Wilkins RM, Gitelis S, et al: The use of a surgical grade calcium sulfate as a bone graft substitute: results of a multicenter trial. *Clin Orthop Rel Res* 382:42-50, 2001.

23. Kim P, Wakai S, Matsuo S, et al: Bisegmental cervical interbody fusion using hydroxyapatite implants: surgical results and long-term observation in 70 cases. *J Neurosurg* 88:21-27, 1998.

24. Kingma MJ, Hampe JF: The behaviour of blood vessels after experimental transplantation of bone. *J Bone Joint Surg* 46B:141-150, 1964.

25. Kline LT, Wolfe SA: Complications associated with the harvesting of cranial bone grafts. *Plast Reconstr Surg* 95:5-13, 1995.

26. Kurtz LT, Garfin SR, Booth RE Jr: Harvesting autologous iliac bone grafts: a review of complications and techniques. *Spine* 14:1324-1331, 1989.

27. Marchesi DG: Spinal fusions: bone and bone substitutes. *Eur Spine J* 9:372-378, 2000.

28. Mirovsky Y, Neuwirth MG: Comparison between the outer table and intracortical methods of obtaining autogenous bone graft from the iliac crest. *Spine* 25:1722-1725, 2000.

29. Moeller KH, Lawrence DP: Hernia through an iliac bone graft defect. *Mil Med* 161:176-178, 1996.

30. Mosdal C: Cervical osteochondrosis and disc herniation: eighteen years' use of interbody fusion by Cloward's technique in 755 cases. *Acta Neurochir (Wien)* 70:207-255, 1984.

31. Rengachary SS, Redford JB: Partial median corpectomy for cervical spondylotic myelopathy. In Wilkins RH, Rengachary SS (eds): *Neurosurgery: Update II.* New York, McGraw-Hill, 1991, pp 356-359.

32. Rish BL, McFadden JT, Penix JO: Anterior cervical fusion using homologous bone grafts: a comparative study. *Surg Neurol* 5:119-121, 1976.

33. Roberston PA, Wray ACF: Natural history of posterior iliac crest bone graft donation for spinal surgery: a prospective analysis of morbidity. *Spine* 26:1473-1476, 2001.

34. Saunders RL: Ventral exposures of the subaxial cervical spine. In Benzel EC (ed): *Surgical Exposure of the Spine: an Extensile Approach.* Rolling Meadows, IL, American Association of Neurological Surgeons, 1995, pp 55-68.

35. Sawin PD, Traynelis VC, Menezes AH: A comparative analysis of fusion rates and donor-site morbidity for autogeneic rib and iliac crest bone grafts in posterior cervical fusions. *J Neurosurg* 88:255-265, 1998.

36. Scott W, Peterson RC, Grant S: Method of procuring iliac bone by trephine curettage. *J Bone Joint Surg (Am)* 31A:1949.

37. Senter HJ, Kortyna R, Kemp WR: Anterior cervical fusion with hydroxylapatite fusion. *Neurosurgery* 25:39-43, 1989.

38. Simmons EH, Bhalla SK: Anterior cervical discectomy and fusion: a clinical and biomechanical study with eight-year follow-up. *J Bone Joint Surg (Br)* 51:225-237, 1969.

39. Smith GW, Robinson RA: The treatment of certain cervical spine disorders by the anterior removal of the intervertebral disc and interbody fusion. *J Bone Joint Surg* 40A:607, 1958.

40. Stevens KJ, Banuls M: Iliolumbar hernia following bone grafting. *Eur Spine J* 3:118-119, 1994.

41. Stevenson S, Emery SE, Goldberg VM: Factors affecting bone graft incorporation: review. *Clin Orthop Relat Res* 324:66-74, 1996.

42. Weikel AM, Habal MB: Meralgia paresthetica: a complication of iliac bone procurement. *Plast Recon Surg* 60:572-574, 1977.

43. White AA, Hirsch C: An experimental study of the immediate load bearing capacity of some commonly used iliac bone grafts. *Acta Orthop Scand* 42:482-490, 1971.

44. Whitecloud TS: Cervical spondylosis: the anterior approach. In Frymoyer JW (ed): *The Adult Spine: Principles and Practice.* New York, Raven Press, 1991, pp 1165-1185.

45. Wittenberg RH, Moeller J, Shea M, et al: Compressive strength of autologous and allogenous bone grafts for thoracolumbar and cervical spine fusion. *Spine* 15:1073-1078, 1990.

46. Wolfe SA, Kawamoto HK: Taking the iliac-bone graft: a new technique. *J Bone Joint Surg* 60A:411, 1978.

47. Wuisman PIJM, Jiya TU, Van Dijk M, *et al:* Free vascularized bone graft in spinal surgery: indications and outcome in eight cases. *Eur Spine J* 8:296-303, 1999.

48. Yonemura KS: Bone grafts: types of harvesting and their complications. In Menezes AH, Sonntag VKH (eds): *Principles of Spinal Surgery*. New York, McGraw-Hill, 1996, pp 151-156.

49. Zdeblick TA, Ducker TB: The use of freeze-dried allograft bone for anterior cervical fusions. *Spine* 16:726-729, 1991.

50. Zileli M, Resnick DK, Benzel EC: Bone physiology and bone healing. In Selman WR and Benzel EC (eds): *Neurosurgical Care of the Elderly*, Rolling Meadows, IL, American Association of Neurological Surgeons, 1999, pp 149-157.

# CHAPTER 94

# Timing of Spinal Surgery: Argument for Elective Surgery

**Jamie Baisden, Dennis J. Maiman, and Thomas B. Ducker**

Little has changed in the past 10 years with respect to management of acute spinal cord injury other than an attempt to standardize steroid protocols, improved radiographic imaging studies, and improved spinal instrumentation. The goals of rapid immobilization, systemic resuscitation, steroid administration, radiographic evaluation, decompression of the spinal cord, restoration of spinal alignment, and spinal stabilization have remained constant.[3,26,37,38,45]

However, the timing of spinal surgery still remains controversial. The national trend toward evidenced-based medicine and outcome studies has once again attempted to develop guidelines for the timing of spinal surgery. Unfortunately, we are left to review a multitude of Class III evidence to develop the guidelines for timing of spinal surgery.

This Class III evidence of therapeutic effectiveness consists of many retrospective case reports, flawed attempts to randomize controlled trials, and much "expert" opinion. Animal studies on spinal cord injury (SCI) have been difficult to analyze due to differences in mechanisms to human trauma.[1,4,8,14-16,48] Practically speaking, it would be extremely difficult for a group of spinal surgeons (e.g., neurosurgeons and orthopedic surgeons) to come to a consensus to design an appropriate methodologic study to determine optimal timing of spinal surgery and to generate enough accurate data for statistical significance. The variability between participating centers would make diagnostic testing reliability and validity almost impossible to determine. This lack of accuracy would also reflect a lack of sensitivity and specificity on both diagnostic interpretation and clinical assessment.

The process of randomization in this type of study in an acute SCI setting also raises the possibility of additional ethical and legal issues in management of patients with SCI. Pharmacologic therapies in acute SCI have been much easier to design studies as compared with surgical studies.[11,20,21,49] Lastly, the difficulty in obtaining informed consent for patients to participate in this type of study makes a definitive study to determine optimal timing of spinal surgery highly improbable.

The pressures of minimizing hospital stays and cost containment have supported early surgical intervention. Often, in reviewing the surgical literature, it is difficult to determine the time frame within which the surgery was performed. Acute surgical intervention is associated with earlier mobilization, briefer hospital stays, and fewer complications related to prolonged bedrest as compared with nonoperative treatment.[12]

Determination of faster neurologic recovery and sustained long-term neurologic outcome in early versus elective surgery is difficult to ascertain due to the lack of a unified definition of *early*° with regard to surgery.[18,41]

Fehlings and Tator[19] provided an evidence-based review of decompressive surgery in acute SCI. This review covered a Medline search from 1966 to 1998 involving the role of surgical decompression in the treatment of SCI. In their review, 59 papers (16 experimental animal studies and 43 clinical studies) were analyzed. Of the 43 clinical papers, there were no Class I (well-designed, well-conducted randomized controlled trials), 5 Class II (prospective cohort studies or controlled studies with well-defined comparison groups), and 26 Class III (case series, retrospective reviews, and expert opinion) evidence-based papers.

A close review of each of the Class II evidence-based clinical papers shows a common theme: no significant difference in neurologic outcome based on timing of surgery. Tator *et al.*[39] studied a group of 208 patients with acute SCI to determine the role of surgery. They measured the time interval from accident to admission into an acute SCI unit. The timing of surgery was compared with complete cord injury and incomplete cord injury. Almost half (48.2%) of the operations were performed in the first week postinjury, and 86.2% of the surgical group had undergone surgery by the end of the fourth week. The conclusion of the study noted no difference between operated and nonoperated patients in length of stay or neurologic recovery. The authors also observed that operative treatment was associated with a lower overall mortality rate (6.1%) than the nonoperative (15.2%) treatment group, despite a higher frequency of thromboembolic complications in the surgical group.

Duh *et al.*[17] used data from the National Acute Spinal Cord Injury Study (NASCIS) II to determine the effectiveness of surgery in patients with acute SCI and its relation to pharmacologic treatment. Five hundred eighty-five patients were studied. The timing of surgery and the approach (ventral versus dorsal) were reviewed. Early surgery was defined as surgery within 100 hours of injury and late surgery as surgery after 100 hours postinjury. Neurologic scores were compared. The results of this study indicated no difference in the neurologic improvement at 1-year follow-up comparing those who underwent surgery with those who had no surgery. The results suggested that either early surgery (at or before 25 hours after injury) or late surgery (more than 200 hours) may be associated with increased neurologic recovery, particularly motor function, and that the results of surgery were equivocal. The authors did observe that the best predictors of improvement in motor score were 25 years of age or younger, incomplete injury, and lower baseline emergency department neurologic

---

°Because of the range of meanings in terms that describe the timing of spinal surgery, definitions of words such as *early, delayed,* and *late* will change throughout the chapter, depending on the context of the study being discussed.

scores (less severe SCI). The authors also concluded that this study does not provide clinically relevant evidence concerning the efficacy of timing or the value of surgery in treating patients with SCI.

The effect of surgery on motor recovery following traumatic SCI was studied by Waters et al.,[45] between 1985 and 1990. Two hundred sixty-nine consecutive traumatic SCI patients were studied, and the methylprednisolone protocols of Bracken et al.[11] (NASCIS) were not used. The motor recovery between 1 month and 1 year was assessed prospectively in the 269 acute SCI patients using the American Spinal Injury Association (ASIA) classification system. This study did not have an early treatment group and included both penetrating and nonpenetrating types of injuries. Among patients who received surgical treatment for their SCI, only those who underwent surgery in the first 3.5 months postinjury were included in the study. Patients were assigned to one of four categories: (1) complete paraplegia, (2) incomplete paraplegia, (3) complete tetraplegia, and (4) incomplete tetraplegia. Within each subgroup, patients were further assigned to one of five categories based on treatment received: (1) no surgery, (2) spine fusion with instrumentation, (3) anterior decompression with or without spine fusion and instrumentation, (4) laminectomy with or without internal fixation and fusion, and (5) bullet removal. The authors determined that motor score recovery between 1 month and 1 year after injury was highly dependent ($\rho \leq .001$) on the level and completeness of injury. Motor recovery did not significantly differ between patients categorized in various surgical subgroups or between those having surgery and those treated nonoperatively.

Vaccaro et al.[42] conducted a randomized prospective controlled study at the Regional Spinal Cord Injury Center of the Delaware Valley between October 1992 and November 1995. They defined early surgery as less than 72 hours after SCI and late surgery as more than 5 days after SCI. Injury mechanisms and surgical approaches and procedures were identified in both the early and late surgical groups. Postoperative days in the acute hospital and in rehabilitation were determined. Average motor scores using Frankel grades on admission, on admission to rehabilitation, on discharge from rehabilitation, and on follow-up were compared between the early and late surgical groups.

The results of this study showed no significant difference in length of acute postoperative intensive care unit (ICU) stay, length of inpatient rehabilitation, or improvement in ASIA grade or motor score between early versus late surgery. The authors concluded the results of this study revealed no significant neurologic benefit when cervical spinal cord decompression after trauma is performed earlier than 72 hours after injury (mean of 1.8 days) as opposed to waiting longer than five days (mean of 16.8 days).

Vale et al.[43] studied 77 patients with acute SCI after 1992. Surgery was performed in 31 of 35 patients with cervical SCIs and in 27 of 29 patients with thoracic cord injuries. Early surgery was defined as occurring within 24 hours of injury and delayed (late) surgery defined as occurring more than 72 hours after injury. Early surgery was performed in 7 of 35 cervical cord injured patients and

4 of 29 thoracic cord injured patients. Nine SCI patients with cervical SCIs and four patients with thoracic cord injuries underwent surgery between 24 and 72 hours after injury. Delayed surgery (more than 72 hours after injury) was performed on 15 cervical (mean of 11 days) and 19 thoracic (mean of 10 days) cord injured patients. Sixty-four patients were followed a minimum of 12 months postinjury with detailed neurologic and functional ability assessments.

The authors found no statistically significant difference between the preoperative neurologic examination and the selection for, or timing of, surgery in patients with cervical or thoracic spinal cord injuries in this series. They also noted that stratification of neurologic recovery at the 12-month follow-up for cervical and thoracic cord injuries revealed no statistically significant effect of the timing of surgery with respect to outcome (cervical $\rho < .985$, thoracic $\rho < .352$ [one-way analysis of variance]).

Each of the five Class II studies reviewed had flaws. Although the studies were prospective, randomization was not performed, and all the studies basically defined early versus late surgery differently and measured severity of injury and neurologic assessment differently. This apparent lack of a consensus in the designs of the studies' methodologies demonstrates the need for further randomized controlled trials to assess the optimum timing of decompressive surgery in acute SCI patients.

In reviewing the Class III evidence of operative management of cervical and thoracolumbar SCI, wide variations in study design and result interpretation are apparent.

## Operative Management of Cervical Spinal Cord Injury

A multicenter prospective study reviewed by Marshall et al.[32] revealed a 4.9% deterioration following acute SCI. Early surgery on the cervical spine when SCI was present was suggested to appear hazardous in multiple early studies.[10,32]

Other studies designed to determine the effectiveness of early spinal surgery have shown no difference in outcome* while other studies have supported a more delayed, scheduled approach to spinal surgery in the SCI patient.[4,5,7-9] No optimal time to surgery or single operative approach has been determined to be superior in the treatment of the acutely injured SCI patient.

A two-part retrospective study by Anderson and Bohlman[2,3] reviewed ventral decompression and arthrodesis of the cervical spine in both incomplete and complete traumatic quadriplegics. Ventral decompression and arthrodesis, even when performed late (1 month to 9 years) after the SCI, improved neurologic function in both upper and lower extremities or primarily the lower extremities in many patients who have incomplete quadriplegia due to fractures or dislocations of the spine.[8] Others have suggested that ventral decompression and arthrodesis of the cervical spine in complete traumatic quadriplegics has shown poor results in both patients older than 53 years of age and patients who had decompression 18 months or more after the injury.[2]

---

*References 10,24,29,39,40,44-46.

Review of both experimental and retrospective clinical studies of facet fracture/dislocation injuries of the cervical spine have advocated early reduction by either nonoperative or surgical means followed by arthrodesis to stabilize the spine in order to maximize root recovery.[22,30,47] Wolf et al.[47] studied 52 consecutive patients with bilateral facet dislocations and noted that the rates of improvement were not statistically significant between those undergoing acute (26.7%) or delayed (18.8%) surgery ($\rho$ = .46). Hadley et al.[22] reviewed 68 patients with acute traumatic cervical facet fracture dislocations. Forty-two percent of the facet dislocation injuries could not be reduced by closed techniques, and neurologic deficits worsened in 11% of the patients; the majority of these subsequently recovered. In the authors' experience, a relative increase in neurologic deficits among patients treated with early open reduction with internal fixation (ORIF) was not observed. Maiman et al.[30] reported their experience in the management of bilateral locked facets of the cervical spine and determined that restoration of the spinal canal and neural foramen was valuable to improve the neurologic status after cervical spine dislocation. In reviewing time frame injury to operation, timing did not affect neurologic outcome.

Improvements in functional recovery for cervical spine fractures operated on electively have been well documented.[4,5,7-9,25] Benzel and Larson[6] studied 99 patients with cervical spine fractures from C4 to C7 with an average interval between injury and operation of 29 days. Their observations did not demonstrate a correlation between the timing of operation and the degree of neurologic return.

Bohlman[7] retrospectively reviewed 300 patients who were hospitalized for acute cervical injuries. He noted the best chance for recovery of neural function and restoration of stability occurred with closed or open reduction followed by dorsal fusion for subluxations or dislocations and ventral decompression and fusion for vertebral compression fractures. However, laminectomy alone resulted in a high mortality rate and loss of motor function.[9]

In Horsey et al's[25] review of early ventral operation in acute cervical spine injuries, the 74 patients who had a ventral procedure underwent operation on an average of 9.1 days after injury or 7.4 days after admission to the hospital, a delayed intervention according to today's standards. None showed deterioration following the procedure, and almost all improved.

## Operative Management of Thoracolumbar Spinal Cord Injury

Thoracolumbar SCI, although probably less urgently taken to surgery than cervical SCI due to the severity of multiple trauma, remains controversial. In the thoracolumbar spine, early surgery is typically within 24 to 48 hours of injury,[13,27,28,34] although there is no evidence the secondary insult is different.

Clohisy et al.[13] treated 22 patients with incomplete neurologic deficits due to spinal fractures at the thoracolumbar junction. The authors determined that early ventral decompression at the thoracolumbar junction was associated with improved rates of neurologic recovery when compared with late decompression, despite lacking

matched controls and having a disproportionate number of patients older than 50 years of age in the delayed surgery group (4 of 9 versus 1 of 11 of the early group). Krengel et al.[27] also retrospectively reviewed incomplete patients with SCI between T2 and T11 and determined early surgical reduction, stabilization, and decompression was safe and improved neurologic recovery in comparison to historic controls treated by postural reduction or late, often inappropriate, surgical intervention, such as laminectomy. This study entailed 14 patients: 12 who underwent surgery within 24 hours of neurologic injury, one at 36 hours, and one at 5 days. Three of the 14 cases of early surgery were taken back for subsequent surgical decompression or instrumentation and fusion. Perhaps if surgery had been performed in a more delayed, considered, or scheduled fashion, a 21% reoperation rate would not have occurred.

Other studies have shown neurologic improvements in patients undergoing delayed operative procedures for thoracolumbar fractures.[4,23,31,33] Benzel and Larson[4] reviewed a series of 105 patients who underwent delayed reconstructive spine surgery consisting of anterior decompression and fusion using the lateral extracavitary approach with or without dorsal instrumentation. All patients were allowed to neurologically plateau. Reconstructive procedures were performed on average of 19.4 to 48.3 days postinjury, depending on their neurologic grade. None of the 34 motor/sensory complete SCI patients recovered any function below the level of the injury. Of the 33 disabling incomplete SCI patients, 17 of 21 patients with minimal neurologic deficit preoperatively improved to a normal neurologic state following elective reconstructive spinal surgery.

McAfee et al.[33] also studied ventral decompression traumatic thoracolumbar fractures in incomplete SCI using a retroperitoneal approach. In this series, operative decompression was performed within 1 year after injury, with an average time interval from injury to anterior decompression of 60 days. Thirty-seven of the 42 patients improved by at least one class in motor strength. Fourteen of 30 nonambulatory patients regained independent walking ability. Twelve of 32 patients with conus medullaris injury demonstrated neurologic bowel and bladder recovery. No patient lost further cord or cauda equina function after the ventral decompression. This study did not show an association between the promptness of surgical decompression and the ultimate level of neurologic function.

Maiman et al.[31] reviewed the cases of 20 patients with previously operated thoracolumbar SCI with residual mass in the spinal canal or development of kyphotic deformity. The lateral extracavitary approach and dorsal instrumentation were used to compress and stabilize the spine. The mean time to the second operation was 6 months for kyphotic deformity and 23 months for canal masses. Seventeen of 20 patients obtained substantial neurologic improvement, with seven of seven in the kyphotic group and 10 of 13 in the canal mass group regaining the ability to ambulate. Although this study was not designed to study the optimal timing of spinal surgery in SCI, it does demonstrate that delayed "elective" ventral approaches for reconstruction of the spinal canal with appropriate stabilization can result in significant neurologic improvement.

In Hanley et al.'s[23] review of fractures of the thoracic, thoracolumbar, and lumbar spine, the authors noted that urgent surgical treatment is not indicated if there is no neurologic deficit or a true complete neural deficit without major spinal column displacement. They recommended a delay of 48 hours after the injury to allow the patient to medically stabilize, repeated examination of the neurologic situation, and planning of operative treatment between 48 and 72 hours after injury in a controlled surgical setting.

Rechtine[35] studied 83 patients with single or multiple thoracolumbar fractures from 1985 through 1992. Thirty-two were treated nonoperatively on a Roto-Rest bed for 4 to 6 weeks with aggressive physical therapy; 20 patients were treated surgically with hook-rod constructs; and 30 were patients with pedicle screw instrumentation and posterior arthrodesis. Significant improvement in neurologic function in some incomplete patients was noted regardless of the treatment. However, more debilitating and greater numbers of complications were observed in the operative group than in the nonoperative group.

## Summary

Intuitively, it seems that early surgical decompression and stabilization (if indicated) of acute SCI would improve the physiologic environment of the spinal cord to allow for maximal neurologic improvement. Unfortunately, the majority of surgical data addressing early versus late surgery is based on Class III evidence, and the Class II evidence reviewed shows major methodological errors to each study.

The optimal time to surgery in acute SCI remains controversial and cannot be determined with the clinical studies published to date. Delayed surgical intervention permits well-planned elective procedures on patients who are neurologically and metabolically stable. Although animal studies regarding the timing of SCI surgery have suggested that early decompression and stabilization enhance neurologic recovery, human clinical studies have failed to support those findings. Large, controlled, randomized prospective studies are needed to settle the controversy of efficacy of early versus late or delayed surgery in SCI.

## REFERENCES

1. Anderson DK, Hall ED: Pathophysiology of spinal cord trauma. *Ann Emerg Med* 22:987-922, 1993.
2. Anderson PA, Bohlman HH: Anterior decompression and arthrodesis of the cervical spine: long-term motor improvement. *J Bone Joint Surg* 74-A(5):683-691, 1992.
3. Baisden J, Maiman DJ: Timing of surgery: argument for delayed elective surgery. In Brunzel EC (ed): *Spine Surgery: Techniques, Complication Avoidance, and Management*, vol 2. Churchill Livingstone, 1999, pp 891-895.
4. Benzel EC, Larson SJ: Functional recovery after decompressive operation for thoracic and lumbar spine fractures. *Neurosurgery* 19(5):772-778, 1986.
5. Benzel EC, Larson SJ: Recovery of nerve root function after complete quadriplegia from cervical spine fractures. *Neurosurgery* 19(5):809-812, 1986.
6. Benzel EC, Larson SJ: Functional recovery after decompressive spine operation for cervical spine fractures. *Neurosurgery* 20(5):742-746, 1987.
7. Bohlman HH: Acute fractures and dislocations of the cervical spine. *J Bone Joint Surg* 61-A(8):1119-1142, 1979.
8. Bohlman HH, Andersen PA: Anterior decompression and arthrodesis of the cervical spine: long-term motor improvement. *J Bone Joint Surg* 74-A(5):671-682, 1992.
9. Bohlman HH, Freehafer A, Dejak J: The results of treatment of acute injuries of the upper thoracic spine with paralysis. *J Bone Joint Surg* 67-A(3):360-369, 1985.
10. Bose B, Northrup BE, Osterholm JL, et al: Re-analysis of central cervical cord injury management. *Neurosurgery* 15(3):367-372, 1984.
11. Bracken MB, Shepard MJ, Collins WF, et al: A randomized, controlled trial of methylprednisolone or naloxone in the treatment of acute spinal cord injury. *N Engl J Med* 322(20):1405-1411, 1990.
12. Chen TY, Dickman CA, Eleraky M, Sonntag VKH: The role of decompression for acute incomplete cervical spinal cord injury in cervical spondylosis. *Spine* 23:2398-2403, 1998.
13. Clohisy JC, Akbarnia BA, Bucholz RD, et al: Neurologic recovery associated with anterior decompression of spine fractures at the thoracolumbar junction (T12-L1). *Spine* 17(suppl 5):S325-S330, 1992.
14. Collins WF: A review and update of experiment and clinical studies of spinal cord injury. *Paraplegia* 21:204-219, 1983.
15. Delamarter RB, Sherman J, Carr JB: Pathophysiology of spinal cord injury. *J Bone Joint Surg* 77-A(7):1042-1049, 1995.
16. Dolan EJ, Tator CH, Endrenyi L: The value of decompression for acute experimental spinal cord compression injury. *J Neurosurg* 53:749-755, 1980.
17. Duh MS, Shepard MJ, Wilberger JE, Brackern MB: The effectiveness of surgery on the treatment of acute spinal cord injury and its relation to pharmacological treatment. *Neurosurgery* 35(2):240-249, 1994.
18. Fehlings MG, Sekhon LHA: Spinal cord injury: update. *Semin Spine Surg* 13(2):116-120, 2001.
19. Fehlings MG, Tator CH: An evidence-based review of decompressive surgery in acute spinal cord injury: rationale, indications, and timing based on experimental and clinical studies. *J Neurosurg* (Spine 1) 91:1-11, 1999.
20. Geisler FH: Past and current human spinal cord injury drug trials in contemporary management of spinal cord injury. In Benzel EC, Tator CH, (eds): *American Association of Neurologic Surgeons*, 1995.
21. Geisler FH, Dorsey FC, Coleman WP: Recovery of motor function after spinal cord injury—a randomized, placebo-controlled trial with GM-1 ganglioside. *N Engl J Med* 324(26):1829-1838, 1991.
22. Hadley MN, Firzpatrick BC, Sonntag VKH, Browner CM: Facet fracture-dislocation injuries of the cervical spine. *Neurosurgery* 30(5):661-666, 1992.
23. Hanley EN, Simpkins A, Phillips ED: Fractures of the thoracic, thoracolumbar, and lumbar spine: classification, basis for treatment, and timing of surgery. *Semin Spine Surg* 2(1):2-7, 1990.
24. Harris P, Karmi MZ, McClemont E, et al: The prognosis of patients sustaining severe cervical spine injury (C2-C7 inclusive). *Paraplegia* 18:324-330, 1980.

25. Horsey WJ, Tucker WS, Hudson AR, Schatz SW: Experience with early anterior operation in acute injuries of the cervical spine. *Paraplegia* 15:110-122, 1977-1978.

26. Krause JS: Spinal cord injury and its rehabilitation. *Curr Opin Neurol Neurosurg* 5(5):669-672, 1992.

27. Krengel WF, Anderson PA, Henley MB: Early stabilization and decompression for incomplete paraplegia due to a thoracic-level spinal cord injury. *Spine* 18(14):2080-2087, 1993.

28. Lemons VR, Wagner FC, Montesano PX: Management of thoracolumbar fractures with accompanying neurological injury. *Neurosurgery* 30(5):667-671, 1992.

29. Levi L, Wolf A, Rigamonti D, *et al:* Anterior decompression in cervical spine trauma: does the timing of surgery affect outcome? *Neurosurgery* 29(2):216-222, 1991.

30. Maiman DJ, Barolat G, Larson SJ: Management of bilateral locked facets of the cervical spine. *Neurosurgery* 18(5): 542-547, 1986.

31. Maiman DJ, Larson SJ, Benzel EC: Neurological improvement associated with late decompression of the thoracolumbar spinal cord. *Neurosurgery* 149(3):302-307, 1984.

32. Marshall LF, Knowlton S, Garfin SR, *et al:* Deterioration following spinal cord injury. *J Neurosurg* 66:400-404, 1987.

33. McAfee PC, Bohlman HH, Yuan HA: Anterior decompression of traumatic thoracolumbar fractures with incomplete neurological deficit using a retroperitoneal approach. *J Bone Joint Surg* 67-A(1):89-104, 1985.

34. Osebold WR, Weinstein SL, Sprague BL: Thoracolumbar spine fractures. *Spine* 6(1):13-34, 1981.

35. Rechtine G: Surgical considerations in acute SCI. In *American Spinal Injury Association Annual Meeting,* Houston, April 1997.

36. Sonntag VKH, Francis PM: Patient selection and timing of surgery in contemporary management of spinal cord injury. In Benzel EC, Tator CH (eds): *American Association of Neurologic Surgeons,* 1995.

37. Tator CH, Duncan EG, Edmonds VE, *et al:* Complications and costs of management of acute spinal cord injury. *Paraplegia* 31:700-714, 1993.

38. Tator CH, Duncan EG, Edmonds VE, *et al:* Neurological recovery, mortality and length of stay after acute spinal cord injury associated with changes in management. *Paraplegia* 33:254-262, 1995.

39. Tator CH, Duncan EG, Edmonds VE, *et al:* Comparison of surgical and conservative management in 208 patients with acute spinal cord injury. *Can J Neurol Sci* 14(1):60-69, 1987.

40. Tator CH, Fehlings MG: Review of the secondary injury theory of acute spinal cord trauma with emphasis on vascular mechanisms. *J Neurosurg* 75:15-26, 1991.

41. Tator CH, Fehlings MG, Thorpe K, Taylor W: Current use and timing of spinal surgery for management of acute spinal cord injury in North America: results of a retrospective multicenter study. *J Neurosurg* (Spine 1) 91:12-18, 1999.

42. Vaccaro AR, Daugherty RJ, Sheehan TP, *et al:* Neurologic outcome of early versus late surgery for cervical spinal cord injury. *Spine* 22:2609-2613, 1997.

43. Vale FL, Burns J, Jackson AB, Hadley MN: Combined medical and surgical treatment after acute spinal cord injury: results of a prospective pilot study to assess the merits of aggressive medical resuscitation and blood pressure management. *J Neurosurg* 87:239-246, 1997.

44. Wagner FC, Chehrazi B: Early decompression and neurological outcome in acute cervical spinal cord injuries. *J Neurosurg* 56:699-705, 1982.

45. Waters RL, Adkins RH, Yakura JS, Sie I: Effect of surgery on motor recovery following traumatic spinal cord injury. *Spinal Cord* 34:188-192, 1996.

46. Waters RL, Sie IH, Adkins RH: Rehabilitation of the patient with a spinal cord injury. *Orthop Clin North Am* 26(1):117-122, 1995.

47. Wolf A, Levi L, Mirvis S, *et al:* Operative management of bilateral facet dislocation. *J Neurosurg* 75:883-890, 1991.

48. Young W: Session 2: secondary CNS injury. *J Neurotrauma* 5(3):219-221, 1988.

49. Young W, Kume-Kick J, Constantini S: Glucocorticoid therapy of spinal cord injury. *Ann N Y Acad Sci* 743: 241-265, 1994.

# CHAPTER 95

# Minimally Invasive Spinal Decompression and Stabilization Techniques I

**Joseph Watson, Sait Naderi, Nevan G. Baldwin, and Maurice M. Smith**

Ideally, minimally invasive techniques should achieve the operative goal with minimal tissue disruption. In spinal stabilization surgery, particularly in the thoracic and lumbar regions, much of the associated morbidity is secondary to the extensive soft-tissue dissection necessary to widely expose the spine for arthrodesis.

Percutaneous fixation of the thoracic and lumbar spine was used as an alternative to invasive surgery in the 1980s. Concomitantly, growing experience with percutaneous discectomy nurtured the development of fusion techniques to accompany decompression. The current widespread use of minimally invasive techniques in thoracic and abdominal surgery has been a catalyst for the development of less invasive ventral approaches to the spine.

The anatomic and biomechanical differences among the cervical, thoracic, and lumbar regions of the spine create completely different issues in the approach to decompression and stabilization of each region. Techniques for minimally invasive treatment are considered for each region separately; however, many of the principles of complication avoidance and management apply to all regions. The experience with techniques in the lumbar spine far outweighs that of the thoracic region. Comparatively little data have yet been brought forth on cervical spine approaches.

The evolution of minimally invasive spinal surgery for decompression of the neural structures began with the uniportal procedures, using the arthroscope for decompression of contained disk herniations. The first laparoscopic lumbar discectomy was reported by Obenheim in 1991.[21] The efficacy of different endoscopic surgical procedures has been documented and led to the development of more complex and biportal arthroscopic procedures for treatment of noncontained herniations.

The use of minimally invasive surgery for fusion of motion segments of the spine occurred at a later date. Magerl introduced this technique for percutaneous external transpedicular fixation of the thoracic and lumbar spine.[14] Percutaneous dorsolateral interbody fusion was also performed successfully by Leu and Schreiber.[12] The likelihood of screw tract infection and discomfort associated with externally placed implants were the drawbacks of these procedures.

Recent advances in the evolution of minimally invasive surgery for fusion and stabilization include: (1) percutaneous interbody fusion during arthroscopic disk surgery; (2) transperitoneal and thoracoscopic placement of the interbody cage implant in the lumbar spine and thoracic spine, as well as placement of the transpedicular screw, combined with temporary subcutaneous plates in the lumbar spine; and (3) the placement of the plates and screws in the thoracic spine. Simultaneously, other researchers developed techniques for fusion without instrumentation.

Mathews[15] was one of the first people to use endoscopy for spinal fusion, both ventrally and dorsolaterally. Endoscopic spinal fusion was performed first in the lumbar spine. Interest in the use of minimally invasive surgery for thoracic spine disease has increased recently. The initial results, using video-assisted thoracoscopic surgery (VATS), are encouraging because this procedure is characterized by less pain and shorter hospital stays.[1,13,30]

Regan et al.[24,26,27] reported their results in thoracic spinal pathology using ventral and dorsal interbody grafting, with and without instrumentation. Rosenthal et al.[28] reported the use of VATS for ventral decompression and stabilization in patients with metastatic tumors of the thoracic spine. Their technique involves endoscopic microsurgical decompression, combined with reconstructive techniques and instrumentation placed through thoracoscopic portals.

## Stabilization and Fusion

### Advantages and Difficulties

The main advantages of endoscopic spine surgery are lower morbidity, attributable to the minimally invasive approach, and cosmetic advantages. Significantly less postoperative pain is experienced by these patients because of the avoidance of extensive muscular incision and removal of ribs. There is also less impairment of pulmonary function after VATS. Dorsolateral endoscopic approaches for pedicular fixation result in less epidural bleeding, a decreased incidence of perineural and intraneural fibrosis, less venous stasis, and less chronic perineural edema.

The most important disadvantage of endoscopic stabilization is that it is time-consuming.. This aspect can be overcome, but there is a considerable learning curve. The technology and equipment costs for this approach also create a large "up-front" investment requirement. It is of note that all endoscopic approaches, especially thoracoscopic approaches, can be converted to open procedures, if necessary, to control bleeding or to deal with excessive adhesions.

### Indications and Contraindications

Although the indications for endoscopic fusion and stabilization are similar to those of the open procedures, the options are more limited. Endoscopic stabilization can be performed after decompression for burst fractures, spinal tumors, spinal deformities (e.g., idiopathic scoliosis and Scheuermann's disease), and for instability secondary to degenerative disease of one or two motion segments.

Contraindications of the endoscopic dorsolateral lumbar spine fusion and stabilization include (1) considerable loss of intervertebral disk height, preventing decortication of the end-plates, (2) severe spinal deformity associated with distorted neural and pedicular anatomy, (3) infection, (4) failed previous operation for interbody fusion, and (5) very large tumors, requiring extensive resection.[8]

Contraindications to VATS include (1) inability to tolerate deflation of one lung, (2) significant respiratory disease, and (3) previous open thoracotomy.[6] Contraindications to laparoscopic transperitoneal lumbar fusion and stabilization include (1) significant abdominal trauma, (2) previous transabdominal lumbar operation, and (3) previous lower abdominal laparoscopic procedure (e.g., hysterectomy).[37]

### Approaches

The anatomic features of different regions of the spine dictate a variety of endoscopic approaches for fusion and stabilization. A thoracic spine endoscopic approach necessitates VATS, whereas a lumbar spine instability requires a ventral approach, a dorsolateral approach, or both. The choice of endoscopic approach in the lumbar spine relies largely on surgeon bias.

### Video-Assisted Thoracoscopic Surgery

VATS is performed using a double-lumen tube for deflation of the ipsilateral lung with the patient under general anesthesia and in the lateral decubitus position (Figure 95.1).

### Method

Instruments required for an open thoracotomy should be readily available for emergency use. A left- or right-sided approach may be used, depending on the eccentricity of the pathology. Some authors prefer a right-sided approach in a case in which the pathology is not lateralized, because there is a greater space lateral to the azygos vein than the aorta. Consideration should be given to the position of the artery of Adamkiewicz if the intervention requires the sacrifice of one or more segmental arteries in the middle to lower thoracic region, especially T9-11 on the left.

The initial trocar should be inserted in the manner of a tube thoracostomy (over the top of the rib) in the anterior axillary line at the sixth or seventh intercostal space. Multiple working trocars may be used for instrument insertion as necessary. Soft trocars are preferred for the portals because they are less traumatic to the neurovascular bundle on the inferior rib undersurface. The size of the instrument is limited only by the intercostal distance.

The surgical levels are identified by counting ribs, preferably with fluoroscopy, and by marking in the disk space. Alternatively, ribs may be counted endoscopically from the first rib down. The rib number corresponds to the lower vertebral body at the disk space (e.g., sixth rib at T5-6). Adequate exposure of the disk space usually requires resection of the rib head, except in the lower thoracic region where the rib head may be well caudal to the disk space, permitting unobstructed access. Attention to the segmental vascular branches in the mid-bodies is

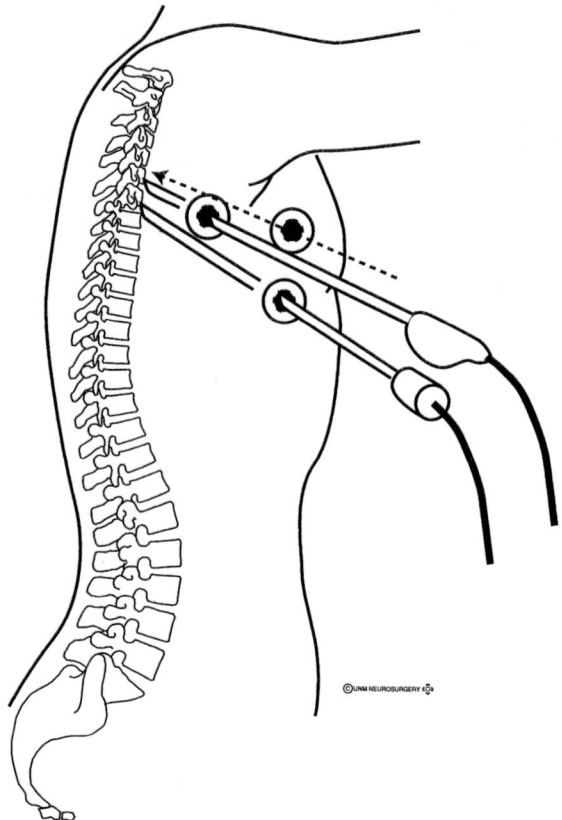

**Figure 95.1** Thoracoscopic spinal surgery. Portal placement varies according to the level of the pathology. More portals may also be required for procedures with instrumentation to allow improved angles for hardware placement and access for retractors and other instruments.

advised. Stabilization across the vertebral body requires the careful division of these vascular structures. The sympathetic chain may also be identified in the surgical field through the parietal pleura. Varying anatomy of the regions of the thoracic spine dictates different exposure techniques. For the upper thoracic region it may be necessary to elevate and support the ipsilateral arm to rotate the scapula away. In the lower thoracic region it may be necessary to retract the diaphragm.

After exploratory thoracoscopy using a 30-degree–angle scope, a second trocar is inserted. If complete atelectasis is not achieved, a brief period of $CO_2$ insufflation may help to collapse the lung. As the thoracic spine is visualized through the parietal pleura, the correct level is identified by counting the ribs. Radiographic confirmation by fluoroscopy or a plain radiograph can also be obtained. The parietal pleura is then divided using monopolar cautery. After the fluoroscopic identification of the correct level, the third and fourth ports are inserted at the level of the pathology. A 0- or 30-degree–angle scope can be used. Generally, 2 to 3cm of rib resection and partial resection of the pedicle is adequate. After using electrocautery to "clean-up" the surrounding soft tissues, a discectomy with decompression is performed. The bleeding at this stage can be controlled by bipolar electrocautery, argon beam coagulation, or packing the area with Gelfoam or Surgicel.

It is of note that uncontrolled bleeding may necessitate conversion to an open procedure. Therefore the availability of an open thoracotomy set-up is advisable.

On completion of the decompression, fusion can be performed using bone chips from rib or harvested from iliac crest. Regan *et al.*[27] described the placement of an interbody cage into the disk space after decompression.

Rosenthal[28] described reconstruction by homologous bone or by injection of semiliquid methyl methacrylate. He used a ventral plate and screw system (Z-plate, Sofamor-Danek, Memphis) for fixation. For this reason, he used special equipment for dilation of the skin incision during the insertion of the plate, and for insertion of instruments for handling the plates and screws in the chest cavity. These techniques allow the surgeon to address pathology resulting from degenerative disease, trauma, or metastatic disease, and then to stabilize the spine with methyl methacrylate struts, cages, or plates.[2,19,28,29]

After completion of the entire decompression and stabilization procedure, a tube thoracostomy is placed and the lung is re-expanded.

## Complications

As with laparoscopic procedures, there is an entire complement of risks associated with the intrathoracic approach. Reported complications are prolonged atelectasis, pleural effusions, intercostal neuralgia, and diaphragmatic injury.[2,19,29] Time of lung collapse (length of operation) is related to the pulmonary morbidity associated with chest procedures. Therefore until familiarity with the thoracoscopic spine procedures is achieved, the operating surgeon may expect longer operating times and some increased morbidity. In one series of thoracic endoscopic discectomies, the complication rate was 14%, which was compatible with the reported complication rate with the open approaches.[25] The use of flexible portals may reduce the incidence of intercostal neuralgia, although this still occurred in two of 17 patients in whom the flexible portals were used.[2] Complications related to the decompression, in a series of 77 patients, were excessive epidural bleeding in one patient and transient paraparesis in another.[19]

Operating at the wrong level is always a concern in the thoracic spine. This may be avoided by ruling out variant anatomy (e.g., accessory ribs), using preoperative radiographs, and by accepting only quality radiographic images intraoperatively.

### Laparoscopic Transperitoneal Surgery for the Lumbar Spine

Laparoscopic transperitoneal fusion is performed with the patient under general anesthesia and in the Trendelenburg position (Figure 95.2). Harvesting of iliac crest graft and packing of the cage with bone can be performed before the main procedure. An incision is made at the umbilicus and an insufflation needle is inserted into the abdominal cavity. After endoscopic inspection of the abdominal cavity, two ports are placed lateral to the epigastric area. After mobilization and retraction of the sigmoid colon and opening of the parietal peritoneum, the correct level is identified and the ventral aspect of the level is dissected. The Trendelenburg position can be used to facilitate the dissection. After dissection of the anterior longitudinal ligament and annulus fibrosus, an endoscopic discectomy is performed and both end plates are decorticated. Intervertebral cage implants are then placed under anteroposterior and lateral fluoroscopy. After hemostasis, the parietal peritoneum and incision sites are closed.

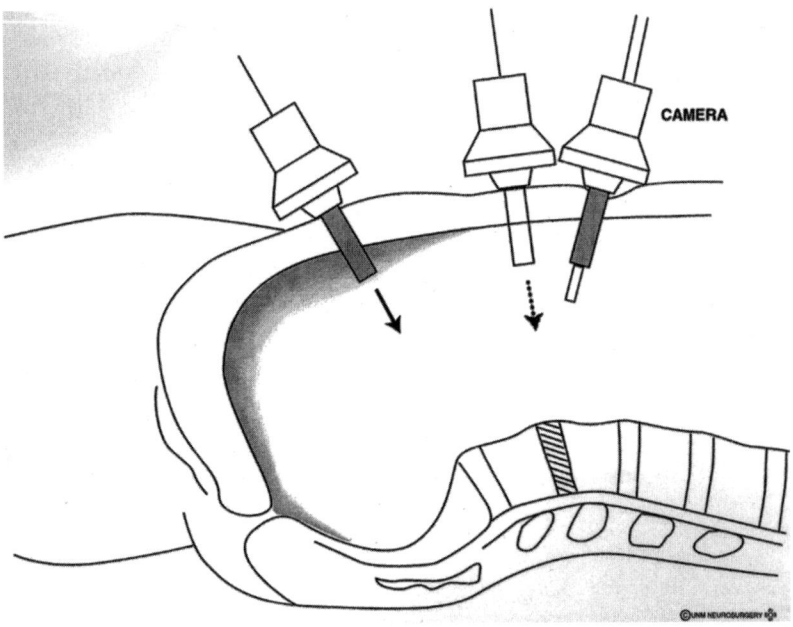

**Figure 95.2** The transperitoneal approach to endoscopic lumbar interbody fusion. Insufflation is maintained through the caudal portal, while dissection and instrumentation are performed through the portal directly aligned with the interspace.

### Dorsolateral Endoscopic Transpedicular Fixation

The dorsolateral approach is performed with the patient under general anesthesia and in the prone position. After a standard arthroscopic discectomy, both end-plates are decorticated. With the use of a pedicular jig, the guide pins are placed in the center of the pedicles under fluoroscopic control. Over the guide wire a cannulated pedicle obturator is placed and the soft tissues surrounding the pedicle are bluntly dissected. Extended-length pedicle screws are inserted under fluoroscopic control. The extensions are connected to the subcutaneous plate.

### Results

Although the total minimally invasive experience in spine surgery is small in comparison with the vast experience with open procedures, the early results are encouraging (Table 95.1). The follow-up of these patients, to date, is relatively short. Mathews et al.[16] reported successful fusion in all of their first five cases. McAfee et al.[18] reported the complications in the first 50 endoscopic procedures in a multicenter study. They did not observe any great vessel complications. The complications reported by other authors include cage extrusion, inferior vena cava laceration, posterior disk extrusion, prolonged ileus, and atelectasis. Zuckerman[38] and Novotny et al.[20] reported the conversions of 2 of 23 and 2 of 8 operated cases to open surgery, respectively.

The first results of the minimally invasive surgery for spine decompression and stabilization are encouraging. However, some problems persist. These include long operation time, the requirement of expensive equipment, and the steep learning curve. With increased experience the rate of complications should decrease. Technologic advances should improve the safety of these operations and may also broaden the indications for the application of these techniques.

### Lumbar Spine Decompression

The large bulk of the dorsal paraspinal muscles, and the anatomic relation to the great vessels ventrally, pose significant impediments to exposure of the lumbar spine for fusion. A commonly accepted approach, the dorsolateral arthrodesis, creates significant lasting muscle trauma and denervation, which may limit recovery.[35] Minimally invasive techniques were developed in an attempt to avoid these difficulties.

There is minimal blood loss associated with minimally invasive approaches; this obviates the need for transfusion and its associated risks. Because these techniques do not directly expose the spinal canal, epidural scar formation is avoided. Some procedures may be performed with the patient under local or spinal anesthesia, thereby avoiding the risks of general endotracheal anesthesia.

### Dorsolateral Interbody Fusion

Percutaneous nucleotomy of the lumbar spine was developed and widely used as an alternative to open discectomy. Experience with the approach to the disk space paved the way for the application of noninstrumented interbody fusion techniques. Placement of bone graft material after percutaneous discectomy with fluoroscopic guidance proved to be feasible.[14] The technique is as follows: with the use of a biportal technique under local anesthesia, the disk is removed and the end-plates are decorticated. Autologous bone graft from the iliac crest, supplemented with frozen bone chips, is packed into the disk space through the percutaneous cannulae. External corset bracing is then used. There are no current outcome or follow-up data for this technique.

A similar technique[10-12,34] uses an endoscopic-assisted, percutaneous posterolateral approach. The procedure differs greatly from that previously described because it is augmented by the preoperative placement, under general anesthesia, of an external spinal fixator. With the patient under local anesthesia, a biportal technique is then used for nucleotomy. The vertebral end-plates are decorticated with a specially designed curette. Autologous bone is then packed into the disk space with the aid of distraction by the external device. The disk space is then placed under compression by the fixator and secured. The external device is left in place for 3 months. Outcome data indicate solid fusion, as defined by plain radiography, in 42 of 50 patients.

The major advantages of this form of arthrodesis are the use of local anesthesia and the lack of blood loss. When

| TABLE 95.1 | | |
| --- | --- | --- |
| **Recently Reported Series of Patients Undergoing Fusion and Stabilization Via Endoscopic Procedures** | | |
| **Author** | **No. of Patients** | **Procedure** |
| Mathews (1991)[15] | 4 | ALIF |
| Novotny et al. (1994)[20] | 8 | TP-ALIF with cage or femoral allograft |
| McAfee et al. (1994)[17] | 10 | TP fusion |
| Mathews et al. (1994)[16] | 5 | TP with iliac crest |
| Kambin and Schaffer (1996)[8] | 25 | Lumbar posterolateral |
| Zuckerman et al. (1996)[37] | 23 | TP with cage implant |
| Rosenthal et al. (1996)[29] | 12 | Thoracoscopic with anterior plate |
| Regan (1996)[25] | 7 | Thoracoscopic with anterior instrumentation |
| Dickman et al. (1996)[2] | 1 | Thoracoscopic fusion |

ALIF, Anterior lumbar interbody fusion; TP, transperitoneal.
Note that cases involving decompression only are excluded from the table.

the procedure is used in conjunction with an external fixator, some of these advantages are lost, because this component of the procedure carries significant risks of infection and nerve root damage. The major disadvantage is the limited exposure that prevents the placement of oversized bone graft into the disk space under compression and prevents placement of ventral instrumentation. The result is limited anterior column support during healing. Furthermore the percutaneous techniques are limited with regard to their ability to decompress the spinal canal and are contraindicated in the presence of a sequestered disk rupture.

## Complications

Complications associated with percutaneous lumbar discectomy are few, but include a 1% to 2% risk of discitis and a 1% to 2% risk of a symptomatic psoas muscle hematoma. An anecdotal risk of injury to the nerve roots or surrounding vascular structures is also present.[3,23,32,33] As is emphasized in Chapter 29, careful placement of the guide wire is crucial for the avoidance of complications with this approach. Theoretically, the risks of infection and injury to the great vessels are increased by the manipulations of bone grafting. However, this has not been demonstrated clinically.

## Ventral Endoscopic Procedures

The ventral endoscopic approach is primarily limited to the L4-5 and L5-S1 disk spaces because of the relation of the aorta and vena cava to the spine. The increased use of minimally invasive abdominal and retroperitoneal procedures with the laparoscope has paved the way for its use as an approach to the spine.

Despite the limited enthusiasm for laparoscopic ventral discectomy for the treatment of simple disk disease,[27] interbody fusion techniques have received a warm welcome, as evidenced by the number of meeting presentations and papers on the topic.* The procedure has evolved from the placement of bone graft in the interspace to the use of titanium interbody distraction cages.

### Technique

The ventral exposure of the lumbar spine from the peritoneal cavity is limited to L5-S1 and variably to L4-5. Laparoscopic exposure is performed in the routine manner, similar to an intraabdominal procedure. This includes a bowel preparation, insertion of a Foley catheter and a nasogastric tube, and preincisional prophylactic antibiotics. The patient is supine in the Trendelenburg position, with the back extended using large rolls under the lumbosacral junction. Insufflation techniques are standard, but a gasless technique is also described, which does not require specially designed instruments.[36] Assistance from a general surgeon comfortable with laparoscopy is advised.

Exposure of the L5-S1 space requires the incision of the parietal peritoneum over the disk in the midline. Fluoroscopy is used to properly identify the disk. The mid-

line sacral artery and vein must be divided. The parietal peritoneum is mobilized using blunt dissection, with bleeding controlled by bipolar electrocautery (rather than unipolar cautery), for fear of injuring the closely related autonomic plexus. At the L4-5 space the exposure can be more difficult, because the disk space often sits at the crotch of the bifurcation of the great vessels. In fact, gentle retraction of the common iliac vein and artery is required, and segmental branches may need to be sacrificed. Exposure may be facilitated by inserting Steinmann pins into the L4 vertebral body to give static retraction of the vessels.

Discectomy is performed by sharp incision of the ventral annulus fibrosus and by radical removal of disk material with curettes and pituitary forceps. Fusion proceeds by distraction of the disk space and insertion of bone graft under compression. Currently popular is the use of a threaded titanium cage, which is cleared by the Food and Drug Administration (FDA) and is commercially available for open procedures. It is also cleared for endoscopic placement from the ventral approach. With the endoscopic placement, the procedure is outlined as follows: an estimate of graft size is made on the basis of the preoperative radiographs and specific templates provided by the manufacturer of the device. The sizes are checked in situ to confirm that adequate exposure is available. Next, a disk space distractor is placed on one side of the midline. On the other side, a circular hole is drilled (under fluoroscopic guidance to ensure a trajectory parallel to the vertebral end plates) to a depth of approximately two thirds of the diameter of the disk space. The hole is then tapped and the titanium implant, filled with autologous bone chips, is screwed into the disk space. The distractor is then removed and the tapping/implant procedure is repeated at the site previously occupied by the distractor. The implants should be sufficiently countersunk so that no aspect comes into contact with the overlying vascular structures. The peritoneum is then reapproximated over the site. The exposure and anatomy may dictate that only one graft be placed. However, this is not as biomechanically sound as two cages, placed side by side, especially in lateral flexion.[9] Currently, other materials such as threaded allograft dowels are also available for transperitoneal endoscopic fusion operations.

A retroperitoneal approach to the ventral aspect of the spine at levels L4-5 and L5-S1 with interbody fusion is also technically feasible. This reduces the chance of postoperative adynamic ileus and intraabdominal adhesions. This approach also provides access to the lateral aspects of level L1-4, although the great vessels prevent midline access at these levels. Previous abdominal surgery is a relative contraindication for the transperitoneal exposure. This is not an issue with the retroperitoneal approach. An experience with 20 cases has been reported.[22]

### Complications

Complications associated with transperitoneal exposure are infrequent. However, they require immediate management by experienced abdominal surgeons. An experience with 17 cases included significant ileus in four patients that required an open laparotomy in two patients for bleeding. In addition, there were two graft donor site infections.[39]

---

*References 9,16,19,20,22,31,39.

In another series of 22 cases, one iliac vein laceration was encountered, as well as two bone donor site infections.[19] In the small series of ventral retroperitoneal fusions, no significant complications were reported.[22] Sexual dysfunction is a dreaded complication of this approach, resulting from disruption of the sacral autonomic plexus. Several cases of transient (3 weeks) retrograde ejaculation were reported in a series using an open anterior lumbar interbody fusion technique.[9] It is recommended that in men the reflection of the parietal peritoneum over the ventral disk space be performed with the aid of bipolar rather than monopolar electrocautery to prevent the spread of current and reduce the risk of damage to the autonomic plexus.[9,36] If Steinmann pins are used, care must be taken during removal, as well as insertion, so that the sharp tip does not lacerate a vessel, particularly the iliac vein. The hazards of the approach and drilling the disk space adjacent to the iliac vessels are ameliorated with special instruments to protect the vessels during drilling. Familiarity with these instruments is imperative.

## Cervical Spine Decompression

Despite advances in available technology and interest in minimally invasive stabilization procedures in the thoracic and lumbar spine, reports on the use of these methods in the cervical spine are relatively few. Percutaneous discectomy and chemonucleolysis of the cervical spine are reportedly effective in selected patients in uncontrolled trials.[4,5] Percutaneous disk access requires a ventrolateral approach. The needle entry is at the medial border of the sternocleidomastoid muscle. With the fingers of one hand acting to separate the carotid sheath and esophagus, the needle is passed under fluoroscopic control into the desired disk space. Although percutaneous decompression has been described, concomitant fusion has not been reported to date.

## REFERENCES

1. Dickman CA, Mican CA: Multilevel anterior thoracic discectomies and anterior interbody fusion using a microsurgical thoracoscopic approach: a case report. *J Neurosurg* 84:104-109, 1996.
2. Dickman CA, Rosenthal D, Karahalios DG, *et al*: Thoracic vertebrectomy and reconstruction using a microsurgical thorascopic approach. *Neurosurgery* 38:279, 1996.
3. Epstein NE: Surgically confirmed cauda equina and nerve root injury following percutaneous discectomy at an outside institution: a case report. *J Spinal Disord* 3:380-382, 1990.
4. Gomez-Castresana F, Herrero CV, Horche JLB, Rodriguez-Navia IM: Cervical chymopapain nucleolysis: MR imaging assessment of chymopapain efficacy. *Neurosurg Clin N Am* 7:1, 1996.
5. Hoogland T, Scheckenbach C: Low-dose chemonucleolysis combined with percutaneous nucleotomy in herniated cervical disks. *J Spinal Disord* 8:228, 1995.
6. Horowitz MB, Moossy JJ, Julian T, *et al*: Thoracic discectomy using video assisted thoracoscopy. *Spine* 19:1082-1086, 1994.

7. Kambin P: Posterolateral percutaneous lumbar interbody fusion. In Kambin P (ed): *Arthroscopic Microdiscectomy: Minimal Intervention in Spinal Surgery*. Baltimore, Urban & Schwarzenberg, 1991, p 117.
8. Kambin P, Schaffer JL: Arthroscopic fusion of the lumbosacral spine. In Margulies JY, Floman Y, Farcy JPC, Neuwirth MG (eds): *Lumbosacral and Spinopelvic Fixation*. Philadelphia, Lippincott-Raven, 1996, p 565.
9. Kuslich SD, McAfee PC, Regan JJ: Spinal instrumentation. In Regan JJ, McAfee PC, Mack MJ (eds): *Atlas of Endoscopic Spine Surgery*. St Louis, Quality Medical Publishing, 1995, p 293.
10. Leu H, Hauser R, Schreiber A: Percutaneous lumbar spine fusion. *Acta Orthop Scand* 64 (suppl 251):116, 1993.
11. Leu HF, Hauser RK: Percutaneous endoscopic lumbar spine fusion. *Neurosurg Clin N Am* 7:107, 1996.
12. Leu HJ, Schreiber A: Percutaneous lumbar restabilization. In Kambin P (ed): *Arthroscopic Microdiscectomy, Minimal Intervention in Spinal Surgery*. Baltimore, Urban & Schwarzenberg, 1991, p 123.
13. Mac MJ, Regan JJ, Bobechko WP, Acuff TE: Application of thoracoscopy for disease of the spine. *Ann Thorac Surg* 56:736-738, 1993.
14. Magerl FP: Stabilization of the lower thoracic and lumbar spine with external skeletal fixation. *Clin Orthop* 189:125-141, 1984.
15. Mathews HH: Presented at the First International Symposium on Lasers in Orthopaedics, San Francisco, September 1991.
16. Mathews HH, Evans MT, Kyles MK, *et al*: Laparoscopic discectomy with fusion. In Proceedings of the 9th Annual Meeting of the North American Spine Society. Minneapolis, October 1994, p 63.
17. McAfee PC, Fedder IL, Geis P, *et al*: Laparoscopic lumbar spine surgery. In Proceedings of the 9th Annual Meeting of the North American Spine Society, Minneapolis, October 1994, p 63.
18. McAfee PC, Regan J, Picetti G: The incidence of complications in endoscopic anterior thoracic spinal reconstructive surgery. A prospective multicenter study comprising the first 50 consecutive cases. In Proceedings of the 9th Annual Meeting of the North American Spine Society, Minneapolis, October 1994, p 64.
19. McAfee PC, Regan JR, Zdeblick T, *et al*: The incidence of complications in endoscopic anterior thoracolumbar spinal reconstructive surgery. A prospective multicenter study comprising the first 100 consecutive cases. *Spine* 20:1624, 1995.
20. Novotney SR, Guyer RD, Regan JJ, Ohnmeiss DD: Laparoscopic-assisted anterior lumbar interbody fusion. In Proceedings of the 9th Annual Meeting of the North American Spine Society. Minneapolis, October 1994, p 61.
21. Obenheim TG: Laparoscopic lumbar discectomy: case report. *J Laparoendosc Surg* 1:145-149, 1991.
22. Ominus M, Papin P, Gangloff S: Extraperitoneal approach to the lumbar spine with video assistance. *Spine* 21:2491, 1996.
23. Onik G, Mooney V, Maroon JC, *et al*: Automated percutaneous discectomy: a prospective multi-institutional study. *Neurosurgery* 26:228, 1990.

24. Regan JJ: Endoscopic applications of the BAK system (L4-5) In Regan JJ, McAfee PJ, Mack MJ (eds): *Atlas of Endoscopic Spine Surgery*. St. Louis, Quality Medical Publishing, 1995, p 321.

25. Regan JJ: Percutaneous endoscopic thoracic discectomy. *Neurosurg Clin N Am* 7:87, 1996.

26. Regan JJ, Mack MJ: Endoscopic thoracic fusion cage. In Regan JJ, McAfee PJ, Mack MJ (eds): *Atlas of Endoscopic Spine Surgery*. St. Louis, Quality Medical Publishing, 1995, p 350.

27. Regan JJ, Mack MJ, Picetti GD: A technical report on video-assisted thoracoscopy in thoracic spinal surgery. Preliminary description. *Spine* 20:831-837, 1995.

28. Rosenthal D: Endoscopic internal fixation of the thoracic spine. In Regan JJ, McAfee PJ, Mack MJ (eds): *Atlas of Endoscopic Spine Surgery*. St Louis, Quality Medical Publishing, 1995, p 333.

29. Rosenthal D, Marquardt G, Lorenz R, Nichtweiss M: Anterior decompression and stabilization using a microsurgical endoscopic technique for metastatic tumors of the thoracic spine. *J Neurosurg* 84:565-572, 1996.

30. Rosenthal D, Rosenthal R, de Simone A: Removal of a protruded thoracic disc using microsurgical endoscopy. A new technique. *Spine* 19:1087-1091, 1994.

31. Sachs BL, Schwaitzberg SD: Lumbosacral (L5-S1) discectomy and interbody fusion technique. In Regan JJ, McAfee PC, Mack MJ (eds): *Atlas of Endoscopic Spine Surgery*. St Louis, Quality Medical Publishing, 1995, p 275.

32. Savitz MH: Same-day microsurgical arthroscopic lateral-approach laser-assisted (SMALL) fluoroscopic discectomy. *J Neurosurg* 80:1039, 1994.

33. Schaffer JL, Kambin P: Percutaneous posterolateral lumbar discectomy and decompression with a 6.9 millimeter cannula. Analysis of operative failures and complications. *J Bone Joint Surg* 73:822, 1991.

34. Schreiber A, Leu H: Percutaneous nucleotomy: technique with discoscopy. *Orthopedics* 14:439, 1991.

35. Sihvonen T, Herno A, Paljarvi L: Local denervation atrophy of paraspinal muscles in post-operative failed back syndrome. *Spine* 18:575, 1993.

36. Transfeldt EE, Schultz L: Approach to the lumbar spine without insufflation. In Regan JJ, McAfee PC, Mack MJ (eds): *Atlas of Endoscopic Spine Surgery*. St Louis, Quality Medical Publishing, 1995, p 137.

37. Zuckerman JF, Hsu K, Implacito D: Instrumented transperitoneal laparoscopic fusion. In Margulies JY, Floman Y, Farcy JPC, Neuwirth MG (eds): Lumbosacral and spinopelvic fixation. Philadelphia, Lippincott-Raven, 1996, p 579.

38. Zuckerman JF, Zdeblick T: Instrumented laparoscopic spinal fusion. In Proceedings of the 9th Annual Meeting of the North American Spine Society. Minneapolis, October 1994, p 66.

39. Zuckerman JF, Zdeblick TA, Bailey SA, *et al*: Instrumented laparoscopic spinal fusion: preliminary results. *Spine* 20:2029, 1995.

# CHAPTER 96

# Minimally Invasive Spinal Decompression and Stabilization Techniques II

**Eeric Truumees, Isador H. Lieberman, Richard G. Fessler, and John Regan**

## Introduction and History

Endoscopic spine surgery refers to a rapidly evolving set of techniques potentially offering equivalent surgical outcomes with lower surgical morbidity. Endoscopic spine surgery does not refer to a single technique but rather a set of tools that may be employed during the approach to the spine. The philosophy behind spinal endoscopy is to target the pathology and apply a therapeutic intervention while minimizing damage to surrounding non-pathologic tissues.[14,54,74] These endoscopic techniques are part of a trend toward less-invasive interventions in patients with spinal disease that include percutaneous and fluoroscopically guided treatment.

Endoscopy employs a fiberoptic camera and light source for visualization and magnification through small percutaneous portals. Endoscopic inspection of the thoracic cavity was initially conceived by Bozzini in 1806.[8] Jacobaeus[48] provided its first clinical application for diagnosing and treating tuberculosis in 1910. In 1991, Lewis popularized VATS (video-assisted thoracic surgery) for pulmonary diseases. Orthopedic applications of endoscopic principles began with the advent and acceptance of knee arthroscopy. Tagaki was the first to describe and Watanabe was the first to advance diagnostic knee arthroscopy in 1918 and 1957, respectively. Cascells in 1970 and Jackson in 1972 are credited with promoting in North America the Japanese experience with arthroscopy. Over a short time, endoscopic techniques have become standard for many abdominal and knee procedures, such as cholecystectomy and meniscectomy.[80] Endoscopic spinal surgery was first performed in the lumbar spine and, currently, experience in the lumbar spine outweighs that of thoracic endoscopy.[17] The first description of VATS for thoracic spinal diseases was published by Mack and others in 1993.[59]

With improved instrumentation and increasing experience, interest in the use of minimally invasive surgery for thoracic spine disease has increased. Regan *et al.* reported their results in diverse thoracic spinal pathology including deformity and degenerative disease. They have successfully employed endoscopic technique to perform interbody grafting and, more recently, instrumentation.[75-77] Rosenthal *et al.*[85] reported the use of VATS for ventral decompression and stabilization in patients with metastatic tumors of the thoracic spine. The initial results with video-assisted thoracoscopic surgery (VATS) are encouraging. Although VATS is characterized by less pain and shorter hospital stays, spinal endoscopy remains in its infancy.[17,18,54,86]

An endoscopy may be placed during posterior approaches to improve visualization of the anterior cord.

This chapter addresses the philosophy of endoscopic spine surgery and its specific applications in thoracic spine. These include anterior and posterior approaches for decompression and stabilization. Relevant indications and contraindications, as well as published results and complications, are discussed.

## Philosophy of Spinal Endoscopy

Vertebral tissues are located centrally in the body. Open surgical approaches therefore involve significant soft tissue dissection that increases surgical risk, recovery time, and long-term functional consequences. Minimally invasive approaches attempt to perform the same operation while decreasing the size of the incision and damage to otherwise normal surrounding tissues. Decreasing the collateral damage to surrounding tissue should decrease the morbidity, pain, and hospitalization while leaving an aesthetically more acceptable scar.

### Ventral Approaches

While no direct, randomized trial has compared endoscopic techniques with thoracotomy or costotransversectomy, there are many theoretical and apparent advantages (Box 96.1).* First, a quality endoscopic video system affords the surgeon improved visualization through outstanding illumination and up to 15× magnification. By manipulating endoscopic portal placement, scope angle, and camera trajectory, a parallel approach to disc space can be maintained even in coronal plane deformity.

Second, VATS requires less muscle dissection and no rib spreading, and therefore decreased incisional pain. Similarly, decreased soft tissue injury results in more cosmetically acceptable scars, lower risk of postoperative infection, and decreased compromise of respiratory and shoulder mechanics. With prone positioning, simultaneous ventral and dorsal procedures may be undertaken. These advantages, taken together, may reduce intensive care unit and hospital stays.

On the other hand, VATS has several disadvantages over open surgery as well.* First, these procedures require substantially different technical skill sets than traditional, open approaches. This surgical novelty has been termed a "steep learning curve" but more correctly represents a flat learning curve in that a significant amount of time must be spent with animal, cadaveric, and proctored cases before proceeding with independent VATS spine surgery. Endoscopy changes the surgeon's binocular vision to monocular video-assisted

---

*References 1,7,13-16,17-20,28,29,33,51,64,65,74-76,80.

vision. This loss of depth perception is compounded with a loss of tactile feedback associated with the long-handled instruments needed to pass through endoscopic portals. Working distance and instrument excursion increases from 4 to 30cm. Visualization and manipulation of sensitive spinal structures also requires triangulation from widely separated starting points on the chest wall to a small thoracic disc space. Prior to embarking on endoscopic thoracic spine surgery, the surgeon must be familiar with open anterior spinal anatomy and surgical techniques. Ultimately, the surgical procedures are the same but the methods are different enough to challenge even the most experienced spinal surgeon. Other disadvantages are more technical in nature. In some centers, VATS is performed with a second, experienced thoracoscopic surgeon. Even if a spine surgeon does not typically employ a thoracic surgeon for open thoracotomy approaches, the additional manpower is increased in VATS procedures in that this specialist or assistants for the entire procedure.

Although the insult to postoperative pulmonary mechanics may be decreased with endoscopic approaches to the thoracic spine, double lumen intubation and single lung ventilation are typically required. Long periods of single lung ventilation are physiologically demanding to the patient and technically demanding to the anesthesiologist.

VATS procedures require additional, expensive, and often single-use equipment. Endoscopic instrumentation is constantly improving and, with these improvements, the technical limitations of thoracoscopy spine surgery are declining. Theoretical technical limitations in the ability to treat intraoperative complications endoscopically remain. In particular, it may be difficult to obtain vascular control of major vessel hemorrhages. Similarly, options for dural repair are limited. Finally, techniques and implants for structural grafting and spinal reconstruction remain developmental. Emerging, innovative technologies are gradually addressing these limitations.

## Dorsal and Combined Approaches

The majority of open thoracic and lumbar spine procedures continue to be performed from posterior approaches. The approaches offer relatively direct access to the bony elements and the spinal canal. However, canal exposure may result in symptomatic epidural fibrosis. The dissection and retraction of the paraspinal muscles may lead to dead space formation and extensor muscle disruption. Such disruption has been referred to as "fusion disease"[104] and may be associated with early fatigability and other long-term symptoms. Endoscopic techniques may allow for less disruption of the posterior musculature and a smaller laminotomy. Dorsal and dorsolateral approaches are also limited by the surgeon's ability to visualize the anterior dura. Use of an angled endoscope may greatly improve visualization while decreasing soft tissue dissection and rib resection.

Combined approaches are being increasingly described in the literature. These approaches include simultaneous anterior and posterior surgery for tumors and deformity.[27,51] Combined approaches may also refer to combining endoscopic and open techniques in "mini-open" or endoscopically assisted spine procedures to exploit the advantages of both techniques.[28,33]

## Relative Indications

In considering the role of endoscopic spine surgery as part of a continuum of spine care, it is useful to remember that the most minimally invasive modality remains non-operative care. Non-operative treatment is appropriate and effective in the vast majority of patients with degenerative conditions of the spine. Non-operative management should remain a consideration for most degenerative conditions, especially those involving axial pain in the absence of neurologic dysfunction. Surgical indications must not be liberalized simply because the procedure can be completed endoscopically.

### Video-Assisted Thoracoscopic Spine Surgery

The majority of endoscopic thoracic spine surgery is directed anteriorly to avoid larger incisions and post-thoracotomy pain. A traditional thoracotomy requires a large incision, division of the shoulder girdle musculature, rib resection, and forcible rib retraction. This approach can result in desiccation of the exposed lungs and vessels, measurable reduction in pulmonary and shoulder girdle function, post-thoracotomy intercostal pain syndrome, and an unsightly scar.[51,54] On the other hand, thoracoscopic approaches visualize the anterior spinal elements from the T1-2 to L1-2 disc spaces from the side of approach to the midline.[18] VATS affords easier exposure of "the extremes" of the thoracic spine than open thoracotomy.[71] For example, a

**BOX 96.1**

## Advantages and disadvantages of thoracic endoscopic spine surgery

**Advantages**
Improved visualization
Decreased postoperative incisional pain
Cosmetically acceptable scars
Opportunity to perform simultaneous anterior-posterior procedures
Reduced blood loss
Reduced infection risk
Decreased compromise of respiratory mechanics and rib splinting
Decreased postoperative shoulder girdle dysfunction
Reduced intensive care and hospital stay

**Disadvantages**
Surgical novelty ("learning curve")
Monocular visualization (triangulation, depth perception)
Loss of tactile feedback (increased working distance)
Need for second surgeon
Technical limitations in treating intraoperative complications
Anesthetic demands of double lumen intubation and single lung ventilation
Currently limited ability to perform endoscopic reconstruction
Currently limited ability to perform dural repair
Specialized, costly, and often single-use instruments

T12 corpectomy can be performed without diaphragmatic take-down, and T3 can be accessed without mobilizing the scapula as would be required with an open technique.

## Indications and Contraindications

Currently, VATS may be employed for a number of pathologies affecting the anterior and middle columns of the thoracic spine (Box 96.2). These include infections, which can be biopsied, débrided, or as in the case of epidural abscess, drained. Similarly, thoracoscopic access is suitable for tumor biopsy or piecemeal excision. A number of authors have described the use of VATS in patients with degenerative conditions of the thoracic spine including excision of herniated thoracic discs and fusion of painful degenerated segments. In trauma, corpectomy/decompression and stabilization procedures have been performed. The largest early experience with VATS in spine patients has been in the correction of deformity.[14] Here, a thoracoscope can be used to assist anterior release surgery in kyphotic or scoliotic deformities. This surgery has included the pediatric patient population as well as those with neuromuscular scoliosis.

Contraindications to thoracoscopic spinal surgery include the inability to tolerate single lung ventilation as in patients with severe or acute respiratory insufficiency.[76] On the other hand, VATS should be considered for patients who are at high pulmonary risk for thoracotomy.[76] Thoracoscopy may decrease many of the detrimental physiologic sequelae of thoracotomy. For example, post-thoracotomy rib splinting leads to atelectasis and decreased functional residual capacity.[53] Thus, while VATS is ideally avoided in patients with severe lung disease, its less deleterious effect on pulmonary mechanics makes it a better option than thoracotomy. Typical patient groups include: patients with COPD or interstitial fibrosis, or those with significant restrictive lung disease from deformity, such as children with neuromuscular scoliosis.

Other contraindications stem from difficulty visualizing and manipulating instruments through a scarred chest cavity. Therefore VATS should not be offered to patients with pleural symphysis, failed prior open ventral surgery, or bullous lung pathology. Relative contraindications include empyema, previous thoracotomy, or previous tube thoracostomy.

## Relevant Anatomy

The rib cage and chest wall form a rigid open space in which endoscopic surgery may be performed. Unlike the abdomen, $CO_2$ insufflation is not required to maintain a working space. Through most of the thoracic spine, ribs articulate at the disc space level. The rib number corresponds to the lower vertebral body at the disc space (e.g., the sixth rib comes off the T5-6 disc space). Because the rib comes directly off the disc space from demi-facets arising on the vertebral body just above and below the disc, rib resection is required for adequate access to the posterolateral corner of the disc. In the lower thoracic region, T11 and 12, the rib head may be well caudal to the disc space, permitting unobstructed access.

The segmental vessels lie in the waist of the vertebral bodies. When approaching the spine endoscopically, it is important not to inadvertently lacerate these vessels. Various spinal procedures, including corpectomy and instrumentation, require sacrifice of the segmentals. Discectomy and ventral release procedures, on the other hand, do not require vessel sacrifice. One cadaver study demonstrated adequate discectomy without sacrifice of the intercostal or segmental vessels once an adequate mobilization of the esophagus and azygos vein had been carried out. The authors concluded that the segmental vessels ought to be preserved to reduce the risk of cord ischemia.[7] In a two-phase goat study, thoracoscopic discectomy and fusion were undertaken both with and without sacrifice of the segmentals.[94] In the first phase, the area of disc excision was slightly higher in the vessel ligated group, but this was not felt to be significant. Operative times were the same. In the second phase, biomechanical testing of the resulting fusion was undertaken and the vessel spared group revealed less flexibility in lateral bending. The authors concluded that the segmental vessels in the thoracic spine can be effectively spared without injury during disc excision and fusion. They noted that while slightly more disc area was excised with ligation of the vessels, sparing the segmental vessels may provide blood supply that aids in fusion. They recommended sparing the segmental vessels in patients with a high risk for cord perfusion-related neurologic injury, such as revision surgery, severe kyphosis, and congenital anomalies.

These studies have been criticized for not adequately modeling the intraoperative conditions of spinal deformity.[3] Many authors report that sacrificing the segmental vessels provides better visualization through improved pleural reflection and more complete discectomy.[3,64,65] In a report of 1197 procedures in which more than 6000 vessels were sacrificed, there were no adverse neurologic consequences.[103] It may be reasonable to employ both vessel-sparing and vessel-sacrificing techniques as a function of the clinical situation. For example, in congenital deformity cases wherein spinal cord blood supplies may be anomalous, vessel sparing may be more important.[64] Also, if the intervention requires the sacrifice of one or

---

**BOX 96.2**

### Indications and contraindications for thoracoscopic spine surgery

**Indications**
Infections: biopsy, drainage, debridement
Tumor: biopsy, excision, cord decompression
Degenerative disease: thoracic discectomy
Trauma: canal decompression and stabilization
Deformity: anterior releases, stabilizations

**Contraindications**
Respiratory problems: insufficiency, inability to tolerate single lung ventilation
Pleural symphysis
Prior anterior surgery: thoracotomy, tube thoracostomy
Bullous lung pathology
Empyema

more segmental arteries in the mid to lower thoracic region, especially T9 to T11, a right-sided approach should be considered to avoid ligation of the artery of Adamkiewicz.

Other important structures include the superior intercostal veins and the sympathetic chain. The veins empty into the azygos circulation at or about the T3-4 interspace.[14] Branches from the sympathetic chain run over the rib heads, just below the parietal pleura.[97] Over the fifth through tenth ribs, these coalesce as the greater splanchnic nerve that courses into the abdomen.

There are critical regional differences in thoracoscopic anatomy that dictate different exposure techniques. In the upper thoracic region, for example, the surgeon should elevate and support the ipsilateral arm to rotate the scapula away. Here, unless there are apical adhesions, the collapsed lung readily falls away from the spine, allowing excellent visualization.[38] In the mid-thorax, there is more available space that allows more variation in placement of the camera and retractor ports. On the other hand, a fan retractor or strategically placed sponges are typically needed to keep the collapsed lung out of the operative field. Similarly, a second retracting port may be needed to move aside a bullous or stiff lung.[38] Tilting the operating table forward may improve visualization with less forceful lung retraction. In the lower thoracic region, it may be necessary to retract the diaphragm, but here, as at the apices, lung retraction is not usually a problem.

## Anesthesia

Safe, close communication with the anesthesia team and a thoracoscopic spine surgery begins with meticulous room and intubation set-up. Selective double lumen endotracheal intubation allows collapse of the lung on the operative side. As the tube may easily migrate, frequent bronchoscopic assessment of tube position is mandatory.[52] In small patients (under 45kg), even the smallest double lumen endotracheal tube may not fit. In these cases, bronchial blockers are required.[64,74] Blockers are technically more difficult to use and have a higher rate of incomplete lung deflation which may seriously impair visualization.[74] Prone positioning in deformity cases may allow single-lumen intubation.[43]

General anesthetic options include: total intravenous technique, isolated volatile agent, or a combination of volatile and intravenous agents. Initially, intravenous technique was recommended because of the potential risk of hypoxic pulmonary vasoconstriction with inhalational agents during single lung ventilation. Recently, however, a series of 85 patients found no difference among these techniques.[52] Hemodynamic monitoring includes a double-lumen central venous catheter. Alternatively, pulmonary artery catheterization may be undertaken.[52] Hypotensive anesthesia should be avoided in myelopathic patients or in those undergoing segmental artery sacrifice.[75]

Once tube position has been confirmed, the ipsilateral lung is deflated by clamping the lumen of its endotracheal tube. Once the chest has been entered with the first portal, the lung should collapse. If inadequate collapse is noted, a short period of positive pressure $CO_2$ insufflation may assist in collapsing the lung. Usually, this insufflation is not necessary.[58]

King et al.[43] describe use of 4mmHg of $CO_2$ insufflation during single lumen intubated prone cases to allow enough atelectasis to develop without fully collapsing the ipsilateral lung. At these pressures, the authors report that no significant mediastinal shift occurs. On the other hand, Krasna et al.[47] found that pressure greater than 12mmHg is associated with mediastinal shift and rapid changes in cardiac output.

For patients with no cardiorespiratory disease, tidal volumes of 10 to 15mL/kg and 100% oxygen content are appropriate.[17,52] The respiratory rate is adjusted to titrate the end-tidal partial pressure to between 35 and 40mmHg. If $O_2$ saturation decreases during the procedure, reassess ET tube position.

## Patient and OR Positioning

A radiolucent operating frame is preferred for either lateral decubitus or prone positioning. Lateral decubitus, identical to open thoracotomy positioning, is most typical for VATS spine surgery. Bean bag or bolsters may be used to maintain laterality. If intraoperative imaging is to be used, assess the location and lucency of the positioning aids. The patient should be well padded and an axillary roll is typically employed.

The patient is belted into place so that the table may be tilted into Trendelenburg or reverse Trendelenburg or even tilted right or left as necessary to improve intraoperative visualization. It is important to ensure the patient stays in a strict lateral position during the initial approach to the spine so as to maintain surgeon orientation. Some surgeons will prefer to "airplane" the table up for portions of the procedure, but given the loss of tactile feedback and three-dimensional information associated with endoscopy, a strict knowledge of the patient's body position in space is necessary. In some settings, particularly in the lower thoracic spine, it may be useful to "jack-knife" the table to improve access to the lateral body wall. In patients with significant spinal cord compression, excessive jack-knifing may increase the risk of iatrogenic neurologic progression.[58]

Prone positioning may be employed as part of simultaneous ventral/dorsal approach.[43,51] Simultaneous surgery eliminates the need to stage the procedures, or the added time and costs for re-positioning, re-draping, and a new operating room set-up. Prone position is particularly advantageous in cases of marked instability. For example, in ankylosing spondylitis, the spine may suddenly translate at the osteotomy site during repositioning. Prone position also allows a gravity reduction of hyperkyphosis.[43] Finally, prone positioning confers the additional advantage of allowing the lungs to fall away from the spine, decreasing the need for retraction.

A large operating room is needed to accommodate the special equipment required in VATS cases.[71] The gowned and sterile team typically includes two surgeons, one assistant, and one scrub nurse. Additional personnel include the anesthesia team, SSEP monitoring personnel, cell saver transfusion technicians, and circulating nursing staff. Beyond the usual complement of anesthesia machines and back tables for instruments and implants, endoscopic spine surgery requires two video monitors, a fluoroscope, and neuromonitoring equipment. The endoscopic surgeon and spine surgeon typically work on same side of the patient (facing the patient in lateral decubitus). Alternatively they can work opposite one another. Video mixers can convert image orientation so that no mirror image instrument manipulation is required.[14] More and more frequently, voice-activated robotics are being used to replace the assistant surgeon in camera positioning. Robotics may improve visualization by providing a steady image.

Instruments for an open thoracotomy should be readily available for emergency use. In the prone position, open access can be achieved with an extended costotransversectomy approach. As the lung has already been mobilized, it is easy to enter the chest. Once in, the surgeon is readily able to access, identify, and control the major vascular structures.[51]

The workhorse of spinal endoscopy is the video equipment. This begins with the endoscope itself. A number of standard 10mm endoscopes are employed, most commonly 0- and 30-degrees. Occasionally, 70-degree scopes are needed. The 0-degree scope is standard for thoracoscopy, but a 30-degree scope decreases instrument crowding and allows better visualization around bony corners.[76,78] Typically a 10mm, 15-inch end-viewing scope is employed; however, in pediatric cases and, with increasing frequency in adults, a 5mm scope may be preferred.[76] The smaller scope provides less illumination but with improvements in high-resolution, three-chip technology is adequate in most cases. Three-dimensional endoscopes are becoming increasingly available and help visualize landmarks and render improved depth perception.[76]

Instruments are introduced into the chest through trocars. Initially, these trocars were hard. Hard trocars may protect the thoracoscope against the rigid fulcrum of the ribcage.[14] More recently, soft trocars have been developed that may be less traumatic to the neurovascular bundle on the inferior rib undersurface. Standard trocars are either 5mm or 10mm and are selected based on the size of instrument to be passed and the intercostal distance, which in adults is less than 12mm.[58]

Typical spine instruments are customized for endoscopic applications by creating an extended shank of uniform diameter to match standard trocar sizes (Figure 96.1). These include long-handled curettes, Cobbs, pituitaries, nerve hooks, and Penfields. High-speed burrs with long extenders are often required, as are more specialized endoscopic equipment such as Endoshears, a bipolar endoscopic electrocautery, the harmonic scalpel, endovascular clips and loop ligatures, and endoscopic fan retractors.

### Initial Surgical Approach

A left- or right-sided approach to the thoracic spine may be used depending on the eccentricity of the pathology (Figure 96.2). With a left-sided approach, the thick resilient aorta is less prone to injury than the large friable tortuous veins of the azygous system. Some authors prefer a right-sided approach when the pathology is not lateralized, because there is a greater spinal surface area lateral to the azygos vein than the aorta.[18] This difference can be assessed with preoperative axial CT or MRI images. Below T9, consider a left-sided approach to avoid the more cranial diaphragm reflection the right.

The initial trocar creates the main viewing portal and is placed in the anterior axillary line at the sixth or seventh intercostal space, giving an unobstructed view of the entire hemithorax. The trocar is inserted in the manner of a tube thoracostomy with blunt dissection with a Kelly forceps just over the top of the rib to avoid damage to the neurovascular bundle or deep structures. A digital exploration is undertaken to exclude adhesions and avoid parenchymal lacerations of the lung. Some recommend Bovie dissection through musculature to prevent bleeding around portal, which can obscure the camera image.[14]

This first portal is the only one to be inserted blindly. Once open to the atmosphere, the lung falls away from the thoracic wall, allowing insertion of the thoracoscope. In patients with marked pleural symphysis, consider aborting thoracoscopy for an open approach. Insert the endoscope and perform an exploratory thoracoscopy. Release minor lung adhesions. If complete atelectasis is not achieved, a brief period of $CO_2$ insufflation may help to collapse the lung.

The camera assistant must maintain the camera orientation and keep operative field centered in view with a steady hand. The camera and instruments should be in the same 180-degree arc to avoid working in a mirror image. The camera assistant and the operating surgeon should work in unison with small movements. The camera should be removed for cleaning at various intervals. It should be reinserted carefully, because the lung may have partially reinflated, and injury to the lung parenchyma is possible.[58] Self-cleaning and defogging arthroscopes are very helpful in this regard.[76]

Manipulate only one object at a time. The camera operator provides zoom-in to the operative site. Then, as new instruments are introduced, pan the camera out to follow the instrument into the operative field, preferably without changing the camera angle. Similarly, remove retractors and other instruments under direct visualization. Fan retractors should be removed in the fully closed position only. Avoid levering instruments on rib cage to decrease pressure on the intercostal nerve.[35]

### Deep Approach

Once in the chest, surgical levels are identified. Operating at the wrong level is always a concern in the thoracic spine. Screen for variant anatomy, such as accessory ribs, with preoperative radiographs, then find the level by counting down from the first rib. The first rib may be difficult to identify. Mark the disc space and obtain radiographic confirmation. A Steinmann pin can be passed directly through the chest wall into the pathologic level.[71] A radiograph confirms level localization and the pin also demonstrates the optimal location for the working portal. Accept only quality radiographic images. Anteroposterior radiographs are typically more helpful than lateral.[97] In some centers, marking beads are placed at each spinal level and radiographs or fluoroscopy are obtained prior to entering the operating suite. The appropriate level bead is maintained on the patient for intraoperative confirmation.[38]

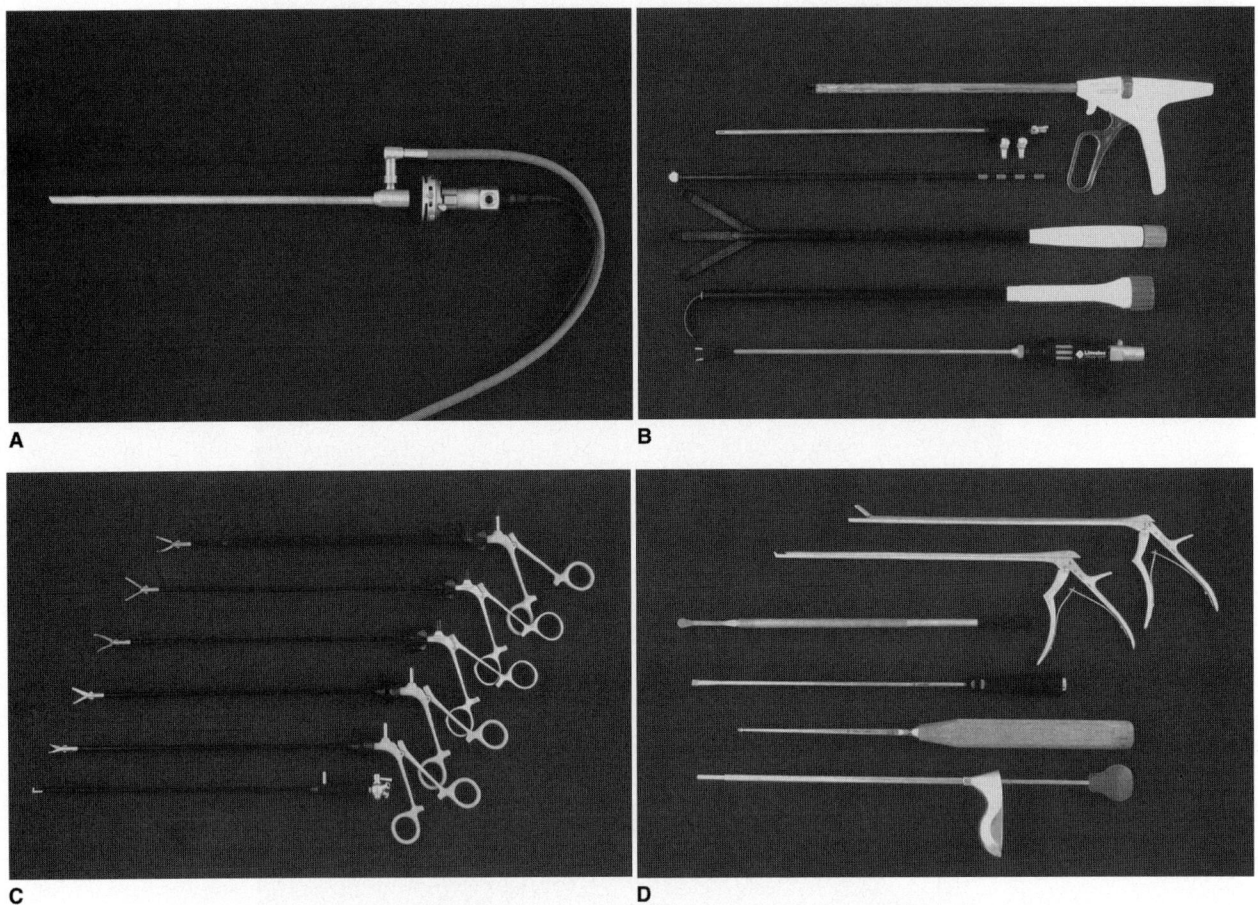

**Figure 96.1** Spinal thoracoscopy benefits from an ever-increasing array of available instruments. Important among these are the **(A)** endoscope itself, **(B)** standard endoscopic instruments (including a fan retractor and auto-suture device), **(C)** endoscopic dissecting tools, and **(D)** typical spine instruments modified for thoracoscopic use with long hands and uniform diameter shafts.

To manipulate the spinal tissues, additional instruments will need to be inserted into the chest through additional trocars. Typically, two working portals are created under direct video visualization with the lung protected. The chest is percussed and by visualizing the percussions from within the chest, additional sites are chosen. As an alternative, 18-gauge spinal needles can be placed through the interspace to verify the level and trajectory. Organize the remaining portals to center the instruments at the level of pathology. A number of portal patterns have been described and are covered in more detail in the sections below. Typically, an L or V shape at the dorsal axillary line 2 interspaces cephalad and caudad to the viewing portal is creating, depending on the chest wall morphology and the intended spinal level. Space portals far enough apart that instruments do not "fence" with each other. The final viewing portal should be far enough away from the lesion to allow a panoramic view and to allow room to manipulate instruments.[74] During the procedure, the instruments and scope are interchanged between the portals to facilitate work at different levels. It is preferable to make another portal perpendicular to the operative level than to operate at an acute angle to the pathology.[38]

When the appropriate portals have been placed and the correct level identified, incise the parietal pleura with monopolar cautery. Alternatively, employ the harmonic scalpel to dissect with less smoke and char.[15,73] Avoid monopolar cautery over the inferior margin of the rib head where electrocautery injury to the intercostal nerve may occur.[58] The degree of pleural dissection depends on the extent of the intended surgery but may include longitudinal approaches parallel to the spine or transverse approaches parallel to each disc space. If the segmental vessels are to be preserved, smaller pleural incisions are created parallel to the disc space. Bluntly dissect the incised parietal pleura proximally, distally, and anteriorly to expose as much of the vertebral margins as is necessary.

Endoscopic visualization amplifies the apparent amount of bleeding. At each step, meticulous hemostasis is required. Control bleeding with mono- or bipolar electrocautery, harmonic scalpel, argon beam coagulation, or hemostatic packing. Uncontrolled bleeding may necessitate conversion to an open procedure.

At the conclusion of the procedure, irrigate out any disc or bony debris. Most authors do not attempt to close the parietal pleura. Some recommend an intercostal bupivacaine block to decrease postoperative pain.[1]

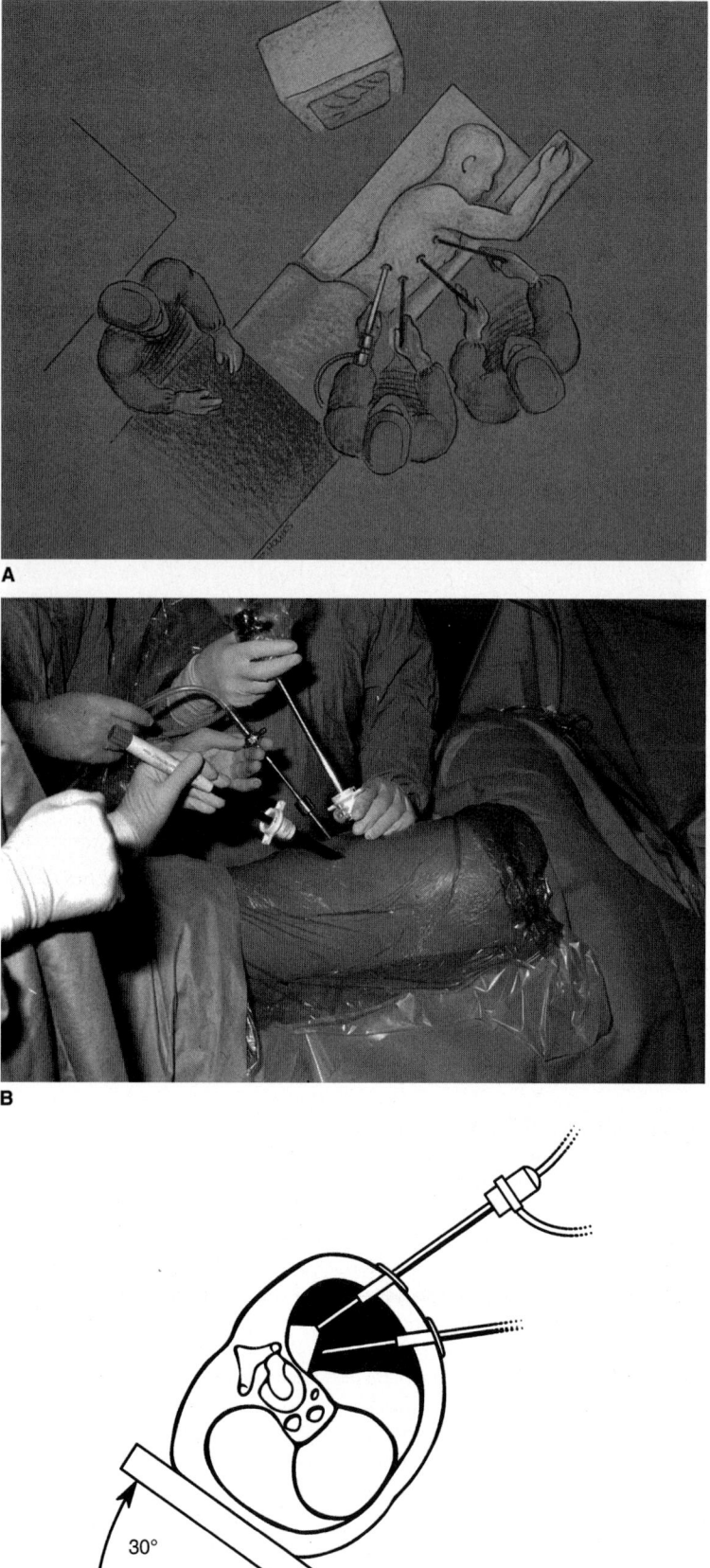

**Figure 96.2** Lateral thoracoscopy. (**A**) Operating room set-up. (**B**) Clinical photograph of lateral thoracoscopy. Note the assistant in the foreground holding the fan retractor. (**C**) Visualization is improved when the lungs fall away from the spine with an anterior tilt of the operating room table of 20 to 30 degrees. (**C** *from Regan JJ, Jarolem KL: Thoracoscopy of the spine. In Herkowitz HN, et al. Rothman-Simeone The Spine, ed 4. Philadelphia, WB Saunders, 1999, p 601.*)

A 20F, 24F, or 28F chest tube is selected depending on patient's size. Insert the tube through the inferior-most portal and run it cranially along the vertebral column. Rosenthal uses two chest tubes, one apical tube for air and a second, basilar tube for effusions.[85] Depending on the nature of the procedure, the tube can be maintained at water seal or at 20cm of water suction. Typically, the tube can be removed 1 to 2 days postoperatively.

In the postoperative period, most patients are extubated immediately. A chest radiograph is obtained in the recovery room to verify full inflation of the lungs.[17] In some settings, a brief period of ICU monitoring is recommended. Aggressive respiratory care is required to prevent "down lung" atelectasis and pneumonia. This may include bronchodilators, deep suctioning, and deep coughing.

## General Results and Complications

Liske et al.[52] described the anesthesia outcomes in their series of 82 patients undergoing thoracoscopic spine surgery under single lung ventilation. The authors found that the anesthesia time was not significantly different than their series of open thoracotomy patients. They noted that VATS required extremely long single lung ventilation times (a mean of 270.2 minutes). Also, the oxygenation index decreased significantly after initiation of single lung ventilation. Despite these physiologic stressors, the authors concluded that VATS was a reasonable alternative to open thoracotomy from the anesthesia perspective because of the clinical benefits of accelerated return to activity and decreased ICU and hospital stays.

One series compared video-assisted thoracoscopic surgery to open thoracotomy in a sheep model. In this series, histologic, biomechanical, and radiographic outcomes were comparable to open surgery. However, endoscopic procedures were associated with steep learning curves, long operative times, increased blood loss, and increased animal morbidity.[16]

The complications associated with thoracoscopically assisted spine surgery are essentially the same as with an open approach and are categorized as incomplete operation, neurologic injury, lung injury, and vascular injury.[20,58,85] For the novice thoracoscopic spine surgeon, endoscopic releases or decompressions may be less complete than open releases. Early in your experience, review postoperative CT scans to determine the adequacy of decompression.

As in any spinal cord level procedure, dural laceration, cord injury or ischemia are possible. Most common, however, is intercostal neuralgia. This may be seen in up to 21% of patients, but it is usually transient.[58] Flexible portals may reduce its incidence, but intercostal neuralgia still occurred in 2 in a series of 17 patients in which these portals were used.[20] Transection of the sympathetic chain causes little or no morbidity, but the surgeon should inform the patient and family of possible temperature and skin color changes below the level of surgery.

A variety of pulmonary complications have been reported. Longer periods of lung collapse increase pulmonary morbidity. To decrease the rate of prolonged atelectasis, the deflated lung should be reinflated for 5 to 10 minutes for every hour of operating time.[17] Trocars or instruments may cause direct trauma to the lungs. Larger air leaks should be repaired with an endoscopic suture ligature. Other common postoperative lung problems include pleural effusions and diaphragmatic injury.

More unusual pulmonary complications may stem from anesthesia or single lung ventilation mishaps. Sucato and Girgis[93] reported a case of an 11-year-old patient with severe scoliosis who developed air in both chest cavities, mediastinum, peritoneum, retroperitoneum, and subcutaneous tissue after intubation with a double-lumen endotracheal tube. While the patient remained hemodynamically stable, bilateral chest tubes were required. The authors note that just as for the surgeon, there is a significant learning curve for the anesthesiologist to become adept at obtaining and maintaining single lung ventilation.

With any ventral thoracic procedure, devastating vascular injuries are possible. The trocars or other instruments may injure the heart, great vessels, azygos vein, esophagus, or segmental arteries. Thoracic duct injury with lymphatic leakage should be closed off with an endoscopic clip applier.

McAfee and others reported their complications with VATS in a prospective series of 78 cases. Transient intercostal neuralgias were noted in 6 patients and atelectasis in 5. One case was converted to open for extensive pleural adhesions. One case of partial neurologic deficit and no deep infections were noted.[58] Huang and co-workers[35] reported their complications in a series of 90 consecutive patients treated with thoracoscopic techniques for a variety of pathologies including infection, fracture, deformity, and degenerative disease. A total of 30 complications were noted in 22 patients (24.4%). Two of these complications were fatal, including one case of massive blood loss and another of pneumonia. One graft dislodgement required revision surgery. The other complications were transient and included 4 cases of intercostal neuralgia, three superficial wound infections, three cases of pharyngeal pain, two cases of atelectasis, and two cases of residual pneumothorax. Four cases were converted to open.

## VATS in Deformity

Endoscopic surgery may directly or indirectly address several of the goals of spinal deformity surgery. These include arrest of curve progression, maximization and maintenance of curve correction, improvement in fusion rate, and decompression and protection of the neural elements[11,41,46,92] (Box 96.3). In scoliosis, morphologic studies demonstrate that the anterior longitudinal ligament migrates to the concavity of the curve. The ALL and concave-side costotransverse ligaments form a structural tether that must be released to gain maximum mobility of the spine.[41] Typically, anterior approaches to the spine in deformity are indicated to release these tethers to allow correction of coronal and sagittal plane deformities.

Indications for endoscopic techniques in spinal deformity are the same as those for thoracotomy.[14,24] The surgeon should consider anterior release in large scoliotic curves greater than 75 degrees and in rigid curves with less than 50% correction on bending films. Anterior epiphysiodesis is typically required to prevent of the crankshaft phenomena in skeletally immature children with curves greater than 50 degrees or in those with progressive con-

## 96.3

### Indications and contraindications to thoracoscopic spine surgery in deformity

**Indications:**

*Same as for thoracotomy*

Curves greater than 60 degrees with less than 50% correction on bending

Curves greater than 75 degrees

Curves requiring rebalancing into the stable zone in either the coronal or sagittal planes

Crankshaft prevention in skeletally immature patients with curves greater than 50 degrees

Kyphotic deformities greater than 70 degrees

Progressive congenital deformities requiring epiphysiodesis

Patients at high risk of pseudoarthrosis from posterior fusion alone

Patients by bone grafting to achieve an interbody fusion

**Additional indications**

Patients with compromised pulmonary mechanics

**Contraindications**

See Box 96.2

Deformity-specific relative contraindications

Narrow anterior posterior chest diameter or other anatomic variants that limit working space in the chest

Significant vertebral rotation at the apex

---

genital deformities within the thorax. Patients with kyphotic deformities greater than 70 degrees or curves that require rebalancing into the stable zone in the coronal or sagittal plane are also candidates for anterior surgery. Interbody fusion techniques are often added to posterior stabilization procedures to minimize pseudarthrosis risk.

Spinal endoscopy should be given particular consideration in the patient with pre-existing pulmonary mechanics compromise caused by the spinal deformity or associated neurologic syndromes (i.e., polio). Here, endoscopic techniques may be indicated to minimize any thoracotomy-related pulmonary compromise. Finally, endoscopic techniques should be considered in any situation in which the cosmetic result is of particular concern to the patient.

Relative contraindications to the use of spinal endoscopy to treat patients with spinal deformity include all of the contraindications to endoscopy in general.[51] Also, special consideration needs to be paid to the relationship of the spine to the thoracic cage. A narrow anterior-posterior chest diameter, significant vertebral rotation at the apex, or thoracic scoliosis curves greater than 75 degrees may preclude safe visualization and instrumentation of the spine. For example, in curves greater than 75 degrees, the chest cavity on the concave side and the rib interspaces are too small to accommodate the 10mm-diameter endoscopic portals and instruments. Also, with spinal rotation the mediastinal organs begin to obstruct exposure. In certain cases, these variables may be overcome by adding more working portals. For the novice spinal endoscopist, however, formal open thoracotomy may be more prudent.

## Technique

During scoliosis correction, the spine may be exposed on the curve's convexity or concavity, depending on clinical circumstances or the surgeon's preference (Figure 96.3). Historically, because the structural tether resides in the concavity, anterior releases through a concave side thoracotomy were recommended by Stagnara.[51] This approach has not gained popularity because of difficulty working deep in the concave portion of the deformity between the narrowed rib spaces. Moreover, the segmental vessels are clumped together and are more likely to be injured. The mediastinal structures, including the aorta, unfold into the concavity of the curve and must be meticulously dissected and mobilized. On the other hand, working in the concavity allows access to more disc spaces with fewer portals and a direct approach to the structural tether in the posterolateral corner of the disc space.

Release on the convexity typically allows easier access to the apex of the curve and has become more common overall. However, complete release and exposure of the concave side posterolateral corner is occasionally difficult at the most proximal and distal levels.[41] Working from the convexity may require more portals to gain parallel access to each disc space. If thoracoplasty is planned, a convex side approach is required. For kyphosis correction, the spine can be approached from either side at the surgeon's discretion.

The lateral decubitus position, mimicking open thoracotomy, is typically selected for spinal deformity procedures.[14,15,54,74,76] However, if a subsequent dorsal stabilization is also required, lateral positioning will require re-positioning and draping.[90] Some authors report simultaneous prone anterior thoracoscopic release with posterior instrumentation[43,51] (Figure 96.4).

In gaining access to the spine, the first portal is created opposite the apex of deformity at the midaxillary line. The lung is retracted, and then the sympathetic chain is bluntly dissected out of the operative field. Incise the anterior longitudinal ligament and annulus. In scoliosis, the aorta may need to be mobilized with blunt dissection, because it frequently lies in the acute angle between the rib head and lateral vertebral body. Once it has been mobilized, place a small sponge or peanut retractor in the interval between the vertebral body and the aorta to protect the great vessels during the preparation of the disc space.

Unlike cord decompression procedures, formal resection of the pedicle is not necessary. Rather, the disc space is incised and the nucleus pulposus is evacuated with rongeurs and curettes down to bleeding subchondral bone end plates (Figure 96.5). Complete this evacuation to the posterior longitudinal ligament. For the scoliosis cases approached from the concavity, the posterolateral corner, costo-transverse ligaments, and rib heads on the concave side are released under direct view to optimize correction. Leave the convex lateral annulus intact as a pivot point to prevent over-distraction during the posterior correction. If working on the convexity, the concave postero-lateral corner must be released to achieve a complete release. For kyphosis releases, incise the entire anterior longitudinal ligament and annulus. During simultaneous front-back cases, the transpedicular instrumentation can be used to

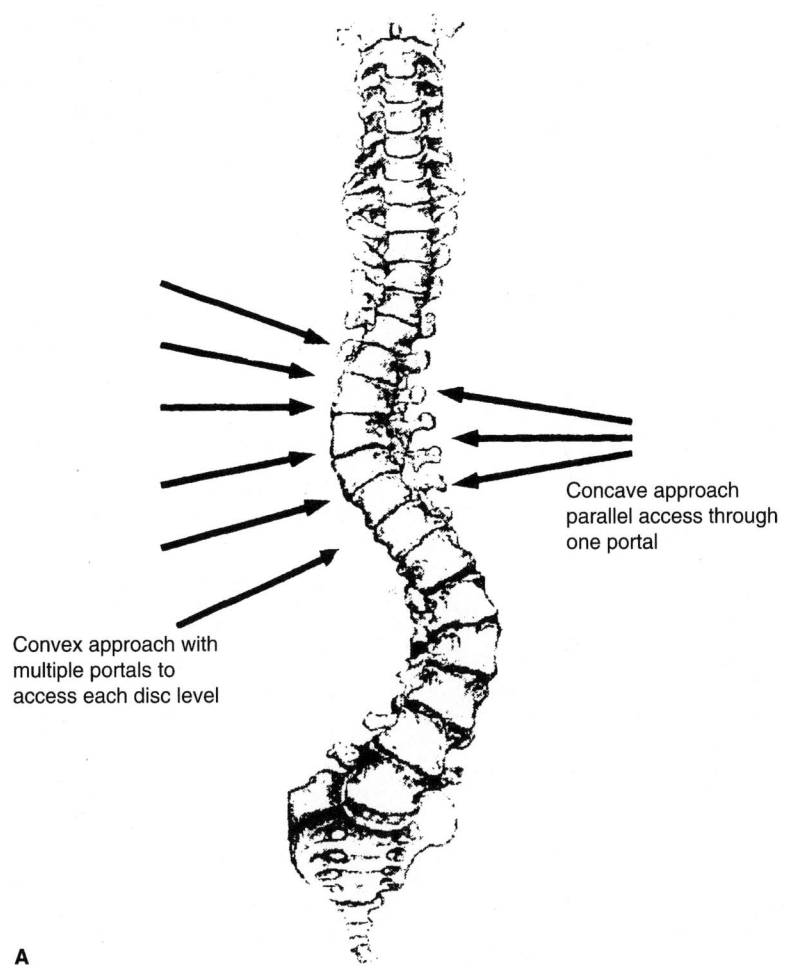

Concave approach
parallel access through
one portal

Convex approach with
multiple portals to
access each disc level

A

**Figure 96.3** Portal placement for lateral thoracoscopy. **(A)** Portal placement will be affected by the presence of coronal plane deformity and the side of approach.

*Continued*

lever the disc spaces open, thereby improving visualization of the PLL.

Once all levels are released, insert a periosteal elevator and rotate slightly to ensure that proper release has been achieved.[14] Then graft the disc spaces with morcellized cancellous iliac crest graft delivered by a funnel. Alternatively, use allograft or autologous rib grafts from an internal thoracoplasty. A structural tri-cortical crest graft or femoral allograft ring may decrease of correction.

Internal thoracoplasty can be performed just after anterior endoscopic release or as an independent procedure as described by Mehlman *et al.*[62] The rib deformity associated with idiopathic scoliosis often represents a significant cosmetic concern to the patient but may not improve significantly after posterior fusion.[101] Preoperatively, ribs to be resected are identified radiographically and by physical examination. From the lateral decubitus position, thoracoplasty is performed on the convex side. Drape the arm free to allow intraoperative scapula mobilization. Tilt the operating room table 15 degrees toward the prone position to help with lung retraction (Figure 96.6).

Plan rib resections as an ellipse to ensure the chest contours are smooth. Work from a cephalad to caudal direction to preserve maximum visibility as the deformity corrects. Expose the ribs to be resected linearly by using a

harmonic scalpel or monopolar cautery. Then subperiosteally strip the segment of rib to be removed with an endoscopic curved elevator. Pay careful attention to the inferior margins of each rib to avoid the intercostal vessels. Insert a high-speed burr through the portal most perpendicular to the rib in question and create medial and lateral osteotomies. Use a metal sucker tip both as a retractor and to protect the vessels below. After ribs are cut with the burr, dissect the segment free with a long handled periosteal elevator and deliver it out of the chest cavity with long-handled forceps. Occasionally, ribs are cut but left in place to ensure adequate thoracic cage stability.[62]

### Results

Wall *et al.*[99] and Newton *et al.*[63] independently reported their results with endoscopic discectomy in an animal model. These authors concluded that the extent of discectomy and quality of release is comparable to open techniques. Published studies describing results of open anterior releases by Kostuik *et al.*,[46] Simmons *et al.*,[92] and Byrd *et al.*[11] reveal that average curve correction ranged from 36% to 48%. The average correction achieved with thoracoscopic techniques appears to be at least equivalent to those reports.[51,64] However, Arlet[3] performed a meta-

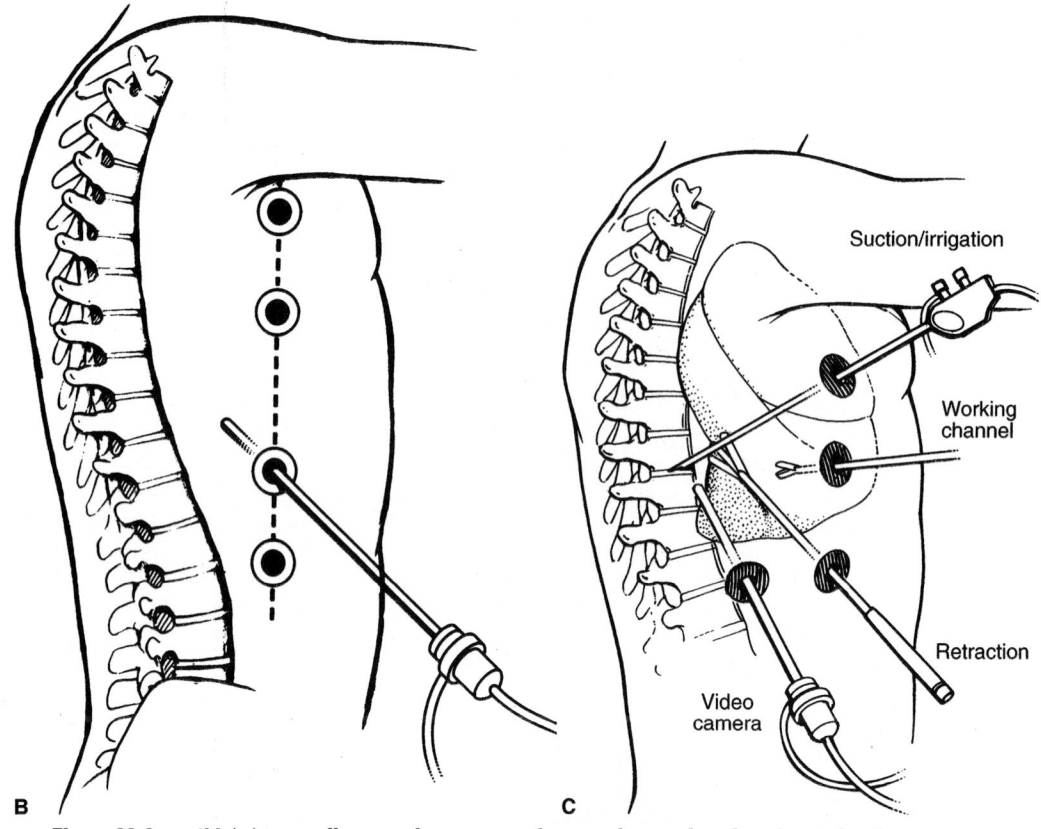

**B**     **C**

**Figure 96.3 *cont'd*** (**B**) Typically, in scoliosis cases, the portals are placed in the midaxillary line. (**C**) For a thoracoscopic decompression, an "L" configuration is often used. (**A** *from Lieberman IH, et al: Prone position endoscopic transthoracic release with simultaneous posterior instrumentation for spinal deformity.* Spine 25:2251-2257, 2000, Fig. 7. **B** *and* **C** *from Regan JJ, Jarolem KL: Thoracoscopy of the spine. In Herkowitz HN et al: Rothman-Simeone The Spine, ed 4. Philadelphia, WB Saunders, 1999, p 606.*)

analysis of the use of VATS in spine deformity surgery. He identified 10 articles comprising 151 procedures. He reported that most authors selected a convex side approach from a lateral decubitus position with four or more ports in the midaxillary line. Four to seven discs were excised and grafted over 2.5 to 4 hours. Most procedures were followed by same-day posterior stabilization. The mean scoliotic curve was corrected from 65 to 35 degrees while the mean kyphosis was corrected from 78 to 44 degrees. Thoracoscopic procedures cost 28% more than thoracotomy. He noted that 7 years after the first report, the literature still contained only 151 patients and no long-term follow-up or significant outcome data in terms of spinal balance, fusion rate, rib hump correction, cosmesis, pain, and satisfaction. Arlet concludes that a more complete discectomy is possible with open technique and that animal studies documenting equivalent discectomies do not account for the visualization difficulties encountered in deformity patients. In his view, the data do not yet support widespread implementation, and the individual surgeon must consider whether he treats enough of the relevant pathologies to make learning the technique worthwhile.

Alternatively, Niemeyer and others[66] evaluated the 2-year clinical results, radiologic correction, and morbidity of anterior thoracoscopic surgery followed by posterior instrumentation and fusion in their series of 29 patients. In the scoliotic patients, a mean preoperative Cobb angle of 65.1 degrees was corrected to a mean 34.4 degrees at final follow-up. In the nine hyperkyphotic patients, the mean preoperative Cobb angle of 81 degrees was corrected to 65 degrees. The average duration of the thoracoscopic procedure was 188 minutes, and this time was noted to decrease as the series progressed. No neurologic or vascular complications occurred. Postoperative complications included four recurrent pneumothoraces, one surgical emphysema, and one respiratory infection. The authors concluded that thoracoscopic anterior surgery is a safe and effective technique for the treatment of pediatric spinal deformity but that a randomized controlled trial, comparing open with thoracoscopic methods, is required.

Newton and others[64] reported a prospective series of 65 consecutive cases of thoracoscopic anterior release with discectomy and fusion performed by one surgeon for the treatment of pediatric spinal deformity. This patient group was 14 ± 3 years old and included patients with idiopathic scoliosis (n = 13), Scheuermann's kyphosis (n = 9), neuromuscular spinal deformity (n = 35), congenital scoliosis (n = 4), and tumor/syrinx (n = 4). The average operative time for the thoracoscopic procedure was 161 ± 41 minutes (range, 50 to 240 minutes), with a slight decrease in the average operative time noted as the series progressed. The average number of discs excised was 6.5 ± 1.5 (range, 3 to 10), and this number increased as the series

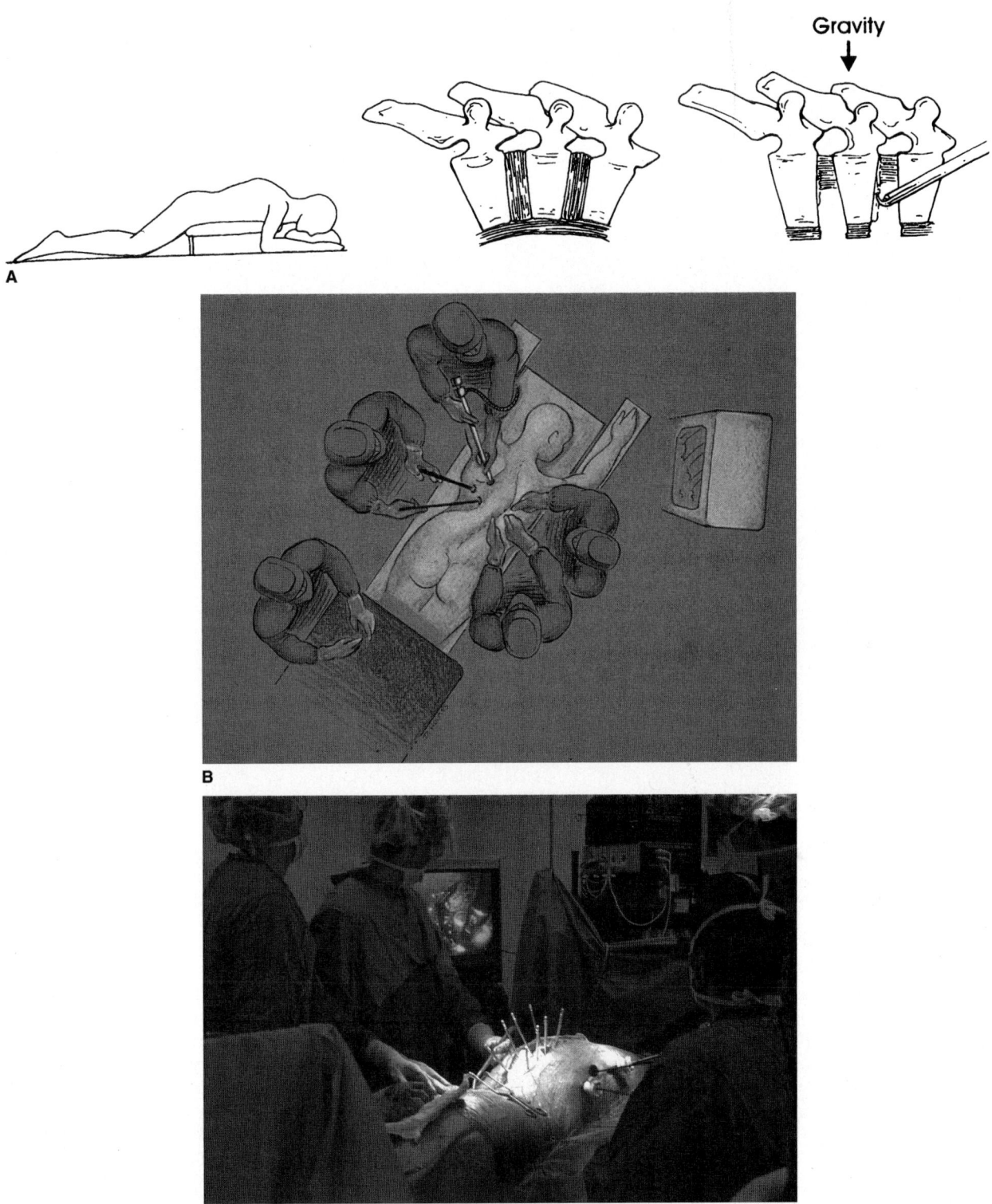

**Figure 96.4** Prone thoracoscopy. **(A)** Prone positioning is especially useful in the treatment of hyperkyphosis, in that gravity will partially correct the deformity. **(B)** OR set-up for prone thoracoscopy. **(C)** Clinical photograph of a simultaneous anterior thoracoscopic release with posterior fusion. (**A** *from King AG, et al: Video-assisted thoracoscopic surgery in the prone position. Spine 25:2403-2406, 2000.*)

progressed. The average operative time per disc was 29.3 ± 7.7 minutes in the first 30 patients, as compared with 22.3 ± 4.7 minutes in the next 35 patients (*P* < .01). The average blood loss during the thoracoscopic procedure was 301 ± 322ml (range, 25 to 2000ml) but did not decrease as

the series progressed. Initial postoperative scoliosis and kyphosis corrections were 59% (from 62 to 25 degrees) and 92% (from 78 to 44 degrees), respectively. Complications occurred in six patients and were evenly distributed throughout the series. Complications included chest tube

*Continued on p. 1293.*

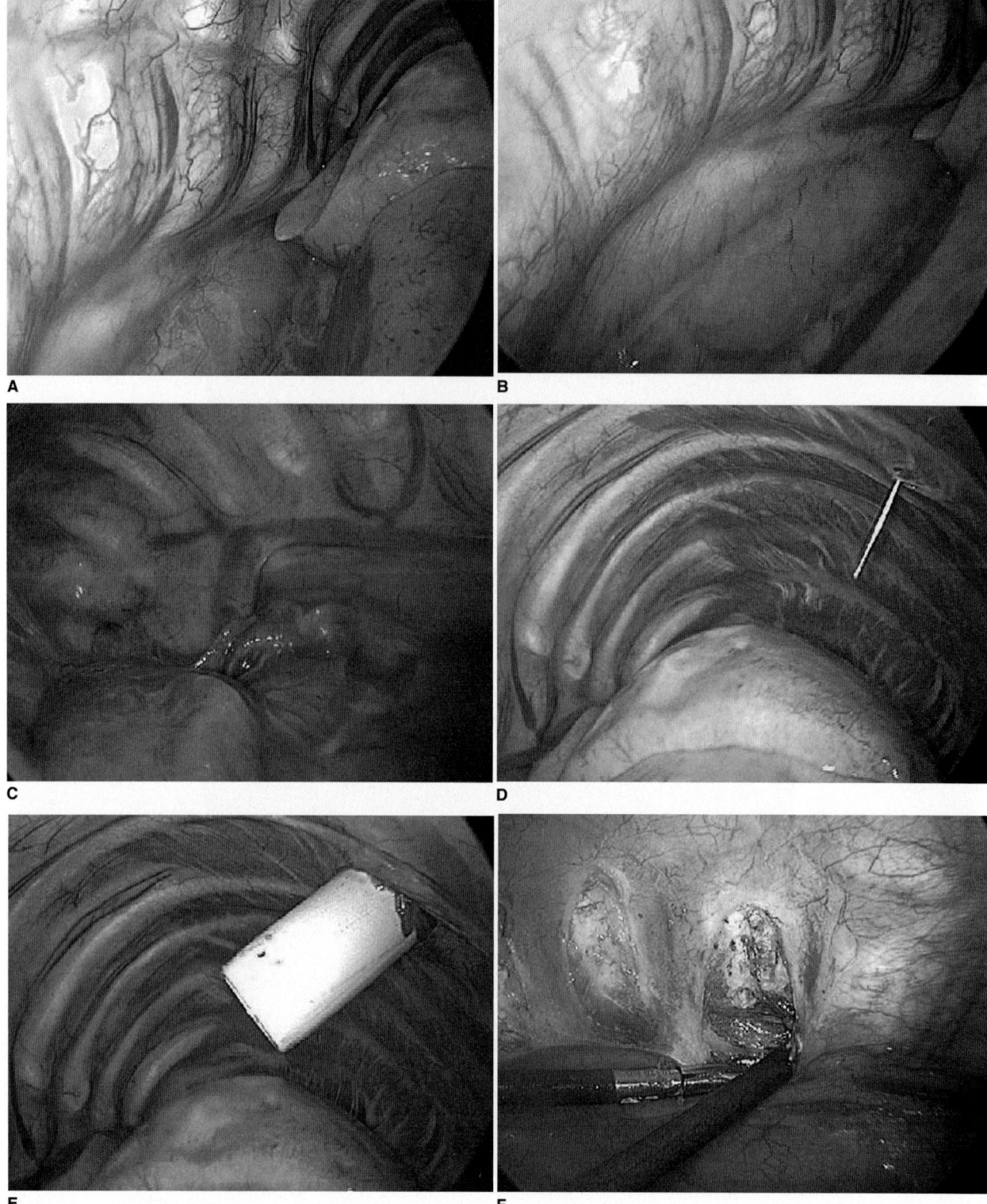

**Figure 96.5** Multiple releases for scoliosis. **(A)** Typical thoracoscopic anatomy. **(B)** Further thoracoscopic exploration of the chest. Note the azygos vein and superior vena cava. **(C)** Here, in the upper thoracic spine, the superior intercostal vein can be seen feeding into the azygos system. **(D)** Further portal placement can be planned with a needle to ensure appropriate alignment. **(E)** Next, the portal itself is inserted. **(F)** An endoscopic dissector is used to take down a portion of the parietal pleura. This view shows three disc levels exposed without sacrifice of the segmental vessels.

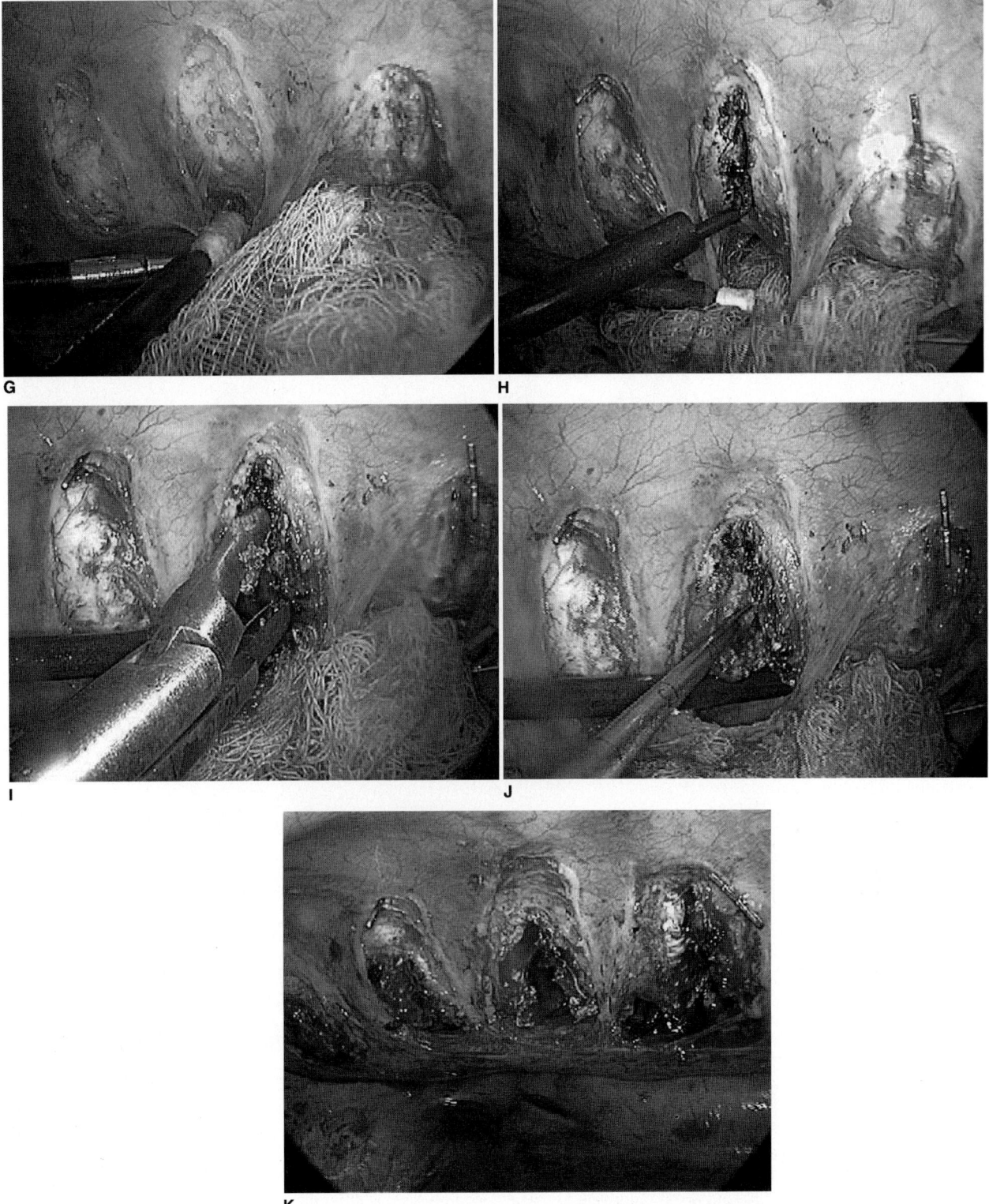

**Figure 96.5 *cont'd*** (**G**) An endoscopic Kidner is used to further dissect the soft tissues from the disc space. (**H**) An annulotomy is then performed. (**I**) More disc material can be retrieved with a pituitary rongeur. (**J**) A long, sharp Cobb is used to dissect the remainder of the annulus and cartilaginous end plates. (**K**) Completed discectomies are demonstrated. Structural or morselized graft can be inserted.

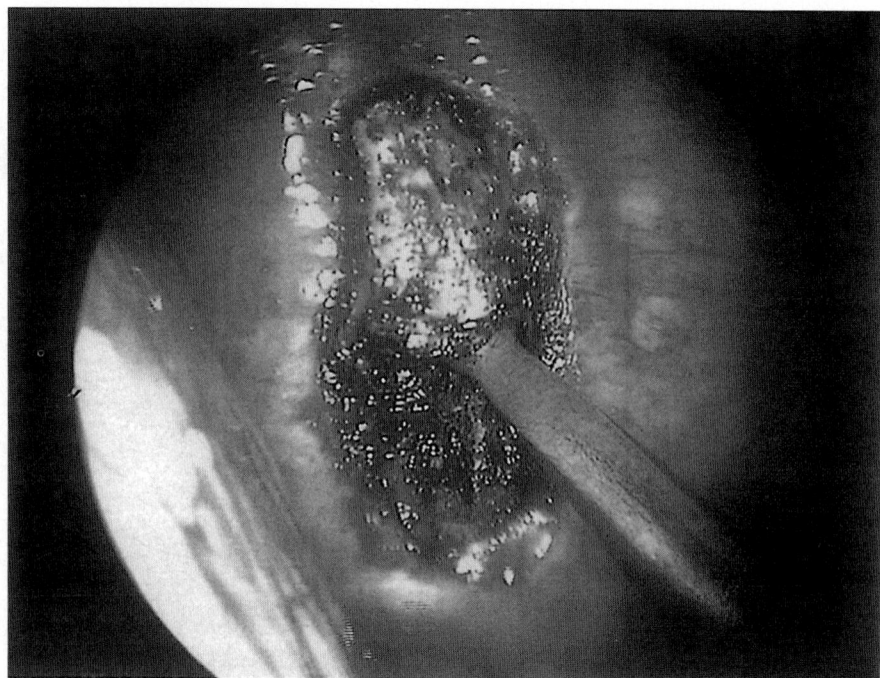

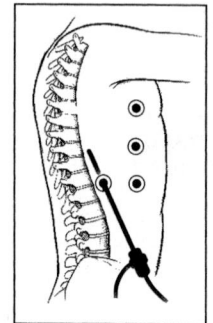

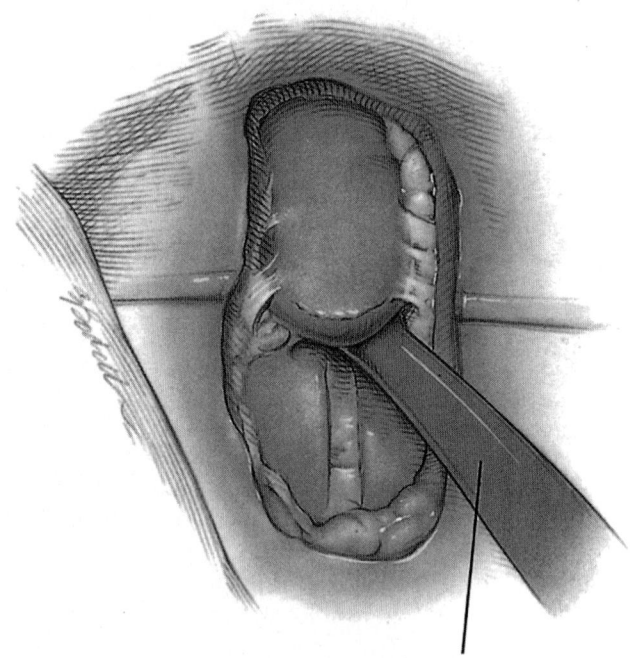

Cobb elevator

**A**

**Figure 96.6** The endoscopic approach for canal decompression is different. Though typically performed at only one or two levels, more dissection of the rib head and pedicle are required to safely visualize the dura. **(A)** After the pleura has been divided over the rib head, the proximal 2cm to 3cm of rib are exposed with a Cobb. The radiate and costotransverse ligaments are cut away from the rib using the Cobb, curettes, and special curved dissectors.

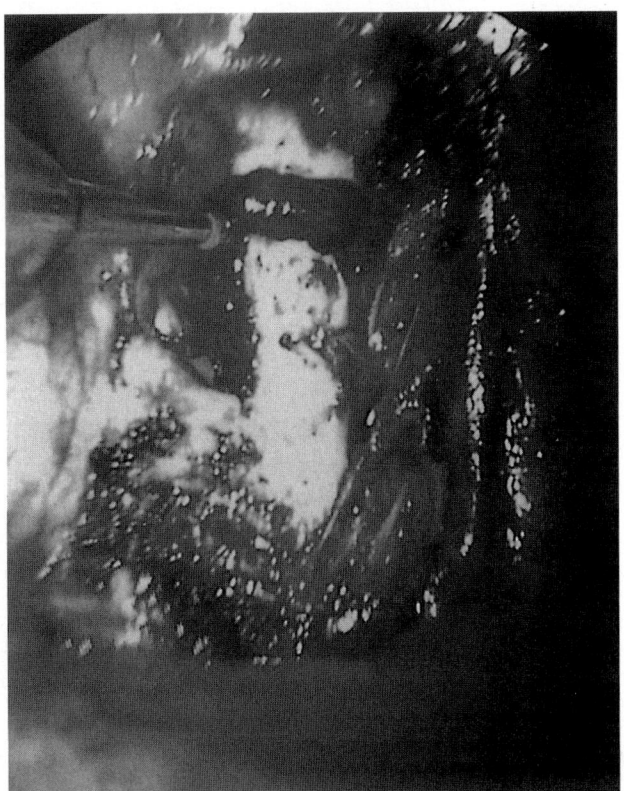

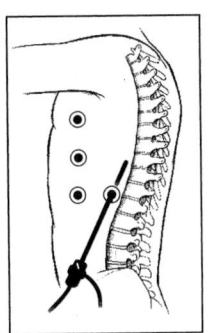

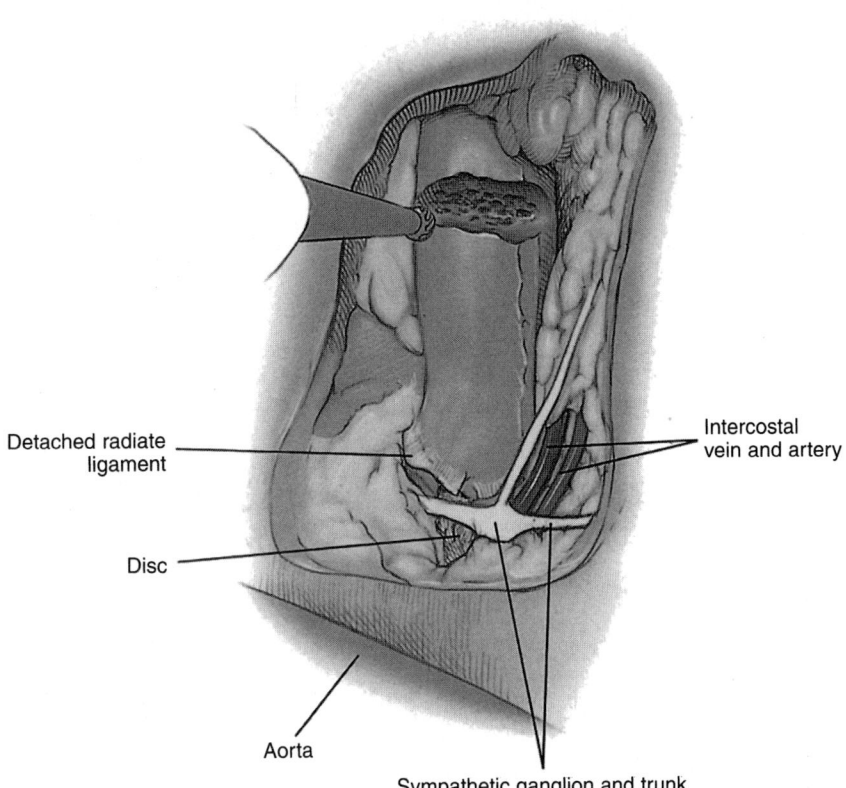

Detached radiate ligament

Intercostal vein and artery

Disc

Aorta

Sympathetic ganglion and trunk

B

**Figure 96.6 _cont'd_** (**B**) A burr is used to divide the rib 3cm from its head. The fragment is grasped with a pituitary and delivered through the port. _Continued_

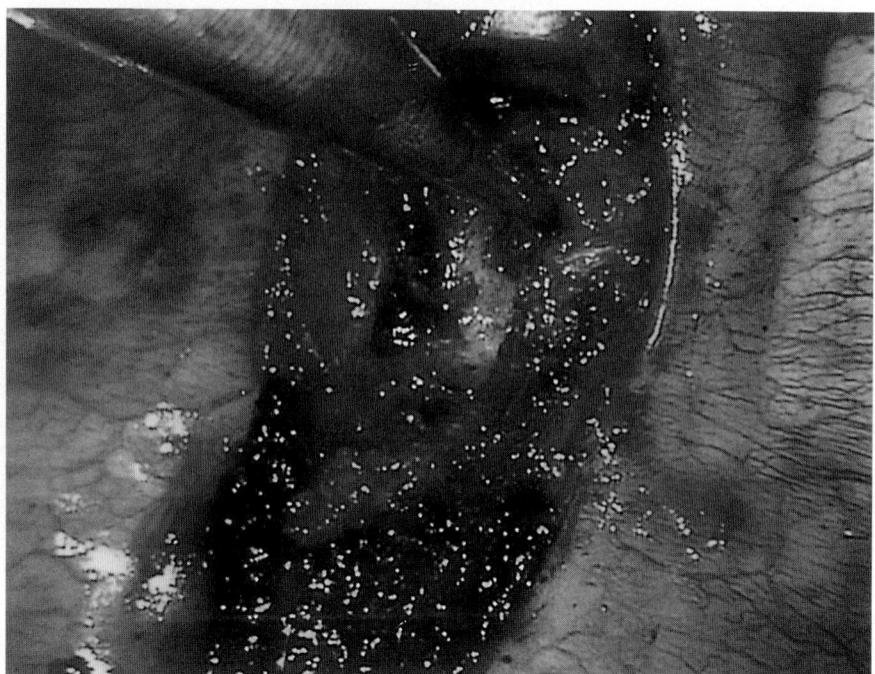

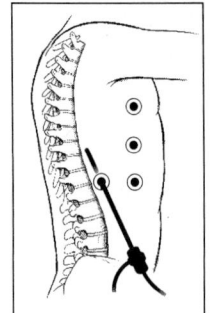

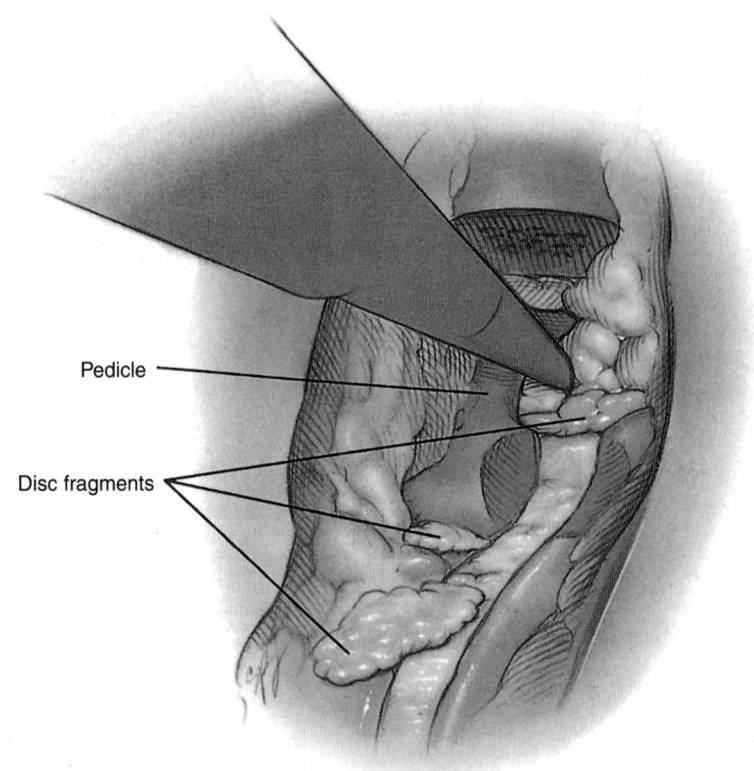

**C**

**Figure 96.6** *cont'd* (**C**) Identify the superior portion of the pedicle and remove it with an angled curette, burr, or Kerrison rongeur.

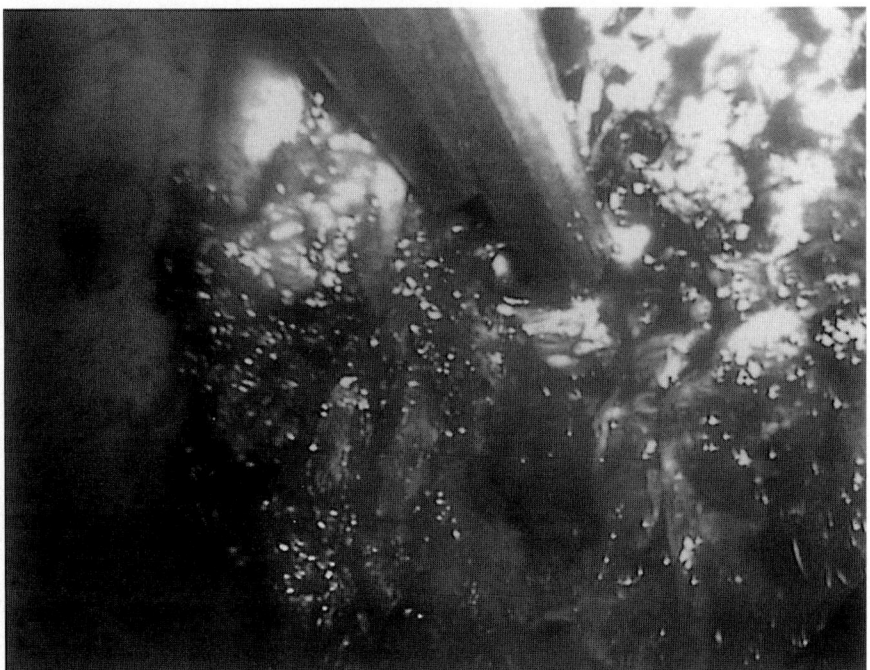

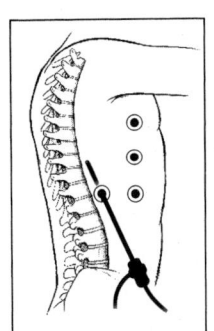

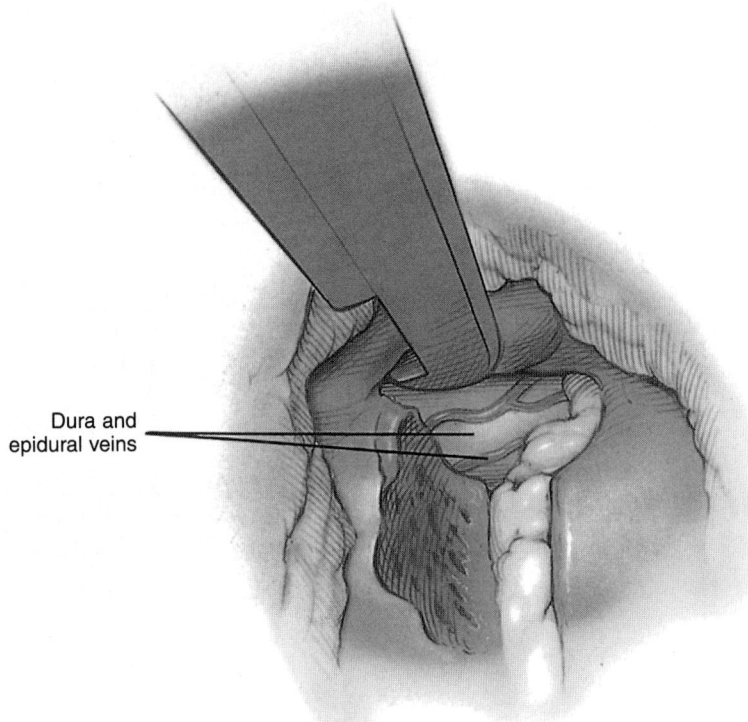

**D**

**Figure 96.6 *cont'd* (D)** Removal of this portion of the pedicle will expose the dura or epidural fat. Thoracic disc herniations can be identified at this point by following the pedicle back to the vertebral body.                                                                                          *Continued*

Dura and epidural veins

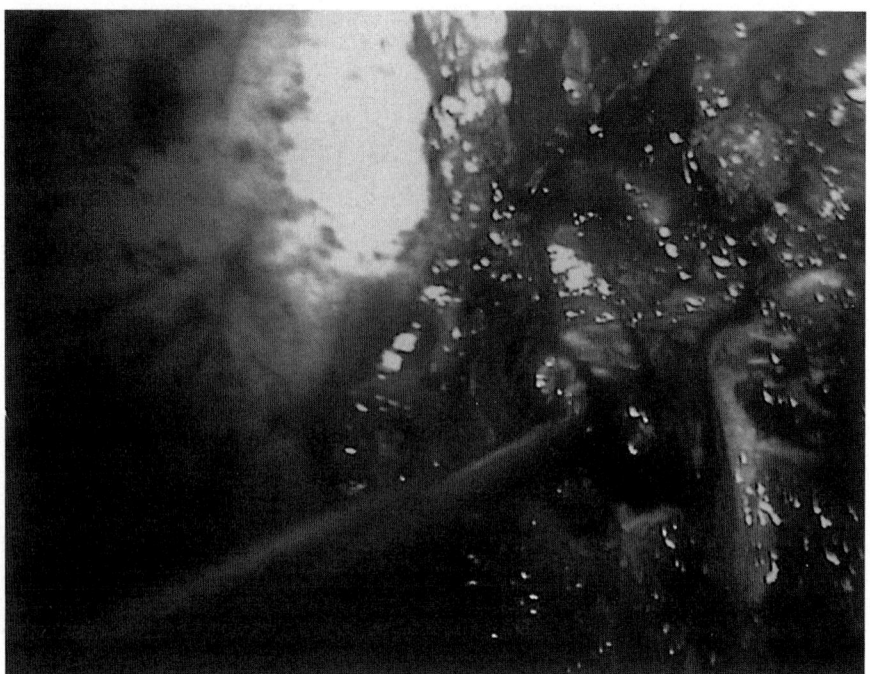

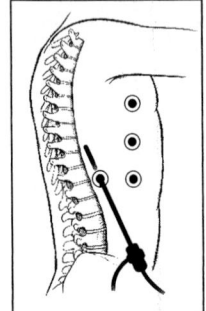

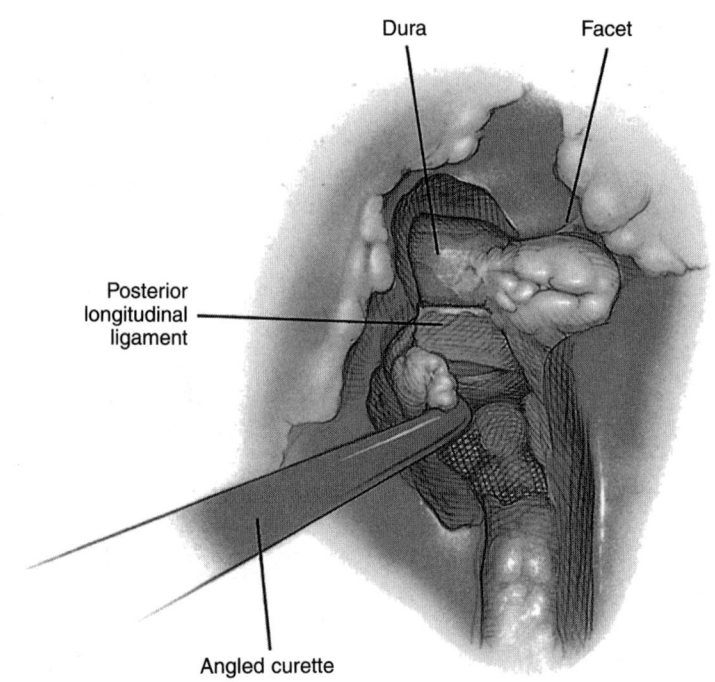

E

**Figure 96.6 *cont'd*** (**E**) Disc or other compressive material is pulled anteriorly with a pituitary or with a curette. (*From Regan JJ*, et al: Atlas of Endoscopic Spine Surgery. *St Louis, Quality Medical Publishing, 1995, pp 168, 170, 173, 175, 177.*)

reinsertion in 3 patients for pleural effusion or chylothorax, conversion to thoracotomy in 2 cases, and 1 case of incorrect levels of fusion. The authors concluded that the learning period for thoracoscopy is substantial but not prohibitive and that the technique provides a safe and effective alternative to thoracotomy in the treatment of pediatric spinal deformity.

In another series, Newton et al.[65] compared their early outcomes and costs between a series of 14 consecutive thoracoscopic releases with 18 open thoracotomies performed the previous year. Percentage of curve correction was similar between the groups, with 56% correction in the thoracoscopic scoliosis group versus 60% in the open group and 88% in the thoracoscopic kyphosis group versus 94% in the open group. Blood loss and complication rates were the same in both groups, but chest tube output was greater in the thoracoscopic group. The length of hospital stay was not reduced and costs of the open procedure were 29% less than for the thoracoscopic procedure.

Holcomb and others[30] reported on their first seven deformity patients undergoing anterior discectomy followed by posterior fusion. These included congenital deformity patients with hemivertebrae. They performed a mean 4 discectomies in an average of 174 minutes. There was only one complication related to excessive bleeding from an intercostal vessel that was immediately controlled with vessel clips.

Rothenburg[87] reported a series of 20 ventral releases performed thoracoscopically in children from 8 to 17 years of age. The thoracoscopic portion of the procedure lasted a mean 106 minutes. All patients underwent subsequent dorsal instrumentation and fusion. Corrections were noted to be acceptable and equivalent to open technique. Earlier extubation, shorter ICU stays, and lower morbidity were reported.

Crawford and colleagues[14] reviewed their experience with video-assisted thoracoscopy in the treatment of children with severe spinal deformities. The authors noted that surgical time was reduced from open thoracotomy. More importantly, tissue damage, blood loss, postoperative pain, and ICU and hospital stays were all reduced. Respiratory and shoulder function were less affected. The authors list possible complications from the procedure, but these are not different from similar complications encountered in open procedures.

The prospective series of Lieberman et al.[51] followed fifteen consecutive adult patients with spinal deformity who underwent simultaneous anterior endoscopic and posterior instrumentations for an average of 31 months (Figure 96.7). There were no intraoperative technical problems with the endoscopic equipment or instruments, and visualization of the anterior spinal column was excellent. No vessel or organ injuries were encountered and no cases were converted to open thoracotomy. No patient complained of postoperative radicular symptoms or chest pain consistent with a post-thoracotomy syndrome, and there were no wound complications at the portal or posterior incisions. There were no immediate, 6-month or 2-year postoperative complications related to the endoscopic component of the procedure. In the scoliosis patients, the average correction was 60%. In the kyphosis patients the average correction was 39%. Total operative time varied from 6 to 10 hours, depending primarily on the complexity of the posterior instrumentation. Average time per disc space evacuation was 20 minutes, with a range of 15 to 35 minutes. Blood loss averaged 1200ml for the entire anterior and posterior procedures. Average hospital stay was 6.5 days, with a range of 5 to 8.

King et al.[43] describe 27 patients undergoing VATS in a prone position for scoliosis or kyphosis. No conversions to open technique were required. Only discs that did not correct to neutral or beyond on bending films were incised. A mean 3.5 disc spaces were treated. In the scoliosis patients, the mean preop Cobb angle of 70.2 degrees was corrected to 22.9 degrees. For kyphotic patients, the mean Cobb angle improved from 82.3 to 48.1 degrees. Complications related to the anterior approach included 1 case of atelectasis and 3 persistent pneumothoraces after removal of the chest tube.

## VATS for Thoracic Spine Degenerative Disease

While the majority of thoracoscopic procedures have been performed for deformity correction, implementation of this technique in patients with tumors or herniated thoracic discs is becoming increasingly common.[54,74,79,84] Overall, the incidence of clinical significant thoracic disc herniation is as low as 1 per million,[12] or 0.25% to 0.75% of all disc ruptures.[2]

For these uncommon lesions, a number of surgical approaches have been described including laminectomy, pediculectomy, costotransversectomy, lateral extracavitary, transverse arthropediculectomy, and transthoracic approaches.[1] Laminectomy alone is ineffective and may be associated with neurologic decline in 50% of patients.[4] Although costotransversectomy and lateral extracavitary approaches have the advantages of being able to decompress and stabilize the spine through a single incision in one stage, they are limited by their time-consuming and technically demanding nature.[81] Each of these has significant potential morbidity (see Table 96.1). Moreover, they confer only a limited view of anterior spinal cord. In one report, anterior approaches were found to have a complication rate ranging from 14% to 31%, while dorsal-approach-related complications ranged from 17% to 51%[81] (Table 96.1). The first application of VATs to degenerative spinal disease was in 1993.[54]

When selecting a patient for endoscopic thoracic discectomy, the surgeon must remember that true radicular or myelopathic symptoms from thoracic disc herniations are rare. A more common scenario is the diffuse mid-thoracic back pain with imaging showing multiple degenerative segments with or without herniations. These patients are typically not ideal candidates for discectomy of any form, either open or endoscopic.

### Technique

Symptomatic thoracic disc herniations amenable to endoscopic transthoracic decompression are typically approached from the side of the herniation. In the context of previous surgery, a contralateral approach may be employed. The first trocar is inserted at the sixth or seventh interspace toward the anterior axillary line. Then insert 2 to 3 additional portals under direct vision. Usually 1 to 2 portals are inserted at the anterior axillary line and 1 at the posterior axillary line. Use

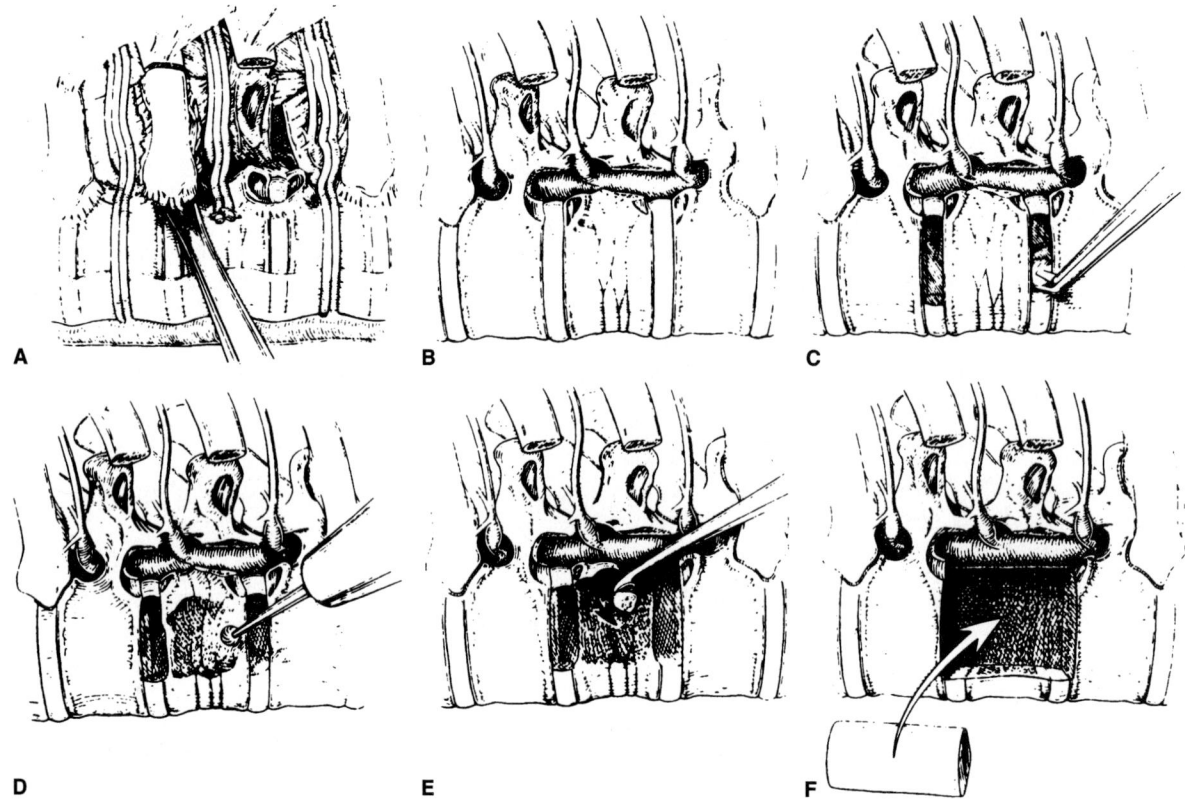

**Figure 96.7** Thoracoscopic vertebrectomy is undertaken in a manner similar to discectomy. **(A)** The ribs of the affected level and level below are removed to expose the pedicles. **(B)** The pedicles are resected to expose the dura. **(C)** With the dura in view, discectomies can be performed. **(D)** A large cavity is created anteriorly with burrs, curettes, and rongeurs. **(E)** The remaining posterior cortex is pulled anteriorly into the defect. **(F)** The defect is reconstructed with a strut graft or cage. (*Reprinted with permission of Barrow Neurological Institute.*)

**TABLE 96.1**

**Comparison of Approaches to Thoracic Disc Herniations**

| Note | Costotransversectomy | Thoracotomy | Thoracoscopy |
|---|---|---|---|
| Direction | Dorsolateral | Vertebrolateral | Vertebrolateral |
| View of cord | Oblique, indirect | Full, direct | Full, direct |
| Incision size | 4-12in | 6-15in | 0.5-1.0in × 3-4 |
| Muscle transaction | Moderate to extensive | Extensive | Minimal |
| Relationship to pleura | Extrapleural | Intrapleural | Intrapleural |
| Chest tube | No | Yes | Yes |
| Access to post elements | Yes | No | No |
| Anterior fixation | No | Yes | Yes |
| Extent of rib resection | 3-7in removed | 6-12 in | 1in of rib head |
| Retraction | Moderate | Extensive | None |
| Postoperative intercostals neuralgia | Uncommon/transient | Common/prolonged | Uncommon/transient |

From Dickman CA, Detweiler PW, Porter RW: Thoracoscopic spine surgery. *Clin Neurosurg* 43:396, 2000.

a 30-degree angled rigid scope to see into the disc space and around the bony edges. Identify the appropriate level and resect the proximal 2cm of rib head, if above T11 (Figure 96.8). Cut the foraminal ligaments from the superior edge of the pedicle. Resection of the superior part of the pedicle will expose the dura. Some authors excise the entire pedicle, particularly for larger and more central herniations.[84]

Next, with the spinal cord continuously visualized to prevent inadvertent entry into the canal, create a cavity in the disc space and vertebral bodies anteriorly. Increase the size of this space for larger or more central herniations. The cavity should be wide enough that the surgeon can visualize normal dura above and below the herniation.[84] The cavity must be deep enough to expose the entire width of the

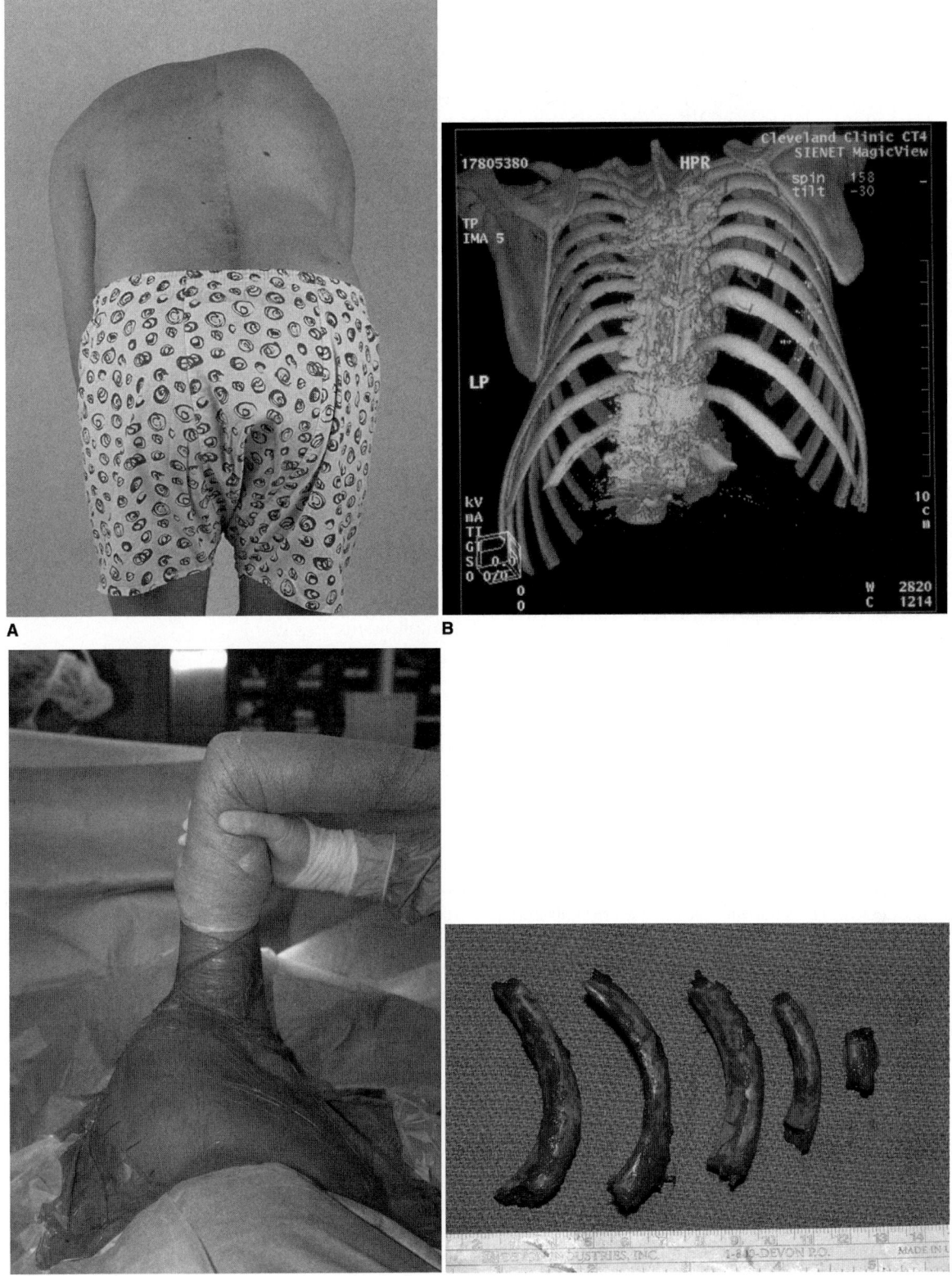

**Figure 96.8** (**A**) This patient had previously undergone posterior spinal fusion for scoliosis but continued to complain of a painful and unsightly rib hump. (**B**) A 3D CT reconstruction of the patient's chest was undertaken and planned rib resections marked. (**C**) Here, the patient is positioned for thoracoplasty with the arm draped free. (**D**) The removed rib sections.

*Continued*

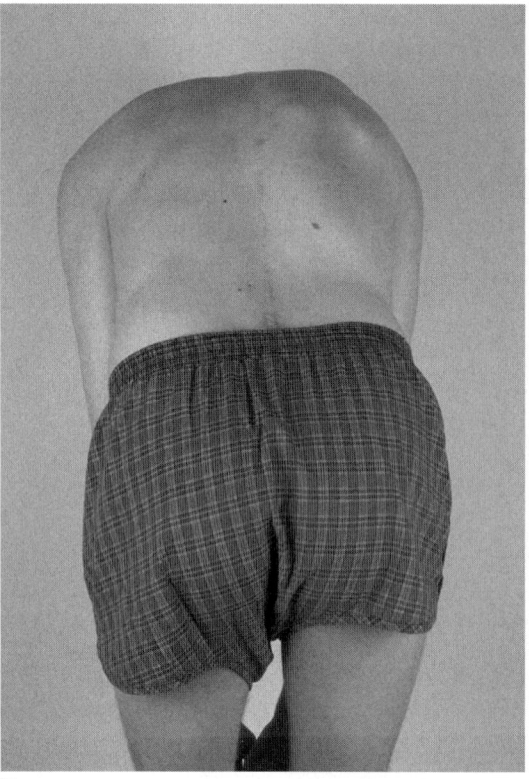

**E**

**Figure 96.8 *cont'd*** (**E**) Postoperatively the patient had significant improvement in pain and body contour.

anterior dura to the contralateral pedicle. A corpectomy may be required for larger or ossified herniations (Figure 96.7).

Find the disc herniation by tracing the superior edge of the pedicle to the vertebral body and disc space. Fine instruments can then be used to pull the disc herniation into the created cavity. Once the decompression has been completed, document its medial-lateral and cranial-caudal extent by placing a Penfield across the intervertebral space and using fluoroscopy or a radiograph.

If a corpectomy was required for adequate decompression, concomitant fusion should be considered. Typically a trough is made with a side cutting burr and a rib fragment or iliac crest wedge is tamped into position across the disc space. Alternatively, Regan *et al.*[77] describe placement of an interbody cage into the disc space after decompression.

## Results

Only a few centers are currently employing endoscopic techniques to decompress thoracic disc herniations, and only a few clinical reports are published. In one series of thoracic endoscopic discectomies, the 14% complication rate was comparable with rates reported for open approaches.[74] Horowitz and others[31] documented their experience with cadavers and a porcine model. At the time of their report, the authors were successful in decompressing the cord in 5 of 7 cadaver disc spaces and 2 of 3 porcine spaces. One dural violation occurred. The authors felt that improvement in instrumentation would allow safer and more complete disc space access.

Rosenthal and Dickman[84] reported outcomes of 55 consecutive patients undergoing video-assisted thoracoscopic discectomy. In their group, 65% presented with myelopathic signs and symptoms caused by spinal cord compression, the remainder had severe thoracic radiculopathy. After surgery, 60% of the myelopathic patients recovered neurologically (22 completely and 5 with improvement, but residual myelopathic symptoms). Seventy-nine percent of the radiculopathic patients recovered completely, and 21% improved. No one worsened. They compared their thoracoscopic patients with patients treated by costotransversectomy or thoracotomy and found that thoracoscopy was associated with 1 hour less OR time, and half the blood loss. Postoperative chest tube output and narcotic usage were significantly lower in the thoracoscopic group.

Regan and others[75] reported 1-year follow-up data on their first 29 patients undergoing video-assisted thoracoscopic excision of herniated discs at 32 levels. In this series, mean operative time was 175 minutes and EBL ranged from 75 to 2500ml. Mean hospitalization was 3.9 days. They found that 75.8% were satisfied with the procedure, 20.1% were unchanged, and 3.4% were worse. Significant improvements in Oswestry scores were noted in radiculopathic and myelopathic patients. There was a 13.8% complication rate but no long-term sequelae from any of the complications.

Subsequently, Anand and Regan[1] reported their results after 117 thoracoscopic discectomy procedures in 100 consecutive patients with an average follow-up of 4 years. Patient presentation ranged from pure axial pain to pure radiculopathy to pure myelopathy with various combinations of these complaints. Mean operative time was 173 minutes and blood loss averaged 259ml. Average ICU stay was less than 1 day, and average hospital stay was 4 days. Minor complications occurred in 21 patients, all of which resolved with no untoward effect. No patient's neurologic status worsened. Clinical success was defined as a modest 20% improvement in Oswestry score at final follow-up. Overall, objective clinical success was observed at final follow-up in 70% of these patients. The greatest gains were noted in myelopathic patients followed by the radiculopathic patients. Axial pain patients exhibited the least postoperative improvement. The authors concluded that video-assisted thoracoscopic surgery appears to be a safe and efficacious method for the treatment of refractory symptomatic thoracic disc herniations.

McAfee[58] reported complications related to a thoracoscopic decompression, in a series of 77 patients, as excessive epidural bleeding in one patient and transient paraparesis in another. A number of other case reports and small series are also available with similar results.[68,98]

## VATS in the Treatment of Spine Tumors

Much as with thoracic disc herniations, the previous standard approach to cord compression from spinal tumors was laminectomy. However, for ventral lesions, the rate of neurologic improvement after surgery has been poor.[25] Over time, more aggressive and more highly morbid approaches such as costotransversectomy and thoracotomy have been

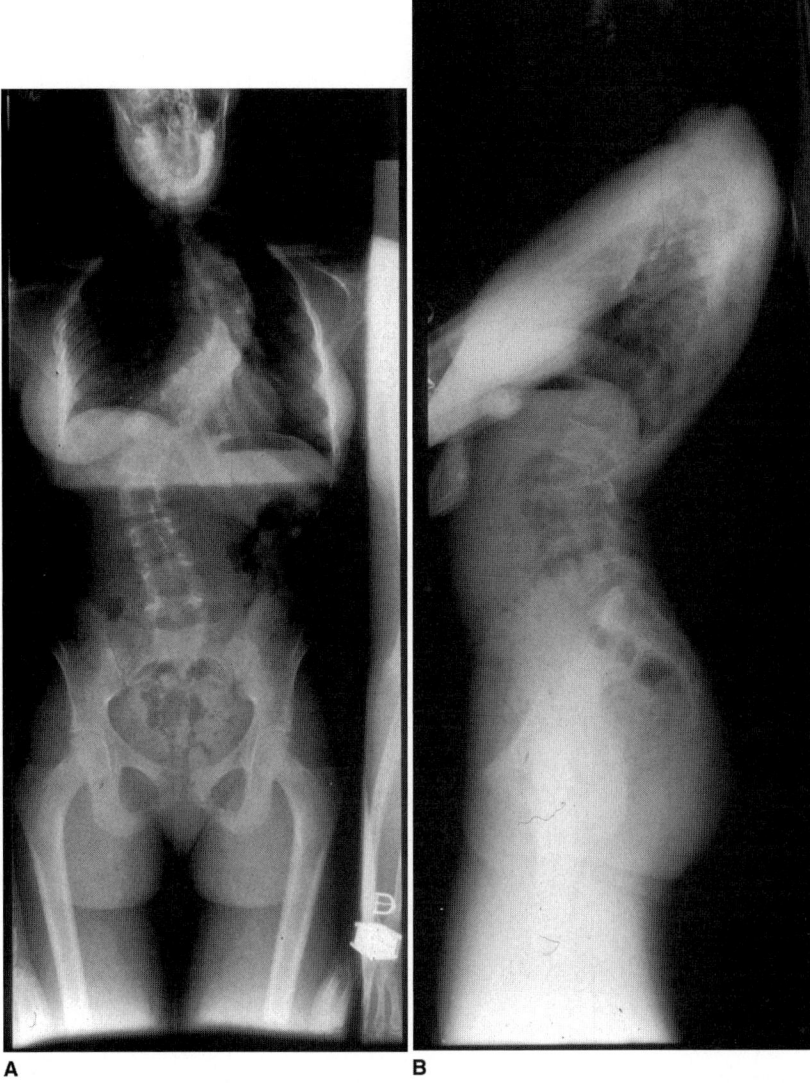

**A**                                           **B**

**Figure 96.9** This patient presented with a progressive, rigid thoracic scoliosis. AP, lateral, and side-bending films are shown (**A**, **B**, and **C**, respectively).

*Continued*

espoused for more complete cord decompression. Yet the desire to limit the invasiveness of an operative approach for neurologic decompression or spinal stabilization is even more acute in patients with spinal malignancy. VATS techniques have been typically employed in intralesional or "piecemeal" tumor debulking procedures. Solitary tumor "en-bloc" resections typically require open approaches.

The technique of decompression in patients with spinal tumors is similar to that in degenerative disease (Figure 96.10). Preoperatively, consider the vascularity of the lesion. In most cases, preoperative embolization is justified. Embolization is critical for most rapidly growing neoplasms, especially renal cell cancer. When removing decompressed tumor material, it may be appropriate to drop the material into a tumor bag before bringing it through the body wall. This will limit exposure of the thoracic cavity to neoplastic cells. Reconstruction techniques in malignancy may be liberalized depending on the anticipated life span of the patient. To avoid the morbidity of graft harvest

and to achieve early stability, Rosenthal described reconstruction by injection of semiliquid methylmethacrylate.[83] The PMMA is injected through a tube into the cavity and allowed to polymerize in situ. For patients with longer anticipated survival, a fusion should be performed. Anterior instrumentation options are improving. In Rosenthal's series, special equipment was used to dilate the skin incision to allow insertion of a ventral plate. Special instruments are used to handle the plates and screws in the chest cavity.

There are few published series describing the results of endoscopic decompression of spine tumors. Rosenthal described outcomes in 4 patients with malignancies of the thoracic spine and progressive neurologic deficits treated with thoracoscopic decompression.[85] At an average of 11 months' follow-up, all patients were free of pain and neurologically improved. In this small series, there were no complications or hardware failures. All patients were braced, and adjuvant chemotherapy or radiation

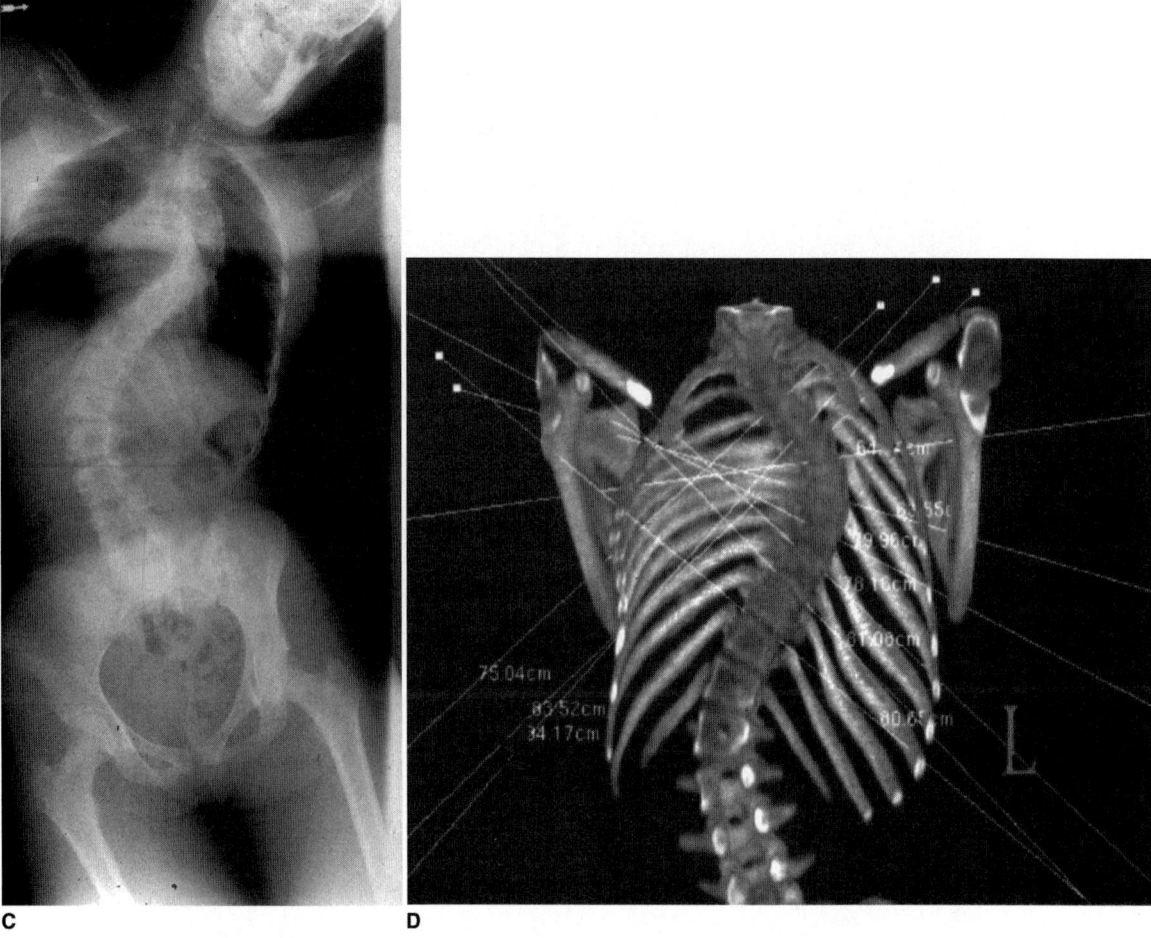

**C**             **D**

**Figure 96.9** *cont'd* 3-D CT reconstructions are useful for surgical planning and portal preparation (**D** and **E**).

therapy was used in several patients. Dickman and others[20] reported on the outcomes of 7 patients undergoing thoracoscopic vertebrectomy for tumor. They found that the operative time and blood loss were similar to that of a similar, open thoracotomy group. On the other hand, narcotic utilization, ICU stay, and hospital length of stay were all dramatically reduced in the thoracoscopic group. Huang and coworkers describe successful cord decompression in three patients with thoracic malignancy and myelopathy through an extended endoscopic/mini-open approach.[32]

One subgroup of spine tumors that has received special emphasis are the so-called Dumbbell Tumors. Up to 10% of neurogenic tumors in the posterior mediastinum extend into the spinal canal.[27] These lesions have previously required resection through open thoracotomy, often with a staged laminectomy. Heltzer and co-authors[27] describe resection of such a "dumbbell lesion" through a staged laminectomy followed by thoracotomy approach. Subsequently, Konno et al.[45] reported a series of 5 patients treated with a similar technique and followed for at least 3 years. In their series, postoperative instability did not develop in any patient. Alternatively, a simultaneous approach may be undertaken.

The intracanal portion of the tumor should be resected prior to resection of the intrathoracic component.

Citow *et al.*[13] described a single-stage, combined laminectomy and thoracoscopic resection of a 4 × 5 × 5 cm mass filling 60% of the spinal canal at the T3 level. The lesion was first detached from the spinal cord by way of laminectomy with medial facetectomy. Then, a three-portal thoracoscopic approach was undertaken in which the parietal pleura was incised and the tumor bluntly dissected and removed through an expanded anterior portal in a specimen bag. The authors noted that a potential limitation to this approach was possible communication between the subarachnoid space with the low-pressure pleural cavity, which would increase the risk of CSF fistula. They recommended an endoscopic suture of the parietal pleura. Further, because of the potential for malignant lesions to encase or invade the mediastinal structures, they suggested distinguishing between benign and malignant lesions prior to proceeding with the endoscopic approach.

Van Dijk *et al.*[96] described another combined technique for solitary spine tumor resection wherein thoracoscopically assisted ventral releases were followed by a dorsal en

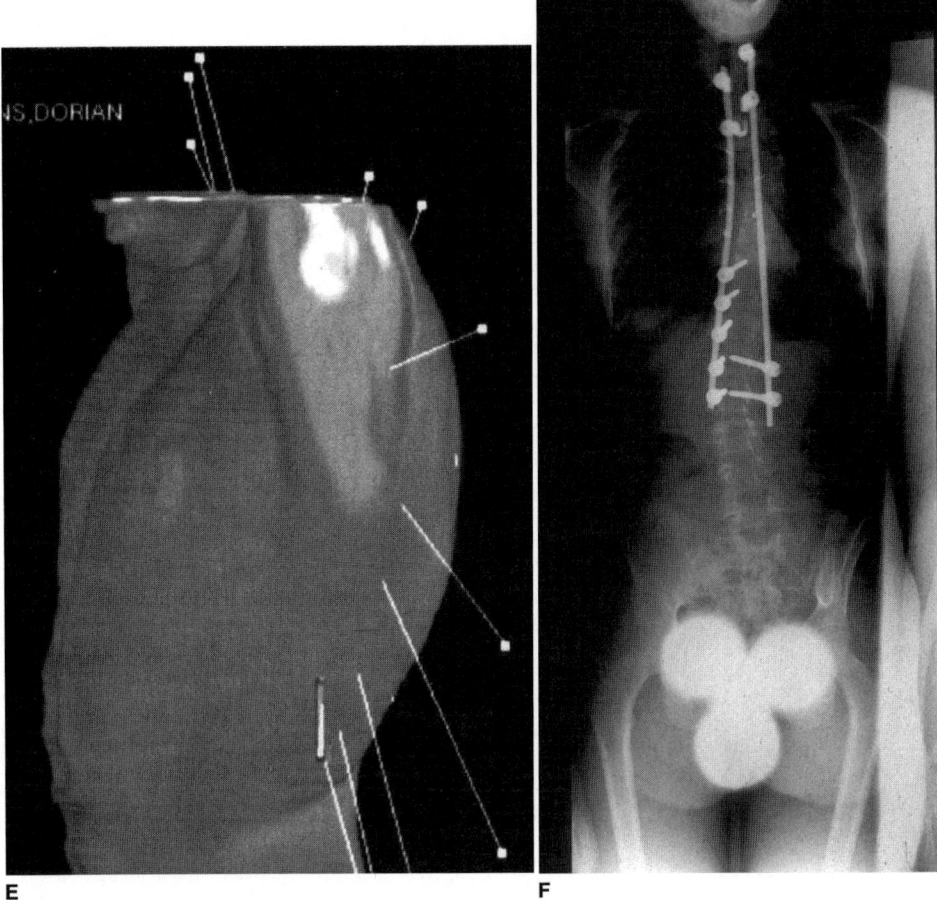

**Figure 96.9 cont'd** A simultaneous anterior release and posterior instrumented fusion were undertaken. Postoperative films are shown (**F** and **G**).

*Continued*

bloc spondylectomy and reconstruction. This approach allowed thoracoscopic access and release of the involved spinal segments to achieve surgical and histopathologic wide margins while avoiding the disadvantages inherent to thoracotomy.

## VATS in the Treatment of Thoracic Spine Trauma

The advantages of a thoracoscopic approach in trauma patients are similar to those in other etiologic groups. Thoracoscopic techniques may be particularly helpful in the decompression of burst fractures in elderly patients who may not tolerate a thoracotomy and diaphragmatic takedown. Similarly, the decreased disruption of shoulder mechanics may be helpful in paraplegic or significantly leg-injured patients to allow earlier rehabilitation and independent transfers.

Trauma applications typically require vertebral corpectomies or osteotomies. These procedures may be performed in the lateral or prone positions depending on subsequent procedures. For prone procedures, dorsal instrumentation can be manipulated to increase intervertebral exposure as with kyphosis correction in deformity patients. The initial trocar is inserted at the seventh ICS in the midaxillary line and the chest is explored. The injured level is easily identified by the subpleural hematoma covering it. After identifi-

cation of the level, a second trocar is inserted ventrally to allow lung retraction toward the mediastinum.

Because a significant portion of thoracic trauma occurs at the thoracolumbar junction, the extended manipulating channel method described by Huang et al.[36] may be useful. For these injuries, an approach from the left is recommended because the aorta lies just left of midline and there is more space available next to vertebral surface. After the initial portal has been made at the seventh ICS, an extended portal 5 to 6cm in length is made at the injured level or slightly behind the posterior axillary line at the T9-10 interspace. A similar length of underlying rib is removed and a small, self-retaining rib spreader is then placed, allowing introduction of larger instruments and direct palpation of the spine. Gently push the diaphragm down with a sponge forceps introduced through the manipulating channel. The approach-side pedicles are key landmarks and are removed at the vertebrectomy level and the next caudal level.[17] The dura mater is exposed, and discectomy of the superior and inferior disc space are undertaken.

With the dura mater exposed and monitored during the remainder of the procedure, damaged disc and bone fragments are removed with forceps and rongeurs. Create a defect in the anterior portion of the vertebral body with a high speed burr or rongeur, then pull compressive pathology, such as the posterior cortex or retropulsed fragments,

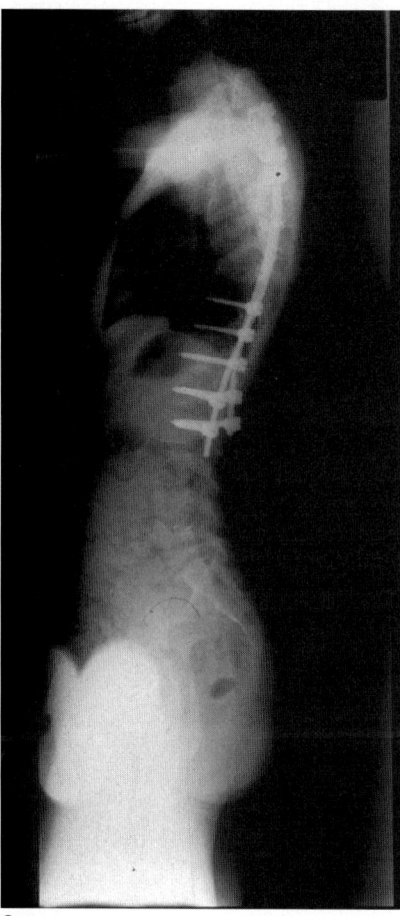

**G**

**Figure 96.9** *cont'd*

away from the dura. Complete decompressive corpectomy requires direct palpation of the contralateral pedicle.

Reconstruction after trauma includes morselized or structural anterior grafting followed by anterior or posterior instrumented stabilization. Morselized bone placed into partial corpectomy defects are typically stabilized posteriorly with short segment transpedicular instrumentation.[28] Alternatively, a corpectomy reconstruction can be completed by negotiating allograft struts, or mesh cages, into the defect, after inserting them into the chest through one of the portals. Then, either anterior or posterior instrumentation is used to stabilize the construct to extension, rotation, and side flexion.

Hertlein *et al.*[28] describe eight cases of staged, anterior thoracic discectomy and bone grafting after posterior transpedicular stabilization. Short segment posterior instrumentation is used to reduce the kyphotic deformity. Then tomograms or sagittal CT reconstructions are obtained to assess the size of the anterior column defect. If large, this anterior defect is directly bone grafted by using thoracoscopic means.

Dickman and others[20] reported on the outcomes of six patients undergoing thoracoscopic vertebrectomy for fracture. They found that the operative time and blood loss were similar to that of a similar, open thoracotomy group.

On the other hand, narcotic utilization, ICU stay, and hospital length of stay were all dramatically reduced in the thoracoscopic group.

Huang *et al.*[32] described their series of anterior decompressions and stabilization in 8 elderly patients when using a modified two-portal technique with a 5cm minithoracotomy incision. Over the mean 30-month follow-up period, no injuries to the great vessels, internal organs, or spinal cord were noted. Complications included one screw migration with graft displacement and transient problems with iliac crest donor site pain and wound hypesthesias. Average neurologic recovery was 1.1 grades on the Frankel scale. The authors concluded that this minimal-access technique with thoracoscopic assistance is an ideal alternative in treating patients with osteoporotic vertebral fractures and neurologic deficits but also that purchase of anterior vertebral screws in the osteoporotic spine was of concern.

## VATS in the Treatment of Spine Infection

Spinal infections are typically divided anatomically into vertebral osteomyelitis, discitis, or epidural abscess.[71] Treatment decisions are based on the sensitivity of the organism, the response of the infection to antibiotic management, the presence of abscess, the presence of neurologic involvement, the progression of spinal instability or deformity, involved spinal levels, and host factors such as age and medical comorbidities. Increased age and cephalad level of infection predispose to neurologic decline and paralysis.[22]

Treatment begins with identification of the offending organism through blood culture or biopsy. Typically, a fluoroscopically or CT-guided biopsy affords adequate diagnostic material. However, when clear identification of the organism is not obtained, consider surgical biopsy. Endoscopic techniques are an ideal, less invasive means to obtain an adequate tissue sample. Tan *et al.*[95] reported the case of an 18-month-old infant with increasing back pain and gait difficulty. Low-grade fever was noted, as was an end plate irregularity of the end plates at T7-8. CT scan demonstrated a soft tissue mass, but attempts at percutaneous needle biopsy were unsuccessful. A standard thoracoscopic approach was undertaken, and a 4mm pediatric biopsy forceps was used to take several samples from the affected site.

After the organism has been identified, institute a course of antibiotics and bracing. Surgery is indicated in any patient with neurologic deficits, failure to improve with medical management, or continued vertebral collapse. In most cases, when spinal cord compression occurs, the pathology is anterior, and wide approaches such as thoracotomy or costotransversectomy are required. Unfortunately, these approaches are highly morbid in this compromised patient population.[71] VATS can be employed in patients with spinal infections in a manner similar to that of tumor patients. That is, VATS can be employed for biopsy, debridement, cord decompression, and reconstruction.

The technical details of VATS for spine infection are similar to those of other indications. Surgical goals include confirmation of tissue diagnosis with biopsy, radical debridement of all necrotic debris, correction of any secondary deformity, and stabilization with autogenous bone

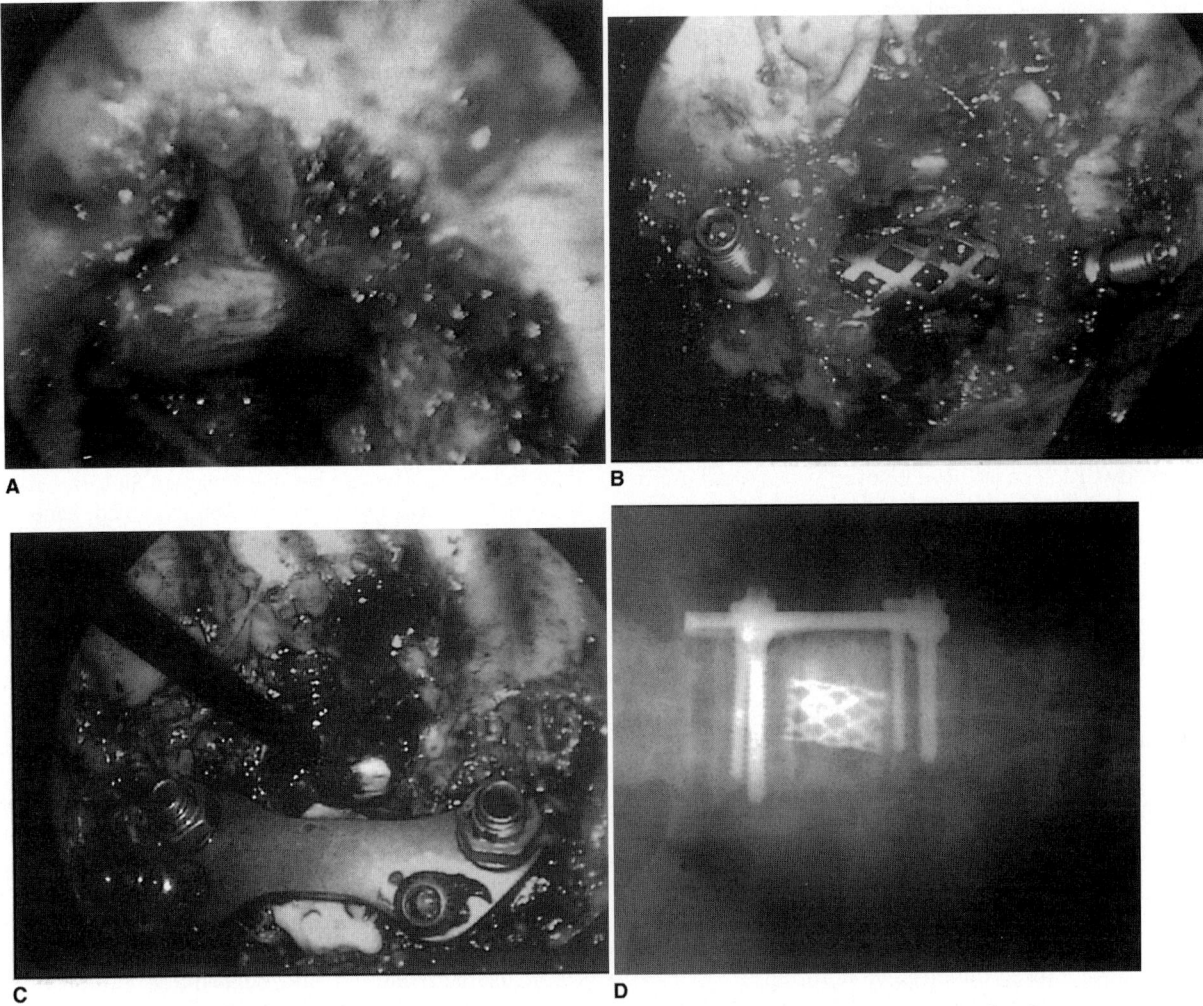

**Figure 96.10** A patient with metastatic breast cancer and a pathologic fracture presented with impending paraplegia. (**A**) A thoracoscopic corpectomy allowed complete decompression of the dura. The exiting nerve root is clearly visible. (**B**) A Harms cage, in this case filled with PMMA, is inserted into the defect. (**C**) Further fixation is afforded by a plate applied over the cage. (**D**) Intraoperative, cross-table anteroposterior radiograph demonstrates satisfactory positioning of the implants. (*From Regan JJ, Jarolem KL: Thoracoscopy of the spine. In Herkowitz HN, et al. Rothman-Simeone The Spine, ed 4. Philadelphia, WB Saunders, 1999, pp. 608-609.*)

grafting.[71] Typically a four-portal technique starting with an initial viewing portal at the T7 level is used. There may be a higher rate of pleurodesis secondary to the inflammation that requires either meticulous thoracoscopic adhesion takedown or a higher rate of conversion to open procedures. For similar reasons, the risk of postoperative air leak is higher as well.

Frequently, a paraspinal subpleural mass is identified. Open the pleura parallel to the spine with careful control of the segmentals at the midbody level. Débride extraspinal extension of necrotic material and identify the disc levels above and below the infected segment. Perform discectomies and prepare the end plates for subsequent fusion. This process affords the surgeon excellent orientation to the spinal anatomy. The pedicles of the affected vertebral bodies are removed. Then the corpectomies themselves are undertaken from disc space to disc space,

progressing in a cranial to caudal direction. As with trauma, begin by creating a hollow in the vertebral body ventrally. Then dorsal cortex and compressive material can be delivered anteriorly with a curette or small Kerrison. The magnification and lighting afforded by the endoscope allows the decompressed dura to be inspected at close range to ensure adequate decompression.

Huang et al.[33] reported their experience with video-assisted thoracoscopic surgery in managing tuberculous spondylitis in 10 patients. At a mean 24-month follow-up, average neurologic recovery was 1.1 Frankel grade. Complications included one lung atelectasis, pleural adhesions requiring conversion to open in one case, and 4 transient postoperative air leaks. The authors concluded that thoracoscopic techniques were a useful adjunct in the management of patients with tuberculous spondylitis for either biopsy or formal decompression and reconstruction.

For debridement and reconstruction, the authors recommended a combination of thoracoscopic visualization and mini-thoracotomy for debridement and instrumentation.

Dickman and others[20] reported on the outcomes of 3 patients undergoing thoracoscopic vertebrectomy for infection. They found that the operative time and blood loss were similar to that of an open thoracotomy group. On the other hand, narcotic utilization, ICU stay, and hospital length of stay were all dramatically reduced in the thoracoscopic group.

### Thoracoscopic Instrumentation

The next major step in endoscopic transthoracic spinal surgery is the development and application of spinal implants capable of stabilization and correction. Threaded cylindrical interbody fusion cages have enjoyed widespread use in the lumbar spine, and this experience is now being extended to the thoracic spine. Threaded cages can be applied in the coronal or oblique plane. Application in thoracic spine may be technically less demanding, but the risks of malposition are clearly more significant. The fusion rates of single cages in the thoracic spine remain to be evaluated.

With some difficulty, existing rod and screw implant systems may be inserted in an endoscopic or endoscopically assisted fashion. These systems have also been modified by using, for example, cannulated screws and combinations of endoscopic and fluoroscopic insertion techniques.[88] From a clinical standpoint there are several concerns with the existing systems.[88]

- In the case of scoliosis, currently available implants and application techniques assuming a two-dimensional correction for a three-dimensional deformity
- The thoracic cage limits access to the implants, thus requiring extensions beyond the chest wall to manipulate the implants. These extensions will be limited in their excursion and correction ability by the chest wall. Further, using these extensions implies that an exaggerated lever arm will be applied to the implant bone interface, which may jeopardize screw purchase and cause premature implant loosening resulting in pseudarthrosis or loss of correction.

Hertlein et al.[29] described their first two cases of thoracoscopic osteosynthesis. After decompression and grafting as described above, AO dynamic compression plates were brought into the wound through the working trocar. The plate was preliminarily fixed to the spine by using two Kirschner wires. A Cardan drill was then inserted into the trocar, and 3.2mm holes of 2cm depth were prepared. Next, 6cm screws were inserted into the plate with a Cardan screwdriver. These patients were not braced postoperatively.

Crawford[14] and Picetti et al.[73] have described similar endoscopic instrumentation techniques in the deformity setting. The authors used circumferential C-arm access to the patient along with a tricannulated pitchfork. The tricannulated pitchfork was used to place guide pins and subsequently screws. The device allows the surgeon to line up the best coronal location for the screw and place a Steinmann pin through the cannula under image control.

The pin is placed in the mid-coronal plane of the vertebra and driven from slightly posterior to anterior starting just anterior to the rib head. Starting at the rib head prevents the surgeon from starting the screw too far posteriorly. The surgeon stands at the patient's back and places the instrumentation from back to front, aiming away from the spinal cord. Once the Steinmann pin has been placed, its external portion is secured to prevent penetration through the body into the opposite hemithorax. A cannulated tap prepares the site for a bone screw. When the screws have been placed, a measuring device for rod length is advanced through inferior portal. The rod is inserted through the inferior portal and seated into the screw heads. Capture screws are seated into screw heads to secure the rod. The bottom screw is tightened first so that all compression projects superiorly toward the top of the thoracic cage rather than inferiorly toward the diaphragm. Once the rod has been fully seated, a compressor is introduced, each set of screws is individually compressed, and the capture screw is tightened and torqued. With present designs, a true rotational maneuver is not possible.

Recently Assaker and co-workers[5,6] studied the feasibility of adding computer guidance to endoscopic spine procedures. In this setting, three-dimensional assessment of instrumentation position would be possible through video monitors by using an extracorporeal fiducial and a CT-based navigational system. This may improve the speed and accuracy of endoscopically performed decompression and instrumentation.

Huang et al.[34] describe a combination thoracoscopic and mini-open approach to decompress and stabilize the spine in a series of four patients with thoracic myelopathy. A 3 to 4cm manipulating channel is created for both endoscopic instrumentation and subsequent tumor removal and reconstruction. Standard reconstructive instrumentation may then be inserted with standard instrumentation.

These techniques are not without potential complications. The greatest of these is malposition of the instrumentation into the spinal canal or vascular structures because of the loss of three-dimensional vision and direct palpation. Roush et al.[88] reported a case of tension pneumothorax during fluoroscopic guide pin placement for a video-assisted anterior scoliosis stabilization procedure. In this case, the guide pin was inadvertently over-advanced 2cm past the contralateral vertebral cortex. Five minutes after this over-advancement was corrected, the patient's heart rate increased with a corresponding decrease in oxygen saturation and blood pressure. Ultimately, a tension pneumothorax was diagnosed and treated with tube thoracostomy of the opposite hemithorax.

### Dorsal Spinal Endoscopy

Direct dorsal approaches to midline neurocompressive thoracic pathology have largely been abandoned because laminectomy alone will not adequately decompress a kyphotic spinal segment. Moreover, attempts to indirectly decompress central pathologies have been unsuccessful, or worse, have resulted in neurologic decline.[37,50] On the other hand, costotransversectomy and lateral extracavitary approaches are associated with large incisions, increased postoperative morbidity, wound healing problems, and difficulty with visualization.[14,17] Smaller, transpedicular approaches from the posterior can utilize small incisions and a 70-degree endoscope to better visualize the anterior dura and avoid the need for postoperative chest tube drainage required of either thoracoscopy or thoracotomy.

### Indications and Contraindications

The role of endoscopic and minimally invasive techniques in treatment of metastatic and degenerative disease is evolving. While ventral approaches to metastatic disease are favored overall, the use of an endoscope to assist posterolateral decompression may obviate the need for a second, ventral surgery in patients undergoing posterior stabilization. This approach is particularly useful in patients with radioresistant metastases of the upper thoracic spine, where thoracotomy is difficult and highly morbid.[59,60] Similarly, dorsal vertebrectomy and decompression techniques must be considered in patients unable to tolerate single lung ventilation or thoracotomy. Contraindications to the currently available techniques include failed prior open surgery and large lesions. Posterior trans-pedicular instrumentation is another area in which endoscopic assistance may allow for smaller incisions and decreased muscle injury. These resection techniques are intralesional and are therefore not indicated in patients with primary neoplasms.[59]

### Anatomy and Technique

Osman and Marsolais[69] described a posterior endoscopic approach to the thoracic disc space in a cadaver. The authors found that above T10, the rib neck was an ideal guide to the disc space and prevented lateral excursion into the lung. The shoulder girdle and transition from thoracic kyphosis to cervical lordosis made accurate insertion at the T1-2 and T2-3 levels difficult. They concluded that this approach would be technically feasible for soft lateral discs. With further development of endoscopic instrumentation, even calcified or adherent central discs could be approached in this manner.

Jho[40] described a minimally invasive posterior approach to thoracic disc herniations employing a 2cm long transverse paramedian incision at the pedicle level of the involved vertebra. Patients are positioned 60 degrees forward inclined to keep the lesion side facing upward. The paraspinal muscles are dissected from the spinous process, lamina, and transverse processes by using a periosteal elevator. A tubular retractor is passed into the wound over the facet and lamina. The medial portion of the facet, the lateral portion of the lamina, and the rostral third of the pedicle are removed with a high-speed burr to gain access to the disc space and to expose the very lateral margin of the spinal cord dura. A 2mm burr removes the bone spurs rostral and caudal to the herniated disc and creates a cavity into which material from the decompression is moved. When an appropriate 1.5cm cavity has been created, a 4mm diameter rigid endoscope with a 70-degree lens is mounted to a custom-made endoscope holder. Surgical decompression of the ventral cord can then be performed by using 90-degree curved surgical instruments. For example, a down-biting curette can be

used to push more osteophyte away from the cord and into the created cavity. Material can be removed from the cavity with a curved pituitary.

McLain's technique for decompression of thoracic metastases is similar, but is undertaken through a longitudinal incision.[59,60] The initial approach mimics costotransversectomy, wherein the proximal rib is removed with the entire pedicle. Here too, a cavity is created anteriorly, and anterior compressive pathology is collapsed into this cavity by using Epstein curettes. After complete decompression, a corpectomy defect is created and the space can be reconstructed by using titanium mesh cages followed by posterior, segmental instrumentation (Figure 96.11).

### Results

Jho[40] reported on a consecutive series of 25 patients undergoing minimal-access thoracic discectomy. Seven patients were myelopathic, 6 presented with myeloradiculopathy, 10 presented with radicular complaints, and two were felt to have segmental pain. He reports the perioperative morbidity of this procedure to be similar to lumbar microdiscectomy, and radiculopathic patients are allowed to go home the same day. In his series, the 2 patients with segmental pain did not note relief of symptoms despite MRI documentation of complete decompression. Of the radiculopathic patients, 9 of 10 had complete relief of symptoms. Twelve of 13 myelopathic or myeloradiculopathic patients had significant relief of symptoms.

McLain[59] described the successful use of an endoscope to complete anterior decompression from a posterior approach in 5 patients by using an endoscope to increase visualization. Mean operative time was 7.25 hours, and mean blood loss was 1800ml. Neurologic recovery was judged excellent.

### Conclusions and Future Directions

Techniques for both anterior and posterior endoscopically assisted access to the thoracic spine are evolving rapidly. With this evolution, it is important to remember that endoscopic spine surgery refers to a change in approach, not in the operation itself. Therefore the indications for operative intervention are not relaxed merely because these procedures may be performed through smaller incisions. As in any spine surgery, careful patient selection is the critical factor predicting successful outcomes.

Endoscopic thoracic spinal surgery confers many proven and potential advantages to both the surgeon and patient, including improved surgical visualization through magnification and lighting, decreased perioperative morbidity, and shorter hospital stays. But these advantages must be counterbalanced with disadvantages of these approaches including lack of familiarity, decreased three-dimensional perspective, and a loss of tactile sense. Initial experience with these procedures should include cadaveric and animal lab work, followed by visits to active centers or proctoring at your center.[17] Preferably these lab sessions and active center visits will include several members of the operating room team. As these procedures are introduced to a new center, a

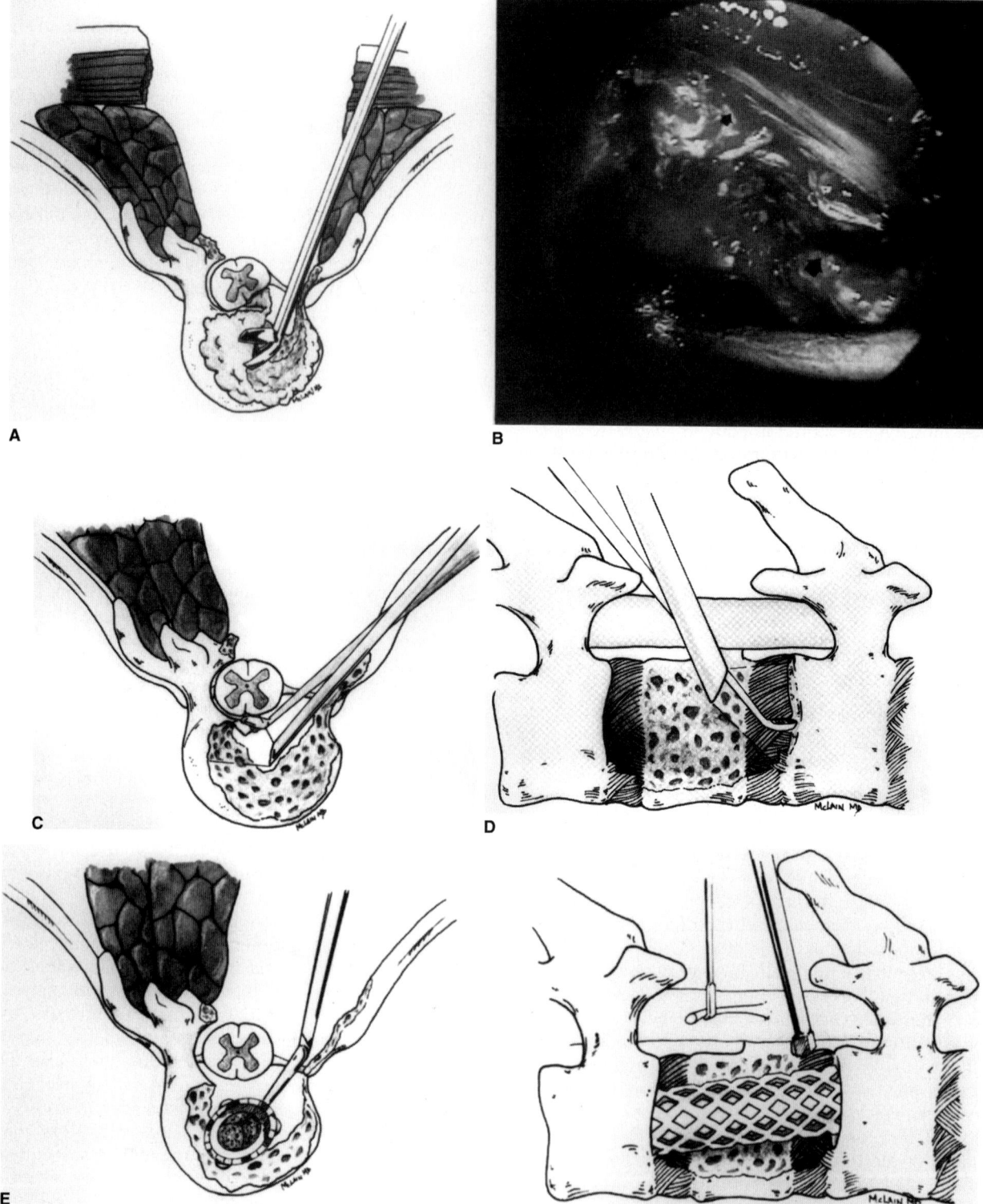

**Figure 96.11** An endoscope may be used to assist posterior spinal decompressions as well. The pedicle and medial rib are removed. This allows decompression of tumor or other compressive pathology to the vertebral midline (**A**). Then, a 70-degree endoscope can be used to visualize the PLL, and the remainder of the posterior cortex can be collapsed into the vertebrectomy defect anteriorly (**B** and **C**). In **B**, the large arrow indicates the interval between the posterior vertebral cortex and dura, and the small arrow indicates the posterior longtudinal ligament. With the decompression completed, the vertebrectomy can be further prepared by removing the adjacent discs and end plate cartilage with a curette or rongeur (**D**). Finally, the defect is reconstructed by using a strut graft or cage (**E**). *(From McLain RF: Endoscopically assisted decompression for metastatic thoracic neoplasms.* Spine 23(10):1130-1135, 1998, Fig. 1-4.)

proctoring surgeon from an active center is helpful, and instruments for immediate conversion to open technique are mandatory. Early cases may be associated with higher complication rates and operating times. Ultimately, a less efficacious technique should not be employed merely because it is endoscopic.

As endoscopic spine surgery techniques are also personnel and equipment intensive, involvement of OR and hospital-wide administrative personnel may smooth the adjustment. A second approach surgeon may be needed for a given endoscopic procedure that might not be required in an open procedure. Specialized and often single-use instruments are required. These additional OR costs may be recouped with earlier patient discharge. However, the potential benefits of a minimal approach are not going to be realized by every surgeon.

There is ample opportunity to study and improve upon these techniques. A randomized clinical trial comparing open with endoscopic techniques is needed, and long-term outcome data are needed. Many of these procedures are promising, but significant advantages over previous techniques remain to be proven.

The current indications for thoracic endoscopy include minimally invasive access to the intervertebral disc, both anteriorly and posteriorly; debridement of tumor and infection; releases for deformity; and anterior interbody fusions. Endoscopic spinal instrumentation is evolving rapidly. Endoscopic procedures will become more commonplace as image-guided and robot-assisted technology is more pervasive and as instrumentation systems are improved.

# REFERENCES

1. Anand N, Regan JJ: Video-assisted thoracoscopic surgery for thoracic disc disease: classification and outcome study of 100 consecutive cases with a 2-year minimum follow-up period. *Spine* 15;27(8):871-879, 2002.
2. Arce CA, Dohrman GJ: Thoracic disc herniation. Improved diagnosis with CT scanning and a review of the literature. *Surg Neurol* 23:356-361, 1985.
3. Arlet V: Anterior thoracoscopic spine release in deformity surgery. A meta-analysis and review. *Eur Spine J* 9 (suppl 1):S17-S22, 2000.
4. Arseni C, Nash F: Thoracic intervertebral disc protrusion. A clinical study. *J Neurosurg* 17:418-430, 1960.
5. Assaker R, Cinquin P, Cotten A, Lejeune JP: Image-guided endoscopic spine surgery: Part I. A feasibility study. *Spine* 26(15):1705-1710, 2001.
6. Assaker R, Reyns N, Pertruzon B, Lejeune JP: Image-guided endoscopic spine surgery. Part II: clinical applications. *Spine* 26(15):1711-1718, 2001.
7. Birnbaum K, Pieper S, Prescher A, Siebert CH: Thoracoscopically assisted ligamentous release of the thoracic spine: a cadaver study. *Surg Radiol Anat* 22 (3-4):143-150, 2000.
8. Bloomberg AE: Collective reviews: thoracoscopy in perspective. *Surg Gynecol Obstet* 147:433-443, 1978.
9. Bohlman HH, Zdeblick TA: Anterior excision of herniated thoracic discs. *J Bone Joint Surg [Am]* 70:1038-1047, 1988.
10. Burgos J, Rapariz J, Gonzalewz-Herranz R: Anterior endoscopic approach to the thoracolumbar spine. *Spine* 23(22):2427-2431, 1998.
11. Byrd JAI, Scoles PV, Winter RB, et al: Adult idiopathic scoliosis treated by anterior and posterior spinal fusion. *J Bone Joint Surg* 69A:843-850, 1987.
12. Carson J, Gumpert J, Jefferson A: Diagnosis and treatment of thoracic disc protrusions. *J Neuro Neurosurg Psychiatry* 34:68-77, 1971.
13. Citow JS, Macdonald RL, Ferguson MK: Combined laminectomy and thoracoscopic resection of a dumbbell neurofibroma. Technical case report. *Neurosurgery* 45(5);1263-1266, 1999.
14. Crawford AH, Wall EJ, Wolf R: Video-assisted thoracoscopy. *Orthop Clin North Am* 30(3):367-385, 1999.
15. Crawford AH, Wolf RK, Wall EJ: *Pediatric spinal deformity.* In Regan JJ, McAfee PA, Mack MJ (eds): *Atlas of Endoscopic Spine Surgery.* St Louis, Quality Medical Publishing, 1995.
16. Cunningham BW, Kotani Y, McNulty PS, et al: Video-assisted thoracoscopic surgery versus open thoracotomy for anterior thoracic spinal fusion. A comparative radiographic, biomechanical, and histologic analysis in a sheep model. *Spine* 23(12):1333-1340, 1998.
17. Dickman CA, Detweiler PW, Porter RW: Endoscopic spine surgery. *Clin Neurosurg* 46:526-553, 2000.
18. Dickman CA, Karahalios DG: Thoracoscopic spine surgery. *Clin Neurosurg* 43:392-422, 2000.
19. Dickman CA, Mican CA: Multilevel anterior thoracic discectomies and anterior interbody fusion using a microsurgical thoracoscopic approach. Case report. *J Neurosurg* 84:104-109, 1996.
20. Dickman CA, Rosenthal D, Karahalios DG, et al: Thoracic vertebrectomy and reconstruction using a microsurgical thorascopic approach. *Neurosurgery* 38:279, 1996.
21. Ebara S, Kamimura M, Itoh H, et al: A new system for the anterior restoration and fixation of thoracic spinal deformities using endoscopic approach. *Spine* 25(7): 876-883, 2000.
22. Eismont FJ, Bohlman HH, Soni PL, et al: Pyogenic and fungal vertebral osteomyelitis with paralysis. *J Bone Joint Surg* 65A:19-29, 1983.
23. Errico TJ, Cooper PR: A new method of thoracic and lumbar body replacement for spinal tumors. Technical note. *Neurosurgery* 32:678-681, 1993.
24. Gonzalez-Barrios I, Fuentes Caparrios S, Avila Jurado MM: Anterior thoracoscopic epiphysiodesis in the treatment of crankshaft phenomenon. *Eur Spine J* 4: 343-346, 1995.
25. Hall AJ, MacKay NNS: The results of laminectomy for compression of the cord and cauda equine by extradural malignant tumor. *J Bone Joint Surg* 55-B:497-505, 1973.
26. Hasnain J, Krasna M, Barker S, et al: Anesthetic consideration for thoracoscopic procedures. *J Cardiothorac Vasc Anesth* 6:624-627, 1992.

27. Heltzer JM, Krasna MJ, Aldrich F, McLaughlin JS: Thoracoscopic excision of a posterior mediastinal dumbbell tumor using a combined approach. *Ann Thorac Surg* 60:431-433, 1995.

28. Hertlein H, Hertl WH, Dienemann H, *et al*: Thoracoscopic repair of thoracic spine trauma. *Eur Spine J* 4:302-307, 1995.

29. Hertlein H, Hartl WH, Piltz S, *et al*: Endoscopic osteosynthesis after thoracic spine trauma: a report of two cases. *Injury* 31(5):333-336, 2000.

30. Holcomb GW, Mencio GA, Green NE: Video assisted thoracoscopic discectomy and fusion. *J Ped Surg* 32(7):1120-1122, 1997.

31. Horowitz MB, Moossy JJ, Julian T, *et al*: Thoracic discectomy using video assisted thoracoscopy. *Spine* 19:1082-1086, 1994.

32. Huang TJ, Hsu RW, Chen YJ: Minimal-access surgery in managing osteoporotic vertebral fractures with neurological deficits: a preliminary report. *Changgeng Yi Xue Za Zhi* 23(9):542-549, 2000.

33. Huang TJ, Hsu RW, Chen SH, Liu HP: Video-assisted thoracoscopic surgery in managing tuberculous spondylitis. *Clin Orthop* 379:143-153, 2000.

34. Huang TJ, Hsu WW, Liu HP, *et al*: Analysis of techniques for video-assisted thoracoscopic internal fixation of the spine. *Arch Orthop Trauma Surg* 117:92-95, 1998.

35. Huang TJ, Hsu RW, Sum SW, Lie HP: Complications in thoracoscopic spinal surgery. *Surg Endoscopy* 13:346-350, 1999.

36. Huang TJ, Scu RW, Hsu KY, *et al*: Video-assisted thoracoscopic treatment of spinal lesions in the thoracolumbar junction. *Surg Endosc* 11:1189-1193, 1997.

37. Hulme A: The surgical approach to thoracic intervertebral disc protrusions. *J Neuro Neurosurg Psychiatry* 23:133-137, 1960.

38. Ikard RW, McCord DH: Thoracoscopic exposure of intervertebral discs. *Ann Thorac Surg* 61:1267-1268, 1996.

39. Islam S, Hresko MT, Fishman SJ: Extrapleural thoracoscopic anterior spinal fusion: a modified video-assisted thoracoscopic surgery approach to the pediatric spine. *JSLS* 5(2):187-189, 2001.

40. Jho HD: Endoscopic transpedicular thoracic discectomy. *J Neurosurg (Spine 2)* 91:151-156, 1999.

41. Johnson JR, Holt RT: Combined use of anterior and posterior surgery for adult scoliosis. *Orthop Clin North Am* 19:361-370, 1998.

42. Kambin P, McCullen G, Parke W, *et al*: Minimally invasive arthroscopic spinal surgery. Instructional Course Lectures. 46:143-161, 1997.

43. King AG, Mills TE, Loe WA, *et al*: Video-assisted thoracoscopic surgery in the prone position. *Spine* 25(18):2403-2406, 2000.

44. Kinnear WJ, Kinnear GC, Watson L, *et al*: Pulmonary function after spinal surgery for idiopathic scoliosis. *Spine* 17:703-713, 1992.

45. Konno S, Yabuki S, Kinoshita T, Kikuchi S: Combined laminectomy and thoracoscopic resection of dumbbell-type thoracic cord tumor. *Spine* 26(6):E130-134, 2001.

46. Kostuik JP, Israel J, Hall JE: Scoliosis surgery in adults. *Clin Orthop* 93:225-234, 1973.

47. Krasna MJ, Mack MJ: *Atlas of Thoracoscopic Surgery*. St Louis, Quality Medical Publishing, 1994.

48. Kuklo TR, Lenke LG: Thoracoscopic spine surgery: current indications and techniques. *Orthop Nurs* 19(6):15-22, 2000.

49. Landreneau RJ, Hazelrigg SR, Mack MJ, *et al*: Post-operative pain-related morbidity: video-assisted thoracic surgery versus thoracotomy. *Ann Thorac Surg* 56:1285-1289, 1993.

50. Larson SJ, Holst RA, Hemmy DC, *et al*: Lateral extracavitary approach to traumatic lesions of the thoracic and lumbar spine. *J Neurosurg* 45:628-637, 1976.

51. Lieberman IH, Salo PT, Orr RD, Kraetschmer BG: Prone position endoscopic transthoracic release with simultaneous posterior instrumentation for spinal deformity: a description of the technique. *Spine* 25(17):2251-2257, 2000.

52. Lischke V, Westphal K, Behne M, *et al*: Thoracoscopic microsurgical technique for vertebral surgery. Anesthetic considerations. *Acta Anaesthesiol Scand* 42:1999-1204, 1998.

53. Logas WG, El-Baz N, El-Ganzouri A, *et al*: Continuous thoracic epidural anesthesia for postoperative pain relief following thoracotomy. A randomized, prospective study. *Anesthesiology* 67:787-791, 1987.

54. Mack MJ, Regan JJ, Bobechko WP, Acuff TE: Application of thoracoscopy for diseases of the spine. *Ann Thorac Surg* 56:736-738, 1993.

55. Magerl FP: Stabilization of the lower thoracic and lumbar spine with external skeletal fixation. *Clin Orthop* 189:125-141, 1984.

56. McAfee PC: Complications of anterior approaches to the thoracolumbar spine. Emphasis on Kaneda instrumentation. *Clin Orthop* 306:110-119, 1994.

57. McAfee PC, Regan JJ, Fedder IL, *et al*: Anterior thoracic corpectomy for spinal cord decompression performed endoscopically. *Surg Laparosc Endosc* 5(5):339-348, 1995.

58. McAfee PC, Regan JJ, Zdeblick T, *et al*: The incidence of complications in endoscopic anterior thoracolumbar spinal reconstructive surgery. A prospective multicenter study comprising the first 100 consecutive cases. *Spine* 14:1624-1632, 1995.

59. McLain RF: Endoscopically assisted decompression for metastatic thoracic neoplasms. *Spine* 15(10):1130-1135, 1998.

60. McLain RF: Spinal cord decompression. An endoscopically assisted approach for metastatic tumors. *Spinal Cord* 29:482-487, 2001.

61. McLain RF, Lieberman IH: Controversy: endoscopic approaches to metastatic thoracic disease. *Spine* 25(14):1857-1858, 2000.

62. Mehlman CT, Crawford AH, Wolf RK: Video assisted thoracoscopic surgery (VATS), endoscopic thoracoplasty technique. *Spine* 22(18):2178-2182, 1997.

63. Newton PO, Cardelia JM, Farnsworth CL, *et al*: A biomechanical comparison of open and thoracoscopic anterior spinal release in a goat model. *Spine* 23(5):530-536, 1998.

64. Newton PO, Shea KG, Granlund KF: Defining the pediatric spinal thoracoscopy learning curve: sixty-five consecutive cases. *Spine* 25(8):1028-1035, 2000.

65. Newton PO, Wenger DR, Mubarak JS, Meyer RS: Anterior release and fusion in pediatric spinal deformity. A comparison of early outcome and cost of thoracoscopic and open thoracotomy approaches. *Spine* 22(12):1398-1406, 1997.

66. Niemeyer T, Freeman BJ, Grevitt MP, Webb JK: Anterior thoracoscopic surgery followed by posterior instrumentation and fusion in spinal deformity. *Eur Spine J* 9(6):499-504, 2000.

67. Ohtsuka T, Ohnishi I, Nakamura K, Takamoto S: New instrumentation for video-assisted anterior spine release. *Surg Endosc* 14(7):682-684, 2000.

68. Oskouian RJ Jr, Johnson JP, Regan JJ: Thoracoscopic microdiscectomy. *Neurosurgery* 50(1):103-109, 2002.

69. Osman SG, Marsolais EB: Posterolateral arthroscopic discectomies of the thoracic and lumbar spine. *CORR* 304:122-129, 1994.

70. Otani K, Yoshida M, Fujii E, *et al:* Thoracic disc herniation. Surgical treatment in 23 patients. *Spine* 13:1262-1267, 1988.

71. Parker LM, McAfee PC, Fedder IL, *et al:* Minimally invasive surgical techniques to treat spine infections. *Orthop Clin North Am* 27(1):183-199, 1996.

72. Pereon Y, Delecrin J, Nguyen S, *et al:* Successful monitoring of neurogenic mixed evoked potentials elicited by anterior spinal cord stimulation through thoracoscopy during spine surgery. *Spine* 24(19):2025-2035, 1999.

73. Picetti G III, Blackman RG, O'Neal K, Luque E: Anterior endoscopic correction and fusion of scoliosis. *Orthopedics* 21(12):1285-1287, 1998.

74. Regan JJ: Percutaneous endoscopic thoracic discectomy. *Neurosurg Clin North Am* 7(1):87-98, 1996.

75. Regan JJ, Ben-Yishay A, Mack MJ: Video-assisted thoracoscopic excision of herniated thoracic disc. Description of technique and preliminary experience in the first 29 cases. *J Spinal Disord* 11(3):183-191, 1998.

76. Regan JJ, Guyer RD: Endoscopic techniques in spinal surgery. *CORR* 225;122-139, 1997.

77. Regan JJ, Mack MJ: Endoscopic thoracic fusion cage. In Regan JJ, McAfee PJ, Mack MJ (eds): *Atlas of Endoscopic Spine Surgery*. St Louis, Quality Medical Publishing, 1995, p 130.

78. Regan JJ, Mack MJ, Picetti GD: A technical report on video-assisted thoracoscopy in thoracic spinal surgery. Preliminary description. *Spine* 20:831-837, 1995.

79. Regan JJ, Mack MJ, Picetti GD, *et al:* A comparison of video-assisted thoracoscopy surgery (VATS) with open thoracotomy in the thoracic spinal surgery. *Today's Therapeutic Trends* 11:203-218, 1994.

80. Regan JJ, Yuan H, McCullen G: Minimally invasive approaches to the spine. *Instr Course Lect* 46:127-141, 1997.

81. Resnick DK, Benzel EC: Lateral extracavitary approach for thoracic and thoracolumbar spine trauma. Operative complications. *Neurosurgery* 43:796-803, 1998.

82. Rogers MA, Crockard HA: Surgical treatment of the symptomatic herniated thoracic disc. *Clin Orthop* 300: 70-78, 1994.

83. Rosenthal D: Endoscopic internal fixation of the thoracic spine. In Regan JJ, McAfee PJ, Mack MJ (eds): *Atlas of Endoscopic Spine Surgery*. St Louis, Quality Medical Publishing, 1995, p 333.

84. Rosenthal D, Dickman CA: Thoracoscopic microsurgical excision of herniated thoracic discs. *J Neurosurg* 89(2): 224-235, 1998.

85. Rosenthal D, Marquardt G, Lorenz R, Nichtweiss M: Anterior decompression and stabilization using a microsurgical endoscopic technique for metastatic tumors of the thoracic spine. *J Neurosurg* 84:565-572, 1996.

86. Rosenthal D, Rosenthal R, de Simone A: Removal of a protruded thoracic disc using microsurgical endoscopy. A new technique. *Spine* 19:1087-1091, 1994.

87. Rothenberg S, Erickson M, Eilert R, *et al:* Thoracoscopic anterior spinal procedures in children. *J Pediatric Surg* 33(7):1168-1170, 1170-1171, 1998.

88. Rouch TF, Crawford AH, Berlin RE, Wolff RK: Tension pneumothorax as a complication of video-assisted thoracoscopic surgery for anterior correction of idiopathic scoliosis in an adolescent female. *Spine* 26(4):448-450, 2001.

89. Schwab FJ, Smith V, Farcy JP: Endoscopic thoracoplasty and anterior spinal release in scoliotic deformity. *Bull Hosp Jt Dis* 59(1):27-32, 2000.

90. Shufflebarger HL, Grimm JO, Bui V, Thomson JD: Anterior and posterior spinal fusion. Staged versus same day surgery. *Spine* 16:930-933, 1991.

91. Sihvonen T, Herno A, Paljarvi L: Local denervation atrophy of paraspinal muscles in post-operative failed back syndrome. *Spine* 18:575, 1993.

92. Simmons EDJ, Kowalski JM, Simmons EH: The results of surgical treatment for adult scoliosis. *Spine* 18:718-724, 1993.

93. Sucato DJ, Girgis M: Bilateral pneumothoraces, pneumomediastinum, pneumoperitoneum, pneumoretroperitoneum, and subcutaneous emphysema following intubation with a double-lumen endotracheal tube for thoracoscopic anterior spinal release and fusion in a patient with idiopathic scoliosis. *J Spinal Disord Tech* 15(2):133-138, 2002.

94. Sucato DJ, Welch RD, Pierce B, *et al:* Thoracoscopic discectomy and fusion in an animal model: safe and effective when segmental blood vessels are spared. *Spine* 15;27(8):880-886, 2002.

95. Tan HL, McMurrick PJ, Merriman TE, Torode IP: Thoracoscopic biopsy of a pathological vertebral body. *Aust NZ J Surg* 64:726-728, 1994.

96. van Dijk M, Cuesta MA, Wuisman PI: Thoracoscopically assisted total en bloc spondylectomy: two case reports. *Surg Endosc* 14(9):849-852, 2000.

97. Vissochi M, Masferrer, Sonntag VKH, Dickman CA: Thoracoscopic approaches to the thoracic spine. *Acta Neurochir (Wien)* 140:737-744, 1998.

98. Waisman M, Saute M: Thoracoscopic spine release before posterior instrumentation in scoliosis. *CORR* 336;130-136, 1997.

99. Wall EJ, Bylski-Austrow DI, Shelton FS, *et al:* Endoscopic discectomy increases flexibility as effectively as open discectomy. *Spine* 23(1):9-16, 1998.

100. Watkins RG: Cervical, thoracic and lumbar complications, anterior approach. In Garfin SR (ed): *Complications of Spine Surgery*. Baltimore, Williams & Wilkins, 1989, pp 211-247.

101. Weatherly CR, Draycott V, O'Brien JF, *et al*: The rib deformity in adolescent idiopathic scoliosis. *J Bone Joint Surg* 69-B:179-182, 1987.

102. Westfall SH, Akbarnia BA, Merenda JT, *et al*: Exposure of the anterior spine. Technique, complications, and results in 85 patients. *Am J Surg* 154:700-704, 1987.

103. Winter RB, Lonstein JE, Denis F, *et al*: Paraplegia resulting from vessel ligation. *Spine* 15;21(10):1232-1233, 1996.

104. Zdeblick TA: A prospective, randomized study of lumbar fusion. Preliminary results. *Spine* 18(8):983-991, 1993.

# CHAPTER 97

# Vertebroplasty and Kyphoplasty

## Daisuke Togawa and Isador H. Lieberman

## Osteoporotic Vertebral Compression Fractures

Osteoporosis is widely viewed as a major public health concern. The National Osteoporosis Foundation (NOF) estimates more than 100 million people worldwide, and nearly 30 million people in the United States, are at risk to develop fragility fractures secondary to osteoporosis. The vertebrae are particularly affected by these fractures, which manifest clinically as vertebral compression fractures (VCFs). In the United States there are 1.5 million fragility fractures caused by osteoporosis annually. Approximately half (700,000) of these fractures affect the spine in the form of painful progressive VCFs, of which more than a third become chronically painful.[5,35] These compression fractures lead to progressive deformity and changes in spinal biomechanics, and are believed to contribute to an increased risk of further fracture. Whether or not the fracture is painful, the resultant spinal deformity impacts health, daily living, and medical costs through loss of lung capacity, reduced mobility, chronic pain, loss of appetite, and/or clinical depression.[*] With each osteoporotic vertebral compression fracture, there is a 9% loss in forced vital capacity, a 23% age-adjusted increase in mortality,[21] and a 5-year survival rate less than that for hip fractures.[6] Osteoporotic VCFs are clearly a clinically significant health problem with continuously increasing economic and social ramifications. The NOF predicts the number of vertebral body compression fractures will double in the next 15 years because of the aging population and our increasingly sedentary lifestyles.

### Nonoperative Management

The medical treatment of osteoporosis starts with prevention. The strategies of prevention include maximizing peak bone mass in adolescence, maintaining bone mass during adulthood, and minimizing postmenopausal bone loss. All individuals require age-matched physiologic doses of calcium and vitamin D. These nutrients are critical for achieving peak bone mass. Pharmacologic management to minimize bone loss includes estrogens, calcitonin, and bisphosphonates. Estrogen is an effective agent for the treatment of postmenopausal osteoporosis and has been shown to reduce hip and spine fractures. Calcitonin is a peptide hormone that reduces osteoclastic bone resorption and has analgesic properties. Bisphosphonates are analogs of

pyrophosphates, but are impervious to enzymatic hydrolysis and alter bone remodeling by reducing bone resorption.

Although narcotic medications are sometimes effective, symptomatic relief of pain can be difficult to achieve in the treatment period of osteoporotic fractures. In many cases physical therapy, rehabilitation, and bracing help achieve pain relief, but unfortunately, these nonoperative treatment regimens for painful fractures do nothing to restore spinal alignment and may compound the problem. Traditionally, VCFs were only rarely treated with surgical modalities. Because of its inherent risks, invasive nature, and the poor quality of osteoporotic bone, surgical treatment of VCFs has been limited to cases in which there is concurrent spinal instability or neurologic deficit.

### Operative Management

The indications for surgery to treat osteoporosis are progressive deformity accompanied by significant pain in the scoliotic or kyphotic patient, an acute osteoporotic fracture with neurologic problems, and osteoporosis in conjunction with spinal instability, most commonly associated with spinal stenosis.[22] Reconstruction with structural bone graft and instrumentation may be performed from a ventral or dorsal approach; however, the success of these techniques is limited by the patient's poor bone quality and general medical condition.

### Vertebral Augmentation

Percutaneous vertebral augmentation ("vertebroplasty"; PVP) was first performed by Galibert et al.[16] in 1984, and initially involved the augmentation of the vertebral body with polymethylmethacrylate (PMMA). PVP was first described in French literature in 1987,[16] but was not performed in the United States until 1994. Originally targeted for osteolytic metastasis, myeloma, and hemangioma, PVP resulted in early appreciable pain relief and a low complication rate.[16,20] Its indications now include osteoporotic vertebral collapse with chronic pain, expanding further to include treatment of asymptomatic vertebral collapse and even prophylactic intervention for at-risk vertebral bodies.[1] Nevertheless, the treatment of acute fractures in ambulatory patients and prophylactic treatment remains controversial.[2] In fact, vertebral augmentation itself is somewhat controversial, with questions concerning a lack of defined indications, expected complications, outcome measures, and the results after long-term follow-up.[15] In addition, the PMMA bone filler has associated problems (e.g., epidural leakage, thermal necrosis, inability to integrate with bone, handling difficulties, and toxicity to patient and operator).[13,15]

Kyphoplasty is a newer, minimally invasive technique with a number of potential advantages over PVP, including lower risk of cement extravasation and better restoration of vertebral body height.[25] The first kyphoplasty was performed in August 1998; up to January 2004, more than 30,000 patients in the United States have had kyphoplasty procedures for more than 40,000 fractures. More than 90% of patients reported significant pain relief. During the procedure, a cannula is introduced into the vertebral

---

[*]References 4,24,27,31,32,37,38.

1309

body, followed by insertion of an inflatable bone tamp (IBT), which when deployed, reduces the compression fracture and restores the vertebral body toward its original height, while creating a cavity to be filled with bone cement. The cement augmentation is therefore done with more control into the low-pressure environment of the preformed cavity with viscous, partially cured cement.

## Indications

Vertebroplasty or kyphoplasty are currently indicated for progressive, painful osteoporotic or osteolytic vertebral body wedge compression fractures. Kyphoplasty may be considered for both acute and chronic fractures. Similar to any other fragility fracture the goals are to restore stability, anatomic alignment, and function as soon as safely possible. Like hip fracture surgery, the results are most predictable with immediate intervention.

The contraindications include any systemic pathology, such as sepsis, local active osteomyelitis, prolonged bleeding times, and other cardiopulmonary pathology, which would preclude the safe completion of the procedure under either conscious sedation or general anesthesia. Other relative contraindications include nonosteolytic infiltrative spinal metastases, vertebral bodies with deficient posterior cortices, and patients presenting with neurologic signs or symptoms. Certain burst or vertebrae plana fracture configurations may be technically difficult, are relative contraindications, and should be assessed on the merits of the case.

## Preoperative Planning

For both vertebroplasty and kyphoplasty procedures the preoperative planning involves diagnostic and technical exercises. Radiographs, computed tomographic (CT) scans, magnetic resonance imaging (MRI) scans, and nuclear medicine bone scans are used to confirm the fracture and define the anatomy. The most reliable tool for diagnosing spinal compression fractures is the MRI. The sagittal MRI cuts with short tau inversion recovery (STIR) sequences highlighting the marrow edema changes associated with the compression fractures. The sagittal and axial CT and MRI scans are particularly important to plan the trajectory for the percutaneous procedure.

## Positioning and Anesthesia

The patient is positioned prone on the operating room table, or in the radiology suite on a spinal frame or cushioned bolsters. If possible, positioning should promote extension of the thoracic and lumbar regions of the spine. Biplane fluoroscopy, a single C-arm or two C-arms (with one positioned for anteroposterior [AP] views and one for lateral views), are positioned and tested to ensure all vertebral landmarks (pedicles and cortices) can be defined. This may be difficult in some patients with severe osteoporosis, or more likely with poor C-arm equipment. In these cases the procedure should not be performed.

Local anesthesia with intravenous conscious sedation, or general anesthesia, may be used on the patient. If the patient has two or more fractures, it may be more reasonable to perform the procedure with the patient under general anesthesia, or to perform multiple procedures at different sessions. Patients typically can tolerate a single-level procedure under local anesthetic with little discomfort. In the medically ill patient local anesthesia may be preferable.

## Approaches

### Transpedicular Approach

A transpedicular vertebral body cannulation (Figure 97.1) can usually be used from T5-L5 when performing a vertebroplasty. With kyphoplasty the IBTs need to be placed medially within the vertebral body, making transpedicular appropriate from T10-L5. With correct placement the pedicle guides the needle into the vertebral body relatively safely. Limitations in using the transpedicular approach include inadequate pedicle width, usually above level T8 (occasionally at the thoracolumbar junction) and lateral angulation of the pedicle, with respect to the vertebral body. Additionally, vertebral body fractures that are compressed to a level below the pedicles may not be treatable with this approach.

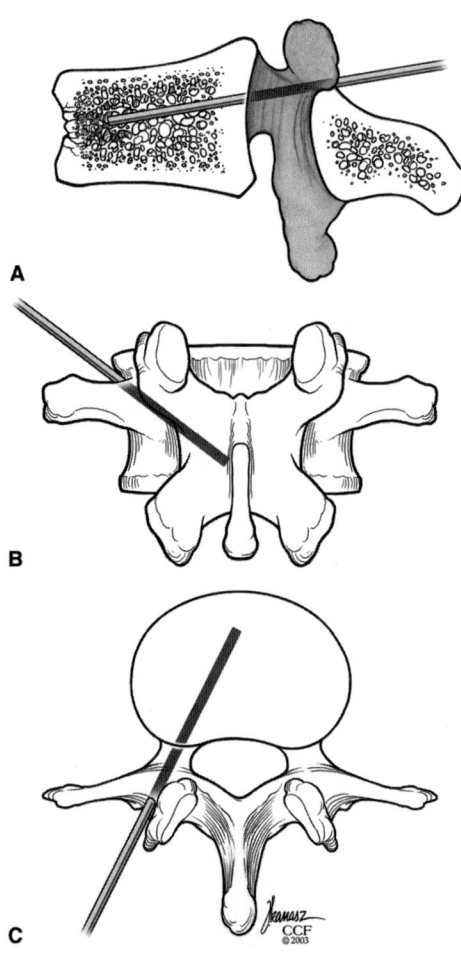

**Figure 97.1** Transpedicular access.

The procedure begins with a small stab wound positioned slightly lateral to the appropriate pedicle. The appropriate spinal needle (11-gauge [2.5mm] biopsy needle) is directed to the posterior, lateral, superior corner of the pedicle (10 and 2 o'clock positions), or centered directly over the pedicle. The former position provides the most flexibility in directing the needle. The needle is slowly advanced toward the vertebral body through bone 1mm at a time with frequent checks on the AP and lateral images. While advancing the needle ensure on the AP image that the needle tip is always lateral to the medial border of the pedicle until the junction of the body and pedicle is reached. At this point the needle tip on the AP film should be just at the medial pedicular ring margin to safely ensure that the canal has not been violated.

A 10-degree en face fluoroscopy (C-arm) view, looking straight down the pedicle, has the advantage that the physician can visualize the edges of the pedicle and determine that the tool is contained within the pedicle. With experience, however, some physicians use just a true AP view for needle placement to decrease C-arm movement during needle placement in the early parts of the procedure. Before advancing the needle anteriorly into the pedicle, the lateral view should be checked to be sure the needle is directed toward the vertebral body. If the patient has a rostral fracture the needle should be placed inferior to the midline. If the fracture is through the caudal end-plate the needle should be placed just superior to the midline. If the height of the vertebral body is 1.5cm or less the needle should be aimed at the midpoint of the anterior cortex on lateral view.

### Extrapedicular Approach

The extrapedicular approach (Figure 97.2) is an alternative for the thoracic vertebral bodies with small pedicles, or for midthoracic vertebral bodies, since a transpedicular approach will result in lateral balloon placement in kyphoplasty. The entry point is immediately rostral and slightly lateral to the pedicle, just medial to the rib head. This may involve actually cannulating the rib head and entering the vertebral body through the rib facet on the posterosuperolateral corner of the vertebral body. Ideally, the guide needle enters the pedicle slightly laterally and then is directed into the vertebral body. With this approach the chest cavity is protected by the rib head laterally, and the docking point on the pedicle is below the equator of the spinal canal (on the lateral image); therefore proper placement has minimal risk. If, on the other hand, the approach is too lateral and/or too proximal and medial, the risks are obvious.

### Posterolateral Approach

In lumbar vertebral bodies with narrow pedicles, or for ease and rapidity of insertion, the dorsolateral approach may be used (Figure 97.3). This is identical to the one described by Ottolenghi[33] for lumbar vertebral biopsies. The skin entry point is 8 to 10cm lateral to the midline, with the needle directed 40 to 50 degrees from the sagittal plane. The entry point in the bone is at the junction of the pedicle and dorsal vertebral body on the lateral radiograph. Often this requires a trajectory through the

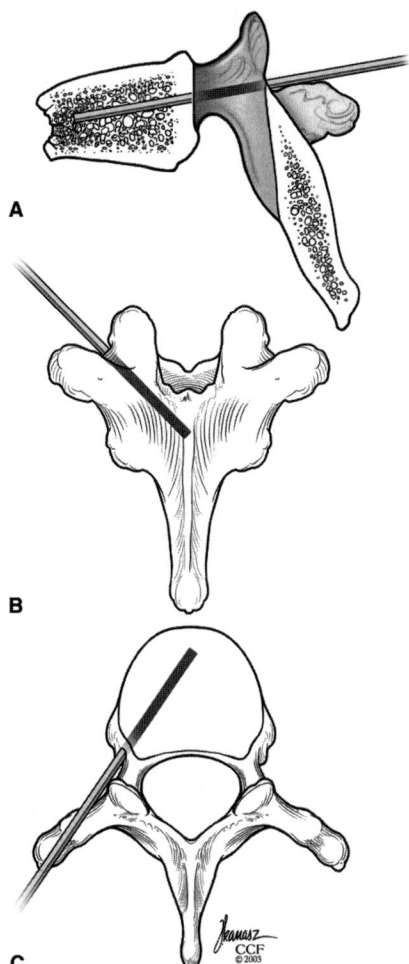

**Figure 97.2** Extrapedicular access.

transverse process. This is a safe zone because the exiting nerves are out of harm's way.

## Techniques

### Percutaneous Vertebroplasty

A transpedicular vertebral body cannulation can usually be used from T5-L5 when performing a vertebroplasty. Once the vertebral body is cannulated, the 11-gauge biopsy needle is advanced into the vertebral body, guided by AP and lateral views. The goal is to remain in the center of the pedicle, bringing the needle within 5mm of the wall of the vertebral body. It is important to image frequently using AP and lateral views to ensure proper needle placement because of the proximity of the pedicle to the spinal canal medially, nerve roots laterally, and other vital structures anterior to the vertebral body. This technique is repeated on the contralateral side. Once appropriately positioned, the center stylets of the needles are removed.

The next step involves the injection of 5ml of contrast medium through the biopsy needle. This will show whether the needle is placed in, or if there is direct communication with the venous sinuses, in which case the needle is advanced or retracted to a safer position to avoid an immediate vascular fill during cement injection. This is repeated on the contralateral side. Many patients find this uncomfortable (describing a stinging sensation), and should be warned if under local anesthesia.

There are currently no commercially available bone cement mixtures with enough barium to allow visualization during cement injection. Therefore additional sterile barium must be added to the mixture. To accomplish this, it is recommended that 6g of sterile barium be mixed with PMMA powder before adding the liquid monomer. Normally, within a minute, the mix goes from powdery to thick to soupy in consistency. When the mix can pour off the spatula in a thin liquid stream, multiple (8 to 10) 1ml syringes (through the top with the plunger removed) are loaded. The plungers are then refitted into the syringes.

The syringes are sequentially attached onto the Luer-Lok of one of the biopsy needles and the cement is slowly injected, under fluoroscopic visualization, into the vertebral body while looking through the lateral view to observe if cement projects dorsally toward the spinal canal. It is critical to perform this aspect of the procedure under real-time fluoroscopy, because maximal hand pressures are usually required to place the bone cement into the vertebral body. Although cement leakage is common, embolization is rare, as are clinically significant canal protrusions.

If cement leaks from the vertebral body as soon as it is introduced, one should wait 30 to 60 seconds, then resume

slowly injecting the cement. (The early injection may occlude crevices, thereby preventing further leakage.) The procedure is finished when: (1) cement has filled the ventral two thirds of the vertebral body, (2) cement leaks, even if one has stopped and reinjected, or (3) cement flows back toward the spinal canal. The procedure is repeated on the other side, if possible. Before moving the patient, intraoperative images are usually obtained to ensure that cement has not entered in the spinal canal. The incisions can be closed with single stitches and sterile bandages. The patient should remain prone for 10-15 minutes until the cement hardens.

## Kyphoplasty (see Figures 97.4 to 97.8)

A biopsy needle is a convenient way to begin a kyphoplasty, following strategically placed 3mm incisions and the careful needle advancement technique with multiple images as described previously. Once the needle is just inside the dorsal cortex, the stylet is removed and the guide pin is inserted down the shaft of the needle until 1 to 2mm of the guide pin tip shows. Placement is checked using a lateral view. While holding the guide pin in place, the needle is removed and guide pin placement is reconfirmed with a lateral fluoroscopic view. The blunt dissector is advanced over the guide pin. If this requires some force, put the T-handle onto the blunt dissector and tap with a mallet. This should be performed with caution, and placement confirmed with lateral images. One should stop advancing when the tip of the guide pin is a few millimeters into the vertebral body. The guide pin is removed and the cannula over the blunt dissector is placed. It is advanced to just beyond the junction of the pedicle and body on the lateral view using hand pressure or gentle mallet tapping. When the cannula is appropriately placed, a drill bit is placed down the cannula. With the use of manual control, the drill bit is twisted to enter the vertebral body. The final position is just dorsal to the ventral cortex. When the drill is halfway across the vertebral body in the lateral view, the AP view is assessed to ensure that the drill bit is approximately halfway between the pedicle and the spinous process. If the drill is too medial on the AP radiograph, the spinal canal may be threatened. On the AP view, if the drill is directed straight ahead without medial deviation, it may advance laterally out of the cortex. On the lateral view it should be within the rostral and caudal edge of the

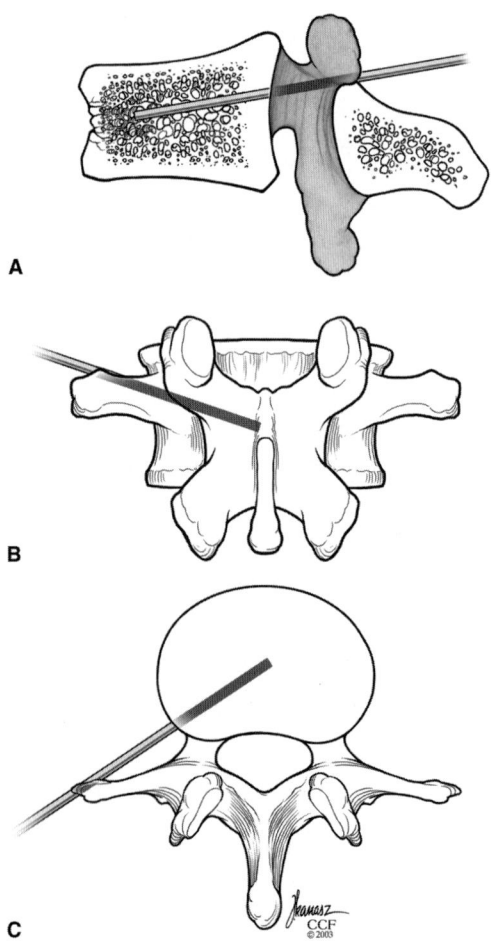

**Figure 97.3** Posterolateral access.

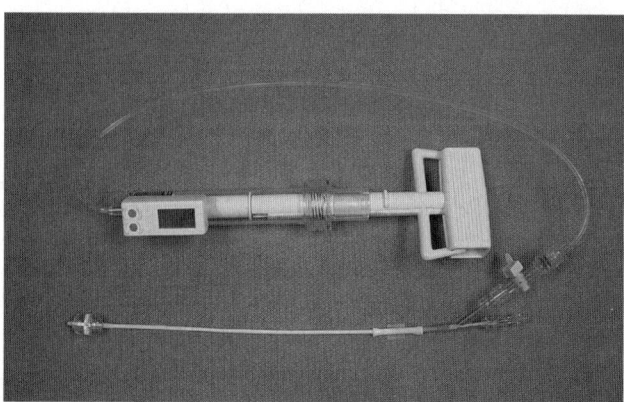

**Figure 97.4** Inflatable bone tamp. (Courtesy KyphX®, Kyphon, Inc. Sunnyvale, Calif.)

pedicle. When the drill bit is positioned appropriately on the image, it should be removed and the IBT should be inserted through the same cannula.

The inflatable bone tamp is prepared with contrast medium (dilution of 60% contrast mixed with saline) to facilitate imaging during inflation. The balloon is inflated using a manometer with a digital pressure gauge. The initial injection holds the balloon in place while the tools are placed in the contralateral pedicle and another balloon inserted. Alternate slow filling of the balloons by adding 1ml or by raising the pressure to 150psi (whichever comes first). There should be a gradual reduction of pressure after the bone expands and the cavity is created. Alternate balloon filling should continue until appropriate pressures are reached and fracture reduction is maximized safely. As

balloon volumes increase beyond 2ml, only 0.5ml or less should be introduced into each balloon until a stopping point is reached.

Fracture reduction using the IBT is guided by: (1) desired reduction, (2) proximity of IBT to cortical walls as observed on AP, lateral, and oblique views, (3) pressure readings remaining at the rated maximum of 220psi, or (4) reaching maximum rated balloon volume (4ml for the 15mm length or 6ml for the 20mm length). With the observations of any of these guidelines, inflation should cease. Inflation should proceed in small volume increments while trading sides. The IBTs should remain inflated with a similar volume. The inflation path and proximity to cortices should be monitored using frequent AP and lateral views.

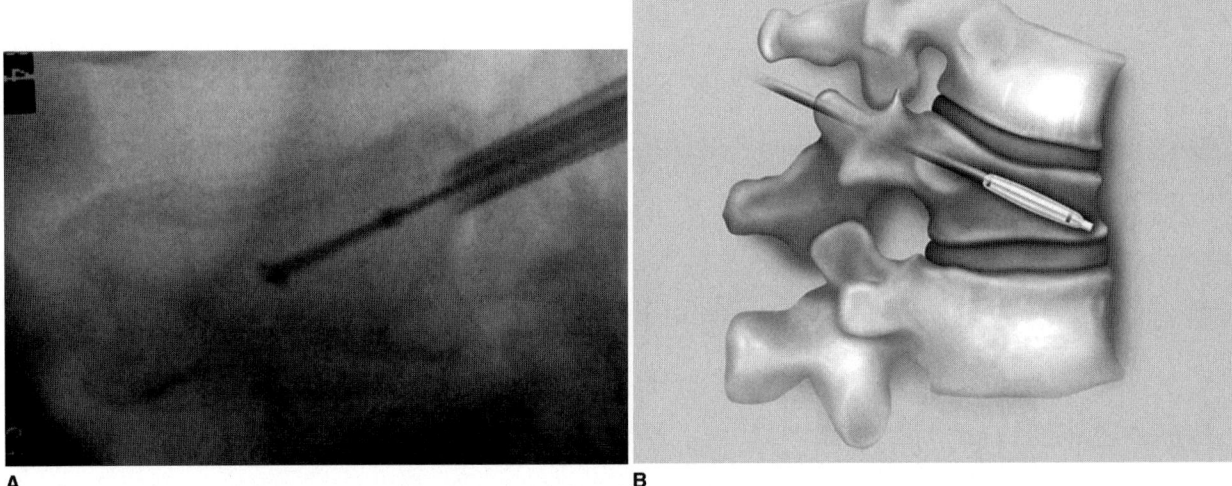

**A**                                                          **B**

**Figure 97.5** Radiograph (**A**) and drawing (**B**) of inflatable bone tamp in position.

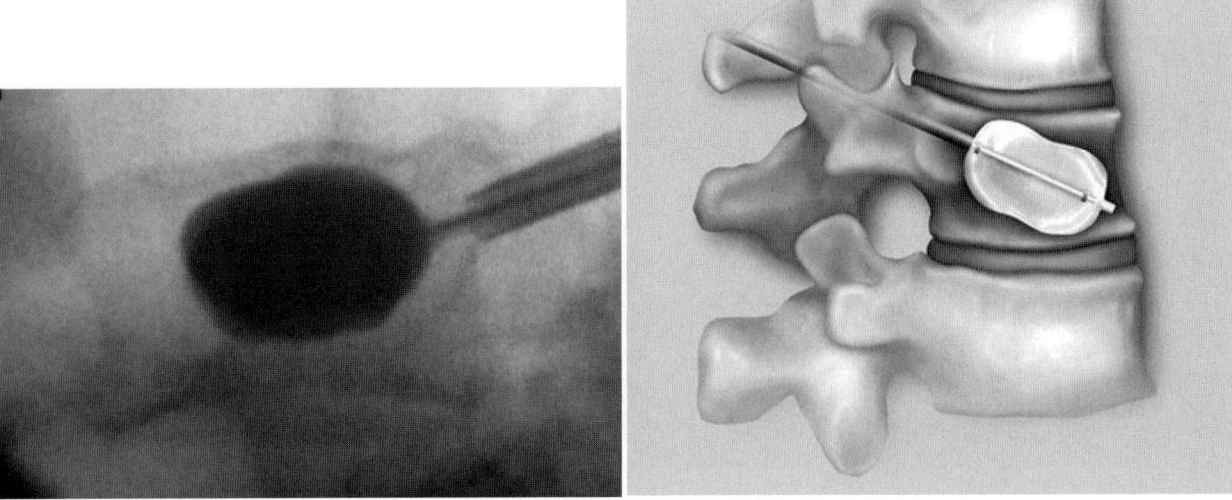

**A**                                                          **B**

**Figure 97.6** Radiograph (**A**) and drawing (**B**) of inflatable bone tamp inflated.

The risks related to balloon failure are generally minimal because the pressure rapidly decays to zero, a small volume of contrast medium and saline often leak out, and the IBT can be safely removed. However, contrast medium sensitivity is a concern. The risks to IBT inflation beyond the cortices are the same as those with a conventional bone tamp, and can be avoided by proper placement and careful monitoring.

Once appropriate volume and reduction have occurred, the IBT is deflated and slowly rotated, and the inflation device is removed. Because the bone is impacted and the patient is prone without gravitational forces loading the spinal column, loss of reduction usually does not occur. However, this has been observed in acute fractures (less than a month) and can be prevented in a bilateral procedure by maintaining inflation of one IBT while stabilizing the other side with PMMA.

If the treating physician chooses PMMA to fill the cavity, the mix ratio and setting times should be trialed before a clinical case, because each cement brand has its own characteristics. The cement is ready for application once it no longer sticks to the surgeon's gloves or drips (by gravity) from the mixing utensil. In any event, 6g of sterile barium powder must be added to enhance visualization during the fill procedure. Once mixed, the cement is poured into a 20ml syringe with the plunger removed. Remove the stylet from the cement cannula and attach the nozzle to the Luer of the 20ml syringe. Each cement cannula holds 1.5ml. Knowing the volume of the void from the volume of inflation medium used in each IBT, the cement cannula is filled to exceed that volume by approximately 1ml.

When ready to fill, one or both IBTs are deflated and, using lateral C-arm guidance, a cement cannula is inserted through the working cannula to the anterior wall of the

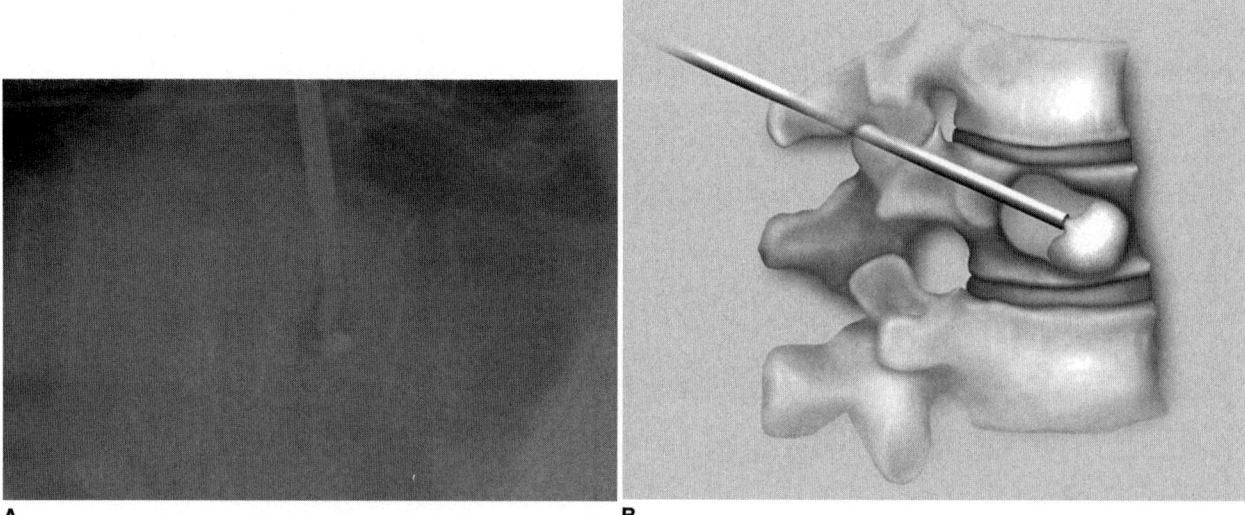

**A**                                                        **B**

**Figure 97.7** Radiograph (**A**) and drawing (**B**) of cement deposition.

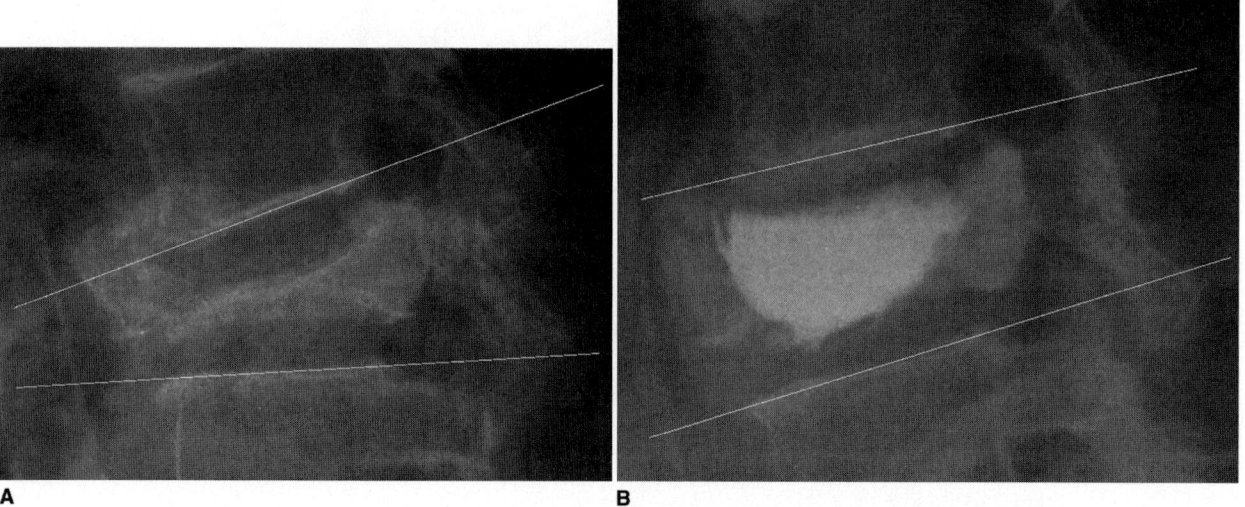

**A**                                                        **B**

**Figure 97.8** (**A** and **B**) Radiographs from a representative case of height restoration. Vertebral height was restored by kyphoplasty procedure. Segmental kyphosis was also corrected.

vertebral body. Confirm placement on AP and lateral images. The cement cannula stylet is used to gently push the selected viscous bone filler from the cement cannula while the cement cannula is withdrawn to the level of the middle of the cavity. With continued filling the volume of the cement grows around the cement cannula as it is held in place in the middle of the void. Leaks generally do not occur, unless the bone filler is too runny or a cortex was violated. If filler begins to escape anteriorly, or through the end plates, stop injecting for at least 90 seconds. Repeat the process from side to side if necessary. Once hardened, the cannula should be twisted to break off any filler on its edges and then pulled out. A final AP and lateral radiograph is obtained to ensure that no filler has escaped into the spinal canal. The patient is left in position on the table until the cement has hardened. Incisions are sutured as clinically indicated.

## Results

### Percutaneous Vertebroplasty

Vertebroplasty data from nearly 400 patients have been reported in several case series.[*] The longest reported follow-up is 3 years; although the first paper on vertebroplasty was published in 1987. Pain has been reported to be reduced in 70% to 90% of patients. There have been no reported cement failures, and only two reported cases of fracture progression in treated vertebral bodies (caused by inadequate cement fill). Barr et al.[2] reported the results of 47 patients treated with vertebroplasty with an average follow-up of 18 months. The report outlines marked to complete pain relief in only 63% of patients with osteoporotic VCFs. Vertebroplasty, however, does not address the spinal deformity. Also, this technique requires a high-pressure cement injection using low viscosity cement, thus

---

[*]References 7,10,12,20,28,41.

increasing the risk of cement leaks through the fracture clefts or the venous sinuses.

## Kyphoplasty

### Clinical Results

In a phase 1 Institutional Review Board approved study,[25] 70 consecutive kyphoplasty procedures were performed in 30 patients over 34 sessions. The mean age was 68.6 years (range 48-86). The indications included painful primary (n = 20) or secondary (n = 4) osteoporotic VCFs for a total of 24 patients unresponsive to nonoperative modalities. Another six patients presented with painful compression fractures caused by multiple myeloma. The mean duration of symptoms was 3.5 months (0.5-12). Outcome data was obtained by comparing preoperative and latest postoperative SF-36 scores. In this study all 30 patients tolerated the procedure well, and improvement in pain and mobility was seen early. Virtually all patients subjectively reported immediate relief of their typical fracture pain, and no patient complained of worse pain at the treated levels. The levels treated ranged from T6 to L5, the majority at the thoracolumbar junction (T11-7, T12-14, L1-9). Seventy percent of the levels treated showed a 47% restoration of the lost height. Thirty percent of the levels treated showed no appreciable height restoration even though generous cavities were created within the collapsed vertebral bodies. SF-36 scores for bodily pain, physical function, vitality and role physical subscales all showed statistically significant improvement. At final follow-up there were five clinically insignificant cement leaks (8% overall), and no major systemic complications or neurologic injuries related directly to use of this technique or the IBT.

### Biopsy *(Figures 97.9 and 97.10)*

A diagnostic bone biopsy can be easily performed during a kyphoplasty procedure and does not affect the safety of the procedure if done appropriately. The authors

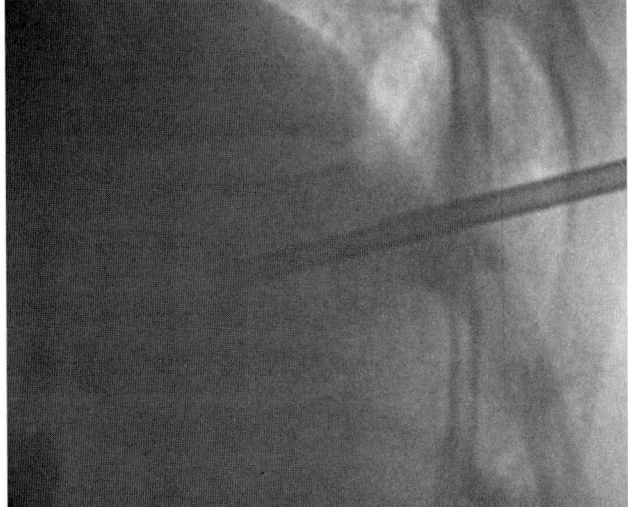
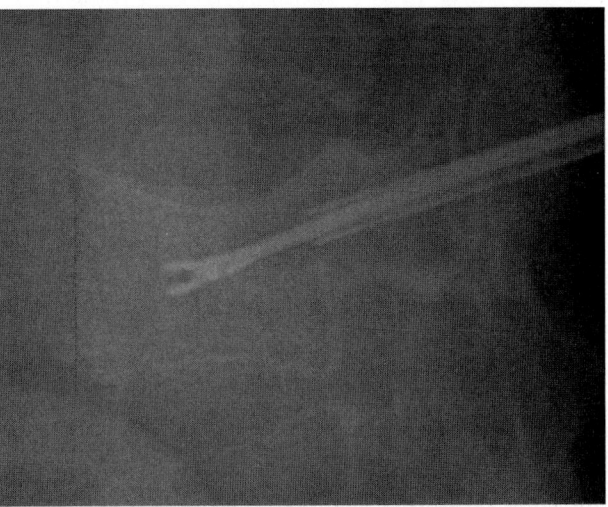

**A**                                                                                              **B**

**Figure 97.9** Intraoperative radiographs showing biopsy procedure. Biopsy trephine (**A**) and pituitary (**B**) can be used to take biopsy before vertebral augmentation.

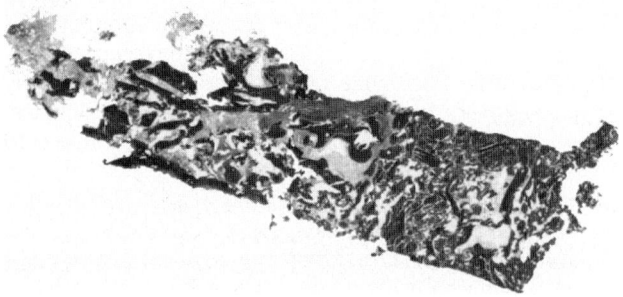

**Figure 97.10** Biopsy specimen obtained from collapsed vertebra (stained with toluidine blue).

histologically evaluated 149 biopsies obtained from 115 patients during 210 kyphoplasty procedures. These biopsies showed partially necrotic fragments of bone as well as areas of fibrosis and variable stages of woven bone, suggesting ongoing fracture healing.[39] Twenty-two (15%) of 149 biopsy specimens showed a marked increase in osteoid in undecalcified sections. These thickened osteoid seams may suggest osteomalacia. Osteoid can be increased either because of increased bone remodeling activity, or because of a mineralization defect. Tetracycline labeling is the only method of distinguishing between these two diagnoses. Careful administration of tetracycline labels may help identify any correlation between vertebral fracture and osteomalacia. Also in this series, the biopsies of four patients provided a definite diagnosis of plasma cell dyscrasia in otherwise unsuspected or unknown spinal lesions. These findings suggest that the biopsy is useful for all the kyphoplasty cases to rule out any occult lesions.

### Human Retrieved Specimens (*Figures 97.11 and 97.12*)

In spite of reported good clinical results, several aspects of the kyphoplasty procedure are controversial, including the optimum methods of mixing and injecting the cement, the potential importance of a foreign body reaction at the cement-bone interface, efficacy of bone tamp usage, the use of relatively high concentrations of radiopaque agents and antibiotics in the cement, and the clinical indications for the procedure. A few histologic documentations of human vertebrae after vertebral augmentation are currently available. Four vertebral bodies from two cases ranging from 1 month to 2 years after cement augmentation were analyzed histologically.[40] In this study the histology of vertebrae treated using the kyphoplasty technique revealed a dense, cancellous shell around the cement mantle. This suggests that the tamping had displaced bone, essentially autografting the space around the cement. Bone immediately around the cement did not show extensive necrosis. However, foreign body giant cells contained material consistent with cement particles and/or barium sulfate. Particles were also identified within vascular spaces. Further histologic evaluation may help clarify the safety and efficacy of kyphoplasty.

### Incidence of Adjacent and Remote Fractures

One theoretical issue continuously raised by the spine community regards the incidence of remote and adjacent

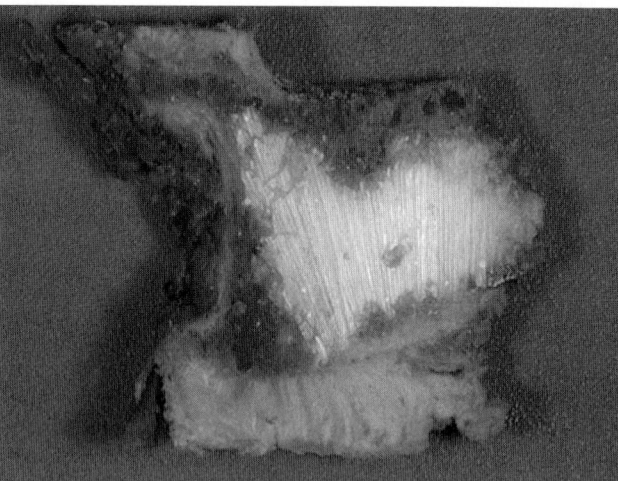

**Figure 97.11** Photograph of a section of human vertebra retrieved during reconstructive surgery. Most of the vertebral body is occupied by PMMA.

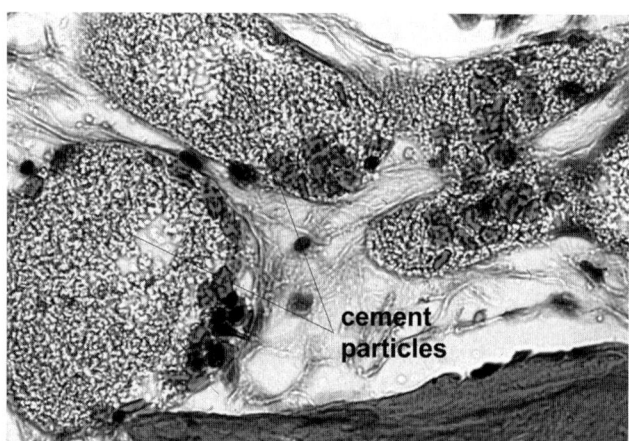

**Figure 97.12** Cement particles and/or barium sulfate were found within vascular spaces of the vertebral body in an autopsy specimen.

level VCFs after an index VCF has been augmented by either vertebroplasty or kyphoplasty. Left untreated the incidence of subsequent vertebral fracture after an index fracture is reported as approximately 20%.[26] One reference reported a 52% rate of remote or adjacent level fractures after vertebroplasty.[17] Harrop *et al.*[18] reported that the incidence of post-kyphoplasty VCFs in the primary osteoporotic patients was 11.25% (nine fractures in 80 patients), whereas the incidence in the steroid-induced osteoporotic patients was 48.6% (17 fractures in 35 patients). These results imply that the intervention—kyphoplasty—in primary osteoporotic patients does not increase the rate of remote or adjacent level fractures compared to the historic natural history reports. These results also imply that the secondary osteoporotic patients are in fact at increased risk for subsequent VCFs compared to primary osteoporotic patients, although there is no natural history benchmark to which we can compare this rate.

## Complications

### Percutaneous Vertebroplasty

Cement leakage rates have been reported to occur in 34% to 67% of cases, but are usually clinically insignificant.[°] Reported major complications caused by cement leaks include increased pain, radiculopathies, pulmonary embolism, and spinal cord compression. Cement leakage that leads to radiculopathy or spinal cord injury is more common after the treatment of pathologic fractures that resulted from metastasis than for osteoporotic fractures.

### Kyphoplasty

In a phase one Institutional Review Board approved study,[25] cement extravasation was seen at six (8.6%) levels. Cement entered the epidural space in one patient, and in the remaining cases cement appeared to leak through the superior endplate or a sidewall crack. No problems were identified clinically as a result of these extravasations immediately after surgery or at final follow-up. In prospective multicenter series there were six (1.1%) major complications, four (0.75%) of which were neurologic complications. These were directly attributable to breach of technique.

## Other Issues

An open question in both PVP and kyphoplasty is the mechanism of pain relief. The most intuitive explanation involves simple mechanical stabilization of the fracture; the cement stabilizes vertebral bodies and offloads the facet joints. However, another possibility is that analgesia results from local chemical, vascular, or thermal effects of PMMA on nerve endings in surrounding tissue.[8,29] Supporting this concept is the lack of correlation between cement volume and pain relief.[9,11] Further evidence against an effect resulting solely from mechanical stabilization is the fact that PVP typically does not restore lost vertebral body height and therefore does not correct altered biomechanics.[2,19]

## Osteolytic Vertebral Compression Fractures

Osteolytic destruction of the vertebral bodies secondary to metastatic disease or multiple myeloma affects up to 70% of patients.[30,36] Pain is the initial complaint in up to 95% of patients, despite the fact that more than 50% of spinal metastases are asymptomatic.[30,36] Only 10% of patients with spinal metastases present with neurologic signs or symptoms on initial presentation.[30] With modern advances in oncologic treatment patient survival has improved to the point where what was once life threatening could now be considered a chronic disease. Unfortunately, the oncologic treatment itself also contributes to the already present osteolytic bone loss. With the increased survival and ongoing bone loss osteolytic VCFs are becoming much more of a clinical and functional problem for these patients. The indications for surgical intervention are reported as being progressive collapse, neurologic deterioration, and intractable pain. However, surgical intervention in this patient group is typically regarded as very difficult by virtue of the comorbid conditions and the poor bone quality. Similar to the scenario with osteoporotic compression fractures, possible complications associated with these osteolytic fractures include cord compression, urinary retention, ileus, and intractable pain, as well as pulmonary compromise (a 9% loss in predicted forced vital capacity with each vertebral fracture).[21,24] Other chronic sequelae include deconditioning, deformity, insomnia, and depression, resulting in substantial physical, functional, and psychosocial impairment. To alleviate these issues, percutaneous, minimally invasive, vertebral augmentation techniques have recently evolved and show promising preliminary results for this debilitated group of patients.

### Multiple Myeloma

Multiple myeloma is a monoclonal proliferation of malignant plasma cells that usually affects the bone marrow. Excessive bone resorption resulting from an increase of proinflammatory cytokines is a characteristic feature of the disease.[23] This tumor is grossly a very soft vascular tumor, as evidenced by the backflow of blood from the working cannulae during kyphoplasty. The near-fluid consistency of the tumor and the lytic nature of the bone make it easy for the IBT to displace tissue in the act of reducing the fracture and creating the cavity. This then results in impressive cement filling of the vertebrae. Dudeney et al.[14] reported satisfying results in the treatment of osteolytic VCFs caused by multiple myeloma. Fifty-five consecutive kyphoplasty procedures were performed over 27 sessions in 18 patients. The mean age of patients was 63.5 (48 to 79) years, the mean duration of symptoms was 11 months, and the mean follow-up was 7.4 months. There were no major complications related directly to use of this technique. On average, 34% of height loss at the time of fracture was restored. After stratifying for those where height was not restored, the remaining vertebral bodies showed an average of 56% height restoration. Asymptomatic cement leakage occurred at 2/55 levels (4%). Significant improvement in SF-36 scores occurred for bodily pain: 23.2 to 55.4 ($p$ = .0008), physical function: 21.3 to 50.6 ($p$ = .0010), vitality: 31.3 to 47.5 ($p$ = .010), and social functioning: 40.6 to 64.8 ($p$ = .014). The authors concluded that the kyphoplasty technique was efficacious in the treatment of osteolytic VCFs caused by multiple myeloma, and associated with early clinical improvement of pain and function, as well as some restoration of vertebral body height in these patients. The effects of potential tumor dissemination, in what is already widespread disease, is not known. Any significant systemic effects are not suspected and have not been noted in the initial study group.[14]

### Other Tumors

In an ongoing evaluation of nonmyelomatous osteolytic collapse the results have remained very favorable. From April 1999 to September 2002, we treated 11 patients of nonmyelomatous osteolytic vertebral collapse (8 breast, 1 lung, 1 pharyngeal basal cell, 1 unknown origin). The patients reported statistically significant improvements in

---

[°]References 3,9,12,20,34,41.

their objective outcome scores. Barr *et al.*[2] reported his results with osteolytic metastatic vertebral collapse in eight patients and revealed that only four patients experienced any pain relief. In this group of patients there was a 6% complication rate.[2]

Other solid organ-type tumors and previously irradiated tumors may not be as compliant to the IBT while reducing the fracture or creating a cavity. Further investigation into various modalities of treatment needs to be performed before a definitive recommendation on indications in other tumor types can be made.

## Summary

Vertebral augmentation by vertebroplasty or kyphoplasty, according to the early studies, are clearly efficacious treatments for painful progressive osteoporotic or osteolytic compression fractures. Using kyphoplasty to create a cavity and realign the spine appears to have significant advantages over vertebroplasty. Kyphoplasty also minimizes the risk of cement leakage by compacting the cancellous bone to the periphery and sealing off the fracture clefts, and by creating a cavity into which cement is poured, as opposed to injected under pressure. This technique may prevent propagation of further fractures by reducing the collapsed vertebral bodies toward its native height and thus normalizing the sagittal spinal alignment. Both techniques have proved to be valuable, and there is no doubt that with future developments other techniques will also evolve.

## REFERENCES

1. Bai B, Jazrawi LM, Kummer FJ, *et al*: The use of an injectable, biodegradable calcium phosphate bone substitute for the prophylactic augmentation of osteoporotic vertebrae and the management of vertebral compression fractures. *Spine* 24:1521-1526, 1999.
2. Barr JD, Barr MS, Lemley TJ, *et al*: Percutaneous vertebroplasty for pain relief and spinal stabilization. *Spine* 25:923-928, 2000.
3. Chiras J, Depriester C, Weill A, *et al*: Percutaneous vertebral surgery. Techniques and indications. *J Neuroradiol* 24:45-59, 1997.
4. Cook DJ, Guyatt GH, Adachi JD, *et al*: Quality of life issues in women with vertebral fractures due to osteoporosis. *Arthritis Rheum* 36:750-756, 1993.
5. Cooper C, Atkinson EJ, O'Fallon WM, *et al*: Incidence of clinically diagnosed vertebral fractures: a population-based study in Rochester, Minnesota, 1985-1989. *J Bone Miner Res* 7:221-227, 1992.
6. Cooper C, Campion G, Melton LJ III: Hip fractures in the elderly: a world-wide projection. *Osteoporos Int* 2:285-289, 1992.
7. Cortet B, Cotten A, Boutry N, *et al*: Percutaneous vertebroplasty in patients with osteolytic metastases or multiple myeloma. *Rev Rheum Engl Ed* 64:177-183, 1997.
8. Cotten A, Boutry N, Cortet B, *et al*: Percutaneous vertebroplasty: state of the art. *Radiographics* 18:311-320; discussion 20-23, 1998.
9. Cotten A, Dewatre F, Cortet B, *et al*: Percutaneous vertebroplasty for osteolytic metastases and myeloma: effects of the percentage of lesion filling and the leakage of methyl methacrylate at clinical follow-up. *Radiology* 200:525-530, 1996.
10. Cotten A, Duquesnoy B: Vertebroplasty: current data and future potential. *Rev Rheum Engl Ed* 64:645-649, 1997.
11. Dean JR, Ison KT, Gishen P: The strengthening effect of percutaneous vertebroplasty. *Clin Radiol* 55:471-476, 2000.
12. Deramond H, Depriester C, Galibert P, *et al*: Percutaneous vertebroplasty with polymethylmethacrylate. Technique, indications, and results. *Radiol Clin North Am* 36:533-546, 1998.
13. Deramond H, Wright NT, Belkoff SM: Temperature elevation caused by bone cement polymerization during vertebroplasty. *Bone* 25:17S-21S, 1999.
14. Dudeney S, Lieberman IH, Reinhardt MK, *et al*: Kyphoplasty in the treatment of osteolytic vertebral compression fractures as a result of multiple myeloma. *J Clin Oncol* 20:2382-2387, 2002.
15. Einhorn TA: Vertebroplasty: an opportunity to do something really good for patients. *Spine* 25:1051-1052, 2000.
16. Galibert P, Deramond H, Rosat P, *et al*: [Preliminary note on the treatment of vertebral angioma by percutaneous acrylic vertebroplasty]. *Neurochirurgie* 33:166-168, 1987.
17. Grados F, Depriester C, Cayrolle G, *et al*: Long-term observations of vertebral osteoporotic fractures treated by percutaneous vertebroplasty. *Rheumatology* (Oxford) 39:1410-1414, 2000.
18. Harrop JS, Prpa B, Reinhardt MK, *et al*: Incidence of remote and adjacent vertebral compression fractures after kyphoplasty. *Spine* 2004 (in press).
19. Heini PF, Walchli B, Berlemann U: Percutaneous transpedicular vertebroplasty with PMMA: operative technique and early results. A prospective study for the treatment of osteoporotic compression fractures. *Eur Spine J* 9:445-450, 2000.
20. Jensen ME, Evans AJ, Mathis JM, *et al*: Percutaneous polymethylmethacrylate vertebroplasty in the treatment of osteoporotic vertebral body compression fractures: technical aspects. *AJNR Am J Neuroradiol* 18:1897-1904, 1997.
21. Kado DM, Browner WS, Palermo L, *et al*: Vertebral fractures and mortality in older women: a prospective study. Study of Osteoporotic Fractures Research Group. *Arch Intern Med* 159:1215-1220, 1999.
22. Kostuik JP, Heggeness MH: Surgery of the osteoporotic spine. In *The Adult Spine*, ed 2, Philadelphia, Lippincott-Raven, 1997, pp 1639-1664.
23. Lecouvet FE, Vande Berg BC, Maldague BE, *et al*: Vertebral compression fractures in multiple myeloma. I. Distribution and appearance at MR imaging. *Radiology* 204:195-199, 1997.
24. Leech JA, Dulberg C, Kellie S, *et al*: Relationship of lung function to severity of osteoporosis in women. *Am Rev Respir Dis* 141:68-71, 1990.
25. Lieberman IH, Dudeney S, Reinhardt MK, *et al*: Initial outcome and efficacy of "kyphoplasty" in the treatment of painful osteoporotic vertebral compression fractures. *Spine* 26:1631-1638, 2001.

26. Lindsay R, Silverman SL, Cooper C, *et al*: Risk of new vertebral fracture in the year following a fracture. *JAMA* 285:320-323, 2001.

27. Lyles KW, Lammers JE, Shipp KM, *et al*: Functional and mobility impairments associated with Paget's disease of bone. *J Am Geriatr Soc* 43:502-506, 1995.

28. Martin JB, Jean B, Sugiu K, *et al*: Vertebroplasty: clinical experience and follow-up results. *Bone* 25:11S-5S, 1999.

29. Mathis JM, Petri M, Naff N: Percutaneous vertebroplasty treatment of steroid-induced osteoporotic compression fractures. *Arthritis Rheum* 41:171-175, 1998.

30. McLain RF, Weinstein JN: Tumors of the spine. In Herkowitz HV, Garfin SR, Balderston RA, *et al* (eds): *The Spine*, ed 4, Philadelphia, WB Saunders, 1999, pp 1171-1206.

31. Nevitt MC, Ettinger B, Black DM, *et al*: The association of radiographically detected vertebral fractures with back pain and function: a prospective study. *Ann Intern Med* 128:793-800, 1998.

32. Oleksik A, Lips P, Dawson A, *et al*: Health-related quality of life in postmenopausal women with low BMD with or without prevalent vertebral fractures. *J Bone Miner Res* 15:1384-1392, 2000.

33. Ottolenghi CE: Aspiration biopsy of the spine. Technique for the thoracic spine and results of twenty-eight biopsies in this region and over-all results of 1050 biopsies of other spinal segments. *J Bone Joint Surg Am* 51:1531-1544, 1969.

34. Padovani B, Kasriel O, Brunner P, *et al*: Pulmonary embolism caused by acrylic cement: a rare complication of percutaneous vertebroplasty. *AJNR Am J Neuroradiol* 20:375-377, 1999.

35. Riggs BL, Melton LJ III: The worldwide problem of osteoporosis: insights afforded by epidemiology. *Bone* 17:S505-S511, 1995.

36. Sundaresan N, Krol G, Digiacinto G, *et al*: Metastatic tumors of the spine. In Sundaresan N, Schmidek HH, Schiller AL (eds): *Tumors of the Spine: Diagnosis and Clinical Management*. Philadelphia, WB Saunders, 1990, pp 279-304.

37. Schlaich C, Minne HW, Bruckner T, *et al*: Reduced pulmonary function in patients with spinal osteoporotic fractures. *Osteoporos Int* 8:261-267, 1998.

38. Silverman SL: The clinical consequences of vertebral compression fracture. *Bone* 13 (Suppl) 2:S27-S31, 1992.

39. Togawa D, Bauer TW, Lieberman IH, *et al*: Occult osteomalacia and myeloma in patients with osteoporotic compression fractures. *Eur Spine J* 12(Suppl 1):S3, 2003.

40. Togawa D, Bauer TW, Lieberman IH, Takikawa S: Histologic evaluation of human vertebral bodies after vertebral augmentation with polymethyl methacrylate. *Spine* 28:1521-1527, 2003.

41. Weill A, Chiras J, Simon JM, *et al*: Spinal metastases: indications for and results of percutaneous injection of acrylic surgical cement. *Radiology* 199:241-247, 1996.

# CHAPTER 98

# The Obese Patient

**Joseph S. Cheng, Meic H. Schmidt, Wade M. Mueller, and Edward C. Benzel**

Obesity and being overweight have been grouped as one of the leading health indicators in healthy people (2001), the nation's health objective for the first decade of the twenty-first century.[34] In 1999 an estimated 61% of U.S. adults were considered overweight or obese and an additional 13% of children and adolescents were overweight. There are now almost twice as many overweight children and three times as many overweight adolescents as compared to 1980, with approximately 300,000 deaths per year in the United States associated with obesity and being overweight.[2] In 2000 the total health care cost of obesity was estimated to be $117 billion, with many of these costs resulting from type 2 diabetes, coronary artery disease, and hypertension.[60] Although obesity has been associated with arthritic changes,[51] the impact of body weight on spinal disorders seems less clear.[27,56] However, it has also been shown that associated medical problems such as venous stasis and sleep apnea can significantly affect the outcome of spinal surgery. This chapter outlines the current management of the obese patient as it relates to spinal disorders and surgery.

## Diagnosis of Overweight and Obesity

The word *obesity* is derived from Latin roots meaning "to overeat," but now has become defined as "a disease of excess body fat."[25] Rather than a simple personality trait, this change in definition characterizes obesity as a complex disorder that develops through a combination of genetic, environmental, psychosocial, and physiological causes. In our current Western society, excess body fat accumulation commonly occurs because of a high caloric diet and low physical activity.

*Overweight* and *obesity* were terms originally used by the insurance industry to determine risk factors associated with an increase in morbidity and mortality, and the diagnosis determined by the amount of excess body fat. Fat is one of the basic components of the human body that is essential for survival, and the normal range of body fat is both age and gender dependent. In general, normal body fat percentage ranges from 13% to 16% in adult men and 20% to 24% in adult women, with being overweight and obesity occurring when these values are exceeded.

The measurement of body fat can be technically challenging. The most accurate method is the underwater immersion technique; however, this is impractical for routine use in patients. In the clinical setting skin fold and waist measurements, along with body weight for height measurements, seem to be the most practicable, but with less accuracy. In 1998 the World Health Organization (WHO), along with the National Institutes of Health (NIH), endorsed the use of the body mass index (BMI) as a measure of obesity, because it appears to correlate better with body fat than any other indicator of height and weight.[26,61]

The BMI, or Quetelet's index, is a mathematical formula in which the body weight in kilograms is divided by the square of the person's height in meters (BMI = body weight [kg]/height [m]$^2$). Over the years, BMI has been tabulated from medical and insurance data to derive standards to determine obesity. In general a BMI of 25 to 29.9kg/m$^2$ is considered overweight and a BMI greater than 30kg/m$^2$ (or a 20% increase over the ideal body weight as determined from actuarial tables) is deemed obese (Table 98.1). Severe or morbid obesity, as defined by Payne in the early 1960s, used an arbitrary definition of greater than 100lb or 45kg above the ideal body weight, but has also been defined as a BMI greater than 35.[25,56] Patients who are morbidly obese have the highest risk for perioperative morbidity and mortality. Further delineation was accomplished with the WHO standard, in which obesity has been classified into three groups with correlation of health risks as denoted by changes in morbidity and mortality (see Table 98.1). Class I obesity is defined as a BMI in the range of 30-34.9 and is associated with moderately increased morbidity and mortality as compared to the general population. Class II obesity is a BMI between 35 and 39.9 and is associated with a severe increase in health risks. Class III obesity occurs when the BMI is greater than 40, and the increased incidence of morbidity and mortality are denoted as very severe.

The BMI is an accurate measurement for most individuals, except for serious bodybuilders who may have a high BMI secondary to increase lean body mass (muscle), and pregnant individuals. In addition, the distribution of excess fat can be important because some patients can have a normal weight but have significant abdominal fat that results in visceral obesity. Abdominal (visceral) obesity has been associated with type 2 diabetes, dyslipidemia, and cardiovascular disease.[11] Measurements of waist circumference can indicate this accumulation of abdominal fat.

## Spinal Disorders in the Obese Patient

Obesity has been linked to osteoarthritis and degenerative joint disease.[51] Studies have indicated a link between excessive weight and osteoarthritis of the knee and hip joints.. Prospective evaluations have shown that the risk of knee osteoarthritis is increased by 15% for each additional kg/m$^2$ of BMI above 27. Non–weight-bearing joints in the hand are also more frequently afflicted by osteoarthritis in the obese. Longitudinal studies indicate that increased weight precedes the presentation of both hand and knee osteoarthritis.

The affect of osteoarthritis and degenerative spine disease is not well defined. Biomechanically, obesity can increase both the direct vertical compressive loads and the ventrally acting loads on the spinal column.[59] In particular, abdominal obesity can increase the stress on back muscles and the facet joint complex, potentially causing

**TABLE 98.1**

| Classification of Body Mass Index (BMI) | |
|---|---|
| **Classification** | **BMI (kg/m²)°** |
| Underweight | <18.5 |
| Normal range | 18.5 to 24.9 |
| Overweight | 25 to 29.9 |
| Obese | ≥30 |
| Obese Class I | 30 to 34.9 |
| Obese Class II | 35 to 39.9 |
| Obese Class III | ≥40 |

°$BMI$, kg/m² or (lbs/in² × 703).

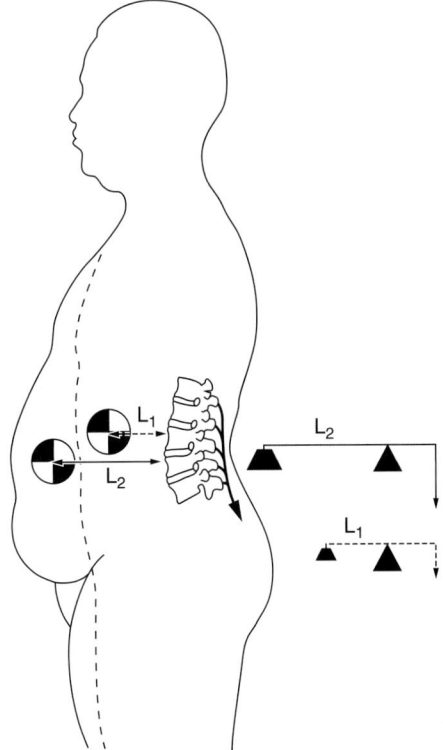

back pain and degenerative spine disease (Figure 98.1). Although obesity has been associated with pain syndromes such as coccydynia and meralgia paresthetica, clinical studies have produced conflicting results regarding spinal disorders and obesity.[12,27,28,31,43] Vertebral osteophytosis appears to be more common in patients with a higher BMI and obesity.[10,35]

Obesity has not been established as a cause of low back pain (LBP). Many authors question whether LBP precedes obesity or vice versa.[12] Clinically, the presentation of LBP in obese patient appears to be more common than in the general population.[7] However, in a systematic review of the epidemiologic literature of 56 journal articles by Leboeuf-Yde,[27] it was demonstrated that only 32% of studies indicate a statistically significant association between body weight and LBP. Because many studies have confounding factors, the authors felt that body weight should be considered a possible weak risk indicator for LBP.

The prevalence of obesity in patients admitted for elective spinal surgery is increased by some reports. Of 256 patients undergoing elective lumbar discectomy, 27% had a BMI consistent with obesity, compared to a prevalence of 16% in the general population in Finland.[7] However, it is unclear if this is directly related to obesity or to the fact that obese patients seek medical care more often than normal-weight individuals. In other studies BMI and patient height have been shown to be associated with those requiring surgery for lumbar intervertebral disc herniations.[19] In a cross-sectional study, Bostman[6] reviewed 1128 patients who underwent lumbar disc surgery as compared to the general population. Increased BMI and tall stature were significantly associated with lumbar disc herniations that required surgery.[6]

Overall, the literature is controversial regarding the cause of LBP and disc herniation in obese patients. In addition, it is not clear if the surgical outcome of LBP or disc herniation is worse than the general population after surgery in obese patients. A small, prospective study (n = 159) comparing lumbar spine surgery in obese and nonobese patients showed that both groups had similar outcomes for decompressive laminectomies, discectomies, and lumbar fusions.[3] This study found no difference in blood loss, operative time, hospital stay, rate of complications, or functional outcome between the two groups.[3] Surgical failure to relieve symptoms of radiculopathy and LBP might be related to patient selection rather than obe-

**Figure 98.1** Spinal load effects of obesity. Vertical axial and ventral loads are increased with obesity, with larger joint reaction forces caused by the longer lever arm induced by the panniculus. (*From White AA, Panjabi MM, Clinical Biomechanics of the Spine, ed 2. Philadelphia, JB Lippincott, 1990.*)

sity. In associated patients with obesity, the presence of diabetic neuropathy may result in poor results.[49] Finally, even morbidly obese patients who have undergone treatment for their weight disorders still maintain risk factors from their prior obesity. Of note, Bano *et al.*[4] have reported osteoporotic changes and reduced bone mineral density in patients who have undergone jejuno-ileal bypass surgery for morbid obesity.

## Health Risks and Medical Issues in the Obese Patient

Even if obesity does not clearly cause spinal disorders, many obese patients still require spinal surgery. The prevalence of obese patients undergoing spinal surgery is increased compared to the general population.[7] Management and attention to obesity-associated medical problems may decrease perioperative complications and increase the potential for successful spinal surgery. Medical disorders that have been associated with being overweight and obesity are summarized in Box 98.1. Many of these disorders have the potential to increase the risk for perioperative medical and surgical complications. Although not all obese patients have significant medical disorders, it is important to understand the health risks and medical disorders associated with obesity.

## Mortality

Epidemiologic studies show an increase in mortality associated with being overweight and obesity. Obese individuals (BMI ≥30) have a 50% to 100% increased risk of premature death from all causes as compared to normal-weight individuals, and are noted to have higher surgical morbidity and mortality.[11,14,48] A study that compared mortality rates for gastrointestinal surgery showed that obese patients have a 6.6% mortality rate compared to 2.2% for nonobese patients.[41] In contrast to the study on spinal operations by Andreshak et al.,[3] obese patients have been shown to have more blood loss, longer operation time, and major complications from orthopedic and other surgical procedures.[9,22,39]

## Pulmonary Function

Obesity is commonly associated with pulmonary dysfunction and difficult airways, and postsurgical pulmonary complications in the obese patient have been reported, ranging from 3.9% to 95%.[37,48] Gas exchange is frequently impaired in obese patients, and obesity significantly increases the risk of difficult endotracheal intubations. This risk is further compounded by smoking, with the literature suggesting that cessation of smoking of at least 8 weeks before surgery, along with weight loss of as little as 10 to 20kg, can significantly improve the chances of reduced postoperative pulmonary complications.[23,44] Obstruction of the upper airways by abundant soft tissue can also produce hypoxemia and hypercarbia. The weight of the torso and abdomen decreases the functional residual capacity and makes diaphragmatic excursion more difficult. The prone position, which is frequently used for spinal procedures, may actually improve some aspects of pulmonary function.[38] However, this improvement may depend on the frame on which the patient is positioned.[36] Late effects have also been reported, with obesity a risk factor for airway obstruction from angioneurotic edema secondary to angiotensin-converting enzyme inhibition postoperatively.[33]

Decreased residual capacity can reduce the time before which hypoxia occurs during intubation. In the obese patient with cervical spine pathology that requires careful intubation, the decreased time to hypoxia, combined with a difficult upper airway structure, may make intubation a challenge. In addition, obese patients have an increased volume of acidic gastric juice, which puts the patient at risk for aspiration.[55] The risk for pulmonary aspiration from gastroesophageal reflux is greatest during bucking or coughing on an endotracheal tube, which can occur more often during awake intubation. All obese patients should be considered at risk for intraoperative and postoperative hypoxia.

## Cardiac Function

Adipose tissue increases the cardiac output by 0.1L/min to perfuse 1kg of fat. Hypertension, cardiomegaly, and left ventricular failure can result from increased cardiac output requirements and can push the heart to its functional limits. Therefore the obese patient often has limited cardiac reserve and poor cardiac stress tolerance induced by hypotension, hypertension, tachycardia, or fluid overload during surgery. Carbon dioxide retention in massively obese patients is called Pickwickian syndrome and is associated with alveolar hypoventilation, somnolence, hypoxemia, right-sided heart failure, and secondary polycythemia. These patients may require more invasive monitoring. Preoperative evaluation should include an electrocardiogram (ECG) and an arterial blood gas analysis to assess the degree of hypoventilation. Often, smoking harms the cardiopulmonary system further, and in these patients, pulmonary function tests and chest radiographs should be obtained.

## Diabetes

Glucose tolerance is frequently impaired in the obese patient. Pancreatic islet hypertrophy and hyperinsulinemia result in a higher prevalence of diabetes and its associated health problems. Diabetes has been shown to be associated with poor outcome after spinal surgery. A study of 62 obese and nonobese patients with diabetes who underwent lumbar spinal surgery demonstrated higher rates of postoperative infection and prolonged hospitalization.[49]

## Thromboembolism

Thromboembolic complications are common after neurosurgical and orthopedic procedures. Obesity may increase the risk of deep vein thrombosis (DVT) and pulmonary embolism (PE).[45] Application of sequential leg compression devices and stockings may be problematic in obese patients. Early ambulation and subcutaneous heparin should be considered for patients, with careful attention to their pulmonary status.

## Wound Healing

Wound complications after dorsal spinal surgery are common. The incidence of wound infections and dehiscence are increased for obese patients.[45]

## Pharmacologic Issues

Pathophysiologic changes in obesity that affect drug distribution include increased cardiac output, blood volume, decreased lean body mass, organ size, and adipose mass.[1,5] In general, hydrophilic drugs are less affected by obesity. However, lipophilic drugs have an increased volume of distribution, slower elimination, and therefore sometimes a slow recovery from many anesthetic drugs. Associated hepatic and renal dysfunction can compound the tendency of slow recovery after anesthesia.

The administration of analgesia can also be affected by obesity. One study demonstrated that obese patients had less need for postoperative analgesics, compared to normal-weight patients.[42] Opioid analgesics might be hazardous in obese patients because of altered pharmacokinetics. Intramuscular injections may not result in predictable opioid blood levels in the obese. Patient-controlled anesthesia (PCA) has been effective in morbidly obese patients.[18,30] However, other reports imply that PCA may be more dangerous in obese patients with obstructive sleep apnea.[54]

## Diagnostic Considerations of Spinal Disorders in the Obese Patient

Evaluation of obese patients with spinal disorders is based on a thorough history and physical examination that is no different than for other patients. Detailed descriptions of the type of pain, its distribution, and associated radicular symptoms are important. The review of systems is critical in identifying potential medical problems associated with obesity. In particular, questions relating to cardiovascular disease, breathing difficulties, sleep apnea, and endocrine abnormalities should be asked. Often, morbidly obese patients are under the medical care of a primary care physician who can assist with a medical work-up, if indicated by the history, physical examination, and review of systems. High-risk anesthesia involvement and the need for a postoperative intensive care unit (ICU) stay should be based on concomitant diseases and length of surgery.[48] Physical examination might be limited secondary to the patient's body habitus. Associated knee and hand osteoarthritis might limit diagnostic maneuvers. Diabetic neuropathy may mask symptoms and signs of myelopathy.

Diagnostic imaging in the obese patient is sometimes challenging. Dynamic flexion and extension plain films are limited, and plain radiographs are frequently of a poor quality secondary to limited penetration. Magnetic resonance imaging (MRI) and computed tomographic (CT) scanning can be difficult to obtain because of size restrictions.[46] Open MRI scanners are less restricting and particularly useful for the obese patient with claustrophobia.

## Surgical Issues in Obesity

Approaches to the surgical management of obese patients with spinal disease should follow the same individualized approach as for nonobese patients. Medical issues associated with obesity may increase the operative risk factors; however, obesity in itself is not a contraindication for elective spinal surgery. Many anecdotal reports have been noted regarding the difficulty and increased postoperative complications related with obesity, but these reports have not been supported by the literature. Institutional experience at the Medical College of Wisconsin notes no clear differences in fusion rates or major complications when comparing the obese and nonobese patient populations. Andreshak and colleagues[3] reviewed a prospective series of 159 obese and control patients and noted that factors such as duration of surgery, blood loss, duration of hospital stay, incidence of complications, and clinical outcome did not differ between the two patient groups undergoing lumbar spine fusion.

### Operative Approaches

The decision of which operative approach to consider is dictated by the anatomy and disease process at hand. Certain approaches, such as ventral approaches, may be complicated by morbid obesity. Factors that include location and size of the panniculus, along with availability of appropriate retractors and instrumentation, may warrant modification of a standard approach that is normally used in nonobese patients. Although the approach is generally based on the anatomic structures that are encountered during dissection toward the lesion, many facets encompass the approach, including preoperative positioning, retraction, and intraoperative imaging studies.

### Patient Positioning

As with nonobese patients the goal of proper positioning remains obtaining optimal exposure and visualization. This is accomplished in conjunction with optimizing cardiovascular and respiratory dynamics, while avoiding blood loss, venous congestion, neurovascular compromise, and pressure point complications. Preparation should also be made to accommodate intraoperative needs that arise, such as localization radiographs, use of retractor systems, changes in patient position, or implantation of spinal instrumentation. Standard operative tables and fixation devices, such as three-point fixation for dorsal cervical procedures, may still be used. There is a significant number of different equipment and tools that may be used, and only a small subset of those readily available are described in this chapter.

## Supine Position

The supine position allows access to the ventral aspect of the patient and approaches, including ventral-cervical, transthoracic, and transabdominal; as well, iliac crest grafts are indications for this position. Arm boards and sleds may be used to help support the upper extremities during positioning, or for cervical procedures the use of a draw sheet to wrap around the patient may offer the arm support needed. Pressure points should all be carefully padded to include those areas within supportive sleds and sheets. If necessary, two operating tables connected with safety straps and cloth tape, and locked into position, may be used to accommodate those patients with substantial girth. Standing stools are then frequently used to assist in reaching the operative site, with care not to lean into the patient.

Exposure for ventral cervical approaches can be effected by a large submandibular panniculus. Visualization may be enhanced by use of a commercial chinstrap or tape, along with a shoulder roll. For dorsal cervical approaches, caudal traction of the shoulders bilaterally with cloth tape on a Reston base may not only smooth out the folds of the caudal neck, but may also provide shoulder traction for localization radiographs. Obesity does not confer protection from pressure point reactions, and during long procedures the problem may be enhanced by hypothermia and vasoconstrictive hypotension.[32]

## Prone Positioning

For patients who need to be positioned prone, a standard Amsco operating table (Amsco 3085 SP Surgical Table, Steris Corp., Montgomery, Ala.) with large, padded chest rolls is commonly used at the authors' institution. After padding the pressure points at the knees, ankles, elbows, and wrists, the patient is immobilized with standard safety straps and cloth tape placed over the Reston base to avoid direct skin contact with the adhesive. If thorough immobilization is needed, as in approaches where the operative table is to be rotated for better visualization, one needs to be cognizant of overconstricting with the straps and tape to avoid neurovascular or respiratory compromise. For cervical procedures, three-point fixation provides better surgical access and the potential for fewer neurovascular or mechanical pressure injuries than with horseshoe or padded facial rests.

Compared to the supine or lateral decubitus positions, there is a greater potential for respiratory compromise and abdominal compression. Signs of this may manifest not only in increased physiologic parameters such as peak airway pressure, but also with increased venous congestion and more difficult hemostasis. Alternatives to the standard chest rolls include use of equipment such as the Jackson table (OSI Corp., Union City, Calif.). This frame design allows specific padding and support placement to allow the abdomen to hang free and decrease the intraabdominal pressure. However, for some morbidly obese patients with a significant abdominal panniculus, it may be necessary to place an adjustable metal stool under the free

hanging abdomen to provide some additional support to prevent excessive stretching (the "Milwaukee brace"). Benefits of the Jackson table also include radiolucency for intraoperative imaging and accommodation of cervical traction and fixation. Although the frame is electric, rotation of the bed is done manually, and positions out of the neutral position are dependent on a friction stop. Weight allowances for the table are up to 350lb, but modifications are available to accommodate patients weighing up to 500lb.

## Lateral Decubitus Position

In cases of severe obesity in which the current operating table is insufficient or when the prone position is contraindicated, such as in patients with prominent renal transplants, the lateral decubitus position can be used.[21]

The lateral decubitus position may also be used in cases where visualization of the ventral or lateral thoracolumbar spine is desired. From this patient positioning, dissection via the transthoracic, retropleural, or retroperitoneal approaches may be applied. This patient position permits accommodation for those with a large thoracoabdominal pannus that may pose a significant technical challenge in the supine position. However, it should be noted that with this position, dorsal midline dissections might be more difficult; especially in the cervical spine, and that this position may also be problematic in the presence of spinal instability. Although spine alignment in the lateral decubitus position may be held with pillow or other flank supports, this position should be used with great caution in this setting.

## Kneeling Position

Other positioning options when the patient is required to be in the prone position include variations of the kneeling position. Manometric studies of inferior vena cava pressures have noted that there is a significant decrease while using the tuck position, compared to a either the Georgia or standard prone positions.[8,14,50,57] The benefit of lowering intraabdominal pressure is evident with better hemostasis, which allows for better visualization and lower intraoperative cardiac and respiratory pressures. However, the benefits of the kneeling position must be weighed against the drawbacks, which include more time-consuming positioning, increased susceptibility to neurovascular and mechanical pressure injuries, lumbar muscular and ligamentous tension, and potential difficulties of altering lumbar curvature during surgery.[8,24,53] These potential complications are generally avoidable, but they warrant careful consideration and an individualized approach.

## Sitting Position

Although the sitting position has been used for dorsal cervical procedures, additional pitfalls are present in using this position on the obese patient, aside from the general concerns of air emboli and cardiovascular or respiratory compromise.[32] The obese patient's large, ventral mass, along with limited flexibility, may make initial positioning much more difficult. Gravity that is beneficial for enhanced visualization, with bleeding draining away from the area of interest in the operative field, may hinder straps and taping efforts to mobilize the shoulders. The obese patient has a tendency to slip downward during a procedure in the sitting position. Gravity also affects the retractors that are used. Larger retractors with deeper blades, such as the Scoville, may require slings made of strung-out sponges and hemostats to help hold them in position. Nonetheless, the sitting position has been used successfully in the obese population. However, the authors generally use the prone positioning instead for dorsal cervical approaches.

### Other Aspects of Positioning

Regardless of the surgical approach and patient positioning strategy used, attention is still required to the basic circulatory and respiratory changes. Padding of the pressure points, application of sequential compression devices (SCDs) to help minimize dependent venous pooling, axillary rolls to prevent compromise of the axillary neurovascular bundle, and careful attention to the ventilatory status for any potential ventilation perfusion mismatches are all required.

## Surgical Equipment

### Operative Tables

At the authors' institution, the Amsco surgical table is used as the basic mobile surgical table providing an electro-hydraulic control of the flexible articulations that assists with patient positioning. The table can sustain up to a 1000lb (452kg) patient in the normal orientation where the base is centered relative to the patient's pelvis, or up to a 500lb (226kg) patient in the reverse orientation where the base is at the level of the patient's knee (Figure 98.2). The reversed position facilitates C-arm and other intraoperative imaging that can be a crucial part of various spinal procedures (see Figure 98.2B). Large, padded chest rolls are used for the patient in the prone position, and adapters for three-point cranial fixation, as well as traction for tongs, are available. However, for larger patients, or those with significant truncal obesity, specialized tables such as the Jackson frame may assist in positioning and abdominal decompression.

By allowing more of the abdomen to hang freely, compared to large chest rolls, the Jackson frame helps to reduce the epidural venous bleeding by decompression of the vena cava (Figure 98.3). The frame composition provides radiolucency while maintaining a load-bearing capacity of up to 500lb. Although this table has 360-degree rotational capabilities (allowing the use of this frame for 360-degree procedures), it lacks the table breaks of the Amsco table to facilitate bending and repositioning of the patient intraoperatively.

### Pressure Point Padding

Appropriate padding and immobilization are significant concerns in the positioning of any patient, but is sometimes more difficult given the large body size of the obese population. When manufacturers' safety straps are inadequate, the judicious use of standard pads and tape to secure the patient must be used. The authors of this chapter are quite liberal with their use of Reston and egg-crate foam pads, as well as cloth tape to secure the patients during surgery. Patients who are latex sensitive can still be secured with the use of copious amounts of plastic tape. The use of towels or sheets to prevent direct contact of the tape to the patient's skin may prevent breakdown and rashes. Taping over the costal margin or femoral head should be avoided to prevent pressure necrosis.

Gel pads supplemented with egg-crate foam pads protect the dependent portions of the patient from pressure sores and necrosis. Axillary rolls made of a saline bag wrapped in Reston, a thick gel pad, or a rolled sheet are used to protect the dependent axillary neurovascular bundle by placement on the ribs to allow the axillary region to be free from compression. The upper extremities may be positioned and padded in a variety of ways, with two-tiered supports or pillows most commonly being used.

## Operative Considerations

### Surgical Exposure

In any surgical procedure obtaining adequate exposure is perhaps the most challenging aspect of the case, and this fact is not lost on spine surgery in obese patients. "Macro incisions for macro people" is an adage that is used to denote that because of the depth of the exposure, a small incision would result in poor visualization of the surgical site given the natural coning effect of the field of view. Optimal exposure is directly dependent on appropriate positioning and type of approach, appropriate incision size and configuration, adequate muscle relaxation, and the use of an appropriate retractor system. Difficulty with any of these factors, along with inadequate lighting and hemostasis, only compounds a suboptimal exposure and hinders the operation.

The choice of operative approach must account for the obese patient's habitus in addition to the usual considerations, because obese individuals vary in terms of fat distribution. For example, many middle–aged, male obese patients carry much of their weight ventrally in the abdomen; therefore a dorsal midline exposure may not require as deep an exposure as may be expected initially. Conversely, ventral or lateral exposures in such patients may be more difficult than in a thin patient.

Adequate decompression is predicated on satisfactory exposure and retraction. The tendency for progressive narrowing of exposure in the depths of a wound can carry over into decompression unless vigilance is maintained. Again, liberal incisions and undercutting or past pointing of the dissection beyond the precise area of interest enhance the deep exposure in the obese patient and help minimize this phenomenon. Precise localization is an additional potential difficulty with obese patients, and thorough preoperative planning and preparation may mitigate this problem. This may include positioning in preparation for the possibility of multiple radiographs and obtaining test radiographs after positioning to ensure adequate visualization before draping. Skin markers may be unreliable because of movement with changes of position and the relatively long distance between the skin surface and underlying spinal region of interest (location of pathology).

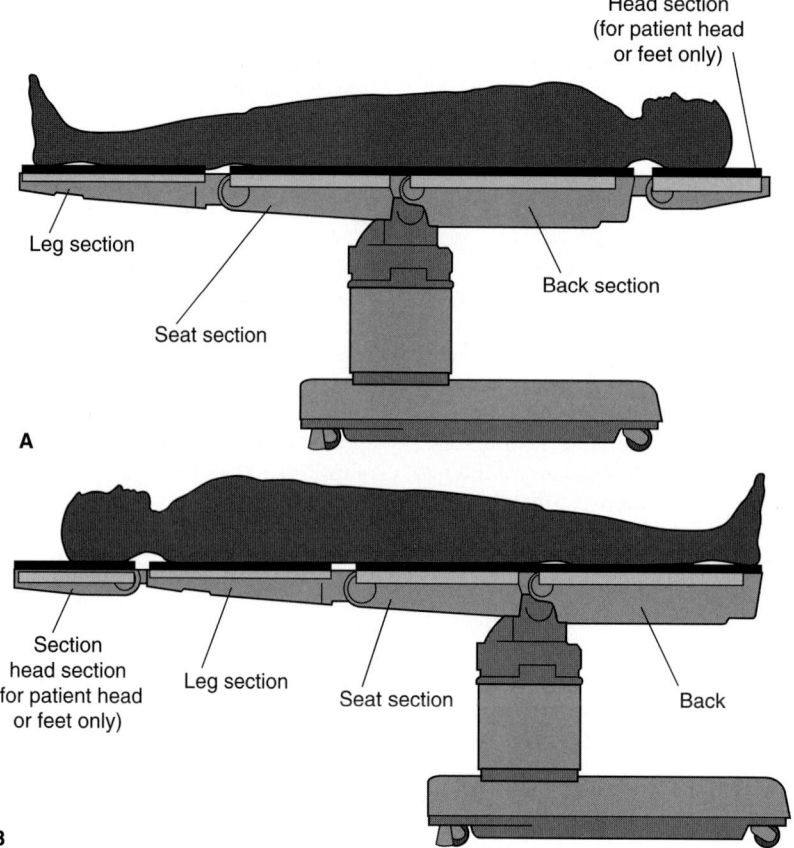

**Figure 98.2** (**A**) Normal orientation of operative table. The normal orientation of the operating table can sustain up to a 1000lb (452kg) patient. The base is centered relative to the patient's pelvis. (**B**) Reverse orientation of operative table. The reversed orientation of the surgical table can sustain a 500lb (226kg) patient where the base is at the level of the patient's knee. This reversed position facilitates **C**-arm and other intraoperative imaging that can be a crucial part of various spinal procedures. (**A** *and* **B**, *Courtesy Amsco 3085 SP Surgical Table Manual, Steris Corp., Montgomery, Ala.*)

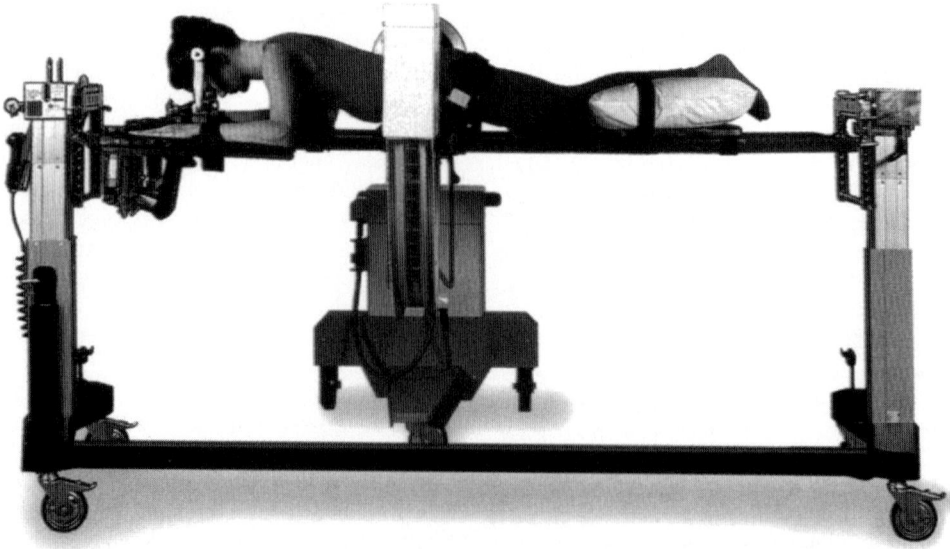

**Figure 98.3** Jackson spinal frame. The Jackson spinal frame allows more of the abdomen to hang freely as compared to the use of large chest rolls, thereby reducing epidural venous bleeding by decompression of the vena cava. The radiolucent frame can hold up to 500lb and allows 360-degree rotation, but lacks table breaks to facilitate bending of the patient. (*Courtesy Orthopedic Systems, Union City, Calif.*)

Lastly, one should not hesitate to extend an incision as necessary to directly visualize a useful landmark or structures, such as the C2 or C7 spinous process, the first rib, or the sacrum.

## Retractor Systems

Adequate exposure of deep structures depends on adequate retraction. A variety of systems are currently available and the choice of retraction systems should be individualized, depending on body habitus, approach, body region, and surgeon preference. Table 98.2 lists some systems that are used at the authors' institution. This list is not intended to be all-inclusive. The authors acknowledge that many other successful methodologies may be used.

Retraction often begins before the surgical preparation. Submandibular and supraclavicular redundant skin folds may be carefully taped away from the incision site. Similarly, the abdominal pannus may be retracted with tape to optimize iliac crest access. A shoulder sling or two Kerlix rolls, looped around the patient's wrists and brought off the foot end of the table, permits downward shoulder traction while obtaining intraoperative radiographs. Continuous shoulder traction with braces or tape may be obviated with such maneuvers. It is emphasized that continuous traction is generally less desirable because of potential brachial plexopathy.

For the most part the combination of the long, straight and large, curved Weitlaner retractors tend to provide adequate exposure. However, in the obese patient in whom the depth of the exposure is increased, there is a tendency to angle the tips of the Weitlaner retractors to the base of the exposure. This causes the handle to ride higher and become an obstacle in the operative field. Specialized side-loading retractor systems with longer blades, such as the TrimLine (Figure 98.4) and the Koros Super-Slide II (Figure 98.5), permit a lower profile with retraction. In the cervical region, side-loading systems such as the TrimLine retractor system with the Caspar distraction pins permit excellent surgical exposure for ventral approaches. Custom-made longer blades are available if a deeper exposure requires a longer reach, and use of a folded sponge underneath one of the blades can assist in proper positioning against the mobile soft tissue. For dorsal lumbar approaches, the authors often use the Koros system, and the use of a custom post on one side with a lone retractor blade on the other can facilitate hemilaminar exposures in large patients.

For ventral or lateral approaches in the thoracic or lumbar spine, the authors have typically used the Thompson table-mounted system (Figure 98.6). Previously used by general surgical colleagues, its use has grown from the ventral abdominal exposures and is adaptable for a variety of spine applications. The initial setup time may be longer than with other systems, but this time is subsequently compensated for by improved deep exposure.[15] The malleable Thompson blades are available in various sizes and permit versatile atraumatic retraction, which is particularly well suited for ventral or lateral thoracolumbar and ventral cervical use. The authors have routinely used customized, enlarged Scoville type articulated retractors with lengthened and angled blades for enhanced purchase and elevation of the paraspinal musculature (Figure 98.7), and customized enlarged and angled cerebellar type retractors for deepened and enhanced retraction without "slip out" at the extremes of a wound (Figure 98.8).

## Implant Modifications and Fusion Techniques

Anecdotal reports on the potentially higher failure rate of internal fixation and fusion in obese patients are prevalent. However, there is no conclusive clinical evidence to support such concerns.[3] Reasons for this speculation may result from the paucity of clinical data and studies that address the issue of morbidity associated with spinal instrumentation and fusion in normal versus obese patients. Although not a direct correlation, inference from data of other load-bearing implants, such as total hip arthroplasty, does not support a significant difference in implant failure or fusion rates in the obese population.[29]

From a biomechanical standpoint the obese patient does present some differences in body configuration and dynamics that may be of some concern in construct design. Variations in body weight and morphology contribute to the individualized spinal loading patterns seen, with obesity representing an extreme. The center of gravity is shifted in the obese patient and both direct vertical compressive loads, as well as the ventrally acting loads, are increased.[59] This shift of the center of gravity ventrally produces a longer lever arm with respect to the spine, with the potential for increasing the stress on pedicle screw cantilever beam type constructs or multisegmental dorsal

| **TABLE 98.2** | | |
|---|---|---|
| **Retraction Systems** | | |
| **Body Region** | **Approach** | **Suggested Retractor System** |
| **Cervical** | Ventral | TrimLine or other side-loading retractors, Caspar system, or table-mounted retractors |
| | Dorsal | Large angled Weitlaner or cerebellar retractors, or Shadow-Line or other side-loading retractors |
| **Thoracic** | Ventral/Lateral | Large angled Weitlaner retractors, Smith Beckman or table-mounted retractors |
| | Dorsal | Combination large straight and angled Weitlaner retractors, Smith Beckman or table-mounted retractors |
| **Lumbar** | Ventral/Lateral | Large angled Weitlaner retractors, Smith Beckman, or table-mounted retractors |
| | Dorsal | Koros or Scoville side-loading retractors, custom-made large cerebellar retractors, or Carlens retractors |

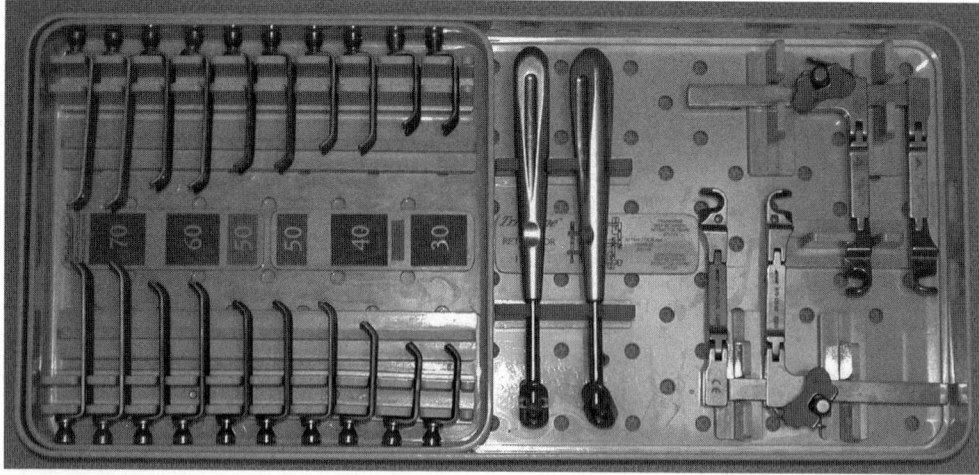

**Figure 98.4** TrimLine Retractor System for cervical procedures. Side-loading retractors such as the TrimLine model are useful for ventral cervical approaches.

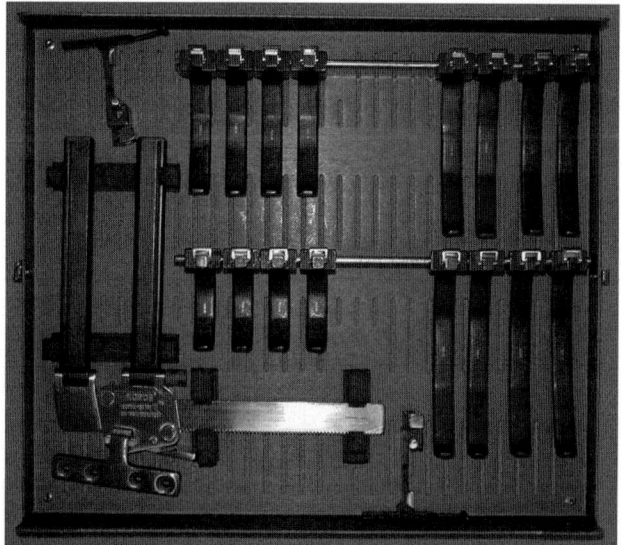

**Figure 98.5** Koros Retractor System for lumbar procedures. Specialized side-loading retractor systems with longer blades, such as the Koros Super-Slide II system, allow for a lower profile with retraction.

constructs[58] (Figure 98.9). Therefore to compensate for this morphology, one might be inclined to use a pedicle screw with a larger diameter and length to theoretically increase the load-bearing capacity and the pull-out strength, as well as to protect the shaft from exposure to higher bending moments. Bicortical sacral fixation may also be necessary to offset the toggle effect caused by the longer moment arm on short segment lumbosacral cantilever beam type constructs. For multisegmental hook and rod construct, as would be used in the presence of a kyphotic deformity, a longer construct with more fixation points should provide an increase in construct stiffness (Figure 98.10). All of these aspects remain theoretical concerns of uncertain clinical significance that probably vary in importance from case to case. Lastly, one should consider the potential limitations of various orthoses in this patient population. What may otherwise be a "stable"

construct in a thin patient with a tight-fitting orthosis may not suffice in a heavier patient with an ill-fitting or misapplied orthosis.

## Wound Closure Techniques

Special consideration to the wound closure of the obese patient is needed, as emphasized by the prevalence of surgical literature pertaining to the increased rates of dehiscence and infection.[15,20,40,52] The relatively poor vascularity of adipose tissue, the overall thickness and lack of strength of the adipose layer for suture retention, and its inability to respond to an inoculum all contribute to the morbidity associated with the wound. Maintaining the concept of minimizing the dead space with a multilayered closure applies not only to obese patients, but also to larger patients in general. Use of a closely spaced, interrupted dermal layer of suture, as well as approximation of the superficial fascia (Camper's) within the adipose layer, may add to the strength of the superficial approximation of the wound. Placement of a drain should be considered if potential dead space is present, despite the multilayered closure, and multilayered drainage may also be helpful in some settings. However, it is the experience of the authors that no clear difference in wound-related complications is present with or without drain use. At the authors' institution a subcuticular suture is often used with a good dermal closure for cosmesis; otherwise, skin sutures or staples are removed in 7 days with placement of Steri-Strips.

Overall, there is still a general tendency toward more frequent superficial drainage or dehiscence in this group.[29] Treatment of this situation follows general surgical techniques with superficial opening, debridement, and packing of the wound. After the wound has been cleaned in this manner, healing by granulation or delayed primary or secondary closure is performed. For deeper subfascial infections, management again follows the general surgical techniques as in nonobese patients. Deeper infections require operative debridement and thorough irrigation, followed by fascial reapproximation and layered drainage, or suprafascial packing with healing by granulation or delayed primary closure.

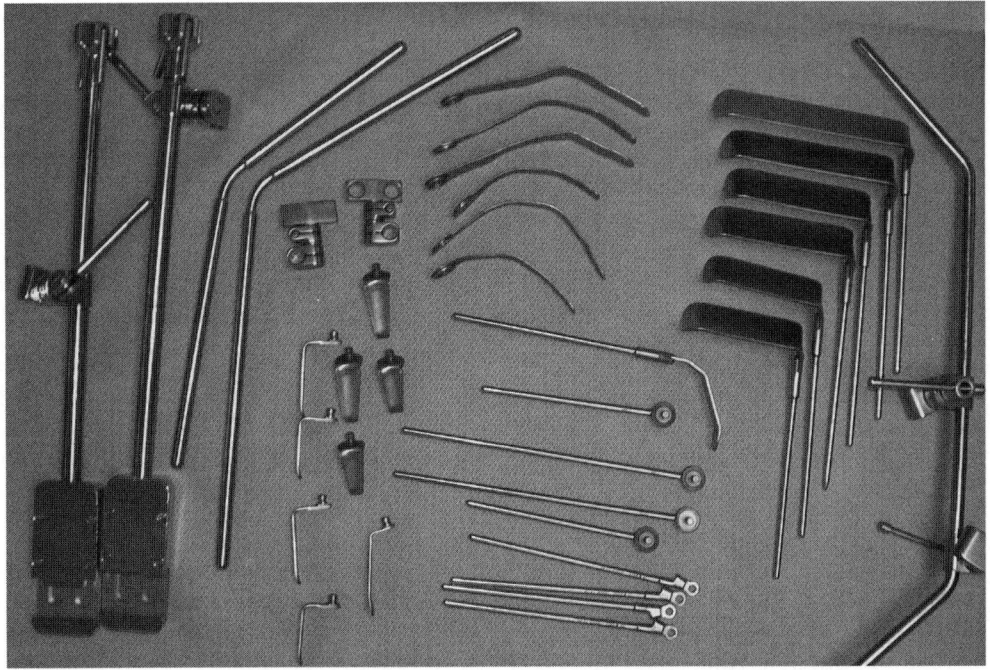

**Figure 98.6** Thompson table-mounted retractor. The malleable Thompson blades permit versatile atraumatic retraction, particularly well suited for ventral or lateral thoracolumbar use, as well as ventral cervical use.

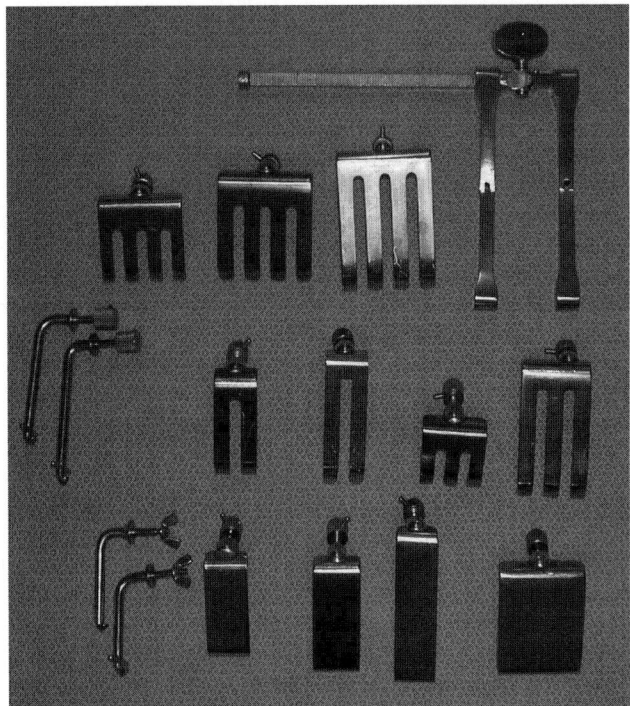

**Figure 98.7** Scoville type articulated retractors. Scoville type articulated retractors with lengthened and angled blades permit enhanced purchase and elevation of the paraspinal musculature.

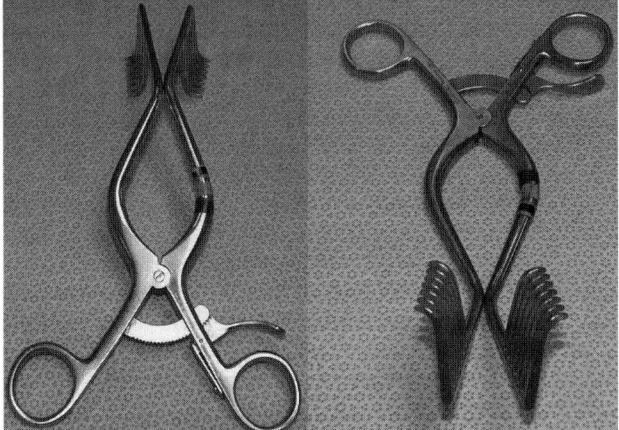

**Figure 98.8** Modified large cerebellar retractors. Customized enlarged and angled cerebellar type retractors permit deepened and enhanced retraction without "slip out" at the extremes of a wound.

superficial infections should be treated by local debridement and antibiotic therapy. Deeper infections require intraoperative debridement and irrigation, followed by a prolonged course of antibiotic therapy. Foreign bodies and materials such as Gelfoam, exposed sutures, and loose bone graft fragments should be removed. However, solidly implanted spinal instrumentation requires removal only in the most severe cases of deep wound infections that are resistant to aggressive drainage and debridement.[20]

## Postoperative Management

Postoperative care is aimed at establishing an optimal recovery period, and management of the obese patient

If debridement of the wound edges and sides is required, large retention sutures or surgical undermining may be helpful for wound reapproximation in such cases.

In general, aggressive surgical management is important when an infection has been identified. Given the poor penetration of antibiotics into adipose tissue, only the most

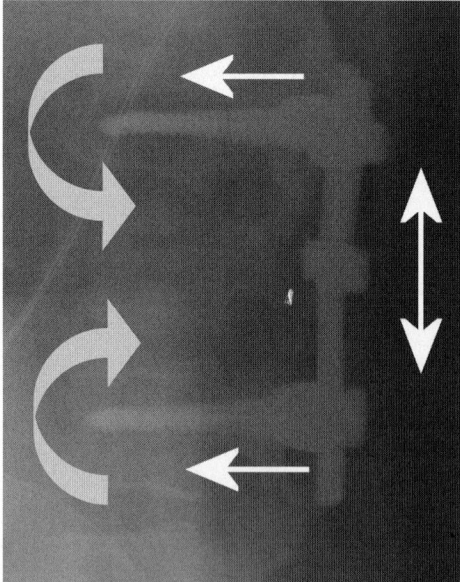

**Figure 98.9** Forces seen by the spinal construct. Diagram of some of the forces seen by the pedicle screw cantilever beam type constructs that are increased with obesity.

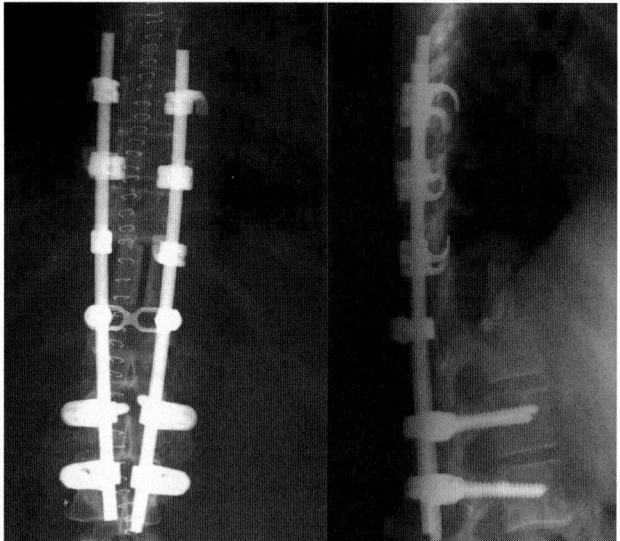

**Figure 98.10** Multisegmental hook and rod construct. Multisegmental hook and rod construct, used in the presence of a kyphotic deformity, requires a longer construct with more fixation points to increase in stiffness of the construct, given the longer ventral lever arm in obese patients.

should not differ significantly from the normal weight population. However, there are factors that are unique to the obese patient that should be taken into account. Pulmonary complications can be prevalent in this group of patients, and those presenting with even mild preoperative hypoxemia may be at significant risk, requiring the use of vigilant postoperative monitoring.[23] For obese patients with evidence of concomitant medical issues, it is generally recommended that they be observed in an ICU during the early postoperative period to provide more careful

monitoring, especially of their pulmonary and cardiovascular status.[10]

The use of aggressive pulmonary toileting is essential to prevent atelectasis and postoperative pneumonia. Early mobilization is frequently used in the nonobese population to decrease the risk of deep venous thrombosis, pneumonia, and to increase the patient's functionality. The elevation of the head of the bed, incentive spirometry, and trapeze bar, as well as early ambulation has been recommended to facilitate recovery and pulmonary function in both the nonobese and obese populations.[23] However, the obese patient may have a significant degree of pulmonary arteriovenous (AV) Z pulmonary shunting, which with early mobilization and upright posture, can cause an increase in hypoxia compared with the recumbent position.[47,58] For this reason oxygen saturation should be monitored by pulse-oximeter. Hypoxia, if present, should be corrected before ambulation is begun.

Other issues include the adequacy of analgesia in the obese population. Studies have debated the amount of medication needed, but in general the larger lipophilic body mass of this group of patients may require the titration of narcotics to account for the increase in body weight. Also, postoperative hemoglobin levels should be maintained in the normal range to prevent anemia, additional cardiac stress, and wound hypoxia. Blood glucose levels should be monitored as well, because the stress of surgery or the use of corticosteroids may result in hyperglycemia, thus increasing the risk of infection and impairing wound healing. The importance of thromboembolic prophylaxis has already been discussed.

Finally, the surgeon must be alert to the possibility of postoperative wound infections that may be difficult to manage in obese patients. The signs and symptoms of a wound infection in the obese population are no different than from those in the nonobese patient. Physical findings of local erythema and tenderness, as well as the presence of leukocytosis and a persistently elevated erythrocyte sedimentation rate (ESR) or c-reactive protein (CRP) are important clues.

## Summary

Obesity in itself is not a contraindication to elective spinal surgery, but does pose its own set of challenges and difficulties to the spine surgeon. Cognizance of the comorbid medical issues that are associated with obesity, as well as the specific patient needs for operative management, are required to optimize treatment of this population of patients. In addition to careful surgical and equipment planning, patient involvement with weight loss and smoking cessation programs, if indicated, may help improve the overall outcome and lower the operative risks.

## REFERENCES

1. Abernethy D, Greenblatt D: Pharmacokinetics of drugs in obesity. *Clin Pharmacokinet* 7(2):108-124, 1982.

2. Allison D, Fontaine K, Manson J, *et al*: Annual deaths attributable to obesity in the United States. *JAMA* 282(16):1530-1538, 1999.

3. Andreshak T, An H, Hall J, Stein B: Lumbar spine surgery in the obese patient. *J Spinal Disord* 10(5):376-379, 1997.

4. Bano G, Rodin DA, Pazianas M, Nussey SS: Reduced bone mineral density after surgical treatment for obesity. *Int J Obes Relat Metab Disord* 23:361-365, 1999.

5. Blouin R, Kolpek J, Mann H: Influence of obesity on drug disposition. *Clin Pharm* 6(9):706-714, 1987.

6. Bostman O: Body mass index and height in patients requiring surgery for lumbar intervertebral disc herniation. *Spine* 18(7):851-854, 1993.

7. Bostman O: Prevalence of obesity among patients admitted for elective orthopaedic surgery. *Int J Obes Relat Metab Disord* 18(10):709-713, 1994.

8. Bostman O, Hyrkas J, Hirvensalo E, Kallio E: Blood loss, operating time, and positioning of the patient in lumbar disc surgery. *Spine* 15(5):360-363, 1990.

9. Bowditch MG, Villar RN: Do obese patients bleed more? A prospective study of blood loss at total hip replacement. *Ann R Coll Surg Engl* 81(3):198-200, 1999.

10. Buckley F: *Anesthesia and Obesity and Gastrointestinal Disorders*. Philadelphia, Lippincott-Raven, 1989, pp 1117-1131.

11. Clinical guidelines on the identification, evaluation, and treatment of overweight and obesity in adults. Public Health Service, National Institutes of Health (NIH), 1998.

12. Cvijetic S, McCloskey E, Korsic M: Vertebral osteophytosis and vertebral deformities in an elderly population sample. *Wien Klin Wochenschr* 112(9):407-412, 2000.

13. Despres J, Lemieux I, Prud'homme D: Treatment of obesity: need to focus on high risk abdominally obese patients. *BMJ* 322(7288):716-720, 2001.

14. Deyo R, Bass J: Lifestyle and low back pain: the influence of smoking and obesity. *Spine* 14(5):501-506, 1989.

15. Dominguez-Cherit G, Gonzalez R, Borunda D, *et al*: Anesthesia for morbidly obese patients. *World J Surg* 22(9):969-973, 1998.

16. Eie N, Solgaard T, Kleppe H: The knee-elbow position in lumbar disc surgery: a review of complications. *Spine* 8(8):897-900, 1983.

17. Foley K, Lee R: Surgical complications of obese patients with endometrial carcinoma. *Gynecol Oncol* 39(2):171-174, 1990.

18. Graves D, Batenhorst R, Bennett R, *et al*: Morphine requirements using patient-controlled analgesia: influence of diurnal variation and morbid obesity. *Clin Pharm* 2(1):49-53, 1983.

19. Heliovaara M: Body height, obesity, and risk of herniated lumbar intervertebral disc. *Spine* 12(5):469-472, 1987.

20. Heller J: *Postoperative Infections of the Spine. Complications of Spinal Surgery*. Philadelphia, WB Saunders, 1992, pp 1817-1837.

21. Hitchon P, Traynelis V: *Lumbar Hemilaminectomy for Excision of a Herniated Disc*, vols 124-129. Chicago, American Association of Neurological Surgeons, 1992, pp 373-379.

22. Holub Z, Jabor A, Kliment L, *et al*: Laparoscopic hysterectomy in obese women: a clinical prospective study. *Eur J Obstet Gynecol Reprod Biol* 98:77-82, 2001.

23. Jackson C: Preoperative pulmonary evaluation. *Arch Int Med* 148(10):2120-2127, 1988.

24. Keim H, Weinstein V: Acute renal failure—a complication of spine fusion in the tuck position. A case report. *J Bone Joint Surg* American volume 52(6):1248-1250, 1970.

25. Kral J: Morbidity of severe obesity. *Surg Clin North Am* 81(5):1039-1061, 2001.

26. Kuczmarski R, Flegal K: Criteria for definition of overweight in transition: background and recommendations for the United States. *Am J Clin Nutr* 72:1074-1081, 2000.

27. Leboeuf-Yde C: Body weight and low back pain. A systematic literature review of 56 journal articles reporting on 65 epidemiologic studies. *Spine* 25(2):226-237, 2000.

28. Leboeuf-Yde C, Kyvik K, Bruun N: Low back pain and lifestyle. II. Obesity: information from a population-based sample of 29,424 twin subjects. *Spine* 24(8):779-784, 1999.

29. Lehman D, Capello W, Feinberg J: Total hip arthroplasty without cement in obese patients. A minimum two-year clinical and radiographic follow-up study. *J Bone Joint Surg Am* 76(6):854-862, 1994.

30. Levin A, Klein S, Brolin R, Pitchford D: Patient-controlled analgesia for morbidly obese patients: an effective modality if used correctly. *Anesthesiology* 76(5):857-858, 1992.

31. Maigne J, Doursounian L, Chatellier G: Causes and mechanisms of common coccydynia: role of body mass index and coccygeal trauma. *Spine* 25(23):3072-3079, 2000.

32. Martin J: *Patient Positioning*. Philadelphia, Lippincott-Raven, 1989.

33. Mchaourab A, Sarantopoulos C, Stowe D: Airway obstruction due to late-onset angioneurotic edema from angiotensin-converting enzyme inhibition. *Can J Anaesth* 46(10):975-978, 1999.

34. Office of the Surgeon General: The Surgeon's General's call to action to prevent and decrease overweight and obesity. Rockville, Md.: Public Health Service, U.S. Department of Health and Human Services, 2001.

35. O'Neill T, McCloskey E, Kanis J, *et al*: The distribution, determinants, and clinical correlates of vertebral osteophytosis: a population based survey. *J Rheumatology* 26(4):842-848, 1999.

36. Palmon S, Kirsch J, Depper J, Toung T: The effect of the prone position on pulmonary mechanics is frame-dependent. *Anesth Analg* 87(5):1175-1180, 1998.

37. Pasulka P, Bistrian B, Benotti P, Blackburn G: The risks of surgery in obese patients. *Ann Intern Med* 104(4):540-546, 1986.

38. Pelosi P, Croci M, Calappi E, *et al*: Prone positioning improves pulmonary function in obese patients during general anesthesia. *Anesth Analg* 83(3):578-583, 1996.

39. Perka C, Labs K, Muschik M, Buttgereit F: The influence of obesity on perioperative morbidity and mortality in revision total hip arthroplasty. *Arch Orthop Trauma Surg* 120(5):267-271, 2000.

40. Polk H: *Principles of Preoperative Preparation of the Surgical Patient*, ed 13. Philadelphia, WB Saunders, 1986, pp 87-98.

41. Postlethwait R, Johnson W: Complications following surgery for duodenal ulcer in obese patients. *Arch Surg* 105(3):438-440, 1972.

42. Rand C, Kuldau J, Yost R: Obesity and post-operative pain. *J Psychosom Res* 29(1):43-48, 1985.

43. Regachary S: *Meralgia Paresthetica*, vol 2. Chicago, American Association of Neurological Surgeons, 1992, pp 373-379.

44. Rochester D, Enson Y: Current concepts in the pathogenesis of the obesity-hypoventilation syndrome. Mechanical and circulatory factors. *Am J Med* 57(3): 402-420, 1974.

45. Rosenbaum M, Leibel R, Hirsch J: Obesity. *N Engl J Med* 337:396-407, 1997.

46. Rothschild P, Domesek J, Eastham M, Kaufman L: MR imaging of excessively obese patients: the use of an open permanent magnet. *Magn Reson Imaging* 9(2):151-154, 1991.

47. Savino J, Del Guercio L: Preoperative assessment of high-risk surgical patients. *Surg Clin North Am* 65(4): 763-791, 1985.

48. Schroder T, Nolte M, Kox W, Spies C: Anesthesia in extreme obesity. *Herz* 26(3):222-228, 2001.

49. Simpson J, Silveri C, Balderston R, *et al*: The results of operations on the lumbar spine in patients who have diabetes mellitus. *J Bone Joint Surg Am* 75(12):1823-1829, 1993.

50. Smith R, Gramberg Z, Valpitta P: Problems related to the prone position for surgical operations. *Anesthesiology* 22:189-193, 1961.

51. Sowers M: Epidemiology of risk factors for osteoarthritis: systemic factors. *Curr Opin Rheumatol* 13(5):447-451, 2001.

52. Strauss R, Wise L: Operative risks of obesity. *Surg Gynecol Obstet* 146(2):286-291, 1978.

53. Summans E, O'Leary P: *Complications of Spinal Surgery for Disc Disease and Spondylolisthesis*. Philadelphia, Lippincott-Raven, 1978.

54. VanDercar D, Martinez A, De Lisser E: Sleep apnea syndromes: a potential contraindication for patient-controlled analgesia. *Anesthesiology* 74(3):623-624, 1991.

55. Vaughan R, Bauer S, Wise L: Volume and pH of gastric juice in obese patients. *Anesthesiology* 43(6):686-689, 1975.

56. Wallace J, Schulte W, Nakeeb A, Andris D: Health problems related to severe obesity. *MCW Healthlink*, 2001.

57. Wayne S: The tuck position for lumbar-disc surgery. *J Bone Joint Surg Am* 49(6):1195-1198, 1967.

58. Weir B: Prospective study of 100 lumbosacral discectomies. *J Neurosurg* 50(3):283-289, 1979.

59. White A, Panjabi M: *Clinical Biomechanics of the Spine*, ed 2. Philadelphia, JB Lippincott, 1990.

60. Wolf A, Colditz G: Current estimates of the economic cost of obesity in the United States. *Obes Res* 6(2):97-106, 1998.

61. World Health Organization. Obesity: preventing and managing the global epidemic. Report of a WHO consultation on obesity, Geneva, 1998.

# CHAPTER 99

# Smoking, the Spine, and Spinal Fusion

**Tunc Oktenoglu, A. Fahir Özer, Scott D. Boden, and Glenn R. Rechtine II**

Habitual tobacco use, particularly smoking, has important and diverse negative health consequences. Chronic cigarette consumption has been linked to a myriad of human ailments and diseases, including stroke, heart disease, emphysema, and cancer.[1,103,151,167,170] Predictably, chronic tobacco use has significant deleterious effects on the health, strength, and metabolism of the vertebrae of the human spinal column.[4,15,44,46] Not only are vertebrae of chronic smokers less healthy and more susceptible to premature degeneration and fracture, but they are also less likely to heal after injury and are associated with higher rates of failure after attempted spinal fusion.[*] This chapter reviews epidemiologic, clinical, and laboratory evidence documenting the deleterious impact smoking has on the human vertebral column. Also, the biologic, physiologic, and mechanical impact of smoking on spinal fusion procedures is discussed.

## Overview

The tobacco plants of commerce—Nicotiana tabacum and Nicotiana rustica—were used in the Western world for a thousand years before European contact. Tobacco cultivation has been widespread throughout the Americas for millennia. Nicotiana tabacum, the species used by Native Americans in Central and South America, is not a natural plant.[2] Genetic studies demonstrated Nicotiana tabacum is a hybrid resulting from two wild species—Nicotiana sylvestris and Nicotiana tomentosiformis. Nicotiana rustica, which has a higher nicotine content than Nicotiana tabacum, was cultivated in North America.

The appeal of these plants is the production of effects on the brain when tobacco is consumed. Nicotine produces these effects, including addiction.[158]

The use of tobacco to create and satisfy nicotine addiction was introduced to Christopher Columbus, a Genoese admiral, by Native Americans on his first voyage to North America. Columbus introduced the tobacco leaf and seeds to Europe, particularly in England, France, Portugal and Spain, where they began growing and using tobacco by the end of the sixteenth century.[96] Portuguese and Spanish ships took tobacco around the world. By the end of the sixteenth century tobacco was introduced to nearly the entire world with the exception of Australia and Antarctica.[26]

Numerous factors played roles in the explosive growth of smoking tobacco. The first factor was the development of automated machine-rolled cigarettes in 1880, which significantly lowered production costs for cigarettes.[90] The second factor that caused the growth of the cigarette industry was the decrease of federal tax on cigarettes. The tax on cigarettes was $1.75 per 1000 cigarettes during the Civil War. In 1883 the federal tax was reduced to $0.50 per 1000 cigarettes, which provided incentive to manufacturers to lower their prices. The third factor was the rapid increase in the U.S. population. Including immigrants, the population nearly doubled between 1880 and 1910. As one might expect, the population of the lower socioeconomic segments, in particular, increased. This resulted in an increase in tobacco addiction. World War I (1914-1918) promoted the habitual use of tobacco all around the world. By bringing together so many individuals from different cultures and socioecenomic segments, the profile of smokers changed. Smoking was popular in poor and lower socioeconomic classes before World War I. However, after the war, cigarettes became so widely used that they became accepted by all social segments.[30] In fact, cigarettes were provided free to American soldiers. Similarly, in World War II (1939-1945) cigarette sales hit record highs. Today, cigarettes are the most widely used addictive agent around the world.

## Tobacco Addiction

Drug addiction is defined as the compulsive use of a psychoactive substance, the consequences of which are detrimental to the individual or society.[113] Nicotine dependence resulting from tobacco use was not classified as drug abuse for many years. This is mostly because the ill effects of smoking on human health were not widely recognized, and also the habit was not associated with obvious intoxication or socially unacceptable behavior. In time, however, the cumulative findings of more than 2500 reports on tobacco were summarized in the U.S. Surgeon General's Report on the Health Consequences of Smoking in 1988.[159] This report concluded that cigarettes and other forms of tobacco are addictive.

The psychoactive component of tobacco is nicotine. The behavioral and pharmacologic processes that determine tobacco addiction are similar to those that determine addiction to other drugs, such as heroin and cocaine. Nicotine is absorbed rapidly from tobacco smoke into the pulmonary circulation and moves quickly to the brain. Nicotine acts on nicotinic cholinergic receptors to produce its effects, which occur within 10 to 15 seconds after the smoker takes a puff. Nicotine is believed to contain positive reinforcing and addictive properties because it activates the dopaminergic pathway, projecting from the ventral tegmental area to the cerebral cortex and the limbic system.

In addition, nicotine causes an increase in the concentrations of circulating norepinephrine and epinephrine and an increase in the release of vasopressin, beta-endorphin adrenocorticotropic hormone (ACTH), and cortisol. These hormones are believed to contribute to the basic stimulatory effects of nicotine on the central nervous

---

[*]References 17,18,28,40,44,57,70,93-97,157.

1333

system (CNS). Dependence on nicotine develops quickly, probably because of the activation of the ventral tegmental area dopaminergic system by nicotine. Cocaine and amphetamines affect the same system. With long-term use of tobacco physical dependence develops as a result of an increased number of nicotinic cholinergic receptors in the brain.*

Withdrawal symptoms from nicotine can develop within 2 hours of smoking the last cigarette, usually peak in the first 24 to 48 hours, and can last for weeks or months. The common symptoms include an intense craving for nicotine, tension, irritability, difficulty in concentrating, drowsiness and paradoxical sleeplessness, restlessness, bradycardia, and hypotension, increased appetite and weight gain, decreased motor performance, increased muscle tension, and in some people, depression.[22,62,78]

Addiction to tobacco is multifactorial, including a desire for the direct pharmacologic actions of nicotine, relief of withdrawal symptoms, and learned associations. Smokers report numerous reasons for smoking, such as pleasure, enhanced vigilance, improved performance, relief of anxiety or depression, reduced hunger, and to control body weight. Additionally, environmental cues such as a meal, a cup of coffee, an alcoholic beverage, or friends who smoke might trigger someone to smoke.

Most tobacco use begins in childhood or adolescence. Risk factors for youth smoking include peer and parental influences, behavioral problems, personality characteristics, and genetic influences.[31,49]

## Harmful Constituents of Tobacco

Tobacco smoke is an aerosol of particles containing water, nicotine and other alkaloids, and tar. Tobacco smoke contains several thousand chemicals, many of which may contribute to human disease. Major toxic chemicals in the particulate phase of tobacco include nicotine, benzo(a)-pyrene, and other polycyclic hydrocarbons, N-nitrosornornicotine, β-naphylamine, polonium-210, nickel, cadmium, arsenic, and lead. The gaseous phase contains carbon monoxide, acetaldehyde, acetone, methanol, nitrogen oxides, hydrogen cyanide, acrolein, ammonia, benzene, formaldehyde, nitrosamines, and vinyl chloride.[13,98] Tobacco smoke may produce illness via systemic absorption of toxins and/or cause local pulmonary injury by oxidant gases. These poisons impair bone metabolism, compromise nutrient bone blood supply, accelerate bone degradation, contribute to poor bone healing after fracture, and increase the likelihood of fusion failure after spinal reconstructive procedures.†

The alkaline pH of smoke from blends of tobacco used for pipes and cigars allows sufficient absorption of nicotine across the oral mucosa to satisfy the smoker's need for this drug. Therefore smokers of pipes and cigars tend to not inhale the smoke into the lung, confining the toxic and carcinogenic exposure mainly to the upper respiratory tract.

The acidic pH of smoke generated by the tobacco used in cigarettes dramatically reduces absorption of nicotine in the mouth, necessitating inhalation of smoke into the larger surface of the lungs to absorb quantities of nicotine sufficient to satisfy the smoker's addiction. This results in increased deposition of smoke in the lung.

## Epidemiologic Data

According to World Health Organization (WHO) reports, there were 1.1 billion smokers in the beginning of 1990s; 300 million (200 million men and 100 million women) of these smokers live in developed countries, whereas 800 million (700 million men and 100 million women) smokers reside in less-developed countries. At the same time the prevalence of smoking among people age 15 and older is estimated to be 42% for men and 24% for women in developed countries. In less developed countries the corresponding rates would be 48% and 7%, respectively.[171]

In 1988 the Surgeon General's Report on the Health Consequences of Smoking: Nicotine Addiction was published.[158] In this report it is stated that nicotine is an addictive drug. The effect of this report and many other public health information campaigns decreased the percentage of smokers in United States from 44% (in 1964) to 27% (in 1991). Currently, about 45 million people in the United States are cigarette smokers (28% of men and 23% of women). Adults age 26 and older were the most likely to have smoked a pack or more of cigarettes per day. Men smoked significantly more than women. The people in nonmetropolitan areas smoked more than the individuals in metropolitan areas.

Currently, habitual tobacco use is higher in uneducated or less-educated people than in well-educated people. Smoking was estimated to cause approximately 3 million deaths per year in the early 1990s.[169] Unfortunately, despite an increase in information about the effects of smoking, the number is expected to reach 10 million deaths per year by 2020 or the early 2030s.[119]

The ill effects of smoking on health cause about 430,000 preventable U.S. deaths annually. A chronic smoker has about a one in three chance of dying as a complication of smoking. Another important fact is that 60% of the direct health care costs in the United States are allocated to treat tobacco-related diseases.[49,112,138]

## Smoking and Spine Disease

Several investigators have documented an increased incidence of back pain, sciatica, disk degeneration, and spinal degenerative disease among chronic cigarette smokers, compared with nonsmokers.* Spinal disorder-related physician visits are more common, and spinal surgical procedures are four times more common among cigarette smokers than among nonsmokers of the same age group.[4,36,44,53,95]

The prevalence of low back and lumbar spine complaints increases with the number of pack years of cigarette consumption.[43,52,100] This appears particularly true of

---

*References 98,114,118,123,150,153,161,163.
†References 23,27,28,33,39,40,42,44,47,55,57,61,64-66,70-73,75,79, 92-94,107,125,136,143,144,146,149,152,157.

*References 3,4,9,15,20,43,52,60,68,99,134,155.

smokers older than age 50 and of those persons engaged in labor-intensive occupations.[20,68] Nicotine abusers have an increased risk of disk degeneration and herniation compared with nonsmokers.[*] Discordant twin studies, in which identical female twins discordant for cigarette consumption were analyzed, reveal a 20% higher incidence of symptomatic lumbar disk degeneration and significantly accelerated vertebral bone mineral density (BMD) deficits in the smoking twins compared with the nonsmoking twins.[9,75] In a recent epidemiologic study, investigators noted a threefold increase in the risk of symptomatic cervical and lumbar disk disease among chronic smokers. These symptoms were dramatically improved among those patients who subsequently were able to stop smoking.[4] Continued smoking appeared to lead to increased patient complaints. When discectomy was performed, the outcomes for persistent smokers were worse than for nonsmokers.

Smoking has a significant adverse effect on vertebral body BMD and bone mineral content.[†] The bone mass of the human spine reaches its maximum in young adulthood and then stabilizes for several decades.[148] At about the age of 40, bone loss begins at a slow rate in both sexes. Women, around the age of menopause and for approximately 10 years thereafter, lose bone at a rapid rate.[6] Smokers of both genders, particularly women, have an earlier, accelerated rate of bony demineralization compared with nonsmokers.[‡] Hopper and Seeman[75] discovered advanced bone degradation and osteoporosis in the vertebral column and pelvis of the smoking twin in studies of female twins discordant for smoking. They noted accelerated bone turnover and quantified significant reductions in BMD and bone mineral content among chronic smokers. They determined that for every 10 pack years of cigarette consumption, the BMD of the lumbar vertebrae was 3% lower than that identified in the nonsmoking twin.

Decreased bone mineral density and decreased bone mass (osteoporosis) are associated with loss of bone strength and an increased risk for long bone and vertebral column fractures.[§] This is in concert with clinical observations of an increased risk of vertebral compression fractures [VCFs]) among postmenopausal smokers, compared with age-matched nonsmokers, after relatively trivial trauma.[40,61,75]

The available epidemiologic evidence suggests that chronic cigarette users suffer from advanced spinal and intervertebral disk degeneration, experience advanced bone demineralization and accelerated osteoporosis, and have less strong and less healthy vertebrae than do their nonsmoking counterparts. The deleterious effects of chronic tobacco use on the aging vertebral column appear to be independent of lifestyle and genetic makeup.

## Clinical Studies of Spinal Fusion

Several surgeons have reported that chronic cigarette users treated with spinal fusion procedures have experienced either delayed bone healing or an increased risk of pseudarthrosis after attempted spinal arthrodesis.[*] To date, little effort has been directed at identifying the causes of these phenomena.

Symptomatic fusion failure of the lumbar spine is three to five times more common among cigarette smokers than among nonsmokers.[18,28,64,94,164] Not only is the risk of fusion failure higher, but the rate of fusion, when it does occur, is also considerably delayed in the chronic smoker.[61,164] The detrimental effects of tobacco use on lumbosacral spinal fusion procedures have been observed, irrespective of the use of internal fixation hardware and the type of fusion substrate used, and appear to be independent of age, gender, and racial origin.[28,61,95]

Cervical spinal fusion procedures also appear to be impacted by chronic cigarette use.[†] Although a few investigators have reported no significant differences in fusion success rates after attempted anterior interbody procedures, and cite "the forgiving nature" of the cervical spine, most contemporary surgical series document higher delayed fusion rates and an increased incidence of fusion failure among chronic cigarette smokers compared with nonsmokers.[5,24,25,44,164] Bishop et al.[17] found a statistically significant difference in fusion success, including maintenance of interspace height and angulation, after attempted intervertebral fusion, between smokers and nonsmokers. This was particularly apparent when allograft bone was used as the fusion substrate. In a review of 26 patients treated for painful cervical pseudarthrosis, Lauryssen et al.[97] identified chronic cigarette use as an important contributor to failure of attempted ventral cervical interbody fusion. In a recent study Hilibrand[70] reported that both fusion rates and clinical outcomes were significantly worse among smokers compared with nonsmokers. Glassman et al.[57] demonstrated the ill effect of smoking on dorsal instrumented fusion. They found a 14.2% nonunion rate for nonsmokers, a 26.5% rate for patients who continued to smoke after surgery, and 17.1% for patients who stopped smoking after surgery. Moreover, return to work was achieved in 71% of nonsmokers, 53% of nonquitters, and 75% of patients who stop smoking after surgery. For a variety of reasons to be explored, chronic tobacco users have more difficulty with bone healing after spinal fusion procedures than do nonsmokers.

## Laboratory Data

A number of experimental studies support the hypothesis that by a variety of mechanisms, chronic cigarette use negatively impacts bone metabolism and bone healing.[‡] Tobacco extract provided to pregnant animals resulted in subsequent fetal bone growth retardation and impaired ossification in a CD-1 mouse model and in a Sprague Dawley rat model.[116,117] Nicotine administration and chronic inhalation of cigarette smoke, in two separate studies, resulted in impaired long bone development and accelerated bony resorption in Fisher rats.[142,147] Chronic

---

[*]References 4,9,46,61,67,88.
[†]References 8,33,42,72,75,80,92,108,136,141,146,152.
[‡]References 3,33,40,65,66,72,74,92,107,149.
[§]References 32,40,71,73,93,166.

[*]References 4,5,17,18,25,28,44,64,95,97,164.
[†]References 4,5,17,24,25,164.
[‡]References 27,39,48,63,74,94,116,133,142,144,157.

nicotine administration caused reduced BMD in a mouse model, resulted in deformities of the toes in a chick embryo model, and depressed long bone length and weight in a rat model.[27,48,133] Daftari et al.[39] noted impaired neovascularization of bone grafts implanted in the anterior chamber of the eye in a rabbit model assessing the effects of nicotine administration on bone graft incorporation. Hambly and Mooney noted significant changes in bone metabolism in a rabbit nicotine exposure model.[63] They documented marked changes in vertebral and intradiscal acidity (lower pH) in nicotine-treated animals, effects that they believe led to impaired intradiscal metabolism and promoted proteolytic enzymatic bone and collagen degradation. Silcox et al.[143] discovered that nicotine significantly impaired bone healing in a rabbit model of dorsal spinal fusion. These authors documented delayed bone growth, less bone formation, and an increased rate of failure of spinal fusion in nicotine-treated animals compared with controls. Bone that formed in the treated animals was found to be weaker and biomechanically inferior to bone formed in nicotine-free animals.

In vitro cell culture studies further define the deleterious effects of cigarette use and smoking on bone metabolism. Nicotine and cigarette smoke extract, independently, have been shown to impair DNA synthesis, collagen synthesis, oxygen consumption, and cellular proliferation in osteoblasts.[47,55,129] This has been confirmed in both UMR 106B01 rat osteoblastic osteosarcoma cell lines and in osteoblasts isolated from chick embryo calvaria.[47,129] Investigators have identified increased DNA degradation and increased collagen turnover in the chemically treated cell lines. Collagen synthesis is impaired and total collagen production is reduced in chick embryo tibiae and calvaria osteoblast cells exposed to nicotine.[55,129] Nicotine administration suppresses cellular proliferation in rat osteosarcoma osteoblasts and results in morphologic changes and

impaired mitochondrial oxidative function in chick embryo osteoblast cell lines.[55] Smokeless tobacco extract and nicotine, in separate studies, have been shown to result in decreased osteoblast metabolism, reduced oxygen use, and increased lactic acid production in osteoblast cell culture studies.[47,55,129] It appears that a variety of the components of cigarette incineration, not just nicotine, play roles in the toxic inhibition of bone metabolism among chronic tobacco users. In a recent study, Theiss et al.[157] showed the effect of nicotine gene expression in the bone fusion process. In an animal model, they found that nicotine inhibits expression of cytokines, thus resulting in low fusion rates.

## Effect of Tobacco on the Human Spine

The specific impact of the individual toxic components of cigarette consumption on the human skeletal system remains incompletely elucidated. Three main mechanisms by which nicotine and other toxic metabolites and by-products of cigarette incineration affect bone have been postulated:

1. Acceleration of osteoporosis
2. Impairment of bone blood supply
3. Inhibition of osteoblastic cellular metabolism and proliferation

### Accelerated Osteoporosis

Chronic smokers show accelerated bone degradation and bone turnover, and accelerated loss of BMD and total bone content compared with nonsmokers (Figure 99.1). Hormonal factors appear to play a major role in the advanced bone demineralization identified in habitual cig-

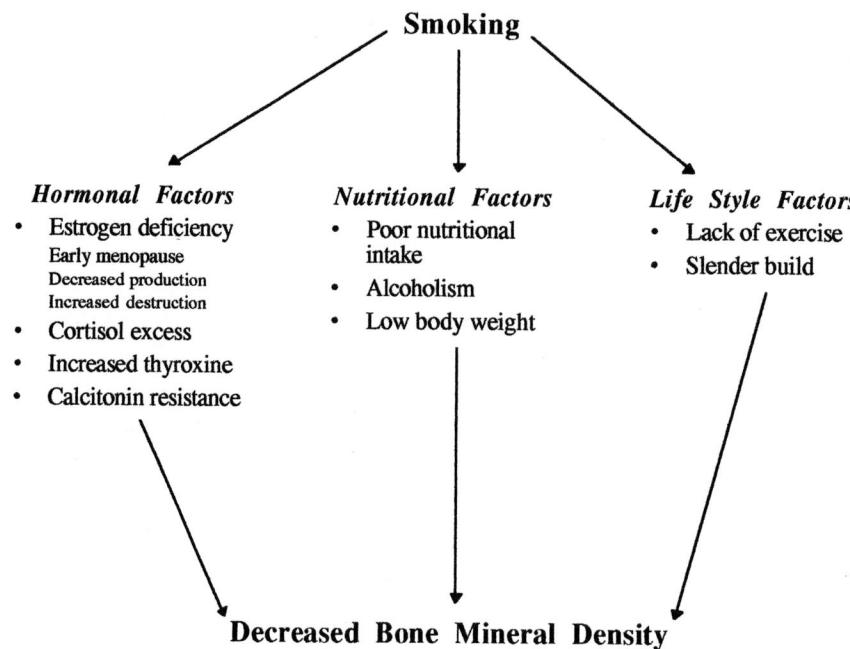

**Figure 99.1** Relationship between tobacco smoking and bone mineral density.

arette users. How nicotine and other noxious components within cigarettes create hormonal imbalances and deficiencies is unknown. Several important imbalances are common among chronic smokers, including hypercortisolism, hyperthyroidism, calcitonin resistance, progesterone deficiency, androgen imbalance, and particularly, estrogen deficiency.[*] All these abnormalities are known to have deleterious effects on bone metabolism and to accelerate skeletal bone demineralization.

The protective role estrogens play in preventing bone degradation and osteoporosis has been particularly well established.[8,109] The serum estrogen concentration has been identified as an important independent predictor of skeletal and vertebral bone mass over time.[146] Estrogen deficiency is associated with accelerated depletion of BMD and bone mineral content, and advanced osteoporosis. Chronic smokers have reduced serum estrogen levels compared with nonsmokers.[75,105,110] This is particularly true of female cigarette users.[75,79,82,105] Women who smoke generally experience earlier menopause compared to nonsmokers and have depressed serum estrogen levels despite exogenous hormone replacement. Investigators have documented increased hepatic metabolism of estrogens and accelerated hydroxy-inactivation of estrogens among habitual smokers.[79,110] These two mechanisms by which estrogen degradation is accelerated help explain the aforementioned phenomena and contribute to the advanced vertebral osteoporosis identified among chronic tobacco users.

Typically, habitual smokers have a thin, lean body habitus.[9] In these persons, extraovarian estrogen production from adipose tissue is almost absent, a circumstance that further compounds the estrogen-deficient state of the chronic smoker.[8,79,136] In contrast, obesity, which generally confers some protection against osteoporosis, provides the smoker with little or no benefit because of increased systemic estrogen breakdown and metabolism.

Nutritional factors play an important role in skeletal health and vertebral bone metabolism. Inadequate or unbalanced nutrition, more common among individuals who smoke, contributes to vertebral osteoporosis.[†] Dietary deficiencies of essential amino acids, essential minerals, and antioxidant vitamins are typical among contemporary cigarette users.[19,34,77] Low levels of zinc and selenium and deficiencies of vitamins C and E and beta carotene contribute to osteoblast vulnerability to free radical oxidative injury.[‡] Because cigarette smoke is an abundant source of toxic oxidant free radicals, chronic cigarette users with less than optimal dietary habits are subject to impaired bone metabolism and accelerated bone degradation.

## Impaired Bone Blood Supply

The adverse impact of chronic cigarette smoking on the cardiovascular and peripheral vascular systems has been well documented.[84,85,102,103] Similar pathophysiologic mechanisms result in compromise of the nutrient blood supply to the human spinal column. These mechanisms chemically induce vertebral vessel constriction, endothelial cell, leukocyte, and platelet damage, and leukocyte and platelet aggregation, all of which alter bone blood rheology and contribute to hypercoagulability, microvascular stasis, and ischemia (Figure 99.2)

Acetylcholine, acting at muscarinic receptors, is a potent vasodilator in bone.[23,38] Administration of nicotine, which acts at nicotinic receptors, causes vessel constriction, effectively reducing bone blood supply.[23,52] In addition, cigarette smoke extract has been demonstrated to significantly attenuate the expected vasodilation caused by acetylcholine administration in a hamster bone blood flow model.[135]

A number of the components of cigarettes, particularly nicotine, result in blood vessel endothelial damage. Damaged endothelial cells release endothelin, a potent vasoconstrictory peptide.[101,102,172] In a canine tibia model, endothelin administration caused marked nutrient vessel vasoconstriction and resulted in a significant reduction in tibial blood flow.[23] It is believed that smoking-induced endothelin release is an important contributor to the reduced bone blood supply identified among chronic smokers.[7,23,115,172,174] The production of prostacyclin, a vasodilator and inhibitor of platelet aggregation, is profoundly impaired among chronic cigarette smokers.[*] Inhibition of prostacyclin synthesis by nicotine has been confirmed in both animal and human studies and is believed to be an important mechanism of the impaired bone blood rheology and blood flow among cigarette users.[7,38,111,121,147]

Habitual cigarette consumption has a variety of detrimental effects on platelet and leukocyte function, fibrinogen and fibrinolysis, and endothelial cell integrity.[†] Cigarette smoking thus leads to impaired bone blood flow, microvascular occlusion, and vertebral body ischemia by a host of mechanisms.[‡]

## Impaired Osteoblast Metabolism

Several of the toxic components of cigarette incineration are damaging to bone-forming osteoblasts.[14,140] Gaseous phase toxins include carbon monoxide, formaldehyde, volatile nitrosamines, and benzene. Particulate phase toxins include nicotine, benzopyrene, cadmium, and tobacco-specific nitrosamines. The precise mechanisms by which osteoblasts are injured by these compounds are not well understood. Proposed mechanisms include impairment of mRNA and DNA synthesis, inhibition of protein synthesis, inhibition of cellular metabolism, and toxic free radical injury.

Nicotine, the best studied toxin in cigarettes, has a direct injurious effect on osteoblastic cells. Aside from its detrimental effect on BMD and bone blood flow, nicotine has been documented to decrease osteoblast cellular proliferation, interrupt collagen synthesis, and inhibit osteoblastic cellular metabolism.[27,47,55,129]

Two types of free radicals identified in burning cigarettes have been associated with oxidative injury to

---

[*]References 3,35,37,50,76,92,108,126,168,169.
[†]References 19,34,45,77,122,124,136,154.
[‡]References 19,34,45,66,77,84,124,154.

[*]References 38,81,111,121,147,165.
[†]References 7,11,21,41,53,54,56,58,102,115,120,132.
[‡]References 12,16,59,83,91,102,104,156.

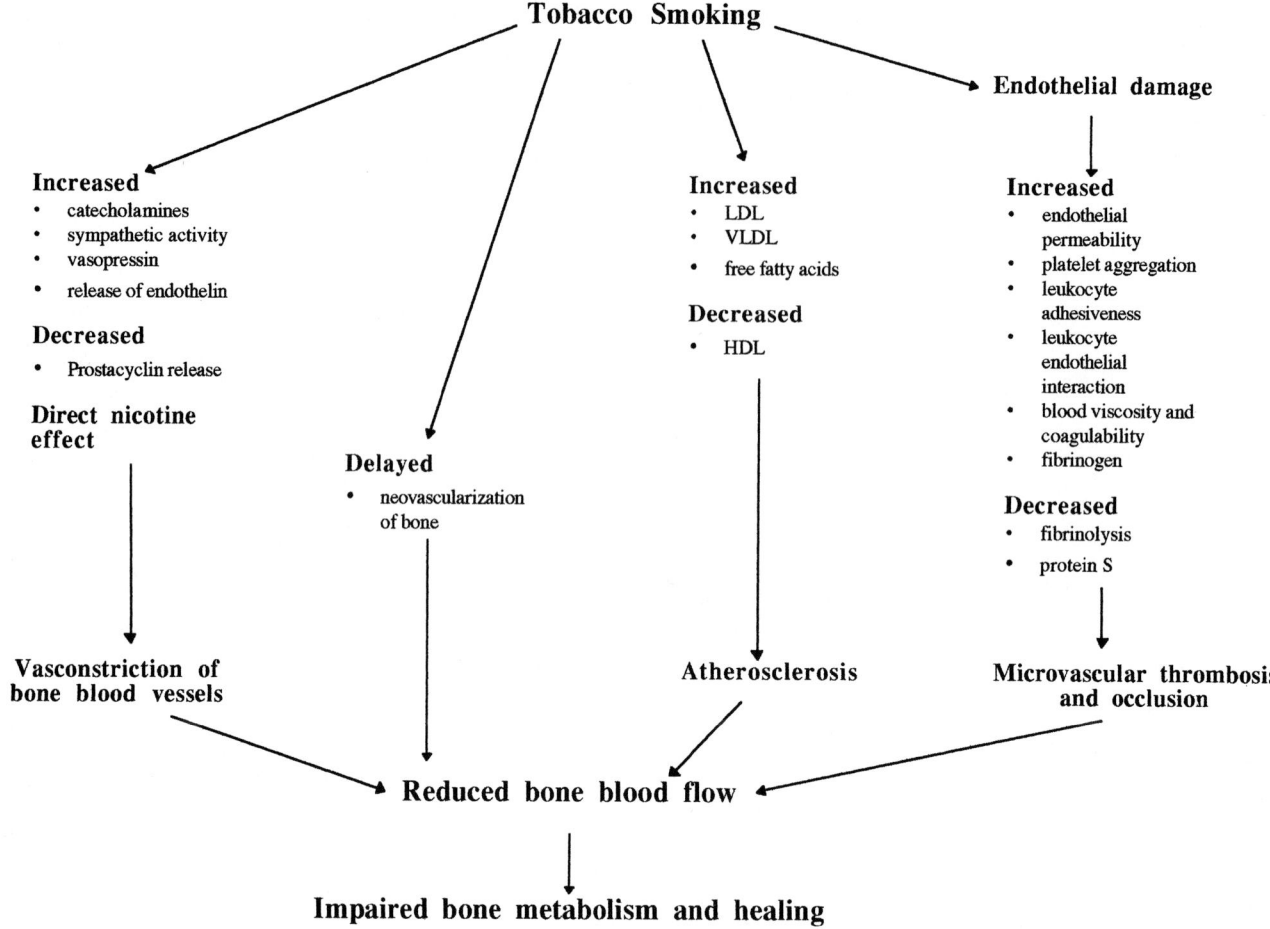

**Figure 99.2** The effects of tobacco smoking in relationship to bone blood flow.

osteoblasts.[108,127,128] Short-lived, highly reactive carbon- and oxygen-centered structures are components of the gaseous (smoke) phase. Long-lived, free radicals of the semi-quinone type are components of the particulate (ash) phase. Osteoblasts, endothelial cells, and leukocytes have been shown to sustain free radical membrane injury from these toxic substances.[83,99,115] In addition to osteoblast membrane destabilization via lipid peroxidation, osteoblast cellular metabolism is compromised by injury to osteoblastic mitochondrial oxidative function.[160]

Cadmium, a component of the particulate phase of cigarette incineration, has an antizinc effect, effectively blocking the ability of zinc to participate in superoxide dismutase reactions, which provide protection to osteoblasts from free radical injury.[124,139] In addition, cadmium reduces the availability of selenium, the lack of which leads to inferior bone production by osteoblasts, which contributes to decreased bone strength, particularly at a site of repair or injury.[137,173]

These cumulative toxic effects on bone-forming cells, combined with reduced bone blood flow, a more acidic and low oxygen tension environment, and accelerated bone degradation, help provide the biologic rationale for the accelerated vertebral osteoporosis, greater propensity for vertebral fracture, and poor bone healing characteristics in chronic cigarette smokers.

## Smoking and Spinal Fusion

Fusion of two or more vertebral segments generally follows a well-defined progression of events over a specific, temporal course. Successful fusion depends on four main factors.[29,61,86,89,125]

1. Preparation of the graft recipient (fusion) site
2. Healing process at the site of fusion
3. Local and systemic responses to the fusion substrate
4. Mechanical principles of motion restriction after attempted fusion

Assuming that the recipient site is properly prepared and that factors 3 and 4 are not detrimental to spinal fusion, the healing process at the site of fusion becomes the major factor for successful bony arthrodesis. The temporal course of spinal fusion is divided into three phases: (1) an early or inflammatory phase lasting 1 to 3 weeks, (2) a middle or reparative phase lasting approximately 6 weeks, and (3) a late or remodeling phase lasting 12 to 18 weeks or longer (Box 99.1).[29,86,89,125,143]

Chronic cigarette use appears to be most detrimental to successful vertebral arthrodesis in the early and middle phase of spinal fusion. It is in these initial 9 weeks after attempted fusion that osteoconduction and osteoinduction

## 99.1

### Phases of spinal fusion

Early phase (inflammatory)
    Duration: 1-3 weeks
    Events:
        Formation of hematoma
        Recruitment of fibroblasts, macrophages
        Infiltration
        Recruitment of osteoid cells
        Early formation of membranous bone
Middle phase (reparative)
    Duration: 6 weeks
    Events:
        Revascularization of graft
        Resorption of graft
        Further recruitment of osteoid cells
        Dedifferentiation into osteoblasts and chondroblasts
        Formation of cartilage and bone
Late phase (remodeling)
    Duration: 12-18 weeks or more
    Events:
        Further formation of bone
        Conversion of cartilage to bone
        Increase in marrow volume
        Reconstruction of bone
        Strengthening
        Remodeling

occur, resulting in vascular ingrowth into the fusion substrate and differentiation into and recruitment of bone-forming cells (pluripotent osteoprogenitor cell and osteoblasts).[32,89,125,143] After initial capillary ingrowth from viable adjacent recipient site bone, complete revascularization of the graft occurs, followed by cartilage and bone formation by recruited osteoid cells, with subsequent remodeling and further bone formation. These processes occur in a delayed and limited fashion in active chronic cigarette users. This is not to say that bony arthrodesis will not occur among cigarette smokers. Fusion will occur in these patients, but failure rates are high, delayed nonunions are common, and bone, when it does form, appears to be weaker than that which forms in healthy nonsmokers.*

The biologic explanation for these phenomena is multifactorial. Applying clinical and laboratory evidence, the authors provide the following hypothesis. The general environment at the site of potential fusion in a chronic tobacco consumer is more acidic and of relatively low oxygen content. The vertebral segments to be fused in the chronic smoker have undergone bone demineralization to a variable extent and have reduced bone blood supply and harbor fewer and less healthy osteoblasts. These vertebrae and their immediate surroundings represent a less than ideal environment for potential bone fusion. Once the graft has been placed, either as an intervertebral, interposition strut, or as dorsal onlay substrate, the viable, decor-

ticated vertebrae to be fused must actively invest the graft and, ultimately, resurrect it as new, remodeled living bone. Assuming that the graft substrate used is suitably osteoconductive, osteoinduction (the process by which the graft substrate stimulates vascular ingrowth and the recruitment of bone-forming cells from the adjacent vertebrae) becomes the critical event in the early and middle phases of the process of spinal fusion. Unfortunately, in chronic tobacco users, compromised vertebrae are less able to mount an effective, productive response to the osteoinductive signals from the bone graft substrate. The vertebrae are less able to develop capillary budding and vascular ingrowth into the graft, and they have fewer, less healthy pluripotent and osteoblastic bone-forming cells available for recruitment. These factors, coupled with the ongoing noxious chemical stimuli from continued cigarette use in the perioperative period, help to explain why smokers are less likely to achieve early and effective arthrodesis after attempted spinal fusion, compared with nonsmokers, and why, when bone forms in chronic cigarette users, it is often less healthy and less strong.

This synopsis also helps explain the especially poor fusion rates reported when allograft bone is employed as the fusion substrate among tobacco users.* Allograft bone has less osteoinductive potential and no osteogenic ability compared with autograft bone, because in the preparation process to reduce the antigenicity of the allograft, all cells (osteoinductive cytokines, trophic factors, and proteins within the allograft), except the few proteins that remain intrinsic to the actual bony matrix, are stripped and rinsed. Allograft bone is biomechanically weaker and of less osteoinductive potential than is autograft bone and is associated with greater collapse and higher fusion failure rates than autograft bone, particularly among persons with a compromised environment for potential fusion (e.g., chronic tobacco users).[17,61,89]

Chronic smokers should be educated and counseled to discontinue tobacco use before elective spinal arthrodesis procedures. Although this may not be critical for a single-level anterior ventral interbody fusion procedure, it is essential for patients anticipating dorsal spinal fusion procedures. It is suggested that complete tobacco abstinence occur 8 weeks before surgery and continue for 12 weeks after surgery. The use of autograft fusion substrate helps maximize the potential for fusion in the chronic smoker. The use of internal fixation hardware and bone growth stimulators, offered as adjuncts to improve fusion success rates among chronic smokers who require vertebral arthrodesis, shows promise, but its efficacy has yet to be proved in randomized, blinded trials.

A commitment on the part of the spine physician to patient smoking cessation cannot be overemphasized. It can truly affect a difference in patient outcome, quality of life, and life expectancy. Nicotine cessation programs are available from a variety of sources, such as The National Cancer Institute of the National Institutes of Health, Bethesda, Md.; The American Academy of Family Physicians, Kansas City, Mo.; The American Center Society, Atlanta; The American Lung Association, New York; and the American Heart Association, Dallas.[130,131]

---

*References 3,5,17,24,44,143,164.

*References 5,17,61,69,106,164.

# REFERENCES

1. Aaron J: Biochemical links between cigarette smoking and pulmonary emphysema. *J Appl Physiol* 55:285-293, 1993.
2. Akuhurst BC: *Tobacco*. London, Longman, 1981.
3. Aloia J, Cohn SH, Vaswani A, *et al*: Risk factors for postmenopausal osteoporosis. *Am J Med* 78:95-100, 1985.
4. An HS, Silveri CP, Simpson JM, *et al*: Comparison of smoking habits between patients with surgically confirmed herniated lumbar and cervical disc disease and controls. *J Spinal Disord* 7:369-373, 1994.
5. An HS, Simpson JM, Glover JM, Stephany J: Comparison between allograft plus demineralized bone matrix versus autograft in anterior cervical fusion. *Spine* 20:2211-2216, 1995.
6. Arnaud CD, Sanchez SD: The role of calcium in osteoporosis. *Ann Rev Nutr* 10:397-414, 1990.
7. Asmussen I, Kjeldsen K: Intimal ultrastructure of human umbilical arteries. Observations on arteries from newborn children of smoking and nonsmoking mothers. *Circ Res* 36:579-589, 1975.
8. Baron JA: Smoking and estrogen-related disease. *Am J Epidemiol* 119:9-22, 1984.
9. Battie MC, Bigos SJ, Fisher LD, *et al*: A prospective study of the role of cardiovascular risk factors and fitness in industrial back pain complaints. *Spine* 14:141-147, 1989.
10. Battie MC, Videman T, Gill K, *et al*: Smoking and lumbar intervertebral disc degeneration: An MRI study in identical twins. *Spine* 16:1015-1021, 1991.
11. Belch JJF: The role of the white blood cell in arterial disease. *Blood Coag Fibrinolysis* 1:183-191, 1990.
12. Belch JJF, Mcardle BM, Burns P, *et al*: The effects of acute smoking on platelet behavior fibrinolysis and haemorheology in habitual smokers. *Thromb Haemost* 51:6-8, 1984.
13. Benowitz N: Clinical pharmacology of nicotine. *Ann Rev Med* 37:21-31, 1986.
14. Benowitz NL, Kuyt F, Jacob P III: Circadian blood nicotine concentrations during cigarette smoking. *Clin Pharmacol Ther* 32:758-764, 1982.
15. Biering-Sorensen F, Thomsen C: Medical, social and occupational history as risk indicators for low back trouble in a general population. *Spine* 11:720-725, 1986.
16. Billimora JD, Pozner H, Metselaar B, *et al*: Effect of cigarette smoking on lipids, lipoproteins, blood coagulation, fibrinolysis and cellular components of human blood. *Atherosclerosis* 21:61-76, 1975.
17. Bishop R, Moore KA, Hadley MN: Anterior cervical interbody fusion using autogenic and allogeneic bone graft substrate: a prospective comparative analysis. *J Neurol Surg* 85:206-210, 1996.
18. Blumenthal SL, Baker J, Dossett A, Selby DK: The role of anterior lumbar fusion for internal disc disruption. *Spine* 13:566-569, 1988.
19. Bolton-Smith C, Woodward M, Brown CA, Tunstall-Pedoe H: Nutrient intake by duration of ex-smoking in the Scottish heart health study. *Br J Nutr* 69:315-332, 1993.
20. Boshuizen HC, Verbeek JHA, Broersen JPJ, Weel ANH: Do smokers get more back pain? *Spine* 18:35-40, 1993.
21. Boutet M, Bazin M, Turcotte H, Lagace R: Effects of cigarette smoke on rat thoracic aorta. *Artery* 7:56-72, 1980.
22. Breslau N, Kilbey MM, Andreski P: Nicotine withdrawal symptoms and psychiatric disorders: Findings from an epidemiologic study of young adults. *Am J Psychiatry* 149:464, 1992.
23. Brinker MR, Lippton HL, Cook SD, Hyman AL: Pharmacologic regulation of the circulation of bone. *J Bone Joint Surg* 72A:964-975, 1990.
24. Brodke DS, Zdeblick TA: Modified Smith Robinson procedure for anterior cervical discectomy and fusion. *Spine* 17:S427-430, 1992.
25. Brodsky AE, Khalil MA, Sassard WR, Newman BP: Repair of symptomatic pseudarthrosis of anterior cervical fusion. Posterior versus anterior repair. *Spine* 17:1137-1143, 1992.
26. Brooks JE: *Tobacco Through the Centuries*. Boston, Little, Brown, 1952.
27. Broulik PD, Jarab J: The effect of chronic nicotine administration on bone mineral content in mice. *Horm Metab Res* 25:219-221, 1993.
28. Brown CW, Orme TJ, Richardson HD: The rate of pseudarthrosis (surgical non-union) in patients who are smokers and patients who are nonsmokers: A comparison study. *Spine* 11:942-943, 1986.
29. Burchardt H: The biology of bone graft repair. *Clin Orthop* 174:28-42, 1983.
30. Burnham JC: *Bad Habits: Drinking, Smoking, Taking Drugs, Gambling, Sexual Misbehavior, and Swearing in American History*. New York, University Press, 1993.
31. Carmell D, Swan GE, Robinette D, Fabsitz R: Genetic influence on smoking: A study of male twins. *N Engl J Med* 327:829, 1992.
32. Carter DR, Hayes WC: The compressive behavior of bone as a two phase porous structure. *J Bone Joint Surg* 59:954-962, 1977.
33. Cheng S, Suominen H, Heikkinen E: Bone mineral density in relation to anthropometric properties, physical activity and smoking in 75 year old men and women. *Aging Clin Exp Res* 5:55-62, 1993.
34. Church DF, Pryor WA: Free radical chemistry of cigarette smoke and its toxicological implications. *Environ Health Persp* 64:111-126, 1985.
35. Cohn SH, Roginsky MS, Aloia JF, *et al*: Alteration in elemental body composition in thyroid disorders *J Clin Endocrinol Metab* 36:742-749, 1973.
36. Cox JM, Trier KK: Exercise and smoking habits in patients with and without low back and leg pain. *J Manipulative Physiol Ther* 10:239-245, 1987.
37. Cryer PE, Haymond MW, Santiago JV, Shah SD: Norepinephrine and epinephrine release and adrenergic mediation of smoking-associated hemodynamic and metabolic events. *N Engl J Med* 295:573-577, 1976.
38. Dadak CH, Leithner CH, Sinzinger H, Silberbauer K: Diminished prostacyclin formation in umbilical arteries of babies born to women who smoke. *Lancet* 1:94, 1981.
39. Daftari TK, Whitesides TE, Heller JG, *et al*: Nicotine on the revascularization of bone graft. An experimental study in rabbits. *Spine* 19:904-911, 1994.
40. Daniell HW: Osteoporosis of the slender smoker: vertebral compression fractures and loss of metacarpal cortex in relation to postmenopausal cigarette smoking and lack of obesity. *Arch Intern Med* 136:298-304, 1976.

41. Davis JW, Shelton L, Eigenberg DA, Hignite CE: Lack of effect of aspirin on cigarette smoke-induced increase in circulating endothelial cells. *Hemostasis* 17:66-69, 1987.

42. de Vernejoul MC, Bielakoff J, Herve M, *et al*: Evidence for defective osteoblastic function. A role for alcohol and tobacco consumption in osteoporosis in middle aged men. *Clin Orthop* 179:107-115, 1983.

43. Deyo RA, Bass JE: Life style and low back pain: the influence of smoking and obesity. *Spine* 14:501-506, 1989.

44. Ducker TB: Cigarette smoking and the prevalence of spinal procedures. *J Spinal Disord* 5:134-136, 1992.

45. Duthie GG, Arthur JR, Jame WP: Effects of smoking and vitamin E on blood antioxidant status. *Am J Clin Nutr* (Suppl 4) 53:S1061-S1063, 1991.

46. Ernst E: Smoking, a cause of back trouble? *Br J Rheumatol* 32:239-242, 1993.

47. Fang MA, Frost PJ, Iida-Klein A, Hahn TJ: Effects of nicotine on cellular function in UMR 106B01 osteoblast-like cells. *Bone* 12:283-286, 1991.

48. Forsyth CS, Frank AA, Watrous BJ, Bohn AA: Effect of coniine on the developing chick embryo. *Teratology* 49:306-310, 1994.

49. Fiore MC: Trends in cigarette smoking in the United States. The epidemiology of tobacco use. *Med Clin North Am* 76:289, 1992.

50. Friedman AJ, Favnikar VA, Barbieri RL: Serum steroid hormone profiles in postmenopausal smokers and nonsmokers. *Fertil Steril* 47:398-401, 1987.

51. Frymoyer JW: Research perspectives in low back pain. *Spine* 14:1384-1389, 1989.

52. Frymoyer JW, Pope MH, Clements JH, *et al*: Risk factors in low back pain. An epidemiological study. *J Bone Joint Surg* 65A:213-218, 1983.

53. Frymoyer JW, Pope MH, Costanza MC, *et al*: Epidemiologic studies of low back pain. *Spine* 5:419-423, 1980.

54. Galante A, Pietroiusti A, Polucci C, *et al*: Influence of acute and chronic smoking on leukocyte aggregation. *Clin Physiol Biochem* 10:33-35, 1993.

55. Galvin RJ, Ramp WK, Lenz LG: Smokeless tobacco contains a nonnicotine inhibitor of bone metabolism. *Toxicol Appl Pharmacol* 95:292-300, 1988.

56. Gillespie MN, Owasoyo JO, Kojima S, Jay M: Enhanced chemotaxis and superoxide anion production by polymorphonuclear leukocytes from nicotine-treated and smoke-exposed rats. *Toxicology* 45:45-52, 1987.

57. Glassman SD, Anagnost SC, Parker A, *et al*: The effect of cigarette smoking and smoking cessation on spinal fusion. *Spine* 25(20):2608-2615, 2000.

58. Gu YD, Zhang GM, Zhang LY, *et al*: Clinical and experimental studies of cigarette smoking in microvascular tissue transfers. *Microsurgery* 14:391-397, 1993.

59. Gudmundsson MD, Bjelle A: Plasma, serum and whole blood viscosity variations with age, sex and smoking habits. *Angiology* 44:384-391, 1993.

60. Gyntelberg F: One year incidence of low back pain among male residents of Copenhagen aged 40-59. *Dan Med Bull* 21:30-36, 1974.

61. Hadley MN, Reddy SR: Smoking and the human vertebral column: A review of the impact of cigarette use on vertebral bone metabolism and spinal fusion. *Neurosurgery* 41:116-124, 1997.

62. Hall SM, Tunstall CD, Vila KL, Duffy J: Weight gain prevention and smoking cessation: Cautionary findings. *Am J Public Health* 82:799,1992.

63. Hambly MF, Mooney V: Effect of smoking and pulsed electromagnetic fields on intradiscal pH in rabbits. *Spine* 16:S83-S85, 1992.

64. Hanley EN Jr, Levy JA: Surgical treatment of isthmic lumbosacral spondylolisthesis. Analysis of variables influencing the results. *Spine* 14:48-50, 1989.

65. Hart DJ, Spector TD: Cigarette smoking and risk of osteoarthritis in women in the general population: the Chingford study. *Ann Rheum Dis* 52:93-96, 1993.

66. Hazes JMW, Dijkmans BAC, Vandenbroucke JP, *et al*: Life style and the risk of rheumatoid arthritis: cigarette smoking and alcohol consumption. *Ann Rheum Dis* 49:980-982, 1990.

67. Heliovaara M, Knekt P, Aromaa A: Incidence and risk factors of herniated lumbar intervertebral disc or sciatica leading to hospitalization. *J Chron Dis* 40:251-258, 1987.

68. Heliovaara M, Makela M, Knekt P, *et al*: Determinants of sciatica and low back pain. *Spine* 16:608-614, 1991.

69. Herron LD, Newman MH: The failure of ethylene oxide gas-sterilized freeze-dried bone graft for thoracic and lumbar spinal fusion. *Spine* 14:496-500, 1989.

70. Hilibrand AS, Fye MA, Emery SE, *et al*: Impact of smoking on the outcome of anterior cervical arthrodesis with interbody or strut-grafting. *J Bone Joint Surg Am* May 83-A(5):668-673, 2001.

71. Hirota Y, Hirohata T, Fukuda K, *et al*: Association of alcohol intake, cigarette smoking and occupational status with the risk of idiopathic osteonecrosis of the femoral head. *Am J Epidemiol* 137:530-538, 1993.

72. Hollenback KA, Barrett-Connor E, Edelstein SL, Holbrook T: Cigarette smoking and bone mineral density in older men and women. *Am J Public Health* 83: 1265-1270, 1993.

73. Hollo I, Gergely I, Boross M: Influence of heavy smoking upon the bone mineral content of the radius of the aged and effect of tobacco smoke on the sensitivity of calcitonin in rats. *Aktuelle Gerontol* 9:365-368, 1979.

74. Holm S, Nachemson A: Nutrition of the intervertebral disc: Acute effects of cigarette smoking: An experimental animal study. *J Bone Joint Surg* 8A:243-258, 1984.

75. Hopper JL, Seeman E: The bone density of female twins discordant for tobacco use. *N Engl J Med* 330:387-392, 1994.

76. Horsman A, Marshall DH, Nordin BEC, *et al*: The relation between bone loss and calcium balance in women. *Clin Sci* 59:137-142, 1981.

77. Hoshino E, Shariff R, van Gossum A, *et al*: Vitamin E suppresses increased lipid peroxidation in cigarette smokers. *J Parenteral Enteral Nutr* 40:300-305, 1990.

78. Hughes JR, Gust SW, Skoog K, *et al*: Symptoms of tobacco withdrawal: A replication and extension. *Arch Gen Psychiatry* 48:52, 1991.

79. Jensen J, Christiansen C, Rodbro P: Cigarette smoking, serum estrogens and bone loss during hormone-replacement therapy early after menopause. *N Engl J Med* 313:973-975, 1985.

80. Jensen EW, Eldrup E, Kelbaek H, *et al*: Venous plasma noradrenaline increases with age: correlation to total blood volume and long-term smoking habits. *Clin Physiol* 13:99-109, 1993.

81. Johnson RA, Morton DR, Kinner JH, et al: The chemical structure of prostaglandin X (prostacyclin). Prostaglandins 12:915-928, 1976.

82. Jick IJ, Purter J, Morrison AS: Relation between smoking and age of natural menopause. Lancet 1:1354-1355, 1977.

83. Kalra J, Chaudhary AK, Prasad K: Increased production of oxygen free radicals in cigarette smokers. Int J Exp Pathol 72:1-7, 1991.

84. Kannel WB: New perspectives on cardiovascular risk factors. Am Heart J 114:213-219, 1987.

85. Kannel WB, D'Agostino RB, Belanger AJ: Fibrinogen, cigarette smoking and risk of cardiovascular disease: Insights from Framingham study. Am Heart J 113: 1006-1010, 1987.

86. Kaufman HH, Jones E: The principles of bony fusion. Neurosurgery 24:264-270, 1989.

87. Kelsey JL: An epidemiological study of acute herniated lumbar intervertebral discs. Rheumatol Rehabil 14: 144-159, 1975.

88. Kelsey JL, Githens PB, O'Connor T, et al: Acute prolapsed lumbar intervertebral disc: An epidemiologic study with special reference to driving automobiles and cigarette smoking. Spine 9:608-613, 1984.

89. Kirkpatrick JS, Hadley MN: Autograft vs. alloimplant bone as substrate for spinal fusion. Persp Neurol Surg 4:38-48, 1993.

90. Kluger R: Ashes to Ashes: America's Hundred-Year Cigarette War, the Public Health, and the Unabashed Triumph of Philip Morris. New York, Alfred A. Knopf, 1996.

91. Koenig W, Ernst E: The possible role of hemorheology in atherothrombogenesis. Atherosclerosis 94:93-107, 1992.

92. Krall EA, Dawson-Hughes B: Smoking and bone loss among postmenopausal women. J Bone Miner Res 6: 331-338, 1991.

93. Kyro A, Usenius JP, Aarnio M, et al: Are smokers a risk group for delayed healing of tibial shaft fractures? Ann Chir Gynaecol 82:254-262, 1993.

94. Lau GC, Luck JV Jr, Marshall GJ, Griffith G: The effect of cigarette smoking on fracture healing: an animal model. Clin Res 37A:312, 1989.

95. Lauerman WC, Bradford DS, Ogilvie JW, Transfeldt EE: Results of lumbar pseudarthrosis repair. J Spinal Disord 5:149-157, 1992.

96. Laufer B: Introduction of Tobacco into Europe. Chicago, Field Museum of Natural History, 1924.

97. Lauryssen C, Moore K, Hadley MN: Symptomatic pseudarthrosis of the cervical spine. J Neurol Surg 1998.

98. Le Houezec J, Benowitz NL: Basic and clinical psychopharmacology of nicotine. Clin Chest Med 12: 681, 1991.

99. Lehr HA, Kress E, Menger MD, et al: Cigarette smoke elicits leukocyte adhesion to endothelium in hamsters: Inhibition by CuZn-SOD. Free Radic Biol Med 14: 573-581, 1993.

100. Leigh JP, Sheetz RM: Prevalence of back pain among fulltime United States workers. Br J Ind Med 46:651-657, 1989.

101. LeMonier de Gouvelle AC, Lippton HL, Cavero I, et al: Endothelin: new family of endothelium-derived peptides with widespread biological properties. Life Sci 45: 1499-1513, 1989.

102. Levenson J, Simon AC, Cambien FA, Beretti C: Cigarette smoking and hypertension: factors independently associated with blood hyperviscosity and arterial rigidity. Arteriosclerosis 7:572-577, 1987.

103. Levy D, Kannel WB: Cardiovascular risks: new insights from Framingham. Am Heart J 116:266-272, 1988.

104. Lowe GDO, Drummond MM, Forbes CD, Barbenel JC: The effects of age and cigarette smoking on blood and plasma viscosity in man. Scott Med J 25:13-17, 1980.

105. MacMahon B, Trichopoulos D, Cole P, Brown J: Cigarette smoking and urinary estrogens. N Engl J Med 307: 1062-1064, 1982.

106. Malinin TI, Brown MD: Bone allografts in spinal surgery. Clin Orthop 154:68-73, 1981.

107. Mazess RB, Barden HS: Bone density in premenopausal women: Effects of age, dietary intake, physical activity, smoking and birth control pills. Am J Clin Nutr 53: 132-142, 1991.

108. McCusker K, Hoidal J: Selective increase of antioxidant enzyme activity in the alveolar macrophages of cigarette smokers and smoke-exposed hamsters. Ann Rev Resp Dis 141:678-682, 1990.

109. Meema S, Bunkler ML, Meema HE: Preventive effect of estrogen on postmenopausal bone loss. Arch Intern Med 135:1436-1440, 1975.

110. Michnovicz JJ, Hershcopf RJ, Naganuma H, et al: Increased 2-hydroxylation of estradiol as a possible mechanism for the antiestrogenic effect of cigarette smoking. N Engl J Med 315:1305-1309, 1986.

111. Nadler JL, Velasco JS, Horton R: Cigarette smoking inhibits prostacyclin formation. Lancet 1:1248-1250, 1983.

112. National Cancer Institute: Changes in Cigarette-Related Disease Risks and Their Implication for Prevention and Control. Smoking and Tobacco Control (Monograph) No 8, USDHHS NIH NCI, (NIH) Publication 97-4213, 1997.

113. National Institute on Drug Abuse: National Household Survey, Highlights, 1991. Washington, U.S. Government Printing Office, 1991.

114. Newhouse PA, Hughes JR: The role of nicotine and nicotinic mechanisms in neuropsychiatric disease. Br J Addict 86:521, 1991.

115. Noronha-Dutra AA, Epperlein MM, Woolf N: Effect of cigarette smoking on cultured endothelial cells. Cardiovasc Res 27:774-778, 1993.

116. Paulson RB, Shanfeld J, Mullet D, et al: Prenatal smokeless tobacco effects on the rat fetus. J Craniofac Genet Dev Biol 14:16-25, 1994.

117. Paulson R, Shanfeld J, Sachs L, et al: Effects of smokeless tobacco on the development of the CD-1 mouse fetus. Teratology 40:483-494, 1989.

118. Perkins KA, Grobe JE, Epstein LH, et al: Chronic and acute tolerance to subjective effects of nicotine. Pharmacol Biochem Behav 45:375, 1993.

119. Peto R, Lopez A, Boreham J, et al: Mortality from Smoking in Developed Countries 1950-2000. Oxford, England, Oxford University Press, 1994.

120. Pittilo RM, Clarke JMF, Harris D, et al: Cigarette smoking and platelet adhesion. Br J Haematol 58:627-632, 1984.

121. Pittilo RM, Mackie IJ, Rowles PM, et al: Effects of cigarette smoking on the ultrastructure of rat thoracic aorta and its ability to produce prostacyclin. Thromb Haemost 48:173-176, 1982.

122. Pocock NA, Eisman JA, Yeates MG, *et al:* Physical fitness is a major determinant of femoral neck and lumbar spine bone mineral density. *J Clin Invest* 78:618-621, 1986.

123. Pomerleau DF: Nicotine and the central nervous system: Biobehavioral effects of cigarette smoking. *Am J Med* 93(1A):2S, 1992.

124. Preston AM: Cigarette smoking: Nutritional implications. *Prog Food Nutri Sci* 15:183-217, 1991.

125. Prolo DJ, Rodrigo JJ: Contemporary bone graft physiology and surgery. *Clin Orthop* 200:322-342, 1985.

126. Prummel MF, Wiersinga WA: Smoking and risk of Graves' disease. *JAMA* 269:479-482, 1993.

127. Pryor WA: Free radicals in biological systems. *Sci American* 223:70-83, 1970.

128. Pryor WA, Church DF, Evans MD, *et al:* A comparison of free radical chemistry of tobacco burning cigarettes and cigarettes that only heat tobacco. *Free Radic Biol Med* 8:275-279, 1990.

129. Ramp WK, Leng LG, Galvin RJ: Nicotine inhibits collagen synthesis and alkaline phosphatase activity, but stimulates DNA synthesis in osteoblast-like cells. *Proc Soc Exp Biol Med* 197:36-43, 1991.

130. Rechtine GR, Frawley W, Castellvi A, *et al:* Effect of the spine practitioner on patient smoking status. *Spine* 25(17):2229-2233, 2000.

131. Rechtine GR, Rechtine JC, Bolesta MJ: Smoking cessation in the spine surgeon's office: A review. *J Spinal Disord* 12(6):477-481, 1999.

132. Renaud S, Blache D, Dumont E, *et al:* Platelet function after cigarette smoking in relation to nicotine and carbon monoxide. *Clin Pharmacol Ther* 36:389-395, 1984.

133. Riesenfeld A: Growth-depressing effects of alcohol and nicotine in two strains of rats. *Acta Anat* 122:18-24, 1985.

134. Roncarati A, McMullen W: Correlates of low back pain in a general population sample. *J Manipulative Physiol Ther* 11:158-164, 1988.

135. Rubenstein I, Yong T, Rennard SI, Mayhan WG: Cigarette smoke extract attenuates endothelium-dependent arteriolar dilatation in vivo. *Am J Physiol* 261: H1913-H1918, 1991.

136. Rundgren A, Mellstrom D: The effect of tobacco smoking on the bone mineral content of the aging skeleton. *Mech Ageing Dev* 28:272-277, 1984.

137. Saldivar L, Luna M, Reyes E, *et al:* Cadmium determination in Mexican produced tobacco. *Environ Res* 55:91-96, 1991.

138. Schelling TC: Addictive drugs: The cigarette experience. *Science* 255:430, 1992.

139. Scherer G, Barkmeyer H: Cadmium concentrations in tobacco and tobacco smoke. *Ecotoxicol Environ Safety* 7:71-78, 1983.

140. Scherer G, Conze C, von Meyerinck L, *et al:* Importance of exposure to gaseous and particulate phase components of tobacco smoke in active and passive smokers. *Int Arch Occup Environ Health* 62:459-466, 1991.

141. Seeman E, Melton LJ III, O'Fallon WM, Riggs BL: Risk factors for spinal osteoporosis in men. *Am J Med* 75: 977-983, 1983.

142. Shevelva GA, Kiriushchenov AP, Sheina NI, Silant'eva IV: Characteristics of the effect of nicotine on the mother-fetus system in exposure over the course of the entire pregnancy. *Pharmakol Toxikol* 47:78-83, 1984

143. Silcox DH III, Daftari T, Boden SD, *et al:* The effects of nicotine on spinal fusion. *Spine* 20:1549-1553, 1995

144. Silcox DH, Boden SD, Schimandle JH, *et al:* Reversing the inhibitory effect of nicotine on spinal fusion using an osteoinductive protein extract. *Spine* 23(3):291-297, 1998.

145. Slemenda C, Hui SL, Longcope C, Johnston CC: Sex steroids and bone mass: a study of changes about the time of menopause. *J Clin Invest* 80:1261-1269, 1987.

146. Slemenda CW, Hui SL, Longcope C, Johnston CC: Cigarette smoking, obesity and bone mass. *J Bone Miner Res* 4:737-741, 1989.

147. Sonnenfeld T, Wennmalm A: Inhibition of nicotine on the formation of prostacyclin like activity in rabbit and human vascular tissue. *Br J Pharmacol* 71:609-613, 1980.

148. Sowers M, Wallace RB, Lemke JH: Correlates of forearm bone mass among women during maximal bone mineralization. *Prev Med* 14:585-596, 1985.

149. Sparrow D, Beausoleil NI, Garvey AJ, *et al:* The influence of cigarette smoking and age on bone loss in men. *Arch Environ Health* 37:246-249, 1982.

150. Srivastava ED, Russell MA, Feyerabend C, *et al:* Sensitivity and tolerance to nicotine in smokers and nonsmokers. *Psychopharmacology* 105:63, 1991.

151. Steinfeld JL: Smoking and lung cancer: a milestone in awareness. *JAMA* 253:2995-2997, 1985.

152. Stevenson JC, Lees B, Davenport M, *et al:* Determinants of bone density in normal women: risk factors for future osteoporosis? *Br Med J* 298:924-928, 1989.

153. Stolerman IP, Shoaib M: The neurobiology of tobacco addiction. *Trends Pharmacol Sci* 12:467, 1991.

154. Subar AF, Harlan LC: Nutrient and food groups intake by tobacco use status: the 1987 National Health interview survey. *Ann NY Acad Sci* 686:311-322, 1987.

155. Svensson H, Vedin A, Wilhelmsson C, Andersson GBJ: Low back pain in relation to other diseases and cardiovascular risk factors. *Spine* 8:277-285, 1983.

156. Tauheed S, Shoaib S, Kamal A: Haemoglobin, haematocrit and plasma fibrinogen in cigarette smokers. *J Pak Med Assoc* 42:162-163, 1992.

157. Theiss SM, Boden SC, Hair G, *et al:* The effect of nicotine on gene expression during spine fusion. *Spine* 25(20):2588-2594, 2000.

158. United States Department of Health and Human Services: The Health Consequences of Smoking: Nicotine Addiction: A Report of the Surgeon General. U.S. Department of Health and Human Services, Public Health Service, Centers for Disease Control, Center for Health Promotion and Education, Office on Smoking and Health, DHHS Publ No (CDC) 88-84-8406, 1988.

159. United States Department of Health and Human Services: The Health Consequences of Smoking Nicotine Addiction (A Report of the Surgeon General). Rockville, Md., Office on Smoking and Health, 1988.

160. Van Jaarsveld J, Kuyl M, Alberts DW: Exposure of rats to low concentration of cigarette smoke increases myocardial sensitivity to ischemia/reperfusion. *Basic Res Cardiol* 87:393-399, 1992.

161. Vaughan DA: Frontiers in pharmacologic treatment of alcohol, cocaine, and nicotine dependence. *Psychiatr Ann* 20:695, 1990.

162. Wallace AL, Wyatt BC, McCarthy ID, Hughes SPF: Humoral regulation of blood flow in the vertebral end plate. *Spine* 19:1324-1328, 1994.

163. Warburton DM: Nicotine as a cognitive enhancer. *Prog Neuropsychopharmacol Biol Psychiatry* 16:181, 1992.

164. Wetzel FT, Hoffman MA, Arcieri RR: Freeze dried fibular allograft in anterior spinal surgery: cervical and lumbar applications. *Yale J Biol Med* 66:263-275, 1993.

165. Whittaker N, Bunting S, Salmon J, et al: The chemical structure of prostaglandin-X (prostacyclin). *Prostaglandins* 12:915-928, 1976.

166. Williams AR, Weiss NS, Ure CL, et al: Effect of weight, smoking and estrogen use on the risk of hip and forearm fractures in post-menopausal women. *Obstet Gynecol* 60:695-699, 1982.

167. Winniford MD: Smoking and cardiovascular function. *J Hypertension* 9:S17-23, 1990.

168. Winsa B, Mandahl A, Karlsson FA: Graves disease endocrine ophthalmopathy and smoking. *Acta Endocrinol* 128:156-160, 1993.

169. Winternitz WW, Quillen D: Acute hormonal response to cigarette smoking. *J Clin Pharmacol* 17:389-397, 1977.

170. Wolf PA, D'Agostino RB, Kannel WB, et al: Cigarette smoking as a risk factor for stroke. The Framingham study. *JAMA* 259:1025-1029, 1988.

171. World Health Organization: Tobacco or Health: First Global Status Report. Geneva, WHO, Tobacco or Health Programme, 1997.

172. Yanagisawa M, Kurihara H, Kimura S, et al: A novel potent vasoconstrictor peptide produced by vascular endothelial cells. *Nature* 332:411-415, 1988.

173. Yang C, Niu C, Bodo M, et al: Fulvic acid supplementation and selenium deficiency disturb the structural integrity of mouse skeletal tissue. *Biochem J* 289:829-835, 1993.

174. Zimmerman M, McGeachie J: The effect of nicotine on aortic endothelium: a quantitative ultrastructural study. *Atherosclerosis* 63:33-41, 1987.

# CHAPTER 100

# The Geriatric Patient

## Robert A. Hart, Mark D. D'Alise, and Edward C. Benzel

When planning either elective or emergent spinal surgery in elderly patients, one must consider the numerous physiologic changes associated with advanced age. Each organ system manifests specific changes that impact surgical decision making, preoperative evaluation, and intraoperative and postoperative management. This chapter addresses the unique aspects affecting spine care that must be considered in elderly patients.

Surgical morbidity and mortality have been shown to be higher in the elderly patient.[42] Although this subset of patients is very heterogeneous, the general decline in physiologic reserve and presence of coexistent disease is primarily responsible for this finding.[14,29] The spine surgeon should be able to recognize specific surgical risk factors and develop an appropriate treatment plan that accommodates the specific needs of elderly patients.

## Organ Systems

### Cardiovascular System

It has been reported that at autopsy 50% of patients older than age 70 have significant cardiovascular disease. The cardiac risk index, a commonly used assessment tool, incorporates myocardial infarction in the past 6 months, uncompensated congestive heart failure, aortic stenosis, nonsinus rhythm greater than 5 premature ventricular contractions (PVCs) per minute, diabetes mellitus, and age older than 70 as major risk factors for postoperative cardiac complications of noncardiac surgery[12] (Box 100.1).

The basic cardiovascular work-up in patients older than age 65 should include a thorough history and physical examination and a baseline electrocardiogram. Myocardial infarction, unaccompanied by recognized symptoms, occurs in as many as 10% of elderly patients.[24] Reports of syncope or dyspnea are the most suggestive symptoms of this event. Peripheral vascular disease is often present with coronary artery disease and may complicate the diagnosis of neurogenic claudication. Absent peripheral pulses or a history of transient ischemic attacks or stroke should lead to a more comprehensive cardiac work-up.

In patients with unstable angina, elective spinal surgery is clearly contraindicated. Patients with well-controlled, stable angina, however, have only a slightly increased risk for perioperative cardiac complications, and may therefore be considered for surgery.[40] Moderate to severe congestive heart failure is associated with a significant perioperative risk.[7,11,25] Jugular venous distension and peripheral edema are suggestive signs, whereas a history of dyspnea on exertion and orthopnea are symptoms of a more severe form of congestive heart failure.

### Respiratory System

Elderly patients are at particular risk for perioperative pulmonary complications for several reasons. Decline in pulmonary function and reserve, underlying chronic obstructive disease and bronchitis, lack of mobility or bed rest associated with spinal surgery, and airway obstruction all can lead to significant morbidity or mortality for these patients.[20,21] In a series of 100 patients older than age 70, approximately 40% of those without a history of lung disease had abnormal pulmonary function.[39] Pulmonary function tests (spirometry) should be obtained for patients older than age 65 or with a history of obstructive lung disease if an anterior approach is being considered.[38]

A forced expiratory volume in 1 second of less than 50% of the predicted value does not suggest an increased risk of postoperative mechanical ventilation, but combined with dyspnea at rest and arterial hypoxemia, it is an established risk factor.[30] Room air arterial blood gas should be tested in elderly patients with lung disease, as well as those with a history of shortness of breath, poor exercise tolerance, orthopnea, and/or excessive smoking. Elevated carbon dioxide tension ($Pco_2$) reflects a loss of pulmonary reserve. A preoperative $Pco_2$ of greater than 45 is associated with an increased incidence of postoperative pulmonary complications,[36] and patients with $Pco_2$ of greater than 50 will often require a period of postoperative mechanical ventilation.[28]

There is no well-defined lower limit of pulmonary function established by any criteria that strictly contraindicates surgery. Optimizing preoperative function certainly helps decrease the overall risks associated with lung disease. Equally important is an aggressive postoperative care plan, including early mobilization, incentive spirometry and coughing exercises, chest physiotherapy with postural drainage and nasotracheal suction, and use of bronchodilators and mucolytics as needed. Finally, an operative plan that avoids thoracotomy in patients with significant pulmonary compromise is well advised.

### Renal System

Decline of renal function in the elderly is more consistent than that of other organ systems.[32] In geriatric patients, serum creatinine levels may be artificially low because of decreased production, caused by a shrinking muscle mass. For this reason creatinine clearance is the preferred test for patients suspected of having significant renal disease. The effect of chronic nonsteroidal anti-inflammatory drug (NSAID) use on the kidney may also contribute to the decline in renal function with advancing age. These drugs can decrease renal blood flow, adding to an already diminished glomerular filtration rate.[10] This has clinical significance in the perioperative patient because water homeostasis may be difficult to achieve in elderly patients, leaving them prone to hyponatremia and volume overload. The use of isotonic fluids, restriction of free water, and careful administration of diuretics may be helpful.

**100.1**

## Cardiac risk index (major risk factors)

Myocardial infarct in past 6 months
Uncompensated congestive heart failure
Aortic stenosis
Nonsinus rhythm greater than 5 PVCs per minute
Diabetes mellitus
Age greater than 70

### Other Sources of Morbidity

Advanced age itself is a risk factor for deep venous thrombosis (DVT).[42] Given the risks associated with bleeding after spine surgery, many surgeons are hesitant to anticoagulate, even with DVT demonstrated by venous Doppler ultrasound. Such patients can be considered for vena cava filter placement or delayed (5 to 7 days postoperatively) anticoagulation. All patients should receive aggressive physical therapy with early ambulation and range-of-motion exercises. Pneumatic compression devices should be used on all patients during their period of bed rest.

Malnutrition is associated with increased morbidity and mortality in elderly surgical patients.[1] Dietary supplements should be added to the hospital diet of patients with reduced postoperative caloric intake to achieve a protein intake of 1 to 2g/kg/day.

Advanced age is also a risk factor for wound infection. A sixfold increase in clean wound infections has been reported in patients older than age 66 compared with patients younger than age 14.[6] The use of routine perioperative antibiotics, minimizing operative times, appropriate postoperative wound care, and attention to nutritional status all may decrease this risk.

Constipation can also be a major problem in elderly postoperative patients. Immobility, decreased gastrointestinal motility, narcotic medications, dehydration, and lack of privacy of the bedridden patient may all contribute to this problem. Stool softeners, fiber-enriched diets, gentle laxatives, and enemas should be used early in the postoperative patient. Perhaps the best method of avoiding postoperative constipation is simply early mobility and physical therapy.

## Spinal Disorders in the Elderly Patient

### Osteoporosis

Osteoporosis is a state of decreased density of mineralized bone. The biochemical make-up and structure of osteoporotic bone is normal, but the volume density of bone is below normal. Bone mass reaches its maximum in the third decade and then begins to decrease.[31] At its peak the maximum surface area of bone crystals of an adult is estimated to be 100 acres.

Bone is a biphasic material consisting of an organic component, osteoid, which is a matrix of collagen and other proteins, and an inorganic component consisting of hydroxyapatite. The mineral component of bone accounts

**100.2**

## Medical treatment of osteoporosis

**Bisphosphates**
Alendronate 10mg daily or 70mg weekly
Risendronate 5mg daily or 35mg weekly
(both with 1000mg calcium plus 400IU vitamin D)

**Selective estrogen receptor modulators (SERMS)**
Raloxifene 60mg daily

**Recombinant human parathyroid hormone 1-34**
Teriparatide 40IU SQ daily for 1 year

**Other treatments**
Conjugated estrogens (postmenopausal women), 0.625mg daily
Calcium carbonate, 400mg bid
Calcitonin (salmon) nasal spray 200IU daily

for the majority of its mechanical strength. Bone is constantly being remodeled by the opposing actions of osteoblasts and osteoclasts. When the balance falls in the direction of osteoclastic activity, net bone resorption occurs. Factors that are predisposed to bone resorption include loss of estrogen and androgens, corticosteroid use, alcohol and tobacco use, and poor nutrition. Bone mineral loss is also associated with increasing age in both men and women. These factors cause depletion of elemental calcium at a rate up to between 30 and 40mg/day from a peak mass of 1000g.

Loss of bone mineral content mainly occurs from trabecular bone because of its increased baseline metabolic activity and greater surface area compared with cortical bone. Hence structures formed of trabecular bone are more susceptible to osteoporosis.[22] In vertebral bodies, trabecular bone accounts for 90% of axial load-bearing resistance. As a result of primary osteoporosis, elderly people may suffer vertebral compression fractures (VCFs) with minimal trauma. Current recommendations for the medical management of osteoporosis are summarized in Box 100.2.

Bone densitometry has been shown to predict risk of osteoporosis.[27] Currently two methods are used to evaluate bone density. Dual energy radiography measures area density ($g/cm^2$) of the spine. This test is simple, accurate, and carries a low radiation dose. It is also well tolerated, with a procedure time of 10 to 15 minutes. Quantitative computed tomographic (CT) scanning is a measurement of true density ($g/cm^3$) via a cross-sectional view of the vertebral body. The precision of this test is excellent, but it can be compromised by patient positioning and movement. The small increase in accuracy provided by this test over dual energy radiography may not justify the expense, discomfort, and added radiation dose.[18] A bone mineral density by dual energy radiography of 1g/cm$^2$ carries a fracture risk over time of 32%, whereas a density of less than 0.8 g/cm$^2$ carries a risk of 50%.[35,41]

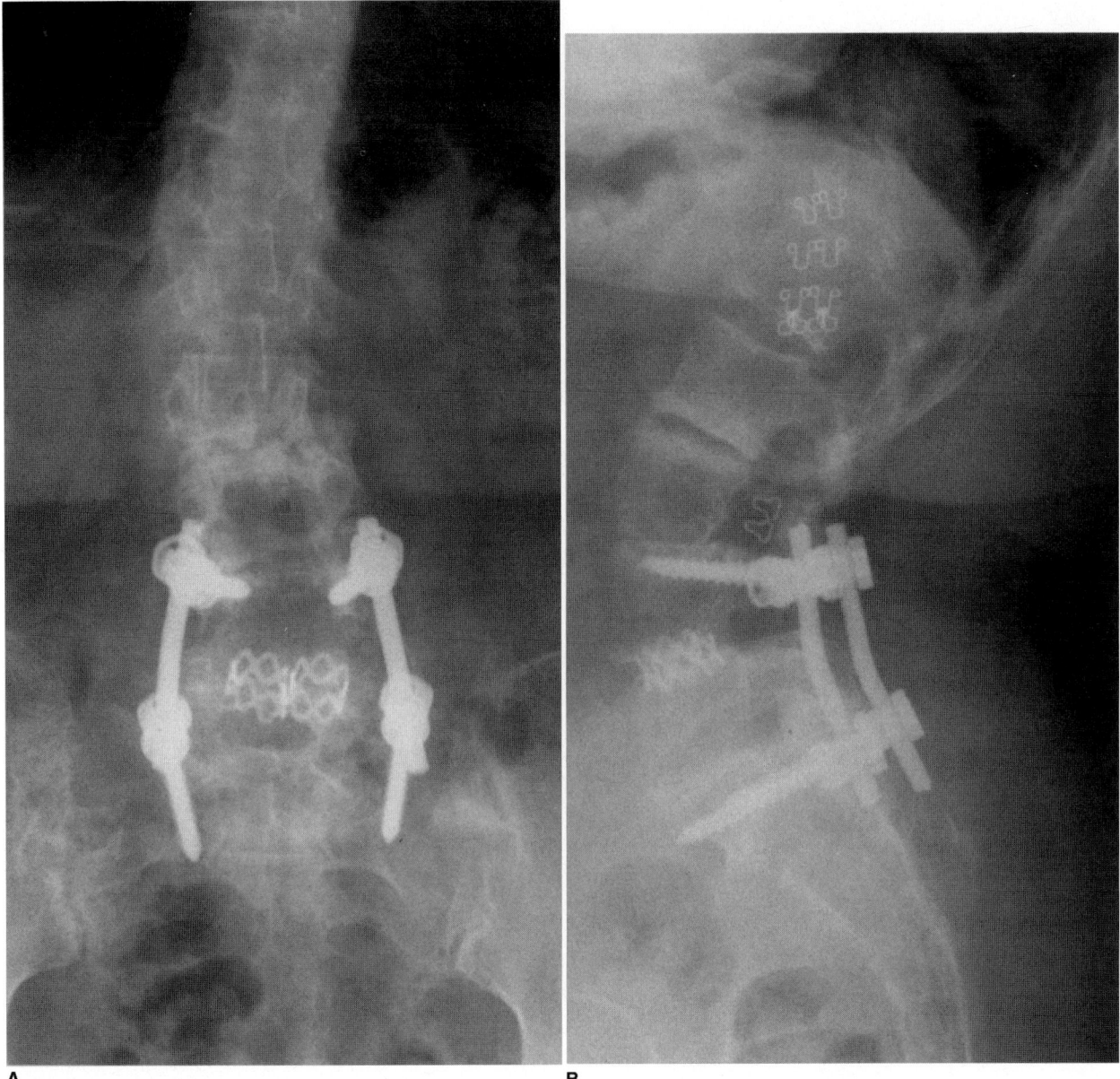

**Figure 100.1** (**A** and **B**) A myelogram of a 76-year-old woman who had undergone a prior fusion from L4 to sacrum with clinical success. Adjacent segment disease had led to a laminectomy above her fused segment at L2 and L3, with resulting segmental instability. At the time of her appearance, she suffered from intractable leg and back pain with severe functional limitations.

*Continued*

Presence of osteoporosis may affect choices regarding instrumentation and fusion for patients indicated for spinal surgery. Obtaining adequate purchase in patients with significant osteoporosis may require using longer constructs to distribute forces and increase numbers of purchase points. In addition, some patients with osteoporosis may be more appropriately treated via uninstrumented spinal fusion or via operative approaches that avoid fusion entirely.

The effect of osteoporosis on vertebrae adjacent to areas of spinal fusion must also be considered. In elderly or osteoporotic patients in whom long fusion constructs are unavoidable, the long-term stability of adjacent vertebral segments is a significant concern. Particularly for areas of high mechanical stress, such as the thoracolumbar junction, consideration should be given to prophylactic enhancement of the strength of vertebrae adjacent to long fusion constructs through procedures such as vertebroplasty (Figure 100.1).

## Osteoporotic Compression Fractures

The most common type of spinal fracture in the elderly is the vertebral compression fracture. These fractures occur not only with higher energy mechanisms but often occur with bending, lifting, or even during normal activity. Management should be directed primarily toward pain control. It should also be recognized that such low energy fractures often are the first indication of underlying

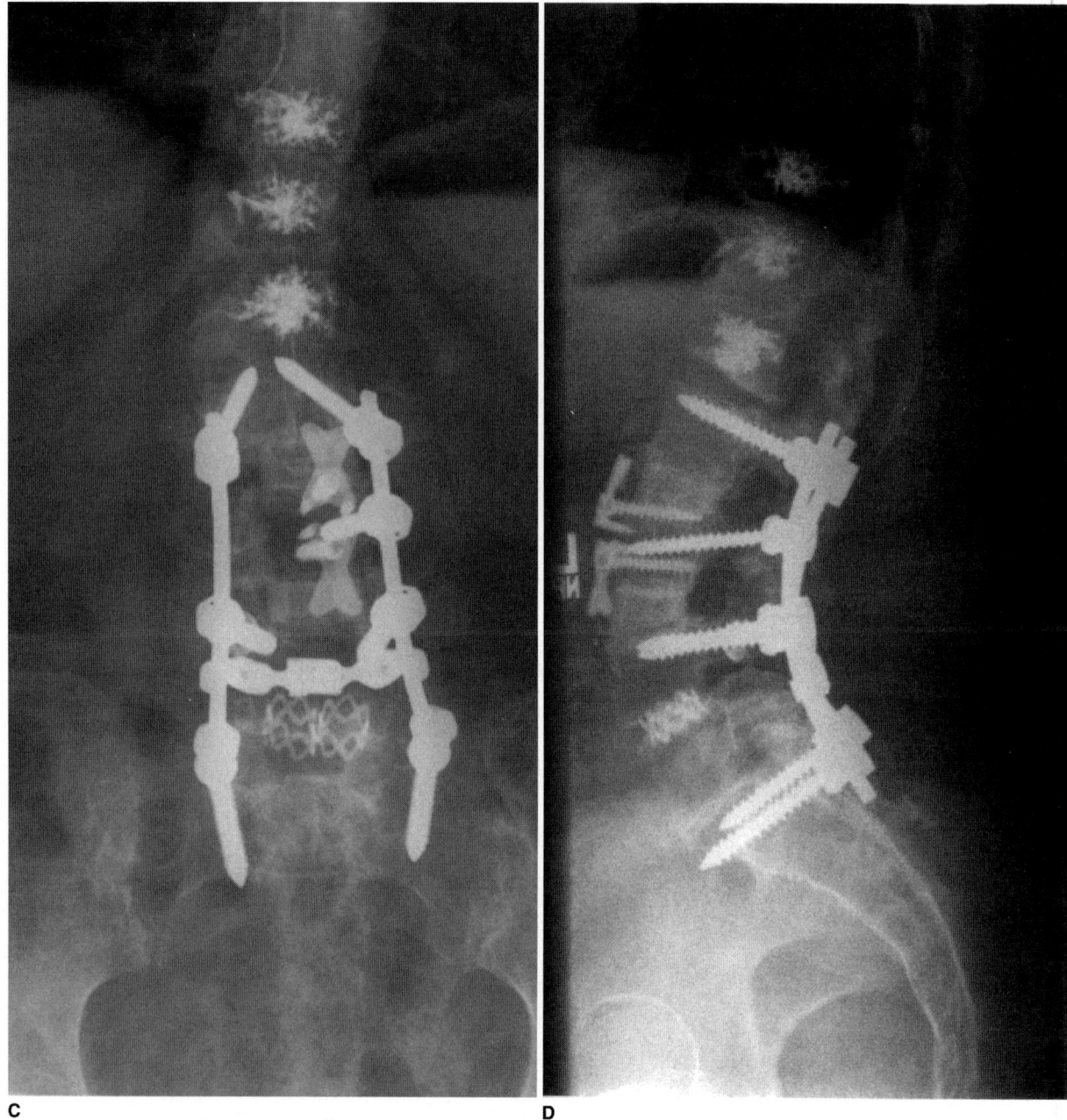

C                                                    D

**Figure 100.1 *cont'd*** (**C** and **D**) Patient underwent a successful ventral/dorsal reconstruction with the revision laminectomies and fusion from L2 to the sacrum. Because of the patient's underlying osteoporosis and advanced age, adjacent vertebral levels were augmented with vertebroplasty. Note postoperative compression fracture of L1 vertebra on lateral view. This fracture did not collapse beyond the appearance shown and remained asymptomatic throughout the postoperative course.

osteoporosis and patients should be started on appropriate medical therapy (see Box 100.2).

Elderly patients with osteoporotic compression fractures who are requiring bed rest or significant narcotic analgesia, or for whom disabling pain has persisted over 4 to 6 weeks, may be candidates for percutaneous stabilization procedures, such as vertebroplasty or balloon-assisted vertebroplasty (kyphoplasty). These procedures are relatively recent additions to the treatment arma-

mentarium for these injuries and are generally well tolerated with success rates of 80% to 90% in terms of pain relief.[16]

## Degenerative Lumbar Spondylolisthesis

Degenerative spinal stenosis results from neurologic impingement by the disc, facet joints, and spinal ligaments. Kirkaldy-Willis *et al.*[19] proposed that biochemical and bio-

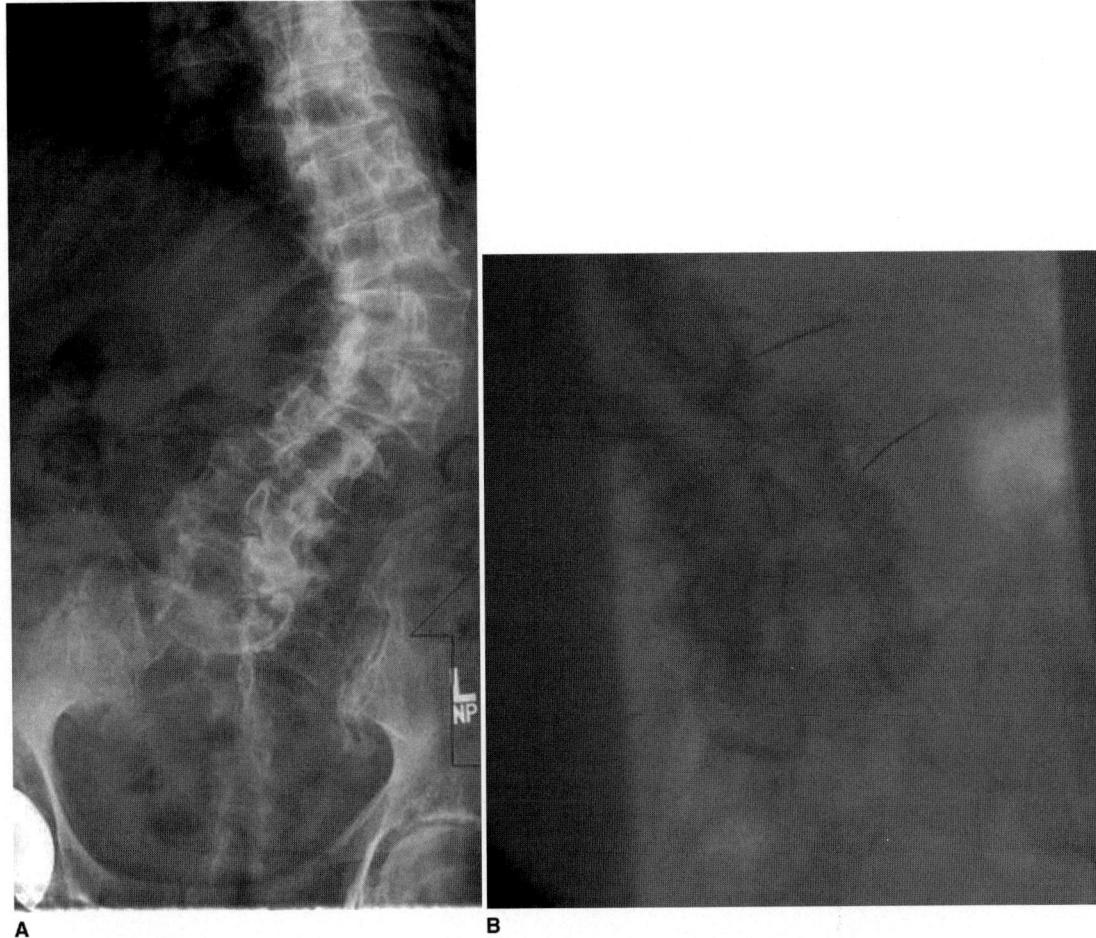

**Figure 100.2** **(A)** A myelogram of an 88-year-old man with severe degenerative scoliosis of the thoracolumbar spine. This amount of curvature likely represents degenerative disease of a preexisting scoliotic curve. **(B)** Patient underwent selective nerve root blocks of the right L3 and L4 nerve roots. Because of the relief experienced after this procedure and subsequent recurrence of symptoms, the patient underwent selective foraminotomies at these levels. He had partial relief of his lower extremity symptoms after this procedure. Given his advanced age and the severity of his deformity, it was felt that reconstruction via instrumented fusion would not be well tolerated by this patient.

mechanical changes associated with age cause increased mobility at a spinal segment, leading to osteophyte formation and joint hypertrophy that reduce spinal canal diameter and local stiffness. The increased joint laxity resulting from facet degeneration leads in some cases to spondylolisthesis between adjacent vertebrae.

For patients with degenerative spondylolisthesis of the lumbar spine, use of instrumentation has not been convincingly shown to improve clinical outcomes after fusion.[5,9,37] Avoiding instrumentation when performing fusion in elderly, osteoporotic patients with degenerative spondylolisthesis is a reasonable option, particularly when facets are oriented relatively in the coronal plane and segmental instability is not present.

### Degenerative Scoliosis

Degenerative scoliosis, unlike idiopathic scoliosis, is an acquired disorder of adult patients for which there is no gender preference. Patients present with symptoms simi-

lar to those of degenerative lumbar stenosis. Nonoperative treatment modalities include physical therapy, muscle relaxants, and nonsteroidal antiinflammatory medications. Surgical options include neurologic decompression via laminotomy or laminectomy. Spinal fusion may or may not be appropriate, depending on the patients' presentation, health status, and expectations from surgery.[2,23,33,34] There are conflicting reports regarding the need for spinal stabilization after decompression for degenerative scoliosis.[2,3,23,33] Patients without lateral listhesis between adjacent vertebrae may be appropriately treated with laminectomy without fusion.

Patients of advanced age with significant scoliotic curves may not be appropriate candidates for the large reconstructive fusion procedures required to treat their spinal deformity. Judicious use of selective nerve root blocks with isolated unilateral foraminotomies may be used to good effect in such patients with limited risk of deformity progression (Figure 100.2). Elderly patients for whom stabilization is required will benefit from efforts to limit the extent of surgery, including use of posterior or transforaminal interbody fusions (PLIFs or TLIFs) in favor of ventral approaches (Figure 100.3).

### Cervical Degenerative Disease

Elderly patients with cervical degenerative disease and spinal stenosis also present a treatment problem significantly different than younger patients with similar condi-

tions. Concerns due to bone quality and physiologic ability to withstand large reconstructive surgery again play a significant role in decision making.

Ventral decompressive surgery via multiple-level corpectomy may prove difficult in this patient population. Although ventral decompression may be appropriate on a neurologic basis because of kyphotic alignment of the cervical vertebrae,[44] reduced mechanical strength of vertebral bodies increases the risk of graft subsidence or

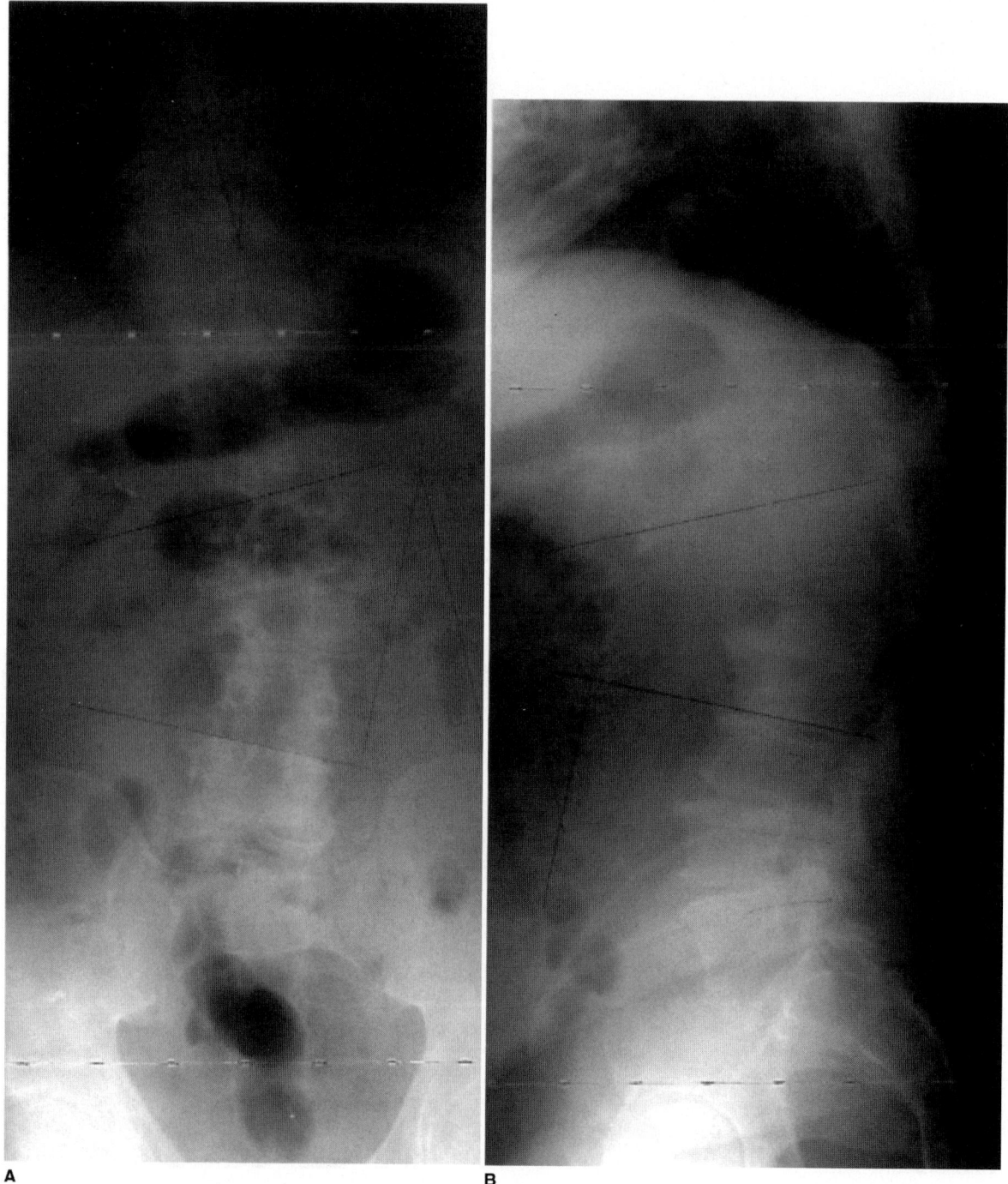

**A**                                               **B**

**Figure 100.3** (**A** and **B**) A myelogram of a 73-year-old man with a longstanding history of degenerative scoliosis and kyphosis. He had undergone prior laminectomies as noted on the anteroposterior (AP) view. This patient was minimally active and wore a TLSO for comfort whenever upright.

dislodgement if an isolated ventral procedure is performed. In addition, the substantial surgery required to accomplish combined ventral-dorsal cervical reconstruction may not be well tolerated by elderly patients.

If ventral decompression is required, multilevel discectomy or combined corpectomy/discectomy procedures may be an appropriate alternative in this age group (Figure 100.4). Patients with central stenosis and neutral or lordotic alignment may be treated via an isolated posterior procedure, such as multilevel laminectomy or laminaplasty.[43] These treatment approaches generally provide satisfactory clinical outcomes while reducing significant complications.

## Spinal Trauma and Spinal Cord Injury

Numerous characteristics of spinal injury are unique in the elderly patient, including injury mechanisms, fracture types, incidence of neurologic deficits, and outcomes. The primary mechanism of injury in young patients is motor vehicle collisions, whereas the leading cause of spine fracture in patients older than age 65 is falls.[17,26] Significant neurologic deficits are also significantly more common in younger patients than in the elderly, possibly reflecting this difference in injury mechanisms.[4,17]

Outcomes from traumatic spinal injuries also differ significantly between elderly and nonelderly adult patients.

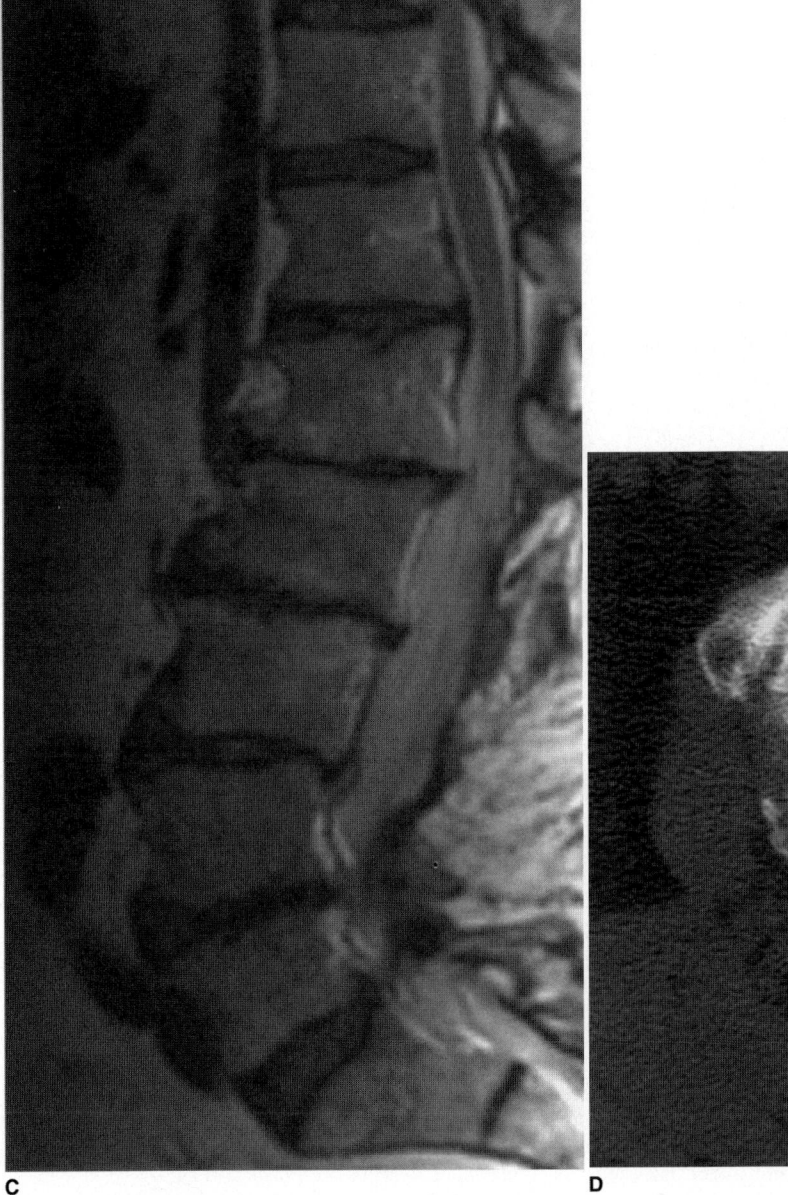

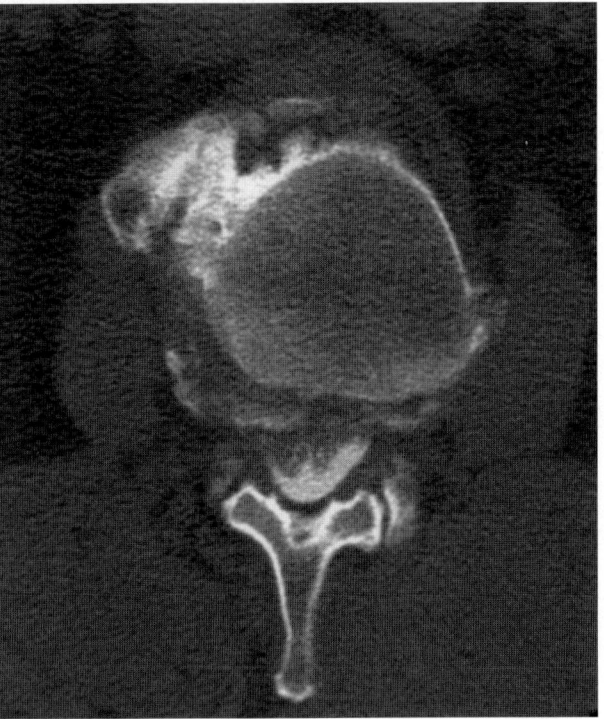

C                                          D

**Figure 100.3 *cont'd* (C** and **D)** Sagittal MRI scan and transverse CT myelogram demonstrate marked degenerative change across the kyphosis with significant residual foraminal and lateral recess stenosis at levels L1-2 and L2-3 despite prior laminectomies.

*Continued*

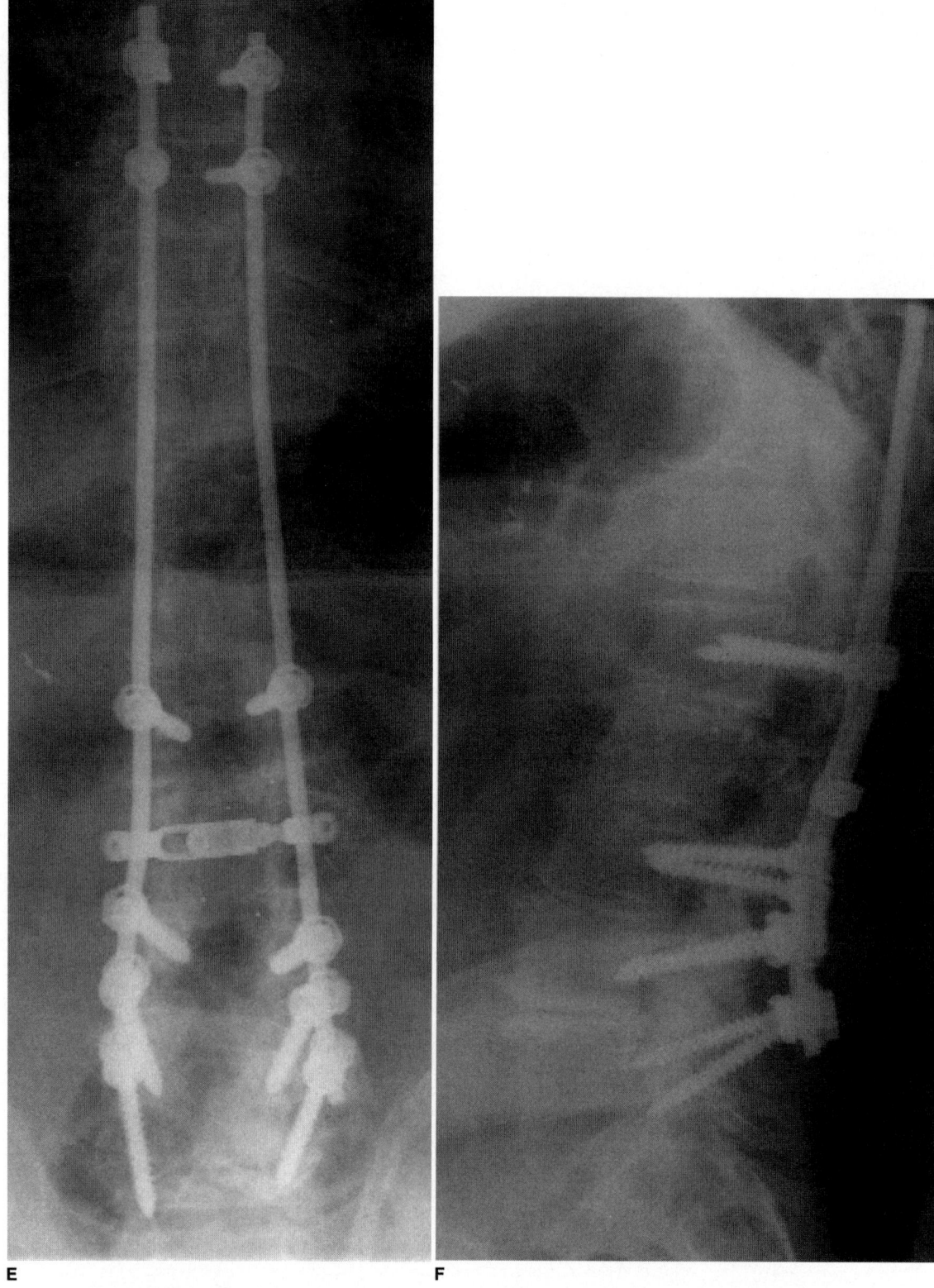

E                                                          F

**Figure 100.3** *cont'd* (**E** and **F**) AP and lateral views after a posterior instrumented fusion and decompression. A transforaminal lumbar interbody fusion (TLIF) procedure was performed at the L1-2 and L2-3 levels using a carbon fiber interbody spacer and iliac crest autograft. By 1 year postoperatively, the patient had experienced excellent relief of both back and leg symptoms and no longer wore a TLSO for routine activities. His functional level was substantially improved and he reinitiated work as a volunteer fireman. Note correction of both the scoliotic curve and kyphotic deformity using this approach.

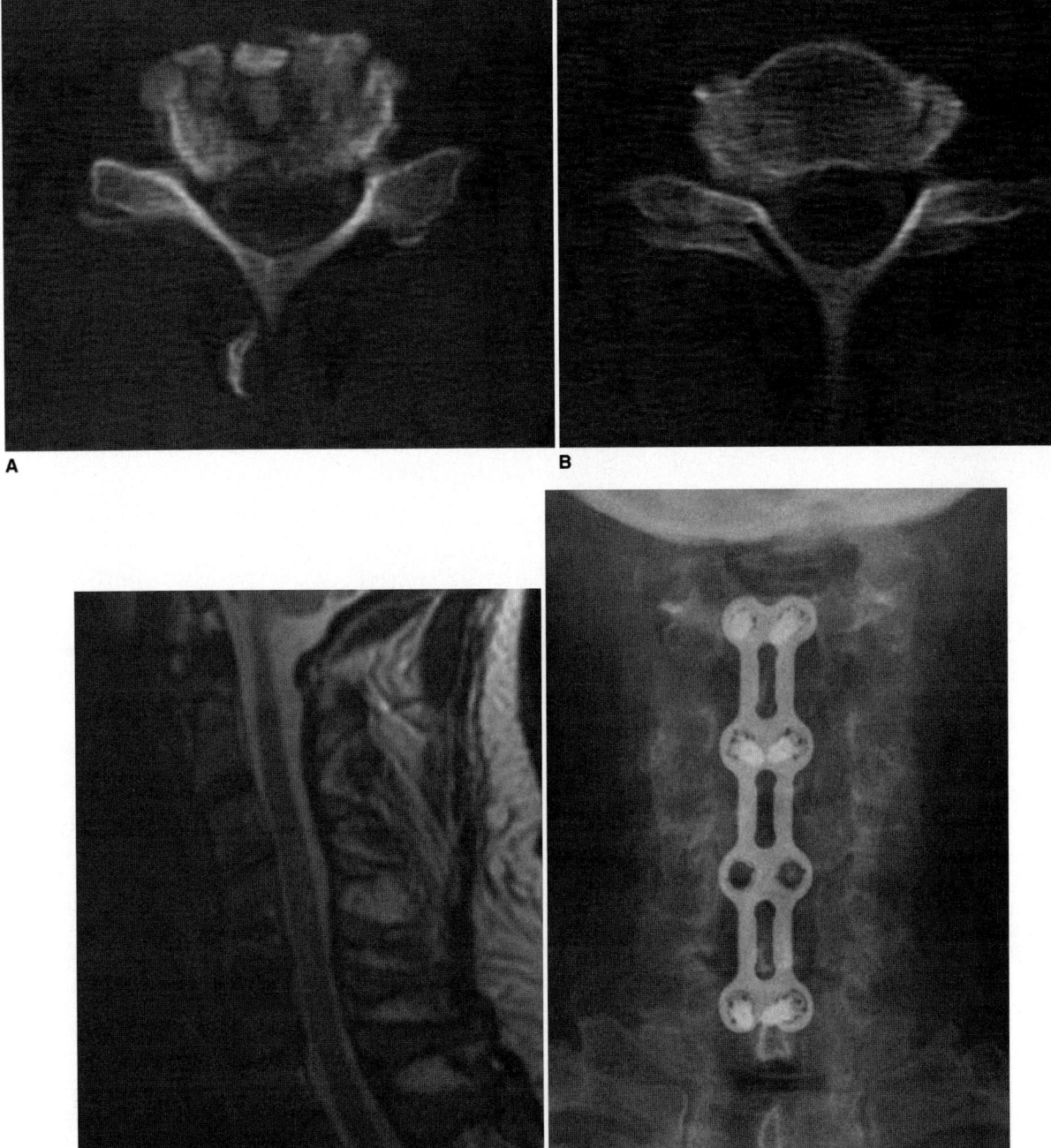

**Figure 100.4 (A-C)** A myelogram of a 65-year-old man who developed recurrent symptoms of radiculopathy after a motor vehicle accident. He had undergone a prior two-level discectomy performed elsewhere with a solid fusion obtained at level C4-5, but a nonunion had occurred at level C5-6. A CT myelogram shows degenerative change and foraminal stenosis at level C6-7 (**B**) and at the nonunion site at level C5-6 (**C**). Note kyphosis across the C3-4 disc demonstrated on sagittal plane MRI.
*Continued*

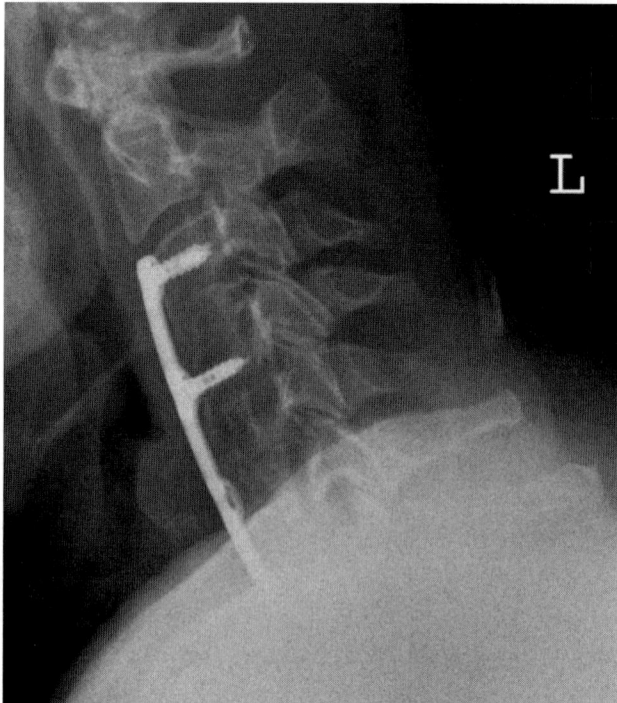

**E**

**Figure 100.4** *cont'd* (**D** and **E**) AP and lateral views demonstrate solid consolidation after a corpectomy of the C6 vertebrae, including resection of the C5-6 nonunion and a discectomy at the C3-4 level with structural iliac crest graft and spanning anterior cervical locking plate. Alternating levels of corpectomy and discectomy, as in this case, allow better anterior column support and segmental fixation with ventral instrumentation.

Elderly patients have a significantly lower survival rate than nonelderly adults, both with and without neurologic injury. Neurologic injury is especially devastating in the elderly, as the 60-day mortality rate for patients older than age 65 with traumatic paralysis approaches 30%.[17]

Understanding these issues may factor significantly in clinical decision making. Families of elderly patients suffering from significant neurologic injuries should understand the high risk of poor outcomes in this age group. Given the significant risk of early mortality, as well as the likely disability resulting from residual neurologic deficits, patients and families may choose withdrawal of support over aggressive interventional treatment.

Finally, injuries appropriately treated with surgical intervention in younger patients may be treatable with minimal intervention in the elderly population. For example, risks associated with nonunion after dens fracture appear to be limited in elderly patients, and it is not clear that surgical stabilization of established nonunions is warranted.[13,16] Treatment decisions for these injuries are best decided on a case-by-case basis, and will depend on patient preferences, health status, and the nature of the injury (Figure 100.5).

## Summary

Elderly patients represent a distinct patient group when planning spinal surgery. Disease and injury mechanisms,

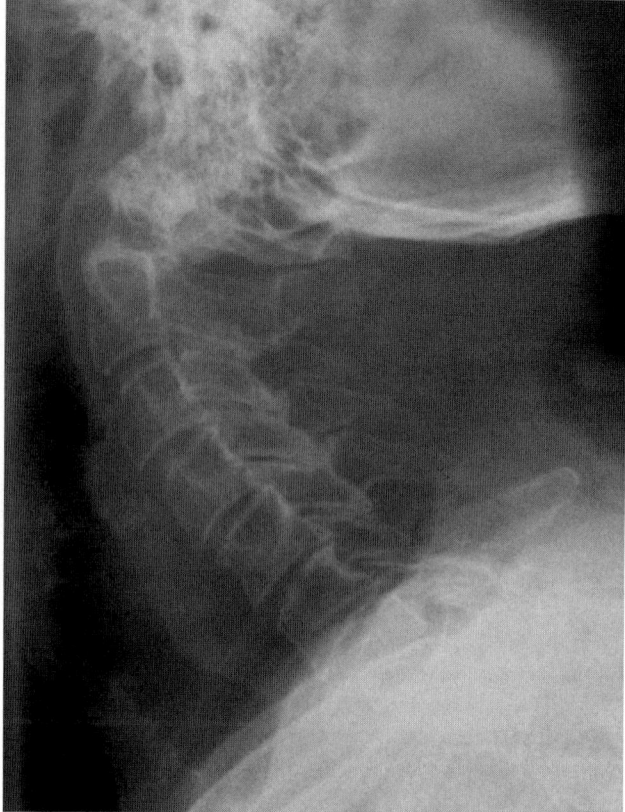

**A**

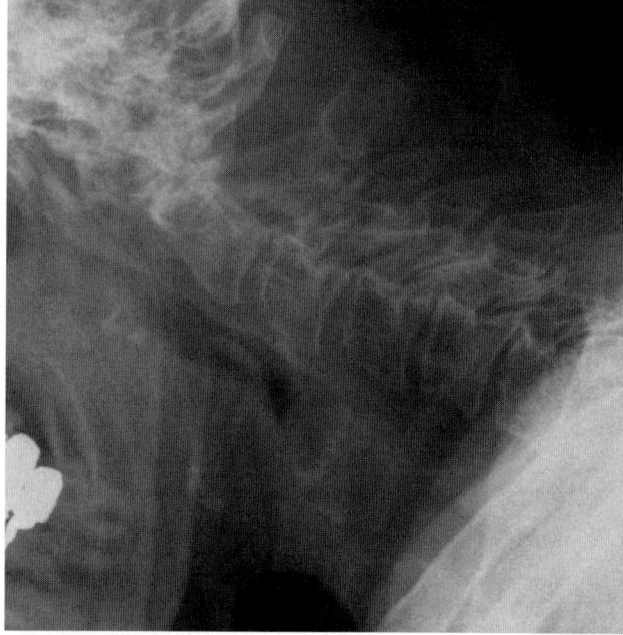

**B**

**Figure 100.5** (**A**) A myelogram of a 97-year-old woman discovered incidentally on admission to trauma service after an MVA to have a mobile nonunion of a prior dens fracture. She was asymptomatic from this, both with respect to neck pain and neurologic symptoms. Work-up did include a CT scan with reconstructions at the time of injury. Space available for the spinal cord (SAC) is 21mm on the extension view (**B**). She was treated with observation without clinical incident at 6-month follow-up.

the ability to withstand significant surgical intervention, and the mechanical effects of osteoporosis all play a role in decision making and treatment outcomes. These issues must be considered on a case-by-case basis, and discussed with patients and families in determining appropriate treatment approaches.

# REFERENCES

1. Bastow MD, Rawlings J, Allison SP: Undernutrition, hypothermia, and injury in elderly women with fractured femur: an injury response to altered metabolism? *Lancet* 1:143, 1983.

2. Benner B, Ehni G: Degenerative lumbar scoliosis. *Spine* 4:548, 1979.

3. Benzel EC: *Biomechanics of Spine Stabilization: Principles and Clinical Practice*. New York, McGraw-Hill, 1995.

4. Bracken MB, Freeman DH Jr, Hellenbrand K: Incidence of acute traumatic hospitalized spinal cord injury in the United States, 1970-1977. *Am J Epidemiol* 113:615, 1981.

5. Christensen FB, Hansen ES, Laursen M, *et al*: Long-term functional outcome of pedicle screw instrumentation as a support for posterolateral spinal fusion. Randomized clinical study with 5-year followup. *Spine* 27:1269-1277, 2002.

6. Cruse PJ, Foord R: The epidemiology of wound infection: a 10-year prospective study of 62,939 wounds. *Surg Clin North Am* 60:27, 1980.

7. Deron SJ, Kotler MN: Noncardiac surgery in the cardiac patient. *Am Heart J* 116:831, 1988.

8. Evans L: *Traffic Safety and the Driver*. New York, VanNostrand Reinhold, 1991.

9. Fischgrund JS, Mackay M, Herkowitz HN, *et al*: Degenerative lumbar spondylolisthesis with spinal stenosis: a prospective, randomized study comparing decompressive laminectomy and arthrodesis with and without spinal instrumentation. *Spine* 22(24): 2807-2812, 1997.

10. Garella S, Matarese RA: Renal effects of prostaglandins and clinical adverse effects of nonsteroidal anti-inflammatory agents. *Medicine* (Baltimore) 63:165, 1984.

11. Goldman L, Caldera DL, Nussbaum SR, *et al*: Multifactorial index of cardiac risk in noncardiac surgical procedures. *N Engl J Med* 297:845, 1977.

12. Goldman L: Cardiac risks and complications of noncardiac surgery. *Ann Intern Med* 98:504, 1983.

13. Hanigan WC, Powell FC, Elwood PW, *et al*: Odontoid fractures in elderly patients. *J Neurosurg* 78:32, 1993.

14. Harbrecht PJ, Garrison RN, Fry DE: Surgery in elderly patients. *South Med J* 74:594, 1981.

15. Hart RA, Saterbak A, Rapp T, *et al*: Nonoperative management of dens fracture nonunion in elderly patients without myelopathy. *Spine* 11:1339-1343, 2000.

16. Hart RA: Percutaneous treatment of osteoporotic spinal compression fractures, *Current Women's Health Reports* 3(1):72-74, 2003.

17. Irwin ZN, Arthur MA, Mullins RJ, Hart RA: Variations in injury patterns, treatment, and outcome for spinal fracture and paralysis in adult versus geriatric patients. *Spine*. (In Press.)

18. Kaplan FS: Prevention and management of osteoporosis. *Clin Symp* 47:2, 1995.

19. Kirkaldy-Willis WH, Paine KW, Cauchoix J, *et al*: Lumbar spinal stenosis. *Clin Orthop* 99:30, 1974.

20. Knudson RJ, Clark DF, Kennedy TC, *et al*: Effect of aging alone on mechanical properties of the normal adult human lung. *J Appl Physiol* 43:1054, 1977.

21. Levitzky MG: Effects of aging on the respiratory system. *Physiologist* 27:102, 1984.

22. Lloyd T, Myers C, Buchanan JR, Demers LM: Collegiate women athletes with irregular menses during adolescence have decreased bone density. *Obstet Gynecol* 72:639, 1988.

23. Lonstein J: Adult scoliosis. In Bradford D, Lonstein J, Ogilvie T, Winter R (eds): *Moe's Textbook of Scoliosis and Other Spinal Disorders*, ed 2. Philadelphia, WB Saunders, 1987.

24. MacDonald JB: Presentation of acute myocardial infarction in the elderly—a review. *Age Ageing* 13:196, 1984.

25. Mangano DT: Perioperative cardiac morbidity. *Anesthesiology* 72:153, 1990.

26. McGlinchey-Berroth R, Morrow L, Ahlquist M, *et al*: Late-life spinal cord injury and aging with a long-term injury: characteristics of two emerging populations. *J Spinal Cord Med* 18:183, 1995.

27. Melton LJ III, Riggs BL: Impaired bone strength and fracture patterns at different skeletal sites. In Unthoff HK, Stahl E (eds): *Current Concepts of Bone Fragility*. Berlin, Springer-Verlag, 1986.

28. Milledge JS, Nunn JF: Criteria of fitness for anaesthesia in patients with chronic obstructive lung disease. *Br Med J* 3:670, 1975.

29. Milzman DP, Boulanger BR, Rodriguez A, *et al*: Pre-existing disease in trauma patients: a predictor of fate independent of age and injury severity score. *J Trauma* 32:236, 1992.

30. Nunn JF, Milledge JS, Chen D, *et al*: Respiratory criteria of fitness for surgery and anaesthesia. *Anaesthesia* 43:543, 1988.

31. Riggs BL, Wahner HW, Melton LJ III, *et al*: Rates of bone loss in the appendicular and axial skeletons of women. Evidence of substantial vertebral bone loss before menopause. *J Clin Invest* 77:1487, 1986.

32. Rowe JW, Andres R, Tobin JD, *et al*: The effect of age on creatinine clearance in men: a cross-sectional and longitudinal study. *J Gerontol* 31:155, 1976.

33. San Martino A, D'Andria FM, San Martino C: The surgical treatment of nerve root compression caused by scoliosis of the lumbar spine. *Spine* 8:261, 1983.

34. Smith OC: Advanced age as a contraindication to operation. *Med Rec* (New York) 72:642, 1907.

35. Smith RW Jr, Rizek J: Epidemiologic studies of osteoporosis in women of Puerto Rico and southeastern Michigan with special reference to age, race, national origin and to other related or associated findings. *Clin Orthop* 45:31, 1966.

36. Stein M, Koota JM, Simon M, *et al*: Pulmonary evaluation of surgical patients. *JAMA* 181:765, 1962.

37. Thomsen K, Christensen FB, Eiskjær SP, *et al*: The effect of pedicle screw instrumentation on functional outcome and fusion rates in posterolateral lumbar spine fusion: a prospective, randomized clinical study. *Spine* 22: 2813-2822, 1997.

38. Tisi GM: Preoperative evaluation of pulmonary function. Validity, indications, and benefits. *Am Rev Respir Dis* 119:293, 1979.

39. Tornebrandt K, Fletcher R: Pre-operative chest x-rays in elderly patients. *Anaesthesia* 37:901, 1982.

40. von Knorring J: Postoperative myocardial infarction: a prospective study in a risk group of surgical patients. *Surgery* 90:55, 1981.

41. Wasnich RD, Ross PD, Heilbrun LK, Vogel JM: Prediction of postmenopausal fracture risk with use of bone mineral measurements. *Am J Obstet Gynecol* 153:745, 1985.

42. Watters JM, McClaran JC: The elderly surgical patient. In *American College of Surgeons: Care of the Surgical Patient*, vol I. New York, Scientific American, 1991.

43. Yoshida M, Otani K, Shibasaki K, Ueda S: Expansive laminoplasty with reattachment of spinous process and extensor musculature for cervical myelopathy. *Spine* 17(5):491, 1992.

44. Zdeblick TA, Bohlman HH: Cervical kyphosis and myelopathy. *JBJS* 71-A(2):170, 1989.

# CHAPTER 101

# Surgery of the Sympathetic Nervous System

J. Patrick Johnson, Saad Khairi,
and William C. Welch

Sympathectomy procedures involve interrupting thoracic or lumbar sympathetic pathways to provide relief from autonomically mediated syndromes. Currently the most common disorder treated is essential hyperhidrosis,[2,35] but sympathectomies have been used extensively in the past to treat various pain syndromes that include complex regional pain syndrome (CRPS), reflex sympathetic dystrophy (RSD), causalgia, vascular insufficiency pain syndromes, and Raynaud's disease.[20,25,33,40] In the recent several years, pain syndromes have been treated less frequently with ablative sympathectomy procedures because of the limited success with sympathectomy and potential improvement in outcomes with neurostimulation techniques.[8,36] This chapter will review the history, anatomy, physiology, surgical indications, techniques of the open and closed sympathectomy procedures, and more recent endoscopic techniques with particular regard to perioperative management, complications, and outcomes of the different sympathectomy procedures performed.

## Historical Background

The earliest known investigations of sympathetic nervous system surgery were described by Francois Parfour du Petit in 1727, reporting on the results sympathectomy in dogs, and Biffi reported similar findings in a doctoral thesis in 1846. Budge and Walker demonstrated the clinical effects of stimulation of the cervical sympathetic chain in humans in 1852. However, it was Claude Bernard, a French physiologist, who published a series of articles in the1850s describing his observations after sectioning and stimulating the cervical sympathetic chain in rabbits that provided a clearer understanding of clinical correlates. A well recognized clinical correlate of Bernard's experimental observations is known as Horner's syndrome, as described by Frederick T. Horner in 1869. However, the first clinical report of a sympathectomy causing the typical ocular changes was reported by Mitchell *et al.* in 1864 that actually predated Horner's description by 5 years. This book also coined the term *causalgia,* a condition that was treated primarily with sympathectomy for many years. Early surgical sympathectomy procedures were promoted by Jaboulay and Johnson, who stripped the periarterial sympathetics to treat exophthalmos, glaucoma, and tic

douloureux, as well as vascular insufficiency. One of Jaboulay's students, Leriche, promoted the use of sympathectomy for ischemic vascular disease; then sympathectomy was used frequently in the 1940s for soldiers sustaining nerve injuries in World War II. Subsequently, various sympathectomy procedures we will review were refined to treat hyperhidrosis and both ischemic and neuropathic pain syndromes.

## Clinical Syndromes: Hyperhidrosis

Palmar and axillary hyperhidrosis are defined as excessive sweating in the upper extremities, particularly the hands and armpits, most often noted during periods of stress. The etiology is unknown, and the incidence is approximately 1% in the Western populations but may be slightly higher in Asian populations. The sympathetic nervous system innervates the eccrine sweat glands via cholinergic fibers arising from the intermediolateral column of the thoracic and upper lumbar spinal cord segments. Sympathetic stimulation causes vasoconstriction to produce cooling of the skin and, when combined with sweating, exacerbates the symptoms. Anesthetic block of the stellate ganglion results in a dramatic drying and warming effect in the ipsilateral hand and armpit caused by decreasing sweating and increased blood flow through cutaneous vessels similar to resection of the sympathetic chain and ganglia in the upper thoracic region that results in lasting relief from hyperhidrosis.

## Clinical Syndromes: Neuropathic and Ischemic Pain

Chronic pain syndromes[6,10] such as causalgia and reflex sympathetic dystrophy (RSD) (now referred to as complex regional pain syndrome [CRPS]), are thought to arise from peripheral nerve trauma that is usually ill-defined. It also includes several other related syndromes (phantom pain, shoulder-hand syndrome, post-traumatic neuralgia). Characteristic symptoms are burning pain and trophic skin changes in the extremity. Ischemic pain syndromes including Raynaud's syndrome and other vasculitic disorders typically have episodes of severe, painful skin blanching, primarily of the hands and fingertips.[34] Cold temperature or emotional response may exacerbate these episodes, and extreme cases may result in ischemia and gangrenous ulceration of the digits. The initial treatment is avoidance of cold and treatment with alpha-adrenergic blocking agents that are useful for less severe cases. Sympathectomy procedures have been used extensively in the past and can provide significant initial relief from severe pain and digital ulcers. However, the long-term outcomes of sympathectomy for relieving the episodic vasospasms associated with chronic pain syndromes and Raynaud's syndrome are less optimal.

## Anatomy and Physiology

The autonomic nervous system includes both the sympathetic nervous system and the parasympathetic nervous systems. The sympathetic system mediates the "fight-or-flight" responses such as pupillary dilation, tachycardia, bronchial dilation, increased muscle blood flow, and the release of adrenergic agents from the adrenal glands. It is a two-neuron disynaptic system in which responses are mediated through autonomic ganglia and the ultimate regulation occurs in the hypothalamus. Outflow from the hypothalamus to spinal levels involves multiple pathways that are not clearly defined. Anatomically, the sympathetic nervous system has outflow in the thoracic and upper lumbar regions of the spinal cord. Preganglionic fibers from the intermediolateral cell column exit the spinal cord through the ventral nerve roots into spinal nerves and enter the paravertebral chain ganglia, coursing through the myelinated white rami communicantes.[20,25] Once in the ganglia, the presynaptic neuron can (1) synapse with a postganglionic neuron and exit as a gray ramus to the viscera, (2) synapse with a postganglionic neuron and exit as a gray ramus in a segmental nerve, (3) travel up or down the sympathetic chain, (4) stimulate the adrenal gland, or (5) exit the sympathetic chain in the splanchnic nerves and enter peripherally located ganglia such as the mesenteric ganglia. Postganglionic fibers travel in peripheral nerves or along arteries to reach their target organs. Afferent autonomic fibers travel from receptors though the dorsal spinal roots to enter the spinal cord, where they can trigger reflexes through spinal cord interneurons and efferent autonomic fibers.

The autonomic ganglia are variable in size, number, and location. There are generally three cervical ganglia (superior, middle, and inferior). The lowest cervical ganglia can fuse with the highest thoracic ganglia to form the stellate or cervicothoracic ganglion.[20,25] Pupillary dilation occurs as a result of sympathetic output from the spinal cord ciliospinal center of Budge. The preganglionic fibers exit the spinal cord at the T1 and T2 levels and travel through the thoracic, stellate, and middle cervical ganglia to synapse in the superior cervical ganglia, then postganglionic fibers enter the sympathetic plexus surrounding the carotid artery and travel along the third, fifth, and sixth cranial nerves to enter the orbit and pass through the ciliary ganglion to the pupillary dilators via the long anterior ciliary nerves. A lesion anywhere along this course is manifested by pupillary miosis, anhidrosis (loss of sympathetic innervation to the sweat glands of the face), ptosis (loss of innervation of the superior tarsal musculature) and, occasionally, enophthalmos. The thoracic ganglia correlate with the corresponding thoracic level, as do the upper lumbar ganglia.

Sexual function and urinary function are also influenced by the autonomic nervous system.[11] Sympathetic efferent innervation to the bladder arises from the lower thoracic and upper lumbar levels. The efferent nerves travel through a series of ganglia in the sacral region, and the postganglionic fibers travel to the vesicular plexus via the hypogastric nerves. There is also sympathetic stimulation involved in both erection and ejaculation in male patients.

The neurochemical aspects are that the presynaptic sympathetic neurons are generally believed to release acetylcholine and peptides that act on muscarinic, nicotinic, or peptidergic receptors of the postsynaptic neurons, which in turn release norepinephrine to achieve stimulatory responses in the innervated organs.

The effects of a sympathetic denervation for the treatment of hyperhidrosis presumably occur by interrupting cutaneous sweating and vasoconstriction mediated by the sympathetic nervous system. The mechanisms of a sympathectomy for treating pain and ischemic syndromes are mediated through less-well-understood pathways from the denervated sympathetic ganglion into the central nervous system, and reducing sympathetic input by a sympathectomy will achieve at least temporary improvement in the pain symptoms.

## Preoperative Evaluation

Patients with autonomically mediated syndromes require thorough diagnostic evaluation and aggressive medical treatment before consideration for surgical treatment. A thorough history and physical examination are necessary to begin the evaluation to consider possible underlying metabolic, infectious, or neoplastic disorders, and radiologic evaluation with plain radiographs and either computed tomography (CT) or magnetic resonance imaging (MRI) of the thorax and brachial plexus may be needed. However, most preoperative diagnostic studies are limited, and imaging studies have not demonstrated any clear diagnostic information. Psychologic evaluation should be considered, particularly in patients with chronic pain disorders.

Diagnostic sympathetic blocks with short-acting anesthetics provide temporary relief, but may cause transient Horner's syndrome. Sympathetic blocks are useful indicators that a sympathectomy will be therapeutically successful. Occasionally, repeated blocks may provide temporary relief of pain syndromes that allow rehabilitation to proceed and preclude the need for a sympathectomy. Anesthetic lumbar blocks for diagnostic and therapeutic effects particularly in lower extremity pain syndromes may be quite useful.

Medical treatment of autonomically mediated syndromes is theoretically useful and may have potential in limited cases. Medications that produce systemic sympathetic blockade include phenoxybenzamine, which blocks the alpha-adrenergic receptors.[18,47] However, there are frequent complications that include hypotension, miosis, and loss of ejaculatory function, but it is an effective test treatment for causalgia-type symptoms.

## Open Sympathectomy Techniques

Open sympathectomy techniques have been used to treat hyperhidrosis effectively but have less efficacy for treating pain syndromes, particularly considering the need for highly invasive procedures. These approaches do not require specialized endoscopic equipment and techniques. The open techniques are generally known to most practicing physicians.

### Cervical and Cervicothoracic Approaches

#### Operative Techniques

Cervical or cervicothoracic sympathectomy procedures can be performed with several techniques. These include ventral supraclavicular or transaxillary approaches or dorsal costotransversectomy approaches.[4,26] Ventral approaches provide good exposure of the sympathetic chain but carry risks of injury to the brachial plexus and pleural cavity.

The most common open approach for upper thoracic and stellate ganglionectomy is the dorsal approach, where a T2 ganglionectomy has been performed for hyperhidrosis and CRPS. The patient is placed in the prone position on the operating table after general anesthesia. A 4 to 5cm midline incision made over T2 and T3 and the paraspinal muscles is retracted to expose and remove the T2 transverse process and proximal rib of T3 (Figure 101.1) with preservation of the intercostal nerves. The lateral surface of the vertebral body is then exposed by elevating the parietal pleura carefully to expose the sympathetic chain. The ganglia are generally clearly visible and easily dissected from the chain, which is then cauterized with bipolar electrocautery above and below the ganglia, and the ganglion is resected (Figure 101.2). The ganglia can be sent to the pathology unit for histologic confirmation. A similar procedure is performed on the opposite side for patients with bilateral palmar hyperhidrosis.

The transaxillary ventral approach was described by Atkins[4] with a patient in a lateral position and the arm extended forward. An incision is made in the second intercostal space from the latissimus dorsi to the pectoralis musculature. The pleural cavity is entered, and the ribs slowly retracted. The lung is partially deflated, the sympathetic chain is located, and the appropriate ganglion is identified and removed. The transthoracic endoscopic approach used in recent years has become the most frequent method used today.

The supraclavicular approach is performed in a supine position, and the neck is placed in hyperextension. An incision is made above the clavicle, and the two heads of the sternocleidomastoid muscle are split. The phrenic nerve is identified and protected, then the anterior scalene muscle is incised and arterial branches of the subclavian artery are sacrificed. The brachial plexus is then identified and the parietal pleura is dissected from the dorsal chest by blunt dissection. The parietal pleura and subclavian artery are retracted caudally, and the sympathetic ganglia are identified and incised.

### Complications

The most common complications after ventral (or dorsal) cervical and thoracic sympathectomy include Horner's syndrome, pneumothorax, pneumonia, wound infection and dehiscence, failure of the procedure to adequately relieve the preoperative symptoms, regrowth of the sympathetic chain, CSF leak, and spinal cord injury. Horner's syndrome is avoided by limiting the resection to the second thoracic ganglion and avoiding injury to the first thoracic and stellate ganglion.[24] Horner's syndrome may be only a temporary effect caused by stretching the chain. Pneumothorax is rare and requires placement of a small tube thoracostomy. Hardy and Bay[20] recommend placement of a 12-Fr red rubber catheter in the pleural cavity if a pleural laceration is noted intraoperatively, and negative suction is applied to the catheter with positive pressure ventilation, then quickly removed and the wound closed.

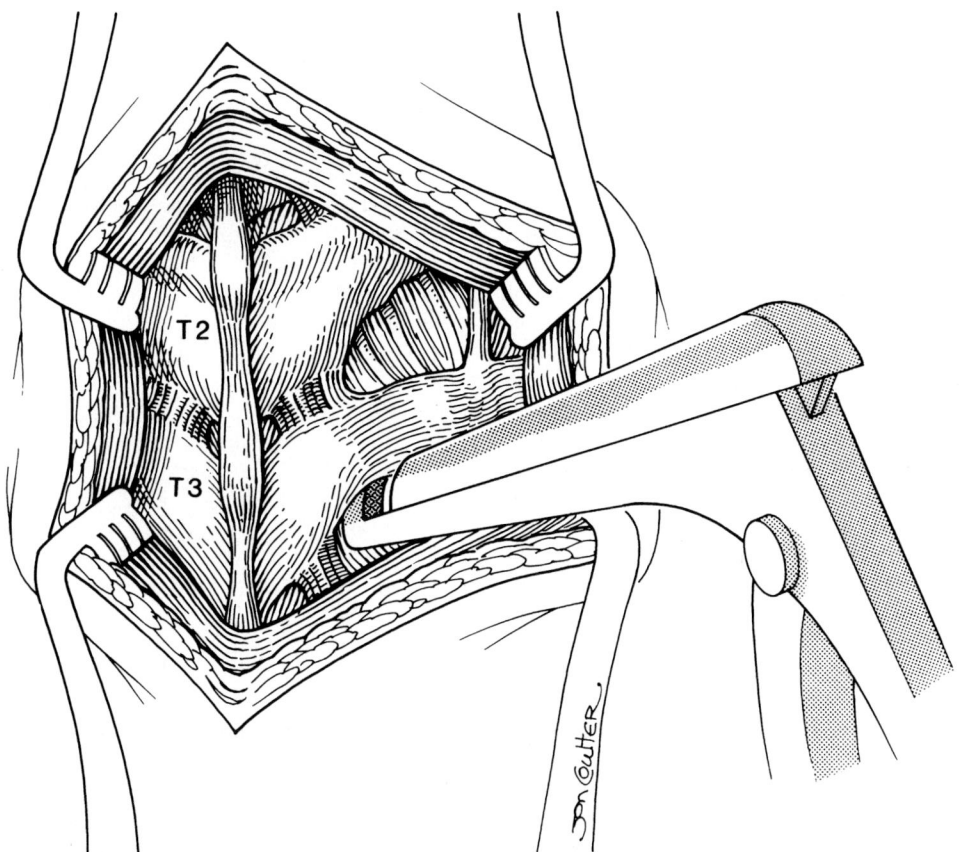

**Figure 101.1** Posterior T2 sympathectomy approach with removal of T2 transverse process and proximal T3 rib.

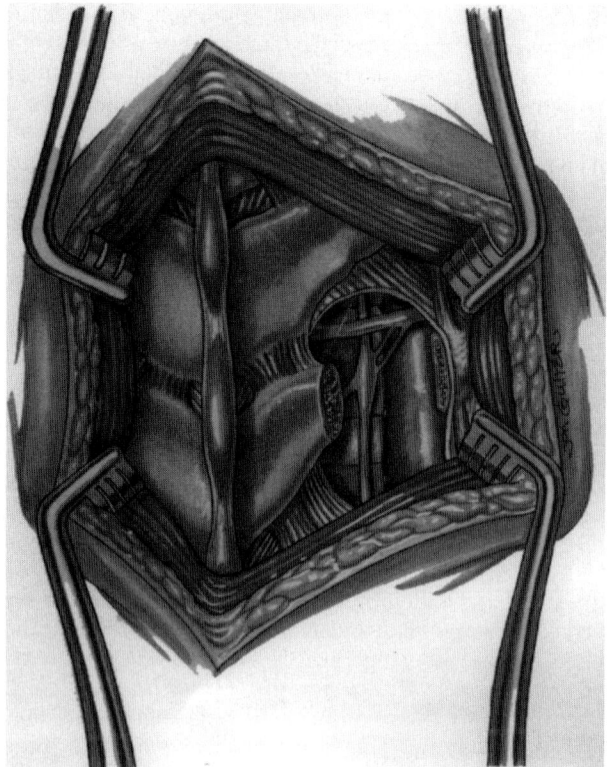

**Figure 101.2** Posterior sympathectomy and removal of the T2 ganglion.

Postoperative chest radiographs should be obtained for all patients to ensure that pneumothorax has not occurred.

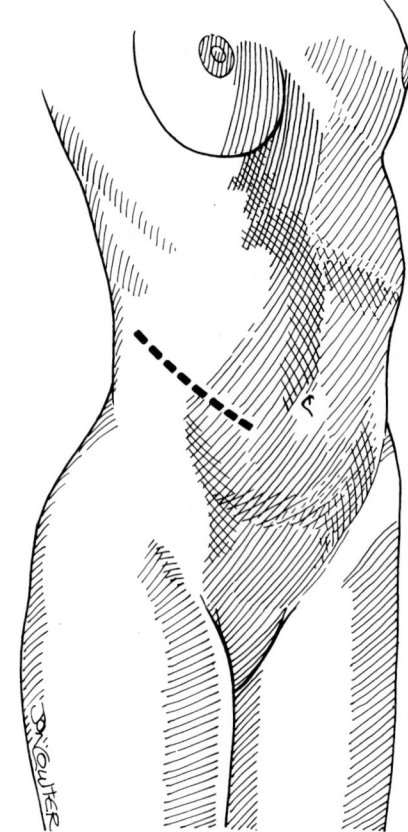

**Figure 101.3** Lumbar flank incision for lumbar sympathectomy.

## Lumbar Approaches

### Operative Technique

The lumbar sympathectomy procedure[5,35] is performed with the patient in the supine position and a 10 to 12cm incision is made in the flank from the tip of the eleventh rib toward the anterior superior iliac spine (Figure 101.3). The abdominal muscles are split longitudinally with the fibers into the retroperitoneal space and the fat is then bluntly divided with digital dissection to the ventrolateral aspect of the spine, where the lumbar sympathetic chain is located in the gutter between the psoas muscle and the spinal column (Figure 101.4). The chain can be tethered by lumbar arterial branches on the left and lumbar veins on the right that must be mobilized and often divided to allow access to the lumbar sympathetic chain. The L2-4 ganglia can then be resected. Occasionally the vena cava must be partially mobilized to gain access to the sympathetic chain on the right side. Closure is obtained by reapproximating the fascia with absorbable suture and the subcutaneous layer and skin.

### Complications

Complications of open ventral lumbar sympathectomy include ileus, infection, injury to intraperitoneal contents, wound complications, impotence, ureteral injury, and vascular injury. Impotence can occur even with uni-

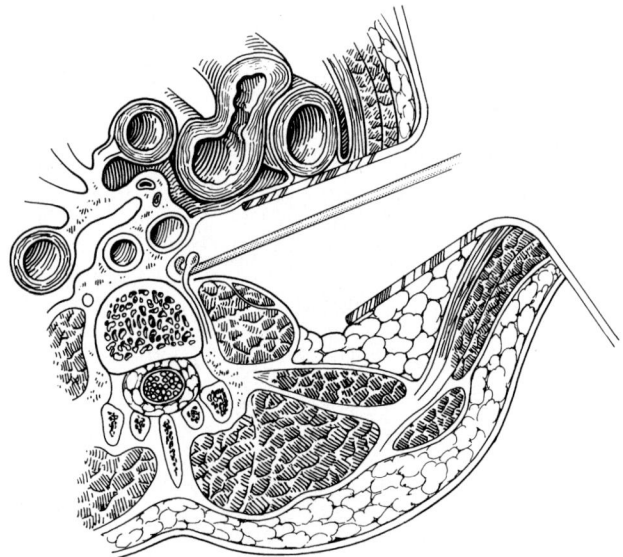

**Figure 101.4** Approach into the lumbar retroperitoneum for lumbar sympathectomy.

lateral disruption or injury to the sympathetic chain, is difficult to predict or prevent, and all male patients should be warned of this potential adverse outcome. The ureter is at risk during all retroperitoneal exposures; however, injury can be avoided by visualizing the ureter, which is usually on the psoas muscle, lateral to the sympathetic chain. Injury to the ureter can be difficult to detect and may result in flank pain and tenderness. Some patients who underwent a lumbar sympathectomy may experience thigh pain for several weeks after the procedure, and the etiology is unclear but may be caused by muscle retraction.

## Endoscopic Sympathectomy Techniques

### Thoracoscopic Approach for Cervical and Thoracic Sympathectomy

Endoscopic thoracic sympathectomy for the upper extremity was originally reported in 1951 by Kux,[27] who described treatment of hyperhidrosis with excellent results. Recently there has been significant interest in these minimally invasive procedures.[17] The interest in minimally invasive treatment of autonomically mediated syndromes affecting the upper extremities is due to the development of endoscopic techniques. The most frequent indication for thoracic sympathectomy is hyperhidrosis.[1,7,12,13,15] Less frequently, RSD, complex regional pain syndrome (CRPS), causalgia, Raynaud's syndrome, postamputation syndrome (phantom pain), and refractory cardiac tachyarrhythmias[16,38,41] are now treated with sympathectomy. Endoscopic techniques provide both a panoramic and magnified view for precise identification for the sympathetic chain and adjacent structures to allow definition of the anatomy for resection of the sympathetic chain. This procedure has become the preferred method of thoracic sympathectomy, and extensive clinical experience has resulted in improvements in patient satisfaction and reduced hospital stays and costs. Since thoracoscopic procedures have a definite learning curve, it is necessary to understand the intrathoracic anatomy and gain endoscopic experience with a thoracoscopic surgeon initially.

Palmar hyperhidrosis is currently the main indication for a thoracic sympathectomy with minimally invasive techniques. Severe axillary sweating (with or without palmar hyperhidrosis) has been treated with good effectiveness. Some patients with facial hyperhidrosis have also been treated successfully with a sympathectomy procedure. The precise sympathectomy procedure for each of these clinical syndromes regarding which ganglia levels are resected remains somewhat speculative. Most authors agree that only a T2 and T3 sympathectomy will effectively treat palmar hyperhidrosis. However, some authors recommend either a T2 or T3 sympathectomy and cite a lowered incidence of compensatory sweating, but this has not been clearly substantiated. Treatment of axillary sweating is generally accepted as best treated with a sympathectomy at T3, T4, T5 for good results. Facial sweating is treated with a T2 sympathectomy just below the stellate ganglion.[29]

Patients with pain syndromes and vasculitis or Raynaud's syndrome may also respond to an endoscopic T2, T3, and/or T4 sympathectomy, but results are less optimal.[3] Recent experience with spinal stimulation appears to have largely replaced sympathectomy procedures for several reasons.[36] These include the following: (1) pain symptoms have a high incidence of recurrence after sympathectomy, (2) stimulation is a non-ablative procedure, (3) stimulation is usually a technically less demanding procedure than a sympathectomy, (4) stimulation is a reversible procedure, and (5) stimulation can be modulated after the procedure is completed.

Patients with cardiac tachyarrhythmias have also been treated with sympathectomy procedures. Studies have demonstrated effectiveness in treating stress-related malignant tachyarrhythmias that may be related to disproportionate left and right sympathetic innervation. Patients treated inadequately with medical therapy can be considered for a left thoracoscopic sympathectomy; however, improved medical therapy has nearly eliminated any patients requiring these procedures.[20,25,33,40]

## Operative Technique

### Anesthesia and Positioning

The patient requires general anesthesia and placement of a double lumen endotracheal tube to allow collapse of the lung on the operated side. The supine position (Figure 101.5) is used, and the head of the table can be elevated and rotated.

### Instruments

The equipment and instruments needed for performing a thoracoscopic sympathectomy procedure are commonly used for laparoscopic surgery. A standard endoscopic video monitor system with either a 5mm (or 10mm) diameter rigid laparoscope (with either a 0- or 30-degree angled lens) is used. The essential endoscopic instruments are (1) 5mm-diameter blunt-tipped (mini-Metzenbaum-type) scissors with a monopolar electrocautery, (2) a 5mm-diameter curved grasper (a hemostat), and (3) a 5mm-diameter suction irrigator.

### Ports And Port Placement

A soft flexible thoracic endoscopic port is inserted through a 2cm chest wall incision that is similar to the placement of a chest tube. A single port (Figure 101.6A), or occasionally two ports (Figure 101.6B), can be used, and both the endoscope and other working instruments can be placed in the port.[21,22,31,44] The port is placed in the third or fourth intercostal space in the midaxillary line while the anesthesiologist deflates the ipsilateral lung.

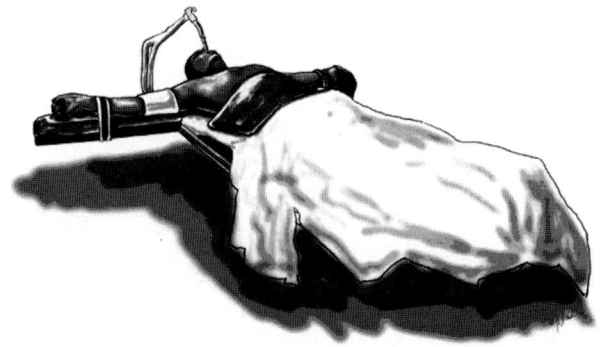

**Figure 101.5** Supine position for bilateral thoracoscopic sympathectomy.

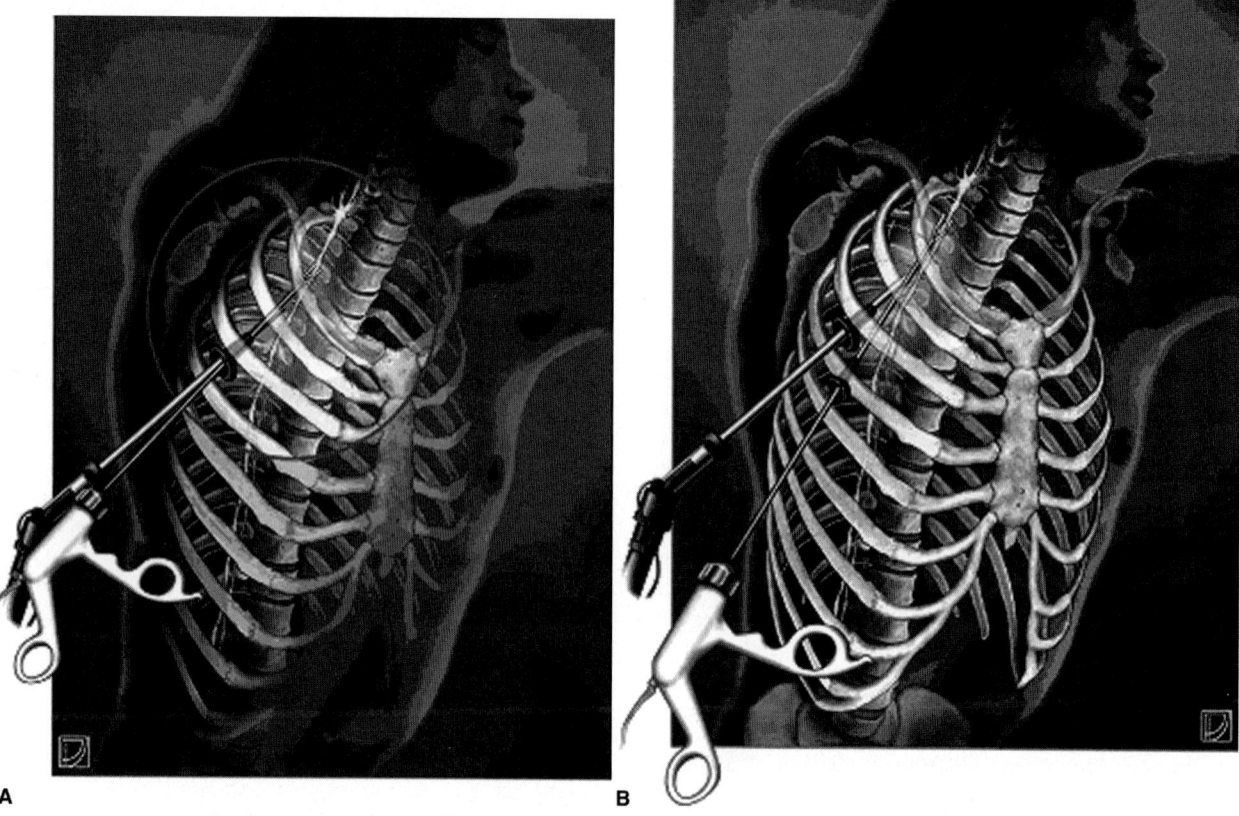

**A**    **B**

**Figure 101.6** Single (**A**) and double (**B**) portal access for right thoracoscopic sympathectomy.

## The Operative Procedure

The endoscope is placed in the chest through the portal and the lung is retracted. The lung can be further retracted with a blunt instrument and rotation of the operating table, which allows the lung to fall forward and away from the vertebral column. The sympathetic chain is visualized overlying the rib heads in the upper thoracic region. The intercostal vessels course over the mid portion of each vertebral body, usually beneath the sympathetic chain. The sympathetic chain appears as a slightly pinkish-white, glistening, raised, longitudinal structure. The rostral aspect of the sympathetic chain extends beneath a fat pad that envelopes the subclavian artery and obscures the first rib and stellate ganglion.

The sympathectomy procedure begins with an incision in the pleura overlying the sympathetic chain at the T3 level with the curved scissors (Figure 101.7). The pleural incision is extended in a rostral direction over the sympathetic chain to T2 (Figure 101.8), and the sympathetic ganglia and chain at T2 and T3 are then cauterized (Figure 101.9). The nerve of Kuntz can often be identified as a large branch arising from the T2 ganglion and courses laterally to the brachial plexus, likely providing much of the sympathetic innervation to the upper extremity. Thus denervation of the T2 ganglion is important.[45] Prevention of Horner's syndrome is best accomplished by avoiding injury or traction to the stellate ganglion that can occur during the dissection and denervation of the T2 ganglion. Once the sympathectomy has been completed, a portion of the sympathetic ganglion

can be sent for pathologic evaluation; then the surgical site is irrigated and hemostasis confirmed. A red rubber catheter is inserted through the port and aspirated while the lung is reinflated by the anesthesiologist and the port is removed; then the incision is closed with absorbable sutures and Steri-strips.

## Postoperative Care

A postoperative chest radiograph is obtained in the operating room to ensure lung inflation. A small pneumothorax will resolve, but a large persistent pneumothorax suggests a parenchymal lung leak that would require chest tube placement until the leak resolves. Oral analgesics are adequate, and the hospital stay is usually only 1 or 2 days.

## Complications

Surgical complications[32,39,42] from thoracoscopic sympathectomy are few, and most do not require intervention. These include (1) pneumothorax, (2) Horner's syndrome, (3) subcutaneous emphysema, (4) pleural effusions, (5) segmental atelectasis, and (6) intercostal neuralgia. Postoperative pneumothorax usually results from inadequate reinflation of the collapsed lung; however, a small apical pneumothorax can be observed and will spontaneously resolve. Horner's syndrome results from injury to the stellate ganglion and is infrequent and usually transient. Injury to the intercostal nerves during port placement or pressure applied during the procedure may result in intercostal neuralgia. The incidence is mini-

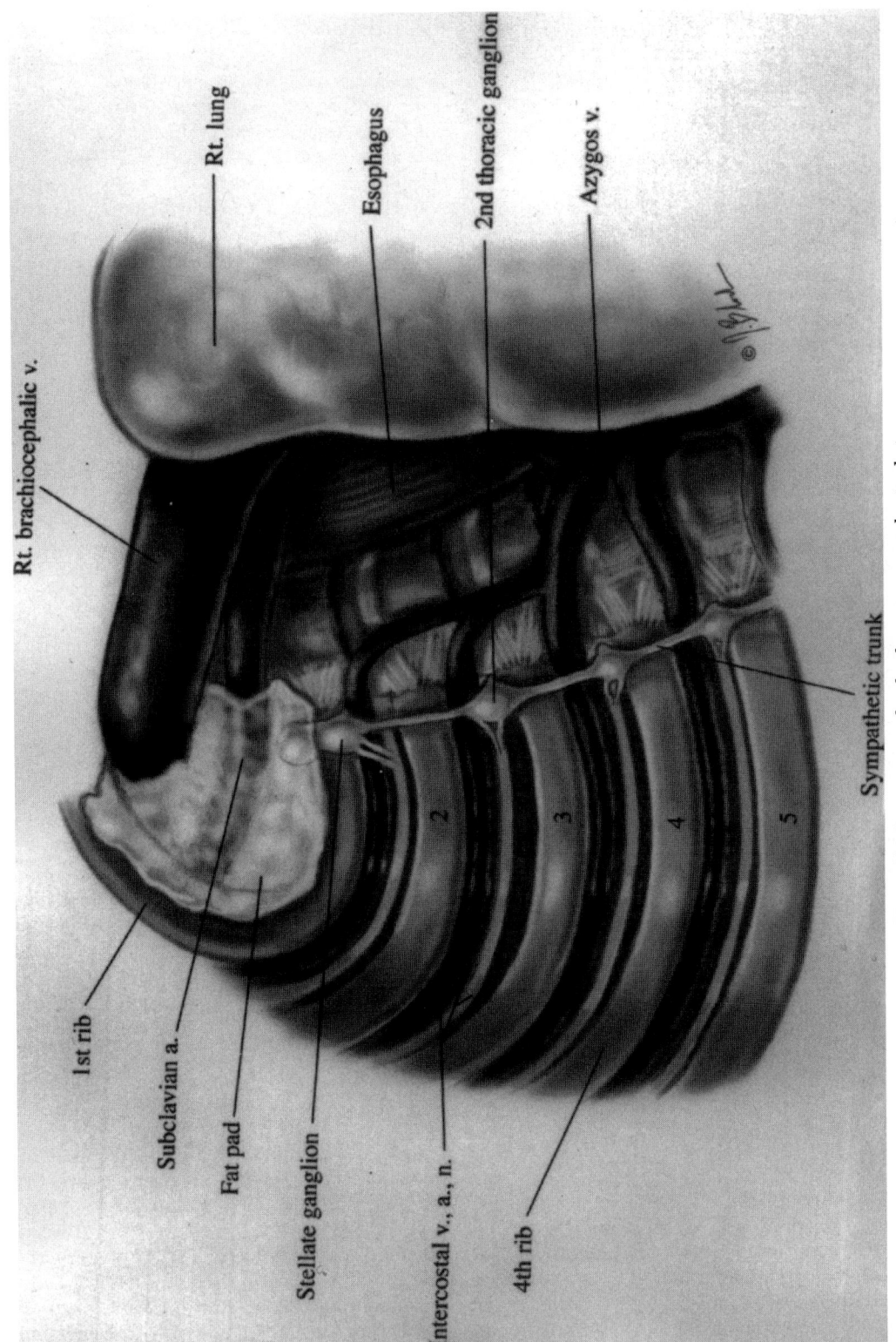

**Figure 101.7** Anatomy of right thoracic sympathetic chain.

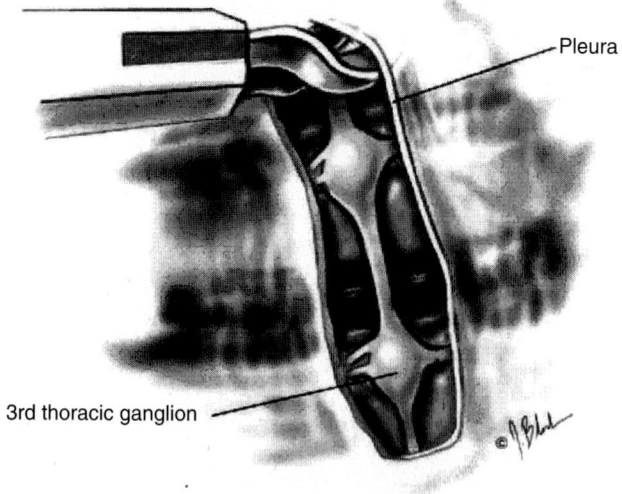

**Figure 101.8** Pleural opening over right T2 and T3 ganglia.

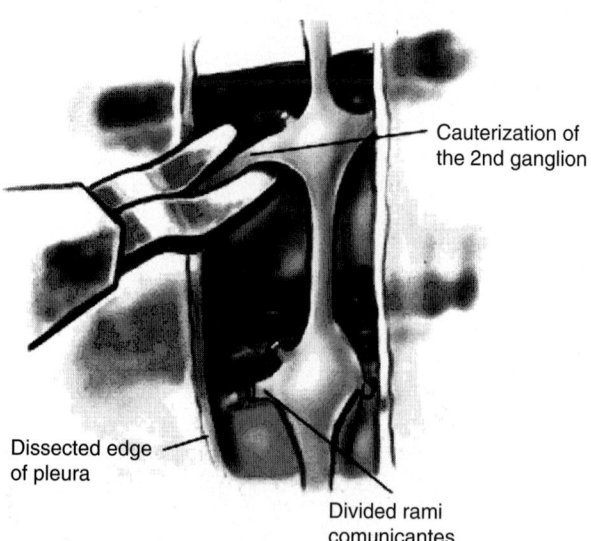

**Figure 101.9** Cauterization and division of right T2 and T3 ganglia.

mized by using soft, flexible thoracic endoscopic ports rather than the rigid laparoscopic ports.

Compensatory hyperhidrosis is increased sweating, usually in the truncal areas, which occur after a sympathectomy procedure.[43] The incidence is probably higher than previously recognized and has been reported to range from 10% to 90%. The severity is highly variable, ranging from mild to severe, and cannot be determined preoperatively. Some authors advocate a more limited sympathectomy of T2 that may reduce the incidence of compensatory sweating, while others claim that only a sympathectomy of T3 reduces the incidence.[28] However, none of these theories have been clearly substantiated. More recently, clipping of the sympathetic chain has been performed in hopes of creating a reversible lesion.[9,30] Reconstruction of the sympathetic chain has been reported, but no long-term data are available.[43]

## Lumbar Endoscopic Sympathectomy

Endoscopic techniques have been used for sympathectomy in the lumbar region and were described by Onimus[37] and others[23,46] more recently; these have similarities to the open lumbar sympathectomy except for a much less invasive procedure (see Figures 101.3 and 101.4). A 1 to 2cm incision is made in the flank below the tip of the eleventh rib, and finger dissection into the retroperitoneum is made. A tissue expander or an optical trocar can dissect in a similar fashion as the open procedure to expose the psoas and expose the lumbar sympathetic chain. An endoscopic portal is inserted, and $CO_2$ insufflation will maintain the space for the procedure. A second portal is placed for an instrumentation portal. The sympathectomy procedure then proceeds similar to the open procedure.

## Radiofrequency and Chemical Destruction of the Sympathetic Chain

Percutaneous placement of a needle into or near a sympathetic ganglion allows destruction of the ganglia with injection of a neurolytic agent (i.e., alcohol, phenol) or else a radio frequency lesion is performed to achieve a sympathectomy. Either fluoroscopic or CT guidance can be used for localization.[14] These techniques can be performed without general anesthesia with local anesthetics and mild sedation in older patients and allow immediate evaluation of the results. They can often be performed on an outpatient basis and obviate the need for expensive and complicated endoscopic technology or large surgical incisions with open procedures. Although some authors have had excellent results with these techniques, not all surgeons can achieve these results, and the short- and long-term results have been less successful than open or endoscopic procedures, presumably because of inadequate denervation.

The percutaneous radio frequency thoracic sympathectomy technique has been well described and documented by Wilkinson.[48,49] The patient is positioned prone on a fluoroscopic table, and a radio frequency lesioning needle is placed in a paramedian location and directed between the ribs with the needle tip at the rib head and the sympathetic ganglion at the T2-3. Stimulation is used to confirm the final needle position, and a radio frequency lesion is generated. A success rate of more than 90% was noted at a 3-year follow-up. The complication rate is low, and complications include pneumothorax.

Chemical sympathectomy with phenol (6% to 10%) has been presented by Gybels and Sweet.[19] It has been used primarily in the lumbar region and placed with fluoroscopic guidance to treat vasoocclusive disease. Most patients obtain fair early relief of pain, but results deteriorate over time. The complications are infrequent and include groin pain and ureteral injuries.

## Summary

The indications for sympathectomy have become clearer throughout 50 years of clinical research. Surgical techniques have become more refined with modern endoscopy and have led to precise minimally invasive procedures. Endoscopy allows less tissue disruption with a magnified and illuminated exposure. The technical challenges and complications of these procedures are now well understood and well defined, where the surgeon can custom-tailor the necessary procedure based on a patient's individual condition for optimal outcomes.

# REFERENCES

1. Adams DCR, Wood SJ, Tulloh BR, *et al*: Endoscopic transthoracic sympathectomy: experience in the south west end of England. *Eur J Vasc Surg* 6:558, 1992.
2. Adar R, Kurchin A, Zweig A, Mozes M: Palmar hyperhidrosis and its surgical treatment. *Ann Surg* 186:34, 1977.
3. Ahn SS, Machleder HI, Concepcion B, Moore WS: Thoracoscopic cervicodorsal sympathectomy: preliminary results. *J Vasc Surg* 20:511, 1994.
4. Atkins HJB: Sympathectomy by the axillary approach. *Lancet* 1:538, 1954.
5. Baker DM, Lamerton AF: Operative lumbar sympathectomy for severe lower limb ischaemia: still a valuable treatment option. *Ann R Coll Surg Engl* 76:50-53, 1994.
6. Bandyk DF, Johnson BL, Kirkpatrick AF, *et al*: Surgical sympathectomy for reflex sympathetic dystrophy syndromes. *J Vasc Surg* 35(2):269-277, 2002.
7. Banerjee AK, Edmondson R, Rennie JA: Endoscopic transthoracic electrocautery of the sympathetic chain for palmar and axillary hyperhidrosis. *Br J Surg* 77:1435, 1990.
8. Barolat G, Schwartzman R, Woo R: Epidural spinal cord stimulation in the management of reflex sypathetic dystrophy. *Stereotact Funct Neurosurg* 53:29, 1989.
9. Beatty RA: The use of clip-suture in thoracic sympathectomy. *J Neurosurg* 81:482, 1994.
10. Bergan JJ, Conn J Jr: Sympathectomy for pain relief. *Med Clin North Am* 52:147, 1968.
11. Burchiel KJ, Burns AS: Summary statement: pain, spasticity, and bladder and sexual function after spinal cord injury [Comment]. *Spine* 26(24 suppl):S161, 2001.
12. Byrne J, Walsh TN, Hederman WP: Endoscopic transthoracic electrocautery of the sympathetic chain for palmar and axillary hyperhidrosis. *Br J Surg* 77:1046, 1990.
13. Chen HJ, Liang CL, Lu K: Associated change in plantar temperature and sweating after transthoracic endoscopic T2-3 sympathectomy for palmar hyperhidrosis. *J Neurosurg* 95(suppl):58-63, 2001.
14. Chuang KS, Liou NH, Liu JC: New stereotactic technique for percutaneous thermocoagulation of upper thoracic ganglionectomy in cases of palmar hyperhidrosis. *Neurosurgery* 22:600, 1988.
15. Claes G, Gothberg G, Drott C: Endoscopic transthoracic electrocautery of the sympathetic chain for palmar and axillary hyperhidrosis. *Br J Surg* 78:760, 1991.
16. Crampton R. Preeminence of the left stellate ganglion in the long QT syndrome. *Circulation* 59:769, 1979.
17. Drott C, Gothberg G, Claes G: Endoscopic procedures of the upper thoracic sympathetic chain: a review. *Arch Surg* 128:237, 1993.
18. Ghostine SY, Comair YG, Turner DM, *et al*: Phenoxybenzamine in the treatment of causalgia: report of 40 cases. *J Neurosurg* 60:1263, 1984.
19. Gybels JM, Sweet WH: Neurosurgical treatment of persistent pain. In Gildenberg PL (ed): *Pain and Headache*, vol 11. Basel, Karger, 1989, p 276.
20. Hardy RW, Bay JW: Surgery of the sympathetic nervous system. In Schmidek HH, Sweet WH (eds): *Operative Neurosurgical Techniques*, ed 2. Orlando, Grune and Stratton, 1988, p 1271.
21. Johnson JP, Patel NP: Uniportal and biportal endoscopic thoracic sympathectomy. *Neurosurgery* 51(5 suppl):79-83, 2002.
22. Johnson JP, Obasi C, Hahn MS, Glatleider P: Endoscopic thoracic sympathectomy. *J Neurosurg* 91(1 suppl):90-97, 1999.
23. Kathouda N, Wattanasirichaigoon S, Tang E, *et al*: Laparoscopic lumbar sympathectomy. *Surg Endosc* 11(3):257-260, 1997.
24. Kisch B: Horner's syndrome, an American discovery. *Bull His Med* 25:284, 1951.
25. Kleinert HE, Norberg H, McDonough JJ: Surgical sympathectomy: upper and lower extremity. In Omer GE Jr, Spinner M (eds): *Management of Peripheral Nerve Problems*. Philadelphia, WB Saunders, 1980, p 284.
26. Kurchin A, Zweig A, Adar R, Mozes M: Upper dorsal sympathectomy for palmar primary hyperhidrosis by the supraclavicular approach. *World J Surg* 1:667, 1977.
27. Kux E: The endoscopic approach to the vegetative nervous system and its therapeutic possibilities. *Dis Chest* 20:139, 1951.
28. Leseche G, Castier Y, Thabut G, *et al*: Endoscopic transthoracic sympathectomy for upper limb hyperhidrosis: limited sympathectomy does not reduce postoperative compensatory sweating. *J Vasc Surg* 37(1):124-128, 2003.
29. Lin TS, Fang HY: Transthoracic endoscopic sympathectomy for craniofacial hyperhidrosis: analysis of 46 cases. *J Laparoendosc Adv Surg Tech A* 10(5):243-247, 2000.
30. Lin TS, Huang LC, Wang NP, Lai CY: Video-assisted thoracoscopic T2 sympathetic block by clipping for palmar hyperhidrosis: analysis of 52 cases. *J Laparoendosc Adv Surg Tech A* 11(2):59-62, 2001.
31. Lin TS, Kuo SJ, Chou MC: Uniportal endoscopic thoracic sympathectomy for treatment of palmar and axillary hyperhidrosis: analysis of 2000 cases. *Neurosurgery* 51(5 suppl):84-87, 2002.
32. Lin TS, Wang NP, Huang LC: Pitfalls and complication avoidance associated with transthoracic endoscopic sympathectomy for primary hyperhidrosis (analysis of 2200 cases). *Int J Surg Investig* 2(5):377-385, 2001.
33. Malone PS, Cameron AEP, Rennie JA: The surgical treatment of upper limb hyperhidrosis. *Br J Dermatol* 115:81, 1986.
34. Matsumoto Y, Ueyama T, Endo M, *et al*: Endoscopic thoracic sympathectomy for Raynaud's phenomenon. *J Vasc Surg* 36(1):57-61, 2002.
35. Munro PAG: *Sympathectomy: An Anatomical and Physiological Study with Clinical Applications*. London, Oxford University Press, 1959.
36. Oakley JC, Prager JP: Spinal cord stimulation: mechanisms of action. *Spine* 27(22):2574-2578, 2002.

37. Onimus M, Papin P, Gangloff S: Extraperitoneal approach to the lumbar spine with video assistance. *Spine* 21:2491, 1996.

38. Ouriel K, Moss AJ: Long QT syndrome: an indication for cervicothoracic sympathectomy. *Cardiovasc Surg* 3:475, 1995.

39. Plas EG, Fugger R, Herbst F, Fritsch A: Complications of endoscopic thoracic sympathectomy. *Surgery* 118:493, 1995.

40. Rutherford RB: Role of sympathectomy in the management of vascular disease. In Moore WS (ed): *Vascular Surgery: A Comprehensive Review*. Philadelphia, WB Saunders, 1993, p 300.

41. Schwartz PJ, Periti M, Malliani A: The long QT syndrome. *Am Heart J* 89:378, 1975.

42. Singh B, Moodley J, Ramdial PK, *et al*: Pitfalls in thoracoscopic sympathectomy: mechanisms for failure. *Surg Laparosc Endosc Percutaneous Tech* 11(6):364-367, 2001.

43. Telaranta T: Secondary sympathetic chain reconstruction after endoscopic thoracic sympaticotomy. *Eur J Surg* 580(suppl):17-8, 1998.

44. Vanaclocha V, Saiz-Sapena N, Panta F: Uniportal endoscopic superior thoracic sympathectomy. *Neurosurgery* 46(4):924-928, 2000.

45. Wang YC, Sun MH, Lin CW, Chen YJ: Anatomical location of T2-3 sympathetic trunk and Kuntz nerve determined by transthoracic endoscopy. *J Neurosurg* 96(suppl):68-72, 2002.

46. Watarida S, Shiraishi S, Fujimura M, *et al*: Laparoscopic lumbar sympathectomy for lower-limb disease. *Surg Endosc* 16(3):500-503, 2002.

47. Weiner N: Drugs that inhibit adrenergic nerves and block adrenergic receptors. In Gilman AG, Goodman LS, Gilman A (eds): *Goodman and Gilman's Pharmacological Basis of Therapeutics*, ed 6. New York, MacMillan, 1980, p 176.

48. Wilkinson HA: Percutaneous radiofrequency upper thoracic sympathectomy: a new technique. *Neurosurgery* 15:118, 1984.

49. Wilkinson HA: Percutaneous radiofrequency upper thoracic sympathectomy. *Neurosurgery* 38:715, 1996.

# CHAPTER 102

# The Value of Surgical Intervention in Spinal Trauma

**Kern Singh, Jennifer Erdos, Alexander Sah, Alexander R. Vaccaro, and Robert F. McLain**

In the United States there are approximately 50,000 new spinal cord injuries reported each year. The estimated cost for the treatment of such persons with spinal cord injury approaches $4 billion dollars annually. Such staggering figures clearly portray a need to delineate what injuries require more aggressive surgical intervention and when that procedure should occur. With improvements in anesthesia, surgical techniques, and spinal instrumentation, many surgeons are now much more confident in their ability to manage selective cases of spinal trauma in an operative fashion. Decreased length of hospitalization, quicker rehabilitation, and earlier entry back into society are all clear advantages of surgical intervention.

With such a myriad of spinal injuries, the precise role of surgery is hard to globally define for the entire spinal column. Nonetheless, a few specific surgical goals can be clearly defined. These include: (1) the establishment of a balanced and stable spine, (2) preservation or improvement in neurologic function, and (3) the return of the patient to an optimal level of functional capacity as quickly and safely as possible.[19] The decision to proceed with surgical management is predicted on a reasonable risk profile and on the potential to achieve the aforementioned goals more efficiently than nonoperative strategies.

The decision for operative versus nonoperative management following spinal trauma is often a subjective choice outside of a clearly unstable neurologic or biomechanical injury. Some clinicians take an extreme position that surgery is not indicated except in the setting of progressive neurologic deterioration or gross spinal instability (Figure 102.1). The majority of spinal care physicians have balanced other factors relating to long-term functional outcome on the need to proceed with operative interventions. These factors include: (1) the ability, with surgery, to accelerate the rehabilitation process, decreasing morbidity for the patient and indirectly the cost of care; (2) the predictable prevention of spinal deformity, which at a later time may manifest as progressive pain, loss of function, and neurologic deterioration; (3) the ability to reduce complications associated with prolonged recumbency/immobilization, particularly in multiply injured patients; and finally (4) the ability to predictably improve modest neurologic recovery, such as spinal cord or nerve root function in the setting of neural compression. Surgeons' improved understanding of the primary and secondary force mechanisms acting on both the spinal column and the spinal cord; improvements in surgical procedures, approaches, and instrumentation; and a better understanding of the anatomy and biomechanics of the spinal column have resulted in much improved surgical outcomes of spinal trauma patients over the last several decades.

## Spinal Stability

Spinal stability is an obscure term poorly understood by many who care regularly for patients following spinal trauma. The spinal column provides support for the musculoskeletal system and houses and protects the spinal cord and cauda equina. An unstable spine may contribute to musculoskeletal or neurologic injury and eventually adversely affect the functional status of the patient. Therefore, surgery in the setting of spinal instability is intended to reestablish the integrity of the spinal osteoligamentous complex and prevent subsequent loss of spinal alignment and its adverse sequelae: pain, deformity, and progressive neurologic injury

Many researchers have proposed mechanistic classification systems designed to prognosticate the degree of spinal instability present. Two and three column theories of stability have been put forth, each with their various proponents. It is clear that the integrity of both the ligamentous and bony constituents of the spinal column contribute significantly to spinal stability. The integrity of the soft tissue stabilizers of the spinal column (i.e., posterior longitudinal ligament, posterior facet capsules, interspinous ligaments) is especially critical in the adult patient where their integrity often determines the need for surgical intervention. In all areas of the spine, complete soft tissue disruption of the supporting ligamentous structures has been shown to result in progressive spinal deformity and in many cases neurologic deterioration.[11] This is clear in specific catastrophic injuries such as occipitocervical dissociation, bilateral facet dislocations, complete distraction extension shear injuries through the intervertebral disc, and pure ligamentous failure of the transverse ligament.[12] There is no argument that surgical intervention is required due to the gross degree of spinal instability present.

The shades of gray in terms of spinal stability and the potential for progressive loss of spinal alignment are those instances of partial ligamentous disruption, or failure, primarily of the bony anatomy, without significant loss of sagittal or coronal alignment (Figure 102.2).

Accurate classification systems reflecting the natural history of immobilized but nonsurgically stabilized fracture patterns are lacking. Gertzbein[9] surveyed the Scoliosis Research Society and found after reviewing approximately 1019 patients, that if a thoracolumbar spinal deformity progresses to greater than 30 degrees of kyphosis, the patient is at risk for chronic pain and disability. One study, examining burst fractures felt to require surgical intervention, synthesized an intricate anatomically based load sharing classification system that quantitates the potential for future deformity if a posterior only approach is selected. This system grades: (1) the amount of comminution/involvement of the vertebral body, (2) the apposition of fragments at the fragment site, and (3) the amount of corrected traumatic kyphosis. A numerical grading system is applied based on a minimum of three points and a maximum of nine points. Scores of six points or less were thought to require adjunctive anterior column support to avoid treatment failure.[14]

Ultimately, in order to determine the need for surgical intervention in the majority of trauma cases, well-designed and often impractical longitudinal cohort studies assessing the long-term outcome of nonoperatively treated injuries that are well classified will have to be performed.

There are many problems with nonoperative strategies used to manage spinal instability in the setting of spinal trauma. Halo devices in the cervical region have been shown to be unpredictable in maintaining alignment in the upper cervical region and at the cervicothoracic junction. Anderson et al.[2] prospectively studied 42 patients with cervical spinal injuries immobilized in halo vests in which radiographs in the supine and upright positions demonstrated significant intervertebral motion. In addition, changes in body posture have been found to translate into compressive or distractive forces at the injury level while in a halo vest. Skeletal traction is a cumbersome and restrictive method of

indirectly providing spinal stability. The majority of patients cannot tolerate long-term bedrest, which traction care requires, not to mention the soft tissue and bony morbidity related to pin placement problems. In addition, McGuire et al.[15,16] has shown that standard nursing techniques such as log rolling and a rotating bed do not adequately prevent motion at the injured segment of unstable spinal injuries. Mirza et al.[17] also demonstrated that surgical stabilization was more predictable and efficacious in terms of functional recovery in a cohort of patients treated with closed spinal reduction than with extended axial-tong traction and rotating bed immobilization. The efficacy of thoracolumbar orthosis in maintaining spinal alignment is also controversial. Many investigators have found that the true value of these braces is primarily through behavioral modification and not skeletal immobilization.

The complex biomechanics of the spinal column, due to its highly regionalized nature, presents unique challenges in the nonsurgical and surgical management of spinal trauma patients. The vastly different biomechanical properties of each region require analysis of each area to understand the potential role of surgical intervention in specific injury patterns.

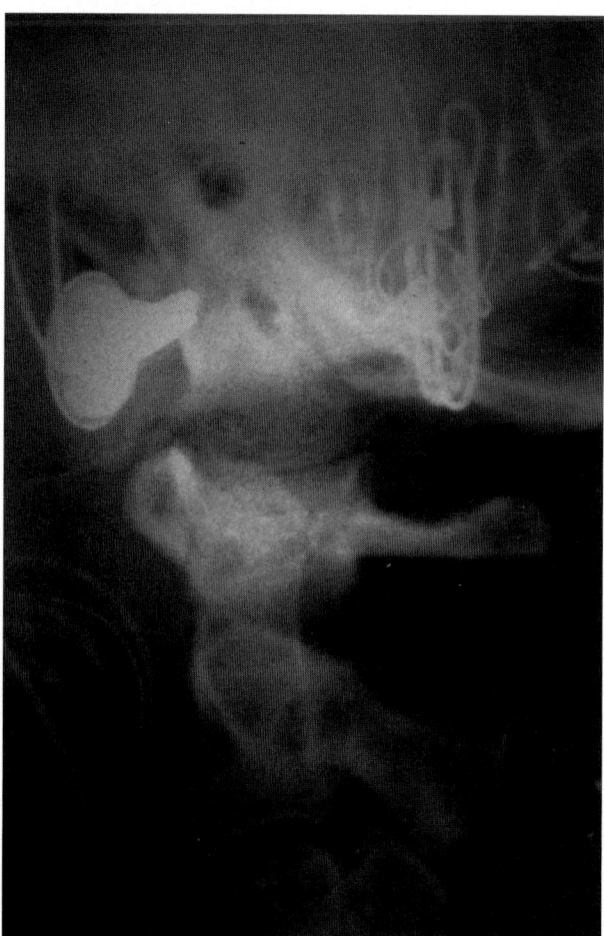

**Figure 102.1** A lateral plain radiograph demonstrating an occipital C1 dissociation.

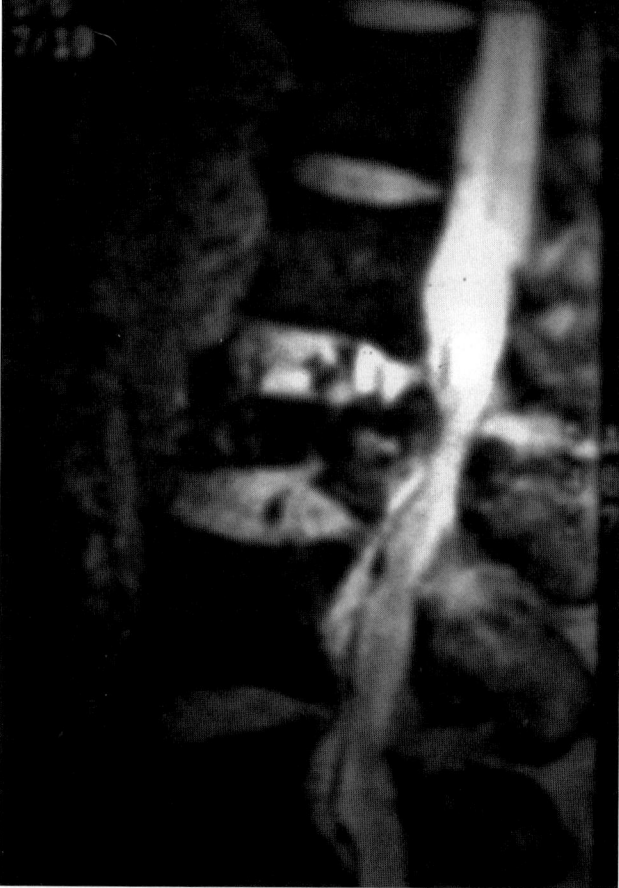

**Figure 102.2** A sagittal MRI of a patient with a lumbar L2 burst fracture. The patient is neurologically intact without significant disruption of the posterior osteoligamentous complex at the fracture level. This patient may be treated nonoperatively with a satisfactory functional outcome although such management is not uniformly accepted by all spinal caregivers.

## Cervical Spine

The substantial range of motion of the cervical region can be attributed to its complex ligamentous and osseous anatomy. The cervical spine, due to its unique anatomy, is often viewed as two distinct regions, the upper (occiput to C2) and the lower cervical spine (C3-T1). The upper cervical spine is highly mobile with the majority of sagittal plane cervical flexion and extension occurring between the occiput and the atlas and the majority of rotation occurring at the atlantoaxial junction. The osseous structures provide little stability in this region and thus the ligamentous attachments play a much more important role in spinal stability.

The lower cervical spine is lordotic and inherently more stable than the upper cervical spine. The space for the neural elements is much smaller in this region than in the upper cervical spine. Therefore, any sudden acute sagittal displacement may result in significant neurologic compromise. There are generally considered only two indications for acute or immediate surgical intervention in the setting of a cervical spine injury. These include: a neurologically incomplete patient with a deteriorating neurologic examination and an associated facet dislocation unreducible by traction, and secondly, a neurologically incomplete patient demonstrating progressive neurologic loss with objective imaging evidence of spinal cord compromise. In the absence of either clinical scenario, immediate surgery has not yet been proven to significantly effect long-term neurologic improvement (Figure 102.3). Grossly unstable spinal injuries such as an occipital-C1 dislocation, a distraction extension injury through the intervertebral disc, or a bilateral facet dislocation, also requires surgical inter-

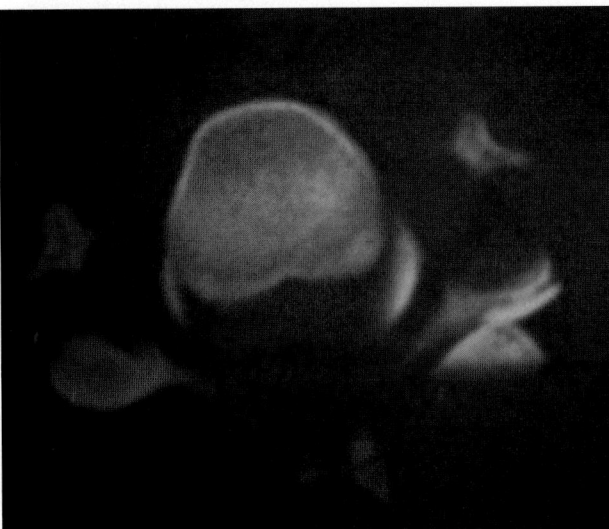

**Figure 102.3** A transaxial CT scan of a cervical unilateral facet dislocation in a neurologically intact patient. In some centers this injury is managed with an immediate closed or open reduction followed by a stabilization procedure. Other centers have chosen to manage these injuries with low weight cervical traction over several days followed if successful with halo or cervical collar immobilization. The method and timing of treatment of this spinal injury in the neurologically intact patient is nonuniform and location dependent.

vention to prevent spinal deformity and the potential for neurologic worsening. The timing of surgical intervention in these clinical scenarios is case specific.

## Thoracic Spine

The thoracic spine (T2-10) normally has a kyphotic alignment and is generally very stable due to the articulating rib cage, sternum, and clavicles. The clinical assessment and treatment of fractures that occur in the thoracic spine are influenced by three factors: (1) the anatomic stability of the surrounding supporting bony structures, (2) the regional kyphosis of the thoracic spine defining the integrity of osteoligamentous spinal environment, (3) and the presence of spinal canal compromise and resultant neurologic profile of the patient. High-energy trauma is often needed to destabilize this region of the spine; and, therefore, surgical intervention is often beneficial to restore spinal stability in a predictable manner.

Most injuries to the thoracic spine are a result of axial loading with flexion. Loss of the anterior height of the thoracic body may occur with insignificant disruption of the posterior and middle column. Indications for operative intervention often include loss of anterior vertebral height greater than 50% with obvious loss of the integrity of the posterior ligamentous support structures, cases of fracture dislocations or flexion distraction injuries or any unstable three column shear injury. The presence of an incomplete neurologic injury in the setting of spinal cord compromise is a relative indication for surgical decompression and stabilization. Nonoperative treatment of incomplete spinal cord injuries in the setting of a thoracic fracture has consistently done poorly. Surgical intervention in this setting has been demonstrated to maintain spinal alignment and potentially improve the neurologic outcome of patients with incomplete neurologic deficits.

## Lumbar Spine

The transition zone at the thoracolumbar junction marks a significant change from a stiff thoracic spine to a mobile lumbar spine. This zone of transition across T10 to L2 is related to the loss of the rib cage as well as the changing orientation of the facet joints. This anatomic zone accounts for approximately 50% of all vertebral body fractures and 40% of all spinal cord injuries.

Again, operative intervention for specific thoracolumbar injuries includes the degree of spinal deformity and therefore the integrity of the posterior osteoligamentous complex. In burst fractures, which represent an injury to the anterior and middle columns, two factors determine the need for operative intervention. These include the patient's neurologic status and the status of the posterior ligamentous complex. Vertebral comminution, reflecting the anterior and middle column's ability to resist axial loads, is a relative indication for surgery. The presence of an incomplete neurologic deficit with residual canal or cord compromise is a relative indication for surgical intervention due to the predictable return of partial or complete neurologic function with surgery (Figure 102.4).

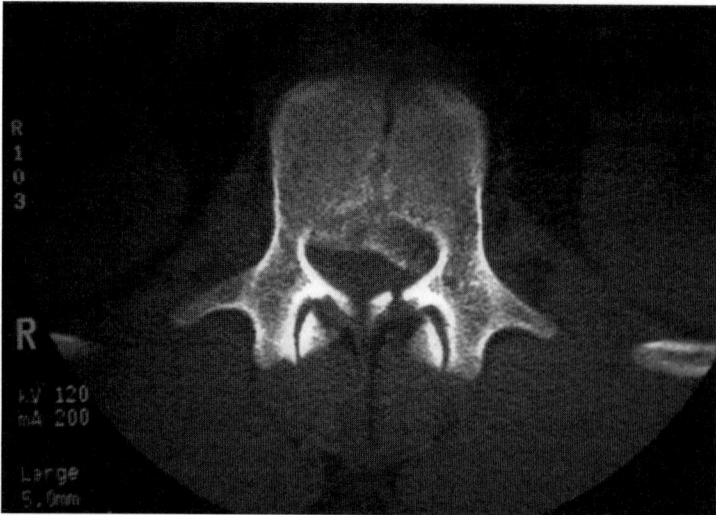

**Figure 102.4** A transaxial CT of a lumbar burst fracture in a patient with an incomplete neurologic deficit. Surgical decompression and stabilization has been found to predictably improve the neurologic profile of a patient with an incomplete neurologic deficit with this fracture subtype.

Once it has been determined that the posterior tension band has been rendered ineffective in resisting the tendency for kyphosis, realignment and surgical stabilization is often beneficial to prevent late onset of instability or deformity. Flexion-distraction injuries range from purely ligamentous to purely bony injuries. The ligamentous and combined osteoligamentous injuries have a significantly less favorable healing rate with nonoperative treatment and are therefore considered unstable injuries. Lastly, fracture-dislocations and three column shear injuries result in disruption of all three columns of the spine. Because of the significant instability present, surgical intervention is almost universally required.

## Neurologic Function

It is a general agreement that patients experiencing a progressive neurologic deficit in the setting of objective neural compression should undergo early surgical intervention. Surgery in this setting may create an environment conducive to neurologic repair and minimize the severity of the secondary cascade of spinal cord injury. In fact, Kiwerski and Weiss found a decrease in mortality in patients with complete spinal cord injuries undergoing surgical decompression and stabilization.[10] Surgery in the setting of a complete lesion has also been shown to accelerate the return of neurologic recovery in a more predictable manner (Figure 102.5). Anderson and Bohlman evaluated the efficacy of anterior surgical decompression and arthrodesis of the cervical spine in quadriplegic patients. A significant number of patients who underwent surgical intervention were noted to recover one or two root levels within the 2 to 3 weeks following surgery.[1]

The timing of surgery may also influence the potential for neurologic recovery following spinal cord injury. Delemarter et al.[4] used an experimental animal model to determine whether the duration of compression and timing of decompression after a spinal cord injury affected the extent of neurologic recovery. He found that early decompression, within 1 hour after the injury, provided the best potential for neurologic recovery and that decompression after 6 or more hours of compression essentially precluded the possibility of neurologic recovery. This study found that there may be a potential for neurologic improvement if surgical intervention is provided on a timely basis. This suggests that the primary mechanism or insult leading to injury may not be solely responsible for the pathologic and clinical findings noted in spinal cord injury.

Mirza et al.[17] investigated the optimal timing of surgical intervention in patients with acute cervical spine injuries and a neurologic deficit. One group of patients underwent surgical intervention within 72 hours while the other group was treated with immediate closed reduction and neurologic observation for 10 to 14 days before surgical stabilization. There was a statistically significant improvement in neurologic recovery in those patients treated with early surgical intervention (within 72 hours of injury). Marshall et al.[13] conjectured that the neurologic response to spinal cord injury was more a reflection of the degree of biomechanical instability and less likely related to the timing of surgery. As such, surgical stabilization, aside from reestablishing spinal stability, may also assist in preventing subsequent neurologic injury. The timing of surgical intervention has not been shown to significantly affect neurologic recovery in any prospective human clinical trial to date as it has in animal investigations. However, early surgical stabilization has significantly decreased acute hospital admission times, ventilation requirements, and outpatient rehabilitation. In an experimental animal spinal cord injury study evaluating the efficacy of surgery and its timing with or without steroid administration, it was found that early surgical intervention (less than 6 hours) resulted in better neurologic recovery than those animals treated with methylprednisolone alone.[7]

Surgical stabilization, preventing excessive motion, has been shown to improve the rate and degree of soft tissue healing in multiple appendicular trauma victims. Franklin et al.[8] demonstrated that skeletal stabilization of appendic-

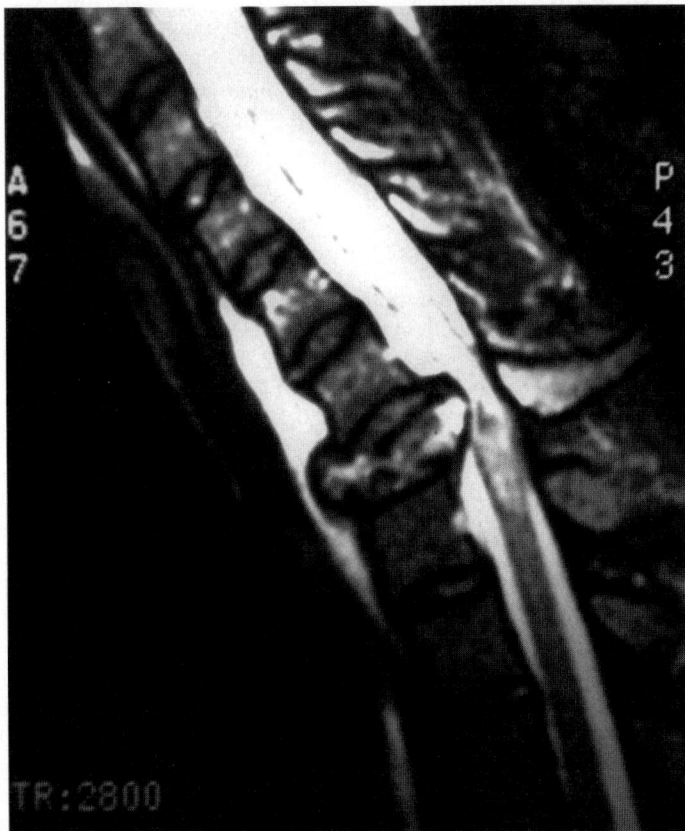

**Figure 102.5** A sagittal MRI of a C7 burst fracture in a patient with a C6 complete spinal cord injury. Surgical intervention in this fracture subtype is controversial. Some surgeons would attempt an anterior decompression and stabilization procedure in this patient in order to improve predictably the chances of root recovery and improved functional status.

ular fractures facilitated associated soft tissue healing and early patient mobilization. An intimate relationship also exists between a patient's neurologic status and the presence of spinal instability. Therefore, excessive motion or repetitive compression or distraction of the level of a compromised spinal cord may impede neurologic recovery or possibly lead to further injury. Therefore, spinal stabilization in the setting of a spinal cord injury may offer a protective effect from additional neural injury and facilitate neurologic recovery. This is supported by Donovan et al.[6] in an investigation of 61 patients following cervical spinal cord injury. It was found that neurologic recovery correlated with the adequacy of spinal alignment, which was more predictably obtained with surgical intervention.

## Primary and Secondary Cascade of Spinal Cord Injury

The primary cascade or initial insult resulting in spinal cord injury may involve a contusion, laceration, blast effect, ischemic event or transient ongoing compression. This insult overwhelms the adaptive ability of the spinal cord and column to absorb and dissipate the energy of impact resulting in a failure of function of the neural elements.[10] This primary injury cascade involves a cascade of complex biochemical events that eventually results in hemorrhage, edema, and ischemia representative of the secondary cascade of neural injury.[4,5] This secondary cascade of spinal cord injury alters the patient's ultimate potential for neurologic recovery. Taken together, many researchers believe in a "window of opportunity" where external manipulation in the form of pharmacologic or surgical intervention may alter the deleterious consequences of these biochemical events.

The value of surgery and its timing has not been resolved primarily due to the lack of good evidence-based medicine evaluating the role of surgery in this clinical setting. Wagner et al.[18] evaluated the role of surgical intervention on neurologic outcome following spinal cord injury. At follow-up, 53% of patients surgically treated were able to walk compared with 23% of conservatively treated patients. However, when patients were stratified as to their presenting neurologic level there was no significant difference between the two groups in terms of neurologic recovery.[18] Surgery, however, appears to be beneficial in the setting of static neurologic compression regardless of the duration of time from injury. Bohlman and Anderson evaluated 51 patients with an incomplete sensorimotor loss below the level of injury who underwent an anterior decompression and stabilization procedure following a remote cervical fracture or dislocation. They found that 50% of patients demonstrated a marked improvement in their functional status illustrating the potential for delayed recovery with late surgical intervention.[3]

## Complications Related to Operative and Nonoperative Care

One of the main historic reasons that surgery was often not chosen in the management of a spinal trauma patient was the belief that surgery resulted in more complications and prolonged recovery of these unfortunate patients. However, as technology has improved in regards to anesthesia techniques, fluid management, and internal fixation, the morbidity related to the surgical procedure is greatly diminished from what it was in the past. In 1983, Whitehill and Schmidt demonstrated that a posterior fusion was safe and effective when compared with other treatments for cervical instability in 22 quadriplegics.[20] Wilmot et al.,[21] in a retrospective study of 106 tetraplegic patients admitted to the Santa Clara Valley Medical Center from August 1981 to September 1983, found that the complications reported in patients who underwent posterior fusion were no greater than patients treated nonoperatively.

Similar findings were also noted by Waters et al.[19] and Mirza et al.[17] in terms of the potential for developing respiratory infections, pulmonary emboli, or bed sores. In fact, Kostuik et al.[11] found that the morbidity from respiratory complications, including the duration of stay in the ICU, was significantly decreased if the unstable spine was operated on in a timely fashion.

## Summary

The role of surgical intervention in the setting of spinal trauma is a complicated issue often argued from experience and myth and rarely from evidence-based medicine. Surgery has several well-supported roles in the setting of trauma. It confers immediate stability to a grossly unstable spine. In the setting of a spinal cord injury, it reduces the period of time in an acute care facility, in an intensive care unit, and accelerates the outpatient rehabilitation. Surgery is also effective in preventing late-onset spinal deformity in the setting of obvious or occult spinal instability. Its role, however, is unclear in the majority of spinal injuries in which the degree of spinal instability is ambiguous or unclear. Only well-designed, controlled, prospective studies can truly answer the value of surgical intervention in these fracture patterns. Although surgery has been found to be effective in improving neurologic recovery in delayed instances of chronic spinal cord compression, its role in early intervention is only conjectured until definitively proven.

## REFERENCES

1. Anderson PA, Bohlman HH: Anterior decompression and arthrodesis of the cervical spine part II—improvement in complete traumatic quadriplegia: long-term motor improvement *J Bone Joint Surg Am* 74:683-692, 1992.
2. Anderson PA, Budorick TE, Easton KB, Henley MB, Salciccioli GG: Failure of the halo vest to prevent in vivo motion in patients with injured cervical spines. *Spine* 16:S501-S505,1991.
3. Bohlman HH and Anderson PA: Anterior decompression and arthrodesis of the cervical spine part I—improvement in incomplete traumatic quadriparesis: long-term motor improvement. *J Bone Joint Surg Am* 74:671-682, 1992.
4. Delamarter RB, Sherman J, Carr JV: Pathophysiology of spinal cord injury. *J Bone Joint Surg Am* 77:1042-1049, 1995.
5. Dohrmann GJ: Experimental spinal cord trauma: a histological review. *Arch Neurol* 27:468-473, 1972.
6. Donovan WH, Kopniky D, Stolzmann E, Carter RE: The neurological and skeletal outcome in patients with closed cervical spinal cord injury. *J Neurosurg* 66:690-694, 1987.
7. Ducker TB, Salcman M, Daniell HB: Experimental spinal cord trauma, III: therapeutic effect of immobilization and pharmacologic agents. *Surg Neurol* 10:71-76, 1978.
8. Franklin JL, Johnson KD, Hansen ST, Jr: Open reduction and internal fixation of open ankle fractures. Report of thirty-eight cases treated with a standard protocol. *J Bone Joint Surg* 66:1349-1356, 1984.
9. Gertzbein, SD: Scoliosis Research Society—multicenter spine fracture study. *Spine* 17:528-540, 1992.
10. Kiwerski J, Weiss M: Neurological improvement in traumatic injuries of the cervical spinal cord. *Paraplegia* 19:31-37, 1981.
11. Kostuik JP: Dysfunction of the spinal stability system and its restabilization. In Holtzman R, McCormick PC, Farcy JC (eds): *Spinal Instability.* New York, Springer-Verlag, 1993, pp 39-44.
12. Levine A, Eismont F, Garfin S, Zigler J: *Spine Trauma.* Philadelphia, WB Saunders, 1998, pp 113-135.
13. Marshall LF, Knowlton S, Garfin SR, et al: Deterioration following spinal cord injury: a multicenter study. *J Neurosurg* 66:400-404, 1987.
14. McCormack T, Karaikovic E, Gaines RW: The load sharing classification of spine fractures *Spine* 19(15):1741-1744, 1994.
15. McGuire RA, Green BA, Eismont FJ, Watts C: Comparison of stability provided to the unstable spine by the kinetic therapy table and the Stryker frame. *Neurosurgery* 22:842-845, 1988.
16. McGuire RA, Neville S, Green BA, Watts C: Spinal instability and the log-rolling maneuver. *J Trauma Inj Infect Crit Care* 27:525-531, 1987.
17. Mirza SK, Krengel WF, Chapman J, et al: Early versus delayed surgery for acute cervical spinal cord injury. *Clin Orthop* 359:104-114, 1999.
18. Wagner FC Jr. and Chehrazi B: Early decompression and neurological outcome in acute cervical spinal cord injuries. *J Neurosurg* 56:699-705, 1982.
19. Waters, RL, Meyer PR Jr, Adkins RH, Felton D: Emergency, acute, and surgical management of spine trauma. *Arch Phys Med Rehabil* 80:1383-1390, 1999.
20. Whitehill R and Schmidt R: The posterior interspinous fusion in the treatment of quadriplegia. *Spine* 8:733-740, 1983.
21. Wilmot CB and Hall KM: Evaluation of the acute management of tetraplegia: conservative versus surgical treatment. *Paraplegia* 24:149-153, 1986.

# CHAPTER 103

# Trauma Nonoperative Management

**Glenn R. Rechtine, Michael Bolesta, and Patrick W. Hitchon**

Injuries to the thoracic and lumbar spine are some of the most common spinal injuries. The treatment remains controversial. Certainly the least invasive treatment method that provides a satisfactory outcome is the treatment of choice. In the majority of instances this will be provided by nonoperative means.

## Initial Evaluation

All spinal injuries are best managed by immediate immobilization. EMS personnel initially accomplish this in the field. There should be a high index of suspicion for these injuries among all personnel at all levels. Unconsciousness, alcohol or drug use, and polytrauma all contribute to delayed or missed diagnosis of spinal trauma.[4,19,39]

## Hospital Evaluation

Immobilization is maintained until spinal stability has been assessed. The ABCs of trauma evaluation are then followed. After life-threatening injuries have been evaluated, the spine itself can be addressed.

## History and Physical Examination

Important indirect information can be obtained from EMS personnel. Even transient paralysis or numbness will be factors in definitive treatment plans. Neurologic evaluation must be done with diligence. Between 15% and 20% of patients with TL fractures will have a neurologic deficit.[1,22,24] Inspection and palpation of the back are done and documented. Abrasions, open wounds, and ligamentous gaps will drastically effect treatment options. After the thorough history and physical have been performed, they are then documented in detail.

## Spinal Radiographs

While still immobilized, radiographic evaluation of the spine is carried out. The cross table lateral cervical spine radiograph must include T1. If the patient is unconscious or unable to cooperate with the exam, the entire spine must be visualized. Upper cervical injuries are common and an open mouth view should be included. If there is unexplained tenderness, definite fracture, or inability to image a particular region with plain radiographs (most often the upper thoracic spine), computed tomography (CT) is indicated.

## Computerized Tomography (CT)

All fractures should be evaluated with a CT scan. Experienced readers on plain radiographs alone misdiagnose approximately 40% of fractures.[11] The combination of displaced laminar fractures and neurologic deficit is associated with entrapped nerve roots. This can change surgical approaches from anterior to posterior.

## Magnetic Resonance Imaging

Magnetic resonance imaging (MRI) is complementary to the CT. It is not required routinely. However, MRI can provide additional information as to the integrity of the ligamentous structures, discs, spinal cord, and nerve roots. It is helpful if the neurologic deficit does not match the noted radiographic injury.

## Classification

After all the studies have been evaluated, the injury is classified. This classification determines the treatment options.

## Anatomic Classification

Anatomic differences make injuries of the upper thoracic spine (T1-9), the thoracolumbar junction (T10-L2), and the low lumbar spine (L3-5) clinically distinct.

### Upper Thoracic

This area is biomechanically reinforced by the rib cage. Minimally displaced injuries are commonly neurologically intact. Displaced fractures and fracture-dislocations tend to be associated with complete paraplegia. There are relatively few incomplete injuries. The combination of an upper thoracic fracture and a sternal fracture is a potentially unstable situation.

### Thoracolumbar Junction

This is the most common area of the spine to be injured. This occurs because of the great forces that are concentrated here by the junction of the stiff thoracic segment and mobile lumbar spine. The neurologic injuries at this level can be very complex because of the spinal cord anatomy at this level. There can be conus (upper motor neuron) or root (lower motor neuron) injuries.

### Lower Lumbar

The lower lumbar injuries (L3-5) usually occur as the result of high-energy trauma such as airplane crashes, parachuting injuries, or high-speed motor vehicle crashes. If seen in the absence of major trauma, the clinician should seek an explanation, such as domestic violence or pathology that weakened the bone.

If a neurologic injury occurs, it is commonly incomplete and has a relatively good prognosis because it is a root injury. Absence of the bulbocavernosus reflex in this region implies a lower motor neuron lesion.

## Structural Classification

### Two or Three Columns?

In 1953, Holdsworth[17] originally described the spine as consisting of two columns, anterior and posterior. Thirty years later, Denis[8] proposed dividing the anterior column of Holdsworth into anterior and middle columns. Denis based this upon CT visualization of the posterior body. It is important to remember that the CT scanner did not invent the burst fracture, it only provided a new way to assess it.

The AO classification differentiates the feasibility of surgical or nonoperative treatment of thoracolumbar injuries.[33] The "A" injuries are axial injuries (compression and burst fractures). The "B" injuries are distraction injuries (flexion-distraction, Chance injuries). The "C" injuries are rotational injuries (fracture-dislocations, shear injuries). The key factor deciding if nonoperative treatment is possible is the integrity of the ligamentous structures. Most A injuries are amenable to nonoperative treatment. The B and C injuries will commonly involve ligament insufficiency, and may require operative stabilization.

## Surgical Indications

### Absolute

An absolute indication for emergent surgery of a thoracolumbar injury is a progressive neurologic deficit in the presence of a surgically correctable compressive lesion or instability. Ligamentous instability is an absolute indication for surgical stabilization, but this usually is not required emergently.

### Relative

The relative indications for surgery of a thoracolumbar injury are a significant motor deficit that is not improving, unacceptable deformity, and inability to cooperate with nonoperative means. There is no clear relationship between canal compromise and neurologic deficit. The mere presence of canal compromise without a neurologic deficit is not a surgical indication.

### Contraindications

The contraindication for surgery for a thoracolumbar injury is mechanically stable injuries with no likelihood of progressive neurologic deficit or deformity.

## Nonoperative Treatment

A more rational approach is to extend the three-column concept proposed by Denis and analyze the degree and type of injury in each column. If a column has primarily bony injury, the fragments are in close proximity, and alignment is good, one can expect that column to heal. It may not bear physiologic loads immediately after injury, but may after 4 to 6 weeks, particularly if protected with a cast or orthosis. If column damage is primarily ligamentous, the injury may be both acutely and chronically unstable, as soft tissue healing yields a biomechanically inferior structure. Therefore, the physician should discern the potential for columns to reconstitute. If this is unlikely, surgical treatment may be indicated. Otherwise, there are more options.[5]

From the ancient Egyptians to the present, nonoperative treatment has been the mainstay of the treatment of spine injuries. There was an increase in operative treatment in the early and mid 1980s. This came about when the CT scan demonstrated previously unrecognized spinal canal compromise. Harrington rods, which had been designed to treat scoliosis, were modified for use in trauma. There may have been overtreatment of many burst injuries.

Recumbency treatment for up to 3 months in spinal fractures was advocated in the work of Ludwig Guttmann[12] and Frankel[10] at the Stoke Mandeville Hospital. Surgical management for fractures was reserved for open fractures, secondary to missile injuries or to fractures with progressive neurologic deficit. In 1949, Nicoll reported on his analysis of 166 thoracic and lumbar fractures in 152 miners in England, the majority of whom were treated with immobilization and bed rest.[26] Good anatomic result did not always equate with a good functional outcome. Postural nonsurgical reduction of thoracic and lumbar fractures was adopted by Bedbrook[2,3] and Davies et al.[7] in Australia and immobilization for 6 to 10 weeks followed by bracing was recommended. Surgery was indicated in the few cases of irreducible fractures, locked facets, gunshot wounds, and neurologic deterioration. In his analysis of 143 thoracic and lumbar fractures, Bedbrook noted that an angulation of 40 degrees was often well tolerated without functional impairment.

Subsequent reports rekindled interest in recumbency in the management of thoracic and lumbar fractures.* This approach was associated with a stable or improved neurologic status, in spite of progression in spinal angulation. In addition, CT scans revealed remodeling of the spine with partial resolution of the compromised canal.

Nonoperative management may consist of bed rest, casting, application of an orthosis, and often, some combination of these. It should be emphasized that nonoperative care requires meticulous attention to detail to be successful and not through benign neglect.[5]

Bohler,[4a] Frankel et al.,[10] and Davies et al.[7] have reported the classic series of nonsurgical treatment. Bed rest of 3 months was standard even in the face of neurologic deficits. The results were reasonable although the complications of decubitus ulceration, pulmonary emboli, and other pulmonary complications were still present. One criticism of bed rest has been deconditioning that may result. A vigorous upper and lower extremity program using range of motion and progressive resistance with rubber bands can counter this. Since the average person takes 17,000 steps each day, the exercise program should simu-

---

*References 6,18,20,21,23,30,34,36.

late the demands of normal walking. This requires a large number of repetitions; specifically we ask our patients to perform 10,000 repetitions per day. In other words, they should be exercising unless they are eating, sleeping, eliminating, bathing, or reading. Compliant patients will be as strong or stronger than they were before injury, even with bed rest of up to 6 weeks. Depending upon the number and nature of other injuries, a fit patient will mobilize quickly after such a program. Although not studied to our knowledge, this exercise may counter the problem of disuse osteoporosis.[5] In 1995, Hartman reported a series of patients treated on a kinetic bed for 4 to 6 weeks with excellent outcomes.[13] By including bony injuries and excluding primarily ligamentous injuries, the kinetic bed provides an environment to allow for bone healing without the risk of anatomic or neurologic deterioration. The costs were found to be comparable between the prolonged hospitalizations required by the Roto-Rest bed treatment and conventional bed rest, which requires a skilled nursing staff. Once the nurses are comfortable with the bed, it is easier to nurse these patients than those in a conventional hospital bed. Prophylaxis against thromboembolism consists of foot, leg, and thigh antiembolism stockings along with mechanical compression devices such as foot pumps or sequential compression stockings. Anticoagulation is avoided in the early postinjury phase to reduce the risk of expanding epidural hematoma with neural compression. Once the patient is stable, physical and occupational therapists are consulted to instruct the patient in exercises to maintain flexibility and strength in all four extremities, modified as necessary by any concomitant injuries.[5]

Rechtine et al.[29] documented the advantage to the patient by avoiding the higher complication rate of surgical management. In the 1999 publication, only the worst-case scenario was considered. Only those patients who had been kept on the Roto-Rest bed for a full 6 weeks were included. Also included in the nonoperative group was a patient who died while awaiting surgical intervention but was canceled five times because he was too ill from his initial injuries to undergo surgery. There were no more decubitus ulcers, pulmonary emboli, or other pulmonary complications in the nonoperative group as compared to the group treated with surgery. The overall infection rate was 8%. In the patients with complete neurologic deficits, the infection rate approached 30%.[29] These are the same patients who will have multiple urinary tract infections over the remainder of their lives. This will predispose them to late spinal infections as well. A complete neurologic deficit is a good indication for nonoperative treatment, as long as it is appropriate for the structural injury. Not all patients are candidates for orthotic or cast treatment. Casts should not be applied over insensate skin. Braces may be used cautiously if skin is inspected frequently. The orthosis is modified or discontinued if there is any erythema or other sign of skin irritation. Emaciated patients are at risk for skin ulceration, regardless of sensibility. This reflects the paucity of soft tissue padding over bony prominences, and in some cases malnutrition. Morbid obesity, coexisting wounds and burns may preclude bracing. Even in patients of normal habitus with intact sensate skin, compliance may be an issue once the discomfort of the trauma subsides. Casts are more challenging for patients to remove, but not impossible. The fit of external devices tends to deteriorate with time, and may require adjustment by the clinician. Thoracic injuries with concomitant sternomanubrial dislocation may not be stable, and these patients may develop kyphosis.[5]

At our center, 66 patients with thoracolumbar burst fractures (T12-L2) were followed prospectively for a mean of over 1 year.[14-16] Twenty-six with a Frankel score of E (intact), and 6 with a score of D (minimal motor deficit), were treated with recumbency (Figure 103.1). Angular deformity measured less than 10 degrees, residual spinal canal on CT

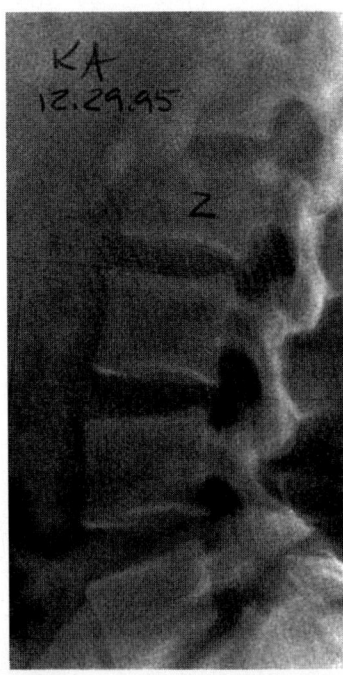

**A**

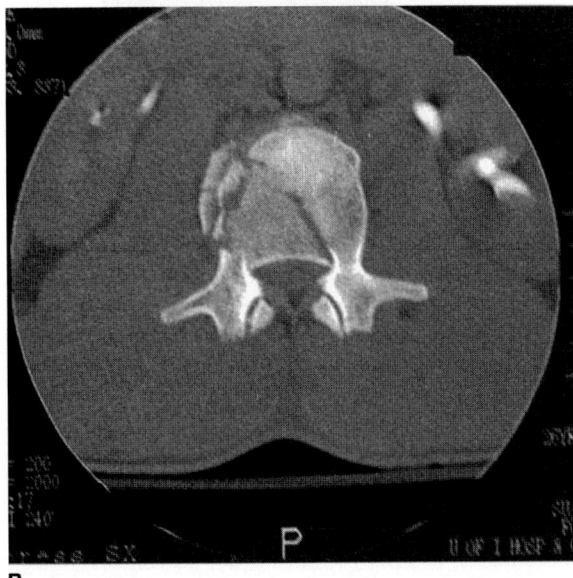

**B**

**Figure 103.1** A 26-year-old man was involved in a single-car accident. He had no evidence of neurologic deficit but had multiple other injuries, including head injuries, bladder laceration, and extremity fractures. **(A)** Lateral radiographs of the spine show a burst fracture of L2 with loss in height. **(B)** CT scan shows the burst fracture of L2 with at least 50% compromise of the AP diameter of the canal.

*Continued*

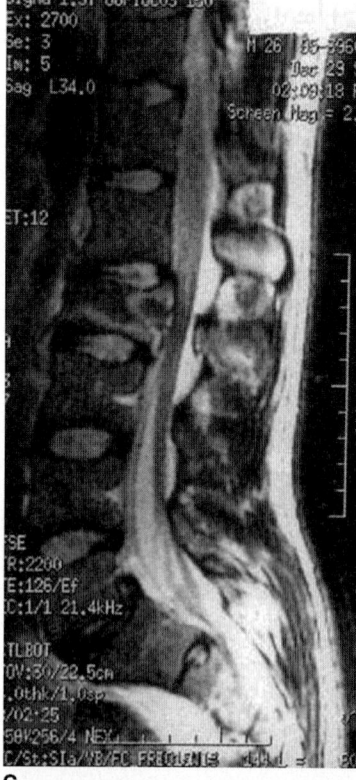

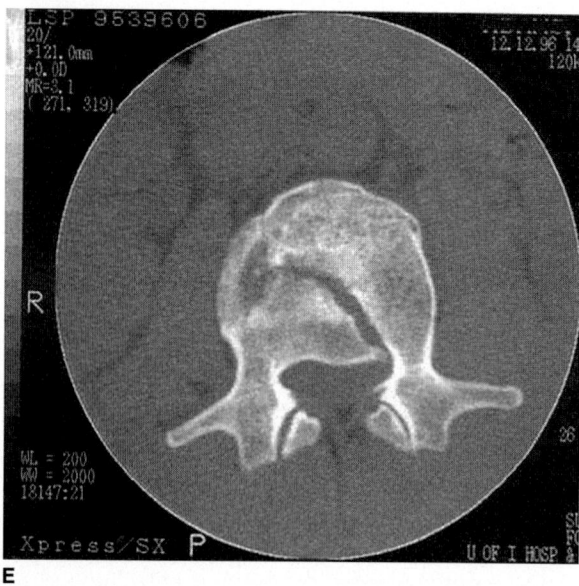

**E**

**Figure 103.1 *cont'd*** (**E**) A follow-up CT scan shows remodeling of the spinal canal with healing of the fractured body. (*From Hitchon P, Torner JC, Haddad SF, Follett KA: Management options in thoracolumbar burst fractures.* Surg Neurol *49: 619-626, 1998.*)

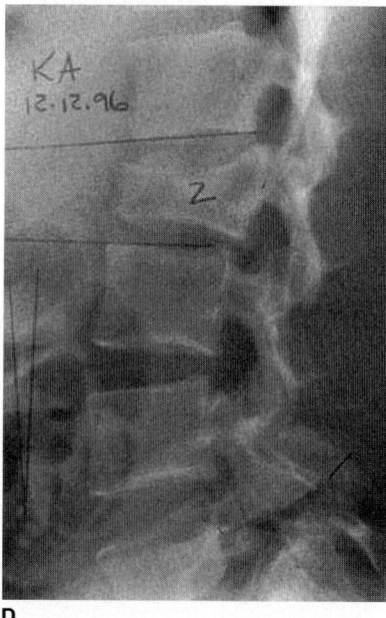

**D**

**Figure 103.1 *cont'd*** (**C**) $T_2$-weighted MRI reveals the burst fracture, with posterior displacement of bone and compression of the later. He wore his customized thoracolumbar orthosis for 3 months. He has since returned to his previous employment without restriction. (**D**) Radiographs obtained 1 year later show an angular deformity at L2 measuring 8 degrees, compared with 5 degrees on admission.

was 50% or more of normal, and an anterior body height greater than 50% of the posterior height. Patients were kept at bed rest for 1 to 3 weeks until their pain resolved. They were mobilized thereafter in thoracolumbar orthosis for 3 to 5 months with sequential radiographs.

Surgery was undertaken in 36 patients. Twenty-six patients had a neurologic deficit with a Frankel score of A (motor and sensory paralysis) in 9 patients, C (partial sensory preservation) in 5 patients, and D (nonfunctional motor preservation) in 17 patients. Only 5 patients were intact. Angular deformity generally measured more than 10 degrees, and the residual spinal canal less than 50% of normal.

Decompression was the prime purpose of surgery and was accomplished via a transpedicular approach in 25 patients, through a costotransversectomy in 7 patients, and through a lateral extraperitoneal approach in the remaining 4 patients. Postoperatively, patients were mobilized in polyester or acrylic thoracolumbar orthoses for 3 to 5 months. The angulation on admission in the surgical group measured 12 ± 7 degrees (range 0 to 25 degrees) was twice that measured in the recumbency group, 5.6 ± 7 degrees (range −1.4 to 16 degrees). This difference was significant ($P = .0035$). The preoperative residual canal at the site of injury measured (means ± standard deviation) 65% ± 18% in the recumbency group versus 42% ± 25% in the surgical group ($P = .0001$). At the time of discharge angular deformity in the surgical group had been corrected to 7.7 ± 6.8 degrees, whereas that in the recumbency group had progressed to 10.7 ± 7.2 degrees ($P = .04$).

The duration of hospital stay was 31.8 days ± 16 days in the recumbency group compared to 31.3 days ± 19 days in the surgical group ($P = .55$). Transfer of our patients to rehabilitation was often delayed owing to lack of funds or inadequate medical coverage. This undoubtedly contributed to lengthier hospital stays in both groups. In the recumbency group, total charges including hospital and physician charges were calculated at $27,000 ± $19,600 per patient. Total charges in the surgical group, including operating room fees and implants, yielded $62,900 ± $38,900 ($P = .0001$). There appeared to be an association between the extent of neurologic deficit and higher cost. The increased cost in the surgical group is not only a reflection of the expenses arising from surgery, but additional expenses are attributed to more severe injuries and a longer stay in the SICU. On the average surgical patients spent twice as long time in the intensive care unit as compared to recumbency patients.

Both groups showed neurologic improvement. Whereas on admission the incidence of deficit in the recumbency and surgical groups was 19% and 86% respectively, these numbers decreased to 3% and 72% respectively at follow-up. At final follow-up angulation progressed to 13.5 ± 8.5 degrees in the recumbency group and to 14.4 ± 10.5 degrees in the surgical group. Where sequential CT scans were obtained, remodeling and an enlargement of the spinal canal were encountered (see Figure 103.1). Not unlike the experience of others,[32,37] an increased incidence of urinary tract infections, pancreatitis, and deep vein thrombosis was noted in our surgical group. This is not entirely surprising owing to the indwelling bladder catheterization mandated by long operative procedures. The postoperative recovery with its pain, stress, and hypercoagulable state can contribute to the development of venous thrombosis and pancreatitis. These complications may in part be responsible for the narrowing of the gap between the two groups in length of hospitalization.

Some individuals do not tolerate rotating bed management but still do not desire surgery. Claustrophobia, boredom, and labile mental status can make kinetic bed treatment challenging. Bony chance fractures, severe compression fractures, and burst injuries without severe comminution can be treated with hyperextension casting treatment if sagittal alignment is restored. However, if there is severe kyphosis, hyperextension casting is less likely to give a good result. A brace should not be considered a substitute for a well-molded hyperextension cast. Finite element analysis suggests that a Jewett brace cannot prevent deformity in single-level three-column injuries.[5]

In a presentation at the AAOS meeting in February 2001, Wood et al. demonstrated similar results in a prospective, randomized study. Fifty-three patients were followed with an average of 47 months follow-up. The nonsurgical patients were mobilized early in casts or braces. There was a greater likelihood of subsequent surgery in the group treated with surgery initially. The outcomes were measured by return to work, pain, Oswestry disability score, Roland-Morris, and SF-36. There was no significant difference in groups although there was a trend for more pain in the surgical group. The costs were five times higher in the surgical group.

## Radiographs

With all nonsurgical as well as operatively treated patients, an upright radiograph should be obtained prior to discharge. When measuring kyphosis, there will be a difference between a supine film with the patient on a board and an upright view in all patients with or without an injury. The deformity is only progressive if it progresses from the original upright lateral view.

## Contraindications of Nonoperative Treatment

Progressive neurologic deficit in the presence of a compressive lesion or instability or the presence of a ligamentous injury are contraindications to nonoperative treatment.

## Remodeling

The development of the CT scanner showed the retropulsed bone in burst fractures. Ten years later the CT scanner has also demonstrated the remodeling that occurs. Multiple studies have shown the posteriorly placed bone resorbs whether there is a surgical fusion or not. This is just another example of Wolff's law in practice. The incidence of neurogenic claudication is extremely low after a burst fracture.[*]

## Summary

Thoracolumbar injuries are very common. The treatment is still controversial. Formerly, bed rest was the only available method. With surgical advances more patients were treated surgically. Recently, we have taken a more critical look at surgical interventions. Surgery should be reserved for those cases in which it provides superior outcome with an acceptable complication rate. The cost effectiveness of treatment options must also be apprised.

The vast majority of traumatic (nonosteoporotic) compression fractures can and should be managed nonsurgically. If there is a progressive motor deficit, ligamentous instability, or progressive deformity, surgery may be indicated.

---

[*]References 9,20,25,27,28,31,35.

## REFERENCES

1. Andresen R, Radmer S, Banzer D: Bone mineral density and spongiosa architecture in correlation to vertebral body insufficiency fractures. *Acta Radiol* 39(5): 538-542, 1998.

2. Bedbrook GM: Spinal injuries with tetraplegia and paraplegia. *J Bone Joint Surg Br* 6(3):267-284, 1979.

3. Bedbrook GM: Treatment of thoracolumbar dislocation and fractures with paraplegia. *Clin Orthop* 112:27-43,1975.

4. Benson DR, Keenen TL: Evaluation and treatment of trauma to the vertebral column. *Instr Course Lect* 39: 577-589, 1990.

4a. Bohler L: *Treatment of Fractures*, ed 4. Translated from the Fourth Enlarged and Revised German Edition. Bristol, John Wright & Sons, 1935.

5. Bolesta MR, Rechtine GR: Fractures and dislocations of the thoracolumbar spine. In Bucholz RW, Heckamn JD (eds): *Rockwood and Green's Fractures in Adults*, vol 2. Philadelphia, Lippincott-Williams & Wilkins, 2001, pp 1422-1426.

6. Chakera TMH, Bedbrook G, Bradley CM: Spontaneous resolution of spinal canal deformity after burst-dispersion fracture. *AJNR Am J Neuroradiol* 9:779-785, 1988.

7. Davies WE, Morris JH, Hill V: An analysis of conservative (non-surgical) management of thoracolumbar fractures and fracture-dislocations with neural damage. *J Bone Joint Surg Am* 62(8):1324-1328, 1980.

8. Denis F: The three-column spine and its significance in the classification of acute thoracolumbar spinal injuries. *Spine* 8:817-831, 1983.

9. Floman Y, Margulies JY, Nyska M, *et al:* Effect of major axial skeleton trauma on preexisting lumbosacral spondylolisthesis. *J Spinal Disord* 4(3):353-358, 1991.

10. Frankel HL, Hancock DO, Hyslop G, *et al:* The value of postural reduction in the initial management of closed injuries of the spine with paraplegia and tetraplegia. Part I. *Paraplegia* 7:179-192, 1969.

11. Garfin S: Can burst fractures be predicted from plain radiographs? *J Bone Joint Surg Br* 74(1):147-150, 1992.

12. Guttmann L: Surgical aspects of the treatment of traumatic paraplegia. *J Bone Joint Surg Br* 3(3):399-403, 1949.

13. Hartman MB, Chrin AM, Rechtine GR: Non-operative treatment of thoracolumbar fractures. *Paraplegia* 33(2): 73-76, 1995.

14. Hitchon PW, Torner JC: Recumbency in thoracolumbar fractures. *Neurosurg Clin N Am* 8:509-517, 1997.

15. Hitchon PW, Torner JC, Haddad SF, Follett KA: Thoracic and lumbar fractures: management analysis. In Hitchon PW, Traynelis VC, Rengachery S (eds): *Techniques in Spinal Fusion and Instrumentation.* New York-Stuttgart, Thieme Medical Publishers, 1995, pp 338-344.

16. Hitchon PW, Torner JC, Haddad SF, Follett KA. Management options in thoracolumbar burst fractures. *Surg Neurol* 49:619-627, 1998.

17. Holdsworth FW, Hardy A: Early treatment of paraplegia from fractures of the thoracolumbar spine. *J Bone Joint Surg Br* 35(4):540-550, 1953.

18. Johnson R, Herrlin K, Hagglund G, Stromqvist B: Spinal canal remodeling after thoracolumbar fractures with intraspinal bone fragments. *ACTA Orthop Scand* 62: 125-127, 1991.

19. Karlsson MK, Hasserius R, Sundgren P, *et al:* Remodeling of the spinal canal deformed by trauma. *J Spinal Disord* 10(2):157-161, 1997.

20. Knight RQ, Stornelli DP, Chan DP, *et al:* Comparison of operative versus nonoperative treatment of lumbar burst fractures. *Clin Orthop* 293:112-121, 1993.

21. Knight RQ, Stornelli DP, Chan DPK, *et al:* Comparison of operative versus nonoperative treatment of lumbar burst fractures. *Clin Orthop* 293:112-121, 1993.

22. Korovessis PG, Stamatakis M, Baikousis A: Unrecognized laceration of main bronchus caused by fracture of the T6 vertebra. *Eur Spine J* 7(1):72-75, 1998.

23. Krompinger WJ, Fredricson BE, Mino DE, Yuan HA: Conservative treatment of fractures of the thoracic and lumbar spine. *Orthop Clin N Am* 17:161-170, 1986.

24. Matsuzaki H, Tokuhashi Y, Wakabayashi K, *et al:* Rigix plate system for anterior fixation of thoracolumbar vertebrae. *J Spinal Disord* 10(4):339-347, 1997.

25. McCormack T, Karaikovic E, Gaines RW: The load sharing classification of spine fractures. *Spine* 19(15): 1741-1744, 1994.

26. Nicoll EA: Fractures of the dorso-lumbar spine. *J Bone Joint Surg Br* 31(3):376-394, 1949.

27. Ponzo L, De Gennaro A, Pavone S, *et al:* Lumbosacral monolateral dislocation. *Chirurgia Degli Organi di Movimento* 79(3):315-319, 1994.

28. Rasmussen PA, Rabin MH, Mann DC, *et al:* Reduced transverse spinal area secondary to burst fractures: is there a relationship to neurologic injury? *J Neurotrauma* 11(6):711-720, 1994.

29. Rechtine G, Cahill D, Chrin AM: Treatment of thoracolumbar trauma: comparison of complications of operative versus nonoperative treatment. *J Spinal Disord* 12(5):406-409, 1999.

30. Reid DC, Hu R, Davis LA, Saboe LA: The nonoperative treatment of burst fractures of the thoracolumbar junction. *J Trauma* 28:1188-1194, 1988.

31. Soderstrom CA, Ducker TB: Increased susceptibility of patients with cervical cord lesions to peptic gastrointestinal complication. *J Trauma* 25:1030-1038, 1985.

32. Tator CH, Duncan EG, Edmonds VE, *et al:* Comparison of surgical and conservative management in 208 patients with acute spinal cord injury. *Can J Neurol Sci* 14:60-69, 1987.

33. Trafton PG and Boyd CA Jr: Computed tomography of thoracic and lumbar spine injuries. *J Trauma* 24:506-515, 1984.

34. Weinstein JN, Collato P, Lehmann TR: Thoracolumbar "burst" fractures treated conservatively: a long-term follow-up. *Spine* 13:33-38, 1988.

35. Willems PC, Nienhuis B, Sietsma M, *et al:* The effect of a plaster cast on lumbosacral joint motion. An in vivo assessment with precision motion analysis system. *Spine* 22(11):1229-1234, 1997.

36. Willen J, Anderson J, Toomoka K, Singer K: The natural history of burst fractures at the thoracolumbar junction. *J Spinal Disord* 3:39-46, 1990.

37. Wilmot CB, Hall KM: Evaluation of acute surgical intervention in traumatic paraplegia. *Paraplegia* 24:71-76, 1986.

38. Wood K, Butterman G, Mehbod A, *et al:* Operative compared with nonoperative treatment of a thoracolumbar burst fracture without neurologic deficit. A prospective, randomized study. *J Bone Joint Surg Am* 85-A(5):773-781, 2003.

39. Zdeblick A, Shirado O, McAfee PC, *et al:* Anterior spinal fixation after lumbar corpectomy. A study in dogs. *J Bone Joint Surg Am* 73(4):527-534, 1991; Erratum in *J Bone Joint Surg Am* 1991 73(6):952, 1991.

# CHAPTER 104

# Complications of Peripheral Nerve Surgery

## Christopher J. Pham, Yong-Jun Cho, and Daniel H. Kim

Any surgical complication can be a horrifying experience, both for the patient and the surgeon, and peripheral nerve surgery is no exception. Evaluating peripheral nerve damage can be difficult if there are injuries to surrounding anatomic structures, such as bones, the lymphatic system, muscle, or vascular structures. In order to avoid complications, the peripheral nerve surgeon must perform a thorough clinical examination to assess motor and sensory deficits, and determine if there is bony fracture involvement before attempting surgical intervention. The inability or failure to recognize peripheral nerve damage can lead to a delay in surgical intervention, thus hindering functional regeneration, which poses serious legal consequences. Other factors that can contribute to surgical complications are misdiagnosis, inappropriate or unskilled surgical technique, and poor infection control. The aftermath of some surgical complications is irreversible; therefore, meticulous attention must be paid to every preoperative and intraoperative detail. Injuries resulting in a complete nerve lesion with sensory overlap and collateral motor involvement can mimic retained function. If this is not recognized, the patient will suffer irreversible loss of nerve function. Spine surgeons need to be aware that both peripheral and cord lesions can coexist and both must be treated.

In order to enhance surgical results, it is important to localize the lesions within the damaged plexus elements, and determine which deficits are complete and which are partial. Understanding the etiology of injury or disease processes is also important. The precise level of the neural lesion must be correctly identified in order to execute an effective treatment plan. Atypical clinical presentations occur from anatomic variants, incomplete lesions, and other medical causes such as diabetes and renal disease. Vague clinical findings warrant additional or repeated examinations with electrical studies, such as electromyography and radiography, which are necessary for serial comparison. Intractable postoperative pain without resolution of neurologic deficits mandates immediate investigation.

This chapter summarizes the complications that can arise from the management of peripheral nerve lesions.

## Preoperative Assessment

The goals of preoperative assessment are to recognize the pathology, to identify the etiology of the disease process, to devise a treatment plan, and to facilitate neurologic recovery. A number of considerations must be ruled out before surgical intervention can be considered. These include immunologic disorders, toxic polyneuropathies, metabolic processes, inflammatory diseases, nutritional deficiencies, drug-induced neuropathies, vasculitis, hormonal etiologies, and connective tissue disorders.[117,131] Therefore, the key to successful surgery is thorough knowledge of normal and variant peripheral nerve anatomy and its relationship to adjacent structures. Additionally, the surgeon must understand the basic concepts of nerve regeneration and intraneural anatomy, which serve as the foundation for surgical intervention.* Inadequate preoperative assessment or misinterpretation of electrodiagnostic studies can obscure a diagnosis, cause one to select an improper surgical intervention, and negatively impact functional recovery.[74,103,116,117,120]

## Clinical Examination

Anatomic variants of the peripheral nerve are frequently encountered. Sensory examination can be confusing in certain areas of nerve distribution. For example, in the Riche-Cannieu anomaly, both branches of the median and ulnar nerves communicate to the thumb, instead of splitting their distribution as would occur normally.[103,108] Another example is a Martin-Gruber anastomosis in the forearm, where there is median to ulnar crossover communication in the nerve.[63,103,108] Misinterpretation of nonspecific sensory findings subsequently leads to inaccurate assessment of the nerve injury, which constitutes a diagnostic pitfall. Clinical examination should begin with a visual inspection and palpation of the region for evidence of any irregularity, tenderness, involuntary or voluntary movement, or atrophy. The patient should be asked to perform a specific motor task. Inability to perform the task will reveal a neurologic deficit, which can be measured. A good diagnostician is able to discriminate between incongruous movements and legitimate pathologies. When there is muscle loss, patients compensate by contracting adjacent muscles.[117]

## Electrodiagnostic Studies

Electrodiagnostic studies help determine the severity of the nerve injury and establish the baseline of the nerve's physiologic status and functional integrity.[88] Sensory testing combined with electrophysiologic studies can confirm suspicious findings, delineate the problem, or predict the possibility of spontaneous recovery and, therefore, should be performed in a timely fashion.[100,103,116,118] Sensory-motor components are influenced by a patient's adaptive response, temperature changes in the pain receptor area, thickness of the myelin sheath, or autonomic conditions.[89-93,95,96]

Nerve conduction velocity (NCV) studies measure the velocity, intensity, and time that it takes an electrical signal to go through the length of the involved nerve. Conduction velocity decreases with age due to degenerative changes in myelin and in the internodal distances[6]; even though conduction tests can show that an injured nerve is abnormal, it does not necessarily mean that the patient has lost

---

*References 18,36,45,58,67,68,80,103,114,115,117.

sensation. For example, a patient who has a sutured nerve that does not fully display nerve conduction during testing may appreciate sensibility for light touch, thus demonstrating progressive improvement.[8] NCV studies are also influenced by the type of instrument being used, the duration and intensity of the stimulation, and the relative distance of the internodes.[9,30,49]

It is best to obtain nerve recordings directly proximal to a nerve lesion. Fluctuations in nerve waveforms can occur if a tourniquet is used or if a nerve is being dissected; therefore, tourniquets should be released 20 minutes prior to recording or dissecting the nerve. Other factors that may invalidate nerve conduction studies include the extensive injuries, neurologic deficits, and the patient's age and associated medical conditions. NCV is inconclusive in some neuropathies because of wallerian degeneration or "dying back" in a portion of an axon. When this occurs, NCV shows slow to below normal values or fibrillations in the distal muscles.[1] The authors advise using nerve stimulation to ascertain if distal segments are innervated prior to surgical exploration.[123-126] Clinical decision making becomes more complex if a neuroma in continuity is discovered, because abnormal nerve conduction can be recorded in an uninjured section of nerve. In the absence of electrical conduction studies, surgical intervention is warranted when there is loss of function in one or more neural elements usually within 3 months of the injury.[103]

### Medical Conditions

Awareness about medical and nutritional conditions associated with peripheral nerve disorders is important because, unrecognized, organic conditions can lead to misdiagnosis and mismanagement. Such conditions include diabetes mellitus, peripheral vascular disease, hypothyroidism, hemophilia, rheumatoid arthritis, and chronic alcohol abuse. For example, alcoholic-nutritional neuropathy causes atrophy and weakness in the involved limb if left untreated.

### Lesion Localization

Localizing a lesion is important to the diagnosis and treatment of peripheral nerve injuries. In brachial plexus lesions, the distal and proximal involvements must be identified. The proximal portion is comprised of spinal nerve and root, but is not readily accessible.[107,112] A myelogram may demonstrate the presence of a pseudomeningocele, which does not necessarily indicate that nerve rootlets are compromised. Intraoperative evoked potential recordings from the spinal nerve rootlets to the cortex may help determine their stability, functionality, and integrity.

## General Complications of Peripheral Nerve Surgery

### Postoperative Wound Infections

Postoperative wound infections may occur, especially if the exposures are large and wounds are exposed for a lengthy period as in brachial plexus repair. Strict adherence to establishing and maintaining a sterile environment throughout the duration of the surgical technique is the simplest and best safeguard against inadvertent postoperative infection. The authors recommend giving the patient a preoperative prophylactic antibiotic, usually a first-generation cephalosporin. During surgery, copious irrigation of the surgical site with an antibiotic solution will further prevent infection. The authors use a mixture of 500,000 units of polymyxin-B with 50,000 units of bacitracin in 1 L of 0.9% NaCl.

Peripheral nerve surgery should be dissected through the intramuscular planes and along the course of the involved nerve. Wound closure must be done with close approximation in order to eliminate dead spaces that can later become infection sites.[48] An antibiotic ointment, such as bacitracin, is applied to the incision area, followed by daily dressing changes. The incision area should also be inspected daily for any abnormal tissue changes. Postoperative antibiotic prophylaxis should not be necessary unless the wound has been seriously contaminated.

### Postoperative Hematoma

Clinically significant postoperative hematoma should also be a rarity. Because postoperative wound hematomas are prime mediums in which bacteria can grow, meticulous attention to hemostasis is important, not only to deter infection, but to reduce the formation of scar tissue. Extensive and repetitive muscle dissection often creates fistula and fascial planes and thus increases the likelihood of postoperative infection and postoperative scar tissue. To reduce risk, the surgeon can use bipolar electrocautery to achieve hemostasis and simultaneously minimize thermal injury to the adjacent neurovascular structures and soft tissues.[103] If the surgeon sees evidence of infected hematomas or other suspicious-looking adjacent tissues (such as drainage, cellulitis, or odor), these tissues must be excised and samples sent to the pathology laboratory for quantitative cultures and stat Gram stains.

### Pulmonary Complications

Pulmonary complications can always occur, especially if general anesthesia is necessary. Complications such as atelectasis, pneumonia, pulmonary embolus, and even acute respiratory distress syndrome can occur.[62] Careful attention must be given to good pulmonary function postoperatively, especially after lengthy nerve operations with the patient under general anesthesia. Pleural effusion, pneumothorax or hemothorax, and diaphragmatic paralysis are more likely with brachial plexus or thoracic outlet procedures and abdominal complications with pelvic plexus procedures.

### Anatomic Variants

Anatomic variants of neural elements and nonneural structures can be encountered in certain areas, such as the infraclavicular brachial plexus.[117] The best safeguard against inadvertent injury to these areas is for the surgeon to be thoroughly knowledgeable about normal and aberrant anatomy. In particular, the nerve to the triceps commonly arises off the dorsal spinal cord of the brachial plexus in the axilla. The subscapular nerve may arise from the posterior cord as part of a common trunk with the nerve to the subscapularis, or from the axillary nerve itself. The musculocutaneous nerve may arise from the median nerve, or can be affixed to the tendon of the pectoralis major muscle, so when retracting, dividing, or reapproximating this tendon, the surgeon should pay close attention to preserving the musculocutaneous nerve.

## Pain or Peripheral Nerve Origin

Pain prevention is essential to the treatment of peripheral nerve problems.[120,125] According to the International Association for the Study of Pain, pain is categorized in three ways: It (1) consists of both emotional and sensory components; (2) cannot be measured objectively because it is a subjective phenomenon; and (3) may occur without evidence of tissue injury, and conversely, tissue injury may occur without pain.

Neuropathic pain is a result of neural injury at any given location within the central or peripheral nervous system. Its characteristics can be described as paresthesia or numbness in the distribution area or even lack of an identifiable source of pain.[21,111] Complete or partial laceration of a cutaneous nerve warrants immediate repair of that nerve. When an intact nerve is identified during intraoperative exploration, neurolysis can successfully relieve pain.[127] Pain is also one of the most debilitating postsurgical complications and if it persists, its cause and etiology should be investigated immediately. It is important to establish the pattern of pain in order to localize precisely a nerve lesion. For example, if there is a stocking distribution of pain, the surgeon should perhaps look for a vascular injury.

Sympathetic involvement following peripheral nerve injury includes paresthesia and intolerance to cold, also termed *posttraumatic pain events*.[56] The sympathetic nervous system maintains a pain syndrome, mostly from a minor injury, termed *reflex sympathetic dystrophy (RSD)*. Pain and cold intolerance associated with RSD is directly related to impaired macrocirculatory and microcirculatory hemodynamics (nutritional deficiency).[56] Nutritional homeostasis is reestablished by addressing the vascular injury. Diagnosis can be aided by evaluating the patient's hemodynamics and thermoregulatory components.[54,55,86]

Vascular injuries can be associated with peripheral nerve injury from trauma, causing claudication, and in those cases must be repaired within 24 to 72 hours to prevent edema. Claudication, however, may be minimal if adequate collateral circulation is present.[53] Thrombosis without adequate collateral circulation may produce segmental ischemia with subsequent neuropathic pain.

Treatment of peripheral nerve pain focuses on immediate pain relief by relieving a local trigger point and maintaining range of motion via therapy. The trigger point of peripheral nerve pain can be identified by gently palpating the involved area, or by introducing a 16-gauge needle into the trigger point. An anesthetic block with 0.5% lidocaine hydrochloride temporarily relieves trigger point pain. If the anesthetic block is ineffective, then a peripheral epineural infusion block can be considered. The authors recommend performing an anesthetic trigger point block using sterile technique. One complication of periodic epineural infusions is that they can irritate the injection site and cause tissue necrosis, which further compromises vascularity. Contraindications of upper-extremity peripheral-epineural infusion are (1) pain persisting for more than 3 months and (2) contralateral pain involvement in an unaffected extremity.

The stellate ganglion is confined in the neck region where it supplies sympathetic innervation to the head, neck, and upper extremities. A nerve block in this area aids diagnosis and treatment for neuropathic pain in the head, neck, and upper extremities. One indication that a stellate ganglion nerve block has been successful is the presence of Horner's syndrome, which is a warm flush of the patient's ipsilateral face. Complications of stellate ganglion block include respiratory depression and hypotension due to local anesthetic injection into a dural cuff. Furthermore, if local anesthetic is injected into a vertebral artery, it precipitates seizure, and in some instances can cause loss of consciousness.[111]

## Complications of Surgery for Traumatic Nerve Injury

Traumatic injuries to the peripheral nerve can cause temporary dysfunction and pain, or more severe wounds can result in complete paralysis of the affected limb and permanent disability. For this reason, it is imperative that the peripheral nerve surgeon immediately and thoroughly assesses the severity and extent of the injury, including surgical exploration and reconstructive surgery if necessary. Until confirmed by intraoperative findings, it is prudent to diagnose traumatic peripheral nerve injuries as neurotmesis.

Most traumatic injuries fall into three categories: (1) laceration of the nerve, caused by knife wounds, car accidents, or work-related injuries; (2) projectile injuries, such as gunshot wounds; and (3) dislocation, fracture, and traction injuries (many are the result of sports injuries). Functional outcomes vary depending on the injury. For example, some peripheral nerves, such as digital nerves, have the capability of regenerating and can regain sensory function to near normal status.[96] Nerve fiber damage is irreversible, however, in cases where ischemia lasts more than 6 hours.[23,67]

### Laceration

In sharp stab wound cases where the nerve is acutely severed and avulsed, the nerve stumps should be secured to the adjacent soft tissues and primary nerve repair delayed. After 2 months, a secondary nerve repair, with or without a nerve graft, may be performed, since normal and aberrant neural anatomy will then be demarcated. Applying too much tension to the nerve ends compromises intraneural physiologic conditions, such as alteration of intracellular nutrition, endoneural fluid pressurization, and infiltration of fibrotic scarring at the suture line.[80-82,87] Repair can be further complicated if the cross-sectional area of the nerve is diminished by high tension. Further, failure to resect the nerve stumps to normal, viable fascicular neural tissue can impair nerve regeneration. Similarly, failure to recognize and resect a neuroma in continuity results in loss of functional recovery. Laceration of the nerve (Seldon's neurotmesis or Sunderland lesion V) can cause complete loss of nerve function and typically does not result in spontaneous recovery. Intraoperative nerve action potential recordings provide the function status of the injured nerve and aid clinical decision making should the injured nerve be resected.

## Projectile Injuries

The consequences of ballistic missile wounds caused by gunshot include crushing and laceration, shock waves, and cavitation as the projectile tears into the body.[109] Handguns typically create low-velocity shock waves, creating neurapraxia and axonotmesis. Shotgun wounds cause a higher percentage of peripheral nerve injuries than do rifle or civilian handgun wounds, because of the extensive damage they inflict on neurovascular structures. Patients with peripheral nerve injuries, in addition to neurovascular damage, have poor prognoses.

Immediate management entails the following four *"Do Nots"*:

1. Do not cut down both saphenous veins, because the other saphenous vein may be needed for vascular grafting.
2. Do not insert intravenous lines into the injured limb.
3. Do not use a tourniquet on the injured limb.
4. Do not attempt to clamp the bleeding wound blindly, because of the risk of severing or lacerating the functioning neurovascular structures.

Wound exploration and fasciotomy is indicated if a severed limb has experienced ischemia for more than 4 hours, or if there is evidence of compartment pressure of more than 40mmHg. Contact wounds, particularly shotgun injuries, are contaminated and often cause extensive soft tissue damage and infection. Intravenous antibiotics, usually a first-generation cephalosporin, should be administered immediately, and continued for a short period of 3 to 5 days.

The functional recovery rate is faster in low-distal extremity injuries than it is in high-proximal extremity injuries. Spontaneous recovery has been observed in 90% of injured nerves 3 to 9 months following an injury, and in some cases has occurred as long as 11 months after an injury.[101] The clinical prognosis in low-velocity gunshot wounds is similar to that of high-velocity injuries, which is a 1- to 4-month recovery period for neurapraxia, and 4 to 9 months for axonotmesis.[94]

## Fracture/Dislocation

Patients presenting with a fracture in an upper extremity must be evaluated for nerve injury involvement, since 95% of upper-extremity fractures result in associated nerve injuries.[42] Humeral fractures frequently cause radial nerve damage, and while it rarely happens, complete resection of the median nerve due to a Colle's fracture is possible.[71] The median nerve is also susceptible to pressure as it courses the carpal tunnel and tends to be entrapped by bony fractures, edema, or hemorrhage. Thus, it is important to look for evidence of any neurovascular deficit fol-

lowing an extremity fracture before attempting surgical reduction, and avoid further damage to the nerves by not applying dressings too tightly.

The time frame for spontaneous recovery of clinical function following a fracture is 1 to 4 months, and 3 to 6 months following a traction injury.[89] Poor chance for spontaneous recovery is related to the severity of the injury and extensive damage of the nerve lesion.[93]

## Timing of Surgery

Timing of surgery is crucial if the surgeon wishes to restore neuronal function, reverse end organ function, and facilitate functional recovery. Because neural regeneration progresses at the rate of approximately 1 inch per month, it is essential that surgical intervention reestablish neuronal connection during this period. Following denervation, the extrajunctional receptors of sensory innervation are maintained for at least 18 months in adults and up to 3 years in pediatric cases. Some pediatric cases have been capable of reinnervation for up to 5 years.[103]

Surgical exploration is immediately warranted when there is evidence of vascular injuries, such as absence of diminished extremity pulses, auscultation of bruits or thrills, or large pulsatile hemorrhage.[97,130] Angiographic investigation can be performed preoperatively for hemodynamically stable patients, and intraoperatively for unstable patients. The peripheral nerve surgeon should be aware of complications related to vascular injuries and be able to handle vascular repairs by consulting with and involving a cohort vascular surgeon. For legal and medical reasons, it is mandatory that a detailed clinical examination be performed, and that neurosensory deficits are carefully documented. An arteriogram should be performed to study vessel properties and exclude the possibility that a pseudoaneurysm is forming. Adequate exposure can be obtained via dissection through the intramuscular planes along the involved nerve in order to avoid injuring adjacent structures. The lesion then can be assessed, evaluated, and surgically removed. Extensive and repetitive dissection often creates multiple pseudo fascial planes and thus increases the formation of scar tissue, which poses a high risk of injury to neurovascular structures, including iatrogenic/traumatic aneurysms or arteriovenous fistulas. Magnetic resonance imaging (MRI) scans should also be obtained to assess adjacent neurovascular structures.

Immediate surgical exploration is also warranted when there is an acute presentation of neurologic deficit. If the nerve is found to be nonviable and transected, nerve repair is indicated in order to permit regeneration. Surgical exploration can be delayed for 8 to 12 weeks in gunshot injuries, provided there is no evidence of neurovascular compromise. During this period, if the patient's neurologic function has deteriorated significantly and displays evidence of complete loss of function in one or more neural elements, intraoperative exploration should be performed.

## Techniques of Nerve Repair

Functional outcomes depend to a large degree on selecting the proper procedure.[13,38,50,79,122] Nerve repair is a delicate procedure and the technique requires minute attention to details. Understanding the axonal regeneration and neurotrophic factors can help surgeons improve the management and outcomes of lacerated peripheral nerves. Recently, tube repair[22,74] (with silicone, collagen, and polyglycolic acid) and allograft nerve transplantation[34,75] have been found to be successful in restoring nerve continuity in humans and experimental animals. Tube repair is based on the hypothesis that neurotrophic factors are synthesized in the injured nerve and accumulate and direct the axonal growth within the tubes. Further, the regenerative potential of the system can be increased by introduction of various neurotrophic agents into the tubes. Tube repair may prove in future as alternative to conventional nerve repair techniques. Nerve allograft transplantation can possibly provide a viable alternative when nerve gap exceeds the lengths that could be reconstructed with available autograft tissue. This technique requires immunosuppression to avoid graft rejection. The indications and relative advantages and disadvantages of commonly used techniques of nerve repair are summarized in Table 104.1.

## Postoperative Management

Postoperative follow-up is vital to good patient care and functional outcomes. The surgeon must assess the wound area for potential infection, the status of the patient's neurologic improvement, and evidence of functional recovery. Ongoing communication and reassurance are important aspects of postoperative management, as they improve the patient's morale during the course of treatment. Postoperative complications mainly arise in the surgical area and its adjacent structures. Routine wound cleansing with hydrogen peroxide followed by an application of an antibiotic ointment can eliminate or reduce the medium for bacteria. The patient is encouraged to mobilize and to increase activities as soon as possible, preferably on the first postoperative day in order to improve circulation, and to prevent soft tissue adhesions. Physical therapy can aug-ment mobilization and functional recovery. Prophylactic use of anticoagulants, such as intravenous dextran, intravenous or subcutaneous heparin, or oral aspirin, may prevent thrombosis at the microsurgical region.[47]

In some patients, pain management can be controlled with nonsteroidal antiinflammatory drugs (NSAIDs). Narcotic pain medications should be prescribed as needed, but discretion should be used if the patient is elderly, or if the physician suspects malingering or addiction.

## Rehabilitation

After a peripheral nerve injury, it is extremely important that patients undergo regular physical therapy to maintain range of motion and to optimize the recovery of motor function as muscle reinnervation occurs. Early mobilization can prevent the formation of tethering adhesions, which can have deleterious consequences, as seen in some orthopedic joint repairs. The need for rehabilitation after the first week of surgery must be assessed on an individual basis. Functional recovery depends on the type and extent of injury, the capability of the nerve to regenerate, associated medical conditions, and the patient's motivation and perseverance. New patterns of motor and sensory innervation continue to reorganize for at least 5 years after recovery. This reestablishment process is slow and may demonstrate considerable variations in neural readjustment. Extensive injuries with multiple nerve lesions require a longer time to improve than do isolated single nerve injuries. If functional recovery is not apparent after an appropriate rehabilitation period, other options such as arthrodesis and tendon transfers should be considered.

## Complications of Surgery for Peripheral Nerve Tumors

Both benign and malignant tumors can affect peripheral nerves.[7,25,29,44] Enlarged peripheral nerve tumors

**TABLE 104.1**

| Techniques of Nerve Repair | | | |
|---|---|---|---|
| Technique | Indications | Advantages | Disadvantages |
| Epineural neurorrhaphy | Primary repair | Simple technique | Increased fascicular malalignment |
| | Proximal plexus lesion | Minimal intraneuronal scarring | |
| | Polyfascicular nerve | | |
| | Monofascicular nerve | | |
| Fascicular neurorrhaphy | Oligofascicular nerve | More precise coaptation than epineural repair | Intraneuronal trauma; cannot resist tension |
| | Distal plexus lesion | | |
| Interpositional graft | Primary coaptation cannot be achieved without tension | Establishes neuronal continuity without tension at suture line | "Suture line" delay at two sites |
| Free vascular graft | Recipient bed cannot maintain donor graft | Experimental evidence for faster axonal regeneration | Complex technique |
| Tube repair | Primary repair | No donor site morbidity | Useful only for short nerve defect |
| | Alternative to nerve graft | Simple technique ?faster repair | Extrusion of tube |
| | Painful neuroma | | Kinking of tube |
| Nerve allograft transplantation | Severe extremity injury | Large nerve defect can be reconstructed | Limited clinical experience |
| | Composite tissue | | Need immunosuppression |

compress adjacent neurovascular structures, causing nerve entrapment and subsequent motor or sensory deficits. Schwannomas and neurofibromas compressing the nerve trunk are encountered most frequently, while neurocutaneous melanosis syndrome and Von Recklinghausen's neurofibromatosis (VRNF) have benign and malignant peripheral nerve tumor characteristics.[7,25,52]

Surgical complications arise when peripheral nerve tumors are not included in the differential diagnosis. During preoperative assessments, the surgeon should be able to distinguish neoplastic malignant transformations from benign tumors, inspect macroscopic and microscopic appearances, and then follow up with histologic, radiologic, and pathologic evaluations to classify the tumor and its cytogenesis. Changes in tumor characteristics are generally indicative that a tumor has become malignant, but it is prudent to consider tumors malignant until confirmed by pathologic examination.

Even when there has been a thorough preoperative assessment, unsuspected peripheral nerve tumors may be discovered during intraoperative exploration. If such cases occur, surgeons inexperienced in managing peripheral nerve tumors should not attempt radical resection, but should abort surgery and refer the patient to a well-known institution that specializes in peripheral nerve management. Poorly performed peripheral nerve tumor resections can lead to neural loss, which is greater with malignant tumors than it is with benign lesions because they adhere to adjacent neural structures and soft tissues such as vessels, muscle, and bone. The patient's long-term outcome is of prime importance; therefore, standards of care should not be compromised.

Intraoperative electrodiagnostic studies are mandatory to assess the viability and integrity of the nerve and to determine whether or not a nerve graft is necessary. When an intraoperative nerve conduction study is performed, long-acting muscle relaxants should not be given to the patient because they interfere with nerve conduction velocity and confound clinical findings.

Surgical management of schwannomas includes complete tumor excision, extending the dissection beyond the entrapment site in order to release compression on adjacent neurovascular structures, and taking care to minimize additional compression caused by postoperative edema. By using a surgical microscope, the operative theater can be visualized and the tumor inspected for peripheral fascicular arrangement. The tumor should then be debulked by gently separating it from the nerve bundles and neural elements, preserving the fascicles unless they are encapsulated and eroded by the tumor or show signs of malignancy.

Neurofibromas can appear to be multiple and fusiform, especially ones that arise from the nerve trunks.[29,52] Surgery is immediately warranted if the patient experiences severe and debilitating pain with deterioration of neurologic function. Resection typically does not result in loss of neurologic function or permanent disability. In cases of resection of a superficial neurofibroma, cutaneous sensation may be temporarily affected.[44]

The postoperative incision area can be padded with soft wound dressings for protection, followed by daily inspection and cleansing to deter infection and facilitate healing.

Splint immobilization of the involved extremity for 1 to 2 weeks is recommended for patients who underwent nerve grafts. Postoperative pain management with appropriate pain medication minimizes discomfort. The patient's anxiety can be managed effectively with open and frank communications.

## Malignant Peripheral Nerve Sheath Tumors

The incidence rate of malignant peripheral nerve sheath tumors is significantly higher in patients who have VRNF than it is compared to those occurring in the general population.[32,52,103] Reliable clinical findings suggesting the presence of a malignant neural sheath tumor are a large tumor mass at initial presentation, followed by a relatively rapid increase in size over a period of weeks to months.[29,69] Initial management should consist of a simple nerve biopsy to provide histologic evidence of malignancy, since frozen section studies are not sufficient for confirming a diagnosis.[44] Do not include specimens from previous biopsy locations or in their vicinities, because fibrotic scarring can make the tissue difficult to distinguish from a neurofibroma.[103]

Radical resection and complete removal of peripheral nerve sheath tumors is advised. Possible surgical techniques include en bloc resection, hemipelvectomy, and amputation of the interscapulothoracic nerve.[119] However, to arrest the intraneural spread of the tumor, radical resection must extend 5 to 10cm beyond the tumor margin in a contiguous nerve.

A lack of surgical experience or lack of understanding about tumor pathology can lead to complications. Successful excision depends on the origin and location of the tumor, and unfortunately, total resection is often impossible to perform without causing severe functional loss. Amputation is seldom warranted at the time of initial surgery because multiple specimens will be needed from several sites in order to confirm a malignancy and assess its invasion into adjacent structures.

## Complications of Surgery for Entrapment Neuropathies

Entrapment syndromes warrant management specific to each particular diagnosis. The cause of an entrapment must be ascertained, the patient treated for pain, the entrapment released, and neurologic dysfunction reversed. While most surgical procedures are routine, complications can occur, resulting in serious morbidity. Inadequate clinical assessment, failure to initiate the proper intervention, and iatrogenic injuries contribute to surgical complications.

### Diagnostic Pitfalls

Inadequate preoperative assessment includes failure to perform a complete and thorough clinical examination, incorrect interpretation of the electrophysiologic studies, or delayed execution of necessary therapeutic or surgical management.[74,117,120] Associated medical conditions such as diabetes, hormonal diseases, connective tissue disorders, rheumatoid disease, arthritis, and metabolic deficiency must be included in the differential diagnosis because these medical conditions may rule out the need for surgical intervention. Additionally, central nervous system pathologies such as syringomyelia and space-occupied intracranial lesions, should also be excluded prior to initiating any surgical intervention.

Misinterpretation of physical signs, such as the Hoffman-Tinel sign, could lead to inappropriate clinical management, especially for surgeons who are inexperienced in peripheral nerve management. For example, a positive Hoffman-Tinel sign (a tingling sensation in the distribution of the median nerve over the hand) has been used to help diagnose carpal tunnel syndrome and indicates axonal regeneration. A negative Hoffman-Tinel sign presents in the early and late stages of nerve entrapment. Another example is Phalen's sign, in which a negative finding suggests severe disruption of neural elements. When a peripheral nerve is entrapped at more than one site, it is termed *double crush syndrome.* This syndrome demonstrates that there is nerve compression at a more distal site, and distal compression is symptomatic. For example, the patient with carpal tunnel syndrome may have a cervical spine pathology; therefore, clinical evaluation should focus on that region in order to rule out the "crush" phenomenon. When nerve compression is symptomatic at more proximal locations, it is termed *reverse double crush syndrome.* In these instances, both "crush" syndromes can be misinterpreted.

Electrodiagnostic studies are often used to confirm peripheral nerve entrapment neuropathies.[103,120] False negative results occur in association with aberrant anatomic variations and ambiguities, associated medical conditions, overlapping sensory innervation, errors in technical skill, and misinterpretation of results. Examples of overlapping sensory innervation include the Riche-Cannieu anomaly (both branches of the median and ulnar nerves communicate) and the Martin-Gruber anastomosis (the median nerve or the anterior interosseous branch communicates with the ulnar nerve), which were discussed in the preceding "Clinical Examination" section. Therefore surgeons must be knowledgeable about diagnostic procedures and electrodiagnostic tests, and interpret them correctly in order to manage peripheral nerve injuries and disorders.

## Surgical Pitfalls

Faultless surgical technique and strict adherence to established guidelines are absolutely imperative if surgical complications are to be avoided. Good functional recovery depends on complete decompression of compressed nerves. If decompression is incomplete, symptoms often reoccur. Adequate surgical exposure can be obtained by dissecting along the course of the nerve distally and proximally until the lesion is well identified. Probing the neural compartment blindly with sharp instruments, such as scissors or scalpels, is not only dangerous, but imprudent. Multiple or widespread dissections cause considerable hemorrhaging, disrupt surrounding tissue, and multiple fascial planes distort the patient's anatomy. Additionally, postoperative hemorrhage consequently produces fibrous scar tissue that then causes recurrent nerve compression; therefore, hemostasis should be carefully controlled.

Despite preoperative electrodiagnostic studies, some lesions are unrecognizable until detected intraoperatively. Furthermore, some anatomic locations are difficult to reach, thus localization of certain compressive lesions, such as entrapments in the brachial plexus and spinal nerve rootlets, may not be feasible. Aggressive radical decompression of these neural elements is not advisable since the risks outweigh the benefits. In these cases, simple external or internal neurolysis is more beneficial to the patient.[73,105]

## Cubital Tunnel Release

Cubital tunnel syndrome is also known as *tardy ulnar palsy,* and can result from traumatic or nontraumatic causes. Since the ulnar nerve is located superficially at the elbow, it is more vulnerable to trauma. Nontraumatic causes of the syndrome are caused by habitually resting the elbow on hard surfaces for a prolonged period, or repetitive elbow extension or flexion motions. Flexion of the elbow elongates the ulnar nerve, accentuating the tethering effect on the nerve and subsequently causing increased intraneural pressure. Cubital tunnel syndrome can also be caused by aberrant bony structures or by space occupied masses such as ganglia, synovial cysts, anomalous muscles, lipomas, or tumors.

Cushioning the arm and positioning the patient properly can reduce surgical complications, especially when the cutaneous ulnar nerve of the medial aspect of the elbow is subjected to direct compression. Postoperative complications of cubital tunnel syndrome are frequently related to technical errors involving transposition procedures.[14,61,76,120] The transposed ulnar nerve is compressed at the entry of the cubital tunnel, at the intermuscular septum, or by fascial slings.[14,103] We recommend dissecting the nerve beyond the distal and proximal ends to permit relaxation of the nerve and to prevent kinking of the transposition. Transposed ulnar nerves can be fibrosed later; therefore, simple ulnar decompression is often preferred over transposition because it is relatively easy to perform and has fewer complications.[20,52,129]

## Thoracic Outlet Syndrome

There are three approaches to thoracic outlet surgery: (1) supraclavicular, (2) dorsal scapular, and (3) transaxillary. The supraclavicular approach is preferred because it provides direct visualization of the brachial plexus roots and trunk, as well as accessory ribs, neural structures, and fibromuscular bands, which is critical to the procedure. An incision is made at the supraclavicular region, separating the anterior scalene from the middle scalene. If the brachial plexus is tethered, the surgeon should make an effort to release the fibrous bands and accessory ribs, using extreme caution as removal of the first rib and scalene muscle can injure the brachial plexus, phrenic nerve, and lung. Other surgical complications include brachial plexopathy and scapular winging from a long thoracic nerve injury. Brachial plexopathy may be caused by a fractured clavicle, callus from a healed fracture, pseudo-aneurysm, or expanded hematoma. Internal fixation is indicated in fractured clavicle cases.

A dorsal subscapular approach is utilized for patients who have a large neck and large cervical ribs. Patients whose brachial plexus was violated by a transaxillary rib approach may benefit from a dorsal subscapular approach.[31] The advantage of this technique is that it allows the surgeon to visualize the spinal nerves at their intervertebral foramina, but conversely, this approach can cause damage to the long thoracic nerve, resulting in scapular wing.

The transaxillary approach is not recommended because it does not permit direct visualization of the plexus. In order to obtain adequate exposure of the brachial plexus, the patient's arm has to be hyperabducted and the neurovascular structures retracted, predisposing the brachial plexus to a greater risk of injury. It also requires the removal of the first rib.

## Standard Open Carpal Tunnel Release (OCTR)

The most common mistake surgeons make in carpal tunnel cases is failure to make a correct diagnosis from the patient's history, clinical examination, and electrodiagnostic studies. Confirmation from electrodiagnostic studies is important because without abnormal electrophysiologic findings, there is little rationale to support surgical intervention. Phalen's maneuver and Tinel's sign can indicate that a patient has the disorder, but abnormal nerve conduction velocity recordings and electromyography (EMG) will confirm it.[43,103,120]

Anatomic variations necessitate the need for meticulous attention to detail, since iatrogenic injuries are common in carpal tunnel surgeries. The transverse carpal ligament curves ulnarly between the hamate and pisiform, and attaches radially between the trapezium and scaphoid. The transverse carpal ligament and the proximal palmar fascia form the flexor retinaculum. The proximal wrist crease exposes the median nerve, which is beneath the flexor retinaculum and serves as an important and reliable guide. Caution should be taken not to injure the ulnar neurovascular bundle when retracting the retinaculum, or damaging the ulnar nerve and artery, which are located radially to the hook of hamate. Injury to the superficial palmar arch during carpal tunnel release can also occur.[65,72]

Persistent wrist pain following a carpal tunnel release indicates an incomplete resection of the transverse carpal ligament, or an injury to the terminal branches of the anterior interosseous nerve.[11,39,72,74] This can be avoided by visualizing and inspecting the extended course of the transverse carpal ligament so that a complete ligamental transection can be performed. The transverse carpal ligament may locate distally and embed with the palmar fascia; therefore, a small incision may not provide adequate visualization. The distal edge of the carpal ligament contains a ramus communicans that is located between the median and ulnar nerves, thus caution should be taken before attempting to resect the carpal ligament.[77] Preservation of the ramus communicans is a must. The motor division of the median nerve occasionally courses along the transligament, and contains a superficial or ulnar origin.[64,117] Injury here can be prevented by maintaining an extended incision along the ulnar aspect of the carpal ligament, and by being particularly aware of the motor branch during dissection.[103] Excessive deviation in the position of the ulnar nerve can result in its laceration, so this must be watched for.[35]

Minor or debilitating postoperative pain may also be caused by the formation of a neuroma. Neuromas occur when an incision is made at the thenar crease or at the wrist transverse.[59,64,72] In these cases, it is prudent to reexplore the wound and remove the neuroma. Other causes of postoperative pain can include injury to the dorsal sensory branch of the radial nerve, to the palmar branch of the digital nerve, or to the palmar cutaneous branch of the median nerve.[60] Since the course of the palmar cutaneous branch is inconsistent, injury to it can occur during wound incision or closure.[117]

Transection of the carpal ligament may create instability in wrist infrastructures like carpal arch widening or flexor tendon bowstringing, which would subsequently affect grip strength.[24,39,72] Instability of bone architecture distorted by ligamental transection compresses and aggravates the small cutaneous or periosteal nerve, causing wrist causalgia.[11,59,65] The free margins of the flexor tendon could be resutured, but the risk of recurrent nerve injury outweighs the benefits.[103] Early splinting of the wrist after surgery prevents this complication.[11]

An injury to the terminal branches of the anterior interosseous nerve results from a retractor that pressurizes the nerve beneath the distal antebrachial fascia.[74] Therefore, care and consideration should be taken when placing the retractor in this particular region. Likewise, Colle's fracture or crush injury to the forearm has profound compressive effects on the distal antebrachial fascia.[117]

Keloid formation is important, not only for cosmetic reasons, but because entrapment of the palmar cutaneous nerve can induce pain. Excision is not practical because further keloid formation can occur, so conservative treatment with cortisone cream, local anesthesia, or pain medications can be used. Reassuring the patient is also very effective. To date, there have been no findings as to which type of incision is best to deter keloid formation.[11,39,113]

## Endoscopic Carpal Tunnel Release (ECTR)

Endoscopic techniques for carpal tunnel release are superior to standard open carpal tunnel procedures because by creating a smaller, less invasive incision, the patient recovers faster, experiences less pain and scar tissue formation, and is able to return to work faster, making the procedure cost effective. However, as with any procedure, there are potential risks due to limited surgical exposure of neurovascular structures, which can result in incomplete resection of the transverse carpal ligament.

Ulnar neuropraxia can also be a potential postoperative problem with endoscopic techniques, particularly with the transbursal approach of the dual portal Chow's technique, which exerts pressure or retraction of the nerve. This can be avoided by using an extrabursal approach (subligamentous dual portal technique) developed by Resnick and Miller.[104] In that approach, the flexor tendon is dissected beneath the transverse ligament. A complete transection of the ulnar nerve can occur in the dual portal Chow's technique as a result of inadvertent placement of the trocar into the

Guyon's canal, especially if the wrist is hyperextended.[83] Therefore, attention to anatomic landmarks is critical. The endoscope trocar should be inserted anterior to the superficial palmar arch and midpalm digital nerve. In order to avoid injuring the median nerve branches, we suggest making an incision at the ulnar margin and utilizing a freer elevator to delineate the median nerve from the carpal tunnel ligament prior to inserting the endoscopic trocar.

The single portal Agee's technique can compromise neurovascular structures because it uses a blind approach during which the knife cannot be visualized as it courses through the carpal tunnel. The later modified single portal Agee's endoscopic system allows the surgeon to visualize the course of the blade, and the risk of neurovascular injuries has been minimized considerably. According to 10 published articles, of 1570 documented procedures using Agee's single portal technique, the complication rate was 1.83%, whereas the failure rate was a mere 1.44%.* Other possible complications associated with Agee's technique include postoperative infection, hematoma, pillar causalgia, laceration of flexor digitorum sublimis, and reflex sympathetic dystrophy.[46] The incidence of reflex sympathetic dystrophy (RSD) associated with carpal tunnel release is relatively high (as much as 5%), and the incidence of RSD increases significantly when carpal tunnel surgery is performed with coexistent Dupuytren's disease.[11,39,60,85]

The Chow's dual portal technique is a widely performed procedure. A classic postoperative complication associated with Chow's technique includes ulnar nerve neuropraxia due to retraction of the ulnar nerve during transbursal approach. Other complications from using Chow's technique include fibrosed tissue scarring, pseudoaneurysm and vascular injury to the superficial palmar arch, median nerve injury, flexor digitorum superficialis laceration, and RSD.[66] In the Brown dual portal technique, common postoperative complications are superficial palmar arch injury, transient paresthesias, and RSD.[15,16,17]

A comprehensive review of 8068 endoscopic carpal tunnel release (ECTR) procedures by Jimenez et al.[46] indicates that complication, failure, and success rates are similar for both endoscopic and standard open procedures. The retrospective questionnaire studied 157 surgeons who performed 6833 ECTR procedures, demonstrating an overall complication rate of 2.6%.[46] Postoperative complications associated with artery, nerve, and tendon injuries were relatively higher in ECTR (1.6%) than in OCTR (0.8%). No statistically significant differences of persistent and recurrent symptoms were found in these two groups (ECTR 7.5% versus OCTR 7.7%).

A successful outcome in ECTR treatment depends on appropriate patient selection, proper identification of anatomic landmarks, and adequate endoscopic visualization. Contraindications of ECTR include fracture pathology, cysts (ganglion or synovial), neuromas, aberrant anatomy, sepsis, and previously failed carpal tunnel release.[46] Lack of formal training in endoscopic technique and unfamiliarity with endoscopic instrumentation must also be taken into account. Surgeons should be prepared to convert ECTR to OCTR when encountering technical dif-

ficulty or if they cannot adequately visualize neurovascular structures. The endoscopic cannula should not be forcefully advanced through the palmar arch, because injury to the superficial palmar arch artery would be imminent.

## Iatrogenic Nerve Injuries

Iatrogenic injuries, those caused by surgical treatment, are the most common complications of peripheral nerve surgery, yet are frequently avoidable. Such injuries can be minor, in which case they may be resolved, or they can be severe and permanently debilitating.

### Tourniquet Injury

Tourniquets are used to control bleeding in injuries of the extremities, especially those that have serious vascular involvement where controlling blood loss is critical. Tourniquets are also used to reduce the presence of blood in the surgical field, which improves visualization. However, the incidence of tourniquet-induced peripheral nerve complications is significant and can occur even if the tourniquet has been applied and used properly, since direct pressure on a nerve causes acute compression and effects intraneuronal physiologic conditions, disrupting motor and sensory innervation.[41,74,103] The most commonly injured nerve in the upper extremity is the radial nerve.[110,117]

The amount of time a tourniquet can be applied is of considerable concern, since prolonged pressure creates considerable compression of the peripheral nerves. Although some surgeons advise releasing tourniquet pressure after 1 to 3 hours of surgery,[84,110,117] 30 minutes of high cuff pressure can produce palsies.[85,110] The authors recommend that tourniquet pressure not exceed 70mmHg above the patient's systolic blood pressure, but it should be sufficient to maintain hemostasis and tourniquets should never be placed below the elbow or knee.[110] Electrophysiologic studies of a pneumatic tourniquet show changes in nerve action potentials and frequent fibrillations 5 to 10 minutes after pressure is applied; therefore, the authors recommend constant monitoring of cuff pressure. Deflation of the cuff for 10 minutes each hourly interval is effective in preventing nerve injury.

Tourniquet-induced peripheral nerve injuries are usually mild and spontaneously resolve within 3 to 6 months. Prognosis varies because tourniquet-induced injuries cannot be assessed accurately and qualitatively.[74,84,110,117] Conservative management includes armrest. Physical therapy can help restore circulation, regain joint motion, and prevent musculature contraction. In cases where there has been serious and irreversible damage to the peripheral nerves due to intraneuronal scarring, or where there is no evidence of functional improvement, surgical exploration is mandatory.

### Patient Malpositioning

Malpositioning predisposes the patient to peripheral nerve injuries and may result in permanent neurologic deficits. This injurious occurrence is preventable if care and consideration are emphasized in properly positioning the

---
*References 2-4,8,16,33,37,46,78,98.

patient for surgery. Positioning the patient improperly during surgery can compress the peripheral nerves against rigid surfaces like aberrant joints or osseoligamentous structures, causing neurologic deficits.[110] There is no correlation between the degree of compression damage and surgical duration. Nerve compression has resulted in surgeries that lasted 1 hour, as well as those lasting up to 4 hours.[5,12,26,99,117] Patients most at risk are those who are particularly thin and have a small stature.[103] Several other factors can predispose a patient to nerve compression, such as bony fractures, aberrant anatomy, compaction of the cervical ribs, associated medical conditions, a history of peripheral neuropathies, anticoagulants, anesthesia-induced skeletal muscle relaxants, or physiologic hypothermia.°

Improper patient positioning such as Trendelenburg's position, where the patient is placed in a steep 30-degree angle, risks damaging both the brachial plexus and the long thoracic nerve.[117] Caution must be used in placing the patient's arm when the patient is in the prone or supine position. Frequent sites of compression occur along the superficial course of the radial and ulnar nerves in relationship to the shaft of the humerus. Therefore, the arms should be secured at the patient's sides and fully padded with foam or soft towels. Improper arm positioning can also occur when the patient is placed in a lateral rotation position, internal rotation, external rotation, abduction, arm-shoulder distraction, pronation, or supination. Do not abduct the patient's arms further than the head for a long period of time, and do not cross the patient's arms,[103] which commonly causes injury to the upper roots of the brachial plexus.

When the patient is placed in a lateral decubitus position, there is significant risk of injuring the peripheral nerves in both the upper and lower extremities. The patient's legs should be placed on soft pillow(s) and secured with a leg strap. The leg strap should be positioned away from the fibular head because the peroneal nerve is superficially localized at this region, making it vulnerable to injury. The femoral cutaneous nerve is located adjacent to the pelvic protuberance and the sciatic nerve is confined within the pelvic outlet region. Similar precautions should be taken to prevent compression of these nerves. Injury to the saphenous and sciatic nerves has been reported in patients who have been placed in a lithotomy position.[120]

If a patient does develop compressive neuropathies, early management must proceed without hesitation in order to facilitate functional recovery. Recovery depends on the severity and extent of postoperative peripheral neuropathies. Complete recovery can be expected within 6 months in 90% of cases.[99] Mild forms of peripheral neuropathy, such as a first-degree conduction block, have better recovery rates than do severe forms like complete neuronal disruption with evidence of hemorrhagic necrosis. If the patient exhibits signs of compressive neuropathies, we advise obtaining a differential diagnosis of coexistent neuropathies, combined with electrodiagnostic studies. If neurologic deficits fail to improve, surgical exploration is indicated.

---

° References 5,12,26,74,99,117.

## Injection Injury

Various pharmacologic agents are used to inject through intravenous, intramuscular, subcutaneous, and even intraarterial routes, but must not be injected directly into the nerve because either the needle or drug can cause permanent nerve damage. The best way to avoid contact with the nerve is to be thoroughly knowledgeable about anatomy and structures adjacent to the nerves, and by paying careful attention to guiding the needle. Particular attention must be paid to epineural, intraneural, and intrafascicular injections, as incorrect techniques for these procedures can have serious consequences.[40,74,117] The radial nerve is commonly vulnerable during arterial line placement and the sciatic nerve is the most commonly injured by intramuscular injections. Careless cannulation of the internal jugular vein during central venous line placement can cause injury to the proximal brachial plexus. The brachial plexus is at risk for injury during central catheter line placement because of its proximity to the internal jugular vein and the subclavian vein. Hematomas can result after sternotomies or placement of internal jugular vein catheters, pressure and/or stretching of the brachial plexus.[106,121] Surgeons need to be aware of these structures to avoid nerve injury: the cervical sympathetic trunk, C5-8 nerve roots, cranial nerve XI, the phrenic nerve, and recurrent laryngeal nerve.

Neurologic sequelae are noticed immediately within minutes of an injection. Causalgia is a typical symptom of an injection injury and can be transient or permanently debilitating. A delayed onset implies that there is injury to the surrounding structures.

If an injection injury results in an incomplete neurologic deficit, conservative management should be initiated within the first 2 months. Surgical intervention is warranted if the neurologic deficit persists, causing functional debilitation and intractable pain. Intraoperative nerve conduction studies should be performed to determine whether the nerves and axons are innervated. Seriously injured nerves require possible graft repair, while minimally or moderately injured nerves can be treated with neurolysis.

## Misdirected Surgical Procedures

During surgical exploration, exposed nerves should be protected and appropriately contained in order to prevent iatrogenic injuries such as stretching or tension injuries. Failure to identify and protect the nerve during surgery may result in nerve laceration or intraneuronal physiologic status damage, which further complicates the patient's functional recovery.

Most iatrogenic injuries are associated with orthopedic, trauma, or hand surgery.[57] For example, during open reduction of a fractured humerus, the surgeon may encounter the nearby radial nerve. Minor surgical procedures, especially lymph node biopsies in the dorsal triangle of the neck, may transect or stretch the spinal accessory nerve.[28] Additionally, various cutaneous sensory nerves are often damaged during surgeries on wrist ganglions, operations at the elbow (antebrachial cutaneous nerves), decompression of the median nerve (palmar cutaneous branches of the median nerve), arthroscopies and surgeries for varicose veins (saphenous nerve and branches), and during surgery to treat Dupuytren's disease (digital nerves).[10]

Positioning retractors may also inadvertently injure the nerve located beneath the blade.[19,26,70] For example, such complications are commonly seen in patients who have undergone gynecologic surgery where the pelvic retractor exerts pressure on the femoral nerve, then the patient later experiences bilateral weakness in that nerve distribution.[57] Such injuries are can be avoided if surgical dissection is performed with attention and care.

Unfamiliarity with anatomy and limited experience of surgical techniques are the common causative factors in peripheral nerve tumor surgeries. Either procedure in relatively inexperienced hands can lead to neural loss, just as with the more benign neural sheath tumors. Loss is more likely with the malignant tumor than with benign lesion, not only because of its more intrinsic nature in relation to the nerve or element of origin, but also, as [MC10]mentioned previously, because of its adherence to adjacent neural structures and other soft tissues such as vessels, muscle, and even bone. A mass that is deeply located is inconspicuously determined until that mass is increased in size considerably and causes compression to adjacent neurovascular structures.

### Medicolegal Aspects of Iatrogenic Injuries

All iatrogenic peripheral nerve injuries have medicolegal implications. Although some iatrogenic injuries are unavoidable, a few result from negligence. Often the principal problem is not with nerve damage itself, but with the manner in which it was subsequently managed. Most frequently, the surgeon has failed to recognize that an iatrogenic injury occurred, followed by a delay in referring the patient to an appropriate specialist for further evaluation and postoperative intervention.[51,128] As a result, the lesions may not be evaluated during the period most critical for repair when outcomes could improve substantially.

The amount of functional recovery that can be expected following iatrogenic lesions, with or without surgical intervention, is often unpredictable. However, some general statements can be made: First, spontaneous recovery is more likely to occur with incomplete lesions than it is with complete lesions, and it is a slow process that may have less than ideal outcomes. Second, if operative intervention is required, it should be performed by a surgeon who specializes in peripheral nerve surgery, and should generally be done within the first 3 or 4 months after injury in order to produce optimal results.[51,128]

### Complications in Nerve Biopsy

A nerve biopsy is the removal of a small sample of nerve for diagnostic purposes in order to determine the cause of severe or progressive neuropathies of unknown etiology.[27] Complications are relatively rare, but they do occur.[102] The most common complaint is persistent paresthesias and hypesthesia. We advise obtaining coagulation tests prior to nerve biopsies, taking precautions that artifacts are not introduced into the specimen that could cause misinter-

| TABLE 104.2 | |
|---|---|
| **Common Complications of Iatrogenic Nerve Injuries** | |
| **Affected Nerve** | **Procedures** |
| Spinal accessory | Lymph node biopsy |
| Transverse cervical or greater auricular | Lymph node biopsy |
| Brachial plexus | Radical neck dissection or mastectomy |
| Median | Carpal tunnel release or removal of ganglion |
| Radial | Arterial puncture or osteosynthesis |
| Ulnar | Removal of ganglion or wrist osteotomy |
| Superficial radial | K-wire placement or removal of ganglion |
| Anterior interosseous | Internal fixation of forearm |
| Posterior interosseous | Osteosynthesis or cast |
| Sciatic | Hip arthroplasty |
| Femoral | Hip arthroplasty or femoral arterial graft |
| Genitofemoral or ilioinguinal | Hernia repair |
| Tibial | Injection or orthopedic procedure |
| Common peroneal | Surgery of the knee or removal of Baker cyst |
| Sural | Vein extirpation |
| Saphenous | Vein stripping |

pretation. Postoperative incisions should be monitored for infection, especially in diabetic patients who are prone to infection and whose wounds require a longer time to heal. For this reason, biopsies for diabetic neuropathies are generally not warranted, although a biopsy would reveal proliferation of basal membranes in the endoneurial capillaries. Other contraindications of nerve biopsy include patients who have a history of coagulopathy disorders or patients who are taking anticoagulants.

### Summary

The perfect surgical paradigm is one without complications. In order to actualize this ideal for peripheral nerve surgery, the peripheral nerve surgeon must:

- Have a thorough understanding of normal and variant anatomy of the peripheral nerve and its adjacent structures.
- Provide a complete clinical assessment.
- Be able to correctly identify and localize lesions and interpret electrodiagnostic studies for surgical planning.
- Anticipate complications that may arise during surgery and know how to manage them.
- Position the patient properly during surgery.
- Execute surgical techniques meticulously.

If the surgeon exercises patience and deliberation during the clinical evaluation, the possibility of surgical complications can be greatly minimized. We owe it to our patients.

# REFERENCES

1. Adams RD, Victor M, Ropper AH: *Principles of Neurology.* New York, McGraw-Hill, 1997.
2. Agee JM, McCarroll HR Jr, North ER: Endoscopic carpal tunnel release using the single proximal incisional technique. *Hand Clin* 10:647-659, 1994.
3. Agee JM, McCarroll HR Jr, Tortosa RD, *et al:* Endoscopic release of the carpal tunnel: a randomized prospective multicenter study. *J Hand Surg Am* 17:987-995, 1992.
4. Agee JM, Peimer CA, Pyrek JD, Walsh WE: Endoscopic carpal tunnel release: a prospective study of complications and surgical experience. *J Hand Surg Am* 20:165-171, 1995.
5. Alvine FG, Schurrer ME: Postoperative ulnar nerve palsy. Are there predisposing factors? *J Bone Joint Surg Am* 69:255-259, 1987.
6. Aminoff MJ: *Electrodiagnosis in Clinical Neurology.* New York, Churchill Livingstone, 1980.
7. Ariel IM: Tumors of the peripheral nervous system. *Semin Surg Oncol* 4:7, 1988.
8. Bande S, De Smet L, Fabry G: The results of carpal tunnel release: open versus endoscopic technique. *J Hand Surg Br* 19:14-17, 1994.
9. Berne RM, Levy MN: *Physiology.* St Louis, Mosby, 1983.
10. Birch R, Bonney G, Wynn Parry CB: *Surgical Disorders of the Peripheral Nerves.* Edinburgh, Churchill Livingstone, 1998.
11. Blair SJ: Avoiding complications of surgery for nerve compression syndromes. *Orthop Clin North Am* 19:125-130, 1988.
12. Bonney G: Iatrogenic injuries of nerves. *J Bone Joint Surg Br* 68:9-13, 1986.
13. Breidenbach WC: Vascularized nerve grafts: an experimental and clinical review. *Ann Plast Surg* 18:137-146, 1987.
14. Broudy AS, Leffert RD, Smith RJ: Technical problems with ulnar nerve transposition at the elbow: findings and results of reoperation. *J Hand Surg Am* 3:85-89, 1978.
15. Brown MG, Keyser B, Rothenberg ES: Endoscopic carpal tunnel release. *J Hand Surg Am* 17:1009-1011, 1992.
16. Brown MG, Rothenberg ES, Keyser B, *et al:* Results of 1236 endoscopic carpal tunnel release procedures using the Brown technique. *Contemp Orthop* 27:251-258, 1993.
17. Brown RA, Gelberman RH, Seiler JG 3rd, *et al:* Carpal tunnel release. A prospective, randomized assessment of open and endoscopic methods. *J Bone Joint Surg Am* 75:1265-1275, 1993.
18. Bunge RP: Some observations on the role of Schwann cell in peripheral nerve regeneration. In Jewett DL, McCarroll HR (eds): *Nerve Repair and Regeneration: Its Clinical and Experimental Basis.* St Louis, Mosby, 1980, p 58.
19. Burkhart FL, Daly JW: Sciatic and peroneal nerve injury: a complication of vaginal operations. *Obstet Gynecol* 28:99-102, 1966.
20. Chan RC, Paine KW, Varughese G: Ulnar neuropathy at the elbow: comparison of simple decompression and anterior transposition. *Neurosurgery* 7:545-550, 1980.
21. Cimino C: Painful neurological syndromes. In Aronoff G (ed): *Evaluation and Treatment of Chronic Pain.* Baltimore, Williams & Wilkins, 1992.
22. Dahlin LB, Lundborg G: Use of tubes in peripheral nerve repair. *Neurosurg Clin North Am* 12:341-352, 2001.
23. Dahlin LB, Shyu BC, Danielsen N, Andersson SA: Effects of nerve compression or ischaemia on conduction properties of myelinated and non-myelinated nerve fibres. An experimental study in the rabbit common peroneal nerve. *Acta Physiol Scand* 136:97-105, 1989.
24. Das SK, Brown HG: In search of complications in carpal tunnel decompression. *Hand* 8:243-249, 1976.
25. DasGupta T: Tumors of the peripheral nerves. *Clin Neurosurg* 25:574-590, 1978.
26. Dawson DM, Krarup C: Perioperative nerve lesions. *Arch Neurol* 46:1355-1360, 1989.
27. Deprez M, Ceuterick-de Groote C, Schoenen J, *et al:* Nerve biopsy: indications and contribution to the diagnosis of peripheral neuropathy. The experience of the Born Bunge Foundation University of Antwerp and University of Liege between 1987 and 1997. *Acta Neurol Belg* 100:162-166, 2000.
28. Donner TR, Kline DG: Extracranial spinal accessory nerve injury. *Neurosurgery* 32:907-911, 1993.
29. Donner TR, Voorhies RM, Kline DG: Neural sheath tumors of major nerves. *J Neurosurg* 81:362-373, 1994.
30. Dorfman LJ, Cummins KL, Leifer LJ: *Conduction Velocity Distributions: A Population Approach to Electrophysiology of Nerve.* New York, Allan R Liss, 1981.
31. Dubuisson AS, Kline DG, Weinshel SS: Posterior subscapular approach to the brachial plexus. *J Neurosurg* 79:319-330, 1993.
32. Ducatman BS, Scheithauer BW, Piepgras DG, *et al:* Malignant peripheral nerve sheath tumors. A clinicopathologic study of 120 cases. *Cancer* 57:2006-2021, 1986.
33. Elmaraghy MW, Hurst LN: Single-portal endoscopic carpal tunnel release: Agee carpal tunnel release system. *Ann Plast Surg* 36:286-291, 1996.
34. Evans PJ, MacKinnon SE, Midha R, *et al:* Regeneration across cold preserved peripheral nerve allografts. *Microsurgery* 19:115-127, 1999.
35. Favero KJ, Gropper PT: Ulnar nerve laceration—a complication of carpal tunnel decompression: case report and review of the literature. *J Hand Surg Br* 12:239-241, 1987.
36. Fawcett JW, Keynes RJ: Peripheral nerve regeneration. *Ann Rev Neurosci* 13:43-60, 1990.
37. Feinstein PA: Endoscopic carpal tunnel release in a community-based series. *J Hand Surg Am* 18:451-454, 1993.
38. Frykman GK, Cally D: Interfascicular nerve grafting. *Orthop Clin North Am* 19:71-80, 1988.
39. Gartsman GM, Kovach JC, Crouch CC, *et al:* Carpal arch alteration after carpal tunnel release. *J Hand Surg Am* 11:372-374, 1986.
40. Gentili F, Hudson A, Kline DG, Hunter DA: Peripheral nerve injection injury: an experimental study. *Neurosurgery* 4:244-253, 1979.
41. Gilliatt RW, Ochoa J, Rudge P, Neary D: The cause of nerve damage in acute compression. *Trans Am Neurol Assoc* 99:71-74, 1974.
42. Goodall RJ: Nerve injuries in fresh fractures. *Tex Med* 52:93-94, 1956.

43. Hope DG, Mulvihill JJ: Malignancy in neurofibromatosis. *Adv Neurol* 29:33-56, 1981.

44. Hudson AR, Gentili F, Kline DG: Peripheral nerve tumors. In Schmidek HH, Sweet WH (eds): *Operative Neurosurgical Techniques,* ed 2. Philadelphia, WB Saunders, 1988, p 1599.

45. Jabaley ME, Wallace WH, Heckler FR: Internal topography of major nerves of the forearm and hand: a current view. *J Hand Surg Am* 5:1-18, 1980.

46. Jimenez DF, Gibbs SR, Clapper AT: Endoscopic treatment of carpal tunnel syndrome: a critical review. *J Neurosurg* 88:817-826, 1998.

47. Jones NF: Intraoperative and postoperative monitoring of microsurgical free tissue transfers. *Clin Plast Surg* 19: 783-797, 1992.

48. Jones NF, Lister GD: Free skin and composite flaps. In Green DP, Hotchkiss RN, Pederson WC (eds): *Green's Operative Hand Surgery,* ed 4. Philadelphia, Churchill Livingstone, 1999, p 1164.

49. Kimura J: Principles and pitfalls of nerve conduction studies. *Ann Neurol* 16:415-429, 1984.

50. Kline DG: Surgical repair of peripheral nerve injury. *Muscle Nerve* 13:843-852, 1990.

51. Kline DG, Hudson AR: Acute injuries of peripheral nerves. In Youmans JR (ed): *Neurological Surgery*, ed 3. Philadelphia, WB Saunders, 1990, p 2511.

52. Kline DG, Hudson AR: *Nerve Injuries. Operative Results for Major Nerve Injuries, Entrapments, and Tumors.* Philadelphia, WB Saunders, 1995.

53. Koman LA, Goldner JL, Smith TL: The effect of extremity blood flow on pain and cold tolerance. In Omer GE Jr, Spinner M, Van Beek AL (eds): *Management of Peripheral Nerve Problems*, ed 2. Philadelphia, WB Saunders, 1988, pp 107-115.

54. Koman LA, Nunley JA: Thermoregulatory control after upper extremity replantation. *J Hand Surg Am* 11: 548-552, 1986.

55. Koman LA, Nunley JA, Goldner JL, *et al:* Isolated cold stress testing in the assessment of symptoms in the upper extremity: preliminary communication. *J Hand Surg Am* 9:305-313, 1984.

56. Koman LA, Smith TL, Poehling GG: Reflex sympathetic dystrophy. *Curr Opin* Orthop 4:85-88, 1993.

57. Kretschmer T, Antoniadis G, Braun V, *et al:* Evaluation of iatrogenic lesions in 722 surgically treated cases of peripheral nerve trauma. *J Neurosurg* 94:905-912, 2001.

58. Kuczynski K: Functional micro-anatomy of the peripheral nerve trunks. *Hand* 6:1-10, 1974.

59. Kulick MI, Gordillo G, Javidi T, *et al:* Long-term analysis of patients having surgical treatment for carpal tunnel syndrome. *J Hand Surg Am* 11:59-66, 1986.

60. Langloh ND, Linscheid RL: Recurrent and unrelieved carpal-tunnel syndrome. *Clin Orthop* 83:41-47, 1972.

61. Leffert RD: Anterior submuscular transposition of the ulnar nerves by the Learmonth technique. *J Hand Surg Am* 7:147-155, 1982.

62. Leffert RD: Surgery of the peripheral nerves and brachial plexus. In Schmidek HH, Sweet WH (eds): *Operative Neurosurgical Techniques,* ed 2. Philadelphia, WB Saunders, 1988, p 1563.

63. Leibovic SJ, Hastings H, II: Martin-Gruber revisited. *J Hand Surg Am* 17:47-53, 1992.

64. Lilly CJ, Magnell TD: Severance of the thenar branch of the median nerve as a complication of carpal tunnel release. *J Hand Surg Am* 10:399-402, 1985.

65. Louis DS, Greene TL, Noellert RC: Complications of carpal tunnel surgery. *J Neurosurg* 62:352-356, 1985.

66. Luallin SR, Toby EB: Incidental Guyon's canal release during attempted endoscopic carpal tunnel release: an anatomical study and report of two cases. *Arthroscopy* 9:382-386; discussion 381, 1993.

67. Lundborg G: The intrinsic vascularization of human peripheral nerves: structural and functional aspects. *J Hand Surg Am* 4:34-41, 1979.

68. Lundborg G: Structure and function of the intraneural microvessels as related to trauma, edema formation, and nerve function. *J Bone Joint Surg Am* 57:938-948, 1975.

69. Lusk MD, Kline DG, Garcia CA: Tumors of the brachial plexus. *Neurosurgery* 21:439-453, 1987.

70. Lusskin R, Battista A, Lenzo S, Price A: Surgical management of late post-traumatic and ischemic neuropathies involving the lower extremities: classification and results of therapy. *Foot Ankle* 7:95-104, 1986.

71. Lusthaus S, Matan Y, Finsterbush A, *et al:* Traumatic section of the median nerve: an unusual complication of Colles' fracture. *Injury* 24:339-340, 1993.

72. MacDonald RI, Lichtman DM, Hanlon JJ, Wilson JN: Complications of surgical release for carpal tunnel syndrome. *J Hand Surg Am* 3:70-76, 1978.

73. Mackinnon SE, Dellon AL: Evaluation of microsurgical internal neurolysis in a primate median nerve model of chronic nerve compression. *J Hand Surg Am* 13:345-351, 1988.

74. Mackinnon SE, Dellon AL: *Surgery of the Peripheral Nerve.* New York, Thieme, 1988.

75. Mackinnon SE, Doolabh VB, Novak CB, Trulock EP: Clinical outcome following nerve allograft transplantation. *Plast Reconstr Surg* 107:1419-1429, 2001.

76. Macnicol MF: The results of operation for ulnar neuritis. *J Bone Joint Surg Br* 61:159-164, 1979.

77. May JW, Rosen H: Division of the sensory ramus communicans between the ulnar and median nerves: a complication following carpal tunnel release. A case report. *J Bone Joint Surg Am* 63:836-838, 1981.

78. McDonough JW, Gruenloh TJ: A comparison of endoscopic and open carpal tunnel release. *Wis Med J* 92:675-677, 1993.

79. Millesi H: Forty-two years of peripheral nerve surgery. *Microsurgery* 14:228-233, 1993.

80. Millesi H, Meissl G: Consequences of tension at the suture line. In Gorio A, Millesi H, Mingrino S (eds): *Posttraumatic Peripheral Nerve Regeneration: Experimental Basis and Clinical Implications.* Philadelphia, Lippincott-Raven, 1981, p 277.

81. Millesi H, Meissl G, Berger A: Further experience with interfascicular grafting of the median, ulnar, and radial nerves. *J Bone Joint Surg Am* 58:209-218, 1976.

82. Millesi H, Meissl G, Berger A: The interfascicular nerve-grafting of the median and ulnar nerves. *J Bone Joint Surg Am* 54:727-750, 1972.

83. Nath RK, Mackinnon SE, Weeks PM: Ulnar nerve transection as a complication of two-portal endoscopic carpal tunnel release: a case report. *J Hand Surg Am* 18:896-898, 1993.

84. Neimkin RJ, Smith RJ: Double tourniquet with linked mercury manometers for hand surgery. *J Hand Surg Am* 8:938-941, 1983.

85. Nissenbaum M, Kleinert HE: Treatment considerations in carpal tunnel syndrome with coexistent Dupuytren's disease. *J Hand Surg Am* 5:544-547, 1980.

86. Nunley JA, Penny WH, III, Woodbury MA, Koman LA: Quantitative analysis of cold stress performance after digital replantation. *J Orthop Res* 8:94-100, 1990.

87. Ochoa J, Marotte L: The nature of the nerve lesion caused by chronic entrapment in the guinea-pig. *J Neurol Sci* 19:491-495, 1973.

88. Omer GE Jr: Continuous peripheral epineural infusion for the treatment of acute pain. In Omer GE Jr, Spinner M, Voorhies RM (eds): *Management of Peripheral Nerve Problems*, ed 2. Philadelphia, WB Saunders, 1998, pp 116-119.

89. Omer GE Jr: Injuries to nerves of the upper extremity. *J Bone Joint Surg Am* 56:1615-1624, 1974.

90. Omer GE Jr: The management of pain. In Lamb DW (ed): *The Paralyzed Hand*. Edinburgh, Churchill Livingstone, 1987, pp 213-216.

91. Omer GE, Jr: Management of pain syndromes in upper extremity. In Hunter JM, Schneider LH, Mackin EH, *et al* (eds): *Rehabilitation of the Hand*. St Louis, Mosby, 1978, pp 341-349.

92. Omer GE Jr: Management techniques for the painful upper extremity. In Terzis JK (ed): *Microreconstruction of Nerve Injuries*. Philadelphia, WB Saunders, 1987, pp 145-159.

93. Omer GE Jr: Present thoughts on the management of pain in the upper extremity. *Clin Plast Surg* 11:85-93, 1984.

94. Omer GE Jr: The prognosis for untreated traumatic injuries. In Omer GE Jr, Spinner M, Van Beek AL (eds): *Management of Peripheral Nerve Problems*, ed 2. Philadelphia, WB Saunders, 1998, pp 365-370.

95. Omer GE Jr: Sensation and sensibility in the upper extremity. *Clin Orthop* 104:30-36, 1974.

96. Omer GE Jr, Bell-Krotoski J: Sensibility testing. In Omer GE Jr, Spinner M, Van Beek AL (eds): *Management of Peripheral Nerve Problems*, ed 2. Philadelphia, WB Saunders, 1998, pp 11-28.

97. Ordog GJ, Balasubramanium S, Wasserberger J, *et al*: Extremity gunshot wounds: Part one: Identification and treatment of patients at high risk of vascular injury. *J Trauma* 36:358-368, 1994.

98. Palmer DH, Paulson JC, Lane-Larsen CL, *et al*: Endoscopic carpal tunnel release: a comparison of two techniques with open release. *Arthroscopy* 9:498-508, 1993.

99. Parks BJ: Postoperative peripheral neuropathies. *Surgery* 74:348-357, 1973.

100. Peterson GW, Will AD: Newer electrodiagnostic techniques in peripheral nerve injuries. *Orthop Clin N Am* 19:13-25, 1988.

101. Rakolta GG, Omer GE Jr: Combat-sustained femoral nerve injuries. *Surg Gynecol Obstet* 128:813-817, 1969.

102. Rappaport WD, Valente J, Hunter GC, *et al*: Clinical utilization and complications of sural nerve biopsy. *Am J Surg* 166:252-256, 1993.

103. Reisner GG, Tindall SC: Complications of peripheral nerve surgery. In Benzel EC (ed): *Spine Surgery*. Philadelphia, Churchill Livingstone, 1999, pp 947-959.

104. Resnick CT, Miller BW: Endoscopic carpal tunnel release using the subligamentous two-portal technique. *Contemp Orthop* 22:269-277, 1991.

105. Rhoades CE, Mowery CA, Gelberman RH: Results of internal neurolysis of the median nerve for severe carpal-tunnel syndrome. *J Bone Joint Surg Am* 67:253-256, 1985.

106. Rieke H, Benecke R, DeVivie ER, *et al*: Brachial plexus lesions following cardiac surgery with median sternotomy and cannulation of the internal jugular vein. *J Cardiothorac Anesth* 3:286-289, 1989.

107. Rorabeck CH, Harris WR: Factors affecting the prognosis of brachial plexus injuries. *J Bone Joint Surg Br* 63B:404-407, 1981.

108. Russell RC, Pribaz JP, Zook EG: Clinical motor function testing—upper extremity. In Omer GE Jr, Spinner M, Van Beek AL (eds): *Management of Peripheral Nerve Problems*, ed 2. Philadelphia, WB Saunders, 1998, pp 39-49.

109. Rybeck B, Janzon B: Absorption of missile energy in soft tissue. *Acta Chir Scand* 142:201-207, 1976.

110. Sanders R: The tourniquet. Instrument or weapon? *Hand* 5:119-123, 1973.

111. Schultz D: Indications for utilization of a pain clinic. In Omer GE Jr, Spinner M, Van Beek AL (eds): *Management of Peripheral Nerve Problems*, ed 2. Philadelphia, WB Saunders, 1998, pp 120-133.

112. Sedel L: The results of surgical repair of brachial plexus injuries. *J Bone Joint Surg Br* 64:54-66, 1982.

113. Semple JC, Cargill AO: Carpal-tunnel syndrome. Results of surgical decompression. *Lancet* 1:918-919, 1969.

114. Smith JW: Factors influencing nerve repair. I. Blood supply of peripheral nerves. *Arch Surg* 93:335-341, 1966.

115. Smith JW: Factors influencing nerve repair. II. Collateral circulation of peripheral nerves. *Arch Surg* 93:433-437, 1966.

116. Smorto MP, Basmajian JV: *Electrodiagnosis. A Handbook for Neurologists*. Hagerstown, MD, Harper and Row, 1977.

117. Sunderland S: *Nerves and Nerve Injuries*, ed 2. Edinburgh, Churchill Livingstone, 1978.

118. Terzis JK, Dykes RW, Hakstian RW: Electrophysiological recordings in peripheral nerve surgery: a review. *J Hand Surg Am* 1:52-66, 1976.

119. Thomas JE, Piepgras DG, Scheithauer B, *et al*: Neurogenic tumors of the sciatic nerve. A clinicopathologic study of 35 cases. *Mayo Clin Proc* 58:640-647, 1983.

120. Tindall SC: Chronic injuries of peripheral nerves by entrapment. In Youmans JR (ed): *Neurological Surgery*, ed 3, vol 4. Philadelphia, WB Saunders, 1990, p 2511.

121. Trentman TL, Rome JD, Messick JM Jr: Brachial plexus neuropathy following attempt at subclavian vein catheterization. Case report. *Reg Anesth* 21:163-165, 1996.

122. Tupper JW, Crick JC, Matteck LR: Fascicular nerve repairs. A comparative study of epineurial and fascicular (perineurial) techniques. *Orthop Clin N Am* 19:57-69, 1988.

123. Van Beek AL: Electrodiagnostic evaluation of peripheral nerve injuries. *Hand Clin* 2:747-760, 1986.

124. Van Beek AL: Intraoperative nerve stimulation and recording techniques. In Omer GE Jr, Spinner M, Van Beek AL (eds): *Management of Peripheral Nerve Problems,* ed 2. Philadelphia, WB Saunders, 1998, pp 251-259.

125. Van Beek AL, Hubble B, Kinkead L, *et al:* Clinical use of nerve stimulation and recording techniques. *Plast Reconstr Surg* 71:225-240, 1983.

126. Van Beek AL, Massac E Jr, Smith DO: The use of the signal averaging computer for evaluation of peripheral nerve problems. *Clin Plast Surg* 13:407-418, 1986.

127. Vrettos BC, Rochkind S, Boome RS: Low velocity gun shot wounds of the brachial plexus. *J Bone Joint Surg Br* 20:212-214, 1995.

128. Wilbourn AJ: Iatrogenic nerve injuries. *Neurol Clin* 16:55-82, 1998.

129. Wilson DH, Krout R: Surgery of ulnar neuropathy at the elbow: 16 cases treated by decompression without transposition. Technical note. *J Neurosurg* 38:780-785, 1973.

130. Wiss DA, Gellman H: Gunshot wounds to the musculoskeletal system. In Browner BD, Jupiter JB, Levine AM et al (eds): *Skeletal Trauma.* Philadelphia, WB Saunders, 1992, pp 367-400.

131. Young HA: Surgical management of peripheral entrapment neuropathy. In Schmidek HH, Sweet WH (eds): *Operative Neurosurgical Techniques,* ed 2. Philadelphia, WB Saunders, 1988, p 1583.

# Spinal

# Instrumentation

# CHAPTER 105

# Basic Biomechanically Relevant Anatomy

**John Butler, Lisa A. Ferrara, and Edward C. Benzel**

Spine biomechanics represents an application of basic engineering and physics principles to a biologic structure, the spinal column. It is an attempt to view the normal physiologic behavior of the spine and pathology of the spine through the eyes of engineers as we attempt to repair it. These concepts are broken down into the simplest, most basic terms. Therefore, it is imperative to understand the language of the engineer and the surgeon. The anatomy of the spine must be placed in biomechanical terms, such that the role of the each structure is understood in relation to the overall structure and function of the spine. The spine is a complex load-bearing structure made up of ligaments, tendons, and bone arranged to effectively dissipate forces and allow a physiologic range of motion, while at the same time protecting the spinal cord.

When injury occurs, when stability is compromised either through trauma or disease, or when years of degeneration culminate in pain and impingement on nerves or the spinal cord itself, surgical intervention may be required. Surgery is a destabilizing process, and often the surgeon must utilize instrumentation to restore stability. Spinal implants are designed to impart force to the spine. In order to apply or design instrumentation, a thorough understanding of the forces at work must be attained. This chapter represents an introduction to the biomechanical anatomy of the spine as well as the basic principles guiding implant and construct design.

## Basic and Biomechanical Anatomy of the Spine

The spine is made up of 33 separate vertebral segments that are interconnected by spinal ligaments, facet capsules, and intervertebral discs. Each bony segment is referred to as a vertebra and each is numbered in a region specific (i.e., cervical, thoracic) rostral to caudal fashion. Thus, there are 7 cervical vertebrae, 12 thoracic vertebrae, 5 lumbar vertebrae, 5 fused sacral vertebrae, and 3 to 4 fused coccygeal segments. There are four normal curves to the spine, all of which occur in the sagittal plane. The cervical and lumbar spine are both lordotic or concave posteriorly, and this is due to the wedge-shaped intervertebral discs. The thoracic and sacral regions are kyphotic or concave ventrally, and, at least in the thoracic spine where the segments are not fused, this is structural and due to the shape of the thoracic vertebral bodies. The anterior vertebral border height is less than the posterior vertebral border height resulting in an anterior or kyphotic curve. These curves function to increase the flexibility and shock-absorbing capacity of the spine. The overall physiologic alignment must be maintained in order to prevent construct failure and accelerated degeneration. Sagittal balance is an indicator of physiologic alignment and is particularly important in lumbosacral procedures. In a normal spine, a plumb line can be dropped from the C7 vertebral body through the lumbosacral junction, and this indicates sagittal balance (Figure 105.1).

## Vertebral Body

The vertebral body is the large bony cylinder that makes up the anterior aspect of each vertebra, except at C1 that has no vertebral body. Each vertebral body consists of an outer rim of cortical bone surrounding a core of softer cancellous bone. The vertebral bodies resist much of the compressive loads placed on the spine in physiologic situations. In general, the height, width, and depth of the vertebral bodies increase as the spine is descended, which seems to account for this increased strength and stress-resisting ability at lower levels in the spine.[29] As previously alluded to, there is a regional variation to the shape of the vertebral body. In the thoracic spine, the anterior border is shorter than the posterior border creating a structural kyphosis in the thoracic spine. The outer shell of cortical bone is more rigid than the softer cancellous core because it is arranged in vertical lamellae to resist compressive forces. The cancellous bone is made up of trabeculae that are arranged to resist a variety of loads. There is greater compressive deformation of the cancellous bone prior to failure than of the cortical bone because of the increased rigidity of the latter.[11,16] Numerous studies regarding the load sharing properties of the cortical and cancellous bone have been done showing that the load carried by the trabecular bone varies anywhere from 35% to 90% depending on age and mineral content of the bone,[18,26] and the strength of the vertebral body decreases with age. Bell et al.[4] have shown that there is a direct relationship between the mineral or ash content of the bone and the strength of the vertebral body. A 25% decrease in mineral content resulted in a greater than 50% decrease in vertebral strength due to loss of the trabecular columns that formed the core of the vertebral bodies. In osteoporosis, the mineral content of the bone is affected and results in loss of the horizontal trabeculae within the vertebral body core thus lengthening the trabecular columns and compromising vertebral body strength.[29] In the thoracic spine the vertebral bodies articulate with the ribs. This articulation with the rib cage significantly augments the strength of the thoracic spine.

The vertebral end plates are formed from the concave, 1 to 2mm thick cortical bone at the rostral and caudal surface of the vertebral body. These are fused to the cartilaginous end plates of the intervertebral disc by a calcified layer of tissue known as the lamina cribrosa, which permits osmotic diffusion of nutrients for the intervertebral disc. In 1957, Perry[25] extensively studied failure of the end plates under compression in and noted that one of three mechanisms of failure occurs depending on the condition of the surrounding discs. Fractures occurred centrally, peripherally, or encompassed the entire end plate. In specimens with nondegenerated discs the fractures typically occurred centrally, and in specimens with degenerated discs the fractures occurred peripherally. At higher loads the fractures encompassed the entire end plate. Because of the presence of nondegenerated nucleus, fluid pressure builds in the center causing deflection of the end plate in the center leading to bending stresses in the same location and ultimately failure.[29] In the degenerated disc, the nucleus lacks water content and there is no buildup of fluid pressure. The load is transmitted primarily through the annulus at the periphery of the disc and end plate resulting in fracture in the same location or in the underlying vertebral body.[29] The strength of the end plate itself has been evaluated as well with regards to resistance to penetration by graft material (subsidence) or disc material (Schmorl's node). Kumar *et al.*[15] determined the greatest resistance to penetration to be within the first 4mm of depth and the end plate to be strongest at the periphery closer to the cortical margin.

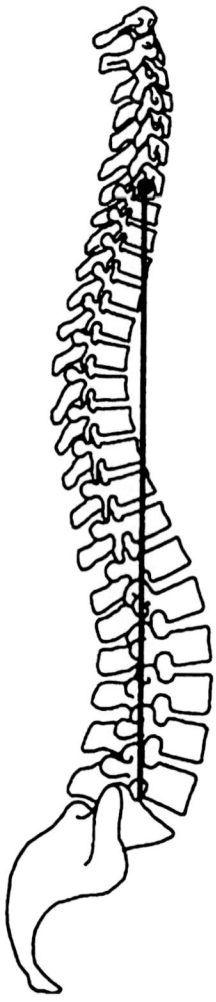

**Figure 105.1** Sagittal balance. A plumb line dropped from the C7 vertebral body in the standing position should pass through the lumbosacral junction when normal sagittal balance is present, as depicted. (*From Benzel EC [ed]:* Biomechanics of Spine Stabilization. *Rolling Meadows, IL, American Association of Neurological Surgeons, 2001.*)

## Intervertebral Disc

The vertebral bodies are separated at each level by the intervertebral disc, which is a viscoelastic structure made up of a central nucleus pulposus, peripheral annulus fibrosus and the cartilaginous end plate of the disc, which separates it from the vertebral bodies above and below. There are 23 intervertebral discs starting between C2 and C3 and ending at L5 and S1. They make up 20% to 33% of the total height of the vertebral column, and there are regional differences that seem to parallel those of the vertebrae. The cross-sectional area of the discs increases in the rostrocaudal direction.

The central nucleus pulposus is composed of mucopolysaccharides and mucoprotein forming a gel with water content ranging from 70% to 90%.[29] The water content is highest at birth and decreases with age.[20] The nucleus pulposus makes up approximately 30% to 50% of the cross-sectional area of the disc, and it seems to lie more posterior in the lumbar spine at the junction of the middle and posterior thirds of the disc in the sagittal plane.[29] The viscoelastic properties of the nucleus pulposus allow it to act as an effective shock absorber for the spine. Surrounding the nucleus pulposus is the annulus fibrosus, which is made up of collagenous fibers in concentric laminated bands with each band oriented 90° to the adjacent bands and 30° to the disc plane (Figure 105.2). The inner fibers of the annulus are attached to the cartilaginous end plates, and the outermost fibers, called Sharpey's fibers, are attached to the cortical bone of the vertebral body. Because of the orientation of the fibers, the intervertebral disc effectively resists rotational, tensile, and shear stresses. The annulus does not resist compressive forces.

With age, the water content of the nucleus pulposus decreases and the nucleus itself becomes less deformable. This results in an overall stiffer intervertebral disc that behaves differently under compressive loads. In a younger disc, the nucleus is compressed, resulting in deformity at the central part of the end plate, but when the nucleus becomes stiffer and less deformable, the load is transmitted through the annular fibers around the periphery with very little central deformation leading to a more evenly

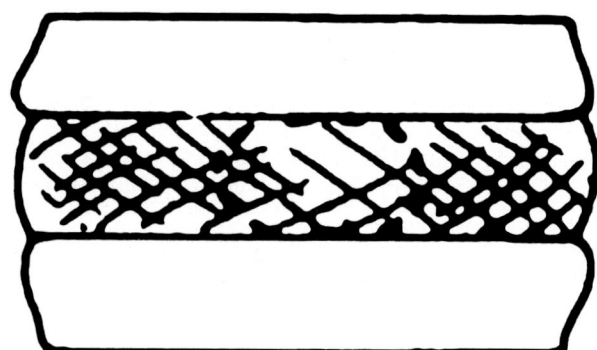

**Figure 105.2** The intervertebral disc. The fibers of the annulus fibrosus are oriented radially and in opposite directions throughout several layers. The nucleus pulposus (*dashed outline*) is contained (in nonpathologic situations) by the annulus fibers. (*From Benzel EC [ed]:* Biomechanics of Spine Stabilization. *Rolling Meadows, IL, American Association of Neurological Surgeons, 2001.*)

distributed load at the end plate. This can result in compression fractures as is commonly observed in the elderly or osteoporotic population. Because of the increased stiffness of the disc and the end plates, overall deformability is less resulting in a smaller elastic zone and lower threshold for failure. The concepts of neutral zone, elastic zone, plastic zone, and failure will be addressed in the next section on biomechanics.

## Facet Joints

The vertebrae articulate with each other at the superior and inferior facet joints, which are diarthrodial joints with a loose synovial capsule located at the superior and inferior aspect of the pars interarticularis. In the cervical spine the facet joints are coronally oriented with an inclination of approximately 45 degrees from the horizontal, and this orientation changes in the thoracic and lumbar spine.[29] The shape, position, and orientation of these articulating surfaces largely determine the pattern of movements throughout the spine (Figure 105.3).

The coronally oriented cervical facet joints face the instantaneous axis of rotation (IAR), which is the axis about which a vertebral segment rotates, and are not particularly restrictive of flexion, extension, rotation, and lateral bending. In the thoracic spine, the inclination of the articulating surfaces is approximately 60 degrees with an additional rotation about the y-axis of approximately 20 degrees toward the midline. The facet surfaces in the lumbar spine are at an inclination of approximately 90 degrees with approximately 45 degrees of rotation about the y-axis directed outwards. The orientations of the facet joints as stated are only approximations with a great deal of variation within the specific regions of the spine.[29] The facets act as important stabilizing structures in the spine with resultant instability following unilateral or bilateral excision.[1]

In the lumbar spine the sagittal orientation of the facet joints allows for substantial resistance to rotation, which is well documented.[1-3] As the facet orientation begins to change from about T7 to L4, the torsional stiffness of the spine increases due to these changes in facet articulation with the peak at T12-L1.[17] In the cervical spine, transaction of the disc and longitudinal ligaments resulted in a 33% increase in horizontal translation with flexion. This increased by 140% following transection of the facets.[24] Removal of thoracic facets resulted in increased flexion and extension in the upper thoracic region and increased axial rotation in the lower thoracic/thoracolumbar region. The capsular ligaments also have a role in maintaining torsional strength.

The facets provide a load-bearing role when the spine is in extension. In dynamic studies with cadaver spines in various postures, the facets have been shown to carry anywhere from 0% to 33% of the load depending on the force vector and position of the spine.[13]

## Dorsal Elements

The remainder of the dorsal elements of the spine includes the pedicle, the lamina, the transverse processes, and the spinous process. Each of these elements varies significantly in morphology between regions of the spine. The pedicle serves as the bridge between the posterior elements and the vertebral body. The importance of pedicle anatomy is due to the major role pedicles now play in

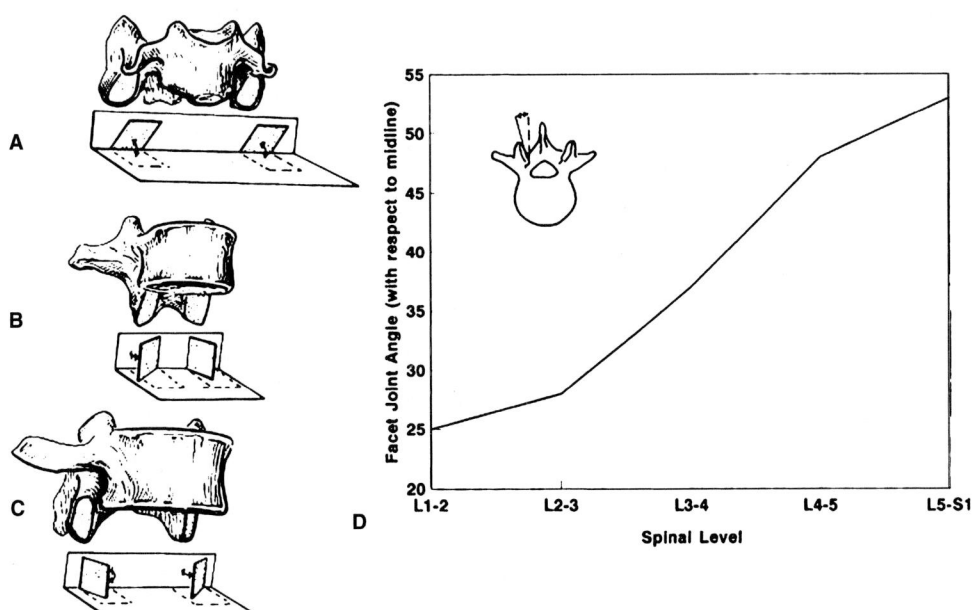

**Figure 105.3** Facet joint orientation. **(A)** The relative coronal plane orientation in the cervical region, **(B)** the intermediate orientation in the thoracic region, and **(C)** the relative sagittal orientation in the lumbar region The facet joint orientation changes substantially in the lumbar region; here the facet joint angle (with respect to midline) is depicted versus spinal level **(D)**. *(From Benzel EC (ed):* Biomechanics of Spine Stabilization. *Rolling Meadows, IL, American Association of Neurological Surgeons, 2001.)*

stabilization constructs. In the cervical spine the pedicles are shorter with greater diameter. From the cervical to midthoracic region, transverse pedicle width gradually decreases then increases from midthoracic to the lumbar region (Figure 105.4).[14,21,32] Sagittal pedicle width increases from the cervical to the thoracolumbar region and then decreases in the lumbar region (Figure 105.5).[14,21,32] From the cervical to the thoracolumbar region the transverse pedicle angle decreases and increases into the lumbar region (Figure 105.6).[14,21,32] The sagittal pedicle angle is a final consideration with regards to pedicle anatomy as it becomes fairly steep in the thoracic and thoracolumbar regions (Figure 105.7).[14,21,32]

The laminae form the dorsal aspect of the neural canal, which contains the spinal cord. The laminae extend from the pedicles to the spinous process dorsally and form the foundation for the spinous processes, provide dorsal protection to the dural sac, and serve as the attachment site of one of the seven spinal ligaments, the ligamentum flavum.[6]

The spinous processes project dorsally and, for the most part, caudally. They form attachment sites for the interspinous ligaments and supraspinous ligaments. The spinous processes from C3 to C7 are bifid and project more caudally as one descends to the midthoracic spine. Further down into the thoracolumbar and lumbar regions the spinous processes project more dorsally.[6]

The transverse processes are located at the junction of the lamina and pedicle and in general extend laterally with some variation in the rostral-caudal dimension depending on the region of the spine. They serve as sites of attachment for the paraspinal muscles. In the cervical spine, the transverse processes are smaller and transmit the vertebral artery through the foramen transversarium from C6 to C1. The transverse processes of the middle to lower thoracic spine become more substantial projecting in a lateral and upward direction. The lower thoracic processes become smaller and more atretic but those of the lumbar spine

become more substantial, extending laterally and ventrally. The transverse processes of the midthoracic and lumbar spine are sizeable enough to serve as sites for hook placement and fusion, but they are limited by a poor blood supply and are easily fractured.[6]

### Ligaments

The ligamentous complex from the occiput to C2 is will be presented separately though much of it represents a continuation of ligaments of the subaxial spine (see Figures

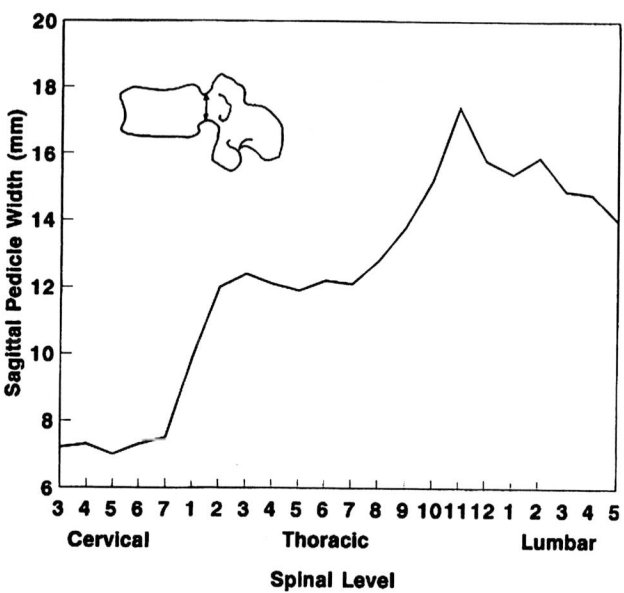

**Figure 105.5** Sagittal pedicle width versus spinal level. (*From Benzel EC [ed]:* Biomechanics of Spine Stabilization. *Rolling Meadows, IL, American Association of Neurological Surgeons, 2001.*)

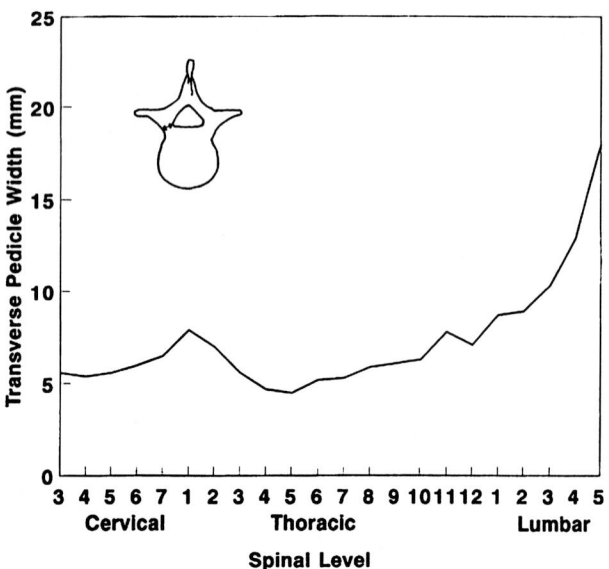

**Figure 105.4** Transverse pedicle width versus spinal level. (*From Benzel EC [ed]:* Biomechanics of Spine Stabilization. *Rolling Meadows, IL, American Association of Neurological Surgeons, 2001.*)

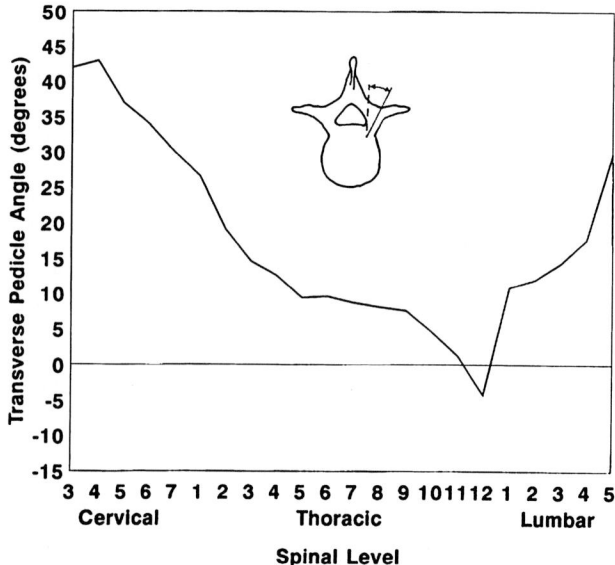

**Figure 105.6** Transverse pedicle angle versus spinal level. (*From Benzel EC [ed]:* Biomechanics of Spine Stabilization. *Rolling Meadows, IL, American Association of Neurological Surgeons, 2001.*)

105.5 to 105.12). The anterior longitudinal ligament begins at the occiput as the atlantooccipital membrane as it passes between the occiput and the anterior arch of C1. The posterior atlantooccipital membrane passes from the posterior arch of C1 to the occiput. When intact, these ligaments offer some advantage in preventing anterior displacement of C1 on C2. The apical ligament stretches from the tip of the odontoid process of C2 to the basion of the skull. The alar ligaments run obliquely from the rostrolateral aspect of the odontoid to the occipital condyles. The cruciate ligament has a vertical and transverse portion. The transverse portion of the ligament attaches to the

tubercles located at the lateral masses of C1 and runs dorsal to the dens. The vertical portion of the cruciate ligament attaches to the occiput immediately dorsal to the apical ligament and descends to intertwine with the transverse portion. The vertical portion then descends to attach to the dorsocaudal aspect of C2. The transverse ligament is the most important ligament of the occipitocervical complex as it prevents horizontal translation of C1 on C2. The tectorial membrane is a continuation of the posterior longitudinal ligament and runs from the body of C2 over the posterior portion of the dens to attach to the anterior foramen magnum (Figure 105.8).

Beyond the occiput–C1-2 complex, there are seven major spinal ligaments that work to stabilize the subaxial spine in its physiologic range of motion. These ligaments also work to restrict the motion of the spine to well-defined limits while at the same time allowing adequate motion and fixed postures in order to protect the spinal cord. Starting anteriorly and moving posteriorly the ligaments are the anterior longitudinal ligament, the posterior longitudinal ligament, the capsular ligaments, the intertransverse process ligaments, ligamentum flavum, the interspinous ligament, and the supraspinous ligament (Figure 105.9). The strength characteristics of the ligaments vary, and the effectiveness of a ligament not only depends on the morphology but also on the length of the moment arm through which it works[22] (Figure 105.10). The moment arm is the perpendicular distance between the force vector and the IAR. A longer moment arm gives a relatively weak ligament mechanical advantage so that it may contribute more to overall spinal stability than a stronger ligament with a shorter moment arm.

The anterior longitudinal ligament begins the entire spinal column from the clivus where it begins as the previously mentioned anterior atlantooccipital membrane to the sacrum. It covers the ventral one fourth to one third of the vertebral body circumference with interdigitizing

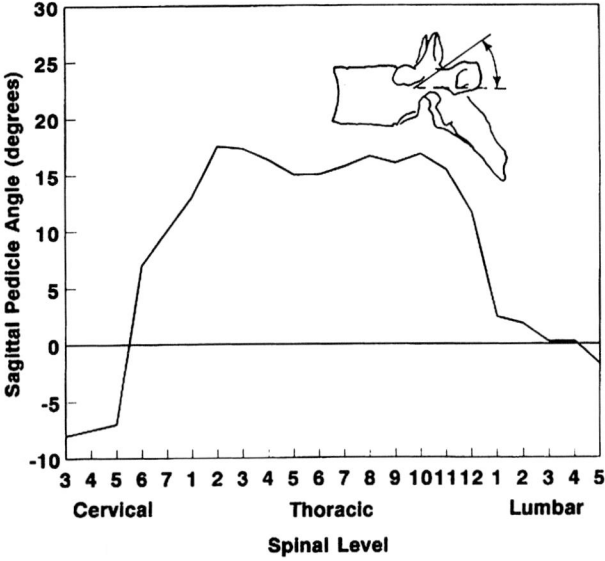

**Figure 105.7** Sagittal pedicle angle versus spinal level. *(From Benzel EC [ed]:* Biomechanics of Spine Stabilization. *Rolling Meadows, IL, American Association of Neurological Surgeons, 2001.)*

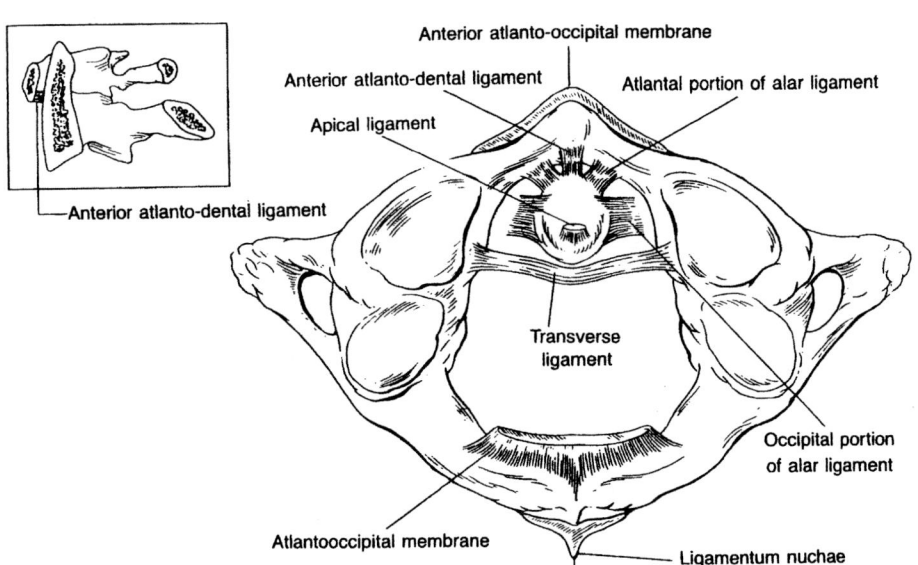

**Figure 105.8** Schematic illustration of the major ligaments involved in the clinical stability of the upper cervical spine. The anterior atlanto-dental ligament has been described recently. *(From White AA, Panjabi MM:* Clinical Biomechanics of the Spine, *ed 2. Philadelphia, Lippincott, 1990.)*

layers of elastin and collagen fibers. The innermost layers bind to the intervertebral discs of adjacent vertebrae. The middle layer binds the vertebral bodies and discs over three levels while the superficial layer extends over four to five levels. Because it is ventral to the IAR, it provides resistance to extension.

The posterior longitudinal ligament starts as the tectorial membrane and also spans the entire length of the spine. It also consists of several layers with the deeper fibers spanning adjacent vertebrae and the more superficial fibers extending over several levels. The posterior longitudinal ligament only marginally attaches to the vertebral body as compared to the anterior longitudinal ligament, which blends into the periosteum at times. The posterior longitudinal ligament is closely adherent to the annulus fibrosus whereas the anterior longitudinal ligament is not. The posterior longitudinal ligament widens in the region of the disc space and narrows as it passes over the vertebral body. It is dorsal to the IAR and has a short moment arm, and, therefore, it is only able to weakly resist flexion forces.

The capsular ligaments are located at the facet joints. These fibers attach to the superior and inferior facets of adjacent vertebrae, and they act as significant stabilizers of the spine, particularly in the cervical spine. The fibers of the facet capsules run in a direction that is perpendicular to the plane of the facet joint. The moment arm (see Figure 105.10) is not substantial but the ligaments are strong enough for the stresses placed upon them, which consist mainly of axial rotation, anterior shear loads and axial loads under certain conditions.

The ligamentum flavum has the highest percentage of elastic fibers of any tissue in the body. The ligamentum flavum is actually a pair of broad ligaments that connect the spinal laminae. They arise from the ventral surface of the caudal lamina and attach to the dorsal border of the

adjacent rostral lamina, and they extend laterally to become confluent with the joint capsules. These ligaments begin at C1-2 and continue caudally to L5-S1. Nachemson and Evans noted that the ligament is in a state of resting "pre-tension" or tension, which is present with the spine in neutral position.[29] This is postulated to lend stability to the spine by keeping the intervertebral discs under a small amount of compression and to keep the ligament from impinging on the spinal cord when the spine is in extension.

The interspinous and supraspinous ligaments simply connect the adjacent spinous processes. The interspinous ligament extends from the base to the tip of each spinous process, and this ligament is present from C2 to S1. The supraspinous ligament begins at the dorsal aspect of C7 attaching to the tip of the spinous process and extends to the lumbosacral region. It is thought to be a continuation of the ligamentum nuchae associated with the dorsal cervical spine. These ligaments effectively resist flexion through long lever arms (see Figure 105.10).

## Musculature

One final consideration regarding the basic biomechanical anatomy of the spine is the surrounding musculature, which lends significant support and stability to the spine. In the cervical region there is a fibrous intermuscular septum previously mentioned known as the ligamentum nuchae, which serves as an attachment to many of the occipitocervical muscles. The splenius capitis muscle arises from lower ligamentum, cervical, and upper six thoracic transverse processes to attach to the occiput. The splenius cervicis muscle arises from the upper six thoracic transverse processes to insert on the posterior tubercles of C1-3. The semispinalis cervicis muscle occupies the next

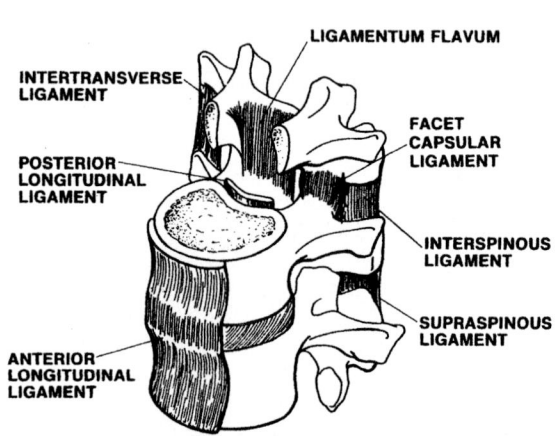

**Figure 105.9** Ligaments of the Spine. Besides the disc, there are seven ligaments that connect one vertebra to the next. Contribution to the spine stability by an individual ligament is dependent upon its cross-section, its distance from the instantaneous axis of rotation (IAR), and its orientation in space. The anatomy of the ligaments is such as to collectively provide stability to the spine in its various physiologic motions. (*From White AA, Panjabi MM: Clinical Biomechanics of the Spine, ed 2. Philadelphia, Lippincott, 1990.*)

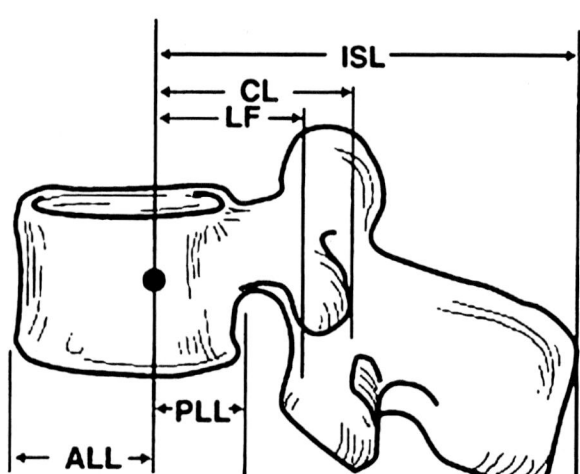

**Figure 105.10** The ligaments and their effective moment arms. Note that this length depends on the location of the IAR. An "average" location is used in this illustration. (*Dot,* IAR; *ALL,* anterior longitudinal ligament; *PLL,* posterior longitudinal ligament; *LF,* ligamentum flavum; *CL,* capsular ligament; *ISL,* interspinous ligament). (*From Benzel EC [ed]:* Biomechanics of Spine Stabilization. *Rolling Meadows, IL, American Association of Neurological Surgeons, 2001.*)

deeper layer and arises from the facets and transverse processes of the upper thoracic spine to insert on the spinous processes of the cervical spine. The semispinalis capitis muscle, occupying the same layer, is more lateral arising from the transverse processes of C3-6 to insert on the occiput. Deeper muscles include the rectus capitis and the capitis obliques, which serve as head extensors. Ventrally, the sternocleidomastoids arise bilaterally from the clavicles and insert on the mastoid processes of the occipital bone. The longus coli occupy a deeper layer in the anterior cervical region arising from the atlas to insert on the transverse processes of C3 to C6.

In the thoracic region, the superficial musculature attaches to the thoracic spinous processes, and in the rostral thoracic region it is made up principally of the trapezius muscle, which inserts laterally on the scapula and medially on the ligamentum nuchae. Lower in the lower thoracic and thoracolumbar region, the superficial musculature is made up principally of the latissimus dorsi muscle, which arises from the transverse processes of the lower thoracic spine and spreads ventrally to the axilla. The rib cage, which articulates with the thoracic spine and lends stability to this region, also possesses its own intrinsic musculature. The intercostal muscles and serratus posterior muscles run between ribs but in opposite directions. In the lower thoracic and thoracolumbar region the lateral muscle groups include the psoas, intertransverse, and quadratus lumborum muscle. The psoas muscles arise from the lateral aspect of the vertebral bodies and insert on the femurs. The intertransverse muscles arise and insert between transverse processes throughout the spine, and the quadratus lumborum muscle arises from the transverse processes and inserts at the lateral ileum.

Ventrally, the lumbar spine is supported by those muscles surrounding the abdominal region, which include the internal and external obliques, the transversus abdominis, and the rectus abdominis. Dorsally, lumbar support is principally from the very prominent paravertebral muscles. These make up the erector spinae muscle group, which begins as a broad tendon attached to the sacrum and iliac crest and extends the entire length of the spine. It is composed of three columns, each of which is composed of shorter fascicles. The lateral column is the iliocostalis muscle, the middle column is the longissimus muscle, and the medial column is the semispinalis muscle. The iliocostalis arises from the iliac crest to insert on the angles of each rib and the cervical transverse processes. The longissimus muscle is the largest and arises from the transverse processes at the lower spinal levels and inserts onto the transverse processes rostrally and onto the mastoid processes of the occipital bone. The semispinalis arises from the spinous processes of the sacrum and inserts onto the rostral spinous processes. Deeper to the erector spinae muscle group is the transverse muscle group, which principally arises from transverse processes and insert onto the spinous processes. The multifidus muscle differs in the cervical and lumbar regions where it arises from the articular joint as opposed to the transverse processes.

Weakness of the muscle groups that support the spine can lead to deformity or pain. The musculature plays a significant role in spine stability. Disuse or denervation atrophy can result in deformity, degeneration, or other painful pathology. The muscular support must be taken into consideration in regards to the biomechanical anatomy of the spine.

## Biomechanics

Biomechanics involves the application of engineering principles to biologic problems. Biomechanics of the spine refers to understanding the normal and the pathologic function of the spinal column with regards to mechanical insult whether it is rapid and sudden or slow and chronic, occurring over a long period of time. Surgery of the spine further disrupts the normal function of the spinal column and a clear understanding of biomechanics is key to restoring normal or near normal pain-free movement and stability.

### Cartesian Coordinate System

The right-handed Cartesian coordinate system is routinely used in spine biomechanics as a system of reference. This system consists of three axes: the x-axis, the y-axis, and the z-axis. Translational and rotational movement can occur along or about these three axes. Translational movements are positive if they occur in the positive direction of the axis and negative in the negative direction. Rotational movements are considered positive in the clockwise direction when viewed from the origin to the positive direction of the axis and negative when counterclockwise from the same viewpoint. The right-handed Cartesian coordinate system as applied to the spine places the x-axis in the dorsal to ventral plane, the y-axis in the right to left plane, and the z-axis in the rostral to caudal plane. This results in positive moments with flexion, left to right lateral bending, and right axial rotation.

### Vectors, Scalars, Bending Moments, and the Instantaneous Axis of Rotation

A vector is a force oriented in a fixed direction in three-dimensional space (as defined by the right-handed Cartesian coordinate system above). It possesses both magnitude and direction, and it may be broken down into its component forces. A scalar is a quantity that is direction independent and possesses only magnitude. A bending moment occurs when a force acts on a lever, or moment arm. A bending moment, when applied to a point in space, will result in a tendency to rotate about an axis. When these principles are applied to a vertebral body, the axis about which a bending moment causes this tendency to rotate is known as the instantaneous axis of rotation (the IAR). The IAR is the axis about which a vertebral segment rotates at any given instant, and the IAR itself does not move during this rotation or translation. It may be considered a fulcrum about which a segment moves. When a body moves in a plane, there is a point in the body or some extension of it that does not move, and the axis that passes perpendicular to the plane of motion and through this point is the IAR as defined by White and Panjabi.[29] The IAR becomes the center of the Cartesian coordinate system used to define the motion. The IAR is dynamic, and as spinal movement occurs the IAR of each involved segment moves. The location of the IAR depends on the manner in which it is determined and the theoretical foundation on which it is based, and it is therefore subject to error.

## Newton's Laws

Spine surgery involves the application of force to the spine. Fundamental to understanding the stresses withstood by the spine is the concept of action and reaction.[6] Newton's laws of motion describe how objects respond to external forces. The first law is the law of inertia, and it states that if an object is subject to no net force, it maintains a constant velocity. The second law is the law of superimposition of forces and it states that the momentum of an object is equal in magnitude and direction to the vector sum of the forces acting upon it. The third law is the law of conservation of momentum and it states that when two objects collide, the overall momentum is constant such that for every action there is an opposite but equal reaction. As the spine is subject to various loads, force couples are created (based on the third law of motion) and the vertebral segments may fail. When applying forces to the spine in order to repair it, these same concepts need to be considered when, for instance, creating compression of adjacent segments in order to cause fusion or tension bands dorsally or ventrally to restore stability.

## Hooke's Law and Stress/Strain Curves

When external forces act on a solid at rest, the solid will be deformed. According to Hooke's law, for small displacements, the size of the deformation is proportional to the deforming force. For solids within the elastic zone, the relationship between deformation and force is linear. In order to make sense of Hooke's law then as it applies to the spine, the concepts of stress/strain curves and deformation need to be expanded upon. Deformation of a solid can be either elastic or plastic. These are defined by recovery once the deforming force is removed, and they exist on a spectrum that can be best illustrated with a deformation curve (Figure 105.11). When a solid is subject to an external or deforming force Hooke's law applies only when the load and deformation occur within the elastic zone of the solid. The elastic zone is defined by elastic deformation, when a solid totally recovers after removal of a stress. Deformation continues to be proportional to the deforming force until the elastic limit of the solid is reached and the linear relationship between force and deformation no longer exists. Beyond the elastic limit of a material is termed the plastic zone, and this is the zone in which the solid acquires permanent deformation and will not completely recover once the stress is removed. As force continues to be applied, eventually the point of failure is reached. On a stress/strain curve as seen in Figure 105.11, the area under the curve represents the amount of energy absorbed and the ultimate strength of a material (the amount of energy required to reach failure). The neutral zone is an area of nonengagement where force is applied but deformation is minimal. It precedes the linear area of the curve.

## Elastic Modulus

The elastic modulus is a constant defined by and characteristic of a given material. It is an indicator of deformability of a specific material. The modulus of elasticity is defined as stress/strain where stress is the force applied to an object, and strain is the response of the object to the force. Strain is linear (normal) or angular (shear) and is manifest as a change in length or angle of an object subjected to a load. It reflects the force-resisting ability of a material, whether it is tensile or compressive forces in normal strain or angular deformation resistance in shear strain. Stress is defined as the force per unit area applied to an object (see equation in next section).

There are three types of elastic moduli, Young's modulus, shear modulus, and bulk modulus. Young's modulus measures the elastic properties of an object when it is stretched or compressed. Shear modulus measures shear deformation that occurs when transverse forces of opposite direction are applied at opposing faces of an object. Bulk modulus measures deformation when a solid is squeezed.

## Section Modulus and Moment of Inertia

The section modulus is a concept that is calculated and used to define the strength of an object. It is applicable here with regards to spinal implants and instrumentation. It is an indicator of the overall strength and more importantly potential failure of an implant. Section modulus is defined by the equation:

$$Z = P \times D^3/32$$

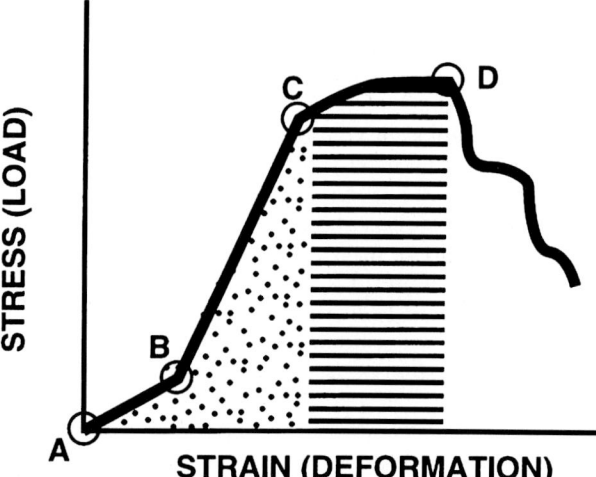

**Figure 105.11** A typical stress/strain curve for a biological tissue, such as a ligament. A-B, the neutral zone. B-C, the elastic zone. When the elastic limit (yield point) C is reached, permanent deformation can occur (permanent set). C-D, the plastic zone where a permanent set occurs. Past D, failure occurs and the load diminishes. Hashed plus dotted area represents strength, whereas the dotted area represents resilience. (*From Benzel EC [ed]:* Biomechanics of Spine Stabilization. *Rolling Meadows, IL, American Association of Neurological Surgeons, 2001.*)

where Z is section modulus and D is diameter. The section modulus or strength of a screw is exponentially related to the diameter of the screw. Other important factors relating to implant failure or potential failure that need to be considered are potential force applications (moment arms, loads, bending moments). Stress defines the relationship of section modulus and bending moment. It represents the force per unit area applied to an object and is defined as:

$$T = M/Z$$

where T is stress, M is bending moment, and Z is section modulus. The bending moment (M) is also defined by an equation.

$$M = F \times D$$

where M is bending moment, F is the force applied, and D is the moment arm through which the force is applied.

The stiffness of an object (implant) is the resistance to deformability. It is also defined by an equation.

$$I = \pi \times D^4/16$$

where I is the moment of inertia and D is the diameter. Therefore, the stiffness is affected to a greater extent by the diameter than the strength and increases more rapidly as diameter increases. This applies directly to screws and rods, which are commonly used implants in the spine.

## Application of Principles to Instrumentation

Surgical implants must be designed with the basic biomechanical principles previously discussed in mind. A clear understanding of the complex forces applied to the spine is necessary when contemplating spinal instrumentation. Important considerations include implant materials, implant bone interface, and the various mechanisms of force application to the spine. Ultimately the forces involved are complex, but they can be broken down into major vector forces. By using vectors and basic biomechanical principles, spinal instrumentation can be systematically analyzed and the appropriate construct applied. Spinal instrumentation is applied for many reasons, and the pathology is beyond the scope of this chapter. Instrumentation and fusion is most often utilized to relieve neural compression and/or to restore stability to the spine and/or to relieve pain.

### Implant Properties

Implants can be made of various materials including metals, nonmetals (i.e., ceramic, glass), and bone. Each material has properties that make it more useful for certain operations, and these specific properties must be kept in mind. An instrumented fusion is essentially a race between fusion formation and instrument failure, and, therefore, certain implants are more suited for this. Metallurgists have produced many alloys, which are now being utilized clinically in spine implants.[6] Stainless steel alloys include 316L stainless steel and 22-13-5 stainless steel, which has the same modulus of elasticity and tensile strength of 316L but twice the ultimate tensile strength.[6] Titanium is available in pure, unalloyed forms, and various alloyed forms.

Pure titanium occurs in several grades (1-4) based on purity and degree of contaminants, and as the oxygen content increases, so does the strength of titanium.[6] The modulus of elasticity remains unaltered but the ultimate strength and 0.2% tensile strength (stress that causes 0.2% deformation) increase with the grade.[7] Titanium may also be alloyed with other elements such as aluminum, vanadium, niobium, and zirconium in specific concentrations resulting in specific properties such as increased resistance to wear.[6] 316L stainless steel and 22-13-5 stainless steel are stiffer than titanium resulting in a smaller transfer of stress from the implant to the bone, termed stress shielding. Elements like chromium and molybdenum present in these alloys provide resistance to corrosion.[6]

Deformability and the ability to resist fatigue are important characteristics of spine implants. Implants do not fail because a static load exceeds the ultimate strength of the implant, they fail because of cyclical loading and fatigue. Fatigue refers to the cumulative damage of cyclical loading that occurs in the form of cracks and corrosion. Titanium performs better than steel at lower frequencies of loading.[27]

Other implant materials include synthetic nonmetals such as polymethylmethacrylate (PMMA), acrylics, ceramics, and glasses. PMMA is most commonly used but only in very specific situations. It has a high modulus of elasticity and is, therefore, very brittle. It has been shown that wire reinforcement, especially with Vitallium, yields a stronger construct.[28]

Finally, bone is commonly used as an implant. Bone graft harvested from the patient (i.e., fibula, iliac crest) is termed an autologous graft while bone graft harvested from a cadaver (and freeze dried or not) is termed allograft. It can be harvested as a strut graft or large piece of bone with both cortical and cancellous bone, which can be cut and shaped to fit into a disc space or to fill the area in which a vertebral body once resided. Bone chips may also be harvested. These consist of cancellous bone, which has been morselized and may come from cadavers or be harvested from the patient. Bone is used to create a fusion, which ultimately lends stability to the spine, and instrumentation will ultimately fail unless fusion and stability are achieved[6]. Bone can be placed ventrally or dorsally in the spine to create a fusion. Ventrally, a bone graft is placed in the weight-bearing part of the spine as an interbody graft, which results in compression and load sharing by the graft. This leads to faster and better healing as dictated by Wolff's law. Wolff explained that internal and external changes in bone architecture occurred according to mathematical laws along with functional changes of bone.[6,30] It has also been shown that electrophysiologic changes occur when bone is placed under compression (i.e., a negative charge is generated).[31] Dorsally, bone is not exposed to the same fusion-enhancing forces as ventral weight bearing grafts. The healing and fusion rates in dorsal fusions are less than in ventral fusions, probably because there is no compression that seems to encourage ventral, interbody fusion.[6,9] The dorsal fusion mass will diminish in volume with time, and it has been shown that a larger volume of initial graft is required for a larger fusion mass at 18 months.[12]

The interface between the implant and bone is important in insuring stability. There are several ways in which implants and bone contact each other. According to Benzel[6] these are: (1) abutting, (2) penetrating, (3) gripping, (4) conforming, and (5) osseointegration. Abutting implants typically include the interbody bone grafts already referred to in the previous paragraph. The role of the interbody implant is to resist axial loads, and this is done most effectively through a large surface area contact between the ends of the bone graft and the adjacent vertebral bodies. Placement of the graft in the IAR is ideal for resisting axial loads, and placement ventral to the IAR will result in a moment arm and some degree of distraction.[6] Penetrating implants include nails, screws, and spikes. The role of the penetrating implant is that of an anchor, and important considerations with regard to these implants include pullout resistance and overall strength when they often function as fixed arm cantilevers.[6] Pullout resistance of screws is enhanced by engaging cortical bone, which markedly resists pullout, and through triangulation (Figure 105.12) or placement of converging or diverging screws optimally at 90 degrees to one another.[5] The bending strength is proportional to the section modulus as discussed above to the cube of the core diameter (i.e., the inner diameter of the screw). The outer diameter and thread depth are important in pullout resistance (Figure 105.13). Hooks and wires are examples of the gripping implants. Wire may be looped around the laminae and spinous processes of adjacent vertebrae and secured via twisting the loops together, and hooks may be placed at the laminae, pedicles, or transverse processes to augment dorsal instrumentation especially screws placed in osteo-porotic bone.[6] They contact cortical bone over a greater surface area and thus may perform better in the setting of osteoporotic bone. Hooks may also be used to augment screw pullout resistance within the same construct.[6] Conforming implants have been mentioned briefly and at this point include PMMA and acrylics. These implants have the unique property of conforming to surrounding bone and are used by some surgeons to augment the screw bone interface.[8,23] The bonding of bone to nonbiologic material is known as osseointegration, and, when this occurs, the load transfer from implant to bone is distributed over a much larger surface area reducing stress risers (focal concentrations of stress).[6] Titanium and a titanium alloy, Ti-13Nb-13Zr (niobium, zirconium), have exhibited potential for osseointegration.[6,10,19]

## Application to Implants

Newton's third law of motion, which states that for every action there is an opposite but equal reaction, governs the placement of spinal implants. Because there is no net movement in the spine when the implant is placed, the forces applied to the spine must occur in pairs such that the net result is zero. No spinal implant is placed in a truly neutral mode because once upright posture is assumed the implant is under some degree of stress, which it then must resist. Implants, when placed dorsally or ventrally, resist these loads dynamically, resulting in load sharing or rigidly resulting in stress shielding. The type of implant is determined by the surgeon when designing the construct, and the surgeon must take into account the region of the spine, the site of fusion (ventral or dorsal), and the forces that will be applied at the site of the implant when the spine is loaded.

Spinal implants impart complex forces on the spine that can be broken down into basic component vectors, and that may be considered separately. Rarely is any one force applied in isolation, and spinal implants function through several of the basic mechanisms of force application. Benzel lists six basic mechanisms of force application: (1) simple distraction, (2) three-point bending, (3) tension-band fixation, (4) fixed moment arm cantilever, (5) non-fixed moment arm cantilever, (6) applied moment arm cantilever.[6] These represent the basic mechanisms by which implants impart force to the spine, and a single implant will often function through several mechanisms at once.

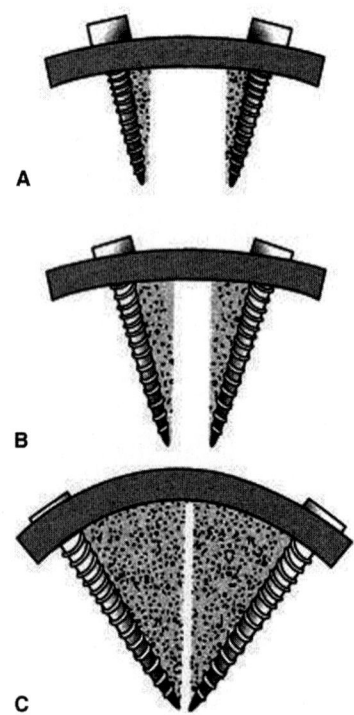

**Figure 105.12** The triangulation effect is proportional to the shaded area subtended by the screw (**A**). The shaded area can be increased by lengthening the screws (**B**) or by altering trajectory (**C**). (*From Benzel EC [ed]: Biomechanics of Spine Stabilization. Rolling Meadows, IL, American Association of Neurological Surgeons, 2001.*)

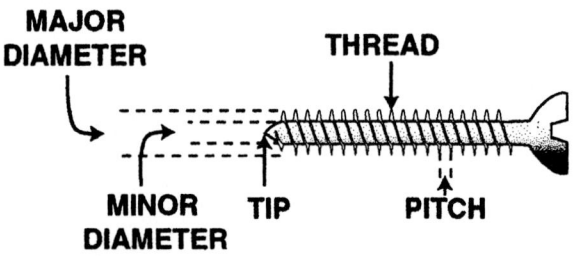

**Figure 105.13** Screw core (minor) and outside (major) diameters, thread depth, and screw pitch. (*From Benzel EC [ed]: Biomechanics of Spine Stabilization. Rolling Meadows, IL, American Association of Neurological Surgeons, 2001.*)

Anterior spine surgery frequently incorporates simple distraction and tension band fixation through nonfixed moment arm cantilever fixation. Three-point bending is also utilized in longer constructs to stabilize the plate and prevent translation. Because surgery in the anterior spine is located ventral to the IAR (the neutral axis is considered in the next section), a bending moment is applied to the instrumented segments. Simple distraction may be applied through ventral placement of an interbody graft (ventral to the neutral axis/IAR) or by placement of a fixed moment arm cantilever in the form of a plate and screws. Plates secured to the anterior spine by screws in distraction are more frequently applied in the cervical spine. They may also be placed in the thoracic and lumbar spine although erosion of the surrounding soft tissue must be considered. Placement of ventral distraction results in extension of the spine, and implants placed in this manner resist axial loads (Figure 105.14). Because these implants bear much of the axial load, failure may occur typically at the screw plate interface. These same implants will resist extension of the spine, and, therefore, act as tension band fixators when the spine is placed in extension. Distraction and compression are forces applied perpendicular to IAR resulting in torque (Figure 105.15). Three-point bending is applied parallel to the IAR and often is accompanied by distraction or compression forces[6] (Figure 105.16). Three-point bending occurs when a fulcrum directs a force vector in a direction opposite to the two terminal force vectors. The force at the fulcrum is equal to the sum of the terminal forces.[6]

Three-point bending requires an intermediate point of fixation between the terminal points of fixation, and when used in a ventral construct will resist translational deformation (Figure 105.17). Ventral compressive implants do not resist axial loads, and the axial load-resisting ability of the spine must be intact or augmented (usually by an interbody graft) when these implants are placed. More recently dynamic ventral systems are being utilized, which allow controlled subsidence and enhanced load sharing by the spine in order to augment bone healing and fusion of interbody grafts, particularly in the cervical spine.

Interbody grafts may be placed in the neutral axis of the spine or the IAR. These implants include autologous bone (i.e., rib, fibula, iliac crest), allograft, acrylic and wire constructs, and cages filled with morselized bone. These implants are usually placed to restore the axial load-bearing ability of the spine, and the principle forces are

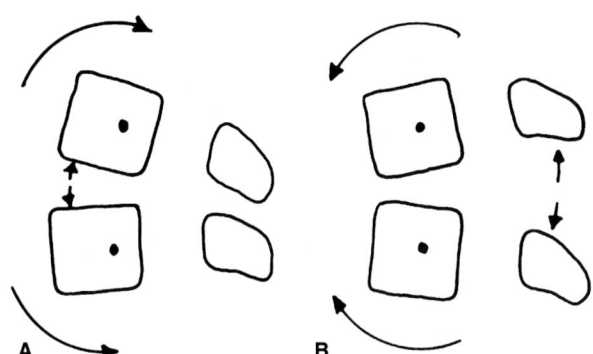

**Figure 105.15** (A) Ventral spinal distraction (*straight arrows*) can cause spinal extension (*curved arrows*) if the distraction forces area is applied ventral to the IAR (neutral axis). (B) Conversely, the application of distraction forces (*straight arrows*) dorsal to the IAR (neutral axis) results in spinal flexion (*curved arrows*) (i.e., in tension-band distraction). (*From Benzel EC [ed]:* Biomechanics of Spine Stabilization. *Rolling Meadows, IL, American Association of Neurological Surgeons, 2001.*)

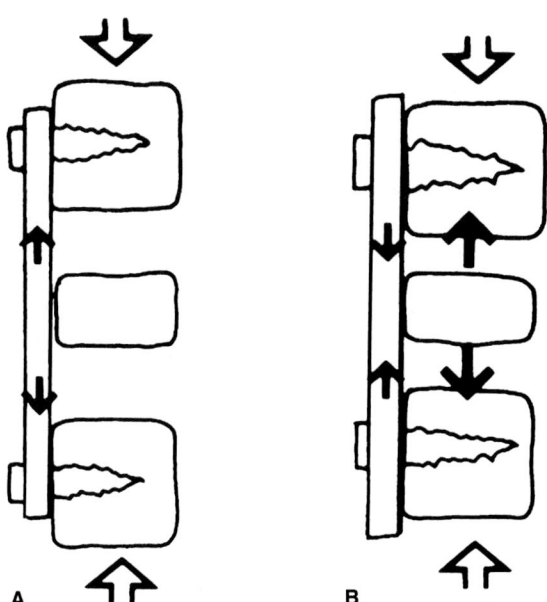

**Figure 105.14** (A) A spinal implant placed in distraction (*thin arrows*). (B) A spinal implant placed in compression (*thin arrows*) shares the axial load (*hollow arrows*) with intrinsic spinal elements (*solid arrows*). The spinal implant is thus unloaded during weight bearing. If enough compression were applied, the spinal implant might conceivably bear no load compression force applied by the implant were equal to the weight of the torso above the implant itself; that is, the case of zero weight bearing. (*From Benzel EC [ed]:* Biomechanics of Spine Stabilization. *Rolling Meadows, IL, American Association of Neurological Surgeons, 2001.*)

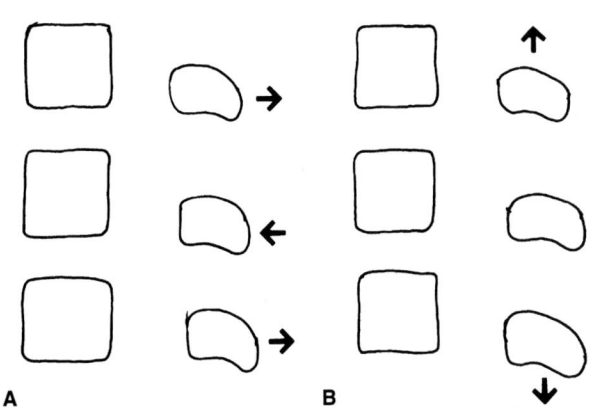

**Figure 105.16** Three-point bending constructs are commonly applied in combination with distraction. These two components, three-point bending (A) and distraction (B), are independent of each other with respect to the forces they apply to the spine. (*From Benzel EC [ed]:* Biomechanics of Spine Stabilization. *Rolling Meadows, IL, American Association of Neurological Surgeons, 2001.*)

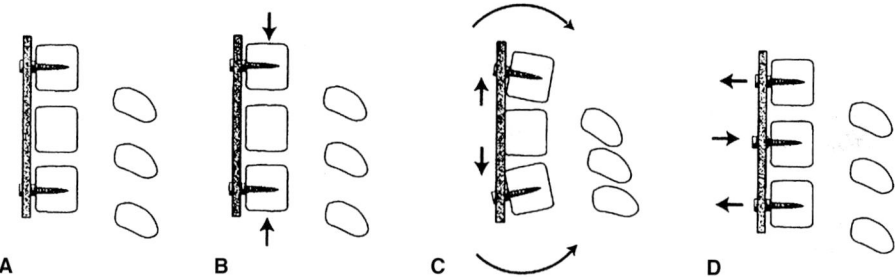

**Figure 105.17** Versatile implants (i.e., implants that can resist a variety of deformations) are optimal. For example, a ventral cervical cantilever beam device **(A)** can resist axial loads *(arrows)* via distraction **(B)** and extension *(curved arrows)* via tension-band fixation **(C)**. If an intermediate point of fixation is used, it can resist translation via a three-part bending mechanism *(arrows)* as well **(D)**. *(From Benzel EC [ed]:* Biomechanics of Spine Stabilization. *Rolling Meadows, IL, American Association of Neurological Surgeons, 2001.)*

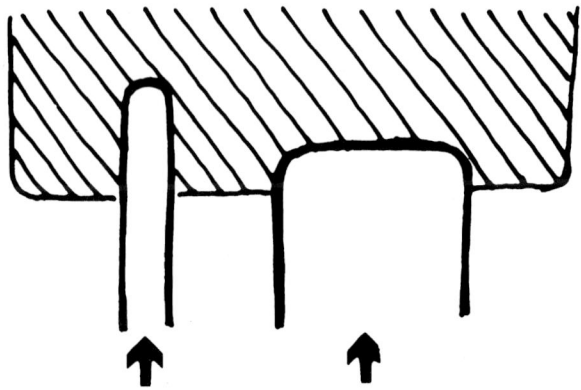

**Figure 105.18** The surface area of the contact surface of interfaces between abutting implants and bone correlates with weight-bearing capacity. A smaller-diameter implant penetrates farther *(left)*, while a larger-diameter implant withstands axial loading more effectively *(right)*. Arrows depict load applied to bone *(hatched area)* by the implant. *(From Benzel EC [ed]:* Biomechanics of Spine Stabilization. *Rolling Meadows, IL, American Association of Neurological Surgeons, 2001.)*

distraction and compression. Removal of a vertebral body (i.e., spondylectomy) or removal of a disc (i.e., discectomy), which incorporates the neutral or weight-bearing axis of the spine, often requires placement of a graft to restore stability. There are several important considerations in placing interbody grafts. Migration of the bone graft into the adjacent vertebral body is known as subsidence. This can be avoided by insuring that the abutting interbody graft occupies a large surface area and is able to withstand axial loads (Figure 105.18). The cortical end plates of the vertebral body may be left intact in order to protect against subsidence as well. The cortical margins of the vertebral body are good buttresses for instrumentation and interbody grafts. Stress shielding occurs when the implant bears more of the axial load than the interbody graft, reducing compressive forces and the chance for fusion by increasing bone resorption. Stress shielding is avoided by placing the interbody graft under compression, which can be achieved by ventral tension band fixation. A final important consideration with regards to interbody grafts is that intact surrounding ligaments as described in the previous section

will add stability when a graft is placed in distraction and the ligaments are placed under tension.

Dorsal instrumentation incorporates distraction, tension band fixation, and three-point bending in order to reduce and stabilize the spine. Often dorsal instrumentation will accompany ventral instrumentation in order to augment the stability of the spine, especially in flexion. Dorsal fixation techniques are numerous and include wires, hooks, screws, and rods. Cross fixation may be added to stabilize the construct and prevent a coronal or sagittal parallelogram deformity (Figure 105.19). Dorsal tension band fixation can be accomplished with laminar wires, clamps, springs, and rigid constructs consisting of lateral mass screws and rods in the cervical spine and pedicle screws, rods, laminar wires, hooks, and cross fixators in the thoracic and lumbar spine. Isolated dorsal compressive constructs are rare. Instrumentation over a number of segments will often employ intermediate points of fixation and three-point bending in order to resist translational deformity (Figure 105.20) . Multisegmented instrumentation insures that the load is distributed over a number of segments. Intact anatomy can be exploited such as in the cervical spine. Dorsal tension band fixation with engagement of the facets results in increased translational stability. At the same time, fusion of the cervical spine can be achieved ventrally and augmented by disruption of the facet joint and subsequent fusion of the lateral masses. As previously stated, axial load bearing by the facet joints is increased when the cervical spine is extended and the joints are engaged. The orientation of the facets resists translational deformity as well.

## Summary

In order to effectively design and place spinal instrumentation, the forces at work must be clearly understood. These are complex, but may be broken down into the most basic components. The process is not straightforward, and results are difficult to predict. Pseudoarthrosis, hardware failure, and failure at the implant bone interface, such as screw pullout, still occur to a significant degree. A clear understanding of the functional anatomy of the spine and good clinical judgment will result in better outcomes.

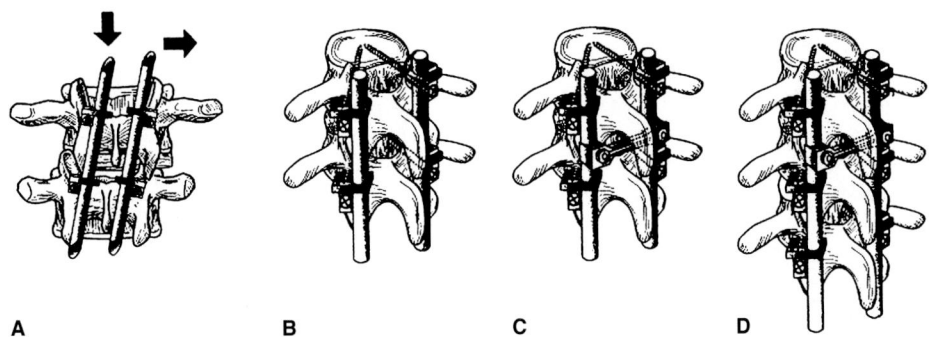

**Figure 105.19** The parallelogram-like effect of lateral translational deformation (**A**) can be prevented by the toeing-in of the screws of the constructs (**B**), providing a cross-fixator (**C**), or increasing the length of the construct to incorporate an additional spine segment (**D**). The latter provides resistance to three-point bending fixation forces in a plane that is lateral to the spine (i.e., coronal plane), as well as in the sagittal plane. *(From Benzel EC [ed]: Biomechanics of Spine Stabilization. Rolling Meadows, IL, American Association of Neurological Surgeons, 2001.)*

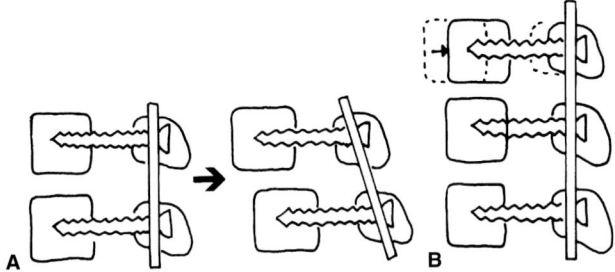

**Figure 105.20** A parallelogram-like translational deformation of the spine in the sagittal plane can occur with nonfixed moment arm cantilever beam constructs (**A**). This untoward occurrence can be minimized by the use of more rigid constructs or the use of a nonfixed moment arm construct over additional caudal segments (**B**). *(From Benzel EC [ed]: Biomechanics of Spine Stabilization. Rolling Meadows, IL, American Association of Neurological Surgeons, 2001.)*

# REFERENCES

1. Abumi K, Panjabi MM, Duranceau JS, Kramer K: Instabilities due to partial and total facetectomies of the lumbar spine. Thirty-Fourth Annual Meeting, Orthopedic Research Society, Atlanta, 1988.
2. Adams MA, Hutton WC: The mechanical function of the lumbar apophyseal joints. *Spine* 8(3):327, 1983.
3. Adams MA, Hutton WC: The relevance of torsion to the mechanical derangement of the lumbar spine. *Spine* 6:241, 1981.
4. Bell GH, Dunbar O, Beck JS, Gibb A: Variation in strength of vertebrae with age and their relation to osteoporosis. *Calcif Tissue Res* 1:75, 1967.
5. Benzel EC, Baldwin NG: Crossed-screw fixation of the unstable thoracic and lumbar spine. *J Neurosurg* 83:11-16, 1995.
6. Benzel EC. *Biomechanics of Spine Stabilization.* Rolling Meadows, IL, American Association of Neurological Surgeons, 2001, pp 1-19.
7. Disegi J: *AO/ASIF Unalloyed Titanium Implant Material,* ed 2. AO/ASIF Materials Technical Commission, 1991, pp 3-25.
8. Duff TA: Surgical stabilization of traumatic cervical spine dislocation using methylmethacrylate. *J Neurosurg* 64: 39-44, 1986.
9. Egger EL, Gottsauner-wolf F, Palmer J, *et al:* Effects of axial dynamization on bone healing. *J Trauma* 34:185-192, 1993.
10. Goodman SB, Davidson JA, *et al:* Histological response to cylinders of a low-modulus titanium alloy (Ti-13Nb-13Zr) and a wear-resistant zirconium alloy (Zr-2.5Nb) implanted in the rabbit tibia. *J Applied Biomaterials* 4;331-339, 1993.
11. Hansson TH, Keller TS, Panjabi MM: A study of the compressive properties of lumbar vertebral trabeculae: effects of tissue characteristics. *Spine* 12:56, 1987.
12. Kim KW, Ha KY, Moon MS, *et al:* Volumetric change of the graft bone after intertransverse fusion. *Spine* 24:428-433, 1999.
13. King AI, Prasad P, Ewing CL: Mechanism of spinal injury due to caudocephalad acceleration. *Orthop Clin N Am* 6:19, 1975.
14. Krag MG, Weaver DL: Morphometry of the thoracic and lumbar spine related to transpedicular screw placement for surgical and spinal fixation. *Spine* 13: 27-32, 1988.
15. Kumar A. Biomechanical testing of vertebral endplate strength: a cadaver study. Presented at the 8th annual meeting of the North American Spine Society, October 20, 1994.
16. Lindahl O: Mechanical properties of dried defatted spongy bone. *Acta Orthop Scand* 47:11, 1976.
17. Markolf KL: Deformation of the thoracolumbar intervertebral joint in response to external loads: a biomechanical study using autopsy material. *J Bone Joint Surg* 54A:511, 1972.
18. McBroom RJ, Hayes WC, Edwards WT, *et al:* Prediction of vertebral body compressive fracture using quantitative computed tomography. *J Bone Joint Surg* 67A(8):1206, 1985.
19. Mishra AK, Bucknell AL, *et al:* In vivo study of anodized commercially pure titanium and diffusion hardened Ti-13Nb-13Zr bone plates in a goat model. Proc Fifth World Biomaterials Congress, Toronto, June, 1996. pp ii-797.
20. Panagiotacopulos, ND, Pope MG, Block R, Krag MH: Water content in human intervertebral discs. Part II. Viscoelastic behavior. *Spine* 12:918, 1987.

21. Panjabi MM, Duranceau J, Goel V, *et al:* Cervical human vertebrae: quantitative three-dimensional anatomy of the middle and lower regions. *Spine* 16:861-869, 1991.

22. Panjabi MM, Greenstein G, Crisco JJ III: Three-dimensional quantitative morphology of lumbar spinal ligaments. *J Spinal Disord* 4:54-72, 1991.

23. Panjabi MM, Hopper W, *et al:* Posterior spine stabilization with methylmethacrylate: biomechanical cement and wire: A clinical review. *J Neurosurg* 68:576-584, 1988.

24. Panjabi MM, White AA, Johnson RM: Cervical spine mechanics as a function of transaction of components. *J. Biomech* 8:327, 1975.

25. Perry, O: Fracture of the vertebral end-plate in the lumbar spine. *Acta Orthop Scand* 25 [Suppl], 1957.

26. Rockoff SD, Sweet E, Bleustein J: The relative contribution of trabecular and cortical bone to the strength of human lumbar vertebrae. *Calcif Tissue Res* 3:163, 1965.

27. Stembough JL, Genaidy AF, *et al:* Biomechanical assessment of titanium and stainless steel posterior spinal constructs: Effects of absolute/relative and frequency on fatigue life and determination of failure modes. *J Spine Disord* 10:473-481, 1997.

28. Taitsman JP, Saha S: Tensile strength of wire-reinforced bone cement and twisted stainless-steel wire. *J Bone Joint Surg* 59A:419-425, 1977.

29. White AA, Panjabi MM: *Clinical Biomechanics of the Spine,* ed 2. Philadelphia, Lippincott, 1990, pp 1-125.

30. Wolff J: *Das Gesetz der Transformation der Knochen,* Berlin, Hirschwald Verlag, 1892.

31. Yasuda I, Noguchi K, *et al:* Callus and electrical callus. *J Bone Joint Surg.* 37A:1292-1293, 1955.

32. Zindrick MR, Wiltse LL, Doornik A, *et al:* Analysis of the morphometric characteristics of the thoracic and lumbar pedicles. *Spine* 12:160-166, 1987.

# CHAPTER 106

# Spinal Implant Attributes: Distraction, Compression, and Three-Point Bending

**Martin W. Weiser, Charles A. Luevano, Vijay K. Goel, Edward C. Benzel, and Nevan G. Baldwin**

Surgeons and engineers who use and design spinal implants must understand the forces acting on the implant and the spine for successful application. These forces are quite complex and constantly change as the patient moves, the spine heals, and the spine-implant interface degrades. This chapter presents a detailed discussion of how various types of distraction, compression, and three-point bending implants carry these forces and redistribute them to the remainder of the spine and related tissues. This information is then used to present strategies that can help prevent overloading any portion of the spine-implant combination (construct) and subsequent failure.

Although the information presented in this chapter is an overview, a more in-depth body of information may be gleaned from a number of sources.[1,5,6,8,9,10-12] Implant-specific information is also available.[2,3,4,7]

## Simple Distraction Fixation

Distraction can be very effective in reestablishing spinal height lost because of compressive fracture. However, it is uncommon to apply distraction alone, via fixation techniques, because it is difficult to apply the forces directly along the neutral axis (the intersection neural surfaces; see Chapter 72) or symmetrically around the neutral axis. The nonsymmetric application of the forces results in the development of a bending moment, as shown in Figure 106.1, since the force is applied at a distance from the instantaneous axis of rotation (IAR). This figure shows the IAR in the disc between the vertebra because the disc is quite flexible and will deform much more than the rigid vertebra at low loads. This bending moment results in compression of the spine on the opposite side of the IAR from the site of distraction force application. The moment of inertia of the structure about the IAR resists this bending moment. The moment (the bending moment that resists deformation and that is usually derived from intrinsic spinal elements—for example, ligaments) can be increased by tensile structures (ligamentous or implant) that are

farther from the IAR than the distraction forces. The moment can be eliminated (no resultant moment) by balancing the distraction and tensile moments as shown in the following equation:

$$F_d \times d_d + F_t \times d_t = 0 \quad (1)$$

where $F_d$ and $d_d$ are the distraction force and lever arm length and $F_t$ and $d_t$ are the tensile force and moment arm length.

The development of bending moments is particularly problematic when the isolated distraction forces are applied dorsal to the IAR. This results in exaggeration of kyphotic deformities (compression of the vertebral body, which is often the site of pathology). The moment of the spine in flexion is quite low, in part because of the low tensile stiffness of the posterior longitudinal ligament. In addition, the anterior longitudinal ligament often limits distraction. Therefore, simple dorsal distraction is uncommonly applied, although it can be combined with three-point bending fixation to impart desirable results.

Simple distraction may be applied to the lateral or ventral portions of the spine. This is because the moment of the spine is higher for extension and in the coronal plane.[11] In addition, these locations are closer to both the IAR and the site of fracture. This results in less compression of the contralateral side of the IAR. It is also easier to align ventral distraction implants with the IAR. This makes them very effective in resisting the bending moments caused by axial loads applied through the center of gravity, which is situated ventral to the spine. These implants can be placed in either an active mode to decompress the fracture or in a neutral mode to resist recompression when the patient assumes an upright posture.

## Three-Point Bending Fixation

A pencil can be placed in three-point bending by placing the thumbs together in the center and the fingers at the ends and pushing on the center of the pencil with the thumbs. The central force vector has twice the magnitude of the sum of the terminal force vectors and the opposite sign. Three-point bending spinal instrumentation applies similar force vectors. They are usually, but not always, applied with an accompanying distraction force by using instrumentation such as Harrington distraction rods or universal spinal instrumentation.

Three-point bending implants usually involve application of dorsal instrumentation over multiple spinal segments (five or more spinal segments).The forces at the rostral and caudal implant-bone interfaces are usually dorsally directed. The central force is usually in the ventral direction. This central force is equal to the sum of the two dorsally directed forces and is normally located over the dorsal surface of the vertebra that requires decompression. If the dorsal surface of this central vertebra is damaged so that it will not resist the application of the force, the location of ventral force application can be moved to the vertebrae above and below the damaged vertebra. This results in *four-point bending fixation*. The effects are very similar to three-point bending fixation, but larger forces or longer moment arms (more spinal segments) are required

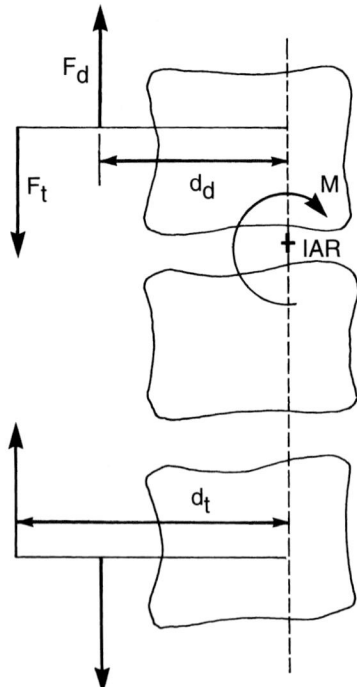

**Figure 106.1** Bending moment $(M)$ resulting from nonsymmetric distraction forces $(F_d)$. The negative moment shown results from the distraction bending moment being larger than the tensile bending moment $(F_t,$ applied by interspinous and other ligaments). $d_d$, Distraction moment arm; $d_t$, tensile moment arm.

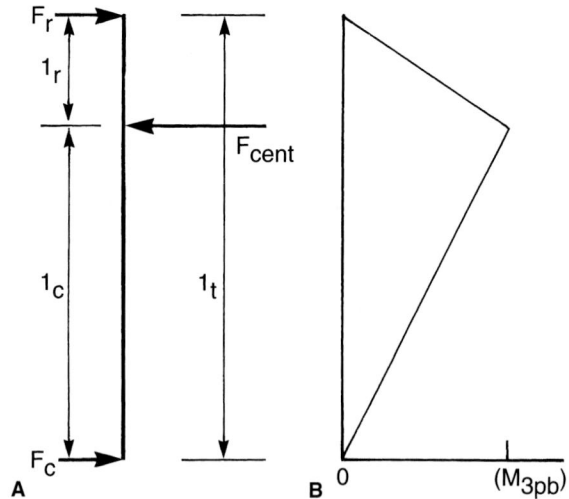

**Figure 106.2** Three-point bending fixation showing **(A)** forces and lengths and **(B)** bending moment as a function of position. $1_t$, Length of construct; $1_r$, length of rostral portion; $1_c$, length of caudal portion of construct; $F_r$, rostrally applied force; $F_c$, caudally applied force; $F_{cent}$, centrally applied force.

to obtain the same bending moment and decompression. This can be visualized by moving the thumbs apart while keeping the fingers in the same location when bending the pencil, as in the example above.

The maximum bending moment, $M_{3pb}$, in three-point bending fixation occurs at the location of the central force and is described by

$$M_{3pb} = F_r \times l_r = F_c \times l_c \qquad (2)$$

where the forces and lengths are as defined in Figure 106.2A, and the system is assumed to be at rest. The requirement that the sum of the three forces be zero can be used to derive the moment in terms of the central force[2] as follows:

$$M_{3pb} = \frac{F_{cent}\, l_r\, l_c}{l_r + l_c} = \frac{F_{cent}\, l_r\, l_c}{l_t} \qquad (3)$$

Examination of this equation shows that the largest moment is obtained when the lengths of the two moment arms, and hence the terminal forces, are the same.

$$F_r = F_c = 0.5 F_{cent}$$

$$l_r = l_c = 0.5\, l_t \qquad (4)$$

$$M_{3pb\ max} = 0.25\, F_{cent}\, l_t$$

Figure 106.2B shows that the moment decreases linearly from the central loading point until it reaches a value of zero at the terminal loading points.

As discussed earlier, it is rare to apply isolated dorsal distraction forces. This is because dorsal distraction also

results in flexion of the spine, because the IAR is ventral to the force application points. Three-point bending fixation opposes this flexion. It is common to combine the two modes of force application. This can be accomplished by bending the rod so that it makes contact with the spine at the location at which the ventral force application is desired or by using a sleeve to increase the diameter of the rod at this location.[7] There are several disadvantages of bent rods. The first is that the rods are difficult to bend to achieve the proper angle. Second, bending fatigues the rod and can result in failure, particularly if multiple bends are necessary to obtain a good fit. Finally, round rods can rotate at the hook interface so that the bend is no longer in the sagittal plane.

Three-point bending fixation can also be used to correct deformities at either termini of an implant as well, particularly deformities in the sagittal plane. The terminal hook applies a dorsal force that can be used to eliminate pressure on the spinal cord by the dorsal surface of the spinal canal. The implant is normally positioned so that the sagittal deformation is at its rostral end. This is because sagittal plane deformations are usually the result of shearing of a vertebra ventrally with respect to the next most caudal vertebra while maintaining normal orientation with respect to the next most rostral vertebra. This deformity can also be corrected by applying a ventral force at the center of the construct and dorsal forces at the ends. However, application of the ventral force by using the rostral terminus is much easier because the vertebra to be moved can be affixed to the rod while the remainder of the rod is used as a lever. In this application, $1_r$ (length of rostral portion) is normally quite short (one segment) and $1_c$ (length of caudal portion) is longer (two to four segments), which allows a large rostral force with application of a small caudal force.

Combined distraction and three-point bending fixation creates a more complex loading state. This is particularly evident at the terminal rod hook, as shown in Figure 106.3

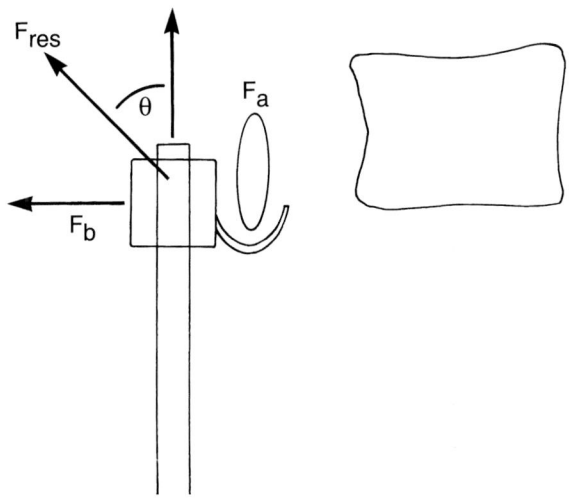

**Figure 106.3** Forces at the rostral end of a combined distraction and three-point bending implant. $F_a$, Distraction force; $F_b$, three-point bending force; $F_{res}$, resultant force.

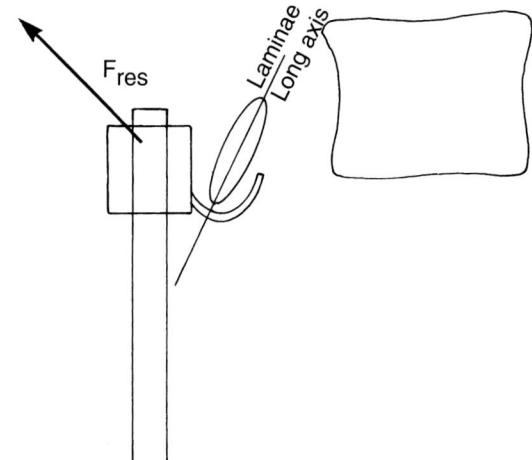

**Figure 106.4** Inclined force at the terminus of a three-point bending construct loading the laminae in a weak direction.

for the rostral terminus. The resultant force at the hook is the vector sum of all of the distraction and dorsal bending forces and is described by the equation

$$F_{res} = F_a + F_b \qquad (5)$$

where $F_a$ and $F_b$ are the distraction and three-point bending forces, respectively, and $F_{res}$ is the resultant force. The magnitude and direction of this force is

$$F_{res} = \overline{\sqrt{F_a^2 + F_b^2}} \text{ (magnitude)} \qquad (6)$$
$$\theta = \cos^{-1}(F_a/F_{res}) \text{ } (direction)$$

where $\theta$ is the angle between the resultant and axial forces.

Combined distraction and bending results in the terminal force vectors being oriented at an angle with respect to the spinal axis. This may be a suboptimal orientation of the force vector for two reasons. First, the inclined force vector can result in loading of the lamina in a weak direction. This is particularly dramatic if the long axis of the lamina cross section is perpendicular to the loading direction, as shown in Figure 106.4. The lamina will carry pure distraction or pure bending loads better than the combined load because its moment of inertia will be higher in these directions. The second reason is that when the rod terminus is being used to correct a kyphotic deformation, the inclined force vector distracts the rostral vertebra and rotates it dorsally. Both problems can be mitigated by clamping the rod to laminae between the center and the terminus. This divides the load between two or more laminae. Careful positioning of the clamps allows the forces on the terminal vertebra to be almost entirely distraction forces or entirely bending forces.

## Tension-Band (Compression) Fixation

Dorsal spinal compression (tension-band fixation) can be applied with many different types of implants that include wires, springs, or rigid constructs such as Halifax clamps, Knodt rods (in compression), Harrington compression rods, or universal spinal instrumentation techniques applied in compression. These techniques all apply spinal compression forces at their point of application, which may be on the dorsal, ventral, or lateral surfaces of the spine.

Tension-band fixation also results in the development of bending moments in the compressed segments that can cause flexion or extension. The magnitude of the bending moment, $M_{tbf}$, for tension-band fixation techniques is

$$M_{tbf} = F_{tbf} \, d_{IARtbf} \qquad (7)$$

where $F_{tbf}$ is compression force applied by the tension-band construct and $d_{IARtbf}$ is the perpendicular distance from the IAR to the applied force, as shown in Figure 106.5. The amount of flexion or extension that results from tension-band fixation depends both on the distance from the IAR and on the flexural rigidity of the segment of the spine to be instrumented. Dorsal application of the tension-band normally results in a larger moment than ventral application because the IAR is ventral to the spinal canal. Typical spinal segments are normally about twice as stiff in extension as in flexion. These factors essentially neutralize each other. Therefore the deformations are about the same for dorsal and ventral applications. However, the flexural rigidity of a damaged segment may be dramatically less than that of a healthy segment; thus, much larger extension and flexion deformations are possible for the same tension-band force.

Normally, it is possible to effectively fix only a few segments with this technique. This is primarily a result of bending of the segments that is a consequence of the compressive force being offset from the IAR. Once the segment bends, the distance between the anchor points is reduced, and a lower force is generated. For most implants the generated force ($F_i$) depends linearly on the displacement in the implant as follows:

$$F_i = S_i \, \Delta l_i \qquad (8)$$

where $S_i$ is the stiffness of the implant and $l_i$ is the length of the implant. For rigid constructs and wires, the force reaches zero with very little decrease in the interanchor

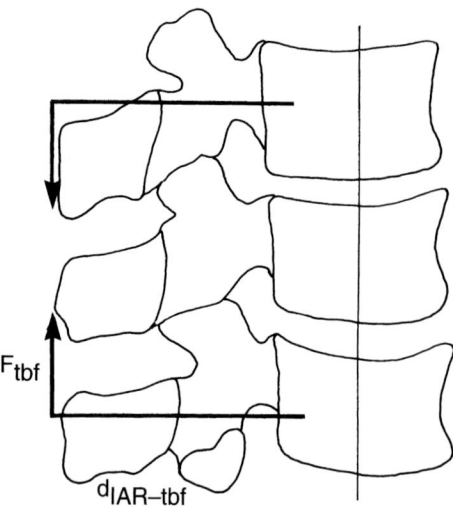

**Figure 106.5** Dorsal tension-band fixation showing the locations of the forces and the IAR.

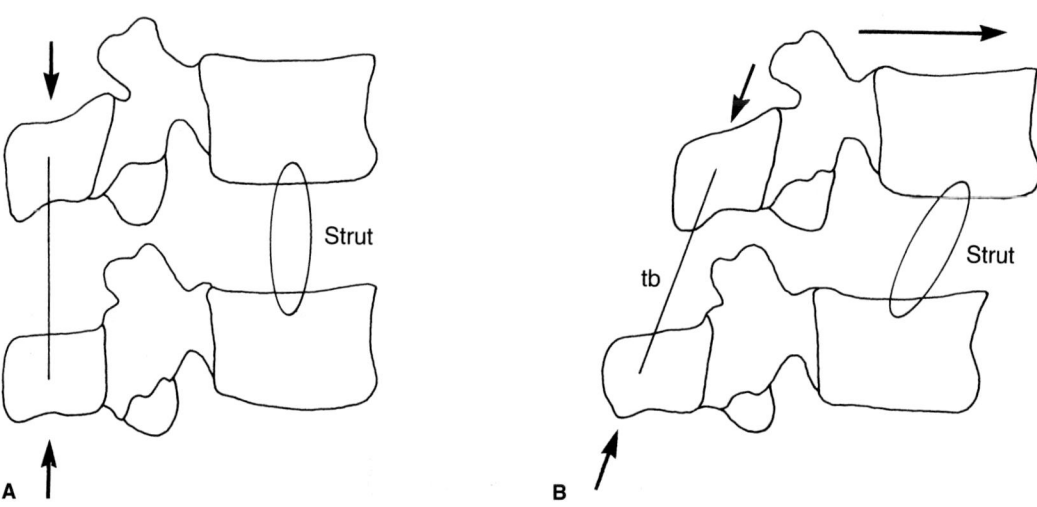

**Figure 106.6 (A-B)** Translation instability of tension-band fixation. The arrows depict applied tension-band fixation forces.

distance. This is because the stiffness of the implant is so high.

$$S_i = \frac{E_i A_i}{l_i} \qquad (9)$$

The above is due to the high elastic modulus ($E_i$) of most implant materials. Springs continue to apply a significant fraction of the initial force because the stiffness of the spring is much lower. Springs are designed to yield a linear force-displacement curve for large displacements.

One problem with tension-band fixation is that extradural masses (bone or disc fragments) can be thrust into the spinal canal during instrumentation application. Therefore decompression procedures may be appropriate before the application of the implant. In addition, tension-band fixation does not control translational movements well, as shown in Figure 106.6. It may even accentuate this motion if this decreases the distance between the insertion points of the tension

band. Therefore, significant spinal integrity must be present when tension-band fixation is used.

## Loading of Rigid or Semirigid Distraction and Compression Constructs

The loading of a construct is much more complex than the simplified models used in the above discussion. All implants are subjected to axial and transverse forces along with bending moments. These forces and bending moments change dramatically when the patient assumes an upright stance and during normal movement. The implant bears part of the load (load bearing) and shares the load with the spine and other structures (load sharing). The fractions of the load that are borne by the implant and shared with the anatomy must be considered each time a spinal implant is used. Neutral constructs (zero load) serve no purpose because the implant must bear a load if it is to correct a spinal deformity or resist deformation. Implants can be placed in a neutral mode, but they will bear a load once the patient assumes an upright posture or moves.

The discussion above of distraction and compression implants assumes isolated axial loads and force applications. However, there are many forces applied by the torso to the implant and by the implant to the spine in the clinical situation. The load on the spine in an upright posture is approximately two to three times the weight of the torso above that section of the spine, as discussed in Chapter 72. The nature of the forces that the implant has to bear will depend both on the mode of insertion (compression, neutral, or distraction) and on the location of the implant.

The center of gravity for the upright body is ventral to the spine. This results in spinal structures ventral to the normal IAR (IAR$_n$) being in compression and structures that are dorsal being in tension during the assumption of the upright posture. Therefore the physiologic loads on the implant depend on the location of the implant. In addition, modifications of the spinal structures during surgery change the flexural rigidity of the functional spinal unit and the location of the IAR. Replacement of a disc or vertebral body with a bone graft (strut) forces the IAR to this location because the axially rigid strut acts as a pivot point for intervertebral motion. The ventrally situated strut shown in Figure 106.7 is then subjected to compressive loads. The dorsal structures of the spine and any implants located in this area will be subjected to lower loads than those applied to normal anatomy. This is because the moment arm available to resist the bending moment (because of the ventral center of gravity) is longer.

Struts that are located dorsal to the normal IAR, as depicted in Figure 106.8A, subject the strut, any dorsal structures, and any dorsal tension band to much larger than normal loads. This is a result of the longer moment arm for the center of gravity and the shorter moment arm for the dorsal structures. A compressive implant can be installed on the ventral side of the normal IAR, as shown in Figure 106.8B, to carry part of the compressive load and move the IAR ventrally to alleviate these large loads.

The net forces on an implant during use are found by a vector summation of the forces resulting from physiologic and surgical loading. For the simple axial loading being considered here, this results in either an increase or a decrease in the forces. The forces borne by distractive implants located dorsal to the IAR and compressive implants located ventral to the IAR will be reduced or will change the sign on application of the physiologic loads. This is because the center of gravity is ventral to the IAR of the spine, resulting in a bending moment that applies a tensile force to dorsal spinal elements and a compressive force to ventral spinal elements. Reduction of the forces borne by the implant is a form of load sharing. It minimizes complications, because the deformation caused by

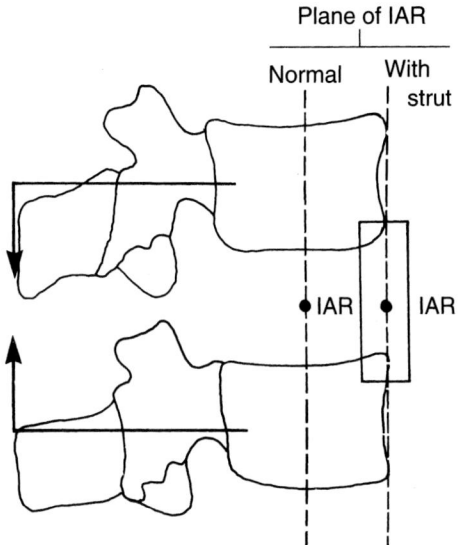

**Figure 106.7** Effect of ventral strut on the IAR and forces resulting from physiologic loading.

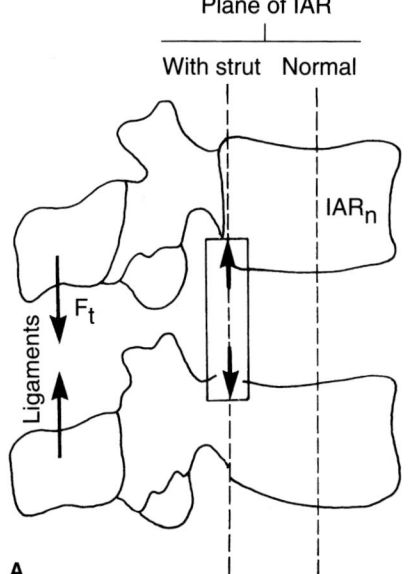

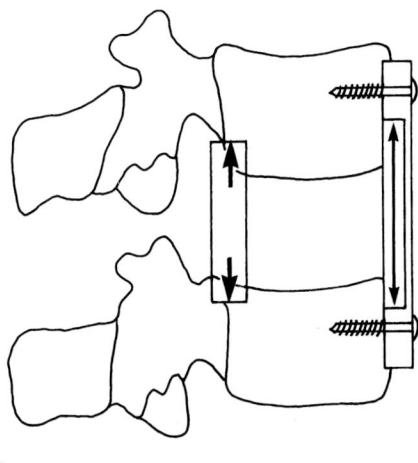

**Figure 106.8** Effect of a dorsal strut on the IAR and forces resulting from physiologic loading. **(A)** Without load sharing. **(B)** With load sharing with a ventral implant.

physiologic loading is in the same orientation as that from the surgical loading (dorsal distraction or ventral compression). However, reversal of the forces borne by the implant can cause problems if the implant is normally designed to bear only one type of load. An excellent example is disengagement of the hooks from the laminae in Harrington distraction rods. This occurs when the distance between the laminae increases in response to the physiologic loading, as shown in Figure 106.9A. This problem can be prevented by placing opposing hooks (claw) around the laminae so that the implant becomes a compressive implant on load reversal, as shown in Figure 106.9B. On the other hand, screw-based implants do not produce this problem, because they are rigidly attached to both the vertebra and the rod.

The forces borne by distractive implants placed ventral to the IAR and compressive implants located dorsal to the IAR increase beyond the surgical loading after physiologic loading. The compressive forces applied to the ventral distractive implants increase dramatically when the patient assumes an upright posture. This is a result of the need both to support the weight of the torso and to resist the bending moment caused by the offset center of gravity of the torso. However, the compressive forces resulting from the bending moment are not as large as for a normal spine, because the addition of the stiff implant moves the IAR ventrally. The tensile forces in the dorsal compressive implant increase to resist the bending moment associated with the center of gravity. However, this increase may be offset by settling of the spine as structures, such as the discs, undergo viscoelastic deformation. These additional forces may be large enough to cause failure of the implants or, more likely, of the interface between the implant and the bone.

## Comparison of Three-Point Bending and Tension-Band Fixation

Both three-point bending and tension-band fixation can be used to generate therapeutic bending moments in the spine. However, the methods by which they generate these moments are significantly different. Three-point bending fixation techniques require the use of either long implants or large forces perpendicular to the spine to generate the necessary bending moments. This is because the bending moment is directly proportional to both the length of the moment arm and the applied perpendicular force as described by Equation 2. The bending moment developed by a tension-band implant depends on the length of the moment arm perpendicular to the spine and the axial force but is independent of implant length as described by Equation 7. Therefore, three-point bending implants are usually employed over more spinal segments (typically five or more) than are tension-band fixation implants (typically two or three segments).

The bending moments present along the spine in a three-point bending construct and a tension-band construct are dramatically different, as observed by comparing Figures 106.2B and 106.5B. For small deformations of a homogeneous body the deformations resulting from these two types of fixation are very similar, as shown in Figure 106.10.

A ventrally directed force is often desirable at the point of spine fracture to move the fractured vertebra ventrally

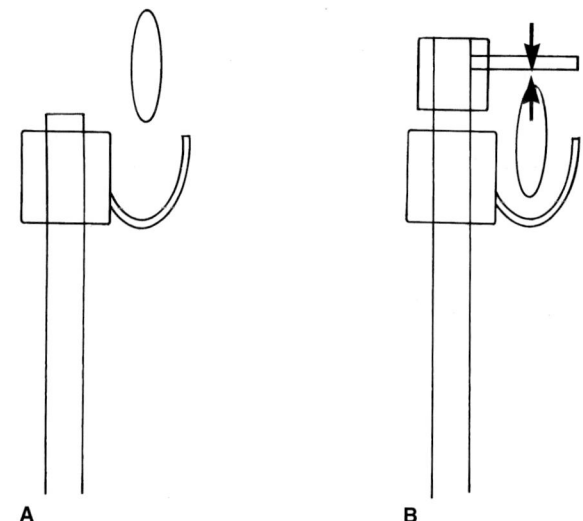

**Figure 106.9** Reversal of loading for dorsal distractive constructs. **(A)** Disengagement of hooks. **(B)** Placement of opposed hooks to prevent disengagement.

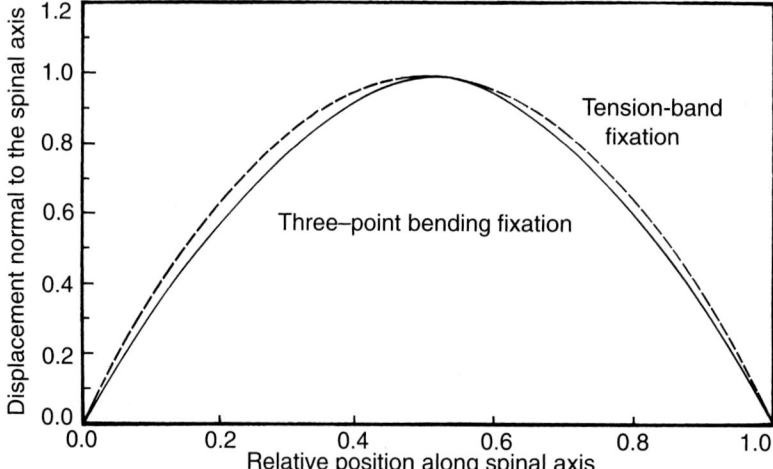

**Figure 106.10** Deformation of a homogenous body because of three-point bending and tension-band fixation.

(since it is often displaced dorsally during fracture). The effective force for the tension-band implant increases with increasing moment arm length ($d_{IAR-tbf}$) but decreases with increasing distance between the attachment points. The product of $F_{tbf}$ and $d_{IAR-tbf}$ is limited by the characteristics of the implant, the compressive strength of the bones or implant at the IAR, and the desire to keep the implant in the body. A long tension-band implant therefore decreases the ventrally directed force. Besides decreasing the ventrally directed force, a long tension-band fixation implant may result in exaggerated extension of the spine. This is a result of either $d_{IAR-tbf}$ increasing as the spine extends or of the spine buckling as the fracture site returns to a kyphotic orientation as shown in Figure 106.11. Therefore, long tension-band fixation should be avoided.[2]

The spine is a very inhomogeneous structure composed of stiff, rigid vertebrae connected through much more flexible discs. In addition, a damaged spine often contains regions with almost no stiffness and rigidity, where portions of one or more vertebrae have been removed. This causes the ventral forces and resulting displacements for tension-band constructs to vary greatly along the construct and from installation to installation. Therefore, if a ventral force is required in a specific location, it is better to use a three-point bending fixture to place this force precisely.

Three-point bending fixation techniques often incorporate distraction forces applied at the terminal (and intermediate) implant-bone interfaces. This increases the stresses applied to the bone as discussed earlier (see Equation 5 and Figure 106.3). However, this does not change the bending moment if the central ventral force and the terminal dorsal forces are not changed. Some authors have advocated using exaggerated distraction forces in conjunction with three-point bending to accomplish spinal column reduction and spinal canal decompression.[5] However, this has not always met with success because of the "sagittal bowstring" effect[2] and fracture of the dorsal fixation site, because the probability of fixation site fracture is increased by the greater total force when both bending and distraction forces are present.

Longer three-point bending implants (more than five spinal segments) can be used to spread the bending and distractive forces over more laminae. They often increase the stability of the construct with regard to physiologic forces because of the greater mechanical advantage and larger number of bone-implant junctures. In addition to increased resistance to the axial and sagittal plane loading discussed above, these constructs are also much more resistant to torsional and translational loads. This is a consequence of connecting more segments, which stiffens the construct with respect to the out-of-plane stresses that create torsional and translational loads. However, such long constructs tend to increase patient discomfort and can result in spinal failure in the segments that are immediately rostral or caudal to the construct. Failure of the spine in these regions is a result of the concentration of the motion (rotation, flexion, and extension) just beyond the ends of the stiff construct.

## REFERENCES

1. Benzel EC: Biomechanics of lumbar and lumbosacral spine fractures. In Rea GL (ed): *Spinal Trauma: Current Evaluation and Management.* American Association of Neurological Surgeons, 1993.
2. Benzel EC: *Biomechanics of Spine Stabilization: Principles and Practice.* New York, McGraw-Hill, 1995.
3. Benzel EC, Larson SJ: Operative stabilization of the posttraumatic thoracic and lumbar spine: A comparative analysis of the Harrington distraction rod and the modified Weiss spring. *Neurosurgery* 19:378-385, 1986.
4. Benzel EC, Kesterson L, Marchand EP: Texas Scottish Rite Hospital rod instrumentation for thoracic and lumbar spine trauma. *J Neurosurg* 75:382-387, 1991.
5. Breig A: *Adverse Mechanical Tension in the Central Nervous System: An Analysis of Cause and Effect: Relief by Functional Neurosurgery.* New York, Almqvist and Wiskell, 1978.
6. Carson WL, Duffield RC, Arendt M, *et al*: Internal forces and moments in transpedicular spine instrumentation. *Spine* 15:893-901, 1990.
7. Edwards CC, Levine AM: Early rod-sleeve stabilization of the injured thoracic and lumbar spine. *Orthop Clin North Am* 17:121-145, 1986.
8. Goel VK, Weinsein JN: *Biomechanics of the Spine: Clinical and Surgical Perspective.* Boca Raton, FL, CRC Press, 1989.
9. Goel VK, Lim T-H, Gwon J, *et al*: Effects of rigidity on an internal fixation device, a comprehensive biomedical investigation. *Spine* 16:S155-S161, 1991.
10. Lindahl O: Mechanical properties of dried defatted spongy bone. *Acta Orthop Scand* 47:11, 1976.
11. White AA, Panjabi MM: *Clinical Biomechanics of the Spine,* ed 2. Philadelphia, Lippincott-Raven, 1990.
12. Yoganandan N, Larson SJ, Pintar F, *et al*: Biomechanics of lumbar pedicle screw/plate fixation in trauma. *Neurosurgery* 27:873-881, 1990.

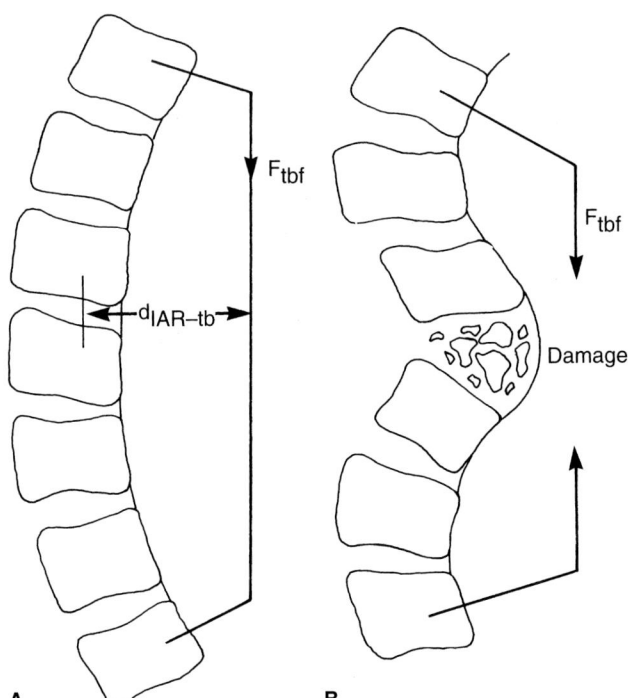

**Figure 106.11** Exaggerated extension in a long tension fixation in an extended spine (**A**) and a "buckled" spine (**B**).

# CHAPTER 107

# Spinal Implant Attributes: Cantilever Beam Fixation

**James P. Hollowell, Narayan Yoganandan, and Edward C. Benzel**

A cantilever is a beam that is attached to an immobile object at one end only. A screw attached to a rod or plate is, therefore, a cantilever beam. It in turn provides cantilever beam fixation. Although long cantilever beam constructs are commonly employed, cantilever beam fixation refers to systems that are typically confined to a single spinal level above and below the area of pathology (short-segment fixation).[3] Clinical failure of this configuration is not uncommon. This emphasizes the importance of a complete understanding of biomechanical principles.[8,12,20,24] The relatively high failure rate of this construct has caused some spinal surgeons to abandon this technique altogether, and others have limited its use to specific situations. Appreciation of the clinical and biomechanical issues permits the safe and effective use of this construct.

The more recent appeal of short-segment fixation is due to several factors. Longer fixation constructs, especially of the lumbar spine, may be associated with excessive pain, suggesting that a shorter construct may reduce pain.[6,14] Shorter constructs require less bone harvest for fusion. Consequently, fusion is readily performed on the entire length of the construct. This eliminates the need for device removal in many patients. Confining instrumentation to the fused levels also avoids the uncertain outcome associated with instrumenting unfused segments. Furthermore, the installation of a short (bilevel) pedicle screw construct requires less soft-tissue dissection and therefore reduces blood loss and operating time. The recent interest has been encouraged by continuing progress in design. Implants capable of withstanding the considerable forces that must be overcome by bilevel fixation have recently been employed.

Several clinical series that used short-segment pedicle fixation have been published.* Whitecloud et al.[31] reported poor results in 4 of 11 patients treated with a variable screw plating (VSP) system for thoracolumbar fractures. This was due to screw breakage and progressive deformity. They concluded that due to the high failure rate, this technique should probably not be performed without ventral interbody grafting. Esses et al.[12] have reported on a multicenter study of 120 patients treated with the AO fixateur interne for thoracolumbar fractures and dislocations.

Eighty-nine patients had a minimal follow-up of 6 months. Only three of the patients underwent ventral surgery. Mean improvement of kyphotic deformity for compression and burst fractures was 14 degrees. In only two cases was this correction significantly lost. Both were associated with hardware loosening.

Lindsey and Dick[20] reported the use of the AO fixateur interne in 80 patients with thoracolumbar fractures and neurologic deficit with a minimum of 2-year follow-up. They averaged 10 degrees of surgical correction of kyphotic deformity but lost all but 1 degree of correction by 2 years. However "formal" fusion was not performed in 70% of these patients, and apparently no ventral surgery was performed. Broken screws were noted in 5 patients, leading to additional surgery in only 1. Early postoperative loss of correction was reported in 3 cases, 2 caused by "extensive vertebral comminution" and 1 caused by malplaced screws.

Daniaux et al.[8] reported short-segment pedicle fixation of 243 patients when using various techniques and devices. They found that rigidly fixed screw and plate systems, without interbody bone grafting, resulted in a 41% rate of screw fracture. If intrabody and interbody grafting was performed with cancellous bone introduced through a funnel, the screw fracture rate could be reduced to 19%. The latter technique resulted in an overall loss of 6 degrees of correction and should not be considered a technique that provides immediate ventral load sharing.

## Cantilever Beam

A cantilever is a large projecting bracket or beam supported at one end only.[3] In the spine, such a construct must support the load of the spinal column or resist deformation in the beam (pedicle screw). It transmits loads through a vertical member (rod or plate), which in turn transmits the load back to the spinal column through another beam (Figure 107.1). The prototype of this construct is a single-level rigid pedicle fixation above and below a pathologic spinal segment (fixed moment arm cantilever beam).[3] The best way to protect such a cantilevered construct from failure is to not use it. Reconstructing the intervening spine element(s) to provide support to the beam (load sharing) is likely to significantly reduce the incidence of device failure, because the inherent weakness of the "cantilever" construct is obviated when the device is no longer cantilevered. The concept of load sharing is more important with cantilevered constructs than any other spinal fixation device.

Other devices, superficially similar in appearance to cantilevered devices (but entirely different in biomechanical properties) have screws that extend through a plate but are not rigidly attached to the plate. These constructs, such as older Luque plates, do not have a rigidly fixed beam, will not support an axial load, and are not cantilevered devices (nonfixed moment arm cantilever beam).[3] With this type of fixation, the pedicle screw experiences a direct tensile "pull-out" force rather than the bending moment of a rigidly fixed device that results in a failure pattern of screw "back-out" rather than proximal screw fracture.[15] Screw back-out was the mode of device failure in 9.3% of 85 cases of lumbar fusion for degenerative disease[16] with a follow-up of 6 years.

---

*References 4,8,9,11,12,22,24,31.

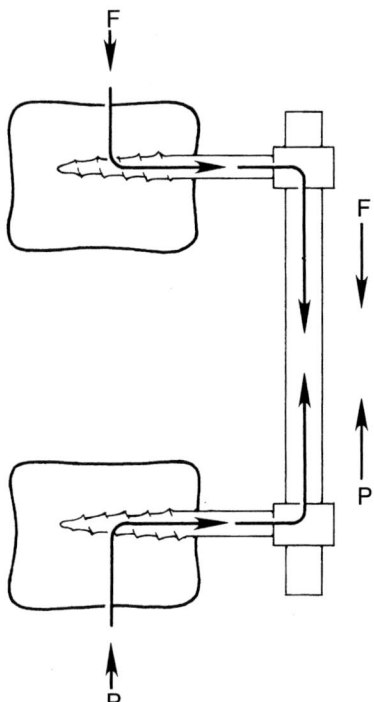

**Figure 107.1** Transmission of loads through a cantilevered short-segment pedicle fixation construct.

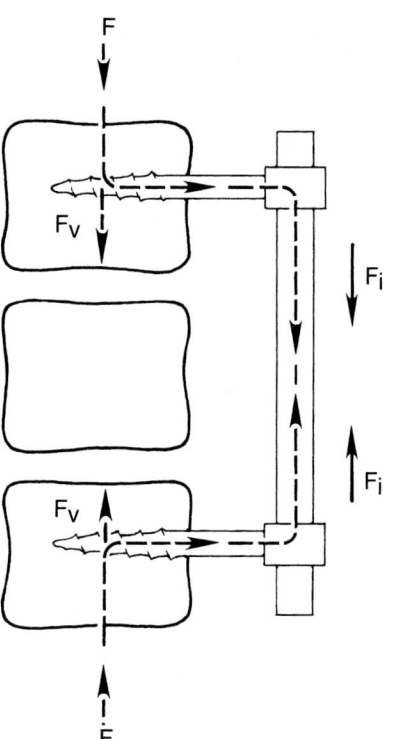

**Figure 107.2** Transmission of loads through anterior spinal column $(F_v)$ and through instrumentation $(F_i)$.

Because these devices are clearly inferior to rigidly fixed pedicle screw systems in their ability to resist an otherwise unsupported axial load, they are not clinically appropriate when such support is required. Other cantilevered devices include ventral spinal plates with rigidly affixed screws used in the cervical and thoracolumbar spine (fixed moment arm cantilevers). Cervical lateral mass plates and many thoracolumbar plates lack fixation of the screw to the plate and are *non-fixed moment arm cantilevers*.

Finally, moment arms can be applied via a cantilevered implant (applied moment arm cantilever). This can be employed to reduce deformation. The AO fixateur interne is an example of this type of implant.[20]

## Loading Path

The loads transmitted through a pedicle screw fixation construct (fixed moment arm cantilever) are depicted in Figure 107.2. The total applied force $(F)$ is transmitted through the vertebra $(F_v)$ and/or through the longitudinal element of the instrumentation $(F_i)$. The entire load of the upper torso can be conceptualized as a force applied at the center of gravity of the torso, which is dependent on the spinal level. The amount of the load that is transmitted through the intervening vertebral body, or reconstructed segment, depends entirely on the integrity of the body, or construct, and hence its ability to "load share." In an extreme case of a traumatic comminution of the intervening body depicted in Figure 107.3, the body is unable to share any load and the entire total applied force $(F)$ is transmitted through the instrumentation $(F_i)$. This situation is clearly the most demanding of the instrumentation,

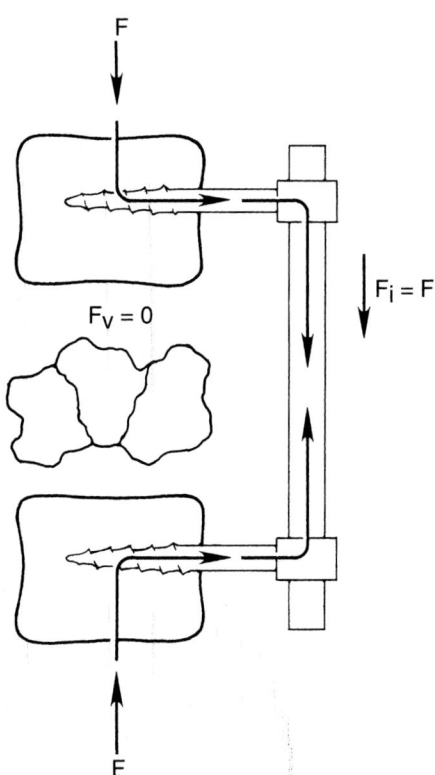

**Figure 107.3** Complete loss of anterior column support $(F_v = 0)$ requiring all load transmission through the instrumentation $(F_i = F)$.

results in the highest rate of instrumentation failure, and should be avoided.

## Bending Moment and Stress

The weak link of the cantilevered device is the proximal shaft of the pedicle screw that experiences the greatest bending moment and stress. All efforts to improve the success of these devices must be focused at reducing this stress or improving the resistance of the screw to this stress. The bending moment ($M$) is the product of the applied force ($F$) and the length of the lever arm of that force. The lever arm is the perpendicular distance from the point of force application (Figure 107.4) ($M = F \times l$). The bending moment increases linearly along the length of the screw, reaching its maximum at the point of connection with the rod. Therefore stress ($S$) is the force per unit area and is largely determined by the diameter ($D$) and length ($l$) of the screw. The equation for stress is $s = F(16l/\pi D^3)$. This calculation has been shown to produce values similar to those measured in experimental conditions with strain gauges.[2] It is the stress rather than the bending moment that predicts the weakest point of the screw at which it is most likely to fail. *The stress is related to the third power of the diameter (D), and linearly to the force or length of the lever arm (l), (i.e., the bending moment). A 20% increase in the diameter of a 5mm pedicle screw to 6mm increases the cross-sectional area and reduces the calculated stress by about 45%. A similar reduction in stress would require a 45% reduction in the applied force (F) or the length of the lever arm over which that force is applied (l).*

## Pedicle Screw

A pedicle screw has several important dimensions, including the inner and outer diameter of the threaded shaft and the diameter of the nonthreaded portion of the shaft. Understanding the transmission of load through the pedicle screw permits optimal screw design for cantilever fixation. Often the inner diameter of the threaded portion of the pedicle screw undergoes abrupt change to the thicker

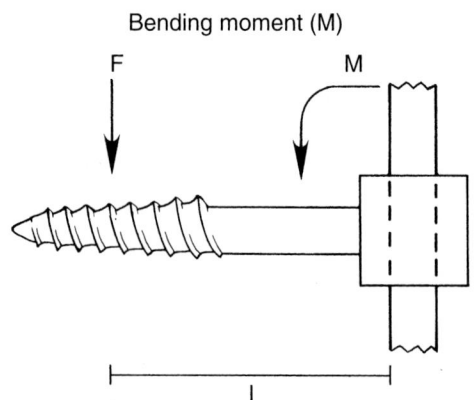

**Figure 107.4** Bending moment ($M$) at proximal shaft of screw is equal to force ($F$) multiplied by length of lever arm ($l$).

diameter of the nonthreaded shaft (collar). The bending moment will be greatest in the shaft at the point of connection to the rod. However, the greatest stress is likely to occur at the thinner diameter of the threaded portion of the screw, thus explaining the frequent site of fracture at the juncture of the threads. By gradually increasing the diameter of the screw at the transition of the threads, the cross-sectional diameter can increase at approximately the same rate as the bending moment, creating a screw without a focal area of weakness (Figure 107.5). If connection to the rod involves transition of the pedicle screw to a smaller diameter machine thread such as a Steffe screw (VSP), this smaller shaft will be exposed to the maximal bending moment, resulting in the highest stress and likely point of failure, as frequently observed for Steffe screws.[7] The Dyna-Lok screw also of Steffe design has acknowledged this vulnerability and increased the diameter of the machine-threaded portion of this screw to approximate the inner diameter of the bone thread. These design factors are now regularly considered in the design of many screws. This has contributed to the reduced failure rate of newer devices.

## Screw Failure

Several techniques of estimating, measuring, or modeling typical transmitted loads have been employed. Duffield et al.[10] have provided finite element analysis of forces and moments acting within a construct. A modified diagram of these data is presented in Figure 107.6. A force of 445 Newtons (N) is depicted at the center of the vertebral body, 51.8mm from the center of the longitudinal member. Because this force is shared between bilateral constructs, each side transmits 222.5N that creates a bending moment of 11.5Nm at the connection of the screw to the rod.

As noted earlier, depending on the screw design and diameter, this moment will create a stress that may or may not be tolerated by a screw. Screws may fail in two ways, either due to a single load to failure, or after repetitive loading (fatigue). Static and cyclic testing of several different pedicle screw constructs has been performed by Cunningham et al.[7] The single maximum axial load to failure for several bilateral constructs in polyethylene blocks is listed in Table 107.1. The calculated maximum moment is also listed in Table 107.1. There is a wide range from the Isola screw (able to withstand a 29-Nm moment) to the Rogozinski screw (able to withstand only 5Nm). Note that this latter screw would not be expected to carry the load successfully modeled in this "worse case scenario" in Figure 107.6 that depicts a bending moment of 11.5Nm.

Cyclic loading data (5 cycles/sec) by the same authors were determined for these same constructs at three loads of 400, 500, and 600N corresponding to 9, 11.25, and 13.5Nm, respectively, shown in Table 107.2. These data reveal that at 9Nm (400N), all systems shown were able to tolerate 1 million cycles, whereas at 13.5Nm (600N) the systems showed tolerance from 47,000 cycles for the Dyna-Lok plate system to 799,000 cycles for the Isola rod system.

For each pedicle screw, static and cyclic load data can be collected to generate a curve as shown in Figure 107.7. This demonstrates that there is a load that will cause screw

Uniform thread depth and inner diameter

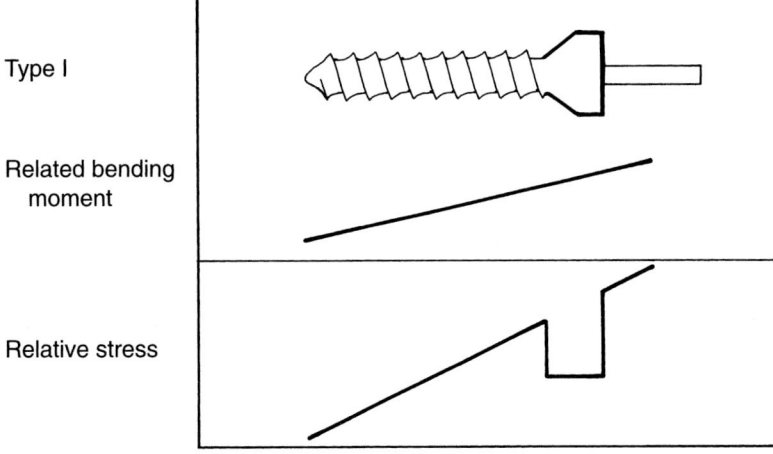

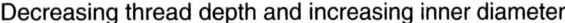

Decreasing thread depth and increasing inner diameter

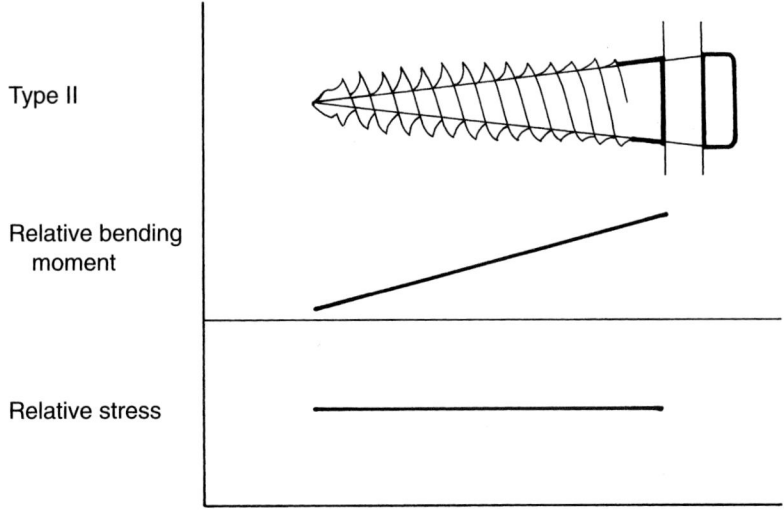

**Figure 107.5** Type I screw with constant inner diameter has greatest stress at junction of cancellous threads with collar and at proximal machine threads. Type II screw has tapering inner core diameter with deep cancellous threads near tip and shallower cortical type threads at junction with collar. Cross-sectional area increases as bending moment increases to create nearly constant stress along screw.

| **TABLE 107.1** | | |
| --- | --- | --- |
| **Compressive Flexural Bending Strength** | | |
| **Construct** | **Mean Force (N)** | **Moment/Screw (Nm)** |
| Isola | 1289.0 | 29.0 |
| Texas Scottish Rite Hospital (TSRH) | 866.5 | 19.5 |
| Steffee (VSP) | 807.8 | 18.0 |
| Compact CD | 753.6 | 17.0 |
| Dyna-Lok | 746.3 | 16.8 |
| AO Fixateur | 609.7 | 13.7 |
| Standard CD | 544.9 | 12.3 |
| Rogozinski | 223.9 | 5.0 |

failure in the first cycle, and as the load is reduced, the screw will survive more and more cycles, until finally a load is reached that is low enough to permit the screw to tolerate cyclic loading essentially indefinitely. This curve clearly depends on the stress the screw experiences, which is a function of the screw design and diameter. Alternatively, the calculated stress (megapascals [MPas] = Newtons/mm$^2$) for a particular screw can be determined as a function of a load $(F)$ at a particular distance (lever arm) to generate a series of curves as depicted in Figure 107.8. These calculated data based on screw dimensions have been found to correlate well with experimental data.[2] The stress endurance threshold for 316L stainless steel (a known constant) is depicted in the graph. As the

**TABLE 107.2**

**Fatigue of Spinal Constructs**

| Construct | Load Moment | | |
|---|---|---|---|
| | 400 N (9 Nm) | 500 N (11.25 Nm) | 600 N (13.5 Nm) |
| Isola | >1,000,000 | >1,000,000 | 799,544 |
| Texas Scottish Rite Hospital (TSRH) | >1,000,000 | >1,000,000 | 624,810 |
| Steffee (VSP) | >1,000,000 | >1,000,000 | 212,960 |
| Compact CD | >1,000,000 | >1,000,000 | 593,566 |
| Dyna-Lok | >1,000,000 | 408,319 | 47,040 |
| AO Fixateur | >1,000,000 | 368,075 | 196,873 |
| Standard CD | >1,000,000 | 202,769 | 135,017 |

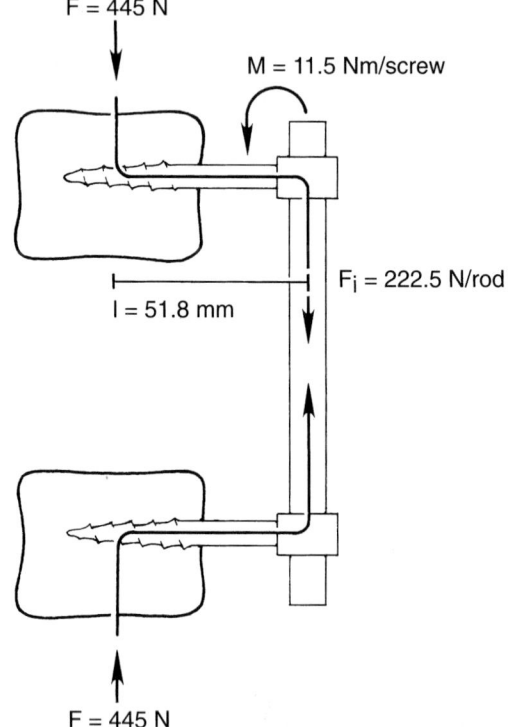

**Figure 107.6**  No ventral load sharing. All of the 445N load passes through bilateral pedicle screws and rods.

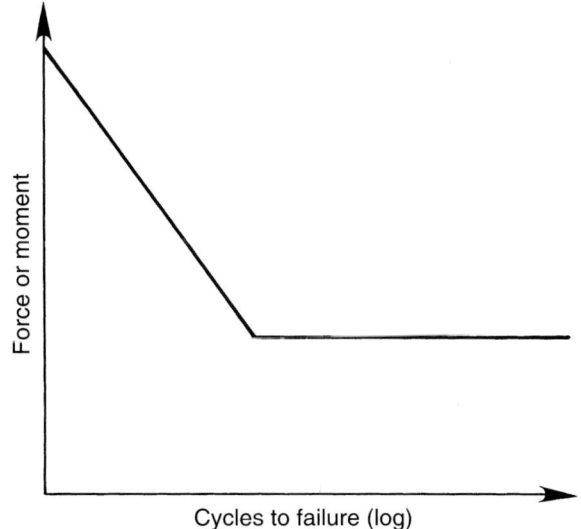

**Figure 107.7**  Fatigue of pedicle screw. As load increases, the pedicle screw tolerates fewer cycles to failure.

calculated stress of a pedicle screw exceeds this limit, fatigue failure is anticipated.

## Load Sharing

It is clear that the expected load that the pedicle screw must bear is near the failure threshold of the screw in a "worst case scenario" when no load is shared by the vertebra. For this reason it is important not to rely on the intrinsic support of the cantilever construct but instead support the beam to reduce the bending moment, and therefore reduce the stress on the proximal shaft of the pedicle screw. The effect of a healthy intervening segment on the predicted load transmission and bending moments of the pedicle construct is depicted in Figure 107.9, as per Duffield et al.[10] It is assumed that the construct has been applied in a "no-load assembly condition." This model predicts that 80% of the load will be transmitted through the vertebral body, leaving only 20% to be transmitted through the bilateral instrumentation (10% through each side). This predicts a bending moment of 2.0Nm on the proximal shaft of the pedicle screw, a reduction of more than 80%. This is well below the strength of even the most vulnerable pedicle screws and explains the relative rarity of pedicle screws fracturing when they are used for degenerative disease compared with their use for fractured and incompetent anterior spinal columns. It also emphasizes that demands on the screw in these different situations are dramatically different. *Pedicle screws that are routinely used successfully for degenerative lumbar fusions should not necessarily be expected to perform equally well for thoracolumbar fractures.*

Several biomechanical studies have demonstrated the improved tolerance of constructs that use ventral load-sharing constructs.[1,10,13,21] The "perfect" ventral reconstruction, from a purely mechanical viewpoint, exceeds the stiffness and load-carrying capacity of an intact motion segment, to approach the stiffness of the vertebral bodies themselves. A diagram of the conceptual relationship between the stress (or bending moment) of pedicle screws

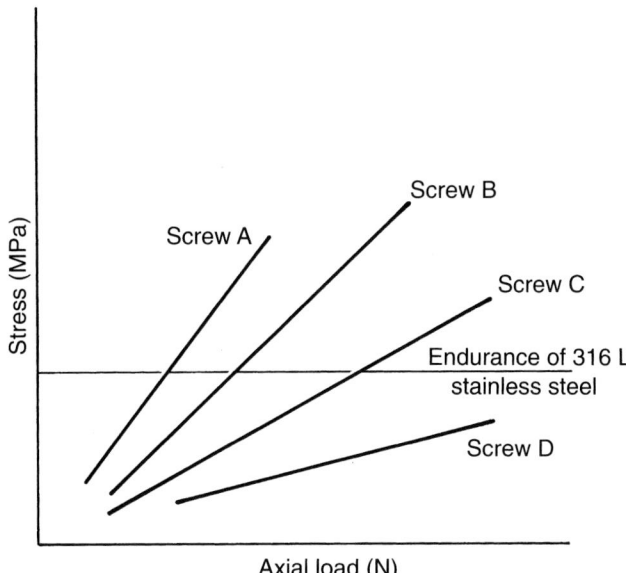

**Figure 107.8** Load versus stress plot reveals that each construct experiences different stress for a given load.

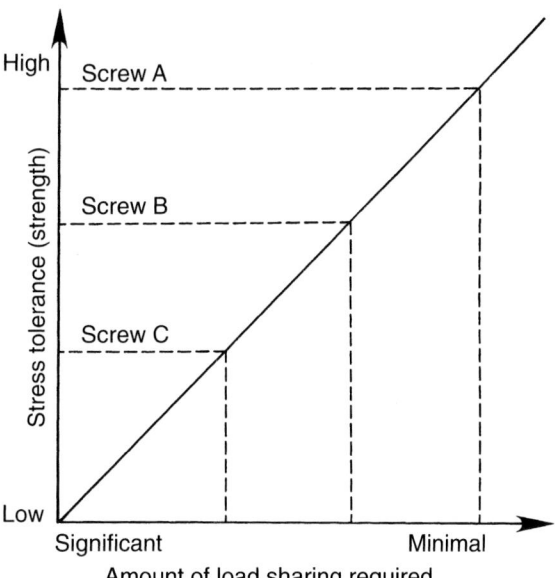

**Figure 107.10** Conceptual relationship between ventral load sharing and stress. Screw A tolerates greater stress and therefore could be used with less load sharing. Screw C tolerates stress less effectively and requires good to excellent load sharing to succeed.

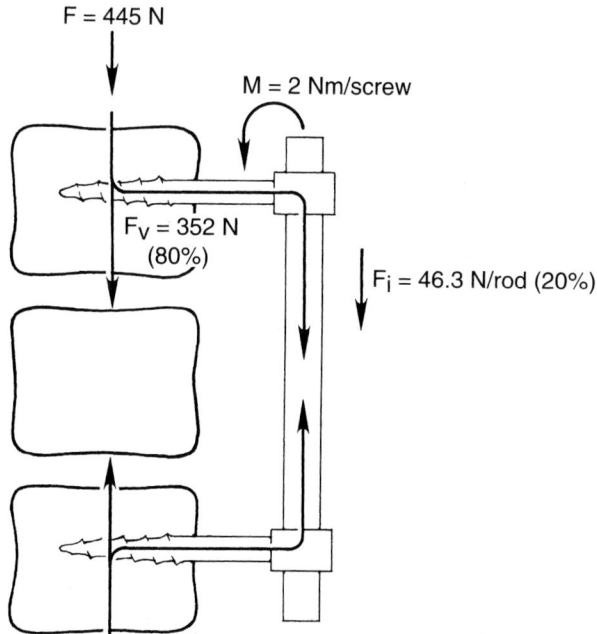

**Figure 107.9** With intact intervening segment, 80% of the load is transmitted through the anterior column (load sharing), leaving only 20% of the load to be divided between the bilateral screws and rods.

and the amount of load shared by an anterior column reconstruction is shown in Figure 107.10. The maximum stress tolerated for the expected in vivo cyclic loading for three different pedicle screw constructs is shown in the graph. Construct A with the highest stress tolerance will be successful even with minimal load sharing. Construct C with the lowest stress tolerance will require at least significant ventral load sharing to prevent failure. An attempt to use construct C, without adequate ventral load sharing, would be expected to result in failure. For each construct

there is a minimum theoretical load that must be shared by the anterior column to prevent device failure. If no ventral load sharing is provided, maximal device strength is required, and risk of failure increases substantially.

It has not been well established what technique creates an adequate ventral reconstruction and provides sufficient load sharing. Techniques and materials vary widely regarding their ability to resist ventral loads. Generally, ventral constructs should have sufficient cross-sectional area to resist subsidence into the vertebral body. This is more readily achieved with iliac autograft, or femur or humerus allograft, than with autologous rib graft, although the use of a three-rib construct has been demonstrated to have axial resistance to graft subsidence that is biomechanically indistinguishable from iliac or humerus grafts.[17] The same study demonstrated that a titanium mesh cage was found to have resistance to subsidence that exceeded any of the bone constructs. Biomechanical superiority of the cage should not suggest clinical superiority of this device.

Although fractures of the vertebra impair the load-bearing capacity of the anterior column, it is difficult to estimate the extent of this impairment. Even comminuted axial compression injuries will support some load. It is not necessary to always reconstruct the anterior column for the use of short-segment pedicle fixation. Several studies have demonstrated the successful use of fixation even with moderate to severe degrees of anterior column compromise.[8,12,20] McLain et al.[24] reported the use of Cotrel-Dubousset (C-D) pedicle screws in 19 patients with thoracolumbar fractures. They found that in 6 patients with preserved or reestablished anterior column, none experienced device failure or kyphotic deformity. Of 13 patients with residual anterior instability, only 3 did not show any evidence of device failure, and the average kyphotic deformity progression was 10 degrees. Devices failed by screw bending in 6, screw fracture in 1, and osseous collapse or translation without device bending in 3 patients. They concluded that residual ventral instability results in a high rate of device failure.

Ebelke et al.[11] reported short-segment fixation with VSP screws and plate fixation for thoracolumbar burst fractures in 21 patients. In 8 patients, ventral bone grafting was performed with cancellous bone through a transpedicular approach. There were no device failures in this group, and only one of these patients developed significant kyphosis. A second group of 13 patients did not have ventral bone grafting, and screw fractures were observed in 5 patients (38%). Patients with failure were found to have vertebral body compression 18% greater than that in the nonfailure group. Although transpedicular grafting provides little if any acute mechanical support, these data suggest that it may provide that support before fatigue failure of the screws can occur.

## Avoiding Failure

Several considerations are important in candidate selection for short-segment pedicle instrumentation. One must establish the integrity of the adjacent vertebral bodies with special emphasis on the pedicles. With only four points of fixation, unlike long universal fixation, the failure of one point of fixation cannot be tolerated. One must confirm that the diameter of the pedicle is sufficiently large to accept a pedicle screw large enough to carry the anticipated load. Generally, the use of screws at least 6mm in diameter is desired. However, as emphasized above, screw design may weigh heavily on this selection. Clearly, there are 6mm screws that are inferior to 5mm screws in load-bearing capacity. Ideally, one should select a screw based on its inner (core) diameter and anticipated stress. For example, the 5mm Schantz screw of the fixateur interne has a relatively short length of threads (3.5cm). The recommended installation technique places the thread-shaft junction at least 1cm deep into the pedicle, thus fully protecting this vulnerable region of the screw. This 5mm screw used in this fashion will likely outperform many 6mm screws with "exposed" thread-shaft junctions.

If a patient has a relatively low body weight, the expected total applied force is reduced, and the stress the pedicle screw is exposed to is correspondingly reduced. In this case, the use of a 5mm screw may be acceptable if moderate ventral load sharing is present or is to be reestablished. However, selection of a 5mm screw in a heavier patient with the same ventral load sharing is likely to result in failure. Although pedicle screws less than 5mm are readily available, their chance of success seems unlikely. Therefore their use should be avoided. In general, the largest pedicle screw that fits safely into the pedicle is used. Misenhimer et al.[25] have demonstrated that pedicle screws greater than 80% of the outer cortical diameter begin to cause plastic deformation of the pedicle and never do obtain cortical purchase within the pedicle. It has been demonstrated clearly that pullout strength is improved by increases in thread depth (outer diameter of the screw).[30] However, because it is screw fracture rather than screw pullout that is the frequent cause of device fail-

ure for a cantilever construct, maximizing the internal diameter of the screw would be expected to reduce failure in most clinical situations. As discussed, an optimal screw has relatively deep threads in the cancellous body, where it is not exposed to significant bending moments, and shallow threads and greater internal diameter as it approaches the longitudinal member (see Figure 107.5; type II screw). There are limited data comparing the variety of pedicle screws. However, Texas Scottish Rite Hospital (TSRH), Isola, Compact and standard C-D, and the fixateur interne are among those implants that are successfully used for fixation of traumatic instability.

The calculated bending moment of 11.5Nm/screw (see Figure 107.6) presumed a lever arm distance of 51.8mm. The bending moment can be minimized by keeping the longitudinal member as close to the dorsal elements as possible. Leaving an unnecessary 10mm of additional exposed screw increases the bending moment on the proximal shaft of the screw by 20%. Pedicle screws should be set as deeply as possible into the pedicle to protect the shaft from exposure to higher bending moments. There have been recent attempts to place percutaneous pedicle screws with longitudinal members in a subcutaneous position. This technique essentially doubles the distance from the point of load and therefore doubles the bending moment. As demonstrated in Figure 107.8, with an intact intervening segment (degenerative disease), the initial bending moment is low (2Nm), and doubling this amount would likely be tolerated. If one starts with an incompetent ventral segment caused by fracture, it is anticipated that this technique would fail unless a distinctly larger screw shaft is used.

Fixation is often provided by four pedicle screws. Losing one point of fixation cannot be tolerated. Loss of fixation on one side places the entire applied load on the intact side. This doubles the bending moment and is likely to result in device failure. Techniques available to reestablish screw "purchase" include infiltration of the pedicle with pressurized or unpressurized methylmethacrylate or increasing the screw size, if appropriate. Both techniques have been demonstrated to return pull-out strength to "normal" under optimal circumstances.[23,32] Pressure infiltration of the pedicle should be performed under direct visualization of the inferomedial walls of the pedicle to minimize the risk of injury to neural elements. Generally, these techniques are not used. If failure of one point of fixation is apparent during placement, the construct should be lengthened to incorporate an additional spinal segment.

As discussed earlier, the entire applied load (F) can be conceptually applied at a single point. This point varies depending on the spinal level and angulation of the spine that affects the center of gravity of the torso. If the spine is abnormally kyphotic, this point of load may shift forward, increasing the lever arm and the bending moment. Figure 107.11A and B show the effect of this conceptual point of load application shifting forward 11.2mm in a kyphotic spine, thus increasing the bending moment more than 20%. Even more important, as the torso moves forward, the measured force at the disc has been found to increase dramatically.[26,28] Nachemson[26] has demonstrated that the intradiscal pressure reflects the load on the spine and increases 200% with 20% forward angulation of the torso. This is due to the center of gravity shifting ventral to the

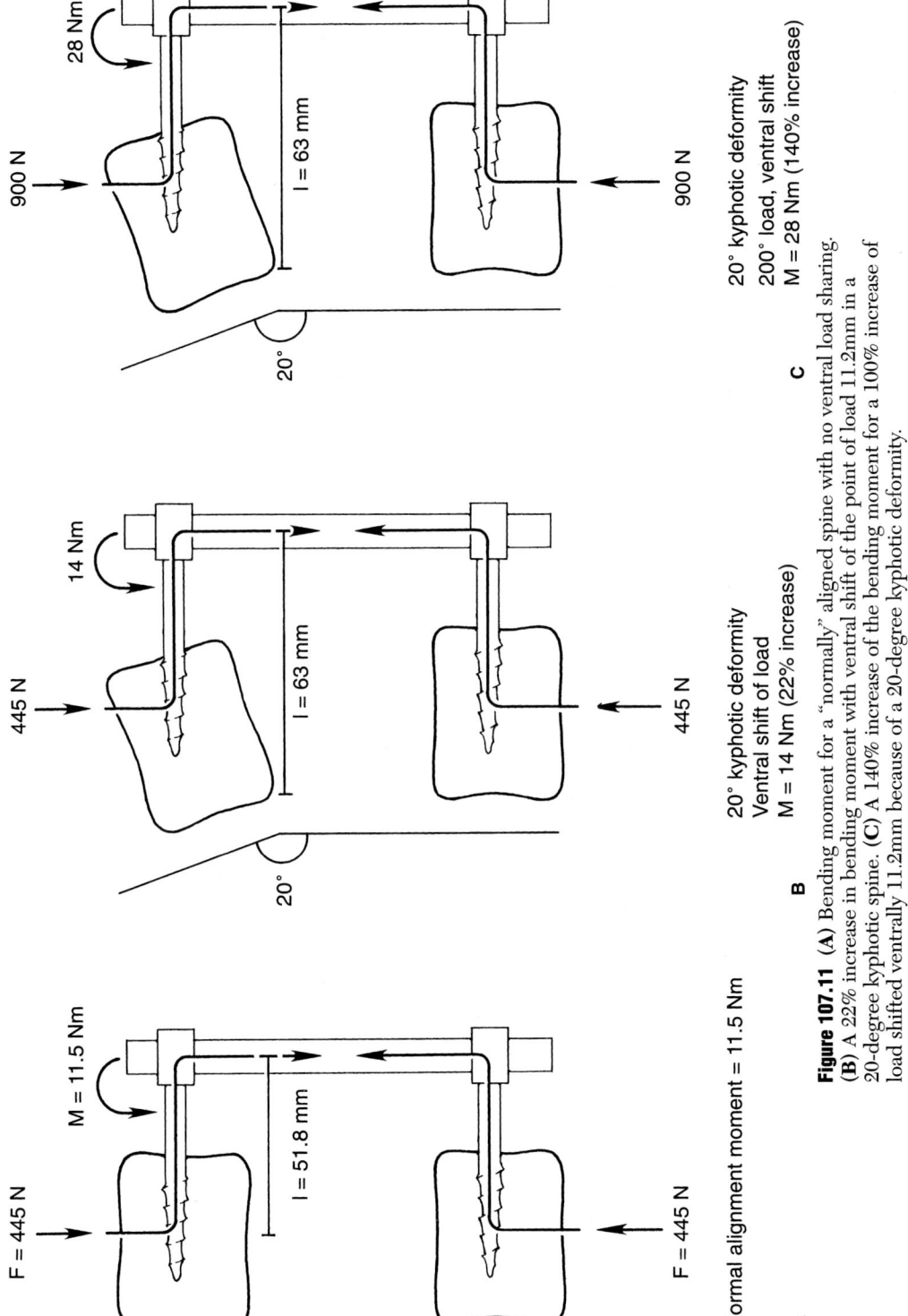

**Figure 107.11** **(A)** Bending moment for a "normally" aligned spine with no ventral load sharing. **(B)** A 22% increase in bending moment with ventral shift of the point of load 11.2mm in a 20-degree kyphotic spine. **(C)** A 140% increase of the bending moment for a 100% increase of load shifted ventrally 11.2mm because of a 20-degree kyphotic deformity.

instantaneous axis of rotation of the vertebral body, thus creating a bending moment on the vertebral body that is opposed by increasing forces of the dorsal extensor musculature. It has not been demonstrated clearly that these same relationships hold true for the stabilized posttraumatic spine. However, it is reasonable to expect that they do. If a kyphotic angulation of the spine results in a 100% increase of load ($F$) at the site of pedicle fixation, the bending moment on the screw increases 140% and likely exceeds its tolerance (see Figure 107.11$C$).

This situation can be avoided by correcting kyphotic deformity at the time of fixation. If neutral spinal alignment is achieved, minimal loads can be expected. Technically, this usually requires the application of a rotational moment of the fixation device in the sagittal plane (extension moment). In this circumstance, the intervening comminuted segment provides no support (load sharing), and thus requires the screws to support the entire load. If ventral load sharing is not reestablished when a kyphotic deformity is corrected, one may create a situation that is even worse than the extra load created by the kyphotic deformity, as depicted in Figure 107.12$A$ and $B$. Note that correction of the deformity increases the bending moment by more than 80%. Careful reestablishment of spinal

alignment without ventral reconstruction to establish load sharing has been clinically observed to result in failure of the fixation device.

Pedicle screws may initially be inserted in a neutral "no-load condition," compressed, distracted, or rotated around the sagittal plane. Screws placed in a "no-load condition" with a patient prone on the operating table must immediately sustain the load of the upper torso in other positions, such as standing or sitting. Similarly, screws initially placed in distraction in the prone position will sustain the load of the upper torso when standing or sitting, as well as the load associated with distraction force application. Use of the screws to reduce a kyphotic deformity does not necessarily increase the bending moment on the screws when the patient is erect, other than by eliminating the load sharing of the comminuted segment. One should not hesitate to restore spinal alignment for fear of "preloading" the construct. However, ventral load sharing should be reestablished.

Even when load sharing and spinal alignment has been optimally reestablished, a patient must be prohibited from forward flexion to protect the pedicle screws. Although an orthotic device may provide little axial support, it is capable of preventing or reminding a patient to avoid forward flexion. Therefore it should be used in all patients for

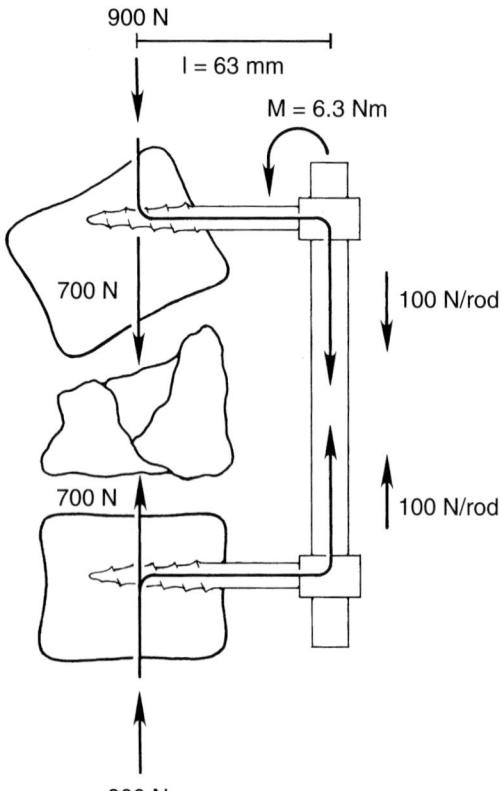

**Kyphotic deformity**
**Significant load sharing**
A    M = 6.3 Nm

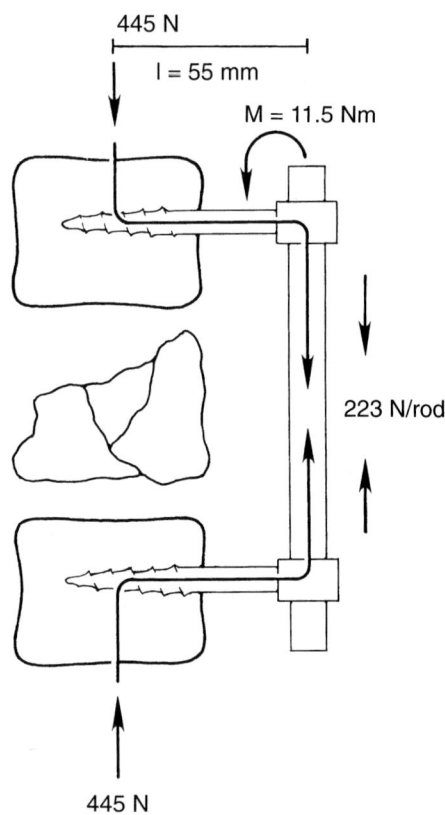

**Deformity reduced**
*No* **load sharing**
B    M = 11.5 Nm (82.5% increase)

**Figure 107.12  (A)** Transmission of a significant portion of the load (78%, 700N) through the comminuted vertebral segment. Although a significant kyphosis exists, the bending moment is relatively small because of load sharing. Correcting the kyphosis without reestablishing ventral load sharing, as depicted in **(B)** directs all of the smaller load through the construct and significantly increases the bending moment and likelihood of construct failure.

3 to 4 months to prevent screws from experiencing large bending moments. Patients should not lift any significant load and should keep all loads close to their body.

Cyclic fatigue data for pedicle screws indicate that in some circumstances the screw has a finite number of cycles before failure. Attempts to reduce the cycling of the screws after implantation may be prudent. Even the soft bounce of a slow gait may significantly increase the axial load (and bending moment) on a device. Nachemson[27] has demonstrated that jumping in place can increase the axial load at L3 from 500 to 700N (40%). Walking 4 miles per day provides more than 10,000 load cycles to the fixation device, after 1 month over 300,000 cycles, and nearly 1 million cycles by 3 months. As Table 107.2 demonstrates, a load of even 600N (13.5Nm) on a bilevel pedicle fixation device cannot be cycled this many times before exceeding the endurance of all systems listed. Exercise in the form of walking is recommended to patients after fusion, but exceptional distances should be avoided.

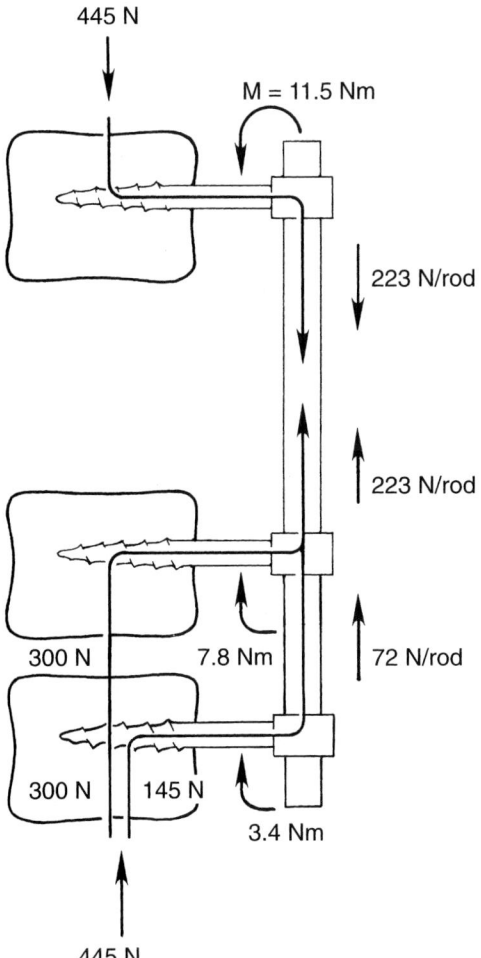

445 N

M = 11.5 Nm

223 N/rod

223 N/rod

300 N     7.8 Nm     72 N/rod

300 N     145 N

3.4 Nm

445 N

**Figure 107.13** Marked reduction in bending moment when additional segment is instrumented. Note that only the one end of the construct is "protected." (*Modified from Duffield RC, Carson WL, Chen L-Y, et al: Longitudinal element size effect on load sharing, internal loads, and fatigue life of tri-level spinal implant constructs. Spine 18:1695-1703, 1993, with permission.*)

The relatively high failure rate of short-segment pedicle fixation has moved some surgeons to avoid it entirely or modify instrumentation in several ways to improve the likelihood of success. One option is to extend the fixation up and down the spine one additional segment, partially eliminating the benefits of short-segment fixation. Figure 107.13 is modified from the work of Duffield *et al.*[10] (using finite element analysis). If two adjacent segments are instrumented as shown, a portion of the load is transmitted from one vertebral body to the next through the intact disc, providing "support" that reduces the load and therefore the bending moment at this level. This effect is dependent on the size and stiffness of the longitudinal members. Figure 107.13 demonstrates a 32% reduction of the bending moment on the first pedicle screw when the longitudinal member is a one-quarter inch rod. This supports the clinical observation that extension of the construct reduces the rate of failure. Note that both ends of the construct are approximately equally vulnerable to screw failure, and extending the construct in only one direction provides no protection to the other end of the construct (which is exposed to the same bending moment). An alternative to providing additional ventral load sharing to reduce the applied load by 30% would be to forego the load sharing and instrument additional adjacent levels.

Other attempts to protect pedicle screws have included the addition of hooks to the terminal or adjacent vertebra. Biomechanical or clinical evaluation of the effectiveness of reducing axial load by these techniques is not available. If the hook is placed in a supralaminar position at the rostral end of the construct on the same vertebra, it is unlikely to carry any axial load and will not protect the screw from bending stress. This technique will offer resistance to axial pullout and rotation, but neither of these is commonly the mode of failure of these constructs. If the hook engages the supra-adjacent vertebral segment in an infralaminar position, it may carry some axial load and thus reduce the bending moment. This configuration would be considerably less effective than a pedicle screw in doing so and also likely to result in the sacrifice of an additional motion segment if instrumentation removal is not planned. Obviously, longer constructs with more points of fixation distribute load and reduce device failure at the price of losing adjacent normal motion segments.

It has been well established that as pedicle screw trajectory is directed medially, a bilevel pedicular construct becomes more stable to laterally directed forces.[5,13] This has been called by some the 4R-4bar mechanism or by others the parallelogram effect. Especially in the lower thoracic and upper lumbar spine, the angle of cannulation of a pedicle is entirely defined by its specific anatomy rather than by surgeon choice. For this reason, one must rely entirely on transverse fixation to resist lateral and rotational forces. Transverse fixation has been demonstrated clearly to reduce lateral instability and rotation and is used routinely.[5,29] A single transverse connector in the middle of the construct has been shown to reduce rotation as much as transverse connectors placed at both ends. The effect of a single central connector on lateral instability, however, has not been well established.[29] When possible, transverse connectors are placed at both ends of the construct for short-segment fixation in unstable conditions. However, a single connector in the middle of the construct may provide nearly the same benefit. Transverse connectors are not found to be necessary in most degenerative conditions.

Screws have been shown to have an increased direct axial pull-out strength in human cadaveric bone with increasing depth of penetration.[18,19] Pullout strength of Vermont Spinal Fixator screws at 50% vertebral body penetration was found to be 75% of that at 80% penetration. At 100% penetration, the pullout strength increases to 124% to 154% as compared with 80% penetration.[18] Screws placed at a depth of 80% extend approximately 50% across the vertebral body. Krag *et al.*[18] have also demonstrated that a screw placed 80% rather than 50% deep has a 32.5% greater resistance to "cut-out" when subjected to rotation in the sagittal plane. Direct axial pull-out or even "cut-out" of rigidly fixed pedicle screws is a rare mode of failure, and attempts to achieve approximately 80% vertebral body penetration, leaving ample room to avoid inadvertent cortical penetration and risk to vascular structures, seem prudent.

## Summary

Short-segment bilevel pedicle fixation confines fixation and fusion to the absolute minimal length of spine adjacent to the injured segment short-segment fixation, thus eliminating the need for routine device removal. Historically, the technique was troubled with a high rate of reported failure. More recently, as a better understanding of the biomechanics has evolved, successful utilization of the technique has become commonplace. Also, recent technologic advances have provided screws with increased resistance to failure. In selected situations, short-segment bilevel pedicle fixation should be considered strongly for thoracolumbar pathology requiring stabilization alone or with ventral decompression and anterior column reconstruction.

## REFERENCES

1. Abumi K, Panjabi MM, Duranceau J: Biomechanical evaluation of spinal fixation devices. *Spine* 14:1249-1255, 1989.
2. Ashman RB, Galpin RD, Corin JD, *et al*: Biomechanical analysis of pedicle screw instrumentation system in a corpectomy model. *Spine* 14:1398-1405, 1989.
3. Benzel EC (ed): *Biomechanics of Spine Stabilization: Principles and Clinical Practice.* New York, McGraw-Hill, 1995.
4. Carl AL, Tromanhauser SG, Roger DJ: Pedicle screw instrumentation for thoracolumbar burst fractures and fracture-dislocations. *Spine* 17:S317-S324, 1992.
5. Carson WL, Duffield RC, Arendt M, *et al*: Internal forces and movements in transpedicular spine instrumentation: the effect of pedicle screw angle and transfixation: The 4R-4bar linkage concept. *Spine* 15:893-901, 1990.
6. Cochran T, Irstam L, Nachemson A: Long-term anatomic and functional changes in patients with adolescent idiopathic scoliosis treated by Harrington rod fusion. *Spine* 8:576-584, 1983.
7. Cunningham BW, Sefter JC, Shono Y, *et al*: Static and cyclical biomechanical analysis of pedicle screw spinal constructs. *Spine* 18:1677-1688, 1993.
8. Daniaux H, Seykora P, Genelin A, *et al*: Application of posterior plating and modifications in thoracolumbar spine injuries: Indication, techniques, and results. *Spine* 16: 125-133, 1991.
9. Dick W: The "Fixatuer Interne" as a versatile implant for spine surgery. *Spine* 12:882-900, 1987.
10. Duffield RC, Carson WL, Chen L-Y, *et al*: Longitudinal element size effect on load sharing, internal loads, and fatigue life of tri-level spinal implant constructs. *Spine* 18:1695-1703, 1993.
11. Ebelke DK, Asher MA, Neff JR, *et al*: Survivorship analysis of VSP spine instrumentation in the treatment of thoracolumbar and lumbar burst fractures. *Spine* 16: S428-S432, 1991.
12. Esses SI, Bosford DJ, Wright T, *et al*: Operative treatment of spinal fractures with the AO internal fixator. *Spine* 16:S146-S150, 1991.
13. Gaines RW Jr, Carson WL, Satterlee CC, *et al*: Experimental evaluation of seven different spinal fracture internal fixation devices using nonfailure stability testing: the load-sharing and unstable-mechanism concepts. *Spine* 16:902-909, 1991.
14. Ginsburg HH, Goldstein LA, Robinson SC, *et al*: Back pain in postoperative idiopathic scoliosis: long-term follow-up study [abstract]. *Spine* 4:518, 1979.
15. Gurr K, McAfee P, Shih C: Biomechanical analysis of anterior and posterior instrumentation systems after corpectomy: A calf-spine model. *J Bone Joint Surg* 70A:1182-1191, 1988.
16. Hollowell JP, Mueller WM, Larson SJ: Lumbar fusion with instrumentation for the treatment of degenerative spinal disorders: A 10 year experience. In Rachidian Society Third Annual Meeting. Kona, Hawaii, 1995.
17. Hollowell JP, Vollmer DG, Wilson CR, *et al*: Biomechanical analysis of thoracolumbar interbody constructs: How important is the endplate? *Spine* 21(9):1032-1036, 1996.
18. Krag MH, Beynnon BD, Pope MH, *et al*: An internal fixator for posterior application to short segments of the thoracic, lumbar, or lumbosacral spine. *Clin Orthop Rel Res* 253:75-98, 1986.
19. Krag MH, Beynnon BD, Pope MH, *et al*: Depth of insertion of transpedicular vertebral screws into human vertebrae: effect upon screw-vertebra interface strength. *J Spinal Disord* 1:287-294, 1989.
20. Lindsey RW, Dick W: The Fixateur Interne in the reduction and stabilization of the thoracolumbar spine fractures in patients with neurologic deficit. *Spine* 16:S140-S145, 1991.
21. Maiman DJ, Pintar F, Yoganandan N, *et al*: Effects of anterior vertebral grafting on the traumatized lumbar spine after pedicle screw-plate fixation. *Spine* 18:2423-2430, 1993.
22. McAfee PC, Weiland DJ, Carlow JJ: Survivorship analysis of pedicle spinal instrumentation. *Spine* 16:S422-S427, 1991.
23. McLain RF, Fry MF, Moseley TA, *et al*: Lumbar pedicle screw salvage: pullout testing of three different pedicle screw designs. *Spinal Disord* 8:62-68, 1995.
24. McLain RF, Sparling E, Benson DR: Early failure of short-segment pedicle instrumentation for thoracolumbar fractures. *J Bone Joint Surg* 75A:162-167, 1993.

25. Misenhimer GR, Peek R, Wiltse LL, *et al*: Anatomic analysis of pedicle cortical and cancellous diameter as related to screw size. *Spine* 14:367-372, 1989.
26. Nachemson A: The load on lumbar disks in different positions of the body. *Clin Orthop Rel Res* 45:107-122, 1966.
27. Nachemson A: Lumbar intradiscal pressure. In Jayson M (ed): *Lumbar Spine and Back Pain.* New York, Grune & Stratton, 1976, pp 257-269.
28. Nachemson A, Morris JM: In vivo measurements of intradiscal pressure. *J Bone Joint Surg* 46A:1077-1092, 1964.
29. Pintar FA, Maiman DJ, Yoganandan N, *et al*: Rotational stability of a spinal pedicle screw/rod system. *J Spinal Disord* 8:49-55, 1995.
30. Skinner R, Maybee J, Transfeldt E, *et al*: Experimental pullout testing and comparison of variables in transpedicular screw fixation: biomechanical study. *Spine* 15:195-201, 1990.
31. Whitecloud TS III, Butler JC, Cohen JL *et al*: Complications with variable spinal plating system. *Spine* 14:472-477, 1989.
32. Zindrick MR, Wiltse LL, Widell EH, *et al*: A biomechanical study of intrapeduncular screw fixation in the lumbosacral spine. *Clin Orthop Rel Res* 203:99-112, 1986.

# CHAPTER 108

# Spinal Implant Attributes: Dynamic Spine Fixation

Steven P. Leon, Denis DiAngelo, Edward C. Benzel, Hansen A. Yuan, and Kevin T. Foley

The benefits of rigid implants (i.e., internal fixation) in the axial skeleton include rigid stabilization, maintenance of alignment, minimal postoperative immobilization, earlier return to function, and potentially enhanced fusion rates.[1] One of the potential shortcomings of rigid implants is that they may stress-shield the bone graft and result in nonunion or implant failure or both. Stress shielding can be defined as an implant-induced reduction of bone-healing–enhancing stresses and loads, resulting in stress reduction osteoporosis or nonunion (Figure 108.1). This hypothesis is in keeping with Wolff's law. Wolff's law postulates that the form and function of bone is a result of changes in the internal architecture according to "self-ordered" mathematical rules.[11] In contemporary terms, this is interpreted to mean that skeletal morphology is substantially controlled by mechanical function and that bone remodeling, both locally and throughout the skeleton, is influenced by the level and distribution of the functional strains within the bone.[9,10] A corollary to Wolff's law is that bone heals optimally under compressive, as opposed to tensile, forces. Experimental studies in the thoracolumbar spine show that a 70% or greater axial load should be transmitted through the spine, not the implant, in order to optimally enhance arthrodesis and provide acute stability.[4]

In an attempt to improve upon the shortcomings of rigid implants, there has been a resurgent interest in dynamic implants, particularly for use in the cervical spine. The concept of dynamic implants is not new. Dynamic hip arthroplasties have been employed for femoral neck fractures with success. They allow for the femoral neck to shorten or collapse along its axis, so that the bone is subject to optimal bone-healing compressive forces.[7] Advocates of dynamic implants hypothesize that implants that permit a limited and controlled type of deformation may be desirable. Some have termed this *controlled dynamism*. In the spine, for example, allowing for some axial deformation but not angular deformation (kyphosis) may be optimal. Occasionally, the failure of a rigid implant may, in fact, permit fusion because the bone graft and vertebral bodies are subsequently exposed to the appropriate bone-healing–enhancing forces. In this case, the implant has "dynamized by failing" (Figure 108.2).

The first ventral cervical plate and screw system was introduced by Bohler[3] in 1964. This ultimately culminated in the development of the Caspar (Aesculap) and Orozco (Synthes) plate systems in the early 1980s. These early anterior cervical plates were dynamic implants and are classified as having unrestricted backout properties (i.e., nonlocking and nonrigid) because of a lack of fixation at the screw-plate interface. These implants permit a significant transfer of load through the bone graft, thereby increasing the likelihood of fusion. The nonfixed moment arm nature of the screw causes degradation of the screw-bone interface with cyclical loading. This effect can be minimized with bicortical screw purchase, which requires C-arm fluoroscopy. The main disadvantage of these plates is that the nonlocking and nonrigid (i.e., variable angle) screws led to high rates of screw backout and screw breakage with graft subsidence (Figure 108.3).

The next generation of ventral cervical plates included CSLP (Synthes) and Orion (Sofamor Danek). The CSLP was developed by Morscher in Europe in the early 1980s and introduced in the United States in the early 1990s. The major advantage of these devices is that they do not require bicortical screw purchase. The CSLP uses a titanium expansion screw that rigidly secures the screw to the plate, thereby greatly reducing the incidence of screw backout. Unlike the Caspar plate where screw angulation could be varied, the CSLP has a predetermined (rigid) screw trajectory: perpendicular at the caudal end and 12 degrees rostrally. It has been suggested that these types of restricted, constrained plate-screw configurations are preferable in trauma cases, where obtaining immediate stability is desired; however, this concept remains unproven.

One of the concerns with rigid plates such as CSLP and Orion is that they are felt to stress-shield the bone graft by reducing the compressive forces that the bone graft experiences and thereby result in increased rates of nonunion (pseudarthrosis).[5] This concern led to the interest in the design of dynamic implants. These newer generation dynamic implants improved upon the Caspar plate design by preventing screw backout while still allowing for some movement at the plate-screw interface, thereby allowing for compressive forces to be shared between the implant and the bone graft. These dynamic implants can be further subclassified into rotational or translational, depending on the type of movement that is permitted at the plate-screw interface.

The original Codman plate system, now called Slim-Loc (Depuy-Acromed), uses screws that are able to "toggle" or "pivot" at the screw-plate interface, thereby increasing the load on the graft and allowing for controlled subsidence. As with the Caspar plate, variable screw trajectories can be used; however, a built-in cam-locking mechanism restricts the screws from backout.[6,8]

The Atlantis ventral cervical plating system (Medtronic Sofamor-Danek) features a floating washer design that prevents screw backout. The Atlantis plate incorporates the most beneficial aspects of several types of cervical plate design. It uses either a variable (i.e., nonfixed) angle cantilever screw or a fixed angle cantilever screw (Figure 108.4). As a result of this flexibility, one can create either a rigid construct (similar to CSLP or Orion) or a pivot rotational construct (similar to the Codman plate), or a hybrid construct with both fixed and rigid qualities. The fixed angle screws using the Atlantis

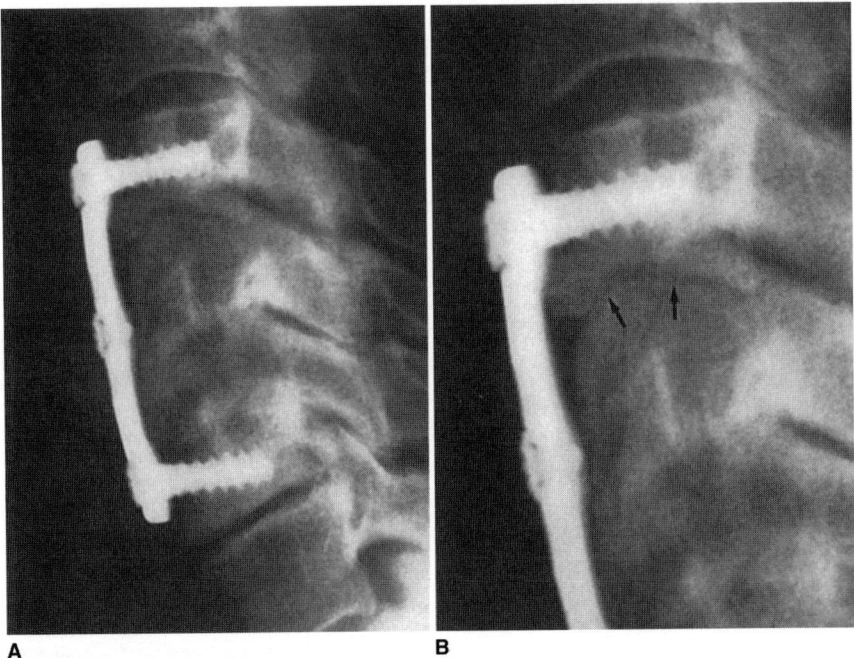

**Figure 108.1** A ventral rigid cervical implant caused stress shielding. This resulted in nonunion (pseudarthrosis) in a patient with preexisting osteoporosis, as depicted. Arrows outline the location of the nonunion. **(A)** Lateral radiograph. **(B)** Close-up. Note pseudarthrosis *(arrows).* *(From Benzel EC:* Biomechanics of Spine Stabilization, *Rolling Meadows, IL, American Association of Neurological Surgeons, 2001.)*

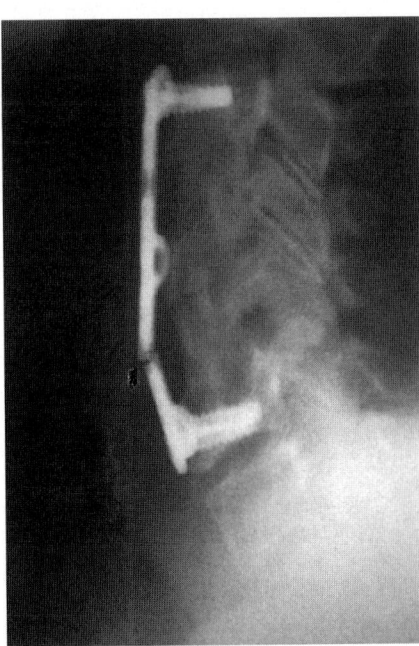

**Figure 108.2** The failure of an implant (by fracture) may allow fusion to occur. In a sense, this implant dynamized by failure, as depicted, thus allowing the bone graft to see bone healing enhancing compression forces. *(From Benzel EC:* Biomechanics of Spine Stabilization, *Rolling Meadows, IL, American Association of Neurological Surgeons, 2001.)*

system are directed 12 degrees rostrally and/or caudally and 6 degrees medially. The hybrid Atlantis construct, fixed angle screws inferiorly, and variable angle screws superiorly may have the advantage of allowing for "controlled subsidence"; the rostral screws are allowed to pivot, while the caudal screws remain fixed. In this way the graft is subjected to compressive forces as the construct settles.

The DOC (Depuy-Acromed) ventral cervical system represents an axial subsidence type of dynamic implant. The screws on the DOC system are not designed to pivot but instead translate, or "slide," along a rail. The screws are rigid at the caudal end, and all cephalad screws have the potential to slide along the rail. This provides axial subsidence and load sharing with the graft while minimizing angular subsidence (kyphosis). This configuration minimizes degradation of the bone-screw interface compared with a device in which screws toggle. Additionally, this system has been demonstrated to be useful for ventral correction of postsurgical cervical kyphosis.

The ABC (Aesculap) and Premier (Medtronic Sofamor Danek) plates allow for both subsidence and pivoting motions at the screw-plate interface. Like the Caspar plate, the ABC and Premier plates allow for variable-angle screw placement but are able to restrict screw backout. With both plates, screws are allowed to subside in a slot and may then pivot after maximum translation. With the ABC plate, all screws can pivot and subside. As with the DOC system the

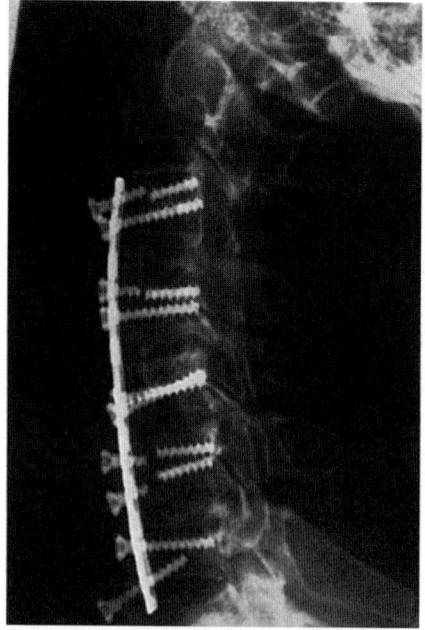

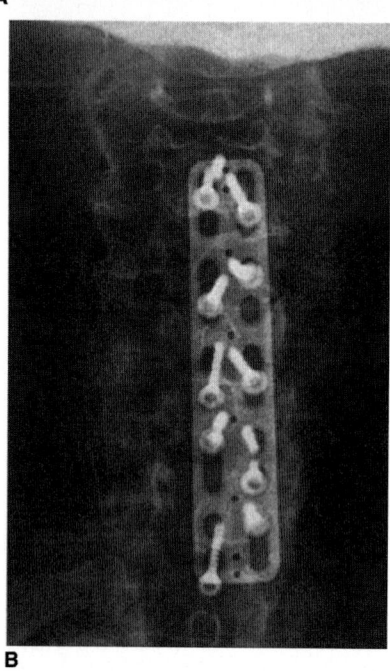

**Figure 108.3** Screws may fracture as a result of excessive stresses placed on them by the subsiding spine, as depicted. (**A**) AP radiograph. (**B**) Lateral radiograph. Note that the screws positioned in holes fractured. They could not axially subside. The screws positioned in slots maintained fixation while dynamizing, thus permitting and encouraging fusion. (*From Benzel EC: Biomechanics of Spine Stabilization, Rolling Meadows, IL, American Association of Neurological Surgeons, 2001.*)

caudal screws of the Premier plate are rigid, and the rostral screws are dynamic, although a version where caudal and rostral screws are dynamic is also available. Despite the purported benefits of the different semiconstrained devices, there is presently a lack of literature directly comparing each of these devices in a clinical setting. Early results with both the ABC and Premier plates are encour-

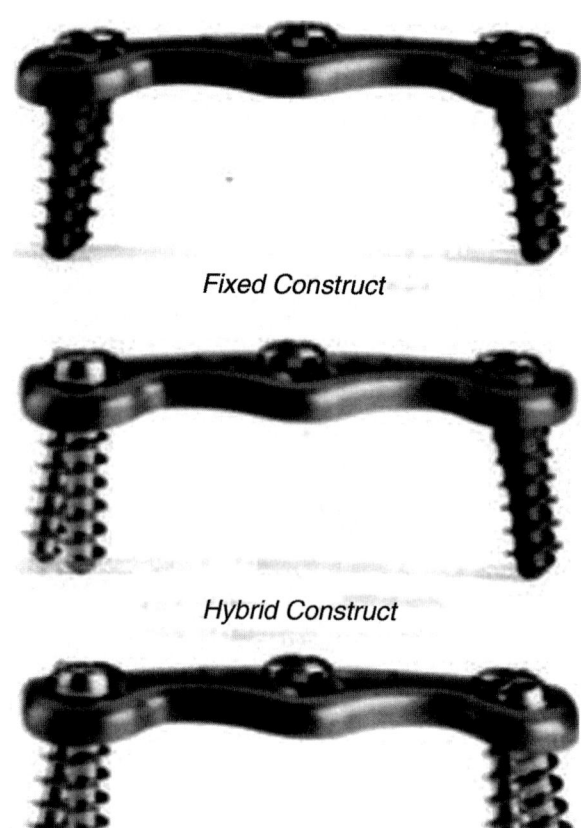

*Fixed Construct*

*Hybrid Construct*

*Variable Construct*

**Figure 108.4** Lateral view of the three types (fixed, hybrid, and variable) of Atlantis constructs. Note that the fixed screws at the caudal end of the hybrid plate act as a buttress, allowing for rotation only at the variable screws at the superior portion of the construct. Additionally, in the variable construct rotation at both ends of the plate is allowed at the plate-screw interface. (*From Haid RW, Foley KT, Rodts GE, Barnes B: The Cervical Spine Study Group anterior cervical plate nomenclature, Neurosurg Focus 12(1): Article 15, January 2002. Available at http://www.aans.org/education/journal/ neurosurgical/jan02/ 12-1-15.pdf.*)

aging, showing that subsidence tends to occur within the first 6 weeks and that there may be a trend toward earlier graft healing.[1,12]

## REFERENCES

1. Abraham DJ, Herkowitz HN: Indications and trends in use in cervical spinal fusions, *Orthop Clin North Am* 29: 731-744, 1998.
2. An HS, Simpson JM: Surgery of the cervical spine. In An H, Simpson J (eds): *Spinal Instrumentation*, London, Marin-Dunitz, 1994.
3. Bohler J, Gaudernak T: Anterior plate stabilization for fracture-dislocations of the lower cervical spine, *J Trauma* 20:203-205, 1980.
4. Craven TG, Carson WL, Asher MA, Robinson RG: The effect of implant stiffness on the bypassed bone mineral

density and facet fusion stiffness of the canine spine, *Spine* 19:1664-1673, 1994.

5. Lowery GL, McDonough RF: The significance of hardware failure in anterior cervical plate fixation. Patients with 2-to 7-year follow-up, *Spine* 23:181-187,1998.

6. Mayr MT, Subach BR, Comey CH, *et al:* Cervical spinal stenosis: outcome after anterior corpectomy, allograft reconstruction, and instrumentation, *J Neurosurg* (Spine 1) 96:10-16, 2002.

7. Mollenhoff G, Walz M, Clasbrummel B, Muhr G: Femoral neck fracture. Osteosynthesis or which endoprosthesis is indicated? *Orthopade* 29:288-293, 2000.

8. Rengachary SS, Sanan A: Anterior stabilization of the cervical spine using locking plate systems. In Wilkins RH, Reganchary SS (eds): *Neurosurgery,* New York, McGraw-Hill, 1996, pp 2983-2986.

9. Rubin CT, Hausman MR: The cellular basis of Wolff's law: transduction of physical stimuli to skeletal adaptation, *Rheum Dis Clin North Am* 14:503-517, 1988.

10. Rubin CT, Lanyon LE: Regulation of bone formation by applied dynamic loads, *J Bone Joint Surg Am* 66:397-402, 1984.

11. Wolff J: *Das Gesetz der Transformation der Knochen,* Berlin, Hirshwald Verlag, 1892.

12. Zdeblick TA, Herkowitz HN: Translational cervical plating: early clinical results (paper no. 39), North American Spine Society, Seattle, WA, 2001.

# CHAPTER 109

# Biomechanics of Mechanical Motion Preservation Strategies

**Robert J. Kowalski, Lisa A. Ferrara, and Edward C. Benzel**

For more than 90 years, surgeons have used spinal arthrodesis to restore ventral column stability in order to alleviate the low back pain resulting from degenerative disc disease. Although this procedure has enjoyed a reasonably high success rate, its mechanism of action may ultimately lead to its obsolescence. By eliminating motion and perpetuating a nonphysiologic state, the normal biomechanics of the spine are altered. Numerous in vitro and in vivo studies have documented the acceleration of the degenerative process at the motion segments adjacent to the fusion mass.[15,24,27] For more than 40 years, researchers have been attempting to duplicate in the spine the success that Charnley observed with his development of total hip replacement.[6] The desire for a more physiologic solution has led to an explosion of interest in motion preservation strategies (e.g., artificial mechanical discs and nuclear replacement strategies) with numerous ongoing research and clinical trials. This focus on motion preservation strategies as a viable alternative to fusion and as an adjunct to discectomy compels one to understand the relevant biomechanical factors. With this knowledge, one can then conceive appropriate design criteria.

## Biomechanics of the Intervertebral Disc

### Structure and Function

The intervertebral disc is a composite structure consisting of a central nucleus pulposus that is surrounded by a multilayered annulus fibrosis. Cartilaginous end plates lie above and below. The nucleus pulposus is about 75% to 80% water. Hydrophilic proteoglycan molecules intermixed with collagen fibers create a gel matrix.

It is convenient, although an oversimplification, to assign responsibility for both the limitation and facilitation of each of the major modes of the range of motion (ROM) to either the intervertebral disc or the facet joints. The intervertebral discs bare the brunt of compression, flexion, and lateral bending, leaving axial rotation and extension to the purview of the facet complex. Once thought of as a simple shock absorber, further study of the viscoelastic properties of the intervertebral disc have shed light on its complexity.[16,18] The normal lumbar disc allows between 8 and 13 degrees of flexion. A similar amount of lateral bending occurs in the upper lumbar region, with considerably less in the lower lumbar spine.[1] The lumbar facet joints provide considerably more resistance to motion, particularly in rotation.

The angled orientation (approximately 30 degrees with respect to the endplate) of the radiating fibers of the annulus fibrosus facilitates a resistance to rotation with relative effectiveness. Compressive loads, however, represent more of a problem, resulting in significant strains on the annulus fibrosus at physiologic loads (Figure 109.1A).[5] A pure axial load results in an even distribution of load over the entire disc (Figure 109.1B). An eccentrically borne load causes the annulus fibrosus to bulge toward the concave side of the spinal curve, while the convex side is subjected to a tension load (Figure 109.1C), as well as paradoxical motion of the nucleus pulposus away from the direction of the disc bulging (Figure 109.1D).[4,23] This explains in part the propensity for dorsal nucleus pulposus herniations with the predominant loading mode of flexion (with axial loading and rotation) in the lumbar spine.

## Pathology

During the progression of disc degeneration, the nucleus pulposus loses its hydrophilic capability and literally deflates. Furthermore, the proteoglycan matrix is altered, and the disc is less able to rehydrate itself efficiently. This results in a cascade of events including loss of disc space height, increased ROM, and instability. The degenerative cascade culminates with a shifting of the load to the annulus fibrosus.

As the disc continues to degenerate, repetitive minor rotational trauma tends to create circumferential tears in the annulus. These may progress and coalesce into radial tears, usually at the dorsal or dorsolateral aspect of the disc, creating an avenue through which the nucleus may herniate.[21] While the direct compression of neural elements by herniated disc material is a common and obvious source of pain and dysfunction, it has been theorized that annular injury alone may be a significant source of axial pain.[7,19] As intradiscal pressures change, the biomechanical parameters alter. This includes, but is not limited to, a shift in load bearing to the perimeter of the end plates and to the facet joints, as well as a shift of the instantaneous axis of rotation.[30] The former seems to be the inciting factor in ligament and facet hypertrophy; the latter is thought to have a more far reaching affect, causing alterations in the biomechanical loads at adjacent vertebral levels and disrupting spinal balance.[20,33,34] The sheer loss of disc space height may be significant enough to allow translation of the superior facet in a rostral and ventral direction, impinging the exiting nerve root in the foramen (Figure 109.2).[21]

## Modes of Disc Interspace Loading

The disc interspace may be loaded along or about each of the three axes of the Cartesian coordinate system in the following manner:

1. Along the long axis of the spine via compression or tension
2. Along the coronal axis of the spine via lateral translations or by flexion or extension

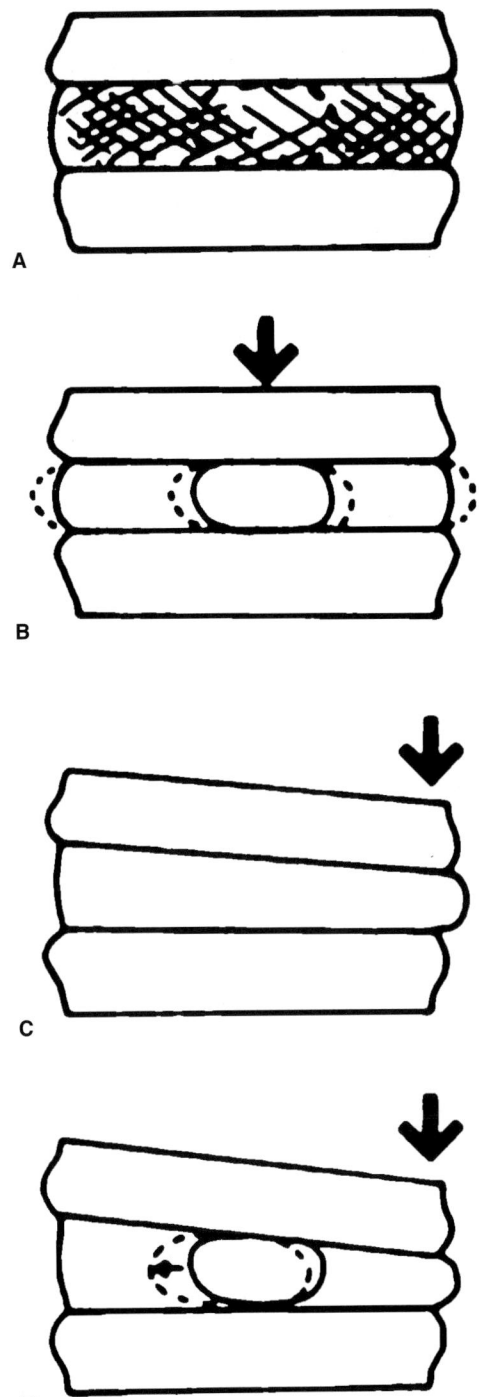

**Figure 109.1** The intervertebral disc. (**A**) The fibers of the annulus fibrosus are oriented radially and in opposite directions throughout several layers. (**B**) The nucleus pulposus (*dashed outline*) is contained (in nonpathological situations) by the annulus fibers. The bearing of an axial load results in an even distribution of force. (**C**) An eccentrically borne load results in annulus fibrosus bulging on the concave side of the resultant spinal curve, and annulus fibrosus tension is present on the convex side of the curve. (**D**) The nucleus pulposus, however, tends to move in the *opposite* direction as the annulus fibrosus bulge when an eccentric load is borne (*solid to dashed outline*).

3. Along or about the sagittal axis of the spine via ventral or dorsal translation or lateral bending (to the right or left).

This, in a sense, provides six types of motion, or six degrees of freedom (Figure 109.3).

It is critical for those who are developing artificial disc technology or for those who are assessing efficacy of an artificial disc or motion preservation strategy to carefully consider each of these types of motions. They have significant short-term and long-term effects on the disc interspace, the ultimate motion preserved or restored, and the structural support of the spine.

Motion about or along the long axis of the spine is a commonly considered movement. Compression of the disc interspace most certainly can lead to excessive loading and failure of disc competence. Failure of a surgical procedure (e.g., a threaded interbody fusion cage, an interbody fusion, or an artificial disc) to effectively replace the disc can compound this loading effect, resulting in failure

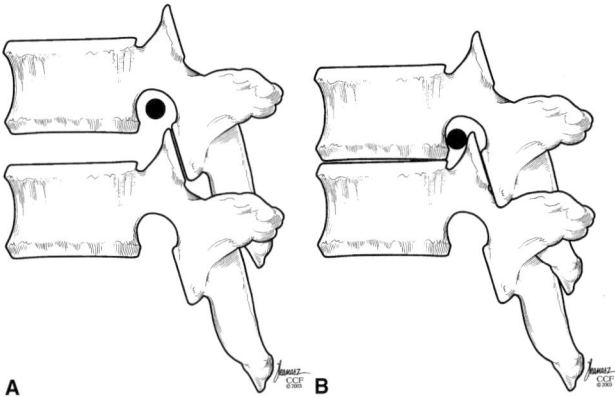

**Figure 109.2** The loss of disc space height from $h_1$ (**A**) to $h_2$ (**B**) causes translation of the superior facet in a rostral and ventral direction, impinging the exiting nerve root in the foramen. (*Copyright Cleveland Clinic Foundation, 2003.*)

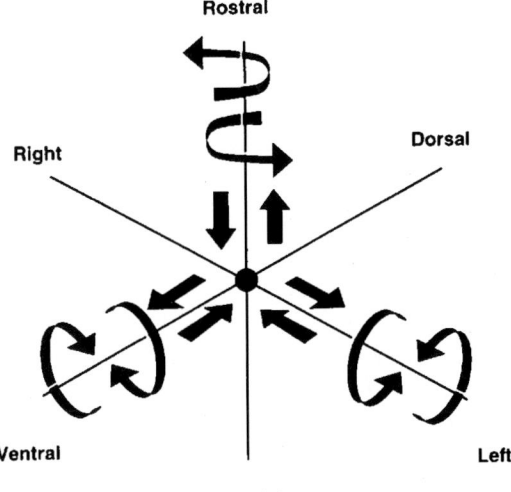

**Figure 109.3** The Cartesian coordinate system with the IAR as the center. Translation and rotation can occur in both of their respective directions about each axis.

at the bone-implant interface. Rotation about the long axis of the spine most certainly complicates this process (Figure 109.4).

Motion about or along the coronal axis involves lateral translation of one vertebral body upon another in the form of translation or rotation about the coronal axis via flexion or extension (Figure 109.5). Although the consideration of all of these motions in the design of a novel artificial disc is imperative, these same motions may contribute to its failure. The sagittal axis motion in the form of ventral or dorsal translation must also be considered. Spondylolisthesis is the common clinical pathologic paradigm for such. Lateral bending must also be permitted (Figure 109.6). These types of motion may contribute to failure of an artificial disc as well.

## Design Criteria

From the outset, a designer of motion preservation strategies is faced with two somewhat disparate goals: mobility and stability. In the intact spine the ROM at each individual joint is both limited and well controlled. If the ROM is restricted too severely, the motion segment approaches the equivalent of an arthrodesis with its aforementioned disadvantages. Likewise, a greater ROM, relative to that of the native disc, leads to hypermobility and possible aggravation of existing pain generators. An extruded prosthesis is as dangerous, if not more so, than a recurrent herniated nucleus pulposus. Therefore, it follows that extrusion rates must be less (much less) than the natural history of reherniation.

Because of both intrapatient and interpatient variabilities in disc space size and shape, manufacturers of disc protheses must provide a mechanism to properly "fit" an implant, as well as provide an adequate variety of sizes and shapes. This is especially important at the cortical margins of the vertebral body, where prosthesis contact points with bone must adequately engage the cortical margin of the vertebral body to take advantage of the boundary effect (i.e., the buttressing effect observed at or near the cortical margin of the vertebral body). The biomechanical properties of the vertebral end plate must also be considered with artificial disc implantation. The circumferential ring of denser end plate bone is termed *ring apophysis,* with the weakest portion of the vertebral end plates centered over the nucleus pulposus. The idea behind cortical margining with the surgical implantation of an artificial disc prosthesis is to achieve the greatest footprint possible while avoiding neurologic compromise. This would allow the denser portion of the vertebral end plate (i.e. the cortical ring along the periphery of the vertebral body) to be utilized to further stabilize the prosthesis. Encompassing the boundary of the vertebral end plate will minimize the risk of implant subsidence and pistoning through the central portion of the end plate.

An implant must provide immediate support and also ensure long-term stability. Furthermore, the implantation procedure must not compromise the critical native spinal elements, such as ligaments and facet joints. Injury of ligamentous structures may lead to spinal laxity and instability and may also enable prosthesis migration. The facet joints are crucial from a stability standpoint; perturbing them may create or exacerbate pain.

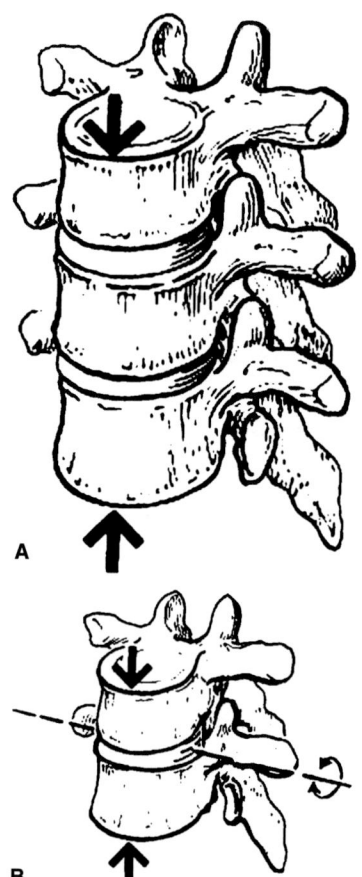

**Figure 109.5** A depiction of the forces (**A**) about a coronally oriented axis of the spine. Rotation about a coronally oriented axis can occur at the level of the disc interspace as well (**B**). Curved arrows depict bending moments. Straight arrows depict applied forces.

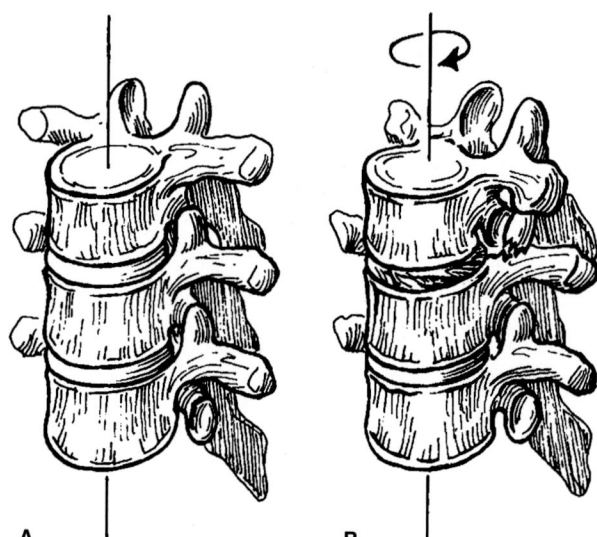

**Figure 109.4** A twisting of the spine about its long axis (**A**) can result in a rotation about the axis (**B**). Curved arrow depicts applied bending moment.

The importance of the bone-implant interface merits special attention. Implant design must consider the ability to achieve both immediate fixation and the promotion of long-term integration to bone (i.e., long-term fixation). Several strategies have emerged to gain immediate fixation and typically involve some combination of screws, staples, or teethlike projections. Long-term fixation is inherently more difficult. Designers have used various coatings and textures to promote bone ingrowth with varying success. Ironically, fixation that is too successful may be disastrous when it comes to revision surgery, if necessary. A significant biomechanical mismatch at this key junction could lead to either bone absorption or deposition, either of which could, in turn, lead to implant failure.

The daunting task of attempting to replicate the multicomponent, multifunctional, and multiplanar intervertebral disc has led some developers to focus on a more manageable number of characteristics. The lumbar disc has the greatest ROM in flexion and extension. This results in sagittal plane motion causing the greatest stress on the disc. This implies that flexion and extension stiffness are the most important mechanical properties of a disc prosthesis. An example of a focused strategy was that employed by Langrana et al.[25] using a design that attempted to duplicate the compressive and torsional stiffness at the cost of flexion, extension, and lateral bending characteristics. Hedman et al.[14] also attempted a more focused device, incorporating a design that consisted of a dorsal hinge with ventral metal springs (Figure 109.7). The result was excessive flexion and extension with minimal lateral bending and rotation. Combinational motions, including bending, compression, and rotation, can place excessive stress on the disc acutely or through repetitive cycling. These combined forces can ultimately fatigue the host bone at the implant-bone interface, thus resulting in prosthesis failure. Therefore, recent advances in disc prosthesis design involve biomechanically compatible materials that possess elastic moduli similar to the natural intervertebral disc. Many of the metal-elastomer-metal designs provide some degree of ROM in all primary directions and in axial compression. However, the exact stiffness and ROM vary greatly with the particular elastomer employed.

After the short-term requirements have been satisfied, two long-term issues must be addressed: creep and fatigue. The presence of any significant nonrecoverable creep jeopardizes one of the fundamental goals of disc space height restoration, ultimately compromising function as well.[2,3] With the expected average age of patients requiring disc replacement at 35 years, a prosthesis should be expected to

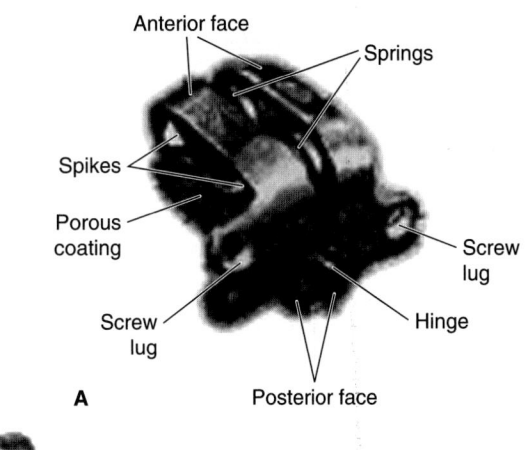

A

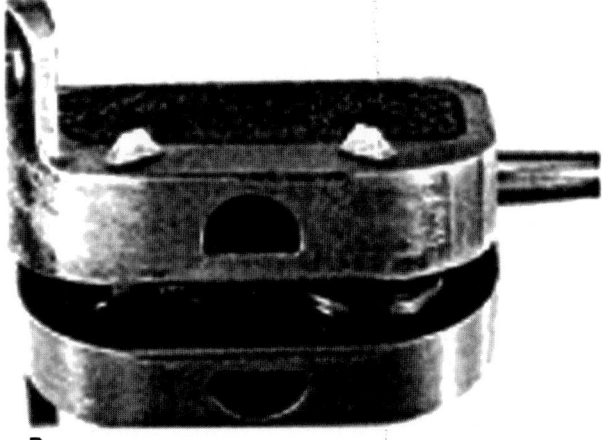

B

**Figure 109.7** (**A**) The Kostuik intervertebral disc prosthesis features a posteriorly located hinge and two titanium (Ti-6Al-4V) springs. (*From Kostuik JP: Intervertebral disc replacement. In Bridwell KH, DeWald RL[eds]: The Textbook of Spinal Surgery, ed 2. Philadelphia, Lippincott-Raven, 1997.*) (**B, C**) The Prosthetic Disc Nucleus (PDN) implant is a nucleus replacement that consists of a hydrogel core constrained in a woven polyethylene jacket. (*Courtesy of Raymedica, Inc., Bloomington, MN.*)

**Figure 109.6** Translation (**A**) and rotation (**B**) about the sagittal axis. (**B**, *Copyright Cleveland Clinic Foundation, 2003.*)

*Continued*

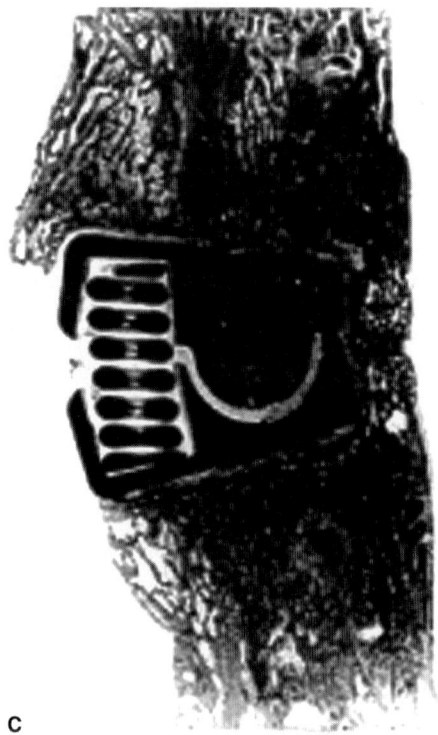

**C**
**Figure 109.7** *cont'd*

last an excess of 50 years. Shortening the disc life span necessitates the need for revision surgery, which, based on current implantation strategies, would be difficult as best. Fifty years of life has been conservatively estimated to equate to over 100 million motion cycles. This does not include minor motions, such as those associated with breathing.[22]

In addition to a high fatigue strength, the material or materials used must also possess additional characteristics, such as biocompatibility; none of the exposed implant components can elicit an inflammatory response. Given the expected longevity of the implant, corrosion and wear debris become significant concerns. In an ideal world, all or at least part of the prosthesis should be visible enough by at least one imaging modality to permit serial assessment of placement and alignment of the prosthesis. In addition, it should not create significant imaging artifact that obscures the prosthesis or surrounding tissues.

In the end, a design must strike a healthy balance between function and simplicity. A design that is too complicated will be difficult to implant surgically and costly to manufacture. Furthermore, a greater degree of design complexity will increase the probability that a given component will fail.

## Indications and Contraindications

The indications and contraindications for a disc prosthesis mirror those of an interbody fusion device, while those for a nucleus replacement device approximate those of a conventional discectomy. For patients with the primary complaint of radicular symptoms, nucleus replacement after discec-

tomy provides the prospect of restored disc height and function. This has been confirmed in numerous biomechanical studies using a human cadaveric model.[11,13,17,29] Patients with low back pain as the major complaint are perhaps more appropriate candidates for a complete disc prosthesis.

Current trials in the United States for lumbar disc prosthesis have been limited to patients who are between 18 and 60 years of age, with a single level of disease at either L4-5 or L5-S1. Patients should have undergone an aggressive conservative treatment trial lasting at least 6 months and should be capable of tolerating an operation that is roughly equivalent to a lumbar fusion.

The most important contraindication is the patient having pathology unlikely to be affected by a disc replacement. This includes those whose pain is not associated with dysfunctional segmental motion. However, this is difficult to define. Furthermore, as with any foreign body placement, the patient should be free of infection. Although there are currently no objective quantitative criteria for osteoporosis and spinal stenosis, there are relative contraindications. Patients who have had any previous lumbar spinal fusion are currently excluded from U.S. trials.

## Implant Types

### Early Attempts

Artificial disc researchers have been attempting to duplicate the success of Charnley[6] with hip replacement. His technology has evolved into a surgical strategy that is associated with significant success, including patient satisfaction. The early pioneers of motion preservation techniques included the work of Nachemson[28] and Fernstrom[12] over 40 years ago. Fernstrom attempted to reconstruct the disc space utilizing stainless steel balls. This strategy fell victim to unacceptably high rates of subsidence (88%). Most subsequent efforts were put on hold, awaiting a better understanding of biomechanics and the degenerative process itself. The development of a large variety of synthetic materials provided designers with a much needed armamentarium.

### Current Strategies

Essentially, three major types of strategies for reconstructing artificial disc space are feasible: (1) biologic reconstruction strategies, (2) nuclear replacement strategies, and (3) total disc replacement strategies (i.e., total disc arthroplasty [TDA]). They are each discussed below.

### *Biologic Reconstruction Strategies*

These strategies should theoretically be able to reconstitute the "youthful disc," or more correctly stated, restore the disc interspace to a more juvenile or youthful form. The young disc is composed of a gelatinous nucleus pulposus well augmented with strong annular fibers surrounding the nucleus. An ideal biologic strategy should, at a minimum, mimic the natural mechanics and anatomy of the intact intervertebral disc. Such strategies are associated with many barriers; perhaps the most significant of these barriers is a diminished potential for disc space

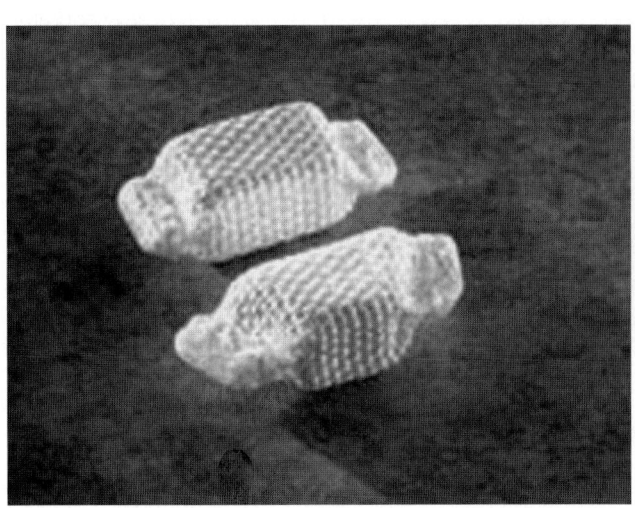
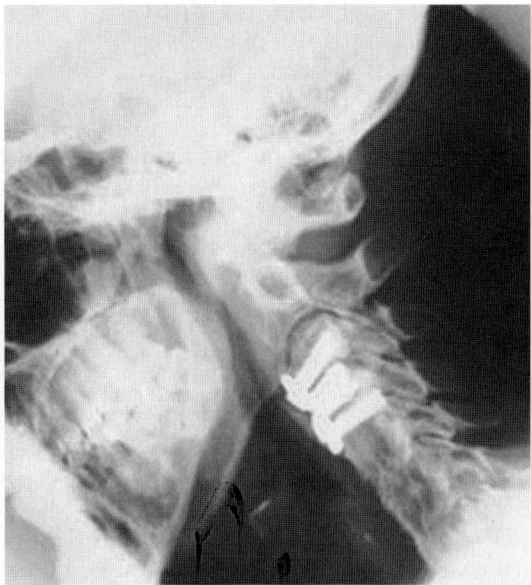

**A**     **B**

**Figure 109.8** **(A)** The cervical disc prosthesis originally developed in Bristol, England, by Cummins. The second generation of the Cummins disc is a ball and socket–type device constructed of stainless steel. It is secured to the vertebral bodies with screws. **(B)** Lateral c-spine x-ray depicting the prosthesis at C3-4.

nutrient delivery, which is vitally important for biologic strategies. Because biologic reconstruction strategies do not constitute a truly mechanical reconstruction process, they are not discussed further in this chapter.

## Nuclear Replacement Strategies

Nuclear replacement strategies involve the replacement of the central disc region (nucleus pulposus) with an artificial material, usually a polymer or similar material that is either prefabricated or is formed in vivo to a "custom fit." "Pillow" technologies, in which the internal material flows (e.g., the Prosthetic Disc Nucleus [PDN] from Raymedica, Inc.), have also been used. Finally, materials that bind with the disc interspace contents (i.e., the nucleus pulposus, annulus fibrosis) via tissue integration are in developmental phases. One distinct advantage to many of the nuclear replacement strategies is the potential for a minimally invasive, percutaneous method of insertion.

The PDN implant is composed of a hydrogel core surrounded by a woven ultrahigh molecular weight polyethylene (UHMWPE) jacket (Figure 109.7,B). When the hydrogel core is dehydrated and compressed, its size can be minimized to the shape of a small pellet, facilitating percutaneous placement. Once in the body, the hydrogel absorbs fluid through the flexible but inelastic UHMWPE jacket, expanding to maximum size over several days. The PDN has undergone extensive in vitro testing with good results. Clinical trials are currently underway in several countries.[31,32]

Other polymeric strategies are under development and investigation. Whether rigid (like a pill) or nonrigid (like a pillow), they all follow the prototypical lead of the Fernstrom ball, perhaps being similarly exposed to many of the problems associated with this strategy.

Nuclear replacement implants present many other challenges such as biocompatibility, extrusion through the annulus, and excessive motion within the discectomized region. Furthermore, repetitive spinal cycling can cause wear and wear debris deposition, as well as excessive motion about the implant. Finally, technologies such as the PDN device currently require an excessive removal of the annulus fibrosus for insertion, thus leading to an increased risk of extrusion. Appropriate annular tissue removal and void sizing within the disc space contributes to the stability of the nuclear replacement device. An oversized centralized void will allow the device to shift and rotate within that space, leading to possible implant migration, extrusion, or subsidence through the end plate. An eccentrically placed void and implant will negatively alter the biomechanics of the disc-implant complex. Therefore, proper host bed preparation is essential for successful implant outcomes.

## Total Disc Replacement Strategies

TDA strategies include artificial discs that require rigid attachments, via an osteointegration-like process, to the end plate. They are composed of two major types or categories: (1) the mechanical artificial disc and (2) the formable/flexible artificial disc. Both of these strategies require a tight bond between the artificial disc complex proper and the bony end plate region of the rostral and caudal vertebrae. Motion is permitted by either a mechanical process (Figures 109.8 through 109.10; also see Figure 109.7) or by a deformation of the formable flexible interface between the end plates (Figure 109.11). Both of these types of deformation are associated with many and significant potential advantages and disadvantages. Disc removal associated with artificial disc insertion requires the removal of at least 75% of the intervertebral disc. Therefore, if osteointegration is insufficient at the bony end plate, the implant is at risk of loosening. This may result in a more extensive revision surgery.

Modern attempts that use a mechanical articulation have included hinged plates and a ball and socket–type device. The Kostuik intervertebral prosthesis used a dorsally placed hinge connecting a set of cobalt-chromium-molybdenum alloy plates with a set of two ventrally placed titanium springs (see Figure 109.7).[14] This design favored flexion and extension over lateral bending and rotation and provided a physiologic range of motion in flexion, between 15 and 20 degrees. Immediate fixation was achieved through securing screws in each plate, while long-term fixation was facilitated by a porous coating on the cranial and caudal surfaces. These surfaces also had spikes to limit translation. The cervical disc prosthesis developed by Cummins (near Bristol, England, hence referred to as the Bristol Disc) uses a stainless steel ball-and-socket mechanism (see Figure 109. 8).[8] Notably, the Bristol Disc has not fallen victim to subsidence. However, total artificial disc implantation at multiple adjacent levels may lead to misalignment issues. This, in turn, would change the biomechanics along the neutral axis of the spine and could augment complications related to motion preservation.

Several artificial disc designs have employed a strategy that uses a formable or flexible core, sandwiched between two metal end plates (see Figure 109.11). The most widely implanted disc, the Charite III, consists of a biconvex UHMWPE spacer between two symmetric oval-shaped end plates made of a chromium-cobalt-molybdenum alloy (see Figure 109.11). Three ventral and dorsal teeth provide immediate fixation, while the end plates are coated with titanium and hydroxyapatite for long-term bony fusion. In the cervical spine the Bryan Disc uses a proprietary elastic nucleus that articulates between two anatomically shaped titanium plates (see Figure 109.10). A flexible membrane creates an enclosed space in which a lubricant bathes the articulating surfaces.

## Vulnerabilities and Complications

Multiple vulnerabilities exist regarding the application of artificial disc strategies to the clinical arena. These include the following:

1. Exposure of the construct to excessive loading
2. Excessive permitted motion
3. Debris from friction and fretting corrosion at motion-segment interfaces
4. Implant failure
5. Failure of osteointegration or tissue integration at the implant-bone or implant-tissue interface
6. Excessive facet joint degeneration
7. Excessive degeneration of the adjacent disc interspaces
8. Hypertrophic ossification
   Discussions of each will follow.

### Excessive Loading

Three fundamental types of loads that can stress the interface between the prosthesis and the end plates include (1) axial loads, (2) translational loads, and (3) angular loads. Excessive axial loading may not be tolerated by the end plate and hence can lead to failure. This usually is the result of an insufficient area of contact or an inadequate quality of surface area contact. The latter may result from the area of contact being located in the region of the end plate where the axial load-bearing ability is not optimal (e.g., in the midportion of the end plate, as opposed to the edges of the end plate [i.e., the boundary effect]) or is related to inadequate end plate integrity (as may be the case with osteoporosis in the aging spine).

Nuclear replacement strategies may suffer as well from inadequate end plate integrity, hence excessive loading is likely due to the small surface area of contact with the end plate. This, however, is obligatory with most nuclear replacement techniques.

Artificial discs of the TDA type differ mechanically from the dynamically changing loading patterns of the aging intact disc. Bone and soft tissue respond to excessive loading by forming more tissue along stress lines. Therefore, mismatched mechanical properties within an aging spine contribute to adjacent segment complications due to excessive loading, as does a solid arthrodesis.

The effectiveness of translation resistance relies on the ability of the prosthesis to solidly engage the end plate, usually via osteointegration (or occasionally via tissue integration). Significant translational stresses are placed on the spine, as is often the case in the low lumbar and lumbosacral regions. These stresses may exceed the ability of the prosthesis to resist translation.

Loading of the ventral end plates during flexion, the dorsal end plates during extension, or the lateral aspect of the end plates during lateral bending results in a significant stress concentration at the convex side of the bend. If the end plate is not capable of resisting such angular loads, failure may occur. Such loading is of greater significance and has a greater impact if a stiff prosthesis is employed. A device that does not absorb a significant amount of angular kinetic energy imparts this energy to the end plate region on the concave side of the bend, thus

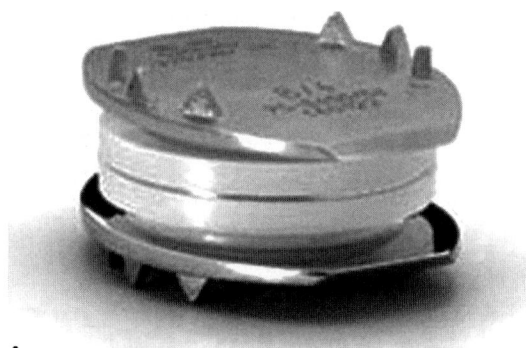

**A**

**Figure 109.9** The most widely implanted disc to date is the Link SB Charité disc (Waldemar Link GmbH & Co, Hamburg, Germany). The Charité III (**A**) consists of a biconvex ultra-high molecular weight polyethylene (UHMWPE) spacer. The end plates are made of casted cobalt-chromium-molybdenum alloy, each with three ventral and dorsal teeth. The device is shown implanted at L4-5 on (**B**) AP and (**C**) lateral lumbar x-rays.

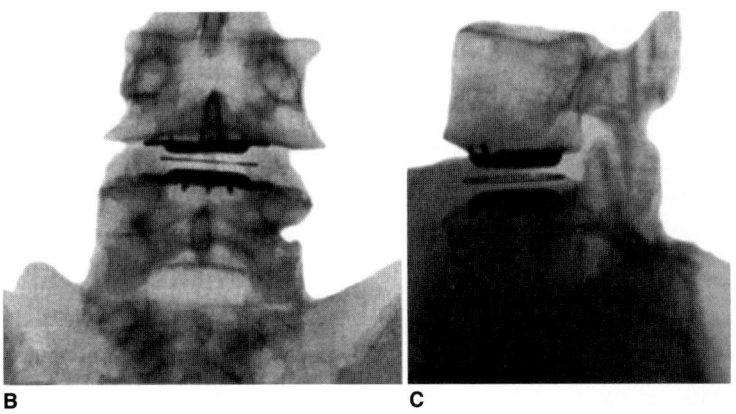

B                                                    C

**Figure 109.9** *cont'd*

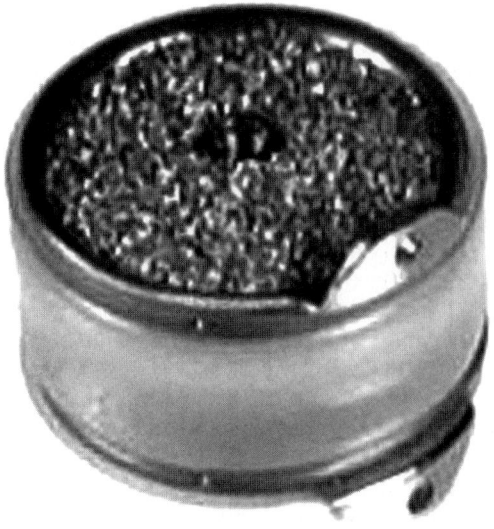

**Figure 109.10** The Bryan Cervical Disc System (Spinal Dynamics Corp, Seattle) is designed based on a proprietary, low friction, wear resistant, elastic nucleus. This nucleus is located between and articulates with anatomically shaped titanium plates (shells) that are fitted to the vertebral body end plates.

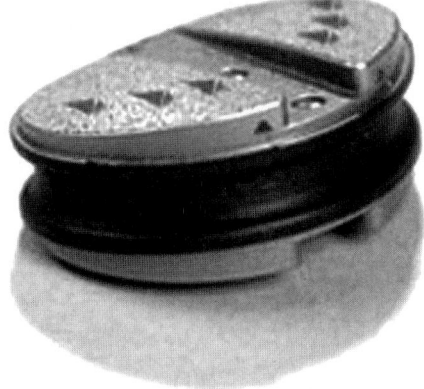

**Figure 109.11** The PRODISC (Spine Solutions, Inc, New York) consists of three implant components utilizing proven implant materials: forged cobalt-chrome–alloy end plate elements and an ultrahigh molecular weight polyethylene inlay element.

potentially creating an unacceptable stress riser at the edge of the implant-end plate interface and resulting in failure.

A question that must be addressed with respect to excessive motion is that of continued facet joint degeneration. It is not currently known if the facet degeneration will be halted, decelerated, or accelerated after artificial disc implantation. Artificial discs certainly can result in an excessive amount of translation, flexion/extension, or lateral bending motion. Obviously some translation, flexion/extension, and lateral bending is appropriate. Physiologic amounts of each is optimal. However, if either too little or too much motion is permitted, the physiologic nature of the motion may induce significant strain on supporting physiologic structures. If excessive motion is allowed, ligamentous supporting structures and paraspinous muscles would be required to compensate for the laxity imposed by the prosthesis. If the prosthesis were too stiff, wear and tear and degradation of the prosthesis-end plate interface may transpire. Obviously, a

homeostatic balance must be sought and ultimately achieved.

## Debris

Friction and fretting between interfaces results in particulate debris formation. This is clearly of concern, not only from a biologic and systemic perspective but also from a local tissue-reaction and propagation-of-corrosion perspective. Implant toxicity must be demonstrated to be zero or near zero. It goes without saying that this applies to local inflammatory and other reactions, as well as to systemic effects. Clinical trials for the first generation Acroflex disc were halted after it was discovered that 2-mercaptobenzothiazole, a chemical that used the vulcanization process for the rubber core, was shown to possibly be carcinogenic in rats.[9] Initial concerns over whether there would be significant wear debris resulting from articulations between UHMWPE and metal, as can be seen with hip protheses, do not seem to have materialized with the Charite III.[26] The makers of the Bryan Cervical Disc System (Spinal Dynamics Corporation, Seattle) have sought to decrease the chance of generation or propagation of wear debris by enclosing the articulating surfaces in a flexible membrane that also holds lubricant (see Figure 109.11).

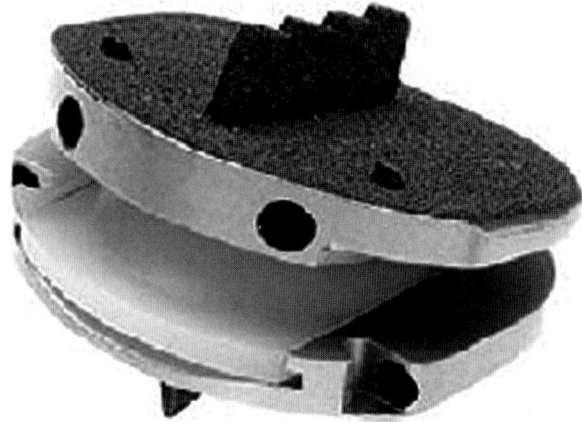

**Figure 109.12** The second generation Acroflex-100 consists of an HP-100 silicone elastomer core bonded to two titanium end plates. (*DePuy Spine, Raynham, MA.*)

## Implant Failure

Nuclear replacement devices, as well as mechanical devices, can migrate both laterally and dorsally (potentially into the spinal canal) or axially (via pistoning or subsiding into or through the end plates). Mechanical devices can fail by simple wear and tear or via other mechanical means at the component interfaces. Extrusion of a nuclear replacement device is a major concern. Under large bending moments and complex loading modes, the device is at risk of extrusion through the insertion tract.

### Failure of Bonding

Osteointegration is required for the success of TDA strategies. Others do not require this integrative process (such as selected nuclear replacement prostheses), whereas others require a bonding to the nucleus pulposus and annulus fibrosis via tissue integration.

### Modes of Failure

Artificial discs can fail in the postoperative period by simple catastrophic failure or migration. They can fail over a subacute period of time (weeks to months) by failing to integrate with juxtaposed tissue or bone (e.g., glacial migration). They can also deteriorate over years by gradual pistoning and failure of the prosthesis-end plate juncture. This may be, in part, attributable to aging and the inevitable osteoporotic and bone-weakening process. Finally, the spine continues to degenerate, even after motion has been restored. Facet joints will continue to degenerate. In fact, they may degrade excessively if an interbody implant permits excessive motion at the disc interspace. Osteophytes may also form at the intervertebral disc. This must be accounted for with respect to the decision to employ such implants.

While the remaining challenges in developing motion preservation strategies are numerous, the potential to improve millions of lives suffering from degenerative disc disease necessitates success. Through hard work and inno-

vation, it may be possible to achieve the same level of success currently enjoyed by knee and hip arthroplasties, two surgical procedures that are among the highest rated in terms of patient satisfaction.

## Published Outcomes and Clinical Trials

Well over 3000 artificial disc surgeries have been performed in Europe, primarily in the United Kingdom, France, Germany, and the Netherlands. In 1997, Lemaire et al.[25] published a series of 105 cases performed in France with the SB Charite III. Patients were followed for an average of 8 years postoperatively. "Excellent" results were reported for 79% of patients, with 87% returning to work. This included 81% of sedentary workers and 45% of heavy laborers returning to the same job. The first independent review was conducted in 1997 in the United States by Alexis Shelekov, MD, and Jeanette Ahrens, PhD. They retrospectively examined 67 patients who received a total of 91 SB Charite III disc replacements (one or two lumbar levels) in Europe. They utilized radiologic and clinical data and had an average follow-up period of 6 years. There was a significant drop in postoperative analog pain scores, with 70% of patients decreasing or discontinuing their use of pain medication. Sixty-seven percent of patients were able to return to work at the same or a modified level of physical activity. A complication rate of 7% was recorded.

In March of 2000 the first SB Charite III artificial disc was implanted in the United States as part of an Food and Drug Administration study funded by LINK Spine Group, Inc., the manufacturers of the disc. The study is intended to eventually include 10 U.S. medical centers that will perform 400 surgeries on patients that will be randomized to the SB Charite III or interbody spinal fusion with the BAK anterior interbody cages. The patients will be followed postoperatively for 2 years, with possible introduction to the general population as early as 2004. Spine Solutions, Inc., the makers of a competing design called the PRODISC, is in the process of conducting multicenter, prospective, randomized, controlled clinical trial comparing the safety and effectiveness of its disc to spinal fusion. Patients will be randomized, using a ratio of 2 to 1, to the PRODISC and a control group of spinal fusion. Both one and two adjacent levels will be studied, but in separate arms of the study.

Recently, de Kleuver et al.[10] conducted a systematic literature review, yielding only nine case series, and notably no controlled trials, for TDA in the treatment of chronic low back pain. Although these devices have been implanted in Europe for almost 15 years, the authors could not find adequate supporting data that TDA successfully filled their three primary criteria: (1) clinical efficacy, (2) continued motion, and (3) reduced degeneration at adjacent segments. They concluded that TDA, based on the available data, does not appear to be better than arthrodesis. As long-term studies on TDA currently underway are completed, it may well be that this technology is ultimately vindicated, but for now it seems it should remain an experimental procedure relegated to strictly controlled clinical trials. The review concludes with a prophetic warning with regards to finding a solution to the multifactorial problem of chronic low back pain. Despite the emergence of new experimental devices, patient selection remains the paramount factor leading to a successful patient outcome.

# REFERENCES

1. Adams MA, Hutton WC: Mechanics of the intervertebral disc. In Golsh P (ed): *The Biology of the Intervertebral Disc*, vol 2. Boca Raton, FL, CRC Press, 1988, pp 39-72.
2. Bao QB, Yuan HA: New technologies in spine: nucleus replacement, *Spine* 27(11):1245-1247, 2002.
3. Bao QB, Yuan HA: Prosthetic disc replacement: the future? *Clin Orthop* Jan:139-145, 2002.
4. Benzel EC: Biomechanically relevant anatomy and material properties of the spine and associated elements. In Benzel EC (ed): *Biomechanics of Spine Stabilization*. Rolling Meadows, IL, AANS Press, 2001, pp 1-17.
5. Broberg KB: On the mechanical behavior of intervertebral discs, *Spine* 8(2):151-165, 1983.
6. Charnley J: Total hip replacement, *JAMA* 230(7): 1025-1028, 1974.
7. Crock HV: Internal disc disruption. A challenge to disc prolapse fifty years on, *Spine* 11(6):650-653, 1986.
8. Cummins BH, Robertson JT, Gill SG: Surgical experience with an implanted artificial cervical joint, *J Neurosurg* 88:943-948, 1998.
9. Deiter MP: *Toxicology and carcinogenesis studies of 2–mercaptobenzothiazole in F344/n rats and B6C3F mice*, NIH pub no 88–8, National Toxicology Program, technical report series no 322, Washington, DC, 1998, U.S. Department of Health and Human Services.
10. de Kleuver M, Oner FC, Jacobs WCH: Total disc replacement for chronic low back pain: background and a systematic review of the literature, *Eur Spine J* 12:108-116, 2003.
11. Eysel P, Rompe J, Schoenmayr R, Zoellner J: Biomechanical behavior of a prosthetic lumbar nucleus, *Acta Neurochir* 141(10):1083-1087, 1999.
12. Fernstrom U: Arthroplasty with intercorporal endoprosthesis in herniated disc and in painful disc, *Eur J Surg Suppl* 357:154-159, 1966.
13. Garcia A, Lavignolle B, Morlier P, *et al:* Intradiscal polymerization: preliminary results of chemical and biochemical studies. In Brock M, Mayer HM, Weigel J (eds): *The Artificial Disc* Berlin, Springer, 1991, p 39-43.
14. Hedman TP, Kostuik JP, Fernie GR, Hellier WG: Design of an intervertebral disc prosthesis, *Spine* 16(Suppl 6): S256-S260, 1991.
15. Hirabayashi K, Maruyama T, Wakano K, *et al.:* Postoperative lumbar canal stenosis due to anterior spinal fusion, *Keio J Med* 30(3):133-139, 1981.
16. Holmes AD, Hukins DW: Analysis of load-relaxation in compressed segments of lumbar spine, *Med Eng Phys* 18(2):99-104, 1996.
17. Hou TS, Tu KY, Xu YK, *et al:* Lumbar intervertebral disc prosthesis. An experimental study, *Chin Med J (Engl)* 104(5):381-386, 1991.
18. Hukins DW: Disc structure and function. In Golsh P (ed): *The Biology of the Intervertebral Disc*, vol 1. Boca Raton, FL, CRC Press, 1988, pp 1-38.
19. Kaapa E, Holm S, Han X, *et al:* Collagens in the injured porcine intervertebral disc, *J Orthop Res* 12(1):93-102, 1994.
20. Keller TS, Hansson TH, Abram AC, *et al:* Regional variations in the compressive properties of lumbar vertebral trabeculae. Effects of disc degeneration, *Spine* 14(9): 1012-1019, 1989.
21. Kirkaldy-Willis WH, Wedge JH, Yong-Hing K, Reilly J: Pathology and pathogenesis of lumbar spondylosis and stenosis, *Spine* 3(4):319-328, 1978.
22. Kostuik JP: Intervertebral disc replacement. In Bridwell KH, DeWald RL (eds): *The Textbook of Spinal Surgery*, ed 2. Philadelphia, Lippincott-Raven, 1997, pp 2257-2266.
23. Krag MH, Seroussi RE, Wilder DG, Pope MH: Internal displacement distribution from in vitro loading of human thoracic and lumbar spinal motion segments: experimental results and theoretical predictions, *Spine* 12(10):1001-1007, 1987.
24. Lee CK, Langrana NA: Lumbosacral spinal fusion. A biomechanical study, *Spine* 9(6):574-581, 1984.
25. Lemaire JP, Skalli W, Lavaste F, *et al:* Intervertebral disc prosthesis. Results and prospects for the year 2000, *Clin Orthop* 337:64-76, 1997.
26. Link HD: LINK SB Charité III intervertebral dynamic disc spacer, *Rachis Revue de Pathologie Vertebrale* 11: 1999.
27. Lipson SJ: Degenerative spinal stenosis following old lumbosacral fusion, *Orthop Trans* 7:143, 1983.
28. Nachemson AL: Challenge of the artificial disc. In Weinstein JN (ed): *Clinical Efficacy and Outcome in the Diagnosis and Treatment of Low Back Pain*, New York, Raven Press, 1992.
29. Ordway NR, Han ZH, Bao QB, *et al:* A biomechanical evaluation of a hydrogel intervertebral disc nucleus in vitro, *Trans Orthop Res Soc* 20:676, 1995.
30. Pennal GF, Conn GS, McDonald G, *et al:* Motion studies of the lumbar spine: a preliminary report, *J Bone Joint Surg Br* 54(3):442-452, 1972.
31. Ray CD, Schönmayr R, Kavanagh SA, Assell R: Prosthetic disc nucleus implants, *Riv Neuroradiol* 12(Suppl 1): 157-162, 1999.
32. Schönmayr R, Busch C, Lotz C, Lotz–Metz G: Prosthetic disc nucleus implants: the Wiesbaden feasibility study. 2 years follow-up in ten patients. *Riv Neuroradiol* 12(Suppl 1):163-170, 1999.
33. Traynelis VC: Joint replacement in neurosurgery. In *Clinical Neurosurgery*, vol 48., Philadelphia, Lippincott Williams and Wilkins, 2000, pp 82-95.
34. Weinstein PR: Anatomy of the lumbar spine. In Hardy RW (ed): *Lumbar Disc Disease*. New York, Raven Press, 1982, pp 5-15.

# CHAPTER 110

# Upper Cervical Screw Fixation Techniques

**Ronald I. Apfelbaum, Mehmet Zileli, and Charles B. Stillerman**

Internal fixation is often used provide immediate stabilization. This protects the vital neural and vascular elements. It is especially important in the highly mobile cervical spine.

The occipitocervical junction and atlantoaxial complex (upper cervical spine) comprise a transitional region connecting the rest of the spinal column to the cranium. The vertebrae and joints in this area are different from those in the subaxial spine, with special modifications to allow unique degrees of motion. Arguably, the most important of these are at the C1-2 complex, where the flat lateral articulations, absence of an intervertebral disc, and lax ligaments permit appreciable rotation at C1-2 (about 50% of total head rotation) (Figure 110.1).[58] This motion is safely tolerated because the spinal canal is more generous, the instantaneous axis of rotation is located close to the spinal cord (minimizing distortion of that structure), and the vertebral arteries loop laterally (allowing for at least one to remain patent, even at the extremes of rotation). Potentially catastrophic translational movements, which would crush the spinal cord, are prevented by the very strong transverse component of the cruciate ligament (in adults, usually 8 to 10mm in diameter) that contains the odontoid process of the axis in the ventral compartment of the atlas. Disruption of this ligament, with or without bursting of the ring of C1 (Jefferson's fracture) or disruption of the odontoid process, results in gross instability. The remaining ligamentous structures, if intact, may provide some support, but they are too weak intrinsically to protect the spinal cord from even relatively minor trauma.

The restoration of structural integrity is critical. If the instability is caused by bone disruption, healing can occur with proper external immobilization. If it is caused by ligamentous disruption, however, it requires surgery to achieve a bony fusion between previously hypermobile motion segments to protect the spinal cord. For bone healing or fusion to occur, two criteria must be met: (1) the bone graft (or bone fragments) must be touching or in proximity and (2) motion must be eliminated or minimized.

Internal fixation can provide immediate stabilization to optimize bone graft and fragment healing. It does this better than rigid external immobilization (such as a halo vest or Minerva jacket) while avoiding the cost, discomfort, and complications associated with these devices.

To achieve the degree of stability necessary to protect the neural elements, screw fixation is often helpful. Wiring techniques alone or devices that do not constrain rotation are usually not sufficient unless a concomitant external orthosis is used.

## General Considerations

It is of paramount importance to protect the neural elements when instability exists. Before surgery, the patient must be properly immobilized. Depending on the degree of instability, this may be achieved with a rigid cervical collar or it may require skeletal traction, a halo vest, or Minerva jacket. Ongoing spinal canal compromise, if present, should be corrected as expediently as possible, before fusion is attempted. This could involve restoring alignment with carefully applied and maintained cervical traction via cranial tongs or surgical removal of intraspinal masses. The latter may require transoral decompression of a rheumatoid pannus or a retropulsed odontoid process or dorsal resection and elevation of indriven bone fragments. Once the nature of the pathology has been fully investigated and plans for restoration of the spinal canal to normal or adequate dimensions and for spinal realignment have been conceived, the stabilization component of the surgical strategy can be planned. Some of the techniques to be detailed require anatomic integrity in specific regions. This must be assessed carefully during the planning stage. The patient's general medical condition should be optimized and other associated injuries and traumatic situations evaluated and treated as appropriate.

## Anesthetic Considerations

The degree of cervical spine instability and direction of movement that produce subluxation should be conveyed to the anesthesiologist. For example, an odontoid process fracture is often unstable in both flexion and extension, whereas a transverse ligament rupture may be unstable only in flexion. In the former case, an awake fiberoptic intubation may be necessary. In the latter case, routine laryngoscopic techniques can be used. The first author (Apfelbaum) uses C-arm fluoroscopy extensively for intraoperative guidance. It may be set up before inducing anesthesia so that it can be used to monitor spinal alignment during intubation and positioning.

Spinal cord injury patients with significantly reduced vasomotor tone may require substantial intravenous fluid volume replacement or vasopressors to maintain adequate circulatory volume and blood pressure.

## Ventral Approaches

### Indications

Ventral screw techniques are primarily indicated for direct screw fixation of odontoid process fractures. Infrequently, direct screw fixation of C1-2 can be performed ventrally as well. C2-3 ventral fusion and plating may be used for a hangman's fracture.[55] The latter technique is no different from ventral cervical fusion and plating at lower levels other than the difficulty associated with the angle of approach to C2. The retractor system used for odontoid screw fixation may sometimes be useful in this regard.

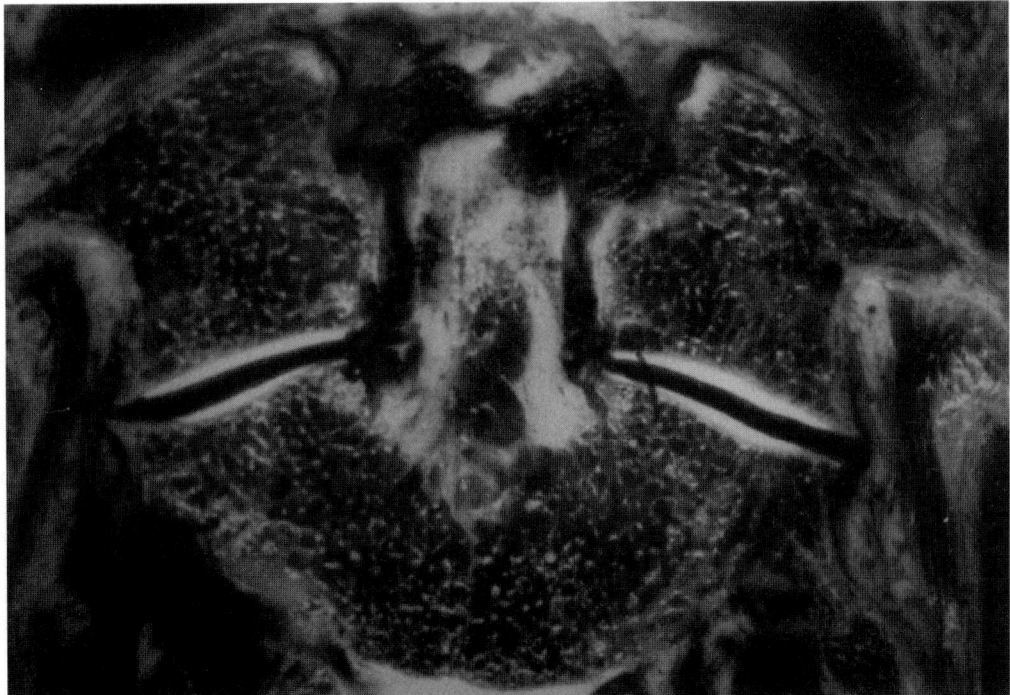

**Figure 110.1** Coronal anatomic section through the atlantoaxial complex at the level of the odontoid process. Note the horizontal axis of the C1-2 articulation and absence of an intervertebral disc that contributes to the degree of rotatory motion at this joint. *(Illustration provided by Dr. Wolfgang Rauschning, Uppsala, Sweden.)*

Odontoid process fractures were classified by Anderson and D'Alonzo[2] as types I, II and III. Type I fractures involve the apical part of the odontoid process, are quite rare, and are usually believed to be stable. However, one report suggests otherwise,[51] and dynamic imaging should therefore be used to assess stability. Type II fractures involve the neck of the odontoid process and are the most common. Type III fractures extend into the body of C2 and generally heal well with immobilization. Benzel et al.,[9] in a very comprehensive review of fractures of the C2 vertebral body, pointed out, however, that the type III fracture described by Anderson and D'Alonzo is not an odontoid fracture at all. They have proposed a classification of C2 body fractures that is more comprehensive and more meaningful in regard to mechanisms of injury.

There is controversy over the optimal treatment of type II fractures. Reported nonunion rates range from 7%[41] to 100%.[43] Nonunion rates of 21% to 45% have been reported frequently,* and there are many other reports of nonunion in the 50% to 63% range.[1,10,36,47,50] Julien et al.,[38] in a thorough literature search, found that for type II fractures, halo vest immobilization produced a fusion rate of 65%, which was only slightly better than traction alone at 57%. This has led some authors to define parameters that predict failure with external immobilization. Extent of dislocation (67% nonunion if dislocation is greater than 6mm[33]; 88% nonunion with dislocation greater than 4mm[8] in two studies), age of patient (higher failure rate if age is greater than 40[8] or 65[23]), and direction of subluxation (higher failure

rate with dorsal subluxation[23]) have all been suggested as predictors, as has a comminuted fragment of bone at the base of the odontoid process (type "IIA").[34] Although these studies fail to agree on many points, they do emphasize the nature of the problem. Degree of offset may be a misleading indicator, because no authors have advocated dynamic studies. Rather, they have made decisions based on single radiographs, which can significantly underestimate the frequency of more serious fractures (Figure 110.2). In a randomized controlled prospective study, Lennarson et al.[39] found a 21 times greater nonunion rate in patients over the age of 50 who were treated with halo immobilization. This study was a key factor leading to a recommendation for surgery in the guidelines for management of acute cervical spine and spinal cord injuries published by the Joint Section of Disorders of the Spine and Peripheral Nerves of the American Association of Neurological Surgeons and Congress of Neurological Surgeons.[32]

The nonoperative treatment of type II odontoid fractures clearly has a high nonunion rate (Figure 110.3). This has led to the development of several alternative methods of surgical fixation. The traditional operative technique for type II odontoid process fractures has been C1-2 dorsal wiring and arthrodesis. A relatively high fusion rate is associated with this technique. However, rigid postoperative bracing for at least 3 months is necessary, and there is a significant reduction in head rotation. The dorsal approach also has an associated traumatic effect on cervical muscles. All these disadvantages can be obviated by using direct ventral odontoid screw fixation techniques.

*References 8,15,22,24,27,32,48,57.

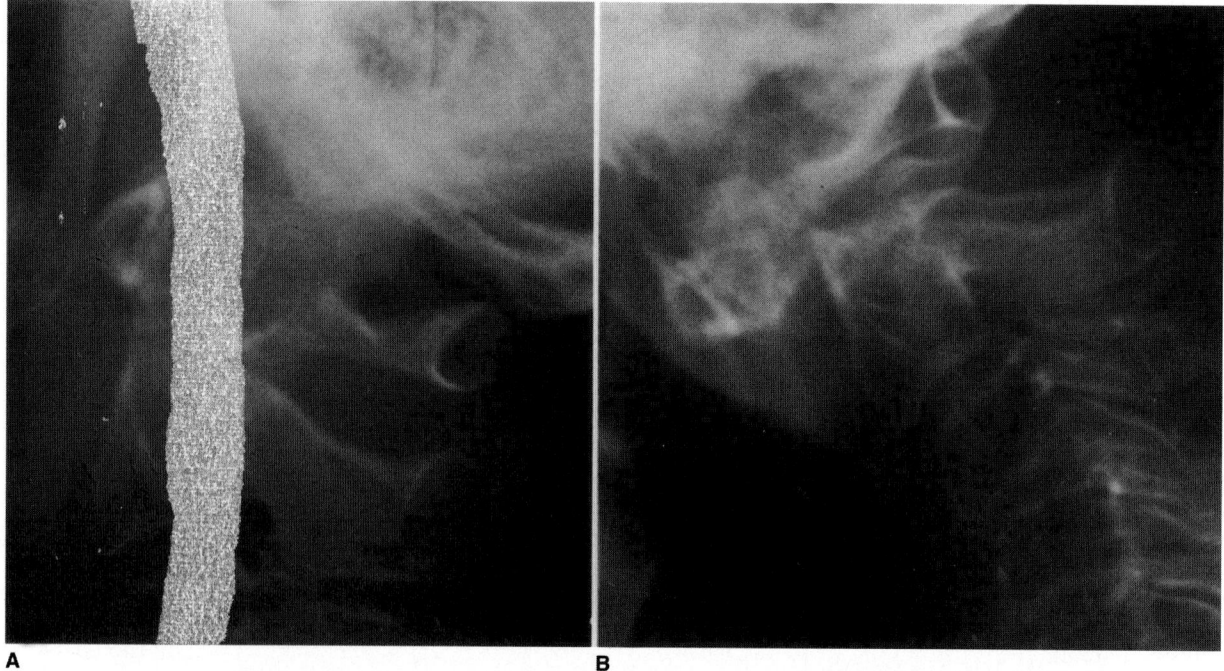

**A**                                                              **B**

**Figure 110.2** **(A)** Patient with unrecognized odontoid process fracture after a fall. **(B)** Flexion film shows severe instability with 100% anterolisthesis, demonstrating the fallacy of relying on a single film to predict the degree of instability.

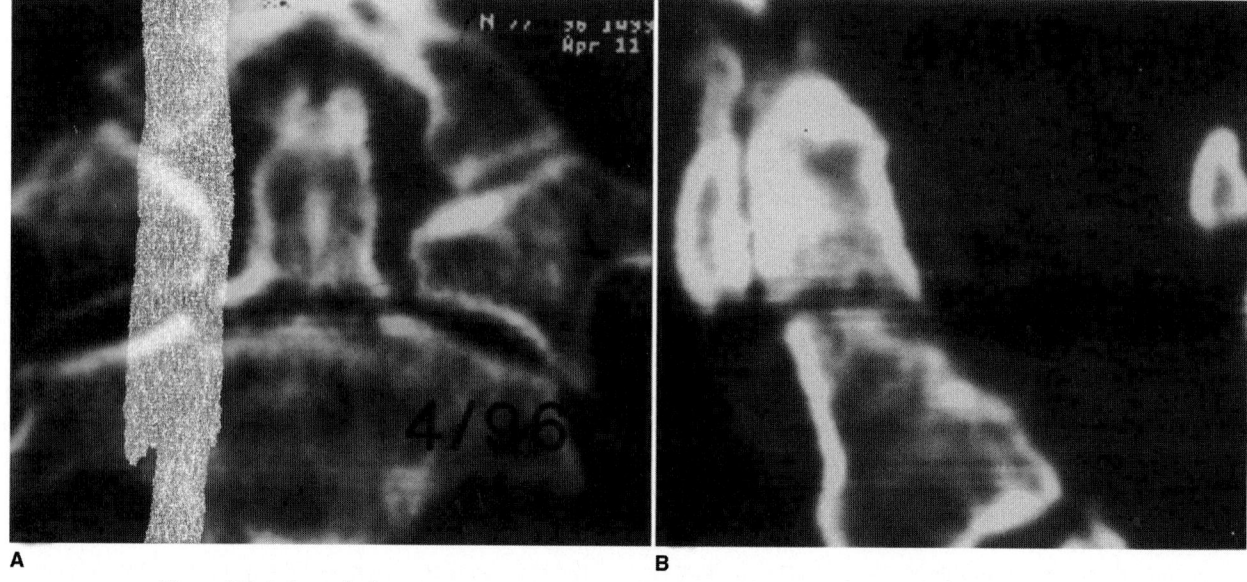

**A**                                                              **B**

**Figure 110.3** **(A** and **B)** Anteroposterior and lateral CT images of a 78-year-old patient with a type II odontoid fracture sustained in a motor vehicle accident. At this juncture he has been in a halo vest for 6 months and has no evidence of union despite being in good alignment.

## Direct Ventral Odontoid Screw Fixation

Direct screw fixation of the odontoid process was first described in 1980 in the Japanese literature by Nakanishi, who began using this technique in 1978.[46] This was followed in 1981 and in 1982 by Böhler, who reported his experience since 1968.[11,12] Lesoin in 1987,[40] Borne in 1988,[13] Geisler in 1989,[29] and Esses in 1991[25] reported their experiences with various approaches to achieve direct odontoid screw fixation. The procedure, however, was not widely accepted. With subsequent developments in instrumentation to refine this technique,[3-5] the procedure has gained popularity. The technique has the advantages of (1) decreased postoperative pain resulting from lack of extensive muscle dissection, (2) avoidance of bone graft harvest, and (3) maintenance of normal anatomy and rotation at the C1-2 joint.[37] Furthermore, many patients require no postoperative immobilization.

Acute type II fractures may be treated this way as the primary approach or after failure to heal after a period of external immobilization. Type II dens fractures with concomitant C1 ring fracture may also be candidates for odontoid screw fixation. However, assessment of transverse ligament integrity is essential preoperatively by magnetic resonance imaging (MRI)[20] and postoperatively by flexion fluoroscopy. If the latter demonstrates continued C1-2 instability, either a ventral or a dorsal C1-2 fusion is necessary. The direct screw fixation technique may also be used in some patients with chronic nonunion of type II odontoid fractures. Candidates should have a relatively small gap between the odontoid process and the C2 body and a reasonably sized odontoid fragment that has not autofused to C1. Chronic malunions that do not meet these criteria rarely fuse and will ultimately fracture the hardware and become unstable. The chance of successful bony union in one small series of such patients with fractures over 18 months of age was only 25%. This sharply contrasted with an 88% fusion rate for type II and high type III fractures of less than 6 months of age. For this reason, we generally recommend posterior C1-2 fusion for chronically nonunited fractures. Unstable type III odontoid fractures that do not extend too far into the body of C2 are also potential candidates for direct screw fixation.

### Contraindications

Absolute contraindications include comminuted fractures of the C2 body and transverse ligament disruption as defined by MRI or suggested by a C1 lateral mass fracture with extensive lateral displacement (greater than 7mm total on anteroposterior radiographs),[53] pathologic fractures, and nonunions of more than 6 to 8 months duration that do not meet the aforementioned criteria. A relative contraindication is severe osteoporosis. In addition, an oblique fracture of the odontoid process, angled caudally and ventrally so that it is parallel to the planned screw trajectory, may not be as suitable for ventral screw fixation because the odontoid process may slide down the fracture plane as the screw is tightened. Such anterior oblique fractures, while accounting for only 16% of the cases in one published series, had a significantly higher failure rate. This is, however, not an absolute contraindication but a relative one. By starting fixation in a slightly retrolisthesed position and augmenting the construct with a rigid cervical collar, successful fusion has been achieved.

A barrel-shaped chest and short neck can render the surgical approach more difficult, but with the instrumentation described below, these are rarely contraindications for the procedure. Finally, two quality C-arms are preferred, and the procedure should not be attempted without at least one.

### Patient Positioning

The patient is placed supine with the neck extended for proper screw trajectory. A folded sheet or blanket is placed under the shoulders. If the neck cannot be initially extended, as judged by careful lateral fluoroscopic monitoring, the head is supported on folded towels in neutral neck alignment. Holter traction with a light weight (5lb)

hung over the Mayfield U-bar attachment to the operative table is very useful for stabilizing the head.

For odontoid or ventral C1-2 screw placement, biplanar fluoroscopy is necessary. The anteroposterior view is obtained transorally. A wine bottle cork, notched for the teeth or gums, is an ideal radiolucent mouth prop. A single fluoroscope can be used if necessary. If so, it must be swung back and forth frequently from the lateral to the anteroposterior position. A triangular space for one side of the C-arm can be walled off with drapes and IV poles to facilitate frequent positioning while minimizing the need to redrape the C-arm. It is best to use a second C-arm fluoroscope. One is placed laterally with the arc horizontally or up to 45 degrees above the horizon. The other can be brought in at a 45-degree angle from the head of the table and positioned for the transoral view (Figure 110.4). Some adjustments may be needed to optimize the views, but once this is achieved, the remainder of the procedure is greatly facilitated. The anesthesiologist remains at the head of the table in the remaining quadrant. This provides optimal access to the patient's head and airway. The surgeon stands on one side of the patient with the assistant on the opposite side. The C-arm monitor should be positioned for optimal viewing by the surgeon.

### Operative Technique

Several screw systems have been used, but all begin with the same exposure. The initial approach to the spine is the same as for a ventral cervical discectomy. The spine is approached at about the C5 level through a unilateral natural skin crease incision. We use a local injection with epinephrine (1:200,000) to minimize skin bleeding and complete hemostasis with bipolar cautery. The platysma muscle is elevated and divided with monopolar cautery. The sternocleidomastoid muscle fascia is opened along the medial side of the muscle with sharp dissection. Blunt dissection then opens the deeper tissue planes medial to the carotid sheath and lateral to the trachea and esophagus to expose the prevertebral space. Dividing the longus colli fascia and the anterior longitudinal ligament in the midline with electrocautery allows the bellies of the longus colli muscle to be elevated bilaterally over approximately one and one-half vertebral segments. Sharp-bladed Caspar retractors are set in place below the muscle and attached to a special retractor holder if the Apfelbaum system (Aesculap Instrument Corporation, South San Francisco, CA) is being used (Figure 110.5) or to a regular Caspar holder with other systems.

The loose areolar tissue in the prevertebral space ventral to the longus colli muscles is easily opened with a Kitner or "peanut" dissector held in a curved tonsil clamp. It is swept from side to side while advancing up to the C1-2 level (monitored with lateral fluoroscopy). The Apfelbaum system has an angled retractor blade that reaches into the space under the mandible and holds open the working tunnel. It attaches to one side of the previously placed lateral retractors. Other systems use different retractors, such as a curved hand-held retractor (Synthes) or small metal hook-shaped retractors (Hohmann) that lock over the shoulders of C2 bilaterally alongside the dens, as initially described by Böhler.[12] The key to the

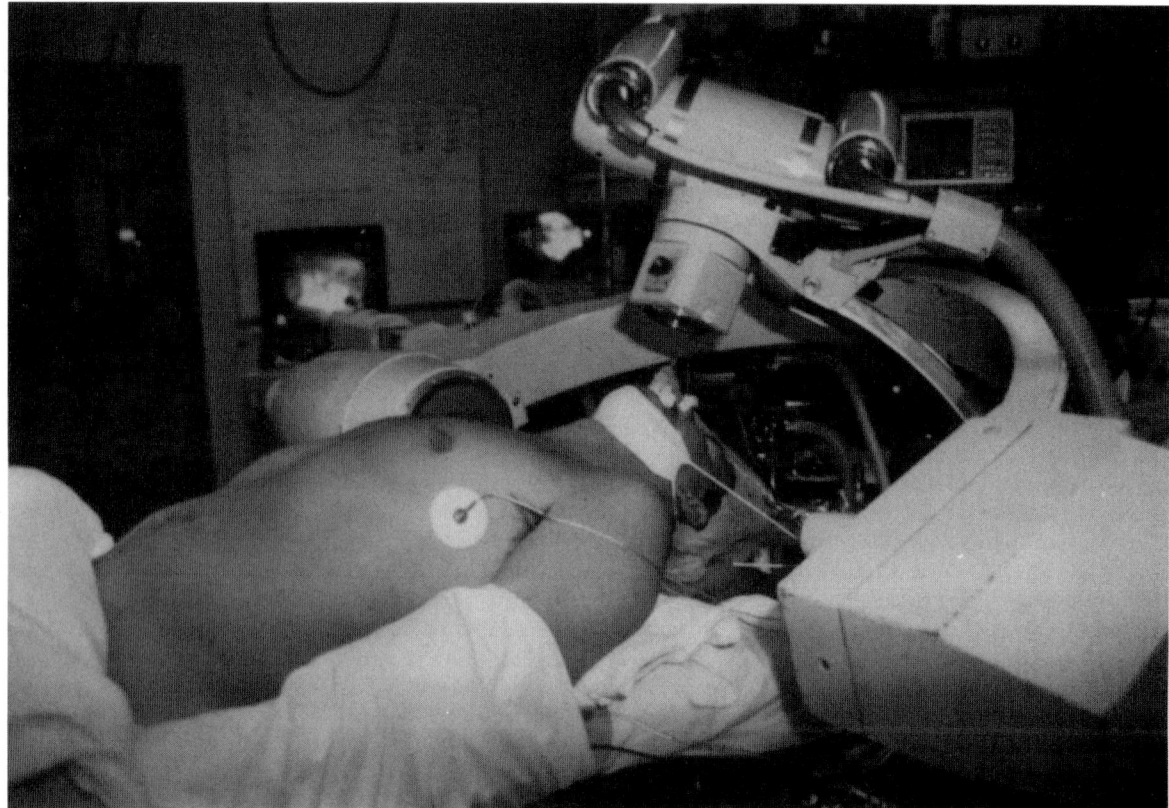

**Figure 110.4** Patient positioned on operating table. Note folded sheet under shoulders to increase neck extension in this patient whose fracture reduced in extension. Note also the placement of two C-arm fluoroscopic units for anteroposterior (transoral) and lateral fluoroscopic control.

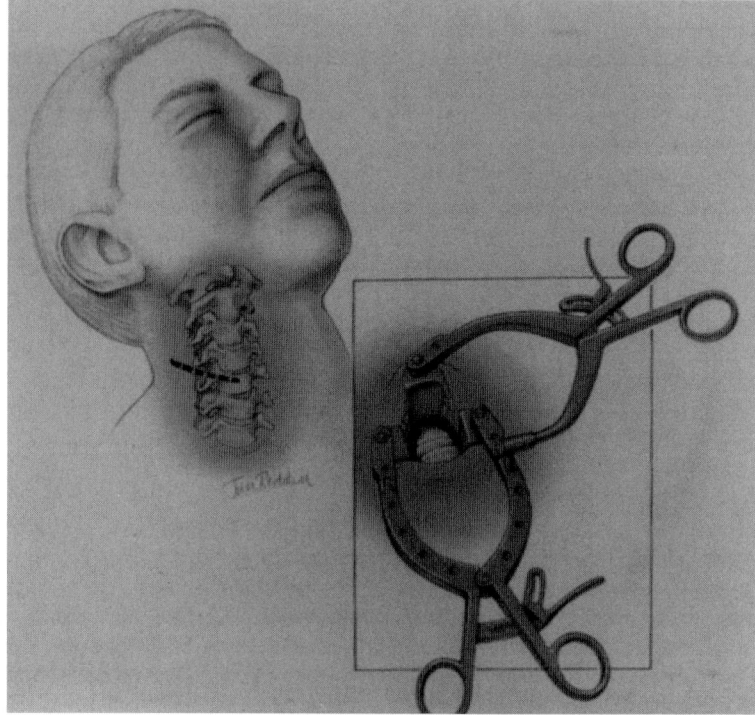

**Figure 110.5** Skin incision in a natural skin crease at about the C5 level. Inset shows retractor in place.

retraction is to create a working tunnel up to the caudal edge of C2, without having any device caudally in the wound that restricts the low trajectory needed for proper screw placement.

At this point, the various systems use somewhat different approaches for placing the screws. The Apfelbaum system has a guide tube system consisting of an outer guide tube with spikes that anchors it to C3 and that can be used to optimize spinal alignment. An inner guide tube, within the outer tube, guides the drilling. Once the pilot hole is drilled, the inner guide is removed, the hole is tapped, and the screws are placed through the outer guide tube. The operative sequence is as follows. First, an entry site on the ventral caudal edge of C2 is selected and a K-wire is impacted into C2 (Figure 110.6A). This is done under biplanar fluoroscopic control. If one screw is to be placed, a midline location is chosen. If two are to be placed, a paramedian location is selected 3 to 4mm from the midline. Care and patience in selecting the entry site and setting the K-wire will be rewarded by the remainder of the procedure being expedited. Once the K-wire is set, a 7mm hollow drill is placed over the K-wire and is rotated by hand to create a shallow trough in the face of C3 and in the C2-3 annulus (see Figure 110.6B-D). No bone is removed from C2. The two guide tubes are then mated together, passed over the

K-wire, and walked up the ventral face of the spinal column until the spikes on the outer tube are over the body of C3. A plastic impactor sleeve allows the seating of these spikes into C3. The inner guide tube is then advanced to the ventral caudal edge of C2 in the trough previously created (Figure 110.7), and the K-wire is removed. Having the guide tube at the entry site prevents the drill from skipping off the edge of the bone and walking up the ventral face of C2. With the guide tube system firmly engaged in C3 and steady, the surgeon can then optimize the C2 alignment by either pushing C2 and C3 dorsally relative to the odontoid-C1 complex or pulling C2 and C3 ventrally. This is performed while monitoring the fluoroscopic images. In the case of a retrolisthesed odontoid process, this realignment can be performed while gradually extending the patient's head and removing the supporting towels beneath it, to obtain an ideal working trajectory.

A pilot hole is then drilled from the ventral caudal edge of C2 to the apex of the odontoid process, advancing the drill slowly under biplanar fluoroscopic control (Figure 110.8). The odontoid process has a dense cortical shell that must be pierced to engage the screw properly and to avoid splitting. The drill enters the odontoid process from the soft cancellous fracture site, and because the odontoid process is firmly held in position by its periosteum and

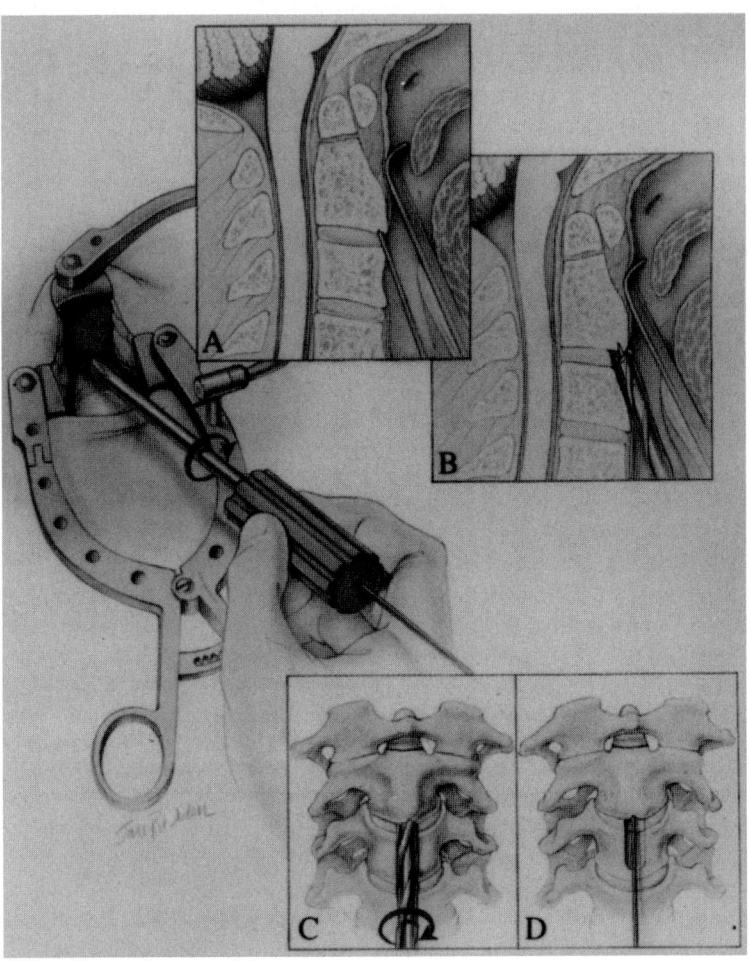

**Figure 110.6** (A) A guiding K-wire in place. (B-D) Hollow hand drill creates trough in face of C3 and C2-3 annulus.

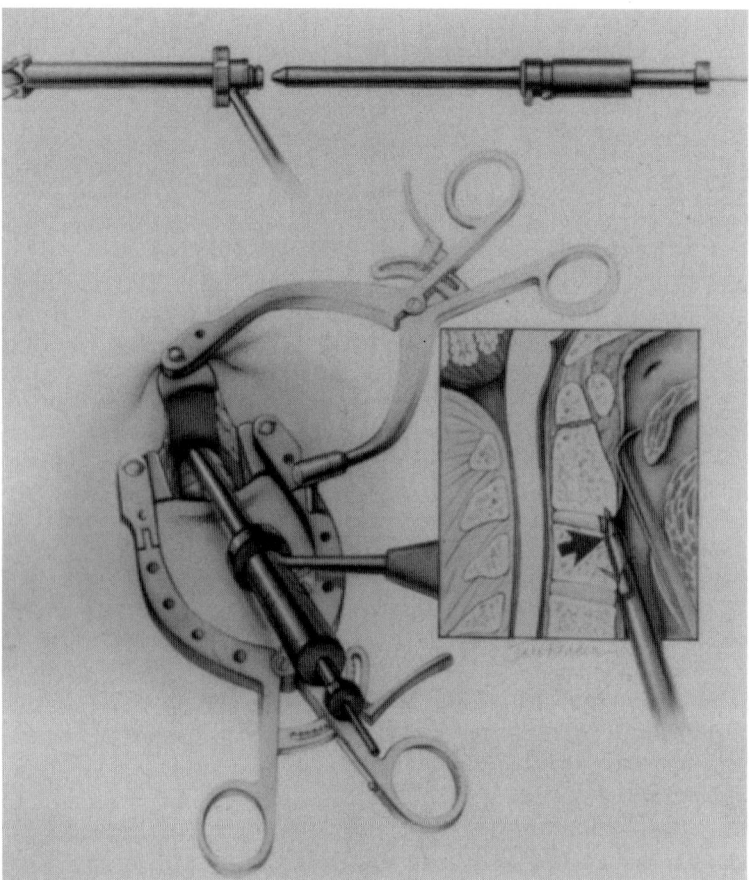

**Figure 110.7** Drill guide system. Inner and outer guide tubes mate together and are placed over the K-wire. The spikes on the outer guide tube are impacted into C3, and the inner guide tube then advances into the previously created trough to the caudal edge of C2.

attached supporting ligaments, it is not displaced by the drill. The angle of drilling is such that the drill can penetrate a substantial distance beyond the apex of the odontoid process into the apical ligaments without threatening the dural or neural structures. If, however, a more dorsal trajectory is needed, greater care must be taken not to penetrate too far into the spinal canal. This is controlled by visualizing the drill's progress on the fluoroscope.

A right-angled (dental-type) drill hand piece is used to avoid interference with the ventral chest wall when drilling. This allows the procedure to be performed even in barrel-chested persons. Once the drill is into the distal odontoid cortex, its depth of penetration is read on the calibrated shaft, and the fluoroscopic image is saved.

The drill is then withdrawn and the inner guide tube is removed. A tap is placed through the outer guide tube and the pilot hole is tapped. This cuts threads in the bone, allowing a more precise bone-screw junction that may reduce bone absorption around the screw caused by pressure necrosis, if a self-tapping screw is used. The tap is then removed and a screw is placed through the guide tube (Figure 110.9). A screw that is a few millimeters shorter than the measured drill depth is chosen to allow for reduction at the fracture site. A partially threaded screw (lag screw) is used to achieve this reduction.

At each of these two steps, the odontoid process-C2 alignment that was achieved initially is easily restored by

comparing the active fluoroscopic image with the stored image taken at the time of drilling. If a second screw is to be placed, the identical series of steps is followed on the contralateral paramedian site, except that either a partially threaded lag screw or a fully threaded screw can be used, because no further lagging action can occur.

After removal of the guide tube, bleeding from C3 can be controlled with bone wax. Lateral fluoroscopy in flexion and extension confirms stability. Closure is routine and is performed in layers, closing the sternocleidomastoid fascia, platysma muscle, and subcutaneous tissue with absorbable sutures and the skin with sterile tape strips. No drains are placed. Unless concern exists regarding the patient's bone quality, external collars are not usually recommended, and patients are allowed to return to work and resume nontraumatic activities promptly.

Several alternative systems have been proposed that are often based on existing long-bone screw fixation techniques. One uses the K-wire to drill and then passes a hollow overdrill over this, followed by a cannulated screw.[25] Theoretically, once the K-wire is placed, it does not have to be removed. This allows precise reentry into the same trajectory. These systems do not appear to have any provision for optimizing alignment with the drill guide, as described above, except by positioning the head and placing additional instruments beside the drill and pushing on C1 or C2.

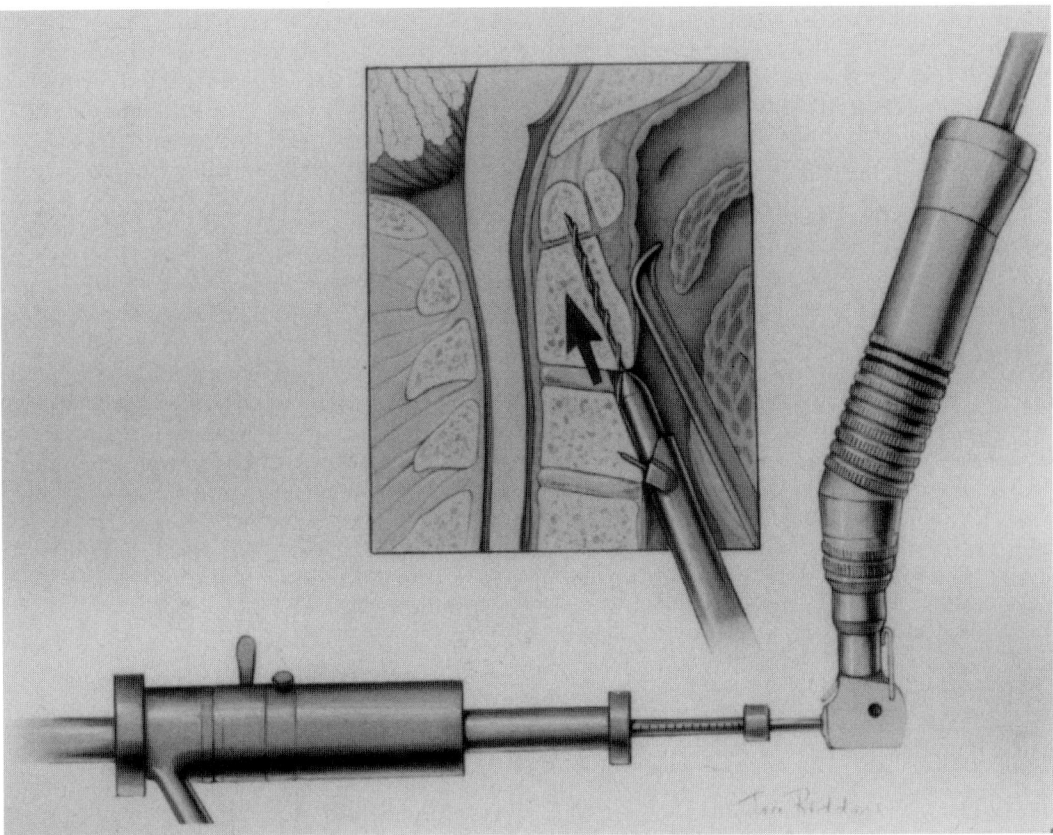

**Figure 110.8** K-wire is removed and replaced with drill, which is guided fluoroscopically to apex of odontoid process after reducing dislocation of the odontoid process.

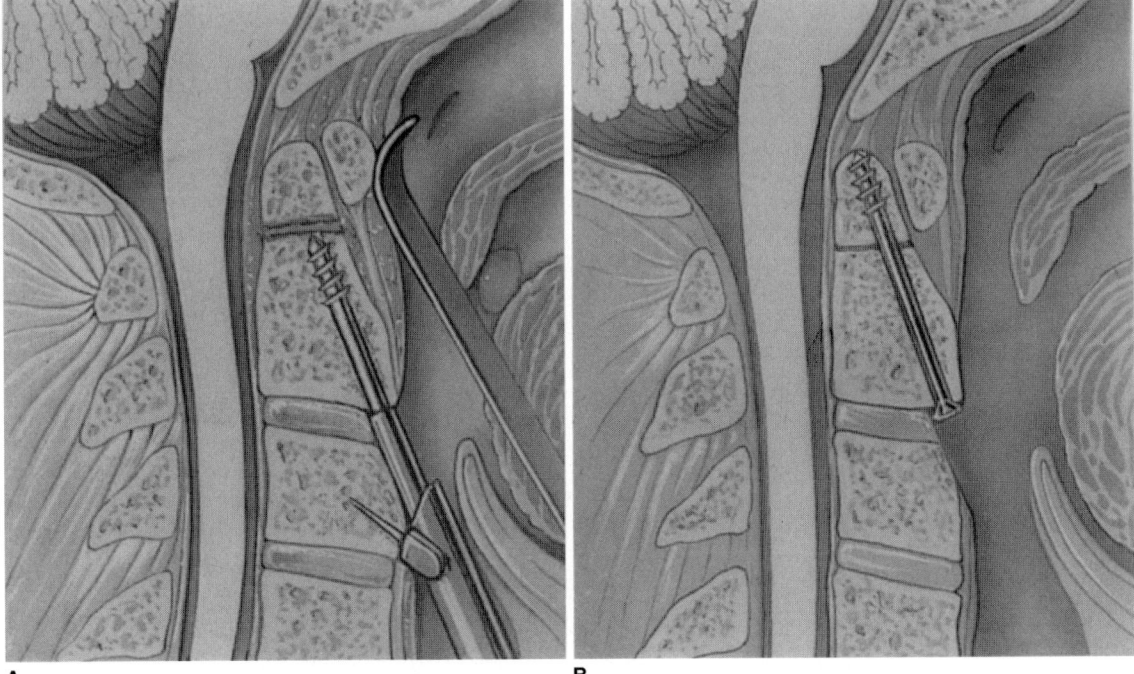

A                                                          B

**Figure 110.9** Lag screw is placed through the guide tube (**A**) and advanced through the tapped pilot hole to its final position (**B**).

Great care must be taken when drilling over the K-wire, because the drill can bind to the K-wire and advance it into the spinal canal or cut the K-wire. This can also occur when placing the screw over the K-wire. Theoretically, K-wires are suboptimal drills because they lack the torsional rigidity of drill bits and can be deflected by irregular densities within the bone. To redirect them, one must remove the K-wire and select a new starting point.[19]

### Controversies

**One-screw Constructs Versus Two-Screw Constructs.** Comparisons between techniques are lacking. theoretically, with one screw the odontoid process could rotate on C2. At least with fresh fractures, the interdigitation of the irregular fracture surfaces usually prevents this. Therefore both techniques have had similar clinical success. Laboratory studies show no greater resistance to screw fracture from bending with one- or two-screw constructs. If a second screw is used, it too should engage the apical odontoid cortex, but it need not be a lag screw. The diameter of the odontoid process should be assessed on the preoperative computed tomography scan to ensure adequate bone volume for a second screw. Some patients may not have a large enough odontoid process to accommodate two screws.[49]

**Screw Size and Type.** Biomechanical data suggest that cannulated screws are quite similar to solid screws in strength, perhaps only 5% to 10% weaker.[19] Various screw diameters have been used. These usually range from 3.5 to 4.0mm and are occasionally larger. The initial experience was with cancellous threaded screws.

These have a deeper thread (smaller minor diameter or core) and are better at resisting pull-out. However, there is little in the way of pull-out forces on odontoid screws. The screw has to resist bending and translational forces primarily. Screw failure, if it occurs, is almost always due to fracture at the level of the bone fracture. Cortically threaded screws (4mm outer diameter) with a larger minor diameter (2.9mm versus the previously used 2.0mm) would therefore seem optimal. Such screws have proven substantially stronger in laboratory tests in which they fail to fracture after 1 million cycles at three times the load at which the older screws fractured at 33,100 cycles. In clinical use, they are also more effective, with no postoperative screw fractures observed in over 400 consecutive screw placements, versus 5% fracture rate in odontoid fixation and 10% fracture rate in C1-2 fixation with the prior screw design. An additional benefit is that the pilot hole is drilled larger (3.0mm versus 2.0mm). This makes the drill hole much more directionally stable, allowing precise correction of pilot hole trajectory to optimize screw placement.

### Results

Type II odontoid fractures less than 6 months old treated with this technique have a high rate of fusion. The combined series of Veres in Hungary and Apfelbaum in Salt Lake City, Utah,[7] encompassed 147 patients whose ages ranged from 15 to 92 years. Successful bony union was achieved in 88% of patients, with an additional 3% achiev-

ing stability via fibrous union. These results agree with other published series with fewer patients.[19,26,29,40,45] The failures that have occurred are usually in elderly patients with poor quality bone. In such circumstances, the screw may fail to hold in C2, particularly if there is an associated fracture in the body of C2. If this complication is recognized early, manipulative realignment and external immobilization has been successful. If not, additional surgery was required. There was one late neurologic complication in which a patient became quadriplegic in the series from Hungary when the construct failed to hold and he subsequently dislocated. There were no other neurologic complications, and other surgical complications are rare.

The high degree of success achieved by using this straightforward, easily mastered technique, with minimal complications, merits its consideration as the primary treatment for many type II odontoid fractures. By allowing the patient to quickly resume normal activity while avoiding the cost and medical and social morbidity of a halo vest, screw fixation appears to be a very cost-effective treatment for this problem.

### Ventral C1-2 Transarticular Screw Fixation

This may be an alternative technique if odontoid screw fixation is not possible, if successful odontoid screw fixation fails to stabilize C2 because of unrecognized concomitant transverse ligament incompetence, or if in rare cases, a dorsal approach is contraindicated. Stabilization is accomplished by placing two screws, each inserted through the lateral masses of C2, into the lateral mass of C1.[18] The entry site is just medial to the vertebral artery, which is placed at risk by this approach. The screws angle laterally about 20 degrees and dorsally at a similar angle. The entry site is selected by following the lateral edge of the vertebral body rostrally from the C2-3 interspace to its junction with the lateral mass, staying as medial as possible in that structure. The drill guide system used for odontoid screw fixation can be used for this as well, although the screw length is considerably shorter.

Although it achieves fixation, this technique does not permit placement of substantial bone graft. Rather, one hopes to achieve long-term stabilization by promoting arthrodesis of the C1-2 lateral articulation, primarily by immobilization. This may be enhanced by curetting the joint, but overall, the construct is less likely to succeed than dorsal screw fixation with dorsal grafting. It should therefore be reserved for exceptional cases.

### Other Ventral Techniques

There are a few reports of using plates and screws transorally.[30] Experience with these is limited because they do not appear to have been widely used. The obvious risk of infection and, to a lesser extent, the limited working space, seem to have deterred most surgeons from these approaches.

## Dorsal Approaches

The dorsal approach is used to stabilize C1 to C2. Rather than providing stabilization and fixation of a fractured bone, it stabilizes what was previously a normal motion segment and provides an optimal environment for bone graft healing. Bone grafting, however, is almost always required for long-term stabilization, because hardware in nonfused segments will ultimately fatigue and fail.

Traditional techniques have utilized a variety of C1-2 wiring strategies with interposed or onlay bone grafting (Gallie,[28] Brooks,[14] and modified[21] fusions). These impart limited stability that deteriorates significantly with cyclical loading.[17] Therefore an external rigid orthosis is usually necessary. Fractured or absent dorsal elements can preclude the use of these techniques. Even in optimal situations, nonunion rates of up to 30% are reported.[17]

Transarticular screw fixation, pioneered by Magerl in 1979,[42] offers immediate stabilization, often without the use of an external orthosis. It optimizes bone graft union and has a high chance of success. It is therefore a major advance in treating instability in this area. The construct can be extended with various devices to include the occiput if needed.

## Indications

This procedure is indicated for atlantoaxial instability from almost any cause be it traumatic disruption of the transverse ligament, rheumatoid or other degenerative diseases, iatrogenic instability after transoral decompression, congenital or acquired absence of a united odontoid process (os odontoideum), ligamentous incompetence associated with various genetic diseases (Down syndrome, Larsen's disease), or chronic odontoid fractures. Occiput-C1 instability can occur from many of the same causes and, if present, can be treated by extending the stabilization and fusion up to the occiput.

## Contraindications

Poor bone quality (osteoporosis) is always of concern during intraosseous fixation and must be evaluated carefully. It is not an absolute contraindication to surgery, but it may necessitate using both internal and external devices. Of paramount importance for transarticular screw fixation is an adequate pathway for the screw that traverses the pars interarticularis (isthmus) of C2 (not the pedicle) to the lateral C1-2 articulation before crossing that joint into the lateral mass of C1. Variations in anatomy and secondary effects of vascular elongation coupled with bone softening can result in the vertebral artery looping up into the pars of C2. This may occur to such an extent that an inadequate pathway remains for safe screw placement. Placing screws in such circumstances has resulted in vertebral artery injury with potentially serious neurologic sequelae. An alternative technique devised by Harms[35] uses screws placed in the lateral masses of C1 and into the C2 pars or pedicle, which are then connected posteriorly with rods. This is applicable in cases in which a safe pathway through the C2 pars to C1 does not exist.

It is therefore critical to evaluate these factors preoperatively before deciding to proceed with transarticular screw fixation. Thin-section computed tomography scans, reconstructed along the planned screw pathway, have

been invaluable in evaluating whether screws can be passed safely (Figure 110.10).

## Patient Positioning

The patient is positioned prone on bolsters with the head supported in a three-pin head holder. This is applied before turning the patient. A cervical collar helps stabilize the patient's neck, but the primary control of this is provided by the surgeon who keeps the patient's neck stable with slight axial traction and in a neutral position as the patient is slowly rolled to the prone position. Final positioning, before securing the head clamp, is performed under lateral fluoroscopic guidance. The best reduction position is often with the neck in extension. This, however, may preclude C1-2 transarticular screw placement in many cases, because lordosis dictates a screw trajectory starting within the thoracic cavity. Instead, the patient should be positioned with the chin slightly flexed and with the head pulled dorsally (Figure 110.11). This has been likened to the posture of military personnel standing at braced attention. This position will often reduce C1-2 dislocations via dorsal translation yet leave the rest of the cervical spine in a flattened or even slightly kyphotic posture. In this position, a feasible screw trajectory is achieved. Also, before securing the skull clamp, one must confirm that the head is not rotated. This can be judged by the symmetry of the ear canals relative to the table or floor. Careful monitoring of the fluoroscopic image facilitates safe positioning. An absolutely perfect position is not necessary; rather, minor residual translational movements can easily be corrected at the time of screw placement.

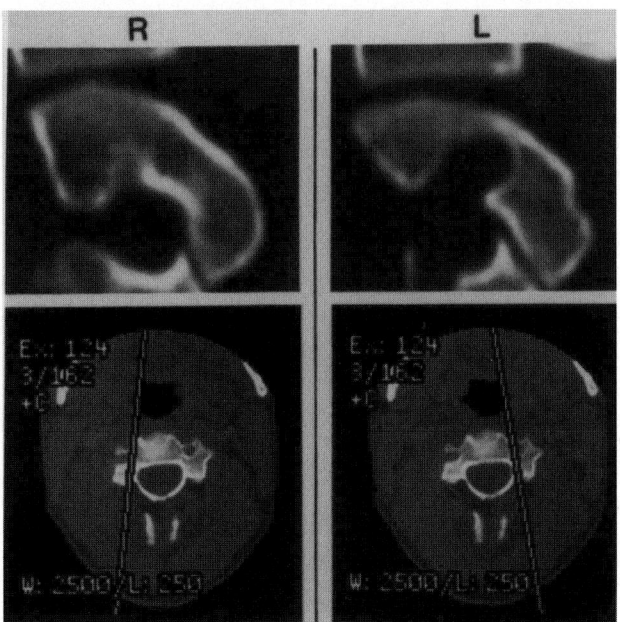

**Figure 110.10** Upper views show CT reconstruction through pars interarticularis of C2 on right and left sides in trajectory shown on axial scout views in lower two panels. Note safe path for screw on patient's right side but abnormally large vertebral artery canal on left with inadequate bony dimensions for safe screw placement on the left. Only one screw was placed in this patient.

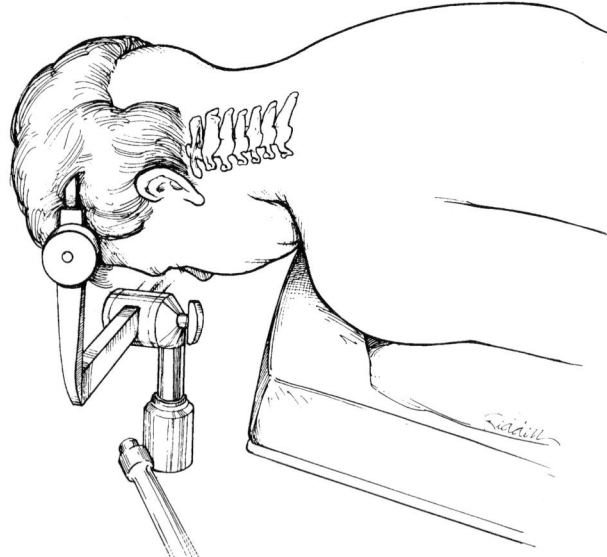

**Figure 110.11** Patient position. Head is fixed in a three-pin head holder. Translating the head dorsally with the chin tucked down reduces atlantoaxial dislocation and allows the lower spine to be kept in a straight or even flexed position. This facilitates the trajectory for C1-2 screw placement. The patient is positioned while monitoring vertebral alignment via lateral fluoroscopy.

The low angle of screw trajectory needed to traverse the C2 pars interarticularis and enter C1 dictates a starting point at about the T1 to T3 level. Magerl's original technique called for an incision and paraspinal muscle retraction down to this level. However, percutaneous tunneling techniques make this unnecessary. In preparation for this, however, the patient's neck and back should be prepared and draped down to about T4 or T5. In addition, the iliac crest donor site is also prepared and draped.

## Operative Technique

A dorsal midline incision extending from just below the inion to C3 is usually adequate (Figure 110.12A). The paraspinal muscles are dissected off the dorsal elements of C1, C2, and the occipital bone and are held back with angled Weitlander retractors. The dissection must be made carefully, the instability of the spine being kept in mind. Therefore this often requires sharp dissection assisted with electrocautery. The full extent of the dorsal elements of C1 and C2 should be exposed, with definition of the lateral aspect of the C2 dorsal elements and the C2-3 facet joint, as well as of the C2 isthmus extending rostrally beneath the C2 nerve root and the associated venous complex (see Figure 110.12B). Bleeding in this area can usually be arrested with small Gelfoam pledgets soaked in thrombin. Also very effective is a slurry made with Gelfoam powder and thrombin. It is not necessary and probably not desirable to disconnect the inferior midline attachments to the bifid C2 spinous process.

Once the anatomic structures are fully exposed, fixation screws are placed. The entry site on each side is just rostral to the C2-3 facet joint and in line with the previously defined pars interarticularis. Standing back from the

wound to reduce parallax, a line representing the inferior extension of the trajectory may be drawn on the drapes. A straight instrument such as a K-wire placed along the patient's neck and manipulated to be superimposed over the desired screw path on the fluoroscopic view provides the intersecting skin coordinates, usually at about T2.

A 1cm to 1.5cm skin incision carried down through the dorsal fascia provides an entry for the drill apparatus (see Figure 110.12A). As with odontoid fixation, a guide tube system (Aesculap Instrument Corporation) may be used. With this system, a smooth tube fitted with a conical tipped obturator is passed from the skin incision up to the drill entry site at the C2-3 junction by pressing firmly in a rostral direction and gently rotating the instrument back and forth to advance it into the surgical field (see Figure 110.12C). Once the guide tube is in place, the obturator is removed and an awl is used to make a starting hole in the C2 laminar bone. An inner drill guide is then placed to support the drill (Figure 110.13). The guide tube assembly allows precise control of drilling direction.

The surgeon must visualize the dorsolateral and medial borders of the pars interarticularis and direct the drill bit accurately between these limits. A tool, such as a small Penfield dissector held by an assistant, can help visualization of this area. Because it is placed on the dorsum of the pars, it serves as a fluoroscopic marker for that boundary. A low-angled trajectory to carry the drill bit just below the dorsum of the pars and across the C1-2 lateral articulation, as far dorsally as possible, engages the maximum amount of the lateral mass of C1. This also keeps the drill dorsal, above the vertebral artery. On the lateral fluoroscopic image the projection of the ventral arch of C1 is a helpful target to aim for, especially at its rostral margin (Figure 110.14). Generally the screw trajectory should be in a straight paramedian direction. Aiming medially results in a smaller area of C1 lateral mass engagement, whereas aiming laterally can jeopardize the vertebral artery. Image-guided stereotactic systems have recently been adapted for this procedure and can assist in accurate screw placement.

When drilling, increased resistance is felt at the cortical margins of the C2 joint surface and then at the C1 joint surface, as well as at the ventral cortex of C1. If necessary, C2 can be translated ventrally or dorsally before drilling across the joint space by grasping the spinous process with a towel clamp, thus assuring optimal alignment.

Once the pilot hole is drilled, the depth is noted on the calibrated drill shaft, and the images are stored. The drill is then removed along with the inner drill guide and is replaced with a tap (Figure 110.15), except in very soft bone. After tapping the hole, a fully threaded screw is placed, because no lag effect is needed. Vertebral alignment is optimized just before crossing the C1-2 articulation by matching the active fluoroscopic image with its stored counterpart.

Bone bleeding may occur, particularly in inflammatory disease. If, however, brisk arterial bleeding ensues from the drill hole, suggesting a vertebral artery injury, placement of one screw for fixation and tamponade is recommended (but do not place a second screw). If this occurs it may be prudent to obtain postoperative angiographic

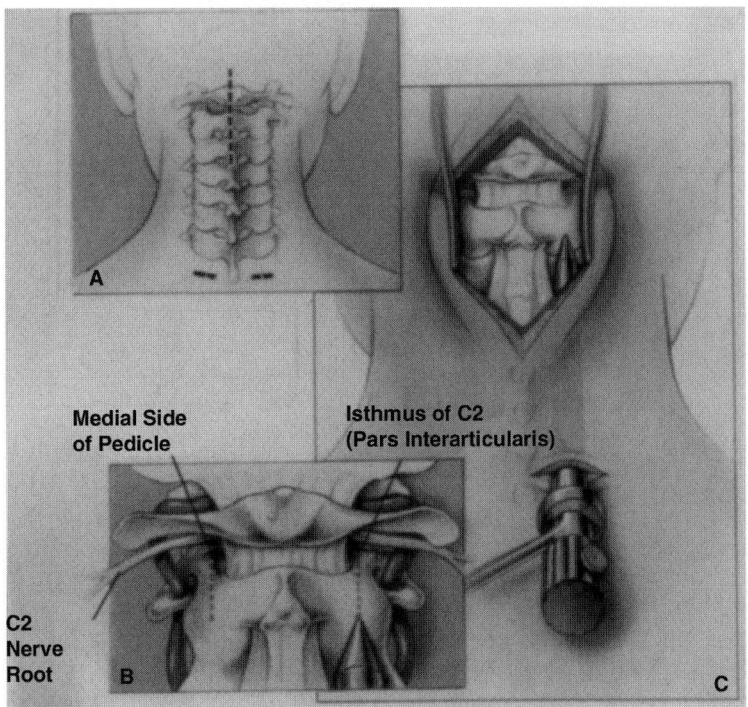

**Figure 110.12** (**A**) Site of surgical incisions. The stab wound sites for placement of the drill guide tube are determined fluoroscopically. (**B**) Details of the surgical anatomy. The desired screw placement is just lateral to the lateral edge of the spinal canal. It will traverse the isthmus of C2 and the C1-2 articulation. The pedicle serves as a positioning landmark (see text), but the screw does not go down the pedicle. (**C**) Placement of guide tube (with obturator) through stab wound and into field.

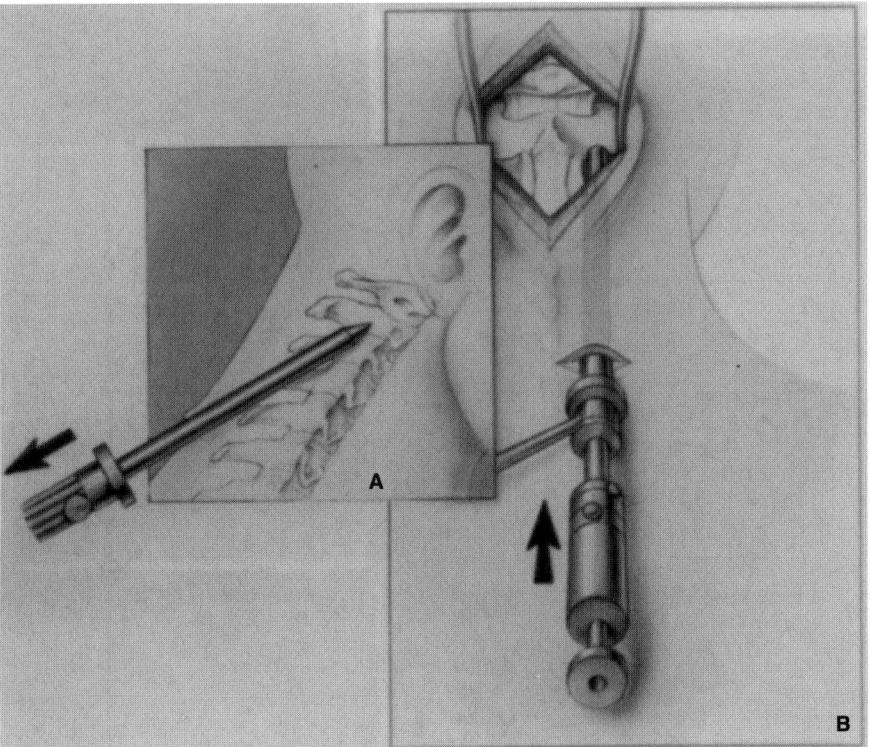

**Figure 110.13** Guide tube in place as seen in sagittal (**A**) and dorsal (**B**) view. Obturator is then removed (**A**) and replaced with inner drill guide (**B**).

images to ascertain the status of the vessel and to detect fistula formation.[16]

Immediately after placing the first screw, significant improvement is observed in patients with gross instability. The same sequence of steps is then repeated on the contralateral side.

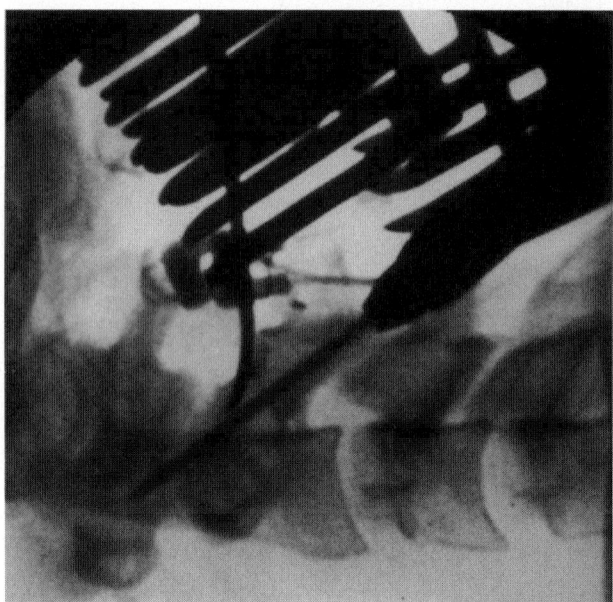

**Figure 110.14** Lateral fluoroscopic view of drilling in process. Note instrument (Penfield dissector) defining the dorsum of the pars, with drill passing just ventral to this structure.

## Bone Grafting

Screw fixation functions as an internal splint. For long-term stability, bone fusion is required because all hardware will ultimately fail without it. Magerl suggested curetting and then packing bone chips into the C1-2 articulation, to encourage arthrodesis. Access to this joint is limited, however, and only a small portion of it can be treated in this manner even in the best of circumstances. Therefore a dorsal fusion construct is often used.

With intact dorsal elements, a modified construct consisting of a combined interpositional and onlay bicortical iliac crest graft is suggested.[21] The graft has ventral and dorsal cortices. However, the cortex is removed at the site at which it contacts the caudal and dorsal surfaces of C1 and the laminar surface and rostral edge of the spinous process of C2. Mating surfaces are denuded with a high-speed burr, and the graft and donor surfaces are contoured for maximum opposition (Figure 110.16). This is secured with a braided titanium cable placed sublaminarly at C1 and around the spinous process of C2, such that the graft is sandwiched between the two layers of cable. This construct provides excellent three-dimensional stability. The screws resist translation and rotation, whereas the graft prevents extension, and the cable prevents flexion. Additional bone chips and curettings may be placed around this construct to enhance fusion.

## Lasso Technique

In the absence of an intact C1 arch, the same construct can be used with a modification, termed the *lasso technique*,

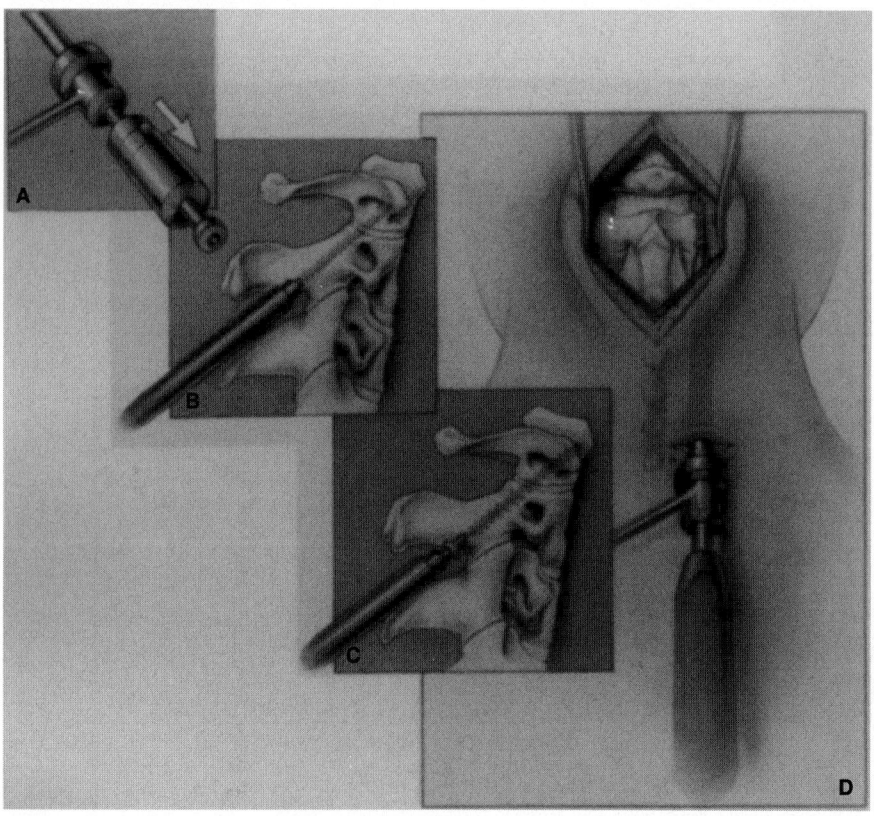

**Figure 110.15** (**A**) Inner drill guide tube is removed. Through the outer guide, the pilot hole is tapped (**B**) and the screw is placed (**C** and **D**).

provided that there are adequate remaining stumps of C1 (Figure 110.17A). As diagrammed in Figure 110.17B, the cable encircles and is cinched to each stump (lasso) to secure it, and the graft is then pulled down to contact the bone (see Figure 110.17C). This technique has been used successfully by the first author (Apfelbaum) in 8 patients. Obviously, for this method to succeed, a wide graft must be harvested, so that it overlaps each cervical arch remnant. The Harm's technique, previously described, is also applicable. Direct fusion at the C1-2 joint can be encouraged by curetting the joint and packing bone chips within it, but access to this joint is limited by the anatomy.

## Extension to Occiput

A longer graft secured in the same manner can be taken up to the occiput and apposed to a denuded area to maximize incorporation potential. A small bone screw inserted through the graft into the occiput can enhance this contact (Figure 110.18).

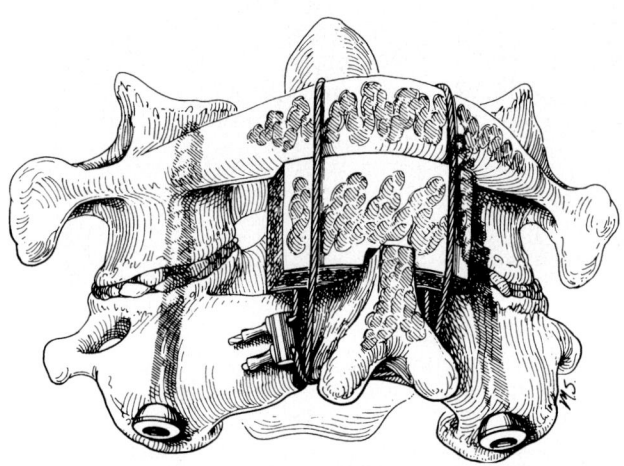

**Figure 110.16** Illustration of completed screw fixation. Unlike this illustration, we notch the graft to contact both the dorsal and caudal edge of the C1 laminar arch to improve the fusion potential at this site. *(From Marcotte P, Dickman CA, Sonntag VKH, et al: Posterior atlantoaxial facet screw fixation. J Neurosurg 79:234-237, 1993, with permission.)*

## Alternative Systems

Drilling with a K-wire and placing hollow cannulated screws is an alternative technique used by some surgeons.[19] The K-wire may be drilled percutaneously or via a similarly placed guide tube. The concerns expressed earlier with regard to inadvertently advancing the K-wire with the drill and to cutting the K-wire pertain here as well.

## Screws

Screws measuring 3.5 to 4.0mm or slightly larger in diameter have been used. Similarly to odontoid screw fixation, there is little pull-out force but significant bending or translational forces. Cortical screws with larger minor diameter, as described earlier in this chapter with regard to odontoid screws, have replaced the smaller minor diameter cancellous screws previously used. This has been a significant improvement that has eliminated screw breakage (Figure 110.19). The screw requires a larger drill (3mm) because of its larger minor diameter. This drill provides more directional control and has resulted in the unexpected benefit of allowing more precise corrections of drill angulation as the drill is advanced.

## Postoperative Care

Some surgeons prefer to use a cervical collar, but unless there is a question of bone quality, or if only one screw is placed, this is probably not necessary. With the immediate elimination of motion, postoperative pain is significantly less, and most patients can be discharged from the hospital in about 2 days. They are followed with serial radiographs until fusion is assured. Nontraumatic activities, including driving, are allowed as soon as the patient is comfortable.

## Results and Complications

Numerous series report excellent stabilization and fusion rates. Magerl's initial series reported a 100% fusion rate,[42] whereas Grob, in 1991, reported a 99% success rate in 161 patients[31]; Stillerman, in 1993, had a 95% rate of successful fusion (21 out of 22 patients)[54]; and Marcotte, in 1993,

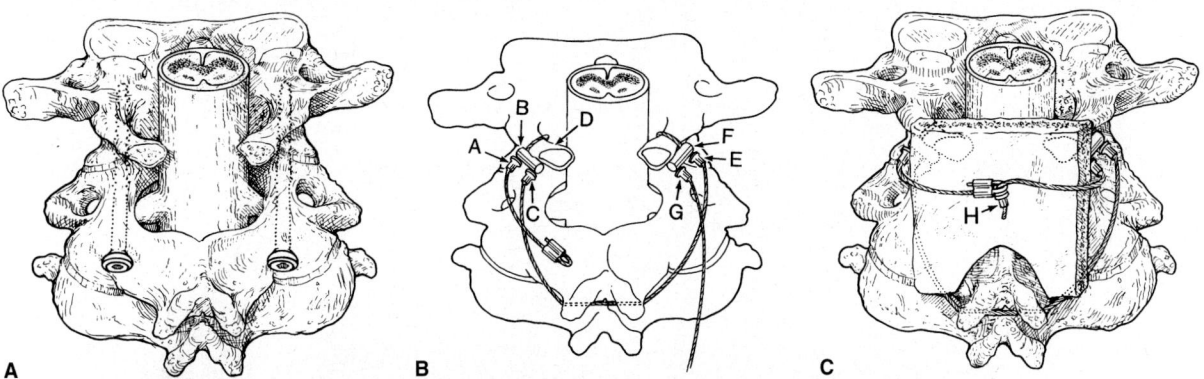

**A**          **B**          **C**

**Figure 110.17** Lasso technique for dorsal grafting in the absence of a C1 arch. **(A)** C1-2 transarticular screws are first placed. **(B)** The remaining stumps of C1 (*D*) are encircled ("lassoed") with a braided titanium cable by cinching (*A* and *C*) around bar (*B*) while tensioning the cable to firmly grasp the stump of C1. A similar sequence on the contralateral side lassoes the other C1 arch. **(C)** An iliac crest graft is then held down by the same cable (*H*) to complete the construct.

had a 100% rate of fusion (in 18 patients).[44] The first author (Apfelbaum) reports only 2 failures in 95 patients.

This procedure is of particular benefit to patients with rheumatoid arthritis who often present with a great deal of pain and who cannot tolerate a halo vest orthosis well. Fusion, in these patients, also takes substantially longer, and the patients have a higher nonunion rate with conventional techniques. With internal screw fixation they are stable, protected, and have good pain relief, as well as an optimum environment for bone healing.

The procedure, however, is technically demanding. It requires a good knowledge of nuances in anatomy and thorough preoperative evaluation via high-resolution computed tomography scans, preferably with reconstruction along the screw pathway. Neurologic complications from direct injury have not been reported. However, vertebral

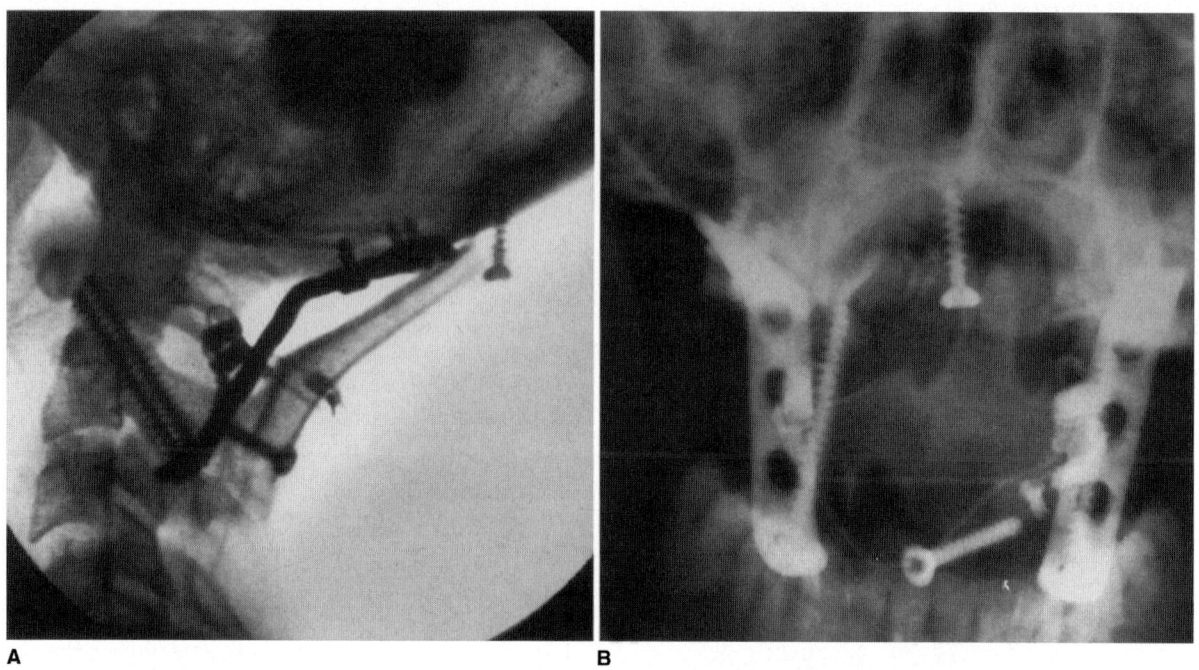

**Figure 110.18** (**A** and **B**) Patient with occiput C1-2 fusion using bilateral fixation. Plates extend from the C1-2 transarticular screw fixation to the occiput, where they are secured with short screws (see text). Note additional screws used to firmly approximate graft to the occiput and C2 lamina.

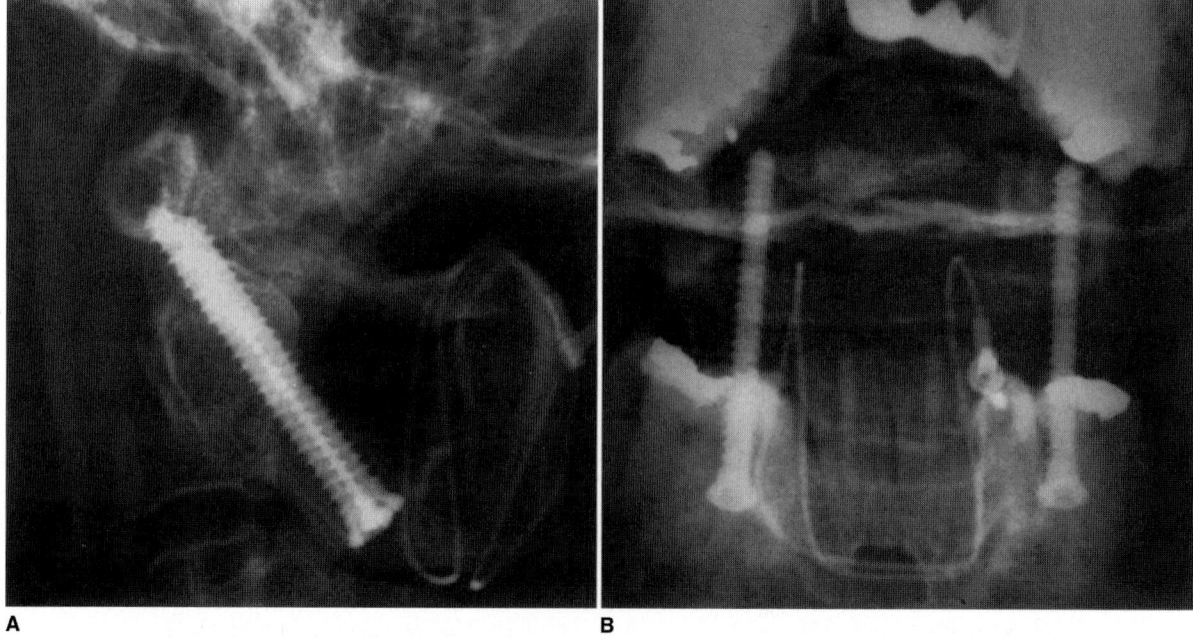

**Figure 110.19** (**A** and **B**) Postoperative appearance of a patient using the cortical screws with a larger minor diameter. Note excellent screw position and interspinous grafting.

artery injuries have occurred, and in one case bilateral vertebral artery injuries eventuated in a fatal brain stem infarction.[6] Unilateral injuries have not resulted in neurologic sequelae but have produced arteriovenous fistulas, one of which presented as a delayed spinal cord compromise from epidural venous engorgement.[16]

Fusion of C1 to C2 will, of necessity, restrict head rotation by about 50%. In a normal patient this leaves a residual motion of ± 45 degrees. Younger patients can regain some of this lost motion, often to a surprising degree, presumably by gaining extra motion at each of the subaxial facet joints. Less limber older patients must learn to compensate by torso rotation, and usually they will do so without difficulty. Paradoxically, some patients have improved motion almost immediately after surgery, because the pain provoked by cervical muscle spasms subsides. Occasionally patients complain of occipital numbness. This is presumably the result of C2 nerve root trauma during surgery and usually resolves within 3 to 6 months.

## Occipitocervical Fusion

Instability or degeneration of the occiput-C1 joint (best evaluated by dynamic radiographs) or basilar invagination may require incorporation of the occiput into an upper cervical fusion.

Two types of screw fixation techniques have been utilized for this in addition to wiring techniques. One approach is to use perforated plates that can be contoured to the occipitocervical contour and that are connected to the cervical spine by the C1-2 transarticular screws, as well as by lateral mass screws below C2 if the fusion needs to be extended subaxially (see Figure 110.18). The cranial ends are secured by small screws into the skull. The graft is also extended up to the occiput between the plates. The calvarium is not very thick over the posterior fossa, especially laterally, so screw purchase is limited and can potentially fail. One approach to this has been to use a special Y-shaped plate in an inverted configuration; the occipital screws are thus placed in the thicker midline bone.[8] A difficulty is that either type of plate must be contoured so that it does not produce a pull-out force on the screw.

Another approach has been to use a "U-loop" (Ohio Medical Instrument Company, Cincinnati, OH)[52] consisting of a titanium rod prebent to the occipitocervical contour. The loop component of the rod is flattened and drilled to allow placement of several occipital screws, both in the midline and in the paramedian locations. The legs of the U-loop may be coupled to the C1-2 transarticular screws by a special device that rotates freely, facilitating alignment of the rod and device (Figure 110.20). Alternatively, cable fixation to the arches of C1 and C2 can be used.

For calvarial fixation, 4.5mm screws can be used in a bicortical manner. In the midline, 10mm to 12mm (or longer) screws may be used, but often only 6mm to 8mm screws can be accommodated laterally. Screw depth is determined by a combination of sensation on drilling (under fluoroscopic control) and of probing the hole with a depth gauge. The construct can be extended subaxially if needed, using lateral mass screws and the same coupling devices.

## Summary

Screw fixation techniques have proven to be safe and extremely effective in the upper cervical spine. This highly mobile area has been difficult to stabilize effectively. Previously used operative and nonoperative techniques

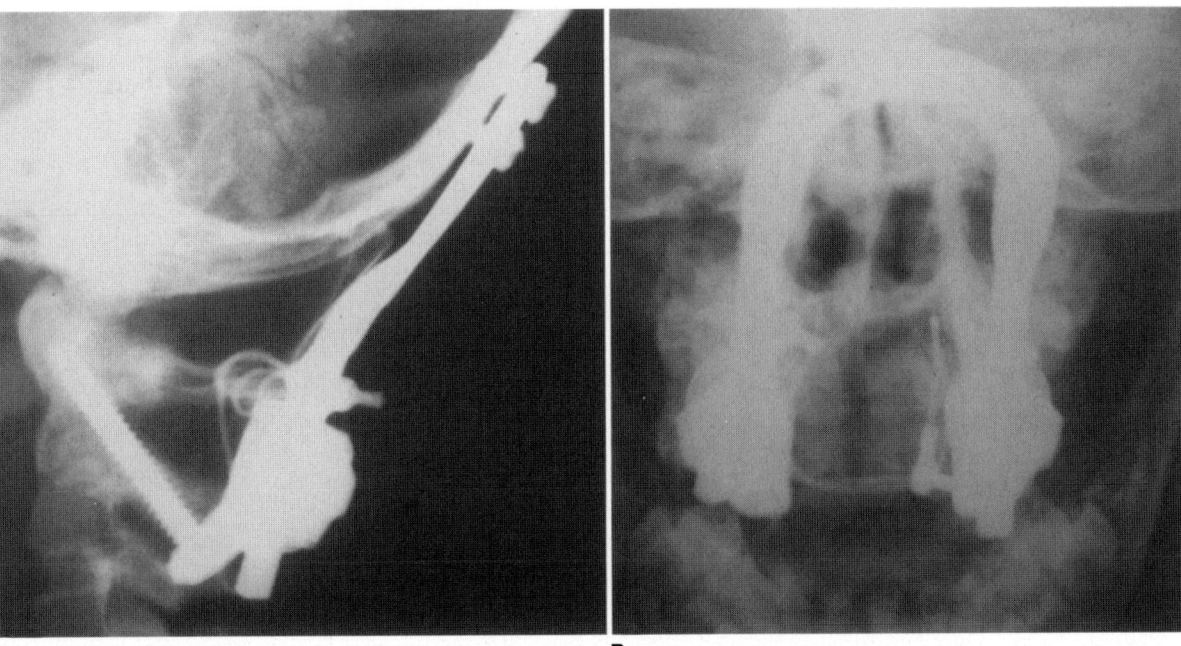

**A**     **B**

**Figure 110.20** (**A** and **B**) C1-2 transarticular screw fixation extended to the occiput using a titanium U-loop secured to the skull with fixation screws and to C1-2 screws with a special coupling device. (*Courtesy Ohio Medical Instrument Co., Cincinnati, OH.*)

have been only partially effective in dealing with the problem. Previous treatments have often resulted in prolonged inability to function normally or have sacrificed normal motion to gain protection for the neural elements.

The two major screw fixation techniques in this region—direct screw fixation of odontoid fractures and C1-2 transarticular screw fixation—are therefore extremely important additions to the surgeon's armamentarium. The available data suggest that these techniques are superior to other approaches.

# REFERENCES

1. Althoff B, Bardholm P: Fracture of the odontoid process. A clinical and radiographic study. *Acta Orthop Scand* 177: 61-95, 1979.
2. Anderson LD, D'Alonzo RTN: Fractures of the odontoid process of the axis. *J Bone Joint Surg* 56A:1663-1674, 1974.
3. Apfelbaum R: Screw fixation of odontoid fractures. In Wilkins RH, Rengachary SS (eds): *Neurosurgery*, vol 2, ed 2. New York, McGraw-Hill, 1996, pp 2965-2973.
4. Apfelbaum RI: Anterior screw fixation for odontoid fractures. In Camins MS, O'Leary PF (eds): *Disorders of the Cervical Spine*. Baltimore, Williams & Wilkins, 1992, pp 603-608.
5. Apfelbaum RI: Anterior screw fixation of odontoid fractures. In Rengachary SS, Wilkins RH (eds): *Neurosurgical Operative Atlas*, vol 2. Baltimore, Williams & Wilkins, 1992, pp 189-199.
6. Apfelbaum RI: Screw fixation of the upper cervical spine: indications and techniques. *Contemp Neurosurg* 16:1-81, 1994.
7. Apfelbaum RI, Lonser RR, Veres R, Casey A: Direct anterior screw fixation for recent and remote odontoid fractures. *J Neurosurg* 93(Spine2):227-236, 2000.
8. Apuzzo MLJ, Heiden JS, Weiss MH, *et al*: Acute fractures of the odontoid process: an analysis of 45 cases. *J Neurosurg* 48:85-91, 1978.
9. Benzel EC, Hart BL, Ball PA, *et al*: Fractures of the C2 vertebral body. *J Neurosurg* 81:206-212, 1994.
10. Blockey NJ, Purser DW: Fractures of the odontoid process of the axis. *J Bone Joint Surg* 38B:794-817, 1956.
11. Böhler J: Schraubenosteosynthese von Frakturen de dens axis. *Unfallchirurgie* 84:221-223, 1981.
12. Böhler J: Anterior stabilization for acute fractures and non-unions of the dens. *J Bone Joint Surg* 64A:18-27, 1982.
13. Borne GM, Bedou GL, Pinaudeau M, *et al*: Odontoid process fracture osteosynthesis with a direct screw fixation technique in nine consecutive cases. *J Neurosurg* 68: 223-226, 1988.
14. Brooks AL, Jenkins EB: Atlanto-axial arthrodesis by the wedge compression method. *J Bone Joint Surg* 60A: 279-284, 1978.
15. Clark CR, White AA: Fractures of the dens. A multicenter study. *J Bone Joint Surg* 67A:1340-1348, 1985.
16. Coric D, Branch CL, Wilson JA, Robinson JC: Arteriovenous fistula as a complication of C1-2 transarticular screw fixation. Case report and review of the literature. *J Neurosurg* 85:340-343, 1996.

17. Dickman CA, Crawford NR, Paramore CG: Biomechanical characteristics of C1-2 cable fixations. *J Neurosurg* 85: 316-322, 1996.
18. Dickman CA, Sonntag FKH, Marcotte PJ: Techniques of screw fixation of the cervical spine. *BNI Quart* 8:9-26, 1992.
19. Dickman CA, Foley KT, Sonntag VKH, Smith MM: Cannulated screws for odontoid screw fixation and atlantoaxial transarticular screw fixation. *J Neurosurg* 83:1095-1100, 1995.
20. Dickman CA, Mamourian A, Sonntag VKH, Drayer BP: Magnetic resonance imaging of the transverse atlantal ligament for the evaluation of atlantoaxial instability. *J Neurosurg* 75:221-227, 1991.
21. Dickman CA, Sonntag VKH, Papadopoulos SM, Hadley MN: The interspinous method of posterior atlantoaxial arthrodesis. *J Neurosurg* 74:190-198, 1991.
22. Dickson H, Engel S, Blum P, Jones RF: Odontoid fractures, systemic disease and conservative care. *Aust NZ J Surg* 54:243-247, 1984.
23. Dunn ME, Seljeskog EL: Experience in the management of odontoid process injuries: an analysis of 128 cases. *Neurosurgery* 18:306-310, 1986.
24. Ekong CEU, Schwartz ML, Tator CH, *et al*: Odontoid fracture: management with early mobilization using the halo device. *Neurosurgery* 9:631-637, 1981.
25. Esses SI, Bednar DA: Screw fixation of odontoid fractures and nonunions. *Spine* 16:S4843-4850, 1991.
26. Etter C, Coscia M, Aebi M: Direct anterior fixation of dens fractures with a cannulated screw system. *Spine* 16S: S25-S32, 1991.
27. Fujii E, Kobayashi K, Hirabayashi K: Treatment in fractures of the odontoid process. *Spine* 13:604-609, 1988.
28. Gallie WE: Fractures and dislocations of the upper cervical spine. *Am J Surg* 46:495-499, 1939.
29. Geisler FH, Cheng C, Poka A, Brumback RJ: Anterior screw fixation of posteriorly displaced type II odontoid fractures. *Neurosurgery* 25:30-37, 1989.
30. Goel A, Karapurkar AP: Transoral plate and screw fixation of the craniovertebral region: A preliminary report. *Br J Neurosurg* 8:743-745, 1994.
31. Grob D, Jeanneret B, Aebi M, Marwalder TM: Atlanto-axial fusion with transarticular screw fixation. *J Bone Joint Surg* 73B:972-976, 1991.
32. Guidelines Committee of the Section on Disorders of the Spine and Peripheral Nerves: Isolated fractures of the axis in adults. In *Guidelines for the Management of Acute Cervical Spine and Spinal Cord Injuries*, Chapter 17: *Neurosurg* 50(3 Suppl):S125-139, March 2002.
33. Hadley MN, Browner C, Sonntag VKH: Axis fractures: a comprehensive review of management and treatment in 107 cases. *Neurosurgery* 17:281-290, 1985.
34. Hadley MN, Browner CM, Liu SS, Sonntag VKH: New subtype of acute odontoid fractures (type IIA). *Neurosurgery* 22:67-71, 1988.
35. Harms J, Melcher P: Posterior C1-2 fusion with polyaxial screw and rod fixation. *Spine* 26:2467-2471, 2001.
36. Hentzer L, Schalimtzek M: Fractures and subluxations of the atlas and axis. A follow-up study of 20 patients. *Acta Orthop Scand* 42:251-258, 1971.
37. Jeanneret B, Vernet O, Frei S, Magerl F: Atlantoaxial mobility after screw fixation of the odontoid: a computed tomographic study. *J Spinal Disord* 4:203-211, 1991.

38. Julien TD, Frankel B, Traynelis VC, Ryken TC: Evidence-based analysis of odontoid fracture management. *Neurosurg Focus* 8:1-6, 2000.

39. Lennarson PJ, Mostafavi H, Traynelis VC, Walter BC: Management of type II dens fractures: a case-control study. *Spine* 15:25(10):1234-1237, 2000.

40. Lesoin F, Autricque A, Franz K, et al: Transcervical approach and screw fixation for upper cervical spine pathology. *Surg Neurol* 27:459-465, 1987.

41. Lind B, Nordwall A, Sihlbom H: Odontoid fractures treated with halo-vest. *Spine* 12:173-177, 1987.

42. Magerl F, Seeman PS: Stable posterior fusion of the atlas and axis by transarticular screw fixation. In Kehr P, Weidner A (eds): *Cervical Spine I.* New York, Springer-Verlag, 1987, pp 322-327.

43. Maiman DJ, Larson SJ: Management of odontoid fractures. *Neurosurgery* 11:471-476, 1982.

44. Marcotte P, Dickman CA, Sonntag VKH, et al: Posterior atlantoaxial facet screw fixation. *J Neurosurg* 79:234-237, 1993.

45. Montesano PX, Anderson PA, Schlehr F, et al: Odontoid fractures treated by anterior odontoid screw fixation. *Spine* 16S:S33-S37, 1991.

46. Nakanishi T: Internal fixation of the odontoid fracture [in Japanese]. *Cent Jpn J Orthop Traumatic Surg* 23:399-406, 1980.

47. Pepin JW, Bourne RB, Hawkins RJ: Odontoid fractures, with special reference to the elderly patient. *Clin Orthop* 193:178-183, 1985.

48. Ryan MD, Taylor TKF: Odontoid fractures: a rational approach to treatment. *J Bone Joint Surg* 64B:416-421, 1982.

49. Schaffler MB, Alson MD, Heller JG, Garfin SR: Morphology of the dens, a quantitative study. *Spine* 17:738-743, 1992.

50. Schatzker J, Rorabeck CH, Waddell JP: Fracture of the dens (odontoid process). An analysis of thirty-seven cases. *J Bone Joint Surg* 53B:392-405, 1971.

51. Scott EW, Haid RW, Peace D: Type I fractures of the odontoid process: implications for atlanto-occipital instability. *J Neurosurg* 72:488-492, 1990.

52. Singh SK, Richards L, Apfelbaum RI, et al: Occipitocervical reconstructions with the OMI loop: results in a multicervical evaluation in 30 cases. *J Neurosurg* 98:(3 Suppl):239-46, 2003.

53. Spence KF, Decker S, Sell KW: Bursting atlantal fracture associated with rupture of the transverse ligament. *J Bone Joint Surg* 52A:543-549, 1970.

54. Stillerman CB, Wilson JA: Atlanto-axial stabilization with posterior transarticular screw fixation: technical description and report of 22 cases. *Neurosurgery* 32:948-955, 1993.

55. Tuite GF, Papadopoulos SM, Sonntag VKH: Caspar plate fixation for the treatment of complex hangman's fractures. *Neurosurgery* 30:761-765, 1992.

56. Veres R, Casey ATH, Crockard HA, Pentelenyi T: Acute fractures of the odontoid process: a critical analysis of anterior screw fixation in 53 cases. Presented at the Sixty-fourth Annual Meeting of The American Association of Neurological Surgeons, Minneapolis, MN, 1996.

57. Wang GJ, Mabie KN, Whitehill R, Stamp WG: The nonsurgical management of odontoid fractures in adults. *Spine* 9:229-230, 1984.

58. White AA, Panjabi MM: The occipital-atlanto-axial complex (C0-C1-C2). In *Clinical Biomechanics of the Spine,* ed 2. Philadelphia, Lippincott-Raven, 1990, pp 92-97.

# CHAPTER 111

# High Cervical and Occipitocervical Plate, Rod, Wire, and Bone Techniques

Noel I. Perin, Nevan G. Baldwin, and Paul R. Cooper

Abnormalities at the craniocervical junction were first reported in the early nineteenth century.[12] Early in the twentieth century, roentgenography was employed. This greatly increased the foundation of knowledge regarding congenital abnormalities and trauma to this region.

The complexity of this region has obstructed progress regarding an understanding of its related pathology. The occipitoatlantoaxial joints are complex, both anatomically and kinematically. Anatomically, two synovial joints are found between the condyles of the occiput and the atlas; four synovial joints are found between the atlas and the axis; and there is a synovial joint between the ventral arch of the atlas and the dens, a second between the dens and the transverse ligament, and two at the dorsolateral joints. The opposing surfaces of the dorsolateral joints are convex and facilitate the rotatory movement.

The occipitoatlantal joints allow 15 to 20 degrees of flexion/extension and 5 to 10 degrees of lateral bending. Head nodding occurs at the occipitoatlantal joint. The atlantoaxial joint allows 47 to 50 degrees of axial rotation, 15 to 20 degrees of flexion/extension, and 15 to 20 degrees of lateral bending coupled with axial rotation.

## Causes of Instability in the Upper Cervical Spine

Instability of the upper cervical spine can be caused by congenital, traumatic, inflammatory, or neoplastic involvement.[3] Of the several congenital abnormalities that occur in the upper cervical spine, basilar impression (or cranial settling) is the most common. Basilar impression may be progressive and lead to cervicomedullary spinal cord compression. Congenital ligamentous laxity in the upper cervical spine (e.g., Down syndrome, Morquio's syndrome) can cause instability and subluxation. Upper cervical spine involvement in patients with rheumatoid arthritis can also lead to atlantoaxial instability and cranial settling, both of which may require surgical decompression and stabilization. Trauma, however, is the most common cause of instability in the upper cervical spine. Most upper cervical spine injuries result from blows to the head (e.g., motor vehicle accidents and falls). The direction of the force vec-

tor determines the type of injury (i.e., blows to the head versus deceleration of the torso). Injuries of the occipitoatlantal junction are usually fatal and are only detected postmortem. Atlantoaxial instability, on the other hand, can result from disruption of the bony or ligamentous elements or both. Bony fractures often involve the dens. Fractures of the odontoid process of C2 are classified into three types: type I, type II, and type III.[1] Type II odontoid fractures are unstable and notorious for nonunion with conservative management. Published reports of nonunion rates for conservatively managed type II odontoid fractures range from 30% to 60%. Type I fractures are always stable, and type III fractures may be unstable in 10% to 15% of cases.

## Instability at the Craniocervical Junction

Several definitions of instability at the craniocervical junction have been proposed. Craniocervical instability can be vertical or horizontal. Vertical instability or cranial settling usually occurs from a congenital or chronic inflammatory process. Destructive arthropathy of the occipital condyles and the lateral masses of the atlas and axis leads to progressive cranial settling in rheumatoid arthritis. Horizontal (ventrodorsal) instability usually results from acute traumatic situations that cause ligamentous disruption and/or bony disruption. A rotary component may or may not be present.

Common radiologic criteria used to document instability at the craniocervical junction include (1) predental distance greater than 5mm in a child (under 8 years of age) and greater than 3mm in adults, (2) separation of more than 7mm of the lateral masses of the atlas on the open mouth view, (3) greater than one third of the rostral dens above the ring of the foramen magnum, and (4) "bare occipital condyles," indicating an occipitoatlantal dislocation.

## Management of Patients With Instability in the Upper Cervical Spine

Patients with instability of the upper cervical spine run the potential risk of fatal injury to the cervical spinal cord. Early recognition, reduction, immobilization, and stabilization are the goals of treatment.

Patients with upper cervical spine instability from congenital causes should be investigated further for other associated congenital defects (e.g., Chiari malformation, spinal dysraphic lesions, and hydrocephalus). A magnetic resonance imaging (MRI) scan should be obtained to assess the soft tissue pathology. In addition, computed tomography (CT) scans and plain radiographs (with or without flexion/extension views) should also be obtained when appropriate.

Patients with rheumatoid arthritis should have an MRI scan to ascertain the presence of inflammatory pannus and/or bony encroachment of the neural elements (Figure 111.1). Patients who have evidence of neural compromise with occipitocervical instability should be considered for a ventral decompressive procedure before undergoing dorsal stabilization.[16]

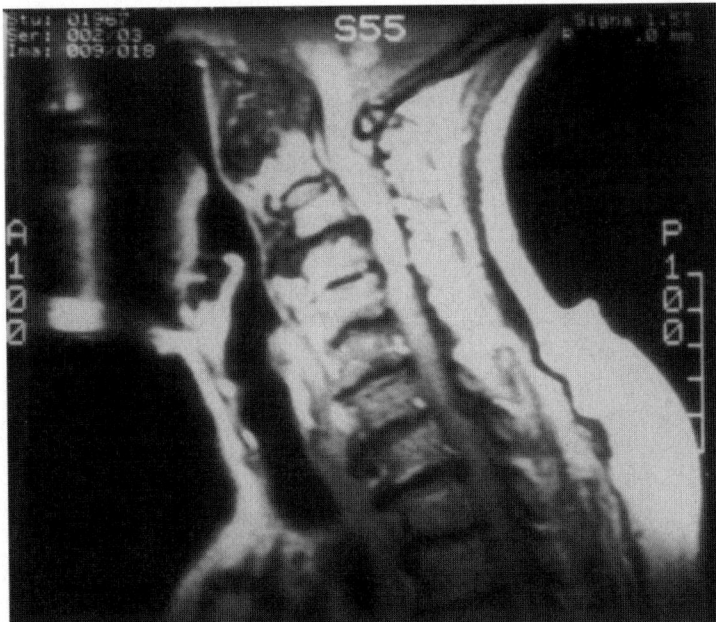

**Figure 111.1** MRI of the cervical spine in a patient with rheumatoid arthritis, showing atlantoaxial instability with pannus formation.

Patients with radiologic evidence of subluxation on neutral radiographs should also be evaluated with dynamic, lateral flexion/extension radiographs to assess the reducibility of the subluxation. Patients with nonreduced subluxations should undergo a trial of cervical traction to reduce the dislocation before a decision is made about the appropriate surgical treatment. Patients with chronic instability should remain in traction for 4 to 5 days with muscle relaxation before being considered for surgical treatment. Patients with a reducible subluxation, reduction achieved with flexion-extension, or with axial traction (Figure 111.2) and without compromise of the cervicomedullary cord may be safely stabilized by a dorsal approach. In contrast, patients who have a ventral spinal cord compression with a nonreducible subluxation may require a ventral transfacial decompression before undergoing occipitocervical stabilization. Usually, patients with instability related to rheumatoid arthritis or with pannus, but without neurologic deficit, can be stabilized from a dorsal approach without undergoing an initial ventral decompression. The pannus typically resolves in 6 to 12 months after abnormal movement has been eliminated.

## Indications for Instrumentation in Occipitoatlantal Instability

The majority of traumatic occipitoatlantal dislocations are fatal. Some patients who arrive in the emergency room are treated effectively in cervical traction followed by occipitocervical instrumentation and fusion. Chronic instability at the occipitoatlantal junction occurs with rheumatoid arthritis and other destructive lesions of the upper cervical region. In patients with chronic instability, erosion of the occipitoatlantal articulation is common and results in cranial settling with associated rotary subluxation. After cranial settling reduction with cervical traction and ventral decompression, these patients often must undergo dorsal occipitocervical instrumentation and fusion. Patients with rheumatoid arthritis, atlantoaxial subluxation, and associated cranial settling are candidates for occipitocervical instrumentation and fusion.

Finally, patients who have a traumatic atlantoaxial subluxation with fractured dorsal elements of C1 and C2 may also be candidates for an occipitocervical fusion because most of the current techniques require intact dorsal elements of C1 and C2 for stabilization.

## Occipitocervical Techniques

Several techniques exist for upper cervical spine stabilization, with or without instrumentation. Bony arthrodesis usually is the long-term goal of these techniques. With occipitocervical junction arthrodesis, a bony ridge must be established between the occiput and the upper cervical spine. Techniques may be divided into those that use bone alone and those that use internal fixation with bone.

In 1959, Perry and Nickel described a simple onlay graft for neck fusion for instability after severe poliomyelitis. In 1969, Newman and Sweetnam[17] described the technique for occipitocervical fusion in atlantoaxial instability. Fusion was achieved by decortication and laying down strips of corticocancellous bone obtained from the iliac crest. Patients were kept in cervical traction for 6 weeks and then placed in a high plastic cervical collar until bone fusion was observed.

The combination of internal fixation with onlay bone grafting has reduced the need for postoperative traction and rigid immobilization. Pseudarthrosis rates in a series of 302 occipitocervical fusions and 98 atlantoaxial fusions have been reported to be as low as 1%.[13]

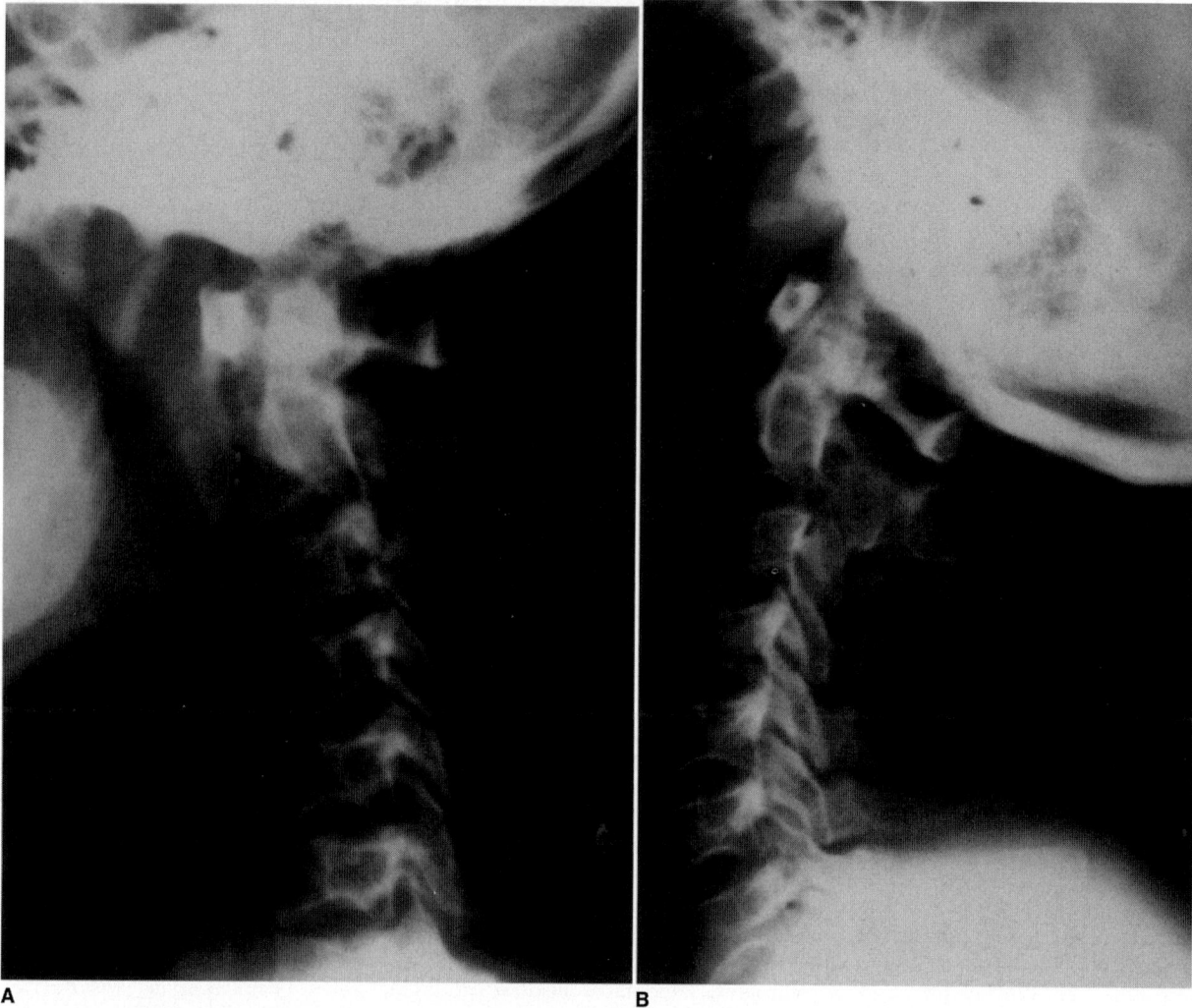

**Figure 111.2** (**A**) Plain lateral cervical spine radiographs in flexion showing ventrolisthesis of C1 on C2. (**B**) Plain lateral cervical spine radiographs in extension showing reduction of the subluxation.

## Perioperative Considerations

Preoperatively, patients remain in traction and are brought to the operating room in their bed. Extension of the neck is usually the position of safety for most patients with upper cervical instability. Thus, oral endotracheal intubation that requires some extension of the neck is usually safe. Patients who achieve reduction when the neck is flexed or in a neutral position are at risk and should be intubated while awake with the aid of the fiberoptic scope, without extension of the neck. After intubation, a firm cervical collar is placed on the patient's neck. Traction on the cervical spine is applied manually by pulling the tongs while turning the patient to the prone position. The patient's head is maintained in a neutral to slightly extended position and supported in a horseshoe headrest or fixed in a three-pin head holder.

## Exposure

A midline incision is made from the inion approximately to the C4 spinous process. The length of the exposure varies,

depending on the length of subaxial spine to be fused. The suboccipital bone around the foramen magnum and the spinous processes and laminae of C1 to C4 are exposed subperiosteally.

## Occipitocervical Fusion

In occipitocervical junction arthrodesis, a bony bridge is established between the occiput and the upper cervical spine. The techniques may be divided into those using bone alone versus internal fixation and bone grafting. A simple onlay graft alone in occipitocervical fusions was used first by Perry and Nickel and later by Newman and Sweetnam.[17] The technique entails decortication and laying down of strips of corticocancellous bone obtained from the iliac crest. The fusion extends from the occipital bone to the atlas and axis. Patients who underwent this procedure were placed postoperatively in a halo-vest for 3 to 4 months until bony fusion was noted on radiologic studies. The authors reported good fusion rates; however, the patients in their series were young and healthy.

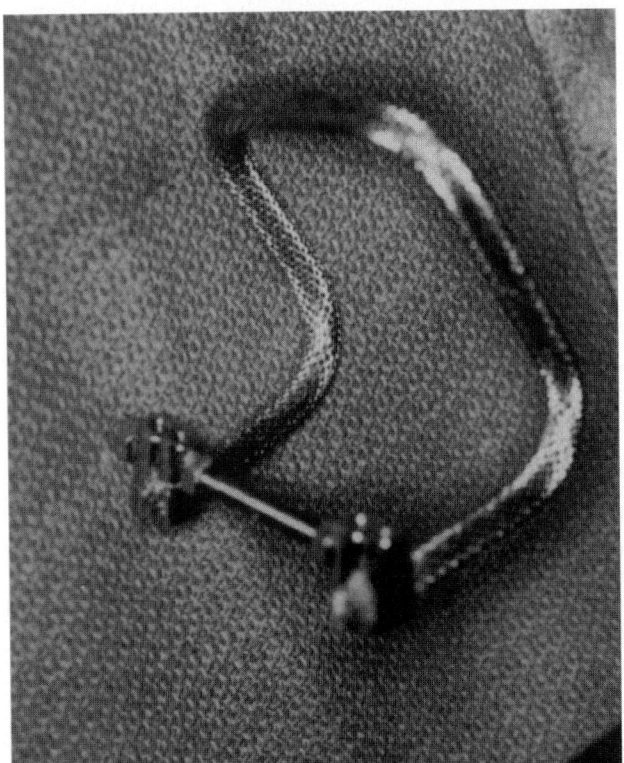

**Figure 111.3** Contoured 5mm Cotrel-Dubousset rod, with cross-fixation linkage.

## Occipitocervical Fusion with Internal Fixation

Rigid metallic implants to obtain immediate fixation with generous onlay bone graft have produced successful fusion without the need for postoperative halo-vest immobilization. Techniques with contoured rods, cables, plates, and screws have been described.

### Contoured Rod and Cable Fixation

Different smooth and threaded rods have been used for internal fixation in occipitocervical fusions. The authors use a titanium rod, contoured similar to the "Ransford loop," with cross-linkage at the caudal end to conform to the craniocervical angle, with the patient's head in a neutral position (Figure 111.3).

Lateral cervical spine radiographs are obtained after the patient is positioned prone, as described previously. The head is maintained in a neutral position. The contoured rod is placed on the back of the occiput, and sites for the burr holes are marked on either side of the occipital portion of the contoured rod bilaterally. Four burr holes are thus made in the suboccipital bone, two on either side of the midline, ensuring an adequate bridge of bone between the burr holes.

The posterior fossa dura mater is separated from the inner table of the bridge of bone between the burr holes, and a double cable is passed from one burr hole to the other. This is repeated on the opposite side of the occiput. The use of a double cable on either side of the occiput provides two cables on either side to hold down the rod. Alternatively, a single burr hole on either side of

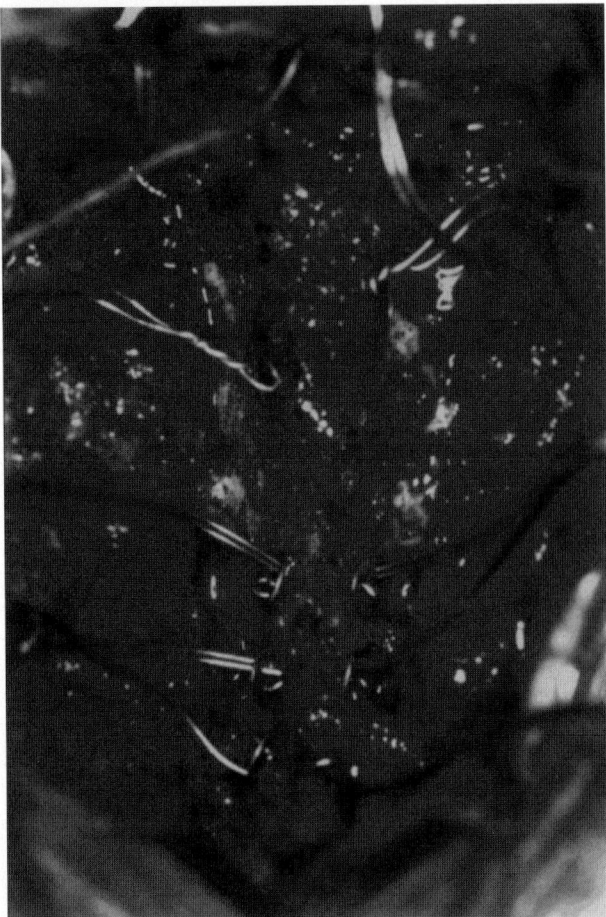

**Figure 111.4** Operative photograph showing the spinolaminar junction wires in place. Note the use of Wisconsin wires and Drummond buttons.

the midline, with the cable passed around the rim of the foramen magnum, can be used.

After cable placement for cranial fixation, sublaminar placement for spinal fixation is achieved by passing a double cable under the dorsal arch of C1 and the lamina of C2. When separated, a single cable is available on either side of the dorsal arch of C1 and C2. At C3 and C4, a hole may be made at the spinolaminar junction using a right-angled drill. Single cables threaded through Drummond buttons are passed from either side of the spinolaminar junction (Figure 111.4). Alternatively, sublaminar cables can be passed with due care under the subaxial cervical spine. The contoured rod is placed in the bed, and the cables are torqued sequentially. The distal end of the rod may be cross-fixed, just caudal to the C3 or C4 spinous process, to increase the rigidity of the construct (Figure 111.5). After decortication, bone graft is obtained through a separate incision from the dorsal iliac crest and is laid as an onlay graft of corticocancellous bone. Care must be taken during head positioning before internal fixation and fusion to obtain the best subluxation reduction with optimal head and neck position, compatible with normal function. Care must be taken to avoid dural perforation during wire passage at the suboccipital burr holes and at C1 or C2. Bevelling the edges of the burr holes and meticulous dissection of the dura mater from the inner table should prevent dural laceration. The leader wire of the single cable should be bent back on itself to present a smooth surface during sublaminar passage. Monitoring the bony surfaces carefully during torquing can help prevent overtightening of the cable. Sequential cable tightening with torque not exceeding 4 to 5 inch-pounds with titanium cables and 8 inch-pounds with stainless steel cables is appropriate in healthy adults. In patients with soft bones and in those patients with rheumatoid arthritis, the torque is reduced as appropriate (i.e., when cable begins to cut into the bone).

All patients are managed postoperatively in a Philadelphia collar for 6 to 12 weeks or until radiologic fusion is observed.

### Plate Fixation

Plates and screws have been used for occipitocervical fixation. However, their limiting factor is the variable thickness of the occipital bone. Heywood *et al.*[12] reported that occipital bone thickness measured 9 to 16mm in the midline and only 3 to 9mm in the lateral suboccipital bone. No room exists between the dura mater and the cerebellum. If the inner table is penetrated, it could lead to cerebellar injury. Therefore, it is possible that with bicortical purchase during plate fixation, especially laterally in the sub-

occipital bone, the tip of the screw could perforate the dura mater and the underlying cerebellum.

With the Y plate system of plate and screws for occipitocervical fusion, the stem of the Y is laid over the midline of the occiput (Figure 111.6). The occipital screws are 2.7mm in diameter and 8 to 10mm long. If subaxial fusion is necessary, transfacet screws are placed in the C1-2 facet joint (Magerl technique) and in the lateral masses of the subaxial spine.

Because of the risk of screws perforating the dura matter and the cerebellum, the use of the Y plate and the lateral occipitocervical plate (Figure 111.7) is limited due to the need to place screws in the lateral suboccipital bone.

## Atlantoaxial Fusion

In 1910, Mixter and Osgood described the first atlantoaxial stabilization procedure using internal fixation. Gallie popularized wiring and bone grafting techniques for dorsal atlantoaxial arthrodesis.[8] A loop of wire is passed beneath the dorsal arch of the atlas from caudal to rostral. The loop of wire is then pulled caudally over the spinous process of C2. The free ends of the wire are run downward and around the spinous process of C2 and are twisted together. The dorsal surfaces of C1 and C2 are decorticated, and onlay bone graft from the iliac crest is placed to achieve bony union. This construct provides minimal rotational stability. In 1978, Brooks and Jenkins modified this

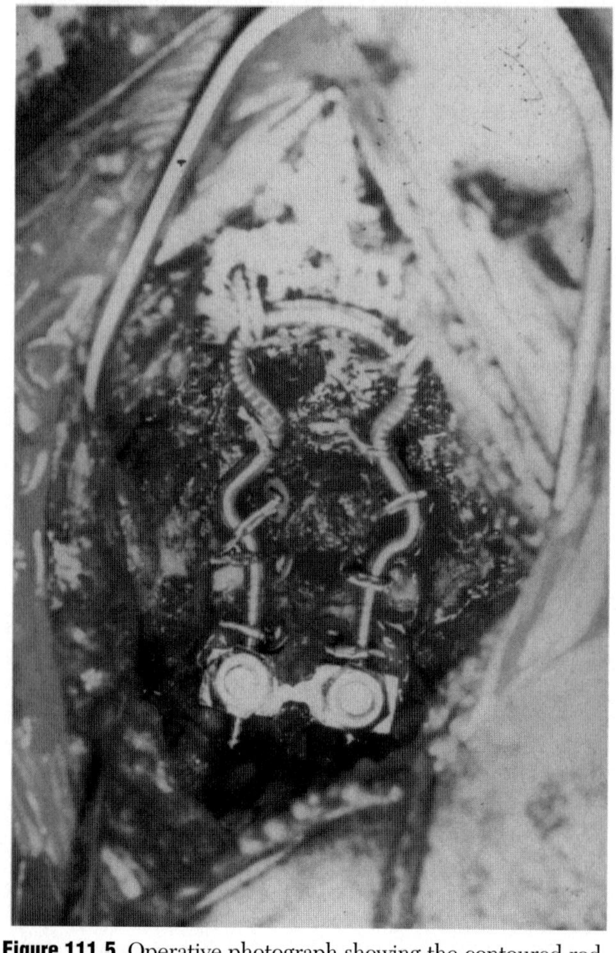

**Figure 111.5** Operative photograph showing the contoured rod in place.

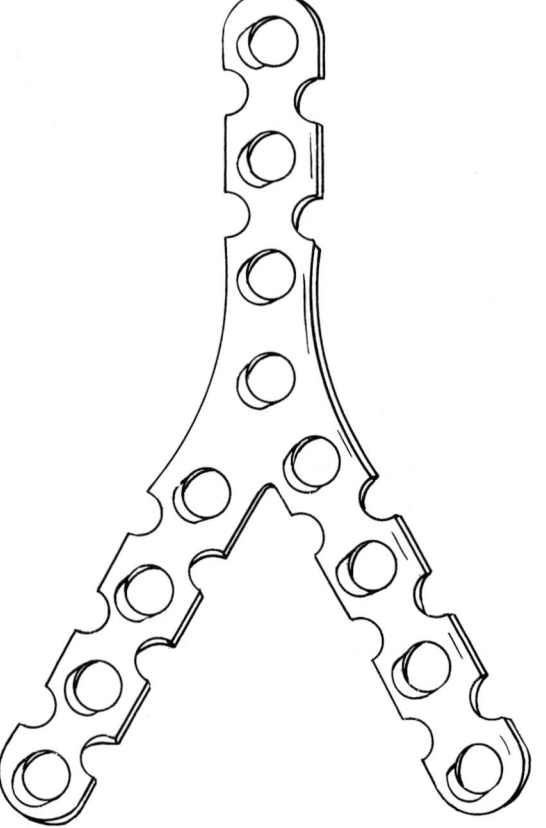

**Figure 111.6** The Y plate, used with the stem of the Y in the midline along the keel of the occipital bone.

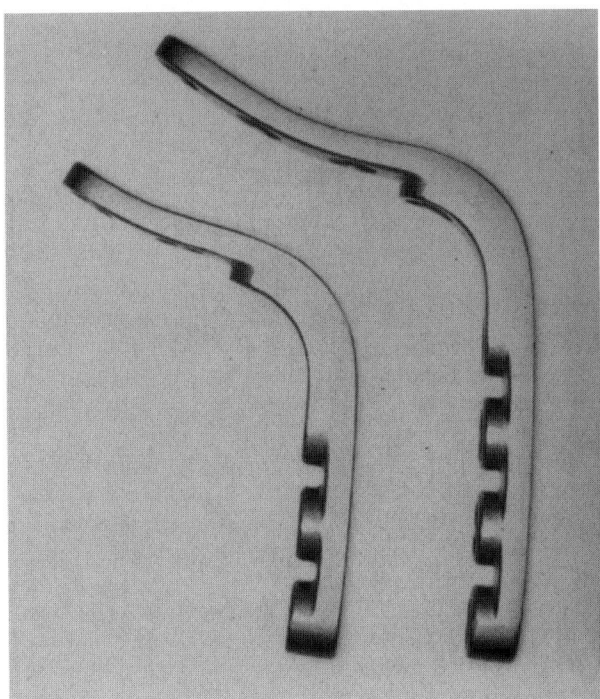

**Figure 111.7** Roy-Camille plate available for lateral occipital fixation.

technique.[4] They described passing two wires on either side, underneath the dorsal arch of C1 and the lamina of C2. Two unicortical wedges of iliac crest bone are placed between C1 and C2. This improves rotational stability. A modification of the Gallie technique described by Papadopoulos et al.[18] uses a bicortical H graft placed between the dorsal arch of C1 and the spinous process and lamina of C2 (Figure 111.8).

Preoperative evaluation and management of patients is identical to that described with occipitocervical fusion. In the modified Gallie technique a loop of cable is passed under the dorsal arch of C1 from caudal to rostral. The caudal edge of the dorsal arch of C1 and the rostral edge of the C2 lamina and spinous process are decorticated. A bicortical graft, notched on its caudal surface to hug the contour of the spinous process and lamina of C2, is placed between C1 and C2 (see Figure 111.8). The cancellous surfaces of the graft abut the decorticated areas of C1 and C2. The cable passes as with the Gallie technique. The loop is dorsal to the graft, and the free ends run ventral to the graft. This ensures that the graft does not migrate dorsally or ventrally while providing the necessary rotational stability. Further decortication and onlay bone grafting of the dorsal surfaces of C1 and C2 is carried out. Overtightening of the cable around the graft can lead to graft erosion and loosening. In the presence of dorsal subluxation of the dens, there is a risk of pulling the dens dorsally into the spinal cord during wire tightening. This risk is minimized by using a larger wedge of bone between the dorsal elements of C1 and C2. The tip of the leader wire

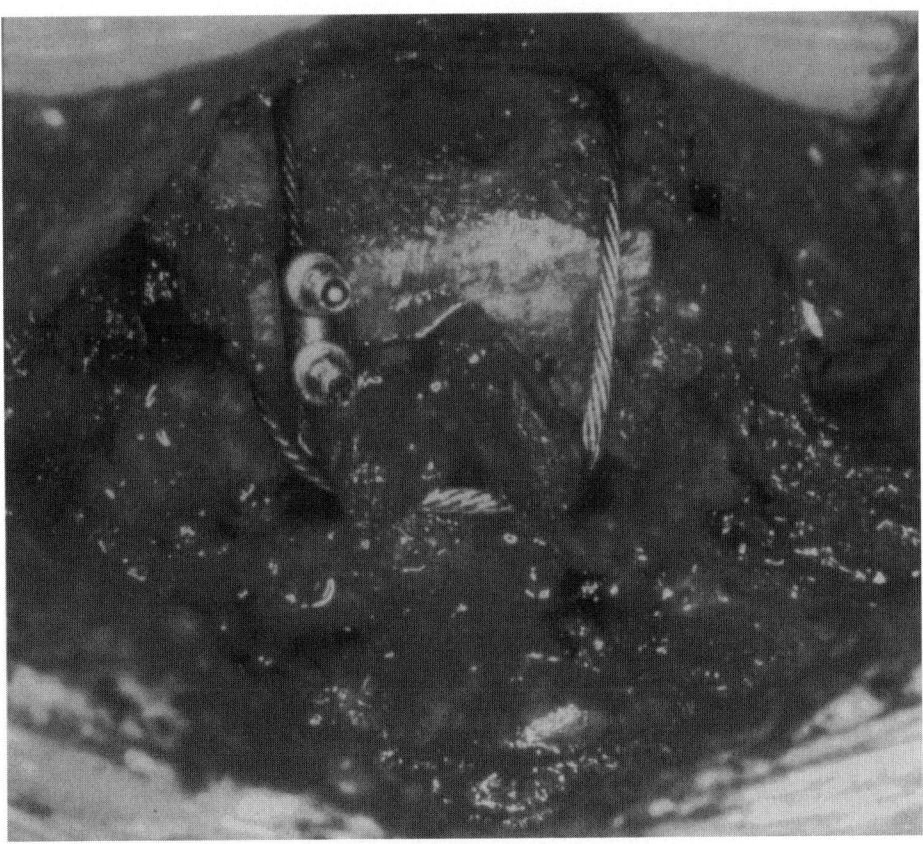

**Figure 111.8** Modified Gallie technique.

should be doubled back to present a smooth surface during sublaminar wire passage to prevent dural laceration.

Several techniques have been described for wiring the atlas to the axis vertebra, with varying degrees of success. The disadvantage for patients undergoing wire and cable techniques alone is that in the presence of significant instability they have to be placed in a halo body vest postoperatively for 3 to 4 months. The patient should undergo transfacet fixation of C1 to C2 when there is significant instability or fractured or absent dorsal elements of C1 or C2 or when a laminectomy of C1 and C2 is indicated.

## Summary

Upper cervical spine stabilization can be achieved using a variety of techniques, depending on the surgical indications. Controversy still abounds regarding the use of occipitocervical fusion versus atlantoaxial fusion in the presence of atlantoaxial instability. Some surgeons continue to perform occipitocervical fusions in patients with instability at the atlantoaxial joint, arguing that the loss of 15 to 20 degrees in flexion/extension by including the occiput in the fusion is negligible. However, the 15 to 20 degrees of movement at the occipitoatlantal joint is responsible for the nodding or chin-tuck movement in the cervical spine, and the loss of this movement may be a cause of significant morbidity. The authors recommend that occipitocervical fusions be reserved for patients with either occipitoatlantal instability or cranial settling, with or without atlantoaxial instability. All other patients with instability at the atlantoaxial articulation alone should undergo the appropriate stabilization technique at C1-2. Rigid internal fixation techniques reduce the need for cumbersome and rigid external orthotics and increase the rate of bone fusion.

## REFERENCES

1. Anderson LD, D'Alonzo RT: Fracture of the odontoid process of the axis. *J Bone Joint Surg Am* 56:1663, 1971.
2. Beighton P, Craig J: Atlanto-axial subluxation in the Morquio syndrome. *J Bone Joint Surg Am* 61:478, 1979.
3. Bohlman HH: Acute fractures and dislocations of the cervical spine: an analysis of three hundred hospitalized patients and review of the literature. *J Bone Joint Surg Am* 61:1119, 1979.
4. Brooks AL, Jenkins EW: Atlanto-axial arthrodesis by wedge compression method. *J Bone Joint Surg Am* 60:279, 1978.
5. Cregan JC: Internal fixation of the unstable rheumatoid cervical spine. *Ann Rheum Dis* 25:242, 1966.
6. Dawson EG, Smith I: Atlanto-axial subluxation in children due to vertebral abnormalities. *J Bone Joint Surg Am* 61:582, 1978.
7. Fielding JW, Hawkins RJ, Ratzan SA: Spine fusion for atlanto-axial instability. *J Bone Joint Surg Am* 58:400, 1976.
8. Gallie WE: Fractures and dislocations of the cervical spine. *Am J Surg* 46,495, 1939.
9. Graham A, Hockley AD, McMillan JJ, Thompson AG: A new method of occipitocervical fusion, using internal fixation. *Neurosurgery* 21:947, 1987.
10. Grob D, Dvorak J, Panjabi M, *et al*: Posterior occipitocervical fusion. A preliminary report of a new technique, *Spine* 16(Suppl 3):S17-S24, 1991.
11. Hadley MN, Sonntag V: Acute axis fractures. *Contemp Neurosurg* 9:1, 1987.
12. Heywood AWB, Learmonth ID, Thomas M: Internal fixation for occipito-cervical fusion, *J Bone Joint Surg Br* 70:708, 1988
13. Menezes AH: Surgical approaches to the craniocervical junction. In Frymoyer J (ed): *The Adult Spine.* New York, Lippincott-Raven.
14. Menezes AH, VanGilder JC, Graf CJ, McDonnell DE: Craniocervical abnormalities: a comprehensive surgical approach. *J Neurosurg* 53:444, 1980.
15. Menezes AH, VanGilder JC: Transoral-transpharyngeal approach to the anterior craniocervical junction: 10-year experience with 72 patients. *J Neurosurg* 69:895, 1988.
16. Menezes AH, VanGilder JC: Abnormalities of the craniovertebral junction. In Youmans J (ed): *Neurological Surgery,* ed 3. Philadelphia, WB Saunders, 1990, pp 1359-1420.
17. Newman P, Sweetnam R: Occipitocervical fusion: an operative technique and its indications. *J Bone Joint Surg Br* 51:423, 1969.
18. Papadopoulos SM, Dickman CA, Sonntag VKH: Atlanto-axial stabilization in rheumatoid arthritis. *J Neurosurg* 74:1, 1991.
19. Pierce DS, Barr JS: Fractures and dislocations at the base of the skull and upper cervical spine. In Cervical Spine Research Society (eds): *The Cervical Spine.* Philadelphia, Lippincott-Raven, 1983, pp 196-205.
20. Rana NA, Hancock DO, Taylor AR, Hill AGS: Atlanto-axial subluxation in rheumatoid arthritis, *J Bone Joint Surg Br* 55:458, 1973.

# CHAPTER 112

# Ventral Subaxial Cervical Fixation Techniques

## David G. Malone and Cary D. Alberstone

In recent years, ventral fixation techniques have been developed to treat a variety of abnormalities of the subaxial cervical spine. All of these techniques involve the use of a ventral cervical plating system with bone screws to lock in the bone graft material. Multiple studies of ventral fixation have been undertaken in patients who have undergone multilevel cervical discectomies with fusion, corpectomies, and strut grafts. No randomized controlled trials with sufficient numbers of patients exist to make definitive statements about the use of fixation in ventral cervical spine surgery. The results of those studies that do exist point out several factors, which include the following:

1. The greater the number of levels fused, the higher the pseudoarthrosis rate.
2. Plate fixation does not conclusively improve patient outcome.
3. Plate fixation does not increase complications.
4. Plate fixation does lessen graft extrusion rates.
5. Plate fixation appears to lessen the rate of pseudoarthrosis and kyphosis.[2,7,15,23-25]

Indications for these ventral fixators include cervical vertebrectomies, multilevel cervical discectomies, cervical fractures, metastatic lesions of the cervical vertebral bodies, traumatic or acquired instability of the cervical spine, and, occasionally, single-level ventral cervical discectomies or infection.[11]

Since the last edition of this text, several new ventral fixation systems have entered the marketplace for fixation of the cervical spine. Other surgical techniques have been implemented to address the problems of subsidence of corpectomy grafts and to eliminate stress shielding of bone grafts. Newer fixation systems now offer dynamic fixation, static fixation, or even a combination of static and dynamic fixation all in one system. Cervical cages are also new since the last edition of this text.

Graft complications occur in 15% of cases and include nonunion, graft extrusion, graft fracture, and graft infection. Ventral cervical instrumentation lessens the incidence of these complications by allowing the surgeon to place the bone graft in compression. This reduces micromotion and may improve fusion. In addition, ventral cervical fixation greatly decreases the incidence of the complication of graft extrusion because the plate acts to secure the graft and may even be mechanically affixed to it.[10]

The ventral approach to the subaxial cervical spine is accomplished via the commonly used surgical approaches. The surgeon must remember that access to the vertebral body above and below the graft site must be obtained to gain access for purchase of the fixation device. A transverse incision may be used and leaves minimal scarring to the skin, but this may limit rostral and caudal dissection. For this reason an incision paralleling the sternocleidomastoid muscle is preferred when four or more cervical discs are to be exposed. When the ventral surface of the spine is reached, the longus colli muscles must be stripped from the midline outward and the disc spaces exposed. It is often helpful, but not mandatory, to identify the disc interspace above and below the vertebral body upon which the fixator is to be attached. This helps the surgeon avoid placing the screws into a disc space. A perhaps faster and simpler solution to the problem of placing screws into the disc space is provided by using fluoroscopic x-ray guidance while placing the screws.

## Multilevel Constructs

Recently, problems have been identified in multilevel constructs with graft subsidence, also known as pistoning or telescoping of the graft into the adjacent vertebral bodies. Biomechanical data reveal that ventral cervical plating excessively loads the graft in extension and may lead to graft pistoning and failure in multilevel constructs.[8] A variety of ventral cervical plates have been developed that offer either dynamic or static (i.e., fixed) interface with the plate. Other operative techniques involving multilevel discectomies with arthrodiesis, sometimes in combination with corpectomies, have been developed to take advantage of the multiple fixation points offered by these new plates. These newer plates minimize or prevent stress shielding of the bone graft.

Biomechanical data comparing dynamic versus static plates are sparse. However, it has been observed that dynamic plates load share more effectively than static plates, especially in a short construct.[3]

Analysis has shown that the caudal end of the construct is the most likely to experience failure by screw loosening or hardware failure. This is thought to occur due to the longer moment arm and increased forces on the caudal end of the construct.[14] This problem may be lessened by (1) maximizing screw purchase at the caudal end of the construct, (2) using dynamic fixation, (3) using meticulous bone grafting and mortising techniques, and (4) constraining the spine with a rigid collar in the first few months after the procedure.

## Technique of Bone Grafting

The proper placement of the bone graft is the key to optimal ventral cervical fixation. Poor grafting technique places increased mechanical stress on the fixation system and may cause the plate or screw to fail. The principles of successful bone grafting include (1) the establishment of good bony contact between the bone and the graft, (2) the placement of the graft in a compression mode, and (3) the immobilization of the bone-graft junction.

Placing a graft that is significantly taller than the height of the interspace can lead to overdistraction of the disc space. Overdistraction of the disc space often leaves the patient with chronic pain in the intrascapular region of the spine and, rarely, neurologic deficits due to overdistraction. This complication can be avoided by careful measurement of the disc space height after the graft site is prepared. The interspace should be measured with an interspace spanner, and the graft is then marked with this spanner, with the cut being made to the outside of the line, making the graft slightly taller than the spanner height.

The technique of bone grafting used with ventral plates is well described by Caspar.[4] Instrumentation to achieve this task is provided by the Caspar system. The graft site is prepared with parallel rostral and caudal edges. All of the disc material is removed, and bone is removed from the end plate until punctuate hemorrhage from the cancellous bone appears. The autologous iliac crest is often the preferred harvest site for a bone graft. The graft site is measured with calipers, and a block graft is harvested that is 2mm longer than the rostrocaudal span of the graft site. The depth and width of the graft is measured. Using an oscillating saw or equivalent technique, the graft is trimmed to the exact width and to a depth approximately 5mm less than the sagittal dimension of the vertebral body. Vertebral body distraction is then used, and the graft is placed 2mm below the ventral surface of the spine. This provides locking of the bone graft and a 3mm safety margin between the graft and the spinal cord. A nerve hook is placed beneath the graft to ensure the absence of impingement of the graft on the spinal cord. A lateral radiograph is obtained to check graft placement dorsally. Graft fracture can be minimized by obtaining a graft of at least 7mm in height and 15mm in depth. Cadaveric bone or methylmethacrylate or other techniques may be used instead of donor bone in cases of malignancy.[4,19]

Controversy has existed as to whether the graft should be placed in the traditional Smith-Robinson configuration with the cortex placed ventrally or in the reversed Smith-Robinson technique with the cortex of the graft placed in the middle column of the spine. High fusion rates are obtained with either technique. It seems that graft extrusion can be lessened with the reverse Smith-Robinson technique; however, the chance of developing kyphosis increases. Biomechanically, loads placed on the spine are resisted better in the classic Smith-Robinson position.[26] When ventral plating is added, the problem of graft extrusion is eliminated and the chance of kyphosis lessened, thus making the choice of graft technique less important.

## Biomechanical Data

Biomechanical studies have demonstrated the characteristics of the Caspar plate when used for trauma. However, there is a sparsity of data that detail the characteristics of the Synthes and the Orion plates. *In vitro* data from cadaveric and animal spine studies demonstrate less rigid fixation of the flexion-injured spine by Caspar ventral cervical spine plates compared with dorsal fixation methods when one motion segment is fixated.[6,13,21]

Additional data comparing *in vitro* fixation between a Caspar plate and dorsal fixation techniques over two motion segments show that ventral plating demonstrated significantly better resistance to extension and lateral bending compared with dorsal wiring and had equal stability acquisition to flexion loading compared with dorsal wiring.[20] Data concerning the need for bicortical purchase of Caspar screws demonstrate no additional significant pull-out resistance to direct axial loads with bicortical purchase.[12] However, bicortical purchase resulted in enhanced stability of the construct under cyclical loading compared with unicortical purchase. Even with bicortical purchase, significant deterioration in the bone-screw junction became evident after cyclical loading.[20]

It is evident that without good bony fusion all fixation devices will eventually fail from either degradation of the bone-implant junction or failure (by fatigue) of the implant itself. The Synthes cervical spine locking plate system and the Caspar plate both provide stability. However, under fatigue cyclical testing, both plates displayed decremental stability, with the Caspar plate retaining greater stability than the Synthes plate. The Caspar plate also is more stable in flexion loading than the Synthes plate. When both plates were tested to failure in the flexion mode, the hardware remained intact, but the vertebral bodies fractured.[5]

### Interference Screw Technique

The interference screw technique uses screws placed between the bone graft and the vertebral body to provide additional resistance to pull-out of the graft. This technique increases pull-out resistance from an average of 58.1N for a Smith-Robinson type graft to 153.9N for two screws and to 217.9N newtons for four screws. Cancellous screws, 14mm in length and 3.5mm in diameter, were used for this study. Problems with this technique include the possibility of screw backout, with esophageal perforation.[22]

### Screw Plate Techniques

A plethora of new plates have entered the marketplace since the first edition of this text was written. Techniques for placing the Caspar plate, Synthesis plate, and Orion plate are left in this edition as illustrative examples of plate placement. The basic techniques of insertion, which have not significantly changed with the introduction of these new systems, include the following:

1. Identification of the midline
2. Removal of ventral osteophytes to allow the plate to lay in contact with the ventral spine
3. Selection of the proper length and hole positions of the plate
4. Measurement of screw length, graft depth, and vertebral body depth prior to placement of screws
5. Selection of screw length to provide maximal unicortical purchase or minimal spinal canal perforation with bicortical purchase
6. Alignment of the plate in the midline, with screw holes positioned over the vertebral bodies

7. Placement of screws into the vertebral body, avoiding the disc space
8. Proper locking of the screws into the plate

Fluoroscopic imaging aids the surgeon in accomplishing the above steps and ensuring proper plate length, screw position, screw length, graft position, and approximation of the plate to the vertebral body.

### Caspar Trapezoidal Osteosynthetic Plate

The Caspar plate uses a trapezoidal-shaped titanium or stainless steel plate of varying lengths, with fixed and slotted holes for fixation with screws. The thickness of the plate is 1.5mm. The screws should be placed to allow bicortical purchase on the ventral and dorsal surface of the vertebral body. If desired, the slotted holes allow placement of unicortical interference screws. There is no true locking mechanism to prevent screw backout with this system. The screw holes in the plate are designed so that additional screws can be placed. Methylmethacrylate adhesive may be placed over the screw heads to provide additional resistance to screw backout. Complications from screws placed too deeply into the spinal canal and esophageal perforation caused by screw backout have been reported.[10]

### *Technique of Placing Caspar Ventral Cervical Plates*

If the Caspar vertebral body distractor is used, the holes placed in the vertebral body should avoid sites to be used as fixation screw placement sites. The length of the plate is selected by both visual and radiographic inspection. The ideal plate provides screw holes directly over the solid bony structures and avoids the soft tissue. No screw should be placed within 2mm of the vertebral end plate. When the proper plate length is selected, the plate should be aligned in the midline and inspected for degree of fit on the ventral surface of the vertebral bodies. If the plate fits poorly, ventral osteophytes should be removed until the plate fits securely.

The plate should only be bent to provide a better fit as a last resort. Plate bending should be performed smoothly to avoid sharp bends. Multiple or sharp bends should be avoided because this weakens the plate and may lead to plate failure. The ventrodorsal distance of the vertebral body is measured from preoperative imaging studies and cross-checked by measurement of the intervertebral ventrodorsal disc space distance. Next, the drill guide is set by the surgeon to a distance 3mm less than the ventrodorsal distance. The plate is held in position with a temporary fixation device. The dual drill guide is then placed into the plate, and the first guide hole is drilled under fluoroscopic guidance. Still under fluoroscopic guidance, a blunt K-wire that is 1.8mm in diameter is used to palpate the drill holes. The drill is then adjusted in 1mm increments, and the holes are periodically palpated with the K-wire until the dorsal cortex is perforated. This process is repeated at all four corners of the plate with the K-wires left in place. Placement of both the plate and the K-wires is rechecked with a lateral radiograph to ensure proper screw-hole placement. Next, the appropriate screw length is measured with the depth gauge, and the ventral cortex is tapped. Blunt-tipped screws that are 3.5mm in diameter and 1mm in length less than the exact measured distance are preferred. The first screw is not fully tightened. The screws are placed and tightened in a diagonal fashion under fluoroscopic guidance. One millimeter of screw thread may penetrate the dorsal cortex without damaging the spinal cord. This is the approximate thickness of the posterior longitudinal ligament. Care must be taken not to overtorque the screws because this may lead to a diminished bony purchase[10] (Figure 112.1).

### Synthes Ventral Cervical Locking Plate System

The Synthes ventral cervical locking plate provides several advantages over the Caspar plate. The Synthes plate is made of pure titanium and uses screws with unicortical purchase, along with a locking mechanism to minimize backout of the screws. The plate interlocks with a drill

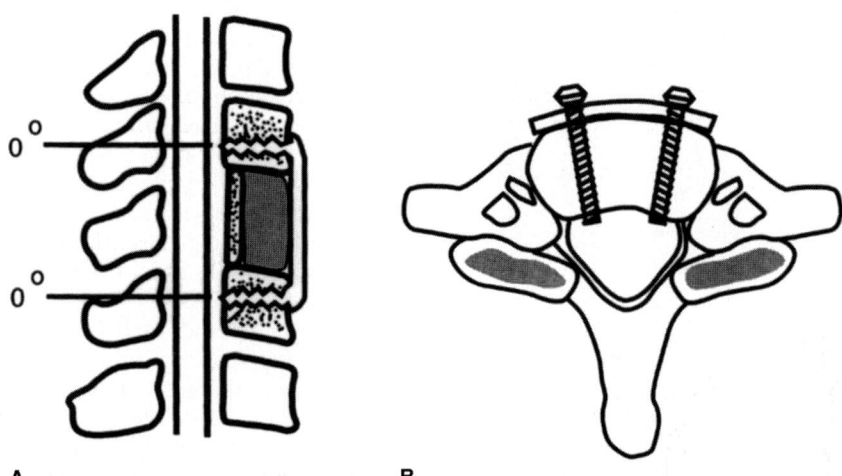

**A**                    **B**

**Figure 112.1** (**A**) Sagittal and (**B**) axial view of the Caspar plate. Note that the screws obtain bicortical purchase. (*Copyright University of New Mexico, Division of Neurosurgery.*)

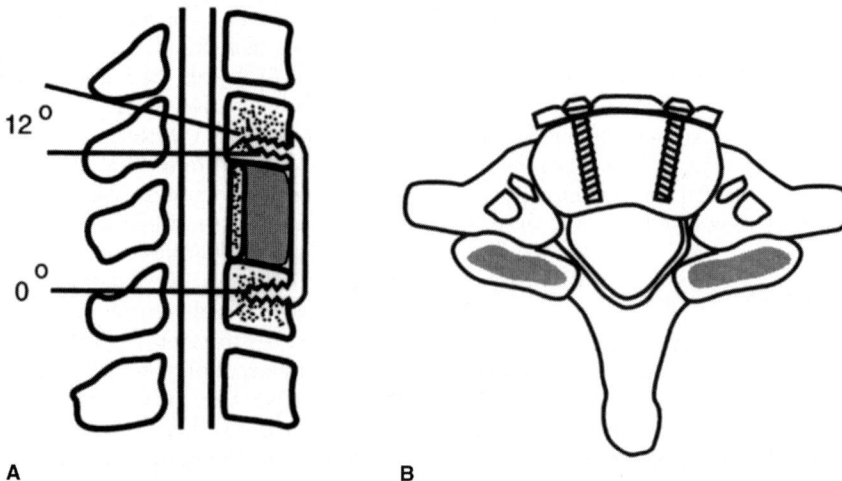

**Figure 112.2** **(A)** Sagittal and **(B)** axial view of the Synthes plate. Note that the rostral screws are angled 12 degrees rostrally, whereas the caudal screws are angled perpendicular to the long axis of the plate. (*Copyright University of New Mexico, Division of Neurosurgery.*)

guide that angles the upper screws on an upward angle of 12 degrees and the lower screws perpendicular to the vertebral body (Figure 112.2). The screw depth is set by the drill guide to 14mm. The plate thickness is 2mm. The screws are designed to countersink into the plate. Locking expansion screws are then placed into the head of the 14mm screw to secure it into the countersunk portion of the plate (Figure 112.3).

Despite these advantages, screw backout, plate fracture, and screw breakage have been reported. Such complications may be minimized by ensuring good bony purchase by the 14mm screws. Other recommendations include avoidance of the fenestrated 14mm screws and avoidance of severe or sharp bending of the plate, which may contribute to the development of metal fatigue.[18]

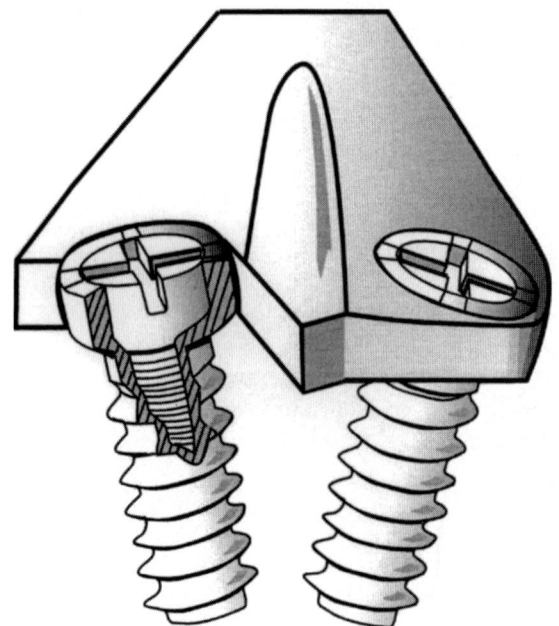

**Figure 112.3** The expansion screw locking mechanism used in the Synthes plate.

## Technique of Placing Synthes Ventral Cervical Locking Plates

Plate length is selected by visual and radiographic inspection. The plate should extend to a point above and below the graft-body juncture so that bone is palpable through the plate holes. When selecting a plate, it is helpful to identify the normal disc space above and below the construct and to select a plate that overlies the middle of the caudal vertebral body and the junction of the caudal and middle thirds of the rostral body. It is important to bear in mind that the trajectory of the rostral screws is angled 12 degrees upward and that the trajectory of the caudal screws is angled perpendicular to the plate (see Figure 112.2).

Using the technique described by Ball *et al.*,[1] K-wires may be placed through the fixation holes of the plate and a lateral radiograph obtained before drilling the guide holes. This technique confirms proper plate length and screw position.

The ventral vertebral bodies may require contouring, or as a last resort the plate may need to be bent to provide a good fit between the ventral aspect of the vertebral bodies and the plate. The plate is then held in position, and using the drill guide and a 3mm diameter drill bit, one hole is drilled to the maximum depth allowed by the stop into the caudal portion of the plate. The drill guide–drill bit combination limits the hole to a maximum depth of 14mm. This hole is then tapped, and one 4mm expansion head screw is placed into the hole, but not fully tightened.

Next, the plate is aligned in the midline, and one rostral hole is drilled using the drill guide and a 3mm drill bit. The hole is tapped, and the 4mm expansion head screw is placed. The other two holes are drilled and tapped in a similar fashion, and 4mm expansion head screws are placed. The expansion head screws are then tightened diagonally, in a sequential fashion, with care taken to avoid overtightening. After these screws are positioned, 1 to 8mm locking screws are placed in the heads of each of the 4mm expansion head screws and tightened fully. Care must be taken to ensure that the expansion head screws fit fully into the plate, otherwise the locking screws will not be able to lock the screws into the plate and may cause fracture of the expansion screw heads. With this type of plate, locking screws may be placed into the graft through the plate, either before or after plate insertion.[10]

## Orion Ventral Cervical Plate System

The Orion ventral cervical plate is made of a titanium alloy (90% titanium, 6% aluminum, 4% vanadium), offers a variety of screw lengths, has a precontoured lordotic curve, and has a locking device to prevent screw backout (Figure 112.4). The plate is designed for unicortical purchase, but due to the variety of screw lengths, bicortical purchase is achievable if the surgeon desires. The plate provides a convergent screw pattern, with the screws angling 15 degrees rostrally and 6 degrees medially for the rostral holes and 15 degrees caudally and 6 degrees medially for the caudal holes (Figure 112.5). Diagonal central slots provide access for the placement of additional screws to further secure the graft. No accommodation is provided for intermediate screws.[12]

### Technique of Placing Orion Ventral Cervical Plates

Plate length is selected using the steps described for the Synthes plate. Note that due to the 15-degree sagittal divergence of the screws at both ends of the Orion plate, it is prudent to choose an Orion plate that is shorter than the appropriate Synthes plate equivalent. The ventral vertebral bodies are contoured to provide good plate contact. Only in rare cases is it necessary to bend the Orion plate to provide a proper fit. After the appropriate plate has been selected, it is held in place by a plate holder so that the plate holes overlie the vertebral body at the junction of the middle and caudal thirds for the upper vertebral body and at the junction of the rostral and middle thirds of the lower body. Proper placement of the plate is facilitated if the disc spaces above and below the construct are identified during the dissection.

Next, the plate is centered over the midline, and the drill guide is inserted into the plate. The Ball K-wire technique, described earlier for the Synthes plate, may be used here as well to confirm proper plate length and screw position. The plate is designed so that the drill guide fits securely into the plate at a 6-degree convergent angle, with a 15-degree rostral and caudal angulation. Several options are available for the selection of hole depth. Although the standard 13mm drill bit with fixed stop is most commonly used, longer screws with drill bits with variable depth stops are available. Great care must be exercised when using these variable bits because the stops may fail under the application of excessive force.

Using a power drill, each of the holes is reamed, starting with a caudal hole. The holes are then tapped, and the appropriate length screw is placed. Most commonly, this is a standard 13mm-in-length, 4mm-in-diameter screw. This first screw is not fully tightened, allowing the plate to be realigned in the midline. The second screw placed is a rostral screw (placed diagonally opposite from the first screw). The last two screws are placed in a similar fashion, and all are tightened sequentially.

The length of each screw should be verified by the surgeon before placement. It is useful to note that the standard 13-mm screw provides 13mm of bony purchase, and with the 15-degree rostral and caudal angulation provided by the plate, the screw end appears flush with the end of the plate in the transverse plane. If bicortical purchase is desired, the ventrodorsal vertebral body dimension should be measured from the preoperative computed tomography (CT) or magnetic resonance imaging (MRI) scan. This dimension should be cross-checked by measuring the ventrodorsal dimension once the disc space dissection has been completed. The drill should be set for 3mm less than the measured dimension, and the holes should be drilled using the same techniques used to drill the holes for the Caspar system (i.e., 1mm at a time under fluoroscopic guidance with palpation of the holes until the dorsal cortex is perforated). The lock screws are then placed, and tightening is begun using the lock screw holder. Once all

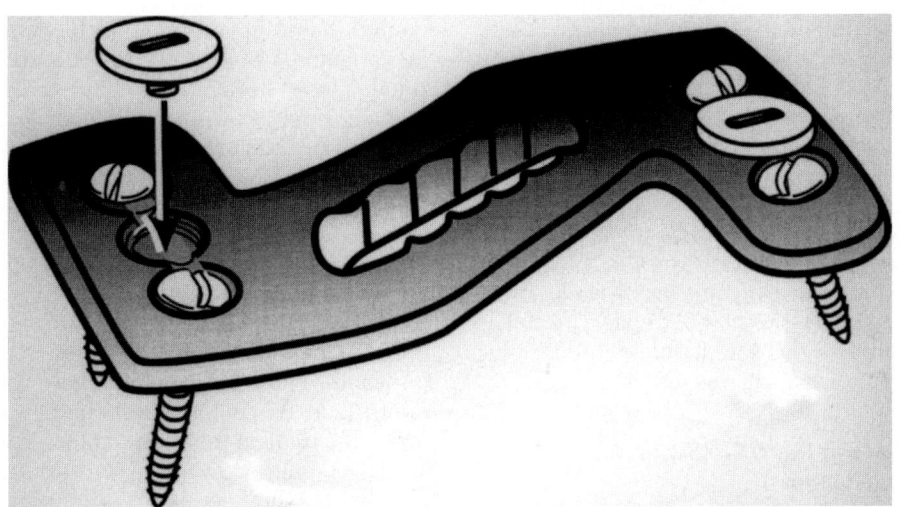

**Figure 112.4** The locking mechanism used in the Orion plate. (*Copyright University of New Mexico, Division of Neurosurgery.*)

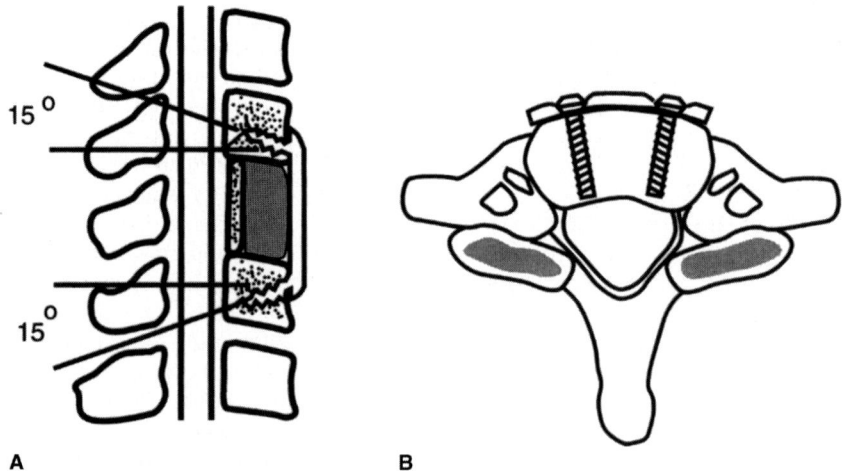

**Figure 112.5** (**A**) Sagittal and (**B**) axial view of the Orion plate. Note that the rostral screws are angled 15 degrees rostrally and the caudal screws are angled 15 degrees caudally. (*Copyright University of New Mexico, Division of Neurosurgery.*)

of the anchoring screws have been adequately placed, an additional screw may then be inserted through the central slot to further secure the graft.

## Cervical Interbody Fusion Systems

Cervical interbody fusion devices are new on the marketplace and have been investigated as part of Food and Drug Administration (FDA) trials of the devices. Randomized controlled trials undertaken as part of an FDA study on ventral cervical cages show that good to excellent results were obtained in 97% of the cage group. A major difference was lack of donor bone graft site pain in the experimental group.[9]

Biomechanical studies have compared autograft-to-ventral plate fixation with cervical cages *in vitro*. These showed the plate construct to limit motion better than the cage device.[16]

## BAK/C Cervical Interbody Fusion System

The BAK/C cervical interbody fusion system is a cage device that is placed either singly or in parallel pairs as determined by the preoperative disc space height and surgeon preference. The device is indicated for single-level radiculopathy of degenerative disc disease in skeletally mature patients treated via a ventral approach from the C3-7 levels. The device is not to be used in cases where there is acute trauma, instability, osteoporosis, infection, rheumatoid disease, myelopathy, active malignancy of the cervical spine, or more than one level to be fused or where there has been previously attempted fusion at the operative level. The system offers advantages in that it avoids bone graft by using local bone and is countersunk into the disc interspace.

### Technique for Placing the BAK/C Cervical Interbody Fusion System

Prior to implantation, the system is templated from plain films, MRI, or CT images. An adjacent noninvolved disc is measured to establish the amount of restoration of disc height desired. The appropriate guide tube is selected from this information, and the size of the implant and instrumentation is generally 2 to 3mm larger than the desired disc height. The patient is positioned as for a standard ventral cervical discectomy. Save all bone removed during the discectomy for use later in the procedure. The discectomy should consist of complete removal of the cartilaginous end plate and disc material, with care taken to remove minimal bony end plate.

Next, select the proper guide tube, and using the guide starter and guide tube, impact it into position in the midline, seating the guide tube. Fluoroscopic guidance facilitates this process. Once the guide tube is in position, remove any additional distraction instruments or traction and remove the guide tube starter. To ensure that the guide-tube teeth do not disengage from the bone, keep downward pressure on the guide-tube holder. At this point, measure the depth of the disc space. This measurement is used in the reaming process. Ideal reaming should be to a depth 2 to 3mm from the posterior cortex. The reamer is adjustable from a depth of 12 to 20mm in 1mm increments. It is vital not to ream too deeply. Reaming should always begin at a depth of 12mm, and if additional reaming is required, it should be done under fluoroscopic guidance in 1mm increments. Once reaming is completed, the reamer is cleaned of any bony material, which is saved for use later in the procedure. The reamed hole is then tapped. Once the positive stop is met, tapping must end, otherwise the tap will strip the threads in the bone. The implant is then selected and is filled with bone harvested from the earlier decompression and from the reamer. The implant driver has color-coded positive stops to allow flush insertion (blue) or recessed insertion (green) of the implant. At this point, select the desired stop level, and rotate the implant into position to the level of the positive stop. Rotating past the positive stop will strip the bony threads, possibly causing loss of fixation of the device. Disengage the implant from the driver and check the implant position with an x-ray.[17]

## Complications

Complications encountered in placing ventral cervical implants are the same as those encountered with any ventral approach to the cervical spine, with several additions. Complications directly attributable to the fixation devices include faulty screw placement into the disc or end plate, excessive screw length, plate malpositioning, screw or plate fracture, and screw backout.[10]

## Radiographic Guidance

Radiographic guidance is helpful for ensuring proper plate and screw position and decreases the amount of time required to place the hardware. With the Caspar system, fluoroscopic guidance is mandatory. It provides visual images of the screws while gaining bicortical screw purchase. Placement of screws without radiographic guidance risks damage to the spinal cord and nerve roots and may allow screw placement into the disc space, leading to poor fixation and hardware loosening. The Synthes system may be placed without radiographic guidance because the system uses only unicortical purchase. However, it is wise to obtain radiographs before closing the wound because it is easy to place screws into the disc space with this system. This may lead to the loss of secure fixation.

The Orion system may also be placed without radiographic guidance because the system only requires unicortical purchase for fixation. Nevertheless, the manufacturer recommends anteroposterior and lateral plain radiographs before screw placement to help ensure proper placement of the screws. All of these systems may be placed under fluoroscopic guidance. This avoids delays associated with waiting for the radiology technician and avoids the repositioning of the system when malposition is detected on the radiograph.[4] Surgeon preference (except with the Caspar system) is the determining factor.

## Postoperative Care

Most patients who have had ventral grafting and plating are immobilized with a hard collar for 8 weeks. In recent years with newer systems, patients who underwent single-level or even multilevel discectomies with fusion have been managed postoperatively without external orthosis if a variety of conditions have been met. An external collar is not required if (1) the bone quality and screw purchase is good, (2) screw fixation has been achieved at each intervening level in a multilevel construct, and (3) no preoperative instability existed. Plain radiographs may be obtained immediately after surgery and at 2 months postoperatively to assess fusion. In the rare event that pseudoarthrosis is present on the 6-month study, consideration may be given to reoperation. This determination is based on the presence and nature of the patient's symptoms, the objective evidence of instability, and the desires of the extensively counseled patient.[4] The majority of corticocancellous grafts have fused 6 months after operation. If fusion does not appear solid, flexion-extension radiographs provide a method of evaluating stability. If plate, screw, or bone graft position is in question, CT scanning or polydirectional tomography may be performed.

## REFERENCES

1. Ball P, Benzel EC, Baldwin NG: A simple method to ensure proper screw position and plate size selection using the Morscher cervical spine locking plate. *J Neurosurg* 80:748, 1994.
2. Bolesta MJ, Rechtine GR II, Chrin AM: Three- and four-level anterior cervical discectomy and fusion with plate fixation: a prospective study. *Spine* 25(16):2040-2044 (discussion 2045-2046), 2000.
3. Brodke DS, Gollogly S, Mohr A, *et al:* Dynamic cervical plates biomechanical evaluation of load sharing and stiffness. *Spine* 26(12):1324-1329, 2001.
4. Caspar W: Anterior cervical fusion and interbody stabilization with the trapezial osteosynthetic plate technique. *Aesculap Sci Info* 12:3, 1993.
5. Clausen J, Ryken T, Traynelis V, Goel V: personal communication, 1994.
6. Coe J, Warden K, Sutterlin C, *et al:* Biomechanical evaluation of cervical spinal stabilization methods in a human cadaveric model. *Spine* 14:1122, 1989.
7. Connolly PJ, Esses SI, Kostuik JP: Anterior cervical fusion: outcome analysis of patients fused with and without anterior cervical plates. *J Spinal Disord* 9(3):202-206, 1996.
8. DiAngelo DJ, Foley KT, Vossel KA, *et al:* Anterior cervical plating reverses load transfer through multilevel strut-grafts. *Spine* 25(7):783-795, 2000.
9. Hacker RJ: A randomized prospective study of an anterior cervical interbody fusion device with a minimum of 2 years of follow-up results. *J Neurosurg* 93(2Suppl):222-226, 2000.
10. Karasick D: Anterior cervical spine fusion: struts, plugs, and plates, *Skeletal Radiol* 22:85, 1993.
11. Lowery G: Orion anterior cervical plate system, *Surgical Technique*, Sofamor Danek, 1994.
12. Maiman D, Pintar F, Yoganandan N, *et al:* Pullout strength of Caspar cervical screws. *J Neurosurg* 31:1097, 1992.
13. Montesano P, Juach E, Anderson P, *et al:* Biomechanics of cervical spine internal fixation. *Spine* 16(Suppl):S10, 1991.
14. Panjabi MM, Isomi T, Wand J: Loosening of the screw-vertebra junction in multilevel anterior cervical plate constructs. *Spine* 24:2383-2388, 1999.
15. Schneeberger AG, Boos N, Schwarzenbach O, Aebi M: Anterior cervical interbody fusion with plate fixation for chronic spondylotic radiculopathy: a 2- to 8-year follow-up. *J Spinal Disord* 12(3):215-220 (discussion 221), 1999.
16. Shimamoto N, Cunningham BW, Dmitriev AE: Biomechanical evaluation of stand-alone interbody fusion cages in the cervical spine. *Spine* 26(19):E432-E436, 2001.
17. *Surgical Technique Sulzer Spine-Tech BAK/C Cervical Interbody Fusion System* (Company monograph).
18. Synthes Spine: *Cervical spine locking plate system*, 1995.
19. Tippets R, Apfelbaum R: Anterior cervical fusion with the Caspar instrumentation system. *Neurosurgery* 22:1008, 1988.
20. Traynelis V, Donaher P, Roach R, *et al:* Biomechanical comparison of anterior Caspar plate and three level posterior fixation techniques in a human cadaveric model. *J Neurosurg* 79:96, 1993.

21. Ulrich C, Woersdoerfer O, Kalff R, *et al:* Biomechanics of fixation systems to the cervical spine. *Spine* 16(Suppl):S4, 1991.

22. Vasquez-Seoane P, Yoo J, Zou D, *et al:* Interference screw fixation of cervical grafts. *Spine* 18:946, 1993.

23. Wang JC, McDonough PW, Endow KK, Delamarter RB: Increased fusion rates with cervical plating for two-level anterior cervical discectomy and fusion. *Spine* 25(1):41-45, 2000.

24. Wang JC, McDonough PW, Endow K, *et al:* The effect of cervical plating on single-level anterior cervical discectomy and fusion. *J Spinal Disord* 12(6):467-471, 1999.

25. Wang JC, McDonough PW, Kanim LE, *et al:* Increased fusion rates with cervical plating for three-level anterior cervical discectomy and fusion. *Spine* 26(6):643-646 (discussion 646-647), 2001.

26. Wang JC, Zou D, Yuan H, Yoo J: A biomechanical evaluation of graft loading characteristics for anterior cervical discectomy and fusion: a comparison of traditional and reverse grafting techniques. *Spine* 23:2450-2454, 1998.

# C H A P T E R   1 1 3

# Subsidence and Dynamic Cervical Spine Stabilization

**Michael P. Steinmetz, Edward C. Benzel, and Ronald I. Apfelbaum**

## Fundamental Concepts

The term subsidence has dual meanings and implications. It can refer to the loss of height that occurs normally with aging as the axial skeleton shortens, but it can also refer to the loss of height at an operative site following surgery on the spine.

The loss of vertical height with aging has been observed for centuries. This process, resulting in humans losing height after the achievement of adult status, is multifactorial. It essentially involves both the loss of disc height and vertebral body collapse.[2] Both of these processes may involve deformation along the neutral axis (axial deformation), but many also involve deformation about an axis of rotation (angular deformation). Both of these deformities, angular and axial, result in loss of vertical height. Gravity and repetitive axial loading contributes to the deformation. Angular deformation most often occurs in the sagittal plane, resulting in kyphosis. Such a kyphosis results in an applied moment arm. As the kyphosis progresses, the moment arm is lengthened, and hence, further deformity progression.[2] This situation is portrayed by the phrase, "kyphosis begets kyphosis." Kyphosis is usually not desired. In the cervical region, it places the cervical musculature at a biomechanical disadvantage and may lead to mechanical neck pain. It may also accelerate adjacent segment degenerative changes.[9,17] If the kyphosis becomes severe, forward gaze and respiration may be adversely affected. Although subsidence occurs in all regions of the spine, its occurrence following surgery is most evident in the cervical spine.

Although angular and axial subsidence can occur during the normal aging process, both may also occur following surgery. Postoperative subsidence can be caused by bone graft absorption with remodeling, graft collapse, or pistoning of the graft into the adjacent vertebral levels. Subsidence in these situations should be considered iatrogenic. Therefore, each of these mechanisms must be addressed.

## Graft Resorption and Remodeling

Graft resorption and remodeling is a normal but complex biologic process. Bone healing occurs by a series of sequential steps that involve an inflammatory phase, with the arrival of inflammatory cells and bone progenitor cells accompanying vascular ingrowth into the graft. This is followed by a repair phase in which osteoclasts begin to absorb the graft while osteoblasts simultaneously lay down osteoid, and mineralization of the osteoid then follows. This begins the process of new bone formation. It continues into the remodeling phase as the bone is remodeled into new living mature bone and necrotic bone is removed by creeping substitution.

Various humoral factors, proteins, growth factors, and mechanical forces mediate this process. The humoral factors include parathyroid hormone, vitamin D, and calcitonin. Proteins and growth factors include a large array of substances including multiple bone morphogenic proteins, insulin-like growth factor, transforming growth factor, platelet-derived growth factor, fibroblast growth factor, and nectins.

Mechanical forces are also very important in this process. As defined by Wolff's law, bone remodeling (and hence its strength) is determined by the load placed on it. This structural adaptation results in bone being formed where stresses engendered by compressive loading or tensile forces occur and is reabsorbed where the stresses do not occur. Therefore, bone or bone graft placed in compression is exposed to "bone healing" enhancing forces as defined by Wolff's law.

As a result of all of the aforementioned processes, bone grafts first partially resorb before being replaced by new living bone. The process results in subsidence of the bone graft following surgery. Again, it bears emphasizing that this is part of the normal biology of bone healing and not a pathologic process. It often is not appreciated in noninstrumented constructs. However, in studies that specifically measure construct height, such subsidence is routinely observed.[5,11,13] The amount of subsidence varies with the type of grafting used and number of levels fused. Thus Bishop *et al.* showed that in uninstrumented ventral cervical discectomies that used iliac crest autograft, the average settling was 1.4mm for a single-level construct and 1.8mm for two-level procedures. The amount of settling increased to 2.4mm for single levels and 3.0mm for two levels when iliac crest allograft was used.

## Graft Collapse

A cervical interbody graft can also collapse prior to its incorporation, also resulting in subsidence. Graft collapse occurs for a number of reasons. If the graft is inadequately sized to handle the loads placed on it, it may collapse. This can occur, for example, if the graft is too narrow in width or depth with respect to the adjacent vertebrae. Such a size mismatch increases the load placed on a graft. A larger graft spreads the load over a larger area, thus reducing the load per unit of surface area. It may therefore be able to more effectively withstand axial loads. Finally, if there is a good match between the contours of the surface of the vertebrae and the graft (so-called "gapless" fusion), the weight-bearing forces are evenly distributed over the region of contact. This diminishes the chance of graft collapse.

The choice of graft material is also important. The gold standard is bone, since living structural bone can respond to stresses placed on it and hence strengthen itself via the aforementioned process and repair itself as needed. Synthetics and allograft bone do not have these properties. It is emphasized that allograft bone preparations are not equal. The techniques of bone handling and processing can affect its structural integrity and strength and hence its suitability as a grafting material.

Allogenic bone used for spine surgery must be sterile. The bone can be sterilely harvested. If sterility is maintained, it may not require further processing. If it is not culture negative or is not sterilely harvested and processed, it may be sterilized with gamma irradiation. "Low-dose" radiation (less than 1.5 to 2 megarads) has been shown to not significantly diminish graft strength. However, high-dose radiation (up to 4 to 5 megarads) used by some laboratories causes significant weakening of the bone. Such grafts have a high collapse rate and should be avoided.

The type of bone, cortical or cancellous, is also important. Cortical bone is significantly stronger than cancellous bone, but its density resists vascular ingrowth and the influx of osteoblasts. Hence it is slower to become living bone via true incorporation. It is neither very osteoconductive nor osteoinductive. As such, osteoclastic activity predominates. This results in progressive weakening of grafts that are primarily of cortical consistency. Therefore, cortical bone provides significant early structural support compared to cancellous bone. Because of the aforementioned properties, true bony incorporation is slow, and hence the weakening of the graft may result in graft collapse or failure prior to the acquisition of solid fusion. Pseudoarthrosis may also result.

Cancellous bone lacks the strength of cortical bone and alone is likely inadequate to support clinical loads. It does however have many favorable properties, including significant osteoconductive activity as well as some osteoinductive capacity. Vascular ingrowth into its loose architecture readily occurs. Cancellous bone incorporates early and more completely. Instrumentation may be used to provide structural support until the cancellous bone fully incorporates and a solid arthrodesis is attained.

An optimal bone graft is one that has the structural integrity of cortical bone and the osteoconductive and inductive properties of cancellous bone. The iliac crest has long been used as a graft source for cervical spine surgery and has both characteristics of an ideal bone graft. It appears to be an excellent choice since it contains a cortical shell that provides structural support and a cancellous core that incorporates quickly. If its size is chosen well, the axial load is shared by the cortical shells of the vertebrae by passing the load onto the cortical walls of the graft. This can minimize pistoning into the adjacent vertebrae (see below).

## Pistoning (Subsidence)

Pistoning refers to failure of the end plate of the vertebrae with impaction of the graft into the vertebral body above or below the graft. Factors that influence pistoning include graft density, graft/donor size mismatches, and donor site preparation. Predominantly cortical implants such as fibula result in a significant graft-to-host density mismatch. The density of the bone graft should be ideally

matched to the vertebrae. For example, fibula (predominantly cortical graft) placed in an osteoporotic spine, results in a significant graft/host density mismatch. This may result in the pistoning of the graft into the vertebra if the stresses placed on the end plates exceed their load tolerance.

The weight or load on the graft is the same whether a small or large graft is used. Greater forces per unit area of contact are applied to a small bone graft because the forces cannot be dispersed over a larger surface area. This load/surface area mismatch can result in end plate failure and pistoning. With a larger graft, the load is dispersed over a large surface area, thus lessening the chance of graft collapse or pistoning. End plate preparation can also influence this. Various types of end plate preparation have been described, as well as various techniques for graft fitting. The goals of end plate preparation must include removal of the cartilaginous end plate to allow bone graft incorporation and the shaping of the end plate to maximize contact with the graft. Beyond these two considerations, considerable variation in techniques exists. Some surgeons have attempted to devise methods of interlocking the grafts and vertebrae when fixation is not used. Other surgeons advocate mortising the graft into the vertebrae; that is, counter-sinking the graft into the cancellous region of the vertebrae beyond the end plates. This minimizes the chance of graft migration or expulsion but at the expense of increasing the chance of subsidence. Others perforate the end plate in various patterns to encourage vascular ingrowth. Unfortunately, extensive violation of the end plate, especially when used with dense cortical bone, will likely increase pistoning. Lim et al.[16] have shown that it is important to preserve as much end plate as possible to prevent graft subsidence into the vertebral body. They found that making one central hole to increase vascular access to the graft rather than multiple smaller holes reduced stresses on the end plate.

## Cervical Plating and the Evolution of Dynamic Fixation
### First-Generation Symptoms

The need to augment cervical spine stability following spine surgery, trauma, or other destructive pathologic processes has led to the development of ventral cervical plating systems. The first generation of these devices included the Orozco plates (Synthes), which were used primarily in Europe, and the Caspar plates (Aesculap), which achieved significant acceptance worldwide. It became evident that such devices offered advantages to cervical spine surgeons and their patients.

The use of such plates helps preserve or restore lordosis, reduces graft extrusion, and improves graft union rates. This use also facilitates the performance of more extensive procedures when indicated by the disease process.* Furthermore, ventral cervical plating allows the surgeon to more liberally use allograft instead of autograft. Allograft success rates have been shown to equal those of autograft when ventral plating was used.[21] This helped

---

*References 8,15,18,20,22,23.

avoid donor site complications, a not-insignificant source of patient morbidity (i.e., pain at the graft harvest site).

The initial ventral cervical implants were not perfect and implant-related complications were observed. The initial Caspar plating system used parallel slots for the screws, which were not locked or constrained to the plate. This was therefore a truly axially dynamic implant. The implant required bicortical screw placement for optimal stability. Despite bicortical placement, screw backout was observed at times. The dynamic nature of the implant permitted axial subsidence. However, this was not recognized at the time as part of the normal biology of bone healing (as already discussed), but instead was felt to be undesirable. Hence the plate was modified so that holes replaced one-half of the slots (Figure 113.1). Rather than preventing subsidence, this led to screw breakage. This virtually always involved the screws placed in the holes, which were subjected to excessive bending moments (Figure 113.2). Fixed in the cortex dorsally and the hole in the plate ventrally, they typically fractured in the middle of the screw at the point of both the maximum bending moment application and maximum stress application (stress = bending moment / strength). The screws placed into the slots were able to toggle and/or slide along the slots and hence did not fracture.

## Second-Generation Symptoms

In an attempt to prevent the aforementioned complications (presumed pathologic settling, screw back-out, and screw fracture), as well as to avoid the need for bicortical screw purchase, a second generation of cervical fixation systems emerged. These devices featured screws fixed to the implant and permitted screw convergence on placement. The cervical spine locking plate (CSLP) from Synthes was the first such device. The ability to "toe-in" the screws secured the plate in part by triangulation and acted to

reduce the chance of screw pull-out (Figure 113.3). Such devices were initially successful, but failures caused by plate or screw fracture, construct pullout, and delayed or nonunions were increasingly recognized. Attempts were made to remedy this by increasing the strength of the plate. The Orion plate from Sofamor-Danek and the Codman Plate are such examples (Figure 113.4). These more-rigid implants reduced hardware fracturing but may have actually increased the incidence of delayed union and pseudoarthrosis caused by stress-shielding (see below).

Despite their shortcomings, second-generation plating systems certainly have achieved better results than noninstrumented fusions; hence they have become quite popular. Multiple variations on this basic theme have been developed as other manufacturers entered the market. Despite the popularity and ease of use of these systems, failures continued to occur. At the time (early 1990s), the spine community did not fully appreciate the reason for these nonunions and failures. Furthermore, since these were often late sequelae, many were not likely recognized, or at least were under-reported. Figure 113.5 illustrates such a case. This patient developed neck pain at 3 years after an apparently successful fusion (Figure 113.5A). The growth of new osteophytes (see Figure 113.5B, *arrows*) was the major clue that a nonunion was present. This was confirmed with flexion and extension films (see Figure 113.5C and D), which demonstrated 8mm of motion at the tips of the spinous processes. None should have been present if indeed a solid fusion was present.

It therefore appeared that rigid implants were working against the biology of bone healing by stress-shielding the graft, at least in some cases. Rather than becoming progressively stronger through bony fusion, these stress-shielded grafts either failed to fully incorporate or did so with suboptimal strength or with failure of fusion.

## Third-Generation Symptoms
### History and Rationale

Benzel and Yuan[4] focused attention on this phenomenon. They used this knowledge to develop the first axially dynamic cervical implant. Although relatively new to the cervical spine (remember the slotted Casper plates), the concept of dynamism has been used in other applications, particularly orthopedic surgery procedures involving the hip and long bones. Dynamic hip arthroplasties have been used for femoral neck fractures with significant success. This construct permits the femoral neck to deform along its axis so that the opposing fracture margins are exposed to optimal bone-healing-enhancing forces. A meta-analysis of 2855 patients showed reductions in cutout (4% vs. 13%), nonunion (0.5% vs. 2%), breakage (0.7% vs. 14%), and reoperation (4% vs. 10%) when dynamic hip pinning was utilized.[7] The Weiss-spring, as modified by Larson, is also a dynamic implant with a spine application. When this is combined with interbody fusion in the thoracic or lumbar spine, subsidence is encouraged and bone healing enhancing forces increased. This increases fusion success.[3]

Understanding the implications of Wolff's Law, as applied to bone healing, and specifically ventral cervical bone grafting, is crucial to understanding the rationale for, and value of, dynamic cervical spine stabilization. Wolff's

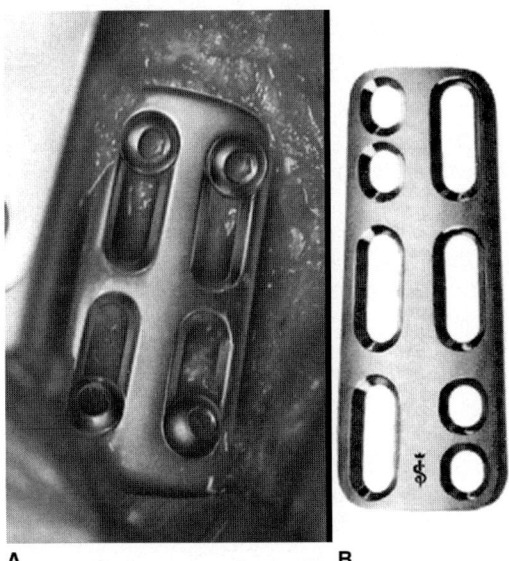

**Figure 113.1** Original Caspar plate (Aesculap) with bilateral slots (**A**), which was modified to have slots alternating with screw holes (**B**) after settling was observed and felt to be undesirable.

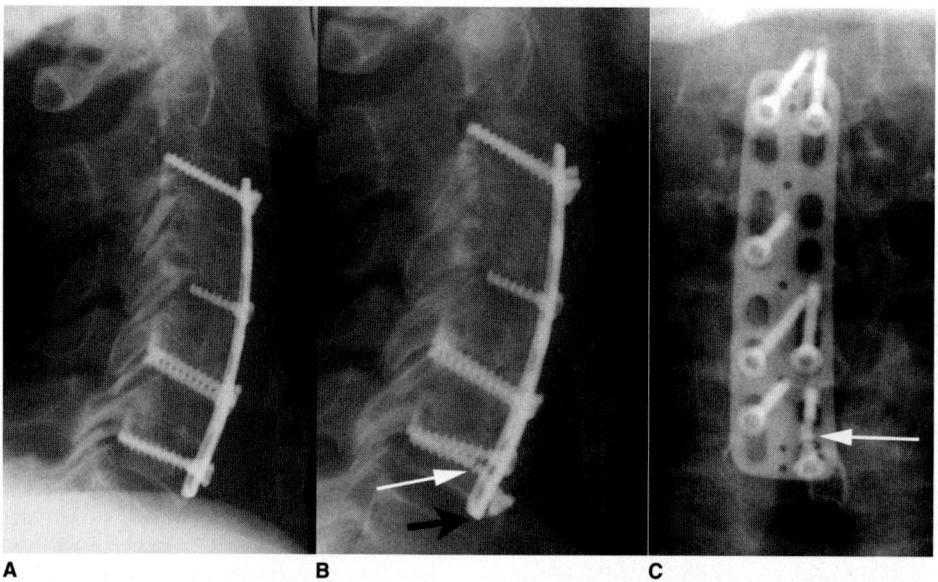

**Figure 113.2** Caspar plate as initially placed **(A),** and with settling **(B and C)**. Solid fusion occurred but the screw in the holes *(white arrow)* fractured as settling occurred as indicated by the plate overlapping the interspace *(black arrow)*.

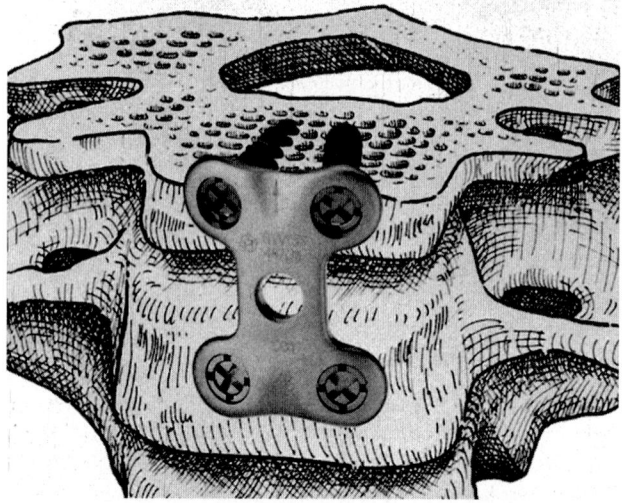

**Figure 113.3** Cervical Spine Locking Plate (CSLP) from Synthes. Triangulation of the locked unicortical screws was utilized to increase pullout strength.

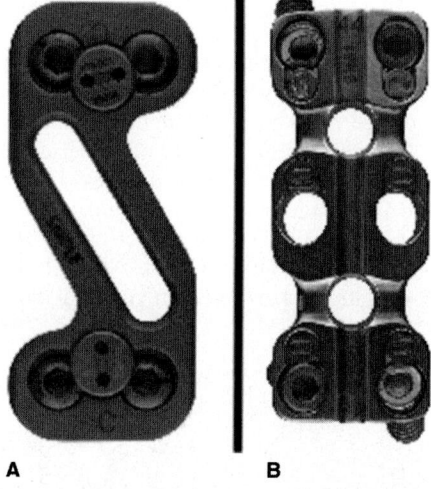

**Figure 113.4** Orion plate **(A)** from Danek and the Codman plate **(B)** were made stronger to try to reduce hardware failures.

Law essentially states that every change in the function of a bone is followed by definite changes in its internal architecture and secondary alterations in its external configuration. This implies that bone is formed where stresses require its presence and is resorbed where stresses do not require it. Thus the load "seen" by a bone to some extent determines its shape and strength. In long-bone fracture fixation with rigid plates, if the plate is not removed after initial healing, late fracture or pseudoarthrosis may occur. If the plate is removed once the initial healing process has occurred, the bone is able to "see" normal weight-bearing forces with resultant maximal healing occurring. This is further illustrated in cases of successful fusion following rigid cervical implant fracture. Fracture of the plate per-

mitted the bone grafts to "see" bone-healing forces and thus encouraged fusion. If the plate had not fractured, a pseudoarthrosis may have developed. This has been referred to as *secondary dynamism by plate fracture* (Figure 113.6).

This logical scenario described by Wolff's law follows the rules of evolution: "ontogeny recapitulates ontogeny." A quadruped requires and has larger and stronger forelimb bones than a biped. On the other hand, if bone growth is excessive or unchecked after fracture or grafting, there would be exuberant overgrowth that could compromise vital structures such as the contexts of the spinal canal. Hence the wisdom of a system in which bone growth responds to the stresses placed on it while regions

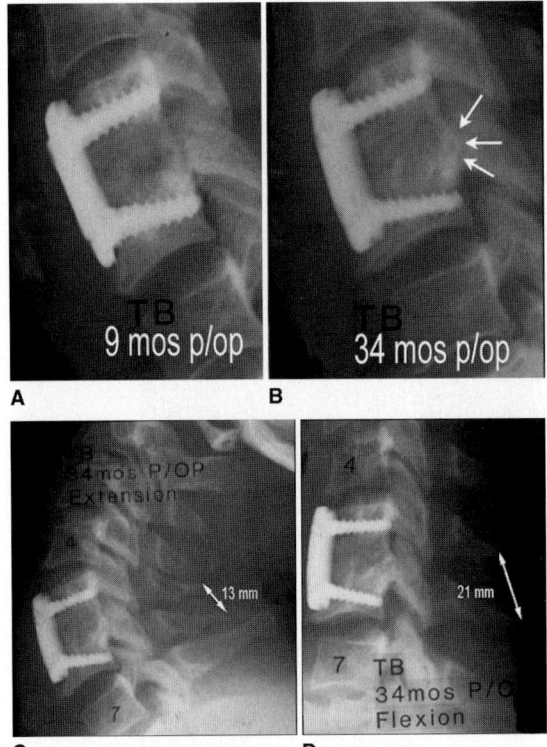

**Figure 113.5** This patient appeared to have a solid fusion (**A**) at 9 months after an ACD/F with an Orion (Sofamor-Danek) plate. At 34 months (**B**) the growing osteophytes (arrows) indicate otherwise, and a nonunion is confirmed by the motion between the spinous processes of the involved vertebrae comparing (**C**) and extension (**D**). This illustrates a late nonunion that could have easily been missed.

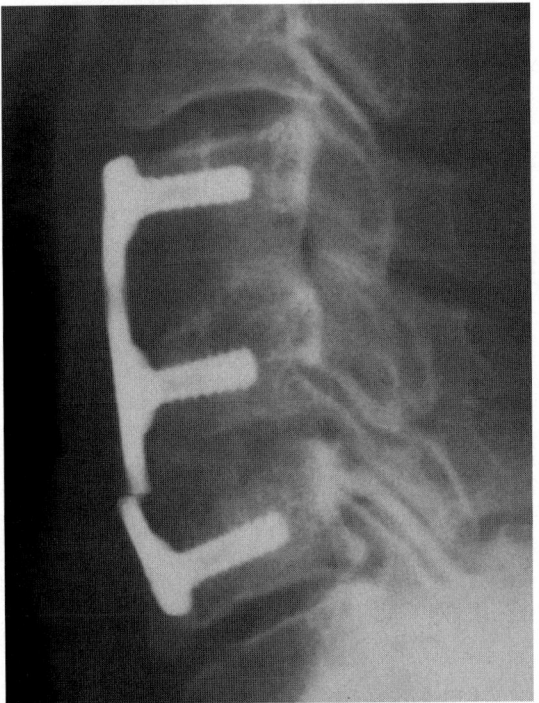

**Figure 113.6** This plate fractured and the pieces overlapped, allowing the graft to again be loaded and the dynamism principle to be applied again. This then went on to solid fusion.

of the fracture or graft that do not contribute to the stress sharing and load bearing are absorbed.

During the evolution of cervical fixation systems, it was recognized that a single fixed screw plate angle was not optimal for all patients. Variable screw angle designs were therefore introduced. Some second-generation systems had the screw locked to the plate to prevent back-out but did not lock the screw angulation when implanted. Thus this angle could change (i.e., toggle). Such designs theoretically could allow some settling as the graft absorbs or subsides. For this to occur, however, the screw must migrate or cut through the ventral cortex or toggle within the vertebrae (Figure 113.7). That this can occur is clear. It is, however, a slow process. This is in contrast to the early subsidence seen with true axially dynamic implants (see below). In some cases, the density of the vertebrae may prevent such screw migration, and screw fracture can occur (Figure 113.8). In addition, such screw migration has the potential of weakening the screw bone interface and may lead to implant failure by pullout. This was observed in the series of Epstein, in which failure occurred with a variable angled screw plate in 16% of her cases.[10]

### The System

The third-generation ventral cervical fixation systems, which provided true axial dynamic stabilization, were pioneered by Benzel and Yuan with the introduction of the "DOC VCSS" system from DePuy AcroMed (Raynham, MA). This plating system was developed after it was perceived that there was a need for a system that would enhance fusion rates, decrease deformity progression, improve deformity correction, and decrease the chance of construct failure. The observation that rigid plates could fracture in patients who were subsequently observed to have a solid arthrodesis provided some additional impetus for the development of an axially dynamic cervical implant. If the plate had not fractured, a pseudoarthrosis may have resulted. These observations led researchers such as Benzel and Yuan to believe that implants that permitted subsidence may be superior for the attainment of cervical fusion.

At the time of this writing, there currently are four axially dynamic ventral cervical plates commercially available in the United States. The DOC VCSS (Depuy-Acromed), the ABC plate (Aesculap), the Premiere plate (Sofamor-Danek), and the C-Tec plate (Interpore Cross). These systems differ regarding the method of implementation of the principle of dynamic spine stabilization and in their geometric and ergonomic design.

The DOC VCSS system consists of platforms that are rigidly affixed to the vertebral bodies via screws. Therefore, toggling the screws in the vertebral body is not permitted. The platforms slide along two rods while a cross fixator rigidly affixed to the rods limits the amount of sliding and, therefore, the amount of subsidence permitted (Figure 113.9). In this manner, axial deformation (subsidence) is controlled. The manufacturer sets this cross fixator at 3mm, but the surgeon may adjust it if deemed necessary. This system is not applicable to single-level constructs.

The ABC system (Aesculap Instrument Corp., Center Valley, PA) permits load sharing by allowing unrestricted subsidence. The plate has slots bilaterally at each level

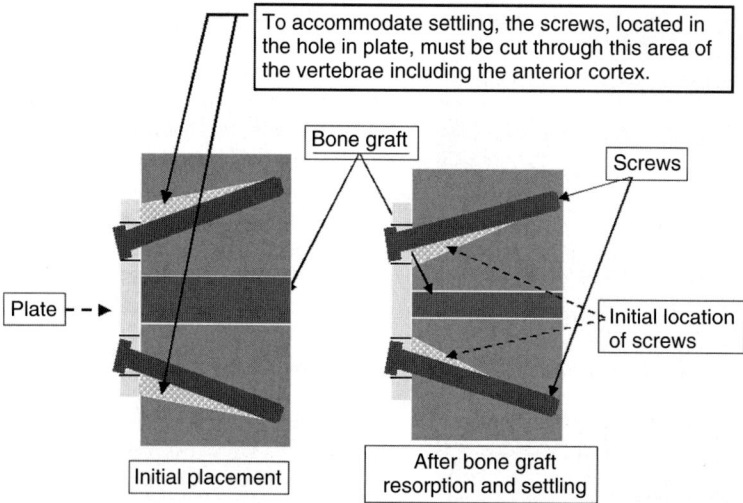

Figure 113.7 Diagram illustrating what occurs at the bone screw interface to accommodate toggling of the screws. To change their angle to allow for graft settling, the screws must cut through the vertebrae as illustrated.

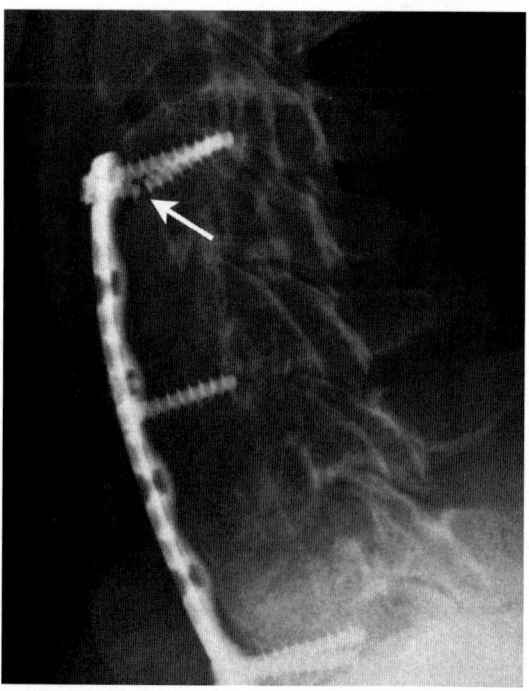

Figure 113.8 As subsidence occurs, screws may fracture *(arrow)* instead of toggling if the bone is strong enough to resist cut through, as this case illustrates.

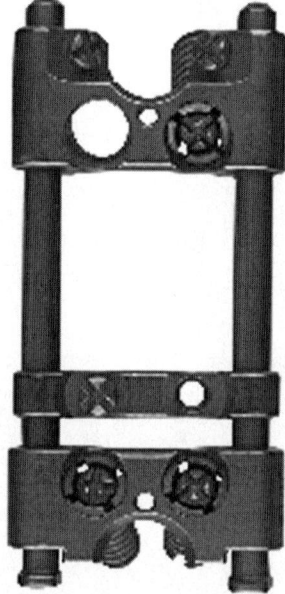

Figure 113.9 DOC VSS plate from DePuy AcroMed. The superior platform slides along the rods to achieve dynamism. The screws are locked to the platforms.

(Figure 113.10). The screws are locked to the plate by a unique internal locking mechanism, which prevents back-out but does not restrict either settling or screw rotation. This is the first implant with this unique design. It is available for single and multilevel constructs. No attempt is made to limit the amount of subsidence, which occurs initially by the screws sliding in their respective slots. If more dynamism is required, screw angulation can occur. This rarely occurs. Indeed, with true load sharing, early and more substantial graft incorporation and maturation is observed so that despite the absence of settling restriction, the extent of settling is not excessive, and often the full

amount allowed by the slot does not occur. This has also been observed with the DOC VCSS system. Even with multiple-level discectomies, less than 3mm of subsidence is the norm.

The Premiere and C-Tec plates have similar slotted designs to allow settling, with a retaining band over the screw heads to prevent back out (Figure 113.11). They functionally differ from the ABC plate in that they do not have a slot in the most inferior (caudal) position but instead have a hole. Whether this restriction of caudal dynamism has a significant effect on outcomes remains unclear, and no clinical series are yet available to answer such questions.

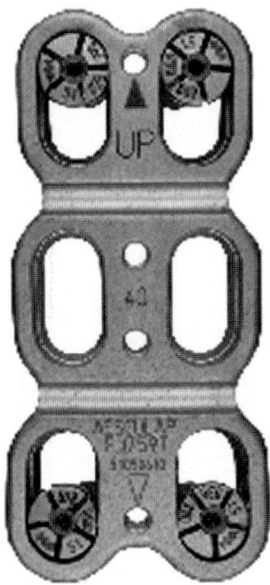

**Figure 113.10** ABC plate from Aesculap. The screws are locked to the plate by a unique internal mechanism that prevents backout, but they are free to slide in the slots and toggle, thereby achieving dynamism.

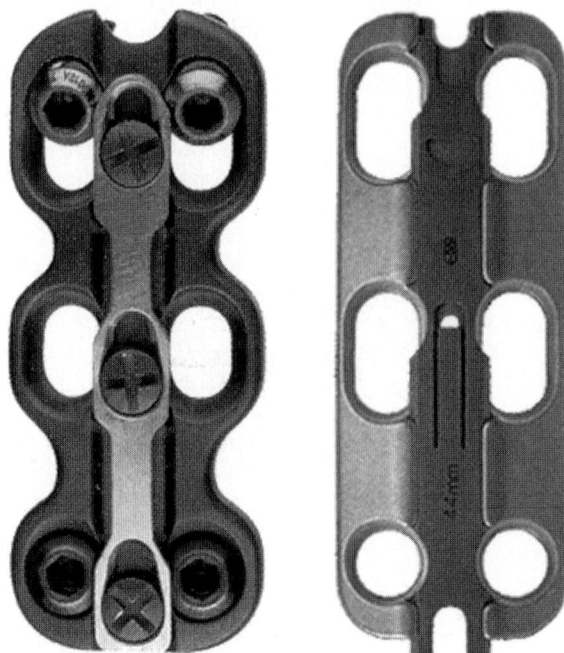

**Figure 113.11** Premier plate (Medtronic-Sofamor-Danek) on the left and C-Tek plate (Interpore Cross) on the right use similar mechanisms to prevent screw back-out while allowing the superior screws to slide in the slot to achieve dynamism.

## Clinical Experience

Clinical series reported with these dynamic systems have shown that they do achieve their goals and offer advantages to spine surgeons and their patients. With the ABC system, early and more substantial graft incorporation has resulted in a very low nonunion rate. A review of nearly 500 patients involving over 800 motion segments has shown that the ABC system effectively stabilizes the spine in a variety of conditions, including surgery for degenerative disease, herniated discs, and trauma.[1] This is true with both corpectomy and interbody approaches, with both allograft and autograft iliac crest bone. Fusion was rigorously defined as absence of motion at the tips of the spinous processes between flexion and extension, in addition to the presence bridging trabecular bone. When using this stringent definition, 67% of the levels (341 of 508) were fused at 3 months, 81% at 6 months (310 of 384 levels), 93% at 12 months (238 of 255 levels), and 100% (69 of 69 levels) at 24 months. Essentially, early trabecular bridging and progressive graft maturation were observed. Measuring the deflection at the tips of the spinous processes magnifies the initial flexibility typically allowed by the weaker new bone. The amount of such movement progressively decreases as the bone graft matures. Most importantly, no regression with increasing motion is observed if the fusion is progressing.

Cobb angle measurements showed preservation of lordosis with minimal losses of 2 to 8 degrees in only 3% to 4% of patients. Kyphotic angulation corrections were maintained within 5 degrees. Dynamic fixation, therefore, did not result in an increased angular deformation reported with uninstrumented fusion.[5,11] The amount of settling observed is consistent with that of uninstrumented fusions, averaging 1.5 to 2.0mm per level, with slightly more settling observed with allograft. Most of the settling occurred within the first month of surgery and virtually all within 3 months. Thus the unrestricted settling allowed by dynamic plating did not cause excessive settling but instead facilitated earlier and more substantial fusion.

Steinmetz et al.[19] reviewed their preliminary clinical experience with the DOC VCSS plate in the treatment of multilevel cervical spondylosis. Thirty-four patients with symptomatic multilevel cervical spondylosis underwent decompression and fusion with the DOC VCSS system. The operations included two-, three-, and four-level ACDFs and one-, two-, and three-level corpectomies. Fusions included both allograft (76%) and autograft (24%). Minimal follow-up was 6 months, with an average of 13 months. The DOC plate did indeed permit subsidence, with an average of 1.7mm of subsidence at 13 months after surgery. The majority of this subsidence occurred within 3 months postoperatively, with 61% of patients demonstrating 2 or more millimeters of subsidence in this early time period.

Following surgery, lordosis was maintained in most patients, with an average of 14 degrees of lordosis observed in the entire patient population. This lordotic configuration was well maintained following surgery. An average change (post-operative compared to latest clinical follow-up) of 0.4 degrees of lordosis was demonstrated at the latest clinical follow-up (13 months following surgery). These results demonstrate that the DOC plate permitted axial subsidence yet prevented angular deformation (kyphosis).

Most significantly, there were no instances of graft or implant failure, although one patient after a motor vehicle accident presented with a collapsed graft and displaced hardware. The overall fusion rate was 91%. A solid arthrodesis was determined if (1) there was no motion across the fusion site on flexion/extension radiographs, (2) trabeculae were observed across each fusion site, and

(3) no lucency was observed at any of the fusion sites or around any of the screws.

With the introduction of dynamic fixation systems, many have expressed concern that "too much dynamism" may not be desirable. In addition, these implants are non-rigid, so there has been concern as to whether they would be adequate to stabilize the spine in grossly unstable conditions. Indeed, initial (appropriately cautious) advice was to restrict their use in cases with a significant instability such as trauma, neoplasia, or multisegmental resections.

Laboratory studies have, however, shown that dynamic systems actually are more stable than their more-rigid counterparts. Brodke et al.,[6] in an instrumented laboratory model, demonstrated that DOC and ABC systems do indeed load share with a simulated subsidence of 10% of the graft height in a corpectomy model. Compared to the CSLP and Atlantis systems, they provide equal initial stability in flexion and extension and lateral bending. Of great significance was the fact that they maintained a much higher level of stability after simulated subsidence. Whereas the CSLP and Atlantis systems lost 80% to 90% of their ability to resist flexion and extension, ABC and DOC maintained most of their initial stiffness. While perhaps counterintuitive, this occurred because the construct was loaded axially, simulating the weight of the head and pull of the neck muscles. With the dynamic systems, the graft-vertebral interface through load-sharing participates in construct stabilization by remaining under axial load and hence imparting stability to the construct. With the more-rigid systems, such axial loading does not load the graft because of stress shielding. The axial forces are cantilevered through the screws to the plate and dorsal aspect of the spine (Figure 113.12). The bone grafts are

shielded from axial loads and therefore are not able to participate in stabilizing the construct. This can result in plate flexion or in a degradation of the screw-bone interface. These data are supported by the laboratory report of DiAngelo and Foley,[9] in which they observed a significant buffering of the loading and unloading of interbody grafts during flexion and extension when axially dynamic fixators were used.

Recent clinical data also support this. Epstein reviewed her series of multilevel corpectomies performed for severe degenerative disease or OPLL with significant myelopathy. She used a ventral fibular strut graft and cervical plates. She augmented this with dorsal wiring and grafting. In 56 consecutive cases, she had a 10% ventral construct failure with Orion rigid plates, 16% construct failure with Atlantis variable-angle plates, but no failures with the 18 ABC dynamic plates. While not a pure ventral plating series, this shows that the dynamic systems are not weaker in these multilevel constructs but rather actually appear superior.[10]

Khoo et al.[14] recently reported a series of 61 patients with cervical trauma, operated on at two large municipal trauma centers over a 5-year period. Four ventral cervical plates were used—CSLP, Atlantis, Codman, and ABC—representing a rigid plate, two variable-angle plates (one of which allowed more screw rotation [the Codman plate]), and a fully dynamic plate (the ABC plate) in conjunction with a variety of constructs including interbody approaches in some and more frequently, corpectomies. In some cases, supplemental dorsal fixation was also used. The follow-up was for a minimum of 12 months. All images were scanned and analyzed by a computerized program, thus ensuring consistent operator-independent measurements. In these grossly unstable spinal injuries, the ABC system substantially performed better than the rigid and semi-constrained variable-angle screw systems with less settling, better preservation of lordosis, and no construct failures. Screw pullout was observed in 13% of CSLPs, 20% of Atlantis, 31% of Codman's, but 0% in ABC. The construct failed in 13% of CSLP and 7% of Atlantis-plated cases. The graft dislodged in 17% of CSLP, 7% of Atlantis, and 15% of Codman cases, but again, no such failures occurred with the ABC-plated cases. The loss of graft height and lordosis was also measured. At 18 months following surgery, the cases in which the Codman plate was used averaged 37% loss of graft height compared with 32% with CSLP, 19% with Atlantis, and 10% with ABC. At 12 months, 7.31 degrees of lordosis was lost with the Codman system, 6.84 with CSLP, 4.3 with Atlantis, and 3.2 with ABC.

These results again point to the advantage of load sharing by the graft, making it an integral part of the construct. The construct thus consists of the plate and screws as well as the graft and vertebral bodies sharing the load. This provides the stability needed to maintain alignment and protect the neural elements while restoring and preserving lordosis. When such load sharing does not occur, late failure of the construct is observed with an increasing amount of settling and/or lordosis.

True dynamic systems (axially dynamic) therefore appear to offer substantial advantages over prior-generation rigid plating systems.

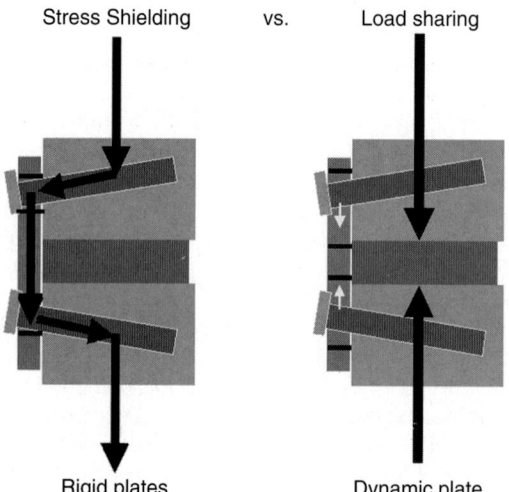

**Figure 113.12** The bold arrows depict the pathway of the major axial loading forces in both static (rigid) and dynamic plating systems. In the rigid system the load is cantilevered around the graft, traveling through the screws and plate. This shields the graft, which sees relatively little of the axial loading forces. Dynamic systems transfer most of the axial load to the graft, since the screws are free to slide in the slots in the plate (*small arrows*). This keeps the graft loaded and allows the principle of Wolff's law to act, resulting in earlier and more substantial fusions.

## Summary

"Subsidence" occurs naturally as part of the biology of aging. Subsidence after ventral cervical spine surgery may indicate construct failure caused by poor carpentry or suboptimal implant choices. Subsidence also refers to the normal graft absorption associated with osteoclastic activity, which is a major component of normal bone healing. Such subsidence is a natural consequence of the normal biology of bone healing. It is a desirable effect that is seen in successful uninstrumented fusions. It cannot be prevented without interfering with successful fusion.

True dynamic fixation systems permit such normal subsidence while still stabilizing the spine. They essentially permit subsidence along an axis defined by the surgeon (via implant contouring) while preventing rotation, translation, and angular deformation. It is emphasized that axially dynamic implants are offloaded axially, thus minimizing the chance of screw, plate, or rod fractures. As such, these systems work with, rather than against, the biology of bone healing, resulting in earlier and more substantial fusions. As a result, fewer instrumentation or construct failures occur. No negative down side to their use has been reported. Thus they would often seem to be the system of choice for ventral cervical stabilization after decompression.

## REFERENCES

1. Apfelbaum RI, Dailey AT, Soleau S, Barbera J: Clinical experience with a new load-sharing anterior cervical plate. In Watanabe K (ed): *Developments in Neuroscience: Proceedings of the 2nd International Mt. BANDAI Symposium for Neuroscience, Spine Section,* Elsevier, 2002, pp 563-580.
2. Benzel EC: *Biomechanics of Spine Stabilization,* ed 2. Rolling Meadows, IL, American Association of Neurologic Surgeons Publications, 2001.
3. Benzel EC, Larson SJ: Operative stabilization of the posttraumatic thoracic and lumbar spine: A comparative analysis of the Harrington distraction rod and the modified Weiss spring. *Neurosurgery* 19:378-385, 1986.
4. Benzel EC, Yuan HA, Weidner A, *et al*: Controlled intervertebral settling in multiple level ventral cervical fusion procedures with a dynamic stabilization implant. The American Academy of Neurologic Surgeons Spine Section Meeting. Rancho Mirage, CA, 1998.
5. Bishop RC, Moore KA, Weidner A, Hadley MN: Anterior cervical interbody fusion using autogeneic and allogeneic bone graft substrate: a prospective comparative analysis. *J Neurosurg* 85(2):206-210, 1996.
6. Brodke DS, Gollogly S, Alexander Mohr R, *et al*: Dynamic cervical plates: biomechanical evaluation of load sharing and stiffness. *Spine* 26(12):1324-1329, 2001.
7. Chinoy MA, Parker MJ: Fixed nail plates versus sliding hip systems for the treatment of trochanteric femoral fractures: a meta analysis of 14 studies. *Injury Int J Care Injured* 30:157-163, 1999.
8. Connolly PJ, Esses SI, Kostuik JP: Anterior cervical fusion: Outcome analysis of patients fused with and without anterior cervical plates. *J Spinal Disord* 9:202-206, 1996.
9. DiAngelo DF, Foley KT, Vossel KA, *et al*: Anterior cervical plating reverses load transfer through multilevel strut grafts. *Spine* 25:783-795, 2000.
10. Epstein N: Anterior approaches to cervical spondylosis and ossification of the posterior longitudinal ligament: review of operative technique and assessment of 65 multilevel circumferential procedures. *Surg Neurol* 55(6):313-324, 2001.
11. Geer CP, Papadopoulos SM: Instrumentation after anterior cervical fusion: the argument for single-level anterior cervical discectomy and fusion with anterior plate fixation. *Clin Neurosurg* 45:25-29, 1999.
12. Geisler F, Herrmann A: Submitted for publication (in review).
13. Hughes SS, Pringle T, *et al*: Multilevel cervical corpectomy and fibular strut grafting. The Cervical Spine Research Society Meeting, Santa Fe, MD, 1995.
14. Khoo LT, Kim A, Laich DT, *et al*: Anterior plating of cervical trauma: the effect of plate design on graft subsidence and the preservation of segmental lordosis. Presented at 2002 American Association of Neurological Surgeons Meeting, Chicago, IL, April 2002.
15. Kostuik JP, Connolly PJ, Esses SI: Anterior cervical plate fixation with the titanium hollow screw plate system. *Spine* 18:1273-1278, 1993.
16. Lim TH, Kwon H, Jeon CH, *et al*: Effect of endplate conditions and bone mineral density on the compressive strength of the graft-endplate interface in anterior cervical spine fusion. *Spine* 26(8):951-956, 2001.
17. Matsunaga S, Yone K, *et al*: Biomechanical changes of the cervical spine after anterior decompression and fusion and magnetic resonance imaging. Cervical Spine Research Society Meeting, Palm Springs, CA, 1997.
18. Shapiro S: Banked fibula and the locking anterior cervical plate in anterior cervical fusions following cervical discectomy. *J Neurosurg* 84:161-165, 1996.
19. Steinmetz MP, Warbel A, Whitfield M, Bingaman W: Preliminary experience with the DOC dynamic cervical implant for the treatment of multi-level cervical spondylosis. *J Neurosurg (Spine 3)* 97: 330-336, 2002.
20. Swank ML, Lowery GL, Bhat AL: Anterior cervical allograft arthrodesis and instrumentation: Multiple interbody grafting or strut graft reconstruction. *Eur J Spine* 6:138-143, 1997.
21. Tippets RH, Apfelbaum RI: Anterior cervical fusion with the Caspar instrumentation system. *Neurosurgery* 22: 1008-1013, 1988.
22. Vaccaro AR, Balderston RA: Anterior plate instrumentation for disorders of the subaxial cervical spine. *Clin Orthop* 335:112-121, 1997.
23. Wang JC, McDonough PW, Endow KK: Increased fusion rates with cervical plating for two-level anterior cervical discectomy and fusion. *Spine* 25:41-45, 2000.

# CHAPTER 114

# Ventral and Lateral Thoracic and Lumbar Fixation Techniques

Gerald E. Rodts Jr., Praveen V. Mummaneni, Regis W. Haid Jr., and Kevin T. Foley

Surgery on the ventral thoracic and lumbar spine began nearly 100 years ago. Ventral approaches for decompression of spinal pathology were first attempted in the early 1900s. Pioneers such as Royle[16] excised hemivertebrae for the treatment of scoliosis. Ito[13] and Hodgson and Stock[11] refined the ventral (transperitoneal) approach to the thoracolumbar spine for the treatment of Pott's disease. These early efforts to decompress ventral spinal pathology were frequently complicated by postoperative mechanical instability and progressive deformity.

The first reports of ventral instrumentation of the spine were from Humphries,[12] who developed ventral interbody fusion with ventral plates and unicortical screws. These devices provided little biomechanical advantage. Most of these cases were transperitoneal approaches for debridement and stabilization in patients with Pott's disease. The transperitoneal approach was eventually replaced by the retroperitoneal or extracavitary approaches for lesions of the lower thoracic and lumbar spine.

Throughout the 1970s, the preferred treatment for traumatic injuries was dorsal fusion/instrumentation, combined with ventral decompression and fusion. The Dwyer[6-8] and Zielke[17] devices were developed as ventrolateral implants that could augment or replace dorsal instrumentation. These consisted of screws that traversed the vertebral body that were interconnected with cable (Dwyer) or threaded rods (Zielke) that could be tightened in tension. These devices had limited ability to fixate two-column traumatic injuries. The Dunn device (developed in the late 1970s) represented a more-rigid instrument for use in burst fractures. This double-screw, double-threaded rod device provided excellent strength but was removed from the market in 1986 after reports of great vessel erosion and rupture.[5]

It wasn't until the 1990s that numerous plate/screw and screw/rod systems were developed. Among the first were the Kaneda, Kostuik-Harrington, the I-plate, and the University Plate. Later products included the Anterior Locking Plate (ALP), the Z-plate, the Texas Scottish Rite Hospital system, the M-8 Dual Rod system and others. Newer systems were developed for lower-profile, rigid ventral fixation of the spine. These systems have the added advantage of easier means of distraction and compression at the moment of plate or rod fixation. Furthermore, shorter segment fusions became more feasible. Some of the early-generation ventral plating systems did not provide for a fully rigid screw/plate interface. Bicortical screw purchase was important and did not eliminate the possibility of screw toggle and possible mechanical failure. Most systems on the market by 2003 provided for a rigid screw/plate or screw/rod interface. To critically analyze the various systems, an appreciation of the biomechanics of the thoracolumbar spine is important. The reader is directed to other chapters outlining more detailed biomechanical information. It is also essential to understand some of the general indications for ventral instrumentation and fusion.

## Biomechanical Considerations

A complex discussion of ventral thoracolumbar instrumentation is beyond the scope of this chapter; however, recognition of several basic concepts is essential to avoid complication. The anterior and middle columns provide the most resistance to axial loads. The ventral approach to spinal pathology has the distinct advantage of allowing for reconstruction of the vertebral body and intervertebral space with autologous or allogeneic bone or synthetic materials (methylmethacrylate, ceramic, etc.). The dorsal tension band—normally provided by the interspinous ligaments, ligamentum flavum, paraspinal musculature, and facet joints—must not be severely damaged if a ventral construct alone is to provide stability, because these devices cannot effectively withstand tremendous flexion forces. Complications arise when a posterior column injury has gone unrecognized or when too much is expected of a ventral construct. Plate and screw constructs can provide resistance against axial load, distraction, and extension. These implants have a higher success rate when axial loads are shared by a sturdy bone graft and the implant.

Certain biomechanical characteristics of implant systems are important to understand. Rigid implants (i.e., Z-Plate, Kaneda, and M-8 Dual Rod system) theoretically allow for greater immobilization of the spine. If the implant bears most of the stress, there is a risk of implant breakage or failure. These plate systems have set screw holes rather than slots, thereby creating a static (nondynamic) condition beginning at the time of plate fixation. Also, stress shielding provided by the rigid fixation may prevent the beneficial compressive forces from enhancing bone fusion (Wolff's law). Because bone is a biologic, deformable material, repeated stress loading may cause bony erosion and failure at the metallic implant-bone interface.

## Indications for Ventrolateral Instrumentation

A variety of infectious, neoplastic, congenital, and traumatic pathologic conditions are suitable for ventral thoracic or lumbar surgery. An initial step in complication avoidance is to determine whether a ventral approach will truly provide the safest and most efficacious means of decompression of the neural structures, reconstruction of the anterior and middle column, application of corrective forces for realignment, and placement of an appropriate graft or spacer/implant construct. Conditions in which dorsal neural compression or posterior column bony/ligamentous damage are the predominant findings are best treated by a dorsal approach. Similarly, lesions with three column pathology may possibly require circumferential treatment.

Anterior and middle column trauma (with preservation of the dorsal elements) may be treated adequately with a ventral approach (Figure 114.1). Failure to recognize significant posterior column injury may result in delayed kyphotic deformity and neurologic deterioration. There are few clinical outcome data to encourage ventral decompression of trauma patients with complete neurologic loss below the level of the lesion. Ventral approaches, however, may be useful in paraplegic patients with a severe kyphotic deformity. Anterior reconstruction may provide better sagittal balance that could be important for long-term pulmonary function, independent transferring, and upper extremity function.

Patients with incomplete spinal cord injury (SCI), severe vertebral body collapse (40% or greater) and kyphosis, and/or significant spinal canal compromise should be considered for ventral decompression and reconstruction. Intact patients with a myelographic block or ventral compression of the spinal cord on magnetic resonance imaging (MRI) may be considered for ventral decompression and stabilization. If the posterior longitudinal ligament is intact on MRI and there is 30% or less loss in height of the anterior and middle column, a dorsal approach with reduction by ligamentotaxis could be considered in the intact or incomplete patient with a burst fracture.

Infection is another indication for ventral decompression, reconstruction, and instrumentation. The primary indication would be severe deformity of the spine, because most spinal infections can be treated without ventral instrumentation. Early ventral approaches for the treatment of Pott's disease have been modified and are still very useful in debridement and stabilization of pyogenic, mycobacterial, or fungal infections. Reconstruction with autologous or allogeneic bone is feasible if a complete debridement of all necrotic tissue is accomplished. The risk of persistent infection or implant failure with instrumentation of infected cases is still largely unknown and must be examined critically.

Metastatic neoplasms commonly affect the vertebral body before the posterior elements and therefore can be palliated with vertebrectomy. The cell kinetics of any malignancy, if known before surgery or determined by frozen section, must be considered when deciding on the material for reconstruction of the axial spine. In cases of a rapidly dividing carcinoma, synthetic spacers such as vertical titanium cages, methylmethacrylate, polyether ether (PEEK) or ceramic can provide immediate stability of the vertebral column in patients with a short life expectancy. In more indolent neoplasms, such as breast or prostate cancer, longer survival can be expected, and autogenous or allogeneic bone can be expected to incorporate, thereby avoiding complications such as methylmethacrylate failure or migration. Use of titanium and other non-ferromagnetic implants allows for long-term follow-up with MRI.

Treatment of other conditions, such as congenital or developmental scoliosis, iatrogenic lumbar kyphosis (flat back), and degenerative lumbar scoliosis may involve a ventral approach. Ventral procedures in adult scoliosis with curves greater than 40 to 50 degrees are associated with a higher rate of fusion than dorsal constructs alone. Ventral fusion and instrumentation may also be useful in patients with deficient laminae, facet joints, or pars interarticulari or extremely severe scarring from prior dorsal surgery.

Inadequate radiographic studies before surgery can lead to intraoperative or postoperative complications. Plain

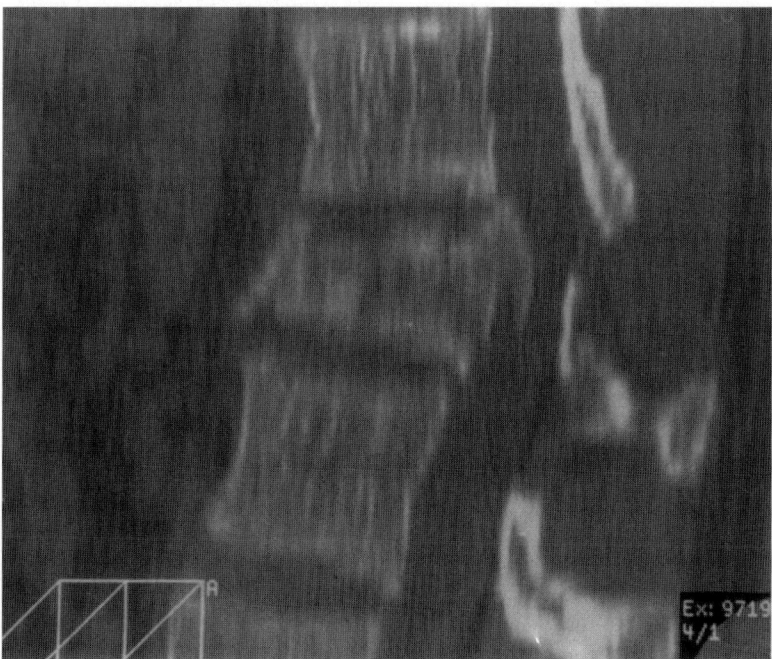

**Figure 114.1** Thoracic burst fracture with retropulsed bone fragment and incomplete spinal cord injury suitable for anterior decompression.

radiographs are essential and should include flexion and extension views when there is any suspicion of mechanical instability. In addition, attention should be paid to the density of bone as well as the sagittal and coronal alignment. Patients with scoliosis should have complete 36-inch standing films to assess overall spinal balance. The value of sagittal reconstruction of computed tomography (CT) scan images is often overlooked, particularly after myelographic dye injection. Axial CT may be preferable over MRI to determine the amount of bony spinal canal compromise in trauma. Sagittal MRI often provides excellent views of the posterior longitudinal ligament. If intact, one may consider use of ligamentotaxis to reduce a burst fracture fragment. MRI has the added advantage of showing signs of soft dorsal tissue injury and hematoma that would commonly go unrecognized with plain radiographs and CT scan alone. Although cost-effectiveness is a primary concern, any patient with complex spinal pathology (and for whom aggressive surgery is contemplated) may require both CT and MRI as part of their workup. We also use three-dimensional computer modeling of the spine to assess complex anatomy and plan surgery preoperatively (StealthStation, Medtronic Sofamor Danek).

## Ventral Surgical Techniques

### Positioning

Complication avoidance in the operating room begins with the simplest of steps. In positioning all patients, the authors place foam rubber padding over ankles and elbows. For the prone position, gel pads are placed over the supports of the Wilson frame or chest rolls. The knees are flexed 45 to 90 degrees. EKG electrodes must not be on areas of the chest or trunk that contact the frame or rolls to prevent pressure necrosis. In females, the breasts must be tucked medially between the supports. Pillows are placed under the feet to provide knee flexion and relaxation of the sciatic nerve. Foam rubber rings are commonly used by anesthesiologists to protect the face and eyes, but one must be careful not to place the neck in too much extension when in the prone position, particularly in patients with diffuse spondylosis. One should double-check the eyes to ensure that there is no direct pressure on the globe. If the arms are not tucked at the patient's side but raised above the head, one should not abduct the shoulders more than 90 degrees nor flex the elbow more than 90 degrees to prevent postoperative shoulder/elbow pain or even peripheral nerve ischemia. Simply asking the awake patients to raise their arms above their head and flex their elbows before surgery takes but a moment and yields important information.

Complications arising from the lateral decubitus position can also be averted with due diligence. The authors place all patients on a bean bag, but the bag must not extend into the axilla of the down arm. A roll (a liter bag of IV solution wrapped in a towel will suffice) is placed above the edge of the bean bag just below the axilla. The peroneal nerve in the down-side leg must be protected with foam and/or gel padding over the fibular head. A pillow is placed between the legs, which are flexed 45 degrees at the hip and knees. The coronal plane of the patient's thorax must be perpendicular to the floor. Wide tape should be used to secure this position to allow rotation of the bed along its long axis ("airplaning"). Establishing this position assists the surgeon in remaining oriented throughout the procedure, especially during the critical steps of decompressing the spinal cord or placing a vertebral body screw. Some tables are equipped with a compass so that the desired neutral position can be recorded and reset by the anesthesiologist if an airplane maneuver is necessary. The perpendicular orientation of the coronal patient plane relative to the floor also allows for more efficient manual reduction of a kyphotic deformity by pressing on the back. The authors routinely "break" or flex the table at the level of the pathology to help open the disc spaces laterally and aid in the insertion of the bone graft (Figure 114.2). Flexing the table also helps open the space between the 12th rib and the iliac crest. Once the bone graft is in place, the anesthesiologist is asked to return the table to the neutral, unflexed position.

The authors routinely administer suitable gram-positive antibiotic coverage (e.g., Ancef 1g or Nafcillin 1g). In cases of severe traumatic canal compromise or cord compression caused by tumor, the authors begin methylprednisolone at least 1 hour before surgery. Using the spinal cord contusion protocol, they begin with a bolus of 30 mg/kg over 45 minutes followed by continuous infusion of 5.4 mg/kg/hr for 23 hours.[2,3]

Paralytic agents are not used after induction to allow for motor response in the event of inadvertent nerve or spinal cord stimulation. The role of somatosensory evoked potential (SSEP) monitoring is debatable. A decrease in SSEP amplitude of more than 50% and limited or absent intraoperative recovery of amplitude are predictors of a postoperative neurologic deficit.[9,10] Despite this reasonable sensitivity and low false-negative rate, SSEP monitoring measures only dorsal column function. False-positives are common and often related to anesthetic considerations that can lead to a dangerous desensitization of the surgeon to warnings of intraoperative injury. SSEPs may be useful in deformity cases in which distractive or compressive forces are anticipated and could be reversed.

Motor evoked potentials (MEPs) may be more accurate than SSEPs in monitoring spinal cord motor function during surgery.[14] This technique is extremely sensitive to anesthetics and requires expertise that is not yet available on a widespread basis.

### Approach and Exposure

The thoracic spine can be approached ventrally by the transmanubrial-trans-sternal approach, conventional thoracotomy, or the thoracoscopic approach. The lumbar spine can be approached by the thoracoabdominal approach, transperitoneal approach, the retroperitoneal approach, laparotomy, laparoscopy, balloon-assisted retroperitoneal endoscopy, or low pelvic approaches. These surgical approaches may be performed by the cardiothoracic, general, or vascular surgeon or by the spine surgeon. Detailed preoperative and intraoperative communication with the surgical colleague (if used) is important to ensure that not only is the pathologic level exposed but also that the exposure allows the spine surgeon to place instruments perpendicular to the axis of the spine for reconstructive and

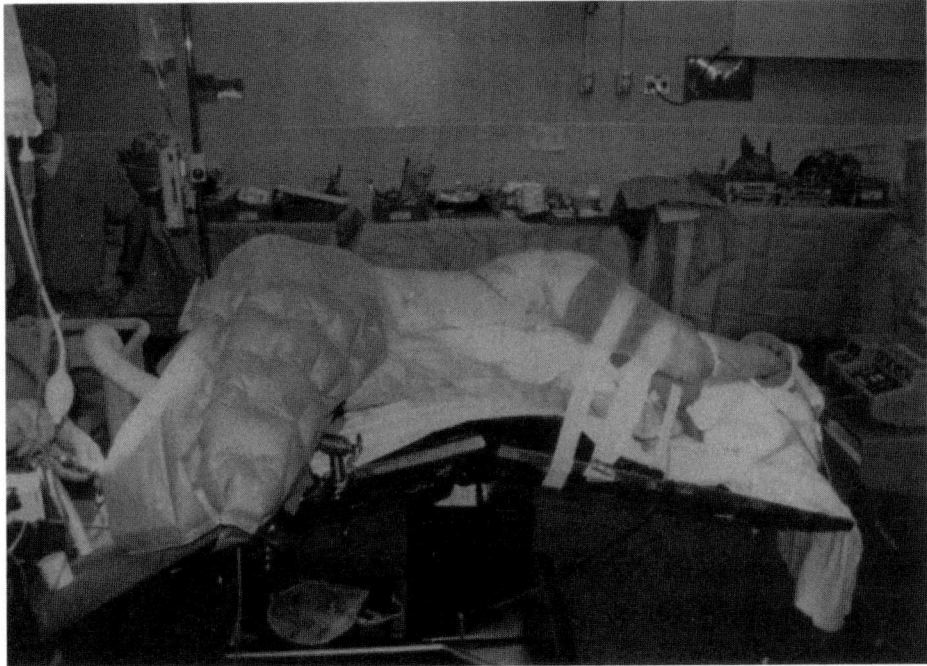

**Figure 114.2** Lateral position for thoracoabdominal or thoracotomy approach with exposed iliac crest harvest site. (Note flexion of table at surgical site.)

fixation techniques. Limited exposure may force a screw trajectory in an unsatisfactory cephalad or caudal direction.

### Upper Thoracic Spine

Ventral exposure of the rostral levels of the thoracic spine is very challenging. The exposure provided by conventional thoracotomy is limited by the scapula. The first and second thoracic vertebrae usually can be approached with a low diagonal or transverse cervical incision. An osteotomy of the medial 2 to 3cm of the clavicle and removal of portions of the manubrium with a rongeur, drill, or osteotome can provide additional exposure down to T2 without sacrificing significant bone. One must be cognizant of the course of the recurrent laryngeal nerve as it emerges dorsal to the brachiocephalic arch to pass between the esophagus and trachea. Although its course is more constant on the left side, low-lying incisions to approach T1 and T2 on the left side put the thoracic duct at risk. This structure is intimately related to the subclavian vein off midline on the left and must be protected. Unrecognized pneumothorax is a complication of this approach because the pleura overlying the medial aspect of the cupola of the lung is adjacent to the spine. Filling the wound with saline and performing a positive pressure inspiration (Valsalva maneuver) at the close of the case is an essential step during closure. An oscillating saw or Gigli saw can be used to remove larger portions of the manubrium, but the retromanubrial space must be palpated to ensure that the brachiocephalic trunk is free. With the patient in the supine position, the upper thoracic spine slopes away from the surgeon, beginning at the T1-2 interspace. It can be difficult to place a ventral plate and screws in this region without a more aggressive removal or splitting of the manubrium or sternum.

Instead of sternotomy, lesions affecting the caudal aspect of T2, T3, T4, and T5 may be approached by a right-sided thoracotomy. The right-sided approach to the upper thoracic spine avoids the aortic arch. One must be cautious, however, to avoid injury to the superior vena cava and supreme intercostal vein. We have found instrumenting the ventral upper thoracic spine to be easier with a high, right-side thoracotomy than a midline sternotomy. This experience is particularly true with severe kyphosis (e.g., Scheuermann's kyphosis) in this region.

The transaxillary approach is familiar to most vascular surgeons and can be considered for lesions affecting the upper thoracic levels. This approach, however, offers a limited exposure at the base of a cone-shaped cavity and should be reserved for small, more ventrolateral lesions not affecting the entire vertebral body and not requiring (complete) corpectomy or when only open biopsy is necessary. Ventrolateral instrumentation is very difficult because of the limited exposure. The transaxillary approach has associated risks to the lower brachial plexus, long thoracic nerve, and thoracodorsal nerve as well as to vascular structures in the axilla. Splitting of the pectoralis major muscle can also be a source of significant morbidity.

The ventral upper thoracic spine can also be accessed via a third-rib approach in which the patient is positioned in the lateral position with the arm elevated on a rest. The right side is preferable because of the straight course of the brachiocephalic artery. A curved incision is made beginning below the caudal angle of the scapula and ending between the medial scapula and the spinous process of C7. The trapezius and latissimus dorsi muscles are divided medially to minimize denervation, and the scapula is retracted laterally. The dorsal 10cm of the second, third, and fourth ribs are resected, and the segmental vessels are ligated. The dorsal 3cm of the first rib can also be dissected for additional exposure, but care must be taken not to injure the T1 motor root. The pleura and upper mediastinal structures can then be bluntly dissected for access to the vertebral bodies. Deflation of the lung with a double-lumen endotracheal tube can be very helpful. This approach requires tube thoracostomy placement at the end of the procedure because the parietal pleura is opened and the lung is exposed.

### Midthoracic Spine

Lesions involving the midthoracic region are best approached via thoracotomy. Thoracic surgeons are very experienced with this approach. It is recommended that a thoracic surgeon perform the thoracotomy if the spine surgeon is not familiar with this approach. The patient is placed in the lateral decubitus position on a bean bag. The bean bag should not be higher than just below the axilla, and an IV bag or other suitable axillary pad should be placed to protect the brachial plexus and vessels. The area of break in the table should be determined before final positioning so that the desired thoracic level can be placed directly over this area to assist in exposure, opening of the disc spaces, and placement of the graft. Pillows may be placed under the down leg to protect the peroneal nerve and between the legs.

The left side is almost always used for the approach because it is safer and easier to visualize, dissect, and mobilize the aorta and segmental vessels than is the vena cava or azygous venous system. It is easier to repair an injured aorta than the vena cava. One should consider obtaining a preoperative axial CT or MRI to assess the location of the aorta. If the aorta is lying very far lateral to the left (Figure 114.3) or if the pathology is strictly right sided, a right-sided approach can be performed. A stan-

dard thoracotomy incision is used beginning approximately two fingerbreadths below the angle of the scapula and coursing ventrally to the midaxillary line. One should select the intercostal space directly over the level of pathology to enter the pleural cavity. We have had satisfactory experience in performing a retropleural thoracotomy. In this procedure, the surgeon separates the endothoracic fascia from the parietal pleura, and the dissection is made down to the rib heads and spine extrapleural. This is technically more difficult but can obtain a transthoracic approach without the need for a postoperative chest tube. A postoperative x-ray in the recovery room is essential to rule out a significant undetected pneumothorax.

In the lower thoracic spine, this usually corresponds to the rib two numbered levels rostral to the desired vertebral body. For instance, a T8 lesion usually corresponds to the horizontal segment of the 6th rib. Commonly, the rib need not be resected unless being harvested for bone graft or if unusually lengthy exposure of the spine is needed. Once the lung is deflated via a double-lumen ETT and the viscera are packed away with moist towels, the ribs are counted from inside the thoracic cavity. The rib identified as at the same level as the pathology is then exposed in a subpleural fashion down to its insertion on the pedicle. The segmental vessels are identified by blunt or scissor dissection in the midportion of each body. The disc spaces represent the "hills" and the midvertebral section (where the vessels are located) are the "valleys." The vessels are ligated with silk suture or metal clips in approximately the midbody. Taking the vessels too close to the aorta risks avulsion during this procedure. Conversely, sacrificing the vessels too close to the neural foramen may interfere with the collateral circulation of the spinal cord. Ligation of the vessels should be performed over the lateral aspect of

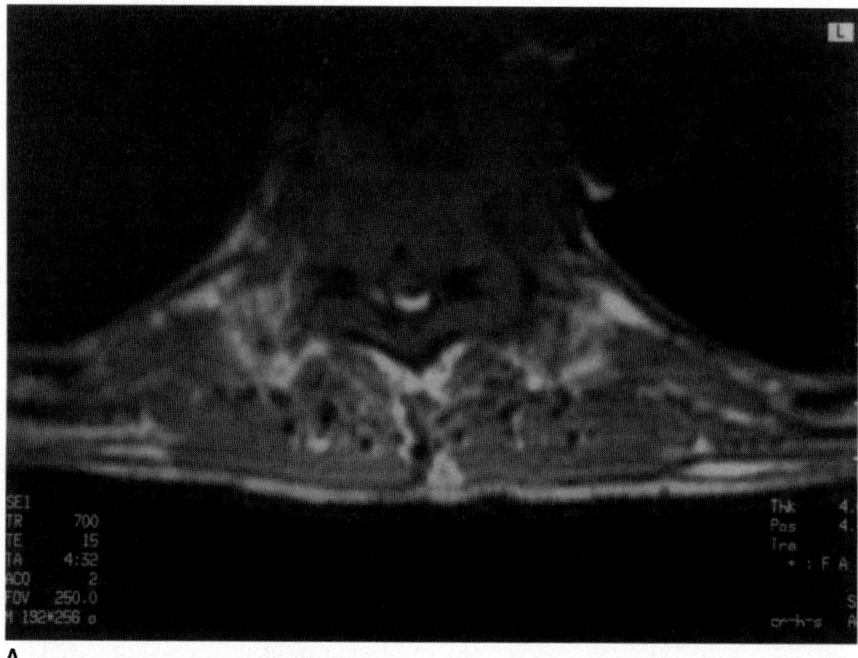

**A**

**Figure 114.3** (A) Laterally located aorta in which a right-sided approach was chosen.

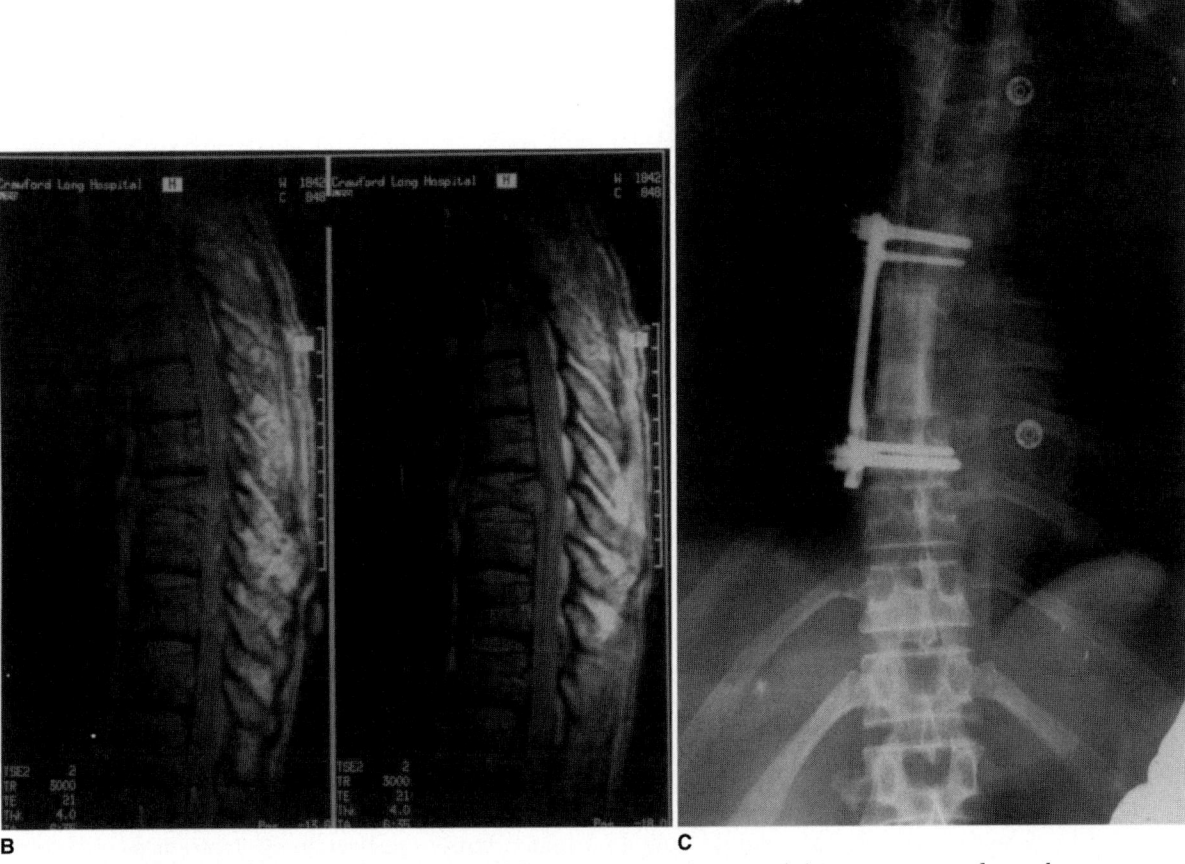

**Figure 114.3** *cont'd* (**B**) Sagittal view of the same metastatic tumor. (**C**) Postoperative radiograph of this case instrumented with a Z-plate and humerus allograft packed with autologous cancellous bone harvested from the iliac crest.

the vertebral body between the aortic branch point and the neural foramen. Most surgeons and the scoliosis literature agree that up to three adjacent segmental arteries may be taken without neurologic sequelae, but the importance of the artery of Adamkiewicz (T10-L2) is still debated. Some surgeons advocate a preoperative spinal angiogram. Once the vessels are ligated and transected, a subperiosteal dissection of the vertebral body is carried out by using an elevator and unipolar cautery. The anterior longitudinal ligament (ALL) is elevated or incised if ventral release is necessary. If left intact during the exposure, the ALL can serve as a tissue barrier between the aorta and the operative site during the procedure. Some surgeons elevate the ALL sharply or use monopolar cautery from the bone and use that potential space to hold a malleable retractor for added safety.

In anticipation of instrumentation to the levels above and below the pathology, the segmental vessels should be taken here as well. Once this step is complete, a periosteal elevator or monopolar cautery is used to complete a subperiosteal exposure of the diseased level and other levels needed for instrumentation. Thus the rostral end plate and disc space of the level above and the inferior end plate and disc space of the level below the pathologic levels must be clearly and completely visualized. Ventrally, the exposure is limited by the aorta, but with careful mobiliza-

tion and retraction (e.g., with large malleable retractors) the cortical bone and disc can be dissected close to (but just short of) the midline. It is critical that a thorough exposure be completed dorsally. The dorsal 2 to 3cm of each rib (level) involved must be removed with a ½- or ⅜-inch osteotome. Rongeurs or a drill may also be useful. Once the heads of the ribs are disarticulated and removed, the pedicles at each level are exposed and the dorsolateral edge of the vertebral body is confirmed by palpation with a Penfield no. 4. Identification of the pedicle and dorsal vertebral body is essential for recognizing the location of the spinal canal and is necessary for safe and accurate identification of landmarks for placement of instrumentation. Frequently there is a large mass of soft tissue, including the ligated ends of the segmental vessels, that has been swept into the area of the foramen. One should not attempt to cut away or use the monopolar to cauterize this tissue; the patent segments of the vessels will often cause annoying bleeding. Shrinking the tissue near the foramen with the bipolar cautery and then placing a single silk suture through the cauterized mass and sewing it in traction to rib periosteum is often useful. This assists in identifying the spinal canal by bringing this tissue more dorsal. Decompression should not be attempted until the limits of the spinal canal are clearly visualized. Catastrophic neurologic injury may result from initially not identifying accurately the borders of the pedicle, foramen, and dorsal vertebral body (i.e., the spinal canal).

### Thoracolumbar Junction

For lesions affecting T10 through the upper lumbar spine (L1), a combined thoracoabdominal approach is necessary. This may be true for lesions at L2 that will require exposure to the T12-L1 disc space for instrumentation. During a standard thoracotomy, the patient is positioned in the right lateral decubitus position with a bend in the table to facilitate exposure. A double-lumen endotracheal tube is used for ipsilateral lung deflation. The incision is commonly made over the 10th rib and carried from the anterior axillary line to the posterior axillary line and extended as needed. The oblique and transversus abdominis muscles are incised, but care should be taken not to enter the peritoneal cavity. A subperiosteal dissection of the rib allows for efficient resection of the rib. The thoracic cavity is entered via the 10th or 11th rib space, and the diaphragm is immediately identified. The parietal pleura and peritoneal sac are bluntly mobilized by using finger and sponge-stick dissection. Avoiding the monopolar cautery for most of this stage can prevent inadvertent entry into the peritoneal cavity, lung, or abdominal viscera. The diaphragm is mobilized from its peripheral attachment to the 11th rib. A 2 to 3cm cuff of diaphragmatic tissue is maintained to allow for reapproximation during closure. The spinal attachments of the diaphragm are taken down sharply or with monopolar cautery. The medial attachment of the lateral arcuate ligament and the lateral attachment of the medial arcuate ligament are divided close to the tip of the transverse process of L1. The crus of the diaphragm is divided 2 to 3cm away from the vertebral body and should be tagged. At this point, large self-retaining chest retractors can be placed to displace the peritoneal contents and diaphragm. Vessels that require sacrifice should be taken as close to the aorta or vena cava as possible to allow for maximal mobilization of these structures. Coagulation near the neuroforamen should be avoided to decrease the risk of compromising important radicular feeders to the spinal cord. The psoas muscle can be sharply dissected with periosteal elevators or monopolar cautery back to the attachments to the pedicle to maximize exposure of the lumbar vertebral bodies. Gentle retraction can allow exposure from T9 through L3.

Although identification of severe fractures or tumor pathology is often easy, localization for less-obvious lesions at the thoracolumbar junction can be difficult. Although usually accurate, counting the ribs should not be relied on to identify the level. Plain radiographs are recommended and should be repeated with different orientation until the desired levels are confidently identified. With the patient in the lateral decubitus position, cross-table anteroposterior and lateral x-rays often are sufficient for accurate localization of the appropriate level.

### Retroperitoneal Approach

The retroperitoneal approach is useful for lesions extending from the inferior surface of L1 to the superior surface of L5. Keep in mind that instrumentation and fusion for pathology that actually extends to either the rostral or caudal limits of this exposure will require longer exposure that may not be provided by the retroperitoneal approach alone. As well, the iliac crest prevents the true lateral access to the L5 vertebral body for transverse screw placement. To fully expose the vertebral body of L1 dissection of some of the crural attachments may be necessary. A pneumothorax is a potential complication. At the caudal end, the L5-S1 interspace can be very difficult to expose fully (particularly in large male patients) because of the bulk of the psoas muscle.

Administration of cathartic agents before surgery, and placement of a nasogastric tube during induction of anesthesia, may facilitate easier retraction of the peritoneal contents during the case. Positioning for the retroperitoneal approach is similar to that for the thoracoabdominal exposure: the patient is in the lateral position with a break in the table at the level of the pathology. Upper lumbar exposure may require resection of the 12th rib. The incision is typically made from the lateral margin of the dorsal longitudinal paraspinal muscles (iliospinalis, sacrospinalis, etc.) and extends ventrally to the lateral border of the rectus abdominis muscles. The external and internal oblique and transversus abdominis muscles are divided with monopolar cautery. Clamp dissection and elevation of these muscles before incision can avoid entry into the peritoneal cavity. Blunt dissection with a sponge-on-a-stick can mobilize the peritoneum away from the spine. Great care must be taken to avoid damage to the ureter, although it is usually safely reflected ventrally with the peritoneal contents. Large, self-retaining table-mounted retractors (Omni, Thompson-Farley, etc.) are used over moist laparotomy sponges to maintain exposure. The transverse processes are palpable through the psoas muscle. This muscle can be dissected from its periosteal attachments by using monopolar cautery. This technique loses less blood than using a Cobb or periosteal elevator. Vigorous attempts at retraction with a Meyerding or similar retractor may cause laceration of the muscle and excessive bleeding. Careful "toeing-in" of the Meyerding or McElroy retractor is all that is usually necessary to put the psoas on stretch and facilitate subperiosteal exposure. Too much stretch, however, may cause postoperative psoas or iliopsoas weakness and pain. Mobilization of this muscle dorsally to the pedicle will allow palpation and visualization of the ventral border of the spinal canal. Key points regarding closure of the retroperitoneal exposure include meticulous closure of the abdominal wall muscular layers to prevent hernia formation. The authors recommend leaving a large Hemovac drain in the retroperitoneal space for 24 to 48 hours, especially when decortication or resection of vertebral bone causes significant oozing of blood still seen at the time of closure. Another potential complication of this approach is intestinal ileus. Nasogastric suction is continued postoperatively until bowel activity is confirmed.

### Transabdominal (Transperitoneal) Approach

Ventral decompression, reconstruction, and fixation of the lower lumbar spine and lumbosacral junction via the transperitoneal approach (open or laparoscopic) is possible.[18-20] Threaded interbody titanium cages, bone dowels, and other synthetic implants are available for interbody fusion/fixation. Typical thoracolumbar bone screws, plates, and rods are difficult to insert from this approach and have a high profile near vascular structures. The exposure tends to be triangular in shape because the field of view limited by the bifurcation of the iliac vessels and the L5-S1 disc space. Direct ventral screw fixation (e.g., buttress screw) of the upper sacrum is possible after a subperiosteal exposure of S1 immediately caudal to the disc space is performed. Use of Steinmann pins or a table-mounted vascular retractor is useful in retracting the iliac veins and arteries. Blunt dissection and avoidance of the monopolar cautery may avoid damage to the superior hypogastric plexus (and associated retrograde ejaculation). The L5-S1 disc space is readily evacuated, and bone graft and/or implants can be inserted.

Exposure of L4-5 is very feasible, but the surgeon must take extra care to immediately identify the iliolumbar vein. Although its origin is variable, this vein usually branches off the lateral aspect of the left iliac vein. Other times it originates directly from the vena cava. The vein courses to the region of the L5 pedicle and foramen. Heavy blood loss can occur if the left iliac vein is retracted to the patient's right before the iliolumbar vein is ligated. One may also consider low-dose heparin administration prior to retraction of the bifurcation and vena cava to help prevent thrombosis. Other helpful pearls include use of Steinmann pins to retract the iliac vessels laterally. The Trendelenburg position can facilitate the approach to the sacral angle. Currently, laparoscopic techniques are under investigation that may improve access to the L5-S1 level and allow for decompression, fusion, and instrumentation.

L5 vertebrectomy has been accomplished via the open, laparoscopic, or retroperitoneal approach, but the procedure is difficult and carries a higher risk than discectomy for vascular injury.[21,22] Furthermore, reconstruction of L5 from the direct anterior transperitoneal approach is also very difficult. Vertebrectomy of L4 is similarly very difficult from the anterior approach and can be more readily accomplished via the retroperitoneal approach. The mid- and upper-lumbar levels (L3-4, L2-3, L1-2) are more difficult to expose via a transperitoneal approach because of the bulk of abdominal contents that must be retracted. The retroperitoneal approach should be considered.

### Decompression

For a vertebrectomy, the discs above and below are incised with a knife blade, or a straight osteotome is used to separate the bulk of the disc from the end plates. One must keep in mind the concave curvature of the dorsal vertebral body in the thoracic spine to avoid the ventral spinal canal. If soft tumor is encountered, large scoop curettes or the ultrasonic aspirator are efficient tools for rapid tissue removal. For stronger bone, a 1- or 2-inch osteotome may be used to make two cuts to remove a large portion of the body. The first cut is 5 to 8mm dorsal to the ventral-most cortex of the vertebral body in the vertical plane (perpendicular to the disc space) and is approximately 15 to 20mm deep (toward the opposite side). The second cut is similarly perpendicular to the disc space and is approximately 8mm ventral to the dorsal cortex of the vertebral body and spinal canal. A curved osteotome or

large curette can then remove a large block of bone, leaving a barrier between the aorta and the decompression site and between the spinal canal and the decompression site. The remainder of bone is then removed either piecemeal with smaller curettes or with a high-speed drill. The Midas Rex (Fort Worth, TX) Am-11 tool is ideal; similar-shaped drill bits are available from Aesculap and Anspach. Drilling may offer a less-traumatic initial removal of bone compared with osteotomy, but blood loss may be less with the faster latter technique. The bone ventral to the canal is the last area to be removed. Once the dorsal cortex and posterior longitudinal ligament have been removed, the dura is decompressed from the ipsilateral pedicle to the contralateral pedicle. The ventral-most and far lateral cortex are preserved as much as possible to help secure the bone graft. One should be able to visually inspect the contralateral pedicle. The epidural space rostral and caudal is palpated with a double-ender (dental or Woodsen) instrument. One must decompress from pedicle to pedicle to fully ensure that there is no spinal cord compression.

The complication of neurologic injury is best avoided by clearly exposing the ventral spinal canal and dorsal body first. The next step is to create a cavity into which the critical bone fragments or tumor (compressing the spinal cord) can be safely reduced. Thus, one should first complete the bulk of the corpectomy or vertebrectomy (depending on the pathology), leaving the portion in the ventral epidural space last. Then the dorsal vertebral cortex, fracture fragments, or tumor in the epidural space is more safely removed via regular or reverse angle curettage. At times, a diamond burr may be useful. Instruments are best manipulated toward the vertebrectomy defect away from the spinal cord during epidural decompression.

### Fracture Reduction

A pathologic or traumatic fracture dislocation can be reduced with several maneuvers. The most direct technique is manipulation of vertebral bodies with a large Cobb elevator or curette. This can be difficult and runs the risk of having the instrument slip into the canal.

With the patient in the lateral position, the surgeon can push on the back at the apex of the kyphotic deformity. This technique is very effective, and the decompression site can be visualized during the manipulation. If the posterior longitudinal ligament (PLL) is intact, then ligamentotaxis can aid to pull fracture fragments ventrally.

Several ventral thoracolumbar instrumentation systems have bolts that (once placed in the adjacent vertebral bodies) can be used with a distractor to accomplish reduction and distraction. Distraction is effective, but the distractor can obscure the surgeon's view and compromise access to the decompression site during placement of the bone graft. Interspace spreaders have the same limitation, although newer models are longer and more streamlined, allowing greater accessibility to the vertebrectomy site during distraction and reconstruction (Figure 114.4). When combined with ligamentotaxis from the PLL, anterior distraction maneuvers can be an effective method to reduce posteriorly displaced fractures.

A fourth method to reduce posteriorly displaced fracture fragments is an eggshell osteotomy. The cancellous

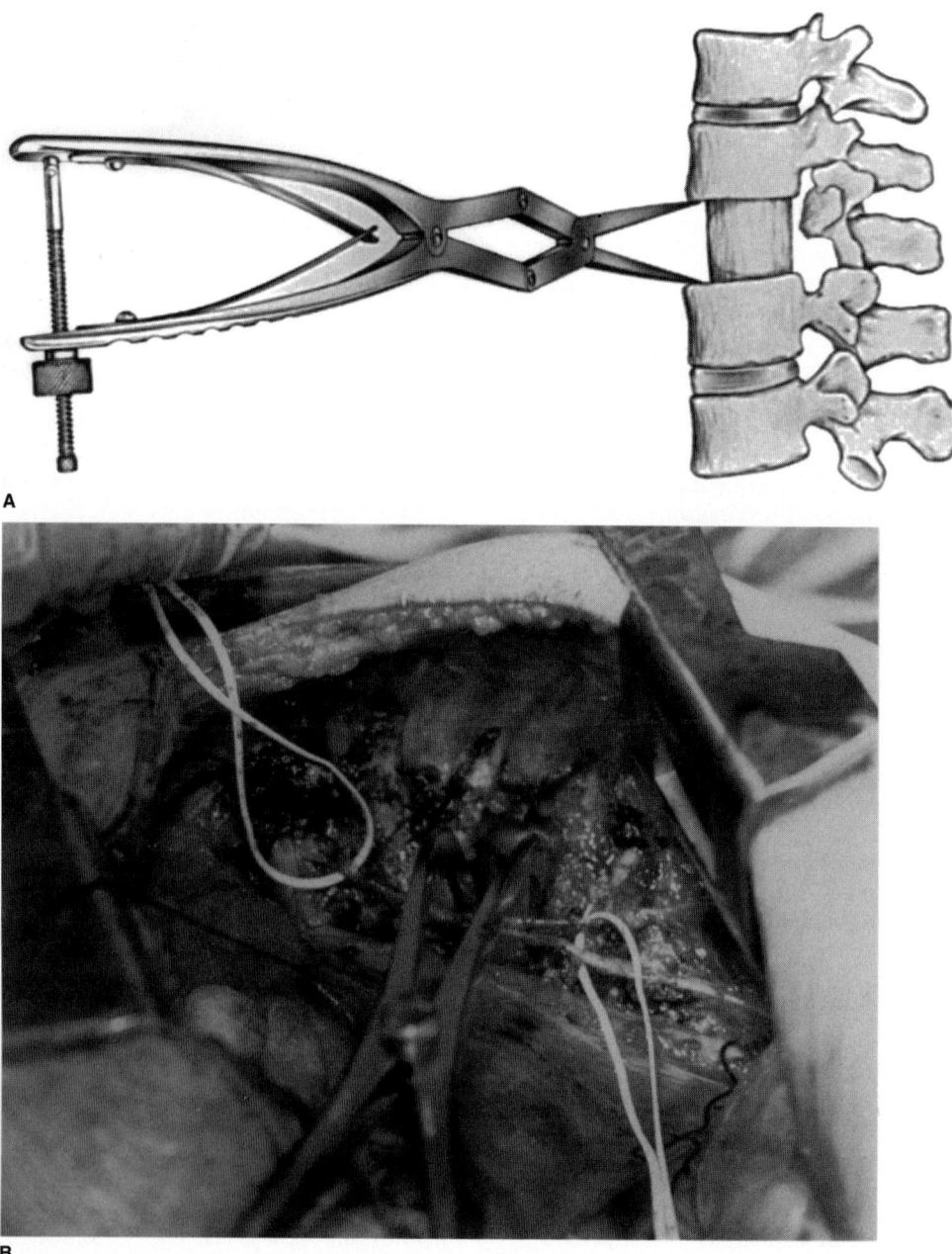

**Figure 114.4** **(A)** Diagram of intervertebral body spreader and bone graft reconstruction. **(B)** Intervertebral body spreader (Synthes) distracting prior to bone graft placement. The thoracic dura is visible posteriorly.

portion of the fractured vertebral body is removed with a high-speed drill, leaving the cortical remnants. The posteriorly displaced cortical fragments can then be pulled anteriorly by using reverse-angle and straight curettes.

## Bone Graft, Vertebral Body Replacements

The choice of bone graft or reconstructive implant depends on the distance the anterior fusion needs to span. The location in the thoracolumbar spine and the patient's underlying pathology are also important. Factors such as

the presence of osteopenia, tumor, previous radiation, diabetes, rheumatoid arthritis, and tobacco use are important. Grafts that span an entire vertebral body length or more must withstand greater axial loads. Allogeneic humerus, tibia, or femur can be used, and they are typically packed with autologous cancellous bone harvested during the vertebrectomy. Rib and iliac crest are also excellent sources of bone to use in and around allograft struts. One should keep in mind that allograft bone takes much longer to incorporate.

Portions of rib tied by suture or cable into a barrel-shaped cylinder can be used as a spacer fusion. Ribs are thought to be high in bone growth factors but provide less strength in resisting axial loads than some of the alternatives.

Autologous tricortical iliac crest provides satisfactory axial support. Harvest of large tricortical graft endangers the peritoneal contents. Great care should be taken during periosteal dissection. Significant morbidity can be associated with harvest of autologous iliac crest bone. The authors typically use a unipolar cautery with the tip angled ventrally to hug the dorsal cortex during stripping of the muscular and fascial attachments. A Cobb elevator is also useful, but care must be taken to avoid plunging into the peritoneum. Vessels perforating the iliac crest must be coagulated or the emissary ostia treated with bone wax to help prevent accumulation of a hematoma. One should always stay one to two fingerbreadths dorsal to the anterior superior iliac spine to avoid injury to the lateral femoral cutaneous nerve. If one desires to reconstruct the defect in the iliac crest, both natural and artificial methods are possible. If rib is available, the ends can be impacted into the harvest site sides of the iliac crest to recreate the superior contour. Steinmann pins or screws (titanium or stainless steel) as a support for methylmethacrylate may be used.[1] If the latter technique is used, a postoperative drain is recommended, as the cement will elicit a collection of serous fluid.

Autologous fibula can also be used. In cases of infection, some surgeons will also perform microvascular anastomosis to the intercostal arteries to preserve graft blood supply. Meticulous surgical technique must be used to avoid the peroneal nerve near the fibular head and to avoid the ankle joint (syndesmosis). A good rule of thumb is to stay 10cm or more away from the ankle joint below and the fibular head above. A preoperative lower extremity arteriogram is useful to define the arterial supply to the fibula.

It is important to emphasize that regardless of the source of autologous bone, all soft tissue (muscular or tendinous attachments, cartilage, fascia, etc.) must be cleanly stripped off before implantation to maximize bone surface area for fusion. Leaving cartilaginous material adherent to the vertebral body end plate can result in pseudarthrosis; thus the vertebral end plates should be meticulously stripped of all disc tissue. Scattered areas of decorticated end plate facilitate fusion, but significant amounts of cortical bone must be spared to allow strong purchase of the bone graft and to prevent impaction of the graft through the end plates during axial loading. Removing (decorticating) too much of the end plate may result in collapse of the bodies above and below with telescoping of the graft. This problem is encountered more often when rigid allograft tibia, fibula, or femur is used.

In addition to autograft or allograft bone, methylmethacrylate and artificial bone spacers are currently being marketed. Ceramic blocks, vertical mesh titanium cages (Pyramesh, Medtronics Sofamor Danek, Memphis, TN; Harms, Depuy AcroMed, Raynham, MA; Synmesh System, Synthes, Paoli, PA), carbon fiber cages (Stackable Cage System, DePuy AcroMed) polyether ether blocks (PEEK, Medtronic, Sofamor Danek), and expandable metallic implants are available (Synex System, Synthes [Figure 114.5]; VertiSpan, Medtronic Sofamor Danek [Figure 114.6].

The benefit of having a break in the table can be enhanced with the use of an interspace spreader or by manual pressure on the dorsal spine to help open the disc space during distraction and bone impaction. When screw-rod systems are used, direct distraction of vertebral body screws allows for efficient placement of the graft. Once all graft material is in place, the table is returned to the neutral position to help lock in the graft. In addition, compression can be applied across the vertebral body screws and maintained by rod attachment.

The importance of meticulous shaping and "carpentry" with the graft during this step cannot be overemphasized. A spinal metal implant is not a substitute or savior for a poorly shaped or fitted bone graft.

## Instrumentation

Ventral or ventrolateral metal implants provide immediate rigidity, allow for compression of bone graft, and help maintain correction of a deformity. Based on individual experience, various amounts of time working with sawbone models or cadavers are needed before use in actual clinical situations. The three basic types of implants are rod, plate, and cable systems.

### General Principles Of Ventrolateral Instrumentation Systems

Whether rods, plates, or cables are being used, all implants in the thoracolumbar region should be placed on the lateral aspect of the vertebral body. The construct

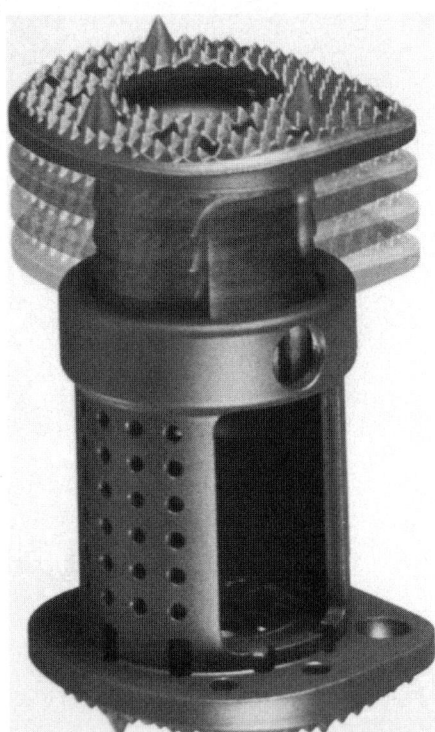

**Figure 114.5** The expandable Synex vertebral body implant demonstrating several possible ratcheted positions of the top metal plate (Synthes, Paoli, PA).

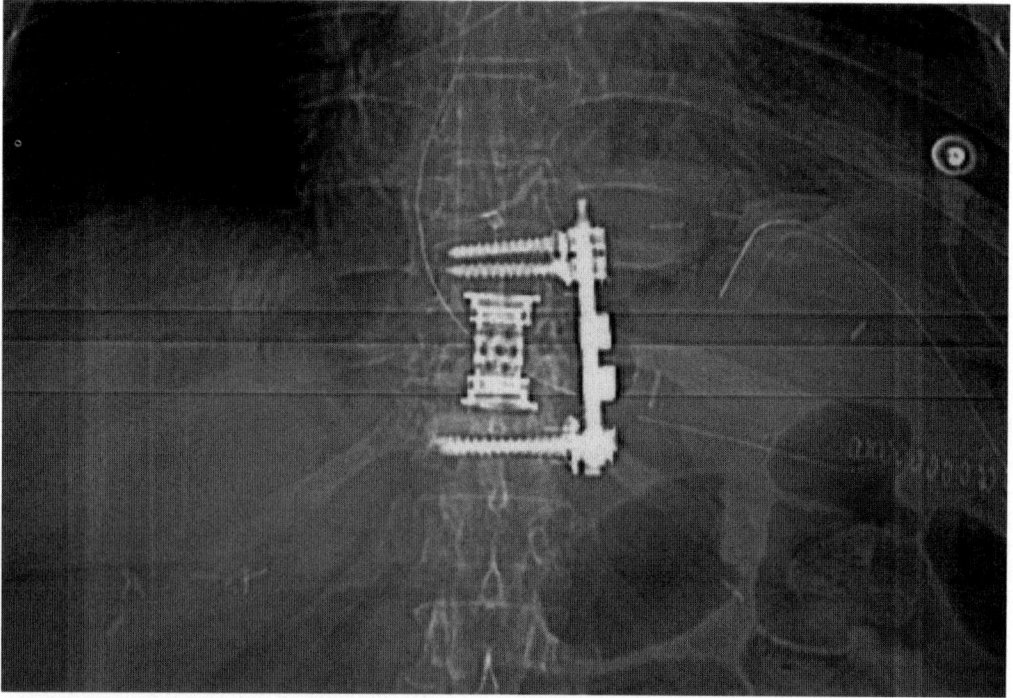

A

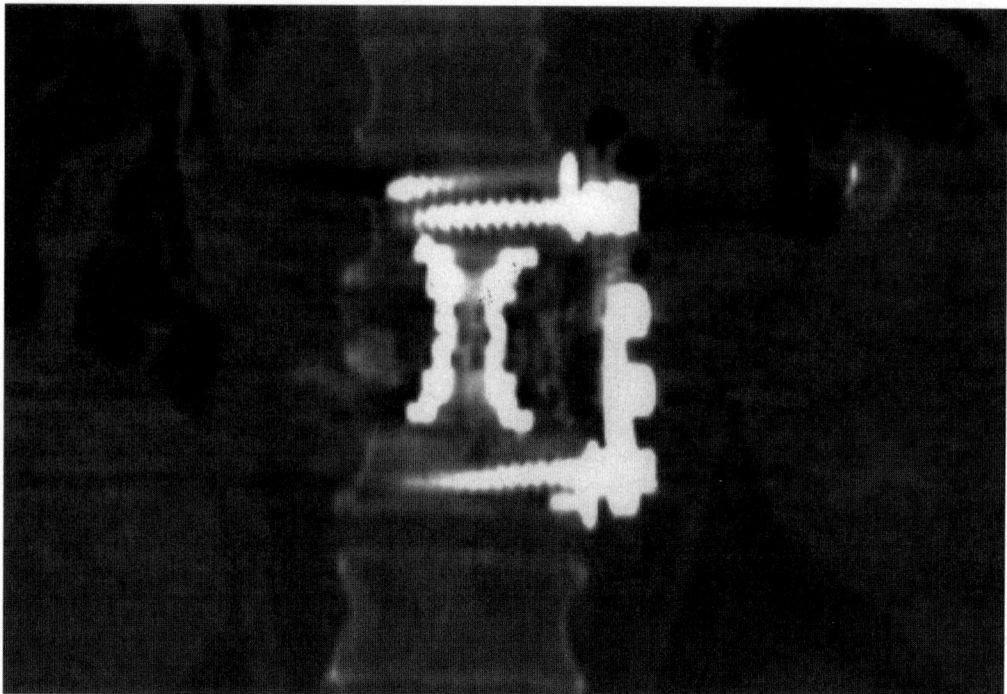

B

**Figure 114.6** **(A)** Immediate postoperative radiograph of the VertiSpan expandable cage system from Medtronic Sofamor Danek (Memphis, TN). **(B)** Immediate postoperative coronal CT scan of the same type of expandable cage. Note the central and peripheral placement of cancellous bone from the iliac crest.

should have a low profile to avoid vascular or visceral injury. To avoid unequal strain and stress on the metallic implant, great care must be taken to maximize the total surface area of metal-to-bone contact. In a method commonly referred to as "gardening" the spine, rongeurs and drills should be used to flatten out the lips of the vertebral end plates, and the heads of the ribs should be removed at all levels to be instrumented. This is particularly important with plate implants.

The dorsal-most points of screw fixation in the vertebral body should be 8 to 10mm ventral and caudal to the dorsal-rostral corner of the vertebral body at the rostral end of the construct or 8 to 10mm ventral and rostral from the dorsal-caudal corner of the caudal body in the construct. A minimum screw trajectory of 10 degrees ventrally away from the spinal canal is necessary to avoid injury. An awl should be used to begin screw or bolt holes to prevent skating of instruments near the spinal canal or the large vessels and viscera. Screw placement is dictated by the desired forces. To correct a kyphosis, the screws should be placed more ventrally with distraction/compression dual rod systems (e.g., Kaneda or M-8 Dual Rod system). With dual-rod systems, the more ventral rod should be longer to correct the kyphosis. The longer segment is distracted initially. One must recognize that even minor distraction forces may cause spinal cord injury via stretch or vascular compromise. In single-rod/cable tension systems used to correct a scoliosis, a ventrally placed screw may be used to produce a relative kyphosis. In general, when correcting scoliosis, tension forces should be applied on the convex side of the curve starting at the apex and directed rostrally and caudally in sequential fashion. Bicortical screw penetration is preferred to provide the strongest purchase of the vertebral body, but care must be taken not to penetrate beyond 2 to 3mm of the distant cortex of the vertebral body.

### Cable Systems

The Dwyer cable system was first developed in the early 1960s for application to the convex side of thoracolumbar scoliotic curves. The basic principle of ventrolateral correction of scoliosis is to shorten the convexity by applying compressive forces. A screw with a staple (to maintain screw position and prevent movement) is placed on the convex side of a curve into the vertebral body on the lateral side. A titanium cable is then connected to the screws and tightened to create a compressive force. Excessive force, however, can produce undesirable thoracic kyphosis or, further caudally in the spine, the flattening of a normal lumbar lordosis. Dwyer reported a 43% complication rate, including screw pull-out and vascular/visceral injuries. This system can be used for degenerative lumbar curves, but it is not recommended in flat back or kyphotic deformities. This particular type of implant system has been abandoned by many surgeons in favor of rod and plate systems.

### Rod Systems

**Zielke USIS.** The Universal Spinal Instrumentation System (USIS) developed by Zielke is a refinement of the Dwyer system and uses flexible rods instead of cables. This system allows for segmental compression or distraction via the ventrolateral approach and provides improved rotational control over scoliotic curves. A device is included that can derotate the scoliotic curve or produce lordosis. A correction of 10% to 15% per level fused can be obtained. This system is well suited for thoracolumbar and lumbar scoliosis but is somewhat limited for other applications because of the limited stability of a single point of fixation per vertebral body.

**Kaneda Anterior Scoliosis System (KASS, DePuy AcroMed).** This screw/rod system corrects scoliosis by securing each vertebral body in the curve with two screws inserted through a vertebral staple. Two contoured rods are placed into the heads of the screws. This system is designed for the correction and stabilization of idiopathic thoracolumbar, lumbar, and thoracic scoliosis. The Frontier Anterior Deformity System is a similar system from the same company that is suited for thoracoscopic scoliosis surgery.

**Kostuik-Harrington (Zimmer, Inc.).** This system is a ventral modification of the dorsal Harrington distraction rod. Vertebral body screws and stabilizing staples are placed at each level ventrally, and a distraction rod is inserted through these screws and used for placement of the strut graft. Compression of the graft is then accomplished with placement of larger Kostuik spinal screws dorsally on the lateral aspect of the vertebral body. These screws hold a heavy ratcheted Harrington compression rod that, in concert with the ventral rod, also provides good rotational control. This system is useful for short segment fixation and allows for distraction to correct kyphotic deformity. Currently this system is no longer in widespread use.

**Kaneda (AcroMed, Inc.).** A unique aspect of the Kaneda system (Figure 114.7) is the tetra-plate with four corner spikes that is initially hammered into the center of the lateral aspect of the vertebral body. One should "garden the spine" to ensure flush contact between the staple-plate and the bone. Two vertebral (preferably bicortical) screws are placed through each plate. The heads of the screws have a channel through which rods are placed. The design of the staple plate is such that the ventral screw holes are more rostral and caudal in the upper and lower plates, respectively. Thus the ventral span of the rod is longer than the dorsal. The heads of these screws can be engaged by a distractor for placement of the strut graft. The Kaneda distraction system is very effective and allows ample working space through which the bone graft can be placed. Cross-fixators are available to enhance the rigidity of this implant. This device is very effective for short (one or two) segment fixation for a variety of pathologies. Sources of complication include failure to achieve maximal surface area contact between staple-plate and bone (by allowing rocking of the metal over a bony prominence) and placement of screws that are either too short or too long. Preoperative axial CT slices (bone windows) can be used to indirectly measure the length of screw needed. One can usually feel the screw engaging the opposite lateral cortex. Inadequate countersinking of the graft may make it difficult to apply a cross-link.

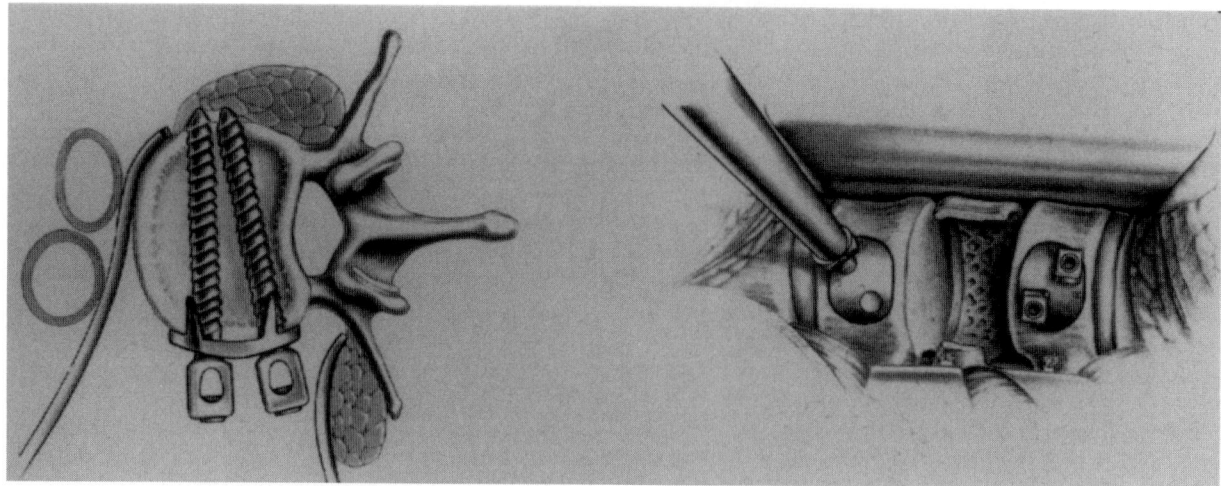

**Figure 114.7** Tetra-plates and eye bolts of the Kaneda system (DePuy AcroMed). Smooth rods are placed through the eye bolts and tightened with a top-loading screw. Like the Z-plate system, the bolts can be used for distraction or compression.

**Anteres Dual Rod System (Medtronic Sofamor Danek).** This system is very similar to the Kaneda system. An anchoring plate with cleats is impacted into the side of the vertebral bodies above and below. Bolts are then placed through holes in the plates and across the vertebral bodies. Rods are then slid into the bolts, compressed, and then locking screws are tightened. Cross-links are available.

**VentroFix System (Synthes).** Also similar to the Kaneda device, the VentroFix system uses plates that are screwed into the spine (as opposed to impacting cleats). Rods then slide through grooves and openings in the anchoring plates. Locking screws fix the rods to the anchoring plates.

**Texas Scottish Rite System (TSRH) (Sofamor-Danek, Inc.).** This implant system of variable angle screws and rods (connected by variable-width offset connectors or eye bolts) is most commonly applied to the dorsal spine but is easily adapted to ventrolateral fixation. Screws of 5.5, 6.5, 7.0, and 7.5mm diameter width and various lengths are available for bicortical purchase. Screws can be placed in a trapezoidal array similar to the Kaneda device so that the longer span is ventral. Rods of 3/16 or 1/4 inch or intermediate 5.5mm diameter are (as with the screws) available in stainless steel and titanium. Distraction and compression forceps are available and connect to the rods below or above the screw-offset connection to apply the desired force. Use of TSRH for ventrolateral fixation should be done with the knowledge that the heads of the variable angle screws are somewhat higher in profile than those of other plate and rod systems. Side-tightening screws may be easier to apply than top-tightening.

### Plate Systems

**Z-Plate (Sofamor-Danek, Inc.).** This system designed by Zdeblick (Figures 114.8 to 114.10) combines the low-profile advantage of plates with the distraction and compression capability of vertebral body screws. Bicortical

purchase is recommended, and a combination of bone screws and bolts are used to rigidly lock to the plate. Dorsally, screws are placed 10 degrees ventrally away from the canal. The starting point for the rostral body is 8 to 10mm inferior and ventral to the upper dorsal corner of the vertebral body on lateral exposure. Conversely, the entry point for the caudal bolt is 8 to 10mm superior and ventral to the lower dorsal corner of the vertebral body. An awl is used to pierce the cortex, but the bone is not tapped. These bolts can be used for distraction and allow for placement of a strut graft and correction of kyphosis. In patients with suboptimal bone strength, it is useful to use (initially) an intervertebral body spreader to apply force over a broader area. When the strut graft is in place, the bolts can be compressed and locked rigidly to the plate. As a last step, cancellous bone screws are placed through the ventral slots in the plate and angled 10 degrees dorsally. These screws are typically 5mm longer than the dorsally placed bolts because of the configuration of the vertebral body. Complications can arise from placing a plate that is too long and that extends above or below, across, or into a disc space. This may accelerate degeneration at that motion segment. The usual risks of bicortical screw placement also apply. One must also make sure that the bolts, and especially the bone screws, are not angled down or up into the graft or adjacent disc. The latest version of the Z-plate allows for rigid fixation of the screw heads to the plate.

**Anterior Thoracolumbar Locking Plate (ATLLP) (Synthes, Inc.).** The Synthes plate system (Figure 114.11) is also low profile and titanium (MRI compatible). It differs from the Z-plate in that distraction forces are not applied to the bolts or screws but are applied directly to the vertebral body end plates. Synthes makes a long-handled distractor with strong but thin blades that allow perhaps the best access to the graft site during placement of the strut. Once the graft is in place, angled screw hole trajectories in the plate cause up to 3mm of compression as the screws are driven into the bone. This system uses

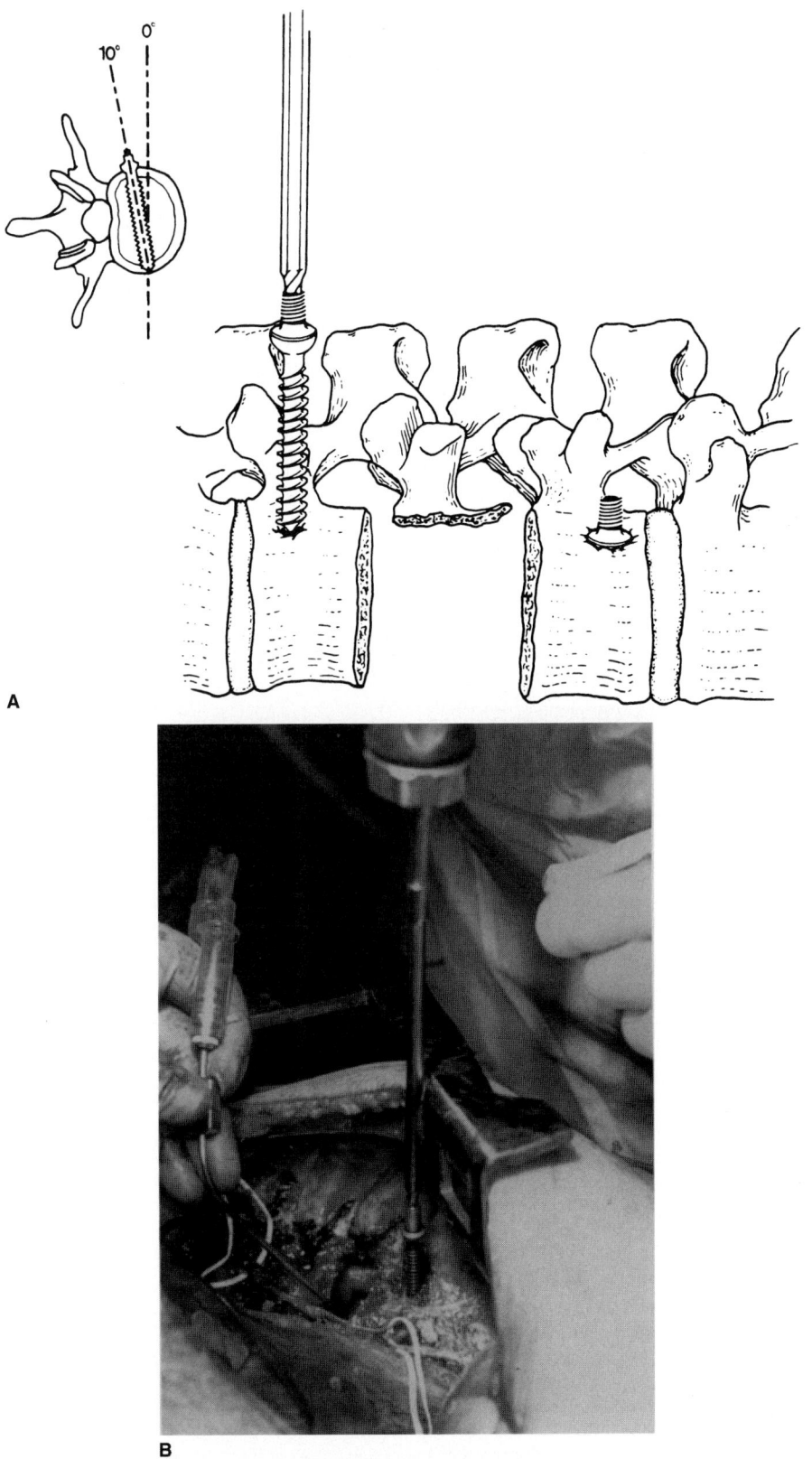

**Figure 114.8** (**A**) Diagram of dorsal bolt trajectory (10 degrees ventral to or away from the spinal canal). (**B**) Placement of Z-plate bolt (Medtronic Sofamor-Danek) at caudal, dorsal corner of lower vertebral body (note dura mater visible through corpectomy defect).

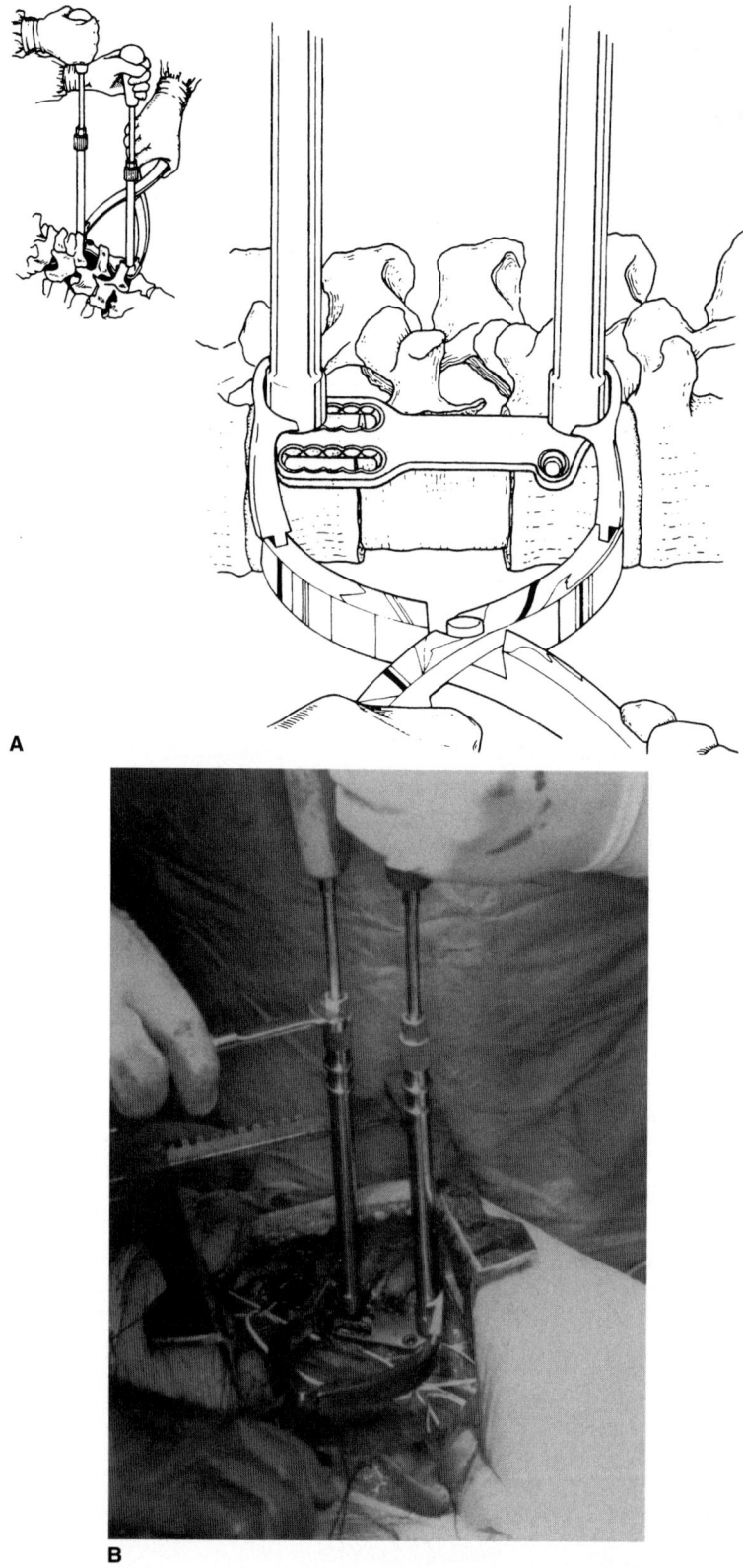

**A**

**B**

**Figure 114.9** (A) Diagram of simultaneous compression across and tightening of bolts to top-loaded thoracic plate (Sofamor-Danek). (B) Operative photograph of tightening of dorsal bolts in Z-plate system with extended wrenches and long compressor (Medtronic Sofamor-Danek).

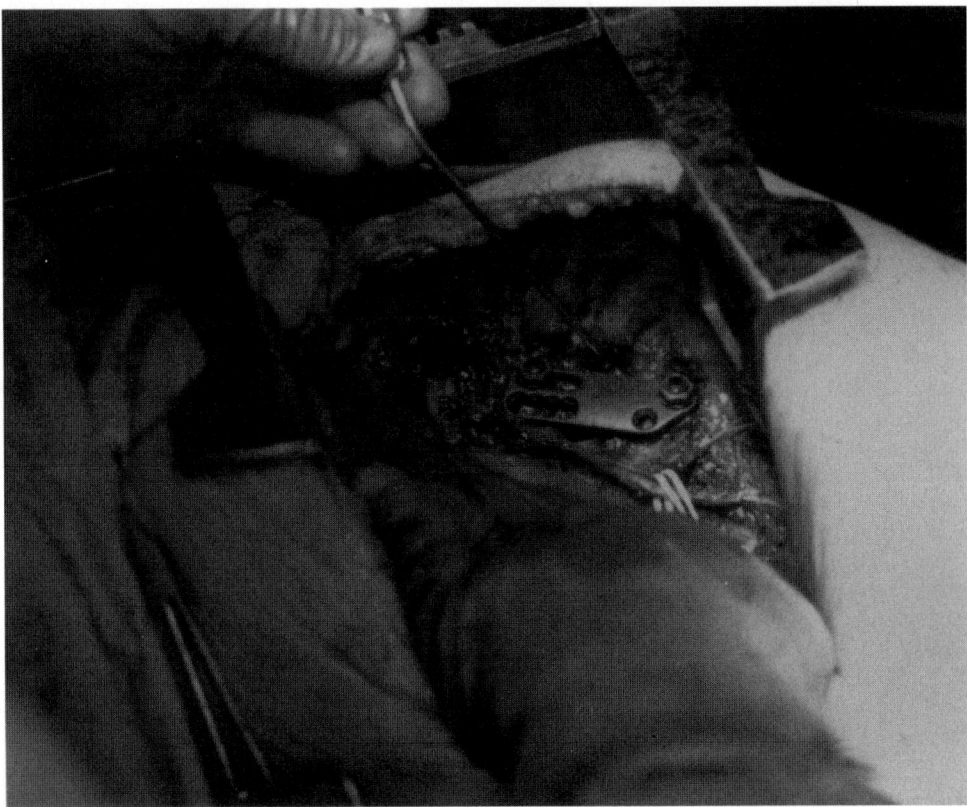

**Figure 114.10** Ventral thoracic plate (Z-plate) with posterior bolts in place just before ventral screw placement. Plastic loops are around the sympathetic chain.

wide, cancellous screws for unicortical purchase, although bicortical purchase is an option. Because placement is unicortical, equal-length screws are used dorsally and ventrally. This system has the advantage of being able to effectively provide distraction and compression, is low-profile, and is perhaps the simplest in design. It is limited in the amount of compression (2 to 3mm) provided by the dorsal compression screws. This system is no longer in widespread use.

**Interbody (Disc Space) Metallic Devices.** Implants have been developed to make interbody (disc space) fixation and fusion easier. These implants can be placed via the ventral approach and are used primarily in the lumbar spine. Both open and laparoscopic placement are possible ventrally. Generically referred to as cages, these cylindrical devices are usually threaded. Currently, implants are available in titanium (Ray cage [Surgical Dynamics]; Harms cage [Moss Systems]; Pyramesh cage, InterFix cage, the lordotic LT cage [Medtronics Sofamor Danek]) or are cut from allograft femur (Cortical Bone Dowels [Sofamor-Danek]). Others are available that are square-shaped and made from carbon-fiber (Brantigan cage [AcroMed]). All of these disc space or interbody implants can be packed with autologous bone to aid arthrodesis. In July 2002, a commercial form of rhBMP2 (InFuse, Medtronic Sofamor Danek) was approved by the FDA for use in anterior lumbar interbody fusion.

Biomechanically, interbody implants offer resistance to axial forces across the ventral and middle columns of the spine and can resist flexion and extension. They are usually placed during distraction of the disc space, allowing for compression of the implant like a screw. The Harms cage and the Pyramesh cage are not threaded. They are hollow titanium cages with teeth along both rostral and caudal surfaces that gain purchase into the end plates during placement into the disc space. This is similar to the fixation afforded by the Brantigan cage. Interbody implants may be used with or without ventral or dorsal segmental instrumentation (plates, pedicle screws, or hooks).

It is difficult to assess fusion in the postoperative state because of the artifact from the implants. CT scans with sagittal reconstruction through the middle of the implants can be useful. Flexion and extension radiographs can determine whether pathologic motion is present but cannot directly assess the degree of arthrodesis. Despite these controversial aspects of interbody fusion devices, long-term success has been reported.[4,15]

## Summary

Ventral approaches to the thoracic and lumbar spine have advanced because of better understanding of the biomechanics of the spine, the importance of sagittal balance, the radiographic and clinical indications for any given approach, better appreciation of subtle anatomy, and

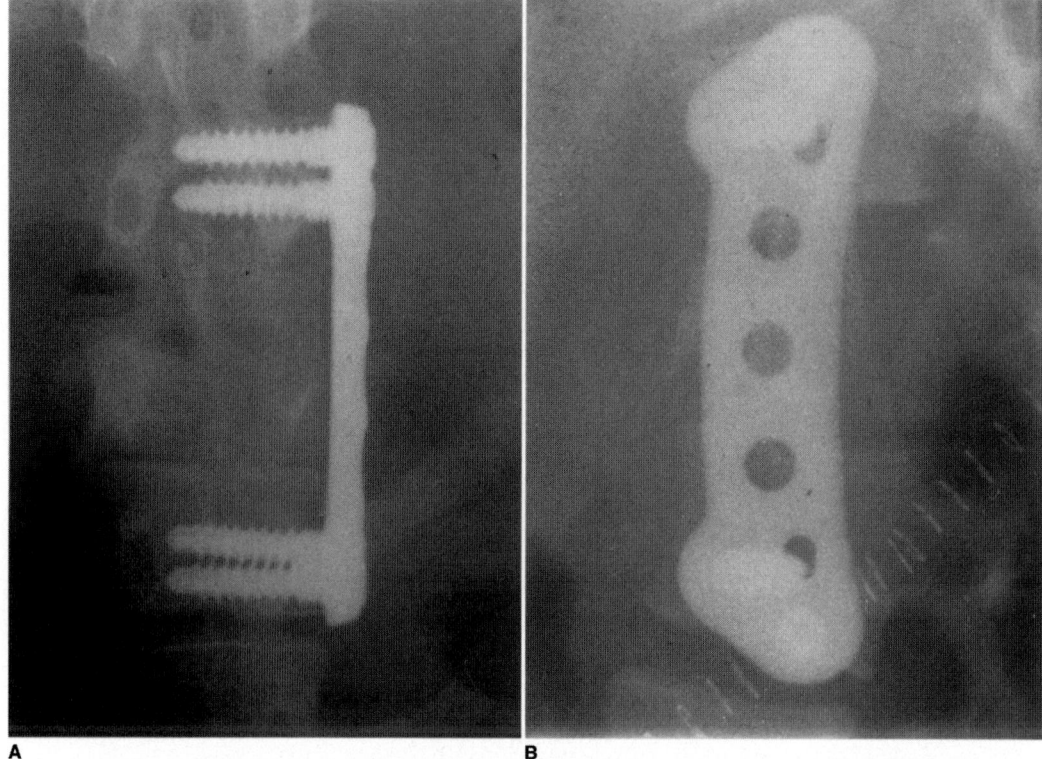

**Figure 114.11** Ventral (**A**) and lateral (**B**) view of the anterior thoracolumbar locking plate (Synthes) with iliac crest bone graft (note convergent path of self-tapping, unicortical screws).

improved implant technology. The recent introduction of commercially available bone morphogenetic protein also ushers in an era of biologic advantage when performing anterior spinal reconstruction and fusion. Compared with more familiar or frequently practiced posterior approaches, there is significant potential for vascular and visceral injury. For surgeons inexperienced in performing thoracotomy, or thoracoabdominal, transperitoneal or retroperitoneal or laparoscopic approaches, consideration of further training may be necessary. Alternatively, working with a thoracic, general, or vascular surgeon allows one to develop an experienced, efficient team for anterior thoracolumbar approaches.

# REFERENCES

1. Alleyne CH, Rodts GE, Haid RW: Corpectomy and stabilization with methylmethacrylate in patients with metastatic disease of the spine. *J Spinal Disord* 8(6): 439-443, 1995.
2. Bracken MB, Shepard MJ, Collins WF, *et al*: A randomized, controlled trial of methylprednisolone or naloxone in the treatment of acute spinal cord injury. *N Engl J Med* 322:1405-1411, 1990.
3. Bracken MB, Shepard MJ, Collins WF, *et al*: Methylprednisolone or naloxone treatment after acute spinal cord injury: 1-year follow up data. *J Neurosurg* 76:23-31, 1992.
4. Brantigan JW, Steffee AD: A carbon fiber implant to aid interbody fusion. *Spine* 18:2106-2117, 1993.
5. Brown LP, Bridwell KH, Holt RT, *et al*: Aortic erosions and lacerations associated with the Dunn anterior spinal instrumentation. *Orthop Trans* 10:16, 1986.
6. Dwyer AP, Newton NC, Sherwood AA: Anterior approach to scoliosis. *Clin Orthop* 62:192-202, 1969.
7. Dwyer AP, O'Brien JP, Seal PP, *et al*: The late complications after the Dwyer anterior spinal instrumentation for scoliosis. *J Bone Joint Surg* 59B:117, 1977.
8. Dwyer AP, Schafer MF: Anterior approach to scoliosis: results of treatment in 51 cases. *J Bone Joint Surg* 56B: 218-224, 1974.
9. Forbes HJ, Allen PW, Waller CS, *et al*: Spinal cord monitoring in scoliosis surgery. *J Bone Joint Surg* 73B: 487-491, 1974.
10. Goto T, Crosby G: Anesthesia and the spinal cord. *Anesthes Clin North Am* 10:493-519, 1992.
11. Hodgson AR, Stock FE: Anterior spinal fusion. A preliminary communication on radical treatment of Pott's disease and Pott's paraplegia. *Br J Surg* 44:266-275, 1956.
12. Humphries AW, Hawk WA, Berndt KL: Anterior fusion of the lumbar spine using an internal fixation device. *J Bone Joint Surg* 41A:371, 1959.
13. Ito H, Tsuchiya J, Asami G: A new radical operation for Pott's disease. *J Bone Joint Surg* 16:499-515, 1934.
14. Levy WJ, York DH: Evoked potentials from the motor tracts in humans. *Neurosurgery* 12:422-429, 1983.
15. Ray CE: Interbody fusion cage instrumentation: Concepts, methods, and results: a comparison of current devices. *J Neurosurg* 82:A351, 1995.

16. Royle ND: The operative removal of an accessory vertebra. *Austr Med J* 1:467, 1928.

17. Zielke K, Stukat R, Beaujean MA: Derotation and fusion-anterior spinal instrumentation. *Orthop Trans* 1:270, 1978.

18. McLaughlin M, Comey CH, Haid RW, *et al:* Laparoscopic anterior lumbar interbody fusion. *Contemp Neurosurg* 20: 1-9, 1998.

19. McLaughlin MR, Zhang JY, Subach BR, *et al:* Laparoscopic anterior lumbar interbody fusion. *Neurosurg Focus* 7(6): Article 8, 1999.

20. Rodts GE, McLaughlin MR, Zhang JY, *et al:* Laparoscopic anterior lumbar interbody fusion. *Clin Neurosurg* 47: 541-556, 2000.

21. Muhlbauer M, Pfisterer W, Eyb R, *et al:* Minimally invasive retroperitoneal approach for lumbar corpectomy and anterior reconstruction. *J Neurosurg* 93(1 suppl):161-167, 2000.

22. Rrajaraman V, Vingan R, Roth P, *et al:* Visceral and vascular complications resulting from anterior lumbar interbody fusion. *J Neurosurg* 91(1 suppl):60-64, 1999.

# CHAPTER 115

# Dorsal Subaxial Cervical Instrumentation Techniques

Vincent C. Traynelis, Kurt M. Eichholz, Joseph F. Cusick, and Regis W. Haid, Jr.

There are many causes of subaxial cervical instability. These include trauma, degenerative disease, neoplasm, and infection. Instability may also develop after spinal canal or foraminal decompression or in conjunction with tumor resection. Historically, the management of such instability first consisted of extended immobilization with traction or an orthosis to maintain proper alignment until bony and/or ligamentous healing transpired. Despite the usefulness of these treatment modalities, they predispose patients to a variety of medical complications. Furthermore, such management does not always result in long-term spinal stability. In 1891, Hadra[16] described the role of spinous process wiring to treat traumatic and inflammatory cervical instability. Subsequently a multitude of cervical fusion techniques that used wires secured to the spinous processes, laminae, and/or facets were reported. Cervical wiring techniques are important in the management of cervical instability.

Sophisticated cervical instrumentation has expanded the surgical capabilities for spinal reconstruction. Cervical fixation devices are particularly useful to treat multiplanar or multisegmental instability. Rigid and semirigid internal stabilization usually provides excellent neural protection until fusion occurs, lessens the number of segments that require fusion, facilitates immediate postoperative mobilization, and minimizes the need for external orthoses. Several dorsal cervical fixation devices have been developed, and each has unique advantages and disadvantages.

This chapter discusses issues pertinent to the application of dorsal cervical instrumentation, including the indications for their use and operative implantation techniques. Specifically, wire fixation, Luque L rod and rectangle constructs, laminar compression clamps, semirigid and rigid lateral mass fixation, hook/rod instrumentation, and pedicle screw fixation are reviewed. Concordant with the overall theme of this text, complication avoidance and management are emphasized here. Although biomechanical concerns are extremely important in the selection of the proper method of stabilization, they are discussed only briefly in this chapter.

## Indications for Surgery

The decision to perform surgery, the operative approach, the need for fusion, and the method by which it is accomplished must be determined on an individual basis. Factors that influence the decision-making process include the patient's overall medical and neurologic condition, the particular pathologic process, the location of the pathology, the degree of instability, and the number of levels affected. These issues, as they pertain to trauma, neoplasia, and degenerative disease, are addressed briefly in this section.

### Trauma

Trauma is a common indication for dorsal cervical stabilization.[1] The primary management of cervical spine injuries consists of realignment (when necessary), decompression of the neural elements (when indicated), and stabilization. In the setting of trauma, if the spine is in good alignment and no decompression is necessary, external immobilization may be all that is required to protect the neural elements while healing occurs. This is particularly true when the major cause of the instability is bony injury. Primary ligamentous instability is much less likely to resolve after immobilization; hence early surgical stabilization is often an appropriate consideration in the management of these injuries.

Instrumentation of the dorsal cervical spine should be considered seriously in all trauma victims who require an open reduction or a dorsal cervical decompression. Persistent dorsal ligamentous instability is most appropriately treated by dorsal surgical stabilization; in fact, it is not unreasonable to offer patients with severe ligamentous injuries internal fixation as an alternative to halo immobilization. Fixation across the afflicted level only is usually successful in achieving long-term stabilization in patients with dorsal ligamentous injuries; however, consideration should be given toward incorporating additional levels into the construct in the setting of severe instability[36] (Figure 115.1). Bony cervical spinal injuries may also be stabilized by using dorsal instrumentation. In particular, lateral mass plates may be used in the presence of laminar and spinous process fractures that often preclude the use of many other types of dorsal fixation.

Extension instability and injuries of the ventral axial spine have been managed successfully by using multilevel dorsal fixation; however, a ventral approach is usually more appropriate. This is particularly true if there is spinal canal compromise from bone or disc fragments or when a burst fracture is associated with 25-degree or greater kyphosis.[13,36]

### Neoplasia

Dorsal cervical instrumentation can be useful in the management of instability associated with neoplasia. If tumor resection is performed via an extensive laminectomy and/or a transpedicular approach, immediate internal stabilization may be accomplished with lateral mass plating. The number of motion segments to be instrumented depends on the location and magnitude of the tumor. In

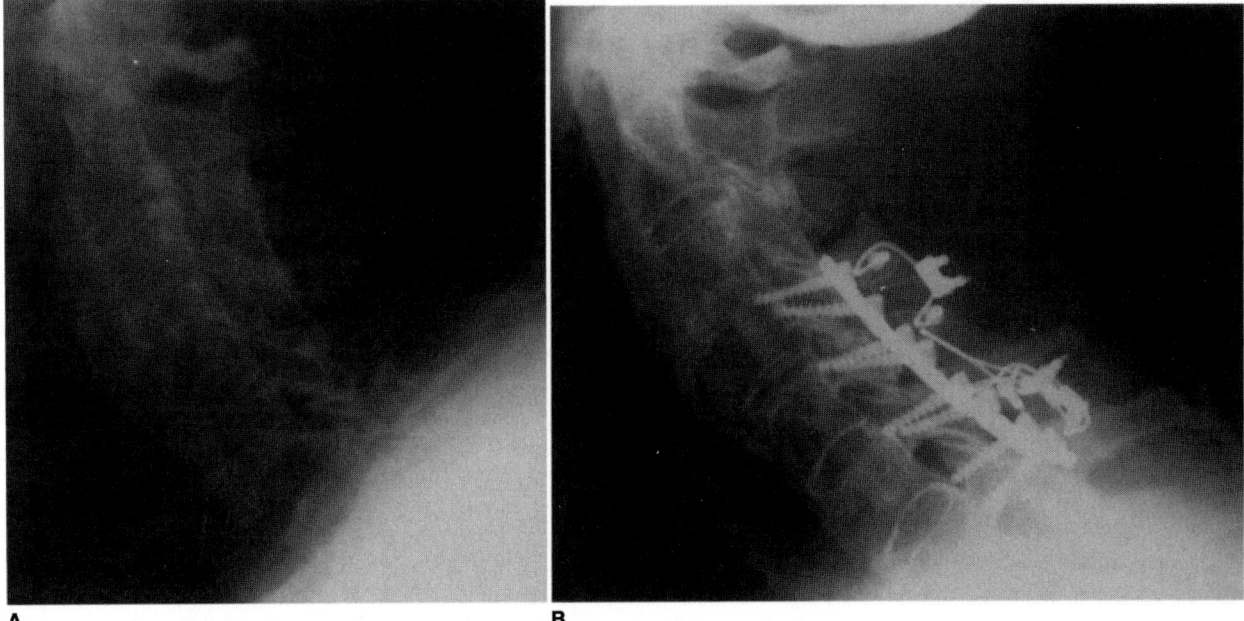

**Figure 115.1** (**A**) Lateral cervical radiograph demonstrating a C5-6 fracture in a patient with ankylosing spondylitis. (**B**) Internal fixation was achieved with lateral mass plates and rib cabled to the spinous processes. The high degree of instability associated with this injury influenced the decision to obtain fixation two levels above and below the injury. Postoperatively the patient wore a rigid orthosis for 2 months. His fusion was noted to be solid 1 year postoperatively.

the setting of malignancy, the surgeon must be certain that solid fixation is achieved well above and below the affected levels. Significant tumor invasion of the vertebral bodies requires a ventral approach not only for decompression but also for stabilization. It should be remembered that the treatment of benign tumors may also result in cervical instability. This is particularly true when preoperative root and/or cord dysfunction is present and a wide exposure is necessary (e.g., with large neurofibromas).

### Spondylosis

Dorsal cervical instrumentation is also useful in the management of spondylotic disease. Proper instrumentation at the time of initial decompression in patients with abnormal segmental motion or absent lordosis markedly decreases their risk of developing postlaminectomy kyphosis. In these cases, instrumentation and subsequent fusion are important to prevent further problems; when a kyphotic deformity has occurred, treatment with dorsal instrumentation alone does not usually provide the optimum result. Almost invariably, ventral spinal reconstruction is the necessary first step needed to correct or halt progressive postlaminectomy kyphotic deformities; dorsal fixation may then be considered as an adjunctive measure in select patients. Dorsal fusion may provide a more successful means of managing patients who experience symptoms from failed ventral arthrodesis than a second ventral surgery.[11,34]

In highly selected cases of severe ventral and dorsal spinal incompetence, a combined or staged "360-degree" operation may be indicated. Generally speaking, such spines are so unstable that reconstruction with instrumentation is preferable to other less-rigid techniques.

### Osteopenia

It is often difficult to maintain alignment and achieve fusion in severely osteopenic patients regardless of the fixation technique. Osteoporosis is a relative contraindication to screw and plate fixation. Osteoporotic spines are also predisposed to wire cutout and instrumentation-associated laminar fractures. The use of rigid external orthotics in such patients aids in maintaining stability while fusion occurs.

## General Considerations

### Imaging

A complete radiographic workup is essential to properly plan and execute any spinal stabilization procedure. This does not mean that every imaging modality must be employed in every patient. Static plain radiographs provide information concerning segmental and overall alignment and bone quality and should always be obtained. Preoperative radiographs also serve as standards against which alignment can be judged after prone positioning and surgery. Dynamic studies (i.e., flexion/extension lateral views) often provide valuable information, particularly in terms of assessing stability. Although dynamic films should be obtained in most patients, they are not universally appropriate, and judgment must be exercised before obtaining flexion/extension radiographs. Specifically, flexion/extension radiographs should not be obtained in the trauma patient until the potential for significant instability has been ruled out with static films and/or scans.

Additionally, the spine should be imaged in the axial plane, and this can be accomplished only by computed tomographic (CT) or magnetic resonance (MR) scans. Such scans can detect bony and ligamentous injuries, assess neural compromise, or identify tumors. They do not just supplement the information gleaned from plain radiographs but are truly instrumental in helping devise and execute the surgical plan.

CT provides better bony detail than MRI and therefore is more useful to define fractures. Instillation of intrathecal contrast markedly enhances the diagnostic value of CT. MR often complements CT in the trauma setting because of its ability to define ligamentous injury.[9] Both modalities are useful to assess the extent of tumor involvement in patients with metastatic malignancies.

Axial images are particularly helpful for determining the best method of dorsal fixation. For example, if relative spinal stenosis is detected, then it is prudent to avoid sublaminar wire or cable passage. Likewise, preoperative information concerning the size of the lateral masses and pedicles and their relationship to the vertebral arteries is useful when considering lateral mass screw fixation.

### Intraoperative Monitoring

If one plans to monitor sensory-evoked potentials and/or motor-evoked potentials intraoperatively, baseline studies should be obtained before surgery whenever possible. The authors rarely employ such monitoring (barring experimental protocols) and question its usefulness in treating cervical pathology other than intrinsic tumors, vascular malformations, or severe deformities.

### Tracheal Intubation

Whenever possible, awake fiberoptic intubations should be performed in patients with significant preoperative instability. Furthermore, this technique allows one to secure the airway with minimal manipulation of the cervical spine and facilitates awake positioning of the patient. Careful intubation under general anesthesia is an alternative to an awake intubation. The head must be held in the neutral position or traction employed if the concern for preoperative instability is real. External orthoses, manual in-line immobilization, and/or axial traction may be used to limit the motion of unstable segments during intubation and positioning.[23,24,29]

### Positioning

The prone position is most frequently used for these operations, and positioning the patient is probably more dangerous, in terms of compromising spinal alignment, than intubation. Awake positioning is a reasonable method of minimizing risk during turning; however, this technique is not advised for uncooperative patients. The surgeon should be responsible for maintaining proper cervical alignment while turning. When the final position is achieved, the neurologic evaluation is repeated immediately. Neurologic deterioration after positioning warrants prompt physical reappraisal of cervical alignment, evaluation of the amount and direction of axial traction, and radiographic examination. It may be preferable to position uncooperative or pediatric patients under general anesthesia. As always, the turn should be performed in a deliberate and controlled manner with care taken to maintain proper cervical alignment. Unstable patients positioned under general anesthesia should have lateral cervical spine films taken immediately after positioning.

Occasionally the sitting position is desired; in fact, it can be particularly advantageous for obese or pregnant patients. Air embolism detection monitoring may be indicated when using the sitting position, and precautions to minimize the risk of air embolism must be taken during positioning and throughout the surgical procedure. This includes the placement of a central venous catheter as well as precordial Doppler. The dorsal cervical spine is effectively exposed when using a midline approach. After the proposed incision is inscribed and the skin is prepared and draped, the dermis and superficial tissue may be infiltrated with epinephrine solution to effect vasoconstriction and thereby facilitate hemostasis. The incision is carried sharply to the ligamentum nuchae. The spinous processes and laminae are exposed via a subperiosteal dissection. The cervical spine should always be exposed gently, and delicate technique is particularly important in the setting of instability or dorsal element fractures.

### Surgical Exposure

The surgical opening should provide adequate visualization, but care should be taken to expose only the levels necessary to safely perform the procedure. Specifically, exposure of articular joints at additional segments should be avoided. It is particularly important to preserve the large ligamentous attachments to the spinous process of the axis whenever possible. These large ligaments are key in preventing postsurgical kyphosis. This will not only reduce the length of the procedure and postoperative discomfort but will also lessen the chance of inadvertently creating instability at an additional, unwanted level. Any dorsal supporting structures, such as the interspinous and supraspinous ligaments, should be left intact whenever possible.

### Bony Fusion

Fusion is always part of a cervical instrumentation procedure, and the segments to be fused should be properly prepared. This entails complete removal of the soft tissues and periosteum from all surfaces that one desires to fuse. The cortex should be scraped with a curette or may be eburnated with a burr. If a drill technique is used, the burr should be of cutting design rather than a diamond. Copious irrigation should be employed while drilling to prevent scorching temperatures, which may inhibit bony fusion. The facet joint is frequently the site of fusion when using dorsal instrumentation. Each facet joint is prepared for fusion by removing all cartilage and scraping or burring the bony joint surfaces. If a dorsal decompression is to be performed as part of the operative procedure, the facet joint is dissected and denuded of cartilage before the laminectomy (or laminectomies) is performed. Theoretically, the longer the spinal cord is protected by the bony and ligamentous dorsal elements, the less the chance of inadvertent intraoperative trauma. Approximation of the bony articular surfaces will result in a successful arthrodesis, but frequently this space is packed with autogenous bone to facilitate fusion.

Corticocancellous bone may be obtained from the cervical laminae if a laminectomy is performed. If spinal canal decompression is not warranted, adequate bone for a facet fusion may be obtained from the cervical or upper thoracic spinous processes. Another alternative is to harvest bone from the dorsal iliac crest or a rib.[30] Corticocancellous bone may also be placed over the dorsal elements.

## Hemostasis

After the fusion construct (graft plus instrumentation) has been placed, intraoperative radiographs may be obtained to ensure proper alignment and document hardware position. Before closure, every reasonable effort should be made to achieve hemostasis. In lieu of bone wax, which inhibits bony fusion, thrombin-soaked Gelfoam (Upjohn, Kalamazoo, MI) can be pressed into denuded bone surfaces. This maneuver can be a great aid for achieving hemostasis and may not decrease the likelihood of achieving a successful fusion. Epidural venous bleeding can be controlled with bipolar electrocautery. Thrombogenic substances such as Surgicel (Johnson & Johnson, Arlington, TX), autogenous muscle, or thrombin-soaked Gelfoam may be placed in the epidural space, but care must be taken not to compress the neural elements.

## Cerebrospinal Fluid Leak

If cerebrospinal fluid (CSF) is noted at any time during the procedure, the site of the leak should be determined. Ideally, all dural defects are closed primarily. If a dural violation cannot be directly repaired, such as may be the case if the defect is located laterally or ventrally, fibrin glue may help seal the leak.[31] If a watertight dural closure is not achieved, wound drains should be avoided. In some situations, lumbar CSF drainage will help decrease the risk of developing a CSF fistula or a pseudomeningocele.

## Wound Closure

The wound should be closed in layers with interrupted suture. Removal of the dorsal portion of a prominent C7 and/or T1 spinous process can be extremely helpful for limiting wound tension in slender patients. If local irradiation has been performed or is anticipated, nonabsorbable suture should be considered, at least for the fascial closure. It may be wise to close the entire wound with such suture in these patients. Wound drain placement should be individualized. A dry wound needs no drain; however, if there is oozing from the raw bone surfaces, it may be prudent to place a drain. This is particularly important if a laminectomy has been performed. All wound drains should be tunneled and exit via a separate stab incision.

## Dorsal Subaxial Cervical Instrumentation Techniques

### Luque Instrumentation

Stainless steel pediatric Luque L rods and Luque rectangles (Zimmer, Warsaw, IN) may be used to stabilize the cervical spine.[26] The rectangular construct provides greater torsional stability than the L rods and is therefore preferable. These devices are not indicated for one- or two-level fixation but rather multilevel stabilization procedures. Ideally, both the rods and the rectangles are segmentally secured to every level traversed; however, this is not always necessary. Luque instrumentation can be used to bridge dorsal element defects such as may occur with metastatic malignancies; however, when using this technique, at least two levels of segmental fixation must be obtained above and below the incompetent region. These devices are most useful for fixation extending to the upper cervical spine or crossing the cervicothoracic junction.

For insertion, the majority of the facet should be exposed at each level one wishes to instrument. It is important to choose a rod or rectangle of correct length. The device should not extend above or below the segments at which arthrodesis is desired. When the proper size is selected, the instrumentation is bent to conform to the normal cervical lordotic curve. After contouring is performed, the surgeon should verify again that the length is appropriate. Luque instrumentation can be secured by using wires or braided cables. Cable is stronger and easier to work with than wire. An effort should be made to obtain segmental fixation at every level to undergo arthrodesis.

Laminar, facet, or spinous process purchase may be used. Cervical sublaminar cables are relatively easy to pass, but their use is associated with risk of neurologic injury. Sublaminar wires should be passed with trepidation in the region of the cervical enlargement of the cord; therefore, sublaminar fixation is often limited to the upper cervical segments (C1, C2), C7, and the upper thoracic spine. Spinal canal stenosis is an absolute contraindication to the use of sublaminar wires and cables. Safe passage of sublaminar wires requires opening the ligamentum flavum and directly visualizing the dura mater.

Sublaminar wires and cables should be passed very carefully by using two hands to push and pull simultaneously. When the wires or cables are passed, they should be held taut with heavy clamps hung over the side of the wound. These maneuvers minimize the risk of ventral displacement of the wire or cable. All wires and cables should be passed without the Luque rods or rectangle in the wound. Some epidural bleeding may occur with the dissection and passage of sublaminar wires and cables, but this often stops as the cables or wires are tightened. If the epidural bleeding persists, hemostatic agents such as thrombin-soaked Gelfoam or oxidized cellulose should be employed.

If sublaminar fixation cannot be obtained, Luque instrumentation may be secured to the lateral masses or the spinous processes. Fixation of Luque instrumentation to an articular mass requires removal of the facet cartilage, entry into the joint space, and drilling of the lateral mass. After removal of the cartilage, a dissector such as a Penfield 1 or a Freer is inserted into the facet joint and a small drill hole made in the inferior articular process at each level to be instrumented. This hole should be placed at midposition of each inferior facet and be oriented perpendicular to the dorsal articular surface. A wire or cable is passed through this hole and the ends secured outside of the wound with a heavy clamp. Before the wires are tightened over the instrumentation, the facet joint is packed with cancellous bone chips. Alternatively, the instrumentation may be secured to the spinous processes with either wires or cables alone or in conjunction with Wisconsin buttons.

Securing the Luque instrumentation to the spine is performed in steps. First, the precontoured device is carefully introduced into the wound, and the previously placed cables or wires are positioned around it. L rods are placed such that the short arm of each L lies beneath the end of the opposite long arm (Figure 115.2). The wires or cables are tightened sequentially. Tightening is done gradually so that opposing levels are tightened concurrently, thereby minimizing torsional forces. Cables can generally be tightened to 6 to 8 inch-pounds of torque, but this value should be individualized. Excess wire or cable should be trimmed

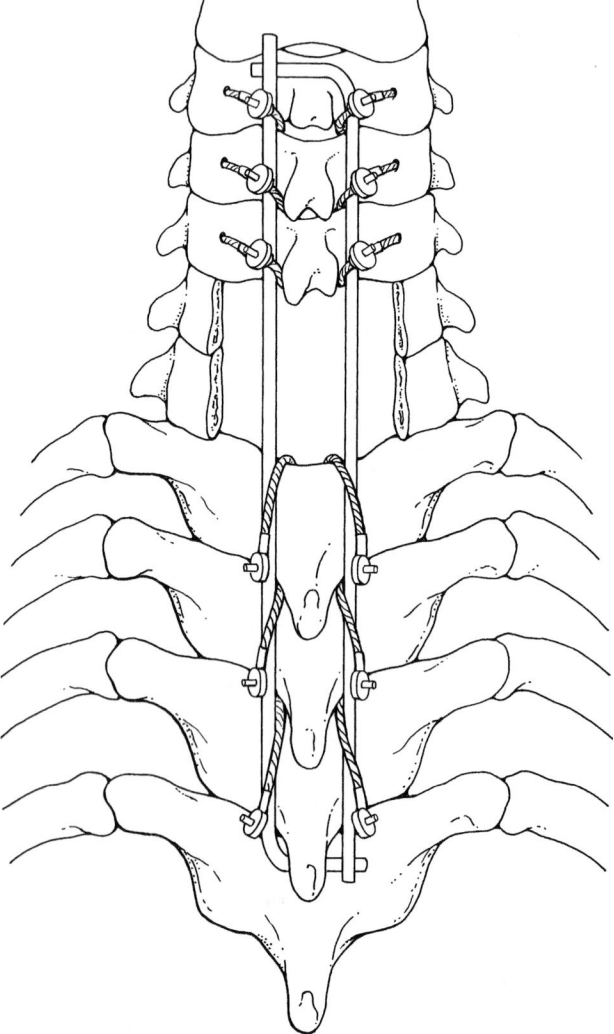

**Figure 115.2** Illustration of the use of Luque L rods for stabilization. This figure depicts a wide two-level laminectomy, as may be performed to remove a metastatic lesion, and subsequent stabilization with Luque L rods. Note how the short arms of the rods are placed under the long arm to improve rotatory stability. Also note that the instrumentation extends several levels above and below the unstable segment and that sublaminar cables are used to secure the thoracic segments while interfacet cable fixation is employed in the cervical region.

appropriately before closure to avoid future wound problems (Figure 115.3). Before closure of the wound, bone grafts may be laid on the laminae and/or the lateral masses.

## Compression Clamps

Another method of internal fixation that requires intact laminae to stabilize adjacent levels across one or two motion segments is the interlaminar compression clamp. These devices include the Halifax clamp (American Medical Electronics, Inc., Richardson, TX) and Apofix (Medtronic Sofamor Danek, Memphis, TN).[5,32] One of the few indications for placement of this device is isolated dorsal ligamentous instability. Although their use in patients with facet injuries and even linear laminar fractures has been reported, they may not be indicated if there is any significant bony injury.[1] There are other contraindications to placement of laminar compression clamps: they should not be used if there is a significant vertebral body injury or in the presence of facet fractures. Lack of ventral column support should be treated with ventral reconstruction, and loss of facet integrity will predispose the cervical spine to rotatory instability that this device is incapable of correcting.

Lateral exposure need only be carried to the medial or central portion of the facet. The pertinent laminae, spinous processes, and dorsal surface of the facets are denuded of periosteum and their bony surfaces prepared, as mentioned previously. The ligamentum flavum is detached from the laminae to be instrumented. For the Halifax instrumentation, appropriately sized clamps are selected and placed temporarily into the wound to estimate the minimal amount the jaws must be opened to pass over the laminae to be instrumented. The clamps are removed from the wound and adjusted accordingly. This maneuver saves time and decreases the amount of "fiddling" within the wound itself. A piece of corticocancellous bone is fashioned such that the dorsally placed clamps will tightly wedge it against the laminae. The clamps are tightened in a controlled, alternating fashion. Although unilateral implantation of cervical laminar compression clamps has been reported, optimum results can only be expected with bilateral fixation.[5]

The Apofix device is somewhat easier to implant. Each sublaminar hook extends into the tubular longitudinal member. The longitudinal tubes are of slightly different diameters, which allows one to telescope into the other. The hooks are set into position, and bone grafts are placed either between the Apofix instrumentation and the laminae or between the spinous processes. A compression instrument is applied, and the clamps are squeezed together. The tubes are secured in the compressed position by a crimper. The excess tube length is trimmed. The Apofix should be implanted bilaterally. Its construct design makes it less likely to rotate out of position than the Halifax clamp.

The bony implant is an extremely important part of the construct. It optimizes the chance of obtaining a successful fusion, which is necessary to avoid delayed instrumentation failure. Biomechanically, the interlaminar or interspinous position of the graft enables the entire construct to resist extension. Although compression clamps

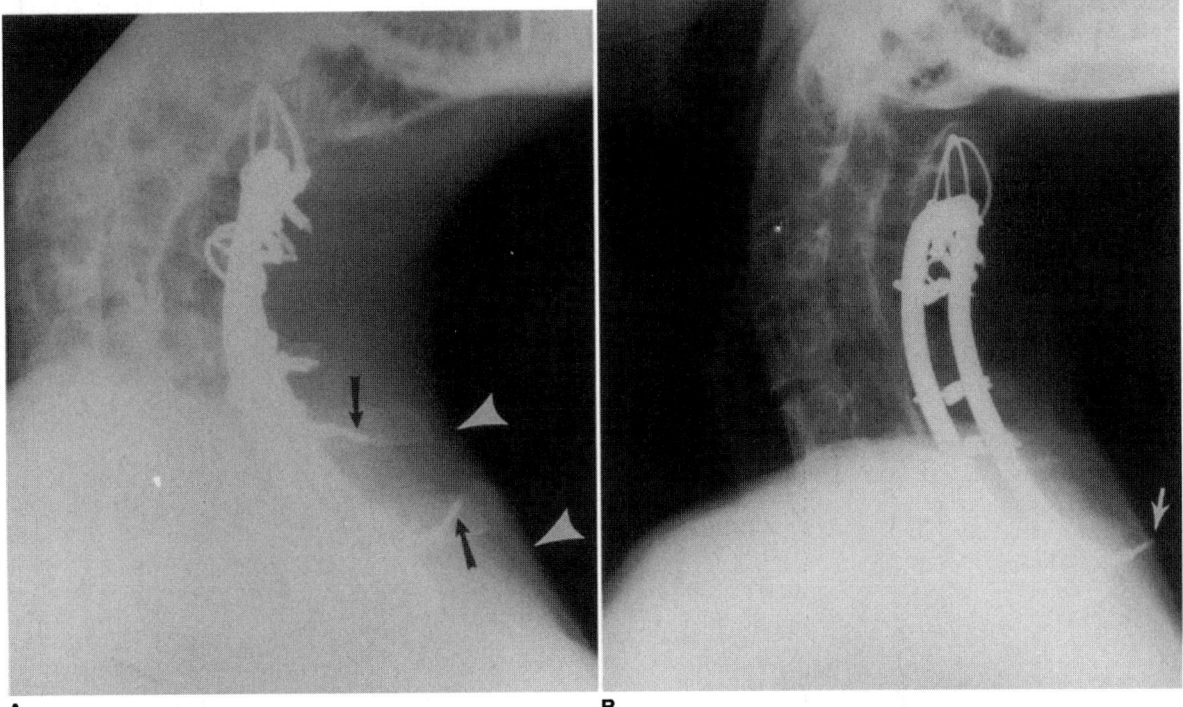

**Figure 115.3** (**A**) Immediate postoperative radiograph of a patient with ankylosing spondylitis and a fracture who was stabilized with a Luque rectangle. Note that the cables are not trimmed flush with the crimps (*arrows*) but they do not reach the surface of the skin (*arrowheads*). (**B**) One year later the inferior cable eroded through to the skin (*arrow*), necessitating a second procedure to trim the cable ends.

provide a resistance only to flexion (tension-band fixation), if some effort is not made to limit extension at the instrumented segment, they can lose their purchase when the patient extends. The graft also helps maintain proper alignment by acting as a "spacer" between the laminae as the clamps are tightened.

The complication rate for these devices is higher at the atlantoaxial level than in the subaxial cervical spine.[5] This is probably due to the large amount of axial rotation that occurs at this level. However, because of the risks of laminar fracture, device dislodgement, and screw loosening associated with laminar compression clamp fixation, the authors believe that if possible, other more effective methods for subaxial dorsal cervical instrumentation should be used.

### Hook/Rod Systems

Immediate multilevel fixation may be achieved by using the hook/rod type systems that have been traditionally applied to the thoracolumbar spine. These devices may be used successfully in select cases of cervicothoracic instability.[8] Recently, rod systems have been developed specifically for the cervical spine. These systems primarily achieve rigid fixation by using lateral mass screws attached to the rods. These rods can also be attached to hooks sized to fit the cervical and upper thoracic laminae.[20,27] Avoidance of hook/rod construct complications in the cervical spine begins with a careful and thoughtful assessment of the true need to place such instrumentation.[15,19,37]

Unlike the thoracolumbar spine, hooks are not usually attached to the pedicles and transverse processes, and cervical fixation is therefore limited to the laminae. When used in the cervical region, these devices are most often applied in compression or as "claw"-type constructs. Pure distraction mode will predispose the cervical spine to kyphosis and is therefore not used.

The application of laminar hooks is described in detail elsewhere in this text. The laminar edge is prepared and a hook inserted. Rods bent to match the cervical lordotic curve are attached to the hooks. Whenever possible, the construct should be cross-linked to increase torsional stability. When instrumenting multiple segments, levels not secured with a hook should be fixed to the rods with sublaminar, facet, or spinous process wires. Care should be taken when designing a hook/rod construct for the cervical spine to avoid crowding the spinal canal significantly with the instrumentation.

### Lateral Mass Plates and Screws

Stabilization of the subaxial cervical spine with lateral mass plates has gained popularity for a variety of reasons.[7,12,13,35] They may be applied from C2 to the upper thoracic spine, and fixation is not dependent on intact laminae or spinous processes. These devices provide superb flexural stability and resist torsion and extension significantly better than wiring constructs.[14] In experienced hands, fusion with lateral mass plates requires significantly less operative time than segmentally wiring rib, iliac crest, or rods to the articular masses. The excellent stability achieved with lateral mass plating can decrease or eliminate the need for postoperative orthotics. Lateral mass plates and screws are more expensive than wire, but this cost may be recouped in decreased operative time and the diminished need for extensive orthotics. They probably also lead to improved patient outcomes.

The disadvantages of lateral mass plate stabilization include the potential for nerve root and vertebral artery injury. As with all cervical plate/screw instrumentation, this instrumentation must be used cautiously in osteoporotic patients, and adequate spinal alignment must be achieved before insertion. Lateral mass plates cannot correct kyphotic deformities, significant translation, or subluxation; therefore, normal lordosis or at least neutral alignment should be achieved before instrumentation. It must always be remembered that these devices are only internal fixators and as such, they are not capable of exerting forces of sufficient magnitude to correct spinal deformities or malalignments.

The standard midline approach described previously is expanded so that the entire lateral mass is exposed at each level to be plated. This is necessary to accurately determine proper screw trajectory. Dislocated facets must be reduced prior to application of instrumentation. The joint space is prepared for fusion as previously described. Occasionally the facet joints may be lax and partly separated. Often this occurs in conjunction with posttraumatic ligamentous instability. In these cases, simple interspinous process wiring approximates and preloads the facet joints, thereby rectifying this problem. If an interspinous process wire is used, it can be left after plating to augment flexural stability. If the dorsal elements are incompetent, approximation of separated facets should be attempted with positional adjustments, if possible.

At this point, a plate is selected for implantation. When using plating systems with different sized plates, the smallest plate that will allow a screw to be inserted into each of the lateral masses to be instrumented should be chosen. Symmetric plates should be placed bilaterally and contoured to match normal cervical lordosis when possible. If normal lordosis cannot be achieved and the spine is in neutral alignment, the plates are inserted without bending. They should never be bent into kyphosis. When a three-hole plate is used to bridge a fractured facet joint or pedicle, no hole or screw is placed at the injured site. If the contralateral facet is not fractured, the middle screw should be placed on that side.

Next, screw holes are drilled into the lateral masses. Several screw trajectories have been used. Based on anatomic, biomechanical, and clinical observations, the authors believe the best trajectory begins 1mm medial to the midportion of the lateral mass and is oriented 15 degrees rostral and 20 to 30 degrees lateral (Figure 115.4). Although a screw may be placed into C7 by using the above angles, the lateral mass of this vertebra is very small. If C7 lateral mass fixation is desired, it may be more appropriate to drill by using trajectories that are slightly more rostral and lateral. It is often preferable to obtain pedicle fixation at C7 (as well as at T1). The pedicle may be entered 1mm caudal to the facet joint. Drilling may continue in a directly ventral course, but a trajectory that

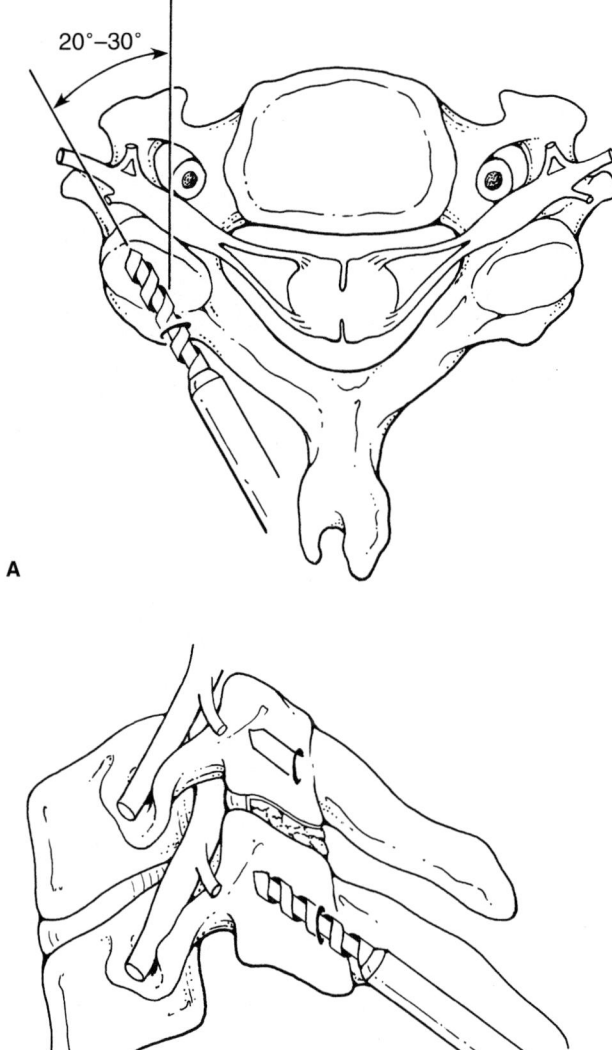

**Figure 115.4** (A) Lateral trajectory for subaxial articular mass drilling. (B) Sagittal trajectory for articular mass drilling. Note that the facet joint is packed with autogenous bone.

angles medially 25 to 30 degrees is more consistent with the anatomic position of the pedicle. The orientation is perpendicular to the long axis of the spine at C7, T1, and T2[6,10] (Figure 115.5). It is the author's practice to verify the position of the pedicle by palpation through a small laminoforaminotomy prior to drilling in all cases.

Screws may also be placed into the pars interarticularis of the axis. This technique is more difficult than placing lateral mass screws, and precision is required to avoid vertebral artery injury. The drill entry site is high and medial on the articular mass. The trajectory is as great as 15 degrees from the medial plane and is about 35 degrees from the long axis of the spine[6,28] (Figure 115.6). Fluoroscopy is not necessary for subaxial lateral mass drilling and screw placement, but should be used when instrumenting the C2 pars.

The authors believe that each hole should be optimally positioned in the lateral mass. This means that the holes are made with reference to the patient's individual anatomy

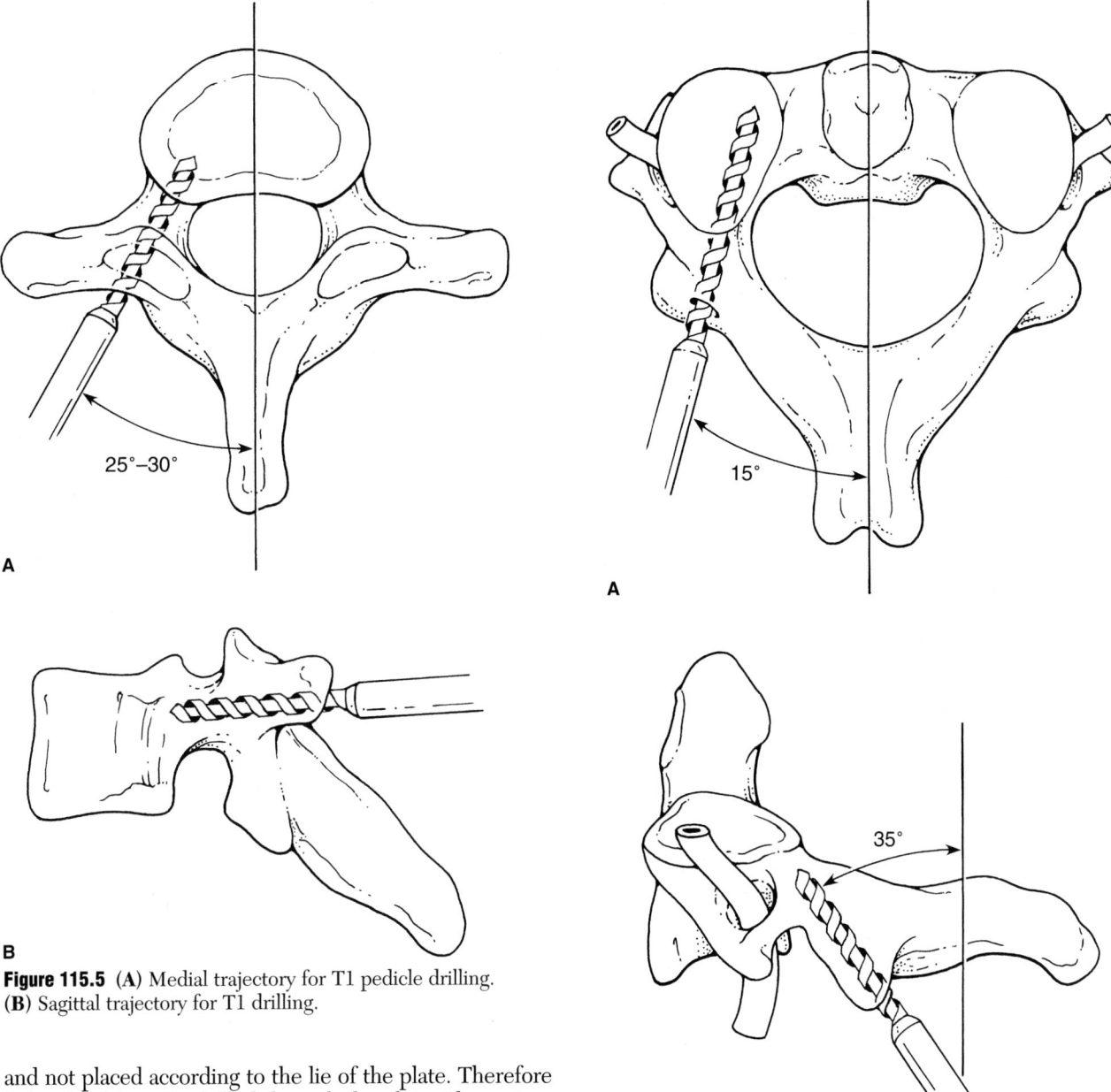

**Figure 115.5 (A)** Medial trajectory for T1 pedicle drilling.
**(B)** Sagittal trajectory for T1 drilling.

**Figure 115.6 (A)** Medial trajectory for drilling of the C2 pars interarticularis. **(B)** Sagittal trajectory for drilling the C2 pars interarticularis.

and not placed according to the lie of the plate. Therefore holes should not be drilled through the plate. The various plate designs accommodate properly placed screws. The dorsal cortex of the lateral mass is perpendicularly pierced with an awl or drill bit to facilitate initial drilling and limit the potential for deviation from the proposed trajectory. One should use a drill bit that incorporates a depth stop, usually at 15 to 16mm. The diameter of the drill bit must comply with the manufacturer's recommendation for the particular screw to be implanted. Drilling is performed in a precise and steady manner to limit vibration and inadvertent creation of an irregular or oversized hole. Occasionally the drill bit will be felt to penetrate the ventral cortex before its entire length is used. In this situation, drilling should stop. All of the holes on one side should be drilled and prepared and a plate placed before drilling the opposite side. The screws used for lateral mass fixation are most frequently 3.5mm in diameter. Cancellous screws provide better purchase than those with cortical threads. The specific screw type used, however, is generally dictated by the plate system used. If the screw is not self-tapping, at least

the dorsal cortex should be tapped before screw insertion. Safe bicortical fixation is usually achieved with 15 to 16mm screws. Only rarely are longer screws necessary, and shorter screws are appropriate for smaller patients. Although bicortical fixation is considered superior to unicortical fixation, it is not mandatory. The plate is secured to C2 with 4mm diameter cortical screws.[28,33] Primary pedicle fixation may be achieved with 4mm screws.

After drilling all of the appropriate levels on a single side, the plate is secured to that side. The screws are secured as symmetrically as possible, with care taken to not tighten any screw greater than 80% before placing the contralateral plate. When one plate is secured, the contralateral side is drilled, the second plate placed, and final screw tightening performed. Inadequate screw purchase may result from osteoporosis, an excessively large hole secondary to inadvertent toggling during drilling, or stripping of threads in the corticocancellous bone during tapping or screw placement. Frequently, in these cases, a "rescue" screw of slightly larger diameter will improve bony purchase.[25] These are not placed without risk, however, because they may result in a fracture of the lateral mass. Alternatively, a small amount of polymethyl methacrylate may be placed in the hole before screw tightening. Cervical transfacet screws are an excellent choice for salvaging fixation if a lateral mass screw strips. The purchase achieved by these screws is excellent.[22]

In selected cases, one may wish to place additional graft material over the dorsal elements after denuding their periosteum and burring the dorsal cortical surface.

### Subaxial Rod Fixation

Recently, rods have been rigidly secured to the lateral masses of the cervical spine.[27] The rods may be attached to either fixed or polyaxial screws. The screws are placed either in the lateral masses or the pedicles as described previously. These systems are a little more difficult to implant than lateral mass plates, but they offer several advantages. Optimal screw positioning is guaranteed. Some systems have cross-links and hooks. The cross-fixators increase the overall rigidity, and placing a hook at the caudal level will minimize the chance of screw backout at that vertebral segment.

Rods may also be secured to cervical pedicle screws, and a number of surgeons have reported excellent results with pedicle screw fixation. Because lateral mass fixation is successful in almost all patients and has little risk, we do not advocate pedicle fixation from C3 to C6 except in unusual circumstances.[2-4]

## Postoperative Care

Thoughtful preoperative planning and strict adherence to meticulous surgical technique limit complications; however, complications invariably occur, even in the hands of the most careful and experienced surgeon. Some particular considerations are important to address complications in patients who undergo dorsal cervical fusion.

Immediate postoperative radiographs may be obtained to ensure proper cervical alignment and hardware position. If there is any deterioration in the patient's neurologic condition after surgery, a complete work-up is indicated. Although titanium alloy hardware is compatible with radiographic and magnetic imaging, these constructs still cause some artifact and may obscure pathology. If there is any question regarding postoperative spinal canal or neural foraminal compromise or hardware complication in a patient with neurologic deterioration, it may be prudent to obtain a myelogram or CT or reexplore the wound.

Postoperatively, patients should be mobilized in a progressive but cautious manner. Frequent radiographic assessment should be performed to ensure stability of the spinal construct. Appropriate external orthoses should supplement the internal fixation if there is preoperative instability or the bony purchase is suboptimal. If instability in a single plane of motion exists preoperatively and the surgeon is confident that the fixation is solid, then either no bracing or a cervical collar may be appropriate. A 360-degree procedure or more rigid external orthosis such as a halo vest may be needed when dealing with gross multiplanar instability or when the integrity of the construct is in question. The duration of external cervical immobilization is also individualized.

## Complication Management

Postoperative complications may be subdivided into the following groups: general, neurologic, and spinal. Postoperative hematomas, CSF leaks, and wound infections are examples of general complications.

### General Complications

Large postoperative wound hematomas can cause significant neurologic impairment. Smaller clots predispose the patient to infection by acting as a culture medium. Before closure, every effort must be made to achieve adequate hemostasis. Avoidance of hypertension, wound elevation, and correction of coagulopathies help limit intraoperative hemorrhage. Thrombin-soaked Gelfoam can help decrease bone bleeding. Epidural venous hemorrhage may occur after a laminectomy or after passage of sublaminar wires. Whenever possible, it should be controlled with bipolar coagulation and hemostatic agents. Epidural bleeding associated with sublaminar instrumentation is usually self-limited and stops prior to wound closure. In very rare cases, such bleeding is brisk and does not cease, in which case one should consider exposing the spinal canal and directly attacking the source of hemorrhage.

Maintenance of a subperiosteal dissection plane minimizes muscle bleeding. Most significant muscular bleeding comes from violation of small and medium-sized veins. Bleeding from these vessels can be controlled by the pressure exerted by wound retractors. When the retractors are removed, the wound must be irrigated several times and a Valsalva maneuver performed by the anesthetist so these potential sources of postoperative hemorrhage may be identified and cauterized. If a small amount of wound oozing continues despite all efforts to stop it, and there is no CSF leak, then postoperative drainage should be used.

Frequent and regular wound inspection in the early postoperative period allows for the early identification of complications such as a wound infection or CSF fistula. Wound infections should be treated as soon as they are recognized. Antibiotic coverage is guided by Gram stain and culture results. Any fluid accumulations should be drained. Areas of loculated infection or regions of devitalized tissue should be treated surgically. If an infection occurs, it may not be necessary to remove implanted hardware, particularly if expeditious treatment is rendered. When an infection persists despite antibiotic coverage, or if the construct integrity is threatened or compromised by significant osteomyelitis, it may be necessary to remove the instrumentation. If the instrumentation must be removed, immobilization, external orthosis, or traction may be used to manage instability. Rarely, a ventral stabilization procedure may be useful in these cases. It should be noted that metallic instrumentation may not be threatened by infection and does not usually need to be removed. This is particularly true when the infection remains superficial to the fascia.

The management of intraoperative CSF leaks has been discussed. Postoperative leakage of CSF from the wound should be treated aggressively with surgical reexploration accompanied by lumbar CSF drainage. The possibility of a wound infection must always be considered and definitively ruled out in these patients.

## Neurologic Complications

Neurologic complications may be immediate or delayed. The workup of new postoperative neurologic deficits should proceed with great urgency. The possible causes of immediate deficits are numerous. Many instrumentation-related causes of neurologic deficit may be determined radiographically, but the evaluation of these patients must be individualized. Delayed neurologic complications are more likely to be due to instrumentation failures, loss of reduction, or infection. Although evaluation of delayed deficits is dictated by the specific clinical presentation, all such cases should be promptly investigated and appropriate treatment instituted.

Placement of instrumentation may result directly in neurologic compromise. Spinal cord injuries secondary to sublaminar fixation almost invariably present in the immediate postoperative period. The only effective treatment for such injuries is prevention. Sublaminar wires should not be passed over the cervical enlargement or in patients with stenotic canals, and great care must be taken when sublaminar wires or cables are placed in the upper or lower cervical segments.

Lateral mass screws have the potential to compress or injure the nerve roots, spinal cord, and vertebral artery. Spinal cord injury secondary to lateral mass screws has not been reported to our knowledge. Anatomic studies support the concept that the spinal cord is not placed at any great risk from lateral mass screw placement. The direction of drill trajectory and screw placement is important for limiting the risk of arterial or root injury. Roy-Camille et al.[28] advocate a screw position that begins at the center of the lateral mass, is oriented perpendicular to the long axis of the spine, and is angled 10 degrees laterally. The Magerl technique involves placement of the screw 2 to 3mm medial and rostral to the center of the lateral mass and a trajectory that runs parallel to the facet joint and is angled 25 degrees laterally.[21] Anderson et al.[7] suggest screw placement 1mm medial to the center of the lateral articular mass with trajectory parallel to the facet joints and oriented 10 degrees laterally from the sagittal plane, whereas Cooper et al.[12] recommend placement of the screws 1mm medial to the center of the lateral articular mass and oriented 10 degrees laterally but perpendicular to the long axis of the spine.

Overall, there seems to be a general agreement that the screw trajectory should be at least 10 degrees laterally and oriented no more rostral than the articular surface of the facet joint to minimize the risk of inadvertent injury to the nerve root or vertebral artery.[6,17] Cadaveric studies that use such a trajectory suggest that the predicted rates of injury to the nerve roots and vertebral artery would be 3.6% or less and 0%, respectively.[17] The actual clinical incidence of nerve root injury secondary to screw placement is much less. In a review of 704 lateral mass screw placements in 79 patients, Heller et al.[18] reported a 0.6% rate of nerve root injury.

Nerve root injury is usually not appreciated at the time of drilling and screw placement. Somatosensory-evoked potential monitoring of the ulnar and median nerves may help provide intraoperative feedback in the future. Currently, however, the overlap in nerve root innervation of these nerves hampers the sensitivity of this method. Intraoperative root stimulation is another technique that may become useful in the future. Patients with postoperative radiculopathy secondary to malpositioned screws usually improve significantly with removal of the offending screw.

Despite the fear of vertebral artery injury with lateral mass screw placement, it has not been reported with certainty that this has occurred. Lateral angling of the screws is important to minimize the risk of vascular compromise. Vertebral artery injury may or may not be recognized at the time of surgery. There is usually bleeding from the drill hole in the lateral mass, and at times the flow may seem brisk; however, it should never be pulsatile or appear to be under high pressure. When arterial hemorrhage is noted after lateral mass drilling, an attempt may be made to control the hemorrhage by placement of thrombogenic substances and bone wax in the drill hole. A screw may be placed in the hole to control bleeding. Screw placement is not unreasonable if one assumes that (if vertebral artery injury has indeed occurred) the drill has already significantly lacerated the vertebral artery. If the bleeding is refractory to these measures, it may be necessary to expose the vertebral artery for primary repair or occlusion. No contralateral drilling or screw placement should be performed if a vertebral artery injury is suspected intraoperatively, and the patient must be examined immediately on conclusion of the procedure. Vertebral artery injury or occlusion may not be apparent immediately. The development of delayed posterior circulation deficits should alert the surgeon to this possibility. The authors recommend prompt angiographic evaluation of suspected vertebral artery injuries.

## Spinal Complications

Postoperative spinal complications usually, but not always, concern failure to maintain immediate or long-term stability. Poorly conceived stabilization procedures probably account for most dorsal cervical construct failures (Figure 115.7). Instrumentation should be applied judiciously in osteoporotic patients, and in such individuals a 360-degree approach or postoperative external immobilization is very important. Preoperative evaluation and planning are important to ensure that the proposed construct is biomechanically appropriate for the clinical situation.

When dealing with trauma, the operative approach should be designed to counteract the predominant force vectors that resulted in the original injury. For example, one

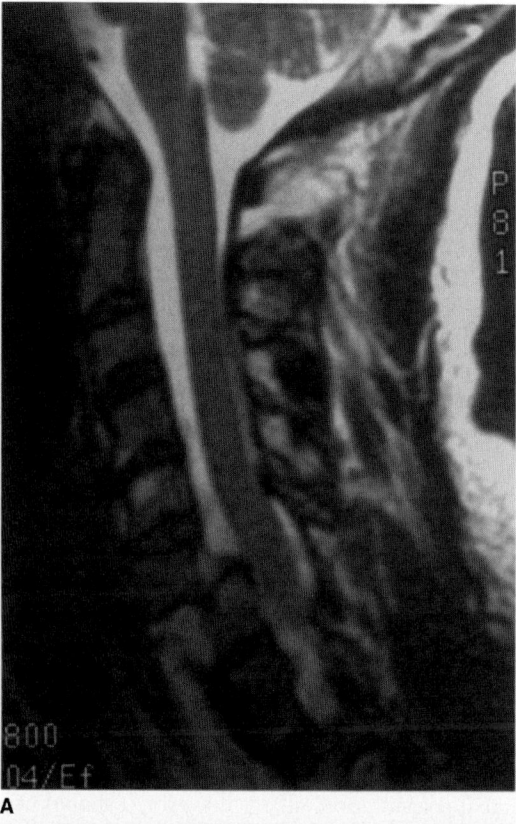

**A**

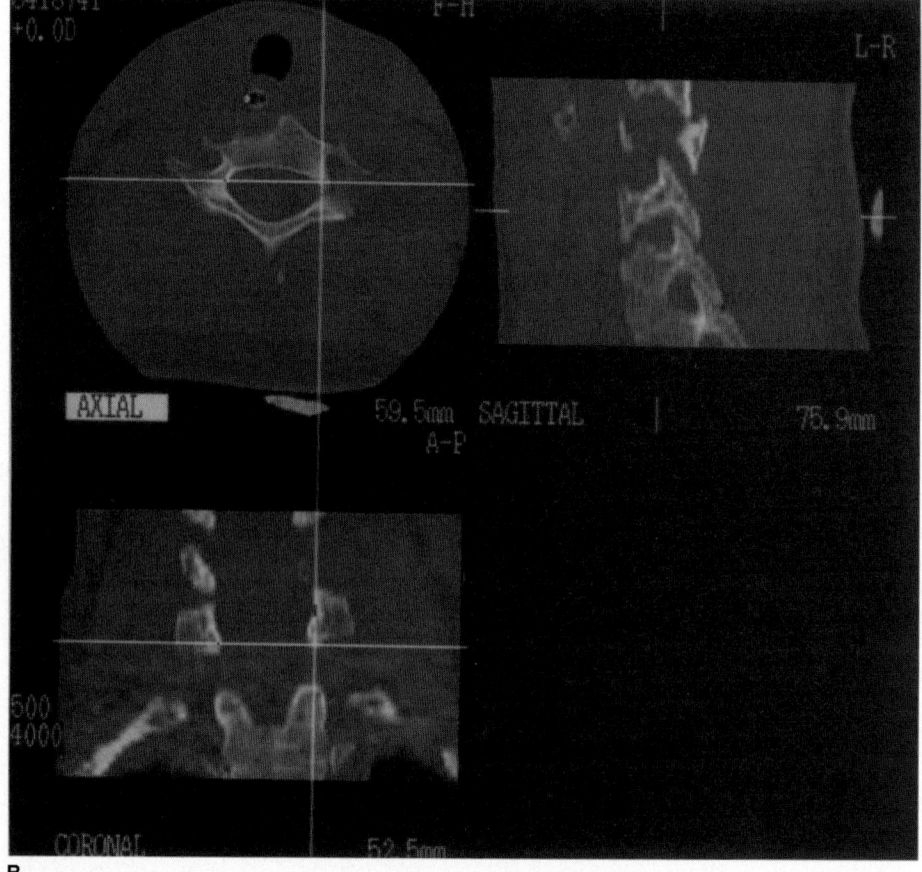

**B**

**Figure 115.7** Severe C6-7 fracture dislocation in a patient with only minor neurologic deficit. (**A**) MR scan on admission demonstrates significant ventral and dorsal injury. (**B**) Reconstructed CT images demonstrate complete loss of left C6 facet integrity.

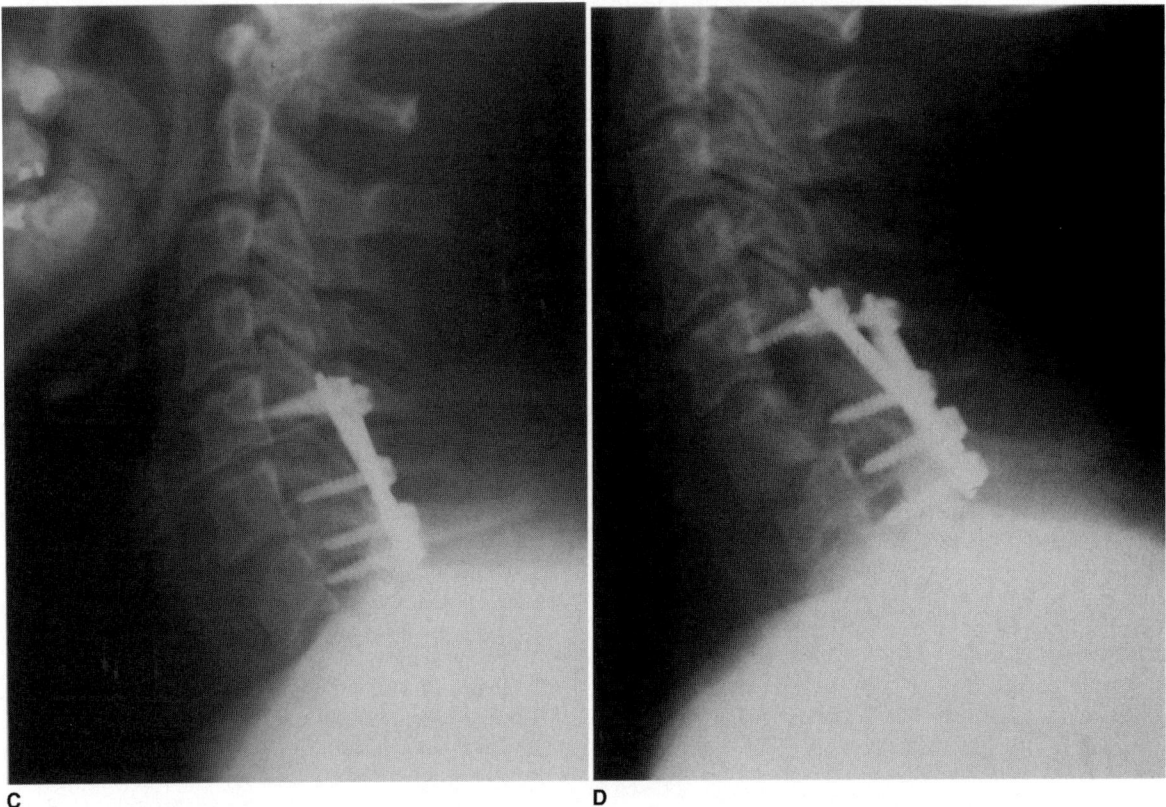

C D

**Figure 115.7 *cont'd* (C)** After realignment, lateral mass plate stabilization was performed and the patient was immobilized in a halo for 3 months. **(D)** Lateral radiograph after halo removal demonstrates resubluxation. This loss of reduction could probably have been prevented by either a 360-degree stabilization procedure or by extending the levels of dorsal fixation.

would not wish to impose additional extension forces by the use of compression clamps in a patient who had incurred mainly an extension type of injury irrespective of whether this was associated with compression or distraction.

Instrumentation failure may occur without clinical consequence.[36] Heller *et al.*[18] observed a 1.3% rate of plate breakage over an average follow-up of 1.5 years. In the same review, the following incidences of screw complications were noted: breakage 0.1%, avulsion 0.1%, and loosening 0.9%. Minor instrumentation failures (i.e., 1mm screw loosening) or those that occur many months after surgery (i.e., single wire breakage) often do not require treatment. Significant or early postoperative instrumentation failures and loss of reduction must be addressed. The management options include institution of rigid external immobilization, bed rest, and/or cervical traction during healing, or reoperation (either repeat dorsal approach or ventral instrumentation). The decision for appropriate treatment must be made on an individual basis, taking into consideration the patient's condition and prognosis, degree of bony union and instability, and rationale for initial choice of dorsal surgical stabilization.

## Summary

Dorsal cervical instrumentation systems that are appropriately selected for the clinical problem, and properly implanted, generally produce excellent results and enjoy a low rate of complication. As with all surgical procedures, the complication rate is related to experience. Before using any of the techniques mentioned in this chapter, surgeons should acquaint themselves fully with the instrumentation and obtain adequate preoperative instruction if they are unfamiliar with the proposed procedure.

Some of the instrumentation systems described in this chapter are currently categorized as Class III devices by the United States Food and Drug Administration. Surgeons should be aware of the classification of the instrumentation to be implanted and relay this information to the patient during the preoperative discussion. Most internal fixation devices are classified as temporary devices. Temporary is defined as intended to be implanted more than 30 days but not intended to be implanted permanently. The Orthopedic Surgical Manufacturer's Association recommends that, whenever possible and practical, bone fixation devices should be removed when their service as an aid to healing is completed; however, the general clinical opinion is that cervical instrumentation that leads to successful fusion without complication does not need to be removed. Each patient should receive preoperative counseling concerning this difference of opinion. When patients understand the risks of repeat surgery yet request removal of hardware after bone fusion has occurred, every attempt should be made to comply with their wishes.

# REFERENCES

1. Abdu WA, Bohlman HH: Techniques of subaxial posterior cervical spine fusion: an overview. *Orthopedics* 15:287, 1992.

2. Abumi K, Kaneda K: Pedicle screw fixation for nontraumatic lesions of the cervical spine. *Spine* 22(16):1853-1863, 1997.

3. Abumi K, Kaneda K, Shono Y, Fujiya M: One-stage posterior decompression and reconstruction of the cervical spine by using pedicle screw fixation systems. *J Neurosurg* 90(1 Suppl):19-26, 1999.

4. Abumi K, Shono Y, Ito M, *et al*: Complications of pedicle screw fixation in reconstructive surgery of the cervical spine. *Spine* 25(8):962-969, 2000.

5. Aldrich EF, Crow WN, Weber PB, Sagnolia TN: Use of MR imaging-compatible Halifax interlaminar clamps for posterior cervical fusion. *J Neurosurg* 74:185, 1991.

6. An HS, Gordin R, Renner K: Anatomic considerations for plate-screw fixation of the cervical spine. *Spine* 16:S548, 1991.

7. Anderson PA, Henley MB, Grady MS, *et al*: Posterior cervical arthrodesis with reconstruction plates and bone graft. *Spine* 3:S72, 1991.

8. Ashman RB, Herring JA, Johnston CE II, *et al*: TSRH *Universal Spinal Instrumentation*. Dallas, Hundley and Associates, 1993.

9. Benzel EC, Hart BL, Ball P, *et al*: Fractures of the C-2 vertebral body. *J Neurosurg* 81:206, 1994.

10. Borne G, Bedou G, Pinaudeau M, *et al*: Treatment of severe lesions of the lower cervical spine (C3-C7). A clinical study and technical considerations in 102 cases. *Neurochirurgia (Stuttg)* 31:1, 1988.

11. Brodsky AE, Khalil MA, Sassard WR, Newman BP: Repair of symptomatic pseudarthrosis of anterior cervical fusion. Posterior versus anterior approach. *Spine* 17:1137, 1992.

12. Cooper PR, Cohen A, Rosiello A, Koslow M: Posterior stabilization of cervical spine fractures and subluxations using plates and screws. *Neurosurgery* 23:300, 1988.

13. Fehlings MG, Cooper PR, Errico TJ: Posterior plates in the management of cervical instability: long-term results in 44 patients. *J Neurosurg* 81:341, 1994.

14. Goel VK, Traynelis VC, Smith DW, Scifert JL: In vitro quasi-static and cyclic biomechanics of a cervical posterior plate vs facet wiring in a laminectomy model. Presented at the International Mechanical Engineering Congress & Exposition, Anaheim, CA, November 1998.

15. Graham AW, Swank ML, Kinard RE, *et al*: Posterior cervical arthrodesis and stabilization with a lateral mass plate. Clinical and computed tomographic evaluation of lateral mass screw placement and associated complications. *Spine* 21:323-329, 1996.

16. Hadra BE: Wiring the vertebrae as a means of immobilization in fractures and Pott's disease. *Trans Am Orthop Assoc* 4:206, 1981.

17. Heller JG, Carlson GD, Abitbol J-J, Garfin SR: Anatomic comparison of the Roy-Camille and Magerl techniques for screw placement in the lower cervical spine. *Spine* 16:S552, 1991.

18. Heller JG, Silcox H, Sutterlin C III: Complications of posterior cervical plating. Presented at the 22nd Annual Meeting of the Cervical Spine Research Society, Baltimore, MD, November/December 1994.

19. Heller JG, Silcox DH III, Sutterlin CE III: Complications of posterior cervical plating. *Spine* 20:2442-2448, 1995.

20. Horgan MD, Kellog JX, Chestnut RM: Posterior cervical arthrodesis and stabilization: an early report using a novel lateral mass screw and rod technique. *Neurosurgery* 44:1267-1272, 1999.

21. Jeanneret B, Magerl F, Ward EH, Ward J: Posterior stabilization of the cervical spine with hook plates. *Spine* 16:S56, 1991.

22. Klekamp JW, Ugbo JL, Heller JG, Hutton WC: Cervical transfacet versus lateral mass screws: a biomechanical comparison. *J Spinal Disord* 13(6):515-518, 2000.

23. Lennarson PJ, Smith DW, Sawin PD, *et al*: Cervical spinal motion during intubation: efficacy of stabilization maneuvers in the setting of complete segmental instability. *J Neurosurg (Spine 2)* 94:265-270, 2001.

24. Lennarson PJ, Smith D, Todd MM, *et al*: Segmental cervical spine motion during orotracheal intubation of the intact and injured spine with and without external stabilization. *J Neurosurg (Spine 2)* 92:201-206, 2000.

25. Lovick DS, Ryken TC, Traynelis VC, Dexter F: Assessment of primary and salvage lateral mass screw insertion torque in a cadaveric model. *J Spinal Disord* 10:431-435, 1997.

26. Maurer PK, Ellenbogen RG, Ecklund J, *et al*: Cervical spondylotic myelopathy: treatment with posterior decompression and Luque rectangle bone fusion. *Neurosurgery* 28:680, 1991.

27. Mummaneni PV, Haid RW, Traynelis VC, *et al*: Posterior cervical fixation using a new polyaxial screw and rod system: technique and surgical results. *Neurosurg Focus* 12(1): Article 8, 2002.

28. Roy-Camille R, Saillant G, Mazel C: Internal fixation of the unstable cervical spine by a posterior osteosynthesis with plate and screws. In Sherk H, Dunn E, Eismont F, *et al* (eds): *The Cervical Spine,* ed 2. Philadelphia, Lippincott-Raven, 1989, p 390.

29. Sawin PD, Todd MM, Traynelis VC, *et al*: Cervical spine motion with direct laryngoscopy and orotracheal intubation: an in vivo cinefluoroscopic study of subjects without cervical abnormality. *Anesthesiology* 85:26-36, 1996.

30. Sawin PD, Traynelis VC, Menezes AH: A comparative analysis of fusion rates and donor-site morbidity for autogeneic rib and iliac crest bone grafts in posterior cervical fusions. *J Neurosurg* 88:255-265, 1998.

31. Shaffrey CI, Spotnitz WD, Shaffrey ME, Jane JA: Neurosurgical applications of fibrin glue: augmentation of dural closure in 134 patients. *Neurosurgery* 26:207, 1990.

32. Statham P, O'Sullivan M, Russel T: The Halifax clamp for posterior cervical fusion: initial experience in the United Kingdom. *Neurosurgery* 32: 396, 1993.

33. Sutterlin CE III: Axis fixation system for posterior cervical reconstruction. In Hitchon PW, Rengachary SS, Traynelis VC (eds): *Spinal Fusion and Stabilization*. New York, Thieme Medical Publishers, 1995, p 159.

34. Swank ML, Lowery GL, Vega J, *et al*: Salvage reconstruction of failed anterior cervical surgeries. Presented at the 22nd Annual Meeting of the Cervical Spine Research Society, Baltimore, MD, November/December 1994.

35. Swank ML, Sutterlin CE III, Bossons CR, *et al*: Rigid internal fixation with lateral mass plates in multilevel

anterior and posterior reconstruction of the cervical spine. *Spine* 22:274-282, 1997.

36. Traynelis VC: Anterior and posterior plate stabilization of the cervical spine. *Neurosurgery* 2:59, 1992.

37. Wellman BJ, Follett KA, Traynelis VC: Complications of posterior articular mass plate fixation of the subaxial cervical spine in 43 consecutive patients. *Spine* 23:193-200, 1998.

# CHAPTER 116

# Dorsal Thoracic and Lumbar Screw Fixation and Pedicle Fixation Techniques

**Andrea L. Halliday, Mehmet Zileli, Charles B. Stillerman, and Edward C. Benzel**

The popularity of pedicle screw fixation has significantly increased in the last two decades. Pedicle screw fixation is the only spinal fixation strategy that engages all three columns of the spine. The pedicle screw-bone junction provides the strongest point of attachment of instrumentation to the spine. Thus, pedicle screw fixation systems can resist motion in all planes.[1] In addition, pedicle screw systems do not require the presence of intact dorsal elements. A historic cohort study with the participation of 303 surgeons and 3498 patients has shown that the use of pedicle screws is a safe and effective form of treatment for spinal disorders.[56]

## History

Toumey[52] in 1943 and King[27] in 1944 provided the first descriptions of the use of bone screws to obtain internal fixation at the time of fusion. Their techniques for lumbosacral fusion involved passing a screw from medial to lateral across the facet of the involved level bilaterally. Their screws were short and designed to cross the facet joint only. Pseudarthrosis rates were unacceptably high with this method of fixation.[44] For this reason, Boucher[8] modified their technique by using a longer screw that crossed the facet joint into the pedicle and body of the vertebra below. Boucher[54] was the first to use pedicle screws. The pseudarthrosis rate for this technique, including multilevel fusions, was 14% to 17%.[22,44] Magerl[34] introduced another variation of facet screws in which a screw was passed from one side of the spinous process into the opposite lamina between its two tables, across the facet joint to the base of the transverse process. One disadvantage of the Magerl technique was that it required intact laminae.

Harrington[23] initially used facet screws at multiple levels to correct scoliosis in polio patients but found that this instrumentation eventually failed. This failure led to the development of Harrington instrumentation. Harrington[24] first used screws inserted into the pedicles of L5 attached to Harrington distraction rods by heavy stainless steel wire for the reduction and stabilization of spondylolisthesis. Roy-Camille[47] was the first to use pedicle screws connected to a dorsal plate. Beginning in 1963, Roy-Camille[47] used pedicle screw fixation in the thoracic and lumbar spine for fractures, instability after the resection of vertebral tumors, and in lumbosacral fusions. A biomechanical study by Panjabi and colleagues[43] demonstrated that facet screw fixation stability was relatively low in flexion/extension and lateral bending in comparison with pedicle screw fixation systems. Because pedicle fixation systems proved to be biomechanically superior for segmental fixation, numerous variations were developed.* The first system that used both screws and hooks, connecting them with rods or plates (i.e., universal spinal instrumentation) was introduced by Cotrel and Dubousset.[13]

## Pedicle Screw Fixation

The pedicle is the sole bridge between the posterior column and the middle and the anterior columns. Hence, pedicle screws traverse all three columns and as such can rigidly stabilize both the ventral and dorsal aspects of the spine. However, hook-rod systems are affixed only to the posterior spinal elements. For these reasons, pedicle screw fixation systems, at least in the lumbar spine, are more commonly used than hook-rod systems. Commonly used implant systems are listed in Box 116.1.

### Advantages of Pedicle Screw Fixation

The nature of the pedicle screw-bone junction is much more secure than the wire- or hook-bone junction. A single screw provides stability in five planes of motion.[1] With transverse connection to the other side, stability is achieved in all six planes of motion.[1] The rigidity of pedicle fixation allows for the incorporation of fewer normal motion segments to achieve stabilization of an abnormal level. Because the pedicle represents the strongest point of attachment to the spine, significant forces can be applied to the spine without failure of the bone-metal junction.

Pedicle screw fixation systems are superior in restoring and maintaining spinal alignment. Because they traverse all three columns of the spine, they provide a longer lever arm through which the longitudinal member can transmit greater corrective forces than are achieved with spinal fixation systems that attach to the posterior elements alone. Just as pedicle fixation systems resist loads in multiple planes, they are able to apply multidirectional corrective forces.

Another advantage of pedicle fixation systems is that they do not require intact dorsal elements. Thus they can be used after laminectomy or traumatic disruption of the laminae, spinous processes, or facets. Pedicle fixation systems also avoid placement of instrumentation in the spinal canal, in contrast to sublaminar wires and hooks. Additionally, postoperative bracing requirements may be less than with earlier, biomechanically inferior fixation devices. Finally, fusion rates are thought to be improved with the pedicle screw systems compared with earlier devices,[50,51,58] as well as with noninstrumented fusions.[31,50,51,58]

---

*References 1-3,13,17,18,21,25,29,32,33,39,45,49-51,54.

## Disadvantages of Pedicle Screw Fixation

A steep learning curve is required for the safe implantation of pedicle screws. Caudal or medial penetration of the pedicle cortex can result in durotomy or neural injury. Implantation of pedicle screws requires extensive tissue dissection to expose the entry points and to provide the required lateral to medial orientation for optimal screw trajectory. Lengthy operations with significant blood loss and an increased risk of infection are not uncommon. Significant osteoporosis is a relative contraindication to the use of pedicle screws because a solid screw purchase is difficult to achieve. Postoperative imaging techniques (especially magnetic resonance imaging [MRI]) are, in part, obscured by the implant. Rigid fixation can accelerate adjacent motion segment degeneration. These are costly procedures.

## Pedicle Anatomy

The pedicle is a very strong, cylindrical, anatomic bridge between the dorsal spinal elements and the vertebral body. It is composed of a strong shell of cortical bone and a core of cancellous bone.

Pedicle size and angulation varies throughout the spinal column. The transverse pedicle width is narrower than the sagittal pedicle width (pedicle height) except in the lower lumbar spine.[4] Pedicle width is more important than pedicle height for pedicle screw placement (Figure 116.1A). The transverse pedicle width increases from L1 to S1.[59] Most of the pedicles below T10 are greater than 7mm in transverse diameter, and most below L1 are greater than 8mm in diameter.[29] In a study measuring the pedicle diameters with computed tomography (CT), Bernard and Seibert[7] found that 20% of pedicles were less than 7mm at L2, 15.6% at L3, and 1.9% at L4. There were no pedicles less than 7mm in diameter at L5 and S1. They concluded that all surgeons should perform preoperative CT scans when instrumenting pedicles above L4.[7]

The transverse pedicle angle or coronal plane angulation (Figure 116.1B) decreases as one descends caudally in the spine until the lumbar region. The angle increases as the lumbar spine is descended. The sagittal pedicle angle (Figure 116.1C) is steep throughout the midthoracic spine and in the upper lumbar spine.[4]

The intrathecal nerve roots course along the medial aspect of the pedicle. At T12, the dural sac is 0.2 to 0.3mm

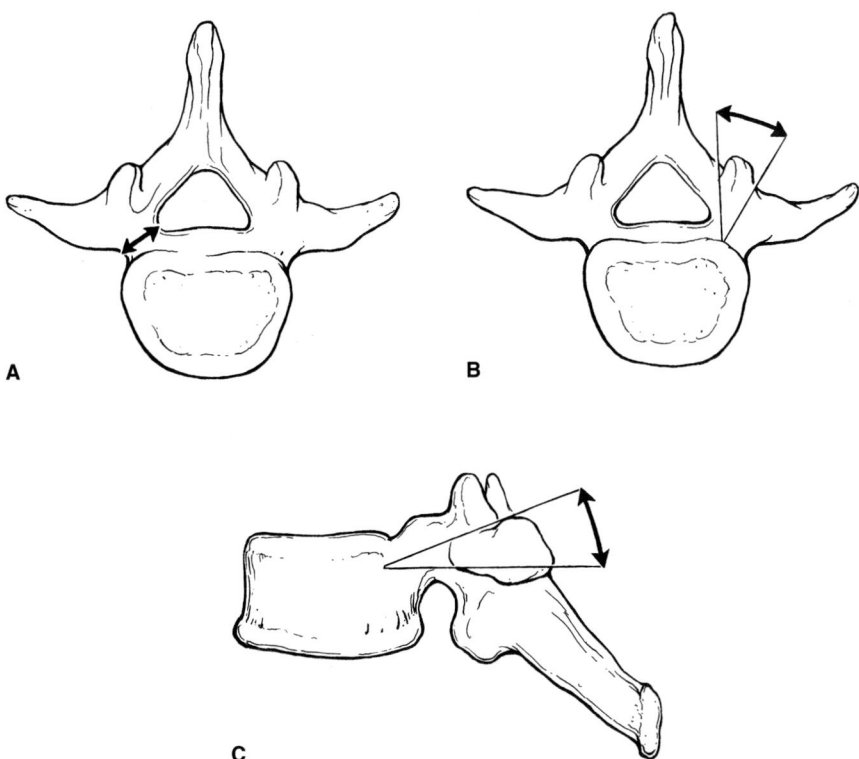

**Figure 116.1** Diagram illustrating the pedicle width (**A**), the transverse or coronal pedicle angle (**B**), and the sagittal pedicle angle (**C**).

away from the pedicle.[4] Below L1, the medial side of the pedicle is almost touching the cauda equina. The nerve root occupies the ventral and rostral one third of the foramen. As a result, violation of the medial or caudal cortex of the pedicle risks injury to the nerve root.

## Biomechanics

Rigid pedicle fixation techniques, such as rigid plate or screw-rod combinations, apply force to the spine by fixed moment arm cantilever beam fixation.[6] A cantilever is a projecting beam that is supported at one end only. It resists axial loads by rigidly buttressing the spine. In the absence of load sharing with the anterior column, significant stress occurs at the screw-plate or screw-rod junction. These constructs tend to fail by screw fracture at the screw-rod or plate junction.[57] However, modifications of the spinal implants (as discussed below) have reduced the incidence of screw breakage.

Pedicle screw fixation systems in which the screws are not rigidly affixed to the plate allow toggling of the screws (Figure 116.2A). These systems constitute nonfixed moment arm cantilever beam fixation.[6] They are unable to resist axial loads without the assistance of an anterior column, which is capable of axial load bearing. Because these systems allow toggling of the screws, they may fail by screw-pullout (Figure 116.2B).[6] For this reason, a fixed moment arm system more effectively resists sagittal translation.

Pedicle screw fixation can be applied with either a flexion component or an extension component to the applied moment arm, which is usually a rigid pedicle fixator.[6] These constructs are used to reduce deformities. Extension moment arm application is their most common mode of application in this regard.

Pedicle fixation techniques may fail during axial loading. This is in part due to a tendency toward the development of a parallelogram-like translational deformity. Toeing-in of the screws and the use of transverse connectors help to prevent this mechanism of construct failure.[30]

The most frequently encountered problems with pedicle screw fixation are hardware failure or failure at the screw-bone junction. Screw pullout, breakage, and toggle are often the result of biomechanically inappropriate applications.

## Screw Characteristics

Most pedicle screws have a cancellous thread pattern. In general, screw outside diameters range from 4.5 to 7mm. Screw lengths are measured from the tip of the screw to the base of the screw head. Pedicle screw lengths range from 30 to 55mm with 5mm increments. There are two predominant types of pedicle screws: (1) self-tapping and (2) nontapping screws. With nontapping screws, a separate tap is used to cut threads into the pedicle.

Screw strength is proportional to the cube of the core (minor) diameter.[5] The larger the minor diameter, the greater the resistance to screw bending or breakage. The outside (major) diameter is an important factor in screw pullout resistance. Other important components of pullout resistance are the thread depth, pitch, and shape. Thread pitch is the distance from one point on the screw thread to

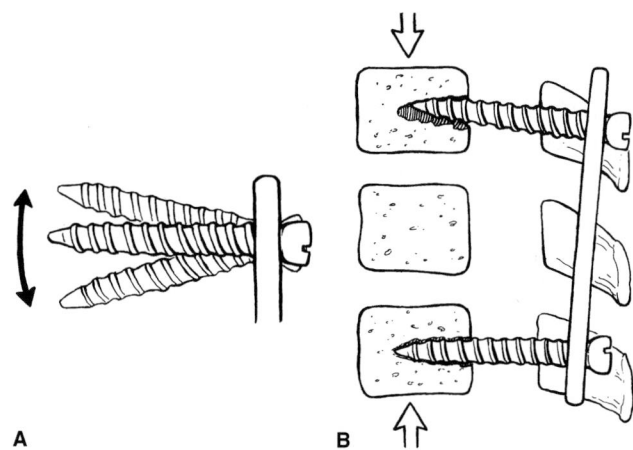

**Figure 116.2** Pedicle fixation systems in which the screws are not rigidly affixed to the plate allow toggling of the pedicle screws (**A**). These systems may fail by screw pullout (**B**).

the corresponding point on the adjacent thread. Pullout resistance is directly proportional to the volume of bone between the threads that is determined by the thread depth and pitch. The angle or shape of the thread can affect the interthread volume and hence the pullout resistance.[5]

Some systems (e.g., compact Cotrel-Dubousset [C-D]) have a smooth extended neck without threads. The diameter of this portion of the neck is greater than the tip and the body. This construction increases the strength of the neck of the screw where most breaks occur. Some systems use screws with a conical inner diameter. This conical shape minimizes screw fracture by increasing the diameter of the screw where it is most likely to fail.

## Preoperative Planning and Surgery

Usually, preoperative plain radiographs and a CT scan should be examined to determine bone quality, pedicle transverse diameter, and screw trajectory. Because intraoperative radiographs are usually necessary, preoperative planning should include preparation for anteroposterior (AP) and lateral radiographs. Lateral radiographs can usually be obtained without difficulty whether either a table or frame is used. Special radiolucent spinal frames are useful, particularly for AP radiographs.

The patient is placed prone on rolls, frame, or on a table with the abdomen hanging as freely as possible to indirectly decompress the epidural venous plexus. A midline incision is used and carried down to the level of the spinous processes. An adequate incision length facilitates proper trajectory during screw hole preparation and screw placement. All soft tissue is dissected off subperiosteally to minimize blood loss. Muscle dissection should allow for a lateral exposure of the transverse processes on both sides, leaving the intertransverse membrane intact at all levels of the planned instrumentation. A crank retractor helps to maintain the lateral exposure. Release of the retractor every 30 minutes reduces muscle necrosis and thereby decreases the risk of infection. The spinal level is identified either anatomically or radiographically and a decompressive laminectomy is performed if appropriate.

After placement of the pedicle screws, the dorsolateral bone graft bed is prepared by decorticating the lateral aspect of the facet joints and the transverse processes with a combination of a high-speed drill with a cutting burr and sharp cupped curettes. The synovium can be removed from the facet joints that are included in the fusion and packed with cancellous bone. The importance of meticulous decortication to achieving bony fusion cannot be overstated.

## Pedicle Screw Entry Sites and Trajectory

Every spine surgeon should have a thorough knowledge of pedicle anatomy, including the coronal and sagittal plane angulation of the pedicle (see Figure 116.1). The sagittal pedicle angle increases in the thoracic spine from an average of 0 degrees at T1 to 10 degrees at T8 and then decreases to 0 degrees at T12.[37] Usually the L4 sagittal pedicle angle is 0 degrees, and subsequent rostral and caudal levels are associated with progressively greater sagittal angles. The lordotic curvature of the lumbar spine produces a rostral angulation for upper lumbar screws. The L5 pedicle is 5 to 10 degrees caudally inclined. Coronal plane angulation decreases from the cervical spine to the thoracolumbar region and then increases as the lumbar spine is descended. The coronal plane angulation at T1 is 10 to 15 degrees and at T12 is 5 degrees.[37] A 10-degree medial angulation is satisfactory at L1. A wider angle in the coronal plane is necessary to avoid lateral penetration of the pedicle in the lower lumbar spine. The coronal plane angle increases approximately 5 degrees per level from L1 to the sacrum.[30]

In the thoracic spine, the transverse process commonly does not align directly with the pedicle in the axial plane. For this reason, the anatomic landmarks that are used for lumbar pedicle screw insertion cannot be used in the thoracic spine.[37] The transverse process is rostral to the pedicle in the upper thoracic spine and caudal to the pedicle in the lower thoracic spine. The crossover occurs at T6-7.[37] Because of the variability of the relationship of the pedicle to the transverse process, fluoroscopic guidance or direct vision and palpation of the pedicle via a laminotomy is recommended for insertion of thoracic pedicles. At T1 to T3 levels, Louis suggests the use of 4.5mm diameter screws that are 25 to 30mm in length.[33] At T4 to T10 levels, screws are usually 4.5mm in diameter and 30 to 35mm in length.[33]

The conventional entry site for pedicle screw placement in the lumbar region is at the junction of the lateral facet and the transverse process (Figure 116.3). Although the midline of the transverse process corresponds to the location of the pedicle at L4, this relationship does vary at different lumbar levels. Above L4 the midline of the transverse process is rostral to the pedicle, at L5 it is an average of 1.5mm caudal to the pedicle.[16]

Several nuances should be considered for accurate cannulation of the pedicle, as well as to enable proper screw trajectory. The muscle dissection is performed as lateral as possible to allow palpation of the transverse processes. The lateral aspect of the pedicle is palpated with a nerve hook over the transverse process. If a decompressive laminectomy is not being performed as part of the operative procedure, a small laminotomy may be performed to palpate the medial aspect of the pedicle and its rostral and caudal borders. Palpation of the pedicle helps to guide

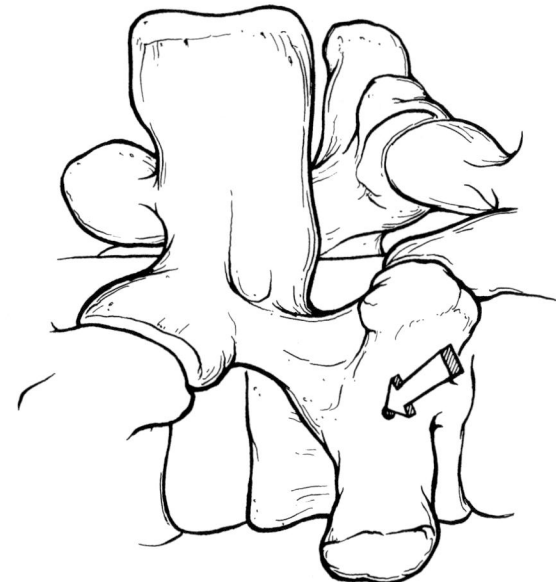

**Figure 116.3** The junction of the lateral facet and the transverse process is the conventional pedicle screw entry site in the lumbar spine.

accurate placement of the screw into the pedicle and increases the safety of the placement. It is strongly recommended for placement of pedicle screws at the level of the conus medullaris and above.

## Screw Insertion

The entry site is decorticated by using a burr and a high-speed drill or a rongeur. A burr or awl is also used to penetrate the dorsal cortex of the pedicle. A curved or straight pedicle probe is used to develop a path for the screw through the cancellous bone of the pedicle into the vertebral body. The advancement of the pedicle probe should be smooth and consistent. A sudden plunge suggests breaking out of the pedicle laterally. An increase in resistance indicates abutment against the pedicle or vertebral body cortex. After cannulation of the pedicle and vertebral body with the pedicle probe, the pedicle sounding probe is then placed into the pedicle that is then palpated from within to make sure there is not a medial, lateral, rostral, or caudal disruption in the cortex of the pedicle. The sounding probe should also be used to determine that there is bone at the bottom of the pilot hole, verifying that penetration of the ventral cortex of the vertebral body has not occurred.

After the pedicles have been probed, different length Steinmann pins or K-wires are placed bilaterally into the pedicular hole at each level. Using different length pins on each side helps to distinguish right and left on the lateral plain radiograph in case the pedicle hole trajectory or depth needs to be corrected. A lateral and an AP radiograph or fluoroscopic image is used to verify the trajectory of the pins. This, however, does not guarantee accurate screw placement.[17] With slightly oblique AP views, a pin located in the middle of the pedicle has a characteristic "target sign." Direct AP views demonstrate the lateral to medial orientation of the screws. Excessive medial orientation of the screws seen on an AP film raises the concern of medial penetration of the pedicle by the screw. Lateral imaging is useful to view the depth of penetration into the vertebral body and the sagittal angulation of the trajectory. Ventral screw penetration is usually between 50% and 80% of the AP diameter of the vertebral body. Ventral screw penetration greater than 80% of the vertebral body on a lateral plain radiograph raises the concern of ventral penetration of the vertebral body cortex because of the convex shape of the vertebral bodies. To avoid vascular and visceral injury, the ventral cortex of the vertebral body is not penetrated, although this would enhance the overall strength of the construct.

After confirmation of correct placement of the K-wires or Steinmann pins, the pedicle screw path is tapped if non-self-tapping screws are used. Some tapping screws are hollow and are slid over K-wires into the pedicles. This helps guide the tap along the same trajectory that the pedicle was previously probed. The screw is then guided into the pedicle by its purchase of the threads tapped into the pedicle. However, tapping is less desirable in cancellous bone because tapping weakens the implant-bone junction.[5] It is of questionable value in the insertion of pedicle screws because pedicle screws rarely obtain cortical purchase within the pedicle.[40] To maximize the bone purchase of the permanent screws, a tap that is smaller in diameter than the screw is used. Tapping is usually not performed at a greater depth than the pedicle.

After tapping of the pedicles, the permanent screws with the largest diameter that will not fracture the pedicle are placed. The length of the screw is determined by measuring the length of the Steinmann pin or K-wire from the pedicle entry site to a depth of 50% to 80% of the vertebral body. Screws in the lumbar spine usually have a 4.5 to 7mm diameter and a 35 to 50mm length. Next, the transverse processes and lateral aspect of the facet joints are decorticated. The screws are connected to a longitudinal member, usually a rod. Bone graft is then placed on the previously prepared fusion bed.

## Complications and Avoidance

Complication rates are as high as 25%. However, most are without permanent clinical consequence. Intraoperative complications occur at a 0.2% to 5% rate.[19] According to a cohort study, the complications are usually implant failures (approximately 7%), pedicle fractures (1%), vertebral body penetration (less than 0.5%), or neurologic deficit (less than 0.5%).[19]

In general, early complications after transpedicular stabilization of the spine are unusual and are infrequently associated with permanent morbidity. There is, however, a high proportion of postoperative radiographic failures. Ohlin *et al.*[41] have reported a 40% radiographic failure rate after surgery. Most of them were screw loosening, angulation, or fracture. Implant removal was required in about 15% of the cases within a year after operation.

### Misplaced Screws

Misplaced screws represent the most frequent pedicle screw complication. The misplacement rate ranges from

1.2% to 28.8% in different series.[20,28,47,53] A rostral breach of the pedicle cortex leads to penetration of the intervertebral disc with resultant poor screw fixation. A caudal misplaced screw risks injury to the dura mater and nerve root. Disruption of the medial cortex leads to violation of the spinal canal, which can cause injury to the dura, spinal cord, or nerve roots. Lateral screw placement risks injury to the segmental vessels and poor screw purchase.[10,53] A laterally placed screw hole can lead to possible retroperitoneal penetration by the pedicle probe because slippage of the probe off the side of the vertebral body occurs from the sudden lack of resistance to advancement of the probe. Although with postoperative CT approximately 15% of the screws have been reported to be suboptimal,[20] nerve root or spinal cord injury is uncommon because of the theoretical safe zones or spaces around the pedicle.

Intraoperative radiographic confirmation of correct screw placement, including the use of fluoroscopy, has still resulted in a high incidence of misplaced screws.[42] Therefore, other methods have been developed to ensure accurate placement of screws within the pedicle. Screw placement can be checked electrophysiologically with direct stimulation of the pedicle probe or screw producing an electromyogram (EMG) response peripherally. If this response occurs below the threshold expected for intact cortical bone, the screws may be redirected or removed. Stimulation can be intermittent[11,14,42] or continuous.[9,46] Spontaneous EMGs are also monitored, which may alert the surgeon to nerve root irritation from retraction during decompressive procedures, stretching during deformity reductions, or impingement by a pedicle screw.

Interactive frameless stereotaxy with surface reference landmarks has been successfully applied to pedicle fixation of the spine. Preoperative axial CT images of the appropriate spinal segments can be manipulated to assist the surgeon in determining the correct entry point, sagittal and coronal angulation, screw diameter, and length for each pedicle, thus reducing pedicle screw misplacement.[26] Frameless stereotactic guidance of pedicle screw placement is particularly useful when the planned exposure does not allow for palpation of the pedicle at the time of screw insertion (e.g., when a lumbar decompression is not planned).

### Nerve Root or Spinal Cord Injury

Neurologic injury during pedicular screw placement is reported to occur in about 2.5% to 7.5% of cases.[17] Nerve root injury may result either from improper screw placement or from correction of a deformity with traction on the nerve root or migration of the screw into the neuroforamen or spinal canal. If the symptoms caused by screw malpositioning do not resolve, the instrumentation should be removed or repositioned. In most cases, the radiculopathy improves after removal or repositioning of the misplaced screw.[41]

### Pedicle Fracture

A break in the cortex of the pedicle can result from a misplaced screw, as discussed above, or the use of too large a screw. The transverse width of the pedicle is the most narrow dimension of the pedicle and determines the largest diameter screw that can be used.[5,50]

## Cerebrospinal Fluid Fistulae

The incidence of dural tears is less than 2.5%.[10] These are due to spinal canal or neuroforamen penetration. Primary repair of the durotomy, if possible, lessens the risk of a cerebrospinal fluid leak through the wound or pseudomeningocele formation.

## Infection

In general, the infection rate after instrumentation is higher than with other spine operations because of longer operative times, extensive surgical exposures, and the placement of a foreign body. For these reasons, prophylactic antibiotic usage and vigorous irrigation of the wound with antibiotic solutions should be performed. Frequent relaxation of the paraspinous muscle retraction reduces the amount of muscle necrosis and lessens the risk of infection. Necrotic muscle should be débrided before closing the wound.

## Damage to Retroperitoneal Structures

The retroperitoneal structures may be damaged as a result of ventral cortex penetration. In upper lumbar spine, the aorta and vena cava lie ventral to the vertebral bodies. At L4-5 and caudally, the iliac vein and artery lie ventral (and ventrolateral) to the spine. Penetration of the ventral cortex is avoided by understanding that intraoperative imaging can be misleading regarding the distance from the tip of the pin to the ventral cortex because of the convex shape of the vertebral body. It can also be avoided by sounding the anterior cortex with a probe and measuring this distance that should not be exceeded by the length of the screw.

## Hardware Failure

Mechanical failure has been reported to be between 5% and 31% in different series.[41]

### Screw Breakage

The reported incidence of screw breakage is 0.8% to 24.6%.* The incidence of screw breakage and bending is higher in patients in whom major deformity reduction and multilevel fusions were attempted.[15,36,41] Rostral screws are more prone to breakage than their caudal counterparts.[36] Matsuzaki et al.[35] have reported that rostral screw breakage is more common in multilevel fusions but caudal screw breakage is more common in single-level fusions. Screw breakage after solid fusion is usually asymptomatic and may not require reoperation. However, screw breakage may indicate a pseudarthrosis.[10,15,33]

The following measures can be taken to avoid screw breakage: (1) choose the largest diameter screws that the pedicle can accept[59]; (2) the upper portion of a construct should be longer if nonrigid fixation systems are used; for fractures in the thoracolumbar junction, fixation to two levels above the fracture site is suggested[28]; (3) if the anterior column is severely disrupted, the pedicle screw construct bears all of the load. This places significant stress at the screw rod junction and can result in breakage of the screw at this point. In this situation, a ventral interbody fusion may be required to share the load with the pedicle screw construct[38,54] (Figure 116.4).

### Screw Pullout

Screw pullout increases with decreasing bone mineral density.[55,57] A solid screw purchase in osteoporotic bone is not

---

*References 10,15,32,33,35,36,41,47.

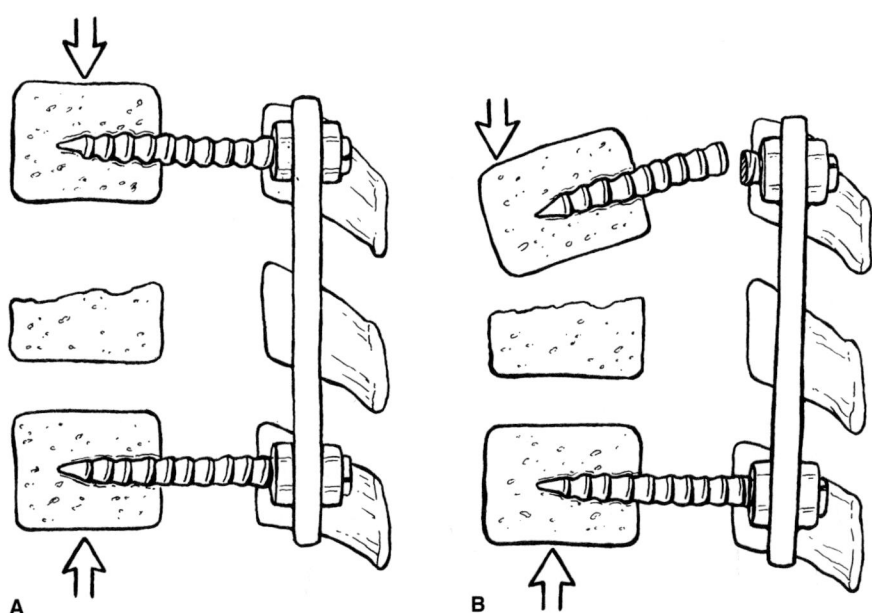

**Figure 116.4 (A and B)** If the anterior column is severely disrupted, the pedicle screw construct bears all of the load and rigid pedicle fixation systems may fail by screw breakage at the screw-rod interface.

easily achieved, and therefore osteoporotic bone is a relative contraindication to the use of pedicle screws. Hooks or wires provide superior pullout resistance as compared with pedicle screws in osteoporotic bone. This is due to the greater cortical bone-metal surface contact.[12] Instrumentation in patients with osteoporosis should include "extra" levels, with multiple points of fixation.

The length of the screw is important regarding screw pullout. Lumbar screws should be placed approximately to a depth of two thirds of the vertebral body on the lateral radiographs. This maximizes depth of penetration without risking bicortical purchase in the lumbar area.[39]

The outer diameter of a screw, particularly with an associated large thread depth and pitch (distance between threads), helps minimize the risk of pullout. However, a larger diameter screw may also cause the pedicle to fracture.

The use of pedicle screw fixation systems that rigidly connect the screw to the plate or rod resist screw pullout by not allowing toggling of the screws.[6] Screw toe-in results in greater pullout resistance and translational deformity prevention if the two sides of the construct are rigidly affixed to each other. In this configuration, the screw pullout is prohibited by its toed-in counterpart.[48]

Placement of a sublaminar hook caudal to a pedicle screw increases the pullout resistance of the construct. This configuration is made possible by the location of the lamina approximately one-half segment below the pedicle. The pedicle screw-sublaminar hook construct resists pullout while maintaining the rotation, flexion, and extension-resisting capabilities of the pedicle screw.[12,48] This is not appropriately applied at the most caudal segment of the construct.

### Screw Loosening, Plate or Rod Breakage

Screw loosening is relatively rare and is often a delayed complication. It is diagnosed by the presence of a lucency seen around the screw on a lateral plain radiograph. It often indicates a fusion delay or pseudarthrosis. It may also be the result of inadequate screw purchase or diminished bone mineral density from osteoporosis. Plate or rod breakage rarely occurs. It is often an indication of pseudarthrosis.

### Loss of Correction

Loss of correction may occur after the reduction of a traumatic or congenital kyphosis, particularly if overdistraction or forceful correction was performed during the operation. The strength of the anterior column is important. If there is significant compromise of the anterior column, ventral grafting and fusion should be added. Otherwise, a loss of correction (kyphosis) may develop, resulting in screw angulation or breakage at the screw-longitudinal member junction (see Figure 116.4).[39,54]

### Wound Breakdown

In thin patients, bulky implants may be felt under the skin. They can cause wound breakdown, especially at the sacral level.[17,54] For this reason, low-profile constructs should be used in thin patients. Painful bursa may also develop over prominent parts of the instrumentation.

## Universal Spinal Instrumentation Systems

Universal spinal instrumentation (USI) systems were developed for the treatment of scoliosis through application of multiple corrective forces at different points on a rod. These systems have proved readily adaptable to the treatment of a wide variety of spinal disorders. USI systems use both pedicle screws and hooks as anchors to the spine. The screws and hooks are interconnected by a rod. A major difference between the systems is the manner in which the rods are coupled to the anchors. The reasons for the selection of rods versus plates in modern systems are (1) rods are more versatile than plates for connection with anchoring devices, and (2) a larger area for grafting is available when rods are used.

The first USI prototype was the Cotrel-Dubousset (C-D) device.[13] This was followed by the Texas Scottish Rite Hospital (TSRH)[3,25] and the Isola[2,44] systems. The C-D system has been updated via the compact Cotrel-Dubousset (CC-D)[21] and the C-D Horizon spinal systems. The characteristics of the C-D, CC-D, TSRH, and Isola systems, as well as their advantages and disadvantages, are depicted in Tables 116.1 and 116.2.

### Cotrel-Dubousset System

C-D instrumentation is the oldest of the universal systems. It was designed by Cotrel and Dubousset in France between 1978 and 1982. It was first designed for correction of pediatric scoliosis.[13] This system provides a rigid three-dimensional short segment fixation without the need for sublaminar wires in the spinal canal. It uses hooks and screws as anchors, coupled to a rod by a set screw. In the first version of the C-D system, set screws of the closed body type were broken (twisted off) at the end of the instrumentation. This makes the revision or removal of the instrumentation very difficult.[39] The C-D system uses self-tapping pedicle screws, whereas the other systems use nontapping screws. The C-D system has a lateral connector that facilitates screw-rod connection in the presence of coronal plane deformities (Figure 116.5).

### Compact Cotrel-Dubousset System

The original C-D instrumentation presented disadvantages such as an unnecessary number of implant components and a permanent implant locking system. Therefore a new version, the CC-D, was developed. The instrument set and the implants were streamlined, and an improved locking system enabled easy removal.[21]

### Cotrel-Dubousset Horizon

The C-D Horizon system is designed to be lower in profile. A recent addition to the C-D Horizon system are polyaxial screws, which minimize rod contouring.

**TABLE 116.1**

**Specifications of Screws and Longitudinal Members of USI Systems**

| | Cotrel-Dubousset | Compact Cotrel-Dubousset | Texas Scottish Rite Hospital | Isola |
|---|---|---|---|---|
| Screw diameters | 6-7mm | 5-6mm | 5.5-6.5-7.5-8.5mm | 5.5-6.25-7mm |
| Screw length | 30-35-40-45-50mm | 35-40-45mm | 25-75mm (5mm increments) | 25-50mm (5mm increments) |
| Screw types | Closed<br>Top opening<br>Side opening | Top opening (all screws have a smooth extended neck with 10mm length and 5-6mm diameter.) | Fixed angle head type<br>Variable angle head type<br>Top opening<br>Side opening | Closed<br>Top opening (a machine-threaded portion with 23-33mm lengths to aid sagittal plane disparity correction) |
| Titanium | — | — | + | + |
| Screw tapping style | Self tapping | Self tapping | Nontapping | Nontapping |
| Sacral screws | NA | 7mm diam./35-40-45mm length<br>Closed body type<br>Top opening type (all have extended necks) | NA | 8.5 mm diam. /30-35 mm length (most are not threaded) |
| Iliac screws | NA | Iliac extension device and sacral screw are inserted into the iliac wing | NA | 6.25-7mm diam/60-80mm length |
| Rods | Knurled rod (0.2mm) 5mm and 7mm diam | Knurled rod (0.2mm) 5-6-7mm diam | Smooth rod<br>¼ inch rigid rod<br>¼ inch flex rod<br>³⁄₁₆ inch flex rod | Smooth rod<br>4.76 mm and 6.35mm<br>Standard length 46 cm |
| Rod-screw Rod-hook anchorage | Blockers for open body type screws<br>Set screws for closed body type screws | Closed body sacral screws have 6mm threaded plug<br>Open body screws have 10mm threaded plug and washer | Eye bolt and nut assembly<br>(a) for fixed screws, side loading eye bolts<br>(b) for variable screws, side loading eye bolts<br>(c) for variable screws, top loading eye bolts | Slotted connector<br>V-groove hollow ground (VHG) design allows maximal rod contact within the hole<br>Rod anchorage: set screws are loaded from the top<br>Screw anchorage: a tapered nut and a locking nut are tightened over the pedicle screw over a slotted connector. |
| Transverse connector | Device for Transverse Traction (DTT)<br>A threaded rod with nuts and set screws | Transverse Linking Device (TLD)<br>A bar and two hooks with closed body type locking | Device for Transverse Traction (DTT)<br>Small diameter threaded rod with nuts and set screws | Transverse rod connectors<br>Split connector jaws are connected with a long threaded rod and fixed with hex nuts |
| Unique specifications | | Sacral Chopin block is unique to the CC-D system. A double screw (7mm diameter, 35-60mm length) can be introduced in divergent directions | The radial serrated splines on the variable angle screw heads facilitate connection between screws oriented in different planes. This allows fixation without rod bending | (1) A machine threaded portion of the screw provides the ability to correct sagittal plane disparities. They are cut at the end of the operation<br>(2) V-groove hollow ground design |

Abbreviation: NA, not applicable.

**TABLE 116.2**

**Main Advantages and Disadvantages of USI Systems**

| | Cotrel-Dubousset | Compact Cotrel-Dubousset | Texas Scottish Rite Hospital | Isola |
|---|---|---|---|---|
| Main advantages | Knurled rod | Knurled rod<br>Fewer parts<br>Removal is easier<br>Double sacral screw fixation | Rod contouring is minimized<br>Fewer parts<br>Removal is easier<br>Titanium available<br>Top and side loading available | V-groove attachment is an easy and strong construct<br>Top loading is easy<br>Titanium available |
| Main disadvantages | Extensive rod contouring is necessary<br>Revision and removing is impossible without drilling or cutting the implanted parts<br>Multiple parts are confusing | Fitting the rod inside the open body screws is difficult | Eye bolts should be preplanned and applied before connecting to screws and hooks<br>Top loading hooks are difficult to use | Adapters for connection can introduce points of movement |

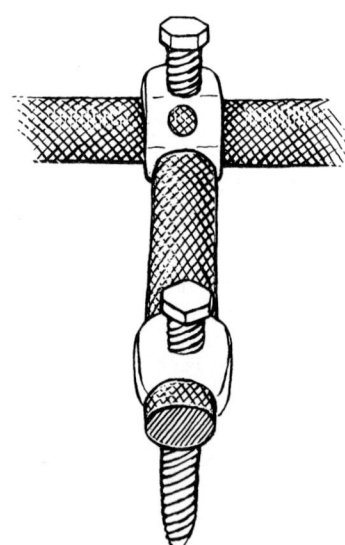

**Figure 116.5** Diagram of the C-D lateral connector that facilitates coupling of the screw to the rod in the presence of coronal plane offsets.

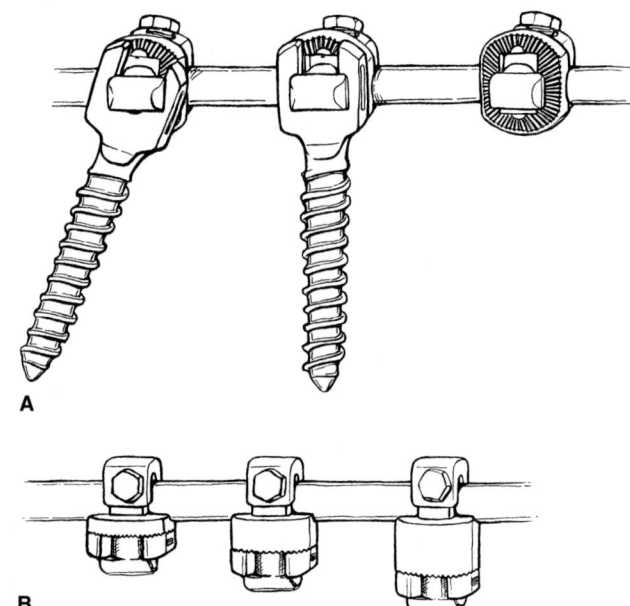

**Figure 116.6** The radial splines on the TSRH variable angle screws facilitate screw-rod connection regardless of the angle of screw insertion (**A**). The top-loading couplers are available in three widths, which helps to accommodate coronal plane offsets (**B**).

## Texas Scottish Rite Hospital System

Perhaps the most important and unique feature of the TSRH system is the variable-angle screw that facilitates coupling to the rod regardless of the angle of screw insertion (Figure 116.6A). The top-loading couplers are available with varying thickness, which accommodates coronal plane offsets and minimizes the need to contour the rod in this dimension (Figure 116.6B).

## Isola System

The Isola system is one of the newest of the USI fixators. A unique feature of the screws of the Isola system is a machine-threaded portion that allows the correction of sagittal deformities by placing straight or angled washers over the threads.[21] Slotted plate connectors couple the rods to the screws. The connectors are first placed on the rods, and then the slotted portion of the plate is placed over the machine-threaded portion of the screw. Plate lengths vary. This minimizes the need to contour the rod to accommodate coronal plane deformities (Figure 116.7).

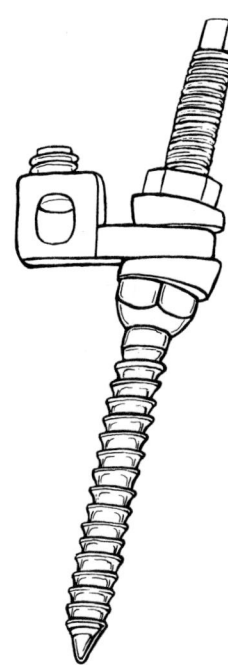

**Figure 116.7** Coronal plane deformities are accommodated by slotted plate connectors of varying lengths that couple the rods to the screws.

## REFERENCES

1. Asher MA: Lumbopelvic fixation with the Isola Spinal Implant System. In Margulies JY, Floman Y, Farcy JC, Neuwirth MG (eds): *Lumbosacral and Spinopelvic Fixation*. Philadelphia, Lippincott-Raven, 1996, pp 215-238.

2. Asher MA, Strippgen WE, Heinig CF, Carson WL: Isola spinal system: principles, design, and applications. In An HS, Cotler JM (eds): *Spinal Instrumentation*. Baltimore, Williams & Wilkins, 1992, pp 325-351.

3. Benzel EC, Baldwin NG, Ball PA: Texas Scottish Rite Hospital hook-rod spinal fixation. In Hitchon PW, Traynelis VC, Rengachary SS (eds): *Techniques in Spinal Fusion and Stabilization*. Thieme Medical Publishers, 1995, pp 229-239.

4. Benzel EC: Biomechanically relevant anatomy and material properties of the spine and associated elements. In Benzel EC (ed): *Biomechanics of Spine Stabilization: Principles and Clinical Practice*. New York, McGraw-Hill, 1995, pp 3-16.

5. Benzel EC: Implant-bone interfaces. In Benzel EC (ed): *Biomechanics of Spine Stabilization: Principles and Clinical Practice*. New York, McGraw-Hill, 1995, pp 127-134.

6. Benzel EC: Mechanical (quantitative) attributes of spinal implants: constructs types. In Benzel EC (ed): *Biomechanics of Spine Stabilization: Principles and Clinical Practice*. New York, McGraw-Hill, 1995, pp 151-162.

7. Bernard TN, Seibert CE: Pedicle diameter determined by computer tomography: its relevance to pedicle fixation in the lumbar spine. *Spine* 17: S160-S163, 1992.

8. Boucher HH: A method of spinal fusion. *J Bone Joint Surg* 41-B:248-259, 1959.

9. Calancie B, Madsen P, Lebwohl N: Stimulus-evoked EMG monitoring during transpedicular lumbosacral spine instrumentation. *Spine* 19: 2780-2786, 1994.

10. Chozick BS, Toselli R: Complications of spinal instrumentation. In Benzel EC (ed): *Spinal Instrumentation*. Park Ridge, IN, American Association of Neurological Surgeons, 1994, pp 257-274.

11. Clements DH, Morledge DE, Martin WH, Betz RR: Evoked and spontaneous electromyography to evaluate lumbosacral pedicle screw placement. *Spine* 21:600-604, 1996.

12. Coe JD, Warden KE, Herzig MA, et al: Influence of bone mineral density on the fixation of thoracolumbar implants: a comparative study of transpedicular screws, laminar hooks, and spinous process wires. *Spine* 15:902-907, 1990.

13. Cotrel Y, Dubousset J, Guillaumat M: New universal instrumentation in spine surgery. *Clin Orthop* 227:10-23, 1988.

14. Darden BV II, Wood KE, Hatley MK, et al: Evaluation of pedicle screw insertion monitored by intraoperative evoked electromyography. *J Spinal Disord* 9:8-16, 1996.

15. Davne SH, Myers DL: Complications of lumbar spinal fusion with transpedicular instrumentation. *Spine* 17: S184-S189, 1992.

16. Ebraheim NA, Rollins, JR, Jr Xu R, Yeasting RA: Projection of the lumbar pedicle and its morphometric analysis. *Spine* 21:1296-1300, 1996.

17. Esses SI, Botsford DJ, Wright T, et al: Operative treatment of spinal fractures with the AO internal fixator. *Spine* 16:S146-S150, 1991.

18. Fessler RG, Sturgill M: Utilization of the Texas Scottish Rite Hospital Universal System for stabilization of the thoracic and lumbar spine. In Fessler RG, Haid RW (eds): *Current Techniques in Spinal Stabilization*. New York, McGraw-Hill, 1996, pp 273-285.

19. Garfin SR: Summation. *Spine* 19:2300S-2305S, 1994.

20. Gertzbein SD, Robbins SE: Accuracy of pedicular screw placement in vivo. *Spine* 15:11-14, 1990.

21. Gillet P: Utilization of the compact Cotrel-Dubousset system for stabilization of the thoracolumbar and lumbar spine. In Fessler RG, Haid RW (eds): *Current Techniques in Spinal Stabilization*. New York, McGraw-Hill, 1996, pp 297-308.

22. Graham CE: Lumbosacral fusion using internal fixation with a spinous process for the graft. *Clin Orthop* 140:72-77, 1979.

23. Harrington PR: The history and development of Harrington instrumentation. *Clin Orthop* 227:3-5, 1988.

24. Harrington PR, Dickson JH: Spinal instrumentation in the treatment of severe progressive spondylolisthesis. *Clin Orthop* 117:157-163, 1976.

25. Johnston CE II, Herring A, Ashman R: Texas Scottish Rite Hospital (TSRH) universal spinal instrumentation system. In An HS, Cotler JM (eds): *Spinal Instrumentation*. Baltimore, MD, Williams & Wilkins, 1992, pp 127-165.

26. Kalfas IH, Kormos DW, Murphy MA, et al: Application of frameless stereotaxy to pedicle screw fixation of the spine. *J Neurosurg* 83:641-647, 1995.

27. King D: Internal fixation for lumbosacral fusion. *J Bone Joint Surg* 30A:560-565, 1948.

28. Krag MH: Biomechanics of thoracolumbar spinal fixation: a review. *Spine* 16:S84-S99, 1991.

29. Krag MH, Beynnon BD, Pope MH, et al: An internal fixator for posterior application to short segments of the thoracic, lumbar, or lumbosacral spine: design and testing. *Clin Orthop* 203:75-98, 1986.

30. Krag MH, Weaver DL, Beynnon BD, Haugh LD: Morphometry of the thoracic and lumbar spine related to transpedicular screw placement for surgical spinal fixation. *Spine* 13:27-32, 1988.

31. Lorenz M, Zindrick J, Schwaegler P, *et al*: Comparison of single level fusions with and without hardware. *Spine* 16:S455-S458, 1991.

32. Louis R: Fusion of the lumbar and sacral spine by internal fixation with screw plates. *Clin Orthop* 203:18-33, 1986.

33. Louis R: Application of the Louis system for thoracolumbar and lumbosacral spine stabilization. In Fessler RG, Haid RW (eds): *Current Techniques in Spinal Stabilization*. New York, McGraw-Hill, 1996, pp 399-407.

34. Magerl FP: Stabilization of the lower thoracic and lumbar spine with external skeletal fixation. *Clin Orthop* 189:125, 1984.

35. Matsuzaki H, Tokuhashi Y, Matsumoto F, *et al*: Problems and solutions of pedicle screw plate fixation of lumbar spine. *Spine* 15:1159-1165, 1990.

36. McAfee PC, Weiland DJ, Carlow JJ: Survivorship analysis of pedicle spinal instrumentation. *Spine* 16:S422-S427, 1991.

37. McCormack BM, Benzel EC, Adams MS, *et al*: Anatomy of the thoracic pedicle. *Neurosurgery* 37:303-308, 1995.

38. McCormack T, Karaikovic E, Gaines RW: The load sharing classification of spine fractures. *Spine* 19:1741-1744, 1994.

39. McCormick PC: Utilization of the Cotrel-Dubousset instrumentation system for stabilization of the spine. In Fessler RG, Haid RW (eds): *Current Techniques in Spinal Stabilization*. New York, McGraw-Hill, 1996, pp 287-296.

40. Misenhimer GR, Peek RD, Wiltse LL, *et al*: Anatomic analysis of pedicle cortical and cancellous diameter as related to screw size. *Spine* 14:367-372, 1989.

41. Ohlin A, Karrlson M, Duppe H, *et al*: Complications after transpedicular stabilization of the spine. A survivorship analysis of 163 cases. *Spine* 19:2774-2779, 1994.

42. Owen JH, Kostuik JP, Gornet M, *et al*: The use of mechanically elicited electromyograms to protect nerve roots during surgery for spinal degeneration. *Spine* 19:1704-1710, 1994.

43. Panjabi MM, Yamamoto I, Oxland TR: Biomechanical stability of five pedicle screw fixation systems in a human lumbar spine instability model. *Clin Biomech* 6:197-205, 1991.

44. Pennal GL, McDonald GA, Dale GG: A method of spinal fusion using internal fixation. *Clin Orthop* 35:86-94, 1964.

45. Rengachary SS, Flores E: Segmental fixation of the lumbosacral spine using the Isola/VSP system. In Fessler RG, Haid RW (eds): *Current Techniques in Spinal Stabilization*: New York, McGraw-Hill, 1996, pp 367-378.

46. Rose RD, Welch WC, Balzer JR, Jacobs GB: Persistently electrified pedicle stimulation instruments in spinal instrumentation. Technique and protocol development. *Spine* 22:334-343, 1997.

47. Roy-Camille R, Saillant G, Mazel C: Internal fixation of the lumbar spine with pedicle screw plating. *Clin Orthop* 203:7-17, 1986.

48. Ruland CM, McAfee PC, Warden KE, *et al*: Triangulation of pedicular instrumentation. A biomechanical analysis. *Spine* 16:S270-S276, 1991.

49. Steffee AD: The variable screw placement system with posterior lumbar interbody fusion. In Zin PM, Gill K (eds): *Lumbar Interbody Fusion: Principles and Techniques in Spine Surgery*. Gaithersburg, MD, Aspen Press, 1989, pp 81-93.

50. Stillerman CB, Gruen JP: Universal spinal instrumentation fixation. In: Benzel EC (ed): *Spinal Instrumentation*. Park Ridge, IN, American Association of Neurological Surgeons, 1994, pp 147-174.

51. Stillerman CB, Gruen JP, Roy R: Thoracic and lumbar fusion: techniques for posterior stabilization. In Menezes A, Sonntag VKH (eds): *Principles of Spinal Surgery*. New York, McGraw Hill, 1996, pp 1199-1224.

52. Toumey JW: Internal fixation in fusion of the lumbosacral joint. *Lahey Clin Bull* 3: 188-191, 1943.

53. West JL III, Ogilvie JW, Bradford DS: Complications of the variable screw plate pedicle screw fixation. *Spine* 16: 576-579, 1991.

54. Whitecloud TS III, Butler JC, Cohen JL, *et al*: Complications with the variable spinal plating system. *Spine* 14:472-476, 1989.

55. Yamagata M, Kitahara H, Minami S, *et al*: Mechanical stability of the pedicle screw fixation systems for the lumbar spine. *Spine* 17:S51-S54, 1994.

56. Yuan HA, Garfin SR, Dickman CA, Mardjelko SM: A historical cohort study of pedicle screw fixation in thoracic, lumbar and sacral spinal fusions. *Spine* 19: S2279-S2296, 1994.

57. Yoganandan N, Larson SJ, Pintar F, *et al*: Biomechanics of lumbar pedicle screw/plate fixation in trauma. *Neurosurgery* 27:873-881, 1990.

58. Zdeblick TA: A prospective, randomized study of lumbar fusion. *Spine* 18:983-991, 1994.

59. Zindrick MR, Wiltse LL, Widell EH, *et al*: A biomechanical study of intrapedicular screw fixation of the lumbosacral spine. *Clin Orthop* 203:99-112, 1986.

# CHAPTER 117

# Dorsal Thoracic and Lumbar Simple Hook-Rod, Wire, and Wire-Rod Techniques

## Bernardo Jose Ordonez

The first internal fixation device was designed by Paul Harrington in 1947, a period in which the number of patients with poliomyelitis-induced scoliosis was growing and there was dissatisfaction with the current management of corrective casting. The device was aimed at correcting the scoliotic curvature and halting the progression of cardiopulmonary compromise in affected patients. Initial attempts consisted of screw fixation of facet joints in the corrected position. The results appeared promising, but early beneficial results were short-lived. Facet screw failure led to the development of a hook-and-rod construct, in which hooks were attached to the dorsal elements and held in place with a combination of distraction and compressive forces. The clinical results of Harrington's new system were published in 1962.[9-11,18,23]

The Harrington system offered the first internal fixation device for the correction of scoliotic deformities. The system was quickly adopted by spine surgeons and was rapidly applied to various other conditions including trauma, neoplastic disease, fixed deformities, and degenerative disorders.[10,13,18,23,24]

The Harrington system, although versatile, was plagued with inherent problems, and it has been modified over the years. The system was limited in its design, which allowed for only two points of fixation. Failure at any single hook site led to failure of the entire system.[18]

In the early 1970s, Eduardo Luque was faced with an impoverished community in which postoperative bracing was impossible. From these circumstances arose the concept of segmental spinal instrumentation. The Luque system consisted of straight, L-shaped or rectangular rods attached to lamina via sublaminar wires.[16,17] The advent of segmental spinal instrumentation addressed the main problem of the Harrington system that had only two points of fixation. Initially, sublaminar wires were used to supplement the Harrington system.[13,18,21,23,24] This was followed by interspinous wiring techniques such as Wisconsin wires and Drummond buttons.[5,23,24] The original Harrington rod was rigid and difficult to contour, and the rounded caudal tip failed to prevent rotation. This shortcoming led to the development of the square-ended Moe rod that allowed rod contouring and also prevented rotation.[*] The three-point bending force, which a con-

toured rod provides, was further enhanced by the development of the Edward sleeve.[6,7,18] The Harrington system, although often replaced by newer universal spinal instrumentation systems, can be used to stabilize thoracic and lumbar fractures that result from axial loading and in which the anterior longitudinal ligament is intact.[†]

## Harrington Distraction Fixation

### Technique

The patient is placed in the prone position, either on laminectomy rolls or on a specialized frame. All pressure points are inspected and adequately padded. Surgical site preparation should include at least one iliac crest. A midline incision is made to expose at least three levels above and two levels below the lesion. A subperiosteal dissection is performed and is carried laterally over the transverse process. An intraoperative radiograph can be obtained to verify the location of the lesion. The upper hook site is then prepared. Typically, this is located three levels above the injury site, and at this level, the inferior facet is exposed. The caudal tip is amputated with either a ¼-inch osteotome or a small Kerrison rongeur. The caudomedial margin of the lamina and underlying ligamentum flavum are excised. The lamina is conformed to allow seating of the rostral ratcheted hook, typically a no. 1253 hook. A no. 1251 hook can be used as a starter hook, which can then be replaced by a no. 1253 hook, a keeled hook, or a bifid no. 1262 hook. The hook is inserted to follow the angle of the facet joint and is then gently tapped into position. A well-seated hook should lie orthogonal to the spine (Figure 117.1). The caudal hook site is generally located two levels below the level of the injury. The interlaminar region at this level is enlarged with a Kerrison rongeur. The ligamentum flavum is excised, and the rostral margin of the lamina is conformed to accommodate the caudal hook, usually a no. 1254 round hole hook or a no. 1201 square hole hook (Figure 117.2). Square-hole caudal hooks are most commonly used because they allow contouring of the rods and minimize rotation. A construct undergoing distraction is depicted in Figure 117.3.

### Segmental Fixation

Segmental fixation of the Harrington system has been shown to increase stability.[13,18,21,24] Segmental fixation can use either sublaminar wires or cables or interspinous techniques (e.g., Wisconsin wiring technique).[5,24] When sublaminar fixation is chosen as a means of segmental fixation, consideration should be given to the use of cables, which are stronger and more flexible and which may decrease the incidence of neurologic complications. Placement of sublaminar wire or cable can be accomplished by removing the interspinous ligament and performing an interlaminar laminotomy along the midline at each level that is to be instrumented. The ligamentum flavum is removed with a Kerrison rongeur, and the dura mater or epidural fat is visualized. Adequate removal of the ligamentum flavum

---

[*]References 1,3,13,18,23,24.
[†]References 2,4,6,7,13,18,23,24.

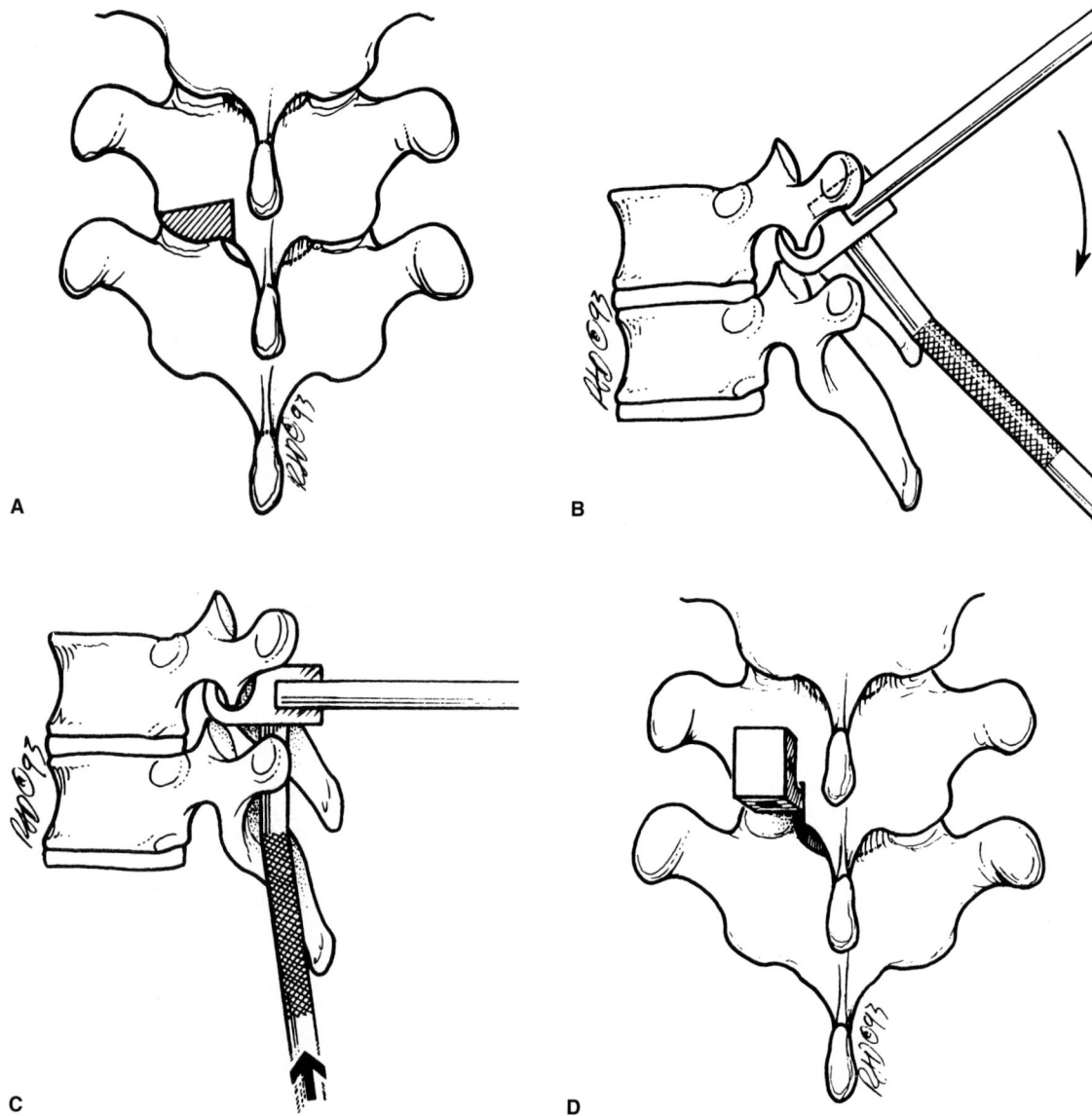

**Figure 117.1** Harrington fixation, upper hook site. (**A**) Preparation. (**B-D**) Insertion.

ensures easy passage of the sublaminar wire or cable. A 16- or 18-gauge wire is doubled and formed into an S or a fishhook shape. Alternatively, a cable can be used, in which case the cable leader is bent into an S or fishhook shape. The leader or wire is then passed beneath the caudal edge of the lamina gently by hand, without any downward pressure being used. This avoids injury to underlying neural elements. Once the tip of the wire or leader is visualized, it is grasped with a clamp, and constant upward pressure is maintained on the wire or cable to minimize canal compromise. Once the wire is passed, it is bent over the lamina to guard against inadvertently displacing the wire into the spinal canal. The cable leaders are cut at this point to create two single cables. Sublaminar wires or cables can also be placed at each level to be stabilized. Laminotomies are performed at each interlaminar space with a Kerrison rongeur. The underlying ligamentum flavum is excised and the dura mater or epidural fat is visualized. Wires or cables are then passed as described.

## Interspinous Segmental Instrumentation

Interspinous segmental instrumentation can also be used to supplement the strength of the construct.[5,24] A single hole is made at the base of each spinous process to be instrumented, with a curved awl, a bone tenaculum, or a drill. Beaded Wisconsin wires, with attached Drummond buttons, are passed through the base of the spinous process from each side. Once it is through the base of the spinous process, the beaded Wisconsin wire is passed through the contralateral Drummond button. The Wisconsin wires are then pulled tight until the Drummond button fits snugly against the base of the spinous process. The beads are then cut. Once the rods are in place, the wires are tightly secured to the rods, and the excess wire is removed. The free wire ends are then bent to provide a low profile (Figure 117.4).

A square-ended rod is then chosen, with an appropriate length of rod that allows one ratchet to be visualized

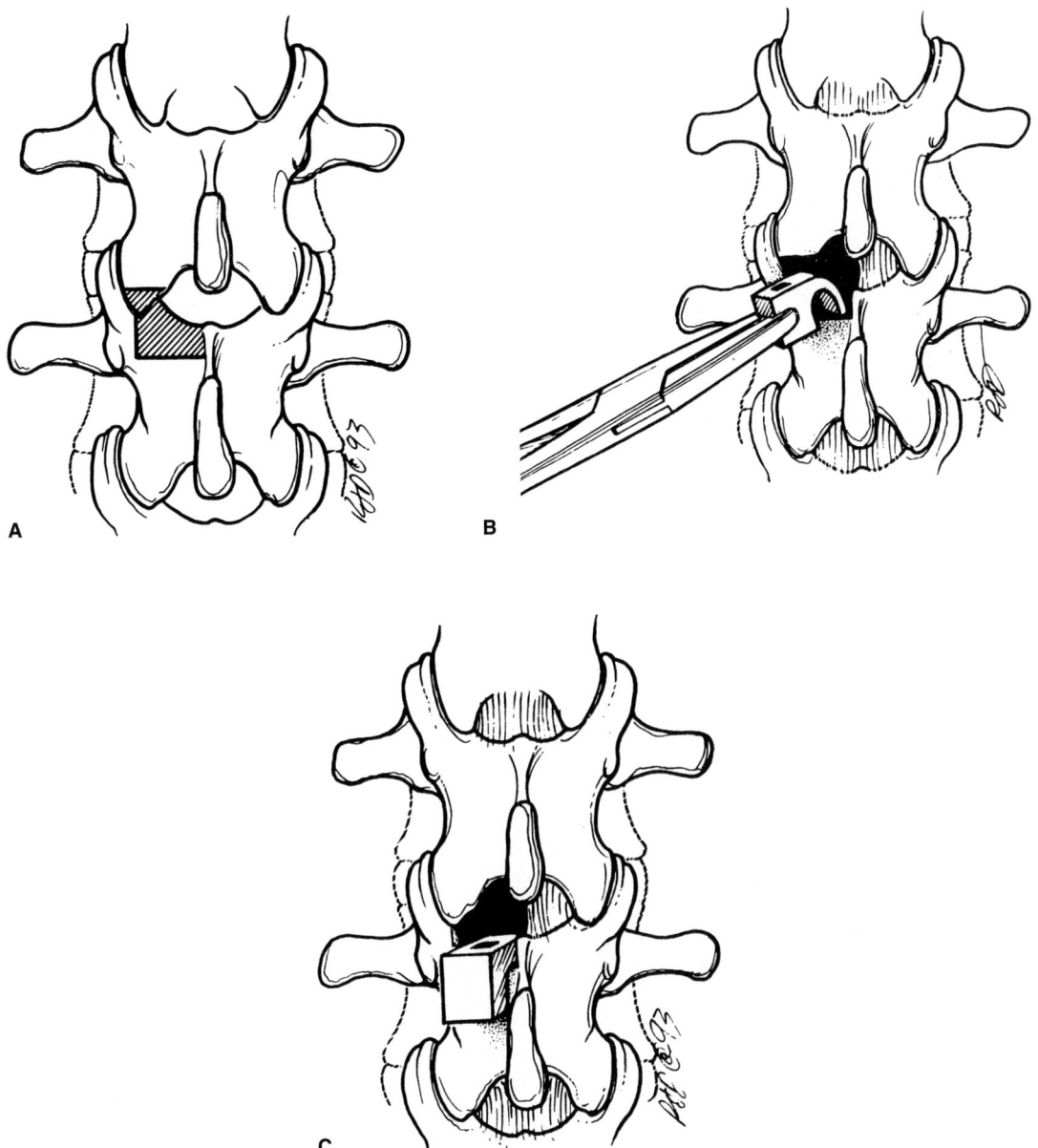

**Figure 117.2** Harrington fixation, lower hook site. **(A)** Preparation. **(B** and **C)** Insertion.

beneath the rostral hook. The rod is then contoured to maintain normal spinal alignment. Edward sleeves can also be used to enhance reduction of kyphotic deformities.

## Rod Sleeves

Rod sleeves are designed to provide reduction of kyphotic deformities.[6,7,18,24] They are made of high-density polyethylene with barium sulfate for radiodensity. Rod sleeves are made in various sizes: small 2mm sleeves for use in the thoracic spine, medium 4mm sleeves for use between T10 and L1, large 6mm sleeves for use between T12 and L2, and elliptical sleeves for use in the lumbar region (Figure 117.5). The rod is inserted into the rostral hook, and the rod sleeve is then advanced along the rod until it overlies the apex of the deformity. The caudal end is grasped with a hook holder, and the distal rod is held with a rod holder. The

deformity is reduced by applying constant ventral pressure. The rod is then moved caudally until the distal tip engages the caudal hook, and distraction is then applied with the rod distractor. The second rod is placed in a similar fashion. Overdistraction is prevented by obtaining intraoperative radiographs. C-clamps are applied to the ratchet below the upper hook to avoid loss of distraction. Sublaminar wires or cables or interspinous wires are then secured to the rods. Excess wire is cut and the free ends are bent toward the midline to offer the construct a low profile. The facet joints to be fused are denuded, the spine is decorticated, and autologous bone graft is placed dorsally and dorsolaterally. A drain may be placed at this point and brought to the skin through a separate stab incision. The wound is then closed by using 0 or 2-0 absorbable suture to approximate the fascia and 2-0 or 3-0 absorbable suture to approximate the subcutaneous tissue. The skin edges are closed according to the

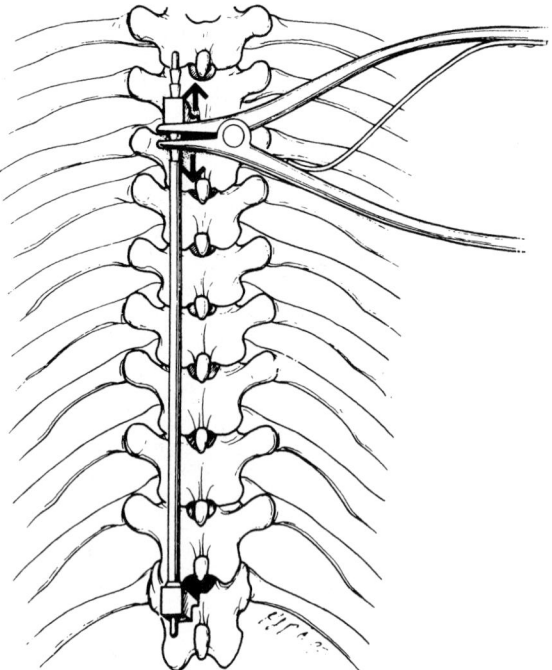

**Figure 117.3** Distraction rod insertion.

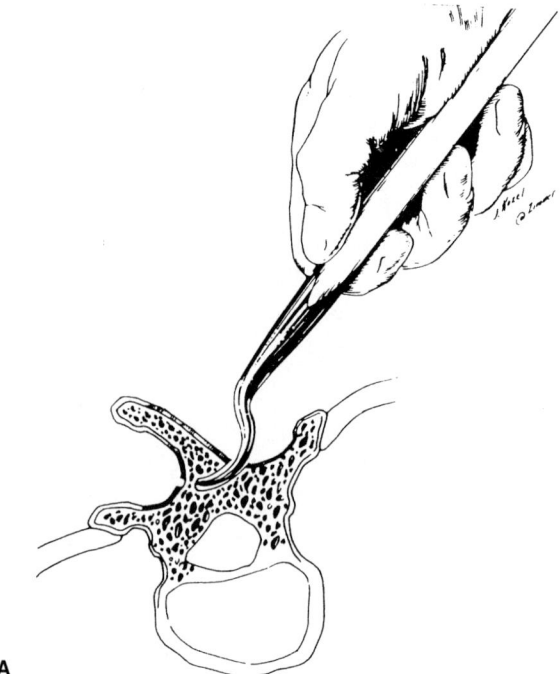

A

**Figure 117.4** Placement of interspinous segmental instrumentation using Wisconsin wires and Drummond buttons.

surgeon's preference. If a drain is used, it is removed after 24 hours. The patient is mobilized as soon as a molded brace is available. Radiographs are obtained with the patient in an upright position to assess the stability of the construct. Provided these films show a stable construct, the brace is continued for 12 weeks or until a fusion mass is evident.

## Luque Segmental Wire Fixation

Luque instrumentation has been largely replaced by universal spinal instrumentation. Whereas the Luque system offers good stability against rotational and transitional forces, it provides less resistance to flexion-extension and little or no resistance to axial loading. The Luque system may still be used to treat slice fractures, in which the middle column fails because of shearing forces. It may also be useful in cases in which long fixation is required for correction of paralytic scoliotic deformities or in traumatic or neoplastic lesions that lead to flexion-compression fractures. The Luque system may be beneficial in patients with poor bone quality who require spinal stabilization.[12,16-18,20,23,24]

### Technique

The technique for patient positioning and exposure is similar to that used for Harrington instrumentation. The technique for passage of wire or cable is as previously described for sublaminar wire or cable placement. An appropriate Luque rod is chosen and contoured to conform to the curvature of a normal spine. Alternatively, a Luque rectangle can be used.

Luque rectangles confer rotational and migrational stability to the construct. Sublaminar wires or cables are secured to the appropriately contoured Luque rod or rectangle (Figures 117.6 to 117.8). The short limb of the L-shaped Luque rod should be secured beneath the long limb of the contralateral L-shaped Luque rod (Figure 117.9). Interspinous wiring techniques described for Harrington instrumentation can also be used with L-shaped Luque rods. The interspinous wiring technique, although safer to perform than placement of sublaminar wires or cables, creates a weaker construct; also, it cannot be used with Luque rectangles because the Luque rectangle cannot be adequately approximated to the spinous process.

The Luque system, although originally designed for neutral fixation of the spine, can be used to reduce kyphotic deformities. In this situation, the rostral end of one L-shaped Luque rod and the caudal end of the contralateral L-shaped Luque rod are attached and can be used to reduce kyphotic deformities. In this situation, the rostral end of one L-shaped Luque rod and the caudal end of the contralateral L-shaped rod are attached via sublaminar or interspinous wires or cables. The free ends of the rods are then used as levers to reduce the existing kyphotic deformity (Figure 117.10). Once reduced, the wires or cables are sequentially tightened, ensuring lasting reduction. Excess wire or cable is cut, and the free ends are contoured to allow a construct of low profile. Closure is performed as described for Harrington instrumentation, and postoperative care is also identical to that used with Harrington instrumentation.

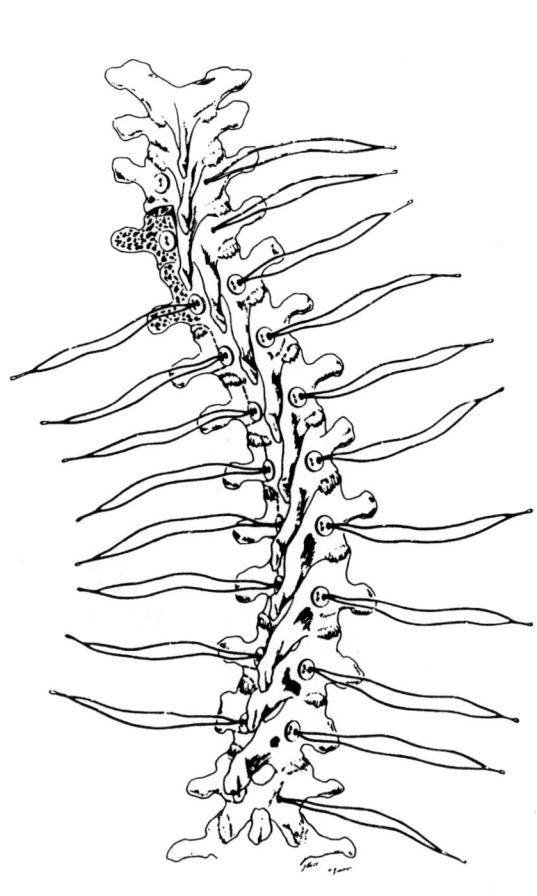

**B**

**Figure 117.4** *cont'd*

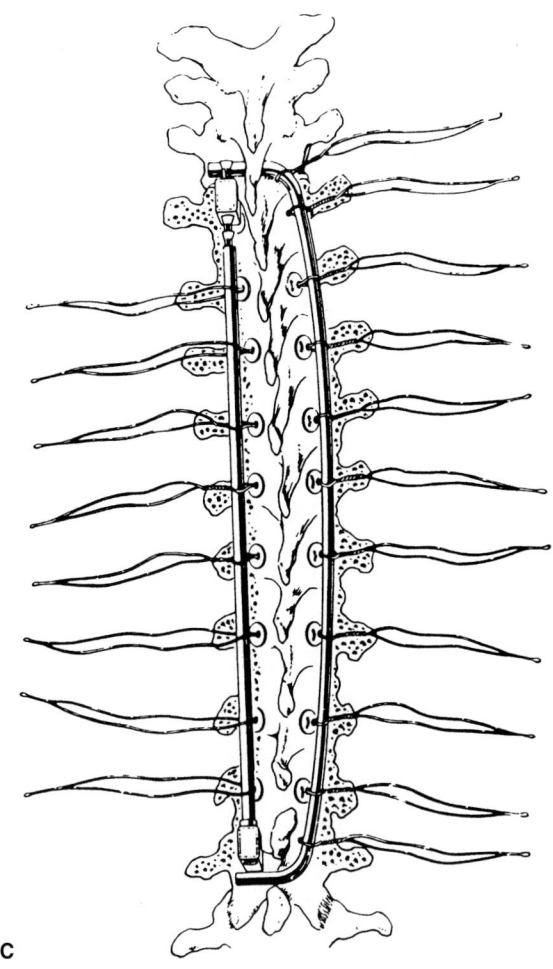

**C**

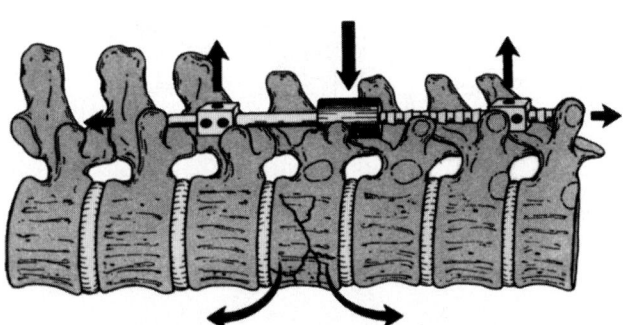

**Figure 117.5** Placement of Edward sleeves.

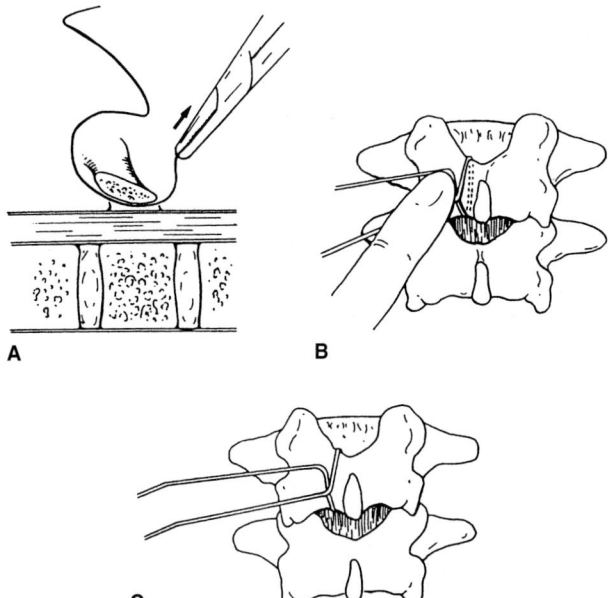

**A**        **B**

**C**

**Figure 117.6** Placement of sublaminar wires via midline laminotomy (**A**). Crimping prevents spinal cord encroachment (**B** and **C**).

## Scott Wiring Technique

Wiring techniques for the spine were first described by Hadra in 1889.[8,15] Numerous techniques have since been proposed, used, and gradually replaced by newer, more versatile universal spinal instrumentation. Few indications remain for the use of spinal wiring in the lumbar spine. One such indication is symptomatic lumbar spondylolysis with or without grade I spondylolisthesis in a patient younger than 25 years who has failed conservative therapy.

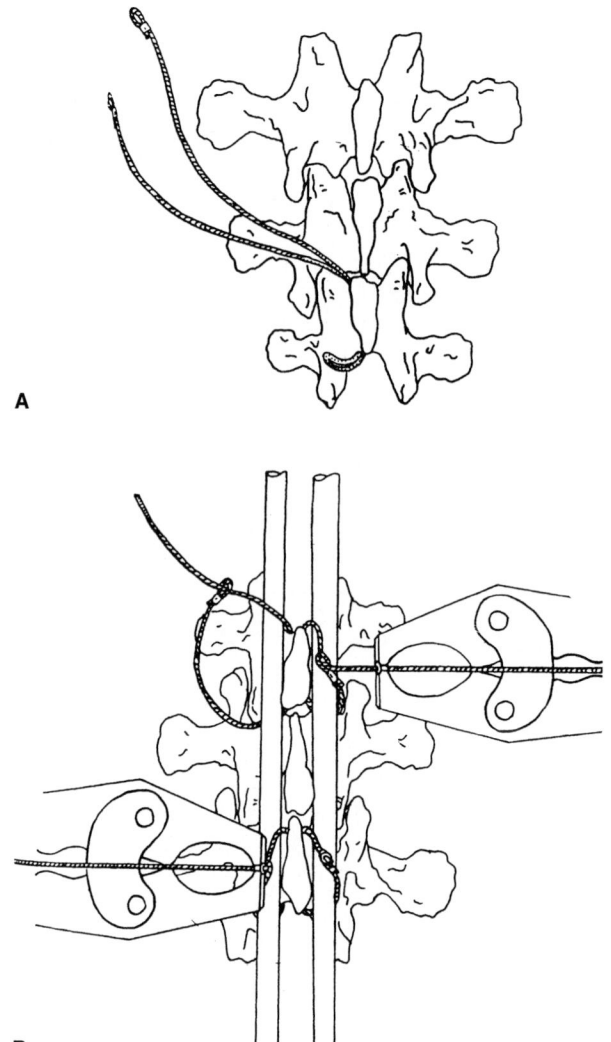

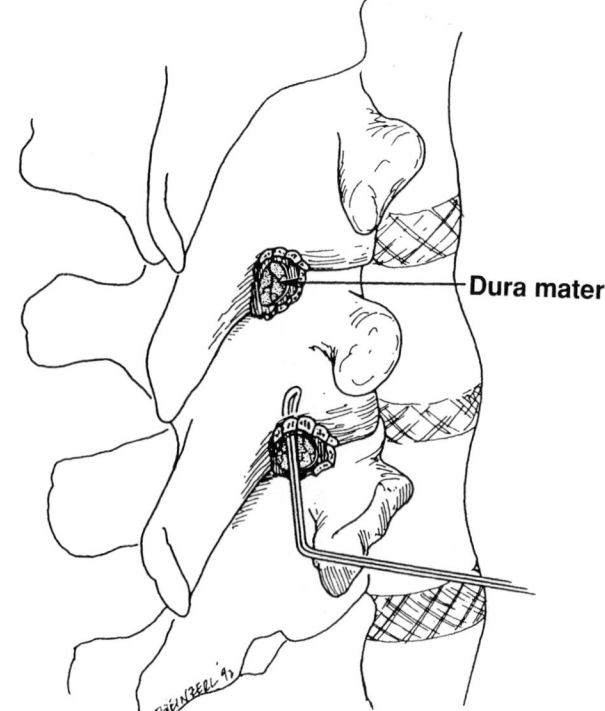

**Figure 117.8** Placement of sublaminar wires via bilateral laminotomies.

**Figure 117.7** Placement of sublaminar multistrand cable via midline laminotomy (**A** and **B**).[22]

This wiring technique for direct repair of spondylolysis was described by Nicol and Scott[19] and later modified by Johnson and Thompson.[14] The Scott wiring technique consists of wiring the transverse process to the spinous process.

### Technique

The patient is placed prone, supported on laminectomy rolls or a frame. Pressure points are inspected and adequately padded. A midline incision is made overlying spinous processes adjacent to the level of interest. A subperiosteal dissection is performed and carried laterally, extending over the transverse processes. Bilateral pars interarticularis fractures are readily identified by the increased mobility of the affected segment. The defect is freed of any overlying or intervening fibrous tissue. The bony margins of the defect, base of the transverse process, and adjacent lamina are decorticated. Originally, a wire was passed around the transverse process bilaterally, and the free wire was passed beneath the subadjacent spinous

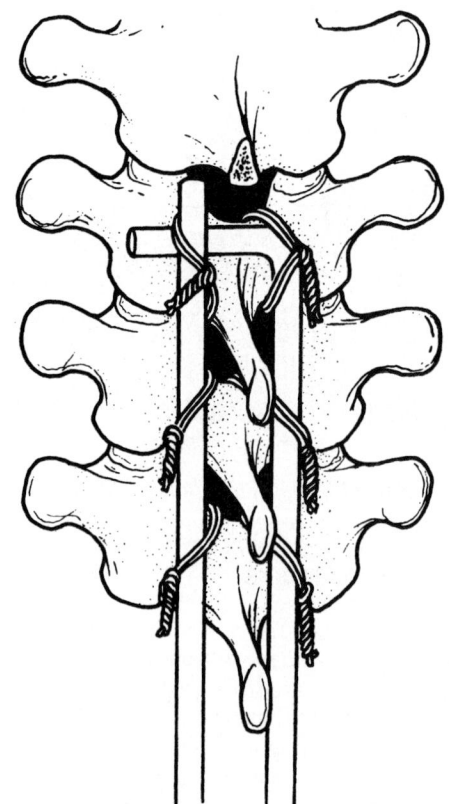

**Figure 117.9** Luque L-rod configuration at termini of construct.

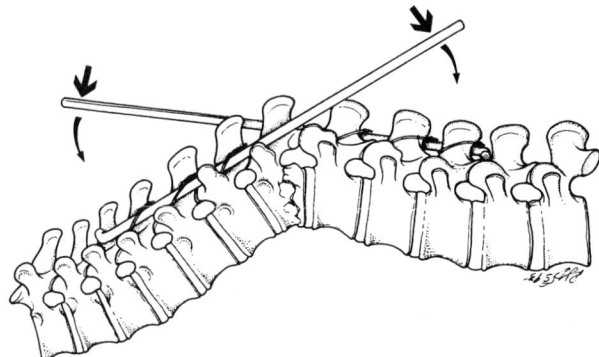

**Figure 117.10** Harrington placement of Luque L-rods used in reduction of kyphotic deformities.

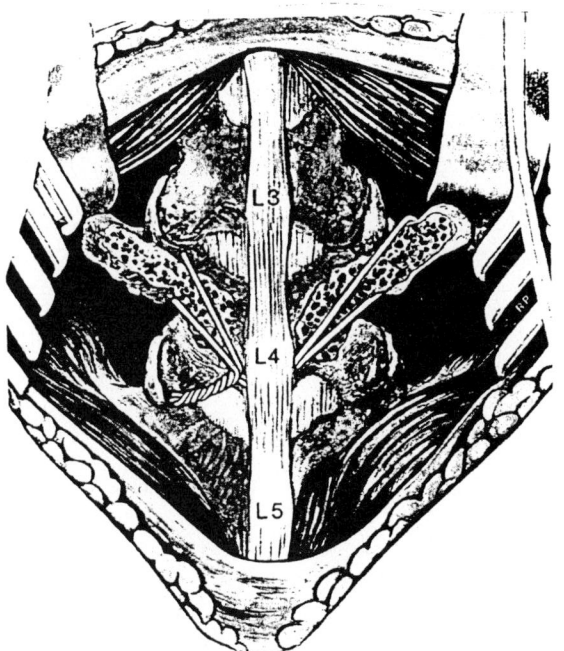

**Figure 117.11** Scott wiring technique.

process and was secured (Figure 117.11). This technique was later modified to minimize the incidence of nerve root injury. With the modified technique, a hole is drilled at the base of the transverse process and the spinous process. A wire, or alternatively, a multistrand cable is passed through the hole at the base of the transverse process and then through the drill hole at the base of the spinous process, forming a figure-eight configuration. Autologous cortico-cancellous strips are placed over the pars interarticularis defect and decorticated transverse process and lamina. The bone grafts are secured into position by tightening the wire or cable. The wound is then closed as previously described. A removable brace is worn for 12 weeks. The patient can resume normal activities once a radiograph reveals a solid fusion.[14,19]

## Summary

Simple hook-rod, wire, and wire-rod techniques for the dorsal stabilization of the thoracic and lumbar spine have been available since the early 1960s. A testament to their utility is their longevity. These techniques provided the basic principles from which modern spinal instrumentation techniques have evolved, but they have been largely replaced by universal spinal instrumentation techniques. However, they are still used for indications such as thoracic and lumbar instability, fixed deformities, neoplastic diseases, and degenerative disorders.

## REFERENCES

1. Akbarnia BA, Fogarty JP, Tayob AA: Contoured Harrington instrumentation in the treatment of unstable spinal fractures: the effect of supplementary sublaminar wires. *Clin Orthop* 189:186-194, 1984.
2. Anden U, Lake A, Nordwall A: The role of the anterior longitudinal ligament in spinal fractures. *Spine* 5:23-25, 1980.
3. Denis F, Ruiz H, Searls K: Comparison between square-ended distraction rods and standard round-ended distraction rods in the treatment of thoracolumbar spinal injuries. *Clin Orthop* 189:162-167, 1984.
4. Dickson JH, Harrington PR, Erwin WD: Results of reduction and stabilization of the severely fractured thoracic and lumbar spine. *J Bone Joint Surg* 60A:799-805, 1978.
5. Drummond DS: Harrington instrumentation with spinous process wiring for idiopathic scoliosis. *Orthop Clin North Am* 19:281-289, 1988.
6. Edwards CC, Levine AM: Early rod-sleeve stabilization of the injured thoracic and lumbar spine. *Orthop Clin North Am* 17:121-145, 1986.
7. Gokaslan ZL, McCormick P: Surgical techniques: thoracic and lumbar. In Benzel EC, Tator C (eds): *Contemporary Management of Spinal Cord Injury*. Park Ridge, IL, American Association of Neurological Surgeons Publications Committee, 1995, pp 153-166.
8. Hadra BE: The classic wiring of the vertebrae as a means of immobilization in fracture and Pott's disease. *Clin Orthop* 112:4-8, 1975.
9. Harrington PR: Treatment of scoliosis: correction and internal fixation by spinal instrumentation. *Bone Joint Surg* 44A:591-610, 1962.
10. Harrington PR: Technical details in relation to the successful use of instrumentation in scoliosis. *Orthop Clin North Am* 3:49-67, 1972.
11. Harrington PR: The history and development of Harrington instrumentation. *Clin Orthop* 93:110-112, 1973.
12. Hitchon PW, Follet KA: Luque instrumentation for the thoracic and lumbar spine. In Hitchon P, Traynelis V, Rengachary S (eds): *Techniques in Spinal Fusion and Stabilization*. New York, Thieme Medical, 1995, pp 198-203.
13. Hitchon PW: Harrington distraction rods for thoracic and lumbar fractures. In Hitchon P, Traynelis V, Rengachary S (eds). *Techniques in Spinal Fusion and Stabilization*. New York, Thieme Medical, 1995, pp 204-208.
14. Johnson GV, Thompson AG: The Scott wiring technique for direct repair of lumbar spondylolysis. *J Bone Joint Surg* 74B:426-430, 1992.

15. Krag MH: Spinal fusion: overview of options and posterior internal fixation devices. In Frymoyer JW (ed): *The Adult Spine: Principles and Practice*. Philadelphia, JB Lippincott, 1991, pp 1919-1945.

16. Luque ER: The anatomic basis and development of segmental spinal instrumentation. *Spine* 7:256-259, 1982.

17. Luque ER, Cassis N, Ramirez-Wiella G: Segmental spinal instrumentation in the treatment of fractures of the thoracolumbar spine. *Spine* 7:312-317, 1982.

18. McCormick PC: Dorsal distraction and neutral segmental fixation of thoracic and lumbar spine: Harrington and Luque techniques. In Benzel EC (ed): *Spinal Instrumentation*. Park Ridge, IL, Publications Committee of the North American Association of Neurological Surgeons, 1994, pp 125-141.

19. Nicol RO, Scott JHS: Lytic spondylolysis repair by wiring. *Spine* 11:1027-1030, 1986.

20. Parsons JR, Choski BV, Lee CK, *et al*: The bio-mechanical analysis of sublaminar wires and cables using Luque segmental spinal instrumentation. *Spine* 22:267-273, 1997.

21. Silverman BJ, Greenberg PE: Idiopathic scoliosis: posterior spine fusion with Harrington rod and sublaminar wiring. *Orthop Clin North Am* 19:269-279, 1988.

22. Songer MN, Spencer DL, Meter PR, Jayaraman G: The use of sublaminar cables to replace Luque wires. *Spine* 16(suppl):418-421, 1991.

23. Stillerman CB, Gruen JP, Roy R: Thoracic and lumbar fusion: techniques for posterior stabilization. In Menezes A, Sonntag V (eds): *Principles of Spinal Surgery*. New York, McGraw-Hill, 1996, pp 1199-1223.

24. Richardson WJ, Hardaker WT Jr.: *Management of Thoracic and Lumbar Spinal Instability*. In Wilkins R, Renegachary S (eds): *Neurosurgery*. New York, McGraw-Hill, 1996, pp 2998-3001.

# CHAPTER 118

# Dorsal Thoracic and Lumbar Universal Spinal Instrumentation Techniques

## Daniel K. Resnick and Sait Naderi

The treatment of traumatic, neoplastic, and degenerative disorders of the spine has evolved over the last several decades. A significant advance in the treatment of spinal disease has been the use of universal spinal instrumentation (USI). The term "universal" refers to the applicability of the construct throughout the thoracic and lumbar spine as well as to the variety of configurations with which it may be applied. These systems may be applied to the spine by using a variety of hooks and screws, alone or in combination. Multiple systems are currently available, and each has its own strengths and weaknesses of design. This chapter discusses the history of dorsal fixation techniques and the basic biomechanical principles used during the application of universal instrumentation systems. The techniques of implant insertion and the similarities and differences between several of the most commonly used systems are discussed.

## History

Reports of wire and screw fixation of the thoracic and lumbar spine appeared in the medical literature in the late 1800s. In 1891, Hadra[17] described a procedure performed in 1887 in which Wilkins attempted fixation of T12-L1 in a neonate by using silver wire. Lange[23] contemporaneously described the (unsuccessful) use of nonfixed steel rods for the treatment of spinal deformity. Instrumentation of the thoracic and lumbar spine was restricted to wiring techniques and the occasional use of the facet screw until 1962, when Harrington introduced his spine instrumentation system. This system was the first that allowed for significant correction of spinal deformity and rigid fixation of the diseased spine.[6,18]

In the early 1970s, Luque[24] introduced segmental spinal instrumentation with sublaminar wires. The use of sublaminar wires provided multiple points of fixation, and when combined with closed loops instead of rods, or with the Harrington distraction system, provided significant resistance to flexion, extension, and lateral bending.[5] Continued modification of the Luque and Harrington systems through the 1970s laid the groundwork for the introduction of universal instrumentation in the early 1980s.

Pedicle screw fixation devices were introduced by Roy-Camille[31] in the 1980s. These devices use rods, plates, or fixators as longitudinal members. Pedicle screw fixation allows for the creation of rigid constructs. This rigidity has led to the advent of short segment fixation. Because of the strength and the geometry of the systems, it is possible to allow for greater preservation of segmental motion at adjacent segments. Cotrel and Dubousset[8] introduced the first "universal" spine fixation system in the late 1980s. This system used pedicle screws as well as multiple hooks. The latter were specifically designed to engage the pedicle, lamina, or transverse process. This allowed the application of the device throughout the thoracic and lumbar spine. Furthermore, the use of a combination of components allowed for the application of a variety of forces (compression, distraction, three-point bending). This in turn allowed for the efficacious correction of spinal deformities.[5,6] Recently the advent of frameless stereotaxic techniques has led to an increased popularity in the use of thoracic pedicle screws. The use of thoracic pedicle screws allows for rigid fixation of the thoracic spine without the need for intracanalicular instrumentation.

## Surgical Indications

The indications for thoracic and lumbar dorsal instrumentation are evolving. Zdeblick,[40] Mardjetko,[25] and others have demonstrated that instrumentation improves the rate of fusion in traumatic and degenerative conditions. In addition to increasing fusion rates, the stabilizing effect of dorsal universal instrumentation allows for earlier mobilization of patients with traumatic or neoplastic spinal instability. Although no benefit regarding neurologic outcome has been demonstrated, the ability to allow patients to ambulate soon after injury or surgery substantially lowers morbidity and allows for a more rapid rehabilitation.[19,38] The most common current use for thoracolumbar universal instrumentation systems is in the setting of degenerative lumbosacral instability.

Several models and point systems currently exist for the determination of acute traumatic instability.[11,37] Subacute and glacial instability may be objectively demonstrated with serial and dynamic radiographs. Regrettably, the great majority of patients with back pain do not exhibit such clear-cut indications for surgery. The role of fusion and instrumentation for the treatment of "dysfunctional motion segments" remains somewhat controversial. The decision to use any of these systems for the treatment of back pain without clear radiographic evidence of instability is based solely on the clinical judgment of the surgeon.[5,15,33]

## Biomechanical Forces Imparted by Thoracic and Lumbar Spinal Implants

The human spine is subject to a variety of stresses on a daily basis. The upright posture necessitates significant load bearing by the thoracic and lumbar spine. In addition, normal activity results in flexion, extension, lateral bending, and axial rotation of the spine. Each of these maneuvers results in the application of forces to the spinal elements.

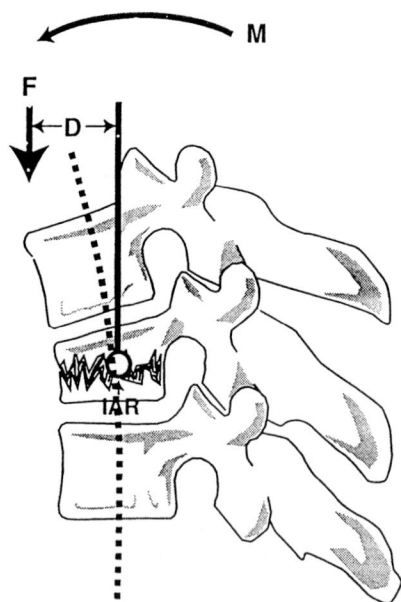

**Figure 118.1** Biomechanical considerations. The forces acting on the thoracic and lumbar spine are depicted here as well as the effective kyphosis of the thoracic spine. An axial load (*F*) acts via a lever arm (*D*) to produce a bending moment (*M*) about the instantaneous axis of rotation (*IAR*). Forces that are transmitted within the neutral axis (*dotted line*) cause no bending moment. (*Copyright University of New Mexico, Division of Neurosurgery.*)

The intact spine, to paraphrase White and Panjabi,[37] resists these forces in such a manner as to avoid neural injury and deformation. When supraphysiologic forces are applied (such as in a motor vehicle accident) or when the integrity of the spinal elements is compromised (tumor or infection), deformation of the spine and possibly neural element damage results. A description of the forces acting on the spine is provided by clinical biomechanics. An understanding of these forces is helpful in planning corrective surgery.

Forces acting on the spine can be broken down into component vectors. A vector is a force that has both a magnitude and a fixed direction in three-dimensional space. A force vector may act directly on a point in space, causing translation (movement in the same plane as the vector). Alternatively, a force vector may act via a lever (moment arm), causing rotation about an axis. When a force vector acts via a moment arm, a bending moment is applied. The axis, or fulcrum, about which this bending moment causes rotation is termed the *instantaneous axis of rotation* (IAR). The IAR may be defined as the axis about which a given vertebral body rotates when acted on by a bending moment.[5,37] In the normal spine, the IAR is located in the region of the dorsal aspect of the vertebral body (middle column of Denis[11]). The bending moment (M) is defined as the product of the force (F) applied and the moment arm (D) or the perpendicular distance from the IAR (M = FXD). The neutral axis is defined as the longitudinal axis that encompasses the IAR of adjacent vertebral bodies. Forces transmitted along the neutral axis cause no significant bending moment[37] (Figure 118.1).

Newton's third law of motion, the law of conservation of momentum, states that interactions between objects result in no net change in momentum; thus for every action there is an equal (in magnitude) and opposite (in direction) reaction. In the present context, this implies that the spine (when at rest) exerts forces that are equal in magnitude and opposite in direction to the axial loads and bending moments applied. The ability of the normal spine to resist these forces is dependent on the material properties of the vertebral bodies and supporting bony, muscular, and ligamentous structures. When spinal instrumentation is applied, the construct may function simply as a replacement for a damaged spinal element (tension-band fixation) or may apply forces to the spine in a relatively unique and complex fashion (three-point bending).[5,37]

## Distraction

Dorsal distraction fixation, usually applied with sublaminar hooks, has been used for short segment distraction for deformity correction and foraminal stenosis. This mode of application has not found widespread use, however, because of a tendency for exaggeration of kyphotic deformity (Figure 118.2).[5]

## Tension Band Fixation

Dorsal compression fixation, also applied with hooks, is used for tension-band fixation in the case of dorsal ligamentous insufficiency. This technique depends on the integrity of the load-supporting capacity of the ventral elements as well as the preservation of the relevant dorsal bony elements. This type of fixation should never be applied without adequate ventral spinal canal decompression. Tension-band fixation may be used as a short segment fixator, since the applied bending moment is independent of construct length (Figure 118.3). Tension band constructs do not, in general, resist translation and should not be relied on as stand-alone constructs when significant resistance to translation is required. When multiple segments are to be instrumented with this technique, multiple points of fixation should be used to prevent terminal bending moments.[5]

## Three-Point Bending

Three-point bending forces are applied when translational forces are applied at both ends of a construct that are equal in magnitude but opposite in direction to a translational force applied to the fulcrum of a pathologic curvature. These constructs are usually applied in a distraction or neutral mode. The prototypical three-point bending construct is the Harrington distraction rod, especially when augmented with sleeves. The application of three-point bending forces depends on the physical contact between the longitudinal member with the fulcrum of the kyphotic deformity. These constructs, when placed dorsally, result in a dorsally directed force at both termini and a ventrally directed force at the fulcrum of the kyphotic curve (Figure 118.4).[5] Three-point bending constructs must, by definition, traverse at least three spinal segments. Because the bending moments applied by a three-point bending implant are proportional to the length of the construct, multiple segment instrumentation is frequently used to

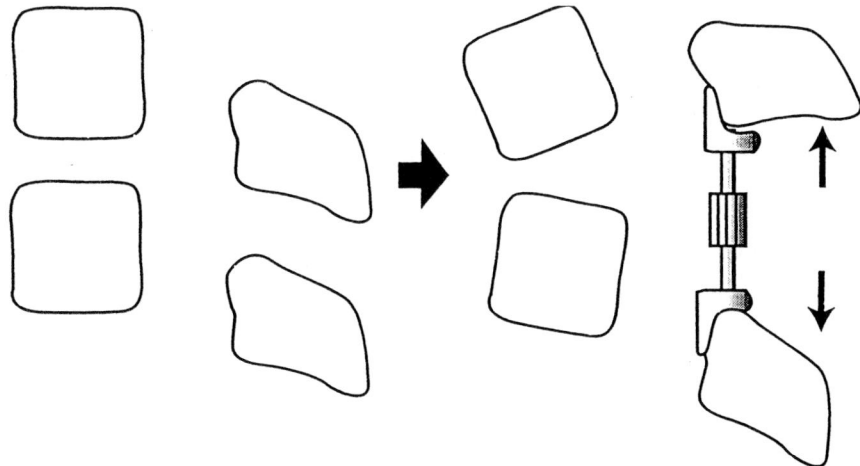

**Figure 118.2** Dorsal distraction fixation may lead to kyphotic deformation, especially if used at or above the thoracolumbar junction. Use of distraction fixation in the lumbar spine may lead to a painful "flat back" syndrome. (*Copyright University of New Mexico, Division of Neurosurgery.*)

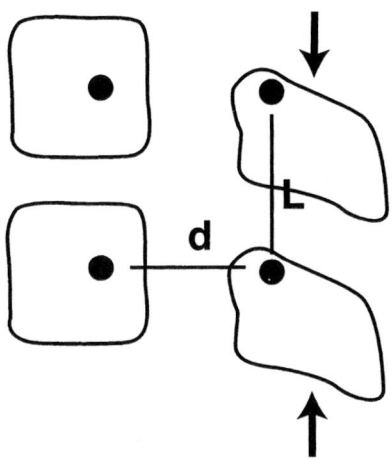

**Figure 118.3** Tension band fixation of the dorsal spine is used most effectively when adequate ventral support is present. The bending moment applied is proportional to the distance between the implant and the IAR (*d*) and is independent of the length of the construct (*L*). Therefore, significant corrective forces may be applied with short segment instrumentation. (*Copyright University of New Mexico, Division of Neurosurgery.*)

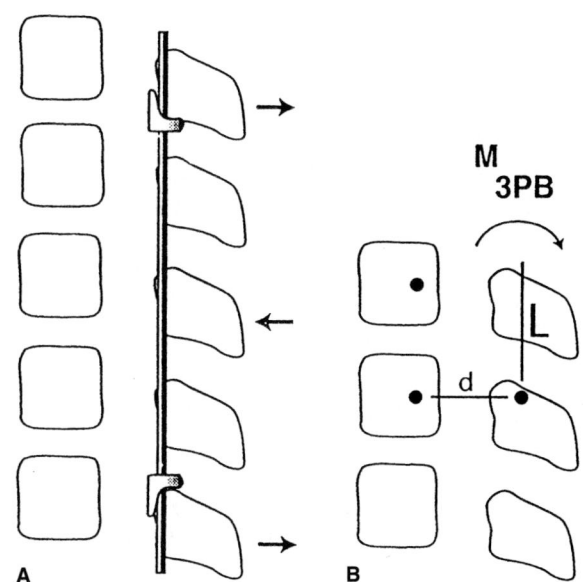

**Figure 118.4** Three-point bending constructs (**A** and **B**) rely on contact between the implant and the apex of a kyphotic curvature to produce forces perpendicular to the long axis of the spine. Forces are directed dorsally at the termini and ventrally in the center of the construct. These forces are equal in magnitude but opposite in direction. In the case of three-point bending implants, the bending moment ($M_{3PB}$) applied is directly proportional to the length of the construct (*L*). Therefore, since there is a limit to the dorsally directed forces that will be tolerated at the terminal implant/bone junctions, longer constructs are generally required for significant deformity correction. Alternatively, increasing the ability of the terminal interfaces to resist dorsally directed forces (e.g., using a claw configuration) will allow for the application of greater corrective forces with shorter segment instrumentation. (*Copyright University of New Mexico, Division of Neurosurgery.*)

correct significant deformity. Because of the strong dorsally directed forces at the termini of the construct, three-point bending constructs are often applied by using hook/lamina fixation. This maximizes the area of contact between the implant and bone. However, sublaminar instrumentation placement carries a risk of injury to the neural elements. Pedicle hooks, transverse process hooks, and hook/screw combinations may be used in many cases to avoid sublaminar placement of hooks. USI systems allow for the application of these constructs in a neutral mode by using hook "claws," which are able to engage the lamina without the significant distractive forces required by the Harrington rod system. Use of the "claw" technique allows for shorter segment fixation, since greater stresses may be born at the hook/hook/lamina junction.[5]

## Cantilever Beam Constructs

The final mode of application of dorsal universal instrumentation systems is cantilever beam fixation. A cantilever beam is simply a beam supported at one end, such as a balcony or awning support. These constructs are applied by using pedicle screws as the beams. Cantilever beams may be applied in one of three fashions. The great majority of cantilever beam constructs applied to the thoracic and lumbar spine are fixed moment arm cantilever beams (Figure 118.5A). A fixed moment arm cantilever beam is one in which the pedicle screw is rigidly affixed to the longitudinal member. This type of construct allows for load bearing (when placed in a neutral or distractive mode) or load sharing (when placed in a compressive mode in conjunction with adequate ventral support).

Nonfixed cantilever beam constructs, in which the pedicle screw is not rigidly affixed to the longitudinal member, are rarely used in the thoracic and lumbar spine because of their inability to bear loads (like a hinged awning) and poor performance as tension-band constructs (caused by screw toggling and pullout) (see Figure 118.5B). In the cervical spine, lateral mass plate/screw systems are commonly applied non-fixed moment arm cantilever beam constructs that work well. These systems take advantage of the anatomy of the cervical facet, which tends to resist translation.

The final cantilever beam construct is the applied moment arm cantilever beam. This type of construct allows for the application of flexion or extension forces at the time of implant placement. Using long screws (Schanz type), a bending moment is applied to the spine. Once the desired corrective forces have been applied, the implant is fixed in place (see Figure 118.5C).[5] Obviously the application of these forces places great stress on the implant. This may result in failure of the implant, particularly if osseus union does not occur in a timely fashion.

## Biomechanical Properties of Universal Spinal Implant Systems

All universal spinal implant systems consist of screws, hooks, and longitudinal members. The composition, shape, and size of the implants vary to some extent. However, all conform to the constraints placed on them by the anatomic configuration of the bony spine. Some of the basic properties of the components and the impact that changes in these basic properties, such as the particular alloy of stainless steel used in a longitudinal member or the profile of the minor diameter of a screw, have on the performance of a given system are discussed below.

### Metallurgy

USI systems are composed of stainless steel, titanium alloy, or pure titanium. Stainless steel implants are, in general, stronger than similar-sized titanium implants and have excellent corrosion resistance. The most commonly used alloy is 316 stainless steel, which contains 17% chromium, 13% nickel, and 2.25% molybdenum. A newer alloy, 22-13-5 (referring to percentages of chromium, nickel, and manganese, respectively) has even greater strength and surface hardness.[3] Stainless steel implants are ferromagnetic and thus interfere with MRI imaging. Furthermore, osteointegration, or the ingrowth of bone into steel screws or rods, does not occur. A final caveat regarding the use of stainless steel is that it should not be used in patients with cutaneous nickel allergies. Dermal patch testing can rule out significant reaction to the alloy if there is a question regarding hypersensitivity.[3]

Titanium alloys have the advantages of being highly biocompatible and of minimally interfering with MRI. The most common titanium alloy is Ti-6-4, a combination of titanium, aluminum, and vanadium. This particular alloy has tensile strength that approaches 316 stainless steel. It is quite brittle, however.[3] Titanium may also be used in its unalloyed, or "pure" form.[7] "Pure" titanium is available in several grades (1 through 4), depending on the amount of impurities found in the metal. The less-pure grades (2 through 4) have tensile and elastic properties that approach 316 stainless steel. Titanium is more resistant to corrosion than steel[5] and also allows for osteointegration,

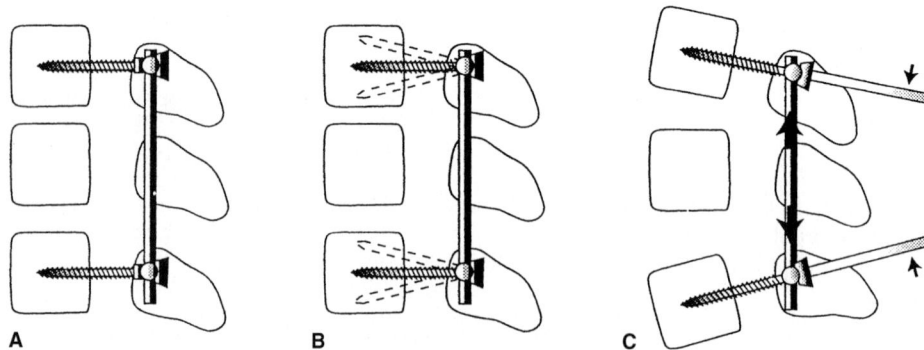

**Figure 118.5** Cantilever beam constructs. There are three types of cantilever beam constructs. Fixed moment arm (**A**) cantilever beam constructs employ constrained linkages between pedicle screws and longitudinal members and allow significant load bearing by the implant. Nonfixed moment arm (**B**) cantilever beam constructs do not allow load bearing and function poorly as tension band constructs because of problems related to toggling and screw pullout. Currently these types of constructs are rarely used in the thoracic or lumbar spine. Applied moment arm (**C**) cantilever beam constructs allow for the application of significant forces to the lumbar spine through the use of long screws. Because of the forces involved, screw breakage is likely to occur in the absence of strong bony fusion. (*Copyright University of New Mexico, Division of Neurosurgery.*)

both of which should decrease the incidence of implant failure.[3]

In addition to the composition of the metal used to create a spinal implant, the processes used to forge the metal and the surface characteristics of the implant affect performance. For example, cold working of a metal implant produces a harder, stronger material than does annealing. Also, shot peening, a surface treatment in which the implant is hardened by firing small particles against it, increases fatigue resistance. Any surface irregularity will increase the rate of corrosion of any implant. Finally, metals in implant construction should not be mixed, to avoid a galvanic current between the implant components. Such a current could, theoretically, increase the rate of corrosion and weaken the implant.[5]

## Hook Design

Hooks used for universal instrumentation may be placed in a variety of positions. Laminar hooks may be placed facing rostrally or caudally. Pedicle hooks are placed outside of the spinal canal and face rostrally, abutting the pedicle. Transverse process hooks are placed facing caudally over the transverse processes of the thoracic spine. Manufacturers have responded differently to the multiple locations and orientations of the hooks. Some systems, such as TSRH, provide a wide variety of hooks specially designed for placement at a specific site and with a specific orientation. Other systems, such as the Isola system, use similar hooks for all applications (Figure 118.6). The choice of the system used depends on surgeon preference. More choices, in terms of hook configuration, obligate less bone contouring. However, more choices also obligate a more cumbersome instrumentation set.[34]

Hooks may be open-ended, allowing top loading of the rod onto the hook, or alternatively, they may be closed to slide the rod through a circular aperture. Closed hooks are theoretically stronger and should in general be used at the terminus of a construct where applied forces are the greatest. Open-ended hooks are best used at sites of intermediate fixation, within the center of the construct, because of their ease of application.[34] In reality, the incidence of hook failure caused by failure of the hook/rod interface is extremely low in modern USI systems.

## Pedicle Screws

Pedicle screws are used for fixation of spinal implants when the lamina or transverse processes are not present (after decompression or trauma) or when significant load bearing by the implant is desired. Pedicle screw design incorporates several biomechanical principles. The minor diameter of a screw is defined as the minimal (inner) diameter of the screw (base of one thread to the base of the opposite thread). The strength, or resistance to bending and breaking, of a screw is proportional to the third power of its minor diameter. Therefore, small increases in the minor diameter of a screw are associated with large increases in strength. Obviously, the anatomic configuration of the pedicle and design constraints limit the minor diameter. Because the region of the screw subject to the greatest strain is the screw/plate or screw/rod junction,

tapered screws have been developed to maximize strength where it is needed without sacrificing pull-out resistance.[3]

The pull-out resistance of a screw is related to the amount of bone that can be incorporated between the threads of the screw. The distance between the threads (pitch), major diameter, and thread shape all influence the pull-out resistance of a screw. Osteointegration should significantly increase resistance to screw pullout. The most important factor in determining screw pullout resistance, it is emphasized, is bone quality. Osteopenic bone and low-density medullary bone provide poor purchase for even the best designed screws. Severe osteopenia may be considered a contraindication for screw fixation. A screw diameter should be selected such that the relatively dense cortical bone of the pedicle walls is partially engaged by the threads of the screw to maximize pull-out resistance.

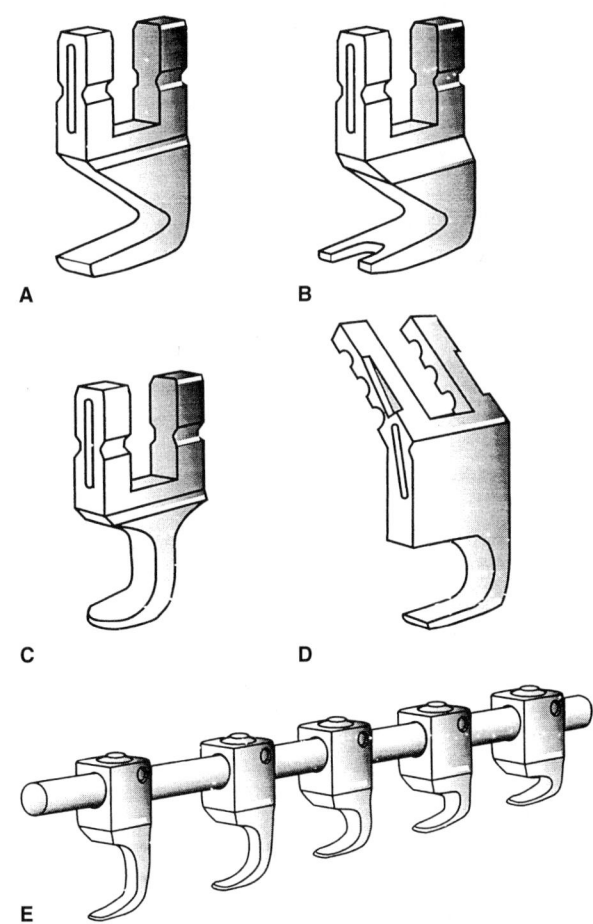

**Figure 118.6** Hook design spinal hooks are available in a variety of configurations for placement under the lamina (**A,** CTSRH laminar hook), abutting the pedicle (**B,** CTSRH pedicle hook), or over the transverse process (**C,** CTSRH transverse process hook). An offset hook (**D**) allows for less rod contouring. Note the throat shape of the laminar hook (**A**), which causes dorsal movement of the hook away from the spinal canal when this caudal facing hook is compressed against the lamina. The bifid blade design of the TSRH pedicle hook (**B**) aids in engagement of the pedicle. The Isola System (**E**) provides hooks that share a common design but vary in size. This may obligate more bone contouring but results in a more streamlined instrumentation set. (*Copyright University of New Mexico, Division of Neurosurgery.*)

Screw length should be selected so that at least one half to two thirds of the vertebral body is engaged. This allows the screw to function as a load-bearing component in all three columns of the spine. Screws may be self-tapping, a property achieved through fluting of the first several threads to allow for the displacement of cut bone.

Like hooks, screws may be attached to longitudinal members in a variety of ways. The great majority of screw/longitudinal component junctions available for use in the thoracic and lumbar spine are constrained (rigid), allowing for the creation of fixed moment arm cantilever beam constructs. End-loading, top-loading, side-loading, and through-the-plate connections are available. Multiaxial coupling systems may significantly simplify construct application. The ability to compensate for small discrepancies in sagittal and coronal alignment decreases the need for three-dimensional rod bending. However, the mechanical strength of these coupling mechanisms must be appreciated by the surgeon prior to application.

### Longitudinal Members

The longitudinal components of USI systems consist of rods or plates. Surface characteristics of the rods vary to maximize component/component junction strength (such as the knurled surfaces of C-D rods) and/or implant corrosion resistance (smooth surfaces of the TSRH rods). Two factors that weaken any longitudinal member are stress risers and notching. Stress risers result from the application of focal stress, usually during contouring of the rods or plates. Notching is an injury to the surface of an implant that may result in significant alterations of structural integrity. A 1% notch (e.g., a 3.6mm rod with a notch 36μm deep) reduces fatigue resistance of 316L stainless steel wire by 63%.[26] Titanium is known to be especially sensitive to the effects of notching.[5,32]

### Component-Component Junctions

USI systems use different mechanisms for component-component junctions. The mechanism of engagement and the surface characteristics of the implants affect the durability and strength of the construct as a whole. The most commonly used mechanisms for attaching component hooks and screws to longitudinal members are the three-point shear clamp, lock screw connectors, circumferential grip connectors, constrained and semiconstrained screw/plate connectors, and semiconstrained hook/rod connectors.[5] Three-point shear clamp connectors use a three-point bending force applied to the longitudinal member (rod) to tightly approximate the components. The majority of TSRH connectors are of this type. A lock screw connector uses a screw to drive the rod into a contoured bed, as with the Isola V groove hollow ground system. Tangential application of the screw appears to have some mechanical advantage.[5]

Circumferential grip connectors provide both halves of a pincer to provide truly circumferential force application (such as in the Synthes locking screw plate connector) or only half of the pincer (Isola VHG).[5] Constrained bolt-plate connectors do not allow toggling of the screw or hook at the component/component junction. The Steffee

plate/pedicle screw connector is an example of this type of connection. The only example of a semiconstrained connector (that allows movement in at least one plane) used in the thoracic or lumbar spine is the Harrington rod/hook connection, which allows for rotation and some toggling of the hook about the rod.[5]

Surface characteristics of the component-component junction are important. Friction enhancers such as knurled surfaces, radial spokes or grooves, or a grid pattern increase friction between the components. Knurled surfaces should not be mixed with smooth surfaces, because this can result in poor surface contact.

## Technical Aspects of Implant Application

USI placement techniques have been described.[4,5,31,34] What follows is a brief overview of the techniques used for the placement of dorsal spinal instrumentation.

### Pedicle Screw Insertion

The pedicle is the strongest portion of the vertebra. It consists largely of cortical bone. The transverse width of the pedicle is the limiting factor in terms of screw size and may be determined by preoperative CT. The transverse pedicle angle increases from near 0 degrees (straight dorsal-ventral) at L1 to nearly 30 degrees (dorsolateral to ventromedial) at L5. The sagittal angle of the pedicle also varies somewhat, but in a narrower range (5 degrees craniocaudal at L1 to 15 degrees at L5).[4,22,37] Preoperative radiographic studies aid in the determination of optimal screw placement angles. Alternatively, recent advances in frameless stereotaxy allow facile comparison of surgical anatomy with preoperative axial imaging studies. A caveat to the use of these systems is that the images displayed are not real time. Therefore the quality of the information provided to the surgeon is completely dependent on the accuracy of registration of the vertebral body involved. Alternatively, fluoroscopy or fluoroscopy-based frameless stereotactic systems may be used to provide feedback to the surgeon regarding hidden anatomy. The main limitation to the fluoroscopy-based frameless stereotactic systems is the quality of the source images. The use of frameless stereotaxy has been reported to improve the accuracy of pedicle screw placement in the lumbar and thoracic spine.[1,21,39] The use of such systems does not appear to degrade the fluoroscopic information and may in fact provide better feedback than live fluoroscopy because of the ability to use multiplanar imaging[29] (Figure 118.7).

The dorsal aspect of the lumbar pedicle is localized by using the junction of two lines. The first line is a straight rostrocaudal line drawn along the lateral border of the superior articular facet. The second line is a transverse line through the center of the transverse process (Figure 118.8). The lateral aspect of the pedicle may be palpated with a dissector placed over the rostral border of the transverse process and when practical, the medial aspect of the pedicle may be exposed by laminectomy or laminotomy. The screw entrance site (dorsal aspect of the pedicle) is decorticated with a drill or rongeur, and the pedicle is probed with a blunt-tipped pin or small curette.

Intraoperative radiographs are used to check the accuracy of pin placement and trajectory. Once adequate placement of the pins has been confirmed, the pins are removed and the holes prepared for screw placement. Alternatively, the pedicles may be cannulated with a 2.5mm drill. This technique is largely used in conjunction with a frameless stereotactic system or with real-time fluoroscopy. Gentle pressure and a slight "tapping" motion help to keep the drill bit within the confines of the pedicle. This technique is especially useful in sclerotic pedicles or in very small pedicles (such as in the thoracic spine, see below). Hole locations are marked with radio-opaque markers and verified with intraoperative radiographs or fluoroscopy.

Reliable anatomic landmarks used for the placement of thoracic pedicle screws probably do not exist. Unfortunately, there is a substantial amount of variability in pedicle location, size, and angle between individuals and between levels in the same individual.[35] As such, pedicle cortex violation is relatively common with blind insertion. One such series reported a 47% rate of pedicle breach.[2] Special aiming devices have been manufactured but have not been subject to critical review.[20] The use of frameless stereotactic techniques has improved accuracy of screw placement in several series[1,21,39] and is the method used by the authors of this chapter. An alternative technique, the performance of laminotomies to directly palpate the pedicle for the placement of thoracic pedicle screws, has also been described as improving accuracy.

When necessary, the holes are tapped with successively larger taps until a desired diameter is reached. The walls of the pedicle should be palpated from within after each tap to verify the integrity of the cortical bone. Intraoperative electrophysiologic stimulation has been used by some authors for the purpose of increased sensitivity to cortical violation.[9,30] Screws should be placed with as much lateral-to-medial angulation as possible so as to maximize the beneficial effects of triangulation on screw pullout and parallelograming.[5] Screw placement lateral to the pedicle may allow for increased triangulation without significantly degrading pull-out resistance. The author reserves this technique for salvage following pedicle stripping or fracture. Screw length should be selected such that the ventral two thirds of the vertebral body is engaged. Because of the constrained linkages between

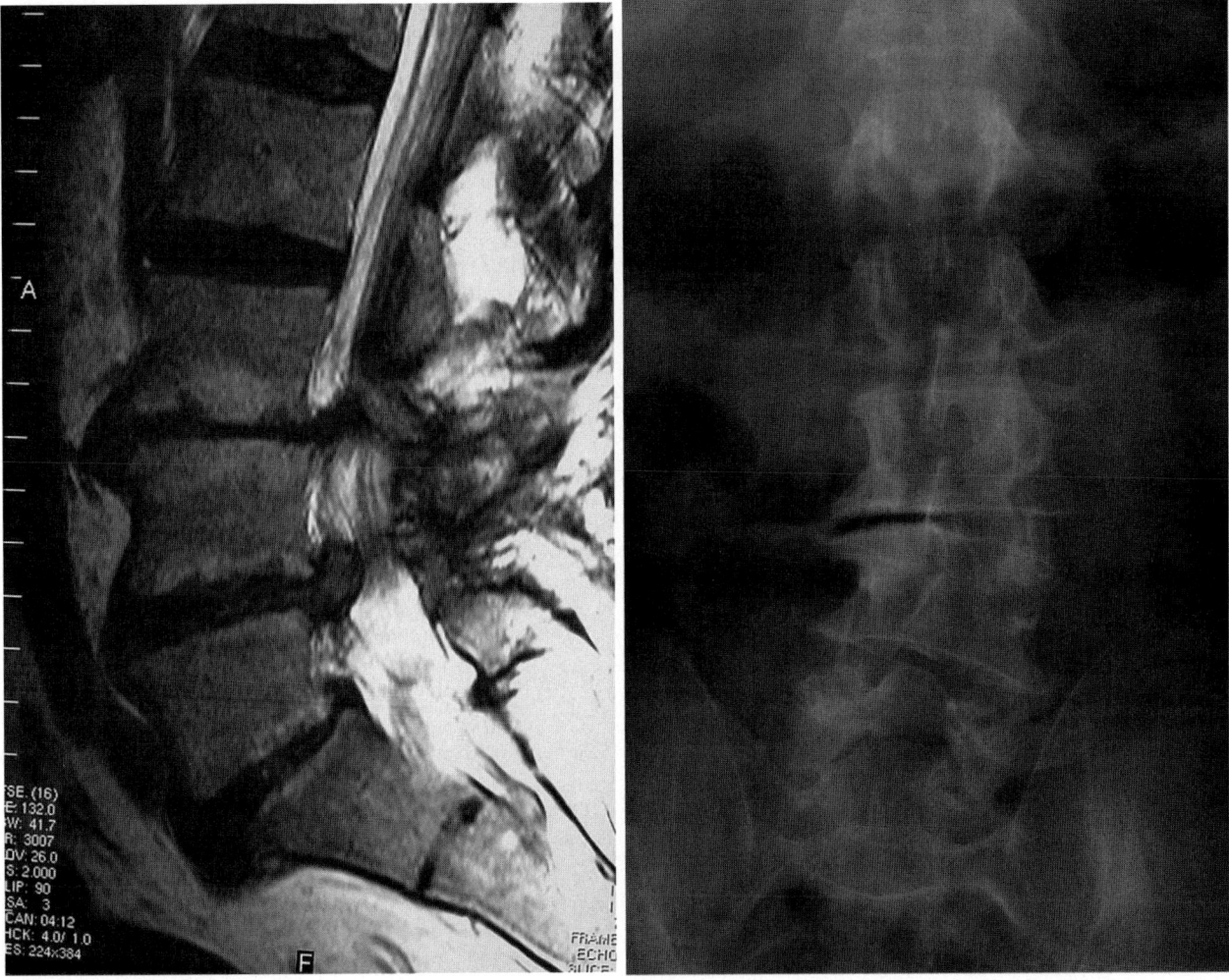

**A1**                                                                                     **A2**

**Figure 118.7**  In this patient with degenerative stenosis instability of the lumbar spine, a significant coronal plane deformity exists (**A1** and **A2**).

*Continued*

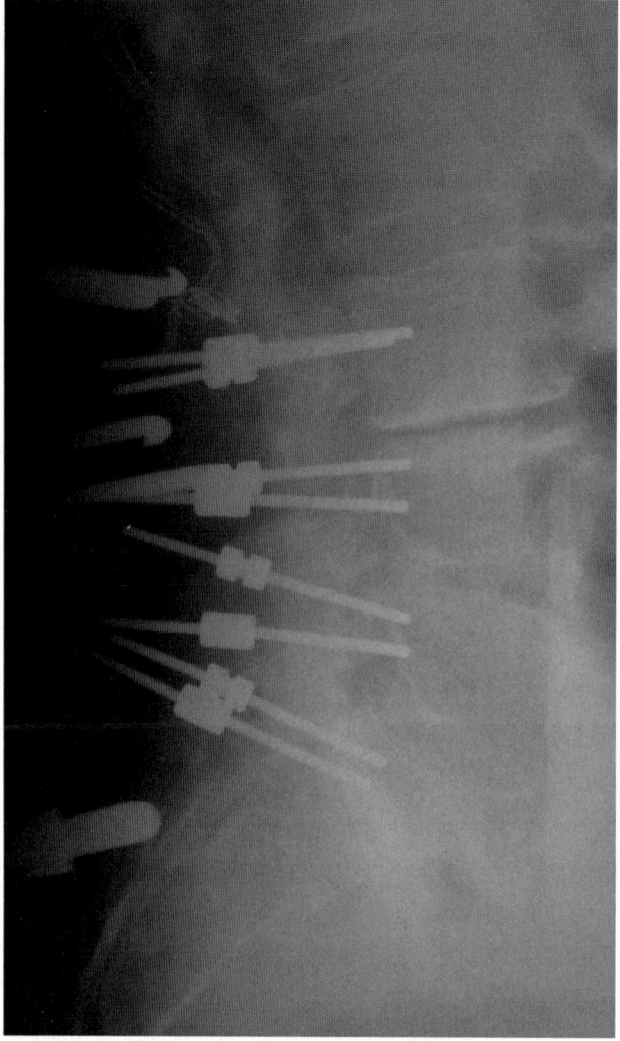

**B**

**Figure 118.7** *cont'd* A lateral radiograph obtained after pin placement may or may not demonstrate optimal screw position (**B**).

the screws and the longitudinal member in all thoracolumbar USI systems, no significant advantage is gained by penetration of the ventral cortex. A final intraoperative radiograph is obtained before linkage to the longitudinal member.

### Laminar Hook Insertion

Laminar hooks are designed to be placed under the lamina, facing either rostrally or caudally. The use of laminar hooks in the lumbar and sacral spine is universally accepted, whereas use of such hooks above the level of the conus medullaris is more controversial. Inspection of preoperative imaging studies is useful to determine the adequacy of the spinal canal for sublaminar hook placement. If a relative stenosis exists at a particular level, that level should be avoided and fixation obtained at another level or by another means. In all cases, care must be taken to prevent encroachment on neural elements by the hooks. Laminotomies are performed, removing the caudal por-

tion of the lamina above and the rostral portion of the lamina below the level of hook application (Figure 118.9). The ligamentum flavum is removed, and in some cases, medial facetectomies are performed. A laminar tester is used to verify the adequacy of the sublaminar dissection. The largest hook that can be placed at a given level should be selected to maximize the bone/implant junction. It is often possible to "stagger" hooks from side to side so as to avoid placing two hooks under the same lamina. The hook must closely appose the laminar surface to avoid encroachment into the spinal canal. If an appropriately contoured hook is not available, the lamina should be contoured for an exact fit. Once a hook is placed, it should be compressed against its lamina to prevent migration into the spinal canal. Special care must be taken when hooks are used as intermediate points of fixation with three-point bending constructs (Figure 118.10), because the hooks may be driven into the spinal canal by the application of such forces if not tightly apposed to their respective lamina.[5,34]

### Pedicle Hooks

Pedicle hooks are placed beneath the caudal articulating surface of the thoracic facet. Pedicle hooks are placed outside of the spinal canal and therefore are used throughout the thoracic spine, with the exception of the thoracolumbar junction. The more sagittal orientation of the lower thoracic facet joints makes hook application difficult at these levels. Most USI systems use bifid hooks, which make pedicle purchase more secure. However, placement of nonbifid hooks is aided by the "sandwiching" effect of the superior and inferior articulating surfaces of the facet joint.

Thoracic pedicle hooks are placed between the superior and inferior articulating surfaces of the facet. The caudal portion of the inferior articular process is removed by using a drill or osteotome. The amount of bone removed is critical, because if too little bone is removed, the hook does not engage the facet (Figure 118.11). Transverse migration may not be prevented (with bifid hooks). Conversely, if too much bone is removed, the hook may cut into the pedicle, thus decreasing the strength of the pedicle/inferior articulating process connection. Frequent trial placements of the hook may be helpful in determining the optimal hook size and amount of bone removal necessary for good purchase.[5,34]

### Transverse Process Hook Insertion

The transverse processes may be used for hook purchase in the thoracic spine. These hooks are usually placed facing caudally in conjunction with a rostrally facing pedicle hook. The costotransverse ligament is stripped off the transverse process by using a specially designed stripping tool, and the hook is placed over the rostral border of the transverse process. Offset hooks are frequently useful, as there is a substantial distance between the transverse process hook and pedicle hook fixation points in the coronal plane. Use of these hooks at the thoracolumbar junction is limited, since the transverse processes of T11 and T12 are usually too small to provide substantial purchase strength.[34]

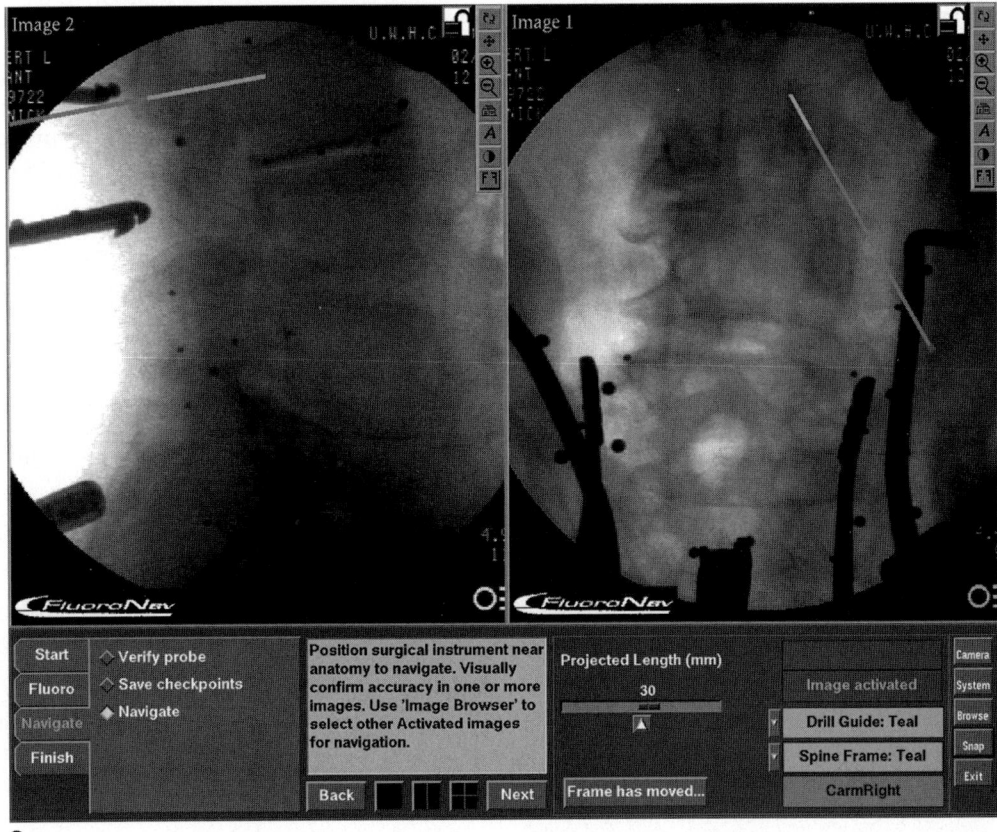

**C**

**Figure 118.7 cont'd** The use of frameless stereotaxy (**C**) allows for multiplanar imaging.

*Continued*

## Cross-Fixation

Cross-fixation increases the stability of a construct by preventing rotation or translation (coronal or sagittal) of the longitudinal members with respect to each other. The torsional stability of an implant is increased substantially by the use of a single cross-fixator (44%) and further increased with the use of two cross-fixators (an additional 26% gain in stability).[12] Screw pull-out resistance is also markedly improved with the use of rigid cross-links combined with toeing in of the screws. A lateral translational deformity caused by "parallelograming" is resisted by the use of cross-fixators.[5] Cross-fixators should be placed at the junctions of the middle third of the implant with the rostral and caudal thirds. No significant biomechanical advantage is gained by the use of more than two cross-fixators. Although some USI cross-fixators are easier to apply than others, it is important, in general, not to mix sets or metals because of the potential for galvanically enhanced electrolytic corrosion caused by contact between dissimilar metals.

## Complication Avoidance and Management

The use of dorsal thoracic and lumbar USI systems is associated with a number of potential complications. The most significant short-term complications relate to loss of bony purchase, immediate implant failure, cerebrospinal fluid (CSF) fistula formation, and neural element injury.[7,10,27,36]

Techniques for the prevention and management of these types of events are discussed below.

## Complications of Hook Fixation

The use of three-point bending forces to reduce deformity may be associated with excessive force application at the terminal bone/implant junctions. This situation most commonly occurs with the use of the Harrington hook/rod system in which substantial translational forces are borne by the terminal hook/bone junctions. Hook cut-out at the rostral terminus is a common complication of these types of constructs. Use of a clawed construct lessens the risk of implant/bone junction failure by increasing the surface area of metal/bone contact. Furthermore, the use of clawed implants allows for the placement of the implant in a neutral mode (in contrast to distraction) with the immobilization of fewer motion segments.

Hooks placed in the spinal canal (laminar hooks) must tightly appose the ventral surface of the lamina to prevent neurologic injury. The use of such hooks above the level of the conus medullaris is possible but certainly carries with it a higher risk for neurologic injury. Great care must be taken with the use of laminar hooks as intermediate points of fixation in a three-point bending implant. The ventrally directed force at the center of such an implant may drive the hook blade into the spinal canal (see Figure 118.10).

Pedicle hooks that are placed outside of the spinal canal may migrate during implant manipulation and may

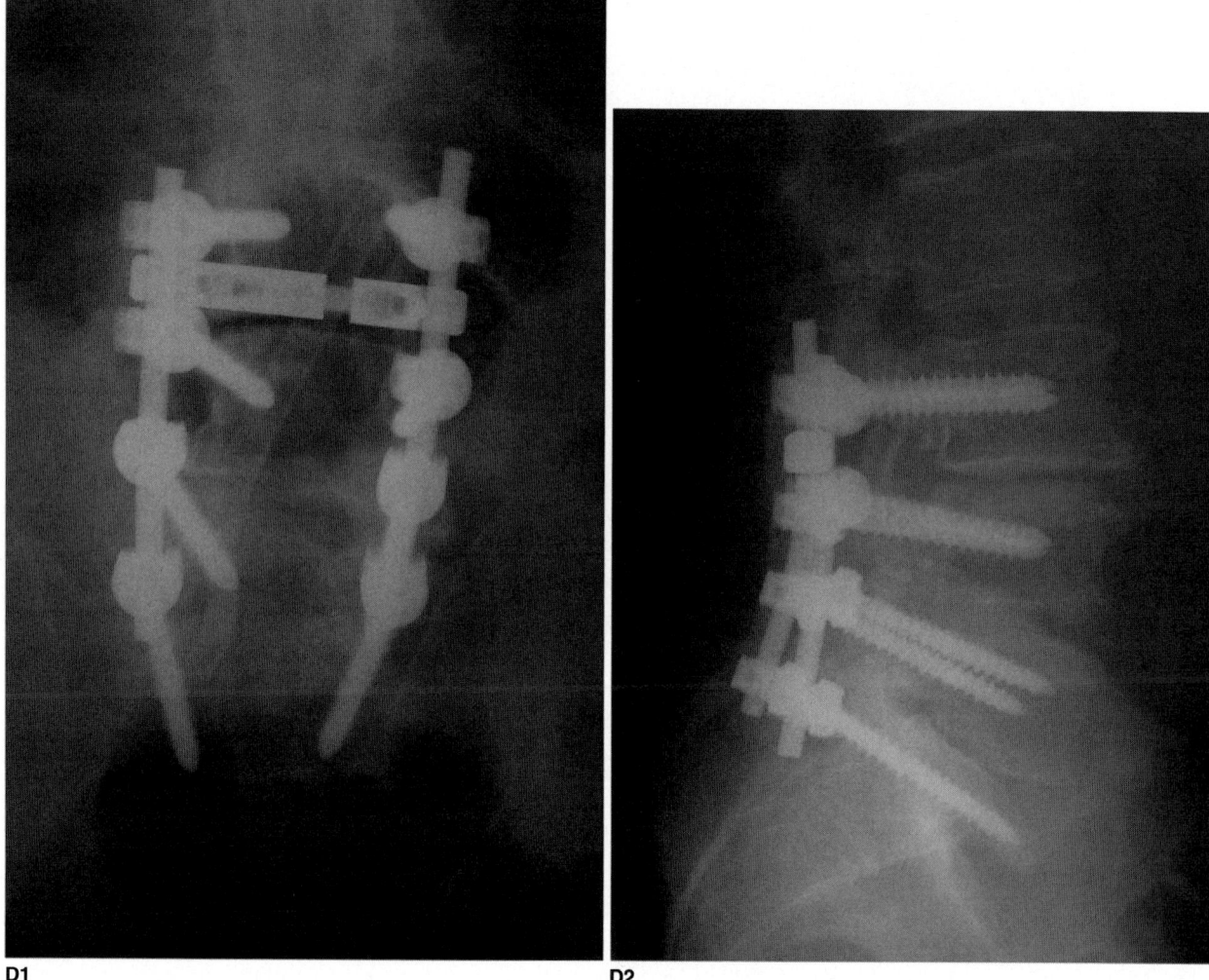

**D1**                                                    **D2**

**Figure 118.7** *cont'd* This ability greatly facilitated screw placement in this case (**D1** and **D2**).

encroach on the spinal canal or neural foramina. Bifid hooks may lessen the risks of this complication. It is important to remove an appropriate amount of bone from the inferior articulating process of the facet before pedicle hook placement. Inadequate or overzealous bone removal may lead to malposition of pedicle hooks in the sagittal plane, which may lead to hook loosening or to pedicle fracture. Frequent use of hook testers will help to determine the correct amount of bone to be removed from the inferior articular process of the facet (see Figure 118.11).

## Complications of Transpedicular Fixation

Complications of pedicle fixation result from technical difficulties with implant application and from improper preoperative planning. The most common technical error in the placement of pedicle screws is malpositioning of the screw, resulting in pedicle fracture.[7,10,13,14] Pedicle fracture may occur if the pedicle screw entry site is inappropriate, the angle of screw placement is off, or the screw selected is too large in diameter. Depending on the location of the pedicle fracture, the consequence may be loss of purchase, CSF fistula, or neural injury. Preoperative studies

must be obtained and reviewed to determine the correct size of screw and angle of insertion (sagittal as well as coronal). Although intraoperative radiography is helpful, screw malposition in the axial plane may still occur despite radiographically acceptable positioning in the operating room.[14] The use of intraoperative electrophysiologic monitoring[9,30,28] and frameless stereotaxy may provide improved feedback to the surgeon for more accurate screw placement.[1,21,39]

As already stated, should pedicle fracture occur, possible sequelae include loss of purchase, CSF fistula, and neural injury. In the instance of loss of purchase, incorporation of an additional spinal segment may be necessary. CSF fistula should be repaired primarily when possible. When impossible or impractical, the pedicle defect may be packed with Gelfoam soaked in thrombin or fibrin glue in an attempt to minimize CSF egress. Screws that are known to have perforated the medial cortex of the pedicle should be repositioned immediately. Screws that are found to be misplaced at the time of follow-up study may be well tolerated by the patient, as there may be up to 4mm of a "safe" zone medial to the lumbar pedicle cortex.[16] This safe zone may not exist in the thoracic spine.[35] Patients

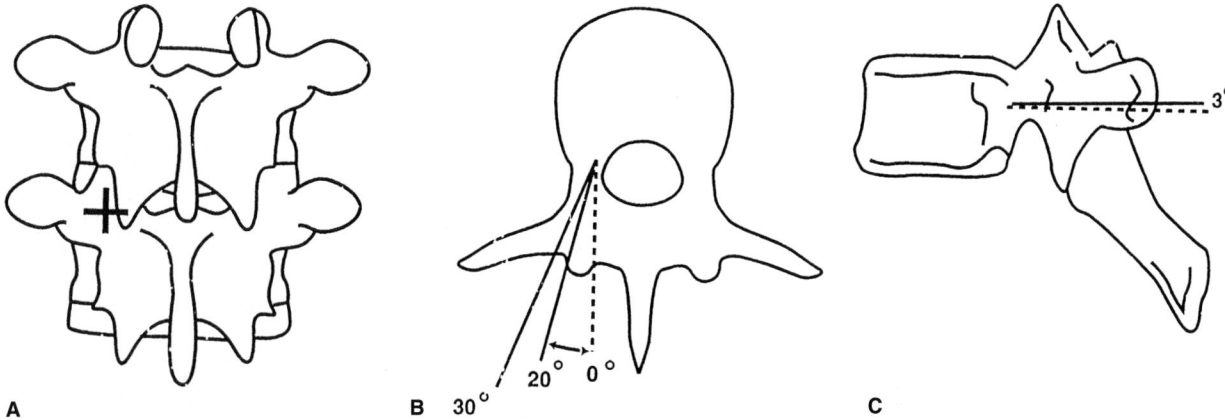

**Figure 118.8** Pedicle screw placement. **(A)** The entrance point for pedicle screw placement is at the junction of the rostrocaudal lateral facet line and the transverse mid transverse process line. **(B)** Axial representations of pedicle screw placement in the L4 and L5 vertebra. Note the difference in the angle of placement with the L4 screw oriented at a 20-degree angle from the sagittal plane and the L5 screw oriented at a near 30-degree angle from the sagittal plane.[22,37] **(C)** Sagittal view of pedicle screw placement in L4 and L5. Differences in the sagittal angulation of the pedicles of the lumbar vertebra are not as pronounced as in the axial plane. Note slight difference in the angulation with the L4 screw placed parallel to the axial plane and the L5 screw placed at a 3-degree angle with respect to the axial plane.[22,37] *(Copyright University of New Mexico, Division of Neurosurgery.)*

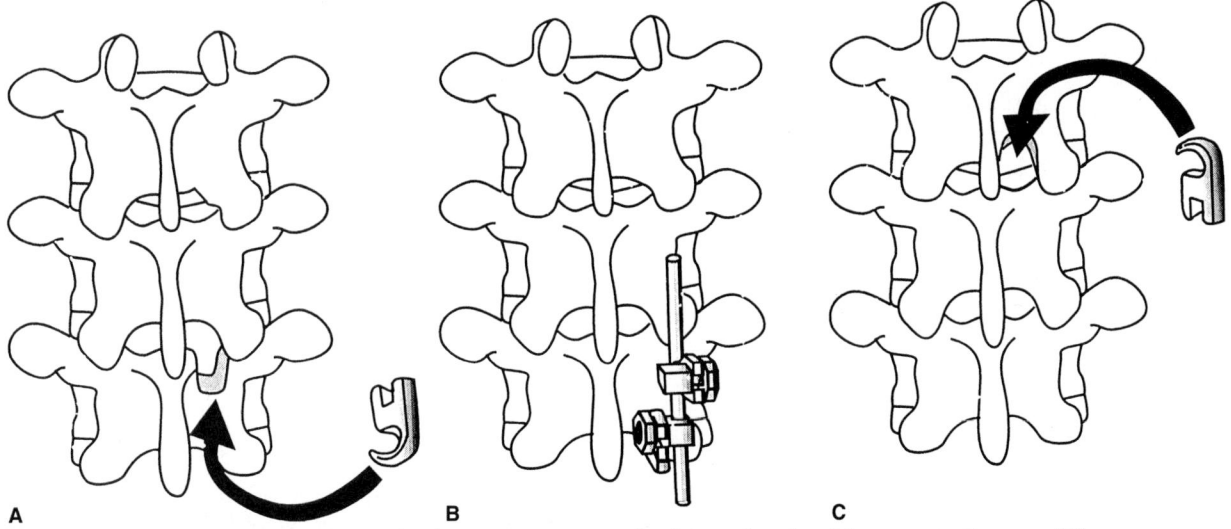

**Figure 118.9** Laminar hook insertion. Laminar hooks may be placed facing rostrally or caudally. For placement of a rostral facing hook, a small laminotomy of the superior portion of the lamina below the level of fixation may be required **(A)**. Because of the width of the lumbar lamina, it is often possible to affix a rostrally directed hook to the lamina of a vertebral body in conjunction with a pedicle screw **(B)**. This configuration aids resistance to screw pullout in cantilever beam constructs without incorporating additional motion segments **(C)**. Caudally directed hooks are placed following a laminotomy of the inferior portion of the lamina above the level of fixation. Caudally facing hooks cannot be placed on the same vertebra as a pedicle screw because of the apposition of the screw and hook connectors. *(Copyright University of New Mexico, Division of Neurosurgery.)*

with medial cortex fractures may develop late erosion of the screw threads into the neural foramina or spinal canal, which may cause nerve root injury. If symptomatic, such screws should be removed. Nerve root irritation may also result from caudal breaches of the pedicle cortex, where the exiting root is vulnerable to impingement or lateral pedicle breach, where the lumbosacral plexus may be irritated. Finally, perforation of the ventral cortex may result in significant vascular or visceral injury.

Postoperative complications related directly to implant failure may be avoided to some extent through proper preoperative planning and construct design. For example, application of three-point bending constructs should usually not be attempted with screws as the terminal fixators. Although screw pull-out resistance may be maximized by the toeing-in of the screws (triangulation) and the use of cross-fixators, hooks still provide a greater resistance to

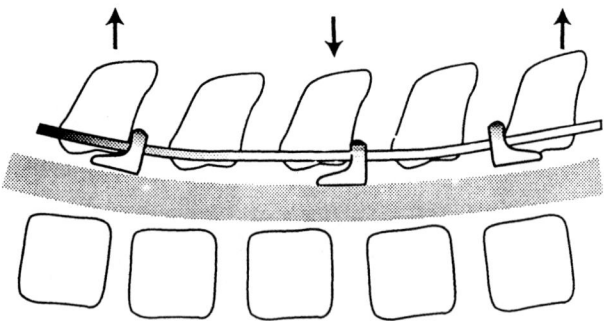

**Figure 118.10** Hook use in three-point bending. Hooks are ideally suited for use as terminal components of three-point bending constructs because of the increased bone/implant contact surface area compared with screws. This increased surface area helps resist the dorsally directed forces at the termini. Because the forces generated at the apex of a kyphotic curvature are directed ventrally, caution must be exercised if hooks are used as intermediate points of fixation. The ventrally directed forces may act to drive the blade of the hook into the spinal canal, as depicted. (*Copyright University of New Mexico, Division of Neurosurgery.*)

translational forces. Similarly, when significant corrective forces are required, a sufficiently long construct should be used so as not to overly stress the implant/bone or screw/rod junction.[4] Dorsal instrumentation cannot be relied on to replace the ventral load bearing capacity of the spine, and attempts to do so are likely to fail.

Pedicle screw fracture may occur at the time of implant application, during attempted removal of instrumentation after fusion, or spontaneously in the months to years following implantation. The decision to remove implants in patients with persistent back pain after thoracic or lumbar fusion must be made on an individual basis. When there is evidence of implant failure, such as a broken rod or screw, medico-legal implications may prompt the surgeon toward attempted removal. If a screw is fractured such that it cannot be removed by using standard techniques, a screw extractor kit may be used to remove distal screw fragments. A carbide-tipped drill is used to drill a hole in the screw fragment and then a left-handed tap is inserted into the hole ("Easy-Out"). As the left-handed threads of the tap engage the screw, the screw begins to back out. Copious irrigation is required to remove fragments of metal, which will obscure postoperative imaging. The author recommends a hand drill as opposed to a pneumatic drill, as even a slight deviation from a coaxial trajectory may result in a violent removal with inadvertent pedicle fracture.

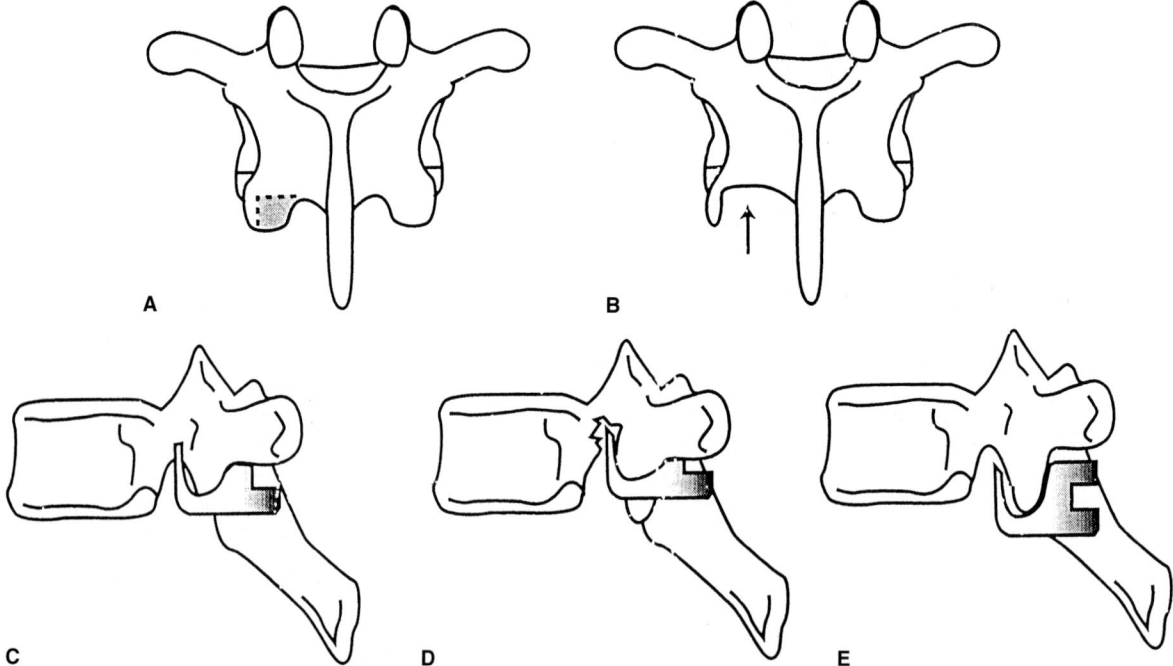

**Figure 118.11** Pedicle hook insertion. Dorsal view of thoracic facet demonstrating the inferior articular process before (**A**) and after (**B**) bone removal (with an osteotome) for placement of a pedicle hook. (**C**) Lateral view of pedicle hook in place, demonstrating appropriate bone removal. Note how the bifid hook properly engages the pedicle. (**D**) If too much bone is removed, the pedicle may migrate rostrally and cut into the pedicle (if hook/rod connection is constrained) or toggle out of position (if hook/rod position is nonconstrained). (**E**) If too little bone is removed, the hook will not engage the pedicle, and mediolateral hook migration may occur with manipulation of longitudinal members. The sandwiching effect of the facet joint will help hold the hooks in position to some extent. The stabilizing effect of pedicle purchase will be less significant with nonbifid hooks. (*Copyright University of New Mexico, Division of Neurosurgery.*)

## Summary

Dorsally applied USI increases the rate of bony fusion after surgery for traumatic, neoplastic, or degenerative conditions of the spine. By providing immediate stability to the spinal column, appropriately designed constructs allow for earlier mobilization, and hence, quicker rehabilitation of patients with spinal disorders. The safe and efficacious application of these systems is based on a clear understanding of the spinal anatomy and the particular pathology being addressed. Multiple systems are now available that differ in coupling mechanisms, metallurgic composition, screw and hook design, and cost. The surgeon must choose the appropriate system for a given patient and the associated pathology. This should be based on a clear understanding of the patient's pathology as well as an understanding of the strengths and limitations of USI systems.

## REFERENCES

1. Amiot LP, Lang K, Putzier M, Zippel H, Labelle H: Comparative results between conventional and computer assisted pedicle screw installation in the thoracic, lumbar, and sacral spine. *Spine* 25:606-614, 2000.
2. Belmont PJ Jr, Klemme WR, Dhawan A, Polly DW Jr: In vivo accuracy of thoracic pedicle screws. *Spine* 26:2340-2346, 2001.
3. Bennett GL: Materials and materials testing. In Benzel EC (ed): *Neurosurgical Topics: Spinal Instrumentation*. Park Ridge, IL, American Association of Neurological Surgeons, 1994, pp 31-46.
4. Benzel EC: Construct design. Benzel EC (ed): *Neurosurgical Topics: Spinal Instrumentation*. Park Ridge, IL, American Association of Neurological Surgeons, 1994, pp 239-256.
5. Benzel EC: *Biomechanics of Spine Stabilization: Principles and Clinical Practice*. New York, McGraw-Hill, 1995.
6. Benzel EC, Ball PA: *History of Spinal Instrumentation*. Benzel EC (ed): *Neurosurgical Topics: Spinal Instrumentation*. Park Ridge, IL, American Association of Neurological Surgeons, 1994, pp 3-10.
7. Chozick BS, Toselli R: *Complications of Spinal Instrumentation*. In Benzel EC (ed): Neurosurgical Topics: Spinal Instrumentation. Park Ridge, IL, American Association of Neurological Surgeons, 1994, pp 257-274.
8. Cotrel Y, Dubousset J, Guillaumat M: New universal instrumentation in spinal surgery. *Clin Orthop* 227:10, 1988.
9. Darden BV, Hatley M, Owen JH: A comparison of impedance and EMG procedures in detecting the presence of pedicle wall breakthrough. *J Neurosurg* 86:414A, 1997.
10. Davne SH, Myers DL: Complications of lumbar spinal fusion with transpedicular instrumentation. *Spine* 17:S184-S189, 1992.
11. Denis F: The three column spine and its significance in the classification of acute thoracolumbar spine injuries. *Spine* 8:817-837, 1983.
12. Dick JC, Zdeblick TA, Bartel BD, Kunz DN: Mechanical evaluation of cross-link designs in rigid pedicle screw systems. *Spine* 22:370-373, 1997.
13. Esses SI, Sachs BL, Dreyzin V: Complications associated with the technique of pedicle screw fixation. A selected survey of ABS members. *Spine* 18:2231-2238, 1993.
14. Farber GL, Place HM, Mazur RA, et al: Accuracy of pedicle screw placement in lumbar fusions by plain radiographs and computed tomography. *Spine* 20:1494-1499, 1995.
15. Frymoyer JW, Selby DK: Segmental instability: rationale for treatment. *Spine* 10:280-286, 1985.
16. Gertzbein SD, Robbins SE: Accuracy of pedicle screw placement in vivo. *Spine* 15:11-14, 1990.
17. Hadra BE: The classic wiring of the vertebrae as a means of immobilization in fracture and Pott's disease (reprinted from original). *Clin Orthop* 112:4-8, 1975.
18. Harrington PR: Treatment of scoliosis: correction and internal fixation by spine instrumentation. *J Bone Joint Surg* 44A:591-610, 1962.
19. Jacobs RR, Asher MA, Snider RK: Thoracolumbar spine injuries: a comparative study of recumbent and operative treatment in 100 patients. *Spine* 5:463, 1980.
20. Jang JS, Lee WB, Yuan HA: Use of a guide device to place pedicle screws in the thoracic spine: a cadaveric study. Technical note. *J Neurosurg* 94(2 suppl):328-333, 2001.
21. Kim KD, Johnson PJ, Bloch BS, Masciopinto JE: Computer assisted thoracic pedicle screw placement: an in vitro feasibility study. *Spine* 26:360-364, 2001.
22. Krag MH, Weaver DL, Beynnon BD: Morphometry of the thoracic and lumbar spine related to transpedicular screw placement for surgical spinal fixation. *Spine* 13:27-32, 1988.
23. Lange F: The classic support for the spondylitic spine by means of buried steel bars attached to the vertebrae (reprinted from original). *Clin Orthop* 203:3-6, 1986.
24. Luque ER: The anatomic basis and development of segmental spinal instrumentation. *Spine* 7:256-259, 1982.
25. Mardjetko SM, Connolly PJ, Shott S: Degenerative lumbar spondylolisthesis. A meta-analysis of the literature 1970-1993. *Spine* 19S:2256-2265, 1994.
26. Oh I, Sander TW, Treharne RW: The fatigue resistance of orthopaedic wire. *Clin Orthop Rel Res* 192:228-236, 1985.
27. Ohlin A, Karlsson M, Duppe H, et al: Complications after transpedicular stabilization of the spine. *Spine* 19:2774-2779, 1994.
28. Reidy DP, Houlden D, Nolan PC, et al: Evaluation of electromyographic monitoring during insertion of thoracic pedicle screws. *J Bone Joint Surg Br* 83:1009-1014, 2001.
29. Resnick DK: Comparison between virtual fluoroscopy and fluoroscopy for the placement of lumbar pedicle screws. *J Spin Disord* 16:254-260, 2003.
30. Rose B, Welch WC, Balzer JR, Jacobs GB: Persistently electrified pedicle stimulation instruments (PEPSI) in spinal instrumentation. *Spine* 22:334-343, 1997.
31. Roy-Camille R, Saillant G, Mazel C: Internal fixation of the lumbar spine with pedicle screw plating. *Clin Orthop* 203:7-17, 1986.
32. Scuderi GJ, Greenberg SS, Latta LL, et al: A biomechanical evaluation of MRI compatible wire for use in cervical spine fixation. Presented at the Cervical Spine Research Society Meeting, Palm Springs, Fl, 1992.
33. Sonntag VKH, Marciano FF: Is fusion indicated for lumbar spinal disorders? *Spine* 20:138S-142S, 1995.
34. Stillerman CB, Gruen JP: Universal spinal instrumentation. In Benzel EC (ed): *Neurosurgical Topics: Spinal*

*Instrumentation.* Park Ridge, IL, American Association of Neurological Surgeons, 1994, pp 147-174.

35. Ugur HC, Attar A, Uz A, *et al:* Thoracic pedicle: surgical anatomic evaluation and relations. *J Spinal Disord* 14:39-45, 2001.

36. West JL III, Ogilvie JW, Bradford DS: Complications of the variable screw plate pedicle screw fixation. *Spine* 16: 576-579, 1991.

37. White AA, Panjabi MM: *Clinical Biomechanics of the Spine,* ed 2. Philadelphia, Lippincott-Raven, 1990.

38. Willen J, Lindahl S, Nordwall A: Unstable thoracolumbar fractures: a comparative clinical study of conservative treatment and Harrington instrumentation. *Spine* 10:111, 1985.

39. Youkilis AS, Quint DJ, McGillicuddy JE, Papadopolous SM: Stereotactic navigation for placement of pedicle screws in the thoracic spine. *Neurosurgery* 48:771-778, 2001.

40. Zdeblick TA: A prospective, randomized study of lumbar fusion. Preliminary results. *Spine* 18:983-991, 1993.

# CHAPTER 119

# Dorsal Thoracic and Lumbar Combined and Complex Techniques

## Parley W. Madsen III and Nevan G. Baldwin

This chapter addresses indications advocated for, and techniques of, combined ventral and dorsal procedures for decompression, fusion, and instrumentation of the thoracic and lumbar spine. It must be acknowledged, however, that most data remain anecdotal and that the controversy over indications for surgical management is almost unaltered from the positions expressed by Cooper and Bell nearly two centuries ago. Sir Astley Cooper (1839) was an advocate of surgical intervention for spine injuries, whereas Sir Charles Bell's (1824) disdain of surgery as additional iatrogenic injury was widely accepted: "laying a patient upon his belly and by incision laying bare the bones of the spine, breaking up these bones and exposing the spinal marrow itself, exceeds all belief...."[20,55] Surgical treatment of spinal cord injury (SCI) continues to be the subject of significant debate.[76]

Gaines and Humphreys[47] lamented that "an assessment of plain roentgenograms, tomograms, and CAT scan and an understanding of the anatomy of the fracture site provide essential, but insufficient, data for clinical decisions ... about surgical stabilization ...." These authors wrote that, "the only absolute indication for surgical internal fixation of the spine" is the "situation in which spinal column healing may not be anticipated with fair reliability ...." This situation is the injury, "generally associated with complete neurologic injury in which there is extremely poor or absent apposition of the fracture fragments."[47] This rare clinical occurrence was compared to a femur fracture with quadriceps muscle interposition that will never heal even with external mobilization because of the lack of bony apposition.[2,23] All other indications for surgery were believed to be dependent on, "other variables of the patient's general situation ...."[47] The other situations in which surgical intervention was advocated were accompanying head injury or poor patient judgment, other organ system injuries that make complete bed rest with careful log rolling and full spine immobilization impossible, failure of conservative management, and the presence of a complete neurologic injury. Acknowledging that most American surgeons will surgically remove bone or disc fragments that compress the spinal canal, Gaines and Humphreys[47] also noted that the scientific soundness of this concept had not been proved in "matched sets of patients."[23,28,78,95]

## Historical Perspective

The Egyptians in the third millennium BC were the first to diagnose and to recommend a treatment for spine and SCI. The remarkable papyrus acquired by and named for Edwin Smith included a detailed description of cervical spine injuries, accompanied by the prognosis of the injured patient and recommended therapy. The latter consisted of dressing of the wound with various materials and good nutritional support, but there was no description of surgical intervention. This unprecedented work was somatotopically organized and abruptly terminated with only a cursory description of a thoracic spine injury; lumbar spine injuries were not addressed. The work was believed to have been written by Imhotep, a high priest and advisor to Pharaoh Djoser, but later reviews of the papyrus opined that the original author was an experienced but otherwise undistinguished laborer, one of the 100,000 persons who, according to Herodotus, worked on the Great Pyramid of Egypt.[9] It appears that this unknown Egyptian was not formally educated in contemporary medical theory but was a very keen observer of persons suffering trauma at the construction site. His lack of formal medical education kept him unbiased and he produced a remarkable, unprecedented clinical treatise of traumatology, unfettered by the need to reconcile clinical observation with mystical explanations and to begin the process of definition of the pathophysiologic basis for clinical disorders.[9,64]

Although Hippocrates' clinical observation was not as keen as the unknown Egyptian, he described the clinical consequences of a thoracic spine injury and recommended an external method of reducing the gibbus often associated with these injuries that would be followed for the next two millennia.[50,64] The pessimistic prognosis pronounced on a cervical spine dislocation with a complete SCI by the unknown Egyptian, "an ailment not to be treated," remained the same at the time of Hippocrates.[9] However, in writings attributed to Hippocrates, a scamnum (a rack-like traction device) was recommended to align the bony abnormalities of thoracolumbar spine fractures.[50] The patient was extended in the prone position with leather straps at the hips and under the shoulders while a reduction force was placed over the site of the kyphosis by manual manipulation or with a lever. This device was advocated as an alternative to the use of succussion that involved tying the patient upside down to a ladder-like device that was suddenly dropped, extending the spine in an attempt to reduce the spinal deformity. Hippocrates did not approve of succussion. No consideration of internal reduction was rendered in any of the many works attributed to Hippocrates.[90]

Paulus of Aginea in the seventh century used the scamnum to reduce spine fractures and then placed an external fixation device made of thin sheets of wood to secure the reduction. He was the first clinician to record his suspicion that laminar fragments pressing on the spinal cord were a source of pain and to advocate a laminectomy for debridement of the fracture site.[55] Although he recommended spine surgery, it is not certain that a surgical debridement was ever attempted during his career.[4]

Ambrose Paré was a sixteenth-century French barber-surgeon who, by careful observation of the treatment of battlefield injuries, devised some effective treatments. His clinical success gained him political power as a counselor to the French monarchy and averted his death as a Protestant in a Catholic country.[73] He was the first to accurately describe the clinical symptoms of a thoracic spinal column and cord injury. Paré revealed, in a treatise on the management of "luxation" of the spine (as he described the deformities associated with trauma), his fascination with these lesions. He acknowledged the stability the rib cage afforded the thoracic spinal column; he stated that the vertebra of the "rack-bones of the back" could be forced from a normal position only with "a great deal of violence" and "the breaking of the ties and ligaments," the result of a "fall from high upon some hard body, a heavy and bruising blow." A ventral dislocation was recognized by the "depressed cavity of the spine," whereas a dorsal dislocation was characterized by a "bunch on the back." Paré clearly outlined the neurologic deficit that accompanied a ventral dislocation, pronounced it a "deadly" disorder without hope, and lamented that he could "not through the belly, force it into its place." He recognized that a ventral "luxation" was more often associated with a neurologic injury than was a spine that was "dislocated outwards."[10]

### Surgical Therapy

Although Paré was acquainted with the poor prognosis assigned these lesions in the writings of Hippocrates and his followers, he advocated and described in detail a dorsal surgical debridement of the injury site for the removal of the "splinters of the broken vertebrae which, driven in, press the spinal marrow in the nerves thereof" in an apparent attempt to lengthen the patient's otherwise shortened life span. There was no description or mention of a ventral approach to the spine.[4] Paré was also the first to use external fixation with a metal orthosis constructed of lead sheets that were placed on the lateral aspect of the torso, leaving the midline over the spinal column open. This orthosis was not dissimilar to the modern thoracolumbosacral orthosis (TLSO) and was used to maintain the reduction of fractured vertebral bodies, which he achieved by first placing the patient into extension and then by gentle manipulation of the deformity.[10]

Isolated reports of successful surgery for spinal injuries appeared before the mid-20th century, including the removal of a bullet from the thoracic spine in 1774 by Antoine Louis. M'Donnell[89] reported a 1864 laminectomy that he performed on a patient rendered paralyzed by a fracture-dislocation. The fragments of the dorsal arch were removed approximately 1 month after the initial injury, and the patient recovered neurologic function. Although the author reported that the patient became pain free postoperatively, the operative subject expired suddenly in the perioperative period. The prognosis continued to be poor for spinal-injured patients as late as World War I, and Cushing reported that survival was less than 2 weeks for 80% of American soldiers so injured.[21] The prognosis for the SCI patient remained dismal until the post-World War II era, and the generally accepted pessimistic outlook for the paraplegic patient was reflected in a 1924 report of the Medical Research Council

(reported by Sir Ludwig Guttmann): "The paraplegic patient may live for a few years in a state of more or less ill-health." These patients would succumb to the ravages of sepsis as a result of infections of the urinary tract or decubitus ulcers within 2 to 3 years of the initial injury.[55]

### Treatment of Spinal Fractures

As late as the 1950s, textbooks on the treatment of fractures stressed early closed reduction of spinal fractures to ensure a favorable outcome; indeed, Sir Watson-Jones[109] stated, "perfect recovery is possible only if perfect reduction is insisted upon; even slight degrees of wedging of the vertebrae may cause persistent aching pain . . . ."[5] Guttmann[54] agreed that alignment of the spine was desirable; however, he disagreed with the methods used to obtain and maintain the reduction. He saw little difference between the use of slings, hanging, or frames for reduction of fractures and the reduction obtained with the ancient scamnum described by Hippocrates. The plaster casts used to maintain the spinal alignment caused pressure sores and interfered with the rehabilitation of the patient. Guttmann also disagreed with Magnus, who renounced fracture reduction and placed patients flat in bed in the supine position. Instead, he advocated a postural reduction of the spinal fractures, accomplished by meticulous positioning of the patient with pillows and sorbo-rubber packs and by laborious manual repositioning of the patient every 2 hours. Nicoll,[92] however, demonstrated that this bias to obtain anatomic alignment was without scientific basis; he reported his experience with coal miners suffering thoracolumbar fractures. Without an attempt to reduce their bony abnormality, many returned to heavy work after the fractures healed, in spite of the continued abnormal alignment of their spinal column.

Many surgeons advocated immediate surgical intervention, and from the time of Paré, surgical treatment was restricted to laminectomy. This intervention did not consistently offer the SCI patient any significant gain in neurologic function but was rather often associated with a deterioration in function because of increased instability of the body column with removal of the posterior elements in this misguided attempt to "decompress" the injured cord.[91] Guttmann[53,54] deplored the iatrogenic injury to the supporting trunk musculature and the subsequent negative effect on the eventual rehabilitation of the spinal-injured patient. Holdsworth and Hardy[63] strongly disagreed with Guttmann on the effectiveness of surgical therapy.

### Internal Fixation

Sir Frank Holdsworth[61] advocated early internal reduction and fixation for spinal injuries. Although advocates of internal fixation reported that rehabilitation could commence more rapidly and safely after surgical stabilization, early incidental attempts at internal fixation of the spine, usually with single segment wiring, were generally unsuccessful. Holdsworth used spinal process plate fixation for stabilization, but other authors noted that the procedure was complicated, with a high failure rate.[47,63] The first truly effective internal fixation system for the spine was introduced by Harrington in the 1960s, but the need for an external plaster orthosis postoperatively resulted in a continuing problem with pressure sores.[54,57,58]

Although multiple devices are now used for fixation of the unstable spine, the Harrington system with modifications by Moe, Edwards, and others remains the "gold standard" to which all other systems must be compared and on which other systems depend for approval for clinical use in the United States.[85,100] Although these newer universal fixation devices may successfully treat the instability induced by a laminectomy, the iatrogenic injury to the trunk-stabilizing musculature deplored by Guttmann[53] has not been obviated. With postural reduction championed by Guttmann[55] and Frankel et al.,[45] spine-injured patients achieved remarkable functional status, but there was considerable controversy over the need for surgical therapy. In spite of increasingly more-sophisticated internal fixation devices, there has not been a significant increase in the magnitude of the return of neural function after surgical intervention. Krengel et al.[75] reported that early stabilization and decompression of incomplete thoracic lesions was associated with improved neurologic function when compared with historic controls, and there are marginal data suggesting that this decreased the length of hospital stay. However, early initiation of rehabilitation and the prevention of bony deformity was associated with early internal fixation. A multicenter study of spinal fracture initially designed to determine the optimal treatment (nonoperative versus ventral versus dorsal surgical procedures) was not able to resolve this issue.[8,19,48,66]

### Anterior Approaches

Paré's wish for a ventral approach to the spine was realized by Hodgson and Stock in 1956. Their techniques of transthoracic decompression and fusion were first used to treat tuberculosis of the spine, but they suggested that this technique would be useful for treatment of other spinal deformities.[59,60] They reported that, "the region from C6 to T4 is reached without undue difficulty" through a third rib resection, and they advised using a rib resection above the level of the lesion in T4 to lumbar levels because, "it is much easier to work downwards than upwards on the spine." The resected rib was available for reconstructive fusion that was not supplemented with instrumentation.[60] This was possible because the disease tended to involve the vertebral body and the ventral paravertebral region differentially, sparing the dorsal aspect of the spinal column. Their guidelines continue to be valid.[33] The introduction of the Dwyer instrumentation was credited with increasing the popularity of ventral approaches to the spine to correct spinal deformities.[31,43] Eismont et al.[33] credited Paul and associates[97] with the first reported use of this technique for decompression and fusion of a traumatic injury of the thoracic spine, and Chou and Seljeskog[17] described "transthoracic osteotomy" for a variety of lesions. Bohlman et al.[7] demonstrated that ventral transthoracic decompression was more effective than conservative therapy or laminectomy in the return of the incompletely injured thoracic spinal cord patient's ability to ambulate. Maiman et al.[87] had reported that a ventral decompression, even when performed months after a

spinal injury, could be associated with neurologic improvement. Esses et al.[37] reported that there were no significant differences in neurologic recovery and reduction of the injury kyphosis in a prospective study of the ventral versus the dorsal treatment of burst fractures. Clohisy and associates[18] reported significant neurologic recovery in patients suffering spine fractures at the thoracolumbar junction who were decompressed ventrally. In a multicenter prospective study of the management of spinal fractures, Gertzbein[48] reported that ventral treatment of spinal injuries had been shown to be of benefit in patients who deteriorated neurologically before initial surgical intervention, in the return of bladder function, and in the treatment of delayed kyphotic deformities. In a retrospective study, Dansia et al.[22] could find no significant differences between ventral and dorsal treatment of unstable burst fractures.

### Hybrid Approaches

Approaches to the spine from a more lateral direction may permit surgical access to both the ventral and dorsal aspects of the spine from a single incision. The lateral extracavitary approach, although technically a dorsal approach, is an excellent technique for decompressing the spinal cord in many cases of ventral pathology. Likewise, the retropleural thoracotomy, described by McCormick et al.,[83] gives excellent exposure of the ventral aspect of the spine. With further dissection in the subcutaneous tissues, the dorsal spine can be exposed either to address pathology or to instrument the spine.

### Treatment of Scoliosis

The treatment of scoliosis has evolved with the development of surgical approaches and instrumentation systems. The introduction of the Harrington instrumentation procedure to stabilize the surgically treated kyphoscoliotic spine of pediatric polio patients was a significant technical advance but was not without limitations.[57] Instrumentation was subject to failure if a dorsal fusion was not performed or did not consolidate within 12 to 18 months. The importance of a concurrent dorsolateral fusion was not initially recognized and resulted in failure of the instrumentation.[58] When using only a dorsal approach, it is not surgically feasible to correct semi-rigid or rigid curves or kyphotic deformities, especially if the disorders are of a longstanding nature.[43] Therefore Hodgson and Stock ventral approaches were used.[43,94] As noted above, Dwyer instrumentation increased the popularity of the ventral approach for scoliosis, but this system also has limitations. O'Brien and Yau[94] found that the ventral treatment of paralytic scoliosis, even when combined with the Dwyer instrumentation, was not adequate to treat the disorder. The authors stated that there was an unacceptably high incidence of pseudoarthrosis, progression of the kyphotic deformity, and occurrence of scoliosis adjacent to the treated vertebral levels. An unacceptably high rate of ventral strut graft failure was observed in patients suffering from tuberculosis treated by ventral decompression and fusion, but without instrumentation. The rate of pseudoarthrosis was dramatically increased if the strut graft spanned greater than two vertebral levels.[99]

Ventral procedures were also shunned by some practitioners because of the lack of an effective ventral instrumentation that allowed ventral grafts to slip, especially when the dorsal aspect of the vertebral column or the associated ligaments were injured.[67] The Dwyer and Zielke devices were not able to effectively fix an unstable spine.[29] The Dunn device was the first ventral fixation device that allowed ventral stabilization of unstable fractures and thereby obviated the need for multilevel dorsal fixation.[29] Although the author who developed the device reported only minor complications, the device was withdrawn because of erosion of the great vessels.[11,69] Kaneda et al.[70] reported a ventral fixation device that was of lower profile and avoided inadvertent vascular injury. Both clinical and experimental evidence substantiated the ability of this device to stabilize otherwise unstable spinal injuries without a dorsal fixation device. Although Dunn warned about the use of a short segment ventral fixation device in the presence of severe osteoporosis, the Kaneda device has been used effectively in this clinical situation.[29,71] The only case in which Kaneda et al.[71] used a combined ventral/dorsal approach to the spine was when the device could not be attached to the distal vertebral body because of the location of the common iliac artery.

### Staged Combined Posterior/Anterior Approaches

Whitesides suggested that a ventral subtotal corpectomy (ventral two thirds of the vertebral body) with fibula and rib strut fusion could be considered for treatment of a significant kyphotic deformity as a result of a "severe" compression fracture, but only after reduction of the kyphosis with halo femoral or hoop traction. Total corpectomy with fusion was recommended for the treatment of stable burst fractures associated with neurologic deficit only after a dorsal Harrington procedure and the demonstration of residual spinal canal compromise on postoperative myelography. Whitesides[111] warned that a ventral decompression of an "unstable" burst fracture was dangerous to perform before dorsal stabilization and, "may occasionally be in order" if a partial neurologic deficit and canal compromise continued after the dorsal treatment. Durward et al.[30] treated thoracolumbar and lumbar spine fractures with a ventral decompression and fusion, after postprocedure computed tomography (CT) scans revealed the failure of the dorsal distraction instrumentation to adequately clear vertebral body fracture fragments from the spinal canal. DeWald[27] also treated thoracolumbar burst fractures first with a dorsal hook/rod construct and then postoperatively evaluated patients who had suffered significant compression of the vertebral body with CT scans. Postreduction fractures that demonstrated a large gap in the injured vertebral body were treated with a ventral decompression and fusion. DeWald did not provide a quantitative measure of the disruption of the vertebral body deficit but instead stated that, "in a clinical situation it can almost be predicted which body will need ventral grafting by the amount of compression initially present."

Other authors also advocated combined ventral and dorsal surgical procedures for the treatment of scoliosis. O'Brien and Yau[94] supplemented ventral interbody fusion and Dwyer instrumentation for paralytic scoliosis with a dorsal Harrington procedure for additional fixation and fusion. The surgical procedures were separated by 6 or more weeks, and the combined therapy was justified by the increased correction of the deformities that could be obtained: 86.6% in the primary deformity and 88% of the secondary curve. No long-term follow-up was given, and the authors reversed the order of the procedures in the latest case of the report. Enslin[35] reported that because of limited correction of a semirigid scoliotic curve that could be safely obtained with dorsal instrumentation, he combined the dorsal treatment with ventral discectomies, interbody fusions, and fixation. In the earliest cases, the dorsal and ventral treatments were staged several weeks apart, but the last 45 patients were treated with combined approaches performed in a single anesthetic setting.

O'Brien et al.[93] extended their experience with combined procedures for scoliosis to patients with intractable low back pain, some of whom had failed previous surgery. Although the title suggests that the procedures were performed simultaneously, the approaches were staged, but completed at the same anesthesia. The first 55 patients were treated initially with a Harrington procedure followed by repositioning for the ventral approach for fusion. The order of the procedures was reversed on the remainder of the 150 patients in the report. The authors noted that placement of the dorsal distraction system first significantly decreased the lumbar lordosis, while normal lordosis of the lumbar spine was maintained when the ventral fusion was performed before the dorsal fusion and fixation. Gertzbein chose to treat unstable spinal fractures ventrally when the patients deteriorated neurologically preoperatively or failed to improve in the "first few days" after the injury because dorsal distraction instrumentation did not reliably reduce spinal canal compromise, and also because of anecdotal reports of neurologic deterioration when distraction was attempted with large intracanalicular fragments.[49] Kostuik et al.[74] treated patients who needed lumbosacral fusion because of lumbar scoliosis accompanied by degenerative disease with a staged ventral procedure combined with a dorsal fusion and fixation. The authors believed that the combined procedure significantly enhanced the fusion rate. A dorsal fusion was also recommended for osteoporotic patients undergoing ventral fixation with a Zielke system. Schnee and Ansell[106] treated thoracolumbar burst fractures with vertebral body or canal compromise of at least 40%, kyphosis of 15 degrees or greater, and three-column instability with ventral decompression and fusion followed by dorsal segmental fixation at the same anesthesia. Danisa et al.[22] reported a comparison of two groups of patients with spinal burst fractures treated either with a ventral or a dorsal approach. The authors found no difference between the treatment groups and suggested that ventral surgical therapy be reserved for patients with a neurologic deficit and persistent spinal canal compromise after dorsal reduction or persons who develop a late kyphosis. Combined procedures were condemned as substandard treatment.

### Simultaneous Combined Approaches

Fountain[44] reported 17 cases with disorders of the thoracolumbar spine that he treated with combined dorsal and ventral approaches. Included were cases of tumor, infection, and fracture-dislocation. Using a right and occasionally a left lateral decubitus positioning, he first placed a Harrington distraction rod construct and dorsolateral fusion, and then without repositioning the patient, decompressed the spinal canal ventrally through a lateral thoracotomy. The dorsal procedure was performed first, to stabilize the spine before beginning the ventral decompression. Only in cases of fixed deformity was the order of the procedures reversed because of difficulty in mobilization of the kyphosis before the ventral release. Spencer and DeWald[107] reported their experience with 14 cases in which simultaneous ventral and dorsal surgical approaches were used to treat complex spinal deformities that required circumferential osteotomy, correction, fixation, and fusion. Included in this series were patients with fixed spinal deformities from ankylosing spondylosis, neurofibromatosis, and isolated hemivertebra, and other patients with ventral and dorsal spinal instability as a result of vertebral osteomyelitis treated with laminectomy and fracture-dislocations. The patients were also placed in the lateral decubitus position and the back, chest, flank, and iliac crest were draped in the field. Both procedures were performed without repositioning the patient. The authors were able to perform the thoracotomy and dorsal fixation in 3 hours by using two surgical teams. Kostuik et al.[74] reserved simultaneous ventral and dorsal approaches to the spine for cases of iatrogenic lumbar stenosis "flat back syndrome," refractory to conservative management. Because the patients have been previously fused, a wedge osteotomy must be performed dorsally through the dorsolateral fusion mass and may be necessary ventrally. The simultaneous ventral and dorsal exposure allows closure of the dorsal osteotomy under direct visualization before ventral grafting. Farcy[38,39] recommended simultaneous ventral/dorsal approaches to the spine for short segment pathology including unstable fractures of the spine and fixed kyphotic deformities that are often the result of trauma.

### Trauma as the Paradigm for the Surgical Treatment of Spinal Deformity

Trauma is the most common etiology of spinal deformity that requires intervention. To properly intervene in cases of traumatic spinal deformity, the surgeon must possess a sound knowledge of all aspects of deformity surgery. The applicable principles of biomechanics must be considered and the issue of instability must be taken into account. A plan for the surgical approach and the strategy for correction of the deformity must be developed. These same considerations apply to all cases of spinal deformity. Because trauma usually results in a relatively focal deformity, and because treatment of those deformities involves the application of principles from all aspects of spine surgery, trauma should be viewed as the paradigm for treatment of spinal deformity. Although other types of spinal deformity such as scolioses, degenerative conditions, and infection all have some particular nuances, they still may be properly treated by considering and applying the principles used to treat traumatic spinal deformity.

## Indications for Surgical Treatment

The controversy over the indications for spinal surgery continued to the present era with no consensus regarding the indications for specific surgical intervention in spinal injuries or other disorders affecting the spinal complex.[37,47,48] The development of ventral approaches to the spinal column and effective ventral and dorsal instrumentation has greatly increased the ability to safely address lesions of all levels of the spinal column, including correction of malalignment and stabilization of the vertebral bodies. What has not been answered is what the long-term effects of specific interventions are.[47] This lack of information is crucial and significantly complicates the determination of the optimal treatment for a given spinal abnormality. The avoidance of unnecessary iatrogenic injury to patients with spinal disorders depends on proper patient selection, but the dearth of scientifically valid information complicates this process. Advocates of surgical treatment of spinal fractures should remember that Guttmann[54] and Frankel[45] maintained that patients managed with postural reduction of the thoracolumbar spine fractures had an improved functional outcome as compared with patients who were treated surgically. In a more recent study of the treatment of thoracolumbar burst fractures, patients could be treated with early ambulation in a thoracolumbar orthosis. Cantor et al.[15] treated patients with kyphotic deformities as large as 26% and with 60% loss of vertebral body height and documented an average of 2 degrees of progression in the kyphosis and less than 5% loss of vertebral body height at 19 months after injury. Spinal canal compromise was reduced by an average of 50% at 1 year; in one patient with a 60% spinal canal stenosis, a follow-up CT scan documented complete resorption of the intracanalicular fragments. Nicoll's 1949 report that none of the patients who came under his care after surgical fusion returned to work remains a sobering reminder that outcome data from specific interventions are lacking.[47,92] The multicenter study of spinal fracture coordinated by Gertzbein[48] found little objective data to suggest that surgical therapy is preferable to nonoperative management. The rate of complication in the nonoperative patients was 3%, as compared with a 25% complication rate in the operative treatment group.

## Spinal Instability

Correction of spinal instability to prevent additional injury to the spinal cord and to allow early mobilization has been cited as justification for surgical treatment of spinal fractures with internal fixation instrumentation.[66] The determination of spinal instability is a complex subject and difficult to precisely ascertain. Clinical instability has been defined as the loss of the ability of the spine under physiologic loads to maintain its pattern of displacement so that there is no initial or additional neurologic deficit, no major deformity, and no incapacitating pain.[110] In a subsequent paper, Panjabi[96] stated that clinical stability is related to the mechanical integrity of the spine, because if the vertebral column is unable to limit its intervertebral displacement, neural structures are subject to injury. This definition is very inclusive but is of limited utility to the clinician needing to make a decision of the optimal treatment for a patient with a given spinal lesion. In the case of spinal fractures, various authors have tried to define stability and recommend treatment based on the presumed injury mechanism.[24,42,66] The definition of instability advocated by one group was extremely inclusive, because they considered any injury of the thoracolumbar spine associated with a neurologic deficit to be unstable for early ambulation. The authors believed any injury that "may result in neurologic injury" was also unstable. In addition, they proposed the existence of a state of "chronic instability" that they defined as spinal injuries with no initial neurologic injury and with virtually no chance that a neurologic injury would have occurred in the immediate postoperative period. In this group of injuries, the authors believed that there was a potential for neurologic damage to develop as a consequence of late progressive deformity. When using these definitions, all thoracolumbar spinal injuries in their report were "unstable."[66]

In 1949, Nicoll[92] attempted to define stable versus unstable fractures by using an anatomic classification in a series of 166 fracture or fracture-dislocations of the thoracolumbar spine. In his view, the major determinant of stability was the integrity of the interspinous ligament. Holdsworth introduced the first modern classification and attempted to correlate radiographic patterns of spinal fractures with early, as well as late, instability. Early instability was characterized by the immediate risk of additional injury to the nervous tissues by the fragments of the bony column, whereas late instability was characterized by slowly progressive deformity of the spinal column.[61] This classification was based on a two-column theory of spinal column stability that was a biomechanical interpretation of injury mechanisms based on the radiographic findings. The integrity of the dorsal bony elements and the posterior ligamentous complex, including the interspinous and supraspinous ligaments plus the ligamentum flavum, was the major determinant of stability. The flexion-rotation injury was the most unstable of spinal column injuries because it disrupted both the bony and ligamentous elements of the dorsal spinal column. Holdsworth acknowledged that his proposed classification system was flawed and that some compression injuries, which according to his classification should be stable, were associated with major neurologic deficits.[62]

## Three-Column Theory of Spinal Stability

Experimental data did not support the assertions by Nicoll or Holdsworth that disruption of the dorsal ligamentous structures alone resulted in instability of the spinal column.[3,61,92] Denis[24] reviewed imaging studies of 412 thoracolumbar fractures and modified the two-column theory of Holdsworth by dividing the anterior column into anterior and middle columns; the latter consisted of the posterior longitudinal ligament and the dorsal half of the vertebral body (Figure 119.1). CT scans of the spine were used to establish the integrity of the newly defined middle column, and "compression" fractures that were associated with disruption of the dorsal vertebral body were named

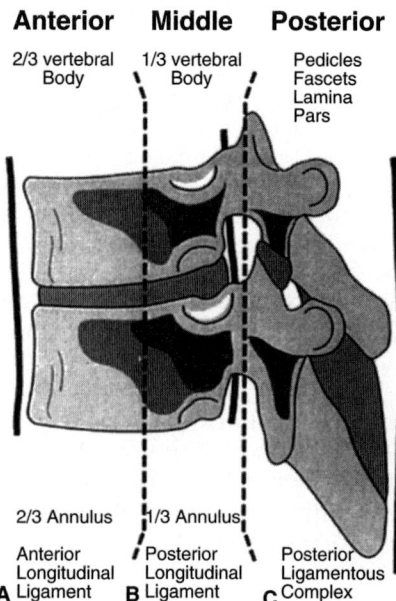

## COLUMNS

**Anterior    Middle    Posterior**

2/3 vertebral    1/3 vertebral    Pedicles
Body             Body             Fascets
                                  Lamina
                                  Pars

2/3 Annulus    1/3 Annulus    Posterior
Anterior       Posterior      Ligamentous
Longitudinal   Longitudinal   Complex
**A** Ligament  **B** Ligament  **C**

**Figure 119.1** The three-column theory of Denis[23] and Ferguson and Allen[41] divides the spine into three columns. (**A**) The anterior column consists of the anterior two thirds of the vertebral body, the anterior two thirds of the annulus fibrosus, and the anterior longitudinal ligament. (**B**) The middle column consists of the dorsal one third of the vertebral body, the one third of the annulus fibrosus, and the posterior longitudinal ligament. (**C**) The posterior column consists of the dorsal neural arch and associated ligaments.

*burst fractures.* This fracture was distinguished from the more common ventral wedge compression fractures where the dorsal cortical rim from the pedicle laterally and the dorsal vertebral body ventrally remained intact. Ferguson and Allen[42] redefined the middle column as only the dorsal third of the vertebral body and associated annulus fibrosus. The middle column became the basis of a new classification of stability, as an injury to the anterior and the middle or the posterior and the middle columns would result in an unstable fracture.[24] Maiman and Pintar[88] have raised objections to the validity of this classification based on biomechanical considerations. They cited experimental evidence that suggested that posterior ligamentous injury can occur with a flexion-compression force on the spinal column before vertebral body failure occurs, and they also raised objections to the use of static radiographs to assess the integrity of the ligamentous structures. McAfee *et al.*[79] separated burst fractures into stable and unstable types; the latter type was associated with disruption of the ligamentous and/or bony posterior column. James *et al.*[68] have also challenged the three-column theory and provided experimental data that the middle column adds little to the stability of the classical burst fracture. These authors also supported the assertion of Holdsworth that the posterior column is the "second, crucial column."[61] Panjabi *et al.*[96] provided the first biomechanical validation of the three-column theory of spinal stability. Using high-speed trauma models of thoracolumbar spinal fracture, axial compression, and flexion/compression injuries, the authors demonstrated that the integrity of the middle column correlated best with eight of nine flexibility parameters.

## Classification of Spinal Fractures

In the papers on the three-column injury model of thoracic and lumbar fractures, Denis also classified fracture types.[24,25] These classification systems continue to be widely accepted classification systems in use today, but at least two other classification systems based on the mechanism of injury need to be considered: (1) that of Ferguson and Allen[41] reported in 1984 soon after the initial report of Denis,[24] and (2) that of Magerl,[86] which was published in 1991. Ferguson and Allen used the three-column (or *regions,* as they preferred to refer to these redefined anatomic areas) to analyze the effects of excessive loading, which resulted in the failure of the spinal column. They used plain, tomograph, and CT imaging studies to assess the injury mechanism and then classified the resultant injury according to the mechanisms deduced from the radiographic findings of compression, tension, torsion, translation, or a combination of loading forces.[41] Using the knowledge of the mechanism that resulted in the failure of the spinal column, the authors developed an algorithm to assist in the selection of the appropriate fixation system to render the spinal column stable.[42]

Magerl's classification system was also based on the mechanism of failure of the spinal column. The original system was extremely complex but has been recently modified for use in research by a committee of members of the major spine societies.[49,86] There are three types of spinal column injuries: type A, compression; type B, distraction; and type C, multidirectional injuries with translation (Figure 119.2). Each type is subdivided into three groups numbered 1 through 3 based on the injury mechanisms. The classification arranges fractures in order of increasing severity of the resultant spinal injury and increasing severity of instability of the spinal column. This particular classification system provides assistance in the determination of the necessity for, and in the selection of, the type of fixation system employed. Type A injuries are compression injuries primarily involving the vertebral body and result from axial loading with or without a flexion load. This type of injury involves the loss of vertebral height but does not involve the dorsal soft tissues. Although there may be a vertical split of the dorsal arch, this dorsal fracture does not significantly influence the overall stability of the vertebral column. There is no translation of one vertebral body on another. The subdivision into groups include: (1) the impaction or wedge compression fracture, (2) the split fracture in which there is a coronal or sagittal split in the vertebral body, and (3) the burst fracture with varying degrees of communication and displacement. Injuries classified in the latter group are more likely to be unstable than are the group 1 injuries. If stability needs to be restored, an instrumentation system that allows distraction will be necessary. Type B injuries are caused by a distractive force that involves both the dorsal and ventral elements. As in the type A fractures, there is minimal or no translation of the vertebral bodies. The subdivision into

groups is based on the transverse disruption of the spinal complex: (1) the dorsal soft tissues, (2) the dorsal bony arch, (3) the ventral disc. Subluxation may occur if the disc space is disrupted or a compression-type injury similar to the type A injuries will occur with ventral axial loading. The group B3 injury is associated with a ventral distractive force and will result in an extension spondylolysis (as illustrated in Figure 119.2[B3]) or in a dorsal subluxation when the dorsal soft tissues, rather than the bony arch, are disrupted. In general, the type B injuries are more likely to be unstable as compared with the type A fractures and may often be corrected with a short segment compression construct. The group B3 injuries may require more extensive fixation construct to restore spinal column stability. The type C injuries involve the dorsal and caudal elements and can be distinguished from the type B injuries by the presence of significant translation that reflects the increased instability of this type of injury. Group C1 fractures are characterized by translation in the ventrodorsal sagittal plane that often results in ventral or dorsal dislocations. If there is an accompanying axial load, a vertebral body compression similar to the type A injury will result. Obviously, the presence of the translation distinguishes the injuries. In the group C2 injury, the translation is caused by lateral shear coronal plane forces and may be accompanied by side flexion. In group C3 injuries, the primary injury mechanism is a rotational force. If there is an associated axial load with compression of the vertebral body, a rotational burst fracture will result, whereas distraction will produce an injury similar to type B. If the rotational shear forces extend obliquely through the vertebral body and are accompanied by dorsal element disruption, a slice fracture, first described by Holdsworth and Hardy, will result.[63] Type C injuries with multiplanar instability need a multilevel (two or more levels on either side of the injury) fixation system, and in some cases combined ventral and dorsal approaches with fusion and stabilization may be necessary. This injury classification system is simple and open ended compared with earlier classification systems. Although the system can be used as a guide for spinal fracture management, it holds greater promise as a research tool; this may allow optimal treatment for specific spinal injuries to be determined.[49]

## Pedicle Screw Fixation

The introduction of pedicle screw fixation afforded an additional tool for the spine surgeon to fix the unstable spinal column and promised to allow less lengthy fixation constructs compared with the Harrington distraction rod fixation.[103,104,108] Fixation of three vertebral body levels rostral and two or three levels caudal to the injury level were advocated for the latter construct based on experimental as well as clinical data.[72,98] The ability to include only the immediately adjacent vertebral levels in the fixation construct is of particular advantage in the lumbar spine.[104,108] Enthusiasm for short segment fixation in the thoracolumbar and lumbar spine was tempered by reports of early construct failures. McLain and associates[84] reported that 13 of 19 patients suffering an unstable spinal fracture treated with a short fixation construct that used a

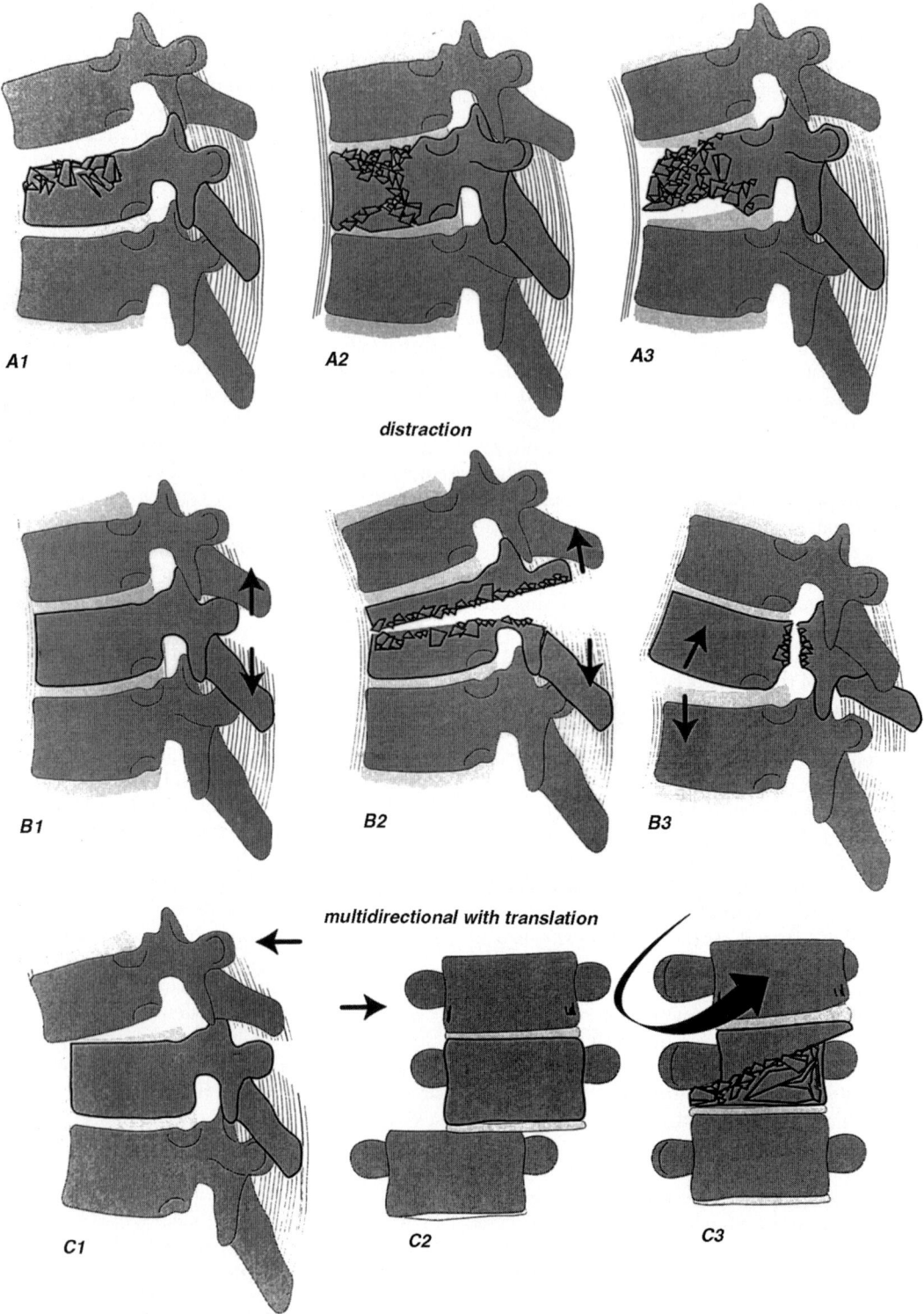

*distraction*

*multidirectional with translation*

**Figure 119.2** The fracture classification system as proposed by Magerl[86] and modified as per Gertzbein.[49] Fractures are divided in types according to major injury force: **(A1-3)**, compression; **(B1-3)**, distraction; **(C1-3)**, multidirectional with translation. Each type is subdivided into three groups (see text for details). The classification system is arranged in order of increasing severity: **A1** is the most stable, while **C3** is the least stable. The classification system can be used to determine the need for instrumentation and the optimal type of fixation. It represents a uniform method of classification of fractures for clinical research.

universal system with pedicle screws had progressive angulation of the kyphosis greater than 10 degrees postoperatively. The authors were puzzled by the results because experimental data in an acute injury model demonstrated that the pedicle screw construct provided torsional, flexural, and compressive rigidity comparable to longer hook/rod constructs of the same system.[51,52] A later clinical report that used the longer fixation construct (three levels above and two levels below) had documented excellent results in the treatment of similar fractures.[81] After analysis of their clinical data, McLain et al.[84] noted that in the 6 patients in whom the short segment constructs did not fail, the anterior column was either reconstructed via a ventral fusion or had not been subjected to a significant axial load (fracture-dislocations or flexion-distraction injuries with compression of the vertebral body.

Ebelke et al.[32] also noted that all failures of another short segment fixation system occurred in patients who did not undergo ventral grafting and that no patient undergoing a transpedicular grafting of the anterior column had a fixation construct failure. McCormack et al.[82] also noted screw fracture of short segmental pedicle screw fixation constructs in 10 of a group of 26 patients. The authors suspected that the instrumentation failures were related to

the fracture anatomy and to the inability of the injured vertebral bodies to load share, as DeWald[27] had reported that even dorsal long rod constructs would fail if there was a significant gap in the reduced vertebral body fragments. McCormack et al.[82] then conducted a retrospective analysis of the fracture anatomy of a consecutive series of patients on whom internal fixation was performed. This review demonstrated a relationship between the characteristics of the most injured vertebral body and failure of dorsal short segment pedicle fixation. Using CT and plain radiographs of the fracture sites, the authors developed a scoring system based on three types of assessment of the severity of the fracture anatomy (Figure 119.3): (1) the amount of vertebral body comminuted by the injury as assessed with preoperative sagittal reconstructions (see Figure 119.3A); (2) the degree of dispersion of the vertebral body fracture fragments as assessed by an axial CT (see Figure 119.3B); and (3) the amount of correction of the kyphotic deformity measured by the comparison of preoperative and postoperative plain radiographs (see Figure 119.3C). Each of the above characteristics was divided into three groups and assigned a numeric value based on the degree of severity: 1 for mild, 2 for moderate, 3 for severe. A total score was generated for each patient's fracture, and the score

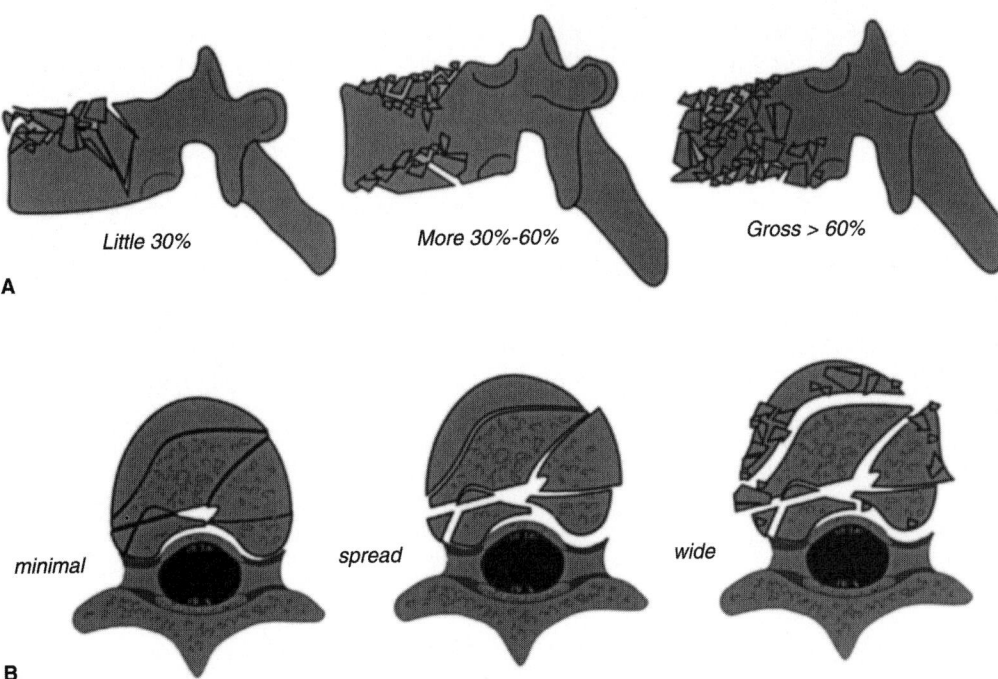

**Figure 119.3** A classification system of fracture anatomy based on three characteristics of the vertebral body injury and used to determine axial load-sharing capability of anterior and middle columns of the injured spine. (**A**) Degree of comminution or percentage of the vertebral body fractured as estimated on sagittal CT reconstruction images. There are three subgroups: (1) little with less than 30% of the vertebral body comminution; (2) greater than or equal to 30% but less than or equal to 60% involvement; and (3) gross involvement, greater than 60%. (**B**) Apposition of vertebral body fragments as determined on axial CT images: (1) minimal, less than 2mm of spread of the fragments; (2) spread of greater than or equal to 2mm of less than 50% of the body area; and (3) wide spread of the fracture fragments greater than or equal to 2mm or greater than or equal to 50% of the body.

*Continued*

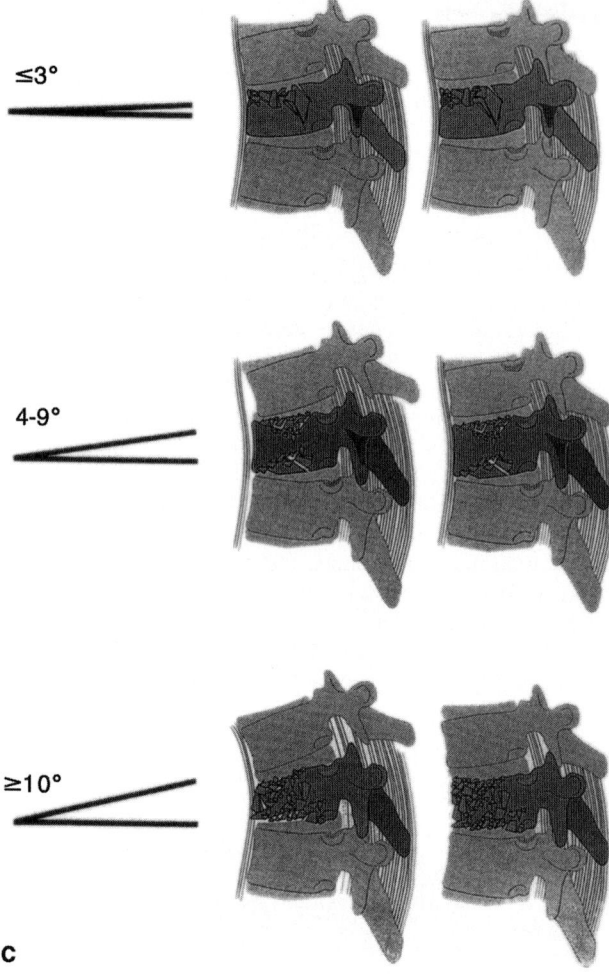

≤3°

4-9°

≥10°

**C**

**Figure 119.3 *cont'd* (C)** The degrees of kyphosis reduction expected with the initial deformity assessed by plain films: (1) little correction, less than or equal to 3 degrees; (2) more correction, 4 to 9 degrees; and (3) most correction, greater than or equal to 10 degrees. Each fracture characteristic is assigned a numeric score based on the subgroup into which a given fracture is assigned. The numeric values of the three subgroups (one from each characteristic) are added to obtain an injury score. The greater the number, the less likely the injured vertebral body is to resist an axial load and more likely a posterior, short segment fixation construct is to fail. *(Redrawn from McCormack T, Karaikovic E, Gaines RW: The load sharing classification of spine fractures. Spine 19:741, 1994.)*

reflected the severity of the injury: 3 for a mild injury and 9 for the most severe (Table 119.1). The authors found that all instrumentation failures occurred in patients with a severity score of 7 or greater. The authors noted that the above classification system did not take into account ligamentous injuries and therefore was not useful as a guide to determine between nonoperative and surgical treatment for an individual patient but was useful to determine the type of operative approach and fixation technique once the decision for surgical treatment had been made. The degree of kyphosis correction expected was estimated from the preoperative plain radiographs of a given frac-

ture. The system was unique as it was not based on injury mechanism.

The authors concluded that the best candidates for short segment dorsal fixation were patients who suffered flexion-distraction injuries or "mild" burst fractures or fracture-dislocation with scores of 6 or less. Patients suffering burst fractures or fracture-dislocations with severe comminution of the vertebral body resulting in point scores of 7 or greater were poor candidates for short segment posterior fixation. McCormack *et al.*[82] recommended that patients with burst fractures with a severity score of 7 or greater be treated via a ventral approach with short segment vertebrectomy, strut fusion, and stabilization with a Kaneda device. Long segment dorsal fixation was reserved for patients with fracture-dislocation injuries who could not make use of the early mobilization possible with a dorsal short segment fixation or patients who were unable to tolerate a two-stage dorsal/ventral procedure because of cardiopulmonary embarrassment. For all other patients with a severe fracture-dislocation injury, dorsal short segment pedicle screw construct with fusion was recommended, followed by a second-stage ventral vertebrectomy and strut fusion.

## Treatment Algorithm

Farcy *et al.*[40] developed an algorithm for the treatment of thoracolumbar fractures that was based on a sagittal index and an instability grade (IG) and used the algorithm in a prospective study. The sagittal index was defined as the measurement of segmental kyphosis at the injury level that is then adjusted for the baseline sagittal contour (Table 119.2). The IG was based on the three-column theory of Denis (discussed above) and considered ligamentous damage in addition to bony element injury in the determination of instability (see Figure 119.1). One point was given for injury to bone and another point for injury to ligamentous structures associated with each column. A total disruption of the bony and ligamentous elements results in an IG of 6 (Table 119.3). Based on a prospective study, the authors determined that a thoracolumbar spine injury with a sagittal index of less than 25 degrees and an IG of less than 3 can be treated without surgery[38-40] (Table 119.4). Farcy recommended that spine injuries with a sagittal index of greater than 25 degrees and less than 35 degrees and/or with an IG of greater than 3 but less than 5 be treated with dorsal reduction and instrumentation. A simultaneous ventral/dorsal approach was recommended for a sagittal index greater than 35 degrees and/or an IG greater than or equal to 5.

## Surgical Technique

### General Principles

Patients with unstable fractures are often nasotracheally or orally intubated awake in a supine position and carefully log-rolled into the prone position on a table or a specialized frame for dorsal or dorsolateral approaches, or to a lateral decubitus position for transthoracic or retroperitoneal approaches. This awake incubation technique is

## TABLE 119.1

### Load-Sharing Classification*

**A. Comminution**

|  | Little | More | Gross |  |
|---|---|---|---|---|
|  | <30% | ≥30% and 60% | >60% |  |
| Score | 1 | 2 | 3 | 1-3 |

**B. Apposition of Fragments**

|  | Minimal | Spread | Wide |  |
|---|---|---|---|---|
|  | Minimal | ≥2 mm; <50% | ≥2 mm; >50% |  |
| Score | 1 | 2 | 3 | 1-3 |

**C. Deformity Correction**

|  | Little | More | Most |  |
|---|---|---|---|---|
|  | ≤3° | 4°-9° | ≥10° |  |
| Score | 1 | 2 | 3 | 1-3 |
| Total score |  |  |  | 3-9 |

*A scoring system for quantitating the ability of the injured vertebral body to share axial loading. The system assesses three characteristics of the injured spine: (A) comminution of the vertebral body as estimated on sagittal CT reconstruction images; (B) apposition or spread of the vertebral body fragments as assessed on an axial CT scan; (C) expected deformity correction that will be obtained with fixation instrumentation expressed as degrees of change in the kyphotic deformity. A numeric value is assigned for each characteristic (1 through 3) and added to determine the total, which is related to the ability of the vertebral body to load-share (see Figure 119.3). (From McCormack T, Karaikovic E, Gaines RW: The load sharing classification of spine fractures. *Spine* 19:741, 1994, with permission.)

## TABLE 119.2

### Sagittal Index*

|  | Vertebral level | | |
|---|---|---|---|
|  | Thoracic | Thora-columbar | Lumbar |
| Local kyphosis | X° | Y° | Z° |
| Baseline curve | 5° | 0° | 10° |
| Sagittal index | SI° = X° − 5° | SI° = Y° − 0° | SI° = Z° − (−10°) |

SI, Sagittal index.
*Sagittal index is based on the measurement of the local kyphotic deformity occurring in a spine injury adjusted for a correction factor that depends on the level of the involved vertebral body. The correction factors subtracted from the measurement of the deformity on plain lateral x-ray films are (1) 5° for the thoracic region; (2) 0° for the thoracolumbar spine; (3) −10° in the lumbar region. (Data from Farcy JP, Weidenbaum M, Glassman SD: Sagittal index in management of thoracolumbar burst fractures. *Spine* 15:958, 1990.)

## TABLE 119.3

### Instability Grade*

|  | Anterior Column | Middle Column | Posterior Column |
|---|---|---|---|
| Bone | Dorsal 2/3 vertebra[†] | Dorsal 1/3 vertebra[†] | Dorsal arch[†] |
| Ligament | Anterior longitudinal[†] | Posterior longitudinal[†] | Dorsal complex[†] |

*Instability grade is based upon the three-column theory of spinal stability, but injury to the bony and ligamentous elements of each column are independently assessed (see Figure 119.1). The grade is determined by giving a point for an injury to bone and one for an injury to a ligamentous structure in each column and adding the total. This score is used with the sagittal index to guide selection of the surgical procedure to treat a spine fracture (see Table 119.2).
[†]One (1) point for injury to either bone or ligament in each column: 0 = uninjured spine (maximum stability); 6 = maximum injury to spine (maximum instability). (Data from Farcy JP, Weidenbaum M, Glassman SD: Sagittal index in management of thoracolumbar burst fractures. *Spine* 15:958, 1990.)

## TABLE 119.4

### Treatment of Spinal Fractures*

| Treatment | SI° | IG |
|---|---|---|
| Brace | <15 | <2 |
| Closed reduction/cast | ≥15 and <25 | >1 and <3 |
| Posterior instrumentation | ≥25 and <35 | ≥3 and <5 |
| Simultaneous anterior/ posterior approach | ≥35 | ≥5 |

IG, Instability grade; SI, sagittal index.
*A treatment algorithm based on the SI and IG proposed by Farcy (see Tables 119.2 and 119.3). (From Farcy JP: Unstable fractures of the lumbar spine: discussion. *Spinal Frontiers* 3:4, 1996, with permission.)

evoked waveforms.[13] In prone positioning, the authors prefer the Relton-Hall scoliosis operating frame (Imperial Medical Ltd, Markham, Ontario) and are careful to avoid malpositioning to eliminate brachial plexus injuries or meralgia paresthetica and to aid closed reduction of the spinal injury. To allow optimal positioning and to prevent injuries to the eyes, patients are placed into the Mayfield Skull Clamp (Ohio Medical Instrument Co., Cincinnati, OH). A Cell Saver system (Haemonetics, Raintree, MA) is often used to minimize total blood loss, and hemostasis is maintained intraoperatively with powdered Gelfoam (Upjohn Co., Kalamazoo, MI). Controlled hypotension is not recommended because of the deleterious effect of hypoperfusion on the compromised nervous system tissue. Sequential Compression Sleeves (Kendall Healthcare Products, Mansfield, MA) are also used intraoperatively to reduce the incidence of complications from venous stasis.

### Fusion

Internal fixation devices are only temporary and will universally fail if an adequate bony fusion is not performed. The authors use cadaveric grafts only in the reconstruction of ventral decompression and use copious autologous bone graft whenever possible. If an allograft is placed, it is supplemented with bone salvaged from the vertebral body at

especially important in patients with incomplete neurologic deficits, with grossly unstable spinal columns.

Once properly positioned, the baseline neurologic assessments are repeated to ensure that no deterioration has taken place. Anesthesia (usually nitrous-narcotic balanced) is used in cases where spinal cord monitoring is essential, because even rather low concentrations of inhalation anesthetic can significantly alter or obliterate the

the time of the decompression. For dorsal constructs, autologous graft is harvested from the dorsal iliac crests and is combined with facet arthrodesis and decortication of the transverse process, lamina, and pars interarticularis.

## Staged Ventral and Dorsal Approaches

Ventral transthoracic decompression can be used to treat fractures of the thoracic and lumbar spine that impinge on the ventral canal and spinal cord. The authors use this approach for patients who are neurologically intact, have an incomplete spinal cord lesion, or have a fixed kyphotic deformity from a remote spine injury. In the thoracic area, this procedure, when combined with ventral grafting, can be the only treatment rendered. With a dorsal column injury, the decrease in the strength of the reconstructed ventral spinal column, after a ventral strut grafting procedure, usually requires dorsal fusion and fixation for adequate stabilization of the spinal column, because an effective ventral stabilization device for the upper thoracic (T10) region does not exist. Gurr *et al.*[52] have demonstrated that the strength of a spine is markedly reduced after a corpectomy when compared with an intact spine in axial, flexion, or rotational loading. The addition of a ventral iliac graft still allowed three times the displacement with axial loading, while torsional stiffness was less than one third that of an intact spine. Uninstrumented ventral decompression should be reserved only for patients with significant ventral spinal canal compromise and minimal instability. The postoperative use of thoracolumbar orthosis is recommended by the authors.

For lesions in the upper thoracic area, T10 or above, a double lumen endotracheal tube is efficacious and allows the collapse of the ipsilateral lung to enhance exposure. The spine can be exposed with the patient in either the left or right lateral decubitus position. The left lateral decubitus is most often used for the uppermost region of the thoracic spine, while the right lateral decubitus position is used for mid- and lower-thoracic regions. Either side can be used if necessary to obtain adequate exposure of the lesion.

An axillary roll is used to prevent a stretch palsy of the lower brachial plexus, and the superior arm is held in a neutral position with an arm support, with the arm held in a forward flexion of no greater than 90 degrees at the shoulder to minimize risk of the upper brachial plexopathy. Wide adhesive tape can be used to secure the position of the patient and should be placed at the level of the greater trochanter and across the shoulder. The tape should be securely affixed to the table. Although some surgeons prefer to use a bean bag under the patient, the authors prefer not to because it limits dorsal exposure. A bean bag is useful when simultaneous ventral decompression and dorsal stabilization are necessary. Care should be taken to prepare an adequate area of skin: to the midline ventrally, beyond the midline dorsally, to just caudal to the axilla, to rostral to the iliac crest.

The skin incision is made over the rib, one to two vertebral levels rostral to the level of the lesion when dealing with lesions from T6 to T10. At the most rostral thoracic levels, the skin incision should extend caudal to the tip of the scapula and halfway between the medial border of the scapula and the midline spinous processes (Figure 119.4). The incision should be extended to the subcutaneous tissues down to the deep fascia and muscles that are divided in line with the skin incision. The rib to be resected is then stripped subperiosteally and divided with a rib cutter. The inner rib bed is divided to expose the chest cavity.

When exposing the uppermost levels in the thoracic region, care should be taken not to injure the long thoracic nerve that runs in the midaxillary line from the axilla to the

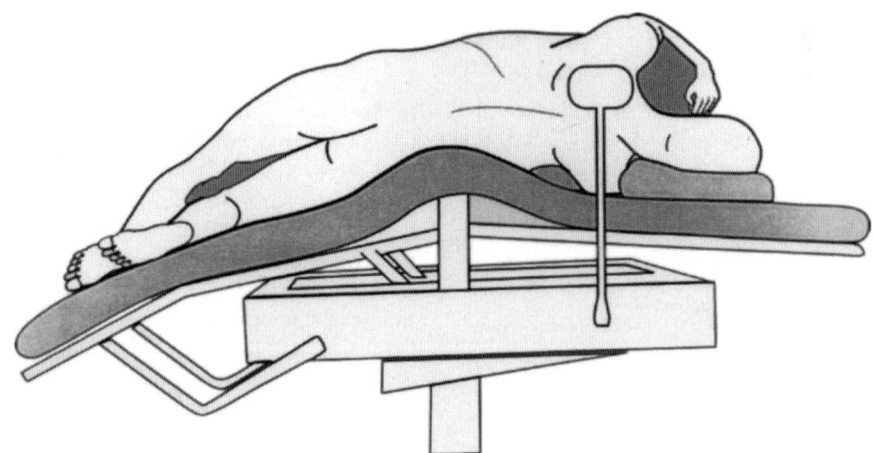

**Figure 119.4** An illustration of the positioning of a patient for a ventral decompression via a lateral thoracotomy or a simultaneous ventral and dorsal approach to the spine. The patient is placed on a mattress and a surgical table with a kidney brake or positioned so that the table can be flexed to facilitate the ventral decompression of the spine. Note the positioning of the superior arm. It is important to securely fix the patient to the bed with braces (seen above the midline incision or tape so that lateral alignment is maintained). (*From Farcy JP: Simultaneous anterior and posterior procedures for short segment spine pathology. Video tape 23112, American Academy of Orthopaedic Surgeons, 1993, with permission.*)

serratus anterior. It is preferable to detach the muscle from the ventral chest wall to avoid cutting the long thoracic nerve. With mobilization of the scapula by dividing the dorsal scapular muscles, rhomboids and trapezius, the third rib is more easily visualized and a greater area visualized with the thoracotomy.

Once the ribs have been counted from inside the thoracic cavity and the level of the rib verified, a self-retaining retractor is then inserted over moist laparotomy sponges. With deflation or packing of the lung, the spine can be visually or tactually identified. The bony column is covered with a thin layer of parietal pleura. The proximal portion of the resected rib can be followed to the vertebral column, where it inserts onto the rostral portion of the vertebral body of the same level. With this localization, the disc space(s) can be identified and a spinal needle placed. A cross-table portable radiograph is used to verify the level.

The parietal pleura is then divided between the rib insertions on the vertebral body and the great vessels until one level rostral and caudal to the levels of the pathology is exposed. The segmental vessels are then identified in the midbody region, clamped, divided, and tied. A spinal angiogram to identify the artery of Adamkiewicz is usually unnecessary. Vascular embarrassment of the spinal cord can nearly always be prevented by maintaining normal blood pressure and by the avoidance of the use of the cautery at or near the neural foramina.[12,101,106] An extraperiosteal dissection of the soft tissues overlying the vertebral body can be performed by using Kitner dissectors or a small Cobb. The dissection can be carried across the ventral midline of the vertebral body and a malleable retractor placed to protect the great vessels and the esophagus (Figure 119.5A).

The proximal portion of the rib inserting at the level of decompression is removed to expose the pedicle and neural foramina. The disc spaces immediately rostral and caudal to the vertebrectomy site should be removed by using a scalpel and rongeurs. A small Cobb elevator is useful to detach the cartilaginous end plate, which can aid in the disc removal. An osteotome is then used to remove a portion of the vertebral body, taking care to leave the ventralmost portion of the vertebral body attached to the anterior longitudinal ligament. The dura can be exposed by using a power burr, rongeurs, curettes, and osteotomes after first identifying the dura at the neural foramina after a partial resection of the pedicle (see Figure 119.5B,D). The dissection should be extended across the full width of the canal until the pedicle on the distal side is identified. Measurements of the vertebral body width from the preoperative imaging studies are valuable. One must explore

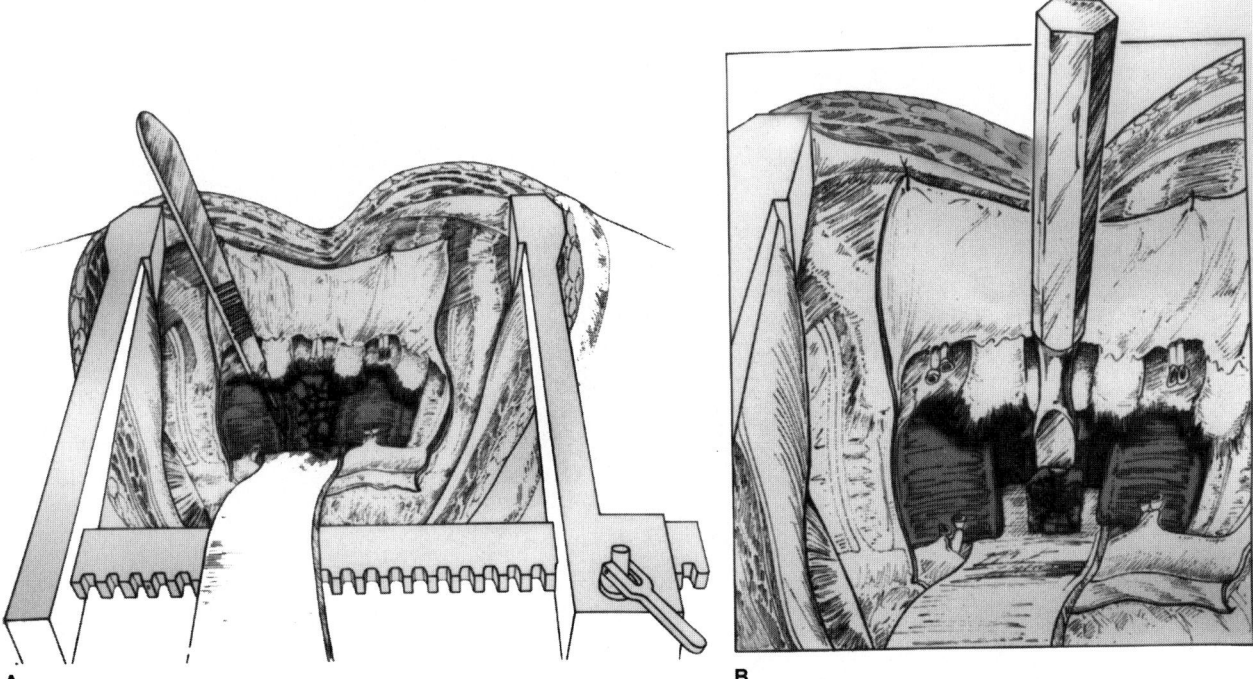

**A**          **B**

**Figure 119.5** Ventral decompression and fusion of the thoracic or lumbar spine via a lateral thoracotomy exposure. **(A)** The opening in the thoracic cavity is held open with a retractor. The segmental vessels at the injury site and at the adjacent vertebral levels have been ligated at the midvertebral body level and well away from the neuroforamen. The parietal pleura has been dissected in the extraperiosteal plane. The dissection has been continued over the distal lateral surface of the spine. Small lap sponges are placed over the great vessels, and a malleable retractor placed over the sponges; the pleura is retracted to allow access to the vertebral discs and body as necessary. One to two centimeters of the proximal rib head is resected to allow the spinal canal to be identified. The annulus is divided sharply above and below the injured vertebra.

*Continued*

the rostral disc space to verify that bony fragments attached to the annulus have been removed from the canal. If there is any question of residual bony fragment having penetrated the posterior longitudinal ligament, the ligament must be divided, or a window cut to allow exploration of the epidural space.

The vertebrectomy site should be grafted to reconstruct the spinal column. The iliac crest can be harvested, but the authors have used tibial allograft struts packed with salvaged fragments of the resected vertebral bodies. The rostral and caudal vertebral bodies are notched to lock the graft in place. The notching of the adjacent vertebral bodies helps to prevent dislodging of the graft during positioning for the dorsal fusion. Mechanical pressure in the midline of the back over the corpectomy site can assist with graft placement by extending the space. The space between the strut and the anterior longitudinal ligament is packed with more autologous vertebral body fragments or morselized rib. A rib strut may also be used if there is minimal instability. There should be sufficient space between the strut graft and the dural covering of the neural ele-ments; the graft should be locked in the rostral and caudal vertebral bodies to prevent dorsal migration into the spinal canal (see Figure 119.5E-G).

Hemostasis should be obtained before closure and after the malleable retractor is removed. An attempt to close the parietal pleura should be made, and a tube thoracostomy placed. Pericostal sutures are placed and tied after approximation of the ribs. The overlying tissues are closed in layers and the skin closed with staples.

The patient is then moved to the second surgical table with a padded fracture frame in place. The patient should be log-rolled into the prone position, taking care to avoid flexion of the spine. A dorsal fusion and fixation can be performed. The authors use hook/rod constructs at T9 and above.

### Simultaneous Ventral and Dorsal Approaches

The patient is positioned in the lateral decubitus position as described above. A padded mattress is placed under the patient. A kidney brake (see Figure 119.4) is preferred by

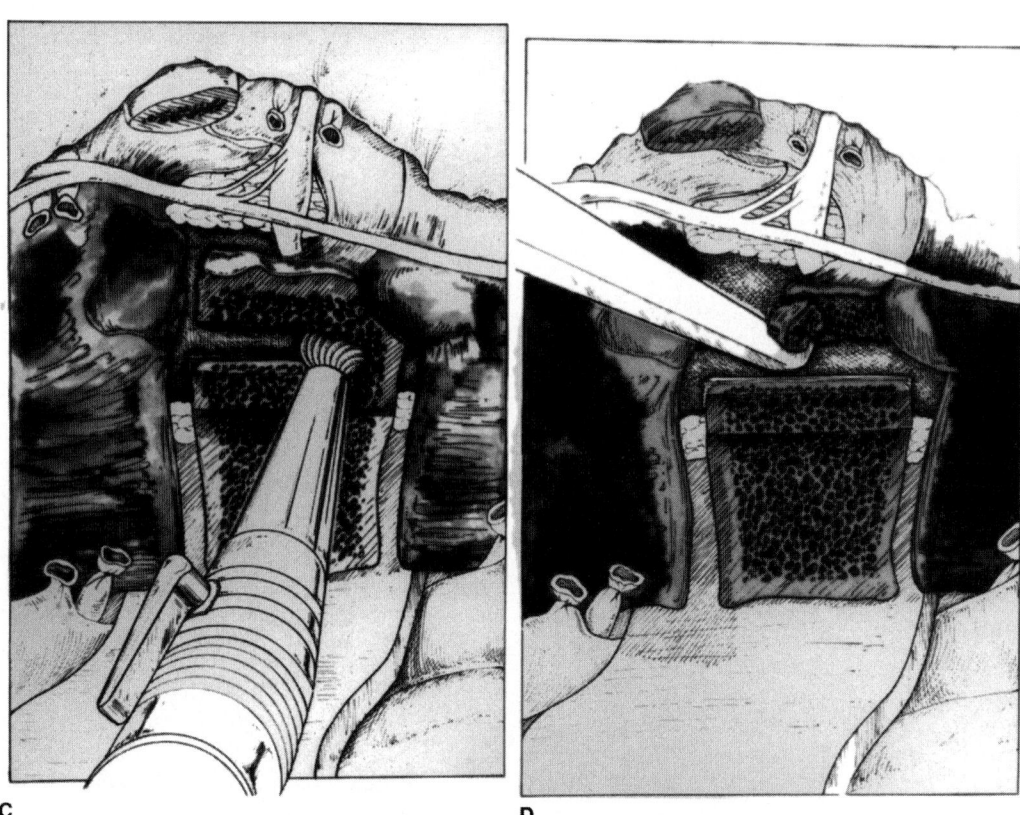

C                                                    D

**Figure 119.5 _cont'd_ (B-D),** Osteotomes, a high-speed drill equipped with a burr, or rongeurs are used to accomplish the vertebrectomy and discectomies. The author normally resects the vertebral body with an osteotome; care is taken to remove 1mm slices of bone when the most posterior aspect of the vertebral body is removed. The previous identification of the spinal canal allows this part of the procedure to be accomplished without injuring the neural contents of the canal. Once the posterior longitudinal ligament (PLL) is identified, long-handled curettes are used to complete the decompression. The anterior longitudinal ligament and immediately adjacent vertebral body are usually left. The full width of the PLL is dissected free. If intradural pathology is suspected, the PLL is opened and the dura inspected under direct visualization. The PLL is explored at the completion of the bone dissection to minimize the venous hemorrhage from epidural, intracanalicular veins.

some surgeons. The patient should be positioned so that lateral bending can be effected. The patient's back should be positioned near the edge of the table. Braces attached to the table can greatly assist in the maintenance of the proper positioning during the procedure. Farcy believes that a ventral brace on the superior thigh is particularly important. The superior arm position is also important to allow room for the surgeon but should not be flexed greater than 90 degrees. Care must be taken to not have

the thoracotomy and midline dorsal incisions intersect. It is not necessary for the thoracotomy incision to extend beyond the angle of the rib, and to extend dorsally will only compromise blood supply to the adjacent skin.[107] The ventral thoracotomy can be extended caudally and medially to allow access to the retroperitoneal region and the lower lumbar spine.

The dissection for the exposure of the spine can continue as outlined above. If the lumbar area is to be

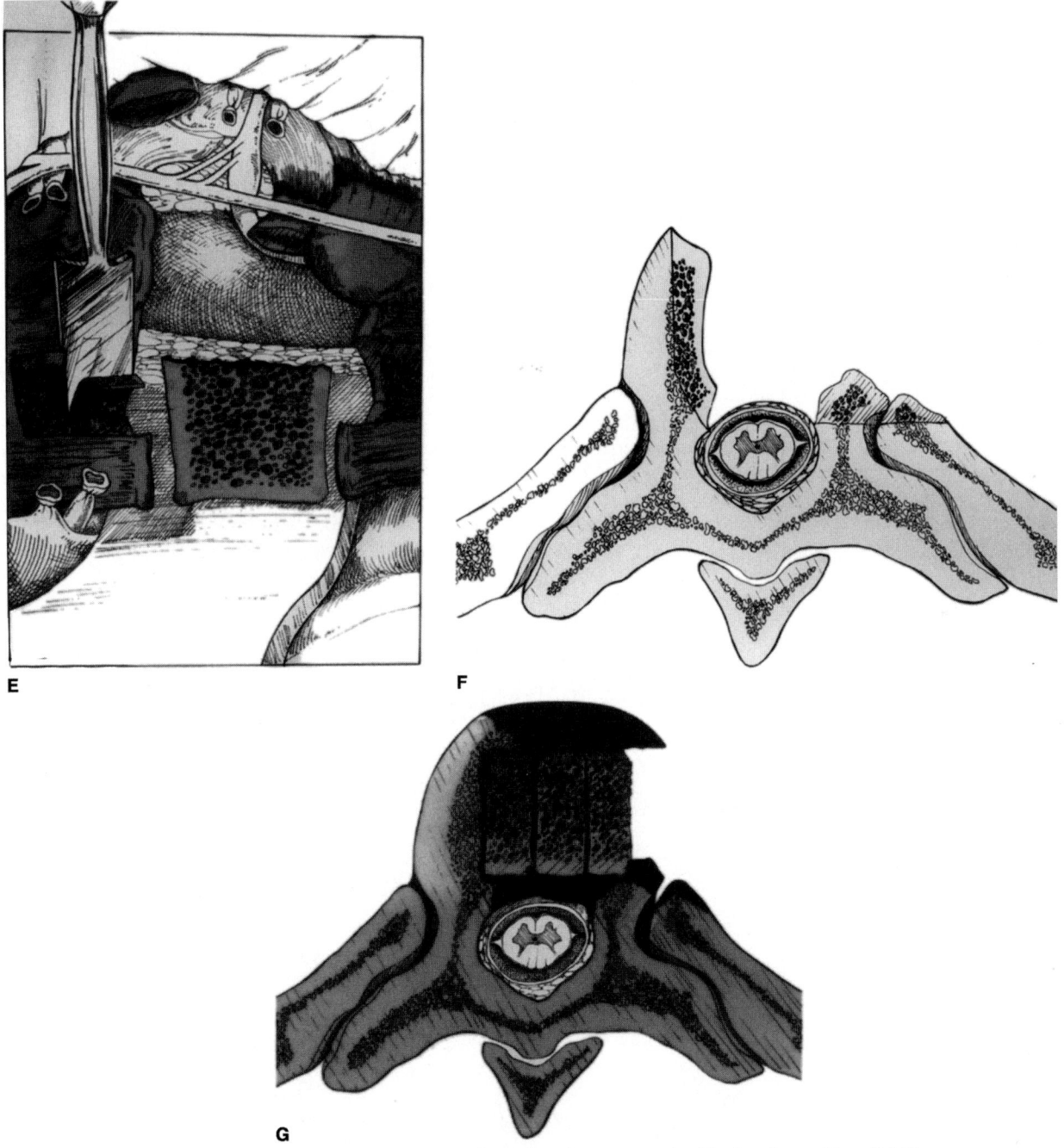

E

F

G

**Figure 119.5, *cont'd* (E)**, Grooves are made in the adjacent vertebral bodies for grafting. **(F)** The cross-section of the spine at the level of the dissection prior to grafting. **(G)** The same view as seen in **(F)** after placement of the fusion material. *(From Eismont FJ, Garfin SR, Abitol J: Thoracic and upper lumbar spine injuries. In Browner BD, Jupiter JB, Levine AM, et al. (eds): Skeletal Trauma, vol I. Philadelphia, WB Saunders, 1993, pp 729-803, with permission.)*

exposed, the T10 rib is dissected free and disarticulated at the costochondral junction. The cartilage is then divided and marked with sutures. The retroperitoneal fat can be seen under the divided cartilage. The diaphragm can be isolated after the pleural cavity is exposed by using blunt dissection. The diaphragm can then be mobilized sharply, leaving a 1 to 2 cm cuff on the chest wall. The crus can be divided; watch for oblique segmental vessels.

A dorsal midline incision can be used to expose the dorsal spine. If the simultaneous combined procedures are being performed for a fixed kyphotic deformity, it may be necessary to perform a chevron osteotomy. After a subperiosteal dissection of the dorsal elements, including the transverse processes, has been accomplished, a V-shaped resection of bone can be made in the dorsal elements (Figure 119.6). The osteotomy extends through the spinous process of the abnormal vertebral body and the caudal portion of the immediately caudal, adjacent level and continues to the transverse processes. Care must be taken to open the foramen completely to prevent trapping the segmental nerve roots. The remaining position of the rostral lamina should be undercut to avoid encroachment on the dura mater.

Farcy recommends that contoured rod be secured by hooks in a claw configuration around the lamina of the second and third rostral vertebral level. By not using a rostral-directed hook at the immediately rostral level, encroachment on the spinal canal at the pathologic level is avoided. Pedicle screws can then be fixed to the vertebral body immediately caudal to the pathologic level, and a second pair placed in the next adjacent level if needed. The rods can be attached to the pedicle screws without reduction of the local kyphotic deformity. This will allow stabi-

lization of the spine while the ventral corpectomy is completed.[39] The edge of the rostral vertebral body should be undercut to avoid compression of the underlying dura mater. Once the osteotomies are completed, the rods can be carefully moved into position and the dorsal osteotomy closed by tightening the connecting nuts. A lamina spreader can be used to distract the corpectomy defect and assist in the realignment of the spine. Once the dorsal construct is in final position and the spine realigned, a ventral strut graft as described above can be fitted into the corpectomy site and a dorsal lateral graft harvested from the iliac crests can be placed (see Figure 119.6C). Farcy originally placed hooks into the lamina in a claw configuration to protect the pedicle screws but now uses pedicle screws for a short segment dorsal construct.[40] The authors prefer to use rostral hooks in the thoracic level. Low-profile hooks with extended threads can be used instead of the pedicle screws if the pedicle anatomy will not allow safe cannulation. A claw can be configured at a single lamina, but biomechanical studies have documented increased strength of claws incorporating two levels.[102]

## Alternative Procedures

Alternative procedures are available that can treat both the ventral and dorsal aspects of the spine from the dorsal approach. Ito et al.[65] reported a ventrolateral decompression of the thoracic vertebral column in cases of Pott's disease. He performed a three-level costotransversectomy to allow ventrolateral decompression of the vertebral column. The authors lamented the fact that the fusion technique described by Albee[1] required a second procedure after a 3-week period of immobilization. Instead of plac-

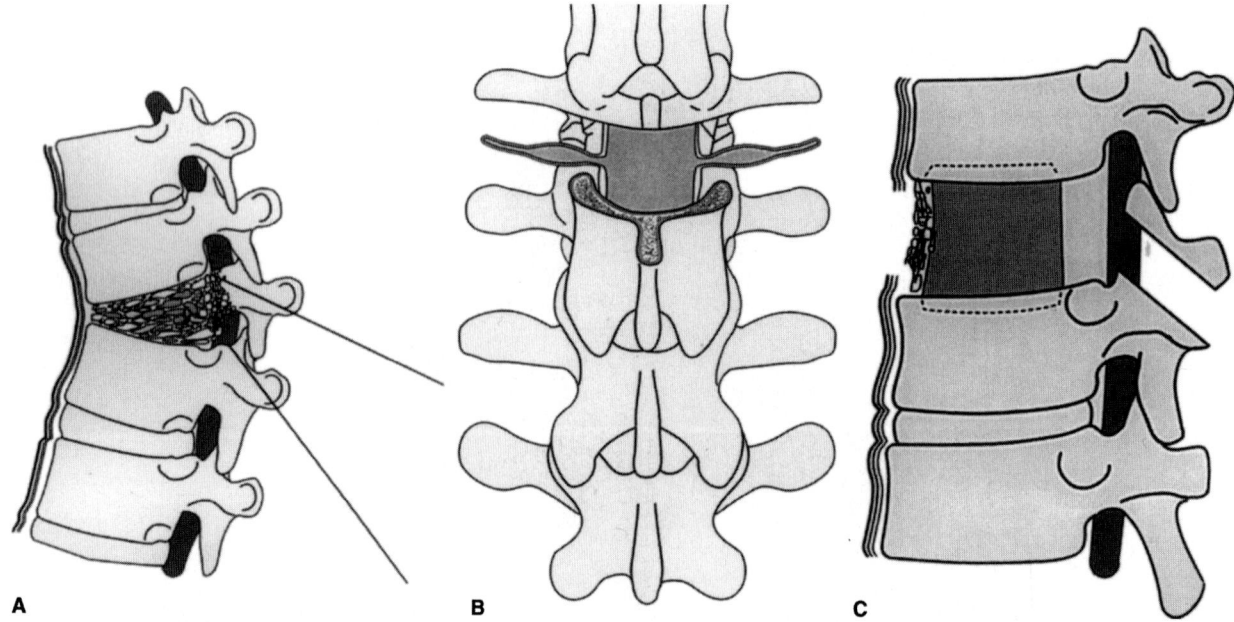

**A**    **B**    **C**

**Figure 119.6** Illustrations of a chevron osteotomy. (**A**) A sagittal view of the injured spine and the line demonstrate the angle of the osteotomy incision. (**B**) A dorsal view of the spinal column after the osteotomy. Note that the nerve roots are exposed and that the dura is tented posteriorly by the retropulsed fragments of the vertebral body. (**C**) A sagittal view of the spine after the osteotomy is closed and a fusion graft has been placed.

ing the tibial graft into the spinous process, the authors created a groove in the adjacent vertebral bodies. They then placed tibial graft or portions of the resected ribs as a strut graft into the grooves. Ito *et al.* reported clinical success with this technique. They reported that they had found a slender fibular strut graft satisfactory to reconstruct the corpectomy site in an experimental animal model.

Larson *et al.*[77] reported the use of a lateral extracavitary approach to the fractures of the thoracic and lumbar spine and credited Capener[16] with the initial description of the procedure. The latter author used a "lateral rhachotomy" to treat Pott's disease. This dorsal approach to the spine allows debridement of a vertebral body fracture, placement of an interbody fusion, and dorsal fixation and fusion to be accomplished through a single incision. The visualization of the ventral structures is obtained by resection of 8 cm of two adjacent ribs and the associated transverse processes, facet joints, and pedicles. In the thoracic region, the dissection is extrapleural, and segmental vessels are divided during the dissection. In the lumbar region, the dissection is between the erector spinae muscles and the quadratus lumborum; the retroperitoneal space is not entered. The authors reported that the ventral aspect of the spinal canal could be safely cleared of encroaching fragments from the dorsal portions of the vertebral body fracture.[77]

Schmidek *et al.*[105] performed a single pediculectomy to approach the fractured vertebral body for thoracolumbar fractures and referred to the technique as anterolateral decompression. The authors reported that with this approach the spinal canal retropulsed fragments during dorsal treatment that included fusion and instrumentation. An air drill with a diamond bit was used to undermine the retropulsed bone. When only a thin rim of the fragment remained, a curette was used to move the residual bone into the created defect.

## Dorsolateral Decompression

In the cases where delayed operative treatment of a fracture is required, dorsolateral decompression may be indicated if significant residual compression remains after reduction with dorsal instrumentation (Figure 119.7). This technique was described for thoracolumbar fractures treated with Harrington distraction rod constructs but has been used successfully with a universal spine system by the current authors.[33,36,46,80] Although this technique allows for a ventral decompression at the time of dorsal stabilization, there are disadvantages. These include the need to remove dorsal elements that may adversely affect long-term stability and the blind removal of the bone fragments causing the ventral compression (the dura mater and neural elements obstruct direct visualization).

Intraoperative ultrasonography can minimize the latter disadvantage. Eismont *et al.*[34] reported on the effectiveness of dorsolateral decompression assessed intraoperatively with ultrasonography. In a series of 23 patients with thoracic or lumbar fractures, 12 required dorsolateral decompression for continued compression of the neural elements. Of those 12 patients, 8 were evaluated by postoperative CT scan. The spinal canal size was demonstrated

to be adequately restored. The only treatment failure was a patient with a second area of compression that was not appreciated preoperatively. Garfin *et al.*[46] also evaluated the effectiveness of dorsolateral decompression in nine patients with residual compression with postoperative CT scan that revealed that only 1 patient had residual bone in the canal. No patient suffered neurologic deterioration because of the procedure. Hardaker *et al.*[56] used a bilateral approach via both pedicles at the injury level.

Dorsolateral decompression is performed at the time of dorsal instrumentation and stabilization. A preoperative CT scan is performed to determine the side of maximal neural compression that will be used for the approach for decompression. Instrumentation is placed on the opposite side. A laminotomy is performed at the site of the maximal neural compression that is usually the area between the pedicles of the fractured vertebral body. This window is used for intraoperative ultrasonography (see Figure 119.7A).

The laminotomy should be extended to expose the pedicle, which will then be "cored" with a curette or power burr, taking care not to penetrate the cortical margins (see Figure 119.7B). The medial margin of the pedicle is then removed with a curette, taking care to not injure the exiting nerve root (see Figure 119.7C). A 1 cm trough is then cut into the vertebral body ventral to the medial portion of the pedicle and the compressing fragment undermined. Reverse angle curettes and pituitary rongeurs can then be used to remove the retropulsed fragments decompressing the ventral spinal canal (see Figure 119.7D,E). This can be done under ultrasonic guidance.

This technique allows lesions just lateral to the midline to be removed, and if the ultrasound reveals lateral compression from residual fragments, the procedure can be repeated on the contralateral side. A fixation rod is place on the decompressed side and the initial instrumentation removed. The rostral disc can also be removed and bone graft impacted into the defect in the body and disc space with this technique. The instrumentation and the dorsolateral fusion are then completed.

A relatively new instrumentation system, GDLH (Sofamor-Danek, Memphis, TN), facilitates the reduction of nonfixed spinal deformities, specifically those associated with trauma (Figure 119.8A-C). The long treated hook posts (see Figure 119.8A,C) allow the hooks to attach to the rod before reduction of the spinal deformity. Figure 119.8A, showing the middle and lower spines, demonstrates the reduction of the deformity of the spine that can be facilitated by drawing the "hook claws" to the rod. The configuration of the hooks permit single-level "claws" to be formed, although as previously mentioned, claws spanning two or more levels have been demonstrated as more secure.[102]

## Clinical Cases

### Case 1

A 34-year-old Southeast Asian immigrant presented to her private practitioner with a week-long history of neck discomfort. When the patient developed paresis, she was admitted to the hospital. Her condition significantly deteriorated before an MRI examination revealed multilevel

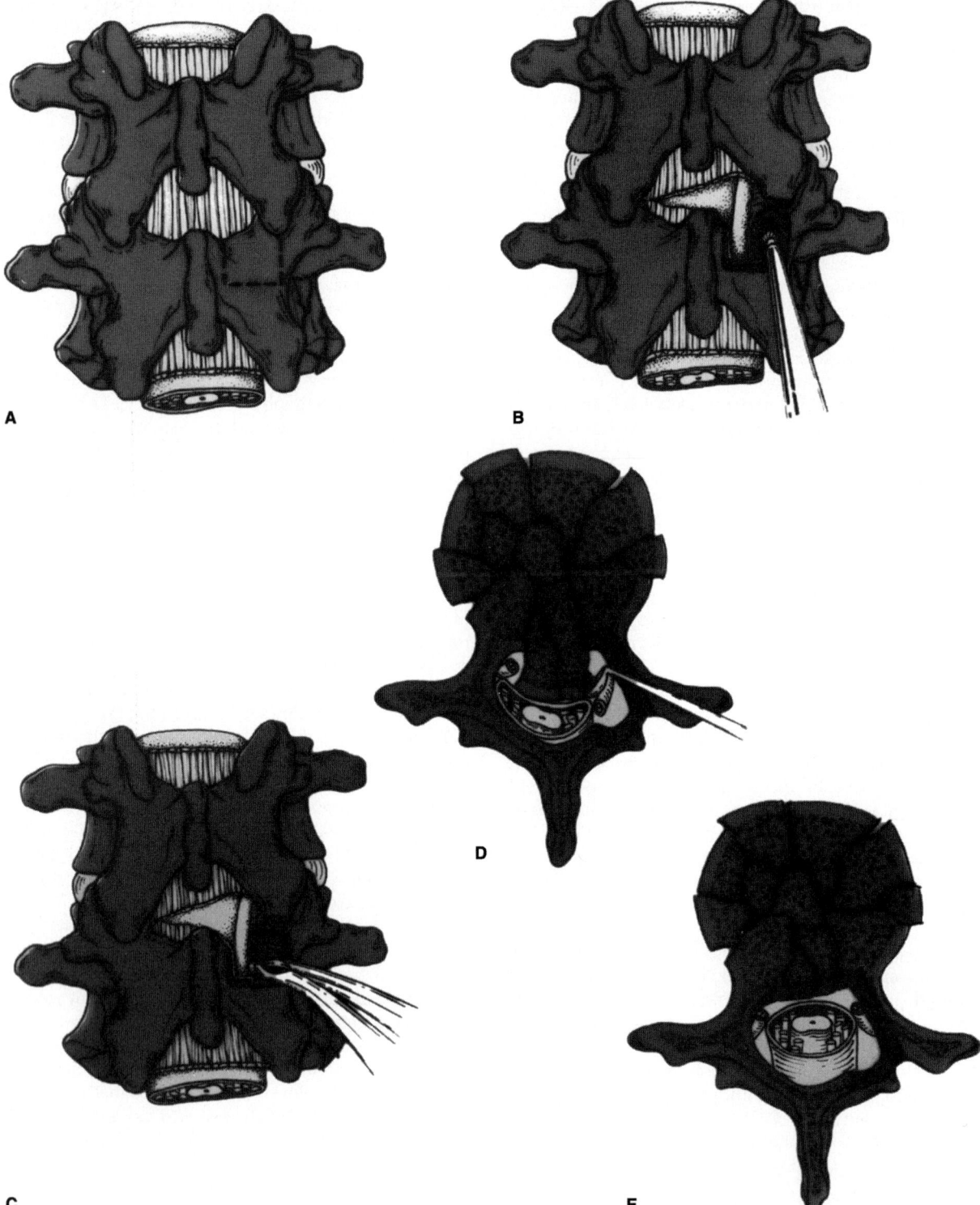

**Figure 119.7** A diagram of dorsalateral decompression of retropulsed vertebral body fragments.
**(A)** A laminotomy is performed to expose the lateral aspect of the spinal canal and the pedicle.
**(B)** A burr or curette is used to approach the vertebral body fragments via the pedicle. **(C)** After
the fragment has been undermined, the medial aspect of the pedicle can be removed and the
remaining rim of the displaced fragment can be driven from the spinal canal **(D)**. **(E)** The spinal
canal is free of bone fragment at the completion of the process. If the canal is not completely
cleared of bony encroachment, the transpedicular decompression can be repeated on the
contralateral pedicle. *(From Eismont et al., with permission.)*

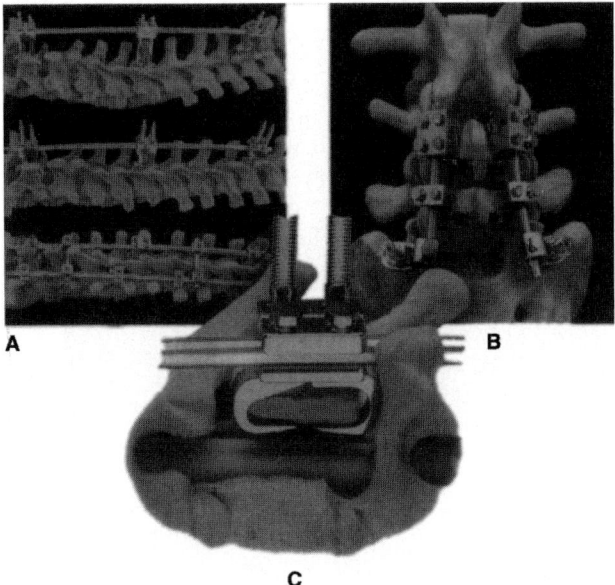

**Figure 119.8** The GDLH dorsal spinal system from Sofamor-Danek (Memphis, TN). **(A)** Reduction of a spinal column deformity in increments (upper to lower spines). **(B)** The hooks can be combined with pedicle screws for additional flexibility in fixation construct configuration. **(C)** A single level "claw" can be constructed because of the low profile and tapered hook shoes.

high signal abnormalities with distortion of the spinal cord (Figure 119.9). The patient was taken to surgery, where a right-sided thoracotomy was performed with a corpectomy; multiple discectomies and strut and morselized rib grafts were placed. Pathologic examination of intraoperative biopsy material revealed caseating granuloma, which ultimately grew tuberculous bacilli. The patient was placed on appropriate antibiotic therapy and returned for dorsal fixation with a universal hook/rod fixation system and dorsolateral fusion. Postoperatively, the patient was placed in a TLSO and transferred to the rehabilitation service. The patient recovered neurologically uneventfully.

## Case 2

A 28-year-old laborer from South America presented with a 3-day history of low back pain. A gibbus deformity was noted on physical examination. Neurologic examination revealed mild lower extremity weakness. Radiographs revealed an impressive deformity of the thoracolumbar spine (Figure 119.10A,B). MRI and CT scans revealed extensive vertebral body destruction and large collections of purulent material (see Figure 119.10C-E). Both T12 and L1 had collapsed. The patient was taken to surgery for a ventral exposure of the spine and drainage of paravertebral abscesses, debridement of the spinal column, and a two-level corpectomy (T12-L1). The vertebral bodies adjacent to the corpectomy site were involved in the infection, and it was not possible to correct the kyphotic deformity without destruction of these bodies. Reconstructive fusion was accomplished with an allograft tibial strut

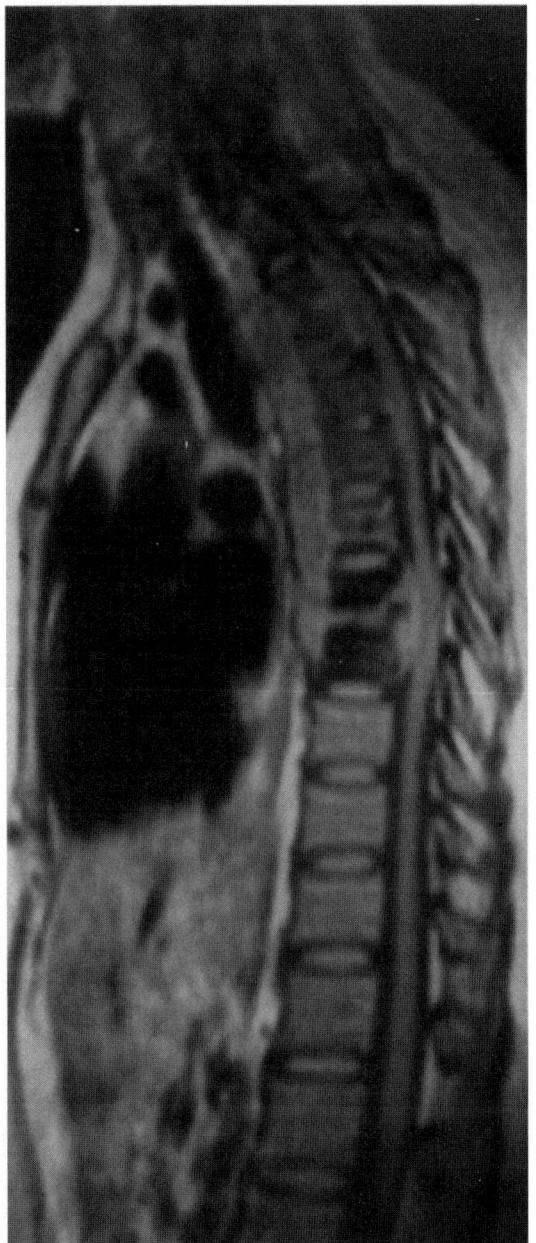

**Figure 119.9** A T1-weighted image after contrast enhancement of a case of Pott's disease. Note the high-intensity collections of material anterior to the vertebral column and the extensions dorsally at T3-4 and T8-9. The spinal cord is significantly distorted at the lower levels. The patient was treated with stage ventral and dorsal approaches. Both areas were débrided and grafts placed through a right-sided T6 lateral thoracotomy. The patient was returned to the operative suite 7 days later for dorsal fixation and fusion.

packed with the resected rib (see Figure 119.10F). It was not possible to stabilize the manual reduction of the spinal column because of the involvement of the adjacent vertebral bodies. The patient was returned to surgery for a dorsal osteotomy, fixation, and dorsolateral fusion with autologous iliac crest fusion. Hook fixation was used because of the involvement of the adjacent vertebral bodies. A three-level claw was used rostral to the

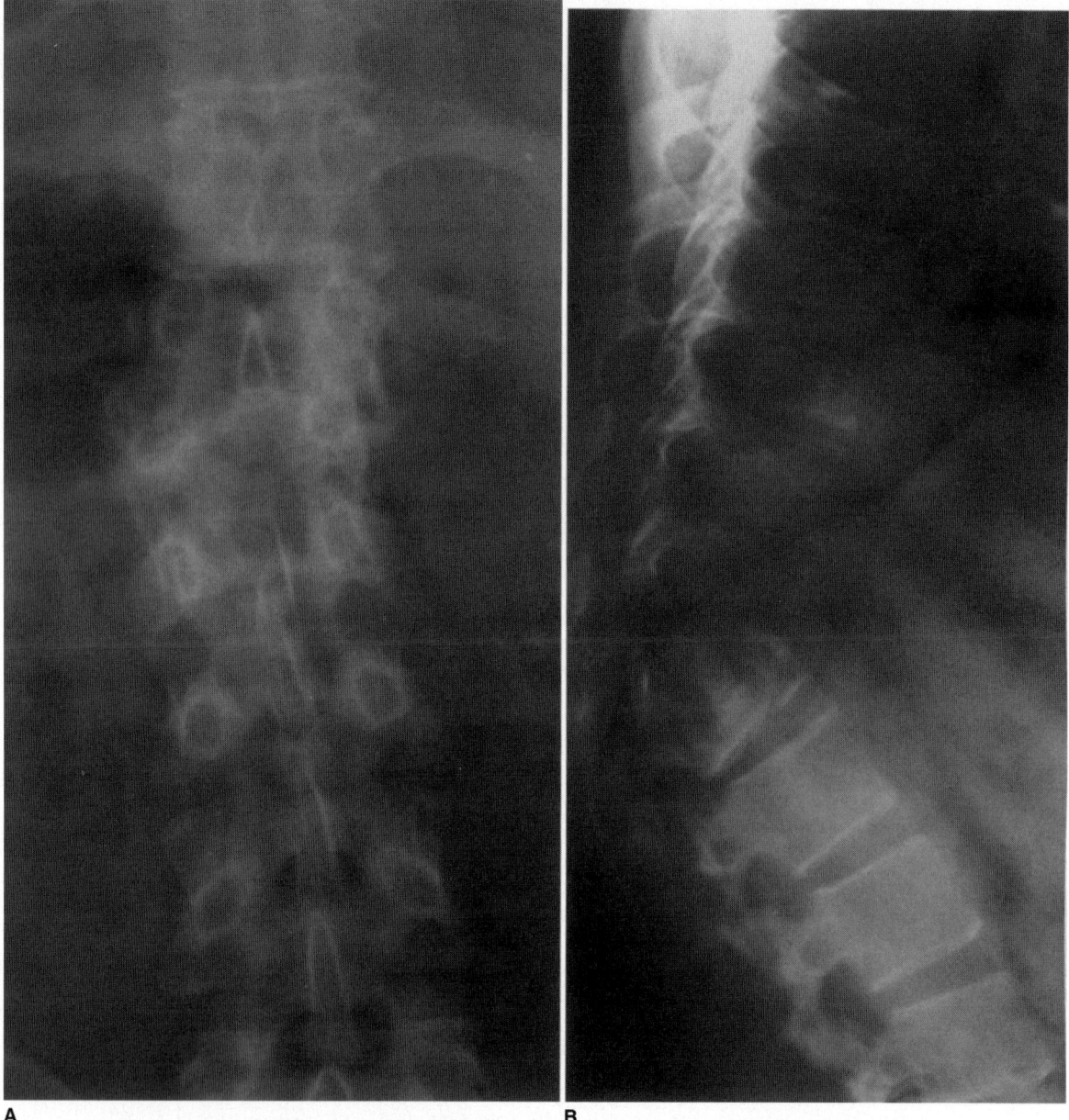

A                                    B

**Figure 119.10** The patient was a 28-year-old construction worker from South America who presented with 3 days of lower back pain but was able to ambulate without difficulty. Plain (**A**) AP and (**B**) lateral radiograph of the thoracolumbar spine revealed destruction of the vertebral bodies with kyphosis and scoliosis.

osteotomy and a two-level claw caudally (to preserve lumbar motion segment). The spine was aligned without difficulty, but the patient complained of left lower extremity pain and was noted to have dorsiflexor weakness in the same extremity. When the patient's pain complaints did not resolve in the immediate postoperative period, a myelogram was performed that revealed encroachment of the lamina on the lateral recess. The patient was returned to surgery for removal of the offending lamina. Good relief of pain and resolution of the neurologic deficit ensued. The patient was placed on long-term antibiotic therapy for Pott's disease.

## Case 3

A 14-year-old female was ejected from a vehicle after a high-speed rollover. On neurologic examination there was no sensation in the lower torso or extremities. There was no motor strength in the lower extremities except a trace of movement in the right great toe. Plain films and an MRI were obtained that demonstrated a Magerl type C3 fracture involving T7 and 8 (Figure 119.11). The patient was placed on a Roto-Rest bed and taken to surgery electively on the seventh postinjury day. Neurologic examination was unchanged except for some slight increase in distal lower extremity motor function. A right T5 thoracotomy and a

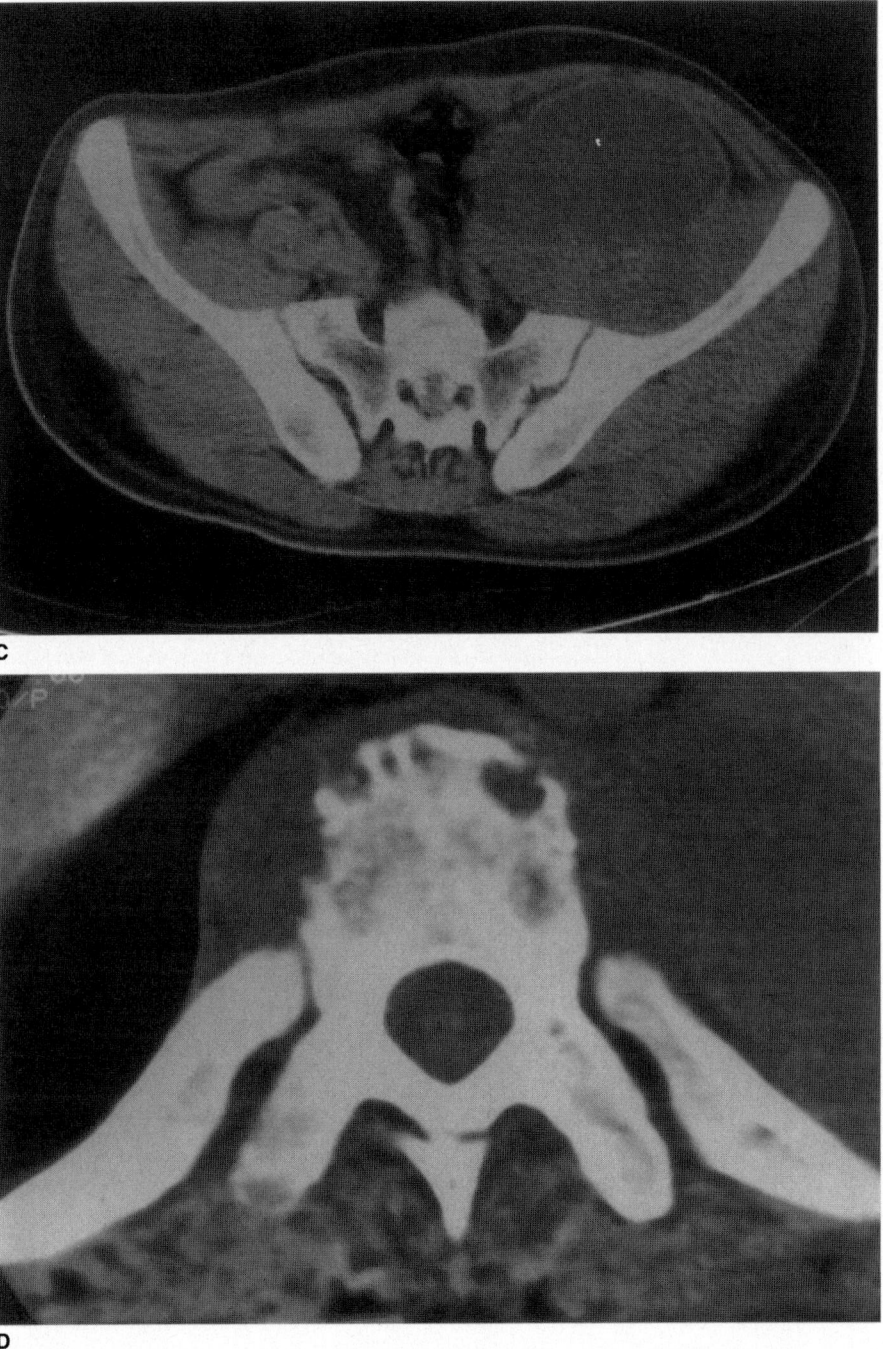

**Figure 119.10 *cont'd*** **(C)** A CT scan of the pelvis demonstrated large bilateral psoas fluid collections. **(D)** A CT scan of the spine revealed a paravertebral mass with destructive vertebral body lesions.

*Continued*

two-level corpectomy were performed. A segment of allograft tibia strut, packed with autologous rib and salvaged vertebral body, was placed. Reduction of the spinal fracture was not possible, and considerable rotation of the spine at the injury site continued after the corpectomy. The malalignment of the spine necessitated cutting grooves in the adjacent vertebral bodies to allow the graft to rotate without displacement. The patient was returned to the surgical suite after 7 days for dorsal debridement of the injury site, realignment, and fixation of the spine with a long titanium universal hook/rod fixation system and a dorsolateral autologous iliac crest graft fusion (see Figure 119.11*B*). The patient's neurologic status rapidly improved and she became able to ambulate within 2 weeks in a TLSO. At 3-year follow-up the fusion had matured and alignment of the spine was maintained. The patient regained bowel and bladder function and ambulates with a slightly spastic gait with tightened heel cords.

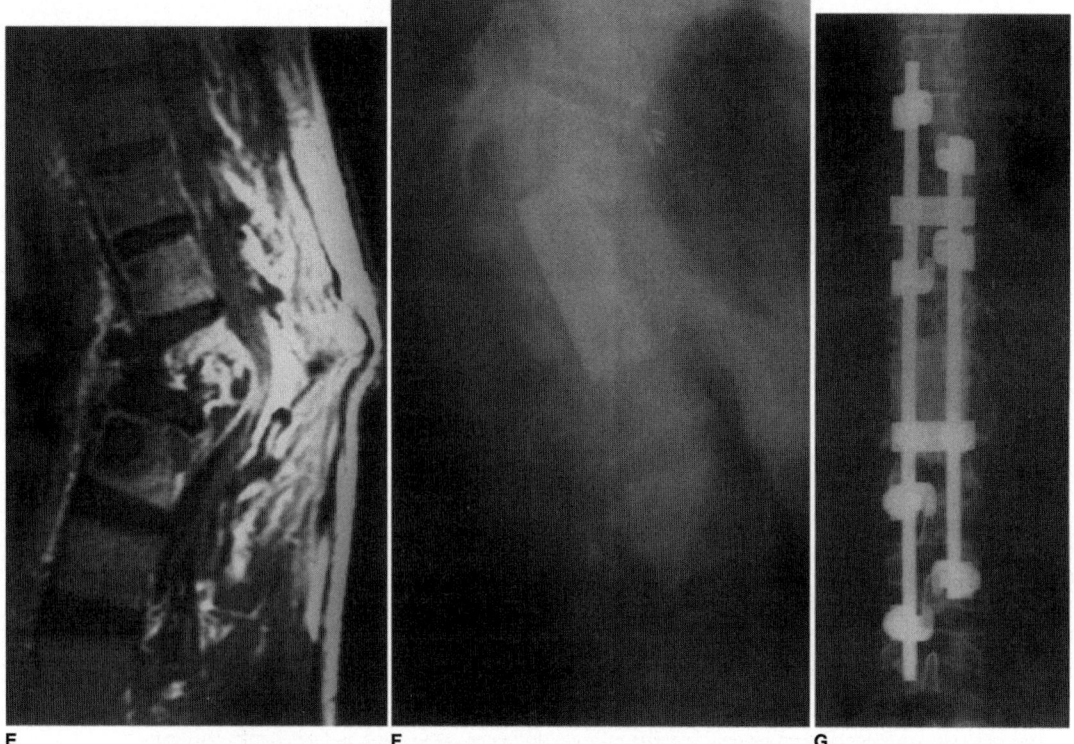

E        F        G

**Figure 119.10** ***cont'd*** **(E)** An MRI study helped to define the anatomy and documented the collapse of T12 and L1. Note the low-density lesion seen in the T11 body. There is considerable compromise of the spinal canal from retropulsed vertebral body fragments with distortion of the spinal cord. **(F)** A lateral plain radiograph of the spine and graft prior to the second procedure. **(G)** An AP plain x-ray of the instrumentation after the posterior approach and placement of fixation instrumentation.

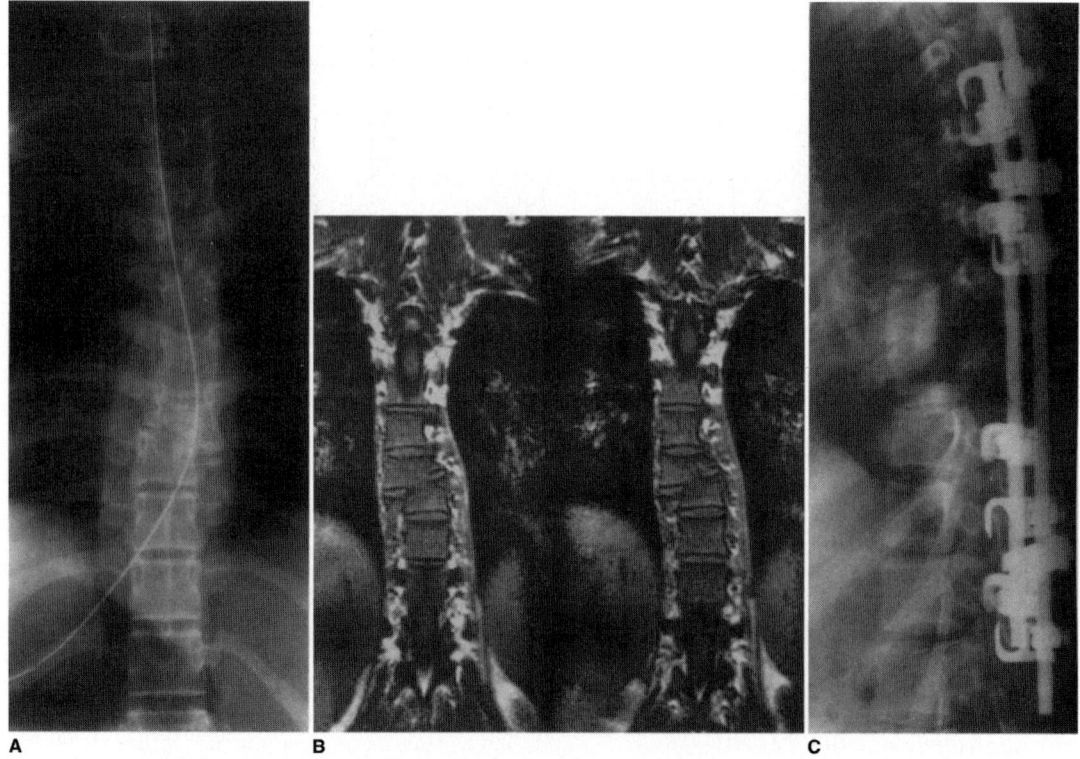

A        B        C

**Figure 119.11** A teenager who was ejected from a vehicle during a high-speed rollover sustained a Magerl C3 fracture. **(A)** An AP plain film revealed translation and rotation which was corrected after stage anterior thoracotomy and posterior stabilization. **(B)** Coronal MRI images of the fracture. **(C)** A lateral plain postoperative radiograph.

# REFERENCES

1. Albee FH: Transplantation of a portion of the tibia into the spine for Pott's disease: a preliminary report. *JAMA* 57:885, 1911.
2. Bedbrook G: Treatment of thoracolumbar dislocation and fractures with paraplegia. *Clin Orthop Rel Res* 112:27, 1975.
3. Bedbrook GM: Stability of spinal fractures and fracture dislocations. *Paraplegia* 9:23, 1971.
4. Bick EM: *Source Book of Orthopaedics*. Baltimore, Williams & Williams, 1948.
5. Bohler L: *The Treatment of Fractures*. Baltimore, W. Woods Company, 1935.
6. Bohlman HH: Treatment of fractures and dislocations of the thoracic and lumbar spine. *J Bone Joint Surg* 61A:165, 1985.
7. Bohlman HH, Freehafer A, Dejak J: The results of treatment of acute injuries of the upper thoracic spine with paralysis. *J Bone Joint Surg* 67A:360, 1985.
8. Braakman R, Fontijne WPJ, Zeegers R, *et al*: Neurological deficit in injuries of the thoracic and lumbar spine: a consecutive series of 70 patients. *Acta Neurochir* 111:11, 1991.
9. Breasted JH: *The Edwin Smith Papyrus*. Chicago, University of Chicago Press, 1930.
10. Brockbank W, Griffiths DL: Orthopaedic surgery in the sixteenth and seventeenth centuries: luxations of the spine. *J Bone Joint Surg* 30B:556, 1948.
11. Brown L, Birdwell KH, Holt RH, Jennings J: Aortic erosions and lacerations associated with the Dunn anterior spinal instrumentation. Presented at the 20th Annual Meeting of the Scoliosis Research Society, San Diego, 1985.
12. Burrington JD, Brown C, Wayne ER, Odom J: Anterior approach to the thoracolumbar spine: technical considerations. *Arch Surg* 111:456, 1976.
13. Calancie B, Klose KJ, Baier S, Green BA: Isoflurane-induced attenuation of motor evoked potentials caused by electrical motor cortex stimulation during surgery. *J Neurosurg* 74:897, 1991.
14. Calancie B, Madsen PW, Lebwohl N: Stimulus-evoked EMG monitoring during transpedicular lumbosacral spine instrumentation. *Spine* 19:2780, 1994.
15. Cantor JB, Lebwohl NH, Garvey T, Eismont FJ: Nonoperative management of stable thoracolumbar burst fractures with early ambulation and bracing. *Spine* 18:971, 1993.
16. Capener N: The evolution of lateral rhacotomy. *J Bone Joint Surg* 36B:173, 1954.
17. Chou SN, Seljeskog EL: Alternative surgical approaches to the thoracic spine. *Clin Neurosurg* 20:306, 1973.
18. Clohisy JC, Akbarnia BA, Bucholz RD, *et al*: Neurologic recovery associated with anterior decompression of spine fractures at the thoracolumbar junction (T12-L1). *Spine* 17:317, 1992.
19. Convery FR, Minteer MA, Smith RN: Fracture dislocation of the dorsal lumbar spine: acute operative stabilization by Harrington instrumentation. *Spine* 3:160, 1978.
20. Cooper A: *The Lectures of Sir Astley Cooper on the Principles and Practice of Surgery*, ed 5. Philadelphia, Haswell, Barrington, and Haswell, 1839.
21. Cushing H: Care of head injuries and injuries to the spine and peripheral nerves in the forward hospitals. In *The Medical Department of the United States Army in World War*, Vol. 11, Pt. 1 (Surgery). Washington, DC, U.S. Government Printing Office, 1927.
22. Dansia OA, Shaffrey CI, Jane J, *et al*: Surgical approaches for the correction of unstable burst fractures: a retrospective analysis of treatment outcomes. *J Neurosurg* 83:977, 1995.
23. Davies WE, Morris JH, Hill V: An analysis of conservative (non-surgical) management of thoracolumbar fractures and fracture-dislocations with neural damage. *J Bone Joint Surg* 62A:1324, 1980.
24. Denis F: The three column spine and its significance in the classification of acute thoracolumbar spinal injuries. *Spine* 8:817, 1983.
25. Denis F: Spinal instability as defined by the three-column spine concept in acute spinal trauma. *Clin Orthop* 189:65, 1984.
26. Denis F, Armstrong GWD, Searls K, *et al*: Acute thoracolumbar burst fractures in the absence of neurological deficit. *Clin Orthop* 189:142, 1984.
27. DeWald RL: Burst fractures of the thoracic and lumbar spine. *Clin Orthop Rel Res* 189:150, 1984.
28. Dickson JH, Harrington PR, Erwin WD: Results of reduction and stabilization of the severely fractured thoracic and lumbar spine. *J Bone Joint Surg* 60A:799, 1978.
29. Dunn HK: Anterior spine stabilization of thoracolumbar injuries. *Clin Orthop Rel Res* 189:116, 1984.
30. Durward QJ, Schweigel JF, Harrison P: Management of fractures of the thoracolumbar and lumbar spine. *Neurosurgery* 8:555, 1981.
31. Dwyer AF, Newton NC, Sherwood AA: An anterior approach to scoliosis. *Clin Orthop Rel Res* 62:192, 1969.
32. Ebelke DK, Asher MA, Neff JR, Krake DP: Survivorship analysis of VSP spine instrumentation in the treatment of thoracolumbar and lumbar burst fractures. *Spine* 16:428, 1991.
33. Eismont FJ, Garfin SR, Abitol J: Thoracic and upper lumbar spine injuries. In Browner BD, Jupiter JB, Levine AM, *et al* (eds): *Skeletal Trauma*, vol I. Philadelphia, WB Saunders, 1993, pp 729-803.
34. Eismont FJ, Green BA, Berkowitz BM, *et al*: The role of intraoperative ultrasonography in the treatment of thoracic and lumbar fractures. *Spine* 9:782, 1984.
35. Enslin TB: Combined anterior and posterior instrumentation and fusion in scoliosis [abstract]. *J Bone Joint Surg* 59B:255, 1977.
36. Erikson DL, Leider LL, Brown WE: One-stage decompression-stabilization for thoracolumbar fractures. *Spine* 2:53, 1977.
37. Esses SI, Botsford DJ, Kostuik JP: Evaluation of surgical treatment for burst fractures. *Spine* 15:667, 1990.
38. Farcy JP: Simultaneous anterior and posterior procedures for short segment spine pathology. Video tape 23112, American Academy of Orthopaedic Surgeons, 1993.
39. Farcy JP: Unstable fractures of the lumbar spine: discussion. *Spinal Frontiers* 3:4, 1996.
40. Farcy JP, Weidenbaum M, Glassman SD: Sagittal index in management of thoracolumbar burst fractures. *Spine* 15:958, 1990.

41. Ferguson RL, Allen BL: A mechanistic classification of thoracolumbar spine fractures. *Clin Orthop Rel Res* 189:77, 1984.

42. Ferguson RL, Allen BL: An algorithm for the treatment of unstable thoracolumbar fractures. *Orthop Clin* 17:105, 1986.

43. Floman Y, Michell LJ, Penny NJ, *et al*: Combined anterior and posterior fusion in seventy-three spinally deformed patients: indications, results and complications. *Clin Orthop Rel Res* 164:110, 1982.

44. Fountain SS: A single-stage combined surgical approach for vertebral resections. *J Bone Joint Surg* 61A:1011, 1979.

45. Frankel HL, Hancock DO, Huslop G, *et al*: The value of postural reduction in the initial management of closed injuries of the spine with paraplegia and tetraplegia. *Paraplegia* 7:179, 1969.

46. Garfin SR, Mowery CA, Guerra J, Marshall LF: Confirmation of the posterolateral technique to decompress and fuse thoracolumbar spine burst fractures. *Spine* 10:218, 1985.

47. Gaines RW, Humphreys WG: A plea for judgment in management of thoracolumbar fractures and fracture-dislocations: a reassessment of surgical indications. *Clin Orthop Rel Res* 189:36, 1984.

48. Gertzbein SD: Scoliosis Research Society: multicenter spine fracture study. *Spine* 17:528, 1992.

49. Gertzbein SD: Spine update: classification of thoracic and lumbar fractures. *Spine* 19:626, 1994.

50. Griffiths DL, Brockbank W: Orthopaedic surgery in the sixteenth and seventeenth centuries: traction apparatus: The Vidian pictures. *J Bone Joint Surg* 31B:313, 1949.

51. Gurr K, McAfee P, Shih C: Biomechanical analysis of posterior instrumentation systems after decompressive laminectomy: an unstable calf spine model. *J Bone Joint Surg* 70A:680, 1988.

52. Gurr K, McAfee P, Shih C: Biomechanical analysis of anterior and posterior instrumentation systems after corpectomy: a calf spine model. *J Bone Joint Surg* 70A:1182, 1988.

53. Guttmann L: Surgical aspects of the treatment of traumatic paraplegia. *J Bone Joint Surg* 31B:399, 1949.

54. Guttmann L: Spinal deformities in traumatic paraplegics and tetraplegics following surgical procedures. *Paraplegia* 7:38, 1969.

55. Guttmann L: *Spinal Cord Injuries: Comprehensive Management and Research*. Oxford, Blackwell Scientific Publications, 1973.

56. Hardaker WT, Cook WA, Friedman AH, *et al*: Bilateral transpedicular decompression and Harrington rod stabilization in the management of severe thoracolumbar burst fractures. *Spine* 17:162, 1992.

57. Harrington PR: Treatment of scoliosis. *J Bone Joint Surg* 44A:591, 1962.

58. Harrington PR, Dickson JH: An eleven-year clinical investigation of Harrington instrumentation: a preliminary report on 578 cases. *Clin Orthop Rel Res* 93:113, 1973.

59. Hodgson AR: Correction of fixed spinal curves. *J Bone Joint Surg* 47A:1221, 1965.

60. Hodgson AR, Stock FE: Anterior spinal fusion: a preliminary communication on radical treatment of Pott's disease and Pott's paraplegia. *Br J Surg* 44:266, 1956.

61. Holdsworth FW: Fractures, dislocations and fracture-dislocation of the spine. *J Bone Joint Surg* 45B:6, 1963.

62. Holdsworth FW: Fractures, dislocations and fracture-dislocation of the spine. *J Bone Joint Surg* 52A:1534, 1970.

63. Holdsworth FW, Hardy A: Early treatment of paraplegia from fractures of the thoracolumbar spine. *J Bone Joint Surg* 35B:540, 1953.

64. Hussein MK: An ancient Egyptian treatise on traumatology: 2000 B.C. *J Bone Joint Surg* 31B:309, 1949.

65. Ito H, Tsuchiya J, Asami G: A new radical operation for Pott's disease: report of ten cases. *J Bone Joint Surg* 16:499, 1933.

66. Jacobs RR, Asher MA, Snider RK: Thoracolumbar spinal injuries: a comparative study of recumbent and operative treatment in 100 patients. *Spine* 5:463, 1980.

67. Jacobs RR, Casey MP: Surgical management of thoracolumbar spinal injuries: general principles and controversial considerations. *Clin Orthop Rel Res* 189:22, 1984.

68. James KS, Wenger KH, Schiegel JD, *et al*: Biomechanical evaluation of the stability of thoracolumbar burst fractures. *Spine* 19:1731, 1994.

69. Jendrisak MD: Spontaneous abdominal aortic rupture from erosion by a lumbar spine fixation device: a case report. *Surgery* 99:631, 1986.

70. Kaneda K, Abumi K, Fujiya M: Burst fractures with neurologic deficits of the thoracolumbar-lumbar spine: results of anterior decompression and stabilization with anterior instrumentation. *Spine* 9:788, 1984.

71. Kaneda K, Asano S, Hashimoto T, *et al*: The treatment of osteoporotic posttraumatic vertebral collapse using the Kaneda device and a bioactive ceramic vertebral prosthesis. *Spine* 17:S295, 1992.

72. Keene JS, Wackwitz DL, Drummond DS, *et al*: Compression-distraction instrumentation of unstable thoracolumbar fractures: Anatomic results obtained with each type of injury and method of instrumentation. *Spine* 9:895, 1986.

73. Keynes G: Editor's introduction. In Keynes G (ed): *The Apologie and Treatise of Ambroise Paré Containing the Voyages Made into Divers Places with Many of his Writing upon Surgery*. London, Falcon Educational Books, 1951.

74. Kostuik JP, Errico TJ, Gleason TF: Techniques of internal fixation for degenerative conditions of the lumbar spine. *Clin Orthop Rel Res* 203:219, 1986.

75. Krengel WF, Anderson PA, Henley MB: Early stabilization and decompression for incomplete paraplegia due to a thoracic-level spinal cord injury. *Spine* 18:2080, 1993.

76. Kuhn WG: The care and rehabilitation of patients with injuries of the spinal cord and cauda equina: a preliminary report on 113 cases. *J Neurosurg* 4:40, 1947.

77. Larson SJ, Holst RA, Hemmy DC, Sances A: Lateral extracavitary approach to traumatic lesions of the thoracic and lumbar spine. *J Neurosurg* 45:628, 1976.

78. Lewis J, McKibbin B: The treatment of unstable fracture-dislocations of the thoraco-lumbar spine accompanied by paraplegia. *J Bone Joint Surg* 56B:603, 1974.

79. McAfee P, Yuan H, Fredrickson B, *et al*: The value of computed tomography in thoracolumbar fractures. *J Bone Joint Surg* 65A:471, 1983.

80. McAfee P, Yuan H, Lasada NA: The unstable burst fracture. *Spine* 2:365, 1982.

81. McBride GG: Cotrel-Dubousset rods in spinal fractures. *Paraplegia* 27:440, 1989.

82. McCormack T, Karaikovic E, Gaines RW: The load sharing classification of spine fractures. *Spine* 19:741, 1994.

83. McCormick PC: Retropleural approach to the thoracic and thoracolumbar spine. *Neurosurgery* 37:908, 1995.

84. McLain RF, Sparling E, Bensen DR: Early failure of short-segment pedicle instrumentation for thoracolumbar fractures. *J Bone Joint Surg* 75A:162, 1993.

85. Madsen PW, Lee TT, Eismont FJ, Green BA: Diagnosis and management of thoracic spine fractures. In Youmans JR (ed): *Neurological Surgery*. Philadelphia, WB Saunders, 1995, pp 2043-2078.

86. Magerl F, Harms J, Gertzbein SD, *et al*: A new classification of spinal fractures. *Orthop Trans* 15:728, 1991.

87. Maiman DJ, Larson SJ, EI-Ghatit AZ: Neurological improvement associated with late decompression of the thoracolumbar spine. *Neurosurgery* 14:302, 1984.

88. Maiman DJ, Pintar FA: Anatomy and clinical biomechanics of the thoracic spine. *Clin Neurosurg* 38:296, 1990.

89. M'Donnell R: Case of fracture of the spine: in which the operation for trephining was performed, with observation [reprint]. *Clin Orthop Rel Res* 189:3, 1984.

90. Mettler CC: *History of Medicine*. Philadelphia, Blakiston, 1947.

91. Morgan TH, Wharton GW, Austin GN: The results of laminectomy in patients with incomplete spinal cord injury. *Paraplegia* 9:14, 1971.

92. Nicoll EA: Fractures of the dorso-lumbar spine. *J Bone Joint Surg* 31B:376, 1949.

93. O'Brien JP, Dawson HMO, Heard CW, *et al*: Simultaneous combined anterior and posterior fusion. A surgical solution for failed spinal surgery with a brief review of the first 150 patients. *Clin Orthop Rel Res* 203:191, 1986.

94. O'Brien JP, Yau AC: Anterior and posterior correction and fusion for paralytic scoliosis. *Clin Orthop Rel Res* 86:151, 1972.

95. Osebold WR, Weinstein SL, Sprague BL: Thoracolumbar spine fractures: results of treatment. *Spine* 6:12, 1981.

96. Panjabi MM, Oxland TR, Kifune M, *et al*: Validity of the three-column theory of thoracolumbar fractures: A biomechanical investigation. *Spine* 15:1122, 1995.

97. Paul RL, Michael RH, Dunn JE, *et al*: Anterior transthoracic surgical decompression of acute spinal cord injuries. *J Neurosurg* 43:299, 1975.

98. Purcell GA, Markolf KL, Dawson EG: Twelfth thoracic-first lumbar vertebral mechanical stability of fractures after Harrington-rod instrumentation. *J Bone Joint Surg* 63A:71, 1981.

99. Rajasekaran S, Soundarapandian S: Progression of kyphosis in tuberculosis of the spine treated by anterior arthrodesis. *J Bone Joint Surg* 71A:1314, 1989.

100. Riebel GD, Yoo JU, Fredrickson BE, *et al*: Review of Harrington rod treatment of spinal trauma. *Spine* 18:479, 1993.

101. Riseborough LJ: The anterior approach to the spine for the correction of deformities of the axial skeleton. *Clin Orthop Rel Res* 93:207, 1973.

102. Roach JW, Ashman RB, Allard RN: The strength of a posterior element claw at one versus two spinal levels. *J Spinal Disord* 3:259, 1990.

103. Roy-Camille R, Saillant G, Berteaux D, Salgado V: Osteosynthesis of thoraco-lumbar spine fractures with metal plates screwed through the vertebral pedicles. *Reconstr Surg Traumat* 15:2, 1976.

104. Sasso RC, Cotler HB, Rueben JD: Posterior fixation of thoracic and lumbar spine fractures using DC plates and pedicle screws. *Spine* 16:S134, 1991.

105. Schmidek HH, Gomes FB, Seligson D, McSherry JW: Management of acute unstable thoracolumbar (T-11-L-1) fractures with and without neurological deficit. *Neurosurgery* 7:30, 1980.

106. Schnee CL, Ansell LV: Selection criteria and outcome of operative approaches for thoracolumbar burst fractures with and without neurological deficit. *J Neurosurg* 86:48, 1997.

107. Spencer DL, DeWald RL: Simultaneous anterior and posterior surgical approach to the thoracic and lumbar spine. *Spine* 4:29, 1979.

108. Steffee AD, Biscup RS, Sitowski DJ: Segmental spine plates with pedicle screw fixation: a new internal fixation device for disorders of the lumbar and thoracic spine. *Clin Orthop Rel Res* 203:45, 1986.

109. Watson-Jones R: *Fracture and Joint Injuries*, ed 3. Baltimore, Williams & Wilkins, 1943.

110. White AA, Panjabi M: *Clinical Biomechanics of the Spine*, ed 2. Philadelphia, Lippincott-Raven, 1990.

111. Whitesides TE: Traumatic kyphosis of the thoracolumbar spine. *Clin Orthop Rel Res* 124:78, 1977.

# CHAPTER 120

# Complex Lumbosacropelvic Fixation Techniques

**Nevan G. Baldwin, Matthew B. Kern, and David W. Cahill**

Diseases of the sacrum and lumbosacral junction (LSJ) lead to clinically complex problems for surgical treatment and biomechanical stabilization. Trauma, infection, degenerative disease, and scoliosis (congenital or acquired) are among the common entities affecting the sacrum and LSJ. Although they are not common, neoplasms of this area often are especially challenging for post-resection reconstruction. The sacrum and dorsal pelvis are also important points of fixation in the treatment of similar disorders at higher spinal regions in which long instrumentation constructs are required.

## Anatomic and Biomechanical Considerations

The LSJ is a unique spinal level in several respects.[21] In the sagittal or flexion-extension axis, it has the largest range of motion of any thoracic or lumbar level, averaging 17 degrees of total movement. In the axial plane and during rotation and lateral (coronal plane) bending, the LSJ has the most limited range of motion of any spinal level, averaging 1 degree of rotation and 3 degrees of bending.[48] Because of the normal lordotic curvature of the lumbar spine, the slope of the lumbosacral intervertebral disc (L5-S1) is usually the steepest of any disc, with respect to the true horizontal. The summation of spinal load vectors results in exposure of the lumbosacral disc to the largest loads encountered throughout the spine. The large loads carried and the angular position of the disc at the LSJ produce unique load-bearing characteristics, including the highest level of translational shear force in the entire spine (Figure 120.1).[14,17,21]

## The Sacrum

The sacrum is formed from five fused vertebrae in which the specially adapted and large transverse processes merge into thick lateral masses, the alae. The sacral spinal canal has four pairs of dorsal and ventral foramina. The subdural and subarachnoid spaces terminate as the thecal sac tapers at the caudal margin of S2. The filum terminale internum is an extension of the pia arachnoid of the conus medullaris, extending from the tip of the conus to the end of the subdural space. At the termination of the subdural space, the thecal sac tapers to invest the filum terminale internum and form the filum terminale externum. The filum terminale externum extends to the end of the sacral canal and attaches to the rostral portion of the coccyx.

## Structures Adjacent to the Sacrum

For the safe placement and attachment of instrumentation constructs in the lumbosacropelvic region, a thorough knowledge of the anatomic relationships of the neural, vascular, and visceral structures in the region is important. The common iliac arteries begin at the aortic bifurcation (L4 level) and pass along the lateral surface of the L5 vertebral body. They then bifurcate at the level of the LSJ, giving rise to the internal and external iliac arteries. The iliac arteries lie ventral and lateral to the iliac veins and therefore do not actually make contact with the spine. The internal and external iliac arteries pass ventral to the sacral alae. The internal iliac arteries pass close to the bony surface of the ala, whereas the external iliacs are separated from the bony surface by the psoas muscles.

The lumbosacral trunk is formed by the ventral branches of the L4 and L5 nerve roots. It is joined by the sacral nerves located on the ventral surface of the alae between the iliac veins and the sacroiliac joint (SIJ). The sigmoid colon is also found in approximation to the ventral surface of the sacrum. It loses its mesentery and becomes far less mobile as it reaches the ventral aspect of the S3 vertebral body.

## Sacroiliac Joint

The SIJ is formed by the interdigitating surfaces of the sacral alae and the iliac bones. It is predominantly a fibrocartilaginous amphiarthrodial (no synovial capsule) joint. There is a small diarthrodial (synovial capsule present) portion located at the ventral aspect of the SIJ. The interdigitation and matching contours of the iliac and sacral alar surfaces create an interlocking mechanism to help stabilize the joint. The wedge-like shape of the sacrum helps to stabilize the SIJ and serves to transfer loads from the spine to the pelvis (Figure 120.2).

The SIJ is essentially an immobile joint that functions as a shock absorber for the spine. In studies on fresh cadavers, there was minimal motion in pediatric specimens, with none in adults.[47] Another cadaveric study has demonstrated that in adults over 50 years of age, autofusion of the joint is observed in 75% of specimens.[9]

The major biomechanical function of the pelvis is that of transferring loads from the SIJ to the hip joints. The stable transfer of these loads is dependent on the ligaments connecting the lumbar vertebrae and the sacrum to the pelvis. The ligamentous structures spanning the SIJ include the interosseous, dorsal, and ventral sacroiliac ligaments (Figure 120.3). The interosseous, sacroiliac, and dorsal sacroiliac complex provides the major stabilization for the SIJ.

The iliolumbar ligament passes from the transverse process of the L5 vertebra to the iliac crests. A less substantial part of the ligament may span to the transverse process of L4 as well. The position of this ligament allows a wide range of motion in flexion and extension across the

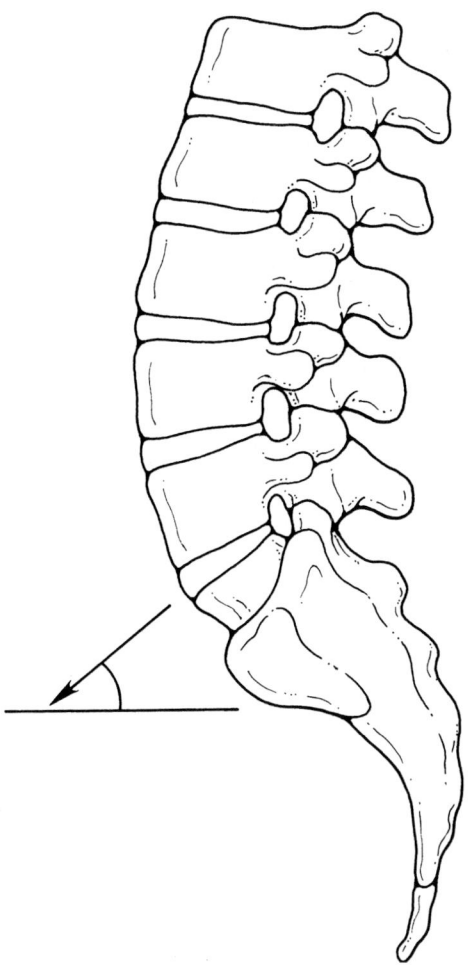

**Figure 120.1** The L5-S1 disc space is the most vertically oriented of any disc space in the spine (arrow depicts approximate angle formed by the disc space). This predisposes the L5-S1 level to unique load-bearing characteristics.

LSJ, but it severely restricts lateral bending and axial rotation.

The force vector of axial load from the spine is located ventral to the SIJ. This causes a ventral rotational tendency of the sacrum at the level of the SIJ. The center point of this rotational vector is located near the center of the S2 vertebral body (Figure 120.4). The sacrospinous and sacrotuberous ligaments pass from the lower sacrum to the ischial bones. The position of these ligaments creates a long moment arm through which they are able to resist sacral rotation and are thereby able to maintain the lordotic lumbosacral posture despite the gravitational sagittal plane vector.

### Muscular Interactions

The musculature of the lumbosacropelvic region acts on the spine in a complex multidirectional fashion. The muscles and the weight of the upper body act in many instances via long moment arms and may place substantial forces on the spine. An example of such action is the force exerted on the spine by the rectus abdominis musculature. These muscles act by a moment arm extending from the

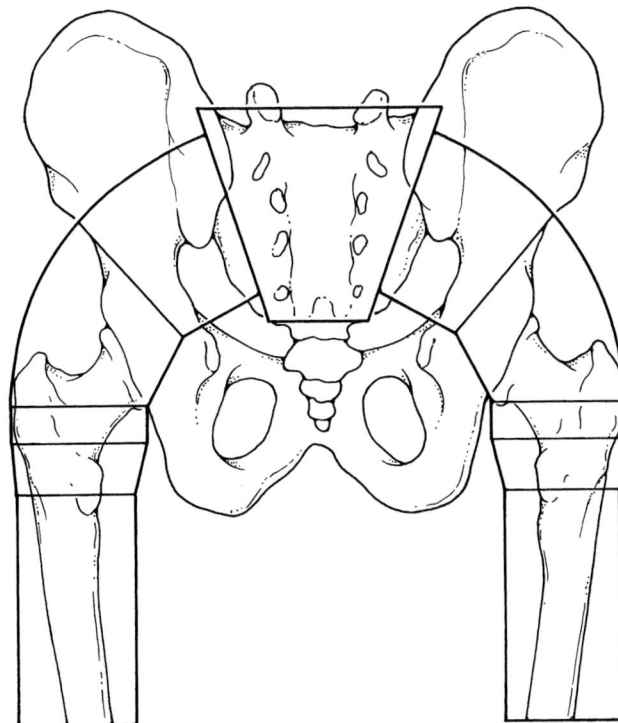

**Figure 120.2** The keystone configuration of the pelvis allows the transfer of weight from the spine to the pelvis and ultimately to the lower extremities.

pubic symphysis to the sternum, producing a spinal vector toward kyphosis. A pendulous abdomen does the same in providing a constant exaggerated spinal load in the upright position and to some extent during sitting.

In the resection of sacral tumors, stability of the sacropelvic region can be jeopardized because portions of the sacrum and possibly the SIJ are removed. Resection of the caudal portion of the sacrum up to the S1-2 interspace and removal of up to one third of the SIJ can be performed with only a 30% loss of weight-bearing capacity. The lower half of the S1 body and up to one half of the SIJ can be resected with a 50% loss of weight-bearing stability.[49] Preservation of 50% of weight-bearing capacity is adequate for early ambulation in the postoperative period, and further stabilization is not likely to be necessary.

### Indications for Lumbosacropelvic Fixation

In short-segment cases and in the absence of osteopenia, sacral fixation with a single pair of bone screws is adequate. In longer segment cases (such as scoliosis, postsacrectomy reconstruction, and multisegmental lumbosacral fusion) or with osteoporotic bone, more substantial segmental fixation is required to achieve rigidity. Rigidity is a crucial element in these constructs because fusion rates are directly related to use of rigid instrumentation, and better outcomes clearly correlate with the acquisition of a solid fusion.* If a long instrumentation construct is placed, the sacral attachment is usually subjected to large cantilevered forces that may lead to screw pull-out (Figure 120.5).

---

*References 7,22,24,25,30,31,37,51.

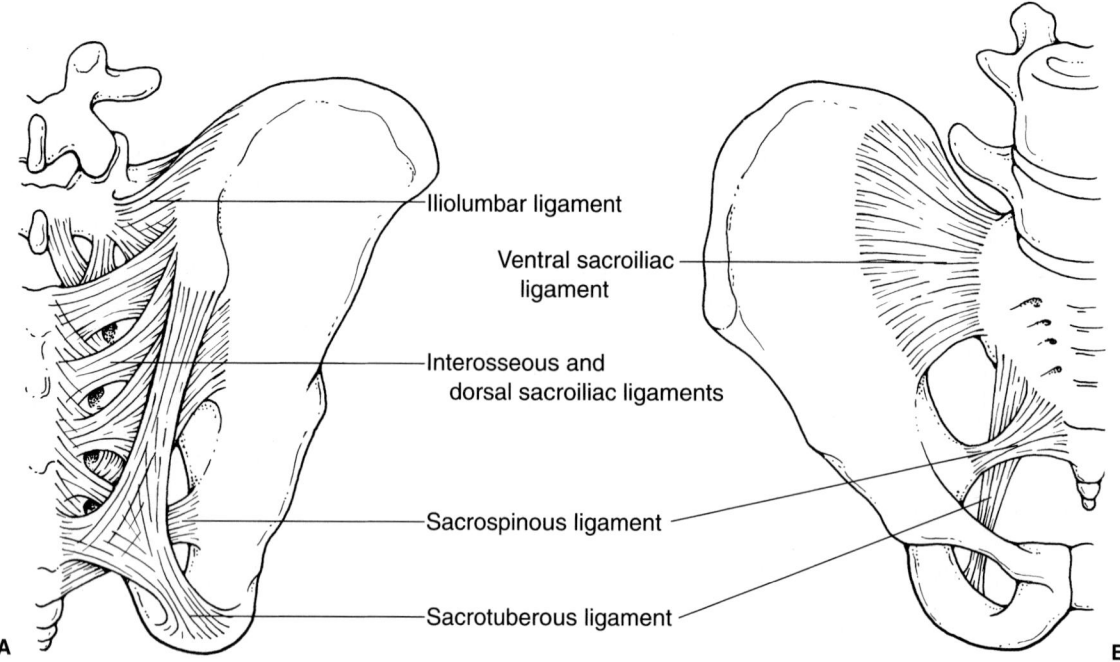

**Figure 120.3** (**A** and **B**) Dorsal and ventral views of the major ligamentous attachments of the sacroiliac joint.

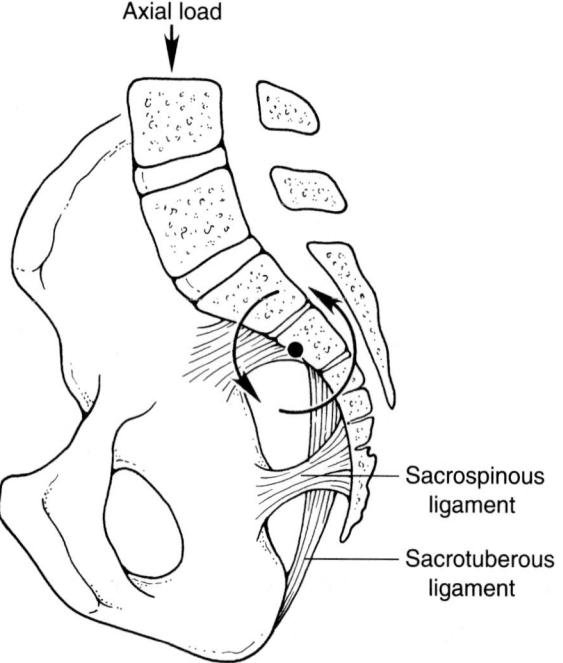

**Figure 120.4** The center point of the rotational vector is located near the center of the S2 vertebral body. The diagram depicts the rotational tendency of the sacrum about this point. It is through the long lever arms created by the sacrospinous and sacrotuberous ligaments that this rotational tendency is counteracted and the sacrum is stabilized.

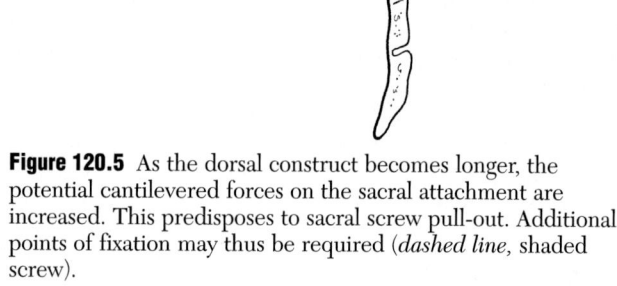

**Figure 120.5** As the dorsal construct becomes longer, the potential cantilevered forces on the sacral attachment are increased. This predisposes to sacral screw pull-out. Additional points of fixation may thus be required (*dashed line,* shaded screw).

Additional points of sacral or sacropelvic fixation may prevent complications in such cases.

Instrumentation may be used in compression or distraction to reduce deformity. This (particularly distraction) may place a substantial stress on the implants, in addition to the physiologic loads that will be exerted by the daily activities and movements of the patient. This stress constitutes implant preload. Instrumentation that will bear a significant preload may require either further sacral fixation points or attachments that cross the SIJ. If the preload is not symmetrically distributed, as in the case of scoliosis correction, the additional instrumentation does not necessarily need to be placed bilaterally but should be included on the side that will bear the larger load. If significant pelvic obliquity is present, as occurs commonly with scoliosis of neuromuscular origin, the construct should cross the SIJ in most instances and should be symmetric.

The SIJ is autofused in many adults over 50 years of age. Long-term follow-up study of patients with instrumentation constructs crossing the SIJ has demonstrated no adverse effects relating to the presence of the implants.[26] Therefore, if it is necessary for additional security of fixation in the lumbosacropelvic region, placement of instrumentation across the SIJ is a rational approach for providing spinal stability.

## Lumbosacral Pivot Point

In a study of the biomechanics of sacropelvic fixation, McCord *et al.* described the concept of the lumbosacral pivot point.[33] This is the axis of rotation at the lumbosacral junction. During flexion, the portions of L5 and the sacrum that are ventral to this pivot move toward one another. Likewise, the portions of L5 and the sacrum located dorsal to this pivot point will move apart during flexion (Figure 120.6). Anatomically, the lumbosacral pivot point is marked by the intersection of the middle osteoligamentous column and the lumbosacral (L5-S1) disc. In constructs that cross the SIJ, only those devices that pass ventral to this point provide a significant biomechanical advantage regarding rigidity of fixation.

## Complex Techniques of Sacral Fixation

Many lumbosacral fusions can be adequately immobilized with placement of bone screws into the sacral pedicles. These screws, however, obtain their thread purchase in the broad cancellous channel of the sacral pedicle. Therefore bone screws in the sacral pedicles are subject to failure because of the relative porosity of the sacrum, the manner in which stress tends to be concentrated at the termini of a fusion construct, and the large flexion moments to which these constructs are subjected.[16,39] Sacral screws may fail by pull-out or by fracture.[16] In cases in which it is believed that the use of a single pair of bone screws may not be adequate for stabilization, the use of more complex techniques is warranted.

With regard to injuring structures ventral to the sacrum, cadaveric studies have shown that the widest margin of safety is found at the medial safe zone (Figure 120.7).[35] Therefore, at the S1 or promontory level, placing the screws in a medial or toed-in direction is preferred. Some authors have advocated bicortical purchase of sacral screws to enhance pull-out resistance, which affords some pull-out strength advantage, although this involves additional risk.° Zindrick *et al.* found that bicortical purchase with a 6.5mm diameter screw resulted in an increase in pull-out strength of about 30%.[52] Penetrating an excessive

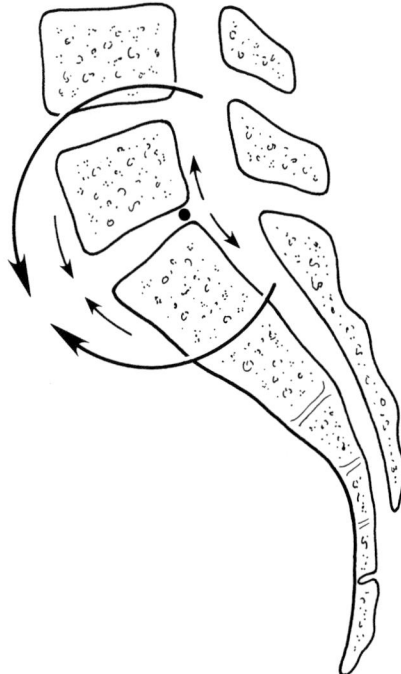

**Figure 120.6** As the lumbosacral joint is flexed, those points located ventral to the pivot point (dot) will move toward each other, whereas those dorsal to it will separate.

distance beyond the ventral cortex carries the risks of neurologic deficit, chronic pain from lumbosacral trunk injury, sympathetic chain injury, peritonitis, sepsis, and hemorrhage,[29,35] although these risks are minimal if the screw penetrates 1cm or less.

### Fixation with Sublaminar Devices

The addition of sublaminar devices such as hooks, wires, or cables at the sacrum is a simple means of enhancing fixation. It should be borne in mind that the sacral laminae are often quite thin and may not provide substantial strength to hold such devices. All of these devices, including hooks, are tension-band fixators. Dorsally placed tension-band constructs provide limitation of flexion but do not provide substantial torsional stability or resistance to extension. With fusions at the LSJ, it has been shown that fixation with sublaminar devices alone does not improve the fusion rate when this rate is compared with that of noninstrumented fusions.[38] Therefore sublaminar devices should be used at the LSJ only in conjunction with other devices.

Although the bony thickness at the sacral lamina is meager, at the nearby dorsal foramina the bone stock is usually quite substantial. The dorsal foramina are therefore excellent sites to place hooks for the purpose of enhancing construct strength. When added to a sacral pedicle screw construct, this technique has been shown to significantly increase rigidity.[45]

### Fixation with Screws

A number of simple techniques use bone screws to enhance sacral fixation. Screws provide rigid three-dimensional

---

°References 11,20,27,29,35,52.

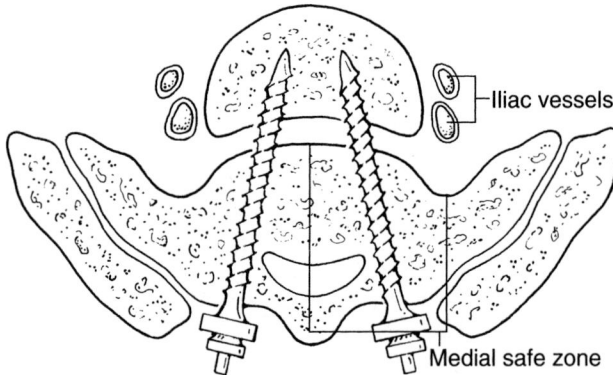

**Figure 120.7** Depiction of the safe medial zone at the portion of the sacrum that lies lateral to the neural canal and medial to the iliac vessels. Sacral pedicle screws therefore need to be "toed in" to avoid these vascular structures.

stabilization and can be used for short-segment fixation at the LSJ. Shorter constructs provide a major advantage because immobilization of long segments of the spine increases the load not only at the immediately adjacent segment but also at more distal segments.[36]

Directing screws medially or laterally and then rigidly attaching them to the rod or plate greatly enhances pull-out resistance. Studies are in conflict regarding which of these two methods is better, but both offer a substantial biomechanical advantage over a straight sagittal-plane trajectory.[12,52] Oblique trajectories dramatically increase the cross-sectional area of bone that resists screw dislodgement via the cantilevered forces applied by the spine in flexion. If the longitudinal members are then linked with cross-members, a triangulation effect is created. This enhances both the rigidity of the construct and its pull-out resistance.[13,41,52] Torsional stability is particularly enhanced by cross-fixation of the rods.[4,13,40]

Perhaps the easiest method for enhancing sacral fixation with screws is the placement of an additional pair of laterally directed bone screws into the sacral alae below the S1 level. This method provides a biomechanical advantage over a single pair of pedicle screws.[31,33] These screws are easily added to a construct without the need for pre-planning or special devices, and fluoroscopy is not required. For this method, a type of screw whose attachment site to the rod is somewhat narrow is optimal. Screws with a broad attachment site may be difficult to place sufficiently close together for the optimal trajectory of the screws to be attained (Figure 120.8).

The placement of screws into the S2 and even the S3 levels has been advocated to enhance the security of sacral fixation. Biomechanical testing has demonstrated that these screw placement sites do not add sufficiently to the security of fixation to warrant their use.[33,52] The thickness of the sacrum in the sagittal plane diminishes at the lower sacral levels. Therefore, inadvertent penetration of the ventral surface of the sacrum with such screws is more likely, and injury to the anatomic structures immediately adjacent to the ventral cortical surface may occur.

Recently, the pedicular transvertebral screw fixation technique has been described for treatment of lumbosacral spondylolisthesis.[1] This technique involves place-

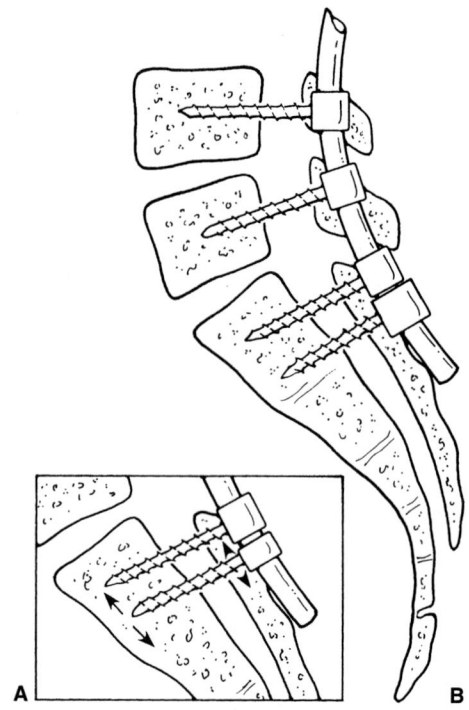

**Figure 120.8** If the site of attachment of the second screw is narrow, sufficient latitude is present to allow proper trajectory (**A**). If the attachment is too broad, it impedes proper placement of the screw (**B**).

ment of a long screw through the pedicle of S1, passing through the rostral end plate of S1 and into the caudal end plate of the L5 vertebral body. When combined with screws in the L4 pedicles, this provides a unique biomechanical construct. It appears to be a simple method for stabilizing high-grade spondylolisthesis. The simplicity of this technique is attractive, and the clinical results appear to be encouraging (Figure 120.9).

Along with placement of screws spanning from vertebra to sacrum, fibular bone struts can be applied in a similar manner. Placement of fibular grafts to act as dowels can be performed from a dorsal or ventral approach.[23,32,43,44,50] The procedure has been reported in use with autografts, allografts, and even with vascularized autografts.[19,32,34,43] Transvertebral fibular dowels should always be augmented with screw fixation.

Along with screw placement, sacral fixation can be supplemented by insertion of the rods directly into the lateral sacral bony masses. Jackson has described a method whereby screws are directed through the S1 pedicle, and cortical purchase is obtained in the vertebral end plate of S1 as well. The rods are then passed into the lateral sacrum toward the SIJ and affixed rigidly to the screws.

## Devices for Sacral Fixation with Multiple Screws

A number of devices especially designed for sacral and sacropelvic fixation have been marketed. The two basic types are those that cross the SIJ and those that affix directly to the sacrum only. The sacral fixation devices are generally plate-like structures that are secured to the sacrum with screws. One early example of these was

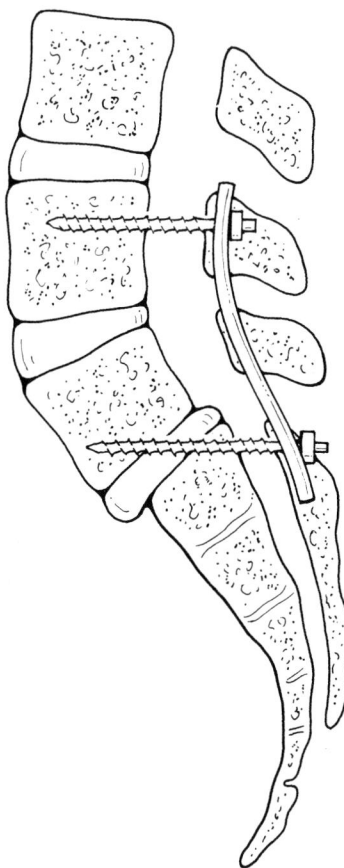

**Figure 120.9** With the pedicular transvertebral screw fixation technique, the sacral screw passes through the pedicle of S1 and into the inferior portion of the end plate of the L5 vertebral body. The upper end of the construct consists of L4 pedicle screws.

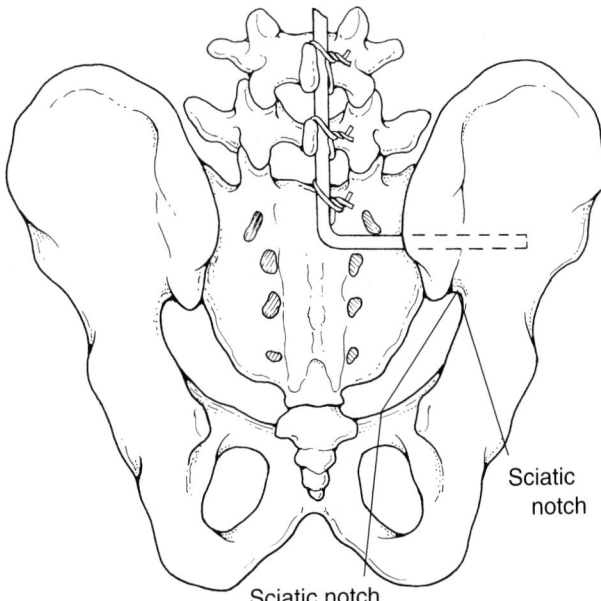

**Figure 120.10** The Galveston technique for sacropelvic attachment uses angled rods that are placed into the iliac bones along the transverse bar of the ilium. The rods are passed into the cortical bone above the sciatic notch.

described by Asher and Strippgen.[5] It is called the Isola plate because of its butterfly shape (and is named after a species of Rocky Mountain butterfly). This design contained holes for the passage of multiple sacral screws. Placement of the screws was dictated by the position of the holes, and spacing of the holes was based on anthropometric sacral measurements taken in male and female cadavers.

The Tacoma plate (Sofamor-Danek, Memphis, TN) is designed to direct the additional screws to the sacral ala rather than to the pedicles. It is available in a two-screw and a three-screw model. Such devices are easily attached without special training beyond that required for pedicle screw placement.

### Fixation Across the SIJ

The most commonly used method for sacropelvic attachment is the Galveston technique or a variation of it. The procedure was originally described by Allen and Ferguson for the treatment of scoliosis.[2,3] It is accomplished by inserting angled rods into the iliac bones and passing them into the hard cortical bone above the sciatic notch (Figure 120.10). This technique is useful for providing extremely rigid fixation in difficult cases, such as reconstruction after tumor resection or patients with lumbosacral agenesis.[18]

In conditions of large preload, such as the correction of pelvic obliquity in neuromuscular diseases, loss of correction can occur because of the slippage of one rod relative to the other. Several manufacturers have developed cross-fixation devices that attach to both rods and prevent such slippage and markedly enhance the rigidity of the constructs. Although the attachment mechanism, ease of use, and biomechanics of these devices differ substantially, they all enhance construct rigidity and lessen the risk of failure in multi-level constructs.

Placing Galveston rods into the ilium can be cumbersome and technically difficult. Therefore, specialized screws for iliac insertion have been developed (Isola iliac screws; AcroMed, Raynham, Mass). Iliac screws are placed by using fluoroscopy, and the rods are then either directly attached or joined to the screw by a connector fitting. These devices markedly enhance the rigidity of lumbosacral instrumentation constructs. The increases in rigidity are similar for both the iliac screws and the Galveston rods.[33] Multiple studies have confirmed that iliac fixation provides the most effective means to supplement sacral screws.[15,28]

### Bicortical Iliac Screw Fixation

A simple method of sacropelvic fixation is the placement of long, variable-angle bone screws obliquely through the iliac bones (Figure 120.11). When combined with additional sites of fixation at the sacrum, this technique creates a tripod effect for load sharing. This method has not been studied for its biomechanical characteristics, but early clinical results appear satisfactory.[8]

Bicortical iliac fixation is a simple technique to perform and does not require preplanning or specialized devices. It is important to pay strict attention to the screw trajectory

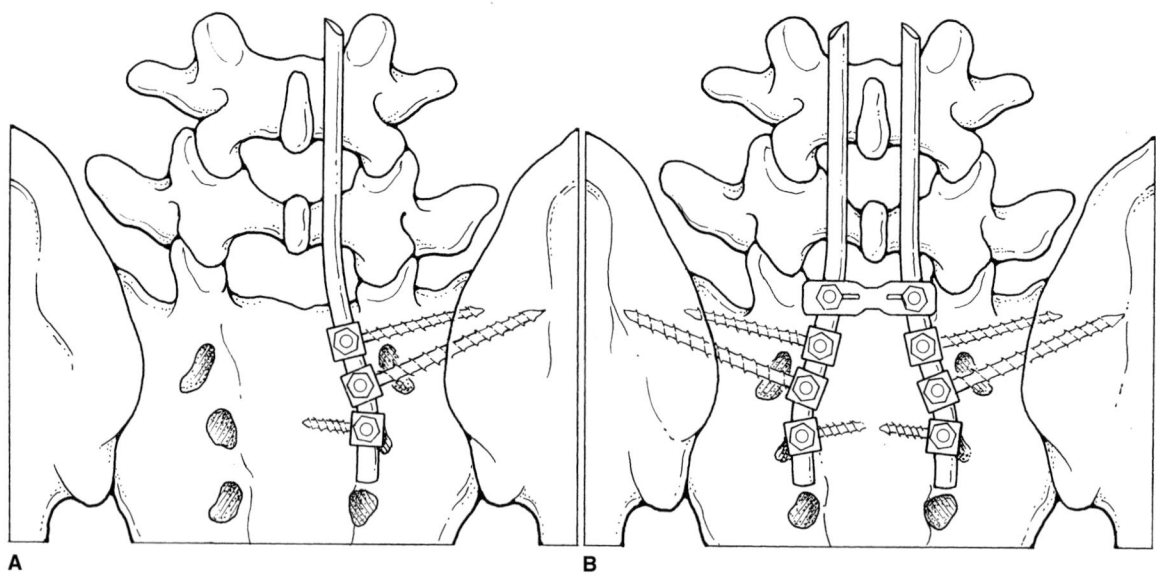

**Figure 120.11** The tripod geometry of variable angle screws that are passed obliquely through the iliac bones as well as the sacrum provides an increased load-sharing capability of the implant (**A**). Adding a rigid cross-member increases the rigidity and stability of the construct (**B**).

and to ascertain that the screw tip will pass ventral to the lumbosacral pivot point. Also, a small section of the dorsal sacroiliac ligamentous complex must be removed to allow the screw to be placed in a low-profile configuration.

## Complications of Complex Lumbopelvic Fixation

The majority of complications associated with complex instrumentation constructs are similar to those of any other spinal fixation procedures. Infection remains a common adverse sequela of these operations, occurring in 3% to 5% of cases, even in experienced hands.[10] Problems such as blood loss, neurologic deficits, and poor bone quality should be managed with the same measures as would be used in any other implant case.

Accurate placement of sacropelvic instrumentation is crucial for optimal results. If difficulty is encountered in visualizing the necessary anatomy with fluoroscopy, further dissection should be undertaken to directly visualize the structures to be instrumented. Dissection along the lateral aspect of the ilium allows easy access for palpation of the sciatic notch, and placement of a Galveston rod above the notch is thereby simplified. Similarly, the sacral ala can be exposed for placement of alar screws. Screw sites should always be probed carefully before tapping or screw insertion. This aids in identifying inadvertent ventral cortical penetration or, if such penetration is desirable, in determining optimal screw length. Screw length can also be confirmed by measuring the appropriate region on a computed tomography scan, although the obliquity of the placement may make this difficult.

### Revision Surgery

One of the major complications of lumbosacropelvic instrumentation is loosening or failure of hardware. In some cases,

however, such loosening or failure may not prevent solid bony fusion. Therefore it is a matter of judgment about when these constructs should be revised. Patients with loosened hardware should be followed closely with serial radiographic studies. Reparation is recommended if evidence of either progressive unacceptable deformity or symptomatic pseudoarthrosis is observed. Because late healing may occur, it is advisable to delay revision surgery until it is certain that an acceptable result will not occur without revision.

Revision surgery of instrumentation constructs should address the reason for the failure. If there is a fractured implant, more fixation points should be included to improve load sharing. If screw pull-out is observed, the use of larger diameter or longer screws provides greater thread purchase. If the pull-out appears to be largely due to poor bone quality, pressurized injection of polymethylmethacrylate may improve screw pull-out resistance.[52]

In general, surgery for failed spinal instrumentation involves the implantation of more hardware. For failed sacral fixation, creation of a construct that spans the SIJ is advisable. Further bone grafting should always be performed by using autologous bone, if possible. Harvest of iliac crest bone may not be possible because many of these patients will have had a previous harvest at the iliac sites. One limited alternative is the use of rib grafts. If iliac harvest is performed in patients with iliac fixation sites, the harvest sites should be placed as far ventrally as possible.

In cases of Galveston rod failure, additional fixation points can usually be secured. These rods tend to loosen by pull-out because they do not have purchase into the deep portion of the iliac bones. Further fixation should be attempted by placement of screws into the sacral pedicles or alae and attachment to the rod. Also, rigid cross-members should be added if these are not already present in the construct.

An alternative surgical approach may also be required for revision surgery. An interbody fusion is sometimes a reasonable alternative to augment a dorsolateral fusion. Ventral fusion at the lumbosacral junction may be accomplished by using interbody grafts after ventral discectomy or vertebrectomy for tumor, infection, or grade III or IV spondylolisthesis. Allograft bone is the usual substrate for grafting in cases of interbody fusion, but newer interbody cage devices that allow the use of autograft will soon be available. Because no rigid ventral stabilization device can be easily applied to the sacrum, either ventrally or laterally, such interbody grafts or cages should be supplemented with dorsal hardware, unless the decompression consisted of only simple lumbosacral discectomy in the absence of pathology in the posterior elements.

Screws may be placed through the sacral promontory retrograde into the S1 pedicles, but the bulk of the attached hardware usually produces risks of iliac vessel injury that outweigh any potential benefits. Because of this anatomic stumbling block, interbody cages should be viewed as supplemental devices rather than as primary stabilization hardware in any case of complex lumbosacral reconstruction. Many different types of interbody devices have been developed for placement via either open or endoscopic techniques (BAK cage, Ray cage, Brantigan device, Novus device, Harms cage). Some of these have received clearance by the Food and Drug Administration and others are seeking clearance.

At the lumbosacral junction it is far easier to place interbody grafts or devices via a true ventral (transperitoneal or extraperitoneal) approach or via a dorsal lumbar interbody approach than by a lateral (retroperitoneal) approach. The crossing iliac veins ventral to L5, the bony iliac wing that blocks the view, and the bulky psoas muscle at this level make the lateral approach to the lumbosacral junction uncomfortable at best. The ventral approach usually sacrifices the sympathetic plexus over the sacral promontory, sometimes producing ejaculatory dysfunction in males, and it may occasionally require sacrifice of one or both internal iliac vessels. The dorsal interbody approach usually involves the sacrifice of some or all of both facet complexes at L5-S1 and has a relatively high risk of nerve root injury. Regardless of which approach is chosen for interbody fusion at the lumbosacral junction, a good working knowledge of the pertinent anatomy and potential complications is critical.

Postoperatively, patients who have undergone revision surgery should be placed in thoracolumbosacral orthoses. The addition of a hip extension device to these orthoses has traditionally been recommended. However, it has been shown that spinal motion is not reduced by the addition of this cumbersome and uncomfortable attachment.[6]

In the management of sacral tumors, involvement of the S1 segment is often the only impediment to what might otherwise be a potential surgical cure. Particularly in chordomas, the most common of sacral tumors, complete surgical resection with margins is usually considered curative because the tumor is usually indolent, metastasizing beyond its site of origin only very late in its course. Many such tumors are detected only when they are quite large, although they are still localized. The ability to perform a total sacrectomy for cure is impaired by the difficulty of re-establishing spinopelvic stability in the absence of the sacrum.

In a few cases such stability has been accomplished by attaching ventral allograft bone struts to transpelvic plates at the lower end and to the remaining lumbar vertebrae above.[42] Pelvic rim stabilization with transverse plates and stabilization with oblique allograft struts from the dorsal iliac wings to the telescoped lumbar vertebrae have also been attempted with some success.[46] Graft positioning oblique to the primary ventral rotational force vector in the upright posture is the main clinical and theoretical impediment to the success of these techniques.

Research continues regarding new techniques of lumbopelvic reconstruction after total sacrectomy. In cadavers, whole allograft sacral transplants may be plated between the iliac wings ventrally to re-establish anterior column support and pelvic ring integrity. The transplants are supplemented with iliolumbar rods (Galveston technique) dorsally and generous volumes of autograft bone. Much work remains, however, before this technique can be considered for clinical use. A number of manufacturers are also offering advanced plating and connector devices for enhancement of fixation in these very difficult cases.

## Summary

Lumbosacropelvic fixation methods are technically challenging and carry significant risk. Such techniques can, however, be used to manage a variety of complex spinal disorders. As with all surgery, strict attention to detail is the key to avoiding complications.

## REFERENCES

1. Abdu WA, Wilber RG, Emery SE: Pedicular transvertebral screw fixation of the lumbosacral spine in spondylolisthesis. A new technique for stabilization. *Spine* 19:710-715, 1994.
2. Allen BL Jr, Ferguson RL: The Galveston technique for L rod instrumentation of the scoliotic spine. *Spine* 7:276-284, 1982.
3. Allen BL Jr, Ferguson RL: The Galveston technique of pelvic fixation with L-rod instrumentation of the spine. *Spine* 9:388-394, 1984.
4. Asher M, Carson W, Heining C, et al: A modular spinal rod linkage system to provide rotational stability. *Spine* 13: 272-277, 1988.
5. Asher MA, Strippgen WE: Anthropometric studies of the human sacrum relating to dorsal transsacral implant designs. *Clin Orthop* 203:58-62, 1986.
6. Axelsson P, Johnsson R, Stromqvist B: Lumbar orthosis with unilateral hip immobilization. Effect on intervertebral mobility determined by roentgen stereophotogrammetric analysis. *Spine* 18:876-879, 1993.
7. Balderston RA, Winter RB, Moe JH, et al: Fusion to the sacrum for nonparalytic scoliosis in the adult. *Spine* 11: 824-829, 1986.
8. Baldwin NG, Benzel EC: Sacral fixation using iliac instrumentation and a variable angle screw device. *J Neurosurg* 81:313-316, 1994.
9. Brooke R: The sacroiliac joint. *J Anat* 58:297-301, 1924.
10. Cahill DW: Infections of the spine. *Contemp Neurosurg* 15:1-8, 1993.

11. Camp JF, Caudle R, Ashmun RD, et al: Immediate complications of Cotrel-Dubousset instrumentation to the sacro-pelvis. A clinical and biomechanical study. *Spine* 15:932-941, 1990.

12. Carlson GD, Abitbol JJ, Anderson DR, et al: Screw fixation in the human sacrum. An in vitro study of the biomechanics of fixation. *Spine* 17:S196-S203, 1992.

13. Carson WL, Duffield RC, Arendt M, et al: Internal forces and moments in transpedicular spine instrumentation. The effect of pedicle screw angle and transfixation: The 4R-4bar linkage concept. *Spine* 15:893-901, 1990.

14. Colombini D, Occhipinti E, Grieco A, et al: Estimation of lumbar disc areas by means of anthropometric parameters. *Spine* 14:51-55, 1989.

15. Cunningham BW, Lewis SJ, Long J, et al: Biomechanical evaluation of lumbosacral reconstruction techniques for spondylolisthesis: an in vitro porcine model. *Spine* 27:2321-2327, 2002.

16. Devlin VJ, Boachie-Adjei O, Bradford DS, et al: Treatment of adult spinal deformity with fusion to the sacrum using CD instrumentation. *J Spinal Disord* 4:1-14, 1991.

17. Dietrich M, Kurowski P: The importance of mechanical factors in the etiology of spondylolysis. A model analysis of loads and stresses in human lumbar spine. *Spine* 10:532-542, 1985.

18. Dumont CE, Damsin JP, Forin V, et al: Lumbosacral agenesis. Three cases of reconstruction using Cotrel-Dubousset or L-rod instrumentation. *Spine* 18:1229-1235, 1993.

19. Esses SI, Natout N, Kip P: Posterior interbody arthrodesis with a fibular strut graft in spondylolisthesis. *J Bone Joint Surg (Am)* 77:172-176, 1995.

20. Esses SI, Botsford DJ, Huler RJ, et al: Surgical anatomy of the sacrum. A guide for rational screw fixation. *Spine* 16:S283-S288, 1991.

21. Farfan HF, Kirkaldy-Willis WH: The present status of spinal fusion in the treatment of lumbar intervertebral joint disorders. *Clin Orthop* 158:198-214, 1981.

22. Hanley EN Jr, Levy JA: Surgical treatment of isthmic lumbosacral spondylolisthesis. Analysis of variables influencing results. *Spine* 14:48-50, 1989.

23. Heller JG, Ghanayem AJ, McAfee P, Bohlman HH: Iatrogenic lumbar spondylolisthesis: treatment by anterior fibular and iliac arthrodesis. *J Spinal Disord* 13:309-318, 2000.

24. Kim SS, Denis F, Lonstein JE, et al: Factors affecting fusion rate in adult spondylolisthesis. *Spine* 15:979-984, 1990.

25. Kornblatt MD, Casey MP, Jacobs RR: Internal fixation in lumbosacral spine fusion. A biomechanical and clinical study. *Clin Orthop* 203:141-150, 1986.

26. Kostuik JP, Errico TJ, Gleason TF: Luque instrumentation in degenerative conditions of the lumbar spine. *Spine* 15:318-321, 1990.

27. Krag MH, Van Hal ME, Beynnon BD: Placement of transpedicular vertebral screws close to anterior vertebral cortex. Description of methods. *Spine* 14:879-883, 1989.

28. Lebwohl NH, Cunningham BW, Dmitriev A, et al: Biomechanical comparison of lumbosacral fixation techniques in a calf spine model. *Spine* 27:2312-2320, 2002.

29. Licht NJ, Rowe DE, Ross LM: Pitfalls of pedicle screw fixation in the sacrum. A cadaver model. *Spine* 17:892-896, 1992.

30. Lorenz M, Zindrick M, Schwaegler P, et al: A comparison of single-level fusions with and without hardware. *Spine* 16:S455-S458, 1991.

31. Louis R: Fusion of the lumbar and sacral spine by internal fixation with screw plates. *Clin Orthop* 203:18-33, 1986.

32. Majd ME, Holt RT: Anterior fibular strut grafting for the treatment of pseudoarthrosis in spondylolisthesis. *Am J Orthop* 29:99-105, 2000.

33. McCord DH, Cunningham BW, Shono Y, et al: Biomechanical analysis of lumbosacral fixation. *Spine* 17:S235-S243, 1992.

34. Meyers AM, Noonan KJ, Mih AD, Idler R: Salvage reconstruction with vascularized fibular strut graft fusion using posterior approach in the treatment of severe spondylolisthesis. *Spine* 26:1820-1824, 2001.

35. Mirkovic S, Abitbol JJ, Steinman J, et al: Anatomic consideration for sacral screw placement. *Spine* 16:S289-S294, 1991.

36. Nagata H, Schendel MJ, Transfeldt EE, et al: The effects of immobilization of long segments of the spine on the adjacent and distal facet force and lumbosacral motion. *Spine* 18:2471-2479, 1993.

37. Nagel DA, Kramers PC, Rahn BA, et al: A paradigm of delayed union and nonunion in the lumbosacral joint. A study of motion and bone grafting of the lumbosacral spine in sheep. *Spine* 16:553-559, 1991.

38. Ogilive JW, Bradford DS: Sublaminar fixation in lumbosacral fusions. *Clin Orthop* 269:157-161, 1991.

39. Pashman RS, Hu SS, Schendel MJ, et al: Sacral screw loads in lumbosacral fixation for spinal deformity. *Spine* 18:2465-2470, 1993.

40. Pintar FA, Maiman DJ, Yoganandan N, et al: Rotational stability of a spinal pedicle screw/rod system. *J Spinal Disord* 8:49-55, 1995.

41. Ruland CM, McAfee PC, Warden KE, et al: Triangulation of pedicular instrumentation. A biomechanical analysis. *Spine* 16:S270-S276, 1991.

42. Shikata J, Yamamuro T, Kotoura Y, et al: Total sacrectomy and reconstruction for primary tumors. Report of two cases. *J Bone Joint Surg* 70A:122-125, 1988.

43. Smith JA, Deviren V, Berven S, et al: Clinical outcome of trans-sacral interbody fusion after partial reduction for high-grade l5-s1 spondylolisthesis. *Spine* 26:2227-2234, 2001.

44. Smith MD, Bohlman HH: Spondylolisthesis treated by a single-stage operation combining decompression with in situ posterolateral and anterior fusion. An analysis of eleven patients who had long-term follow-up. *J Bone Joint Surg (Am)* 72:415-421, 1990.

45. Stovall DO Jr, Goodrich JA, Lundy D, et al: Sacral fixation technique in lumbosacral fusion. *Spine* 22:32-37, 1997.

46. Tomita K, Tsuchiya H: Total sacrectomy and reconstruction for huge sacral tumors. *Spine* 15:1223-1227, 1990.

47. White AA, Panjabi MM: Clinical instability of the spine. In Evarts CM, Burton RI, Cofield RH, et al. (eds): *Surgery of the Musculoskeletal System*. New York, Churchill Livingstone, 1990, pp 2151-2173.

48. White AAI, Panjabi MM: *Clinical Biomechanics of the Spine*. Philadelphia, Lippincott-Raven, 1990.

49. White AAI, Panjabi MM: The problem of clinical instability in the human spine: A systematic approach. In White AA, Panjabi MM (eds): *Clinical Biomechanics of the Spine*. Philadelphia, Lippincott-Raven, 1990, pp 277-378.

50. Whitecloud TS 3rd, Butler JC: Anterior lumbar fusion utilizing transvertebral fibular graft. *Spine* 13:370-374, 1988.

51. Zdeblick TA: A prospective randomized study of lumbar fusion: Preliminary results. *Spine* 18:983-991, 1993.

52. Zindrick MR, Wiltse LL, Widell EH, *et al*: A biomechanical study of intrapeduncular screw fixation in the lumbosacral spine. *Clin Orthop* 203:99-112, 1986.

# CHAPTER 121

# Iatrogenic Spine Destabilization

Mehmet Zileli, Nevan G. Baldwin, and Edward C. Benzel

An increased understanding of spinal mechanics, spinal cord physiology, anesthesia, critical-care, and spinal instrumentation devices has allowed surgeons to approach the spine ventrally, dorsally, laterally, and circumferentially without excessive morbidity. However, these complex interventions often exaggerate spine instability.

The instability that exists after a spinal operation may arise from pathologic (intrinsic) or iatrogenic (surgical) processes. Iatrogenic destabilization can result from a variety of sources, such as the destruction of ligaments, muscles, or bone, and the denervation of muscles (Table 121.1).[5]

## Biomechanical Considerations

Spinal stability is often viewed in terms of support "columns" in the spine. Various systems for evaluating stability consider varying numbers of columns and the fact that the anatomic components of a given column, such as the anterior column, may differ from one system to the next. Also, a column may or may not have a true anatomic correlate.

One method that is commonly used for evaluating stability is the three-column method of Denis.[8] The anterior column is the ventral half of the vertebral body and the anterior longitudinal ligament (ALL). The dorsal half of the vertebral body and the posterior longitudinal ligament (PLL) constitute the middle column. The dorsal column consists of the facet joints and all ligaments dorsal to the spinal canal.

Using the method of Denis,[8] significant instability is considered highly likely if two or more columns have suffered substantial injury. The posterior column has true anatomic boundaries, whereas the anterior and middle columns arbitrarily consider halves of a single vertebral body. Many systems for evaluating stability have been devised, but Denis's method is an example of such a system that is easy to use and widely accepted for clinical application.

## Ligamentous Disruption

Iatrogenic ligamentous instability can be assessed by intra-operative traction/distraction maneuvers, such as distraction, application of vertebral body spreaders, and implant manipulation. These maneuvers may help to determine whether an instrumented fusion is necessary.

### Ventral Surgery

The anterior and posterior longitudinal ligaments and the annulus fibrosis contribute significantly to the stability of the spine.[2,24,38] The PLL is weaker than the ALL and is often intentionally destroyed during dorsal, ventral, or lateral spine surgery. However, the ALL is often not totally disrupted, even with a wide ventral exposure. It is a strong and wide ligament and provides a significant proportion of spinal stability in extension. This function may be considered as a tension band that limits extension. As a result, ventral decompressive spine surgery (e.g., corpectomy), which adequately decompresses the dural sac, generally causes a disruption of the PLL, with preservation of at least a portion of the ALL. The width of the PLL significantly narrows in the middle portions of the vertebral body, thus making it susceptible to surgical disruption. In conjunction with existing bony disruption, surgical decompression usually causes significant instability of the spine. The extent of this destabilization can be assessed via intra-operative manipulation, such as vertebral body distraction. If significant instability is iatrogenically created, an inter-body strut graft is necessary, with or without supplementation by instrumentation. The PLL limits flexion and distraction.

### Dorsal Surgery

Resection of the interspinous ligaments may lead to instability. Although the interspinous ligaments are relatively weak, their long moment arm (i.e., distance from the instantaneous axis of rotation [IAR] to the ligament attachment site) provides a mechanical advantage with regard to their function as a tension band.[5] The capsular ligaments are strong. Although they function through a short moment arm, their relative strength allows them to provide a significant stabilizing effect, if they are intact.

## Bone Destruction
### Ventral Surgery

Bone destruction and additional surgical bone removal have a significant impact on spinal stability. Both the amount of vertebral body destruction and its location play an important role in the surgical destabilization process (Figure 121.1). The first issue is the extent of ventral bony destruction. A complete vertebrectomy causes an obvious instability (see Table 121.1). The extent of instability is closely related to the amount of bone removed.

White and Panjabi[38] used a three-column model to explain the effects of element disruption on spinal column stability. To determine the effect of a partial vertebral body resection on spinal stability, Benzel[5] used a hypothetical design that divides the vertebral body into 27 equal, small cubes (Figure 121.2). In this regard, resection of the ventral portion of the vertebral body affects spinal stability more than does a corresponding resection of the middle or dorsal portion of the vertebral body (Figure 121.3). This is because the largest force to which the spine is subjected is that of flexion. The more ventral portion of the vertebral body will be farther from the IAR, and it will therefore exert its resistance through a longer

**TABLE 121.1**

**Spine Destabilization: Etiology and Management**

| Surgery | Reason for Instability | Recommended Management |
|---|---|---|
| Extensive cervical laminectomy | Tension-band destruction<br>Facet joint destruction | Laminoplasty or lateral mass plating plus fusion |
| Extensive lumbar laminectomy | Tension band destruction<br>Facet joint destruction | Controversial<br>Possibly dorsolateral fusion<br>Possibly dorsal instrumentation |
| Cervical corpectomy | Bony destruction<br>ALL/PLL destruction | Ventral fusion<br>Ventral instrumentation<br>External orthosis |
| Thoracic-lumbar total corpectomy | Bony destruction<br>ALL/PLL destruction | Ventral reconstruction plus ventral instrumentation or dorsal instrumentation |
| Corpectomy plus dorsal decompression or total spondylectomy | Extensive bony destruction + ALL/PLL destruction<br>Facet joint destruction | Circumferential fusion and instrumentation<br>Equal ventral and dorsal instrumentation |

*ALL,* Anterior longitudinal ligament; *PLL,* posterior longitudinal ligament.

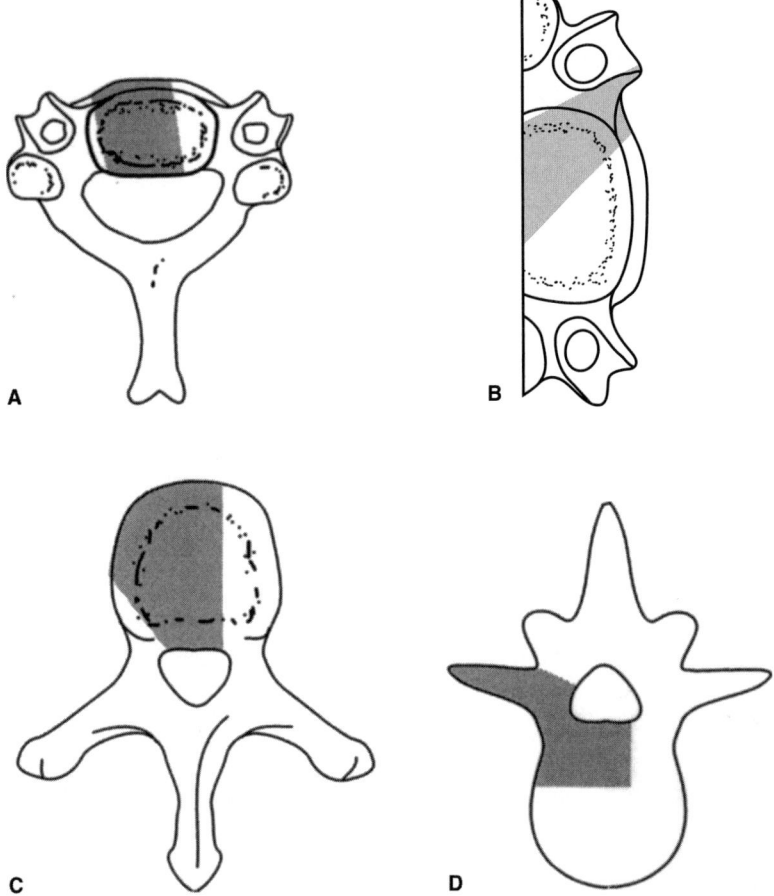

**Figure 121.1** Resection portions of the ventral vertebral body in most frequently performed ventral spine surgeries. **(A)** Cervical corpectomy—resection of the middle horizontal section of the body. **(B)** Oblique cervical corpectomy; resection of the lateral and dorsal sections of the vertebral body. **(C)** Ventral thoracic or lumbar surgery. **(D)** Lateral extracavitary surgery. In the latter two approaches, resection of the posterolateral portion of the body is more extensive in ventral surgery. *(Copyright University of New Mexico, Division of Neurosurgery.)*

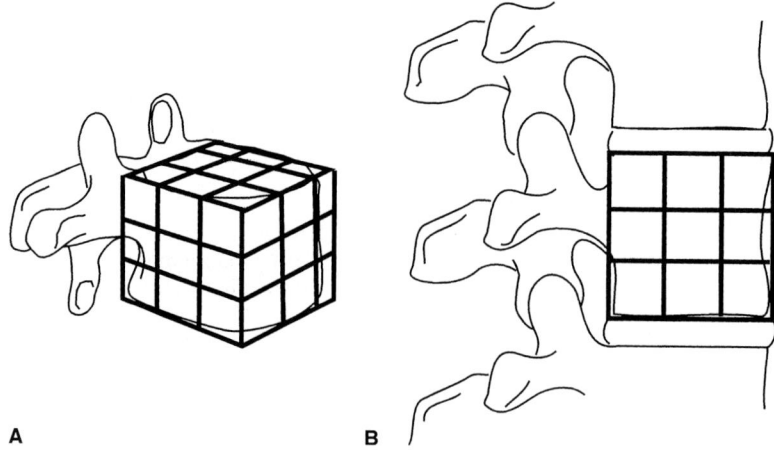

**Figure 121.2** A vertebral body seen, for theoretical purposes, as a cube composed of 27 equal, small cubes (3 × 3 × 3). **(A)** Oblique view, **(B)** Lateral view. *(From Benzel EC:* Biomechanics of Spine Stabilization: Principles and Clinical Practice. *New York, McGraw-Hill, 1995.)*

moment arm in resisting flexion. Also, resection of the middle horizontal section of the vertebral body affects stability more than does resection in the middle vertical sections (Figure 121.4).

Minimizing bone removal helps to decrease postoperative instability. To reach this aim, vertebral body resection in cervical corpectomy should be carefully determined. In this regard, oblique corpectomy is an approach that does not significantly interfere with the stability of the spine.[11,35] This approach protects the ventral portion of the vertebral body, but sacrifices the dorsal and lateral aspects (see Figure 121.1*B*).

As an aside, the uncovertebral joints add stability during extension, lateral bending, and torsion[20] In general, if the following sections of the vertebrae remain intact, a significant instability does not develop: (1) the anterior longitudinal ligament, (2) the ventral section of the vertebral body, (3) dorsal column integrity, and (4) dorsal column ligaments.

### Dorsal Surgery

A laminectomy can cause instability because of destabilization of the spine. The frequency of iatrogenic instability is proportional to the width of the laminectomy.[1,27] Often the extent of the injury is not readily apparent shortly after surgery. The prediction of its subsequent occurrence is even less obvious. If a ventral (vertebral body) lesion already exists, the incidence of postlaminectomy kyphosis is even higher.

Laminectomy often creates distortion of the dura mater and spinal cord, with flexion and distraction over the ventral fulcrum (Figure 121.5). Even in the absence of the ventral pathology, the disruption of the laminae, facet joints, and dorsal ligamentous complex may result in progressive deformity, the so-called postlaminectomy kyphosis (Figure 121.6). Postlaminectomy kyphosis occurs more commonly in the more mobile portion of the spine—the cervical spine. Laminoplasty may preserve a portion of the dorsal tension-band, and thereby diminish the insta-

bility observed after laminectomy.[3] Another alternative that minimizes the destabilizing effect of laminectomy is the addition of a stabilization strategy, such as dorsal fusion or external orthosis.

In summary, there are three important issues that should be addressed during decompressive laminectomy: (1) The presence, or absence, of ventral spinal instability, (2) the extent of resected laminae and facet joints, and the extent of ligamentous disruption, and (3) the location of the laminectomy (i.e., cervical, thoracic, or lumbar spine); the cervical spine is more prone to instability after laminectomy.

The contribution of the facet joints to dorsal column stability is very important. With axial loading the anterior and middle columns transmit only 36% of the applied load, whereas each pillar (facet) transmits 32% of the total applied load.[25] Therefore regardless of the region of the spine involved, excessive facet joint resection can result in instability. In the cervical spine the tolerable limit of resection is one third to one half of the facet joint.[27] In the lumbar spine facet resection may often result in glacial instability. However, the value of fusion and instrumentation after partial facetectomies for spinal stenosis is controversial.[28]

The shape and angulation of the facet joints are also important. A ventral translational deformity is more likely to result if vertically oriented joints and a hyperlordotic posture are present. The L4 and L5 facet joints are sagittally oriented, whereas L5-S1 joints are coronally oriented (Figure 121.7). Therefore L5-S1 joints resist translational deformity, whereas L4-5 joints can easily glide on a sagittal plane. Degenerative listhesis frequently involves this level.

## Clinical Considerations

The major indications for spine surgery are decompression and stabilization. Perhaps the most important indication is decompression. Whether the decompression is ventral or dorsal, it decreases spinal stability.

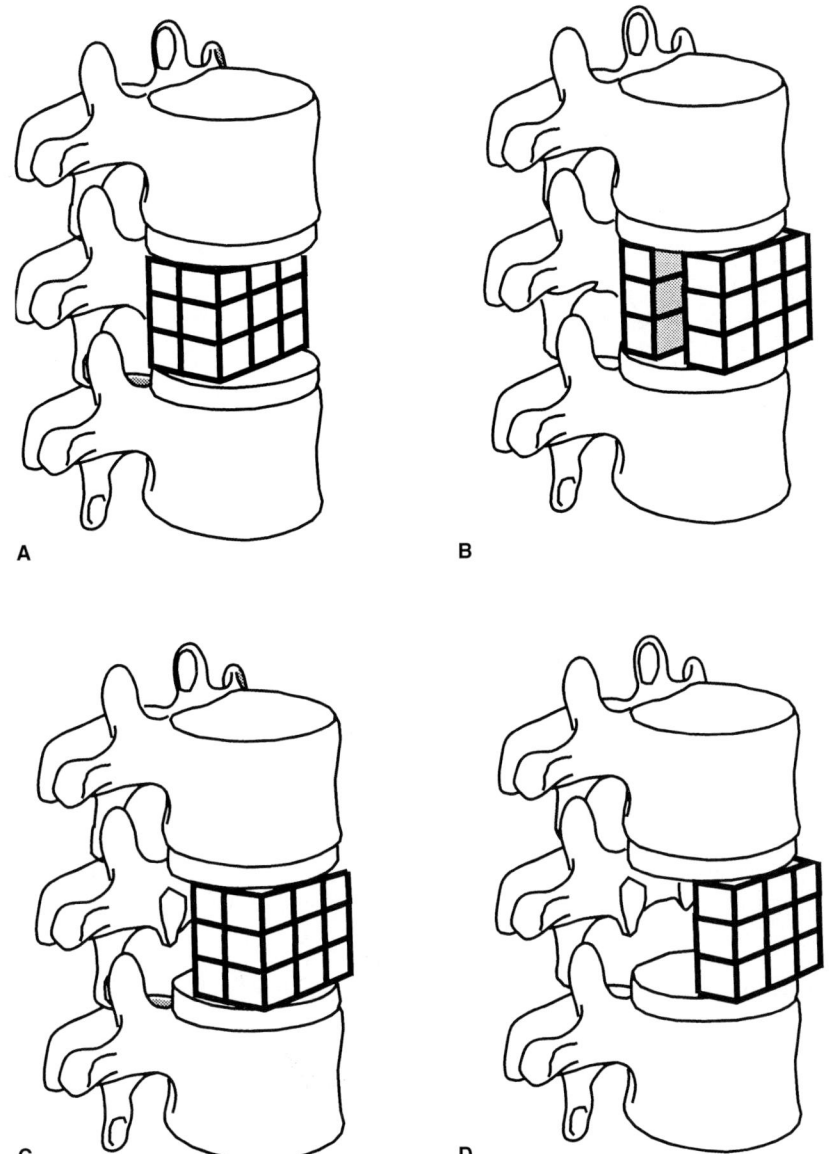

**Figure 121.3** Resection of the components of the cubic vertebral body. Partial vertebrectomy involving removal of the (**A**) ventral component in the coronal plane of the vertebral body affects the stability more than resection of the middle (**B**) or dorsal portion (**C**) in the coronal plane. (**D**) Resection of both the middle and the dorsal third of the vertebral body (in the presence of an intact posterior column and an intact ventral third of the vertebral body) may not significantly disrupt spinal integrity. (*From Benzel EC: Biomechanics of Spine Stabilization: Principles and Clinical Practice. New York, McGraw-Hill, 1995.*)

### Trauma Surgery

Because trauma itself causes instability, additional iatrogenic instability caused by a decompression operation may be catastrophic. Therefore most operations for spine trauma include a stabilization component.

The site of decompression (ventral vs. dorsal) is usually dictated by the type and location of the pathology. Spine stabilization can also be achieved from the same orientation.

### Tumor Surgery

An important issue that the spine surgeon cannot avoid is the iatrogenic instability created by radical tumor surgery.

Until recently the surgical treatment of spinal tumors was accomplished predominantly via laminectomy, despite the fact that the neural compression was often ventral to the spinal cord. However, laminectomy was often ineffective. Ventral surgery is often the procedure of choice for treating most bone tumors of the spine.[9,19,32] Because the pathology in most patients with these bone tumors lies ventral to the spinal canal, attempts at tumor resection can cause loss of ventral spinal integrity.

Tumors involving both ventral and dorsal elements cause even greater instability. For oncologic tumor surgery, extramarginal resection of bone tumors of the spine is desirable. Although the spinal cord and nerve roots do not allow such a resection in many instances, there is an

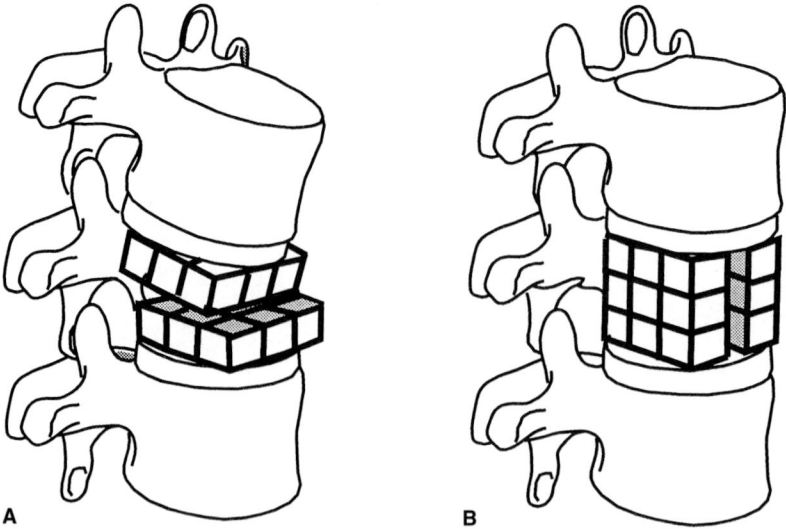

**Figure 121.4** Resections of portions of the cubic vertebral body. (**A**) Resection (or disruption) of the middle axial (horizontal) third of the vertebral body in its sagittal dimension, as may occur after trauma. (**B**) Resection of the middle (vertical) third of the vertebral body. (*From Benzel EC:* Biomechanics of Spine Stabilization: Principles and Clinical Practice. *New York, McGraw-Hill, 1995.*)

increasing trend toward accomplishing total spondylectomies by only a dorsal approach,[9,19,37,39] or by circumferential surgery.[23,29] Because the iatrogenic destabilization of the spine is so significant in these cases, radical measures to reconstruct and stabilize the spine are mandatory.

Preoperatively, the extent of tumor spread is the main determinant of stability. Instability is often not the sole reason for operation. The extent of neurologic deficit, the biology of the tumor, its radiosensitivity, and its sensitivity to chemotherapy are also important reasons. In selected cases radiotherapy of a radiosensitive tumor and external bracing may be suitable.

## Degenerative Spine Surgery

Cervical spondylotic myelopathy is often treated via a decompressive operation. Ventral and dorsal operations both may cause significant iatrogenic spine destabilization. This is similarly true for the thoracic and lumbar spine.

Ventral decompressive surgery of the cervical spine causes bony destruction, and also some form of ligamentous disruption. The PLL is intentionally removed during ventral osteophyte excision for cervical spondylotic myelopathy. In this case interbody strut graft stability, or "clamp down," that would have been phenomenon provided by an intact ligament, is not realized.

Ventral cervical plates can help to resist the distractive forces caused by the disruption of ligamentous resistance.

The annulus fibrosis contributes to the spinal stability in a similar manner on the posterior and anterior longitudinal ligaments. Its disruption in degenerative conditions may cause transitional instability.

### Adjacent-Level Spondylosis

It is common to observe degenerative changes above or below the level of a multilevel fusion. This type of instabil-

ity is obviously iatrogenic. To avoid this, the use of more flexible (dynamic) fixation devices has been proposed.[5] Short segment fixation and fusion may minimize the incidence of this complication. Another technique for dealing with this problem is to create a "transitional" level by using instrumentation that is less rigid at the first segment adjacent to the fused segments. For example, an L3 burst fracture might be treated by the use of rigid screw instrumentation, along with bony fusion from L2 to L4. The "transitional" segment might then be created by the use of laminar hooks (hooks are less rigid than screws) at L1.

Segmental fixation with the use of pedicle fixation systems can be very rigid. Although increasing rigidity may improve fusion rates, it also increases the rate of degeneration of adjacent segments.[16,26] Rahm and Hall[26] have reported an incidence of adjacent segment degeneration of 35% in cases with lumbar fusion and internal fixation. They also noted that the degeneration was associated with increasing patient age, use of interbody fusion, and worsening of clinical results with time.

## Postlaminectomy Instability

Although a dorsal approach is convenient and appropriate for most spine lesions, it causes a significant defect in the structural integrity of the posterior column, as well as a loss of the dorsal tension band.

After cervical laminectomy in children the incidence of kyphosis is very high.[14,18] The important factors that affect cervical instability after laminectomy are (1) the patient's age, (2) the number of laminae excised, (3) the curvature of the cervical spine, and (4) the degree of facet joint violation.[14] Although the relative incidence of instability after cervical laminectomy is controversial, there is a tendency to not perform multilevel laminectomies in pediatric patients and to provide additional stabilization measures in patients with cervical spondylotic myelopathy undergoing laminec-

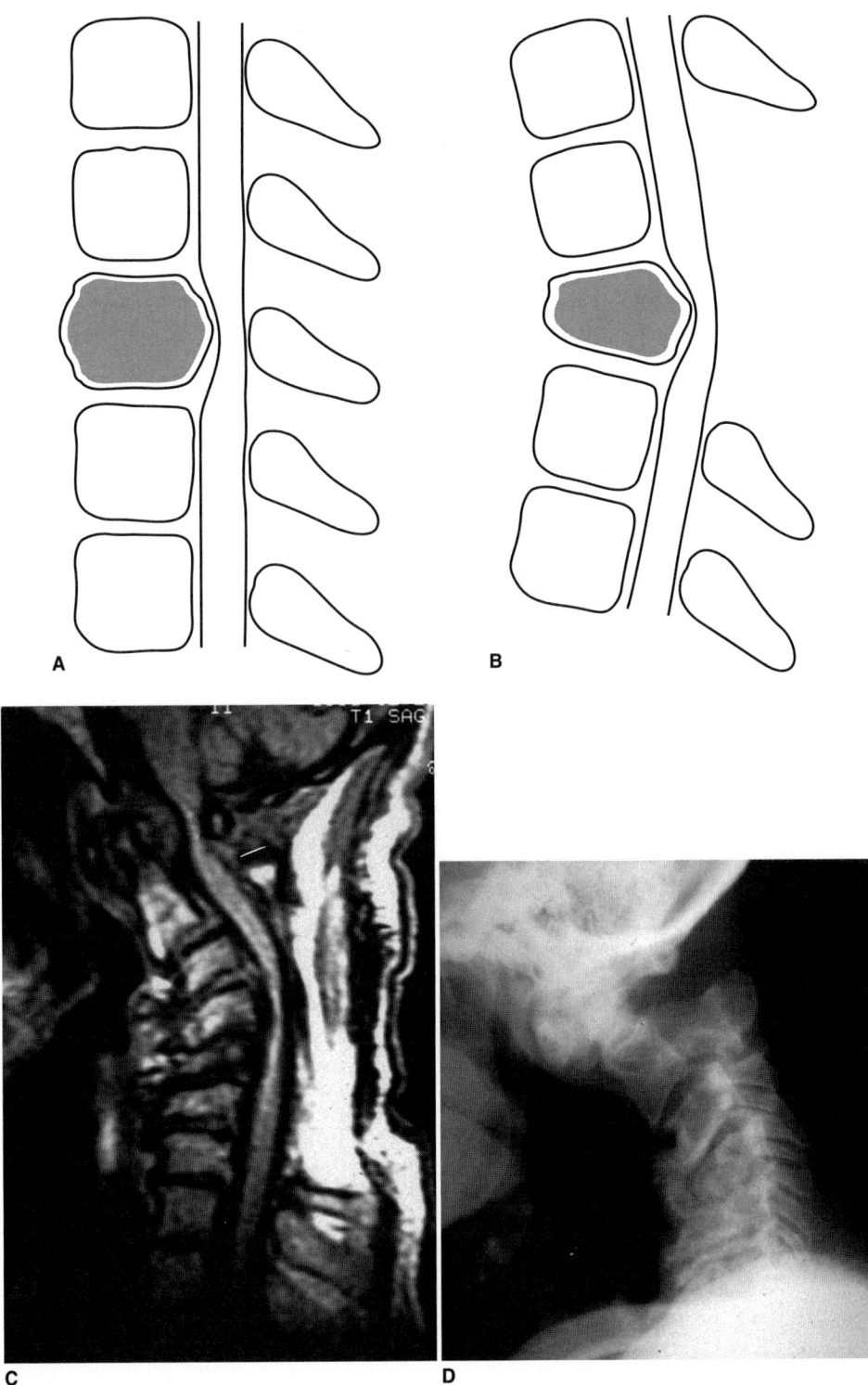

**Figure 121.5** The development of postlaminectomy kyphosis. In the case of preexisting ventral pathology laminectomy (**A**) can cause severe kyphotic deformity (**B**). In the cervical spine, even in the absence of ventral pathology, progressive kyphosis may develop (**C** and **D**).

tomy.[11,14] In patients with cervical spondylotic myelopathy, these measures may either be a laminoplasty or fixation (e.g., lateral mass plating) and fusion after laminectomy.

Extensive lumbar laminectomy is often necessary for patients with spinal stenosis. Because of the nature of the compression, this procedure often includes a partial facetectomy. Although the exact incidence of instability after extensive lumbar laminectomy for lumbar stenosis is not well known, some surgeons have suggested the use of bilateral hemilaminectomies and partial facetectomies, without destruction of interspinous ligaments, while preserving the majority of the laminal and spinous process. Performing a fusion, with or without instrumentation is, however, controversial.[5,15,30]

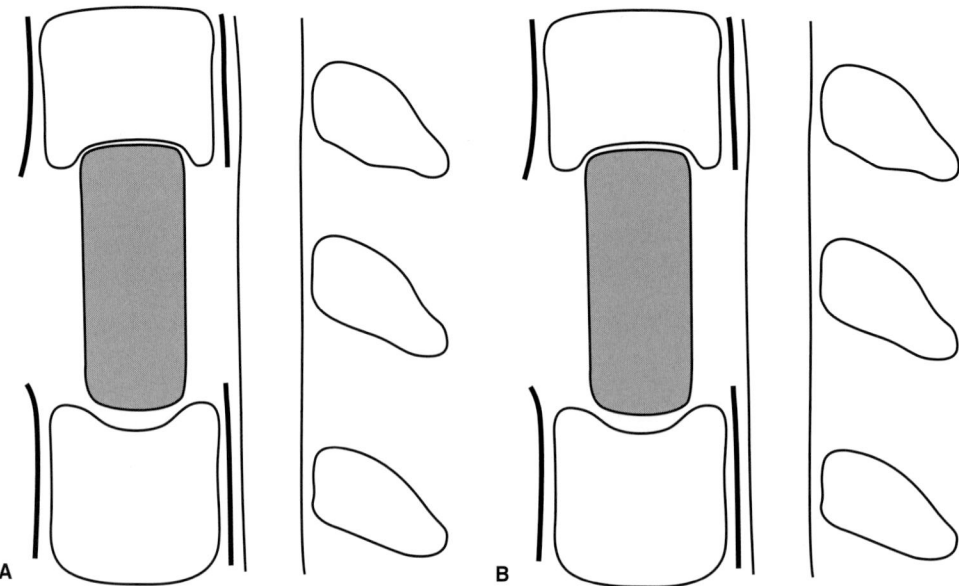

**Figure 121.6** The "clamping down phenomenon" in the cervical spine. If the PLL and ALL are intact, the graft firmly fits into the mortises of both end plates (**A**). If the ligaments are destroyed, their contribution to resisting distraction is lost, and the graft will not fit into the mortises firmly (**B**).

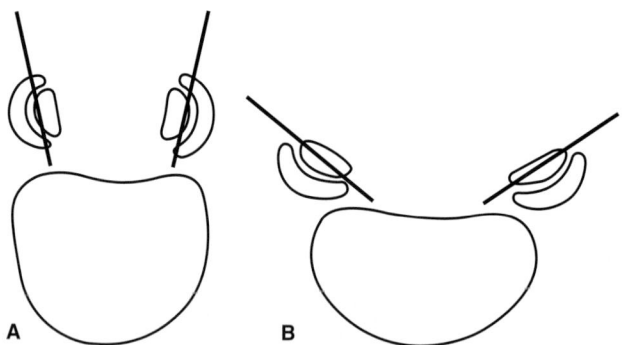

**Figure 121.7** Facet joint angles at the L4-5 and L5-S1 levels. (**A**) The L4-5 facet joints are sagittally oriented and do not resist translation. (**B**) The L5-S1 facet joints are coronally oriented and resist translation well.

### Bone Graft Harvesting

Instability related to bone graft harvesting is a rare but important problem. It was first reported in 1962 by Lichtblau,[21] who observed that dorsal iliac crest graft harvesting can cause dislocation of the sacroiliac joint.

## Prevention and Management of Iatrogenic Spinal Instability

For the management of spinal instability, one or a combination of the following three maneuvers is frequently performed: (1) external bracing with spinal splints, which provides time for healing of bone and ligaments, (2) ven-

tral bone grafts or instrumentation, or (3) dorsal instrumentation or fusion.

### Cervical Spine

Iatrogenic destabilization is most often caused by multi-level decompressions for spondylosis. This may be via a multilevel corpectomy or discectomy, or via laminectomy. Multilevel corpectomy or discectomy is usually accompanied by fusion. Therefore stability is addressed by the fusion. A multilevel central corpectomy injures or destroys the anterior and posterior longitudinal ligaments and also affects bone integrity. In this circumstance the destabilizing effect results from destruction of ligaments and bone.

### Thoracic and Lumbar Spine

Because of the widespread use of ventral surgery for spinal tumors, more reconstruction materials and stabilization problems are discussed. In general, if the lesion is strictly ventral, and the operation has destroyed only the anterior and part of the middle columns, ventral reconstruction and stabilization would be adequate. For single- or two-level lesions in the upper and middle thoracic spine, only a ventral reconstruction can be used. However, for lesions below level T10, ventral instrumentation, in addition to reconstruction, may be necessary. If, however, two or three columns are involved in lesions below level T10, supplemental dorsal instrumentation may be used after ventral reconstruction and ventral stabilization.[7]

Some surgeons perform *en bloc* resections of the dorsal and ventral elements of the spine from a dorsal route.[30] Tomita *et al.*[37] have described this approach as "total *en bloc* spondylectomy." From an oncologic point of view, this method is superior to traditional spinal tumor surgery,

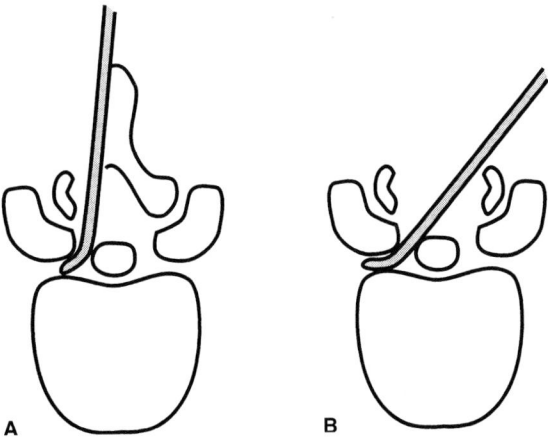

**Figure 121.8** (**A**) Trajectory to the lateral recess achieved via a laminotomy. Note that the Kerrison punch cannot adequately decompress the lateral recess without significant bone removal. (**B**) Trajectory to the lateral recess achieved via a laminectomy. Note that a more optimal trajectory is achieved. An undermining of the lateral recess and foramina may thus be achieved without significant facet disruption. (*Copyright University of New Mexico, Division of Neurosurgery.*)

| TABLE 121.2 |  |
| --- | --- |
| **Resection Levels and the Need for Reconstruction in Sacral Tumor Surgery** | |
| **Resection Level** | **Reconstruction** |
| One sacroiliac joint | Can usually compensate well with external support |
| Partial sacrectomy below S2 (most of the sacroiliac joints are preserved) | Not necessary |
| Total or subtotal sacrectomy above S2 (most of the sacroiliac joints are lacking) | Obviously necessary with instrumentation crossing the sacroiliac joint |

**BOX 121.1**

**Indications for reconstruction of the sacroiliac joints**

Resection of more than 50% of the sacroiliac joints.
Bilateral resection of the sacrum above S2.
Total resection of the sacroiliac joint on one side associated with ventral pelvic disruption or deficiency.

From Bridwell KH: Management of tumors at the lumbosacral junction. In Marguiles JY, *et al* (eds): *Lumbosacral and Spinopelvic Fixation*. Philadelphia, Lippincott-Raven, 1996, pp 109-122.

curettage, and intralesional removal. They have used a reconstruction material and additional dorsal fixation with instrumentation. It can be used in one stage and one position only. However, its disadvantage is the risk of spinal cord ischemia, resulting from bilateral occlusion of the segmental arteries.

Limiting the extent of dorsal element removal or disruption during laminectomy can minimize spine destabilization by limiting the disruption of the dorsal tension band (e.g., by performing multilevel laminotomies instead of laminectomy). Laminotomy, theoretically, restricts the amount of important bone and soft tissue removed. However, laminectomy provides a trajectory advantage that most likely outweighs the laminotomy advantage (Figure 121.8).

## Lumbosacral Spine

The sacrum is a transitory structure between the vertebral column and pelvis. The sacroiliac joint is the immobile joint that functions as a shock absorber for the spine. The pelvis itself transfers loads from the sacroiliac joints to the hip joints, with the help of strong ligamentous structures. White and Panjabi examined the weight-bearing capacity of the sacroiliac joint. They found that, despite the lower half of the S1 vertebral body and half of the sacroiliac joint being resected, only 50% of weight-bearing capacity was lost. This, in fact, is adequate for ambulation, and there is no need for stabilization in most cases (Table 121.2).[38] If the sacral lesion is a primary tumor, and complete tumor removal with extra marginal resection is desired, combined ventral and dorsal approaches, with significant amount of bone and ligamentous tissue destruction, is necessary. In this case an adequate reconstruction is required.[31,33,34,39]

The key point for reconstruction is whether the sacroiliac joints are involved.[6,13] If the tumor is not large and the sacroiliac joints are preserved, stability is not lost. However, involvement of one or both joints dictates the need for internal fixation and fusion. Kostuik and Esses[19] suggest surgical reconstruction if 50% or more of the sacroiliac joint is removed.

If the sacrum above the S2 segment is resected with some of the ilium, the L5 vertebral body will drop into the pelvis.[10,39] In this case an implant connecting the lumbar spine to both sides of the ilium is necessary. Three alternatives for the implant procedure are described in Box 121.1. Because the defect is so massive, the patients' own bones do not allow an autograft fusion, and allograft bone is usually used. The forces from the lumbar spine are distributed to both lower extremities via the sacrum and pelvis. This complicates the lumbopelvic instrumentation decision-making process.[12,36]

Because the sacrum is a transitory structure between the vertebral column and the pelvis and lower extremities, adding the sacrum into the long segment fixations for deformity correction is also an important point.[1,22] Achieving strong lumbosacral fixation and fusion poses unique problems because of the shape of the sacrum and the presence of a large amount of cancellous bone. For this reason, different adaptations, such as use of larger-diameter screws, application of multiple screws, and insertion of the rod into the iliac cristae after significant bending (Galveston technique), have been recommended (Table 121.3).[1,2,4,22]

**TABLE 121.3**

**Methods of Sacropelvic Fixation and Reconstruction**

| Technique | Reference |
|---|---|
| **With Sacrum Preserved** | |
| Isola plate | Asher and Strippgen[2] |
| Galveston technique | Allen and Ferguson[1] |
| Isola iliac screws | |
| **With Sacrum Resected** | |
| Fusion of L5 to the ilium | Shikata et al.[31] |
| Autogenous grafting of residual lumbar vertebral bodies to residual pelvis and sacrum | Kostuik and Esses[19] |
| Massive structural allograft reconstruction (allograft sacropelvis) | |

The modified Galveston L-rod technique is a reasonable reconstructive method after total sacrectomy.[12,17] It prevents caudal migration and axial rotation of the spinal column. Adding a threaded transiliac rod can prevent the open-book phenomenon, and provides stability around the horizontal axis of the spinal column, while also preventing rotation around this axis.

# REFERENCES

1. Allen BL Jr, Ferguson RL: The Galveston technique for L rod instrumentation of the scoliotic spine. *Spine* 7:276-284, 1982.
2. Asher MA, Strippgen WE: Anthropometric studies of the human sacrum relating to dorsal transsacral implant designs. *Clin Orthop Relat Res* 203:58-62, 1986.
3. Baisden J, Voo LM, Cusick JF, et al: Evaluation of cervical laminectomy and laminoplasty. *Spine* 24:1283-1289, 1999.
4. Baldwin NG, Benzel EC: Sacral fixation using iliac instrumentation and a variable angle screw device. *J Neurosurg* 81:313-316, 1994.
5. Benzel EC: *Biomechanics of Spine Stabilization: Principles and Clinical Practice*. New York, McGraw Hill, 1995.
6. Bridwell KH: Management of tumors at the lumbosacral junction. In Marguiles JY, et al (eds): *Lumbosacral and Spinopelvic Fixation*. Philadelphia, Lippincott-Raven, 1996, pp 109-122.
7. Cooper PR, Errico TJ, Martin R, et al: A systematic approach to spinal reconstruction after anterior decompression for neoplastic disease of the thoracic and lumbar spine. *Neurosurgery* 32:1-8, 1993.
8. Denis F: The three column spine and its significance in the classification of acute thoracolumbar spine injuries. *Spine* 8:817-831, 1983.
9. Errico TJ, Cooper PR: Transthoracic and translumbar decompression and stabilization for spine tumors. *Contemp Neurosurg* 15:1-6, 1993.
10. Gennari L, Azzarelli A, Quagliuolo V: A posterior approach for the excision of sacral chordoma. *J Bone Joint Surg Br* 69:565, 1987.
11. George B, Zerah M, Lot G, et al: Oblique transcorporeal approach to anteriorly located lesions in the cervical spinal canal. *Acta Neurochir* 121:187-190, 1993.

12. Gökaslan ZL, Romsdahl MM, Kroll SS, et al: Total sacrectomy and Galveston L-rod reconstruction for malignant neoplasms: Technical note. *J Neurosurg* 87:781-787, 1997.
13. Gunterberg B, Romanus B, Stener B: Pelvic strength after major amputation of the sacrum. *Acta Orthop Scand* 47:635, 1976.
14. Heller JG, Whitecloud TS: Post-laminectomy instability of the cervical spine—etiology and stabilization technique. In Frymoyer JW (ed): *The Adult Spine: Principles and Practice*, vol 2. New York, Raven Press, 1991, pp 1219-1240.
15. Herkowitz HN, Kurz LT: Degenerative lumbar spondylolisthesis with spinal stenosis: a prospective study comparing decompression with decompression and intertransverse process arthrodesis. *J Bone Joint Surg* 73A:802-808, 1991.
16. Hsu KY, Zucherman J, White AH, et al: Deterioration of motion segments adjacent to lumbar spine fusions. Presented at the Annual Meeting of the North American Spine Society, Colorado Springs, CO, 1988.
17. Jackson RJ, Gokaslan ZL: Spinal-pelvic fixation in patients with lumbosacral neoplasms. *J Neurosurg* (Spine 1) 92:61-70, 2000.
18. Katsumi Y, Honma T, Nakamura T: Analysis of cervical instability resulting from laminectomies for removal of spinal cord tumor. *Spine* 14:1172-1176, 1989.
19. Kostuik JP, Esses SI: Sacral destabilization and restabilization—causes and treatment. In Frymoyer JW (ed): *The Adult Spine: Principles and Practice*, vol 2. New York, Raven Press, 1991, pp 2172-2173.
20. Kotani Y, McNulty PS, Abumi K, et al: The role of anteromedial foraminotomy and the uncovertebral joints in the stability of the cervical spine. A biomechanical study. *Spine* 23:1559-1565, 1998.
21. Lichtblau S: Dislocation of the sacro-iliac joint: a complication of bone-grafting. *J Bone Joint Surg Am* 44:193, 1962.
22. Louis R: Fusion of the lumbar and sacral spine by internal fixation with screw plates. *Clin Orth Relat Res* 203:18-33, 1986.
23. Ma YZ, Tang HF, Chai BF, et al: The treatment of primary vertebral tumors by radical resection and prosthetic vertebral replacement. *Clin Orthop Relat Res* 215:78-90, 1987.
24. Mirbaha MM: Exposure of the vertebral bodies of the proximal lumbar segments. Some anatomic points. *Spine* 3:329-335, 1978.
25. Pal GP, Sherk HH: The vertical stability of the cervical spine. *Spine* 13:447-449, 1988.
26. Rahm MD, Hall BB: Adjacent-segment degeneration after lumbar fusion with instrumentation: a retrospective study. *J Spinal Disorders* 9:392-400, 1996.
27. Raynor RB, Pugh J, Shapiro I: Cervical facetectomy and its effect on spine strength. *J Neurosurg* 63:278-282, 1985.
28. Rosenberg NJ: Degenerative spondylolisthesis. Surgical treatment. *Clin Orthop Relat Res* 117:112-120, 1976.
29. Selby DK, Henderson RJ: Circumferential (360 degree) spinal fusion. In Frymoyer JW (ed): *The Adult Spine: Principles and Practice,* vol 2. New York, Raven Press, 1991, pp 1989-2006.
30. Shenkin HA, Hash CJ: Spondylolisthesis after multiple bilateral laminectomies and facetectomies for lumbar spondylosis: follow-up study. *J Neurosurg* 50:45-47, 1979.

31. Shikata J, Yamamuro T, Kotoura Y, *et al*: Total sacrectomy and reconstruction for primary tumors. Report of two cases. *J Bone Joint Surg Am* 70:122, 1988.

32. Sundaresan N, DiGiancinto GV: Surgical considerations and approaches. In Sundaresan N, Schmidek HH, Schiller AL, *et al* (eds): *Tumors of the Spine: Diagnosis and Clinical Management.* Philadelphia, WB Saunders, 1990, pp 358-379.

33. Sung HW, Shu WP, Wang HM, *et al*: Surgical treatment of primary tumors of the sacrum. *Clin Orthop* 215:91, 1987.

34. Stener B, Guntenberg B: High amputation of the sacrum for extirpation of tumors: principles and technique. *Spine* 3:351, 1978.

35. Takayasu M, Hara M, Takagi T: Osteoplastic anterolateral vertebrotomy without fusion for multilevel cervical ossification of the posterior longitudinal ligament. *Neurosurgery* 45:500-507, 1999.

36. Tomita K, Tsuchiya H: Total sacrectomy and reconstruction for huge sacral tumors. *Spine* 15:1223-1227, 1990.

37. Tomita K, Yoribatake Y, Kawahara N, *et al*: Total en bloc spondylectomy and circumspinal decompression for solitary spinal metastasis. *Paraplegia* 32:36-46, 1994.

38. White AA, Panjabi MM: The problem of clinical instability in the human spine: a systematic approach. In White AA, Panjabi MM (eds): *Clinical Biomechanics of the Spine.* Philadelphia, JB Lippincott, 1990, pp 277-378.

39. Zileli M, Sabah D, Hoscoskun C: Surgery of the sacrum tumors. Presented at the Eurospine 96 Meeting, Zurich, Switzerland, October 1996.

# CHAPTER 122

# Cervical Spine Construct Design

Paul D. Sawin, Vincent C. Traynelis,*
Kurt M. Eichholz, and Vijay K. Goel

## Fundamental Concepts

The successful application of cervical spinal instrumentation depends on several factors, including the nature and extent of the disease process, bone quality, and the technical expertise of the surgeon. One of the most crucial, but often overlooked, elements in this process is determined well before the operative procedure is undertaken. This is construct design.

The term *construct* is a neologism that has become entrenched in the spinal literature. For the purpose of this discussion, a construct denotes the aggregate of biologic and/or nonbiologic materials that are implanted for the purpose of providing stability to an unstable region of the spine. Construct design, then, is the process of contriving such an implant. For the most part the design of constructs composed of bone and instrumentation for application in the subaxial cervical spine is addressed.

Without a sound construct design strategy, cervical fixation systems are doomed to failure. The meticulous technical application of a poorly conceived construct is a futile exercise, as prone to failure as the correct system improperly applied. Despite its importance, relatively little emphasis has been placed on this element of the procedure. This chapter presents a strategy to aid in the selection of certain instrumentation systems designed for specific clinical problems of cervical spine instability. The specific advantages and shortcomings of each type of construct are also discussed.

Benzel[7] described an excellent method for preoperative mapping of thoracic and lumbar instrumentation procedures, using a "construct blueprint." This approach is practical in this region of the spine, because the choice of implant components that may be applied here is vast. The design of thoracolumbar constructs entails selection of the longitudinal member, cross-fixation mechanism, and implant-bone junction fixators. Each element may be different at various levels of a long construct, adding to the complexity of the system.

Additionally, the modes of construct application that may be used in the thoracolumbar spine are extensive. This refers to the desired forces that are applied by the

surgeon at the implant-bone junction. Constructs may be placed in compression, distraction, neutral, translation, flexion, extension, and lateral bending modes.[8] In a single thoracolumbar construct, several modes of application may be required, depending on the structural demands at any given level. A systematic approach to the formulation of an operative plan is essential when designing constructs with this degree of complexity. The construct blueprint is a concise format capable of communicating complicated surgical strategies to all members of the operative team.

The options concerning surgical approaches and types of fixation devices are more limited in the cervical region. The mode of application here is also less variable, because most cervical constructs are applied in the neutral mode. Although this simplifies the cervical construct design scheme, the need for cogent preoperative planning is just as essential. The format used to communicate the operative strategy is less important than the intellectual process of visualizing the biomechanical requirements of a given lesion and formulating an appropriate construct that satisfies these requirements.

The fundamental steps for appropriate construct design are to determine the need for instrumentation, select the construct best suited to solve the instability problem, and ascertain the need for postoperative orthotic stabilization to supplement the implant.

## Indications for Cervical Construct Application

White and Panjabi[34] outline four general indications for spinal stabilization: (1) to restore clinical stability to a spine in which the structural integrity has been compromised, (2) to maintain alignment after correction of a deformity, (3) to prevent progression of a deformity, and (4) to alleviate pain. Cervical spinal instrumentation may be applied in conjunction with a bone fusion in all of these scenarios. In rare instances instrumentation may replace bone fusion as the principal means of cervical stabilization.

Optimally, internal fixation provides immediate postoperative stability to the region before the development of osseous fusion. This is beneficial in two respects. Instrumentation protects the neural elements from trauma and the spine from deformity, until the bony fusion matures and can assume this role. Internal fixation also obviates, or at least significantly reduces, the requirement for postoperative external immobilization while the fusion mass heals. This technique improves patient comfort, which encourages accelerated mobilization after surgery. Additionally, this may enhance the probability of attaining successful bone fusion by ensuring compliance with postoperative immobilization.

Internal fixation may allow a reduction in the number of levels that require fusion by adding intrinsic strength and load-sharing properties to the construct. A shorter fusion facilitates the preservation of cervical motion, and limits the resultant moment arm created by the fusion mass.

### Clinical Instability

The most frequent indication for cervical instrumentation is instability. To paraphrase an oft-quoted general

---

*Corresponding author.

definition, instability requires the loss of spinal biomechanical integrity such that the spine is unable to prevent initial or additional neurologic deficit, major deformity, or incapacitating pain under physiologic loads.[34] The precise definition of spinal instability is difficult to establish, and may vary according to the specific clinical setting. A more comprehensive discussion of what constitutes cervical instability has been presented previously.

In practice it is essential to determine precisely the nature and extent of spinal instability. The *nature of instability* refers to the status of specific structures that normally confer stability on each motion segment in the cervical region. This concern addresses the competency of the ligamentous structures, bony elements, and annulus fibrosis of the intervertebral disc. Identification of the incompetent elements allows the severity of segmental spinal instability to be estimated. The *extent of instability* denotes the number of unstable motion segments, as well as whether the instability is predominantly ventral, dorsal, or both. Defining these concepts precisely is of fundamental importance, having an impact on the decision to instrument the spine and also dictating the selection of an appropriate construct.

The etiology of spinal instability is important. Symptomatic cervical instability may result from trauma, degenerative disease, neoplasia, or infection. Iatrogenic instability may also occur, particularly after cervical laminectomy for spondylotic disease. Construct design is influenced by the nature of the disease process that produced the instability. The long-term structural demands placed on a construct are often determined by the progression or remittance of the underlying disease. Posttraumatic instability may demand the least of a construct. Short-term immobilization is often all that is required to promote adequate healing. After the injury heals the load-bearing and load-sharing properties of the construct are no longer required to maintain stability. Spondylotic and iatrogenic instability may require more from a construct, owing to the slowly progressive nature of the process. Instability arising from spinal neoplasia often mandates long-term participation by the instrumentation to maintain structural integrity. Bone fusion may not be attainable because of the rapid progression of disease. In these situations the instrumented construct must be designed to bear physiologic loads for the remainder of the patient's life.

## Maintenance of Alignment

Cervical constructs are often required to maintain spinal alignment. Internal fixation may be indicated to prevent deformity from occurring, or to preserve normal alignment after reduction. Unlike thoracolumbar instrumentation, cervical constructs are generally applied in the neutral mode. Thus deformity reduction is essential before stabilization. This is often accomplished by applying axial skeletal traction. Many constructs designed for use in the thoracolumbar spine can apply significant compressive, distractive, translatory, and rotatory forces to a region of spinal deformity, thus affecting reduction. As a rule most cervical instrumentation systems cannot apply the magnitude of force required to reduce a deformity.

Internal cervical fixation may be used to maintain reduction, but application of reductive forces with these constructs should be avoided in most instances.

Prevention of spinal deformity may also be accomplished by the timely use of internal fixation. Progressive kyphosis or spondylolisthesis may result from spinal decompression procedures. If individuals at risk for this complication are identified preoperatively, cervical deformity may be preventable. Patients exhibiting a loss of the normal cervical lordotic configuration are prone to develop postlaminectomy kyphosis.[4] This complication may be avoided by proper internal stabilization at the time of decompression. Similarly, operative resections that compromise principal load-bearing elements may render the spine incompetent to withstand physiologic loads. Progressive postoperative deformity may be prevented by spinal reconstruction, using bone graft and instrumentation to reconstitute the axial spine.

## Pain Management

Spinal stabilization may be indicated to relieve incapacitating pain by reducing motion between spinal segments. This concept has been applied more extensively in the lumbar spine, particularly for treatment of mechanical low back pain arising from spondylolysis and subsequent degenerative spondylolisthesis. Fusion of the cervical spine purely for amelioration of axial pain may benefit selected patients greatly. Such a procedure should be carefully considered, and only performed after conservative treatment measures have failed.

## Construct Selection

Cervical constructs should be designed to solve case-specific problems of spinal instability. This requires an understanding of the nature, extent, and causes of instability; load-sharing and load-bearing demands; bone integrity; and biomechanical attributes of various internal fixation systems. Implant cost and facility of application are also important concerns. Constructs may fail as a result of poor design, usually because biomechanical expectations of the implant were unreasonable. Two general rules help guide the selection of a cervical construct, and limit unrealistic expectations: (1) the graft and implant must correct the specific preoperative instability, and (2) the long-term success of a cervical construct ultimately relies on the quality of the osseous fusion.

## General Considerations

In most cases cervical constructs are used to maintain clinical stability. This may be accomplished most efficiently by matching the implant with the major site of instability. That is, if the instability is primarily dorsal in location, a dorsal construct should be considered for stabilization. Similarly, ventral instability, created by incompetence of the anterior longitudinal ligament (ALL), vertebral body, or intervertebral disc complex, is most effectively treated by the application of a ventral construct. It is unreasonable to expect that a construct will function with optimal stability when implanted in a biomechanically disadvantageous position.

Internal fixation systems provide immediate postoperative stability to the instrumented region, but do not provide long-term stability due to the "plastic" properties of bone at the implant-bone interface. As with most biologic materials, bone deforms and reforms when stress is applied.[9] Eventually, even the most rigid construct allows a small degree of motion. Repetitive loading gradually increases the amount of movement and can ultimately lead to implant failure, unless bony fusion occurs. The long-term stability of all constructs is thus dependent on osseous fusion. No internal fixation system currently available can compensate for a poorly designed bone graft.[30]

Cervical spinal implants may be considered as rigid, semirigid, or dynamic.[9] Rigid implants attempt to achieve complete immobilization of the instrumented motion segments. Ventral plate systems, with locking screws and dorsal rod and hook/rod systems, provide rigid fixation. Luque rods and rectangles (Zimmer; Warsaw, IN), secured with segmental sublaminar or facet wires, and most lateral mass plate devices are examples of semirigid cervical implants. Rigid immobilization is potentially detrimental to bone fusion because of stress shielding and stress-reduction osteopenia.[9,20] This concern has led to the development of dynamic instrumentation, such as nonfixed moment arm cantilever beam screw-plate implants and axially dynamic ventral fixators.[19]

## Modes of Application

The modes of application available for cervical constructs are more limited than those available for use in other spinal regions. Thoracolumbar implants may be placed in distraction, compression, neutral, translation, flexion, extension, and lateral-bending modes. In contrast, cervical spine constructs are generally applied in the neutral mode. This is not universally true, because certain cervical plate systems and wire constructs may provide a modest degree of compression. Theoretically, cervical rod/hook devices can be placed in the compression or distraction modes as well. However, the vast majority of cervical constructs in clinical use are applied in the neutral mode at the time of surgery. Biomechanical conditions change as the spine is loaded after surgery. Most "neutral" implants must resist axial compression when the upright posture is assumed. These constructs then function in a distraction mode.[9]

Cervical construct designs are also more limited in their mechanism of load bearing than their thoracolumbar counterparts. Generally, cervical constructs conform to one of five fundamental load-bearing types: (1) distraction fixation, (2) tension-band fixation, (3) three-point bending, (4) fixed moment arm cantilever beam, and (5) nonfixed moment arm cantilever beam fixation.[8] Applied moment arm cantilever beam fixation, a technique occasionally applied in the thoracolumbar spine, is not used in the cervical spine. Assigning an implant to one of these fundamental load-bearing types is somewhat artificial, because a given construct may exhibit features of several mechanical types. However, it permits classification of implants by their principal biomechanical attributes.

### Simple Distraction

Simple distraction fixation occurs when a distraction force is applied by a cervical construct, usually from a ventral, interbody location.[8] Interbody strut grafts, with or without ventral plate instrumentation, are examples of this type of fixation. These devices principally resist axial loads. Dorsally applied distraction fixation is rarely used because it is prone to create a kyphotic deformity.

### Tension-Band Fixation

Tension-band fixation is accomplished by any device that reconstitutes the ventral or dorsal tension band, thereby preventing distraction, and also possibly angulation, in the opposite direction. This type of fixation may be applied dorsally with interspinous wires or cables, sublaminar wires or cables, facet wires or cables, interlaminar clamps, or lateral mass plates. A hook/rod construct, applied in compression, also produces tension-band fixation. These dorsal devices resist flexion most efficiently, because the flexion moment is coupled with dorsal distraction. Ventral tension-band fixation is accomplished principally with ventral cervical plate systems. These implants reconstitute the ventral tension band, thereby resisting ventral distraction and providing sound biomechanical stabilization of extension injuries.[30]

### Three-Point Bending

Three-point bending fixation occurs when forces are applied to the spine at three or more sites along the length of the construct.[8] Dorsally directed forces are applied at the rostral and caudal ends of the construct. An equal but opposite ventrally directed force is applied at the fulcrum, usually in the center of the construct. Three-point bending instrumentation is only applied dorsally in the cervical spine, and must fixate multiple motion segments. This type of fixation may be accomplished with Luque rods and rectangles secured with sublaminar wires or cables, lateral mass rib-wire constructs, hook/rod implants, and, to a lesser degree, with lateral mass plates.

### Cantilever Beam Fixation

A cantilever is formed by a projecting beam supported at one end only.[8] When the cantilever is rigidly attached to the supporting longitudinal member, a fixed moment arm cantilever beam is created. This variety of load bearing is accomplished by ventral cervical plate systems secured with locking screws and rigid lateral mass rod/screw instrumentation. A fixed moment arm cantilever beam device contributes some axial load-sharing properties to the construct. Nonfixed moment arm cantilever beam fixation employs a dynamic attachment of the cantilever to the longitudinal member. Lateral mass plates and nonfixed moment arm cantilever beam screw-plate implants and axially dynamic ventral fixators are representative of this type of load bearing.

The classification of spinal implants by mechanism of load bearing is somewhat artificial. In practice a single implant may function by using several of the fundamental load-bearing mechanisms simultaneously. For example, the lateral mass plate is capable of stabilization by three such mechanisms. Dorsal tension band, three-point bending, and nonfixed moment arm cantilever beam fixation are all accomplished by this device.

## Construct Materials

A variety of biologic and prosthetic materials have been used for cervical spine stabilization. Most constructs are composed of a bone graft, coupled with a metal prosthesis. Occasionally, bone and/or metal components may be supplemented or replaced by methyl methacrylate.

### Bone Grafts

Autograft and allograft bone have both been used extensively in spinal stabilization. Some studies report that fusion rates with allograft bone are comparable to those obtained with autograft bone.[12,22,35] Other studies have maintained that autograft bone is superior.[29,30,34] This is particularly evident with dorsal cervical constructs, in which the bone graft is not placed under compression. Certainly, fusion rates with autograft bone meet or exceed those reported with allograft. The use of autograft bone eliminates the concern of infectious disease transmission that may be associated with allograft bone, including human immunodeficiency virus (HIV) and hepatitis virus transmission.

The iliac crest provides a versatile and abundant source of bone graft material for incorporation into cervical spine constructs. Favorable attributes of this type of graft include ease of procurement in both the supine and prone positions, strength, and relative expendability of the donor site.[33,34] The tricortical structure of the iliac crest is responsible for much of the strength inherent in this graft, thereby providing excellent axial load-bearing capability. The abundant cancellous bone provides ample substrate for osseous remodeling. Although all commonly used configurations of iliac crest grafts can sustain high compressive loads, the Smith-Robinson type graft is probably superior to other styles of grafts in this respect.[35] The principal disadvantage associated with iliac crest harvest is donor site morbidity, which may be substantial. Complications include pain, wound hematoma, infection, meralgia paresthetica, hip dislocation, and fracture of the anterior superior iliac spine.

Fibula is another commonly used graft material. It is particularly well suited for multilevel ventral reconstruction procedures, because the thick cortical bone in this graft resists high axial compressive loads. The relatively small amount of cancellous bone present in the fibula graft may delay bone remodeling, however. This may be partially overcome by packing additional cancellous bone in the center of the graft, as well as surrounding the outer cortical surface with the cancellous bone. Donor site morbidity arising from graft harvest may be significant, because one sixth of body weight is borne by the fibula.[9] This may be principally a theoretical concern, as fibula has been used quite successfully in many cases of spinal reconstruction.

Rib grafts have also been used, particularly with dorsal cervical constructs. The native configuration of rib is advantageous because it conforms well to the cervical lordotic curve. There is minimal morbidity in harvesting rib as compared to iliac crest. This is an excellent graft to use for dorsal fusions.[27]

Many interbody allograft products are currently available. The overall fusion rate with these materials is similar to that of autograft, if instrumentation is used.

### Implants

Currently most spinal implants are fashioned from metal. Stainless steel has been used extensively for the manufacture of wires, cables, plates, screws, hooks, and rods used in spinal constructs. This material possesses a relatively high tensile strength while retaining a reasonable degree of malleability. The latter permits custom implant modification, which is often required to tailor a component to anatomic specification. Recently, titanium alloys have replaced stainless steel for use as cervical spine implants. These alloys are strong, biocompatible, and facilitate postoperative magnetic resonance imaging (MRI) and computed tomographic (CT) imaging.

Regardless of the material used, compatibility of the implanted components is essential. All metal implants should be made of the same material. This eliminates the theoretical possibility of internal current generation that may cause corrosion. The size of implanted components should also be compatible. Fixators at the implant-bone junction should be of appropriate diameter, length, and configuration to match the longitudinal member.[30]

Methyl methacrylate has been used to supplement or replace bone, metal components, or both. This material is simple to apply, relatively safe, and inexpensive. Long-term stability of any cervical construct requires osseous fusion. Therefore the ultimate stability of a construct with methyl methacrylate cannot be guaranteed, because no provision is made for bone fusion.

The integrity of the patient's native bone is an important factor. Bone quality can have an impact on construct selection, the biomechanical stability of a construct, and the need for postoperative external immobilization. Osteoporosis is detrimental to all forms of spinal fixation. It influences systems that rely on screw fixation most substantially. Hooks and sublaminar wires are less prone to pull-out than screws, and thus may be more suited for use in the osteoporotic patient.[7] Poor bone quality may necessitate incorporation of additional levels into a construct to promote load sharing and enhance stability.

It is difficult to accurately assess bone quality. A general impression of bone mineralization may be gleaned from plain cervical radiographs. Dual-energy x-ray absorptiometry and quantitative CT provide an objective determination of bone mineral density. The clinical use of this technology is limited by the lack of cervical spine standards available for comparison. Also, the influence of bone mineral density on screw fixation biomechanics is poorly understood. Currently it is not possible to predict the holding strength of fixators at the implant-bone junction from preoperative studies.

## Construct Application

Cervical spine integrity may be restored by either ventral or dorsal stabilization techniques. The application of both may be indicated in cases of severe instability, creating a "360 degree" construct. The rationale for selecting one approach over another is case-dependent and relies on the degree and extent of instability. If the site of major instability is ventral, a ventral construct should be created to restore structural integrity to the ventral spine. Dorsal instability is treated most effectively through dorsal stabilization. This general rule is valid for all causes of cervical instability. The underlying disease process does influence the selection of specific construct components and the method by which they are applied.

Neural compression often accompanies cervical instability and must be alleviated before stabilization. Neurologic deficit may result from direct neural compression by the disease process itself, or by attendant spinal instability. Decompressive procedures may exacerbate segmental instability as a result of key load-bearing structures. This is particularly important when disease involvement is extensive. The underlying pathology may predispose to postoperative instability by rendering other load-bearing elements incompetent.

The requirements of neural element decompression influence the approach that is selected for stabilization. Generally, ventral compressive or invasive pathology should be dealt with via a ventral approach. If dorsal neural compression is encountered, a dorsal decompressive procedure is indicated. Internal fixation techniques should attempt to restore the structural integrity of the elements made incompetent by the disease process or the operative resection.

The surgeon must be wary and avoid exacerbation of neural compromise by the process of spinal stabilization. For example, dorsal tension-band fixation may increase ventral neural compression resulting from traumatic intervertebral disc herniation or neoplastic disease. This may produce additional neurologic deficit. Constructs must be designed with consideration for the structural alterations that they may induce, and the effect that this may have on the neural elements. If this is not appreciated, disastrous consequences may follow.

## Ventral Constructs

Ventral cervical spine constructs are designed to restore stability to the ventral spine when the osseous and/or ligamentous structures are incompetent. Intervertebral strut grafts without instrumentation have been used for more than 40 years to reconstitute the ventral load-bearing column of the cervical spine. Methyl methacrylate may be used as an alternative to bony fusion in this region.

Ventral stabilization is usually performed, in conjunction with a ventral decompressive procedure. The corollary of this observation is also true. Ventral decompression is seldom undertaken without subsequent ventral stabilization. This differs from most dorsal decompression or stabilization procedures, which are often performed independently. Dorsal decompression (i.e., cervical laminectomy) is frequently undertaken without stabilization, and dorsal fixation may not require decompression.

A variety of cervical constructs may be applied via the ventral approach. The following review is not exhaustive, but represents the majority of techniques currently used for ventral cervical stabilization.

### Interbody Strut Graft

By definition, a simple interbody strut graft implanted after a ventral cervical discectomy constitutes a ventral cervical construct. Larger grafts are often used for vertebral body replacement after corpectomy for trauma, neoplasia, and spondylotic disease. Ventral strut grafts function predominantly in the simple distraction mode, reconstituting the ventral load-bearing column of the cervical spine. This construct offers excellent resistance to axial compressive loads (Figure 122.1). It also imparts

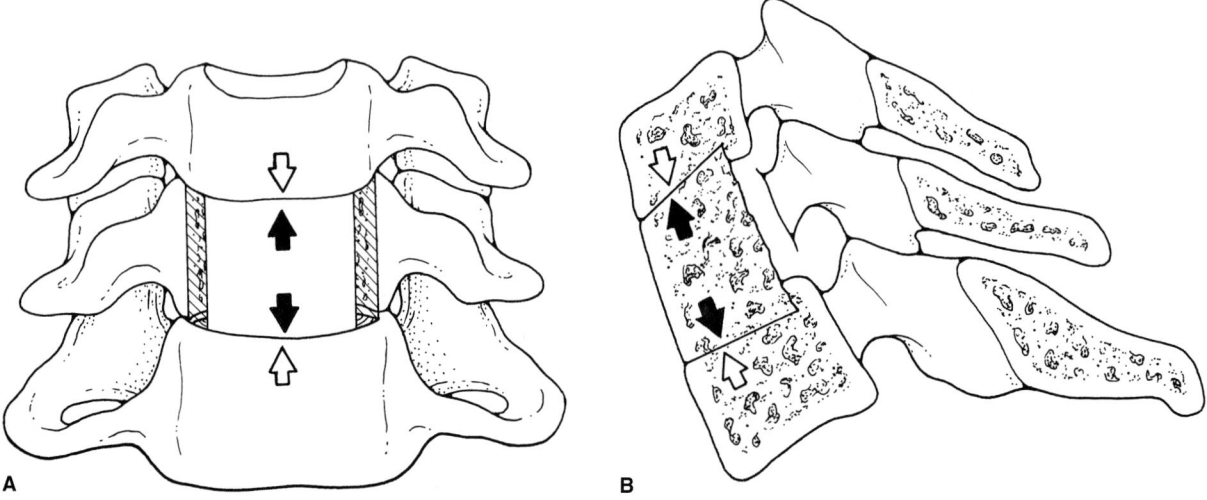

**Figure 122.1** (**A**) Coronal and (**B**) lateral views of an osseous strut graft. This construct functions in a simple distraction mode (*solid arrows*), providing resistance to axial compression (*open arrows*).

some stability in flexion, extension, axial rotation, and lateral bending.[28] In most cases, however, immediate postoperative stability is not provided with a simple strut graft.

Some means of fixation, whether external or internal, is usually required to provide temporary stability while awaiting osseous fusion. The extent of supplemental fixation is dictated by the degree of instability that remains after placement of the bone graft. The instability created by a single-level ventral cervical discectomy may be managed adequately with interbody strut graft placement and immobilization in a cervical collar. More significant instability requires more rigid fixation while the fusion matures. This may be accomplished internally with instrumentation, or externally with an orthosis. In the setting of multilevel corpectomy, some studies suggest that ventral corpectomy with instrumentation be supplemented with dorsal instrumentation to prevent postoperative graft and instrumentation complications.[23,32] However, this is a point of controversy; others have advocated ventral cervical fixation as sufficient for multilevel corpectomy up to four levels.[16]

## Ventral Cervical Plate and Screw Constructs

Ventral cervical plate and screw constructs were developed to provide immediate internal stability before osseous integration of a strut graft. When used in this context, these devices often eliminate the need for postoperative external bracing. All ventral plate constructs reconstitute the ventral tension band, thereby stabilizing most significantly in extension.[14] Some of these devices also provide fixed moment arm cantilever beam fixation, thereby sharing some of the axial load with the strut graft. Rigid implants with locking screw mechanisms function in this capacity. Plating systems that use nonlocking screws are more dynamic implants, and provide less axial load sharing. These devices act as nonfixed moment arm cantilever beam fixators, in addition to their tension-band attributes (Figure 122.2). Dynamic implants such as these

also allow for the graft to be exposed to continuous axial loading. This may facilitate bone fusion.[19]

Biomechanical studies have demonstrated that ventral plates can restore stability to the injured spine in essentially all motion planes, although this is most significant in flexion and extension.[28,31] An interbody bone graft must supplement the instrumentation to effectively stabilize an injured motion segment. The load-bearing capacities of ventral cervical plates are temporary, so all plated segments must be fused to achieve long-term stability.

Ventral cervical plates are affixed with screws at the implant-bone junction. Some devices use screws with bicortical purchase, whereas others use unicortical fixation. Bicortical screw purchase confers greater holding strength to the construct.[25] Placement of bicortical screws is more perilous than unicortical screws, because the dorsal cortex of the vertebral body must be drilled to accept these screws. Caution is required to avoid drilling into the spinal canal and traumatizing the spinal cord. Bicortical screw placement must be monitored with fluoroscopy to minimize the incidence of this complication.[11]

Unicortical screws may be applied with less hazardous results. Fluoroscopy is not mandatory because the dorsal cortex is not violated. Imaging, however, is recommended as a confirmatory intraoperative study.

Indications for ventral cervical plating are extensive. Traumatic lesions that produce persistent instability may require operative stabilization. Unstable injuries involving the vertebral body or intervertebral disc are managed most efficiently by ventral stabilization. This is particularly important when there is compromise of the ventral spinal canal by bone fragments or herniated intervertebral disc material. Cervical burst fractures may require ventral decompression and internal fixation. A strut graft for vertebral body replacement and a ventral plate for immediate internal stability are appropriate construct designs for this indication. Ventral plates should be applied to intact vertebral bodies above and below the involved levels, spanning the instability.

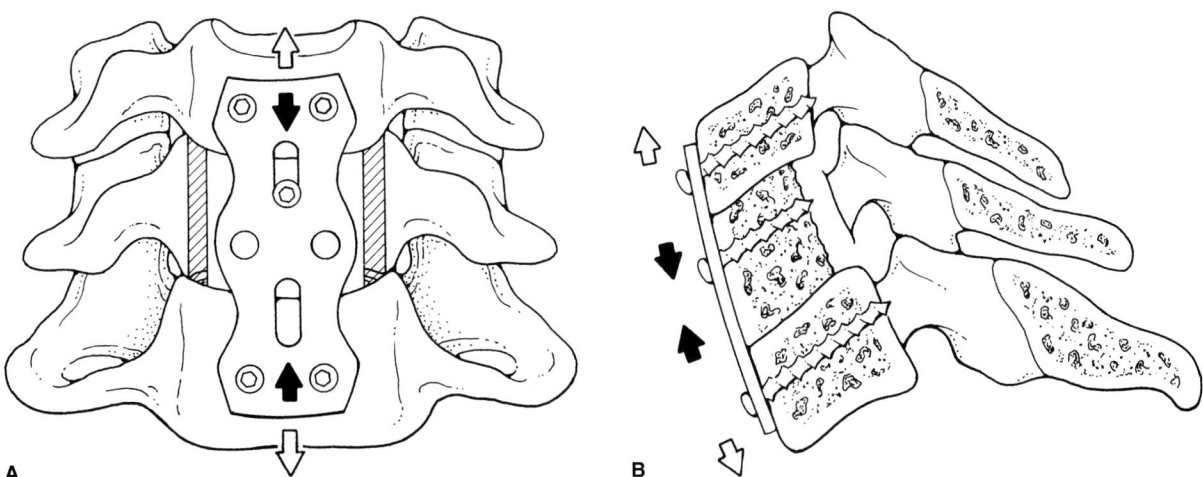

**Figure 122.2** **(A)** Coronal and **(B)** lateral views of a ventral cervical plate (bicortical, unlocked) construct. The plate/screw device reconstitutes the ventral tension band *(solid arrows)*, thereby resisting ventral distraction and extension *(open arrows)*. Axial compressive forces *(not shown)* are resisted by the strut graft, as depicted in Figure 122.1.

Other traumatic lesions may be stabilized ventrally. Irreducible facet dislocations are generally approached dorsally. However, when facet dislocation is complicated by concomitant disc herniation, decompression and reduction may be undertaken via a ventral approach. Stabilization is then accomplished with an interbody bone graft and a ventral plate. Neural decompression must precede reduction of the spinal deformity, thereby minimizing the risk of producing or exacerbating a neurologic deficit.

Spinal neoplasms often involve the vertebral body, potentially causing spinal instability and neurologic dysfunction. Ventral cervical plates may be applied after decompression to reconstruct the axial spine. In these instances screw fixation must be performed in vertebrae that are free of disease.

Cervical spondylotic disease may also be treated by ventral decompression and stabilization, using ventral plates. Kyphotic deformities, regardless of etiology, should be approached ventrally. Corpectomy, strut grafting, and ventral plate stabilization should be considered first-line therapy for this type of spinal deformity.

Ventral cervical plate systems are extremely versatile. They provide substantial immediate postoperative stability, limit the extent of instrumentation, and facilitate aggressive reconstruction of the ventral spine. They may enhance fusion rates and permit early patient mobilization. However, these devices are relatively expensive and require special equipment for installation. Screw and/or plate fracture may occur, resulting in failure of the construct. As with all devices that use screw fixation, ventral plating systems perform poorly in osteoporotic bone.

Cervical cages are another means of stabilizing the anterior column. These devices may be made of titanium, carbon, or other materials. Threaded cages appear to provide greater initial stiffness than the nonthreaded devices.[6,18,26] This fact, however, may be misleading, since subsequent subsidence may lead to a subsequent decrease in stiffness.

## Dorsal Constructs

Dorsal constructs are designed to restore stability to the spine when the dorsal osseous and/or ligamentous structures are incompetent. Several different constructs may be applied via this approach. Basic wiring techniques, incorporating the spinous processes, laminae, or articular facets with or without a bone graft, are time-tested methods used to treat spinal instability. Luque L rods and rectangles have also been used with success in this region. More recently, lateral mass osteosynthetic plates have gained widespread acceptance for dorsal cervical stabilization. Hook/rod devices and interlaminar clamps have also been used for specific applications in the posterior cervical spine.

### Wire Constructs

Dorsal stabilization with wire or braided cables usually entails incorporation of the spinous processes or articular facets, with or without bone autograft. These constructs function primarily by reconstituting the dorsal tension band (Figure 122.3). Dorsal wire constructs provide some stability in flexion, minimal stability in extension, and add little to rotatory or translatory stability.[24] If translational instability exists, dorsal tension-band fixation implants may be inadequate to prevent the "parallelogram effect."[34] This may result in translatory displacement and further spinal deformity. Wiring, alone, does not provide sufficient immediate internal stability in most cases. It must be supplemented with bone graft, methyl methacrylate, or external bracing to augment the construct until bony fusion

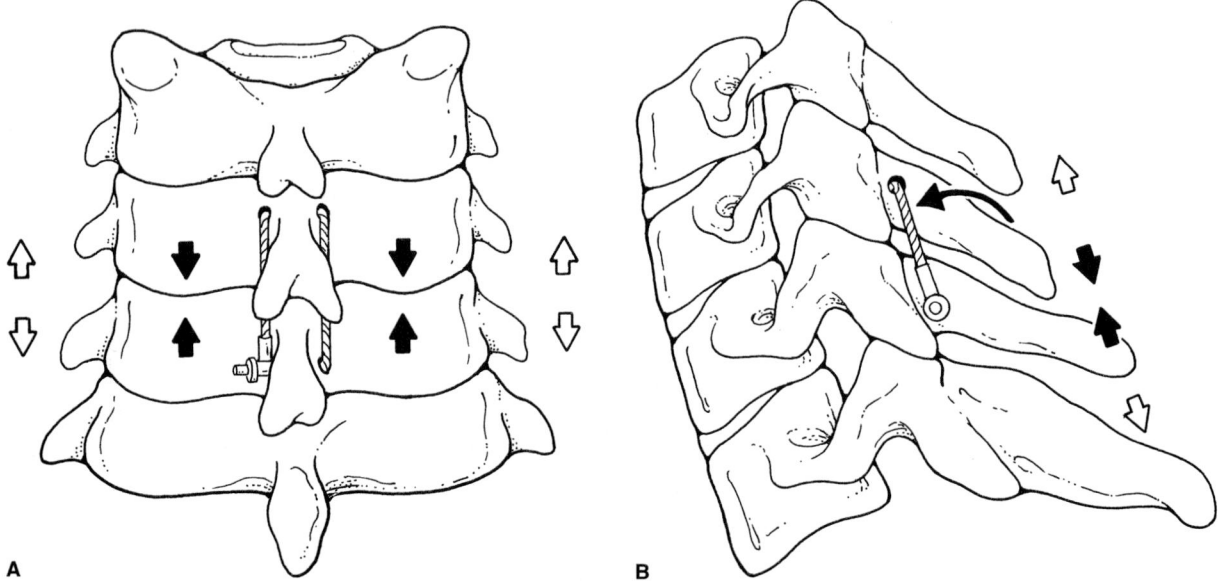

**A**　　　　　　　　　　　　　　　　　　　**B**

**Figure 122.3** **(A)** Coronal and **(B)** lateral views of interspinous cable fixation. This construct reconstitutes the dorsal tension band *(solid arrows)* and resists dorsal distraction *(open arrows)*. As flexion and dorsal distraction are coupled the flexion moment *(curved arrow)* is resisted across the fixed level.

occurs. Still, this is an inexpensive, rapid, and relatively safe method to reconstitute the dorsal tension band, particularly in cases of isolated dorsal ligamentous injury.

Wire constructs may be created with single-strand wire, twisted wire, or braided cables. The latter have the advantage of higher tensile strength, relatively uniform distribution of applied tension, and ease of application. Braided titanium alloy cables are available, and these produce less CT or MRI artifact. Titanium cables are more expensive than wire, although the aforementioned advantages may justify the added cost in many situations.

## Interlaminar Clamps

The dorsal tension band may also be re-created by application of interlaminar clamps. These devices are used rarely, because they are somewhat unwieldy to apply and may be hazardous.[9] These clamps function by reconstituting the dorsal tension band, and may be adequate to restrict flexion. No stability is provided in extension or axial rotation. Extension is prevented by placing the bone graft between the spinous processes. Interlaminar clamps require intact laminae at the levels to be instrumented. They are also prone to experience the parallelogram effect if translatory instability is present.

## Luque L Rods and Rectangles

Originally used for thoracolumbar instability, Luque L rods and rectangles may also be incorporated into dorsal cervical constructs. These devices are usually applied over multiple spinal segments and are secured with sublaminar or facet wires. Alternatively, braided cables may be used to affix the construct at the implant-bone junction. They act principally as rigid implants, reconstructing the dorsal tension band. Additionally, they provide a significant degree of three-point bending fixation (Figure 122.4). These implants stabilize in flexion, extension, and lateral bending modes.

The use of a rectangle rather than two L rods is biomechanically advantageous, because of the strong cross-fixation provided by the rectangle configuration. Torsional

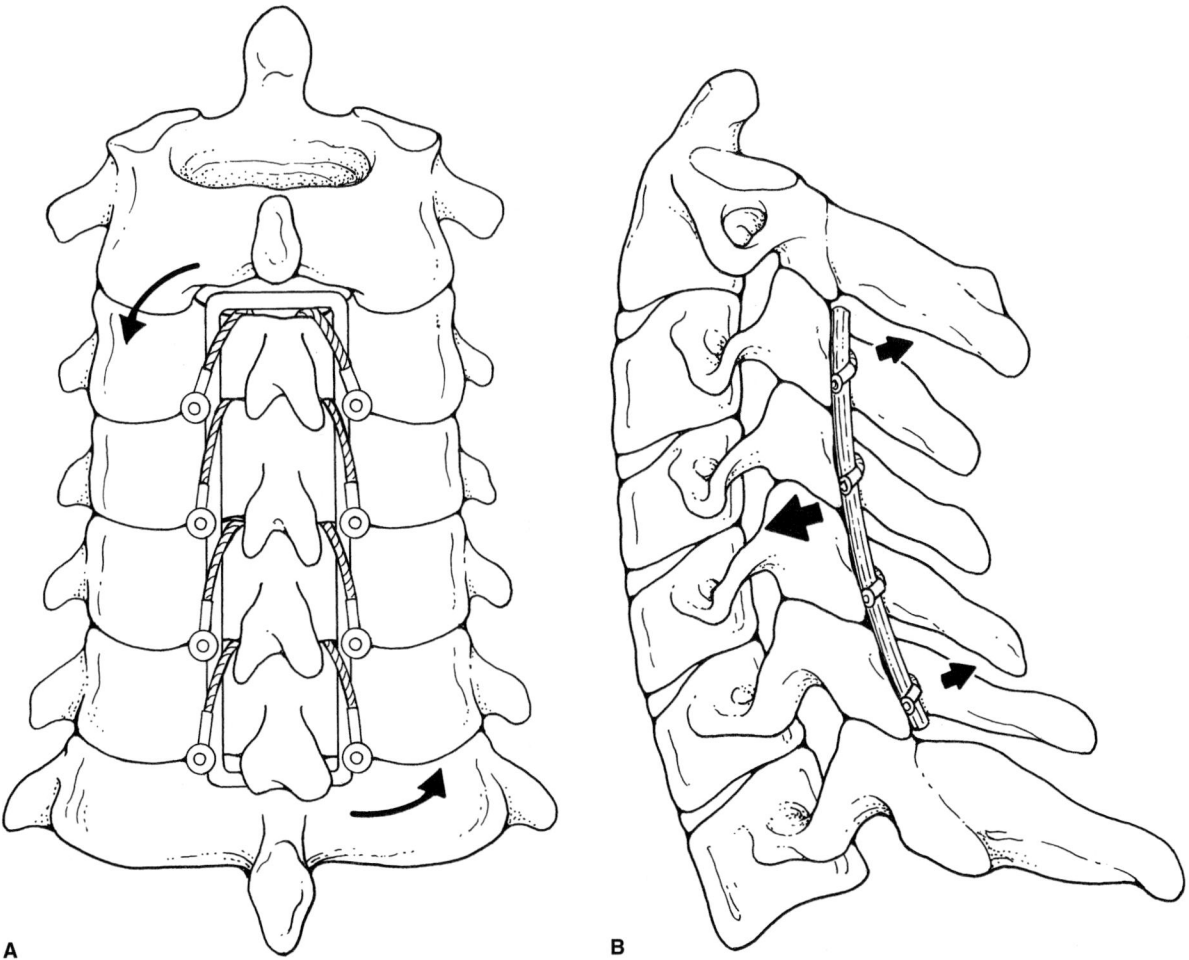

**A**                                                                 **B**

**Figure 122.4** (**A**) Coronal and (**B**) lateral views of a Luque rectangle construct. This device provides three-point bending fixation. Dorsally directed forces are applied at both ends of the construct, with an equal but opposite force applied at the fulcrum (*straight arrows*). Torsional stability (*curved arrows*) is imparted by the strong cross-fixation of the rectangle. Distraction and flexion are also resisted, as this device reconstructs the dorsal tension band. Although the illustration depicts fixation with sublaminar cables, the authors do not recommend sublaminar cable passage in the midcervical spine.

stability is enhanced by this design, and "telescoping" is less likely. These concerns may be partially alleviated by cross-fixation of L rod constructs.

Luque L rods and rectangles are used frequently for the treatment of instability from spinal neoplasia. After dorsal neural decompression, a Luque construct may be applied, if instability or progressive spinal deformity is anticipated. Additionally, this type of construct may be advantageous in patients with poor bone quality. They are fairly simple to apply, inexpensive, and require no special instrumentation to install. However, Luque constructs must often incorporate several motion segments to achieve an adequate biomechanical advantage, thus creating a long fusion. The risk of passing sublaminar wires in the subaxial cervical spine should not be underestimated, particularly if the canal diameter has been further compromised by spondylotic disease, traumatic injury, or neoplasm. In such cases fixation to the spinous processes, facets, or lateral masses is preferable.

### Lateral Mass Plate Fixation

Dorsal cervical stabilization has been revolutionized by the development of lateral mass plate and screw fixation systems. These devices provide a high degree of immediate internal stability, often eliminating the need for postoperative external immobilization or bracing. Lateral mass plates are dynamic implants, and behave primarily as non-fixed moment arm cantilever beam fixators. They also provide some dorsal tension-band fixation (Figure 122.5). Biomechanical studies have demonstrated the ability of these devices to restore stiffness to the injured spine in flexion, extension, and torsion.[13,17] Similar to other constructs that restore the dorsal tension band, lateral mass plates are probably weakest in extension.[5,24]

Lateral mass plates may be used to treat instability from C2 to T1. Posttraumatic instability provides the most common indication for the use of lateral mass plates.[15,30] Dorsal ligamentous injury and irreducible unilateral or bilateral facet dislocations may be stabilized effectively with this type of construct after reduction of malalignment. In these cases instrumentation across the affected segment alone is usually adequate to restore stability. A longer construct may be required if instability of a single motion segment is severe, or if the dorsal elements at the level of instability are not intact. Multiple segments of instability may also mandate instrumentation of additional levels to achieve an adequate biomechanical advantage.

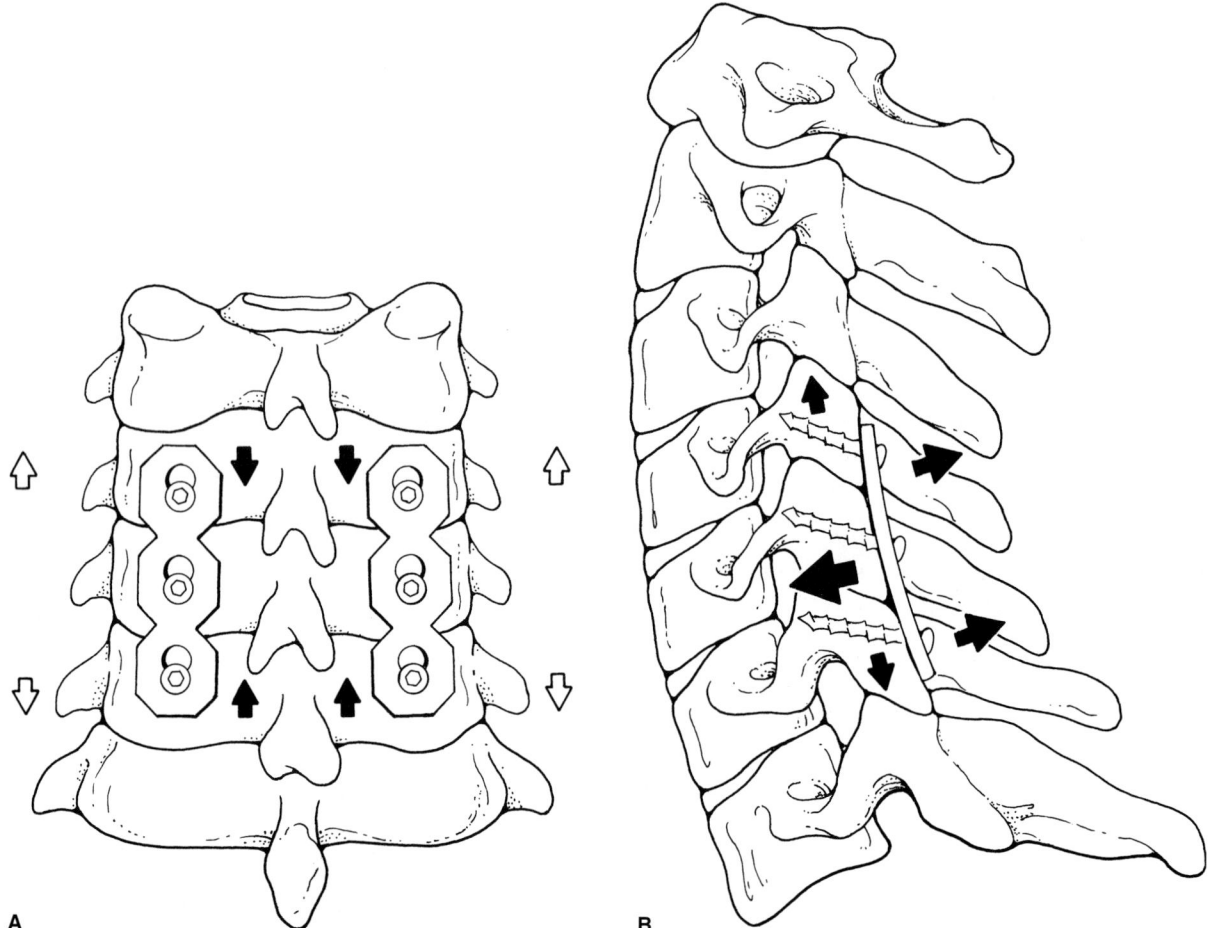

**A**     **B**

**Figure 122.5** (**A**) Coronal and (**B**) lateral views of a lateral mass plate construct. This device provides stabilization in all motion planes, using tension band (*solid, large vertical arrows* in **A**), three-point bending (*solid horizontal arrows* in **B**), and cantilever beam fixation (*solid, small vertical arrows* in **C**).

Unstable fractures of the dorsal cervical elements may be treated with lateral mass plates or hook/rod constructs. Fractures of the articular facet, pedicle, and/or lamina at a given level usually require a multilevel construct to restore stability. An intact level above and below the site of injury should be instrumented. Instability arising from vertebral body fractures has been successfully treated with lateral mass plates, usually incorporating multiple levels into the construct. This should only be attempted when the articular facets at that level are intact, because they must contribute to axial load bearing in this situation. In most cases of vertebral body injury a ventral approach is indicated. Certainly, if ventral spinal canal compromise is present, decompression and stabilization with a ventral construct should be considered.

Lateral mass plating may also be used to re-establish stability after spinal tumor resection. The extent of instrumentation depends on the size and site of the tumor, but in general, several segments above and below the affected levels should be incorporated.[30] Lateral mass screws should be placed only in bone that is free of disease.

Instability created by degenerative disease may be treated with lateral mass plates. This is particularly effective when the dorsal load-bearing elements are incompetent. Additionally, these devices may be applied at the time of laminectomy to prevent progressive kyphotic deformity in patients who are deemed to be at risk. This is more effective than attempting to treat an established kyphotic deformity with dorsal instrumentation, because lateral mass plates are at a mechanical disadvantage in the latter. Ventral decompression and stabilization should be considered in this situation.

Excellent results have been reported using lateral mass plates without fusion.[15,24] However, long-term structural stability is augmented by incorporating bone graft into the construct. This may be accomplished by denuding the articular processes at the unstable level(s) and packing cancellous bone graft into the joint space. Often, adequate material for bone autograft may be obtained from adjacent spinous processes or from bone removed during decompression.

Advantages of lateral mass plates over other dorsal construct designs include superior biomechanical stability in essentially all planes, and applicability to a variety of clinical settings. These devices may be applied in the presence of extensive laminectomies or dorsal element fracture. They provide immediate postoperative stability without passage of sublaminar wires. Their installation may prolong the operative procedure somewhat, and requires special equipment and technical expertise. Use of these devices should be avoided in patients with inferior bone quality, because screw fixation systems perform poorly in this setting. If screws are used in this situation, postoperative immobilization in a halo vest or Minerva apparatus should be considered.

Recently developed cervical hook/rod systems have many of the same advantages of lateral mass plates, while being easier to install. Polyaxial screws allow the lateral mass screws to be applied in the appropriate trajectory, with the appropriately conformed rod applied after screw application. This is in contrast to lateral mass plates, in which the shape of the plate and placement of screw holes can occasionally dictate screw placement. These systems provide rigid fixation that is biomechanically superior to that of the semirigid lateral mass plates.[21]

Cervical pedicle screws have also been shown to provide appropriate dorsal stabilization for the cervical spine.[1-3] However, cervical pedicle screws are significantly more difficult to place than lateral mass screws, and they carry a higher risk of injury to the nerve root and the vertebral artery. Lateral mass screws are probably equally effective in biomechanical stabilization, and are safer in most situations.

## 360 Degree Constructs

Occasionally, cervical spinal instability will be so severe that it warrants both ventral and dorsal stabilization, creating a "360 degree" construct. This approach is usually reserved for situations of ventral and dorsal instability. A 360 degree construct may also be indicated when extensive instability is anticipated from progression of underlying disease. This may be encountered in cases of advanced malignancy or extensive degenerative disease. To justify a 360 degree procedure, there must be a reasonable concern that instability will persist or recur, despite stabilization via an isolated ventral or dorsal approach.

Constructs that use wire-reinforced methyl methacrylate may be used for treatment of instability created by neoplastic disease. The biomechanical stability of methyl methacrylate reconstruction is optimized when a 360 degree construct is applied. Ventral stabilization is usually performed after decompression.

A methyl methacrylate strut may be used as a vertebral body replacement. More commonly, fibular strut grafts are used ventrally to span multiple vertebral levels. Struts function in a simple distraction mode, effectively resisting compressive axial loads (Figure 122.6A). This can be supplemented by threaded Kirschner wires (K-wires), which are embedded into the vertebral bodies above and below the involved region. These devices prevent strut migration and provide some resistance to translatory forces.

A dorsal polymethylmethacrylate (PMMA) or fibular strut construct should be applied, in conjunction with ventral stabilization, which completes the 360 degree construct. Several techniques have been described for application of this material to the dorsal cervical spine. With one such method, K-wires are passed through the spinous processes, are bent, and then are encased in PMMA. These wires provide an increased surface area for interdigitation junction bonding between bone, wire, and cement.[34] The net result is an increase in the tensile load-bearing capacity of the construct.

The dorsal methyl methacrylate-wire construct functions primarily as a dorsal tension-band fixator (see Figure 122.6B and C). Some three-point bending fixation is also provided. When applied in this manner, 360 degree methyl methacrylate constructs provide a substantial degree of immediate internal stability in virtually all motion planes.[34] It must be remembered that, in contrast to an osseous fusion, the strength of a methyl methacrylate construct is maximal initially and decreases over time. This type of construct is generally reserved for treatment of cervical instability associated with progressive spinal

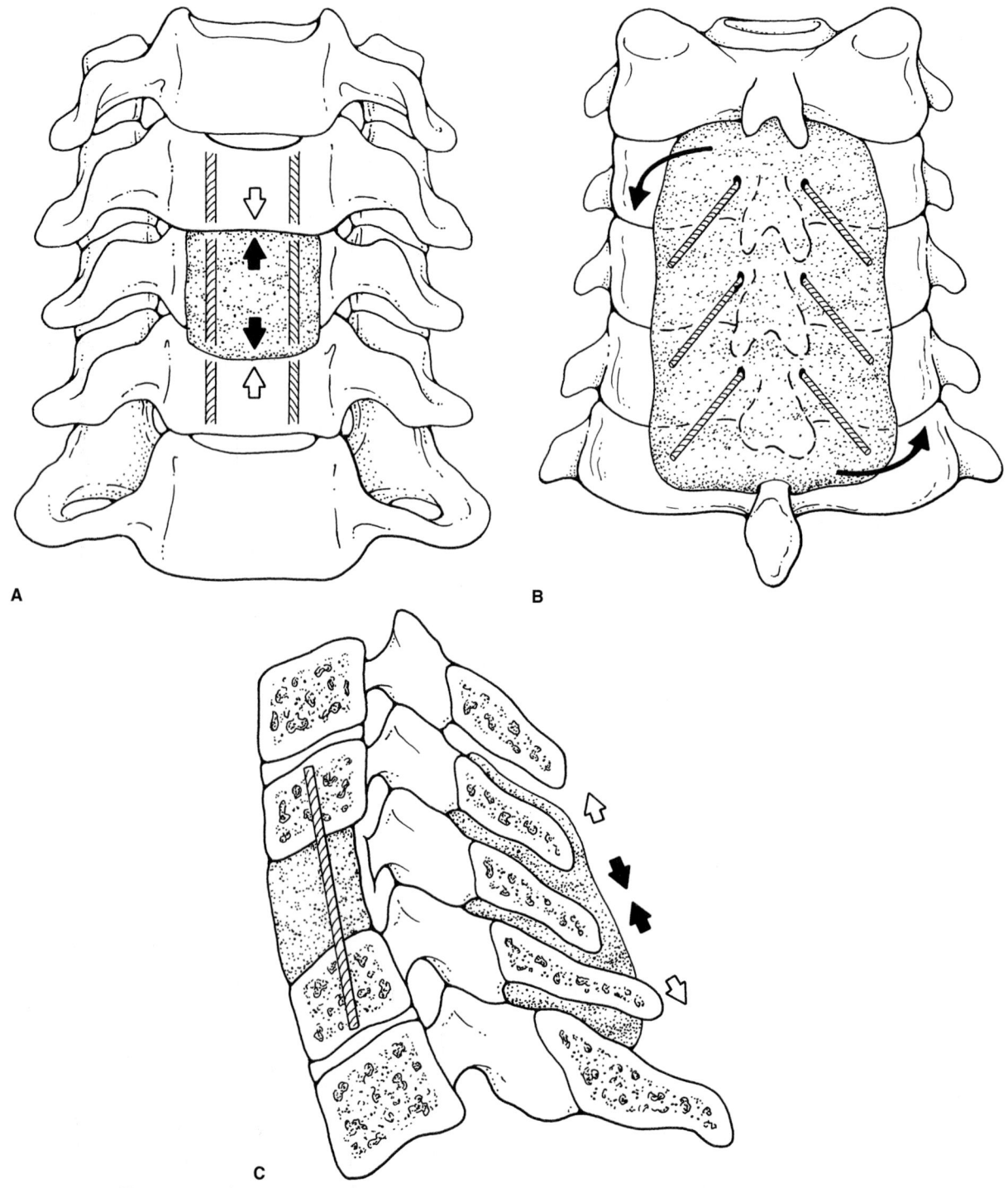

**Figure 122.6** **(A)** Ventral, **(B)** dorsal coronal, and **(C)** sagittal views of a 360 degree wire-reinforced methyl methacrylate construct. The ventral strut provides simple distraction fixation *(solid arrows)*, resisting axial compressive loads *(open arrows [**A**])*. The dorsal construct imparts torsional stability *(curved arrows [**B**])*. It also functions as a dorsal tension band *(solid arrows)*, resisting distraction and flexion *(open arrows [**C**])*.

malignancy. This is a purely palliative procedure, and is not intended for long-term stabilization. It should be used only in patients with a limited life expectancy. Methyl methacrylate has been used for the treatment of traumatic instability,[10] although this material probably should be avoided because other constructs are superior in this context.

Methyl methacrylate constructs are relatively simple and safe to apply. They provide significant immediate internal stability in multiple planes. Special instrumentation is not required, and the materials used are inexpensive. The major shortcoming of this construct is that its long-term stability is suspect. There is no attempt to create an osseous fusion. As a result, the full extent of load bearing must be assumed indefinitely by the cement-wire construct.

A 360-degree construct is occasionally used for treatment of instability created by benign disease. If the nature and extent of instability are such that a single approach would not adequately restore structural integrity, a 360 degree construct must be considered. This situation is occasionally encountered with multilevel procedures when there is preexisting instability and/or deformity. When an osseous strut graft is internally stabilized with a ventral plate, only two motion segments are actually fixed. The intervening motion segments may require dorsal fixation to provide optimal stability to the construct in cases of extreme instability.

Ventral and dorsal cervical plating systems may be applied concurrently, in conjunction with appropriate bone grafting. In most cases these devices should confer an optimal biomechanical advantage to the construct, providing immediate internal stability in all motion planes. Other constructs may be devised if screw fixation is contraindicated by poor bone quality. These situations are rare and necessitate individualized management. However, fundamental construct design concepts should guide the selection and application of hardware systems, just as in less complex problems of instability.

## Economic Considerations

Historically, economic considerations have not been major determinants in the process of construct design. This is no longer true because rising health care costs and declining reimbursement mandate some fiscal responsibility. Material costs represent only a fraction of the expense accrued with spinal instrumentation. Surgeons' fees, operative time, anesthesia support, and fluoroscopy costs (if required) all reflect the complexity of a stabilization procedure. Thousands of dollars may be expended to apply a single construct. With this in mind, it is financially irresponsible to implant an elaborate, costly system when a less expensive alternative could suffice. However, the structural integrity of a construct should not be compromised for purely economic concerns. The spinal surgeon must use restraint in the construct design process, minimizing expenses when possible.

## Supplementary External Immobilization

The need for postoperative external immobilization may be reduced or eliminated when internal fixation provides immediate stability to a construct. Orthoses are selected in accordance with the nature and extent of preoperative instability, quality of the construct, cause of instability, and extent of residual disease. Young patients with isolated dorsal instability can be managed in a soft cervical collar for 4 weeks after most instrumentation procedures. Patients with more severe instability or residual disease require more aggressive postoperative bracing. A hard cervical collar is probably adequate in most cases. Those with osteoporosis, severe preoperative instability, and/or

biomechanically inferior constructs that do not provide sufficient immediate internal stability require postoperative halo vest or Minerva immobilization.[30] Regardless of the bracing method, all patients should be assessed often with serial examinations and radiographs until an osseous fusion is attained.

## REFERENCES

1. Abumi K, Kaneda K: Pedicle screw fixation for nontraumatic lesions of the cervical spine. *Spine* 22: 1853-1863, 1997.
2. Abumi K, Kaneda K, Shono Y, et al: One-stage posterior decompression and reconstruction of the cervical spine by using pedicle screw fixation systems. *J Neurosurg* 90 (1 Suppl):19-26, 1999.
3. Abumi K, Shono Y, Ito M, et al: Complications of pedicle screw fixation in reconstructive surgery of the cervical spine. *Spine* 25:962-969, 2000.
4. Albert TJ, Vacarro A: Postlaminectomy kyphosis. *Spine* 23:2738-2745, 1998.
5. Anderson PA, Henley MB, Grady MS, et al: Posterior cervical arthrodesis with AO reconstruction plates and bone graft. *Spine* 16:S72-S79, 1991.
6. Assietti R, Beretta F, Arienta C: Two level anterior cervical discectomy and cage-assisted fusion without plates. *Neurosurg Focus* 12(1):Article 3, 2002.
7. Benzel EC: Construct design. In Benzel EC (ed): *Biomechanics of Spine Stabilization: Principles and Clinical Practice*. New York, McGraw-Hill, 1995, pp 163-172.
8. Benzel EC: Mechanical (quantitative) attributes of spinal implants: construct types. In Benzel EC (ed): *Biomechanics of Spine Stabilization: Principles and Clinical Practice*. New York, McGraw-Hill, 1995, pp 151-162.
9. Benzel EC: Qualitative attributes of spinal implants. In Benzel EC (ed): *Biomechanics of Spine Stabilization: Principles and Clinical Practice*. New York, McGraw-Hill, 1995, pp 135-150.
10. Branch CL, Kelly DL, Davis CH, et al: Fixation of fractures of the lower cervical spine using methylmethacrylate and wire: technique and results in 99 patients. *Neurosurgery* 25:503-513, 1989.
11. Caspar W: *Anterior Cervical Fusion and Interbody Stabilization With the Trapezoidal Osteosynthetic Plate Technique*. Aesculap Scientific Information. Tuttlingen, Germany, Aesculap-Werke-AG, 1986.
12. Cloward R: Gas-sterilized cadaver bone grafts for spinal fusion operations. A simplified bone bank. *Spine* 5:410, 1980.
13. Coe JD, Warden KE, Sutterlin CE III, et al: Biomechanical evaluation of cervical spinal stabilization methods in a human cadaveric model. *Spine* 14:1122-1131, 1989.
14. de Oliveira JC: Anterior plate fixation of traumatic lesions of the lower cervical spine. *Spine* 12:324-329, 1987.
15. Fehlings MG, Cooper PR, Errico TJ: Posterior plates in the management of cervical instability: long-term results in 44 patients. *J Neurosurg* 81:341-349, 1994.
16. Fessler RG, Barua M, Traynelis VC: Anterior cervical plate stabilization following multilevel corpectomy. Presented at the Cervical Spine Research Society, Monterey, CA, November 2001.

17. Gill K, Paschal S, Corin J, *et al*: Posterior plating of the cervical spine. A biomechanical comparison of different posterior fusion techniques. *Spine* 13:813-816, 1988.

18. Hacker RJ, Cauthen JC, Gilbert TJ, *et al*: A prospective randomized multicenter clinical evaluation of an anterior cervical cage. *Spine* 25:2646-2655, 2000.

19. Haid RW, Foley KT, Rodts GE, *et al*: The Cervical Spine Study Group anterior cervical plate nomenclature. *Neurosurg Focus* 12(1):Article 15, 2002.

20. McAfee PC, Farey ID, Sutterlin CE, *et al*: Device-related osteoporosis with spinal instrumentation. *Spine* 14: 919-926, 1989.

21. Mummaneni PV, Haid RW, Traynelis VC, *et al*: Posterior cervical fixation using a new polyaxial screw and rod system: technique and surgical results. *Neurosurg Focus* 12(1):Article 8, 2002.

22. Nasca RJ, Whelchel JD: Use of cryopreserved bone in spinal surgery. *Spine* 12:222-227, 1987.

23. Riew KD, Sethi NS, Devney J, *et al*: Complications of buttress plate stabilization of cervical corpectomy. *Spine* 24:2404-2410, 1999.

24. Roy-Camille R, Saillanr G, Mazel C: Internal fixation of the unstable cervical spine by posterior osteosynthesis with plates and screws. In The Cervical Spine Research Society Editorial Committee (eds): *The Cervical Spine*, ed 2. Philadelphia, Lippincott-Raven, 1989, pp 390-404.

25. Ryken TC, Goel VK, Clause JD, *et al*: Assessment of unicortical and bicortical fixation in a quasistatic cadaveric model. Role of bone mineral density and screw torque. *Spine* 20:1861-1867, 1995.

26. Salame K, Ouaknine GER, Razon N, *et al*: The use of carbon fiber cages in anterior cervical interbody fusion. Report of 100 cases. *Neurosurg Focus* 12(1):Article 1, 2002.

27. Sawin PD, Traynelis VC, Menezes AH: A comparative analysis of fusion rates and donor-site morbidity for autogeneic rib and iliac crest bone grafts in posterior cervical fusions. *J Neurosurg* 88:255-265, 1998.

28. Schulte K, Clark CR, Goel VK: Kinematics of the cervical spine following discectomy and stabilization. *Spine* 14: 1116-1121, 1989.

29. Stabler CL, Eismont FJ, Brown MD, *et al*: Failure of posterior cervical fusions using cadaver bone graft in children. *J Bone Joint Surg* 67A:370-375, 1985.

30. Traynelis VC: Anterior and posterior plate stabilization of the cervical spine. *Neurosurgery* 2:59-76, 1992.

31. Traynelis VC, Donaher PA, Roach RM, *et al*: Biomechanical comparison of anterior Caspar plate and three level posterior fixation techniques in a human cadaveric model. *J Neurosurg* 79:96-103, 1993.

32. Vaccaro AR, Falatyn SP, Scuderi GJ, *et al*: Early failure of long segment anterior cervical plate fixation. *J Spinal Disord* 11:410-415, 1998.

33. White AA, Hirsch C: An experimental study of the immediate load bearing capacity of some commonly used iliac bone grafts. *Acta Orthop Scand* 42:482-490, 1971.

34. White AA, Panjabi MM: Biomechanical considerations in the surgical management of the spine. In White AA, Panjabi MM (eds): *Clinical Biomechanics of the Spine*, ed 2. Philadelphia, Lippincott-Raven, 1990, pp 511-639.

35. Zhang ZH, Yin H, Yang K, *et al*: Anterior intervertebral disc excision and bone grafting in cervical spondylotic myelopathy. *Spine* 8:16-19, 1983.

# CHAPTER 123

# Thoracic and Lumbar Spine Construct Design

## Darrel S. Brodke, Setti S. Rengachary, and Edward C. Benzel

Construct design is a process that formulates a specific blueprint for an orderly and thoughtful assembly of implantable spinal instrumentation, designed to correct instability and/or deformity of the spinal column.[3] It requires specific understanding of the deformity or instability and the biomechanical forces acting on the pathologic alignment. In addition, an understanding of corrective forces, and where they must be applied, is required. A keen knowledge of the anatomy and pathoanatomy is required to preserve neuralgic function and avoid adjacent segment injury. Although skillful assembly of the mechanical construct is a definite prerequisite, what determines the ultimate success is the orderly thought process for designing the construct, based on personal experience, experience of others, and laboratory data. Creating a preoperative plan, or blueprint, can focus this design process. Spine instrumentation surgery must not be assumed to be strictly "mechanical" or "routine"; rather, it requires serious and meticulous planning to ensure success.

## Nomenclature

The nomenclature of spinal instrumentation is somewhat complex and often confusing at the start. Factors that contribute to this complexity are the numerous components that constitute assembly, the numerous choices for purchase sites in the spine, and the variations in the mode of assembly of the hardware. There are four major categories: (1) *anchors*, devices that attach the construct to the bony spine (e.g., pedicle screws, cables, hooks), (2) *longitudinal members* (e.g., rods or plates), (3) *connectors*, devices that connect anchors to the longitudinal members or connect two longitudinal members (cross connectors), and (4) *accessories* (e.g., washers or spacers). Most spinal instrumentation systems have all four of these components. The skill in designing a construct is reflected in the optimal choice of implants that result in a biomechanically stable architecture.

## Indications for Spinal Instrumentation

Spinal implants may be considered as internal supports that immobilize the spine until bony fusion occurs. Unlike external orthoses that serve similar functions, spinal implants provide direct control of spinal segments, and have a much broader scope.

The goals of spinal instrumentation are threefold. The first goal is the immediate restoration of stability, such that the patient may be prepared for early rehabilitation efforts. Immediate stability often decreases pain and may improve early function. It may also increase the success of bone union or fusion. The second goal of instrumentation is indirect decompression of neural structures, often accomplished by controlled distraction. The instrumentation may also be used to restore or maintain physiologic alignment of the spine. The third goal of spinal instrumentation is the correction of deformity to prevent pain or neurologic compromise, and the neutralization of pathologic, deforming forces. Surgeons designing a spinal instrumentation construct should clearly delineate which of the aforementioned goals, or which combination of goals, they are attempting to achieve.

## Construct Types (Modes of Force Application)

The six fundamental construct types are simple distraction, three-point bending, tension-band fixation, fixed moment arm cantilever beam fixation, nonfixed moment arm cantilever beam fixation, and applied moment arm cantilever beam fixation (Figure 123.1).

## Development of Construct Blueprint

Preoperative development of a blueprint for implant placement, based on the composite information obtained from clinical assessment and imaging studies, ensures a definitive plan and saves time in the operating room. Some plasticity in this plan may be required after surgical exposure of the bony spine, as a result of unexpected findings. For instance, minor fractures at the implant-anchor site may necessitate deviation from the original plan.

A simple scheme should be used that provides: (1) information about the level of the lesion or the level of the unstable segment(s), (2) the types of implants to be used (anchors, longitudinal members, and cross connectors), (3) the length of stabilization required on either side of the lesion, and (4) the mode of load bearing by the construct. The scheme guides selection of the appropriate implant components in advance, improves the intraoperative communication between surgeons and assistants, and enhances the chances of success.

Although the concept of construct design encompasses similar principles in all anatomic regions of the spine, designing a thoracolumbar construct poses more challenges than most cervical constructs. A variety of constructs, using a variety of anchors in various bony landmarks, each used in a variety of mechanical modes (i.e., compression, distraction, neutralization, distraction followed by compression, or distraction and compression at different segmental levels), may be placed in a successful construct. In consideration of these complex decision-making dilemmas, this chapter focuses on thoracic and lumbar fixation design strategies.

### Line Drawing of the Proposed Construct

A simple dorsoventral and/or lateral line drawing of the spine provides a framework for the clear definition of

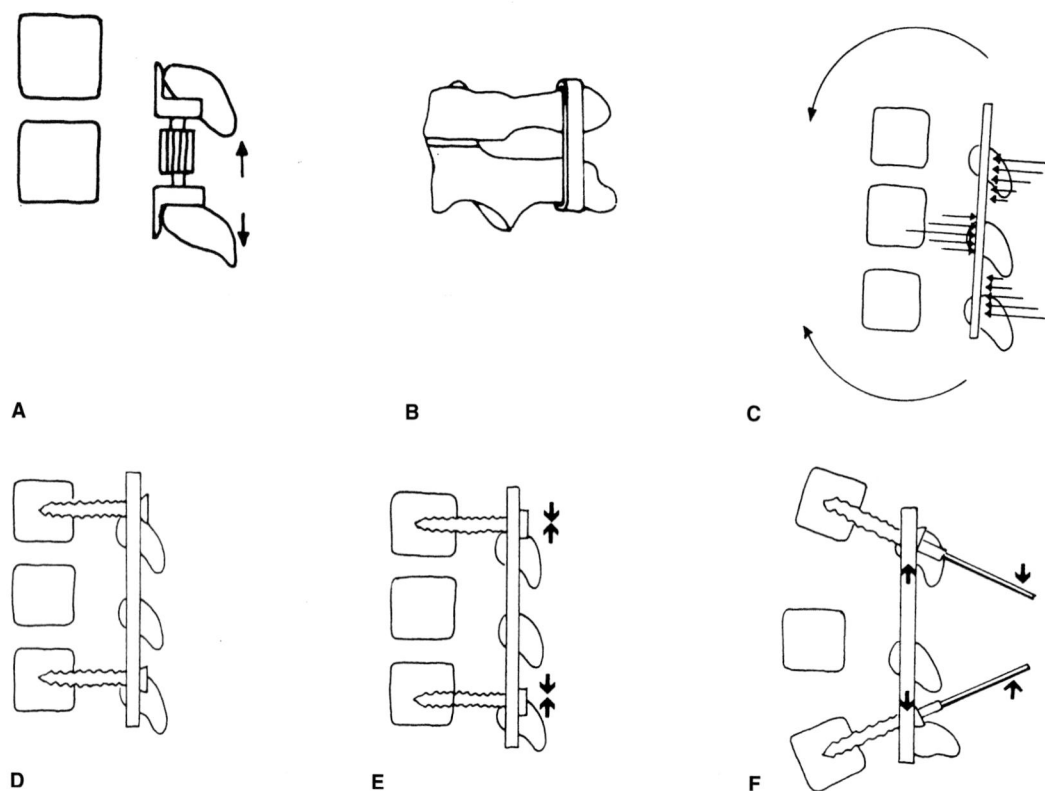

**Figure 123.1** The application of forces to a construct can be broadly categorized into **(A)** *simple distraction* (e.g., Knodt rod), **(B)** tension-band fixation (e.g., spinous process wiring), **(C)** three-point bending using the middle point as a fulcrum (e.g., Harrington rods), **(D)** nonfixed moment arm cantilever design in which axial load cannot be resisted because of nonrigid fixation between the screw and the longitudinal member (e.g., lateral mass plates), **(E)** fixed moment arm cantilever design in which axial loading forces can be resisted because the screws are rigidly fixed to the longitudinal member (e.g., locking cervical plate systems), and **(F)** applied moment arm cantilever design in which complex forces can be applied (e.g., universal spinal instrumentation).

the operative plan. Often only a dorsoventral drawing is necessary, although clear consideration of any sagittal plane deformity is vital. The line drawing provides the blueprint for surgery (Figure 123.2).[4]

The convention used in this chapter, with regard to dorsoventral line drawing, dictates that the left side of the drawing portrays the left side of the patient (i.e., the drawing portrays the patient as viewed from behind). This is in accordance with the most common surgical approaches for complex instrumentation constructs, and decreases the chance for confusion.

### Level of Lesion and Level of Fusion

The designation for the level of the lesion or location of instability, the levels to be fused, and the type of fusion should next be placed on the line drawing. The level(s) of instability or lesion is designated by an "x," and the precise extent of proposed bony fusion is designated by a hatched outline. The number of unstable motion segments should be assessed carefully, as should associated deformity. These factors determine the number of levels to be spanned with the construct. The choice of implants also plays into this decision.

Hook constructs, often used in the past throughout the spine and still currently used in the thoracic region, should incorporate three spinal levels above and two spinal segments below the limits of the lesion (3A-2B rule). If the patient has a marked angular kyphotic deformity, and if three-point bending is considered in an attempt to reduce the deformity, then inclusion of four or more spinal levels above the lesion is common (4A-2B rule) and may provide a more functional lever arm. It is emphasized that such long constructs are suited mostly for lesions in the middle and upper thoracic regions, although thoracic pedicle screws are gaining in popularity, even in these regions.

In the lower thoracic spine (T8-10), the thoracolumbar junction (T11 to L1), and the lumbar region (L2-5), pedicle screw constructs are often preferred. The size of the pedicles, and the increased stiffness these screws provide, make them an ideal choice. Short-segment fixation, with the inclusion of only one vertebra immediately above and below the lesion, is appropriate if the anterior, load-bearing column is intact and kyphotic deformity is not present. The bone structure must also be of sufficient strength. With increasingly sophisticated fixation choices available, it must be remembered that a rigid, stable

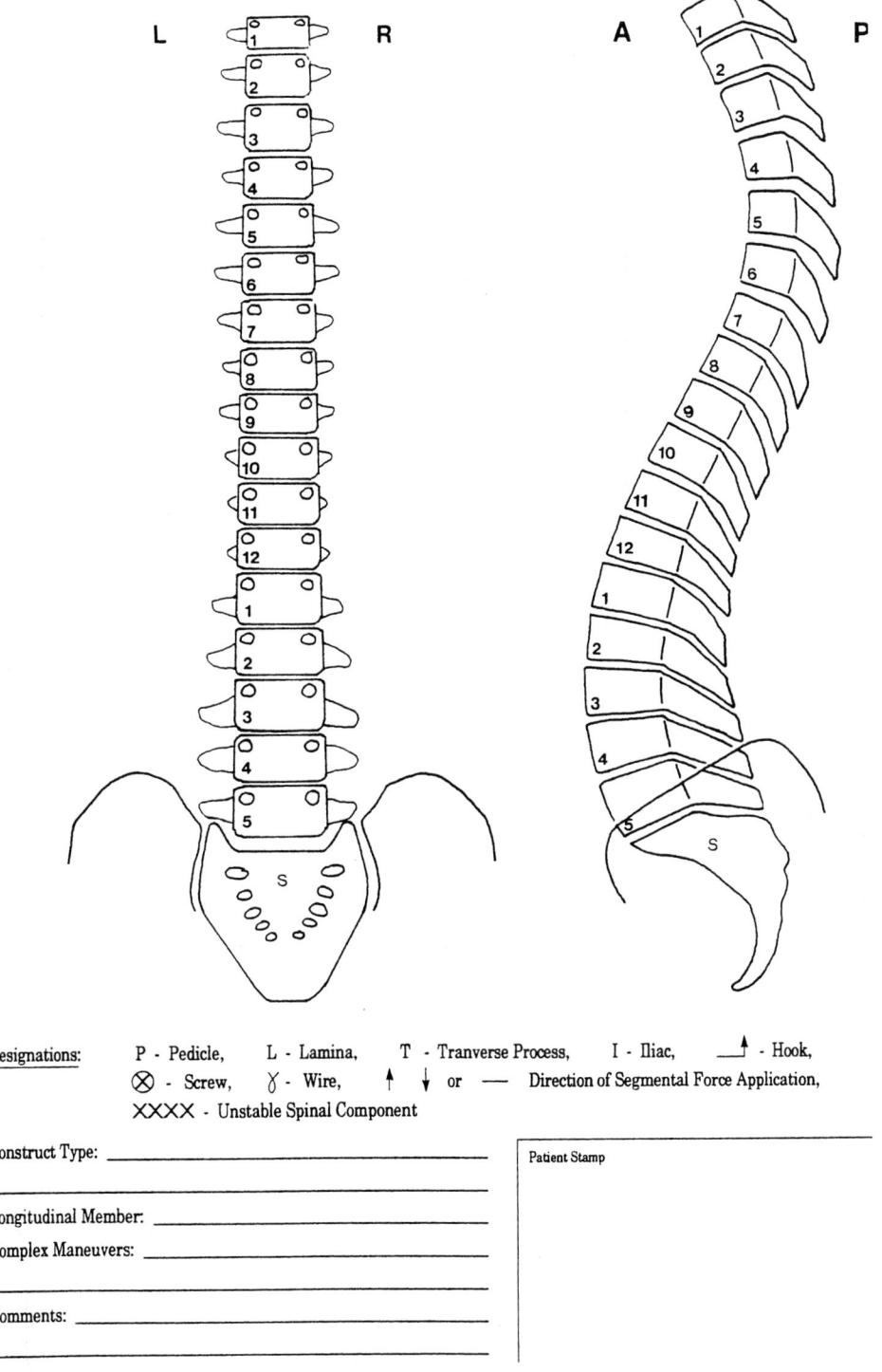

Designations: P - Pedicle, L - Lamina, T - Tranverse Process, I - Iliac, ⌐↑ - Hook,
⊗ - Screw, ૪ - Wire, ↑ ↓ or — Direction of Segmental Force Application,
XXXX - Unstable Spinal Component

Construct Type: _____

Longitudinal Member: _____

Complex Maneuvers: _____

Comments: _____

Patient Stamp

**Figure 123.2** A blueprint of the proposed surgery is helpful in clarifying the treatment plan for both the surgeon and operating team. *(From Benzel EC: Construct design. In Benzel EC (ed): Spinal Instrumentation. Chicago, AANS Publications, 1994, pp 239-256.)*

construct is the goal, and biology and biomechanics surrounding the implants must be taken into account.

## Depiction of Implant Components

The type of implant components used in the instrumentation construct should be delineated clearly on the blueprint. The implant component at each implant-bone juncture may be a cable, hook, or screw. The convention used here is to designate hooks by a right-angled arrow, with the arrowhead pointing in the direction of the orientation of the hook. The purchase site, and therefore the type of hook, is further designated by "P" (for pedicle), "L" (for laminar or sublaminar), or "T" (for transverse process). Screws are designated by an "x" surrounded by a circle and placed over pedicles. Cable (or wire) is depicted as a loop.

The mode of axial load application (distraction, compression, or neutral) at each implant-bone juncture is depicted as an arrow. The arrow points in the direction of force application for distraction and compression, or a horizontal line for neutral. Bending moments are difficult to depict accurately on the line drawing and are described. 

The modes of application of each segmental level are depicted with arrows and lines, as previously described. These are drawn lateral to the designations of implant types. If sagittal plane forces are to be applied, they are depicted on the lateral line drawing. Finally, cross-fixator locations can be designated by rectangles with circles.

## Mechanical Attributes of Spinal Implants: Construct Type

The mechanism that the construct uses (types of construct) to bear loads is also designated. There are six methods of load bearing that are associated with the six construct types: distraction, three-point bending, tension-band fixation, fixed moment arm cantilever beam, non-fixed moment arm cantilever beam, and applied moment arm cantilever beam. It is difficult to depict this information on the line drawing. Therefore this information may be recorded in the space provided at the bottom of the drawing.

## Construct Design Strategies

Multiple factors should be taken into account in designing a spinal instrumentation construct.[10] Consideration should be given specifically to bony integrity, the location of the unstable spinal segment, the implant length with respect to the unstable segment, the need for cross-fixation, the need for dural decompression, the choice of ventral versus dorsal instrumentation, availability of specific instrumentation, metallic composition of instrumentation, and the surgeon's familiarity with a particular technique. Each factor should be adequately addressed to achieve optimal outcome.

### Bony Integrity

Osteoporosis poses a significant problem in spinal instrumentation. Hooks and cables may resist pull-out better than bone screws.[6,9] A longer construct is often required in osteoporotic bone. More anchors are needed to distribute the load over more segments, thereby decreasing the load at any single site. Interbody stability, either from fully collapsed disks or interbody implants, may protect the posterior construct from cantilever pull-out. If pedicle screws are required in a patient with marked osteoporosis, consideration should be given to filling the screw tracks with polymethylmethacrylate (PMMA). This significantly increases screw pull-out strength, and is accomplished by first placing and then removing the pedicle screw. The pedicle must be carefully assessed to be sure no cortical penetration has occurred that would allow the methacrylate to leak. The PMMA is then placed, using a large syringe, under minimal pressure, and the pedicle screws are rapidly reinserted. The spinal canal should be inspected to make certain the methylmethacrylate has not inadvertently extruded into the canal with potential compression of neural elements. The instrumentation construct is then completed.

## Location of the Unstable Spinal Segment

The transition zones in the spine are key locations. They include the junctions of the occiput and cervical spine, the cervical and thoracic spine, the thoracic and lumbar spine, and the lumbar spine and sacrum. Each transition has a change in anatomy, a change in the orientation of facets, and a change in inherent rigidity. Ideally, the construct should not end at an intermediate junction (e.g., cervicothoracic and thoracolumbar junctions). Ending the construct and the fusion at an intermediate junction may lead to higher loads on the implants, higher failure rates, and a greater likelihood of adjacent segment problems.

The closer the lesion or unstable segment is to the occiput or sacrum, the shorter the applied lever arm is to the terminal end of the construct. More rigid fixation is therefore required at the terminal end of the construct.[18] Often multiple points of fixation are used in the sacrum or occiput. Long constructs that end at the sacrum have a high rate of pseudarthrosis at the terminal end (L5-S1).[11] There is a very high flexion-extension bending moment on the S1 screws, which leads to loosening of the screws. The addition of iliac screws, alar screws, or S2 pedicle screws to the construct significantly decreases the bending moment on the S1 pedicle screws and increases the fusion rate.[1,11]

## Implant Length

As a general rule the shortest construct that provides adequate stability is preferred. This preserves as much motion as possible in the normal segments of the spine above and below the construct. Long constructs may also place undue stress on the inferiormost aspect of the construct and the immediately adjacent motion segment. Although long constructs in the relatively immobile thoracic spine will not jeopardize physiologic motion, they should still be avoided, if possible. A relative exception to this is the presence of gross instability.

A long construct may be required to provide greater purchase of adjacent segments, and thus greater stability. In the treatment of gross spinal instability or long curvatures (scoliosis or kyphosis), longer constructs may apply greater force overall and less force at each individual segment. Adding bone anchors, rod diameters, or both, can significantly increase overall stiffness.[14]

Specific issues arise as to the length of instrumentation in circumstances in which it is desired to keep the fusion short. Two options are available: (1) use longer instrumentation, a short fusion, and remove the instrumentation later or alternatively, (2) keep the fusion and the construct short.

### Instrumentation Fusion Mismatch ("Rod Long, Fuse Short")

This describes the discrepancy between the number of spinal levels incorporated within an instrumentation construct and the number of spinal levels undergoing bony fusion. It was particularly popular in the past, when only less rigid anchors were available. Consequently, construct length was increased to gain stability. As a general rule only the spinal segments immediately adjacent to the unstable segment are fused. The rationale for this approach is that a long instrumentation construct is used to achieve reduction and correction of deformity, while fusing only the minimum number of segments necessary. The hardware is later removed (after 1 year), when the fractures have healed and the fusion has consolidated, thus releasing the instrumented, but not fused, segments from immobilization. There is some concern and controversy that the facet joints included within the instrumented non-fused segments may undergo degenerative arthropathy.[8] An additional disadvantage of the rod long, fuse short construct is the potential for the implants to loosen. Hooks and cables allow more movement at this juncture than screws and may not pose as great a problem. This design has generally fallen out of favor. If this mode of construct is desired, screws should not be used as anchors in the nonfused segments.

### Short-Segment Fixation

As a general rule, hook and cable constructs require long constructs, three above and two below (3A-2B) the lesion. This provides a longer and more efficient moment arm, and thus a stronger construct.[2] The 3A-2B configuration is a logical compromise between the problems associated with longer constructs and the shorter moment arm achieved with the shorter constructs, and has been shown to provide good stability. Pedicle screws may allow for shorter constructs and fewer fusion segments, a single level above and below the lesion (1A-1B). Short-segment fixation provides an increasingly popular alternative, particularly when applied in a compression mode. Because of the limited fixation there may be a higher rate of failure.[13] This is particularly true if the screw purchase is poor (osteoporosis) or if the loads are too great, secondary to a loss of anterior column stability. In the very unstable spine without significant anterior column loss, and rotational and shear fractures, pedicle screw fixation with two above and two below should provide adequate stability in most circumstances.

### Cross-Fixation

Cross-fixation between longitudinal members generally improves the torsional stability of longer constructs, as well as the lateral bending stiffness (Figure 123.3).[5,7,15] It is not as critical to use cross-fixation in short-segment constructs. For a short-segment rod construct with a skipped level (nonsegmental fixation), a cross-fixing device improves torsional stability to that of segmental fixation.[7] There is little effect of cross-links on flexion-extension stiffness.[5] When using long rod constructs with hook anchors, cross-fixation is essential to improve hook stability and torsional and lateral bending stiffness. Interconnecting the hooks on the two longitudinal members with cross-links significantly increases the fixation rigidity and decreases the failure rate. When the distal end is anchored by pedicle screws, the torsional and bending stiffness is much greater and not significantly different with cross-links.[17]

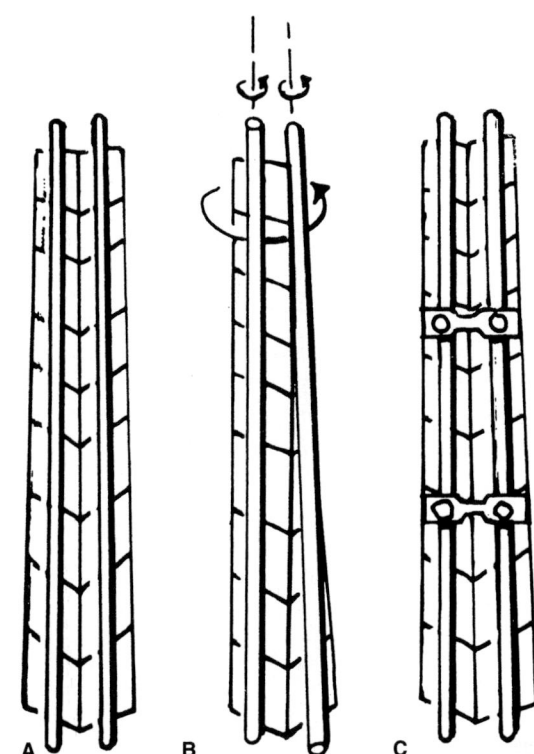

**Figure 123.3** Cross-fixation can effectively resist torsional forces on the rods. (**A** and **B**) Rods without cross-fixation are free to rotate, with respect to one another. (**C**) Cross-fixation prevents the rotation.

With long constructs, when cross-fixation is deemed necessary, two cross-fixators are optimal, creating a box construct. Further cross-links do not offer an advantage. Ideally the links should be placed at the junction of middle and terminal thirds of the construct.

### Axial Load-Bearing Capacity of the Instrumented Spine

One of the main goals in the reconstruction of an injured spine is to restore its ability to carry axial loads. The construct should be so designed that the axial load is transmitted through the reconstituted bony spine, along the axis of the vertebral body rather than through the metallic implants inserted through the pedicles. The latter design may lead to stress risers within the implant, resulting in its ultimate failure.

Two clinical examples may be cited to illustrate this point. In a case of grade 1 degenerative spondylolisthesis, there is a long-standing translational deformity (glacial instability), but no problem with axial load bearing. The role of instrumentation is to reduce the deformity, align the spine, and rigidly stabilize the motion segment to facilitate bony fusion. On the other hand, in a patient with a severe burst fracture of the L1 vertebral body with some loss of bone substance, axial load bearing is not effective. This may be corrected by resection of the vertebral body, replacement with a strut graft, and short-segment stabilization with a locking plate or dual-rod device. Thus the goal of spinal reconstruction in the latter case is to restore load-bearing ability, and to decompress and stabilize the spine.[16] If a short-segment pedicle screw construct is used in such a case without vertebral body reconstruction, there may be significant axial loading of the screws, and they may fail.[12,13]

Regardless of the approach used, if a spinal implant is placed in a compression mode, the dural sac should be decompressed first. Potentially, doing otherwise will result in additional compression of neural elements.

## Nature of Instability

A basic principle used for the correction of a deformity with instrumentation is to apply forces opposite of those that created the deformity. Specific maneuvers for the correction of some specific deformities are given in the following paragraphs.

### Kyphotic Deformity

Kyphotic deformities of the spine may be corrected in one of two ways:(1) with a dorsal approach, using a three-point bending maneuver through a long rod construct, or (2) via a ventral approach, with the resection of a vertebral body, interbody grafting, and application of a plate or dual rod device (Figure 123.4). If the deficit is in the anterior column, such as with compression or burst fracture, then the ventral approach may be more appropriate. If the posterior tension-band is lost, which leads to kyphosis, then

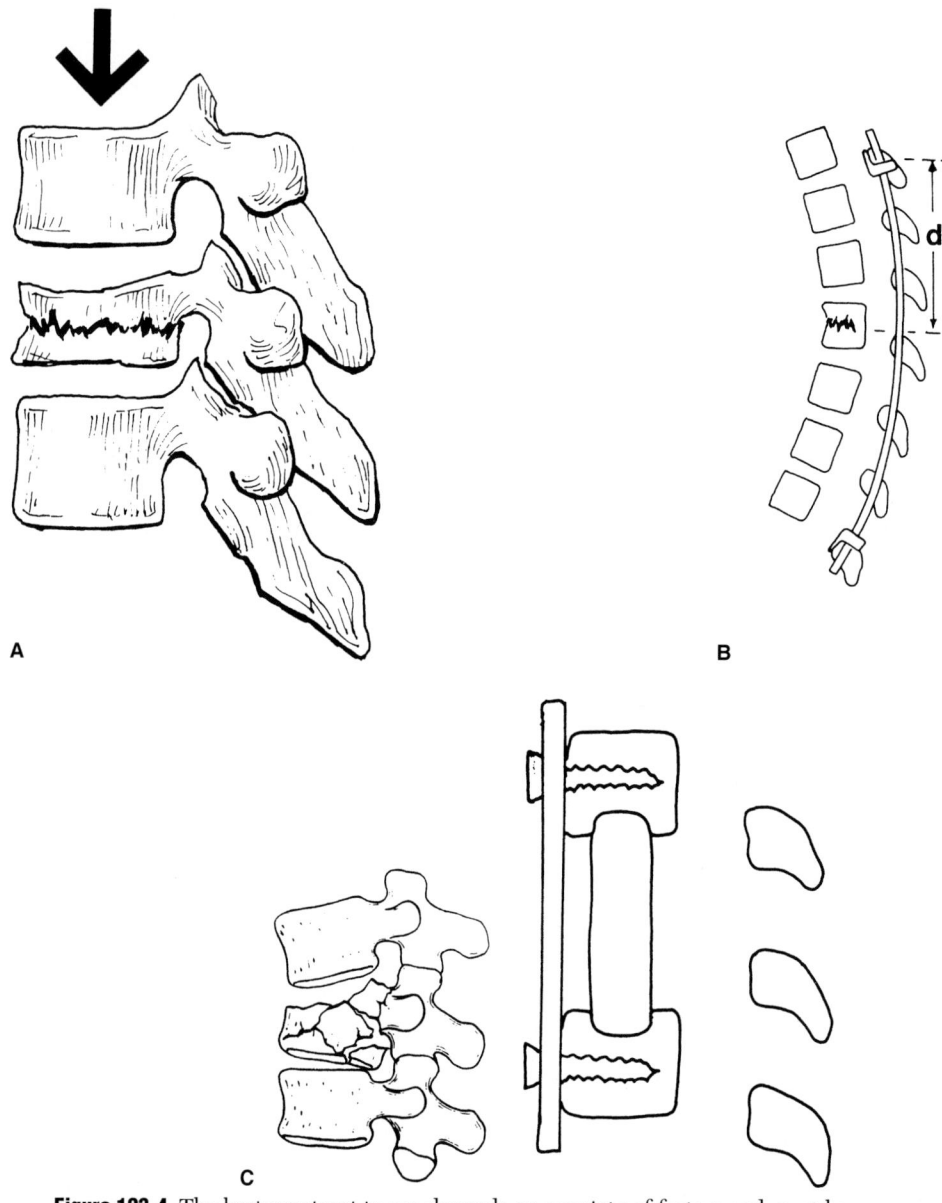

**Figure 123.4** The best construct to use depends on a variety of factors and must be individualized. For example, even the same fracture may require different constructs, depending on the severity of the injury. **(A)** Mild burst fractures can be treated with a dorsal construct **(B)**, using a distraction combined with three-point bending maneuver **(C)**. The more severe burst fracture should be treated with a ventral construct, using a cantilever design.

the dorsal approach may work best. Both approaches may be required if the bone quality is poor.

### Translational Deformity

Translational deformities (e.g., fracture dislocation resulting from trauma) are generally corrected from a dorsal orientation. Distraction and three-point bending with long hook-rod constructs often work well, as do shorter constructs (two above and two below) with pedicle screws. Translational deformity of a glacial type from degenerative spondylolisthesis is generally easily reducible by mere positioning or with a pull-back technique, using pedicle screws, though adding an interbody implant significantly improves the overall stability. Translational deformity resulting from isthmic spondylolisthesis is much more difficult to correct. It requires complete discectomy and intervertebral distraction, followed by pull-back with screws. Great care must be taken with any reduction maneuver, and electromyography (EMG) monitoring of the exiting nerve roots is recommended.

### Axial Loading Deformity (e.g., Burst Fracture)

In milder forms of fracture, distraction and extension via pedicle screws will restore the alignment. In severe burst fractures with considerable bone loss, the preferred treatment is anterior excision of vertebral body, strut grafting, and plating to reconstruct the anterior column.

### Flexion Distraction (SeatBelt) Deformity

This deformity is best corrected by compression and then stabilization. This may be accomplished via a dorsal approach and usually requires only short segment fixation.

### Scoliotic Deformity

Distractive force is applied on the concave side of the deformity, and compression is applied on the convex side of the deformity. Spinal cord monitoring is essential, because distraction may place the cord at risk. Attention should also be paid to the rotational malalignment, which can often be improved with segmental fixation, using screws, hooks, or wires.

### Need for Dural Sac Decompression

As emphasized in previous sections adequate spinal canal decompression before the placement of a compression instrumentation construct is essential. Either ventral or dorsal decompressive operations, particularly in the setting of trauma, result in further destabilization of the spine, and therefore should always be followed by rigid internal stabilization.

### Armamentarium of the Surgeon

The surgeon should be prepared to use alternative stable constructs when a primary (most desired) construct is not feasible for any specific region. For example, the inability to decompress ventral compressive lesions dictates that a dorsal compression instrumentation construct not be applied, or an inability to place pedicle screws because of an anatomic or pathologic state dictates that hooks or wires be required. These limitations force the surgeon to be versatile and thoughtful in the management of complex spinal disorders.

## REFERENCES

1. Alegre GM, Gupta MC, Bay BK, et al: S1 screw bending moment with posterior spinal instrumentation across the lumbosacral junction after unilateral iliac crest harvest. Spine 26(18): 1950-1955, 2001.
2. Benzel EC: Short segment compression instrumentation for selected thoracic and lumbar spine fractures: the short-rod–two claw (SRTC) technique. J Neurosurg 79: 335-340, 1993.
3. Benzel EC: Construct design. In Benzel EC (ed): Spinal Instrumentation. Chicago, AANS Publications, 1994, pp 239-256.
4. Benzel EC (ed): Construct design. In Biomechanics of Spine Stabilization: Principles and Practice. New York, McGraw-Hill, 1995.
5. Brodke DS, Bachus KN, Mohr RA, Nguyen BN: Segmental pedicle screw fixation or cross-links in multilevel lumbar constructs: a biomechanical analysis. Spine 1:373-379, 2001.
6. Butler TE, Asher MA, Jayaraman G, et al: The strength and stiffness of implant anchors in osteoporotic spines. Spine 19:1956-1962, 1994.
7. Dick JC, Jones MP, Zdeblick TA, et al: A biomechanical comparison evaluating the use of intermediate screws and cross-linkage in lumbar pedicle fixation. J Spinal Disord 7:402-407, 1994.
8. Gardner VO, Armstrong GWD: Long-term lumbar facet joint changes in spinal fracture patients treated with Harrington rods. Spine 15:479-484, 1990.
9. Halvorson TL, Kelley LA, Thomas KA, et al: Effects of bone mineral density on pedicle screw fixation. Spine 19:2415-2420, 1994.
10. Krag MH: Biomechanics of thoracolumbar spinal fixation. Spine 16:S84-S99, 1991.
11. Kuklo TR, Bridwell KH, Lewis SJ, et al: Minimum 2-year analysis of sacropelvic fixation and L5-S1 fusion using S1 and iliac screws. Spine 26(18): 1976-1983, 2001.
12. Mann KA, McGowan DP, Fredrickson BE, et al: A biomechanical investigation of short segment spinal fixation for burst fractures with varying degrees of posterior disruption. Spine 15:470-478, 1990.
13. McLain RF, Sparling E, Benson DR: Early failure of short-segment pedicle instrumentation for thoracolumbar fractures. A preliminary report. J Bone Joint Surg 75A: 162-167, 1993.
14. Orchowski J, Polly DW Jr, Klemme WR, et al: The effect of kyphosis on the mechanical strength of a long-segment posterior construct using a synthetic model. Spine 25(13):1644-1648, 2000.
15. Ruland CM, McAfee PC, Warden KE, et al: Triangulation of pedicular instrumentation. A biomechanical analysis. Spine 16:S270-S276, 1991.

16. Shono Y, McAfee PC, Cunningham BW: Experimental study of thoracolumbar burst fractures. *Spine* 15: 1711-1722, 1994.

17. Wood KB, Wentorf FA, Ogilvie JW, Kim KT: Torsional rigidity of scoliosis constructs. *Spine* 25(15):1893-1898, 2000.

18. Zindrick MR, Wiltse LL, Windell EH, *et al*: A biomechanical study of intrapeduncular screw fixation in the lumbosacral spine. *Clin Orthop* 203:99-112, 1986.

# CHAPTER 124

# Fundamentals of Spine Deformity and Correction

**Lawrence G. Lenke, Eric J. Woodard, and Edward C. Benzel**

Spine deformity results from a variety of causes, each creating an imbalance regarding spinal structural support. This imbalance may result from an abnormality or asymmetry of innervation, an asymmetry of structural integrity of the spine and its supporting elements, and/or a preexisting spinal deformity of "idiopathic" (unknown) cause. This chapter outlines the fundamentals of clinically relevant spinal deformity, reviewing its various causes and principles of correction.[1,9]

## Definitions and Terms

Specifying a distinct nomenclature for spinal deformity helps to define precisely the deformity type, its magnitude and direction, and other clinically relevant aspects that are essential in clinical decision making.[4] By definition, spinal deformity involves a curvature or altered alignment that exceeds normal limits for a particular spinal region. Curvature in the sagittal plane is termed a *kyphosis* when its concavity is directed ventrally and a *lordosis* when the concavity is directed dorsally. Frontal plane curvatures are *scolioses,* occurring either to the right or the left. Curve *direction* is named according to the side of the convexity. The magnitude of spinal curvatures is determined by the method of Cobb, which requires identifying the *end vertebrae* and noting the subtended angle between their end-plates. End vertebrae are defined as those that are maximally tilted toward the concavity of a curve (kyphosis, lordosis, or scoliotic curves). Axial plane deformity is described only as degrees of axial vertebral rotation from the frontal or sagittal planes. Thus a curve may be described according to its spinal region, the plane of involvement, its direction, and its magnitude (e.g., "a 45-degree right thoracic scoliosis" represents a thoracic region frontal plane curvature with right-sided convexity measuring 45 degrees between the distal end plates of the end vertebrae). Because of the coupling phenomena, most curves have abnormalities in all three planes that are characteristic of the deformity type.

Balance in the sagittal and/or frontal planes is typically maintained actively on a subconscious level through inner ear, proprioceptive, and visual mechanisms to preserve postural equilibrium. Balance requires that mobile portions of the spine compensate for regional spinal deformi-

ties to keep the head centered over the midsacrum in the frontal plane, and over the sacral promontory in the sagittal plane. The term *structural curve* is used to denote a rigid, inflexible curve that does not itself contribute to spinal compensation. This is usually the largest or *major curve* of a deformity and is closely related to the inciting pathology responsible for the deformity. *Compensatory curves* are mobile segments of the spine that form in response to structural curves to maintain postural balance. Compensatory curves, also termed *minor curves,* are usually smaller in magnitude than major curves. Their mobility may be determined on dynamic spinal bending radiographs, such as flexion/extension, or lateral side-bending views. When deformities exceed compensation ability, trunk imbalance occurs. This requires additional balancing mechanisms, such as hip and knee flexion and/or gait modification, to maintain an upright posture.

## Origins of Spinal Deformity

### Congenital Spine Deformity

Congenital deformities are precipitated by defects in embryologic development of the spine that result in failure of either (1) vertebra formation (2) segmentation, or (3) commonly, both. Vertebral formation occurs by a condensation of mesoderm into paraxial aligned somites that eventually form the structural components of the spinal column and its supporting elements. Mesoderm from adjacent halves of the lateral somites coalesces into individual vertebrae, a process known as *segmentation*, guided about a notochordal remnant that itself becomes the intervertebral disc. Defective formation or organization of somitic mesoderm can lead to inadequate development or loss of a portion of the vertebrae, resulting in asymmetrically shaped, partially formed structures, termed *hemivertebrae*. These may occur ventrally, dorsally, or laterally, resulting in kyphosis, lordosis, or scoliosis, respectively. Resulting deformities depend not only on the position of the hemivertebra, but also on its segmentation with adjacent vertebrae.

Defects in the segmentation process produce fused portions of vertebrae, or "bars," that may occur in a ventral, lateral, or dorsal position. The unsegmented bar inhibits longitudinal vertebral growth and results in vertebral asymmetry caused by uninhibited growth of the opposite side of the vertebrae. Resulting deformities include congenital scoliosis, kyphosis, lordosis, or a combination of scoliosis with kyphosis or lordosis. The majority of congenital defects involve some degree of both altered formation and segmentation and can be classified into three groups: (1) the unilateral unsegmented bar, which is a "pure" segmentation defect, (2) the free-segmented hemivertebra, which is a partial defect of formation with normal segmentation of both adjacent vertebrae, and (3) the semisegmented hemivertebra, which is a partial defect of formation associated with one adjacent normal disc space and one adjacent defect of segmentation. Additional combinations and multiple occurrences of the aforementioned defects are possible. Clinically, congenital deformities are usually apparent at a young age because of the significant spinal distortion they produce. They can lead to severe, often life-threatening, progressive deformity of the chest wall and proximal appendicular skeleton. Appropriate early recognition and characterization of these types of deformities are important for the prediction of progression and early intervention by the surgeon (by means of growth plate arrest by fusion). Hemivertebra excision to produce curve correction is often beneficial.

## Degenerative Spine Deformity

Spondylosis is defined as vertebral osteophytosis secondary to degenerative disc disease. Spondylosis should not be confused with inflammatory processes that may also be associated with osteophyte formation. These latter entities are grouped together as arthritides. The osteophytes of spondylosis are associated with degeneration of the intervertebral disc, which is an amphiarthrodial joint that lacks a synovial membrane. Arthritis, on the other hand, typically involves the synovial membranes of diarthrodial joints (e.g., facet joints). Spondylosis is therefore characterized by the presence of noninflammatory disc degeneration. The process of disc degeneration is complex and involves many alterations of normal physiology.

## Intradiscal Hydrostatic and Oncotic Pressure

Persistent elevation of intradiscal pressures may cause narrowing of the disc interspace. This results in annulus fibrosus and facet joint capsule distortion and stretching, which accelerates the degeneration process. Disc degeneration, however, should be considered a component manifestation of the normal aging process. Its pathologic acceleration, or its deterrence, however, is of obvious clinical significance.

As previously stated the water content of the intervertebral disc gradually decreases throughout life, as a result of progressive mucopolysaccharide and glycoprotein breakdown. Shorter and simpler polymeric forms of these major disc components associate with fewer water molecules, resulting in relative dehydration in proportion to the degree of polymer breakdown. In addition, the vascularity of the disc also decreases, ranging from a fully vascularized disc at birth to essentially no vascular supply by age 30. These and other factors contribute to changes in the chemical and anatomic makeup of the disc. In this altered environment fibroblasts produce inferior quality fibers and ground substance, impairing adequate repair functions. Fissures may occur in the cartilaginous plates, creating defects that result in internal herniations (Schmorl's nodes). Mucoid degeneration, an ingrowth of fibrocartilage, and fibrous obliteration of the nucleus fibrosis ensue. Gas may accumulate in the disc with advanced degenerative change (vacuum phenomenon). With these types of change the disc becomes progressively desiccated, mechanically stiffer, and less able to function as a cushion. Generalized disc deterioration results in a relatively unstable segment, caused by loss of disc height and secondary annulus fibrosus tension and bulging, both of which result in pathologic deformations.

Migration of disc material into the spinal canal (disc herniation) occurs predominantly in a dorsal direction, whereas osteophytic spur formation commonly occurs in the ventral or lateral direction. Flexion and lateral bending cause annulus fibrosus bulging and encourage osteophyte formation along the concave side of a spinal curve. Conversely, the relatively thin dorsolateral annulus fibrosus and weak posterior longitudinal ligament (PLL) combine with the migratory tendencies of the nucleus pulposus to encourage dorsolateral disc herniation.

Most disc herniations do not occur immediately after trauma. Presently, laboratory investigations that attempt to determine the mechanism of disc herniation are inadequate at defining the precise mechanical contribution to disc herniation. A high percentage of lumbar discs in the laboratory can be encouraged to herniate, if the disc is degenerated and a specific force pattern is acutely delivered to the motion segment. This force pattern includes (1) flexion, causing dorsal nucleus pulposus migration, (2) lateral bending away from the side of disc herniation, causing lateral nucleus pulposus migration and extreme annular tension, and (3) the application of an axial load, causing an increase in intradiscal pressure.[1]

This complex loading pattern of the intervertebral disc results in (1) the application of tension on the weakest portion of the annulus fibrosus (dorsolateral position; the location of the herniation), (2) migration of the nucleus pulposus toward this position, and (3) an asymmetric increase in intradiscal pressure. A degenerated disc is apparently a prerequisite for this process to occur. These factors, along with the increasing incidence of annulus fibrosus tears with age and the observation of peak nucleus fibrosus pressures in people ages 35 to 55, are among the risk factors related to the high incidence of disc herniation in this age group.[1,6]

### Disc Deformation

Bulging of the annulus fibrosus elevates the periosteum of the adjacent vertebral bodies at the attachment site of Sharpey's fibers. Bony inflammatory reaction (e.g., subperiosteal bone formation) occurs, resulting in osteophyte formation. This process most commonly leads to spinal canal encroachment in the cervical and lumbar regions, but generally spares the thoracic region. This fact may be associated with the significant mobility of the lordotic regions in flexion and extension (relative to the thoracic spine) that tends to produce annular bulging in a sagittal plane oriented toward the spinal canal. The spondylotic process may be controlled by altering excessive or pathologic motion with fusion or immobilization.

Lateral bending deformities, such as scolioses, frequently exhibit osteophyte formation *on the concave side of a curve*, where annulus fibrosus bulging caused by compression is most significant. This is a classic feature of degenerative lumbar scoliosis. The convex side of the curve, however, is the area most predisposed to disc herniation. This discrepancy may be related to the significant role played by annular tension in creating tears or fissures, and the importance of annular tears as predisposing factors in frank disc herniation.[1]

### Deformity Progression

Spine deformities usually progress. Several factors accelerate or exaggerate this process, including asymmetric force application to the spine, preexisting deformity, weakened intervertebral discs, and weakened vertebrae. Asymmetric force application creates a bending moment through the vertebrae, resulting in angulation and deformity progression. Preexisting deformity places the spine at a biomechanical disadvantage via the application of forces to progressively longer moment arms. Weakened intervertebral discs and vertebrae result in collapse of these structures, usually in an asymmetric pattern. These factors, in turn, result in spinal deformity and a commensurate increase in length of the pathologic moment arm that functions as a lever, amplifying the magnitude of forces applied to the spine, which further reinforces this progression cascade.

The degenerative process often begins via the asymmetric collapse of an intervertebral disc, which places an exaggerated force on the spine via the increased length of the "pathologic moment arm." Lesser forces are required to cause further collapse and deformity progression. If a spinal restabilization process (e.g., spondylosis) or an iatrogenic intervention (e.g., fusion) interrupts this degenerative process, progression of the deformity may be arrested.[1]

### Osteoporosis

Decreased bone formation with an associated continued or accelerated bone resorption leads to a relative decrease in bone mass. This is a complex process principally mediated by osteoclast biology that is closely associated with age, hormonal environment, concurrent medical conditions, and mechanical stress. When extensive, this process may lead to collapse of the vertebral body, as is classically observed in advanced osteoporotic spines. In contrast to the Schmorl's node, the collapse is not circumscribed. The presence of thoracic kyphosis may predispose the spine to ventral vertebral body collapse caused by the ventral location of axially directed force from body weight and ventral flexion musculature. Axial loads applied ventrally to the vertebral column create a flexion moment at the axis of rotation (generally located in the dorsal vertebral body) that is proportional to the force and the length of the moment arm. In the thoracic spine this moment becomes greater with increasing kyphosis and subjects the ventral portion of the vertebral body to significantly larger compressive loads. In osteoporosis, weakening of the rib cage, and its resulting loss of support to the spine, may also play a role in concentrating axial force through the vertebral body. Lordotic regions of the spine may better distribute axial loads between ventral and dorsal elements, and are less prone to vertebral body collapse. This principle also applies to general mechanisms of traumatic injuries.

### Scheuermann's Disease

In the developing spine, intradiscal oncotic pressure, or disc turgor, is normally relatively high. Axial trauma can result in focal sites of penetration of the end plate (Schmorl's nodes), with a resulting injury to the growth plate. The preexisting thoracic kyphosis, which is associated with asymmetrically high ventral intradiscal pressures, may lead to the exaggeration of focal end plate penetration in this circumstance. This phenomenon is known as Scheuermann's disease (osteochondrosis), and is associated with a disproportional loss of ventral vertebral body height, the presence of Schmorl's nodes (predominantly ventrally located), irregularities of the vertebral end-plates, and narrowing of the disc interspaces (predominantly ventrally).[8] Although the precise etiology is still unknown, Kramer[6] believes that the developmental disorders of Scheuermann's disease are secondary changes and are caused by increased pressure of the developing disc tissue on the ventral parts of the intervertebral segments in the kyphotic area of the spine. Because of the increased focal pressures exerted, degeneration of the disc is accelerated, epiphyseal growth plates become dysfunctional, and a wedge deformity of the involved vertebral bodies occurs. Fibrosus and ultimately, bony fusion, typically occur, creating a rigid thoracic kyphosis.

### Other Causes of Spine Deformity

Other causes of spine deformity most certainly exist. Their mechanisms are often similar to either or both of the congenital or degenerative deformity mechanisms previously outlined. Of particular note in this regard are inflammatory and posttraumatic spine deformities. Their geometric and biomechanical characteristics are not unlike those of congenital and degenerative situations. Idiopathic and neurogenic spine deformities are individually unique. Bone and soft-tissue deformation, or loss of integrity, is usually not a factor in these cases. Other obviously complex factors play major roles in these deformities and their progression.

## Deformity Correction

A variety of techniques and implants can be used to bring the spine into axial, sagittal, and coronal plane balance. This is accomplished via the application of forces to the spine along one or a combination of the three axes of the Cartesian coordinate system. Forces applied along the long axis of the spine (e.g., distraction) can be used to correct compression deformations, as well as coronal and sagittally oriented translational deformations. Bending moments applied in the sagittal plane are, in general, applied via a three-point bending or related mechanism, although applied moment arm cantilever beam forces may also be applied.

### Three-Point and Four-Point Bending

Three-point and four-point bending are classically applied by Harrington distraction rod and universal spine fixation systems, respectively (Figure 124.1). Crossed rod deformity correction applies these forces to the spine. The bending moment applied is proportional to the long arm of the spine.

Four-point bending of the spine, as defined by White and Panjabi,[9] involves loading a long structure with two transverse forces on one side and two on the other. The bending moment is constant between the two intermediate points of force application if all forces are equal; this is

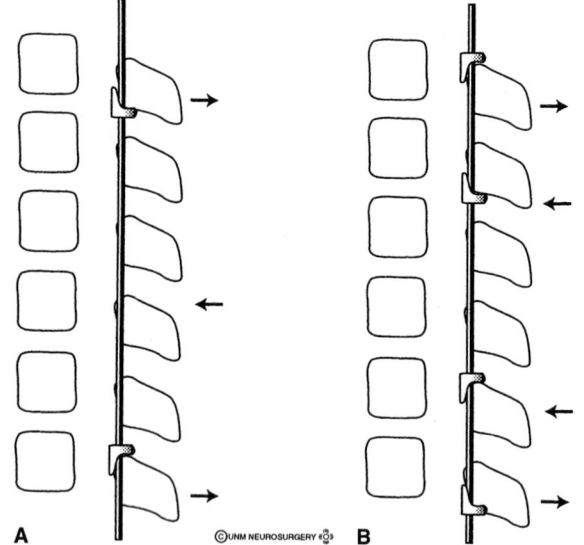

**Figure 124.1** The dorsally and ventrally directed forces (*arrows*) applied by (**A**) three-point bending and (**B**) four-point bending constructs. (*From Benzel EC: Biomechanics of Spine Stabilization: Principles and Clinic Practice. New York, McGraw-Hill, 1995.*)

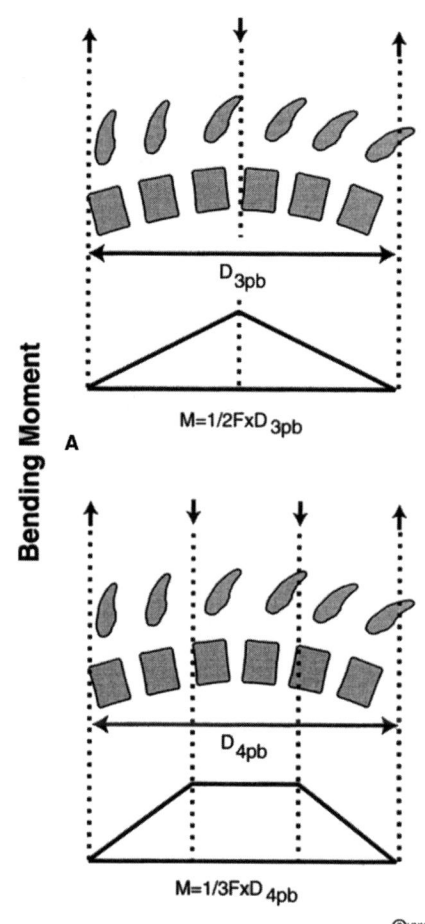

**Figure 124.2** (**A**) Three-point bending and (**B**) four-point bending construct forces and associated bending moments. With the three-point bending construct depicted here, the intermediate force is applied halfway between the terminal points of force application. Therefore the maximum bending moment (M) occurs at the point of intermediate force application (M = 1/2 × $D_{3pb}$). With the four-point bending construct, all forces ($F_{4pb}$) and the distance from the intermediate and terminal points of force application (1/3 × $D_{4pb}$) are equal. In this situation the maximum bending moment, which is constant between the two intermediate points of force application, is defined by the equation $M_{4pb} = F_{4pb}$ 1/3 × $D_{4pb}$. $D_{4pb}$ is the length of the entire construct. Because the forces ($F_{4pb}$) are applied at points dividing the constructs into thirds, the moment arm defining the bending moment is a third of the entire construct length. (*From Benzel EC: Biomechanics of Spine Stabilization: Principles and Clinic Practice. New York, McGraw-Hill, 1995.*)

in contrast to three-point bending in which the bending moment peaks at the intermediate point of force application (Figure 124.2).

## Cantilever Beam Force Application

Applied moment arm cantilever beam constructs are applied in situations in which short-segment constructs are desired for deformity reduction.[5] They are applicable in the thoracolumbar and lumbar regions for the reduction and fixation of traumatic wedge compression and burst fractures. The nature of their application dictates that the construct bears significant loads, both at the time of insertion and during loading (e.g., ambulation). Therefore failure of the construct may become problematic. These constructs can be applied with either flexion or extension bending moments and can use distraction or compression. Frequently, an accompanying ventral decompression and/or interbody bone graft is combined with this type of instrumentation. Cantilever beam constructs can be applied in such a manner that deformity is reduced and an interbody bone graft, if appropriate, is placed in compression (Figure 124.3). These factors may be crucial in optimal construct design. For example, if extension and distraction, without an accompanying interbody fusion, are to be used, screws large enough to withstand significant axial loads must be used. In spite of this, construct failure may result, often at the screw-bone junctures. Cantilever beam fixation may be difficult to achieve in situations when pedicle diameter or geometry dictates the use of relatively small screws. In these situations placing an interbody weight-bearing bone graft (or cage), followed by compression of the construct across the ventral graft and other intrinsic ventral weight-bearing spinal elements, results in the "sharing of the load" among the construct, the spinal elements, and the interbody fusion.

Simultaneously the desired extension bending moment application for deformity reduction is achieved.

The technique of sequentially applying distraction, decompressing the dural sac, placing an interbody strut for fusion, and compressing the construct to achieve load sharing with the ventral spinal elements is termed load bearing-to-load sharing force application. It provides biomechanical advantages of sharing axial loads with the cantilever beam implant to reduce implant failure, and the clinical advantages associated with preloading the

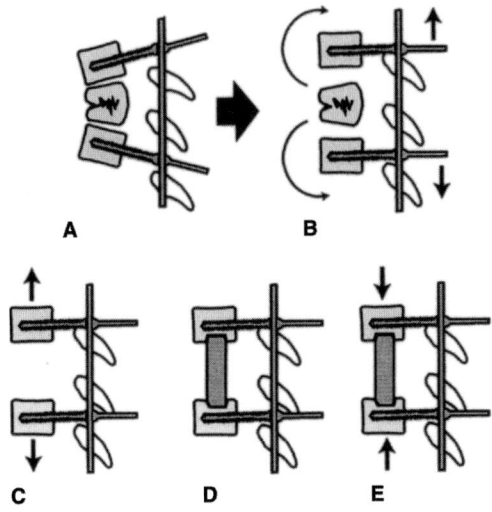

© UNM NEUROSURGERY

**Figure 124.3** (**A** and **B**) An applied moment arm cantilever beam construct that uses distraction and an extension bending moment, without an interbody fusion. This may be associated with a suboptimal success rate.[5,7] Load bearing-to-load sharing force application may minimize this complication by allowing sharing of the load between the implant and the spine (unloading the implant). In this case the spine is distracted (with or without extension or flexion bending moment application) by (**B**) the implant, followed by (**C**) bone graft placement, and (**D**) compression of the implant. This allows for the sharing of the load between the implant and the spine. Straight arrows depict forces; curved arrows depict bending moments. (*From Benzel EC:* Biomechanics of Spine Stabilization: Principles and Clinic Practice. *New York, McGraw-Hill, 1995.*)

interbody graft in compression, a known stimulus for bony fusion (Wolff's law).

## Crossed Rod Deformity Correction

The crossed rod technique is a well-established method for thoracic and lumbar kyphosis correction. It was initially used with Harrington distraction rods and subsequently, more effectively used with multisegmental sublaminar wiring (Luque) techniques.[2] Most recently it has been used with the sequential hook insertion technique with universal spinal instrumentation constructs.[3] Regardless of the construct type, the technique involves the simultaneous application of reduction forces to the spine via moment arms (longitudinal members) affixed at opposite ends of a kyphosis and opposite sides of the spine. Gradual reduction is thus achieved by ventral levering of the rods (Figure 124.4). Pedicle screws used as spinal anchors are an even more powerful means of kyphotic deformity correction.

## Short-Segment Parallelogram Deformity Reduction

Short-segment parallelogram deformity reduction is a rigid, cantilever beam pedicle fixation technique that can be used in the thoracic and lumbar regions for the reduction of lateral translational deformities in the coronal

plane. This method is optimal for circumstances in which short-segment fixation constructs are used. The technique involves (1) placing pedicle screws, (2) decompressing the dural sac, (3) attaching longitudinal members to the screws, (4) applying a lateral rotatory and distraction force to the rods for reduction, (5) maintaining reduction via rigid cross-fixation, (6) placing a fusion (interbody and/or lateral), and finally, (7) compressing the construct to achieve load sharing and secure the interbody bone graft. This applies the load bearing-to-load sharing technique of force application (Figure 124.5).

Short-segment parallelogram deformity reduction is ideally applied in the low lumbar region, because sacral-pelvic fixation points are often suboptimal for long moment arm reduction strategies. Posterior lumbar interbody fusion (PLIF) techniques can also be combined with this method of reduction to attain a ventral interbody fusion mass.

## In Situ Deformity Reduction
### Implant Contouring

Once installed and affixed to the spine, the contouring of the longitudinal member, usually a rod, allows segmental spinal relationships to be altered dynamically. *In situ* contouring is most commonly used for fitting the implant to the contour of the spine. The need for excessive *in vivo* rod contouring should not become a substitute for preinsertion rod contouring and surgical planning. Significant unexpected and untoward forces may be inadvertently applied to the spine via *in situ* deformity reduction techniques, causing acute implant-bone failure. Great caution must therefore be used.

However, the use of *in vivo* implant contouring for deformity reduction is often an effective strategy for the fine-tuning of spinal reduction. For example, a hook-rod universal spinal instrumentation system could be inserted in such a manner that it conforms to a spinal deformity. After insertion the rods could be contoured, along with the attached spine, to achieve an improved alignment. Adequate hook-bone junction security is mandatory. Implant contouring, by its nature, alters the relationships between the implant and the spine. In this case hooks may over-tighten or loosen with respect to their contact with bone, infringe on the spinal canal, or migrate laterally or medially, depending on their orientation (rostrally or caudally facing) and on the orientation of the applied contouring-related bending moment. Rechecking of all hook or implant purchase sites is imperative before final construct tightening and wound closure (Figure 124.6).

## Implant Force Application About the Long Axis of the Spine
### Derotation

The popularization of rod derotation as a therapeutic maneuver is accredited to Cotrel and Dubousset. It can be used in highly complex spine deformations, as well as in cases of simple scoliotic curvatures of the thoracic and lumbar spine. With scoliosis an obligatory rotatory component usually coexists. It is the primary abnormality resulting in the observed two-dimensional deformities

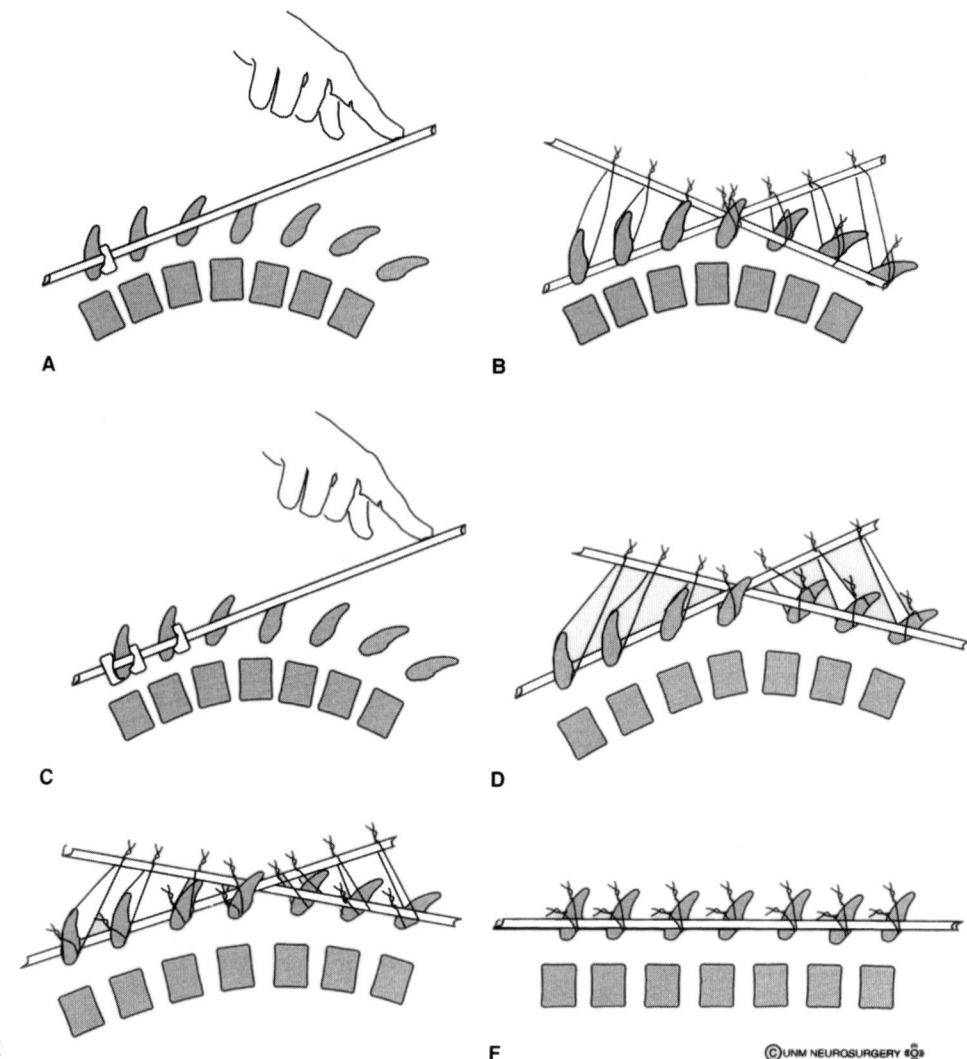

**Figure 124.4** The crossed rod technique of thoracic and lumbar kyphotic deformity correction via the (**A**) Harrington distraction rod, (**B**) Luque sublaminar wiring, and (**C**) universal spinal instrumentation. The latter technique is facilitated by the use of sequential hook insertion (**D-F**). The crossed rod technique involves gradual reduction of the kyphotic deformity, as illustrated serially. (*From Benzel EC:* Biomechanics of Spine Stabilization: Principles and Clinic Practice. *New York, McGraw-Hill, 1995.*)

measured on plain radiography. This is related to the phenomenon termed *coupling*. This rotatory component must be continuously accounted for during implant application and deformity reduction.

Rod derotation essentially is a maneuver whereby a scoliotic curvature is converted to a kyphotic curvature. If the resultant kyphotic curvature is unacceptable, it is then reduced via rod contouring. To accomplish this task the rods are first inserted and attached to hooks, screws, or wires. These are attached in a loose manner (friction-glide tightness) so that rotation can occur at the connection site. The hooks can then rotate about the rod as the rod is rotated. This allows the hooks to maintain their relationship with the spinal attachment site (Figure 124.7). The rods are then simultaneously and gradually rotated 90 degrees to reduce the scoliotic component. If needed, the rods may then be contoured to reduce any unwanted excessive kyphotic curvature and the hook-rod interfaces may be tightened and secured.

It should be remembered that derotation can be performed only on a relatively flexible curve, and care must be taken to perform these maneuvers in a gradual manner. This allows for the continuous assessment and reassessment of the implant-bone relationships. For example, a hook may not be rotating on the rod during rotation of the rod. This, in turn, places a significant amount of stress at the hook-bone junction. Some implants, particularly those using rods with rough surfaces, are prone to this untoward phenomenon. Also, rod derotation maneuvers have been shown to produce minimal true axial derotation to the scoliotic spine.

### Short-Segment Fixation

Implant bending moment application about the long axis of the spine is usually employed in the thoracic and lumbar spine using long-segment implants that apply long bending moments. These moments are applied in either

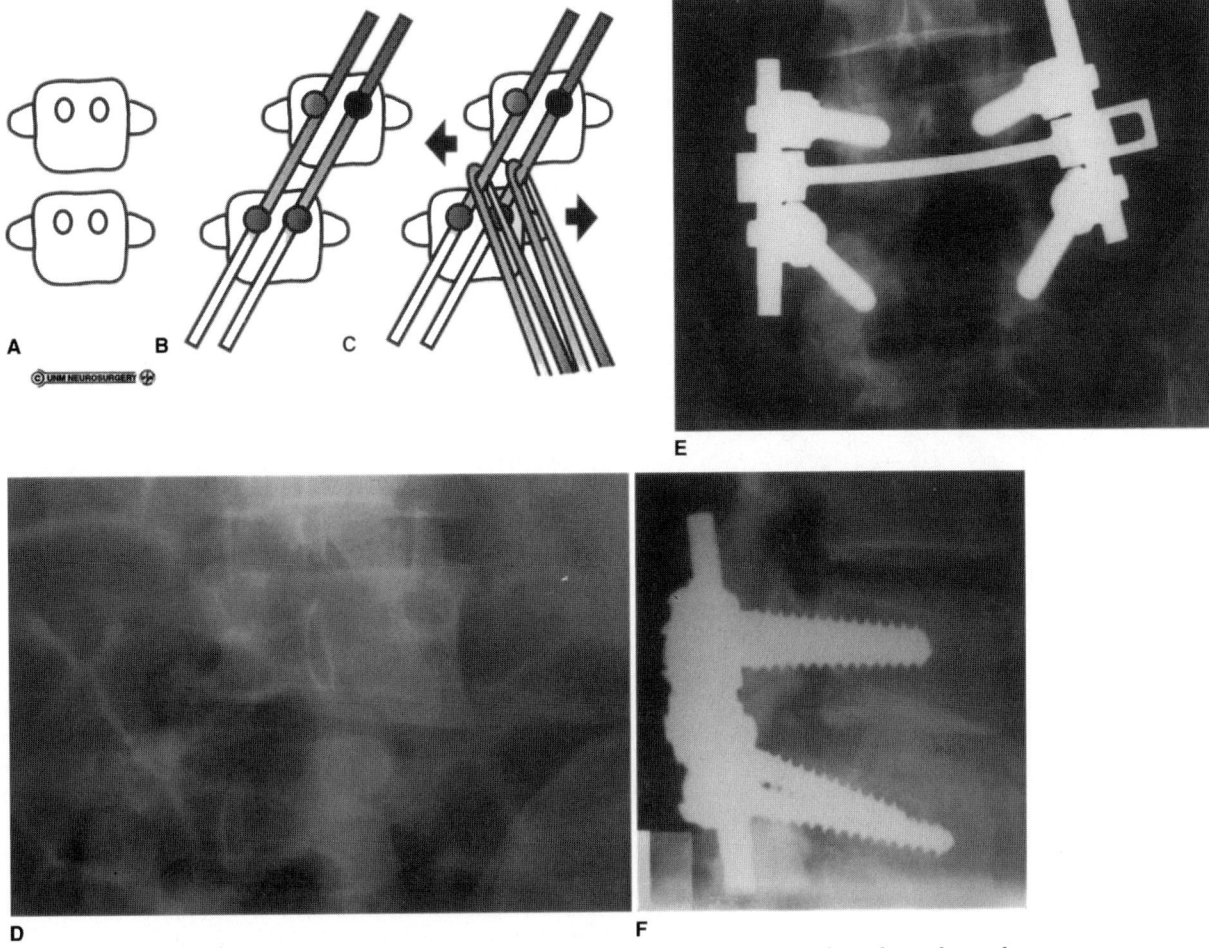

**Figure 124.5** Short-segment parallelogram deformity reduction. **(A)** A lateral translational deformity is observed. **(B)** Pedicle screws are placed and connected by rods. **(C)** Rods are tightened (friction-glide tightness) and a torque is applied to both rods simultaneously via rod grippers to reduce the deformity. **(D)** A clinical example of a lateral L4-5 subluxation (traumatic). The aforementioned technique was used to reduce the dislocation. **(E)** The reduction is maintained via rigid cross-fixation. **(F)** Distraction, followed by interbody bone graft placement and finally, compression, is used to secure the bone graft in place. *(From Benzel EC: Biomechanics of Spine Stabilization: Principles and Clinic Practice. New York, McGraw-Hill, 1995.)*

the sagittal or coronal plane. One- or two-segment scoliotic (coronal plane) deformations (usually lumbar), however, can at least be partially corrected by a short-segment technique. Pedicle screws are inserted, with care taken to consider the rotatory component of the deformation. Rods are then attached to the screws. The concave side of the curvature is distracted (usually 1 to 2cm), and the convex side of the curvature is compressed (Figure 124.8). Cross-fixation to maintain the correction is usually employed. A similar technique may be used on the lateral aspect of the spine (via plates or rods) to achieve a reduction of a sagittal plane deformity.

With distraction or compression of screws associated with any of the techniques mentioned in this chapter, the relationship of the screw to the rod must be carefully monitored to avoid untoward screw-rod relationships (e.g., flexion of the screw on the rod). Only a few screw-rod junctions allow this to occur (e.g., the TSRH [variable angle screw]). Therefore one should carefully consider the type of screw-rod junction (i.e., variable angle vs. fixed angle) to be used. The application of distraction forces to fixed-angle screws results in a cantilevered distraction of the spine without the application of a sagittal plane bending moment to the spine. If, however, a variable-angle screw is used, a cantilevered distraction of the spine may result in screw flexion at the screw-rod junction, thus causing a sagittal plane bending moment to be applied to the spine. This can be prevented by tightening the screw to a friction-glide tightness before applying the distraction forces.

## Cross-Fixation

The rigid connection of each component of dual constructs (e.g., two rods) to each other may result in the substantial augmentation of integrity of the construct. With long constructs, applying cross-fixation can substantially reduce excessive torsional instability. In gen-

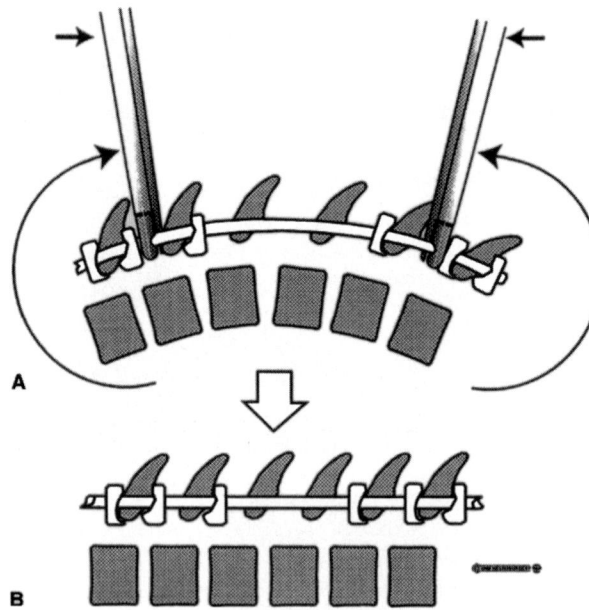

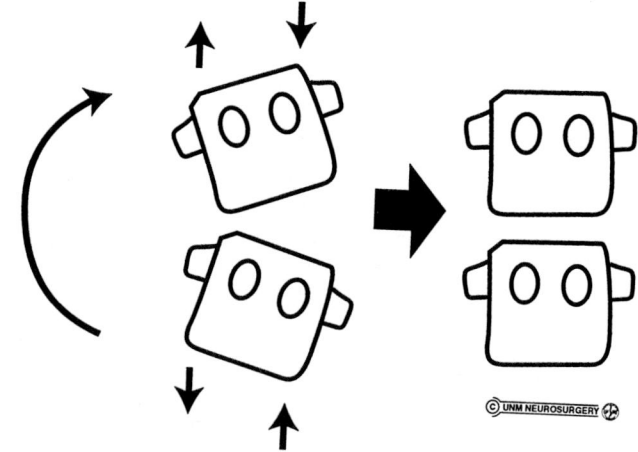

**Figure 124.8** The application of an intrinsic implant bending moment about an axially oriented axis of the spine. Arrows depict forces applied (*straight arrows*) and resultant bending moment (*curved arrow*). (*From Benzel EC: Biomechanics of Spine Stabilization: Principles and Clinic Practice. New York, McGraw-Hill, 1995.*)

**Figure 124.6** Implant contouring. Implant contouring can be used to alter spinal deformity. (**A**) First the implant is inserted, conforming to the deformity. (**B**) Then the implant is contoured *in vivo*. Finally, each component must be checked for purchase site integrity, adjusted, and tightened. (*From Benzel EC: Biomechanics of Spine Stabilization: Principles and Clinic Practice. New York, McGraw-Hill, 1995.*)

eral, short constructs do not significantly benefit torsional stability, from the use of cross-members due to the relationship short moment arm used. However, if deformity maintenance is achieved in part by cross-fixation, it is mandatory.

With longer constructs cross-fixation is biomechanically useful, because it provides a quadrilateral frame construct that is associated with rotatory stability and improved implant-bone junction integrity. In general, two cross-members are stiffer than one, but more than two adds little additional stability. Cross-members should be placed at roughly the "junction of thirds" of the construct length (Figure 124.9).

An additional indication for cross-fixation is maintenance of a desired interrod width. This may prevent lateral pedicle hook migration, the overlapping (medially) of laminar hooks, and screw dislodgement from the ilium.

When cross-members are used for short-segment deformity constructs, very rigid cross-members should be used because of substantial bending moments that are applied at the cross-member rod junction. These can only be resisted by the most rigid of implants.

### Screw Toe-In

Screw toe-in plays an integral role in preventing lateral translational deformity. Screws inserted perpendicular to the coronal plane offer little or no resistance to lateral translation (parallelogramming), because the vertebrae merely rotate around the long axis of the screw. "Toe-nailing" the screw medially orients the screw oblique to the coronal plane, such that translation is resisted more effectively (Figure 124.10). This can also be accomplished by increasing the length of the implant by one segment.

Additionally, screw toe-in (or toe-out) with an accompanying rigid cross-fixation of the right to left component of the system significantly increases pullout resistance. This is because of the increased "volume" of bone that

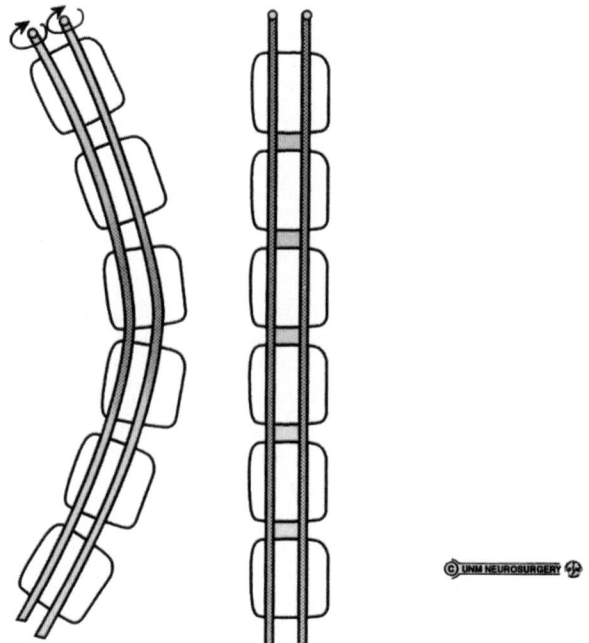

**Figure 124.7** Intrinsic implant bending moment application about the long axis of the spine (i.e., derotation) can be achieved by 90-degree rotation of the right and left rods simultaneously. The rods were initially placed to conform to the scoliosis. A kyphosis results. (*From Benzel EC: Biomechanics of Spine Stabilization: Principles and Clinic Practice. New York, McGraw-Hill, 1995.*)

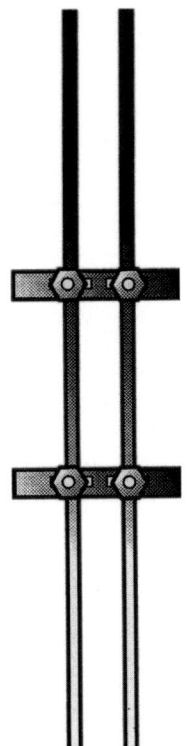

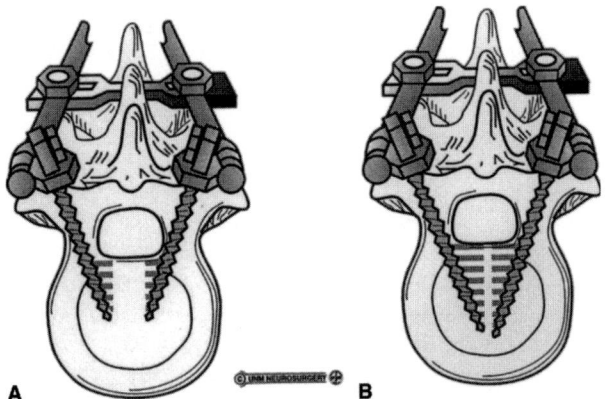

**Figure 124.11** The triangulation of pedicle screws provides additional resistance to pullout. Pullout resistance is proportional not only to volume of bone between screw threads, but also to the triangular area defined by the screw, the perpendicular, and the dorsal vertebral body surface *(shaded area)*. Whereas screw length does not routinely contribute significantly to pullout resistance, it contributes significantly when screws are triangulated (compare **A** and **B**). Increasing the screw angle (toe-in) also increases the size of the shaded area and thus pullout resistance (triangulation). *(From Benzel EC:* Biomechanics of Spine Stabilization: Principles and Clinic Practice. *New York, McGraw-Hill, 1995.)*

**Figure 124.9** A depiction of cross-members placed roughly at the junctions of the middle third with the upper and lower thirds of the construct. *(From Benzel EC:* Biomechanics of Spine Stabilization: Principles and Clinic Practice. *New York, McGraw-Hill, 1995.)*

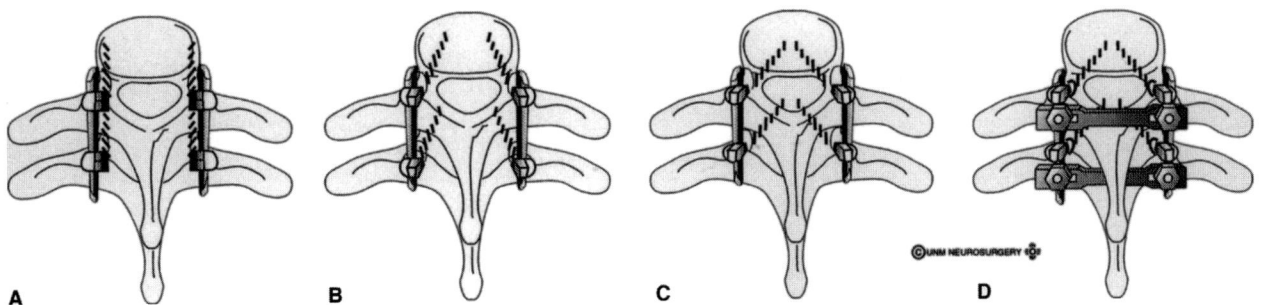

**Figure 124.10** Screw toe-in maintenance results in much greater pullout resistance, translational deformity prevention, and construct security. **(A)** Parallel screws cannot resist translation and resist pullout poorly. **(B)** An intermediate toe-in provides moderate security in these respects. **(C)** Significant toe-in results in even greater security. **(D)** Cross-fixation plus significant screw toe-in provides the optimum in both pull out resistance and translational deformation resistance. *(From Benzel EC:* Biomechanics of Spine Stabilization: Principles and Clinic Practice. *New York, McGraw-Hill, 1995.)*

must be "overcome" by the cross-fixed implant before failure (Figure 124.11).

### Toggle, Cutout, Pullout, and Implant Fracture Prevention

Toggle, cutout, and pullout are undesirable movements at the implant-bone junction, whereas implant fracture usually occurs at the point of the maximum bending moment application through the implant. Applying the principles of load sharing outlined in previous chapters minimizes

the occurrence of each type of construct failure. In general, toggle can be prevented by achieving a bicortical purchase, using rigid fixed moment arm cantilever beam fixation and/or optimizing "load-sharing" principles. Avoiding untoward three-point bending forces and using appropriate screw lengths can minimize screw or hook cutout. By using larger-diameter screws with an accompanying increased thread depth and pitch, screw pullout can also be minimized. Using implants that are structurally sound at points of maximum potential stress, such as the screw shank, minimizes the chance of implant fracture. Irregular or severe implant contouring weakens the implant by creating stress risers and should be avoided, if possible.

## REFERENCES

1. Benzel EC: *Biomechanics of Spine Stabilization: Principles and Clinic Practice*. New York, McGraw-Hill, 1995.
2. Benzel EC: Luque rod segmental spinal instrumentation. In Rengachary SS, Wilkins RH (eds): *Neurosurgical Operative Atlas*, vol 1. Baltimore, Williams & Wilkins, 1992, pp 433-438.
3. Benzel EC, Ball PA, Baldwin NG, Marchand EP: The sequential hook insertion technique for universal spinal instrumentation application. *J Neurosurg* 79:608-611, 1993.
4. Bradford DS, Lonstein JE, Ogilvie JW, Winter RB (eds): *Moe's Textbook of Scoliosis*, ed 3. Philadelphia, WB Saunders, 1995.
5. Dick W: The "fixateur interne" as a versatile implant for spine surgery. *Spine* 12:882-900, 1987.
6. Kramer J: *Intervertebral Disc Disease. Causes, Diagnosis, Treatment, and Prophylaxis*, ed 2. New York, George Thieme Verlag, Stuttgart, 1990.
7. McLain RF, Sparling E, Benson DR: Early failure of short-segment pedicle instrumentation for thoracolumbar fractures. *J Bone Joint Surg* 75A:162-167, 1993.
8. Stoddard A, Osborn JF: Scheuermann's disease of spinal osteochondrosis. Its frequency and relationship with spondylosis. *J Bone Joint Surg* 61B:56-58, 1979.
9. White AA, Panjabi MM: *Clinical Biomechanics of the Spine*, ed 2. Philadelphia, Lippincott-Raven, 1990.

# CHAPTER 125

# Artificial Disc Prosthesis for the Cervical Spine

## Jan Goffin

During the past 30 years, technical advances in the design of large joint reconstructive devices have revolutionized the treatment of degenerative joint disease, arguably transferring the standard of care from arthrodesis to arthroplasty. In spite of this, and with the exception of lateral to far lateral disc herniations where laminoforaminotomy via a dorsal approach,[1,10] or microforaminotomy via a ventral approach,[11] might be alternatives, the only treatment modality currently available to treat degenerative joint disease of the cervical spine remains discectomy (ACD) or discectomy and fusion (ACDF).

The concept that interbody fusion of the cervical spine leads to accelerated degeneration of adjacent disc levels caused by increased motion stress from the fusion is widely postulated. Therefore reconstruction of a failed disc with a functional disc prosthesis should provide the same benefits as decompression and fusion, while simultaneously providing motion. This should protect the adjacent level discs from the abnormal stresses associated with fusion by maintaining physiologic motion and kinematics.

Given the multiple theoretical advantages of functional disc replacement, numerous teams have sought to design a successful intervertebral disc prosthesis. Until recently, most of these efforts have been focused on the lumbar spine. The unique features of cervical spine anatomy, the complex biomechanical loads and motions, and the unique tissue-specific and biomechanical properties may explain, at least in part, this relative lack of interest with regard to cervical spine artificial discs.

## Theoretical Considerations

The success and long-term stability of a prosthesis depends on the prosthetic design and the technique and technology used by the surgeon to implant the prosthesis. It should provide an immediate postoperative stable interface with the vertebral bodies and, ideally, subsequent biologic ingrowth of bone to ensure long-term stability (osteointegration). The device should have significant strength and durability. It should be biomechanically and biochemically compatible, and it should not be associated with excessive subsidence or migration into adjacent bone.[4] Experience with prosthetic large-joint replacements, which are associated with metal-on-polyethylene

or metal-on-metal articulating surfaces, has shown significant problems resulting from wear debris-induced osteolysis. A similar problem might be encountered in the spine. Thus minimal or insignificant wear debris should be produced by the prosthetic joint.[4]

## History

In 1962 Fernstrom,[5] of Uddevalla, Sweden, introduced a spherical intercorporeal endoprosthesis that was designed to be inserted into the center of the evacuated disc space after lumbar laminectomy. The prosthesis consisted of a stainless-steel ball. Fernstrom focused on the lumbar spine, but also used his endoprosthesis in a number of patients with cervical degenerative lesions. The cervical prosthesis had diameters of 6 to 10mm and the ball was 1mm larger than the intradiscal distance of the vertebrae. Eight patients were operated on, and a total of 13 prostheses were inserted in the cervical spine after ventral discectomy. The preliminary results were satisfactory, but follow-up was limited to less than 1 year. Preserved motion of the replaced disc was demonstrated radiographically. The ultimate fate of these patients is not known, but because of hypermobility, migration, and subsidence of the ball into the cancellous bone of the adjacent vertebrae, the technique was eventually abandoned.[4]

In 1964 Reitz and Joubert,[14] both from Durban, South Africa, reported their own experiences with the Fernstrom prosthesis in a series of 32 patients operated on for intractable headache and cervicobrachialgia. A total of 75 cervical disc arthroplasties were performed after removal of the entire nucleus and annulus of the discs via a ventral approach, sparing the posterior longitudinal ligament (PLL). The spherical prosthesis preserved mobility of the intervertebral disc segment, but the reported follow-up of these patients was less than 1 year. There were no neurologic complications. These authors stated that a follow-up study of at least 2 years would be necessary to assess the long-term functionality.

In 1985 Alemo-Hammad[2] reported on the use of in situ cured methylmethacrylate inserted after anterior cervical discectomy in a series of five patients. After discectomy two concavities are made in the end plates of rostral and caudal vertebral bodies adjacent to the disc, after which acrylic is placed into this space and allowed to harden. The resulting concave-lens–shaped mass is said to allow motion. Alemo-Hammad reported satisfactory results at 24 to 36 months' follow-up, although he did not comment on whether motion was preserved.

In 1989 Steffee[17] reported on a patient who received two of his prostheses at the upper and lower levels of a three-level construct in which the central disc level was fused using autograft. The result was satisfactory.

Between 1989 and 1991, the Department of Medical Engineering at Frenchay Hospital in Bristol (United Kingdom) developed an artificial joint, which was designed to be inserted in the cervical intervertebral space after discectomy (the so-called Cummins artificial cervical joint, or the Bristol prosthesis, or the Frenchay prosthesis). This artificial joint is made of stainless steel and represents a "ball-and-socket"–type joint. A stable interface is ensured by mechanical fixation with locking screws placed ventrally and by compression against small ridges in the joint by the vertebral bodies on either side (Figure 125.1A).[4] Cummins[4] has presented his clinical experience a number of times, and he gave a summary of this experience on the occasion of his retirement from the Department of Neurosurgery at Frenchay Hospital in December 1995. In 1998 Cummins *et al.*[4] published their results with a series of 20 patients who were operated on between 1991 and 1996 (see Figure 125.1B). Two of this group of patients received two artificial joints, respectively at levels C3-4 and C6-7, and at C2-3 and C6-7. Seventeen of the patients were myelopathic, two were radiculopathic, one had degenerative disc disease with pain, and three patients suffered from rheumatoid arthritis. Two patients underwent surgery in 1991; two patients each underwent surgery in the years 1992 through 1994, nine patients in 1995, and three in 1996. Therefore the duration of follow-up ranged from 3 to 65 months. At the end of this follow-up period movement of the joint was demonstrated on flexion-extension radiographs in 16 of the patients (80%), with an average flexion-extension range of motion of 5 degrees.

No patient required additional motion segment surgery. Radiologic examination did not demonstrate fusion at the level of the prosthesis in any patient, and the interspace height was preserved in all cases. Further adjacent disc degeneration was absent. Subsidence into the vertebral bodies did not occur, and no wear debris was seen. Osseous incorporation of the prosthesis, however, was not demonstrated.

With regard to pain relief, 16 of the 20 patients reported improvement. Complications occurred in a number of these cases. There were five partial screw pullouts and two broken screws. Because the joints were manufactured in only one size, screw placement was not uniform. The high profile of the ventral flanges of the joint produced dysphagia in most of the patients, and this dysphagia was persistent and significant in four of them.[4]

At the twenty-ninth annual meeting of the Cervical Spine Research Society in Monterrey, CA, held in November 2001, Robertson *et al.*[15] presented a new series of 15 patients with radiculopathy and/or myelopathy, who received disc replacement with the Bristol prosthesis. It is not clear whether these 15 patients reflect a new patient

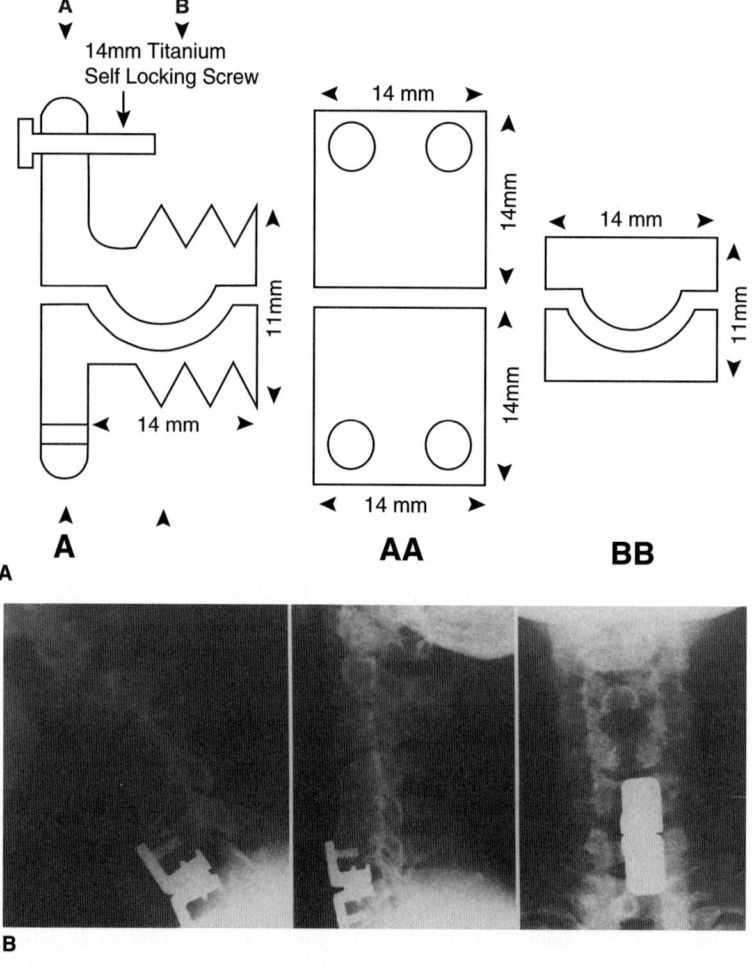

**Figure 125.1** **(A)** Design of Bristol prosthesis. **(B)** Three radiographs showing the Bristol prosthesis at level C6-7 with movement demonstrated on flexion *(left)* and extension *(center)* views; the anterior view *(right)* illustrates artificial joint placement. *(From Cummins B, Robertson G, Gill S: Surgical experience with an implanted artificial cervical joint.* J Neurosurg 88:943-948, 1998.)

group or are part of the previous series of 20 cases. At 2-year follow-up these 15 patients demonstrated satisfactory motion of the artificial disc on flexion-extension radiographic images and a number of them improved with regard to their neurologic signs and symptoms.

In 2002 Wigfield et al.[19] presented a series of 12 patients who received the Bristol prosthesis. The 1-year results were compared to a group of 13 patients who received, during the same period, a classical interbody fusion. The patients who received the artificial cervical joint were most at risk of developing adjacent-level disease (if a standard fusion procedure were to be performed). The indications for cervical joint replacement thus included presentation with radiculopathy and/or myelopathy, with radiologic evidence of neural compression by osteophyte or herniated disc material, and the presence of an adjacent surgically created or congenital cervical fusion. An alternative entry category was for patients with evidence of asymptomatic disc degeneration adjacent to the symptomatic disc targeted for surgery, even if there had been no previous surgery. In the fusion group a significant increase in adjacent-level movement was demonstrated at 1-year follow-up compared with the group of patients in whom artificial cervical joints were placed. The increase of movement occurred predominantly at intervertebral discs that were preoperatively regarded as normal. An overall reduction in adjacent-level movement was observed in patients who underwent disc replacement, although this reduction was compensated for by movement provided by the artificial cervical joint itself. Therefore it remains unknown whether the Bristol-prosthesis has a protective influence on adjacent vertebral discs.

In 2001 Vincent Pointillart,[13] from Bordeaux, France, described his experience with a new low-profile disc prosthesis, implanted after single-level cervical discectomy. The concept of this artificial disc was influenced by the use of unipolar hip replacements. The prosthesis has a titanium base, which is firmly secured by two screws to the caudal vertebral body after all soft and cartilaginous material has been removed from the rostral end-plate of this body. The carbon sliding surface at the rostral side of the prosthesis interfaces with the remnants of disc tissue, which is left in place on the caudal end-plate of the rostral vertebral body. A clinical trial was performed on five male and five female patients, operated on in 1998 and 1999. All patients had radiculopathy, not responding to classical conservative therapy. No collar or brace was prescribed after the intervention. The patients were given a clinical and radiologic follow-up up to 1 year postoperatively. Two of them experienced neck pain, which necessitated removal of the prosthesis and subsequent interbody fusion in one case, with good clinical success 6 months after the first surgery. Radiographically, all mobility of the operated level had disappeared by 1 year postoperatively as the result of spontaneous fusion in all cases.

At the sixteenth annual meeting of the European Section of the Cervical Spine Research Society, held June 2000 in London, André Jackowski, from Birmingham (United Kingdom), presented the results of a number of laboratory tests with his viscoelastic jacketed hydrogel prosthesis. As far as is known this prosthesis has not yet been used in a clinical setting.

Whereas the previously mentioned artificial discs were basically developed as spacers that could also permit motion, a next generation of disc prostheses for the cervical spine has been designed to allow not only motion, but also elasticity.

Since 1997 the Spinal Dynamics Corporation (Mercer Island, WA) has been developing and testing the Bryan Cervical Disc prosthesis. Recently, Spinal Dynamics was acquired by the Medtronic Sofamor Danek Corporation (Memphis, TN).

## Structural and Functional Objectives of the Bryan Cervical Disc Prosthesis

The design objectives were based on established principles and methods that have been validated over the past 10 years for large joint reconstructive devices, including:

- The device should be semiconstrained over the normal range of motion and thus be able to function synergistically with the remaining anatomic structures (e.g., annulus, ligaments, facets and muscles).
- The device should use precise bone preparation techniques, combined with porous bone ingrowth fixation, to be mechanically stable within the interspace.
- The device should provide adequate range of motion in all degrees of freedom to permit restoration of normal function.
- The device should withstand the loads and stresses encountered in the activities of daily living.
- The device should provide long-term useful life in a biologic environment and prevent tissue ingrowth.
- The device should provide elasticity and load-damping properties,
- The prosthesis should be part of a system that includes instrumentation and a surgical technique that ensures accurate placement of the prosthesis with minimal resection of supporting bone and soft tissues.
- The device should use materials with proven success and biocompatibility.
- The device should permit conversion to fusion.

## Description of the Bryan Cervical Disc Prosthesis

Two concave/convex titanium shells capture a proprietary polymer nucleus between them. The external surfaces of the shells fit into concavities in the end plates of the vertebrae that are prepared to fit precisely with the convex surface of the device. This fit is analogous to that of an acetabular cup in the acetabulum, but without a press fit. The convex surface of the shells has a porous coating to facilitate long-term fixation by bone ingrowth and short-term (acute) fixation by high friction. The interior surface of the shells is concave, and highly polished. This surface is designed to articulate with the nucleus via contact occurring over a conforming spherical surface (also referred to as the spherical radius). In the center of the shell's interior surface, there is a post that serves to limit the motion of the shells to the maximum range of motion. There are also holes in the center of the shells, through the posts, which will be discussed later in this chapter.

The nucleus is axially symmetric with an approximately elliptical cross section. There is a hole through the center of the nucleus that fits over the shell posts during the prosthesis assembly process. During normal motion the post and the nucleus hole do not come in contact with each other. The spherical surfaces of the nucleus and the conforming interior surface of the shells articulate during normal motion.

The axially symmetric shape of the nucleus and the shells are designed to permit the coupled motions of the cervical spine; that is, as the vertebrae and shells move in flexion, extension, lateral bending, axial rotation, or combinations of these motions, the nucleus is free to rotate and translate, as required, between the shells. When the device has reached its maximum range of motion, the nucleus concave shoulder contacts the inside rim of the shell, and the shell posts simultaneously contact the nucleus's center hole, thereby stopping the motion.

A sheath is attached to each shell with a wire loop and encloses the nucleus, which creates a closed sealed compartment. The wire is seated in a circumferential groove on the outside of the shell, over the sheath, and is fastened with laser welds.

There is a hole, or port, at the apex of each shell, through the post and into the interior of the closed compartment, permitting access for ethylene oxide gas during device sterilization. Immediately before implantation the device is filled with saline through the ports and the ports are permanently closed with titanium plugs. The saline serves to lubricate the interior of the device, reducing friction and wear (Figures 125.2 to 125.4).

## Biocompatibility of the Bryan Cervical Disc Prosthesis

All materials used in the Bryan Cervical Disc prosthesis and its implantable accessories have a documented history of use in human implants. The metallic materials used in the implant are pure titanium and titanium alloy. The polymer materials are proprietary composites of polycarbonate polyurethanes with silicone modification. These materials have been used in long-term implants since the early 1990s, primarily in cardiovascular devices.

Testing, in accordance with ISO (International Standards Organization) 10993-1, was conducted previously on the raw materials. Additional confirmatory testing, including cytotoxicity, sensitization, genotoxicity, implantation, and chronic toxicity, were also conducted. Confirmatory testing of the finished devices was conducted in accordance with the standard.

## Mechanical Testing of the Bryan Cervical Disc Prosthesis[16]

Cervical spine simulators were developed to evaluate the long-term functionality and durability of the Bryan Cervical Disc prosthesis following 10,000,000 cycles that simulated activities of daily living. The machines simulate normal flex-

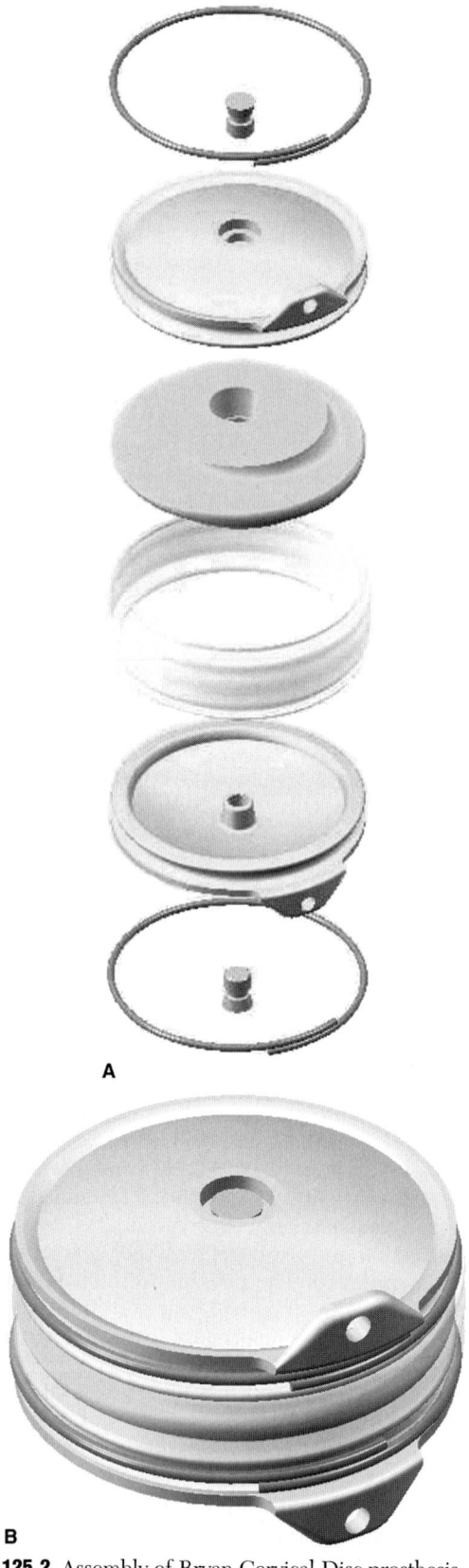

**A**

**B**

**Figure 125.2** Assembly of Bryan Cervical Disc prosthesis. (**A**) Different parts of the prosthesis, from top to bottom: wire loop and shell post; shell with hole for post; nucleus with hole for post; sheath; shell with hole for post; wire loop and shell post. (**B**) Assembly of the different parts.

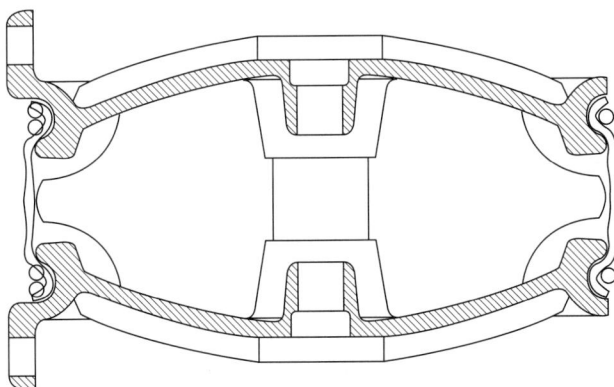

**Figure 125.3** Sagittal section through Bryan Cervical Disc prosthesis.

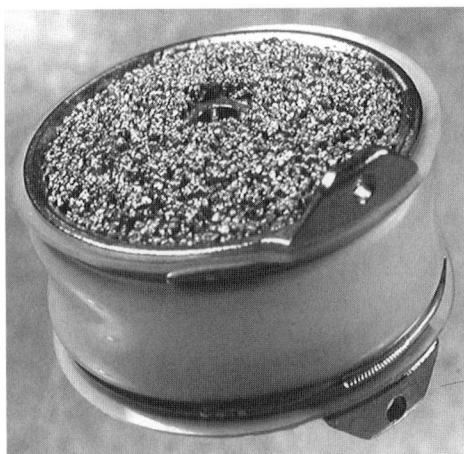

**Figure 125.4** Outer aspect of Bryan Cervical Disc prosthesis.

ion/extension, lateral bending, and axial rotation movements simultaneously under a constant axial compressive load. The average mass lost after adjusting for fluid absorption was 11.5mg. A characterization of the wear debris particles showed that the average particle diameter was 3.89μm. The diameter ranged from 1 to 454.5μm. Particles tended to be granular in shape regardless of particle size.

Additional testing was conducted to ensure that *in vivo* deformation (creep) of the nucleus will not compromise device effectiveness. Nuclei were creep tested at four load levels while submerged in isotonic saline at 37°C (98.6°F). For each of the load levels, nuclei were statically compressed between metal mandrels for a sufficient amount of time to attain the tertiary phase of creep. It was shown that the nuclei demonstrated less than a third of the creep strain that would allow shell-to-shell contact. These results confirmed that nucleus creep is not expected to allow shell-to-shell contact of the implanted prosthesis.

Compression fatigue testing of the nucleus and shell in multiple loading modes demonstrated that mechanical failure of the device should not occur under physiologic loading. Mechanical testing of the porous coating demonstrated that the strength of the coating is mechanically adequate, and characterization shows that it possesses a microstructure appropriate to allow for bony ingrowth.

## Animal Testing of the Bryan Cervical Disc Prosthesis

A first 6-month study assessed the ability of the Bryan Cervical Disc prosthesis to perform as intended when implanted in an adult chimpanzee survivor model, which is similar to human anatomy and biomechanics. Although small anatomic differences were identified between the chimpanzee and the human, these animals have proven to be a good model for the human cervical spine. The use of these animals was quite conservative, because their normal daily activity level is significantly greater than that of humans. The animals were able to move, climb, and resume their normal activities soon after waking from the anesthesia. The results of the study showed that the device performed as intended, and that the devices do not migrate. However, consistent bony ingrowth was not observed in this first study.

After several implant design improvements, an additional 3-month study was conducted. Using fluorochrome labeling techniques, it was demonstrated that the use of a modified porous coating and an improved bone preparation process resulted in bony ingrowth into the coating of the shells. Motion of the device was also demonstrated using dynamic fluoroscopic techniques. Minimal particulate material was observed, and the inflammatory response was indicative of a stable orthopedic implant.

A third animal study has been initiated in goats to evaluate the effect of particulates that may be produced by the device on local and distant tissues. The 3- and 6-month phases of the study have been completed with histologic analysis of periprosthetic tissues, draining lymph nodes, spinal cord, spleen, and liver demonstrating normal tissues. Furthermore no metallic or polymeric particles were identified in any of the tissue samples.

## Operative Technique for the Bryan Cervical Disc Prosthesis

After initial discectomy, surgeons use a simple gravitational referencing system to establish a virtual axis in the intervertebral disc space that is used to position a milling fixture. This fixture precisely controls the powered cutting instruments that prepare the vertebral end plates for placement of the prosthesis. The milled vertebral end plates exactly match the geometry of the implant's convex outer surface, capturing each shell inside a ridge of bone. This tight fit provides immediate anteroposterior (AP) and lateral stability (Figure 125.5).

No restrictive postoperative management (collar or brace) is necessary.

## Preliminary Clinical Experience with the Bryan Cervical Disc Prosthesis

The first implantation of the Bryan Cervical Disc prosthesis was performed at the University Hospital Gasthuisberg, Department of Neurosurgery, of the Catholic University of Leuven, Belgium, on January 5, 2000. This was the beginning of the first prospective multi-center European Clinical

Trial, which also involved centers from the United Kingdom (London), France (Strasbourg and Bordeaux), Germany (Erlangen), Sweden (Gothenburg), and Italy (Rome). This first trial enrolled patients with single-level degenerative disc disease of the cervical spine. The objective was to determine whether the disc prosthesis and the associated decompression can provide relief from objective neurologic symptoms and signs, improve patient functionality, decrease pain, and provide long-term stability and normal range of motion, thereby protecting the adjacent discs from the abnormal stresses caused by interbody fusion. Patients with symptomatic cervical radiculopathy and/or myelopathy were implanted with the Bryan prosthesis after a standard ventral discectomy was performed. The effectiveness of the device was assessed by evaluating each patient's pain, neurologic function, and range of motion at the implanted level during follow-up periods up to 2 years postoperatively.

One hundred and three patients with radiculopathy and myelopathy caused by disc herniation or spondylosis were enrolled, and the enrollment was completed in June 2001. Patients were operated at the C4-5, C5-6, and C6-7 levels. The five available sizes of disc prostheses (14 to 18mm) have been used in the study. The surgical procedure has a learning curve: the first operation, performed in Leuven, required 4 hours' surgical time. Currently, however, it is the time required to complete the discectomy and decompression that indicates the duration of the whole operation. Precision preparation of the end plates and inserting the prosthesis requires only 15 to 20 minutes, leading to normal operation times for one-level cases of 90 minutes.

The preliminary results of this first European trial have been presented at a number of scientific meetings, includ-ing the annual meeting of the European Section of the Cervical Spine Research Society in Turin (Italy) in 2001,[6] the 12th World Congress of Neurosurgery in Sydney (Australia) in 2001,[7] and the annual meeting of the Cervical Spine Research Society in Monterrey (CA) in 2001.[8] A preliminary report has also been submitted to *Neurosurgery* for publication. Up to May 2002, 96 patients had received their 6-month follow-up, 46 were scored for clinical success at 1-year follow-up, and 10 at 2-year fol-low-up. The preliminary clinical results have been very satisfactory and exceeded the targeted success rate at the three follow-up periods. Radiologic analysis shows a flex-ion/extension range of motion of more than 2 degrees in about 90% of the patients at 6 months and 1 year, as well as 2 years postoperatively. The mean flexion/extension range of motion was about 8 degrees at each follow-up point (Figure 125.6). No case of subsidence of the pros-thesis was encountered, and stability has been maintained. A few patients from those who had already reached the 2-year follow-up were chosen at random and asked to undergo a spiral-CT (computed tomographic) examina-tion, which showed bony ingrowth from the adjacent ver-tebral bodies into the porous coating of the shells of the prosthesis (Figures 125.7 to 125.9). At the same time para-vertebral bony deposits were detected in the ventrolateral regions in some of these cases, whereas other had no or almost no such deposits (Figure 125.10). Taking into account their anatomic distribution these deposits proba-bly reflect a type of heterotopic ossification associated with surgical trauma of the longus colli muscles, similar to that frequently observed in total hip-prosthesis surgery, in which prophylactic use of antiinflammatory medication for

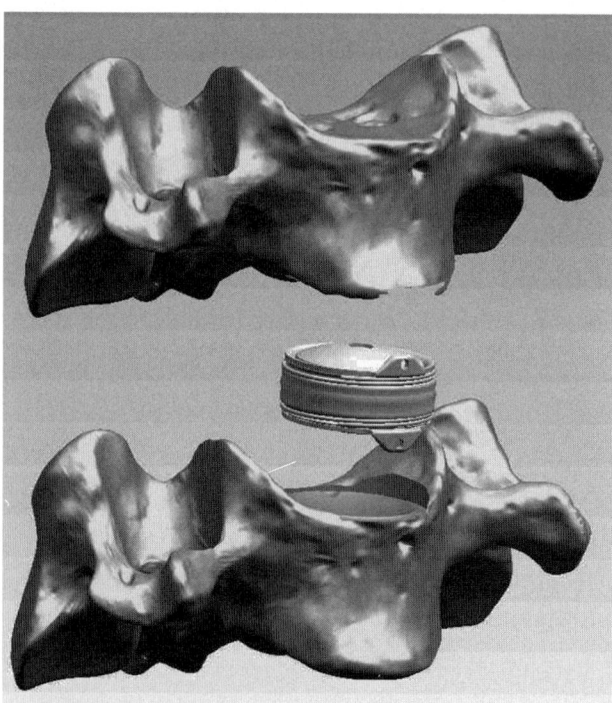

**Figure 125.5** Bryan Cervical Disc prosthesis within specially milled vertebral bodies.

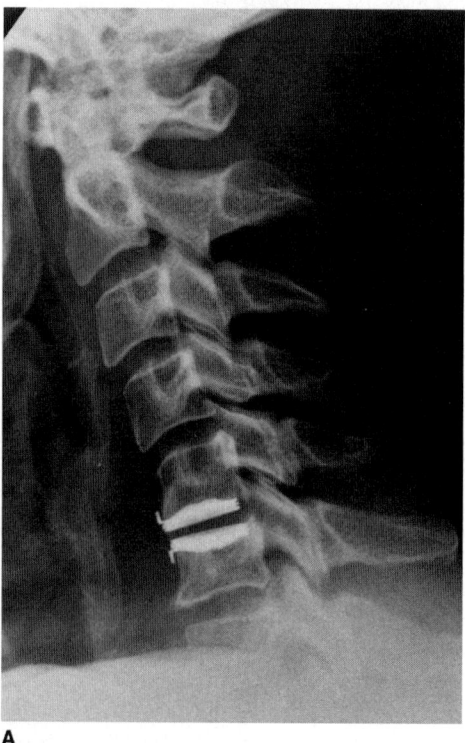

A

**Figure 125.6** Patient with Bryan Cervical Disc prosthesis at 2-year follow-up. Dynamic x-ray films in lateral projection. (**A**) Flexion.

10 to 14 days postoperatively has been effective in reducing or eliminating this bone formation.[3,9,12,18] Further examination of the frequency of this recent finding and its possible functional impact is necessary and has been started, as well as consideration of the prophylactic use of antiinflammatory medications to avoid this ossification. One patient with severe preexisting osteophytosis demonstrated at 1-year follow-up a spontaneous fusion at the operated level. The clinical significance of this finding with regard to the concept of the use of a prosthesis in cases of significant preexisting spondylosis is not clear at this point, nor is its possible correlation with ossification in the region of the longus colli muscles.

In any event, long-term follow-up will be necessary, not only to evaluate the performance of the prosthesis in a clinical setting, which might be different from the situation in the laboratory, but also to assess the impact of the prosthesis on the development of adjacent-level degeneration. Commitments have therefore been made with those patients who were operated on in Leuven to follow them prospectively once every 2 through 10 years postoperatively.

Ten consecutive patients of this initial one-level trial, who were operated on in Leuven, at the C5-6 level, were also examined by videofluoroscopy for flexion-extension motion at 1 year postoperatively and demonstrated normal mobility both at the operated level and at the adjacent disc levels.

Since the middle of 2001 a two-level clinical trial has been ongoing in a number of European centers (Figure 125.11). A very recent extension of the surgical indication, albeit not in the context of a clinical trial, has been symptomatic degenerative disc disease that causes radiculopathy and/or myelopathy, adjacent to a previously fused disc level (Figure 125.12).

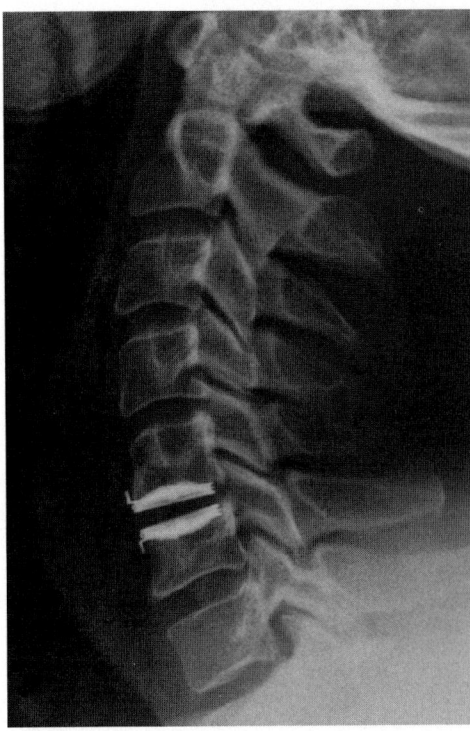

**B**

**Figure 125.6 *cont'd*** (**B**) Extension. The mobility in the sagittal plane is preserved.

## Summary

The preliminary clinical experience with the Bryan Total Cervical disc prosthesis has been very satisfactory, even exceeding the results obtained with interbody fusions. However, long-term follow-up will be necessary, not only to prove continuous motion at the operated level in the long run, but most of all to assess the protective influence of the prosthesis on adjacent-level disc degeneration seen in fusion cases.

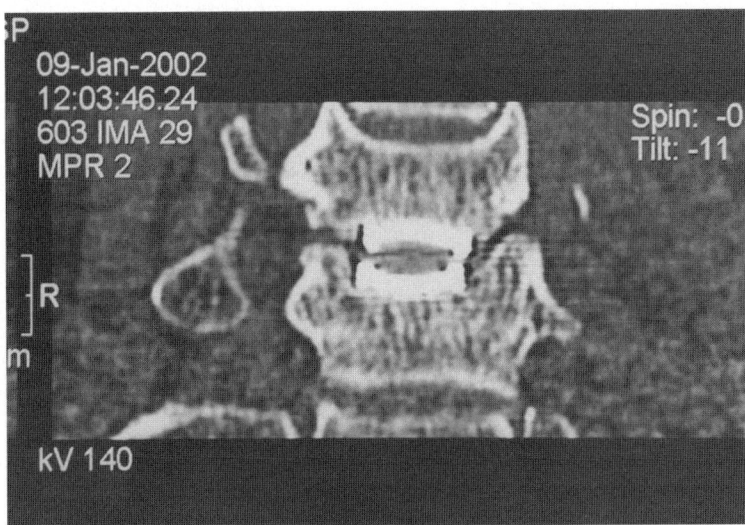

**Figure 125.7** Spiral CT (bone window) of a patient with Bryan Cervical Disc prosthesis at 2-year follow-up. This coronal section shows bony ingrowth into the porous coating of both shells.

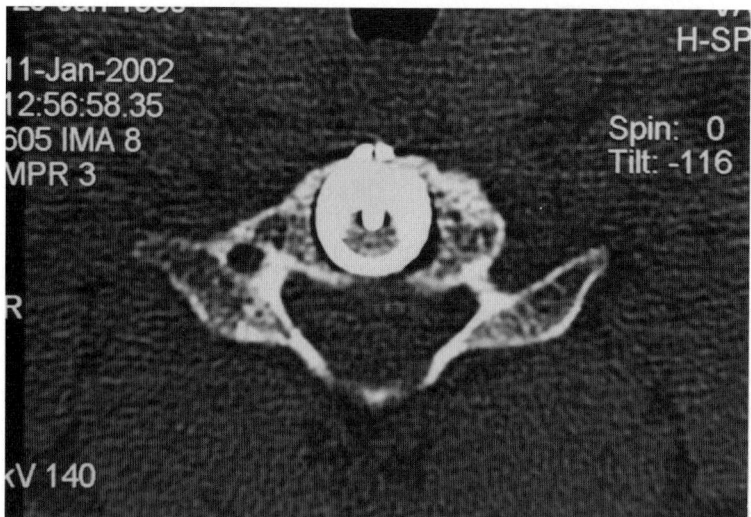

**Figure 125.8** Spiral CT (bone window) of a patient with Bryan Cervical Disc prosthesis at 2-year follow-up (axial section). This is the same patient as in Figure 125.7.

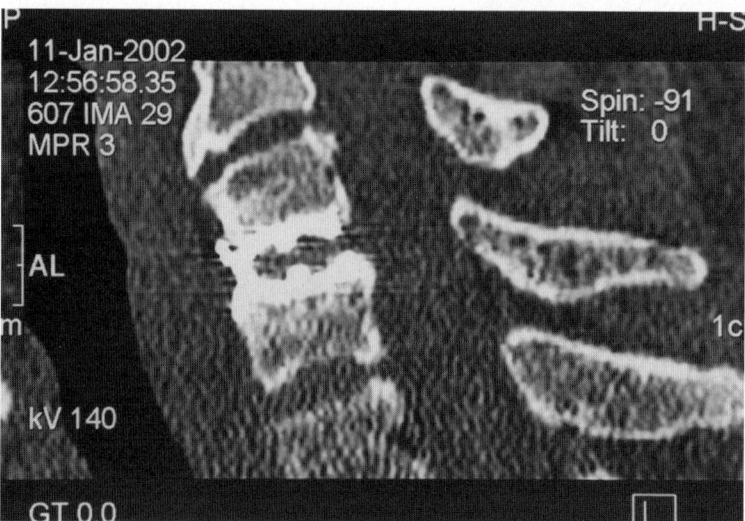

**Figure 125.9** Spiral CT (bone window) of a patient with Bryan Cervical Disc prosthesis at 2-year follow-up (sagittal section). This is the same patient as in Figure 125.7. This view shows bony ingrowth into the porous coating of both shells. The ventral osteophytosis at the rostral adjacent level was preexisting.

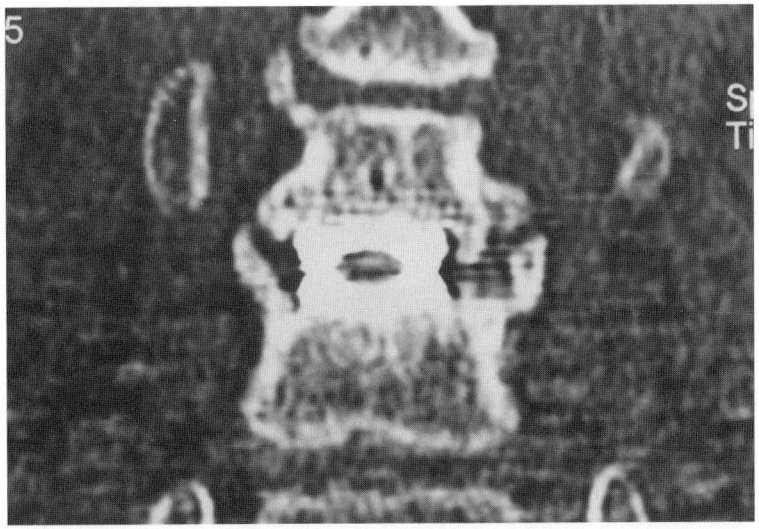

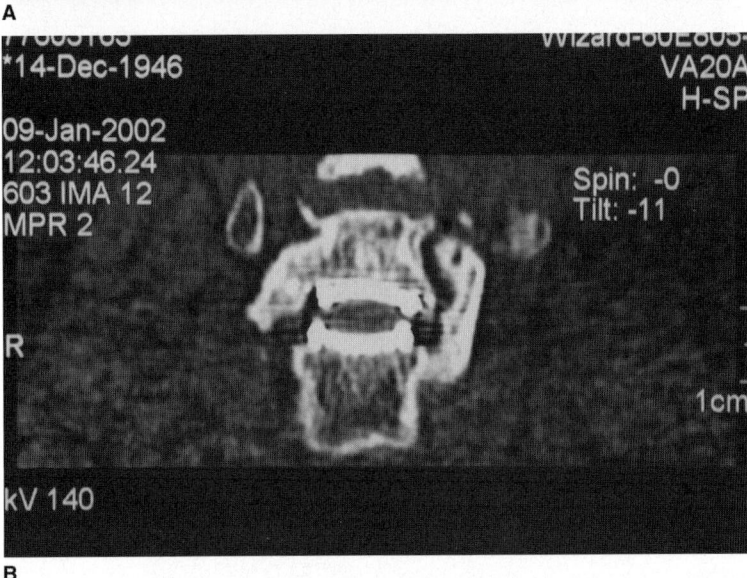

**Figure 125.10** Spiral CT (bone window) of two different patients with Bryan Cervical Disc prosthesis at 2-year follow-up (coronal section). (**A**) Minimal ossification in regions of the longus colli muscles. (**B**) Pronounced ossification in the regions of the longus colli muscles.

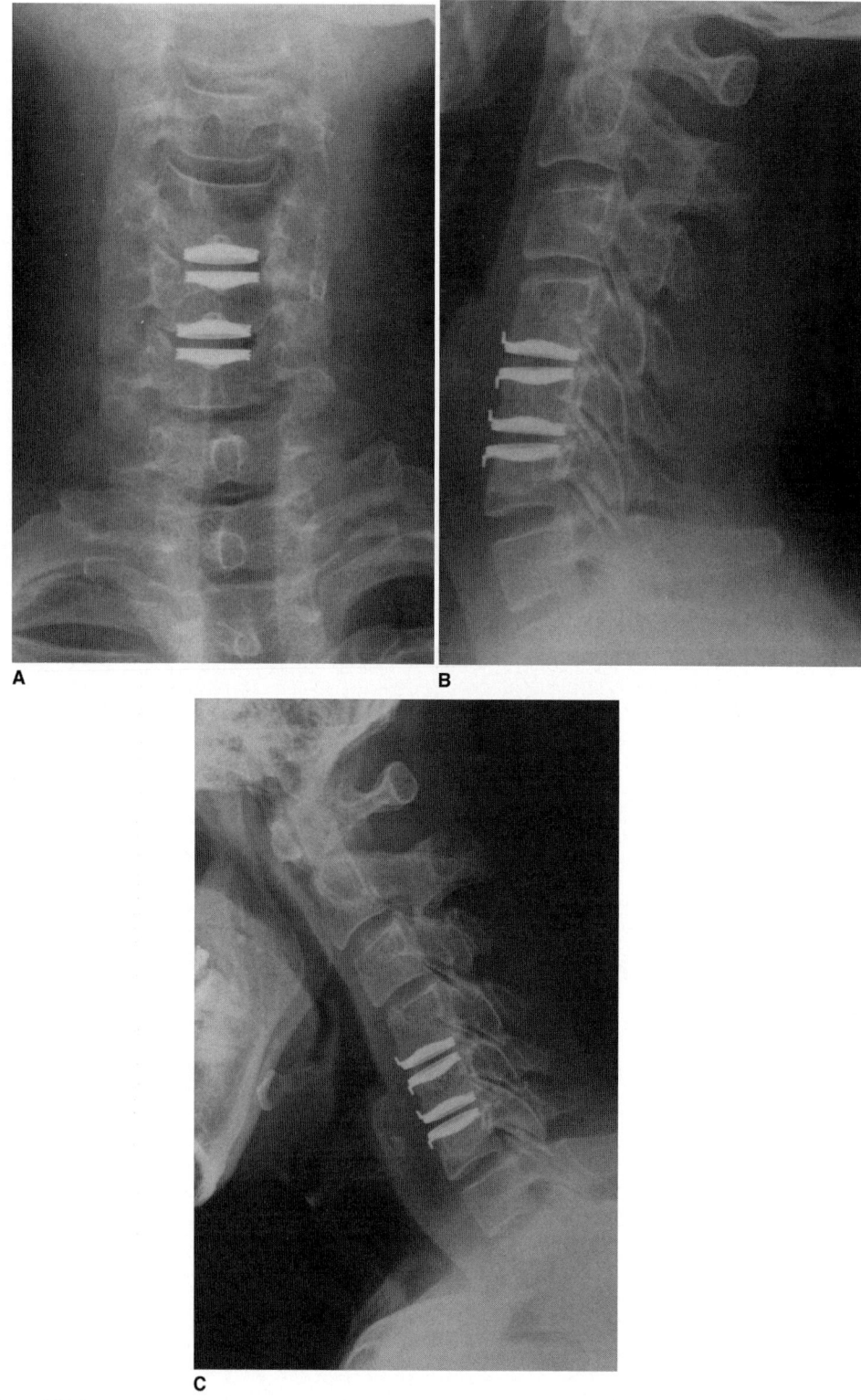

**Figure 125.11** Patient with Bryan Cervical Disc prosthesis at two consecutive levels at 3-month follow-up. Radiographs in (**A**) AP projection, (**B**) lateral projection (flexion), and (**C**) lateral projection (extension).

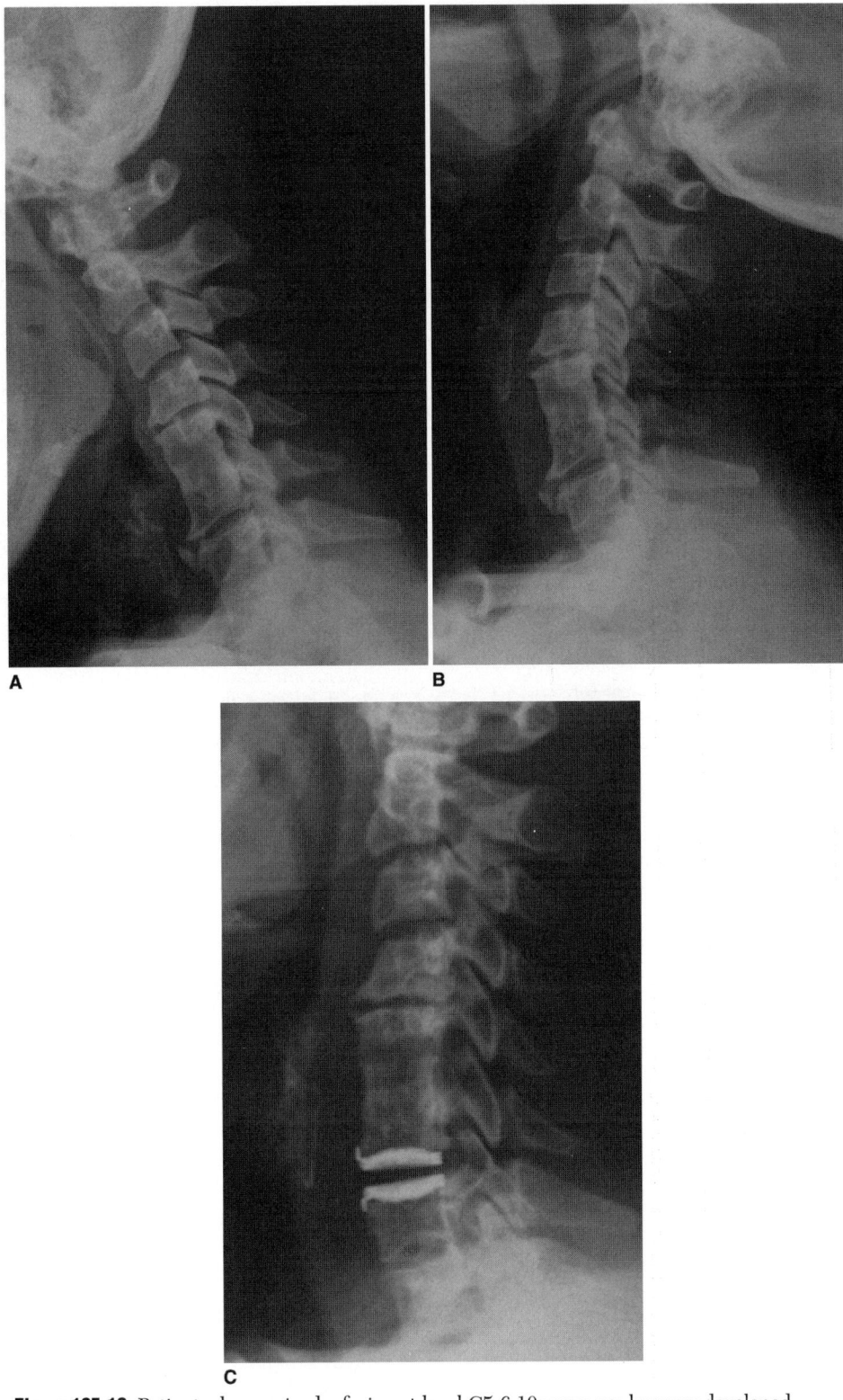

**Figure 125.12** Patient who received a fusion at level C5-6 10 years ago has now developed symptomatic adjacent level disease (radiculopathy) at level C6-7. The C4-5 level is still asymptomatic. (**A** and **B**) Preoperative dynamic radiographs in lateral projection (**A**, flexion; **B**, extension), proving preserved mobility at level C6-7 (**C**). Immediate postoperative x-ray film in lateral projection, showing removal of ventral and dorsal osteophytes and insertion of Bryan Cervical Disc prosthesis at C6-7.

# REFERENCES

1. Adamson T: Microendoscopic posterior cervical laminoforaminotomy for unilateral radiculopathy: results of a new technique in 100 cases. *J Neurosurg* (Spine) 95: 51-57, 2001.

2. Alemo-Hammad S: Use of acrylic in anterior cervical discectomy: technical note. *Neurosurgery* 17:94-96, 1985.

3. Cook S, Barrack R, Dalton J, *et al*: Effects of indomethacin on biologic fixation of porous-coated titanium implants. *J Arthroplasty* 10:351-358, 1995.

4. Cummins B, Robertson J, Gill S: Surgical experience with an implanted artificial cervical joint. *J Neurosurg* 88: 943-948, 1998.

5. Fernstrom U: Arthroplasty with intercorporeal endoprosthesis in herniated disc and in painful disc. *Acta Chir Scand Suppl* 355:154-159, 1966.

6. Goffin J, Casey A, Kehr P, *et al*: Early clinical experience with the Bryan™ cervical disc prosthesis. *Proc Cervical Spine Research Society—European Section* 17:85-86, 2001 (abstract).

7. Goffin J, Casey A, Kehr P, *et al*: Early clinical experience with the Bryan™ cervical disc prosthesis. *Proc World Congress of Neurosurgery* 12:158, 2001 (abstract).

8. Goffin J, Kehr P, Lind B, *et al*: Early clinical experience with the Bryan™ cervical disc prosthesis. *Proc Cervical Spine Research Society* 29:22-23, 2001 (abstract).

9. Günal I, Hazer B, Seber S, *et al*: Prevention of heterotopic ossification after total hip replacement: a prospective comparison of indomethacin and salmon calcitonin in 60 patients. *Acta Orthop Scand* 72:467-469, 2001.

10. Henderson C, Hennessy R, Shuey H, Shackelford G: Posterior-lateral foraminotomy as an exclusive operative technique for cervical radiculopathy: a review of 846 consecutively operated cases. *Neurosurgery* 13:504-512, 1983.

11. Jho H-D: Anterior microforaminotomy for cervical radiculopathy: a disc preservation technique. *Neurosurg Operative Atlas* 7:43-52, 1998.

12. Nilsson O, Persson P-E: Heterotopic bone formation after joint replacement. *Curr Opin Rheumatol* 11:127-131, 1999.

13. Pointillart V: Cervical disc prosthesis in humans: first failure. *Spine* 26:E90-E92, 2001.

14. Reitz C, Joubert M: Intractable headache and cervico-brachialgia treated by complete replacement of cervical intervertebral discs with a metal prosthesis. *S Afr Med J* 38:881-884, 1964.

15. Robertson J, Gill S, Wigfield F, Metcalf N: A two year pilot study of a surgical experience with an artificial cervical joint. *Proc Cervical Spine Research Society* 29:26, 2001 (abstract).

16. Rosler D, Rouleau J, Kunzler A, Conta R: Cervical intervertebral disc prosthesis wear in a cervical spine stimulator. *Proc World Congress of Neurosurgery* 12:158, 2001 (abstract).

17. Steffee A: The development and use of an artificial disc: case presentation. *Camp Back Issues* 2:1-4, 1989.

18. Vastel L, Kerboull L, Dejean O, *et al*: Prevention of heterotopic ossification in hip arthroplasty: the influence of the duration of treatment. *Intern Orthopaedics* 23:107-110, 1999.

19. Wigfield C, Gill S, Nelson R, *et al*: Influence of an artificial cervical joint compared with fusion on adjacent-level motion in the treatment of degenerative cervical disc disease. *J Neurosurg* (Spine) 96:17-21, 2002.

# CHAPTER 126

# Artificial Disc—Lumbar

**Paul C. McAfee and Bryan W. Cunningham**

In the United States there are currently four prospective randomized clinical trials under way to determine the efficacy and safety of lumbar artificial disc replacement—SB Charité, ProDisc, Maverick, and SpineCore.

The objectives of these investigations supported by the Federal Drug Administration (FDA) are to determine if prospective randomized studies of patients with symptomatic degenerative disc disease treated with disc arthroplasty could be safely completed and achieve reproducible results equivalent to traditional arthrodesis. The control group for the SB Charité is stand-alone ventral retroperitoneal Bagby and Kuslich (BAK) arthrodesis, whereas the control group for the other three types of disc replacement is a 360 fusion, dorsal pedicle instrumentation, ventral retroperitoneal femoral ring allograft, and iliac crest harvesting.

Because these are confidential FDA investigations, the focus of this chapter is the 60 patients treated at the author's spine center. Patients with one-level discogenic pain confirmed by plain radiography, MRI, and provocative discography for degenerative disc disease were randomized comparing one third of patients with BAK ventral interbody fusion to two thirds of patients with ventral SB Charité artificial disc replacement.

## Background

The lumbar artificial disc is an alternative to arthrodesis (Tables 126.1 and 126.2). Its purpose is to restore the basic motion of the intervertebral segment and to protect the adjacent levels against unphysiologic loading. Two prostheses with nonrandomized designs placed in uncontrolled studies have over 10-year follow-up results in Europe. Thierry Marney has reported 35 patients with the ProDisc inserted in 50 vertebral levels. Five different investigators, J.P. Lemaire (France), Thierry David (France), Ray Ross (England), Willem Zeegers (Netherlands), and the inventor, Karin Buttner-Janz (East Germany) have each reported large series of SB Charité disc replacement and presented long term follow-up studies.[3] Presented in the next few paragraphs is a representative clinical follow-up study of Lemaire's surgical experience from France.[14]

### Ten-Year European Follow-Up Data

Sixty-four percent of a series of 100 patients had a relative gain of more than 70% (Excellent and Good), ranging from 60% to 70% (Fair) in 27%, and less than 60% (Poor)

in 9%. Conversion of patients having a relative gain of more than 70% to a relative gain between 60% and 70% was explained by intermittent facet pain. After 10 years, good results remain in over 80% of all cases. Poor results were attributed to incorrect indications in four cases: one with facet joint arthritis, thoracolumbar kyphosis superior to the implant site in one case, and extensive postoperative fibrosis in two cases.

Five patients retired, and 82% returned to work; 72.7% had continued the same level activity (91.3% in the sedentary group, 66.6% in the light labor group, 83% in the heavy labor group). Nine percent had a reduced level of activity (19% in the light labor group, 16.6% in the heavy labor group). Nine percent did not return to work (8.7% in the sedentary group, 14.3% in the light labor group).

Fritzell et al.[10] won the 2001 Volvo Award by proving that patients with discogenic pain have better outcomes following successful spinal fusions rather than continued conservative treatment. They performed a randomized controlled trial from the Swedish Lumbar Spine Study Group with 2-year follow-up by an independent observer. There were 294 patients referred to 19 spinal centers—randomized blindly into four treatment groups—nonsurgical groups ($N$ = 72) versus three surgical fusion techniques that were reported together ($N$ = 222).

Disability assessed by the Oswestry Disability Index (ODI) was reduced by 25% in the surgical group versus 6% among the nonsurgical group. The "net back to work rate" was significantly in favor of surgical treatment: 36% versus 13% ($p$ = .002). The early complication rate in the surgical group was 17%. As a result of Fritzell et al.'s study, the current prosthetic disc replacement trials in the United States that randomize and compare results with interbody fusions as opposed to nonoperative care, which would be much more difficult for patients to accept. Table 126.3 lists the current types of implants being evaluated.

## Materials and Methods

This is a report of the SB Charité randomized control trial from the St. Joseph's Medical Center in Towson, Maryland. The primary goal of the study was to determine if the encouraging results of disc arthroplasty in Europe could be reproduced in a prospective randomized controlled study in the United States.[4,12,14,25]

### Inclusion Criteria

- Could be used in males or females
- Age 18 to 60 years, optimally below age 50
- Symptomatic degenerative disc disease (DDD), or lumbar spondylosis with objective evidence of DDD by computed tomography (CT) or magnetic resonance imaging (MRI). Some specific radiographic findings included vacuum disc sign, high intensity zone signal, Modic changes, degenerative cyst formation, and marginal vertebral body osteophyte formation.
- All patients were studied with a provocative discogram performed by an independent radiologist or

anesthesiologist who was not part of the surgical team. To be positive the discogram had to demonstrate concordant pain reproduction and utilize at least one control level that was not painful and did not reproduce the patient's symptoms. Degenerative disc disease was defined as discogenic back pain with degeneration of the disc as confirmed by history and radiographic studies with one or more of the following factors:

1. Contained herniated nucleus pulposus
2. Paucity of facet joint degeneration changes
3. Decrease of intervertebral disc height of at least 4mm and/or
4. Scarring/thickening of annulus fibrosis with osteophytes indicating osteoarthritis

- Only single intervertebral level disc disease at either L4-5 or L5-S1. Note that the ProDisc randomized FDA trial has a treatment arm that allows treatment of two-level disease.
- Nonradicular leg pain or back pain in the absence of nerve root compression (i.e., due to disc herniation) as determined by MRI or CT scan without lateral recess stenosis. The only exception to this is that in carefully selected cases neuroforaminal stenosis could be

corrected by the SB Charité restoring the intervertebral disc height and increasing the neuroforaminal height. So the ideal patient for disc replacement has back pain worse than leg pain. In the future it may be acceptable to treat radiculopathy by two-stage posterior nerve root decompression and anterior disc replacement but this is currently not consistent with ongoing FDA study protocols.

- In all 60 cases an independent nurse practitioner or physician's assistant interviewed the patient and an objective, quantitative pain scale to document the patient's level of pain and functional disability was self-administered. The Oswestry Scale and Visual Analog Scale were both utilized for these prospective studies.[9]
- The disc replacement was used for end-stage type disc disease and symptomatology rather than a primary treatment. All patients exhausted and failed a minimum of 6 months of conservative, nonoperative treatments. These included physical therapy, facet joint injections, epidural steroids, acupuncture, back school, behavior modification, ultrasound, antiinflammatory medications, analgesic medications, muscle relaxants, lumbosacral stabilization therapy, orthotic management, and other

**TABLE 126.1**

**Clinical Results of SB Charité Disc Prosthesis—5-Year Results**

| Work Status | Number of Sedentary Workers (%) | Number of Workers Performing Light Duty (%) | Number of Heavy Workers (%) | Total (%) |
|---|---|---|---|---|
| Same work | 81 | 44 | 45 | 60 |
| Change of work | 17 | 35 | 26 | 27 |
| Unemployed | 2 | 21 | 27 | 13 |

**TABLE 126.2**

**Thierry David's Learning Curve with SB Charité Artificial Disc Replacement***

| Years of Surgery | Number of Patients | Years to Follow-up | Relative Change |
|---|---|---|---|
| 1989-1991 | 43 | 10+ | 27% Fair and Poor, **63% Excellent and Good** |
| 1992-1994 | 57 | 8+ | 3% Fair and Poor, **82% Excellent and Good** |
| 1995-1997 | 44 | 5+ | 2% Poor, 5% Fair, **93% Excellent** |

*From Arrass, France.
Data from Cinotti G, David T, Postacchini F: Results of the disc prosthesis after a minimum follow-up period of 2 years. *Spine* 8:995-1000, 1996.

**TABLE 126.3**

**Current Types of Lumbar Disc Prostheses**

| Name | Year Introduced | Number of Cases (to date) | Type* |
|---|---|---|---|
| SB Charité | 1984 | 6000 | UHMWPE—CoCr, mobile bearing |
| ProDisc | 1991 | 2000 | UHMWPE—CoCr, fixed bearing |
| AcroFlex | 1995 | Clinical trials discontinued | Bion rubber |
| Maverick[†] | 2001 | 700 | Metal-on-metal (CoCr) |
| Takeiron[‡] | 2002 | Pilot studies | Woven UHMWPE fabric and PLLA |

*UHMWPE, ultra high molecular weight polyethylene; CoCr, cobalt chrome; PLLA, polylactic acid.
[†]Used in Europe.
[‡]Used in Japan.

nonoperative attempts at reducing the mechanical back disability.

Patients were excluded if they had undergone a previous attempted fusion procedure anywhere in the thoracolumbar spine. Patients were excluded with osteopenia and high-risk patients in this category such as women status postoophorectomy had to undergo DEXA scans to demonstrate an absence of osteopenia. Other exclusion criteria were (1) objective evidence of nerve root compression, (2) straight leg raise producing pain below the knee, (3) spinal fracture, spondylolysis, spondylolisthesis, scoliosis, spinal tumor, or severe facet joint arthrosis, or (4) being more than one standard deviation greater than normal body weight.

An ideal candidate for an artificial disc replacement is illustrated in Figure 126.1.

Patients with prior discectomy, IDET, or chemonucleolysis were included in this study if there was no leg pain below the knee, and they proved to be excellent candidates for the procedure. Enough of the posterior facets needed to be present to prevent overdistraction. If complete bilateral facetectomies had been performed during the previous surgery, then the patient was excluded, as facet joints are required for rotational stability.

Patients satisfying the above criteria were enrolled in this study according to a prospective randomized design:

two thirds chance for SB Charité disc replacement and one third chance for anterior interbody BAK interbody fusion using autograft. The first five cases to fulfill the above entrance criteria all underwent SB Charité disc replacement as "training" cases so that the remainder of the patients in the randomized design would not be affected by a learning curve or bias pertaining to the surgeon's technical expertise.

All 60 consecutive patients underwent randomization according to a random number generator and had appropriate surgical consent regarding randomization and Institutional Review Board (IRB) approval at St. Joseph's Hospital in Towson, Maryland. Regardless of the treatment arm, BAK interbody autograft fusion or SB Charité disc replacement, the surgical approach was identical—anterior retroperitoneal.

## Surgical Technique

The surgical technique for the SB Charité has been previously reported by this investigative group,[16] including a full-length textbook.[3]

It is worth summarizing several key points, however. First, a complete rather than a "reamed channel" or partial discectomy is required.[20] The lateral circumferential attachments of the annulus fibrosis are preserved. Second, the midline of the spinal column is marked by placing a

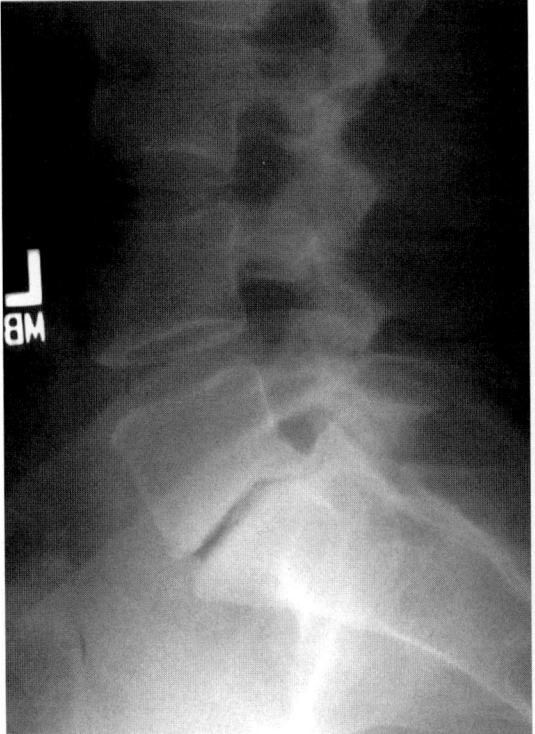

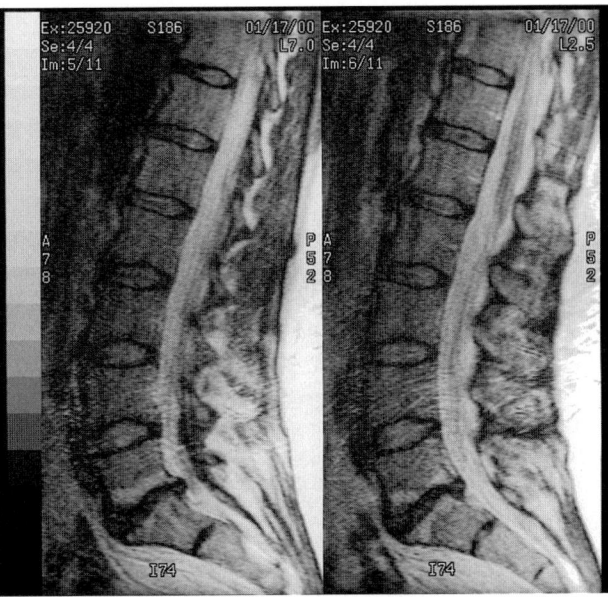

**A**                    **B**

**Figure 126.1** **(A)** A 38-year-old woman with disabling mechanical back pain with L5-S1 disc space narrowing 7 years after L5-S1 discectomy. **(B)** The sagittal MRI demonstrates corresponding Modic changes probably representing bone marrow edema adjacent to the L5-S1 intervertebral disc.                    *Continued*

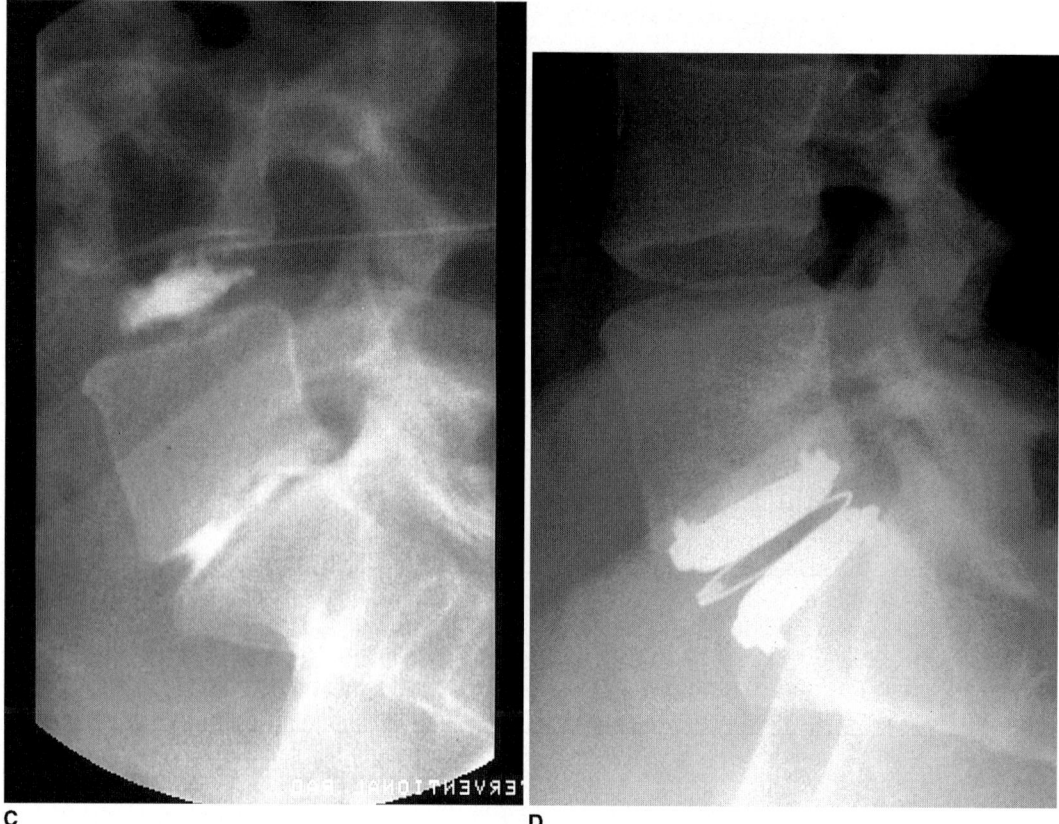

C                                                D

**Figure 126.1 cont'd** (**C**) Discography produced concordant pain reproduction with injection at L5-S1 whereas injection at other levels was nonproductive. (**D**) Two years postoperatively with SB Charité disc replacement her Oswestry Disability Index score improved from 66 to 10 and her Visual Analog Score improved from 99 to 15. She was working full time as a computer programmer.

screw in the vertebral body above the index disc. This needs to be confirmed radiographically by anteroposterior C-arm fluoroscopy immediately after the surgical approach, prior to discectomy. Third, parallel distraction and restoration of the normal intervertebral disc height is accomplished with the use of the central spreader and twisting distracting chisels of graded widths from 7.5 to 9.5mm. Fourth, good coverage of the cross-sectional area of the vertebral end plates is optimized by trying different sizing templates and checking the fit intraoperatively with fluoroscopy. This helps prevent postoperative subsidence. Fifth and most important, the optimal position in the frontal plane is in the midline, but on the lateral image (i.e., midsagittal plane) it is 2mm posterior to the midline. This position reproduces the physiologic instantaneous axis of rotation (IAR), throughout the flexion-extension arc, of the normal disc, as experimentally mapped out by Gertzbein *et al.*[11]

## Results

There were a total of 60 patients enrolled in this prospective, consecutive study—30 males and 30 females. Nineteen patients underwent BAK as part of the surgical control group and 41 patients underwent SB Charité disc

replacement. The mean age was 40.3 years (range: 21 to 56 years). The cases were distributed according to surgical level, 19 cases at L4-5 (Figure 126.2) and 41 cases at L5-S1 (Figure 126.3).

Although it is difficult to measure and compare the technical difficulty and morbidity of the two treatment groups, the surgical anterior retroperitoneal approaches were identical with the exception that the control group patients also underwent iliac bone graft harvesting. Due to the sensitive nature of this innovative study the combined total demographic parameters for the Control group and SB Charité group will be reported together; this is a requirement of the sponsor. The parameters for the BAK group were comparable to that reported by Kuslich et al.,[13,17] in fact, this investigative site was a participant in that prospective protocol for the laparoscopic BAK prospective study. The length of surgery was a mean of 88.4 minutes (range: 57 to 137 minutes) for both groups. The estimated blood loss was a mean of 289.5ml (range: 50 to 1800ml) for the total of 60 patients. The length of hospital stay was a mean of 3.03 days (range: 2 to 6 days) for the total of 60 patients.

The clinical follow-up ranged from 1 to 3 years (Figure 126.4). There were no patients lost to follow-up. There were no patients requiring additional spinal reconstruc-

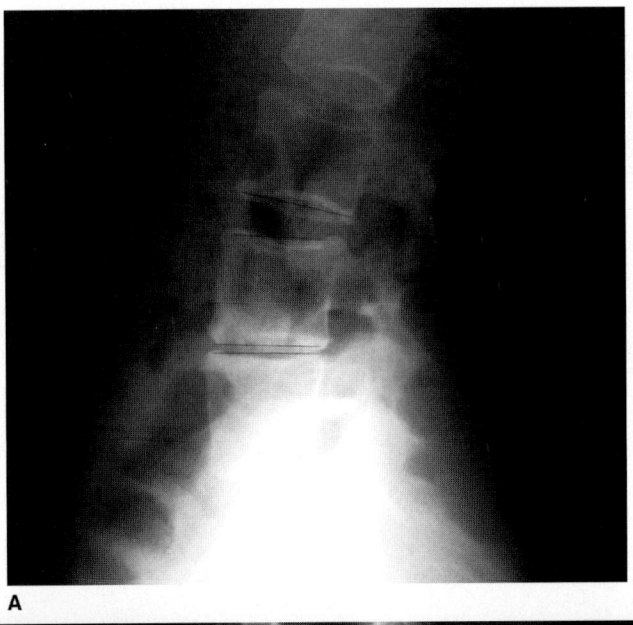

A

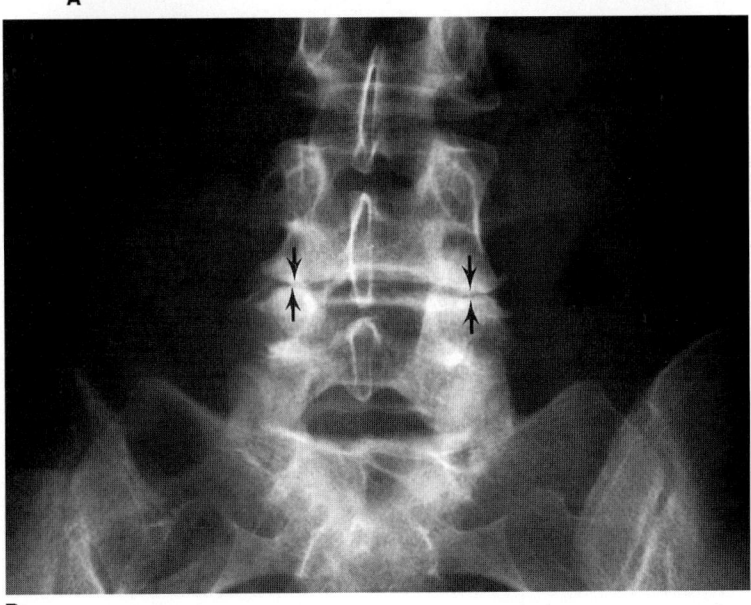

B

**Figure 126.2 (A)** This 42-year-old white female was 3 years after L4-5 laminectomy and discectomy and experienced incapacitating mechanical back pain preventing her from driving her children to school. Her normal disc space height at L3-4 measured 12mm whereas the disc space at L4-5 had been narrowed down to only 2.5mm. **(B)** The corresponding anteroposterior (AP) radiograph documents severe degenerative changes at the level of the prior discectomy at L4-5 *(arrows)* and much more advanced changes than at the adjacent vertebral levels.

*Continued*

tive procedures. There was no dislodgement of the prostheses, no cases of significant subsidence, no evidence of prosthetic loosening, and no late infections.

## Objective Outcome Measures

The preoperative and postoperative Visual Analog Scale (VAS) and Oswestry Disability Index (ODI) objective measures of functional outcome are shown in Figures 126.5, *A* and *B*, respectively. These are compared to the published preoperative and postoperative ODI and VAS from a series of 62 consecutive cases of lumbar spinal stenosis treated by neurologic decompressive surgery reported by Lenke, Riew, and Bridwell's group.[23]

These improvements in outcomes were highly significant ($p < .001$) particularly compared to series of comparisons with pain improvement following prospective randomized trials of interbody fusion cages with BMP-2, which only used a threshold of a 15-point improvement in the ODI as a definition of success. This series of 60 consecutive patients randomized between the BAK, 20-point improvement, and the SB Charité, 25-point improvement

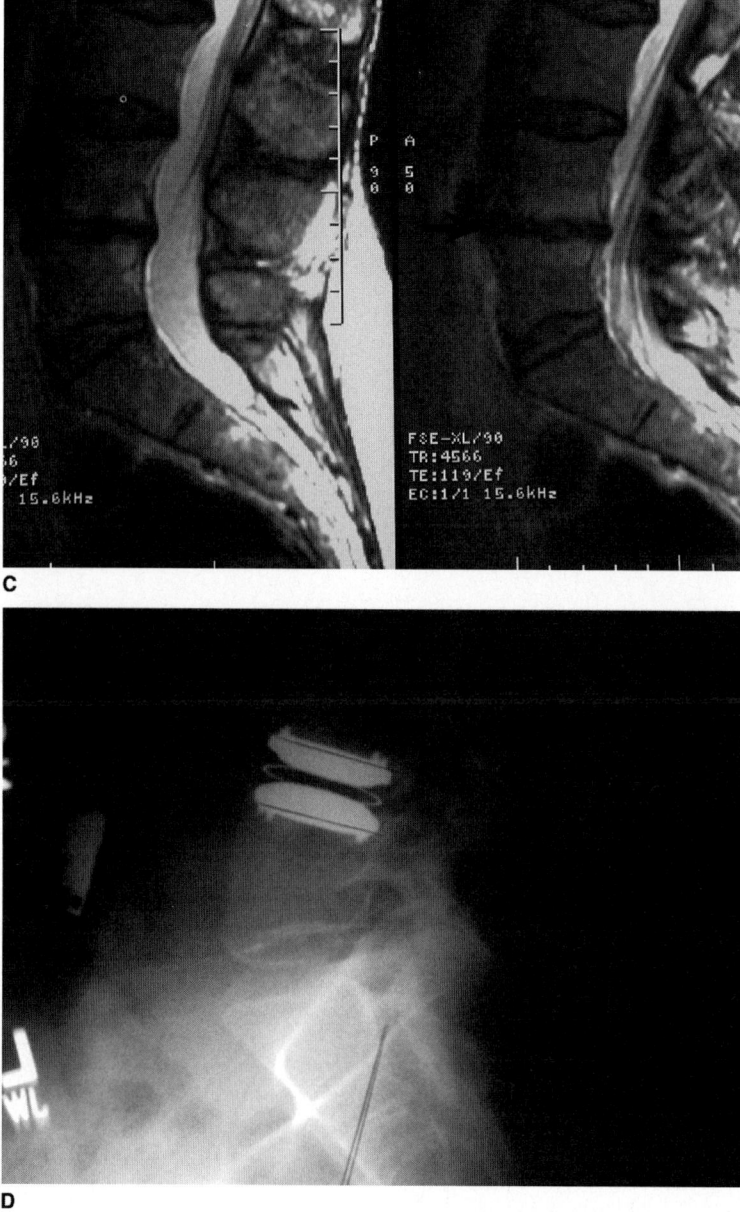

**Figure 126.2 *cont'd*** **(C)** The MRI illustrates a bulging disc at L4-5 and Modic changes with irregular vertebral end plates and increased bone marrow signal. **(D)** Two years following SB Charité disc replacement at L4-5 the lateral flexion radiograph shows restoration of disc space height to 14mm. This is the flexion view with the end plates at 1 degree of angulation.

in the ODI, easily fulfilled the criteria of success in the prior BMP-2 randomized trials.[2,21,24]

## Complications

For the combined 60 patients (i.e., 19 BAK + 41 SB Charité), no implants have been explanted to date.

There was one death unrelated to the spinal procedure.

There was one case of postoperative small bowel obstruction of uncertain etiology. At the conclusion of what was thought to be an uneventful procedure, the left ureter, left and right iliac vessels, the peritoneum, and visceral structures were specifically examined as part of our routine in over 300 consecutive retroperitoneal procedures. There was nothing abnormal noticed by either the access vascular surgeon or the spinal surgeon. Four days postoperatively the patient was admitted with a small bowel obstruction. Emergent exploratory laparotomy revealed adhesions of the greater omentum. Postoperatively there was no deep wound infection or long-term sequelae. The surgeons, in retrospect thought that the sustained retraction of the bowel by a self-retaining Thompson retractor contributed to this condition so its use was subsequently curtailed. The patient is over 30 months follow-up, asymptomatic, and working in the defense industry full time.

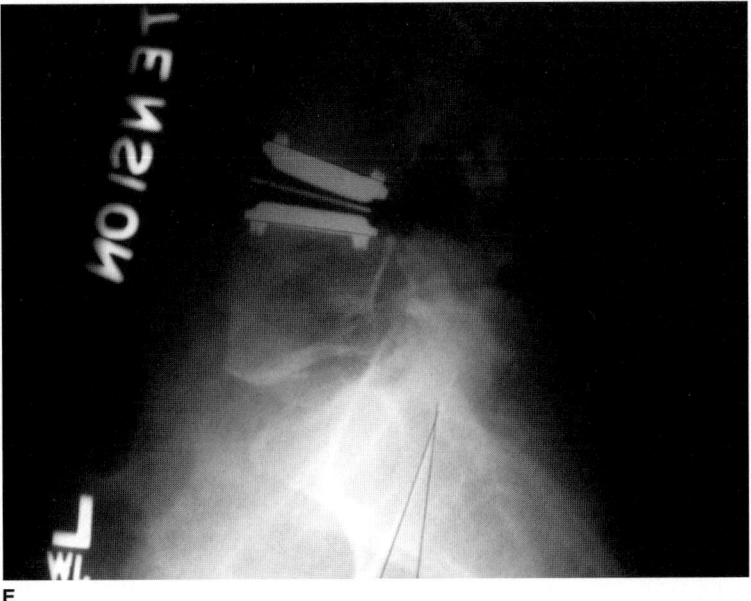

**E**

**Figure 126.2** *cont'd* (**E**) The corresponding extension L4-5 radiograph at 2-year follow-up shows 14 degrees − 1 degree = 13 degrees of flexion-extension movement without instability.
At 2 years postoperatively her VAS had improved from 75 to 8 and her ODI from 58 to 16. She was asymptomatic, she played tennis on a regular basis, and was working as a field hockey coach at a women's preparatory school.

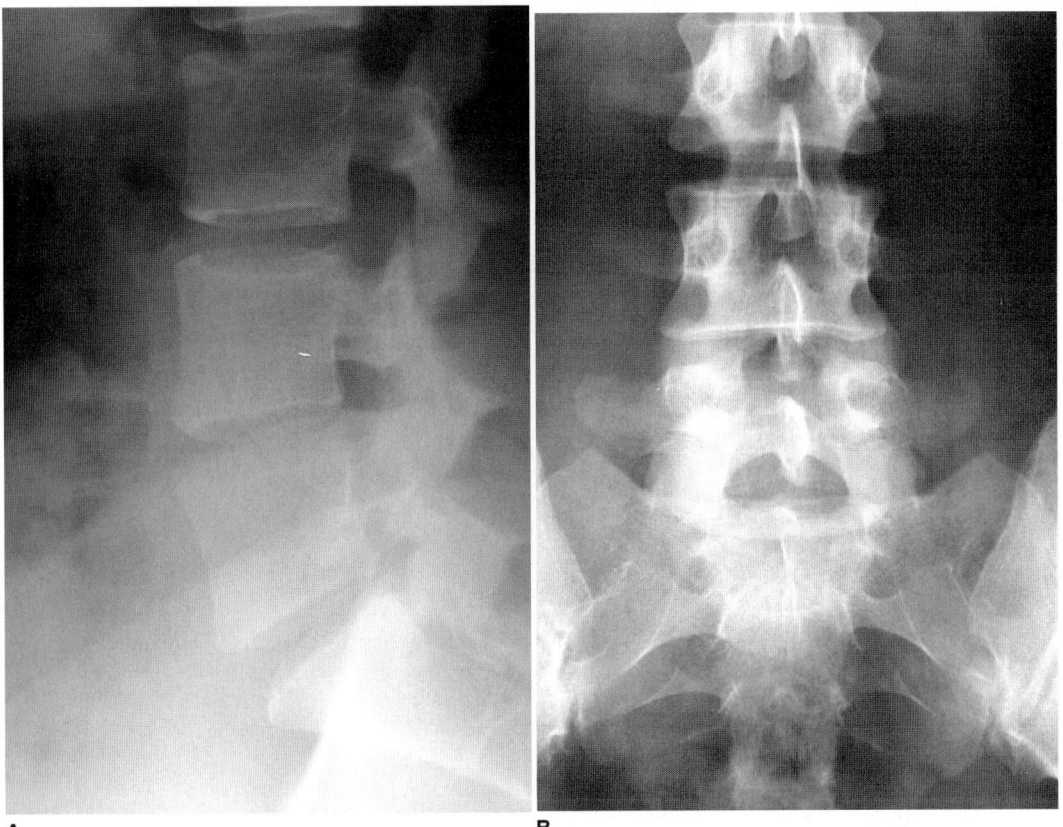

**A**                                        **B**

**Figure 126.3** (**A** and **B**) The lateral and AP radiographs of a 39-year-old woman was unable to play sports or work full time due to L5-S1 discogenic pain. The pain generator at L5-S1 was confirmed and localized by MRI and discography performed by an independent radiologist.

*Continued*

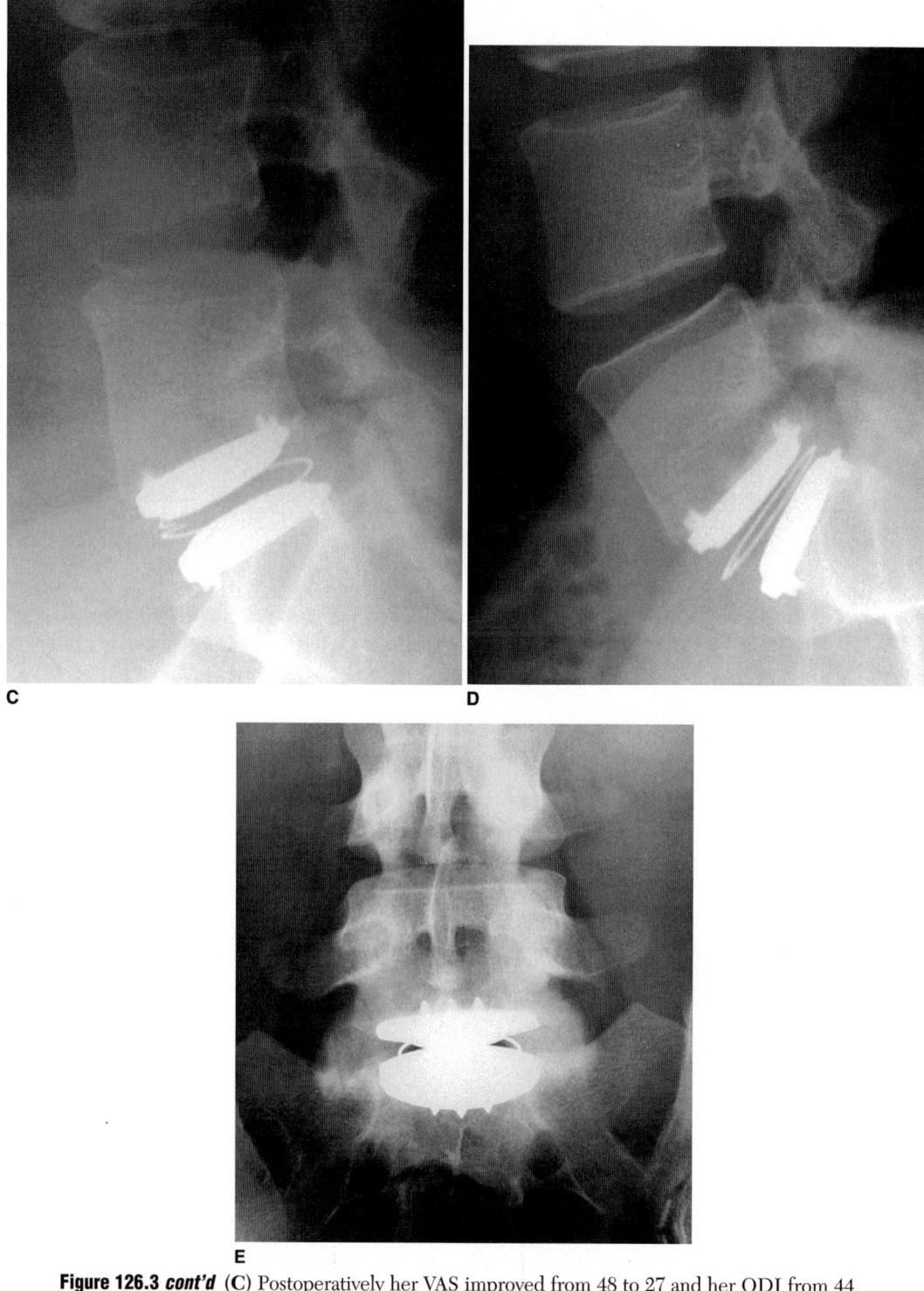

C

D

E

**Figure 126.3 *cont'd*** (**C**) Postoperatively her VAS improved from 48 to 27 and her ODI from 44 to 34. This is the lateral flexion radiograph. (**D**) The corresponding lateral extension radiograph at 2-year follow-up demonstrates 12 degrees of restored mobility at L5-S1. The ideal position on the lateral is to place the prosthesis 2mm dorsal to the middle of the vertebral body in the midsagittal plane. (**E**) The AP radiograph confirms the midline position of the prosthesis, which is ideal.

There was one case of significant postoperative heterotopic ossification and this was specifically looked for in a prospective radiographic evaluation and the subject of another report.[18] This was a Class 2 type of heterotopic ossification, which means there was ectopic bone within the disc space but that it did not affect motion. In fact the patient demonstrated 16 degrees of differential motion at the operative level, L4-5, on flexion-extension radiographs 2 years postoperatively.

One case of each of the following occurred in the total cohort of 60 cases: retrograde ejaculation, depression, adynamic ileus requiring a nasogastric tube, adynamic ileus spontaneously resolving without a nasogastric tube, uri-nary tract infection, epididymitis, lateral epicondylitis, and degenerative changes at the vertebral level above the area of treatment.

## Discussion

### Specific Characteristics of the Disc Replacement Prosthesis

The SB Charité predates any other cobalt-chrome disc replacement by over 10 years. There are five major design parameters of the SB Charité disc arthroplasty: (1) the

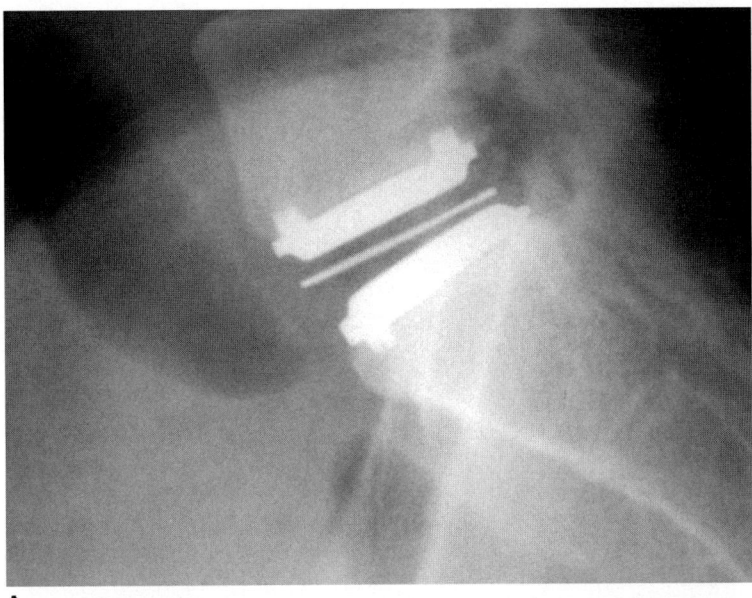

**A**

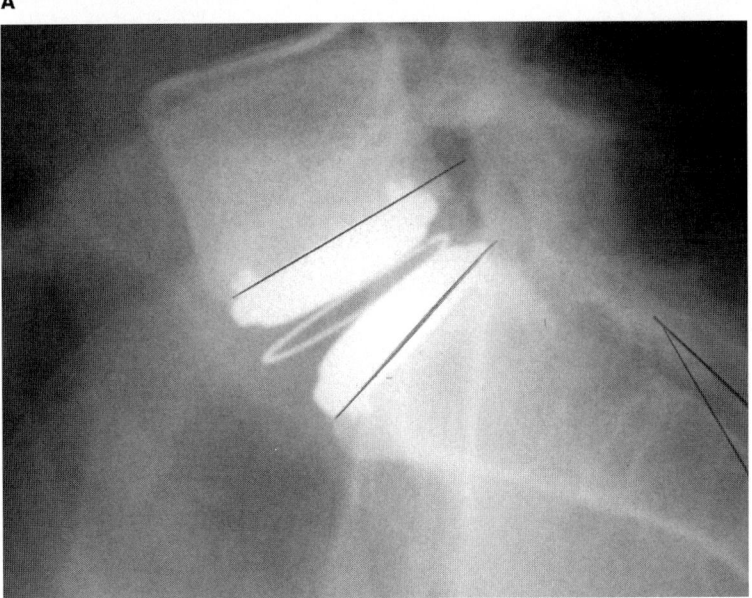

**B**

**Figure 126.4** **(A)** This 39-year-old woman had to quit work due to discogenic L5-S1 mechanical pain exacerbated by flexion, extension, twisting, or prolonged sitting. This is the flexion lateral radiograph showing good position of the prosthesis without loosening or mechanical problems. **(B)** The extension view demonstrates a total flexion-extension arc of 15 degrees of motion at L5-S1. Her VAS improved from 77 to 4 and her ODI from 62 to 10.

*Continued*

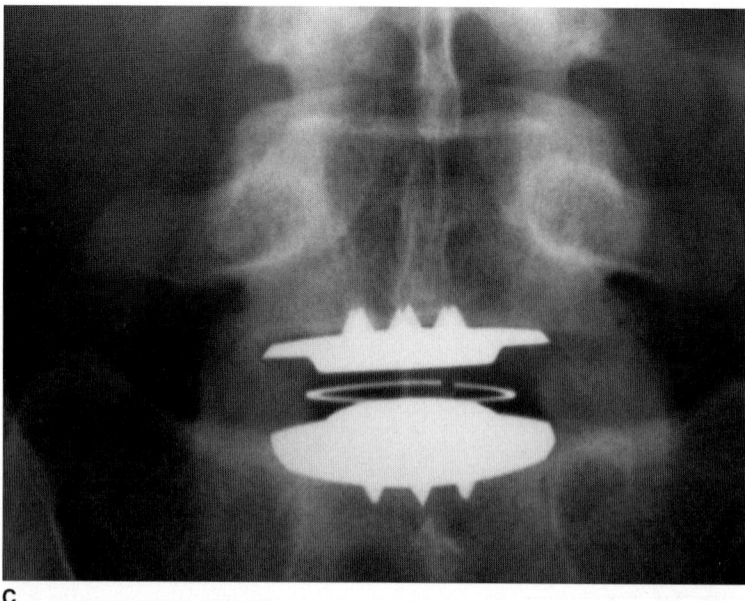

C

**Figure 126.4 *cont'd* (C)** This is the AP view 2 years following SB Charité disc replacement. She had returned full time to work as a photographer lifting up to 40lb of camera equipment on a regular basis.

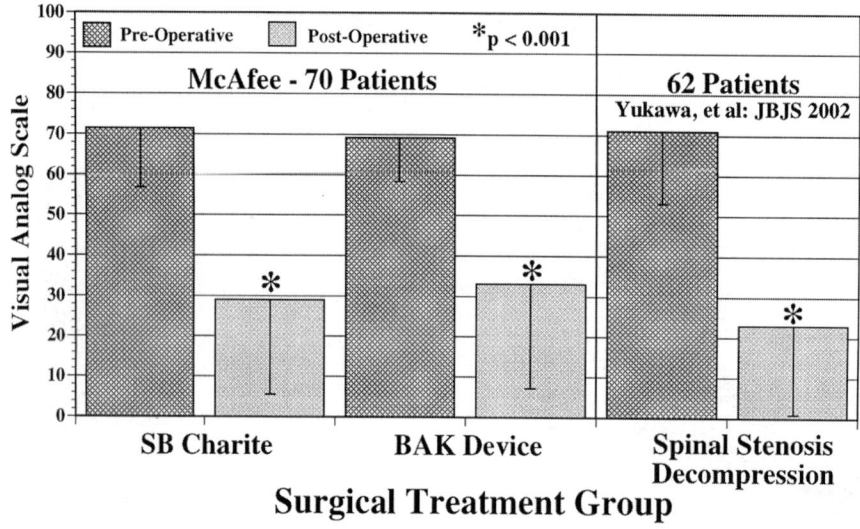

**Figure 126.5 (A)** Visual Analog Scale (VAS) measurement.

biomaterial, ultra high molecular weight polyethylene (UHMWPE)–cast CoCrMo alloy (ISO 5832/IV; ASTM F75-82) articulating bearing surface (rather than metal-on-metal or ceramic-on-ceramic); (2) a mobile bearing design rather than a ball-and-socket design; (3) the porous ingrowth surface used worldwide since 1998 except in the United States[5,19,22]; (4) moderately cross-linked polyethylene by gamma radiation versus highly cross-linked polyethylene,[8] and (5) the maximum preservation of vertebral body bone stock as opposed to cutting a groove into the middle of the vertebral body and insertion of a fin possibly requiring a corpectomy for revision.

## Bearing Surface

The SB Charité articulating surface is cobalt chrome alloy and high-density polyethylene, which has been used since 1987. The calculated wear rate of this type of UHMWPE is less than 0.152mm per year[8] and the thinnest UHMWPE core recommended by the manufacturer is 7.5mm. More favorable wear particulate and incidence of osteolysis has been described with highly cross-linked UHMWPE that is cross-linked either with radiation or peroxidase. The early wear rates of this newer configuration of UHMWPE are improved to 0.015mm/year;

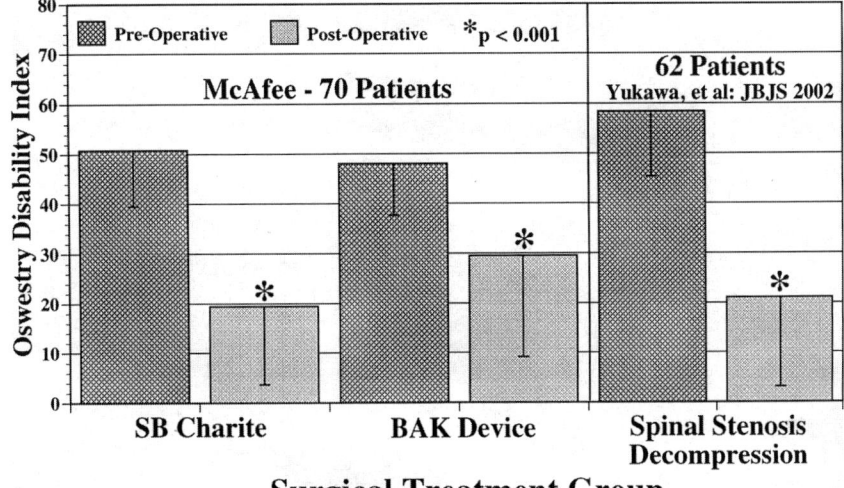

**Figure 126.5 *cont'd* (B)** The Oswestry Disability Index (ODI). **A** and **B** show the total objective outcome measures preoperatively and postoperatively. There were 19 patients randomized for BAK instrumentation with fusion and 41 patients randomized for SB Charité instrumentation and 10 additional patients included with SB III during the continuation phase of the U.S. FDA clinical trial (70 consecutive patients enrolled). For comparison, the corresponding measures for 62 patients with spinal stenosis undergoing spinal decompression (from Yukawa *et al.*[23]) are listed on the right. This is the first study documenting comparable outcome improvements for mechanical back pain as that reported for lumbar neural compression.

however, the highly cross-linked variety requires machining, has a memory, contains microscopic ridges, is more susceptible to impaction (which is why it is currently used for total hip replacement and not total knee replacement), and has more brittle characteristics.

Cold flow of UHMWPE is less of a concern with the SB Charité than any other prosthesis because the prosthetic end plates can be angled into lordosis to ensure that the inner biconvex UHMWPE bearing surface articulates with parallel prosthetic vertebral end plates. The two CoCrMo endplates can be adjusted anywhere from 0, 2.5, 5, 7.5, to 10 degrees. There is greater adjustability of both of the end plates' lordotic angulation than for any other modular prosthesis: 0 to 20 degrees total angulation of lordosis in 2.5-degree increments. The result is less tribologic production of polyethylene wear particulate, less cold flow, and less tangential stress at the metal-bone interfaces.[15]

### Mobile-Bearing Design versus Fixed IAR (Instantaneous Axis of Rotation)

Gertzbein *et al.*[11] have described the physiologic pattern of motion in the normal functioning intervertebral disc as an ellipse rather than a single point (Figure 126.6). The ellipsoid is towards the posterior aspect of the disc space in the same location reproduced by the SB Charité artificial disc. Cunningham et al. have used a pure moment six degree-of-freedom unconstrained biomechanical testing method with image analysis to calculate the variable IAR for the SB Charité prosthesis and it is consistent with the characterization of Panjabi.[6,7] The center of the normal intervertebral disc displaces posteriorly with spinal flexion. This is

only possible without impingement of the zygapophyseal joints if there is an intermediate mobile core between the two prosthetic end plates.[15]

Clinical results of total knee replacements have the longest survival with the lowest incidence of osteolysis if they have a mobile bearing design analogous to the SB Charité. Buechel et al. reported 282 patients with the New Jersey Low Contact Stress total knee replacement surviving a minimum of 10 years.[1] Survivorship of patients who underwent cementless rotating platform knee replacements with endpoints of revision for any reason or a poor clinical knee score was 98.3% at 18 years. The concept of an intermediate bearing of UHMWPE has been borne out in total knee replacements and disc replacements over 10 years.

### Comparison of Spinal Decompression with Back Pain Procedures

The number one parameter responsible for achieving a good result with the SB Charité disc replacement is patient selection.[25] In the past the most successful spinal procedures were the decompression of the cauda equina in relief of neurogenic claudication in lumbar spinal stenosis (i.e., the 90% to 95% success range) whereas surgical procedures, namely spinal fusions, proved successful only 50% of the time if patients presented primarily with low back pain. The comparison of the ODI and VAS outcome measures reported in this study show a quantum improvement in the care of select patients with mechanical, discogenic lumbar pain. This is the first study that shows that improvement of functional outcome measures in a

# Biomechanics

## Translation –
## Importance of unconstrained Sliding Core

In an intervertebral
segment two types
of translation occur
during flexion:

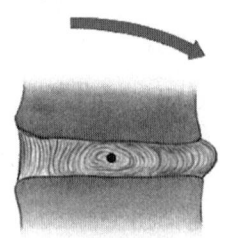

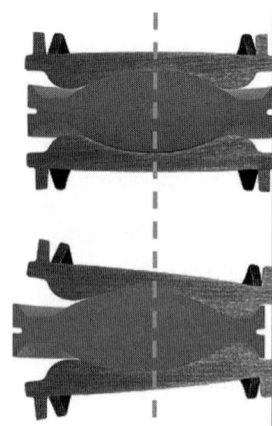

The cranial vertebral body
translates ventrally and the center
of nucleus translates dorsally.

**A**

# Biomechanics

## Vertebrae loaded in Flexion

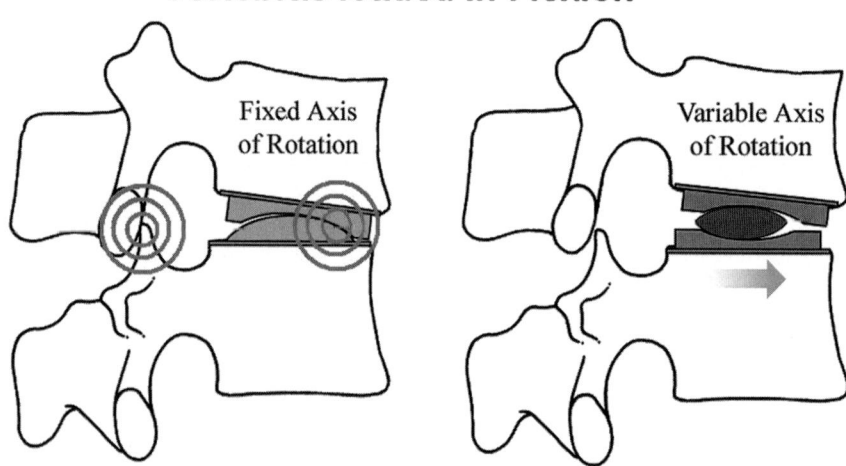

**B**   **Fixed inferior component     Sliding intermediate componen**

**Figure 126.6** A schematic demonstration of the advantages of an intermediate mobile bearing, unique to the SB Charité disc replacement. (**A**) The diagram is oriented so that the anterior aspect of the spine is towards the right side of the page. With normal flexion the anterior corners of the adjacent vertebral bodies move closer together and the center of the intervertebral disc moves dorsally. This is necessary for normal physiologic motion and demonstrates why the center of rotation of a vertebral motion segment is not a point, it is elliptical moving from front to back with spinal flexion. (**B**) If a disc prosthesis is composed of only two fixed components then, by definition, it must behave as a ball-and-socket joint, not as a physiologic disc. On the right the features of an intermediate, mobile-bearing joint prosthesis show that flexion is possible without translation of the upper vertebra. This is important in preventing translation of the posterior longitudinal ligament, neural structures, and obviating impingement of the posterior facet joints. (**A**, *Data from Gertzbein SD, Seligman J, Holtby R, et al: Centrode characteristics of the lumbar spine as a function of segmental instability.* Clin Orthop Rel Res *208:48-51, 1986.*)

prospective randomized design treating primarily mechanical back pain can achieve comparable results to Yukawa et al.[23] in the treatment of lumbar pain for spinal stenosis.

# REFERENCES

1. Buechel FF Sr, Buechel FF Jr, Pappas MJ, D'Alessio J: Twenty-year evaluation of meniscal bearing and rotating platform knee replacements. *Clin Orthop Rel Res* 388: 41-50, 2001.

2. Burkus JK, Transfeldt E, Kitchell SH, *et al:* A prospective randomized study assessing the clinical and radiographic outcomes of patients treated with rhBMP-2 and threaded cortical bone dowels in the lumbar spine. New Orleans, LA, North American Spine Society, 2000, p 114.

3. Buttner-Janz K, McAfee PC, Hochschuler SH: *The Artificial Disk.* Springer-Verlag, 2003.

4. Cinotti G, David T, Postacchini F: Results of the disc prosthesis after a minimum follow up period of 2 years. *Spine* 8:995-1000, 1996.

5. Cunningham BW, Lowery GL, Gonzales V, Orbegoso CM: An analysis of the AcroFlex lumbar disk prosthesis. a non-human primate model. Proceedings of the North American Spine Society, November 3, 2001, Seattle, WA, pp 74-75.

6. Cunningham BW, Orbegoso CM, Dmitriev AE, *et al:* The effect of titanium particulate on the development and maintenance of a posterolateral spinal arthrodesis: an in vivo rabbit model, *Spine* 27(18):1971-1981, 2002.

7. Cunningham BW, Orbegoso CM, Dmitriev AE, *et al:* The effect of spinal instrumentation particulate wear debris: an in vivo rabbit model and applied clinical study of retrieved instrumentation cases. *Spine* 2(5S):69S-70S, 2002.

8. Devane PA, Robinson EJ, Bourne RB, *et al:* Measurement of polyethylene wear in acetabular components inserted with and without cement. *J Bone Joint Surg Am* 79: 682-689, 1997.

9. Egger M, Juni P, Bartlett C: CONSORT Group (Consolidated Standards of Reporting of Trials): Value of flow diagrams in reports of randomized controlled trials. *JAMA* 285:1996-1999, 2001.

10. Fritzell P, Hagg O, Wessberg P, Nordwall A; Swedish Lumbar Spine Study Group: Chronic low back pain and fusion: a comparison of three surgical techniques. A prospective multicenter randomized study from the Swedish lumbar spine study group. *Spine* 27:1131-1141, 2002.

11. Gertzbein SD, Seligman J, Holtby R, *et al:* Centrode characteristics of the lumbar spine as a function of segmental instability. *Clin Orthop Rel Res* 208:48-51, 1986.

12. Griffith SL, Shelokov AP, Buttner-Janz K, *et al:* A multicenter retrospective study of the clinical results of the link SB Charité intervertebral prosthesis. The initial European experience. *Spine* 19:1842-1849, 1994.

13. Kuslich SD Ulstrom CL Griffith SL, *et al:* The Bagby and Kuslich method of lumbar interbody fusion. History, techniques, and 2-year follow up results of a United States prospective, multicenter trial. *Spine* 23:1267-1278, 1998.

14. Lemaire JP, Shalli W, Laveste F, *et al:* Intervertebral disc prosthesis. Results and prospects for the year 2000. *Clin Orthop Rel Res* 337:64-76, 1997.

15. Link HD: History, design, and biomechanics of the link SB Charité artificial disk. *Eur Spine J* 11:S98-S105, 2002.

16. McAfee PC: Artificial disc prosthesis: the link SB Charité. In Kaech DL, Jinkins JR (eds): *Spinal Restabilization Procedures.* Amsterdam-Boston, Elsevier Science, 2002, pp 299-310

17. McAfee PC: Symposium: a critical discrepancy—a criteria of successful arthrodesis following interbody spinal fusions. *Spine* 26:320-334, 2001.

18. McAfee PC, Cunningham BW, Devine JD, *et al:* Classification of heterotopic ossification (HO) in artificial disk replacement. Proceedings of the 17th Annual Meeting of the North American Spine Society in Montreal Canada, *Spine* 2:94S, 2002.

19. McAfee PC, Cunningham BW, Orbegoso CM, *et al:* Analysis of porous ingrowth in intervertebral disc prostheses: a non-human primate model. *Spine* 28:332-340, 2003.

20. McAfee PC, Lee GA, Fedder IL, Cunningham BW: Anterior BAK instrumentation and fusion: complete versus partial diskectomy. *Clin Orthop Rel Res* 389:55-63, 2002.

21. McKay B, Sandu HS: Use of recombinant human bone morphogenic protein-2 in spinal fusion applications. *Spine* 27(16S):S66-S85, 2002.

22. Szmukler-Moncler S, Perin S, Ahossi V, Pointaire P: Evaluation of BONIT, a fully resorbable CaP coating obtained by electrochemical deposition, after 6 weeks of heating: a pilot study in the pig maxilla. In Davidovitch Z, Mah J (eds): *Biological Mechanisms of Tooth Eruption, Resorption and Replacements by Implants.* New York, Springer, 1998, pp 481-485.

23. Yukawa Y, Lenke LG, Tenhula J, *et al:* A comprehensive study of patients with surgically treated lumbar spinal stenosis with neurogenic claudication. *J Bone Joint Surg Am* 84:1954-1959, 2002.

24. Zdeblick TA, Heim SE, Kleeman TJ, *et al:* Laparoscopic approach with tapered metal cages: rhBMP-2 vs. autograft. North American Spine Society. 200, 2001.

25. Zeegers WS, Bohen LMLJ, Laaper M, Vahaegen MJA: Artificial disc replacement with the modular type SB Charité III. 2 year results in 50 prospectively studied patients. *Eur Spine J* 8:210-217, 1999.

# Special

# Topics

# CHAPTER 127

# Surgical Incisions, Positioning, and Retraction

**Mehmet Zileli, Edward C. Benzel, and Glenn R. Rechtine II**

There are a variety of ventral and dorsal incisions used to gain access from the upper cervical to the lower sacral spine. Appropriate positioning plays an important role in minimizing blood loss and providing adequate exposure of the spine. Tissue retraction plays an equally important role. Table 127.1 presents an overview of approaches and corresponding incisions. This chapter focuses on surgical decisions, patient positioning, and retraction techniques to avoid complications during surgery.

## Patient Positioning

Appropriate patient positioning in the operating room is optimally determined by the combined efforts of the surgeon and the neuroanesthetist.

### Sitting Position

An advantage of the sitting position is that it directs blood away from the surgical site (Figure 127.1). The risk of air embolism, however, is a major disadvantage. Furthermore, if the patient is quadriplegic (with a decrease in sympathetic tone), the resulting hemodynamic changes and hypoperfusion associated with the sitting position may compromise the perfusion of the spinal cord. Therefore, the sitting position requires a competent anesthetist as well as right atrial and pulmonary artery catheterization, Doppler ultrasound heart monitoring, and end-tidal $CO_2$ monitoring.

### Ventral Cervical Operations

A bolster beneath the neck and the interscapular region enhances cervical extension. Cervical distraction may be achieved by cervical traction or interbody distraction techniques.

### Lateral Approaches

In the lateral decubitus position, the table may either be neutral or slightly extended to extend the rib cage. In this position, care should be taken to avoid compression of the brachial plexus; therefore, a roll should be placed under the axilla. The upper arm should be abducted no more than 90 degrees. The elbow must be properly padded (Figure 127.2).

## Retractors

Three major types of retractors are used in spinal surgery: hand-held retractors, patient-mounted self-retaining retractors, and table-mounted self-retaining retractors. Because intraoperative radiographs are commonly used in spinal surgery, radiolucent retractors may be very helpful.

### Transoral Retractors

Self-retaining retractors are usually necessary to maintain an open mouth and to depress the tongue. Self-retaining retractor rings are fixed on the upper and lower teeth (Figure 127.3). Table-mounted retractors are attached to the operating table to retract both the palate and the tongue. These retractors may also hold the neck in a fixed position, and thus they may eliminate the need for additional skeletal traction.

### Ventral Cervical Retractors

Hand-held retractors with blunt tips are useful for the dissection phase of the operation. For subsequent phases of ventral cervical operations, the most commonly used self-retaining retractors are the Caspar (Aesculap) (Figure 127.4), Apfelbaum (Aesculap) (Figure 127.5), the Cloward (Codman), and the Farley-Thompson retractors (Figure 127.6).

The transverse blades of self-retaining retractor systems often have teeth that should be placed under the longus colli muscles to avoid damage to the esophagus and carotid artery. The longitudinal blades are smooth.

A modified Caspar retractor has been recommended for ventrolateral foraminotomy, which enables retraction of the longus colli muscle laterally and facilitates vertebral artery retraction.[26]

### Ventral Thoracic and Lumbar Retractors

A crank-type retractor is useful to distract the ribs. The lungs, as well as the diaphragm or retroperitoneal organs are retracted with lung and abdominal hand-held retractors. Although they may narrow the operating space, the placement of laparotomy sponges under retractor blades helps prevent damage to the viscera. The disadvantages of hand-held retractors include the risks of visceral organ damage and the difficulty of manually maintaining sufficient retraction force. Table-mounted systems retract both the rib cage and the lungs.

**TABLE 127.1**

**Classification of Surgical Approaches and Commonly Used Incision Types**

| Region | Exposure | Incision |
|---|---|---|
| **High Cervical Spine** | | |
| Dorsal approaches | Suboccipital craniectomy–C1-2 laminectomy | Dorsal midline |
| | Lateral transcondylar approach | Hockey-stick, retromastoid |
| Ventral approaches | Transoral approach | Midline pharynx |
| | Median labiomandibular glossotomy | Median lower lip, mandible, tongue |
| | Transthyroidal approach | Transverse below hyoid bone |
| | Ventrolateral retropharyngeal approach | T-shaped submandibular or hockey-stick |
| | Retrovascular | |
| | Prevascular | |
| **Subaxial Cervical Spine (C3-T1)** | | |
| Dorsal approaches | Laminoforaminotomy for cervical disc disease | Dorsal paramedian |
| | Laminectomy | Dorsal midline |
| | Laminoplasty | Dorsal midline |
| Ventral approaches | Ventromedial approach | Parallel to skin crests or sternocleidomastoid muscle |
| | Ventrolateral approach—medial to the carotid artery | Parallel to sternocleidomastoid muscle |
| | Ventrolateral approach—lateral to the carotid artery | Parallel to sternocleidomastoid muscle |
| **Cervicothoracic Junction (C7-T3)** | | |
| Dorsal approaches | Laminectomy | Dorsal midline |
| Ventral approaches | Lower ventral-medial cervical approach | Parallel to sternocleidomastoid muscle |
| | Transsternal approach | T-shaped; extending midsternum |
| | Transmanubrial approach | T-shaped; or parallel to SCM extending midsternum |
| | Transverse supraclavicular approach | Parallel to clavicle |
| | Transaxillary extrapleural approach | Subaxillary, parallel to T3 rib |
| | Transpleural-transthoracic approach | Parallel to T3 rib |
| **Thoracic and Thoracolumbar Spine** | | |
| Dorsal approaches | Thoracic laminectomy | Dorsal midline |
| | Transpedicular approach | Dorsal midline |
| | Costotransversectomy | Curved to one side paramedian |
| | Lateral extracavitary approach | Curved to one side paramedian or hockey-stick |
| | Dorsal en bloc total spondylectomy | Dorsal midline |
| Ventral approaches | Transpleural thoracotomy | Parallel to rib |
| | Transdiaphragmatic approach | Flank incision |
| | Ventrolateral retroperitoneal approach | Flank incision |
| **Lumbar and Lumbosacral Spine** | | |
| Dorsal approaches | Lumbar laminectomy | Dorsal midline |
| | Paraspinal approach | Paramedian |
| | Lateral extracavitary approach | Paramedian |
| Ventral approaches | Pelvic brim extraperitoneal approach | Lower flank incision |
| | Transperitoneal approach | Midline/horizontal subumbilical laparotomy incision |
| **Sacrum** | | |
| Dorsal approaches | Dorsal approach | Dorsal midline |
| Ventral approaches | Retroperitoneal approach | U-shaped suprapubic incision |
| | Transperitoneal approach | Midline subumbilical laparotomy incision |

## Dorsolateral Thoracic and Lumbar Retractors

The lateral extracavitary approach to the thoracic and lumbar spine requires significant retraction. A rostral and caudal self-retaining tissue-mounted retractor may be used to medially retract the paraspinous muscles. A wide-diameter, malleable retractor can be used to laterally retract the muscles of the chest wall or the lumbodorsal muscles. Either hand-held or table-mounted retractors may be used.

## Dorsal Approaches to the Upper Cervical Spine
### Midline Dorsal Approach

Either the sitting or the prone position can be used in a midline dorsal approach. If skull traction is required, the prone position with a horseshoe attachment should be considered (Figures 127.7 and 127.8).

The dorsal scalp and cervical regions are prepared for incision. If a fusion is planned, the area for the bone

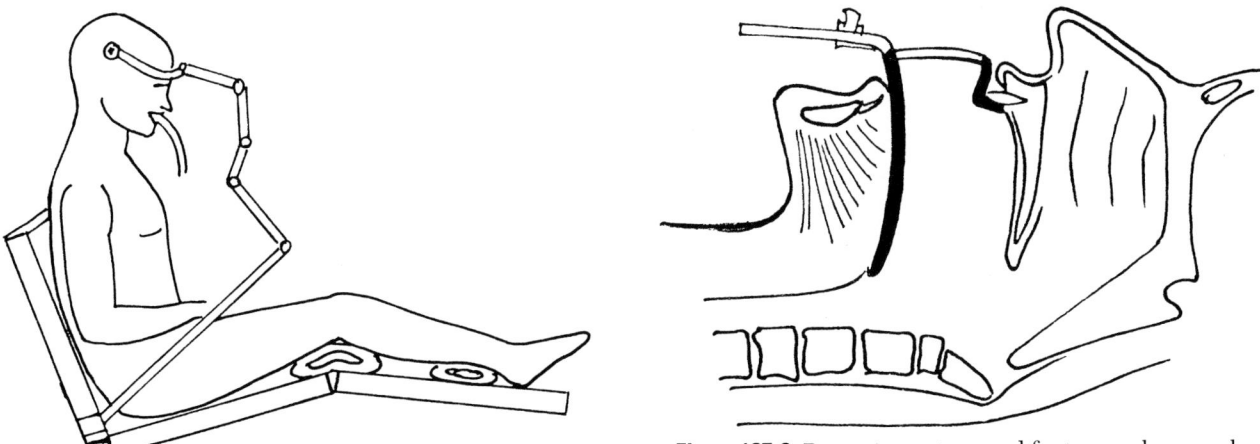

**Figure 127.1** Sitting position.

**Figure 127.3** Retraction system used for transoral approach.

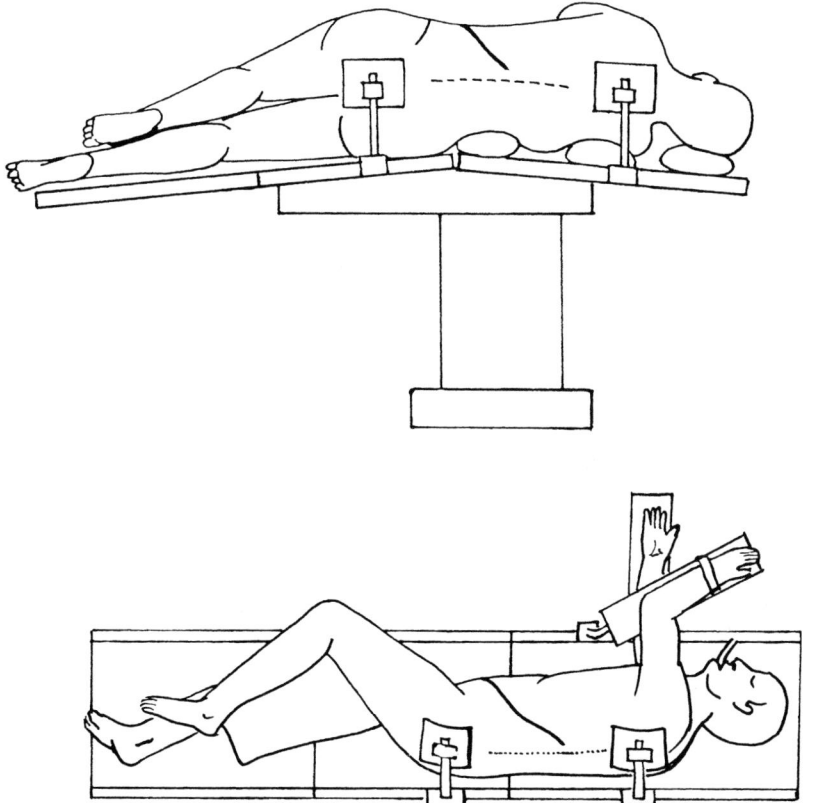

**Figure 127.2** Lateral decubitus position used for thoracotomy or retroperitoneal approach. A pad under the desired vertebral level and another pad under the axilla are placed. Note that the ipsilateral hip is flexed.

harvest (usually the dorsal iliac crest) should also be prepared. A midline incision is made from the external occipital protuberance to the midcervical spinous processes (C5 or C6 or the most appropriate level). Avoid unnecessary dissection, especially interspine and ligaments.

Two deep-seated self-retaining retractors are usually satisfactory. Menezes[48] recommends using two retractors placed at 90 degrees to each other to prevent motion of the occipitocervical and atlantoaxial joints.[48]

## Lateral Transcondylar Approach

The lateral transcondylar approach is also termed the *extreme lateral transcondylar approach* or the *far lateral approach*. With this approach, it is possible to reach the lower clivus, the ventral foramen magnum, and the craniovertebral junction without significant retraction of the lower brainstem, the cervical spinal cord, or the cerebellum.

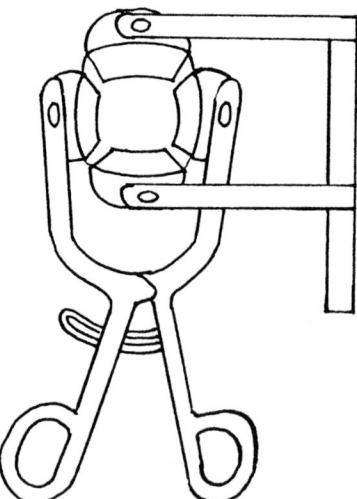

**Figure 127.4** Caspar retractor system for ventral cervical approaches (Aesculap).

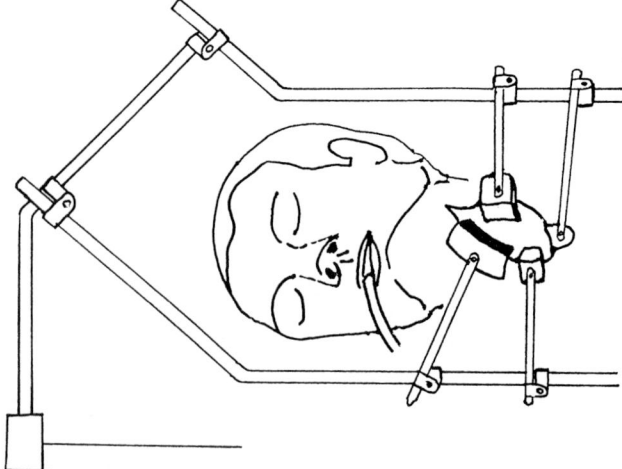

**Figure 127.6** Table-mounted retractor system of Thompson-Farley type.

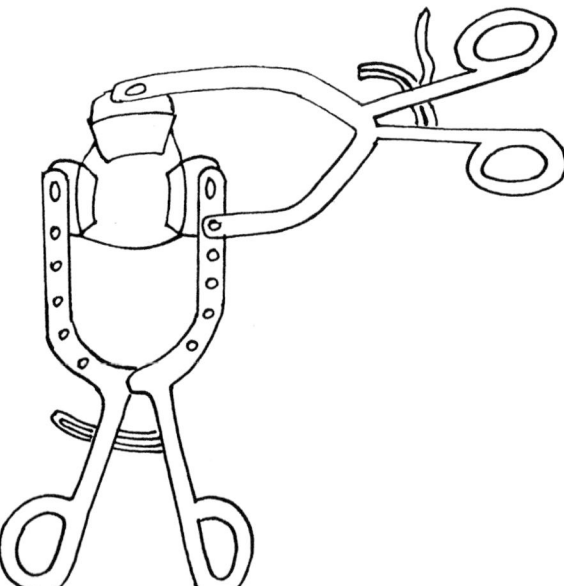

**Figure 127.5** Apfelbaum self-retaining retractor for ventral odontoid screw fixation (Aesculap).

The sitting, the lateral park-bench, or the prone position may be used. In the prone position, the head should be turned to the side of the lesion (at least 20 degrees), and a rigid three-pin head holder should be used. The sitting position provides an excellent exposure, but it carries the risk of air embolism.

The lateral position is a viable option, because the cerebellum falls away from the operating site and venous drainage is optimized. If a modified park-bench position is preferred, the head is rotated downward, flexed, and tilted away from the shoulder.

A straight dorsolateral incision may be used although an inverted J-shaped incision is preferred (Figure 127.9). This incision begins at the mastoid process, extends rostrally and medially, and then caudally in the midline to the level of C6. Because the occipital muscles cover the

craniectomy after the use of an inverted J-shaped incision (compared with a linear incision placed over a craniectomy), this incision is useful in preventing postoperative cerebrospinal fluid leakage.

Hooks are useful for retracting the bulky cervical musculature. A self-retaining cerebellar retractor works well.

One of the most difficult aspects of this operation is the development of a dissection plane along the lateral aspect of C1 and C2, without causing injury to the vertebral artery or associated venous structures.

It is recommended not to remove more than one-half of the occipital condyle to avoid the introduction of occipitocervical instability. The roots of C2 may be sectioned. Only a slight retraction of the vertebral artery, if any, is usually necessary. The cerebellum and the brainstem should not be retracted.

Salas *et al.*[58] have defined four varieties of dorsolateral craniocervical approaches. The *transfacetal approach* is used to treat extradural and intradural lesions ventral to the upper cervical spinal cord. The *retrocondylar approach* is performed for intradural lesions that are located predominantly lateral or ventrolateral to the spinomedullary region or to expose the extradural portion of the vertebral artery. The *partial transcondylar approach* is performed to treat lesions that are located predominantly ventral to the spinomedullary junction. The *complete transcondylar approach* is performed to treat extradural lesions. The *extreme lateral transjugular approach* is performed to supplement the traditional lateral transtemporal approach for the treatment of jugular foramen lesions.

## Ventral Approaches to the Upper Cervical Spine

### Transoral Approach

A standard placement is to have the surgeon at the side, and the anesthetic equipment and anesthetist at the head of the patient. Alternatively, the anesthetic equipment may be placed at the foot and the surgeon may be at the head of the patient. The patient is positioned supine, and intubation is performed with a small endotracheal tube,

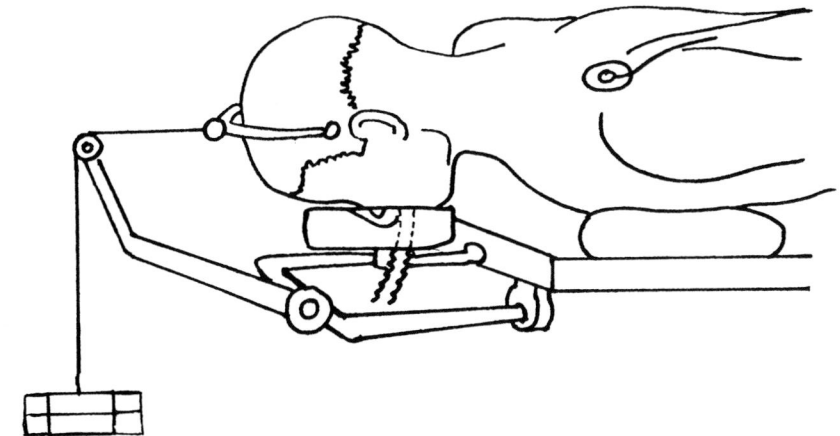

**Figure 127.7** Dorsal midline cervical approach with horseshoe headholder and skeletal traction.

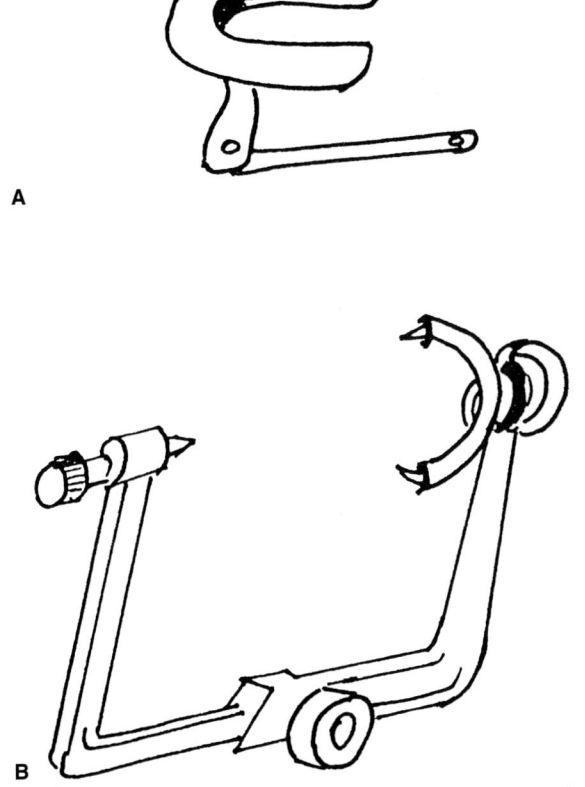

A

B

**Figure 127.8** Two different fixation devices for dorsal cervical operations: (**A**) horseshoe headholder, (**B**) Mayfield-type head clamp with three pins.

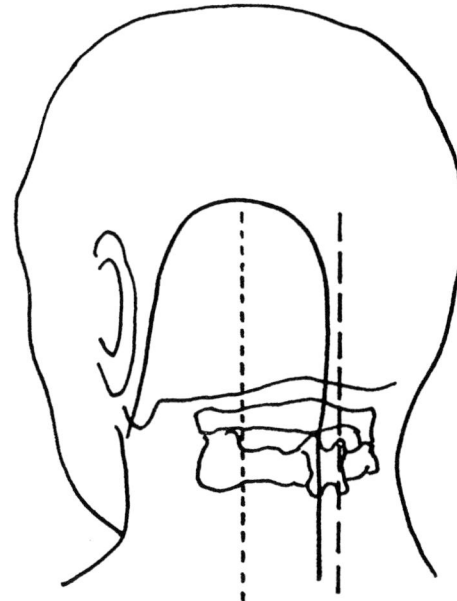

**Figure 127.9** Various incisions used for dorsolateral transcondylar approach. Inverted J-shaped incision (*straight line*), midline dorsal incision (*broken line*), dorsolateral incision (*dotted line*).

which is securely fastened. Intubation when the patent is awake may be necessary, if the spine is unstable. Slight extension facilitates the approach.

Although tracheotomy is not routinely used, if the mouth does not allow adequate space for an endotracheal tube within the operating field, an elective tracheotomy should be considered.

Because the predominant difficulty with the transoral approach is the depth and narrowness of the operative field, a self-retaining retractor is imperative. Retraction of the uvula is also frequently necessary (see Figure 127.3).

The soft palate may be held away from the surgical trajectory by a retractor, or by suturing its border with the uvula to the dorsal palate. Alternatively, a rubber catheter may be passed through the nose and into the mouth. The distal tip of the catheter is sutured to the uvula, and upward traction is applied by gently pulling the catheter through the nose.

An incision is made in the midline of the dorsal pharynx, after infiltration with a local anesthetic containing epinephrine to decrease oozing from the pharyngeal walls. The incision is carried along the tubercle of the atlas to the prominence of the C2-3 disc space. The incision may be extended, if needed, onto the soft palate, and to one side of the uvula.

After dissecting the ventral surfaces of the atlas and axis laterally, a second self-retaining retractor is held to open the dorsal pharyngeal wall along the long axis of the spine.

Stay sutures may be used to provide lateral retraction (see Figure 127.1).

This surgery is relatively straightforward. Once the pharyngeal mucosa and prevertebral muscles have been cleared away, this approach offers an excellent view of the upper ventral cervical spine, which is relatively avascular.

## Median Labiomandibular Glossotomy

Median labiomandibular glossotomy provides a wide ventral exposure from clivus to the lower cervical spine.[3,27,49] A midline vertical incision starts from the lower lip, extends caudally, turns around the chin prominence, and again passes medially in the neck (Figure 127.10). The mandible is cut in a stepwise configuration for subsequent approximation. The tongue is incised longitudinally from the central raphe, and the oropharyngeal mucosa is incised laterally.

When the mandible, mucosa, and tongue are divided, all the medial structures may be retracted laterally, and the dorsal structures, such as the epiglottis and the dorsal pharynx, are visualized.

## Bilateral Sagittal Split Mandibular Osteotomies

This approach is performed in orthognathic surgery to repair a variety of facial and jaw deformities. Because all the incisions made in this approach are intraoral, they are not associated with the cosmetic deformities.[73] It is an adjunct to the transoral approach and the retraction plane

is rostrocaudal instead of lateral. Lingual or inferior alveolar nerve injuries are common complications.

## Transthyroid Approach

The transthyroid approach may provide access to the first four cervical vertebrae.[20] A transverse incision is carried along the upper neck crease, between the hyoid bone and the thyroid cartilage, and is extended laterally (Figure 127.11). The platysma and sternohyoid muscles are divided, and the thyrohyoid membrane detached from the hyoid bone, while protecting the epiglottis.

The internal laryngeal nerves are protected, and the ventral pharynx entered. Rostral retraction of the hyoid bone and caudal retraction of the thyroid cartilage are performed. After incision of the dorsal pharyngeal wall, a self-retaining retractor exposes the vertebral bodies from C1 to C4. Due to the potential for significant morbidity, this approach is infrequently used. It has been associated with damage to the superior and internal laryngeal nerves and involves a significant risk of damaging the epiglottis.[20]

## Ventrolateral Retropharyngeal Approach

The ventral retropharyngeal approach provides access to structures from the clivus to the third cervical vertebrae without entering the oral cavity.[17,45,48,56,75] The advantages of this approach are lowered risks of infection and more extensive exposure of the upper cervical spine.

The patient is positioned supine, and if the incision is on the right side, the head is turned to the left. Moderate extension of the head facilitates the approach to the upper cervical structures.

The upper transverse portion of a T-shaped incision is made just under the mandible. The vertical portion of the incision meets the sternocleidomastoid muscle caudally (Figure 127.12, *A*). Another option is a V-shaped incision (Figure 127.12, *B*).[56]

This ventral retropharyngeal approach may be divided as *retrovascular* or *prevascular* surgery.[40]

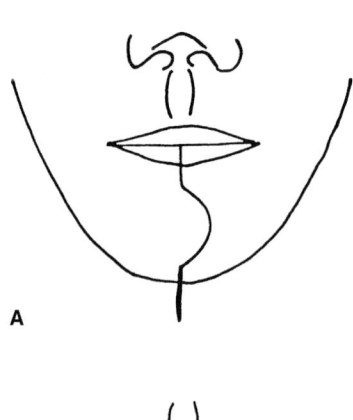

**A**

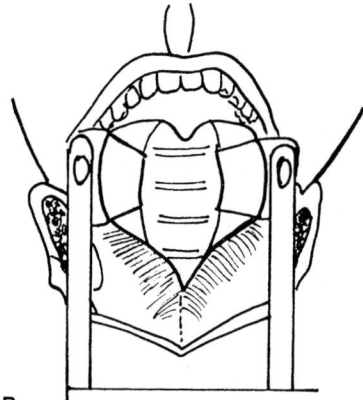

**B**

**Figure 127.10** Mandible-splitting ventral approach to the upper cervical spine: (**A**) incision line, (**B**) retraction and exposure after mandible and tongue splitting.

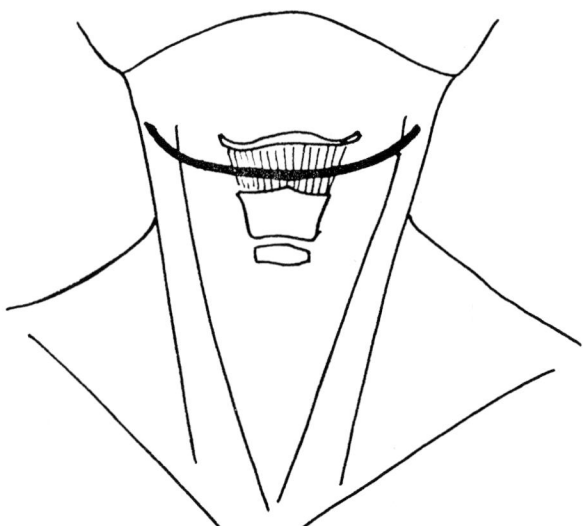

**Figure 127.11** Incision line for transthyroid approach.

## Prevascular Surgery

Prevascular surgery involves an access medial to the carotid sheath and traverses the same fascial planes as in the ventrolateral lower cervical spine surgery[45] (Figure 127.13, *B*).

It allows adequate spinal cord decompression up to the clivus and reconstruction of the anterior column of the spine with strut grafts and internal fixation.

The dissection is medial to the sternocleidomastoid muscle and the carotid artery. The submandibular gland

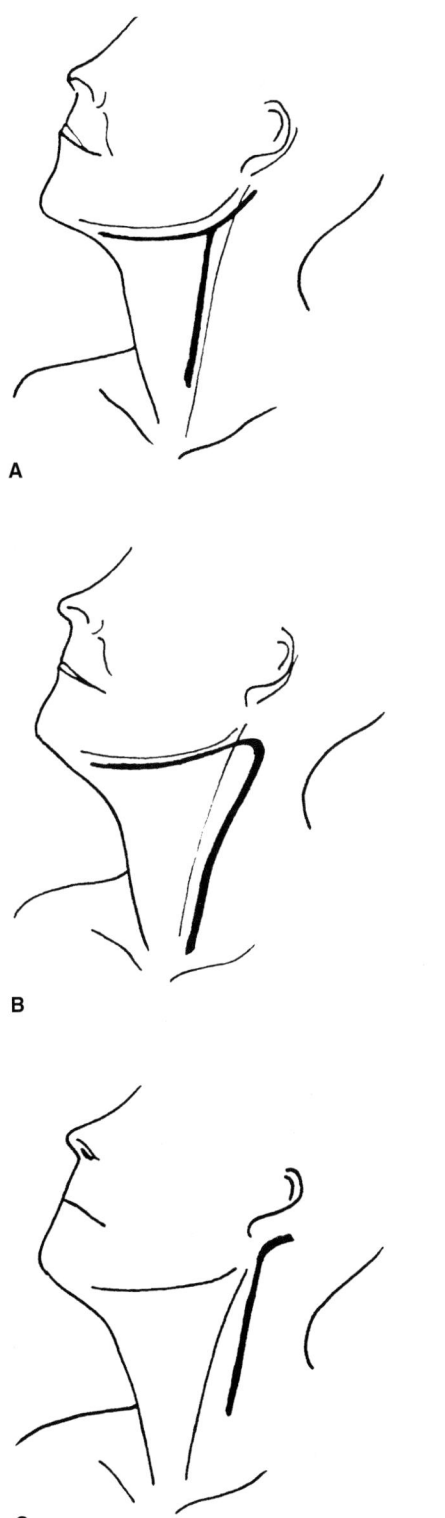

**Figure 127.12** Incision lines used for ventral upper cervical approaches. (**A** and **B**) Ventromedial retropharyngeal approaches: (**A**) T-shaped incision of Schoerbringer; (**B**) incision of Riley; (**C**) ventrolateral approach, incision of Whitesides.

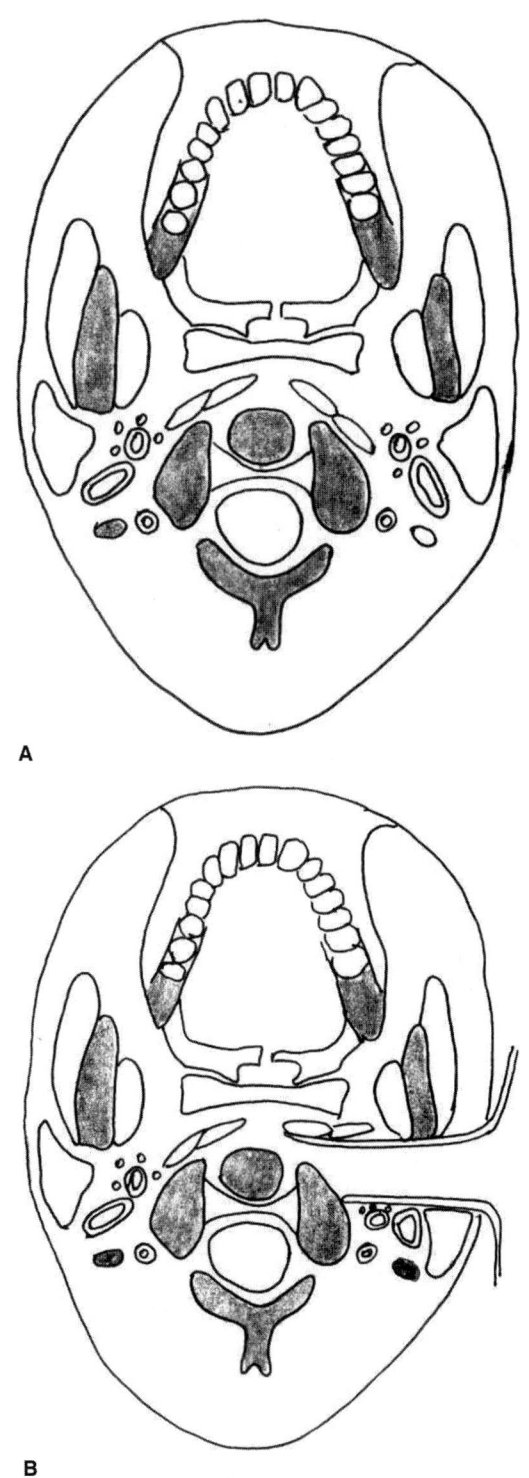

**Figure 127.13** Ventromedial retropharyngeal approach may be accomplished by two different approaches (**A**). The prevascular route is taken medial to the carotid artery and internal jugular vein (**B**). *Continued*

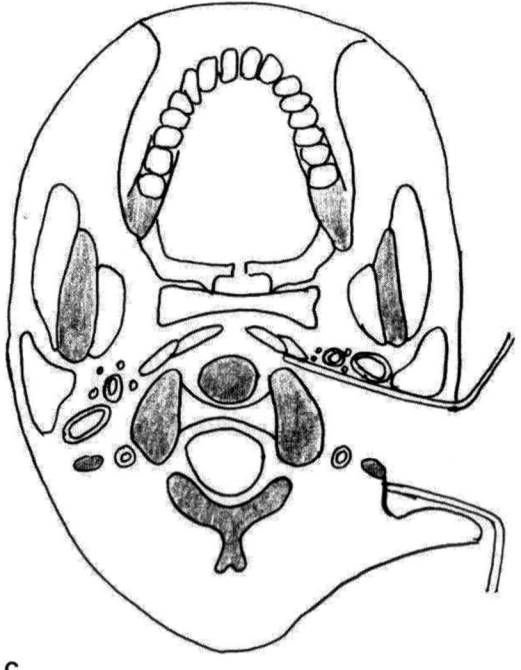

**C**

**Figure 127.13 cont'd** Retrovascular surgery is performed lateral to these vascular structures (**C**). (Redrawn from Laus M, Pignatti G, Malaguti MC, et al: Anterior extraoral surgery to the upper cervical spine. Spine 21:1687-1693, 1996.)

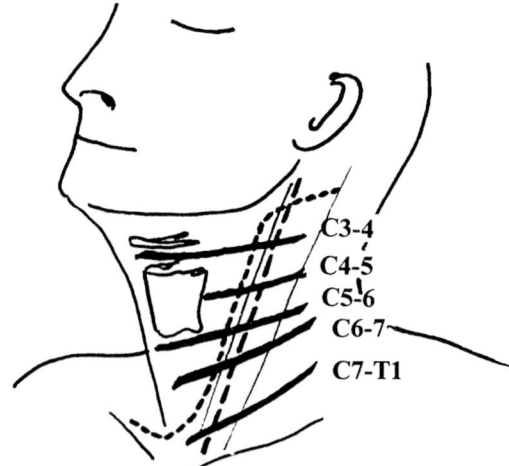

**Figure 127.14** Incision lines used for ventral approaches to the midcervical and lower cervical spine. Straight lines are for transverse incision at different levels, oblique dotted line is longitudinal incision parallel to the sternocleidomastoid muscle, oblique small dotted line is a curvilinear incision for more wide exposure of the multisegmental disease.

may be resected. The facial, lingual, hypoglossal, and superior laryngeal nerves should be identified and protected. After rostral and lateral retraction of these nerves, the hyoid bone and hypopharynx may be retracted medially.

After incising the platysma muscle, the inferior division of the facial nerve and submandibular gland may be divided. The carotid sheath is identified and protected. The dorsal belly of the digastric muscle is traced and transected near its tendon. To retract the larynx, the stylohyoid muscle is transected. The hypoglossal nerve is identified and protected. The retropharyngeal space is opened, and bluntly dissected. After retraction of the longus colli muscles, a self-retaining retractor is positioned.[17,48] It may be difficult to place a self-retaining retractor in this opening. A table-mounted system may be useful in this region.

### Retrovascular Surgery

Retrovascular surgery may also be termed the ventrolateral retropharyngeal approach[MC6]. It is an anatomically complex access that requires sternocleidomastoid muscle eversion; exposition of the spinal accessory nerve and medial mobilization of the jugular vein, vagus nerve, carotid artery, vertebral artery, and cranial nerves XII, IX, VII[59] (Figure 127.14). Although it provides a true lateral access to the upper cervical spine, only limited access is obtained, and neither grafting, nor extensive bony decompression can be achieved. It is also noted to have a significant association with vertebral artery damage.[76]

The major difference between a ventrolateral retropharyngeal approach and a straight ventral retropharyngeal

approach is that the exposure is lateral to the carotid sheath.[34,75,76] The major risk is vertebral artery injury.[76]

The supine position is used. The neck is extended, and the head is turned maximally. Skeletal traction is often useful.

A hockey-stick incision is fashioned along the ventral border of the sternocleidomastoid muscle. The incision begins behind the ear, proceeds caudally over the mastoid process, and extends below the mandibular angle towards the midline (see Figure 127.12, C).

The external jugular vein is ligated and divided. The sternocleidomastoid muscle is divided transversely below the mastoid process. The occipital artery is also ligated. The greater auricular and the accessory nerves are identified and protected. A dissection plane is developed dorsal to the carotid sheath and the retropharyngeal space.[59]

## Dorsal Approaches to the Subaxial Cervical Spine
### Laminectomy and Laminoplasty

The patient position for a midline dorsal cervical approach is similar to that used for posterior fossa approaches. Either the sitting or a prone position may be used.

A longitudinal midline incision is centered over the vertebrae of interest. The occipital ridge must be exposed for occipital fusions.

A bilateral subperiosteal dissection is performed over the laminae with sharp elevators or electrocautery. If no fusion is anticipated, the facet capsules should be preserved. Avoid injury to supraspinous ligaments. To avoid postoperative swelling and excessive injury to the erector spinae muscles, self-retaining retractors should be released periodically.

To decrease the blood loss, packing with sponges may be helpful. Also, the dorsal branches of the segmental arteries that emerge lateral to the facet joints should be preserved to avoid excessive bleeding.

## Laminoforaminotomy for Cervical Disc Disease

In laminoforaminotomy for cervical disc disease three different positions may be used: the prone position, the sitting position, and the lateral or park-bench position.[19] Because lateral muscle retraction is necessary for exposure, hyperflexion and hyperextension should be avoided. If the spine is hyperflexed, the tightened muscles and tendons make lateral retraction difficult. If the spine is hyperextended, the interlaminar spaces close, and interlaminar exposure is difficult.[19]

A midline dorsal or paramedian dorsal incision may be used. The dorsal paramedian incision is used only for one-level laminoforaminotomy.[19] This is a muscle-splitting approach, with only dissection of the muscles from the lamina and facet surfaces. This approach may be used for the keyhole foraminotomy.[61]

The classical midline dorsal approach requires the resection of the muscle attachments from the spinous processes in order to expose the facets and laminae.[62] Only strong lateral retraction is needed to retract the muscles.

## Ventral Approaches to the Subaxial Cervical Spine

### Ventromedial Approach

Exposure of the disc space and vertebral body is usually accomplished by a ventromedial approach.[4,7,15,60] The patient is positioned supine, with the head and neck neutral or slightly extended. Extension of the upper cervical region, with chin retraction, is helpful to reach the C2-3 level. Extension of the mid-lower cervical region is helpful to reach high thoracic region. The head is turned away from the surgeon. In the setting of severe cervical stenosis, extreme extension of the cervical spine may cause spinal cord damage, and therefore, should be avoided.

The sternocleidomastoid muscle is the surface incision landmark for the ventral approach. Either a transverse or a longitudinal incision is appropriate (see Figure 127.14). Rengachary[55] suggests a longitudinal incision for patients with a short neck and kyphotic deformity. The incision begins below the angle of the mandible, extends forward toward the hyoid bone, extends caudally over the sternocleidomastoid muscle, and terminates in the suprasternal notch (see Figure 127.14).[55]

A transverse incision may be used for patients with short necks and limited pathology, whereas a longitudinal incision parallel to the sternocleidomastoid muscle may be used for long thin necks with more extensive pathology. Right-handed surgeons may prefer to use right-sided incisions, although it is usually optimal to approach the patient from the side opposite the most prominent pathology. After the incision of the platysma muscle, the sternocleidomastoid muscle is freed from its attachments.

The carotid sheath is easily identified under the muscle. Both may be retracted laterally by the surgeon's fingers (Figure 127.15, A). Rostrally, the twelfth cranial nerve, and caudally the recurrent laryngeal nerve, should be avoided. Other structures that cross the wound transversely may, if necessary, be sacrificed. These include the inferior and superior thyroid veins and arteries, the facial veins, and the inferior belly of the omohyoid muscle. One should avoid injury to the superior laryngeal and superior thyroid artery.

The three main retraction systems available for ventral cervical surgery are hand-held retractors, self-retaining retractors, and table-fixed retractors (see Figure 127.4). Saunders[59] prefers a table-fixed retraction system, both for the ventromedial and ventrolateral approaches. Retractors themselves may cause injury to the lateral structures, such as the carotid artery, internal jugular vein, cranial nerves 10 and 12, nerve roots, sympathetic chain, thoracic duct, and lung apex. The medial structures, such as the esophagus and the trachea, are also at risk. Manual retraction is usually used at the beginning of the dissection, until the deep cervical fascia is opened, and the longus colli muscles are visualized.

Soft-tissue structures may be placed under significant tension with a self-retaining retractor. The positioning of the medial blades is particularly important. The most common retraction injury is caused by medial retraction of the esophagus; therefore, the retractor blade should be placed under the longus colli muscles. Careful attention must also be given to lateral retraction, which may cause compression of the carotid artery. The ipsilateral superficial temporal artery may be palpated by the anesthesiologist after placement of the retractor to assist with detection of occlusion of the carotid artery. It is prudent to relax the retraction hourly. If necessary, rostral and caudal retraction with blunt-tipped blades may be used.

### Ventrolateral Approach

The lateral approach to the cervical spine from C3 to C7 can be performed via a ventrolateral exposure. However, the lateral exposure of C1 and C2 can only be performed with the dorsolateral transcondylar approach.[1]

There are two variations of the ventrolateral approach. The trajectory of one approach is medial to the carotid artery, whereas the trajectory of the other is lateral (see Figures 127.15, B,C). In the latter approach, the sternocleidomastoid muscle is retracted medially with the carotid sheath. Therefore, retraction of the recurrent laryngeal nerve is avoided.

With either variation, the lateral retractor blade is positioned just lateral to the tubercle of the transverse process, and the medial retractor blade is positioned just medial to the uncinate process (see Figures 127.15, B,C). This exposes the ipsilateral longus colli muscle, which together with the sympathetic chain, is mobilized medially. The muscle insertions to the transverse process are divided. Positioning and incision are the same in the ventrolateral approach as with the ventromedial approach.

For retraction, a medial exposure is made with blunt dissection. The tubercle of the transverse process is then palpated laterally. This tubercle is approximately 1cm lateral to the foramen transversarium. Blunt dissection of the common carotid artery and jugular vein is carefully performed to allow retraction of these structures medially. Extreme care should be taken not to injure the vertebral artery or the sympathetic chain.

A ventrolateral approach medial to the carotid sheath is most frequently used to expose the vertebral artery and the nerve root foramen.[42,72] It is essentially a medial approach, without midline exposure.[44,72] The carotid sheath is retracted laterally as with the ventromedial approach.

Decompression of lateral cervical disc herniations may be done via the same route. This approach may be termed the *ventral cervical foraminotomy*,[33] *ventrolateral transpedicular foraminotomy*,[26] or *microsurgical ventral cervical foraminotomy-uncinatectomy*.[68] The colli muscles are mobilized allowing dissection around the lateral aspect of the vertebral body, a retractor between the vertebral body and the vertebral artery is placed and the lateral portion of the uncovertebral joint is drilled. The herniated disc and uncovertebral osteophytes are

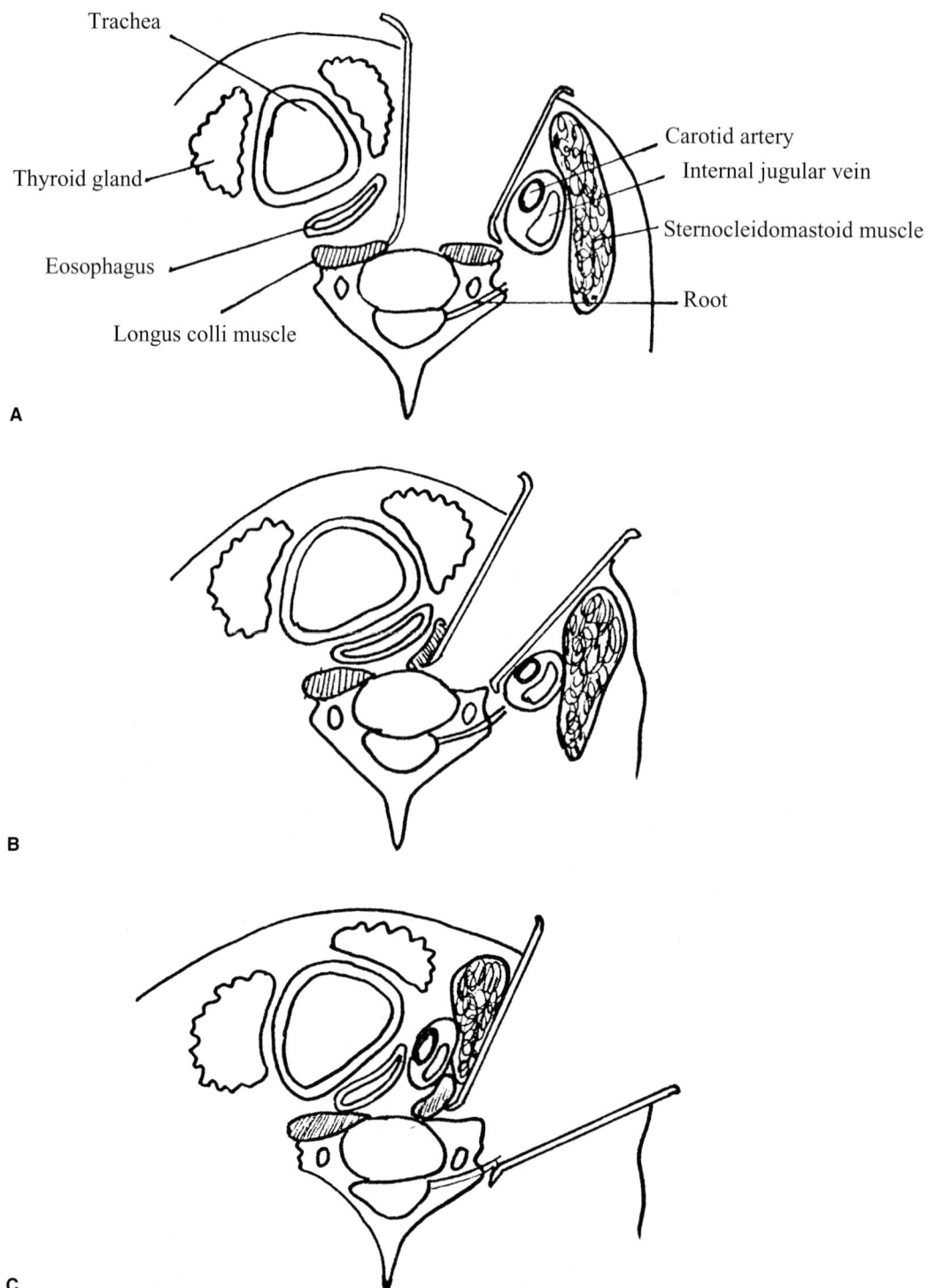

**Figure 127.15** Three basic ventral approaches to the midcervical and lower cervical spine: (**A**) ventral-medial approach; (**B**) ventral-lateral approach, medial to the sternocleidomastoid muscle; (**C**) ventral-lateral approach, lateral to the sternocleidomastoid muscle and great vessels.

removed to decompress the exiting nerve root (Figure 127.16).

A ventrolateral approach lateral to the carotid sheath and sternocleidomastoid muscle is also termed the *oblique cervical approach*.[25] With this exposure, the incision may be fashioned lateral to the sternocleidomastoid muscle. Positioning is similar to the ventromedial approach. The head and neck may be slightly turned to the contralateral side. Both the sternocleidomastoid muscle and the great vessels are retracted medially, together with the trachea and the esophagus. A self-retaining retractor may be used, taking care that the lateral blades do not cause severe retraction of the nerve roots.[2,25]

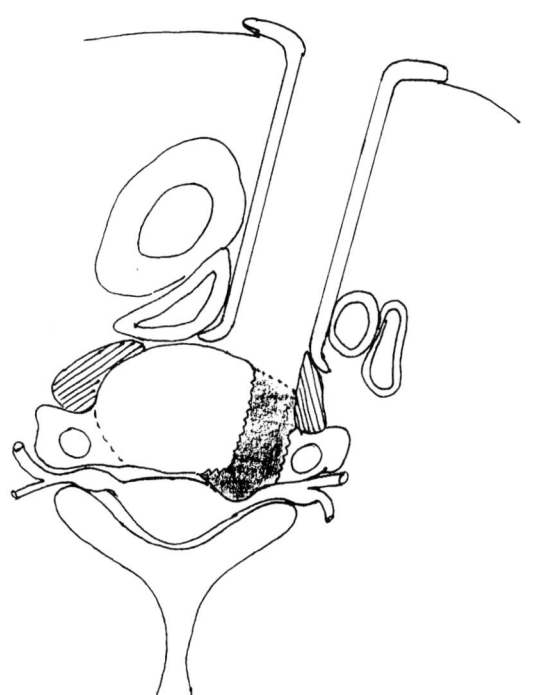

**Figure 127.16** Ventral cervical foraminotomy-uncinatectomy and the amount of bone to be removed.

# Dorsal and Ventral Approaches to the Cervicothoracic Junction

The dorsal approaches are similar to those used for lower cervical dorsal approaches.

The cervicothoracic junction is located between the cervical lordosis and the thoracic kyphosis. The brachial plexus, major vessels, and the lung apex may obstruct approaches to this area. The thoracic cage narrows to reach the thoracic inlet. Therefore, the surgical approach to the ventral cervicothoracic junction is technically demanding. There are six fundamental operative techniques in this region.

### Lower Ventromedial Cervical Approach

The lower ventromedial cervical approach is indistinguishable from that used in the midcervical to lower cervical spine.[54]

### Transsternal Approach

The transsternal approach provides a direct ventral route through a median sternotomy.[13] The morbidity and mortality are high. Hodgson and Yau[30] have reported a 40% mortality rate. Furthermore, it provides little advantage over the transmanubrial approach because the soft tissue structures are the predominant limiting factors.

### Transmanubrial Approach

The transmanubrial approach is a variation of the transsternal approach.[65] It is performed using an osteotomy of the manubrium, with or without a medial claviculotomy.[8,14,30,65,67] Sundaresan *et al.*[66] recommend resection of the medial third of the clavicle along with the creation of a window in the manubrium (Figure 127.17).

The head is positioned slightly contralaterally in the supine position. Most authors recommend a left-sided approach.

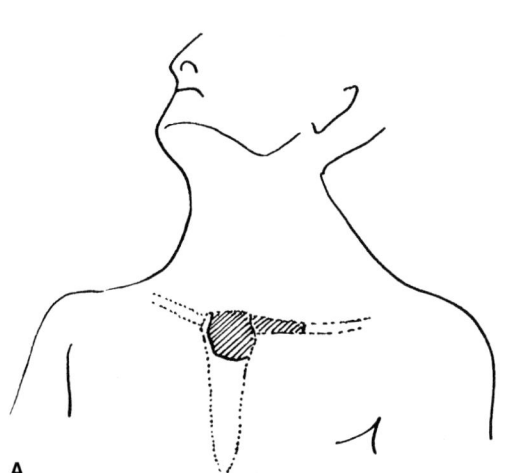
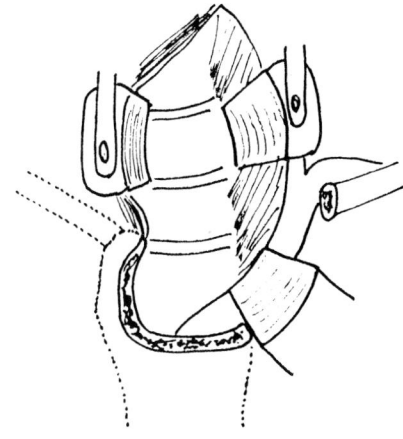

A                                                              B

**Figure 127.17** **(A)** Transmanubrial exposure. **(B)** Resection of the manubrium and the medial part of the clavicle.

Either of two incisions may be used: a T-shaped incision, with the transverse arm 2 cm above the clavicle and the midline vertical arm that extends to the sternum; or a medial sternocleidomastoid incision, extending to the sternum.[16,30] This incision permits a simultaneous ventromedial midcervical approach (Figure 127.18).

The upper outer corner of the manubrium, the first costal cartilage, and the medial third of the clavicle are divided. With this exposure, the great vessels and the lower roots of the brachial plexus are retracted. If connected to a ventromedial cervical exposure, a generous exposure to the cervicothoracic vertebrae from C3 to T4 can be obtained.

The sternocleidomastoid muscle and the omohyoid muscle are divided. The phrenic nerve, the eleventh cranial nerve, the sympathetic chain, and, on the left side, the thoracic duct should be protected. If necessary, the left innominate vein may be divided.[16]

The manubrium and the clavicle may be reattached using wires or miniplates. These bone fragments may be used as bone grafts, without significant deformity or instability in a tumor patient. In a young healthy individual, the clavicle should be replaced.

## Transverse Supraclavicular Approach

The transverse supraclavicular approach was originally described as an exposure for upper thoracic sympathectomy.[50] A transverse incision parallel to the clavicle, and extending beyond the lateral border of the sternocleidomastoid muscle is used.[34,67,74] The sternocleidomastoid muscle, the omohyoid muscle, and the strap muscles are divided. The carotid sheath, the internal jugular vein, and the phrenic nerve are identified and protected. Medial retraction of the neurovascular structures provides a limited exposure lateral to the C7 vertebral body.

## Transclavicular Approach

The transclavicular approach (splitting the clavicle) provides an adequate access to the cervicothoracic junction. This approach is most useful for cervicothoracic spine tumors with paravertebral-plexus involvement. Dividing the clavicle assists in the separation of the intrathoracic components from the lung. A zigzag-shaped incision over the clavicle may be used[37] (Figure 127.19).

## Transaxillary Extrapleural Approach

The transaxillary extrapleural approach is a high thoracic variant of the transthoracic approach. Its advantage lies in the preservation of the pectoral and shoulder girdle muscles.[61] Its disadvantage is that it places the brachial plexus at risk for retraction and stretch injury.

A 60-degree semilateral position is used, with the ipsilateral shoulder and arm abducted. The arm may be fixed in a sling.

A transverse incision is made from the border of the pectoralis muscle to the border of the latissimus dorsi muscle. The third rib is resected, and the dissection is carried through the third rib bed.[10,65,74,78] Retraction is essentially an extrapleural approach. With blunt dissection, the apex of the lung is retracted caudally. A self-retaining retractor may be used.

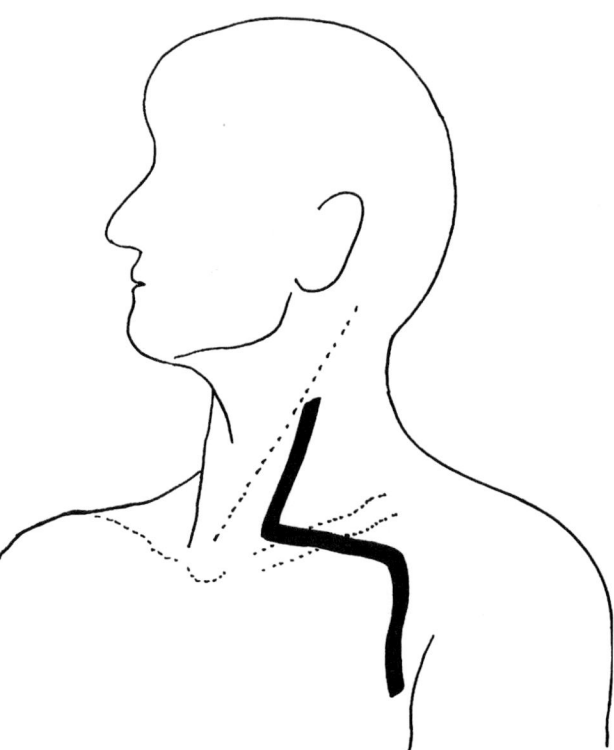

**Figure 127.19** A zigzag-shaped incision for transclavicular approach to cervicothoracic spine tumors with paravertebral-plexus involvement. (*Redrawn from Kubo T, Nakamura H, Yamano Y: Transclavicular approach for a large dumbbell tumor in the cervicothoracic junction.* J Spinal Disord *14:79-83, 2001.*)

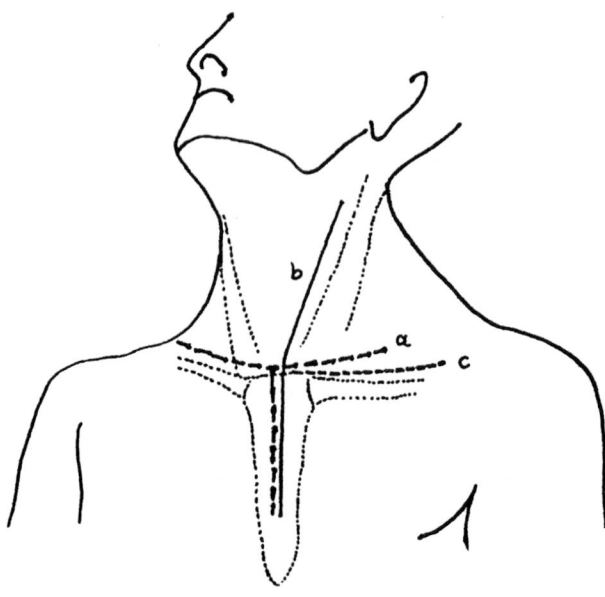

**Figure 127.18** Incisions for ventral cervicothoracic approaches. *a,* T-shaped incision, *b,* ventromedial sternotomy incision, *c,* supraclavicular incision.

## Lateral Parascapular Extrapleural Approach

With this approach, the parascapular shoulder muscles are reflected off the spinous processes to the scapula with preservation of neurovascular structure.[21] The upper dorsal ribs are removed, the rami communicantes of C8 and T1 are transected, and the sympathetic chain is displaced ventrolaterally. This approach provides an easy access to the T2-4 vertebrae.[21]

## Transpleural Transthoracic Approach

With the transpleural transthoracic approach, the upper thoracic vertebrae can be adequately approached through the fourth rib.[71] The left-side-up position is preferred, because it is easier to mobilize the aorta than the vena cava. In the event of vascular injury, it is also easier to repair the aorta than the vena cava. It may be preferred over the extrapleural method, because lung retraction is easier. Unlike the extrapleural approach, however, a tube thoracostomy is required.

Segmental vessels are ligated two levels above and below the level of pathology. This allows retraction of the great vessels.

## "Trap Door" Approach

With this approach, a partial median sternotomy and a ventrolateral approach are added to a standard ventral approach to the cervical spine along the medial border of the sternocleidomastoid muscle.[51] The sternoclavicular joint and clavicle itself are preserved. It provides bilateral ventral approach from C4 to T3. Although it provides a wide exposure and proximal control of important vessels, it is a very morbid operation (Figure 127.20).

# Dorsal Approaches to the Thoracic and Thoracolumbar Spine Junction

The most familiar of all approaches to the spine is the midline dorsal approach. Decompressive laminectomies and dorsal instrumentation procedures are most often accomplished via a midline dorsal incision.

## Thoracic Laminectomy

The patient is positioned prone on a chest frame or on laminectomy rolls that allow the abdominal contents to be free of pressure, thereby reducing venous compression and decreasing blood loss during surgery. Both the pelvis and knees are flexed, to enhance the normal thoracic kyphosis (Figure 127.21). Specialty tables and frames may be used to minimize abdominal pressure. These tables may also facilitate intraoperative radiography.

If an upper thoracic spine exposure is desired, the head should be fixed in the neutral position, either with a Mayfield head holder, or a horseshoe head holder. The patient's arms are positioned at the side.

If a midthoracic or lower thoracic spine exposure is desired, head fixation is not necessary and the patient's arms may be fixed above the head. Care should be taken

to not abduct the arms greater than 90°, to avoid a causing a brachial plexus stretch injury.

The lateral position for thoracic laminectomy is advocated by a few surgeons. This may be particularly useful in the obese patient. A dorsal midline incision is used (Figure 127.22, A).

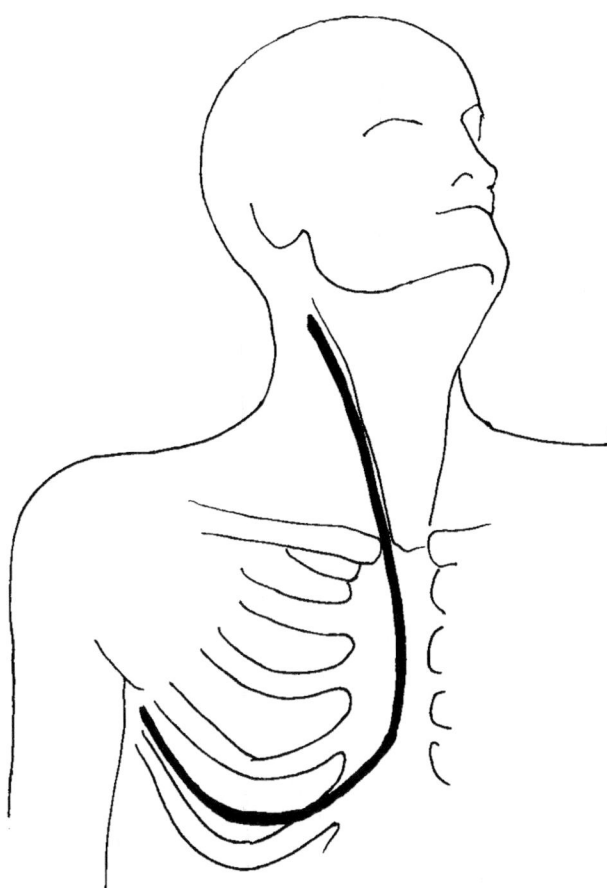

**Figure 127.20** Trap door approach used for extensive cervicothoracic tumors. (*Redrawn from Nazzaro JM, Arbit E, Burt M: Trap door exposure of the cervicothoracic junction: Technical note. J Neurosurg 80:338-341, 1994.*)

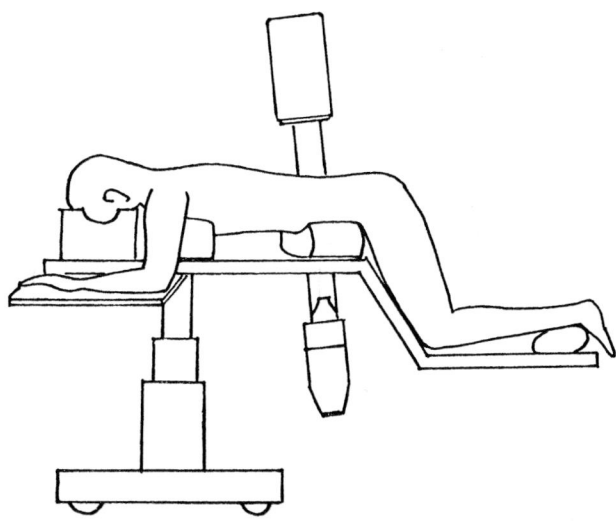

**Figure 127.21** Prone position used for most thoracic, lumbar, and sacral dorsal approaches.

Several self-retaining retractors with blades of varying widths and depths are available (e.g., Weitlaner retractor, crank-type retractor, cerebellar retractor). Hemilaminectomy retractors and table-mounted retractors are also helpful in special situations.

## Transpedicular Approach

The transpedicular approach may be used for thoracic disc removal and vertebral body biopsy.[52] It may also be performed in the cervicothoracic junction. The prone position is used with the transpedicular approach.

A midline vertical incision is performed (see Figure 127.22, A). The paraspinous muscles and the soft tissues are retracted to one side. The facet joint and the pedicle are removed using a high-speed burr. The dorsal aspect of the vertebral body adjacent to the portion of the vertebral body near the rostral intervertebral disc space may be reached through the pedicle.

The exposure provided by the transpedicular approach, however, is limited. It allows only partial tumor or disc removal.

## Costotransversectomy

This approach allows exposure of dorsal and dorsolateral structures, without violating the pleural cavity. It is different from the lateral extracavitary approach, because it involves a midline exposure and a plane of dissection that is medial to the erector spinae muscles. It was first described for drainage of tuberculous abscesses.[47]

The patient is placed prone position and a midline vertical incision is made (see Figure 127.22, A). A modified T-shaped incision has also been described[23] (see Figure 127.22, E). After standard bilateral subperiosteal dissection, a plane of dissection on the ipsilateral side is extended to the tips of the transverse processes and proximal ribs. The 3 to 4cm medial aspect of one or two ribs is then cut, disarticulated from its costotransverse and costovertebral articulations, and resected.

To find the ipsilateral pedicle, the neurovascular bundle is identified under the rib bed, and followed proximally to the neural foramen. After removing the transverse process and the pedicle, the lateral aspect of the thecal sac is visualized. Self-retaining retractors are used.

There is a controversy over the necessity of performing a rhizotomy of the associated nerve root during the procedure. Since the patients whose nerve roots were preserved can show late neuropathic pain, routine transection of the associated nerve root proximal to the ganglion may be desirable.[48]

## Lateral Extracavitary Approach

The lateral extracavitary approach is a modification of costotransversectomy. It was introduced and popularized by Larson et al.,[39] and then used by other surgeons.[6,43,74] The prone position is used frequently although a three-quarter prone position has also been described (Figure 127.23).[6] Several variations of a parasagittal incision are described (see Figure 127.22).[7] Larson et al.[39] uses a midline hockey-stick incision. This approach provides simultaneous access to both the dorsal and ventral aspects of the spine. Dorsal instrumentation may be placed via the same incision used for decompression.

Dissection is carried to the lateral border of the paraspinous muscles. The paraspinous muscles are mobilized in a lateral to medial direction. They may also be transected in a transverse fashion as was originally described by Capener.[12] The lateral exposure reaches 8 to 10cm lateral to the midline. The remaining portion of the operation is similar to the costotransversectomy. It differs from the costotransversectomy, however, because an approxi-

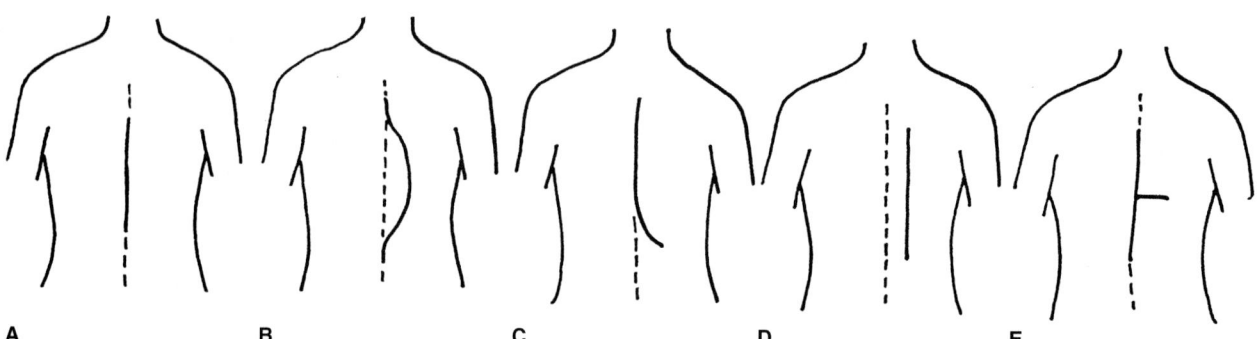

**Figure 127.22** Different skin incisions for dorsolateral exposures of the thoracic and lumbar spine: **(A)** Dorsal midline incision, **(B)** semilunar incision, **(C)** hockey-stick incision, **(D)** straight paramedian incision, and **(E)** T-shaped incision.

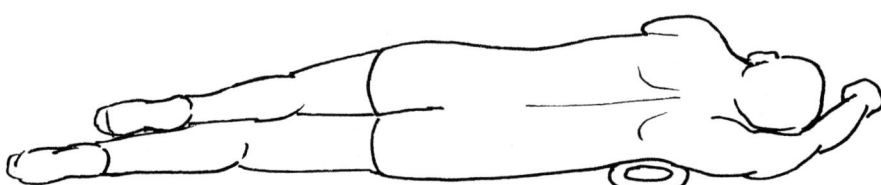

**Figure 127.23** The three-quarter prone position used for lateral extracavitary approach.

mately 15% to 30% ventral angle of exposure is gained by the lateral extracavitary approach (Figure 127.24).

The disadvantages of transpedicular, costotransversectomy, and lateral extracavitary approaches are that they cannot be used for directly ventrally located lesions. Removing the facet joint and pedicle may destabilize the spine.

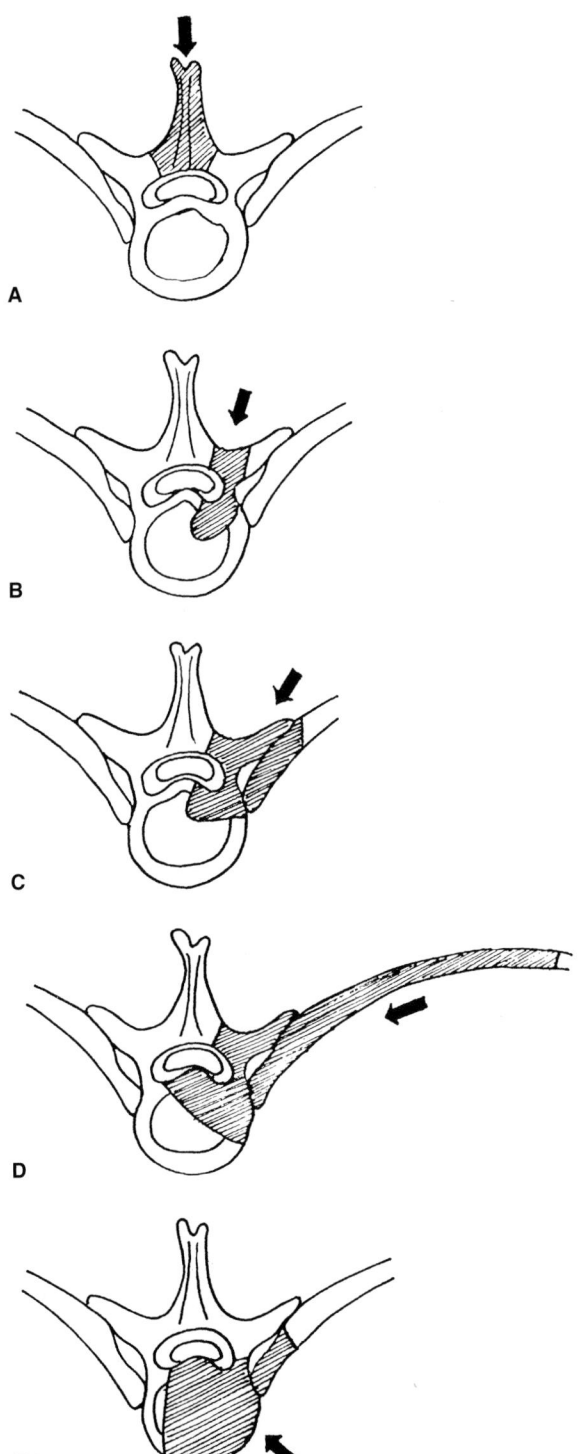

**Figure 127.24** Alternative approaches to thoracic and lumbar spine: (**A**) dorsal laminectomy, (**B**) transpedicular approach, (**C**) costotransversectomy, (**D**) lateral extracavitary approach, and (**E**) ventral intracavitary approach.

## Dorsal En Bloc Total Spondylectomy

En bloc total spondylectomy may be performed by bisecting the affected vertebrae through the pedicles and removing the vertebra en bloc.[1] This method was first introduced by Tomita et al.,[69,70] and then used in other centers.[9,63] There are two variations described in the following paragraphs.[1]

### Single Dorsal Approach: For Lesions from T1 to L2

Tomita[1,69,70] proposed the removal of the dorsal component and lateral components of the spine en bloc by pediculotomy using a fine threadwire saw. If the unilateral pedicle is affected by the tumor, osteotomy may be performed through a neighboring healthy lamina. The involved nerve root occasionally had to be ligated and cut. If the affected pedicle or vertebral body markedly compressed the nerve root, the more severely affected side is sacrificed. Sacrificing both nerve roots in less important areas such as thoracic spine is possible. After the dorsal bony column is removed, the epidural venous bleeding is controlled (Figure 127.25).

After resection of the neural arch, a Gigli saw is inserted to cut the upper and lower levels of the vertebral body or disc into two retractors protecting ventral venous structure and two retractors protecting the spinal dura mater. During the operation, the spinal column is stabilized by connecting unilateral rod to pedicle screws. Then, the affected vertebra is removed dorsolaterally.

This operation is completed by using a long segment dorsal instrumentation and placing a ventral vertebral body prosthesis (i.e., methylmethacrylate, bioactive ceramic, mesh cages, titanium mesh cylinder). Strut and cancellous bone grafts from the resected ribs or fibula were placed around the prosthesis and rods.

### Combined En Bloc Total Spondylectomy: For Lesions from L3 to L5

In the case of large extravertebral tumor, extension or recurrence after radical excision, combined with en bloc total spondylectomy was used, regardless of the level.

The first step is a dorsal approach. The dorsal procedure is similar to the method of Tomita et al.[69,70] After removing the dorsal bony column, the psoas muscles with segmental vessels are dissected as ventrally as possible on the contralateral side of the ventral approach. The posterior longitudinal ligamentum and the dorsal and contralateral part of the adjacent intervertebral disks are cut through the dorsal approach. After dorsal stabilization according to the principle of "one above, one below" using a pedicle screw system, a ventral procedure, including en bloc corpectomy and reconstruction of the ventral column, is performed by replacing the affected vertebral body using a vertebral prosthesis or a titanium cage. This is supported by ventral spinal instrumentation. Bone is also placed around the prosthesis or inside the cages. The ventral fixation construct includes one vertebra above and one below the affected vertebra.

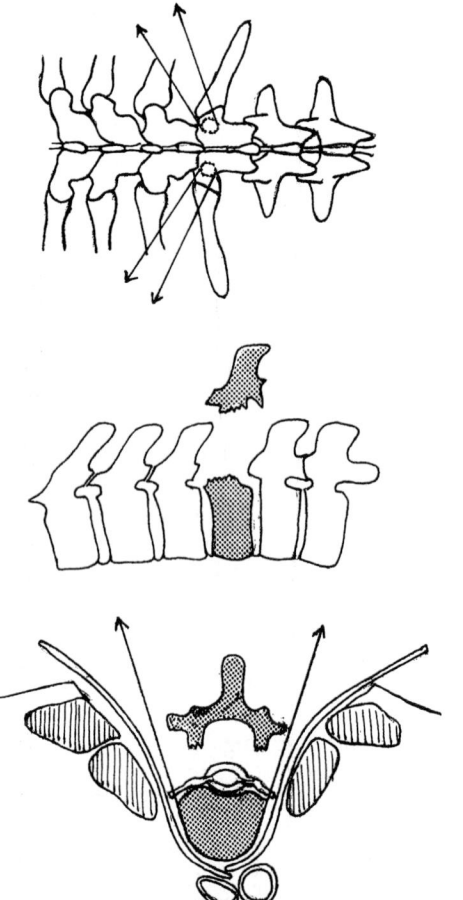

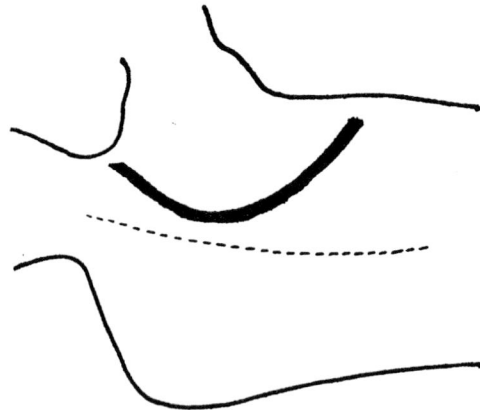

**Figure 127.26** Skin incision for ventrolateral exposure of the upper thoracic spine. The right-side-up position and a curved incision around the scapula finishing at the C7 spinous process are used.

**Figure 127.25** Posterior en bloc total spondylectomy with single dorsal approach is suitable for lesions from T1 to L2. At first bilateral pediculotomy with the aid of a thin Gigli saw and resection of laminar arch is accomplished. After resecting the related nerve roots, and dissection of ventral vascular structures, the vertebral body is removed by cutting through disc spaces. (*Redrawn from Tomita K, Kawahara N, Baba H et al: Total en bloc spondylectomy for solitary spinal metastases.* Int Orthop 18:291-298, 1994.)

## Ventral Approaches to the Thoracic and Thoracolumbar Spine Junction

For levels below T4 to the lower lumbar spine, a direct ventral approach is not possible. For anatomical reasons, a direct ventral approach is possible for cervicothoracic junction and for lower lumbar spine. Thoracotomy and retroperitoneal approaches provides a ventrolateral view of the spine.

### Transpleural Thoracotomy

When a ventrolateral exposure of the spine is required for pathologic processes located rostral to the T12 vertebral body, a transthoracic approach is often appropriate.[7,53,54] It is most useful for the midthoracic segments between T3 and T11.

The main advantage of a thoracotomy is direct access to ventral pathology, multilevel exposure, and ease of ventral instrumentation. The disadvantages of this approach

include violation of the thoracic cavity, the need for a tube thoracotomy, and a relatively weak instrumentation construct (short-segment fixation).

The patient is placed in the lateral decubitus position. Usually the right lateral decubitus position is used. Most surgeons prefer a left-sided approach, because it is easier to mobilize the aorta than the vena cava. In order to open the intercostal and intervertebral spaces on the operative side, a slight break in the table or cushions placed under the contralateral thorax is necessary. The lower arm should be protected by axillary rolls. The upper arm can rest on an arm table or over the cushions. The upper leg is flexed and the lower leg is extended.

A curved incision is fashioned around the medial aspect of the scapula for a thoracotomy in the upper thoracic spine (T2-T5) vertebral lesions (Figure 127.26). For lesions between the T5 and T10, a curvilinear incision is made along the designated rib, extending from the costochondral articulation ventrally, to the lateral aspect of the paraspinous muscles dorsally (see Figure 127.23, A).

The optimal rib to be resected in the thoracic spine is the rib that is located at the level of the surgical pathology in the midaxillary line. Muscle and periosteum may be divided with monopolar cautery. The rib is then dissected subperiosteally with a small periosteal dissector. Resection of the rib is not essential. The pleura is then opened in the bed of the rib. After retraction of the lung, the spine is visualized. Segmental vessels in the desired area are ligated and divided. The periosteum on the ventrolateral spine is incised and retracted.

After collapsing the lung, a self-retaining thoracotomy retractor is used. A malleable retractor with a reversed curve is placed on the ventral aspect of the vertebral body.[57]

### Extrapleural Thoracotomy

An extrapleural thoracotomy approach provides a shorter route to the anterior thoracic spine. Its major advantage is avoidance of pleural cavity violation.[46] Postoperative morbidity, particularly pain and pulmonary complications, are thus reduced.

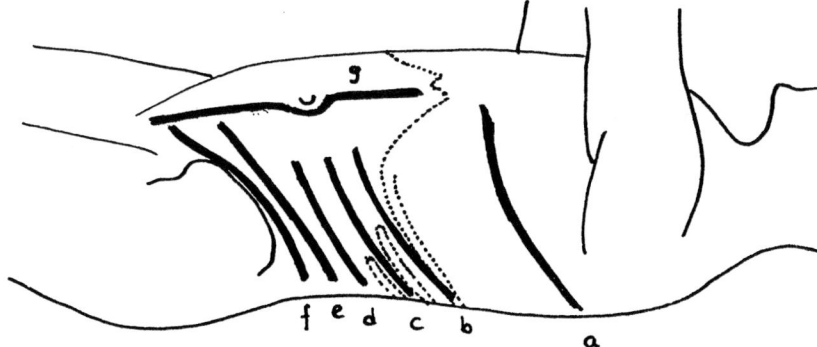

**Figure 127.27** Incision lines for thoracotomy and lumbar ventrolateral retroperitoneal approaches: *a,* lower thoracotomy, *b,* T12-L1, *c,* L1-2, *d,* L2-3, *e,* L3-5, *f,* L5-S1 retroperitoneal approaches, and *g,* transperitoneal approach.

The patient is placed in the lateral decubitus position. As with a transpleural thoracotomy, a curved incision is fashioned around the medial aspect of the scapula.

Intercostal muscles are detached subperiosteally over an 8 to 10cm rib segment.[46] Then, in the resected rib segment, the endothoracic fascia is incised in line with the rib bed. The parietal pleura is widely dissected from the undersurface of the endothoracic fascia with blunt dissectors. After adequate dissection and freeing the parietal pleura over the vertebral body is assured, a self-retaining crank-type retractor facilitates the exposure.

Retropleural approaches are recommended to avoid direct lung trauma and to minimize the need for a tube thoracostomy. In the midthoracic spine, only limited lesions such as thoracic disc herniations may be approached via a retropleural thoracotomy. It is easier to perform an extrapleural operation at thoracolumbar junction. The eleventh or twelfth rib extrapleural-retroperitoneal approach is a prototype for this.[35] The extrapleural space can be expanded to T10 to L2. Some authors have advised to resect the twelfth rib to facilitate exposure.[46]

### Transdiaphragmatic Approach

To approach the T11 or T12 vertebrae, either a supradiaphragmatic or infradiaphragmatic exposure may be possible. However, it is usually necessary to section of the diaphragm to reach the L1 vertebral body.

The diaphragm is a key structure that should be taken into consideration for approaches to the thoracolumbar spine. Its limbs have attachments to the L1 transverse process and vertebral body. It extends laterally over the quadratus lumborum muscle to the tip of the twelfth rib. Because its innervation from the phrenic nerve begins centrally, a peripheral incision is preferred. If a transdiaphragmatic approach to reach the ventral thoracolumbar junction is mandatory, the pleural and retroperitoneal cavities are violated. Because the morbidity of such an approach is higher than a retroperitoneal approach, which violates only one body cavity, it should only be used if absolutely necessary.

The patient is placed in the lateral decubitus position. For thoracolumbar junction, the classical operation is the *"ninth or tenth rib transpleural-retroperitoneal thoracoabdominal approach.* Most commonly, a T10 rib incision is made. The tenth rib may then be resected (Figure 127.27). A self-retaining thoracotomy retractor is used as for thoracotomy. Care must be taken to not injure the spleen on the left side, or the liver on the right side. The major disadvantage of this method is the division of the diaphragm and entering into two body cavities.

Kim *et al.*[35] have recommended using an eleventh rib extrapleural-retroperitoneal approach (Figure 127.28). Since it prevents entering the pleural cavity, thoracic complications should be minimal. However, it is technically demanding, it prolongs the operative time, and the operative exposure is limited.

### Ventrolateral Retroperitoneal Approach

It is possible to reach the lumbar vertebra from L1 to L5 with an extraperitoneal approach. Ventral instrumentation, however, is difficult below L4, because of the constraints of the iliac vessels and overlying iliac crest.

A supine position is appropriate for low ventrolateral lumbar exposure, using a log roll to elevate the operative side. For thoracolumbar approaches, however, a right lateral decubitus position on an ordinary operating table is preferred. Table-mounted retractor systems may help maintain this position during the operation.

The left-side-up position is preferred because it is easier to dissect, mobilize or repair the aorta or iliac artery, compared with the vena cava or iliac vein. The liver, because of its mass and location, is more difficult to retract and mobilize than the spleen. Excessive splenic retraction, however, may result in injury. An adjustable pad is placed at the level of the vertebra of interest.

The skin incision is run obliquely, caudally, and ventrally. This, so-called "flank" incision can be made between the tip of the twelfth rib and the anterior superior iliac spine. It begins dorsally at the edge of the paravertebral muscle, and terminates at the lateral margin of the rectus abdominis muscle. However, the incision may vary based on the spinal level and the surgical indication (see Figure 127.27, *B*).[7]

For an infradiaphragmatic retroperitoneal exposure, subperiosteal dissection of the crus of the diaphragm from its vertebral attachments aids in the visualization of the higher lumbar and lower thoracic vertebral bodies. Resection of the eleventh or twelfth ribs may be used to

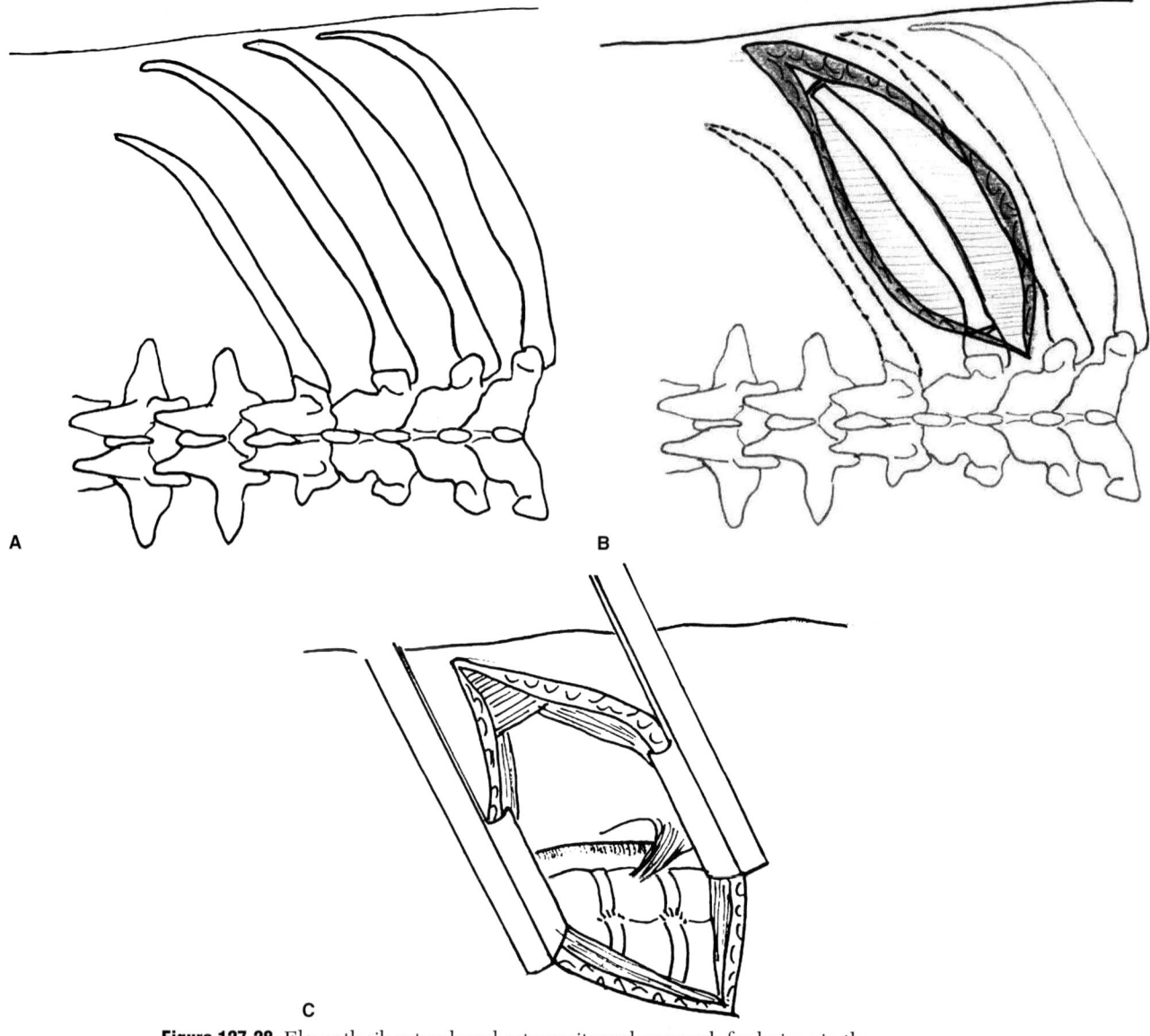

**Figure 127.28** Eleventh rib extrapleural-retroperitoneal approach for lesions in the thoracolumbar spine. A left-sided approach is mostly preferred (**A**). After removing the eleventh rib (**B**), a self-retaining retractor is placed and with blunt dissection ventral vertebral structures are shown (**C**). (*Redrawn from Kim M, Nolan P, Finkelstein JA: Evaluation of 11th rib extrapleural-retroperitoneal approach to the thoracolumbar junction: Technical note.* J Neurosurg 93(1S):168-174, 2000.)

gain access to the thoracolumbar and upper lumbar spine via this approach.[28,29,31]

The exposure to the midlumbar spine is the same approach used for the lumbar sympathectomy. This exposure allows access to the ventrolateral spinal canal from L2 to below the pelvic brim.

The advantages of this approach are its familiarity to all spine and vascular surgeons, and its direct exposure of the midlumbar vertebral bodies. However, it provides a narrow longitudinal exposure that is limited rostrally by the crus of the diaphragm and caudally by the pelvic brim. The psoas muscle also limits the opening of neuroforamina.

It is very important to clearly conceptualize the pathologic levels. For example, if only the L1-2 disc space is to be surgically approached, a subcostal extrapleural, T12 rib resection approach without diaphragm incision should be considered. Excessive left-sided retraction may result in splenic injury. If an L1 corpectomy is needed, a transdiaphragmatic approach may be preferred, depending on the patient's anatomy.

The external oblique, internal oblique, and transversus abdominis muscles are split with cutting diathermy. Retraction of the peritoneal sac ventrally and medially away from the psoas muscle exposes the vessels located ventral to the spine. The attachments of the psoas muscle are dissected laterally and dorsally.

Ligature of the segmental lumbar vessels is necessary. After this ligation, the aorta and the inferior vena cava may be retracted ventrally and medially. Then a malleable retractor may be used to retract the peritoneal sac and the great vessels.

The vascular supply of the spinal cord is worthy of consideration. The most common location of the entrance of the radiculomedullary artery of Adamkiewicz into the spinal canal is on the left, in the midthoracic to lower thoracic region. Generally, the ventrolateral approach is not, however, affected by the location of radiculomedullary arteries, because the angle of the approach does not violate terminal-end arteries. If the surgeon intends to disrupt the soft tissues at the level of the neuroforamina, terminal spinal cord blood flow may be endangered. In this circumstance, an alternative approach should be considered.

## Dorsal Approaches to the Lumbar and Lumbosacral Spine

The dorsal approach to the lumbosacral spine is a standard exposure, and similar to the thoracic dorsal approaches.

### Lumbar Laminectomy and Laminotomy

Because opening of the interlaminar space is important, the patients should not be in extreme lordosis. A standard dorsal midline incision is performed. If a one-level microdiscectomy is planned, the length of the incision may be as short as 2.5cm. An intraoperative radiograph is necessary to confirm the correct level.

Hemilaminectomy retractors are used for two or more level one-sided discectomies. For microdiscectomy, specially designed retractors such as Caspar retractors may be used.

### Paraspinal Approach

The paraspinal approach is used for far-lateral disc herniation[32] or for dorsolateral fusion of the transverse processes.[77] Its main advantage is the decrease in paraspinous muscle retraction.

The patient is placed in the prone position. Wiltse et al.[77] have described bilateral paramedian incisions and a muscle-splitting dissection between the erector spinae and multifidus muscles. If the operation is performed for an extraforaminal disc protrusion, a unilateral small incision is usually sufficient.

The paraspinal approach provides a direct exposure of the intertransverse region and the facet joint. A self-retaining retractor may be used between the muscles.

Jane et al.[32] have described a modification of this approach, which makes it possible to expose the root both from medial and lateral to the facet joint. With this approach, the incision is extended from the midline, but the muscle fascia is incised as an arc, and the spaces first medial to the paraspinous muscles and then lateral to these are exposed.[32]

### Lateral Extracavitary Approach

The lateral extracavitary approach in the lumbar spine is similar to the lateral extracavitary approach in the tho-racic spine. However, it is more important to preserve the lumbar nerve roots. Because there is no rib in the lumbar region, and because the nerve roots pass through the bulky iliopsoas muscle, the lateral extracavitary approach is technically demanding in the lumbosacral region. The obstacle of the iliac crest is another limitation of this approach.[3,10,39,78]

## Ventral Approaches to the Lumbar and Lumbosacral Spine

### Pelvic Brim Extraperitoneal Approach

The pelvic brim extraperitoneal approach provides a limited exposure of the L5 and S1 levels, because of the obstructing iliac vessels and the iliac crest. For this reason, only limited procedures, such as biopsy and simple resections can be performed.

Usually the supine position will suffice with slight elevation on the side of surgery with a log roll. An incision beginning lateral to, and slightly above, the anterior superior iliac spine can be carried medially and caudally. It must be parallel and rostral to the iliac crest and inguinal ligament.

The peritoneum and renal fascia are retracted medially, with great care taken to not injure the retroperitoneal nerves and ureters. This exposure provides a limited view of the vertebrae under the aorta and iliac arteries.

For a minimally invasive exposure of the L4-5 level, a 5 to 8cm horizontal incision through the anterior rectus sheath has been described. The rectus abdominis muscle is then retracted medially. After incision of the posterior rectus sheath, the retroperitoneum is exposed.[6,7,29]

### Transperitoneal Approach

It is possible to reach all the midlumbar and lower lumbar segments, and the sacrum, via the transperitoneal approach.[22,38,57] The transperitoneal approach provides a direct ventral exposure of the lumbar and sacral spine. It is most useful for L5-S1 pathology, when a wide exposure of this region is required.[5] The requirement of a laparotomy and the potential for neural and vascular injury are its disadvantages.

The patient is placed in the supine position. A midline or horizontal subumbilical laparotomy incision is made.

After entry into the peritoneal cavity, the small intestines are packed in the upper abdomen and retracted to the right. A break in the operating table to increase the lumbar lordosis is useful. Care is taken to avoid injury to the bladder. The sigmoid colon is retracted laterally and a longitudinal incision is made in the dorsal peritoneum in the midline. The sacral promontory is an important landmark. The sigmoid colon limits the exposure on the left side, but caudal retroperitoneal structures on the right side are easily identified.

The bifurcation of the iliac arteries and veins do not allow exposure above the L5 vertebral body through the bifurcation. Instead, the approach is to the left of the vessels. Liberal use of epinephrine injection and in males only bipolar electrocautery is used to decrease the risk of presacral plexus injury.

## Dorsal Approaches to the Sacrum

The most common approach to the lumbosacral junction and the sacrum is via a dorsal midline incision. The ventral approach is difficult and requires vascular retraction. With dorsal approaches, there is adequate room for retraction of the cauda equina laterally to expose the ventral sacrum. However, the control of ventral vascular structures is not possible with the dorsal approach.

If a sacrectomy is planned, it is suggested to prepare the patient the day before surgery with repeated enemas. At the beginning of the operation, a vaginal pad is inserted into the rectum.

The patient is placed in the prone position. It is important to keep the abdomen free of pressure, so that bleeding is minimized. If a lumbosacral fusion is to be undertaken and supplemented with internal fixation, the lumbosacral junction should be placed in extension. This can easily be achieved by placing pillows or bolsters under the hips. In the Krause position, the sacrum is prominent, and constitutes the highest point of the table (Figure 127.29).[24]

The incision varies according to the pathology and planned operation. A midline vertical incision, transverse incision, upward arched incision, or downward arched incision may be used (Figure 127.30).

If a sacrectomy or excision of a large tumor is planned, a midline vertical incision is not suitable, because of possible postoperative inflammatory processes and wound dehiscence due to major tissue defect. In addition, a vertical incision could injure the anal sphincter, and does not provide adequate exposure of the lateral sacrum.

Another problem during the sacrum tumor surgery is the necessity for inclusion of the biopsy scar into the excision material. In this case, a T-shaped incision may be most suitable (see Figure 127.30, C).

Wiltse et al.[77] introduced an incision and retraction technique using one or two incisions 5cm lateral to the

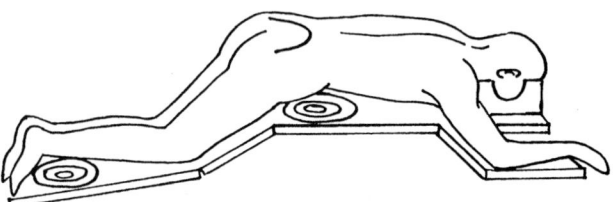

**Figure 127.29** Krause position and inverted U-shaped incision for the exposure of the sacrum.

midline and medial to the posterior superior iliac spine (see Figure 127.30, A). The dissection is deepened to the sacrospinalis muscle and the transverse process of the fifth lumbar vertebrae. Wiltse has used this approach for lumbosacral fusions. Bone grafts from the dorsal iliac crest can easily be obtained with the same exposure.

For midline incisions with restricted operations in the sacrum, a self-retaining retractor is satisfactory. For operations such as sacrectomy, hand-held retractors are more convenient. In this case, skin flaps should be gently retracted.

The ligaments (sacroiliac and sacrotuberalis) and the gluteus maximus muscle are divided as near to the sacrum as possible, because their approximation before wound closure is necessary to avoid ventrodorsal postoperative wound problems.

## Ventral Approaches to the Sacrum

### Retroperitoneal Approach

The retroperitoneal approach is restricted to the sacral pathologies without rectal invasion. Depending on the extent of the pathology, a unilateral or bilateral retroperitoneal dissection may be used.

A supine position with the legs elevated and partly separated (lithotomy position) is advised.[64] If a unilateral dissection is planned, one side of the pelvis may be elevated.

For bilateral retroperitoneal exposure, a large semicircular incision is performed through the skin on the lower abdomen (Figure 127.31, A). The rectus abdominis tendon is severed bilaterally just above the pubic bone. For unilateral exposure, a flank incision without violating the rectus abdominis muscle is satisfactory (Figure 127.31, B).

After dissection and medial retraction of the peritoneum, common iliac arteries and veins with external and internal branches are exposed. Then, dorsal parietal peritoneum, together with the ureter and the superior hypogastric nerve plexus are dissected medially. The right and left dissections meet in the midline. Deep hand-held abdominal retractors are used for retraction of the deep abdominal structures.

### Transperitoneal Approach

The transperitoneal approach is primarily used for L5-S1 ventral fusion operations. It may also be used for the resection of sacral tumors, if the rectum has to be included in the specimen.

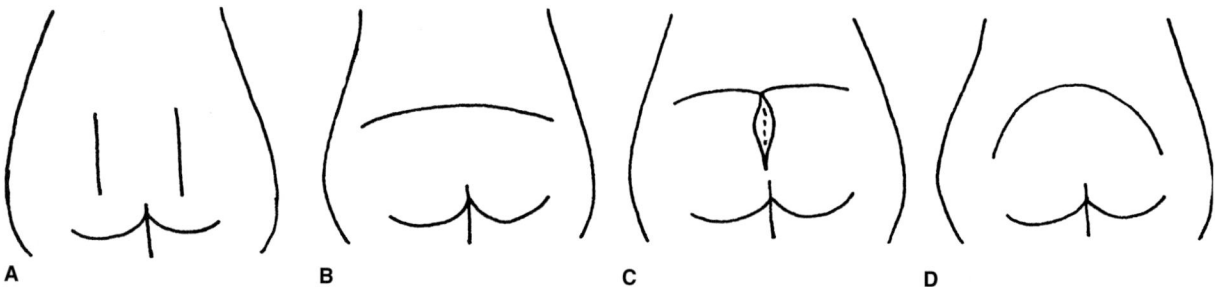

A    B    C    D

**Figure 127.30** Different incisions used for dorsal sacral operations: **(A)** dorsal sacrospinalis splitting approach (Wiltse), **(B)** dorsal transversal incision, **(C)** T-shaped incision including biopsy scar, and **(D)** inverted U-shaped incision.

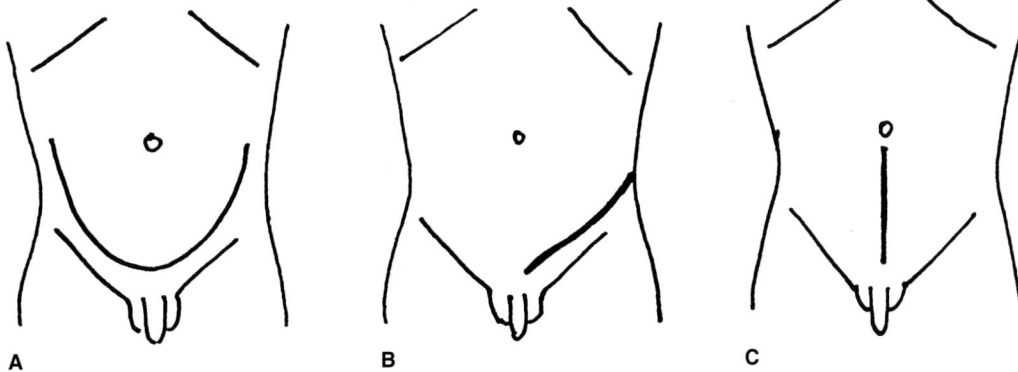

**Figure 127.31** Different incisions used for ventral sacral operations: (**A**) bilateral U-shaped retroperitoneal incision, (**B**) unilateral flank retroperitoneal incision, and (**C**) ventral medial transperitoneal incision.

The patient is placed in the supine position and an inferior midline abdominal incision is made (Figure 127.31, *C*). The median raphe of the rectus abdominis muscle is divided. A suprapubic transverse incision is not recommended, for it requires a rectus abdominis muscle section.

The peritoneum is cut in the midline, and after packing the bowel and small intestines rostrally and laterally, the rectum is released ventrally as far distally as possible.

### Combined Abdominosacral Approach

Total resection of the major primary sacral tumors (i.e., chordoma, chondrosarcoma, giant cell tumor) requires a combined approach, both ventrally and dorsally.[41,65] If the rectum can be preserved, the operation is begun ventrally, and finished dorsally. If not, a ventral, dorsal and ventral approach sequence is advocated.[64]

Some surgeons prefer a dorsal exposure in the prone position. The patient is then placed in the lateral decubitus position, so that a separation of tissue planes from both sides is possible.[11,66] In this case, two surgeons, one from the dorsal and the other from the ventral side may operate simultaneously.

## REFERENCES

1. Abe E, Kobayashi T, Murai H, *et al:* Total spondylectomy for primary malignant, aggressive benign, and solitary metastatic bone tumors of the thoracolumbar spine. *J Spinal Disord* 14:237-246, 2001.
2. Anson JA: Lateral exposures of the cervical spine and vertebral artery. In EC Benzel (ed): *Surgical Exposure of the Spine: An Extensile Approach.* Rolling Meadows, IL, American Association of Neurological Surgeons, 1995, pp 69-81.
3. Arbit E, Petterson RH Jr: Combined transoral and median labiomandibular glossotomy approach to the upper cervical spine. *Neurosurgery* 8:672-674, 1981.
4. Batzdorf U, Batzdorff A: Analysis of cervical spine curvature in patients with cervical spondylosis. *Neurosurgery* 22:827-836, 1988.
5. Benzel EC: Surgical exposure of the lumbosacral plexus and proximal sciatic nerve. In Benzel EC (ed): *Practical Approaches to Peripheral Nerve Surgery.* Rolling Meadows, IL, American Association of Neurological Surgeons, 1992, pp 153-159.
6. Benzel EC: The lateral extracavitary approach to the spine using the three-quarter prone position. *J Neurosurg* 71: 837-841, 1989.
7. Benzel EC: *Surgical Exposure of the Spine: An Extensile Approach.* Rolling Meadows, IL, American Association of Neurological Surgeons, 1995.
8. Birch R, Bonney G, Marshall RW: A surgical approach to the cervicothoracic spine. *J Bone Joint Surg Br* 72:904, 1990.
9. Boriani S, Chevalley F, Weinstein JN, *et al:* Chordoma of the spine above the sacrum: treatment and outcome in 21 cases. *Spine* 21:1569-1577, 1996.
10. Breslau RC: Transaxillary approach to the upper dorsal spine. In Watkins RD (ed): *Surgical Approaches to the Spine.* Springer Verlag, New York, 1983, pp 58-63.
11. Bridwell KH: Management of tumors at the lumbosacral junction. In Margulies JY et al (eds): *Lumbosacral and Spinopelvic Fixation.* Philadelphia, Lippincott-Raven, 1996, pp 109-122.
12. Capener N: The evolution of lateral rhachotomy. *J Bone Joint Surg Br* 36:173-179, 1954.
13. Cauchoix J, Binet JP: Anterior surgical approaches to the spine. *Ann R Coll Surg* 21:237, 1957.
14. Charles R, Govender S: Anterior approach to the upper thoracic vertebrae. *J Bone Joint Surg Br* 71:81, 1989.
15. Cloward RB: New method of diagnosis and treatment of cervical disc disease. *Clin Neurosurg* 8:93-103, 1962.
16. Darling GE, McBroom R, Perrin R: Modified anterior approach to the cervicothoracic junction. *Spine* 20: 1519-1521, 1995.
17. DeAndrade JR, MacNab I: Anterior occipito-cervical fusion using an extra-pharyngeal exposure. *J Bone Joint Surg Am* 51:1621-1626, 1969.
18. Dinh DH, Tompkins J, Clark SB: Transcostovertebral approach for thoracic disc herniations. *J Neurosurgery Spine* 94(1S):38-44, 2001.
19. Ducker TB, Zeidman SM: Cervical disk diseases. Part II: operative procedures. *Neurosurg Q* 2:144-163, 1992.
20. Fang HSY, Ong GB: Direct anterior approach to the upper cervical spine. *J Bone Joint Surg Am* 49:1588-1604, 1962.

21. Fessler RG, Dietze DD, Millan MM, Peace D: Lateral parascapular extrapleural approach to the upper thoracic spine. *J Neurosurg* 75:349-355, 1991.

22. Freebody D, Bendall R, Taylor RD: Anterior transperitoneal lumbar fusion. *J Bone Joint Surg Br* 53:617-627, 1971.

23. Garrido E: Modified costotransversectomy: a surgical approach to ventrally placed lesions in the thoracic spinal canal. *Surg Neurol* 13:109-113, 1980.

24. Gennari L, Azzarelli A, Quagliuolo V: A posterior approach for the excision of sacral chordoma. *J Bone Joint Surg Br* 69:565-568, 1987.

25. George B, Zerah M, Lot G, *et al:* Oblique transcorporeal approach to anteriorly located lesions in the cervical spinal cord. Technical note. *Acta Neurochir* 121:187-190, 1993.

26. Grundy PL, Germon TJ, Gill SS: Transpedicular approaches to cervical uncovertebral osteophytes causing radiculopathy. *J Neurosurg* 93 (1S):21-27, 2000.

27. Hall JE, Denis F, Murray J: Exposure of the upper cervical spine for spinal decompression by a mandible and tongue splitting approach. *J Bone Joint Surg Am* 59:121-123, 1977.

28. Harmon PH: Anterior extraperitoneal lumbar disc excision and vertebral bone fusion. *Clin Orthop* 16:169-198, 1963.

29. Harmon PH: A simplified surgical technique for anterior lumbar diskectomy and fusion: avoidance of complications: anatomy of the retroperitoneal veins. *Clin Orthop* 37:130-144, 1964.

30. Hodgson AR, Yau ACMC: Anterior surgical approaches to the spinal column. In Apley AG (ed): *Recent Advances in Orthopaedics*, Williams & Wilkins, Baltimore, 1969, pp 289-323.

31. Hodgson MB, Wong SK: A description of a technique and evaluation of results in anterior spinal fusion for deranged intervertebral disc and spondylolisthesis. *Clin Orthop* 56:133-162, 1968.

32. Jane JA, Haworth CS, Broaddus WC, *et al:* A neurosurgical approach to far-lateral disc herniation. Technical note. *J Neurosurg* 72:143-144, 1990.

33. Johnson JP, Filler AG, McBride DQ, Batzdorf U: Anterior cervical foraminotomy for unilateral radicular disease. *Spine* 25:905-909, 2000.

34. Johnson RM, Murphy MJ, Southwick WO: Surgical approaches to the spine. In Rothman RH, Simeone FA (eds): *The Spine*, ed 3. Philadelphia, WB Saunders, 1992.

35. Kim M, Nolan P, Finkelstein JA: Evaluation of 11th rib extrapleural-retroperitoneal approach to the thoracolumbar junction. Technical note. *J Neurosurg* 93(1S):168-174, 2000.

36. Kostuik JP: Surgical approaches to the thoracic and thoracolumbar spine. In Frymoyer JW (ed): *The Adult Spine: Principles and Practice*. New York, Raven Press, 1991, pp 1243-1266.

37. Kubo T, Nakamura H, Yamano Y: Transclavicular approach for a large dumbbell tumor in the cervicothoracic junction. *J Spinal Disord* 14:79-83, 2001.

38. Lane J, Moore ES: Transperitoneal approach to the intervertebral disc in the lumbar area. *Ann Surg* 127-130, 1948.

39. Larson SJ, Holst RA, Hemmy DC, *et al:* Lateral extracavitary approach to traumatic lesions of the thoracic and lumbar spine. *J Neurosurg* 45:628-637, 1976.

40. Laus M, Pignatti G, Malaguti MC, *et al:* Anterior extraoral surgery to the upper cervical spine. *Spine* 21:1687-1693, 1996.

41. Localio SA, Eng K, Ranson JHC: Abdominosacral approach for retrorectal tumors. *Ann Surg* 191:555-560, 1980.

42. Louis E, Ruge D: Lateral approach to the cervical spine. In Wiltse LL, Ruge D (eds): *Spinal Disorders*. London, Henry Kimprton, 1977, pp 132-136.

43. Maiman DJ, Larson SJ, Luck E, El-Ghatit A: Lateral extracavitary approach to the spine for thoracic disc herniation: report of 23 cases. *Neurosurgery* 14:178-182, 1984.

44. Manabe S, Tateishi A, Ohno T: Anterolateral uncoforaminotomy for cervical spondylotic myeloradiculopathy. *Acta Orthop Scand* 59:669-674, 1988.

45. McAfee PC, Bohlman HH, Riley LH, *et al:* The anterior retropharyngeal approach to the upper part of the cervical spine. *J Bone Joint Surg Am* 69A:1371-1383, 1987.

46. McCormick PC: Retropleural approach to the thoracic and thoracolumbar spine. *Neurosurgery* 37:908-914, 1995.

47. Menard V: Causes de la paraplegie dans le mal de Pott. *Rev Orthop* 5:47-64, 1894.

48. Menezes AH: Surgical approaches to the craniocervical junction. In JW Frymoyer (ed): *The Adult Spine: Principles and Practice*. New York, Raven, 1991, pp 967-985.

49. Moore LJ, Schawartz HC: Median labiomandibular glossotomy for access to the cervical spine. *J Oral Maxillofac Surg* 43:909-912, 1985.

50. Nanson EM: The anterior approach to upper dorsal sympathectomy. *Surg Gynecol Obstet* 104:118, 1957.

51. Nazzaro JM, Arbit E, Burt M: Trap door exposure of the cervicothoracic junction: Technical note. *J Neurosurg* 80:338-341, 1994.

52. Patterson RH Jr, Arbit E: A surgical approach through the pedicle to protruded thoracic discs. *J Neurosurg* 48:768-772, 1978.

53. Perot PL Jr, Munro DD: Transthoracic removal of midline thoracic disc protrusions causing spinal cord compression. *J Neurosurg* 31:452-458, 1969.

54. Perry J: Surgical approaches to the spine. In Pierce DS, Nickel VH (eds): *The Total Care of Spinal Cord Injuries*. Boston, Little, Brown, 1977, p 53.

55. Rengachary SS: Partial median corpectomy with fibular grafting for cervical spondylotic myelopathy. In *Neurosurgical Operative Atlas*, vol 2, no 6. Rolling Meadows, IL, American Association of Neurological Surgeons, 1992, pp 11-24.

56. Riley LH: Surgical approaches to the anterior structures of the cervical spine. *Clin Orthop* 91:16-20, 1973.

57. Roy-Camille R, Mazel C: Surgical exposures and procedures. In Laurin CA, Riley LH Jr, Roy-Camille R (eds): *Atlas of Orthopaedic Surgery*, vol 1: General Principles and Spine. Paris, Masson, 1989.

58. Salas E, Sekhar LN, Ziyal IM, *et al:* Variations of the extreme-lateral craniocervical approach: anatomical study and clinical analysis of 69 patients. *J Neurosurg* 90(4S):206-219, 1999.

59. Saunders RL: Anterior reconstructive procedures in cervical spondylotic myelopathy. *Clin Neurosurg* 37:682-721, 1991.

60. Saunders RL: On the pathogenesis of the radiculopathy complicating multilevel corpectomy. *Neurosurgery* 37:408-413, 1995.

61. Scoville WB, Dohrmann GJ, Corhill G: Late results of cervical disc surgery. *J Neurosurg* 45:203-210, 1976.

62. Spurling RG, Bradford FK: Neurologic aspects of herniated nucleus pulposus. *JAMA* 113:2019-2022, 1939.

63. Stener B: Technique of complete spondylectomy in the thoracic and lumbar spine. In Sundaresan N, Schmidek HH, Schiller AL, et al. (eds): *Tumors of the Spine: Diagnosis and Clinical Management.* Philadelphia, WB Saunders, 1990, pp 432-437.

64. Stener B, Gunterberg B: High amputation of the sacrum for extirpation of tumors. Principles and technique. *Spine* 3(4):351-366, 1978.

65. Sundaresan N, DiGiancinto GV: Surgical considerations and approaches. In Sundaresan N, Schmidek HH, Schiller AL, et al (eds): *Tumors of the Spine: Diagnosis and Clinical Management.* Philadelphia, WB Saunders, 1990, pp 358-379.

66. Sundaresan N, Galicich JH, Chu FC, Huvos AG: Spinal chordomas. *J Neurosurg* 50:312-319, 1979.

67. Sundaresan N, Shah J, Feghali JG: A transsternal approach to the upper thoracic vertebrae. *Am J Surg* 148(4): 473-477, 1984.

68. Tascioglu AO, Attar A, Tascioglu B: Microsurgical anterior cervical foraminotomy (uncinatectomy) for cervical disc herniation—report of three cases. *J Neurosurg* 94: 121-125, 2001.

69. Tomita K, Kawahara N, Baba H, et al: Total en bloc spondylectomy for solitary spinal metastases. *Int Orthop* 18:291-298, 1994.

70. Tomita K, Kawahara N, Baba H, et al: Total en bloc spondylectomy: a new surgical technique for primary malignant vertebral tumors. *Spine* 22:324-333, 1997.

71. Turner PL, Webb JK: A surgical approach to the upper thoracic spine. *J Bone Joint Surg Br* 69:542-544, 1987.

72. Verbiest H: Anterolateral operations for fractures and dislocations in the middle and lower parts of the cervical spine. Report of a series of forty-seven cases. *J Bone Joint Surg Am* 51:1489-1530, 1969.

73. Vishteh AG, Beals SP, Joganic EF, et al: Bilateral sagittal split mandibular osteotomies as an adjunct to the transoral approach to the anterior craniovertebral junction. Technical note. *J Neurosurg* 90:267-270, 1999.

74. Watkins RG: *Surgical Approaches to the Spine.* New York, Springer Verlag, 1983.

75. Whitecloud TS, Kelley LA. Anterior and posterior surgical approaches to the cervical spine. In JW Frymoyer (ed): *The Adult Spine: Principles and Practice.* New York, Raven, 1991, pp 987-1013.

76. Whitesides TE Jr, Kelly RP: Lateral approaches to the upper cervical spine for anterior fusion. *South Med J* 50:879-883, 1966.

77. Wiltse LL, Bateman JG, Hutchinson RH, et al: The paraspinal sacrospinalis-splitting approach to the lumbar spine. *J Bone Joint Surg Am* 50:919-926, 1968.

78. Woodard EJ. Indications, complications, and comparison of approaches. In Benzel EC (ed): *Surgical Exposure of the Spine: An Extensile Approach.* American Association of Neurological Surgeons, 1995, pp 157-178.

# CHAPTER 128

# Blood Loss

## David G. Malone and Gary L. Rea

Significant blood loss during spine surgery may occur for several reasons, including: dissection extending over multiple levels, bony decortication at the graft and fusion site, long duration of the procedure, and the release of a tamponade on the epidural veins. Blood loss and the resultant need for transfusion are largely affected by surgical techniques including speed of surgery, hemostatic agents, positioning of the patient, and the adjunctive use of hypotension and pharmacologic agents during the procedure. Managing blood loss once it occurs deals with rational planning regarding transfusion needs, the use of antifibrinilytic drugs, replacement of blood through homologous or autologous blood transfusion, and intraoperative or even postoperative blood salvage.

## Preoperative Evaluation

The process of evaluating the patient for spinal surgery includes a complete medical history including medications and bleeding tendencies. If indicated, a hematologic profile with coagulation times, platelet counts, and, in some instances, a bleeding time should be obtained.

### Medication History

Patients with a history of transient ischemic attack, stroke, deep venous thrombosis, heavy bleeding after minor trauma, alcoholism, hepatic dysfunction, and cardiac disease can have increased risk of bleeding. Many patients who undergo spinal surgery take nonsteroidal antiinflammatory drugs (NSAIDs). The NSAIDs inhibit platelet function and may increase bleeding times. The bleeding time often returns to normal within 24 hours of cessation of some NSAIDs, whereas others will require a full 18 days for the drug to be eliminated and new platelets to be produced. Antiplatelet drugs, such as ticlopidine hydrochloride (Ticlid), clopidogrel (Plavix), dipyridamole (Persantine), and aspirin may prolong the bleeding time and must be stopped before surgery.[46] Patients who take coumadin may require cessation or reversal of the anticoagulation. Those rare patients with congenital coagulation deficits may undergo surgery after factor replacement and consultation with a hematologist.[13]

### Preoperative Estimation of Blood Loss

Factors associated with increased blood loss with spinal surgery include tumor, low preoperative hemoglobin level, numbers of levels fused, history of pulmonary disease, less autologous blood available, not using of the Jackson table, and antiplatelet drugs.[37,38,45] When surgery is contemplated for reconstruction in cases of spinal metastasis from renal cell carcinoma, preoperative embolization has been shown to significantly reduce intraoperative blood loss. Therefore, embolization should at least be considered or a preoperative adjunct in all vascular spinal tumors.[31]

The blood loss for a particular operation should be estimated and plans made to ensure that this blood can be replaced if needed. An estimate of 200ml of blood lost per fused segment can be made preoperatively to plan the amount of blood that will be required for replacement.[35] Patients can usually tolerate a loss of 15% of the blood volume before transfusion.[13] In a 70kg patient, estimating 70ml blood/kg body weight, a volume of 735ml would reflect a 15% blood loss.

## Autologous Blood Utilization

Autologous blood donation can be instituted if the estimated blood loss exceeds the 15% blood volume loss. Autologous blood can be obtained in three ways: preoperative donation, intraoperative salvage, and postoperative salvage. Although each requires expensive specialized equipment, a reduction in the potential for the development of chronic liver disease infection transmission may be well worth the cost.[53] One unit of blood can be donated per week if the hematocrit remains above 34%.[51] Other guidelines for autologous donation are for a patient age range of 12 to 70 years,[51] and that the hemoglobin be at least 11mg/dl.[2] Full units can be taken from patients greater than 50 kg and half units from those between 25 and 50 kg. Supplemental iron should be administered when appropriate. In some instances, recombinant erythropoietin can be given to allow increased blood volume for autologous donation.[12,23,47,51] This has been shown to increase blood production significantly both in animal and clinical studies.[12,28]

Consideration should be given as to whether autologous packed red blood cells or whole blood should be transfused. The patients donate whole blood, and in autologous donation it may be best to return whole blood to the patient. Whole blood contains platelets, plasma, and cryoprecipitate, all of which are lacking in packed cells, and these components may help lessen bleeding.[21] Using autologous blood in a community hospital, 95% of the transfusion needs were met for 1600 patients who underwent major orthopedic procedures.[16] Other studies have shown that autologous blood can supply approximately 70% to 80% of the transfusion needs.[2,53] Autologous blood may be cryopreserved or preserved with a storage solution.[39] Cryopreserved blood has a longer shelf life, and the *in vitro* survival of red blood cells is equivalent to that of fresh erythrocytes. There is also no preoperative effect on the hemodynamic status of the patient.[26] Oga *et al.*[39] used cryopreserved cells in patients who underwent scoliosis surgery and solution-stored blood for patients who underwent other spinal procedures. More blood was collected for the scoliosis patients, and the less costly storage method was used for other patients.[39] There are risks to autologous blood transfusion. These include septicemia

1678

from bacterial contamination of the unit, nonimmune hemolytic transfusion reactions, febrile reactions, volume overload, and the possible risk of clerical error resulting in the administration of the wrong unit of blood.[21]

The criteria for returning autologous blood may vary. Albert et al.[1] found that the transfusion of blood during surgery was beneficial for the early postoperative hemoglobin and postoperative patient mobilization. There are different indications for homologous versus autologous blood return. Hemoglobin of less than 7g/dl for homologous, and less than 10g/dl for autologous transfusions are common indicators.[1,2]

Indications for transfusion of homologous blood include a hemoglobin of less than 7.0g/dl in a medically healthy but symptomatic patient, a hemoglobin of less than 10mg/dl in a critically ill patient, a patient with medical risk factors such as cardiovascular disease, cerebrovascular disease, or active hemorrhage. Symptoms indicating hypovolemia, such as tachycardia, tachypnea, or low venous oxygenation, also indicate the need for transfusion.[1,2,20] Other transfusion requirements have been published: hemoglobin less than 8g/dl in an otherwise healthy patient, hemoglobin less than 11g/dl in patients with increased risk of ischemia, acute blood loss with 15% of blood volume lost, or diastolic pressure less than 60mmHg, or systolic blood pressure decrease of greater than 30mmHg, tachycardia, oliguria. Symptomatic anemia with tachycardia, mental status changes, cardiac ischemia, or dyspnea. General transfusion requirements for coagulation products have been listed. Platelet transfusion for platelet dysfunction or thrombocytopenia. Fresh frozen plasma for evidence of coagulation factor deficiencies with prothrombin time and or activated partial thromboplastin time greater than 1.5 times the upper limit of normal. Cryoprecipitate is given for suspected specific factor deficiencies or fibrinogen less than 100mg/dl.[37]

## Homologous Blood

Since the early 1980s, there has been an increasing concern about the risks of blood transfusions. Although the acquired immunodeficiency syndrome virus has been the primary concern, allergic reactions, isosensitization, and the transmission of hepatitis are far more serious in terms of the number of patients affected.

Posttransfusion hepatitis has been reported to occur in as many as 10% of patients after homologous transfusion, with 3.3% developing chronic liver disease.[53]

Since the introduction of tests in 1990 for the detection of hepatitis C, the incidence of transfusion-acquired hepatitis has greatly decreased. The main risk is from donors in the window period of their infection who have donated blood before they have developed antibodies to the virus rendering it impossible to detect the infection. The current risk of hepatitis C transmission is 1 in 103,000 units transfused, and the current risk of hepatitis B transmission is 1 in 63,000 units transfused. The current risk of HIV transmission in tested blood varies with the region of the United States, but is approximately 1 in 450,000 to 660,000 units transfused.[25,48] This estimate of risk assumes a safe, plentiful, well-regulated, and tested blood supply;

unfortunately, this is not universally the case in developing countries.[33]

## Anesthetic Techniques for Lessening Intraoperative Blood Loss

Anesthetic techniques may affect operative blood loss. The uses of specific medications, hemodilutional autotransfusion, and induced hypotension have all been used to decrease intraoperative bleeding.

Randomized controlled trials have shown no difference in the amount of blood loss in patients who received desmopressin as compared to those who did not.[52] Other studies have shown desmopressin to reduce blood loss in spinal surgery by 32.5%.[20] It is administered immediately before surgery at a dose of $10\mu g/m^2$ of body surface area, up to a maximum dose of $20\mu g$. It is prepared by diluting it to a concentration of $0.5\mu g/ml$ in normal saline and infusing over 20 minutes. Desmopressin does lessen bleeding in some subsets of patients such as those with acquired platelet dysfunction such as from aspirin administration, von Willebrand disease, and uremia.[27,37] Desmopressin has been found to decrease partial thromboplastin time, whereas factor VIII coagulant activity and von Willebrand antigen concentrations increased partial thromboplastin time. A Cochrane review found no convincing evidence that desmopressin minimizes perioperative allogenic RBC transfusion in patients who do not have congenital bleeding disorders.[17] Potential postoperative problems include oliguria, which usually responds to furosemide, and hyponatremia due to its potent antidiuretic hormone activity.[24]

Randomized controlled trials of aprontinin in dorsal spinal fusion reveals significant reductions in autologous but not homologous blood transfusion. Aprontinin (Trasylol) has been shown to reduce blood transfusion requirements in cardiac surgery, liver resection, and some orthopedic surgical procedures. The mechanism of action is unknown, but inhibition of fibrinolysis and a protective effect on membrane-binding function has been suggested. The dose administered in the study was 2 million KIU over 20 minutes with the induction of anesthesia, followed by 500,000 KIU/hr continuous drip via infusion pump until skin closure.[26]

E-aminocaproic acid (Amicar) is an antifibrinolytic agent that has been shown to reduce blood loss in cardiac surgery.[11] It has been tested in lumbar spinal fusion and has been shown to reduce autologous blood transfusion in a prospective nonrandomized study by approximately 50%. No complications were noted including thromboembolic or deep vein thrombosis. E-aminocaproic acid was given in an initial dose of 100mg/kg not to exceed 5g over 15 minutes followed by a continuous infusion of 10mg/kg/hr over the remainder of the case with the infusion terminating at skin closure.[8] Aprontin and E-aminocaproic acid were compared in a randomized prospective trial involving adult reconstructive spinal surgery. Aprontin demonstrated a significant reduction in total blood loss as compared to E-aminocaproic acid and control. The doses used in the study were E-aminocaproic acid 5g over 30 minutes followed by a constant infusion of

15mg/kg/hr, and aprontin 1 million KIU load over 30 minutes followed by 0.25 million KIU/hr, and the control group received neither agent.[56] Tranexamic acid is a synthetic antifibrinolytic agent that has been studied as a means to reduce blood requirements in scoliosis surgery. In a double-blinded prospective placebo-controlled study, tranexamic acid, given in an initial dose of 10mg/kg at the time of patient positioning and in a maintenance infusion of 1mg/kg/hr, reduced blood transfusion requirements by 28%.[36]

Acute hemodilutional autotransfusion is another technique used to reduce the need for homologous blood transfusion. After the induction of anesthesia, a venesection is performed and 15% to 25% of the patient's blood volume is withdrawn into a sterile bag containing the anticoagulant citrate. The blood volume withdrawn is then replaced with colloid, on a milliliter for milliliter basis, or crystalloid, on a three-to-one basis. At the conclusion of surgery, the autologous blood is returned to the patient. The patient is then diuresed of excess fluid.[6,42]

Hypotensive anesthesia has been evaluated in patients undergoing scoliosis surgery and fusions for degenerative disease.[30] The hypotension was induced with 25mg of nitroprusside and 125mg of trimethaphan in 500ml of 5% dextrose and infused to maintain a systolic blood pressure between 60 and 70mmHg.[30,51] Enflurane can also be used as a supplement to the general anesthetic agents to induce hypotension. Both methods have been effective in decreasing blood loss in these patients with no adverse sequelae.[41]

A significant concern associated with patients with spinal cord injuries is whether the hypotension can cause neurologic deterioration. Ullrich et al.[55] performed a retrospective study comparing hypotensive and normotensive techniques in patients who underwent fixation of thoracolumbar fractures. There was a significant decrease in blood loss with hypotensive anesthesia, and there was no documented neurologic injury in either group. It is emphasized, however, that hypotensive anesthetic technique, in the presence of a compressive spinal cord lesion, poses at least the potential for further ischemia and adverse neurologic sequelae.

Somatosensory evoked potentials have been used as a monitoring tool in normotensive and hypotensive patients undergoing spinal instrumentation.[14] In the hypotensive group, the systolic blood pressure was maintained between 80 and 90mmHg with nitroprusside alone, or in combination with trimethaphan and/or propranolol. There was a significant difference in blood loss between the two groups. Intraoperative evoked potentials were altered in 5 of 24 patients, with 2 in the normotensive and 3 in the hypotensive group. Wake-up testing revealed satisfactory motor function in all patients, and all 24 patients were neurologically intact postoperatively.

Enderby[7] reported a series of 9107 anesthetics with an overall death rate of 0.1%. However, of the 9 patients who made up the 0.1%, it was believed that only one was due to the hypotensive technique.

Hypotensive anesthesia has the potential for neurologic or systemic complications. With careful cardiac, renal, and pulmonary monitoring and the maintenance of systolic blood pressure greater than 70mmHg, however, many of the complications can be avoided.[29,50] Somatosensory evoked potentials in the normal or incompletely injured patient also offer the ability to monitor physiologic changes during the hypotension and to take corrective measures if indicated.[14] It is also emphasized that the efficacy of such monitoring technique is not proven and that the meaningfulness of the information provided is often in question. This can add to the already confusing nature of the decision-making process.

## Surgical Techniques for Reducing Blood Loss

Appropriate intraoperative technique can reduce blood loss. Less blood is lost if meticulous attention is paid to subperiosteal dissection, hemostasis is controlled at each stage of the operation by cautery and packing, decortication is performed at the termination of the operation, and consideration is given to performing fusion with spinous processes instead of iliac crest bone graft. Infiltrating the skin with a dilute solution of epinephrine (1:500,000) and packing with sponges soaked in dilute epinephrine has been reported to diminish bleeding.[42]

Operative time is important, not only for the minimization of blood loss, but also regarding the diminution of the nonhematologic complication rate.[49] Bostman et al.[4] evaluated blood loss, operating time, and positioning of the patient. In discectomy patients with a shorter operative time, there was less bleeding. Although ascribed to patient positioning, there was a definite correlation between operative speed and blood loss.

Keene and McKinley[22] used spinous processes instead of iliac crest for fusion grafts in patients with thoracolumbar fractures. This eliminated donor site bleeding and decreased operative time with a resultant decrease in blood loss. Bleeding during spine surgery may arise from several sources, including bone, muscle, and epidural veins. Bone wax is effective for bleeding, but will interfere with fusion and bony healing. Gelatin foam (Gelfoam), oxidized cellulose (Surgicel), and microcrystalline collagen (Avitene) have been reported to effectively stop hemorrhage,[29] which all have advantages and disadvantages, but there is some evidence that the microcrystalline collagen is less likely to cause epidural scarring.[19]

Gelatin foam holds clotting factors in place so that clotting is promoted. This process may be facilitated by soaking the gelatin foam in thrombin. Gelatin foam will not function when insufficient clotting factors are present.

Oxidized cellulose promotes clot formation and harbors the additional advantage of possessing antibacterial properties. Microcrystalline collagen causes platelet aggregation and, therefore, is not effective in thrombocytopenia.

### Fibrin Glue

Fibrin glue may be useful in reducing blood loss from decorticated bone. Fibrin glue is formed by combining cryoprecipitate with thrombin and calcium. Thirty milliliters of cryoprecipitate is obtained from the blood bank and is placed in a syringe. In a separate container, 20,000 units of topical thrombin and 1 ampule of calcium chloride are mixed together; this is aspirated into a separate syringe.

Antibiotics are often added to the syringe containing the thrombin calcium chloride solution to diminish the risk of postoperative infection. Equal volumes of the mixture are injected onto the decorticated bone.[54] This fibrin glue recipe can also be used in the treatment of spinal fluid leak. There is a potential risk of infection transmission as the fibrin is derived from donor cryoprecipitate.

## Positioning

Positioning for spine surgery, especially for lumbar surgery, ideally decreases intraabdominal pressure, and subsequently venous pressure. A lower pressure within the inferior vena cava decreases the volume of blood in Batson's plexus. This, in turn, decreases blood loss from epidural veins. Multiple operative frames have been designed to decrease the pressure on the abdomen while in the prone position.[4,15,45,51] Although the kneeling position has been strongly advocated by some authors to decrease abdominal pressure and blood loss, others have shown no relationship between blood loss and vena cava pressure.[34] More recent studies strongly correlate use of the Jackson table with decreased blood loss during spinal surgery.[37,45]

## Intraoperative and Postoperative Blood Salvage

Intraoperative autologous transfusion (IAT) has been shown to be a safe and effective method to reduce the need for homologous blood usage.[3,29,44,51] IAT blood may even have the potential to deliver more oxygen to the tissues than previously stored blood, and have more platelets and clotting factors than bank blood.[7,51] This requires a system that suctions the wound, separates the red blood cells from other blood products and debris, washes the red blood cells, and returns them to the patient.[7,44,51] Flynn et al.[9,10] estimated that approximately 54% of red blood cells were returned to the patient with this technique. To improve this efficiency, they recommended an open tip suction wand with suction pressures below 100mmHg, the avoidance of blood pooling and clotting, the use of fewer sponges, and the rinsing of the sponges to collect the red blood cells.[9,32,40]

Certain precautions, however, should be observed with IAT. If antibiotic irrigation is used, the cells must be washed with large volumes and slow cycle times to remove the antibiotic from the solution. Red blood cell contact with water, betadine, or any solution with a temperature greater than 42°C should be avoided. Excessive hemolysis will result. Collagen powder, collagen sponge, and collagen pads (Avitene, Helistat, and Hemopad, respectively) should not be used with autotransfusion systems. If these collagen products are introduced into the operative field, use of the autotransfusion system should be discontinued, the wound irrigated copiously with saline, and finally, the use of the autotransfusion system reinstituted.

Gelatin foam, oxidized cellulose, and thrombin are safe when intraoperative autotransfusion is used. However, they should not be directly aspirated into the system.

There are some limitations to IAT. Approximately half of the red blood cells are salvaged by standard autotrans-

fusion techniques. It may be contraindicated in patients with systemic infections, gross wound infections, or malignancy, due to the potential for the hematogenous spread of the disease.[51] It also carries a potential for depleting the coagulation factors, if not appropriately replaced. For every 1,000 ml of autologous red blood cells returned to the patient, one unit of fresh frozen plasma should be given. Platelet count should be maintained at greater than 85,000.[9,44]

Pulmonary complications due to tissue debris accumulation and reinfusion are rare.[9] Hemoglobinuria may occur in as many as 5% of the patients. With adequate hydration and urine output (>100ml/hr), these complications should be transient and with minimal or no clinical sequelae.[9,51]

Just as intraoperative blood can be retransfused, so can postoperative blood.[9] It is collected, filtered, anticoagulated, washed, and returned to the patient. Unwashed blood, however, appears to be associated with few complications. This technique has been reported to be safe and may decrease blood bank requirements significantly.[5] Newer postoperative drainage systems have been used in orthopedic surgery and are used to reinfuse blood without filtration directly from the drain into the patient. These systems only return blood lost during the first 8 hours after surgery. These, however, are safe and effective.

## Treatment and Diagnosis of Diffuse Intraoperative and Postoperative Bleeding

Significant hemorrhage rarely occurs. When it does occur, the causative factors may include platelet washout, acute thrombocytopenia, platelet dysfunction, heparin administration, disseminated intravascular coagulation, impaired hepatic function, an undiagnosed hereditary coagulation disorder, or laboratory error failing to detect a coagulopathy. The source(s) of bleeding should be carefully ascertained (e.g., solely from the wound site, from intravenous cannula wounds and other puncture sites, and occult or distant sites). Isolated bleeding from the surgical site may indicate a coagulation disorder or simply poor surgical hemostasis. Bleeding from multiple sites strongly suggests dysfunctional clotting mechanisms; in which case protime, partial thromboplastin time, fibrinogen, D-dimer, complete blood count, platelet count, fibrin split products, and bleeding time should be assessed.

While awaiting these laboratory results, the anesthesia record should be examined to determine if heparin, hypothermia, platelet washout, or dilution of clotting factors are likely causes. Heparin may be reversed with protamine. If hypothermic, the patient should be warmed. Thrombocytopenia may be treated by platelet transfusion, and elevated protimes and partial thromboplastin times may be treated with fresh frozen plasma. Low values of fibrinogen require cryoprecipitate transfusion.

Disseminated intravascular coagulation (DIC) is a syndrome characterized by the generation of thrombin in the peripheral blood. The principal target protein of thrombin is fibrinogen. A delicate balance exists between the synthesis and catabolism of fibrinogen. In DIC, this balance is upset and greatly shifted toward catabolism. DIC can be caused by tissue damaged from spinal surgery. The diagnosis can be confirmed by the observation of an elevated protime, an elevated partial thromboplastin time, a low fibrinogen, and by a positive D-dimer test. Treatment is directed toward clotting factor replacement.[18,43]

The surgeon should be aware during the operation as to whether or not clot exists in the operative site. If there is no clotted blood in the operative site, a coagulopathy probably exists. At this point, coagulopathy screens should be performed. The greater the time that the problem is left uncorrected, the worse it gets; and a vicious cycle begins.

## Summary

The management of blood loss during spine surgery begins well before the patient enters the operating suite. A thorough medical history is obtained, with attention given to medications, and those items indicating hemorrhagic tendencies. For elective surgery, an estimation of potential blood loss is made, and plans for collecting autologous blood are established. The procedure itself should be performed with controlled alacrity and with the use of appropriate hemostatic agents, pharmacologic agents, and surgical and anesthetic techniques.

The transfusion of homologous blood is performed only in patients who have no autologous blood available and who have symptoms of hypovolemia and/or a hemoglobin of less than 7.0mg/dl. Intraoperative autologous transfusion can be used in those patients whose preoperatively estimated blood loss is 2 to 3 units or greater.

The use of hypotensive anesthesia may be considered. This is relative to the individual patient's symptoms and neurologic condition. Patients with a history of hypertension, ischemic cerebral or cardiovascular disease, or other major medical problems should be evaluated carefully before using hypotensive anesthesia. Without the ability to monitor spinal cord function intraoperatively, hypotensive anesthesia should be very cautiously considered.

Thought is given to patient positioning, to avoiding abdominal compression, and to controlling blood loss at each stage of the operation. The surgical procedure is planned so that any available potential bone fusion material, such as laminectomy remnants or spinous process, can be used instead of or in addition to iliac crest. Intraoperative cell salvage and autotransfusion is extremely useful to avoid the use of homologous blood.

Diffuse postoperative and intraoperative bleeding should be aggressively investigated for its cause. It should be treated accordingly. With the use of the aforementioned surgical techniques and technical tools, the use of homologous blood can be significantly decreased.

## REFERENCES

1. Albert TJ, Desai D, McIntosh T, *et al:* Early versus late replacement of autotransfused blood in elective spinal surgery. A prospective randomized study. *Spine* 18:1071-1078, 1993.
2. Bailey TE Jr, Mahoney OM: The use of banked autologous blood in patients undergoing surgery for spinal deformity. *J Bone Joint Surg Am* 69:329-332, 1987.
3. Blevins FT, Shaw B, Valeri CR, *et al:* Reinfusion of shed blood after orthopaedic procedures in children and adolescents. *J Bone Joint Surg Am* 75:363-371, 1993.
4. Bostman O, Hyrkas J, Hirvensalo E, Kallio E: Blood loss, operating time, and positioning of the patient in lumbar disc surgery. *Spine* 15:360-363, 1990.
5. Brown MD, Seltzer DG: Perioperative care in lumbar spine surgery. Review. *Orthop Clin North Am* 22:353-358, 1991.
6. Du Toit G, Relton JE, Gillespie R: Acute haemodilutional autotransfusion in the surgical management of scoliosis. *J Bone Joint Surg Br* 60:178-180, 1978.
7. Enderby GEH: A report on morbidity and mortality following 9,107 hypotensive anaesthetics. *Br J Anaesth* 33:109-113, 1961.
8. Florentino-Pineda I, Blakemore LC, Thompson GH, *et al:* The effect of epsilon-aminocaproic acid on perioperative blood loss in patients with scoliosis undergoing posterior spinal fusion: a preliminary prospective study. *Spine* 15;26(10):1147-1151, 2001.
9. Flynn JC, Metzgar CR, Csencsitz TA: Intraoperative autotransfusion (IAT) in spinal surgery. *Spine* 7:432-435, 1982.
10. Flynn JC, Price CT, Zink WP: The third step of total autologous blood transfusion in scoliosis surgery. Harvesting blood from the postoperative wound. *Spine* 16:S328-S329, 1991.
11. Fremes SE, Wong BI, Lee E, *et al:* Metanalysis of prophylactic drug treatment in the prevention of postoperative bleeding. *Ann Thorac Surg* 58:1580-1588, 1994.
12. Goodnough LT, Rudnick S, Price TH, *et al:* Increased preoperative collection of autologous blood with recombinant human erythropoietin therapy [see comments]. *N Engl J Med* 321:1163-1168, 1989.
13. Green WB, McMillan CW: Surgery for scoliosis in congenital factor VII deficiency. *Am J Dis Child* 136:411-413, 1982.
14. Grundy B, Nash C, Brown R: Deliberate hypotension for spinal fusion: prospective randomized study with evoked potential monitoring. *Can Anesth Soc J* 29:453-462, 1982.
15. Hastings DE: A simple frame for operations on the lumbar spine. *Can J Surg* 12:251-253, 1969.
16. Haugen R, Hill G: A large scale autologous blood program in a community hospital. *JAMA* 257:1211-1214, 1987.
17. Henry DA, Moxey AJ, Carless PA, *et al:* Desmopressin for minimizing perioperative allogenic blood transfusion. Cochrane library. *Cochrane Database Syst Rev* 2:CD001884, 2001.
18. Isselbacher KJ, Harrison TR: *Harrison's Principles of Internal Medicine,* ed 13. New York, McGraw-Hill, 1995.
19. Jacobs RR, McClain O, Neff J: Control of postlaminectomy scar formation: an experimental and clinical study. *Spine* 5:223-229, 1980.
20. James SE, Smith MA: Autologous blood transfusion in elective orthopaedic surgery. *J R Soc Med* 80:284-285, 1987.
21. Janatpour K, Holland P: Blood support for pediatric surgery. Review. *Indian J Pediatr* 68(2):159-165, 2001.
22. Keene JS, McKinley NE: Iliac crest versus spinous process grafts in posttraumatic spinal fusions. *Spine* 17:790-794, 1992.

23. Kickler T, Spivak J: Effect of repeated whole blood transfusions on serum immunoreactive erythropoietin levels in autologous donors. *Spine* 14:358-362, 1989.

24. Kobrinsky NL, Letts RM, Patel LR, *et al:* 1-Desamino-8-D-arginine vasopressin (desmopressin) decreases operative blood loss in patients having Harrington rod spinal fusion surgery. A randomized, double-blinded, controlled trial. *Ann Intern Med* 107:446-450, 1987.

25. Lackritz EM, Satten GA, Aberle-Grasse J, *et al:* Estimated risk of transmission of the human immunodeficiency virus by screened blood in the United States, *N Engl J Med* 333(26):1721-1725, 1995.

26. Lentschener C, Cottin P, Bouaziz H, *et al:* Reduction of blood loss and transfusion requirement by aprotinin in posterior lumbar spine fusion. *Anesth Analg* 89(3):590-597, 1999.

27. Letts M, Pang E, D'Astous J, *et al:* The influence of desmopressin on blood loss during spinal fusion surgery in neuromuscular patients. *Spine* 23(4):475-478, 1998.

28. Levine E, Gould S, Rosen A, *et al:* Perioperative recombinant human erythropoietin. *Surgery* 106:432-438, 1989.

29. Lindop MJ: Complications and morbidity of controlled hypotension. *Br J Anaesth* 47:799-803, 1975.

30. Malcolm-Smith N, McMaster M: The use of induced hypotension to control bleeding during posterior spinal fusion for scoliosis. *J Bone Joint Surg Br* 65:255-258, 1983.

31. Manke C, Bretschneider T, Lenhart M, *et al:* Spinal metastasis from renal cell carcinoma: effect of preoperative particle embolization on intraoperative blood loss. *AJNR Am J Neuroradiol* 22:997-1003, 2001.

32. Mann DC, William MR, Brower EM, Nash CL Jr: Decreasing homologous blood transfusion in spinal surgery by use of the cell saver and predeposited blood. *Spine* 14:1296-1300, 1989.

33. McFarland W, Mvere D, Shandera W, Reingold A: Epidemiology and prevention of transfusion-associated human immunodeficiency virus transmission in sub-Saharan Africa. *Vox Sang* 72(2):85-92, 1997.

34. McNulty SE, Weiss J, Azad SS, *et al:* The effect of the prone position on venous pressure and blood loss during lumbar laminectomy. *J Clin Anesth* 4:220-225, 1992.

35. Murray DJ, Forbes RB, Titone MB, Weinstein SL: Transfusion management in pediatric and adolescent scoliosis surgery. Efficacy of autologous blood. *Spine* 22(23):2735-2740, 1997.

36. Neilipovitz DT, Murto K, Hall L, Barrowman NJ, Splinter WM: A randomized trial of tranexamic acid to reduce blood transfusion for scoliosis surgery. *Anesth Analg* 93:82-87, 2001.

37. Nitu-Whalley IC, Griffioen A, Harrington C: Retrospective review of the management of elective surgery with desmopressin and clotting factor concentrates in patients with von Willebrand disease. *Am J Hematol* 66:280-284, 2000.

38. Nuttall GA, Horlocker TT, Santrach PJ: Predictors of blood transfusions in spinal instrumentation and fusion surgery. *Spine* 2000 25(5):596-601, 2000.

39. Oga M, Ikuta H, Sugioka Y: The use of autologous blood in the surgical treatment of spinal disorders. *Spine* 17:1381-1385, 1992.

40. Osborn JJ, Cohn K, Hait M: Hemolysis during perfusion: sources and means of reduction. *J Thorac Cardiovasc Surg* 43:459-464, 1961.

41. Patel NJ, Patel BS, Paskin S, Laufer S: Induced moderate hypotensive anesthesia for spinal fusion and Harrington-rod instrumentation. *J Bone Joint Surg Am* 67:1384-1387, 1985.

42. Phillips WA, Hensinger RN: Control of blood loss during scoliosis surgery, review. *Clin Orthop* Apr(229):88-93, 1988.

43. Raphael BG, Lackner H, Engler GL: Disseminated intravascular coagulation during surgery for scoliosis. *Clin Orthop* Jan-Feb(162):41-46, 1982.

44. Ray JM, Flynn JC, Bierman AH: Erythrocyte survival following intraoperative autotransfusion in spinal surgery: an in vivo comparative study and 5-year update. *Spine* 11:879-882, 1986.

45. Relton JE, Hall JE: An operation frame for spinal fusion. A new apparatus designed to reduce haemorrhage during operation. *J Bone Joint Surg Br* 49:327-332, 1967.

46. Robinson CM, Christie J, Malcolm-Smith N. Nonsteroidal antiinflammatory drugs perioperative blood loss, and transfusion requirements in elective hip arthroplasty. *J Arthroplasty* 8(6):607-610, 1993.

47. Rothstein P, Roye D, Verdisco L, Stern L: Preoperative use of erythropoietin in an adolescent Jehovah's Witness. *Anesthesiology* 73:568-570, 1990. [published erratum appears in *Anesthesiology* 74(1):206, 1991].

48. Schreiber GB, Busch MP, Kleinman Sh, Korelitz JJ. The risk of transfusion-transmitted viral infections. The Retrovirus Epidemiology Donor Study, *N Engl J Med* 334(26):1685-1690, 1996.

49. Stolke D, Sollmann WP, Seifert V: Intra- and postoperative complications in lumbar disc surgery. *Spine* 14:56-59, 1989.

50. Strumin L: Organ perfusion during controlled hypotension. *Br J Anaesth* 47:173-178, 1975.

51. Tate DE Jr, Friedman RJ: Blood conservation in spinal surgery. Review of current techniques, review. *Spine* 17:1450-1456, 1992

52. Theroux MC, Corddry DH, Tietz AE: A study of desmopressin and blood loss during spinal fusion for neuromuscular scoliosis: a randomized, controlled, double-blinded study. *Anesthesiology* 87(2):260-267, 1997.

53. Thomson JD, Callaghan JJ, Savory CG, *et al:* Prior deposition of autologous blood in elective orthopaedic surgery. *J Bone Joint Surg Am* 69:320-324, 1987.

54. Tredwell SJ, Sawatzky B: The use of fibrin sealant to reduce blood loss during Cotrel-Dubousset instrumentation for idiopathic scoliosis. *Spine* 15:913-915, 1990.

55. Ullrich PF Jr, Keene JS, Hogan KJ, Roecker EB: Results of hypotensive anesthesia in operative treatment of thoracolumbar fractures. *J Spinal Disord* 3:329-333, 1990.

56. Urban MK, Beckman J, Gordon M, *et al:* The efficacy of antifibrinolytics in the reduction of blood loss during complex spinal surgery. *Spine* 26(10):1152-1157, 2001.

# CHAPTER 129

# Imaging: Trauma

**Blaine L. Hart**

## Principles of Imaging Spine Trauma

It is essential to view the entire cervical spine and the junction with the thoracic spine and skull. Incomplete visualization of the cervical spine through the C7-T1 junction is a well-recognized pitfall in acute trauma. If the shoulders obscure the C7-T1 junction on the lateral radiograph, additional imaging must be performed. This may include a swimmers view or a CT scan.

Multiple levels of spine injury are relatively common. Adjacent vertebrae are frequently fractured. In addition, noncontiguous injuries are also common following significant trauma. Detection of one fracture, therefore, should not end the search for spine injury. Especially with the widespread availability of spiral CT, evaluation of the entire cervical spine from craniocervical junction through cervicothoracic junction is very feasible.

Imaging complements the clinical examination. "Clearing" the spine is not a result of completing a set of radiographs or other imaging tests, it must come from a combination of clinical examination and appropriate imaging.

Integrity (stability) of the spine depends on both bone and soft tissue. Although uncommon, it is possible for a patient with no fractures, or seemingly insignificant fractures, to have an unstable spine because of severe ligamentous injury. Even with clearly demonstrated fractures, the outcome may be markedly affected by the extent of accompanying soft tissue injury. Alteration in alignment, worsening neurologic function, or persistent pain may be indications for MRI.

## Techniques for Imaging Spine Trauma

Multiple imaging tools are available for the evaluation of traumatic spine injury. In order to utilize these tools appropriately, it is important to understand the strengths and limitations of the available techniques. The approach to imaging varies, depending on clinical circumstances, availability of imaging tests, and results of any previous imaging.

### Radiographs

Radiographs ("plain films") of the spine, despite the various other imaging tests available, remain the foundation of imaging acute spine trauma. Plain radiography should be readily available at any facility seeing acute spine trauma. Radiographs can be obtained relatively quickly, and they are relatively inexpensive compared to computed tomo-graphy (CT) and magnetic resonance imaging (MRI). Spatial detail is excellent with good technique, although interpretation can be challenging with multiple overlapping structures. One of the strengths of plain radiography is the ability to quickly assess alignment.

There is no universal agreement on the views that should be obtained for acute cervical spine trauma. A lateral view is necessary, and often this is among the first radiographs (along with an anteroposterior [AP] chest radiograph), to be obtained in a multiple trauma victim. As is discussed below, it is essential to view the entire cervical spine, including the junctions with the skull and thoracic spine. A swimmers view may be useful, if needed, to visualize the lower cervical spine. The lateral view is often followed by AP and odontoid views. The odontoid view, in particular, may be difficult with an uncooperative or intubated patient. Additional views may include oblique or pillar views. These can be particularly helpful to assess the dorsal elements. The standard method of obtaining these views involves turning the patient's neck, which is not acceptable in the acute setting. Modified techniques can be used that involve angling the x-ray tube instead of turning the neck; these result in more distortion than a standard view but can still be useful.

AP and lateral views are usually obtained when acute thoracic or lumbar spine injury is suspected. Oblique views have little role in the evaluation of acute lumbar trauma. They add a considerable radiation dose with limited benefit.

Alignment is well assessed with plain films. Soft tissue injury can be inferred from prevertebral soft tissue swelling in the cervical spine. In the lumbar and thoracic spine, paraspinous swelling on the AP view is a sign of acute injury. Otherwise, however, radiographs are insensitive for the detection of significant soft tissue. The sensitivity of plain films for fracture varies depending on the location of the fracture. Vertebral body fractures are usually well visualized on radiographs, but fractures in the dorsal elements can be difficult. Sensitivity of radiographs for dorsal element fractures in the cervical spine has been found to be as low as 50%.[1,41,42] Fractures of the larger vertebra of the thoracic and lumbar spine are usually well visualized on plain films.

### Computed Tomography

Computed tomography (CT) plays an important role in imaging acute trauma. It is frequently used to detect or further characterize spine fractures. Although CT is generally more sensitive for the detection of fractures than plain films, some important limitations exist. The more closely the plane of a fracture lies to the acquisition plane of the scan, the more difficult the fracture can be to see on CT. For example, type II odontoid fractures and Chance fractures may be seen more clearly on plain films than on CT. Reformatted CT views in sagittal, coronal, or other planes are very helpful in such cases, as well as for viewing alignment. Motion during the acquisition of a CT scan can create significant problems. Spiral CT scanning significantly limits the difficulties with motion and permits improved reformation views. Multislice CT adds further possibilities for both speed and thinner slices. Small, nearly isotropic voxels—volume elements that are close to the same size in all three dimensions—permit more accurate reconstructions in sagittal, coronal, or oblique planes, with some cost in greater radiation exposure. As CT increases in speed and technical capability, it has become feasible to incorporate it in a routine manner in the evaluation of major trauma, especially in cervical spine evaluation.[20,22,31]

In addition to planar (2D) reconstruction views, three-dimensional projection views can be useful to evaluate the position of fractures. There is considerable variation possible in reconstruction techniques. The images can be created using surface reconstruction projection or varying degrees of apparent transparency of the reconstructed image. Each has advantages in specific situations, and the user of CT machines should become familiar with the options available. Technologies are being developed for more realistic depth imaging, ranging from true three-dimensional holographic projections to computer-guided models created from CT images. Such advanced techniques may have a role in planning surgery, although the limitations of time restrict the use in the immediate evaluation of acute trauma.

## Magnetic Resonance Imaging

The value of magnetic resonance imaging (MRI) for acute spine trauma may be not obvious. MRI is relatively insensitive for detection of fractures, since cortical bone provides very little signal and appears black on MRI. There are significant limitations of MRI for the acutely injured patient, including challenges in patient monitoring, longer imaging times than with radiography or CT, and difficulties in using standard coils in a patient with spine immobilization. For these practical reasons, MRI is often more suitable in the first few days than the first few hours after trauma. Nevertheless, MRI has unique advantages for assessment of acute spine trauma.

MRI is highly sensitive for soft tissues, especially for edema.[10,30,32] MRI is the best method for visualizing the spinal cord. Compression or deformity of the spinal cord, edema, and hemorrhage are visualized well with MRI. MRI is also excellent for evaluating the intervertebral discs (Figure 129.1). For example, detection of an acute disc disruption may alter plans regarding the surgical approach.[34] Cases have been reported in which the reduction of a dislocation worsened symptoms because of further herniation or displacement of disc material. MRI permits detection of such herniation before surgery. Ligament disruption can occasionally be directly visualized with MRI, especially the anterior and posterior longitudinal ligaments. There is some evidence that suggests that the extent of ligament disruption may correlate with the risk of instability in cervical spine posterior element fractures.

The soft tissues around the vertebra are also visualized with MRI. Extensive edema can serve as a marker for acute injury and the need for further evaluation. Deep, interspinous edema in the setting of acute trauma may be an indication of high risk of instability due to flexion injury. MRI can be helpful in a variety of clinical situations in which the combination of clinical and initial imaging find-

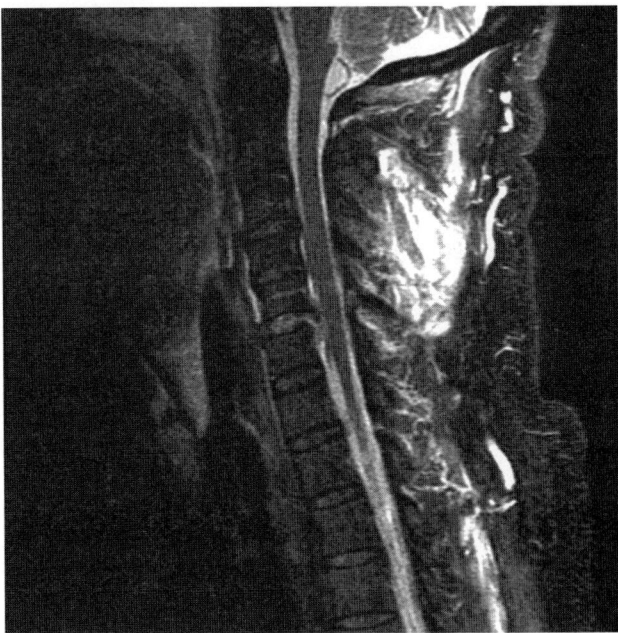

**Figure 129.1** Traumatic disc and ligament disruption. MRI, sagittal fast inversion recovery image, shows disruption of both anterior and posterior longitudinal ligaments at C5-C6 and disc disruption with traumatic disc herniation, and anterior and posterior soft tissue edema. The findings were confirmed at surgery.

ings is ambiguous or nondefinitive. For example, degenerative changes are very common in the cervical spine and can make detection of acute fractures difficult. Although CT can help to identify fractures, subluxation or chronic deformity can still be a challenge. A negative MRI in such situations, showing no evidence of any significant nearby soft tissue edema, makes acute injury unlikely as a cause of subluxation. MRI can be especially helpful in cases in which clinical assessment is limited, such as the obtunded or intubated patient.[4]

Unexpected worsening of neurologic status after spine trauma can be due to a variety of factors. MRI may reveal such causes as epidural hematoma, disc herniation, or spinal cord edema from infarction.

The limitations of MRI mentioned above can be overcome in most cases. Monitoring is essential in the acutely injured patient. MRI-compatible monitoring equipment is available. The patient must be screened for the presence of metallic devices or metal within the body that would preclude MRI. Although standard spine coils may not be usable with a cervical collar, other coils can still permit diagnostic images. Faster imaging techniques continue to be developed for MRI, and it is often not necessary or appropriate to use the same sequences for acute trauma patients that would be used for evaluation of degenerative disc disease, for example. The specific sequences to be used can be tailored to the clinical situation.

Although it is impossible to specify MRI parameters that should be used because of the great variety of manufacturers, machines, and software available, some broad principles apply. A T2-weighted sequence is important to detect edema. Fast-spin echo imaging, in which multiple echoes are acquired during each pulse sequence, are nearly always used in standard spine imaging. Such sequences are much faster than spin echo sequences and produce excellent signal-to-noise and high quality images. Fast spin echo sequences can be excellent for visualization of the spinal cord, for example. However, it is important to note that fat remains very bright on such sequences, even with T2 weighting. Therefore, if adjacent soft tissue edema is to be demonstrated, different sequences must be used that suppress the signal from fat (Figure 129.2). A fat saturation pulse can be added to fast spin echo imaging sequences. Alternatively, inversion recovery sequences (short-tau inversion recovery or STIR) accomplish the same effect of heavy T2 weighting and fat suppression.

Edema within the bone marrow is also well demonstrated with MRI. This appears as low signal (dark) on $T_1$-weighted images, replacing the normally bright signal from fat in the marrow and high signal on fat-suppressed $T_2$-weighted images. Acute fractures, especially those that involve the vertebral body, cause marrow changes, but bone contusions that do not result in cortical bone disruption can also result in marrow edema. Over time, marrow signal intensity usually returns to an appearance close to that of normal vertebral body marrow. Thus, signal intensity in marrow of a compressed vertebral body that matches that of adjacent, normal vertebrae provides evidence for a chronic rather than acute injury.

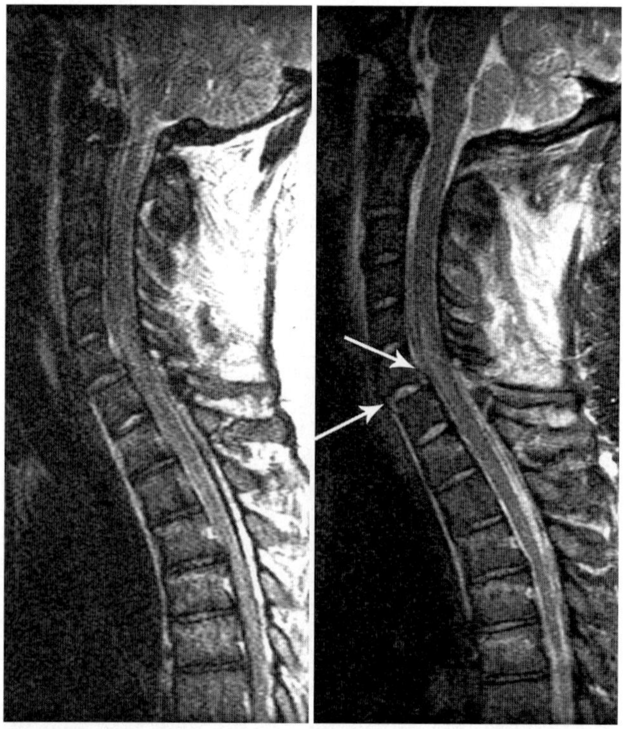

The sensitivity of MRI for acute soft tissue injury depends on several factors. Edema resolves over several days; the precise time-course has not been defined but clearly depends on severity of the original injury. In our experience, soft tissue edema associated with an acute cervical spine injury is likely to be less extensive on MRI in the setting of axial load injuries. Presumably, this is due to less stretching and tearing of the soft tissues. For example, a minimally displaced Jefferson burst fracture may result in very little soft tissue edema. When these limitations are understood, however, MRI can play a very useful adjunctive role in assessing major acute cervical spine trauma.

## Motion Radiography Studies

Radiographs of the spine in different positions, (i.e., flexion and extension views in a lateral position), are excellent for evaluation of stability of the spine in a delayed or chronic setting (Figure 129.3). There are significant limitations of such studies in the acute setting. Most importantly, there are major risks if the spine is in fact unstable. Complications of flexion/extension radiographs are rare but well known. If motion studies are to be undertaken, it is highly desirable that the patient be fully alert, cooperative, and capable of controlling or stopping the motion. If flexion and extension is performed on an obtunded or comatose patient, performing the study under fluoroscopy should improve the safety. The motion can be immediately stopped as soon as subluxation or abnormal movement is visualized. However, data on the safety and accuracy of performing motion radiography on an obtunded patient in

**Figure 129.2** MRI, Fat Suppression for Soft Tissue Evaluation. MRI was performed of a young man with myelopathic symptoms after a motor vehicle accident. (**A**) Sagittal fast spin echo $T_2$-weighted image shows slight subluxation at C6-7, but edema from soft tissue injury is difficult to identify because fat also remains bright. (**B**) On a sagittal fast spin echo inversion recovery image the fat is now dark, but edema in the dorsal soft tissues, in the marrow space of upper thoracic vertebral bodies, and prevertebral space is very conspicuous. Anterior and posterior longitudinal ligaments at C6-7 are stretched (*arrows*).

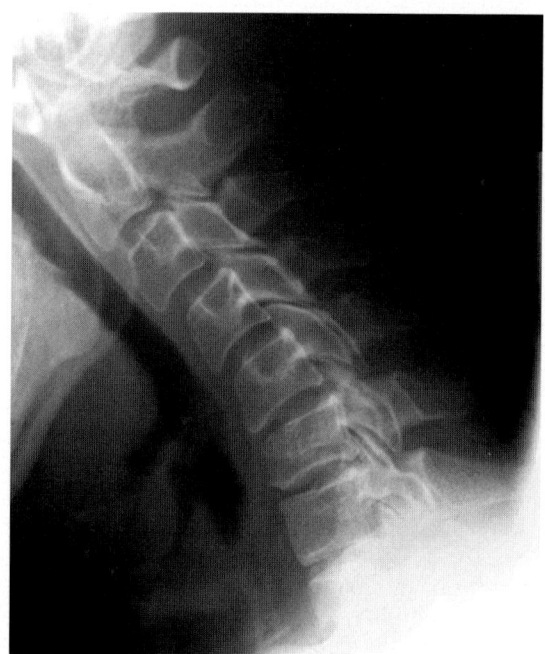

**Figure 129.3** Instability on Flexion Film. Flexion lateral radiograph obtained on a delayed basis after cervical spine trauma shows focal kyphosis and posterior widening. Alignment in neutral position was normal.

the setting of acute injury are very limited. Such studies are often time-consuming, and visualization of the cervicothoracic junction is frequently difficult.

A second limitation in the acute setting is a high incidence of muscle spasm or guarding. From one quarter to one third of patients with acute cervical spine injury may have nondiagnostic results because there is inadequate movement of the neck to assess stability.[6,28] Delayed studies, several weeks after trauma and after muscle spasm has subsided, with the patient cooperative and in control of neck motion, remain the gold standard for evaluating stability of the cervical spine.

## Myelography

Because of the availability of MRI, myelography has a very limited role in the evaluation of spine trauma. There are occasional situations in which patency of the spinal canal must be assessed and MRI is not possible.

## Imaging Findings

### Cervicocranial Junction and Upper Cervical Spine

The upper cervical spine poses challenges for imaging. Upper cervical spine injuries can be multiple, complex, and difficult to identify on imaging.

### C1 Fractures

The Jefferson burst fracture of C1 is a relatively common injury. CT can demonstrate the multiple fractures of the ring of C1 and the extent of displacement (Figure 129.4). Plain films usually show prevertebral soft tissue swelling. Some components of the fractures can be visible on plain radiographs, more so if the fractures are displaced. The lateral masses of C1 are likely to be displaced laterally if the transverse ligament is disrupted. Total displacement of greater than 7mm as seen on an odontoid view has been suggested as a guideline to the presence of transverse ligament rupture.[38] The transverse ligament can be visualized

directly on MRI, and fluid signal in place of the expected low signal intensity of the ligament is evidence of rupture.[14]

The imaging findings above apply to adults. In at least the first 4 years of life, the lateral masses of C1 often project lateral to the lateral margins of C2 on an AP view.[39] Jefferson fractures are uncommon in children, however. CT may be necessary to demonstrate such fractures in children.

Isolated fractures of the posterior arch of C1 can occur with hyperextension injuries (Figure 129.5). In such cases, prevertebral soft tissue swelling would likely be absent, and the posterior arch fracture can be seen on a lateral radiograph. Another type of hyperextension injury at C1 is an avulsion at the anterior inferior ventral arch, at the attachment of the atlantoaxial ligament. In this case the fracture is visible on the lateral view, and there is usually focal prevertebral soft tissue swelling.

### Transverse Ligament Injury

Transverse ligament rupture can be seen in association with a variety of upper cervical spine fractures, and the possibility should be considered in any such injury. In addition, transverse ligament injury uncommonly may occur without other fractures. Loss of integrity of the transverse ligament can result either from rupture in the midportion of the ligament or from avulsion of the ligament at one of the attachments to the lateral mass of C1. In the latter case a small fracture is often visible at the tubercle where the ligament attaches (see Figure 129.26). If the ventral atlantodental space is widened, transverse ligament rupture should be suspected. The ligament itself can be seen directly using MRI. In the case of rupture, fluid signal intensity (bright on $T_2$-weighted images) can be seen in the expected location of the ligament, and fluid is also likely to be present between the dens and anterior arch of C1.

### C2 Fractures

Odontoid fractures can occur from a variety of mechanisms. Anderson and D'Alonzo[2] described three types of

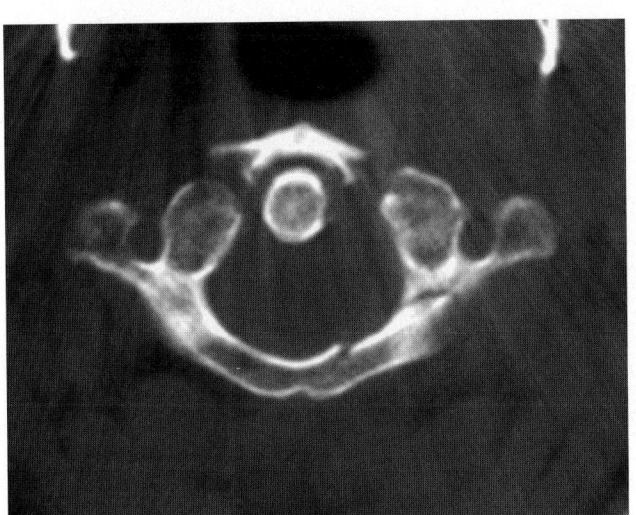

**Figure 129.4** Jefferson Fracture. Patient fell from a ladder onto head. CT shows multiple fractures of the ring of C1.

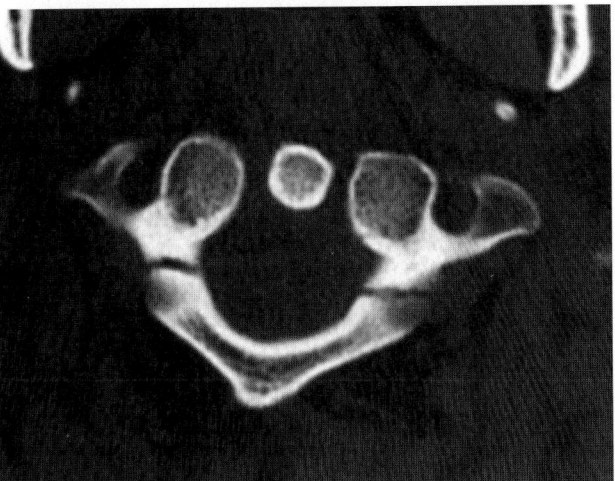

**Figure 129.5** Dorsal Arch C1 Fracture. Extension mechanism: CT shows bilateral fractures through the posterior arch of C1; the ventral arch was intact.

odontoid fractures: type I, an oblique fracture near the apex of the dens; type II, a transverse fracture through the lower third of the dens but above the body of C2 (Figure 129.6); and type III, which is a fracture below the base of the dens and through the body of C2 (Figure 129.7). As with transversely oriented fractures elsewhere, odontoid fractures can be difficult to identify by CT. Axial images may show only a region of lucency or subtle gaps in the

cortical margin. Reconstructed images from thin-slice axial images, especially from rapid spiral acquisitions, can be very helpful to identify odontoid fractures on CT. Plain radiographs should be carefully inspected for signs of odontoid fractures, including prevertebral soft tissue swelling, abnormal angulation of the odontoid process, offset of the dens with respect to the body of C2, and disruption of the cortical margin. The type III fracture

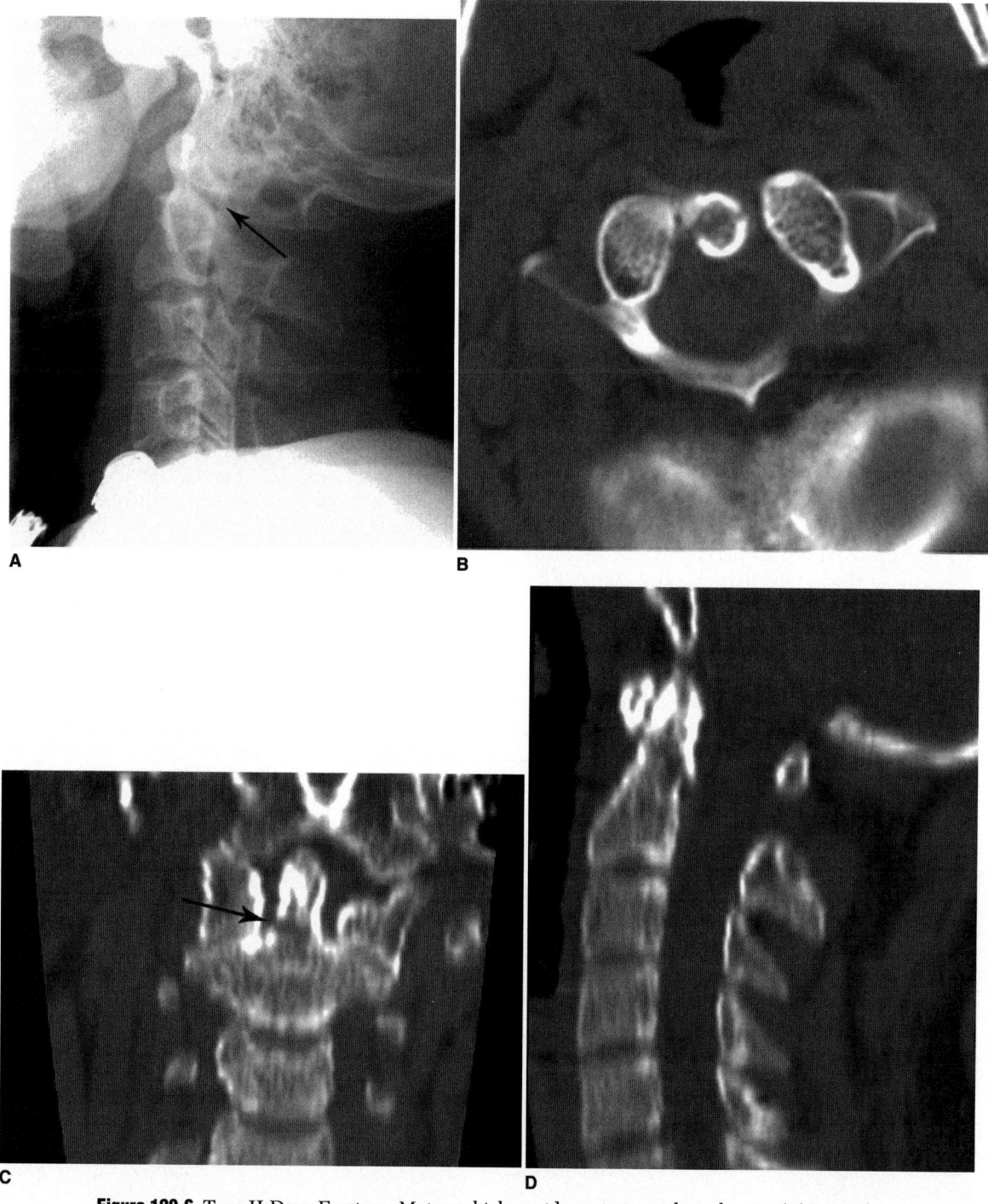

**Figure 129.6** Type II Dens Fracture. Motor vehicle accident victim with neck pain: **(A)** Lateral radiograph shows only mild prevertebral swelling and very subtle lucency at the base of the dens (*arrow*). **(B)** Axial CT discloses a fracture line through the dens. Reconstruction views show the fracture much more clearly, on **(C)** sagittal and **(D)** coronal views. Note in **(A)** that the "ring" appearance over the body of C2 is intact.

(or type 3 C2 body fracture) is a horizontally oriented, rostral fracture at the base of the dens. In such fractures, the lateral radiograph shows a break in the apparent ring that results from the superimposition of densities from the junction of pedicle and body, dens and body, and dorsal cortex of the C2 body.[23] The AP or odontoid view usually shows a fracture with inferior convexity.

Fractures of the body of C2, which have received relatively little attention, include coronally oriented posterior fractures (type 1), which are similar in some respects to the hangman's fracture through the pars interarticularis of C2 (Figure 129.8); oblique, sagittally oriented fractures (type 2), which result from axial loading (Figure 129.9); and the horizontally oriented type 3 fracture

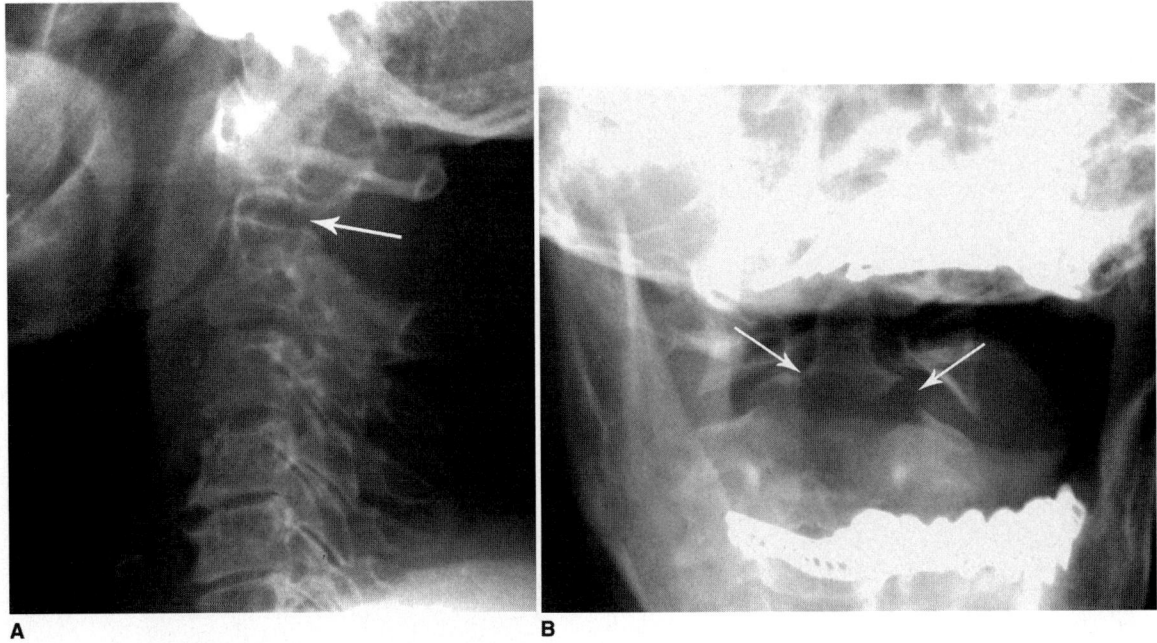

**Figure 129.7** Low Dens (Type III) Fracture. Motor vehicle accident patient: **(A)** Lateral radiograph shows lucency that disrupts the ring appearance *(arrow)*, unlike the type II fracture in Figure 129.6. **(B)** The low fracture, actually a fracture through the rostral portion of the body of C2, is well seen in the AP view *(arrows)*.

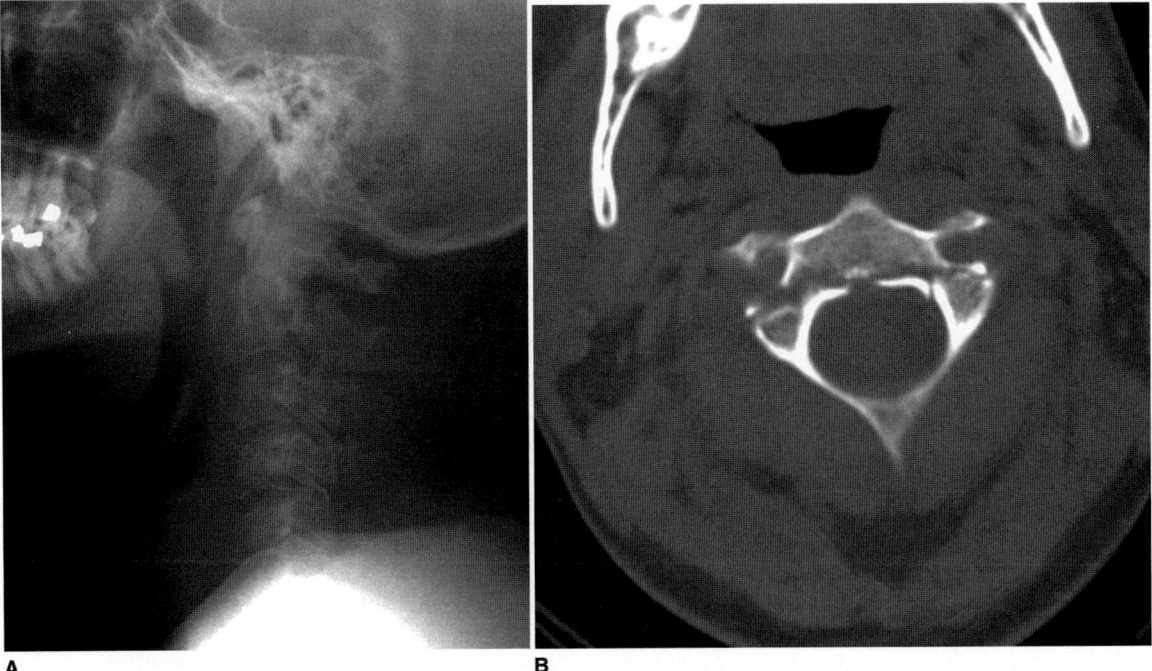

**Figure 129.8** C2 Body Fracture, Type I. **(A)** Lateral radiograph shows lucency in the posterior body of C2, with prevertebral soft tissue swelling. **(B)** CT shows fractures through the dorsal portion of the C2 body.

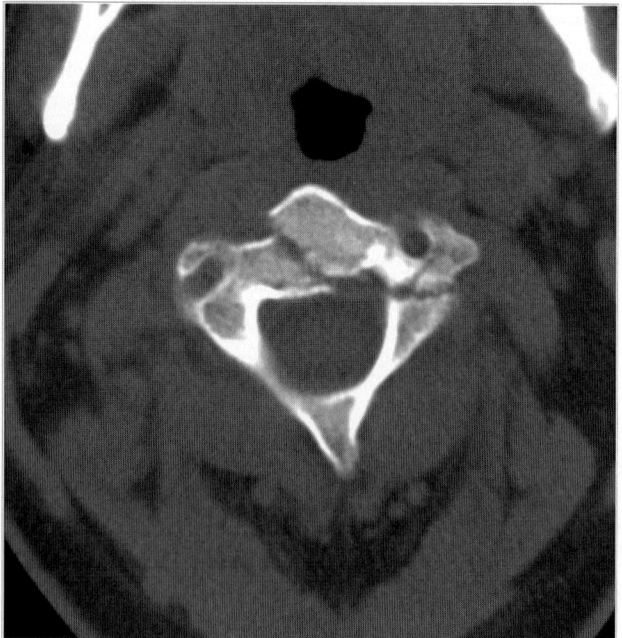

**Figure 129.9** C2 Body Fracture, Type 2. Axial CT of a patient who fell from a ladder onto his head shows an oblique fracture through the C2 body, with an additional fracture through the left lamina.

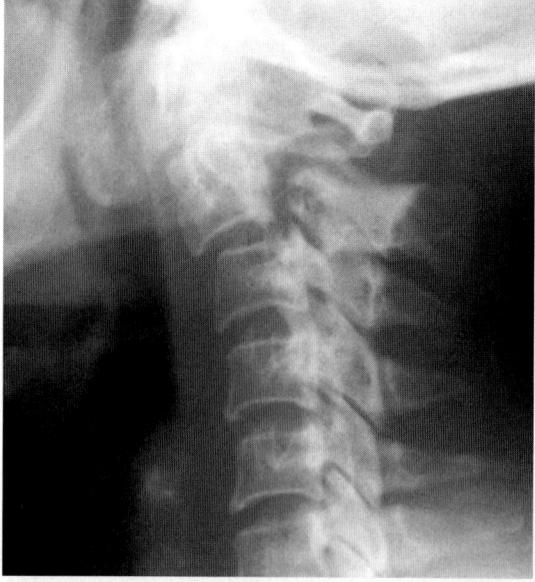

A

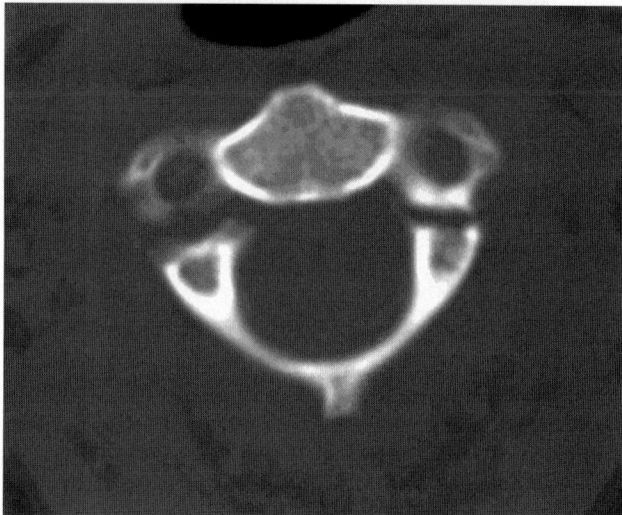

B

**Figure 129.10** Traumatic Spondylolisthesis (Hangman's Fracture). **(A)** Lateral radiograph shows fractures through the pars interarticularis, with ventral displacement of the body of C2 relative to C3 in this case. **(B)** Axial CT in another case shows bilateral fractures through the pars interarticularis.

described above (see Figure 129.7).[3] CT is particularly helpful in C2 body fractures in defining the location and extent of fractures.

The hangman's fracture, or traumatic spondylolisthesis, consists of bilateral fractures through the pars interarticularis (Figure 129.10).[9,13,17] It is usually visible on lateral radiographs as a lucency, with prevertebral soft tissue swelling. The Effendi classification of these fractures is based on the extent of displacement: type I consists of minimal displacement; type II shows anterior displacement and an abnormal C2-3 disc; and type III is anterior displacement of the body of C2 in flexion, with bilateral facet dislocation of C2-3.[16]

The extension teardrop fracture of C2 consists of an avulsion of the ventral caudal corner of the C2 body, at the attachment of the atlantoaxial ligament. There is a characteristic triangular shape on lateral radiographs, usually with accompanying prevertebral soft tissue swelling.

Children can suffer a unique injury of C2, fracture through the subdental synchondrosis. The dens is separated in a sharp, geometric margin from the centrum of C2 below (Figure 129.11).

### Craniocervical Junction

Occipital condyle fractures are especially difficult to identify on plain radiographs. CT with thin slice thickness and reconstruction images is the best imaging tool (Figure 129.12). Occipital condyle fractures have also been classified in three groups. Type I fractures are compression fractures from axial loading. Type II fractures are basilar occiput fractures that extend into the occipital condyle. Type III fractures result from avulsion, a result of lateral

bending and forced rotation. Because of ligamentous injury, type III are the condyle fractures most likely to be unstable.[5,12]

Atlanto-occipital dislocation is often a fatal injury, although less severe forms are increasingly being recognized. Prominent upper cervical prevertebral soft tissue hematoma is nearly always present (Figure 129.13). Several methods of measuring atlanto-occipital dislocation have been proposed. The Powers ratio is the relationship of the distance from basion (B) to the dorsal arch of the atlas (C), compared to the distance from opisthion (O) to midpoint of the dorsal surface of the ventral arch (A).[33] The ratio BC/OA, which is normally less than 1, increases with ventral dislocation. The bony landmarks to determine the Powers ratio can be difficult to identify, and Harris and

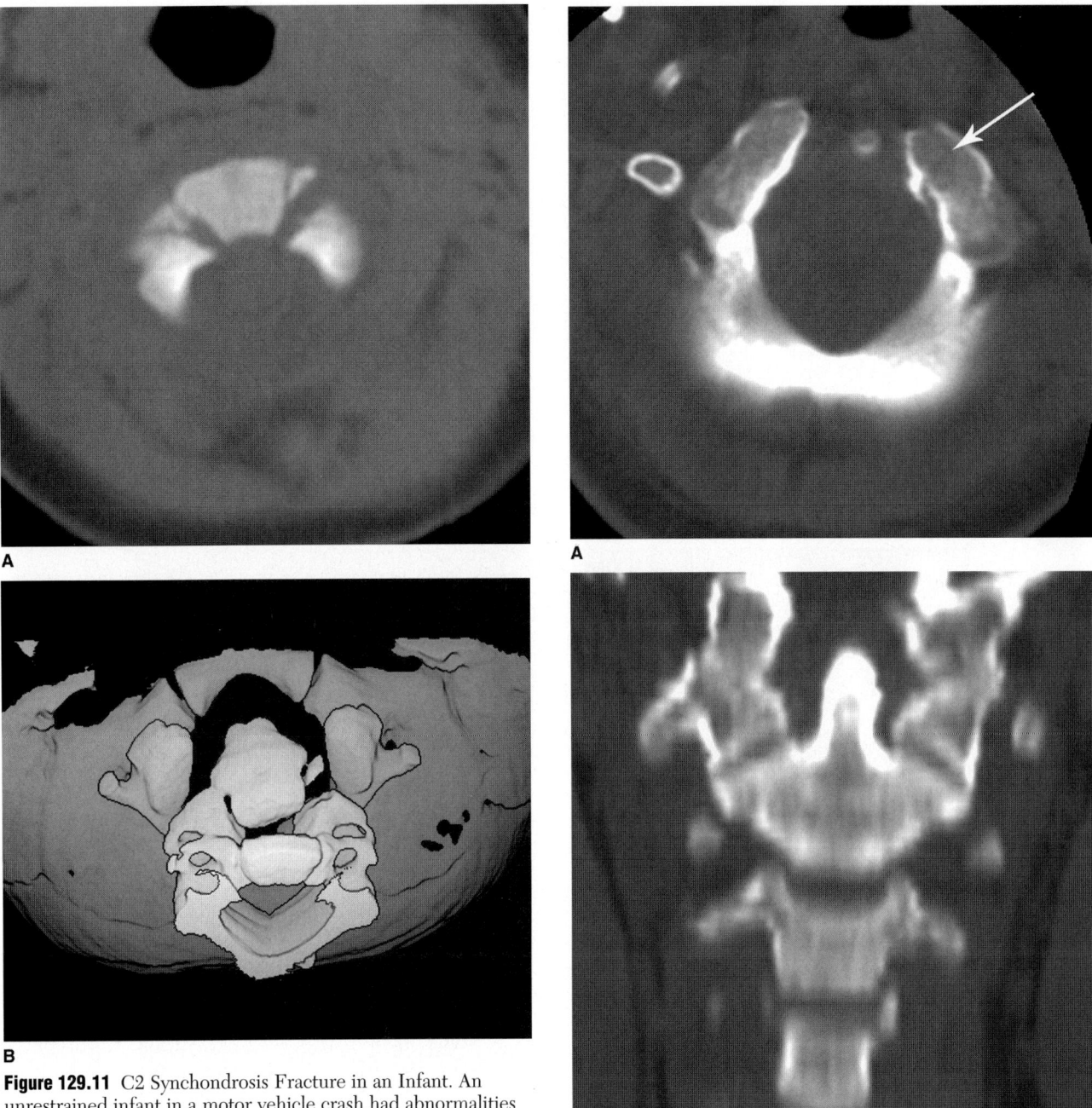

**Figure 129.11** C2 Synchondrosis Fracture in an Infant. An unrestrained infant in a motor vehicle crash had abnormalities at the C2 level on plain film. (**A**) Axial CT shows fractures that mostly involve the neurocentral synchondrosis, separating the body and odontoid from the neural arch. (**B**) A 3D reconstruction from below shows the separation through the synchondrosis. The ventral aspect of the spine, including the ventral arch of C1, has been excluded to allow visualization of C2.

**Figure 129.12** Occipital Condyle Fracture. (**A**) Axial CT shows lucency *(arrows)* in the left occipital condyle. (**B**) Coronal reconstruction demonstrates the oblique left occipital condyle fracture.

colleagues have described two measurements that are easier to perform and less sensitive to the direction of dislocation.[24,25] Both measurements are performed on a lateral radiograph (Figure 129.14). The first is between a dorsal axial line upward from the posterior vertebral body of C2 and the basion. The basion-axial interval should be no less than 6mm or more than 12mm, in both adults and children. The second measurement is between basion and the tip of the dens, the basion-dens interval. This distance should not be more than 12mm. This basion-dens interval depends on complete ossification of the dens and therefore may not be obtainable in children younger than 13 years.

## Subaxial Cervical Spine Injuries

Axial loading injuries in the lower cervical spine result in burst fractures. The basic pattern of the burst fracture is similar throughout the thoracic and lumbar spine, as well.

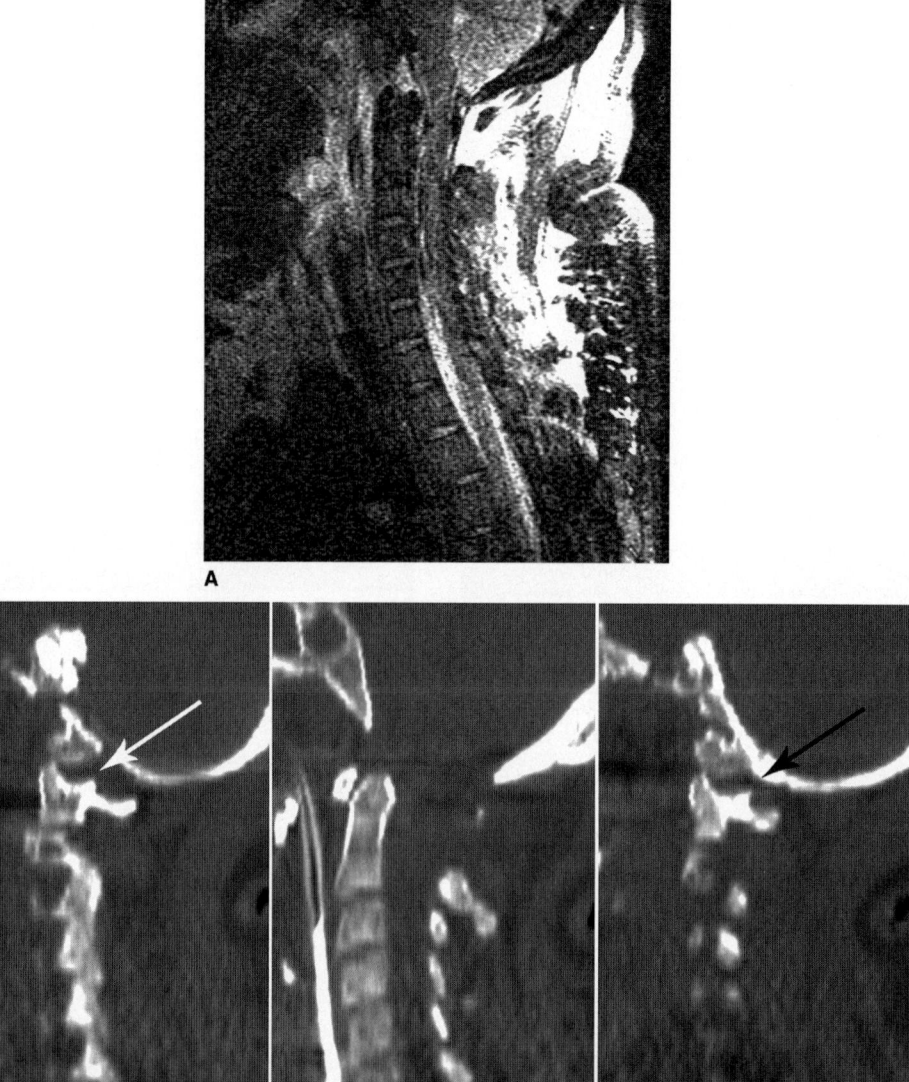

**Figure 129.13** Atlanto-Occipital Dissociation. Other injuries in this passenger in a high-speed motor vehicle accident precluded clinical evaluation of the cervical spine, and plain films were limited. **(A)** MRI sagittal inversion recovery image shows very extensive edema around the upper cervical spine, including the supraodontoid space, with stretching of the ligaments at the cervicocranial junction. There is blood within the spinal canal. **(B)** Sagittal CT reconstruction images, including midline and parasagittal views of both condyles, show subluxation of the occipito-atlantal joints (arrows).

The degree of comminution is variable but there is usually a prominent sagittal component. Dorsal element fractures are common and variable. CT is very helpful is determining the extent of fractures (Figure 129.15). Involvement of multiple vertebrae can occur with more severe injuries. MRI can directly demonstrate the relationship of displaced bone to the spinal cord, spinal cord compression, and spinal cord edema and hematoma, as well as disc disruption.

A variety of flexion injuries can occur in the subaxial cervical spine. Many of these result in a pattern of dorsal widening or fanning of the facets and spinous processes at the level of injury (Figure 129.16). This pattern of flexion injury is an important finding on lateral radiographs.

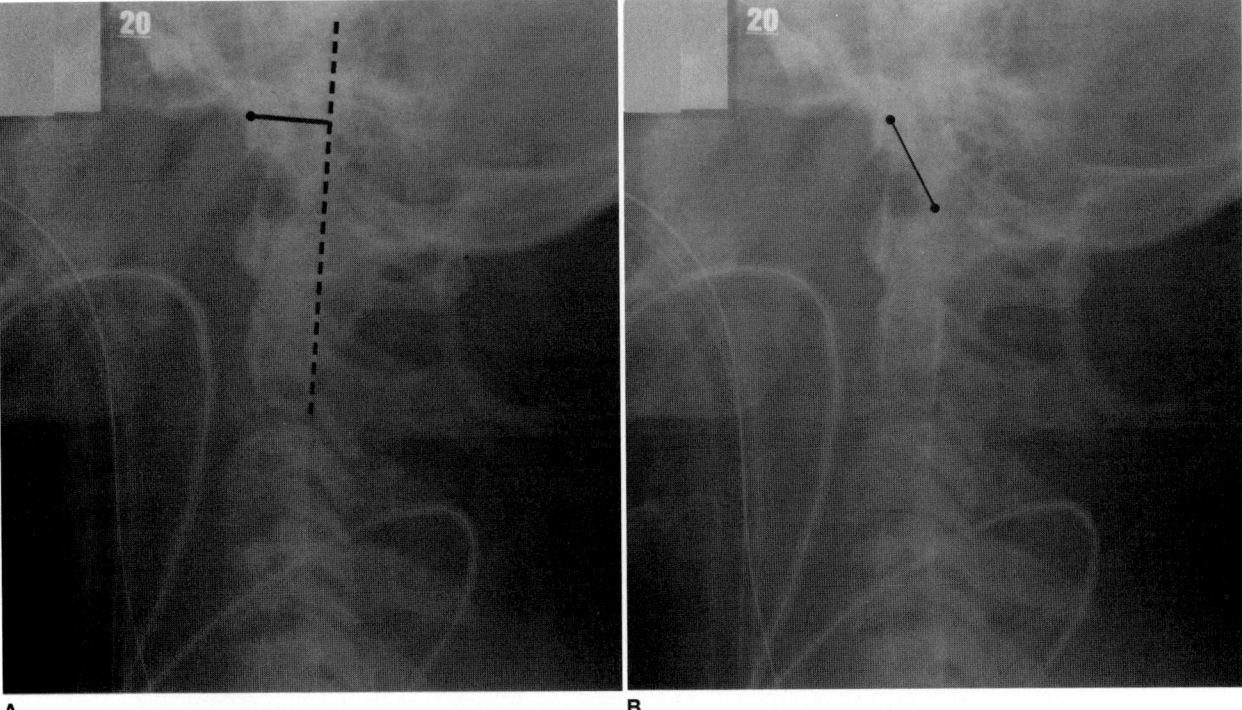

**Figure 129.14** Craniocervical relationships and atlanto-occipital dissociation (AOD). Lateral radiograph of a patient who suffered AOD shows severe prevertebral soft tissue swelling and distraction of the cranium from the spine. Measurements described by Harris *et al.* are illustrated: **(A)** Basion-axial interval, distance from basion to a line extended upward from the dorsal margin of the body of C2. **(B)** Basion-dens interval, distance from basion to the tip of the dens. *(Copyright 2001 University of New Mexico Department of Radiology, Neuroradiology Section.)*

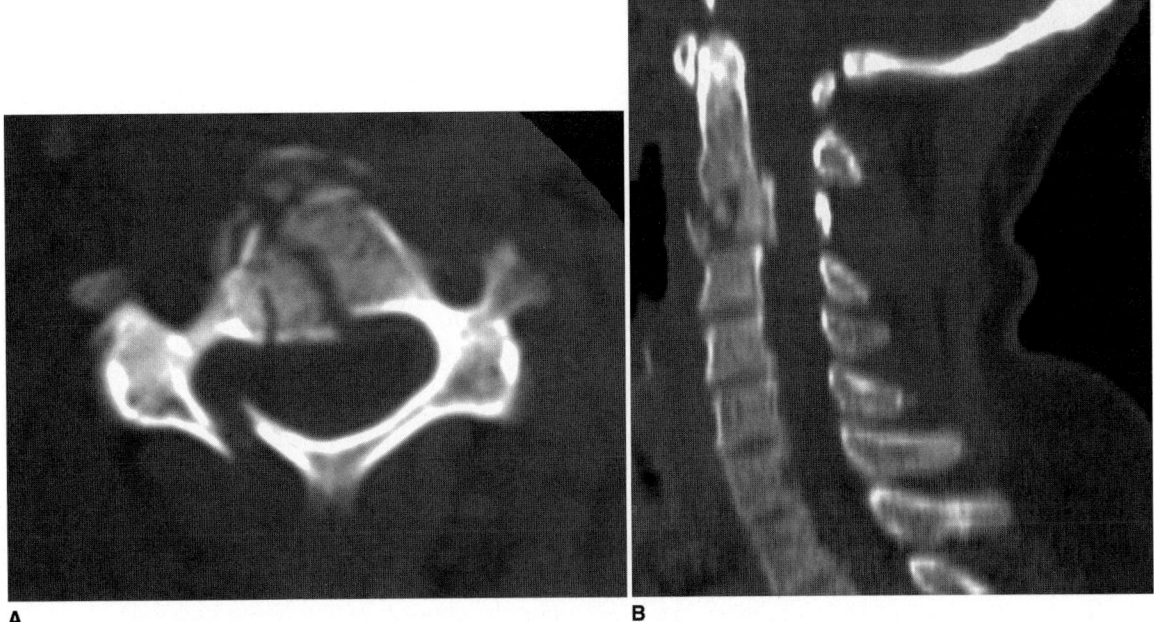

**Figure 129.15** C3 Burst Fracture. **(A)** CT of a patient in a motor vehicle accident through the C3 level reveals comminuted fractures, including the right lamina. **(B)** Sagittal reconstruction shows the displacement into the spinal canal as well as ventrally.

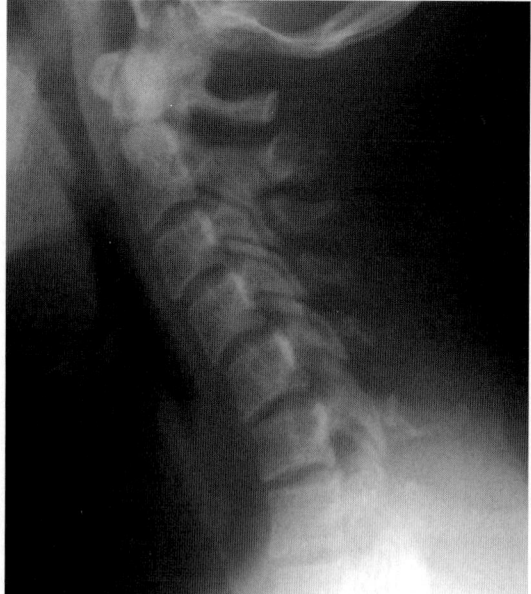

**Figure 129.16** Flexion Sprain. Lateral cervical spine radiograph demonstrates kyphosis and dorsal widening at C5-6 and to a lesser extent at C6-7.

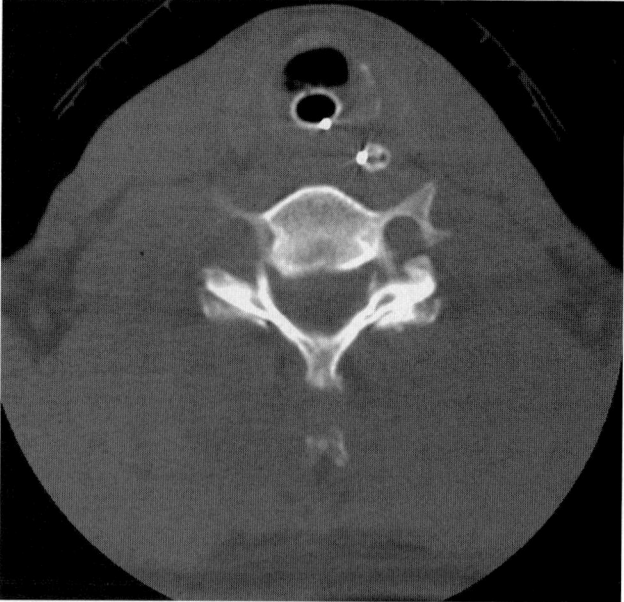

A

**Figure 129.17** Bilateral Facet Dislocation. Patient was quadriplegic after motor vehicle accident. **(A)** Axial CT shows reversal of the normal relationship of the facets bilaterally.

Dorsal ligament injury without fracture can result in instability from flexion sprain. A simple ventral compression fracture results in anterior loss of height of a vertebral body. Dorsal ligament injury may or may not accompany a compression fracture. Focal kyphosis is often observed at the level of compression.[19,26,35] A fairly common pattern of flexion injury in the lower cervical spine is an avulsion fracture of the spinous process, or "clay-shoveler's fracture."

More serious flexion injuries can cause actual disruption of the facet joints and bilateral facet dislocation (Figure 129.17). The vertebra above the level of dislocation is ventrally displaced relative to that below the level of dislocation. Dorsal widening and focal kyphosis are observed. CT often reveals small fractures of the articular processes at the level of dislocation. MRI shows a typical pattern of extensive dorsal soft tissue edema from the level of dislocation and above; and the relationship of the spinal cord to the narrowed spinal canal can be seen on MRI.

A flexion teardrop fracture is one of the most severe flexion injuries of the cervical spine. Lateral radiographs show a large triangular fragment of bone from the anterior inferior corner of the fractured vertebra. Unlike the extension teardrop fracture, there is pronounced flexion of the spine at the level of injury. The typical clinical picture of anterior cord syndrome also distinguishes the flexion teardrop fracture.[36]

Extension mechanisms can cause a variety of cervical spine injuries. Compression of the lamina can cause laminar fractures, visible on lateral or oblique radiographs, and especially CT.

Hyperextension dislocation causes transient dislocation through a disc level and compression of the spinal cord. The usual clinical picture is a central cord syndrome. Radiographic signs are straightening of the cervical spine, diffuse prevertebral swelling, and often an avulsion fracture of the inferior end plate above the level of dislocation (Figure 129.18). Such a fracture is horizontally oriented and is wider than tall. Disc space widening or gas within the disc space are less commonly seen.[15,27] MRI shows the prevertebral edema, abnormal signal in the affected disc space, and edema within the spinal cord. In the author's experience, MRI also often shows dorsal soft tissue edema. Another cause of central cord syndrome resulting from hyperextension was described by Taylor et al.[7,40] In such cases preexisting osteophytes narrow the spinal canal and cause transient spinal cord compression. Diffuse prevertebral soft tissue swelling is lacking in such cases, but MRI shows edema within the spinal cord and the extent of spondylosis (Figure 129.19).

Unilateral facet dislocation results from combined flexion and rotation. There is a typical constellation of imaging findings in such cases (Figure 129.20).[8,43] Lateral radiographs show an abrupt change from a typical lateral appearance below the dislocation to an appearance above that level of an oblique projection. The visualization of both facets on the lateral view just above the dislocation gives a "bow-tie" appearance. On the AP view, there is an abrupt change in the line along the spinous processes. CT shows a reversal of the usual "clamshell" appearance of the facets where they are dislocated. In less severe cases the facets may appear "perched" without frank dislocation, but this finding still implies major ligament and joint disruption.

Fractures involving the lateral masses, pedicles, and lamina, can be very difficult to visualize on plain films. Close inspection of the lateral bony margins seen on AP

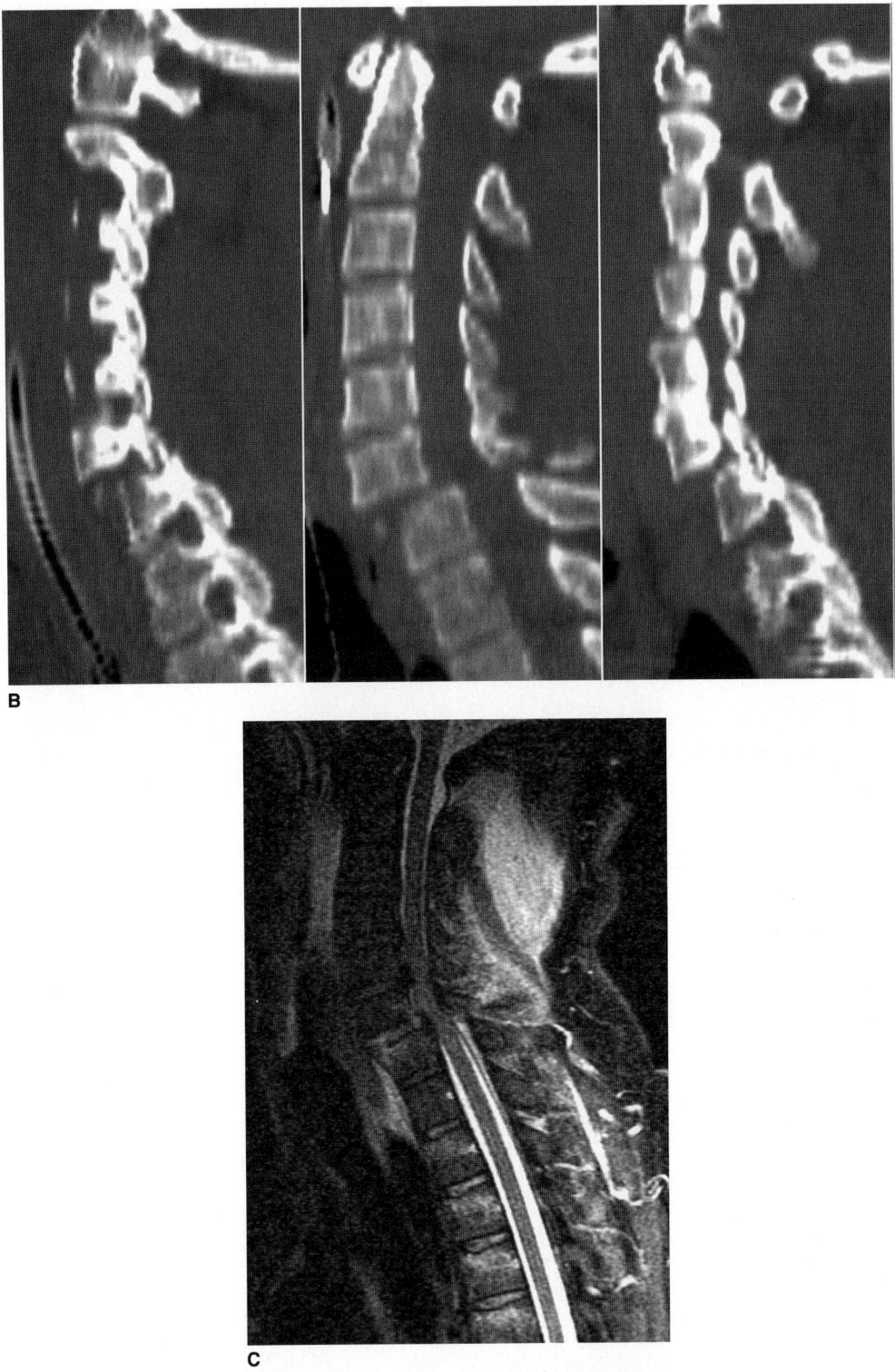

B

C

**Figure 129.17 *cont'd* (B)** Sagittal CT reconstruction views, (parasagittal each side and sagittal) show nearly 50% subluxation of C6 on C7 and bilateral facet dislocation. **(C)** MR sagittal inversion recovery image shows spinal cord compression and edema and extensive soft tissue edema in addition to the subluxation and stretching of anterior and posterior longitudinal ligaments.

views can show irregularity or overlap in some cases. If there is more extensive ligament injury and displacement, there may be rotational displacement that can simulate a unilateral facet dislocation on plain films. However, CT clearly demonstrates the location of fractures (Figure 129.21). Fractures of both pedicle and lamina result in separation of the articular mass from the vertebral body and potential instability. MRI can be helpful to determine the extent of ligamentous injury. This may help predict the risk of instability.[21]

The injuries described above are those seen in some of the more common patterns of cervical spine injury. It is important to remember that fractures commonly occur at more than one level. Identification of a fracture should not terminate the evaluation of the entire cervical spine. Spiral CT can be particularly helpful.

## Thoracic and Lumbar Spine

Along with more restricted movement in the thoracic and lumbar spine compared to the cervical region, there exist fewer patterns of fracture. Compression fractures and burst fractures have similar features to those described for

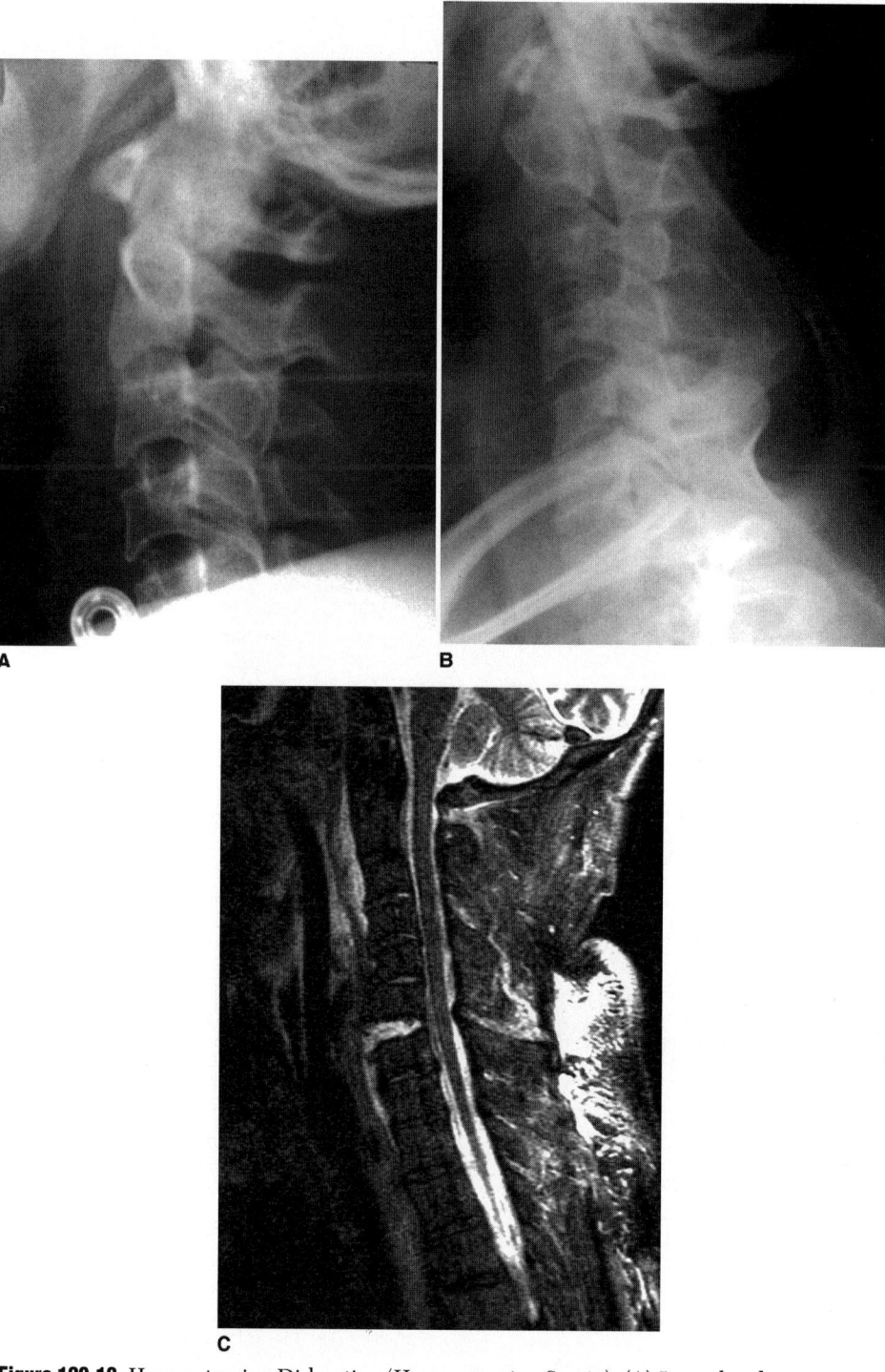

**Figure 129.18** Hyperextension Dislocation (Hyperextension Sprain). **(A)** Lateral and **(B)** swimmers views of this patient who had a central cord syndrome after a motor vehicle accident show straightening of the cervical spine and diffuse prevertebral swelling. **(C)** MR sagittal inversion recovery image of a different patient with hyperextension injury but no spinal cord injury shows disruption of the C6-7 disc space and anterior longitudinal ligament, with both prevertebral and dorsal edema.

the cervical spine. Prevertebral soft tissue swelling is not a very useful plain film finding below the cervical spine, but paraspinal soft tissue hematoma can be visible on AP views, especially in the thoracic spine. With compression fractures, there is ventral loss of height and buckling of the

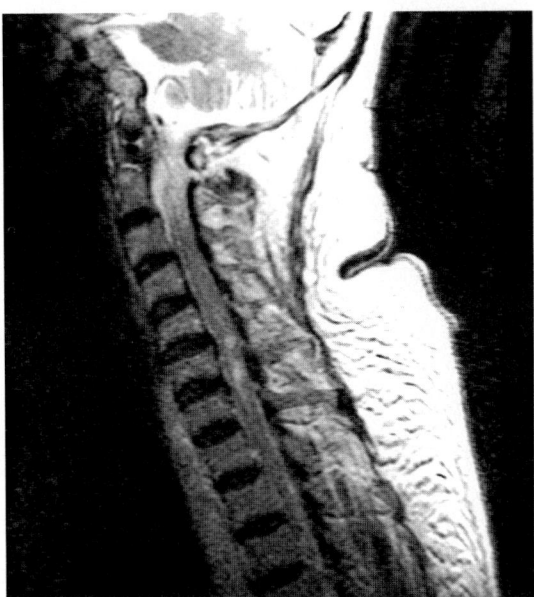

**Figure 129.19** Central Cord Injury from Taylor Mechanism. An elderly woman with relatively minor injury to the forehead and hyperextension injury suffered a central cord syndrome. MR sagittal T$_2$-weighted image shows spondylosis and spinal stenosis in the lower cervical spine and edema in the spinal cord.

superior end plate and ventral cortical margin (Figure 129.22). In more severe cases, some dorsal buckling of the vertebral body is observed. There is usually focal kyphotic angulation. Mild compression fractures are often more obvious on lateral radiographs than on CT. CT may show only subtle lucency along the ventral, superior margin of the vertebral body in mild fractures. If there is uncertainty about whether a fracture is acute or chronic, MRI or bone scan can be helpful. Edema will be seen in the marrow space on MRI in acute fractures; after a period of weeks to months, the marrow signal intensity returns to that similar to adjacent, normal marrow.

Burst fractures are usually visible on plain films, but CT can much more fully characterize the vertebral body fractures, degree of comminution and displacement, and posterior element fractures (Figure 129.23). Fractures of adjacent vertebra are common, so CT should include enough of the nearby spine to ensure that all fractures near the obvious injury have been detected. This is of obvious value in planning instrumentation. MRI yields additional information about the integrity (or loss thereof) of discs and major ligaments as well as spinal cord damage.

Chance-type injuries are characterized by dorsal distraction in combination with anterior flexion. The most common locations are around the thoracolumbar junction. The classic fracture described by Chance extends in a horizontal plane through a vertebral body into the pedicles (Figure 129.24).[11] These fractures are often more easily appreciated on lateral radiographs than on the axial images of CT. Since the fractures lie in the plane of imaging, axial images may be notable only for an absence of bone rather

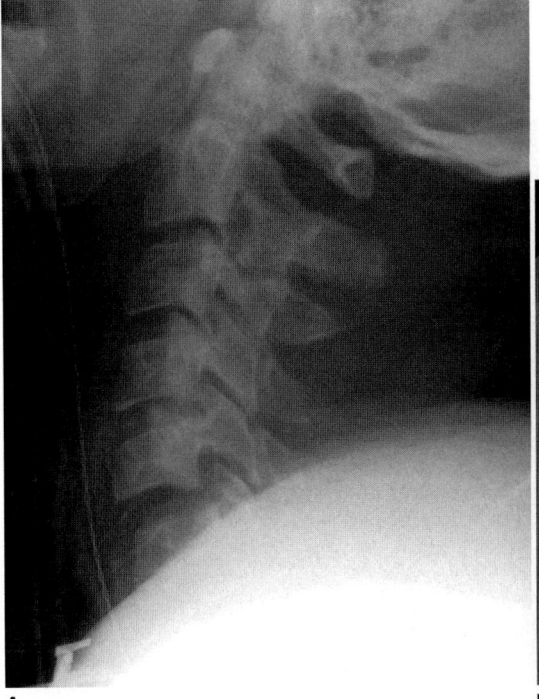

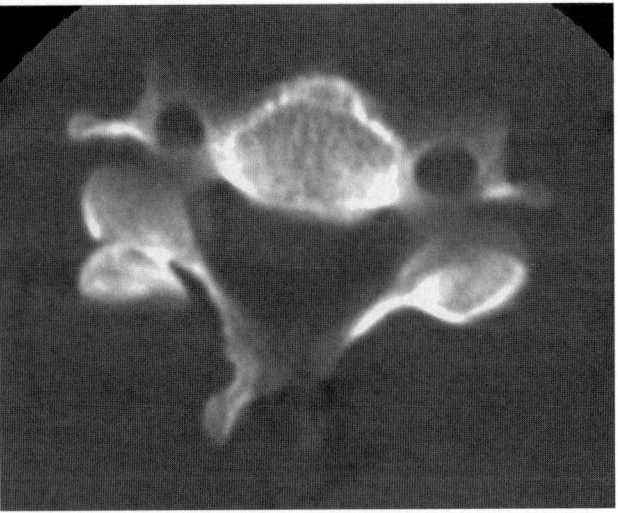

**A**          **B**

**Figure 129.20** Unilateral Facet Dislocation. **(A)** Lateral radiograph of this patient with quadriparesis after a motor vehicle accident shows ventral subluxation of C5 on C6. There is an oblique orientation of the spine above this level and a straight lateral configure below this level. Note the "bow-tie" shape of the articular processes above the level of dislocation. **(B)** CT demonstrates reversal of the normal relationship of the facets at C5-6 on the right side.

*Continued*

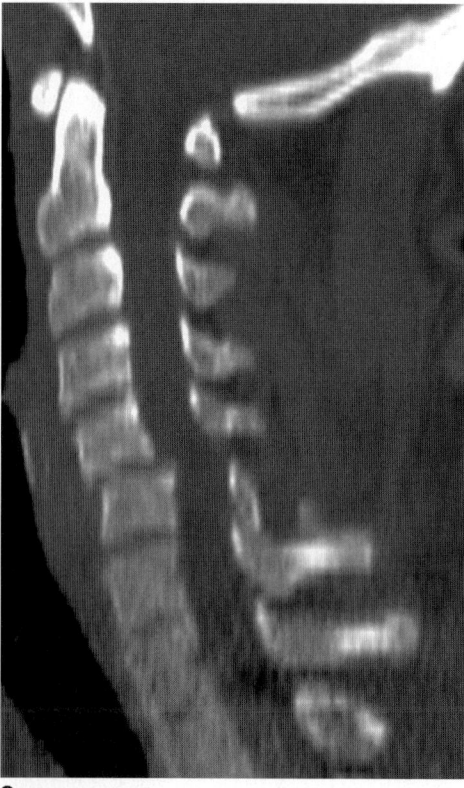

C

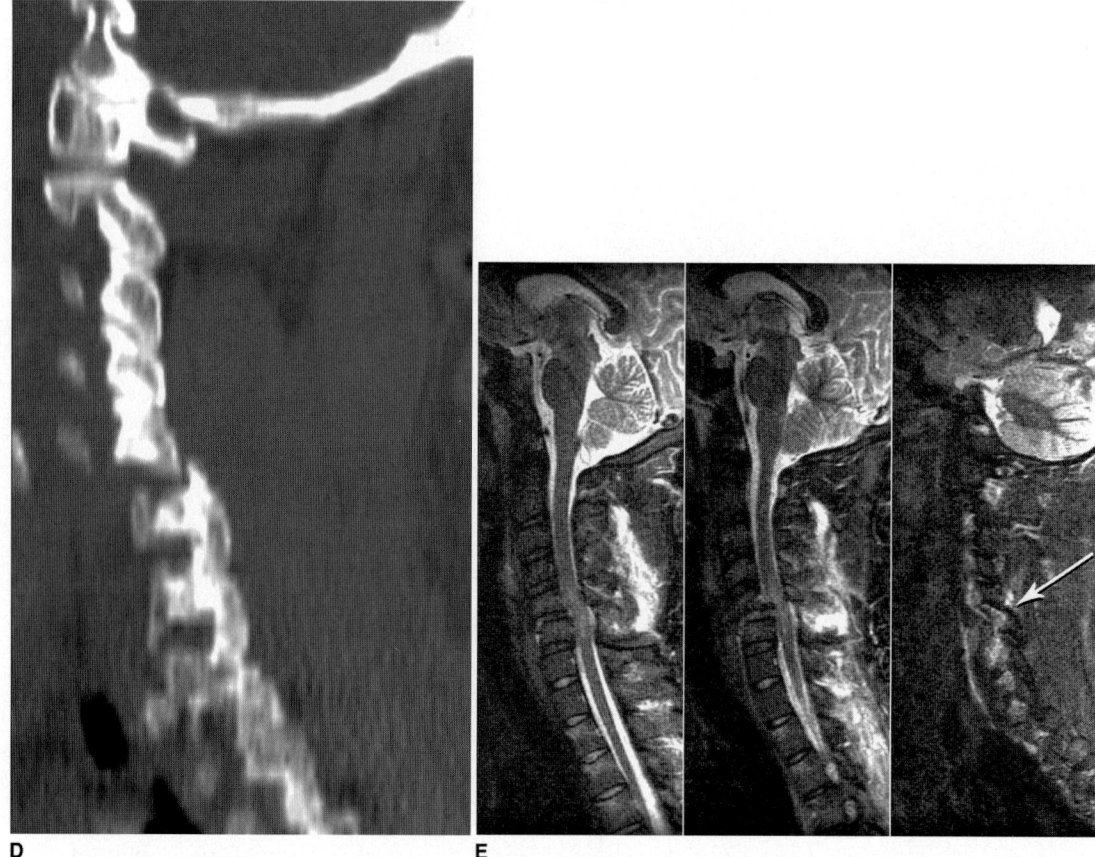

D                                  E

**Figure 129.20** *cont'd* (**C**) Sagittal CT reconstruction shows about 25% ventral subluxation of C5 on C6. A parasagittal (**D**) CT reconstruction through the facets on the right side clearly shows the dislocation. (**E**) The dislocation is also visible on right parasagittal MR inversion recovery image (*arrow*).

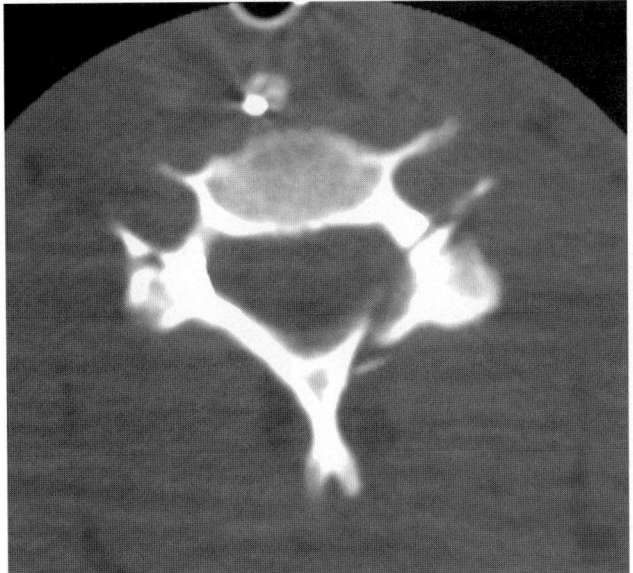

**Figure 129.21** Pedicolaminar Fractures. Axial CT of a patient who was in a motor vehicle accident shows fractures involving the pedicle and lamina on the patient's left side.

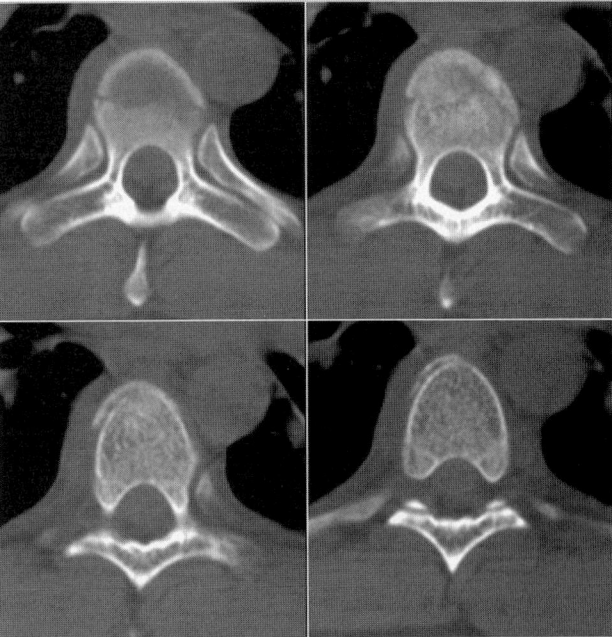

A

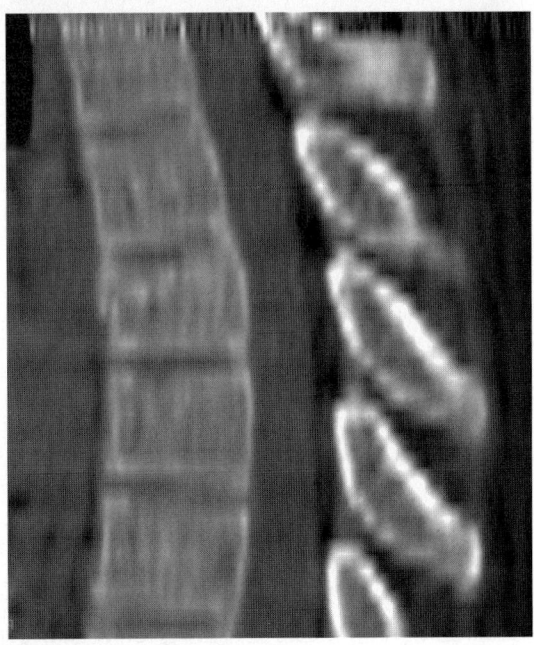

B

**Figure 129.22** Thoracic Compression Fracture. (**A**) Axial CT of T7 shows fractures only in the anterior body. (**B**) Sagittal reconstruction shows mild anterior loss of height.

than distinct fracture lines. Sagittal and coronal reconstruction images show the fractures on CT more clearly than the axial images. However, the category of Chance-type injuries has been broadened to include other injuries that result from a similar mechanism.[18,37] Thus, the horizontally oriented disruption can also occur through an intervertebral disc, and the plane of posterior distraction then typically extends through the facet joints. In any of these patterns, MRI demonstrates localized injury through the dorsal elements and soft tissues. In addition, a Chance injury should always suggest the possibility of associated abdominal injuries. Solid organ lacerations and perforations are present in up to half of patients with Chance-type injuries.

Fracture-dislocation of the thoracic or lumbar spine is the result of very severe injury mechanisms and carries a high risk of spinal cord injury. CT is especially helpful in such cases, and MRI is often also beneficial in evaluating the spinal cord (Figure 129.25). As shown in Figure 129.26, CT is also helpful in evaluating ligament avulsion.

## Nerve Root Injuries

Traction injuries can cause injury to the brachial plexus and/or avulsion of cervical nerve roots as they exit the spinal canal. MRI is especially helpful when such injuries are suspected. Imaging findings include absence of the nerve root in the foramen or lateral recess, a fluid collection (pseudomeningocele) in or lateral to the foramen, and displacement of the thecal sac to the opposite side. Myelography or CT can also demonstrate some of these findings (Figure 129.27). The imaging findings are likely to evolve over time, especially fluid collections.

## Penetrating Injuries

Plain films may be useful initially to assess the location of bullet fragments. Once the level of injury is determined from penetrating injury, CT is especially helpful to evaluate the precise nature of bone injuries and possible involvement of the spinal canal. After it is clear that there is no contraindication such as metal in the spinal canal, MRI can be used to visualize the spinal cord and possible hematomas (Figure 129.28).

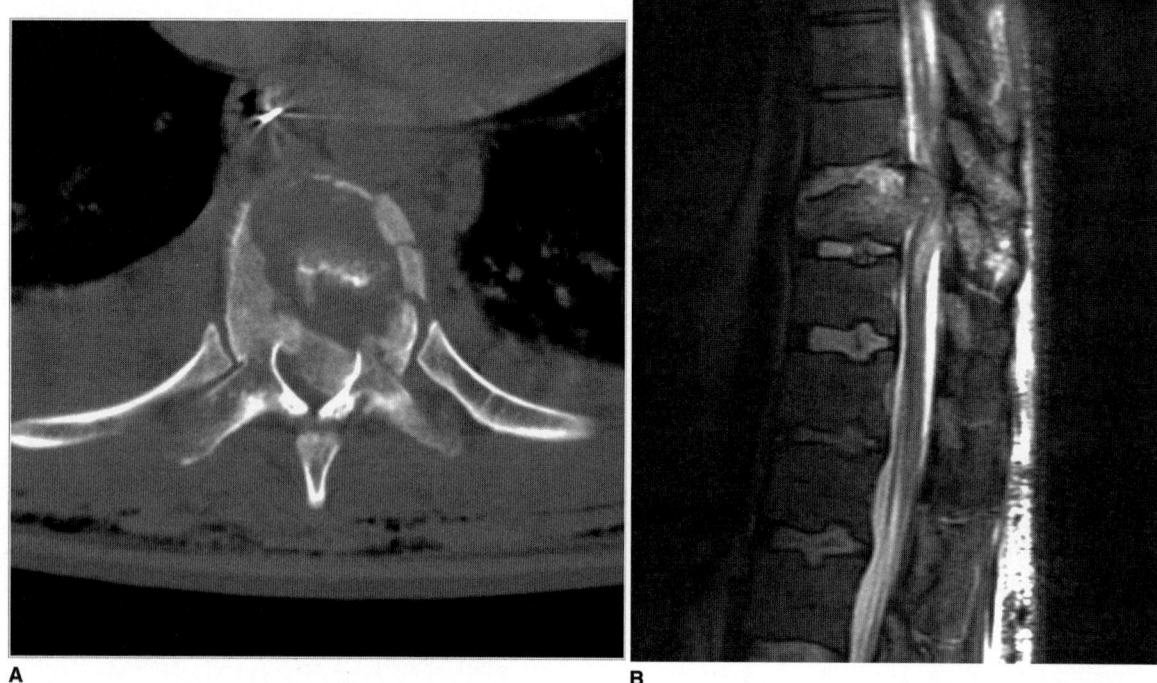

**A**                                                                    **B**

**Figure 129.23** T10 Burst Fracture. **(A)** CT of a paraplegic after motor vehicle accident shows burst fracture of T10, with severe narrowing of the spinal canal from a large bone fragment. **(B)** Subsequent MR sagittal inversion recovery image shows severe spinal cord compression and edema, with relatively little dorsal soft tissue edema. Note the alignment, without the kyphosis often accompanying compression fractures.

## Vascular Injuries

Vertebral artery injuries, ranging from intimal injury, dissection, and frank occlusion, are fairly common in cases of cervical spine injury, especially with fractures of the posterior elements that involve the foramen transversarium. Angiography remains the gold standard for evaluation of the blood vessels, but MRI, MRA, and CT can be of substantial help in many cases. Routine axial MRI images, for example, show lack of signal ("flow void") in normal arteries. The normal black appearance of the artery will be replaced by intermediate or high signal intensity when there is no flow. Slow blood flow in an artery may give a similar appearance. Magnetic resonance angiography (MRA) is a very useful tool for noninvasively evaluating normal and abnormal arteries in trauma patients. Axial MR images and axial source images from MRA may also demonstrate a flap in cases of dissection or blood in the false lumen (Figure 129.29).

## Spinal Cord Injury without Radiographic Abnormality

Spinal cord injury without radiographic abnormality (SCI-WORA) can occur from a variety of mechanisms that result in neurologic injury without fractures. The term dates from earlier reliance on radiographs; MRI nearly always demonstrates imaging abnormalities when neurologic deficits occur.[29] Postulated mechanisms include flexion, transient distraction, compression of the spinal cord, and ischemia.

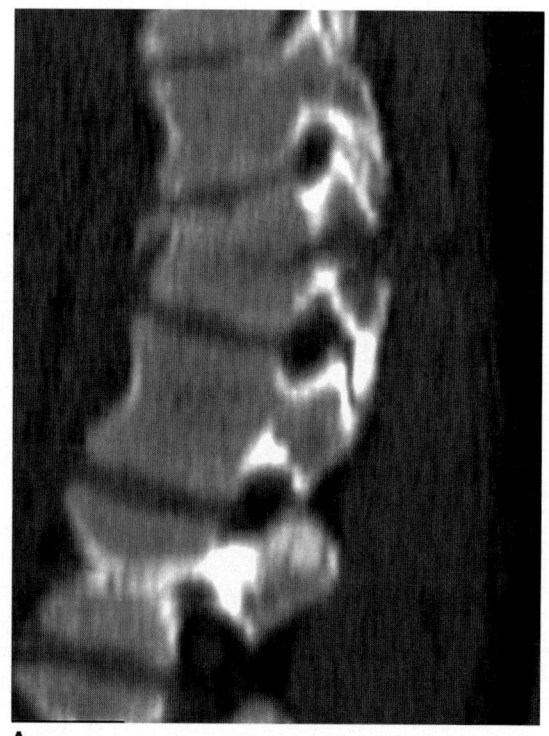

**A**

**Figure 129.24** Severe Flexion-Distraction Injury. **(A)** CT sagittal 2D reconstruction shows T11 ventral compression with dorsal distraction and fracture component through a pedicle.

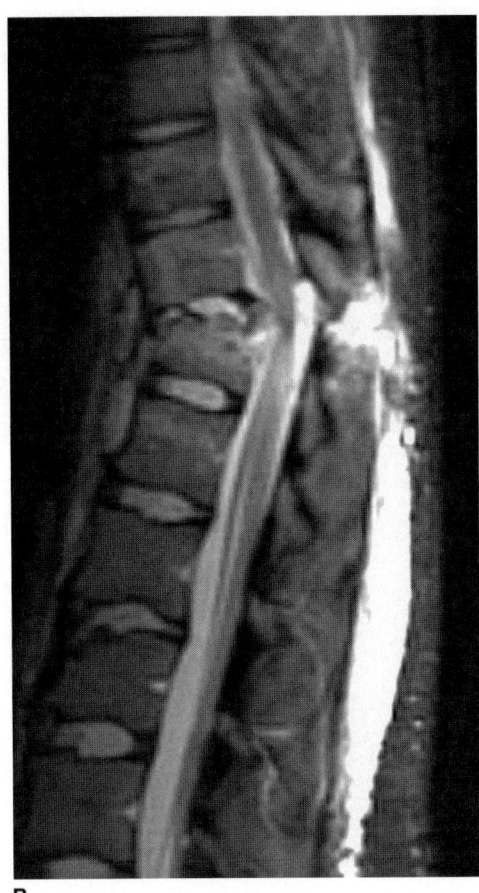

B

**Figure 129.24 *cont'd* (B)** MR sagittal fast inversion recovery image shows fractures, marrow edema within the T11 and T12 vertebral bodies, spinal cord compression, and focal dorsal soft tissue edema.

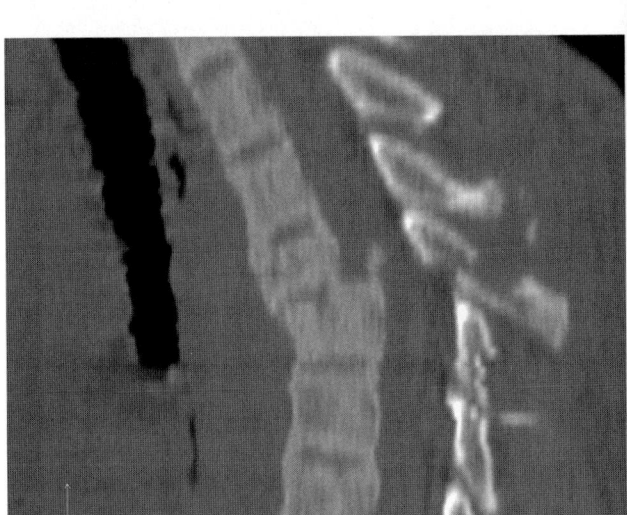

A

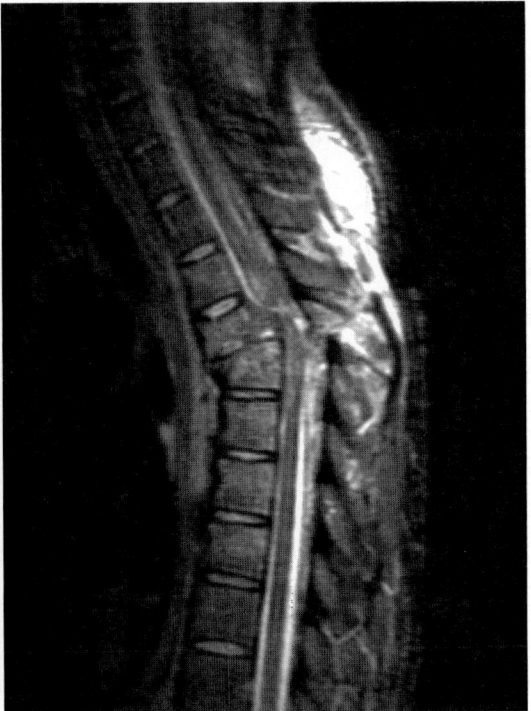

B

**Figure 129.25** Thoracic Fracture-Dislocation. Patient was paraplegic after motorcycle accident. **(A)** Sagittal CT reconstruction shows kyphosis, compression of both T4 and T5, bone fragment in the spinal canal, and posterior element fractures. **(B)** MR sagittal inversion recovery image shows the spinal cord compression.

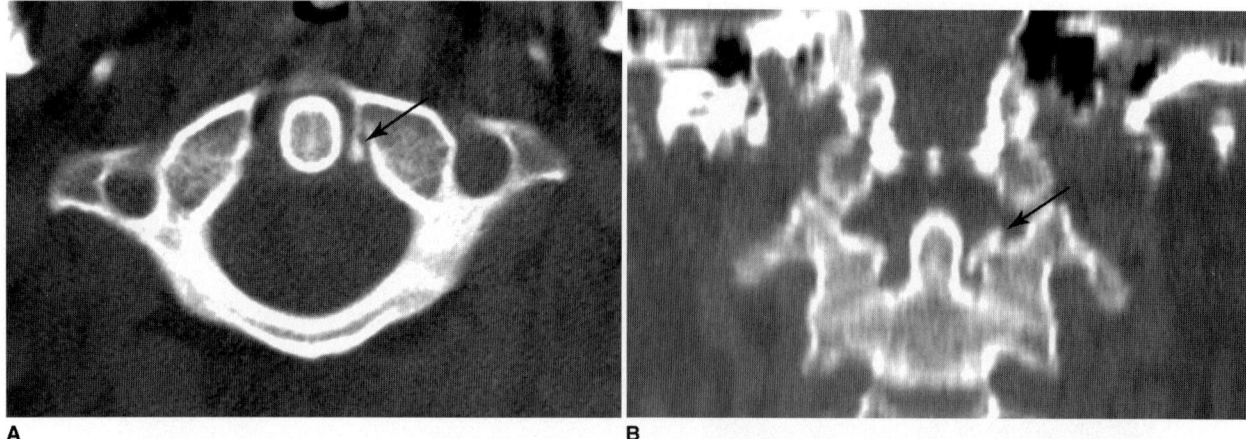

A     B

**Figure 129.26** Transverse Ligament Avulsion. Lateral radiograph demonstrated slight widening of the anterior atlantodental space in this patient after trauma. (**A**) CT shows an avulsion fracture at the site of insertion of the transverse ligament on the left side *(arrow)*. (**B**) Coronal CT reconstruction demonstrates the displaced bone fragment *(arrow)*.

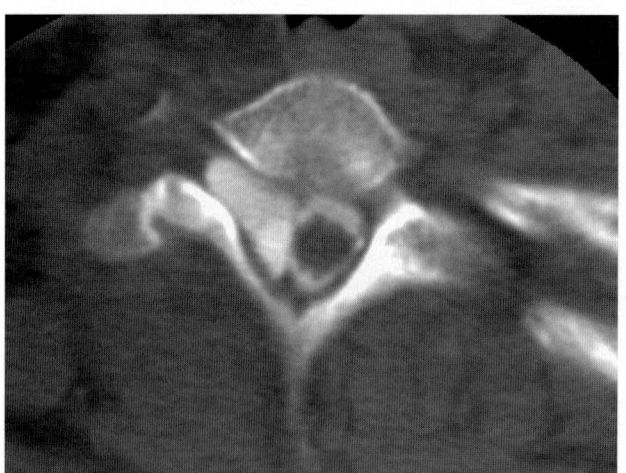

**Figure 129.27** Nerve Root Avulsion. Patient had right upper extremity weakness after a motor vehicle accident. MRI could not be obtained because of orthopedic external fixators. Axial CT after a myelogram demonstrates a collection of contrast material extending into the right neural foramen at the cervicothoracic junction and displacement of the thecal sac to the left.

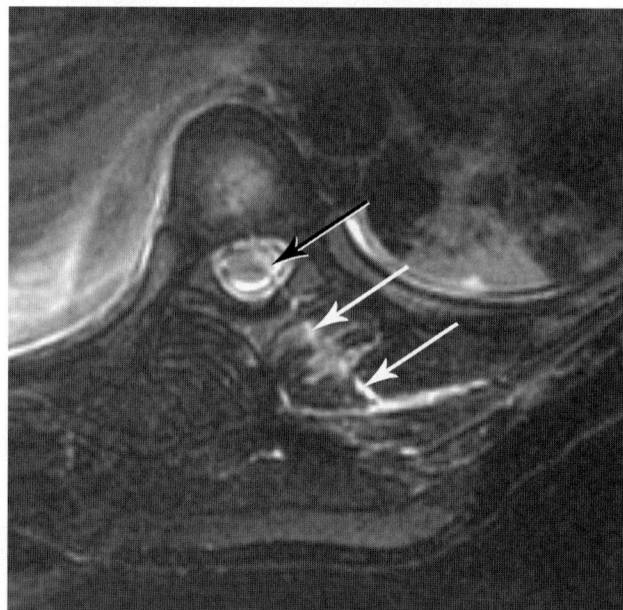

**Figure 129.28** Stab Injury to the Spine. A young adult was stabbed in the back and suffered loss of sensation in left lower extremity; motor function was intact. Axial MR $T_2$-weighted image with fat saturation demonstrates the path of the knife *(white arrows)* in the left lower thoracic spine into the spinal canal, with the knife injury visible in the anterior left side of the spinal cord *(black arrow)*.

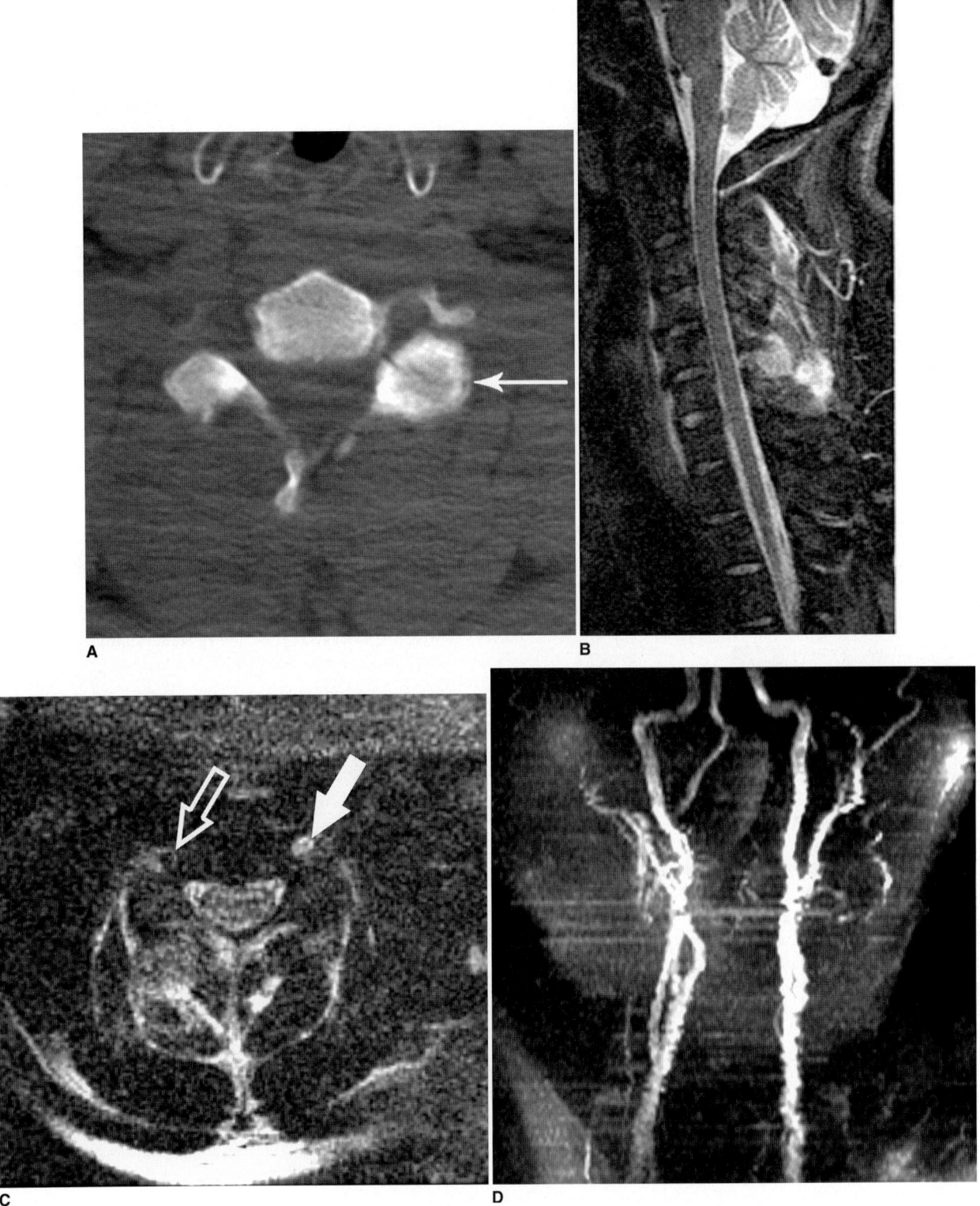

**Figure 129.29** Vertebral Artery Occlusion. The patient had persistent neck pain after a motor vehicle accident. (**A**) CT at the C5-6 level reveals a minimally displaced fracture through the lateral mass and articular processes on the left side *(arrow)*. MRI shows deep, interspinous injury at C5-6 on sagittal inversion recovery image (**B**), and an axial $T_2$-weighted image with fat saturation (**C**) shows normal flow void from the right vertebral artery *(open arrow)* and bright signal from the left *(solid arrow)*. (**D**) MRA of the same patient confirms flow in the right vertebral artery and none in the left vertebral artery.

# REFERENCES

1. Acheson MD, Livingston RR, Richardson ML, Stimac GK: High-resolution CT in the evaluation of cervical spine fractures: comparison with plain film examinations. *AJR Am J Roentgenol* 148:1179-1185, 1987.

2. Anderson LD, D'Alonzo RT: Fractures of the odontoid process of the axis. *J Bone Joint Surg Am* 56:1663-1673, 1974.

3. Benzel EC, Hart BL, Ball PA, et al: Fractures of the C-2 vertebral body. *J Neurosurg* 81:206-212, 1994.

4. Benzel EC, Hart BL, Ball PA, et al: Magnetic resonance imaging for the evaluation of patients with occult cervical spine injury. *J Neurosurg* 85:824-829, 1996.

5. Bettini N, Malaguti MC, Sinitni M, et al: Fractures of the occipital condyles: report of four cases and review of the literature. *Skeletal Radiol* 22:187-190, 1993.

6. Bohrer SP, Chen YM, Sayers DG: Cervical spine flexion patterns. *Skeletal Radiol* 19:521-525, 1990.

7. Borovich B, Peyser E, Gruskiewicz J: Acute central and intermediate cervical cord injury (case V). *Neurochirurgia* 21:77-84, 1978.

8. Braakman R, Vinken PJ: Unilateral facet interlocking in the lower cervical spine. *J Bone Joint Surg Br* 49:249-257, 1967.

9. Brashear HR Jr, Ventera GC, Preston ET. Fractures of the neural arch of the axis. *J Bone Joint Surg Am* 57:869-887, 1975.

10. Chakeres DW, Flickinger F, Bresnahan JC, et al: MR imaging of acute spinal cord trauma. *AJNR Am J Neuro Radiol* 8:5-10, 1987.

11. Chance CQ: Note on a type of flexion fracture of the spine. *Br J Radiol* 21:452-453, 1948.

12. Clayman DA, Sykes CH, Vines FS: Occipital condyle fractures: clinical presentation and radiologic detection. *AJNR Am J Neuro Radiol* 15:1309-1315, 1994.

13. Cornish BL: Traumatic spondylolisthesis of the axis. *J Bone Joint Surg Br* 50:31-43, 1968.

14. Dickman C, Mamourian A, Sonntag VK, Drayer BP: Magnetic resonance imaging of the transverse atlantal ligament for the evaluation of the atlantoaxial instability. *J Neurosurg* 75:221-227, 1991.

15. Edeiken-Monroe B, Wagner LK, Harris JH Jr: Hyperextension dislocation of the cervical spine. *AJR Am J Roentgenol* 146:803-808, 1986.

16. Effendi B, Roy D, Cornish B, et al: Fractures of the ring of the axis: a classification based on the analysis of 131 cases. *J Bone Joint Surg Br* 63:319-327, 1981.

17. Francis WR Jr, Fielding JW, Hawkins RJ, et al: Traumatic spondylolisthesis of the axis. *J Bone Joint Surg Br* 63:313-318, 1981.

18. Gertzbein SD, Court-Brown CM: Flexion-distraction injuries of the lumbar spine: Mechanisms of injury and classification. *Clin Orthop* 227:52-60, 1988.

19. Green JD, Harle TS, Harris JH Jr: Anterior subluxation of the cervical spine: Hyperflexion sprain. *AJNR Am J Neuro Radiol* 2:243-250, 1981.

20. Griffen MM, Frykberg ER, Kerwin AJ, et al: Radiographic clearance of blunt cervical spine injury: plain radiograph or computed tomography scan? *J Trauma* 55:222-227, 2003.

21. Halliday AL, Henderson BR, Hart BL, Benzel EC: The management of unilateral lateral mass/facet fractures of the subaxial cervical spine. *Spine* 22:2614-2621, 1997.

22. Hanson JA, Blackmore CC, Mann FA, Wilson AJ: Cervical spine injury: a clinical decision rule to identify high-risk patients for helical CT screening. *AJR Am J Roentgenol* 174:713-717; 2000.

23. Harris JH Jr, Burke JT, Ray RD, et al: Low (type III) odontoid fracture: a new radiologic sign. *Radiology* 153:353-356, 1984.

24. Harris JH Jr, Carson GC, Wagner LK: Radiologic diagnosis of traumatic occipitovertebral dissociation: 1. Normal occipitovertebral relationships on lateral radiographs of supine subjects. *AJR Am J Roentgenol* 162:881-886, 1994.

25. Harris JH Jr, Carson GC, Wagner LK, Kerr N: Radiologic diagnosis of traumatic occipitovertebral dissociation: 2. Comparison of three methods of detecting occipitovertebral relationships on lateral radiographs of supine subjects. *AJR Am J Roentgenol* 162:887-892, 1994.

26. Harris JH Jr, Yeakley JS: Radiographically subtle soft tissue injuries of the cervical spine. *Curr Probl Diagn Radiol* 18:161-190, 1989.

27. Harris JH Jr, Yeakley JW: Hyperextension-dislocation of the cervical spine. *J Bone Joint Surg Br* 74:567-570, 1992.

28. Lewis LM, Doeherty M, Ruoff BE, et al: Flexion-extension views in the evaluation of cervical-spine injuries. *Ann Emerg Med* 20:117-121, 1991.

29. Matsumura A, Meguro K, Tsurushima H, et al: Magnetic resonance imaging of SCI without radiologic abnormality. *Surg Neurol* 33:281-283, 1990.

30. Mirvis SE, Geisler FH, Jelinek JJ, et al: Acute cervical spine trauma: evaluation of 1.5T MR imaging. *Radiology* 166:807-816, 1988.

31. Nunez DB, Zuluaga A, Fuentes-Bernardo DA, et al: Cervical spine trauma: how much more do we learn by routinely using helical CT? *Radiographics* 16:1307-1318, 1996.

32. Orrison WW, Benzel EC, Willis BK, et al: Magnetic resonance imaging evaluation of acute spine trauma. *Emerg Radiol* 2:120-128, 1995.

33. Powers B, Miller MD, Kramer RS, et al: Traumatic anterior atlanto-occipital dislocation. *Neurosurgery* 4:12-17, 1979.

34. Rizzolo SJ, Piazza MR, Cotler JM, et al: Intervertebral disk injury complicating cervical spine trauma. *Spine* 16:S187-S189, 1991.

35. Scher AT: Anterior cervical subluxation: an unstable position. *AJR Am J Roentgenol* 133:275-280, 1979.

36. Schneider RD, Kahn EA: Chronic neurological sequelae of acute trauma to the spine and spinal cord: part 1. The significance of the acute-flexion or "teardrop" fracture-dislocation of the cervical spine. *J Bone Joint Surg Am* 38:985-997, 1956.

37. Smith WS, Kaufer H: Patterns and mechanisms of lumbar injuries associated with lap seat belts. *J Bone Joint Surg Am* 51:239-254, 1969.

38. Spence KF, Decker S, Sell KW: Bursting atlantal fracture associated with rupture of the transverse ligament. *J Bone Joint Surg Am* 52:542-549, 1970.

39. Suss RA, Zimmerman RD, Leeds NE. Pseudospread of the atlas: false sign of Jefferson fracture in young children. *AJR Am J Roentgenol* 140:1079-1082, 1983.

40. Taylor AR: The mechanism of injury to the spinal cord in the neck without damage to the vertebral column. *J Bone Joint Surg Br* 33:543-547, 1951.

41. Woodring JH, Lee C: Limitations of cervical radiography in the evaluation of acute cervical trauma. *J Trauma* 34:32-39, 1993.
42. Woodring JH, Lee C: The role and limitations of computed tomographic scanning in the evaluation of cervical trauma. *J Trauma* 33:698-708, 1992.
43. Young JWR, Resnick CS, DeCandido P, Mirvis SE: The laminar space in the diagnosis of rotational flexion injuries of the cervical spine. *AJR Am J Roentgenol* 152:103-107, 1989.

# CHAPTER 130

# Degenerative Disease and Infection: Role of Imaging

## Michael T. Modic

The impact of imaging on the management of disorders of the spine is both critical and confounding. The accurate depiction of morphologic abnormalities in conjunction with the history and physical examination is critical to therapeutic decision-making. However, the significance of imaging findings is strongly influenced by the wide range of normal variations, a high frequency of asymptomatic morphologic abnormalities, and the natural history of the disease in question.

## Degenerative Disease

The purpose of a diagnostic test is twofold: first, to provide reliable information about a patient's condition, and second, to influence a physician's plan for management.[136] A necessary component that connects these two purposes is accurate natural history data. Only when this is understood can the results of a diagnostic test be integrated into therapeutic thinking. The relevance of an imaging finding requires knowledge relative to the spectrum of change, prevalence, significance, and behavior with time. This information is critical to developing effective case management guidelines that are based on well-controlled studies rather than history or impression. Before one can assess the value of an imaging study, some type of perspective in which to place the findings is needed. Unfortunately, no good natural history data, only assumptions are usually available. If these assumptions are not accurate, one could be performing tests too soon or too late, both of which could have dramatic counterproductive effects on patient care and costs.

Intervention in a disease condition requires that it be more beneficial, safer, and/or cost-effective, compared with the untreated natural history. In the case of degenerative disease, most episodes of clinical symptoms are self-limited. For patients with low back pain (LBP), with or without radiculopathy, the natural history is not clearly understood. Withholding imaging in these circumstances may not seriously impact patient outcome in most patients and, in fact, may improve conservative management by avoiding the detection of confounding altered morphology.

Because back pain is typically a recurrent problem, physicians and patients should benefit from information related to patient group stratification, prognosis for recovery from acute episodes, and likelihood of recurrence.[28] Traditional practice suggests that there is no role for imaging in patients with back pain unless there are associated signs and symptoms suggestive of a potentially treatable condition related to trauma, instability, infection, or malignancy.

LBP with radiculopathy, on the other hand, is a less diverse group relative to etiology. The symptoms usually suggest nerve root compression. Multiple authors[40,47,80] suggest that an imaging study is indicated for the evaluation of a patient with back pain and associated sciatica when: (1) true radicular symptoms are present; (2) there is evidence of nerve root irritation on physical examination (i.e., positive straight leg raise test); and (3) the patient has failed "conservative management" of 4 to 6 weeks duration. Earlier imaging is considered appropriate if clinical features raise concern regarding malignant or infectious pathology or if neurologic findings worsen during observation. These recommendations are based on several studies of the successful nonoperative treatment of sciatica.[*] Thus, imaging is recommended only for the remaining minority of patients with persistent signs and symptoms who are felt to be surgical candidates or in whom diagnostic uncertainty remains.

Others have suggested the use of diagnostic imaging earlier in the course of a patient's symptoms supported by the following evidence: (1) patients with herniated discs treated surgically have better short-term outcomes than patients treated with conservative management[143]; (2) the earlier the surgery the better the outcome[138]; and (3) surgery is cost-effective compared with conservative management.[85] However, the potential reduction in morbidity from early intervention requires the identification of accurate prognostic indicators, be they clinical or imaging based. Certainly more than morphology is at play. As has been suggested by Postacchini,[113] it seems likely that two needs require respect: (1) protracted conservative treatment may lengthen the time off work and reduce the chances of successful surgical treatment, and (2) a need to avoid surgery in patients with a herniated disc that may become asymptomatic or even disappear within a few months of onset. Thus, the possible benefits of imaging for degenerative diseases of the spine, other than as a presurgical tool, have never been carefully documented and quantified. The cost-benefit ratio of early imaging in patients with radiculopathy needs to be addressed.

Predicting which patients will benefit from imaging is a complicated and controversial subject. Its use as a preintervention planning tool is critical, but its employment for diagnostic information per se is less well accepted and the subject of much debate. Nevertheless, if imaging could be employed to prospectively determine which patients will not do well with surgery or other types of therapy, it would be of great value. Conversely, its use to identify patients undergoing prolonged conservative management who require more aggressive therapy (e.g., surgery) might be equally beneficial. This would save the cost of lost work, medical expenses, and personal discomfort.

---

*References 15,20,23,33,38,57,109,126,144.

Clearly, there is little consensus, either within or among specialties, on the use of diagnostic tests for patients with back pain.[29] The diagnostic evaluation depends heavily on the individual physician, their specialty, and patient socioeconomics in addition to the patient's symptoms.[1,29]

Vertebral osteomyelitis, on the other hand, is a condition with much more dire consequences. Withholding imaging in these cases may prove catastrophic as early and accurate diagnosis has a profound impact on timely management. These two processes illustrate the conundrum of when and what imaging test to employ.

What follows is an effort to describe the advantages and limitations of the most commonly employed imaging tests for the evaluation of the spine, integrated with what is known of the natural history of these disorders and the known confounding morphologic variations.

## Imaging Considerations

The major benefit of imaging is to depict the presence or absence of anatomic derangement and, in the latter case, its impact on adjacent structures. The contrast sensitivity and multiplanar imaging capability of proton magnetic resonance (MR) places the modality in a position to provide a unique noninvasive means of imaging the intervertebral disc, adjacent osseous structures, and associated soft tissues. From an anatomic perspective, it is important to be able to demonstrate the osseous, fluid, and soft tissue interfaces within the three traditional compartments; intramedullary, extramedullary-intradural, and the extradural spaces.

Unlike computed tomography (CT) and conventional radiography, which are dependent on information related to electron density, proton MR signals are influenced by the T1 and T2 relaxation time, proton density, and motion (both macro and micro) to provide greater tissue contrast. Thus, its role may go beyond gross anatomic appraisal to actual tissue characterization of pathology and biochemical change. There are almost limitless potential combinations of pulse sequence parameters, imaging planes, and postprocessing techniques available, which can be used to highlight different aspects of the diskovertebral complex and adjacent spaces. These include, but are not limited to, surface coil technology, cardiac gating, gradient refocusing, paramagnetic contrast agents, saturation pulses, gradient echo volume imaging, TURBO (fast) $T_2$-weighted spin echo, fat suppression, magnetization transfer, STIR, and diffusion techniques. The use of contrast agents is important for the improved depiction of reactive, inflammatory or neoplastic change. Special sequences for the evaluation of the marrow space, 3D data sets and the study of physiologic parameters, such as flow, can also be employed.

Most would agree that the basic examination should include orthogonal imaging, usually sagittal and axial, with both $T_1$- and $T_2$-weighted contrast. Using this approach, the anatomy of the intervertebral disc, spinal nerves, dural sac, and adjacent structures can be clearly depicted. In patients who are postoperative or when there is a suspicion of malignancy or infection, a postcontrast sequence is usually indicated.

## Altered Morphology

The description of altered morphology requires a common set of terms in order to standardize communication. Recently, a multidisciplinary committee endorsed by the North American Spine Society (NASS), American Society of Spine Radiology (ASSR), American Society of Neuroradiology (ASNR), American Academy of Neurology (AAN), Congress of Neurological Surgeons (CNS), and American Association of Orthopaedic Surgeons (AAOS)[99] has proposed a series of definitions based on anatomy and pathology. These are used herein. It must be clearly understood that these terms are descriptive only, and in and of themselves, independent of the test. It cannot be over-emphasized that the following terms do not imply knowledge of etiology, symptoms, prognosis, or need for treatment.

A disc is characterized as degenerated when it exhibits real or apparent desiccation, fibrosis, narrowing of the disc space, bulging, fissuring or mucinous degeneration of the annulus, osteophytes of the vertebral apophyses, and end plate/adjacent marrow changes (Figure 130.1).

In addition to gross morphologic changes related to degeneration, T2W MR is capable of detecting changes in the nucleus pulposis and annulus fibrosus based on a loss of signal intensity. This was initially thought to be secondary to the known changes of hydration that occur with degeneration within the intervertebral disc. However, correlation is not straightforward, as differences in signal intensity appear to be somewhat exaggerated for the degree of water loss noted with degeneration (e.g., ~15%). At this time, the role that specific biochemical changes (e.g., proteoglycan ratios and aggregating complexes) play in the changes of signal intensity is not well understood. In fact, it may not be the total quantity of water, but the state the water is in. Preliminary work at the Cleveland Clinic suggests that there is a positive correlation between the observed attenuation on magnetization transfer contrast images and the percent glycosaminoglycans (GAG) dry weight. This suggests an increase in the amount of bound water with an increase in the amount of GAG. Likewise, sodium images suggest that the signal intensity in the disc on T2 tracks the concentration and regions of highest concentration of GAG. Thus, it seems likely that the health and status of the proteoglycans determine the signal intensity by their effect on the relaxation times.

In the case of severely degenerated disc, where the overall signal intensity is markedly decreased, there may be linear areas of high signal intensity on $T_2$-weighted spin echo images that are thought to represent free fluid within cracks or fissures of the degenerated complex. T1 and gradient echo images are not as sensitive to the signal-intensity changes noted on more $T_2$-weighted images within the disc.

Conventional theory suggests that degeneration and aging are very similar processes, albeit at different rates. It seems likely that all three components of the diskovertebral complex (the annulus and ligaments, the nucleus pulposus, and the cartilaginous end plate and adjacent marrow) can be implicated as well as impacted upon by the process of degeneration.

It has been hypothesized that a normal anatomy and signal intensity of the intervertebral disc implies a normal or normally aging disc, and decreased signal intensity implies a radial tear and degeneration. The contention is that annular disruption is the critical factor in degeneration and when a

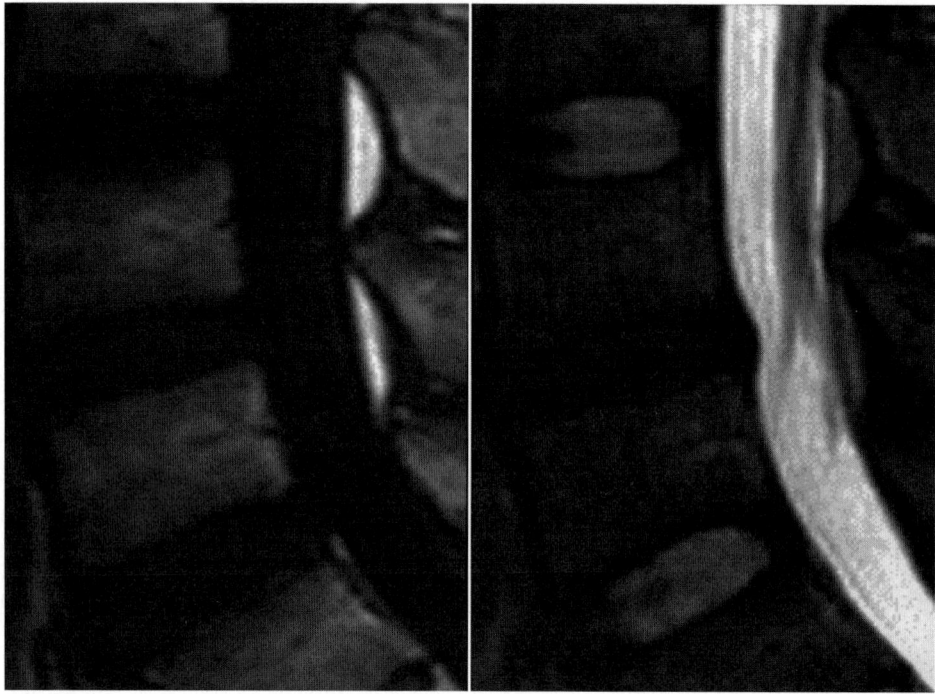

**Figure 130.1** Sagittal T1 and T2 images of the L4-5 disc level. Note the decreased disc height and loss of signal intensity on the $T_2$-weighted images when compared to the L3-4 disc above or L5-S1 disc below.

radial tear develops in the annulus, there is shrinkage and disorganization of the fibrous cartilage of the nucleus pulposus and replacement of the disc by dense fibrous tissue and cystic spaces.[59,148,149] While it has certainly been verified that anular disruption is a sequelae of degeneration, and certainly often associated, its role as the causal agent of disc degeneration has certainly not been proven. To imply that radial tears are anything more than a manifestation of advanced degeneration is unwarranted. This is of pertinence in light of the continuing controversy surrounding the concept of internal disc disruption. Other studies have indicated a genetic predisposition to degenerative disc disease, suggesting a resulting biochemical abnormality within the disc itself, perhaps affecting the GAG or collagen. Still others have suggested that the cartilaginous end plate plays such a critical role in the health of the disc that changes in this area have a secondary effect in facilitating discal degeneration. There is no unifying theory regarding the cause of disc degeneration. It is likely that degeneration and aging are multifactorial processes that encompass a wide spectrum of changes and sequelae of which the radial tear is but one. Disc degeneration may be explained primarily by genetic influences and complex unpredictable interactions of unidentified factors. Previously studied environmental factors that have widely been suspected of accelerating disc degeneration include job type, twisting, sitting, driving, activity level, and smoking.[14]

A host of other degenerative changes can be depicted with magnetic resonance imaging (MRI). The vacuum phenomenon within a degenerative disc is represented on spin echo images as areas of signal void, and may not be seen with the same sensitivity as on plain films or CT. Gradient echo sequences, however, demonstrate the vac-

uum phenomenon better than conventional spin echo sequences, plain radiographs, and CT[16,55] (Figure 130.2). This is due to the magnetic susceptibility effects caused by the intradiscal gas collection and the nature of the gradient echo technique. Magnetic susceptibility effects have been shown to exaggerate the interface between air, blood, or bone in other tissues. At these boundaries, the susceptibility effect manifests itself as a localized static field inhomogeneity, which can have a spatial extent ranging over many pixels. Spin echo and gradient echo sequences differ in their ability to control this inhomogeneity-produced artifact, which dephases the MR signal intensity locally. The gradient echo sequences lack the spin refocusing pulse of spin echo sequences and spin dephasing leads to focal MR signal loss in the vicinity of the susceptibility interface. The longer the echo time (TE) and the gradient echo sequence, the greater is the dephasing or apparent signal loss. While the presence of gas within the disc is usually suggestive of degenerative disease rather than an infectious process, spinal infection may rarely be accompanied by intradiscal or intraosseous gas.[17]

A gas density cleft within a transverse separation of the vertebral body, appearing in extension and disappearing in flexion, is characteristic of a vacuum phenomenon within a region of ischemic vertebral collapse. The region of intraosseous gas may be accompanied by high signal intensity on T2, which is presumably related to fluid within the cleft and can change with position and time. More rarely this phenomenon has been identified with vertebral body neoplasms such as multiple myeloma.[50,73,84,102,120]

Hyperintense intervertebral discs are not an infrequent finding on $T_1$-weighted MRIs of the spine and it has been suggested that the relatively "bright" intervertebral disc

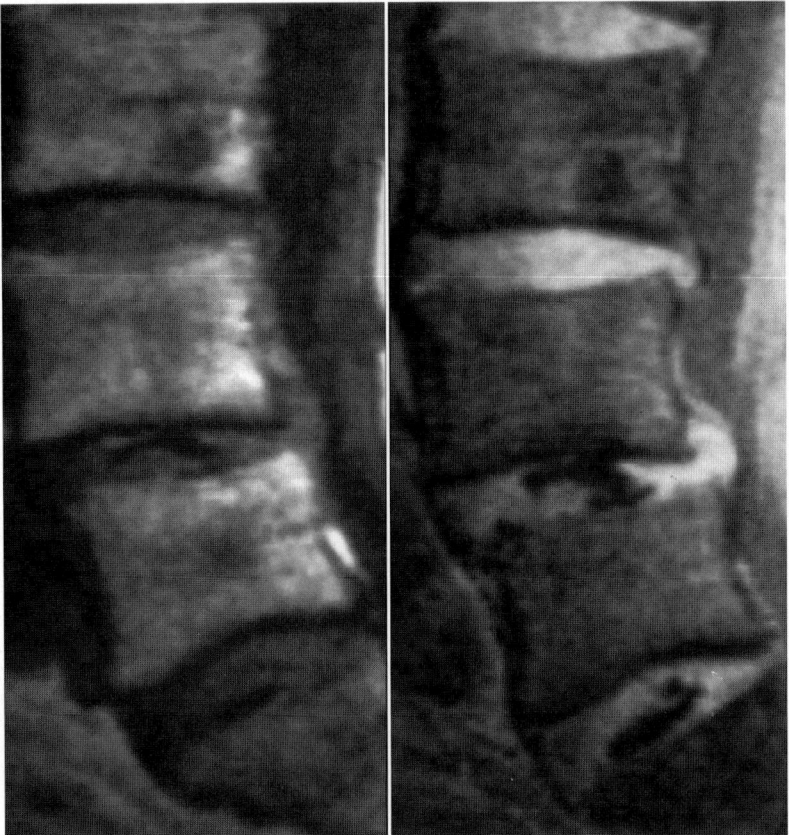

**Figure 130.2** Sagittal $T_2$-weighted and gradient echo images of the lower lumbar spine. On the T1 sagittal image there is a linear area of decreased signal in the L4-5 disc. On the gradient echo images this decreased signal is more obvious and an additional area of decreased signal is now appreciated in the L5-S1 disc. These changes are secondary to vacuum phenomena. These are more conspicuous on the GE image secondary to susceptibility effects.

may reflect diffuse abnormality and loss of normal signal in the marrow of the adjacent vertebral bodies.[27] In the child, there is a greater amount of hematopoietic marrow. This results in a lower vertebral body signal intensity versus the disc. As one ages, the lipid to hematopoietic ratio increases and there is a greater difference in signal intensity between body and disc.

Calcification has usually been described on MRI as a region of decreased or absent signal. The loss of signal has been attributed to a low mobile proton density as well as, in the case of gradient echo imaging, its sensitivity to the heterogeneous magnetic susceptibility found in calcified tissue. Several causes for calcification in the intervertebral disc have been proposed: trauma, infection, congenital malformation, metabolic disorder and degenerative change. Ossification of the embryonic disc cartilage has also been observed. Associations have been reported between calcification of the nucleus pulposus and patent ductus arteriosus, spina bifida, congenital cataracts, mongolism, ventricular septal defects, pulmonary stenosis, renal hypoplasia, adrenal hyperplasia, and fatty metamorphosis of the liver. Calcification and ossification has also been noted in the supporting ligaments.[22,61,75,103]

There is, however, variability of the signal intensity of calcium on various sequences and the type of calcification

and concentration are probably important factors. Multiple examples of a hyperintense signal on $T_1$-weighted spin echo images in areas that contain calcification on CT have been reported in the literature.[58] These hyperintensities have been attributed to the paramagnetic effects of methemoglobin, melanin, and trace elements as well as to the T1 shortening effects of lipids/cholesterol, proteins, and laminar necrosis associated with infarction and calcification. Focal or diffuse areas of hyperintensity on $T_1$-weighted spin echo sequences may also be encountered in the intervertebral disc. A retrospective study of 27 patients who had anecdotally been noted to have one or more hyperintense discs on $T_1$-weighted images demonstrated that there was calcification on plain film and/or CT that correlated with the hyperintense MR signal intensity at levels 26 to 31.[10] The converse was not necessarily true. At some levels, calcification on plain films/CT corresponded to isointense or decreased signal on $T_1$-weighted images. In a subsequent analysis, there was a significant association between signal on $T_1$-weighted images and the degree of calcification on plain films suggesting that heavily calcified discs resulted in an isointense or hypointense signal intensity. This data corresponds nicely to a report that showed particulate calcium could reduce T1 relaxation times by a surface relaxation mechanism. Calcium particles with greater surface areas showed greater T1 relaxation. Reduced proton density and reduced T2 tended to diminish signal intensity, but reduced T1 increased the signal intensity. For concentrations of calcium particulate of up to 30% by weight, the signal intensity on standard T1-weighted images increases but then subsequently decreases. These regions of high signal intensity on T1 are unaffected by fat suppression suggesting that it is a T1 shortening effect rather than the presence of lipid (Figure 130.3).

Hyperintensities have also been noted within intervertebral discs that are affected by fat suppression techniques. These are presumably related to areas of ossification

with the formation of a lipid marrow within the ossified disc space. These also appear calcified on conventional studies.

The term *bulge* is used to describe a generalized extension, greater than 50% of the circumference of the disc tissues to a short distance (<3mm) beyond the edges of the apophyses. A bulge is not a herniation.

Separation between or avulsion of annular fibers from their vertebral body insertions or breaks through fibers that extend radially, transversely, or concentrically through layers of the anular lamellae are referred to as *annular tears/fissures*. On MRI, these changes can occasionally be seen on $T_2$-weighted images as high signal intensity within the outer annulus-PLL complex (Figure 130.4). These

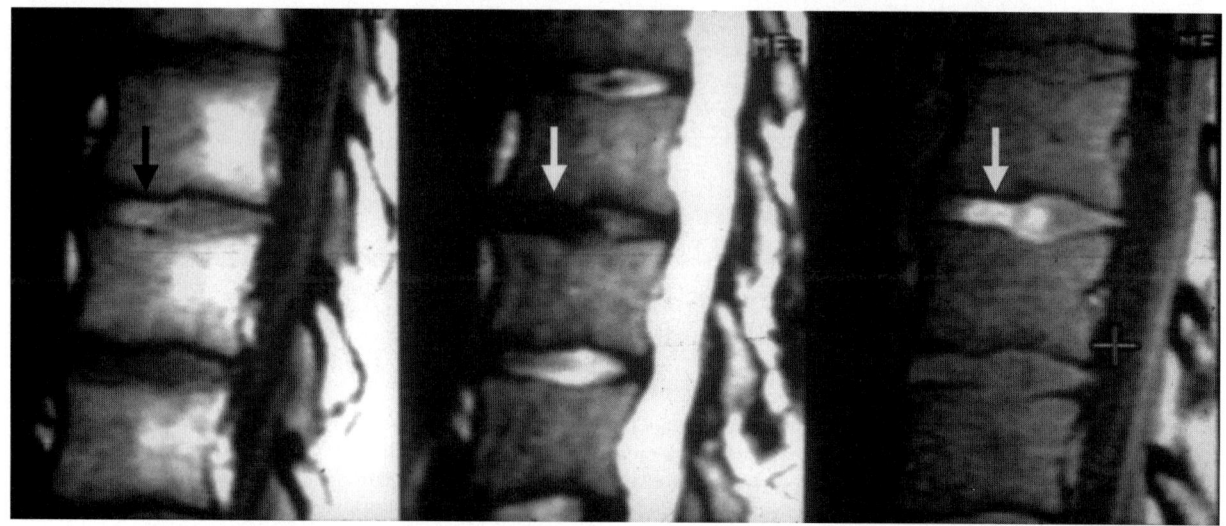

**Figure 130.3** Sagittal, $T_1$-, $T_2$-, and fat suppressed $T_1$-weighted images of the upper lumbar spine. On the $T_1$-weighted images, there is a focus of high signal *(black arrow)*. On the $T_2$-weighted image this same area has a decreased signal *(white arrow)*. On the fat suppressed image the region maintains it high signal while areas which contain fat have decreased *(white arrow)*. The high signal on T1, decreased on T2 and unaffected by fat suppression are indicative of calcification producing T1 shortening.

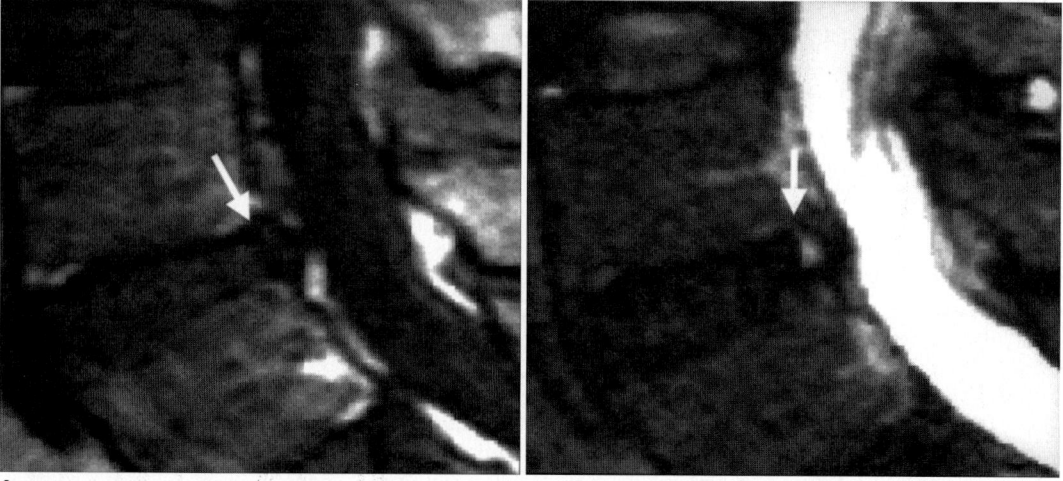

A

**Figure 130.4 (A)** Sagittal T1 and T2 images of the L4-5 disc level. Note the decreased disc height and loss of signal intensity on the $T_2$-weighted images when compared to the L3-4 disc above. There is also a small region of increased signal on the $T_2$-weighted images in the dorsal annulus/posterior longitudinal ligament, which represents an annular tear.

*Continued*

regions may enhance following the administration of paramagnetic contrast, an effect thought to be secondary to reactive reparative tissue (Figure 130.5).

The term *intraannular displacement* is used to describe the peripheral displacement of central, predominantly nuclear tissue into a fissure of the annulus. This is distinguished from disc herniation in that it does not extend beyond the disc space itself.

*Herniations* are localized displacement of disc material beyond the limits of the intervertebral disc space in any direction (Figure 130.6). The disc space is defined in the rostral-caudal direction by the vertebral body end plates and peripherally by the outer edges of the vertebral ring apophyses, exclusive of any osteophytes. If the herniation is less than 25% of the disc circumference, it is referred to as *focal* (Figure 130.7), and if between 25% and 50%, it is referred to as *broad-based* (Figure 130.8).

*Protrusions* are herniations where the greatest distance in any plane between the edges of disc material beyond the disc space is less than the distance between

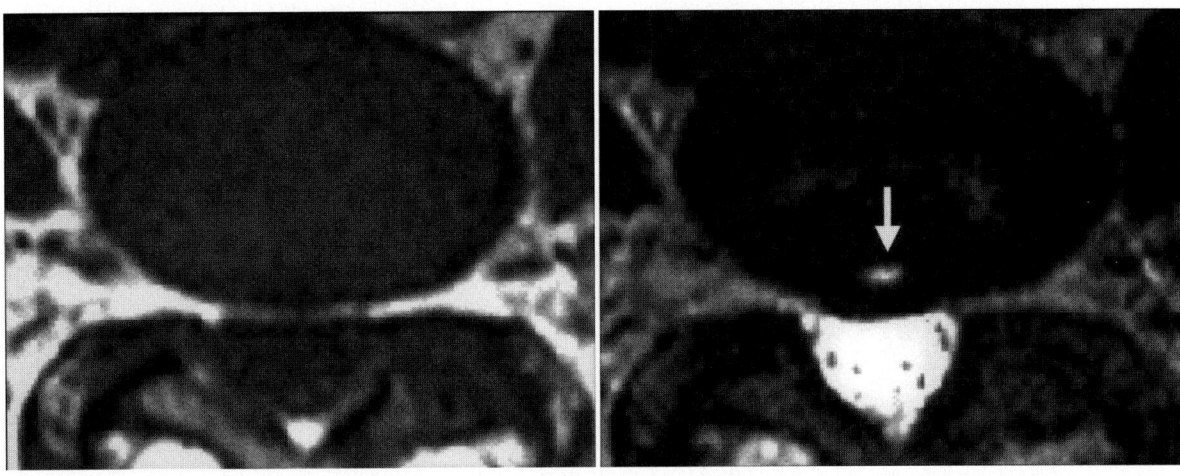

**Figure 130.4 *cont'd*** **(B)** Axial $T_1$- and $T_2$-weighted images through the L4-5 disc. Note the high signal intensity in the posterior margin of the disc on the $T_2$-weighted images indicative of an annular tear.

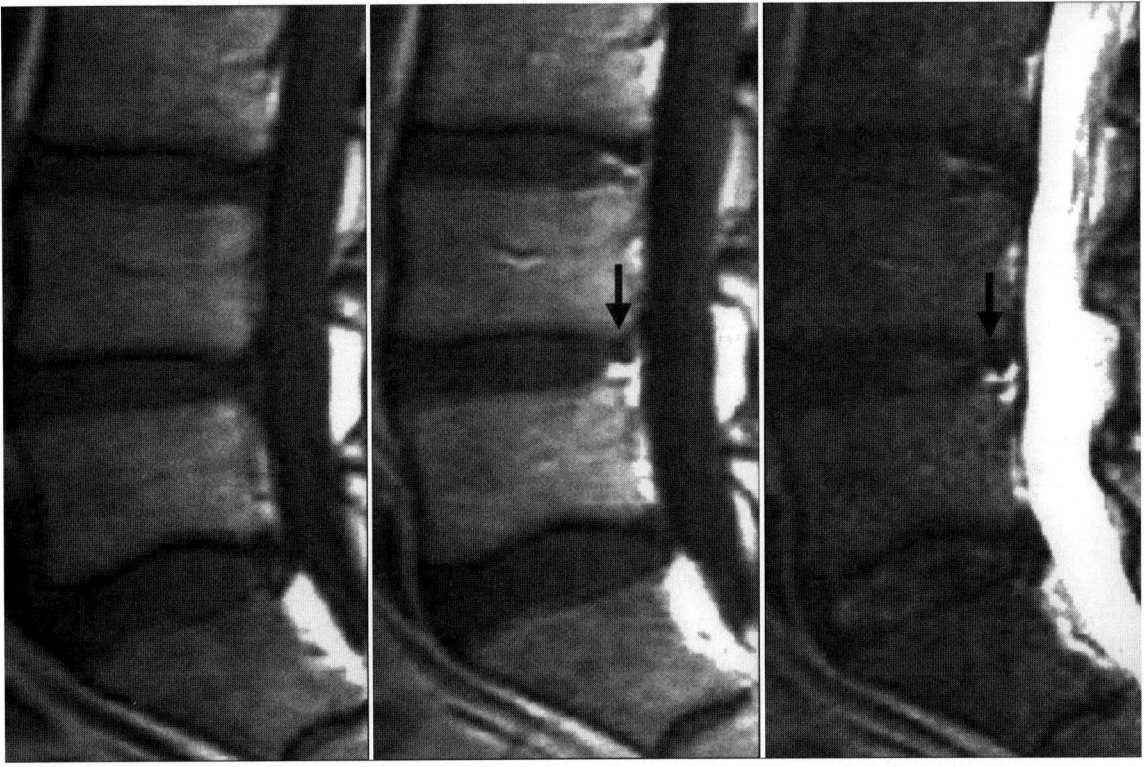

**Figure 130.5** **(A)** Sagittal $T_1$-, $T_1$-postcontrast and $T_2$-weighted images of the lower lumbar spine demonstrating an annular tear of the L4-5 disc.

*Continued*

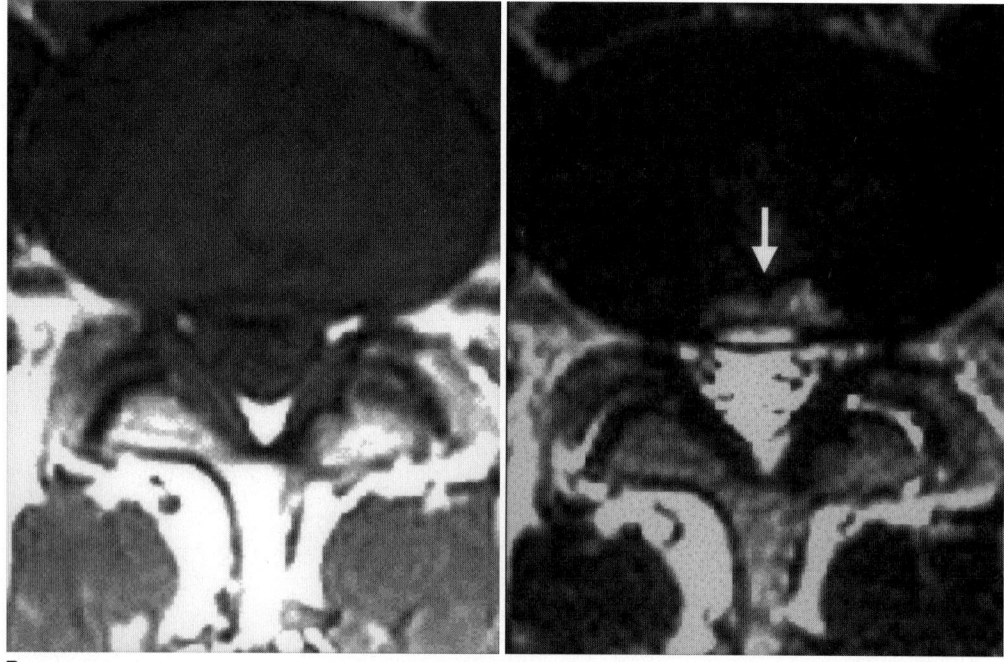

**B**

**Figure 130.5 *cont'd*** (**B**) Axial T$_1$-and T$_2$-weighted images of the L4-5 disc. The sagittal images the T$_1$-weighted demonstrates a mild posterior bulge of the L4-5 disc. The posterior margin enhances following contrast administration *(black arrow)*. This same region demonstrates a high signal on the T$_2$-weighted image *(black arrow)*. On the axial images (**B**) one can again appreciate the mild bulge and high signal *(white arrow)* on the T$_2$-weighted image.

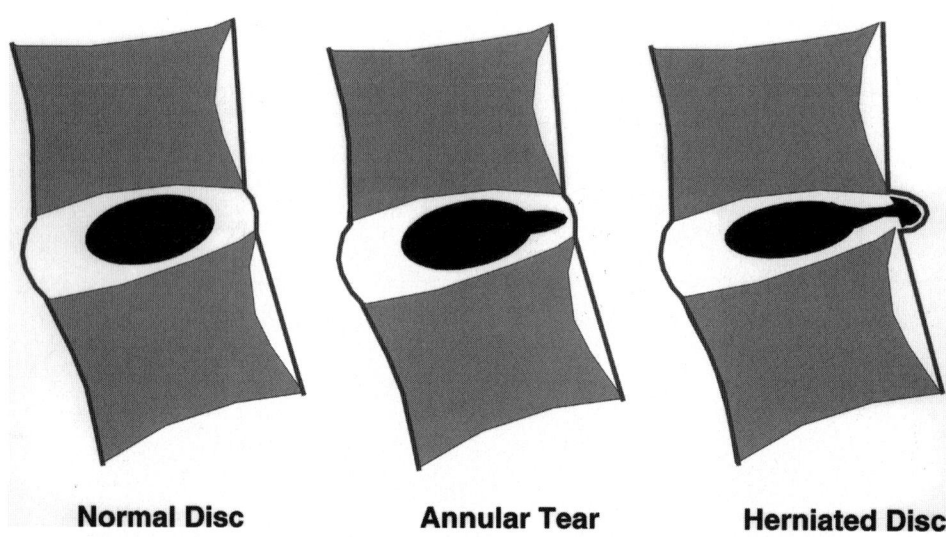

**Normal Disc          Annular Tear          Herniated Disc**

**Figure 130.6** Diagrammatic contrast of a normal disc, one with an annular tear and a herniation.

the edges of the base in the same plane (Figures 130.9 and 130.10).

*Extrusions* are herniations where in at least one plane, any one distance between the edges of the disc material beyond the disc space is greater than the distance between the edges of the base in the same plane (Figures 130.9 and 130.11), or when no continuity exists between the disc material beyond the disc space and that within the disc space. In this latter situation, it is referred to as a *seques-*

*tration* where the displaced material has lost completely any continuity with the parent disc (Figures 130.12 and 130.13). The extrusion is referred to as *migrated* if it has displaced from the site of extrusion, regardless of whether it is sequestrated. The signal intensity of the extruded portion may be increased or decreased on T$_2$-weighted images. There may be associated curvilinear areas of decreased signal intensity on the T$_2$-weighted images, which are related to portions of the annulus and posterior

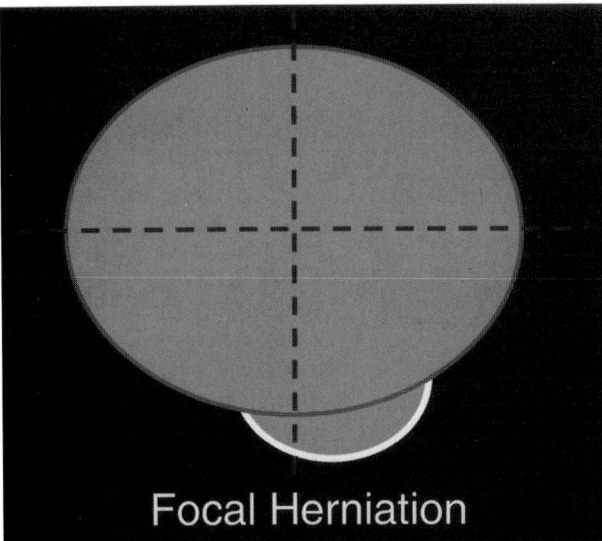

**Figure 130.7** Focal disc herniation, less than 25% of the disc margin.

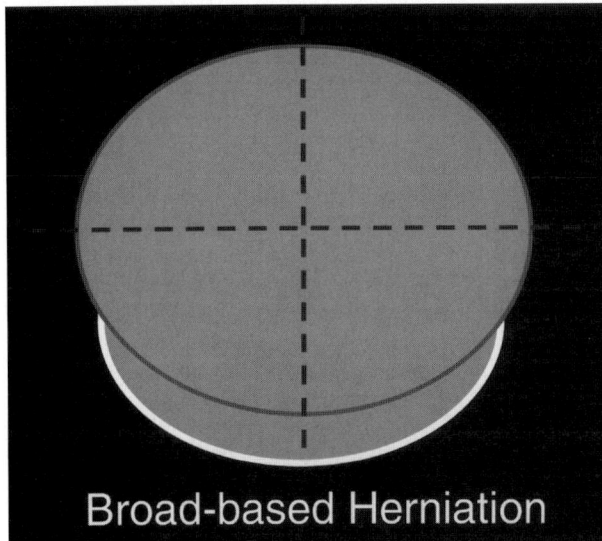

**Figure 130.8** Broad-based herniation, greater than 25% of the disc margin.

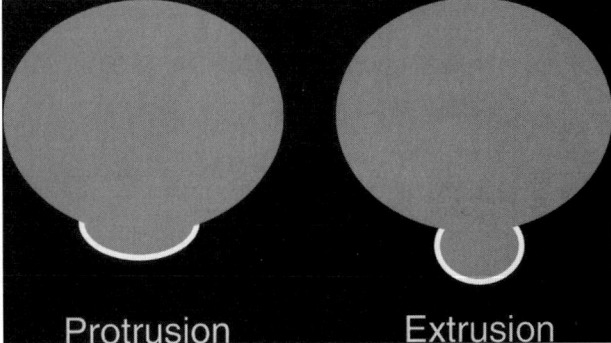

**Figure 130.9** Diagrammatic representation of the difference between a protrusion and extrusion in the sagittal plane. Note that the base of the protrusion is broader than the extent of the disc herniation beyond the margins of the disc. The extrusion on the other hand shows a greater extension beyond the disc margins that the width of the base.

longitudinal ligament. All disc herniations, whether small or large, can be associated with enhancement and as will be discussed later, this enhancement may constitute a large portion of the extradural mass. Sequestered fragments can lie ventral to the posterior longitudinal ligament, especially if they have migrated behind the vertebral bodies where the posterior longitudinal ligament is not in direct opposition, dorsal to the ligament, and even rarely intradural. Nevertheless, there is almost invariably penetration through the posterior longitudinal ligament; either dorsal, where it is fused with the annulus, or rostrally or caudally, where it fuses with the vertebral body margin.

In the majority of patients where sequestered fragments migrate behind the vertebral body, the sequestration usually lateralizes, with disc material pushed across the midline and the leading edge smoothly capped. It has been postulated that this shape is imposed by a midline septum in the ventral epidural space. This space is largest in the lower lumbar region and is delineated dorsally by the posterior longitudinal ligament and laterally attached membranes and ventrally by the vertebral body. It is divided into two compartments by a sagittally aligned septum.

Sequestered fragments within the lateral recess and the neural foramen have been shown to produce eroded cortical bone and expansion of those spaces, and thus, should be considered in the differential diagnosis of a mass arising and expanding the neural foramen and lateral recess. Although uncommon, sequestered fragments may also migrate dorsally in relationship to the thecal sac, and rarely intradural. Intradural disc herniation is rare, with only 52 cases reported. It is most frequent in the lower lumbar spine and the incidence varies between 0.04% and 0.33%. The mechanism is thought to be the development of chronic inflammation leading to adhesions between the dura mater and posterior longitudinal ligament. As the herniated disc penetrates, the ligament extends through the dura instead of pushing it away. Other possible causes are congenital connections between the ligament and the dura or previous surgery.

The characterization of a disc herniation is not always clear-cut and it may appear as a protrusion in one plane and an extrusion in another. If there is displacement away from the disc space in any plane, it should be referred to as an extrusion. *Containment* refers to the integrity of the outer anulus covering the disc herniation. One may view the continuum of herniated disc disease as starting with annular disruption, proceeding on to small focal herniation that is not broken completely through the annulus-ligamentus complex to frank herniation (extrusion), which has dissected through the annulus and posterior ligamentus complex completely. These may show variable degrees of containment, and a line of decreased signal intensity has been reported around sequestered fragments and large extruded discs where there has clearly been disruption of the annulus and ligament. This is thought to be secondary to annular and ligamentus fibers, which are carried away with the disc herniation. The annulus fibrosus and posterior longitudinal ligament are so intertwined at the level of

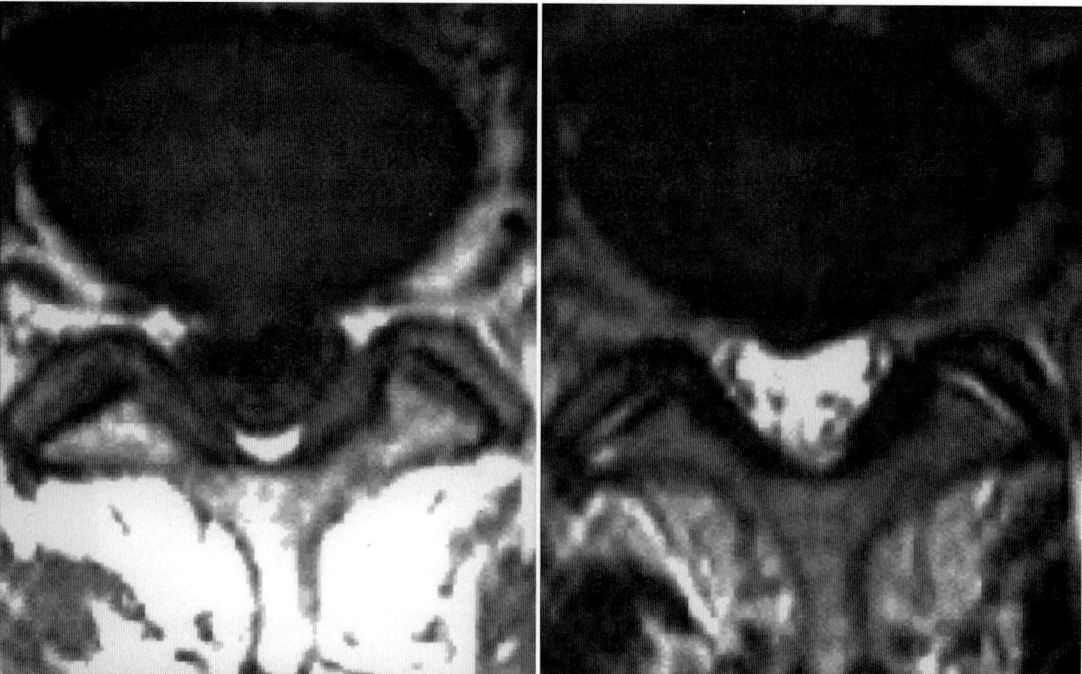

**Figure 130.10** Axial $T_1$-and $T_2$-weighted images of the L4-5 disc. There is a disc protrusion. Note that the base is broader than the dorsal extent of the herniation.

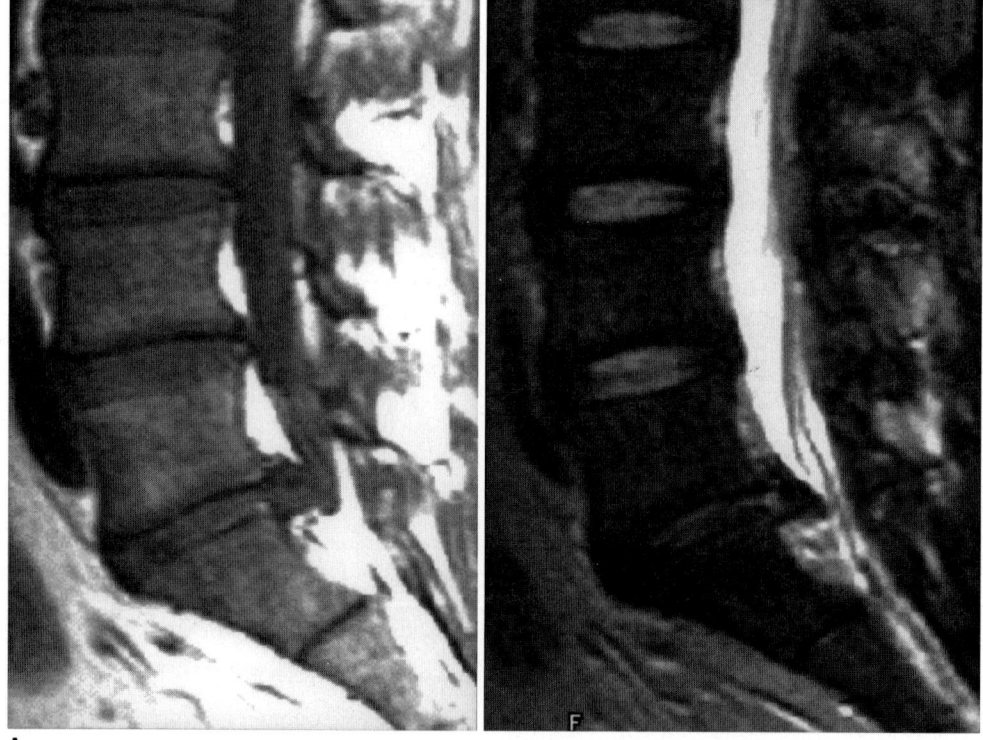

A

**Figure 130.11** Sagittal (**A**) and axial (**B**) $T_1$-and $T_2$-weighted images of a disc extrusion of the L5-S1 disc. Note while broad-based, the dorsal extent of the extrusion is at least as great as the length of the base.

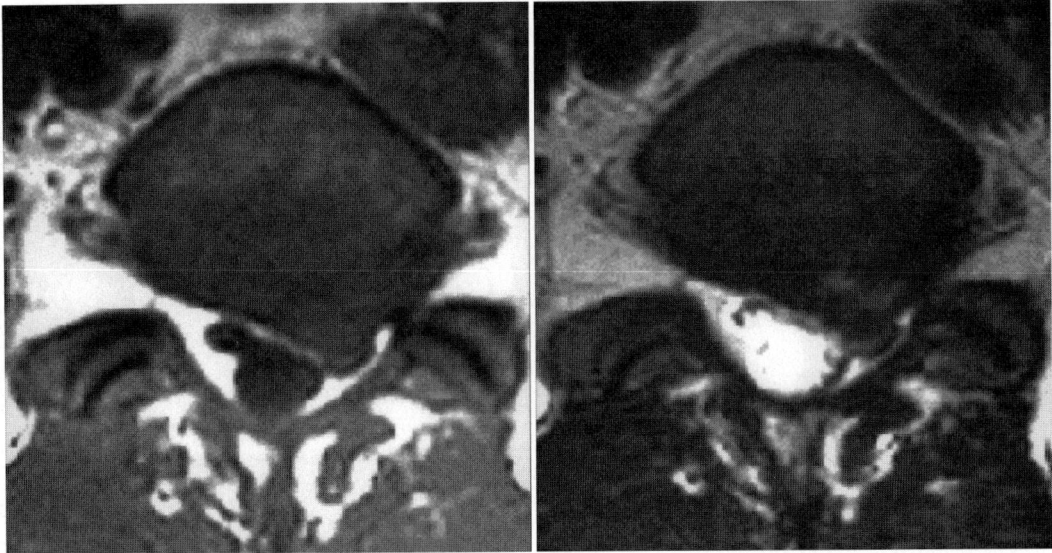

B

**Figure 130.11** *cont'd*

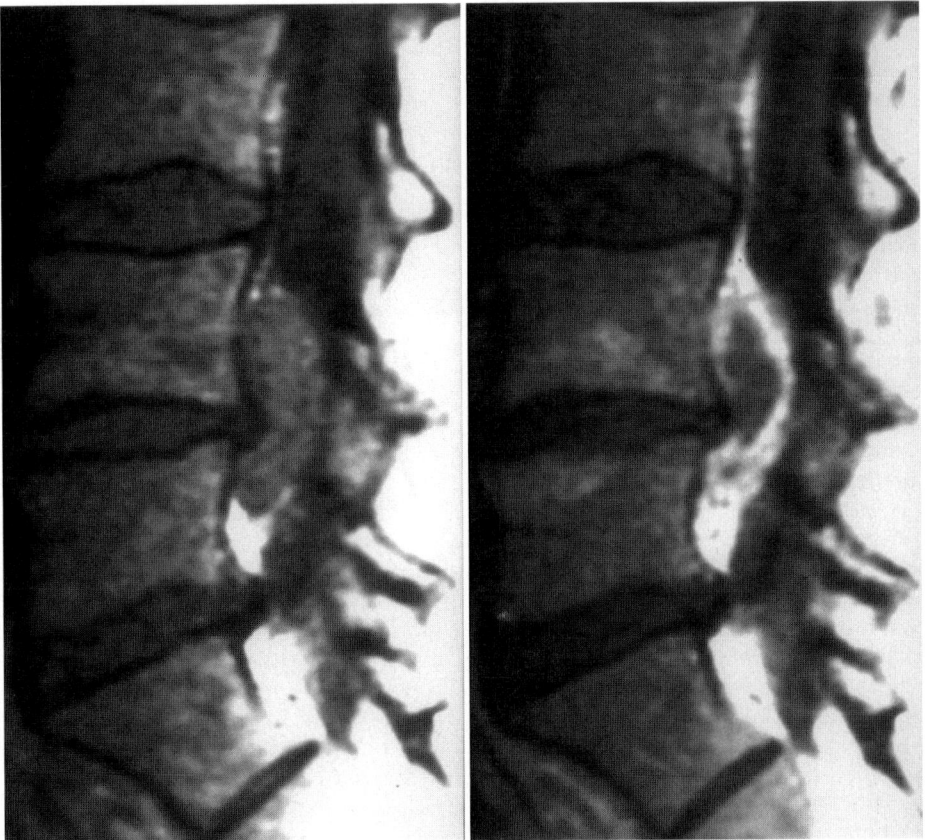

**Figure 130.12** Sagittal $T_1$-weighted precontrasted and postcontrasted images of the lower lumbar spine. Note the large migrated sequestrated disc fragment from the L4-5 level, which has migrated superiorly behind the body of L4. Note that a significant portion of the disc herniation enhances.

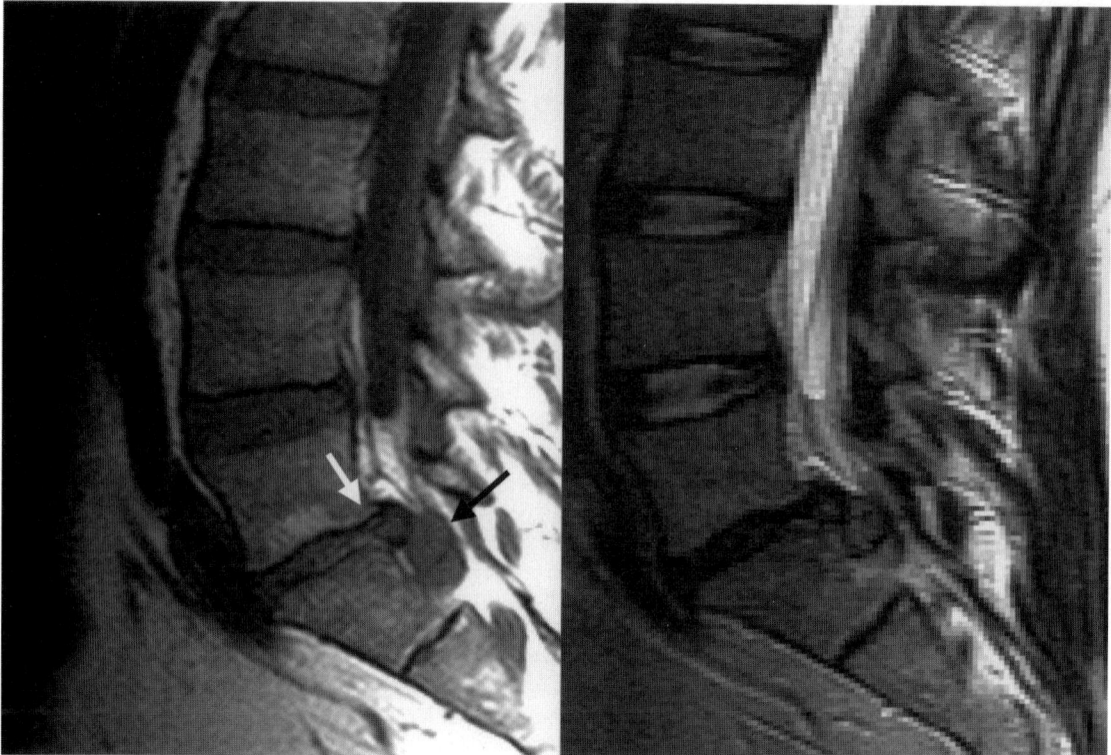

**Figure 130.13** Sagittal $T_1$-and $T_2$-weighted images of the lower lumbar spine demonstrating an extruded and sequestrated disc herniation at L5-S1. There are two portions of this disc herniation. First, an extrusion that is still attached to the disc of origin *(white arrow)* and second, a free fragment that has migrated caudally behind the body of S1 *(black arrow)*.

the disc, that a distinction between the two structures may be impossible or, for that matter, irrelevant. Technical limitations of CT and MRI usually preclude the distinction of a contained from an uncontained disc herniation.

In the transverse plane, the disc abnormality is usually described as *central, right,* or *left central;* and *subarticular, foraminal,* or *extraforaminal (far lateral).* In the sagittal plane, the terms *discal, infrapedicular, suprapedicular,* and *pedicular* are most commonly employed.

While consistent terminology is important for communication, it is not at all clear whether or not these categories of descriptive findings are clinically relevant. Although it has been proposed that it is critical to differentiate between various degrees of herniation, the reality of the situation is that disc herniation most likely represents a spectrum or continuum rather than discrete entities with specific clinical relationships.

The relationship among the vertebral body, end plate, and disc has been studied by using both the degenerated and chymopapain-treated discs as models.[3,39,86,100] Signal intensity changes in vertebral body marrow adjacent to the end plates of degenerative discs are a common observation on MRI. These appear to take three main forms.[100] Type I changes demonstrate a decreased signal intensity on $T_1$-weighted images and an increased signal intensity on $T_2$-weighted images and have been identified in approximately 4% of patients scanned for lumbar disease (Figure 130.14). Type I changes are also seen in approximately 30% of chymopapain-treated discs, which may be

viewed as a model of acute disc degeneration. Type II changes are represented by increased signal intensity on $T_1$-weighted images and an isointense or slightly hyperintense signal on $T_2$-weighted images (Figure 130.15). These were seen in approximately 16% of cases. In both types, there is always evidence of associated degenerative disc disease at the level of involvement. Mild enhancement of Type I vertebral body marrow changes is seen with Gd-DTPA, which at times can extend to involve the disc itself. This enhancement is presumably related to the vascularized fibrous tissue within the adjacent marrow. Histopathologic sections of disc with Type I changes demonstrate disruption and fissuring of the end plate and vascularized fibrous tissues within the adjacent marrow producing prolongation of T1 and T2. Discs with Type II changes also show evidence of end plate disruption with yellow marrow replacement in the adjacent vertebral body resulting in a shorter T1. There appears to be a relationship between these, because Type I changes have been observed to convert to Type II with time, whereas Type II changes seem to remain stable. To date, no attempt has been made to correlate the marrow changes with clinical symptoms or to determine whether they are related to specific biomechanical derangements such as instability.

A third type is represented by a decreased signal intensity on both $T_1$-and $T_2$-weighted images that appears to correlate with extensive bony sclerosis on plain radiographs (Figure 130.16). The first two types show no definite correlation with sclerosis seen at radiography, which

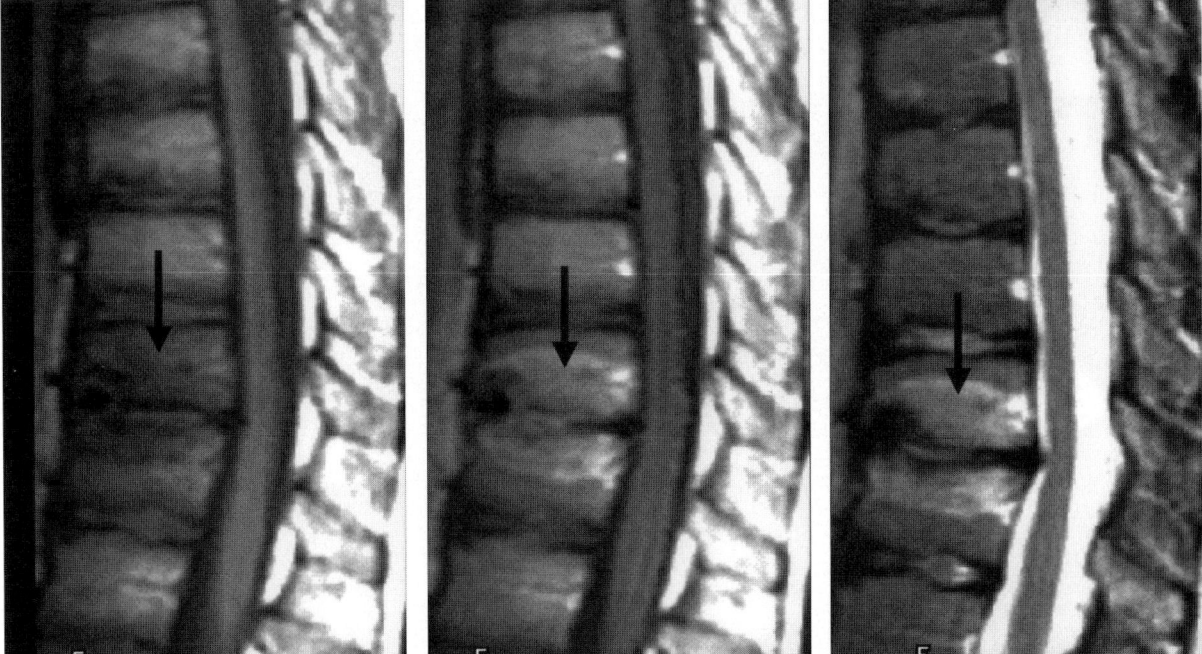

**Figure 130.14** Type I Degenerative Marrow Changes. Sagittal $T_1$, $T_1$ post-contrast and $T_2$-weighted images of the thoracolumbar junction. There is a decreased signal intensity of the opposing portion of the T10 and T11 vertebral bodies adjacent to the end plate. This region enhances after the administration of contrast and demonstrates high signal intensity of the $T_2$-weighted images.

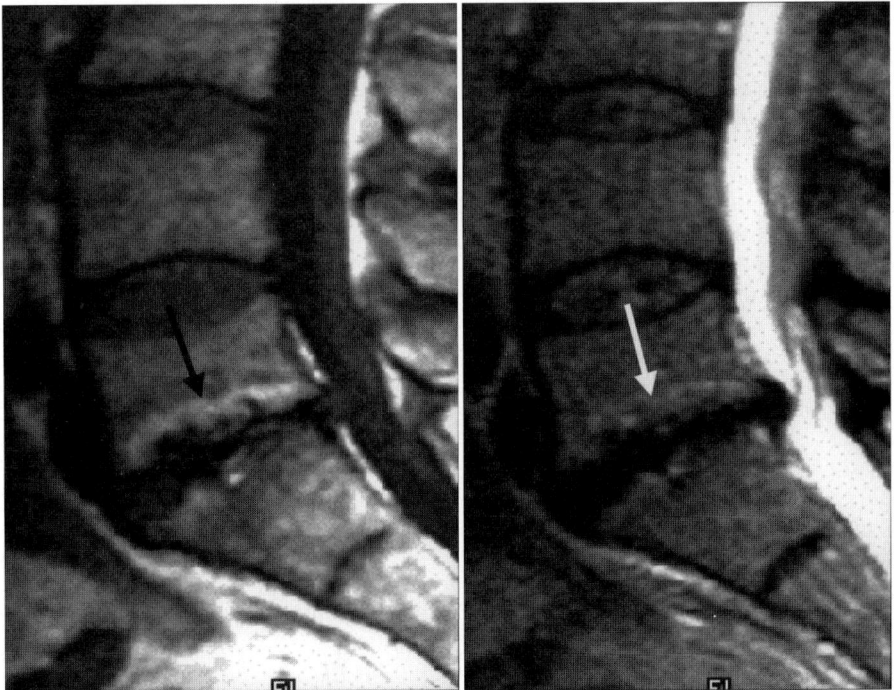

**Figure 130.15** Type II Degenerative Marrow Changes. Sagittal $T_1$-and $T_2$-weighted images of the lower lumbar spine demonstrate high signal on $T_1$-weighted images of the marrow space adjacent to the end plate at the L5-S1 level. This regions shows only a subtle increased signal on $T_1$-weighted images.

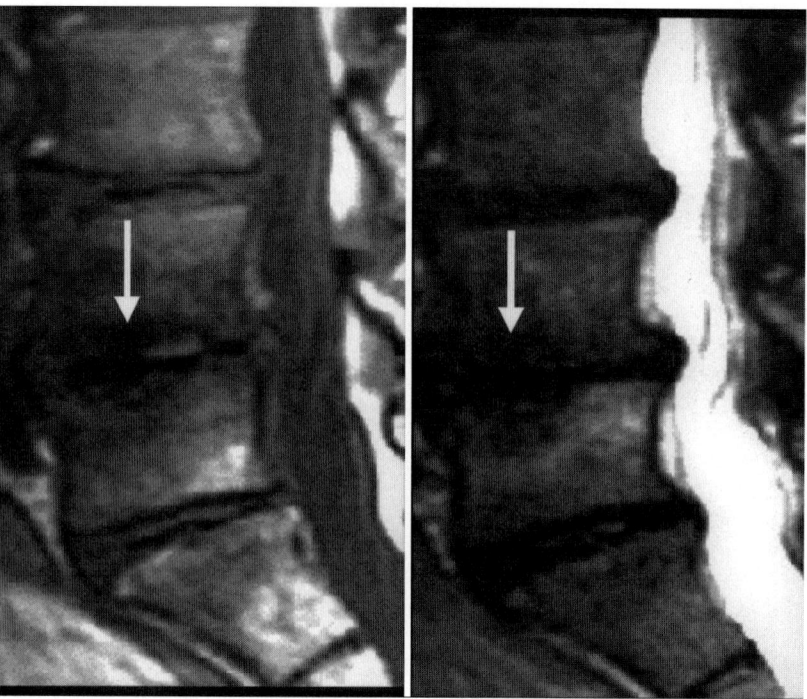

**Figure 130.16** Type III Degenerative Marrow Changes. Sagittal $T_1$- and $T_2$-weighted images of the lower lumbar spine. There is decreased signal intensity of the marrow space adjacent to the end plates on both the $T_1$- and $T_2$-weighted images.

is not surprising when one considers the histology. The sclerosis on plain radiographs is a reflection of dense woven bone within the vertebral body rather than of the marrow elements. The MR signal intensity is more a reflection of the marrow elements, normal hematopoietic tissue, fibrovascular tissue, and lipid (or lack there of) between trabeculae. The lack of signal in the Type III change no doubt reflects the relative absence of marrow in areas of advanced sclerosis. While the signal intensity changes of Type I may be similar to those seen in vertebral osteomyelitis, the distinguishing factor (at least in the adult population) is the involvement of the intervertebral disc, which shows an abnormal high signal intensity and abnormal configuration on $T_2$-weighted images of infection. Discovertebral destruction in ankylosing spondylitis will also cause abnormal signal intensity of adjacent end plates but will usually show decreased signal intensity of the disc region itself on $T_2$-weighted images. Increased signal from the disc may suggest an active inflammatory process. Disc narrowing, sclerosis, and vertebral end plate irregularity suggestive of osteomyelitis have also been demonstrated in long-term hemodialysis and calcium pyrophosphate disease. Classically in the patient with hemodialysis spondyloarthropathy, the intervertebral disc maintains low signal intensity on both $T_1$- and $T_2$-weighted sequences. Crystal disorders should show increased signal intensity on long TE-TR sequences. Exceptions have been noted however where noninfectious spondyloarthropathy has demonstrated an increased signal within the involved interspace.

There are no well-controlled studies documenting the natural history of diagnostic imaging findings in patients with or without radiculopathy. Some information about imaging natural history of herniated disc disease is available. Many have shown that the size of a disc herniation can reduce dramatically in patients undergoing conservative management. Saal et al.[127] evaluated patients with extrusions and radiculopathy in which all patients were treated nonoperatively. Eleven percent of patients had a 0% to 50% decrease in size of the herniations, 36% had a 50% to 75% decrease in size, and 46% had a 75% to 100% decrease in size. Maximum shrinkage of extrusion occurred in the rostra-caudal dimension.

Bush et al.[23] evaluated 165 patients presenting with sciatica. Sixty-four of 84 herniated or sequestered discs showed a degree of, or complete resolution within 1 year, whereas only 7 of 27 bulging discs showed any resolution at 1 year. No correlation was demonstrated between disc resolution and final neurologic outcome.

Maigne et al.[82] evaluated 47 patients with acute sciatica undergoing conservative medical therapy. Follow-up studies demonstrated 9 of the herniations had decreased by 25%, 8 had decreased by 50% to 75%, and 31 had decreased between 75% and 100%. In this study, the large herniations were most likely to decrease in size. These authors do not correlate the time of herniation regression with the regression of signs and symptoms.

Bozzao et al.[20] evaluated 69 patients with MRI-proven lumbar disc herniation. Sixty-three percent of the patients showed a reduction in size of disc herniation (with 48% having reduction of more than 70%), while only 8% demonstrated an increase in size.

In general, these studies were not rigidly controlled and were not able to determine if the change in herniation size is clinically significant, and whether or not it correlates with a favorable outcome.

## Prognostic Value of Morphologic Findings

There is no agreement on the prognostic value of morphologic changes detected by imaging. In fact, recent reviews have stated that MRI has no predictive value.[41,45] Nevertheless, despite the conflicts of opinion and absence of well-controlled studies, most surgeons believe that larger disc herniations do better after surgery than smaller disc herniations. It seems logical therefore to investigate the morphologic information available for modern imaging in an attempt to predict successful outcomes early in the clinical course of radiculopathy or LBP. Instead, investigators have focused on epidemiologic variables such as gender, duration, litigation, compensation status, social-psychosocial history, and so on.

Any attempt to infer prognosis from morphology will be confounded by the high prevalence of morphologic change in the asymptomatic population. Utilizing CT, Wiesel et al.[146] evaluated 52 patients with no history of back trouble. Irrespective of age, 35.4% were found to be "abnormal." Spinal disease was identified in an average 19.5% of those less than 40 years of age, and there was a herniated disc in every instance. In the patients over 40 years of age, there was an average of 50% "abnormal" findings, with a diagnosis of herniated disc, facet degeneration, and stenosis occurring most frequently.

Using MRI, Boden et al.[18] evaluated 67 individuals who never had LBP. In patients less than 60 years old, 20% had a herniated nucleus pulposus and one had spinal stenosis. In patients over 60 years of age, 57% of the scans were abnormal, 37% of the subjects had a herniated nucleus pulposus, and 21% had spinal stenosis. There was degeneration or disc bulge at least at one lumbar level in 35% of the subjects between 20 to 39 years of age.

Jensen et al.[65] evaluated 98 asymptomatic patients by MRI. Subjects ranged in age from 20 to 80 years. All subjects were imaged with MR in a standard fashion. The studies were then read blindly and independently by two experienced neuroradiologists from another institution.

Fifty-two percent of subjects had a disc bulge at one level at least, 27% had a protrusion, and only 1% had an extrusion. Sixty-four percent of the asymptomatic subjects were found to have an intervertebral disc abnormality and 38% were found to have a disc abnormality at more than one level. Nineteen percent of asymptomatic subjects had Schmorl's nodes, 14% had annular defects, and 7% had central canal stenosis. This study emphasizes the importance of correlating the clinical picture with the MRI examination when major surgical or medico-legal decisions are made. In fact, the findings on a lumbar spine MRI examination may be meaningless when considered in isolation. In addition, with only 1% of the sample showing an extrusion, subcategorizing herniations into protrusion and extrusion may be helpful to better characterize asymptomatic versus symptomatic discs.

More recently, the author studied the morphologic alterations at presentation and change in appearance over time in patients with acute LBP only versus those with radiculopathy. One hundred patients (50 with LBP, 50 with radiculopathy) were studied with identical MRI parameters at presentation and again at 6 weeks. Studies were read blind to clinical information and timing by three radiologists. Studies were graded as being normal (N), demonstrating bulges (B) only, protrusions (P), or extrusions (E). The results of the interpretations of the two studies in the same individual were then compared for change. Thirty-one of 50 patients with LBP and 40 of 50 patients with radiculopathy completed both the presentation and 6-week studies. At presentation, 50% of patients with LBP (15N, 10B, 15P, and 10E) and 56% of radiculopathy patients (12N, 10B, 15P, and 13E) had herniations at one or more levels. At 6 weeks, 9% of patients with LBP and 20% of patients with radiculopathy had a significant reduction in the size of the herniation. In patients who had herniations characterized as extrusions, there were significant reductions in size in 60% of patients with LBP and 55% of patients with radiculopathy. The author found that the type and frequency of disc alterations in patients with LBP and radiculopathy at presentation are similar. Discs characterized as extruded showed significant regressions in 55% to 60% of cases in both groups.[95]

Why do some individuals without symptoms show the same morphologic abnormality as those with symptoms? Why do some individuals become symptom free without an obvious change in the morphology of the herniated disc thought to be responsible for the acute event? Why do some individuals show improving symptoms in the face of worsening morphologic changes?

Given the number of questions raised that require good natural history data for further study, the author undertook a small pilot study of 25 radiculopathy patients in order to develop a methodology for assessing the role of imaging. The preliminary observations indicate that there are no characteristics of a disc herniation that are prognostic (i.e., size, location, type, and enhancement). In fact, in this small group, small discs were more likely to fail conservative management than large ones. Only 48% of patients had a 50% improvement in their Roland function score at 6 weeks. This then suggests that 6 weeks might be too soon to image. Unfortunately, due to the small sample size of the study, substantive conclusions about the role of diagnostic imaging could not be made. Enhancement did not seem to be a prognostic indicator in that it was found in virtually all (26 of 28) herniated discs.[99]

Other sequelae of the degenerative process have been studied and ascribed variable clinical significance. This includes annular bulges[87] with annular disruption,[150] facet and ligament degenerative changes, and enhancement on $T_1$-weighted images from scar formation.[122] While no good data exists to clearly support a causal relationship between these degenerative changes and symptoms, annular disruption is important to consider because of a controversial concept of "discogenic pain" and its implications concerning the usefulness of discography for diagnosis. Back pain is thought to occur in some patients without morphologic abnormalities, such as herniation or stenosis—allegedly related to leakage of nuclear material through a disrupted annulus into the epidural space.[89,107]

In general, studies have demonstrated that many morphologic or pathologic findings will enhance, such as the peridiscal scar tissue, annular tears, the intervertebral disc, and nerve roots. However, most of these reports have not correlated enhancement with signs and symptoms or outcome. For instance, nerve root enhancement has been described in association with nerve root compression, but it has been difficult to correlate these changes with clinical symptoms.[66] The significance is further complicated by the observation that normal nerve roots can enhance with high doses of contrast media.

Qualitative morphologic features of the herniated discs in the spinal canal have not proven helpful in predicting outcomes in patients with LBP and sciatica.[26] They do not correlate well with clinical signs and severity of symptoms. More quantitative evaluations, such as disc-to-canal ratios, have shown some correlation with symptoms, but not necessarily with outcomes.

More recently however, a study using quantitative MRI measurements of disc and spinal canal morphology in 188 patients with sciatica indicates a wide range of herniations and canal sizes, with significant differences between men and women.[26] In a cohort of 135 patients followed for more than 2 years, demographic and clinical features appeared to predict outcomes of nonoperative treatment, whereas morphometric features of the disc herniation and spinal canal were much more powerful predictors of surgical outcomes. In particular, the anteroposterior disc length was the most important predictor in the surgical group. This study, however, did not have a patient sample, which was generalizable; it also lacked standardized outcome measures and suffered from dramatic variations in the timing of imaging. Nevertheless, it underscores the potential importance of prospectively studying morphologic changes and their prognostic significance.

Unfortunately, studies to date leave unanswered the question of the significance of the morphologic abnormalities and do not adequately explain the role these changes play in the symptomatic population. As mentioned previously, a standardized classification system would be useful for clinical research studies and for the application of study results to clinical practice. In the Maine Lumbar Spine Study (MLSS), 516 patients were studied to assess the Quebec Task Force Classification Scheme's ability to stratify patients according to severity and treatment at baseline, and to assess changes over time in health-related quality of life including symptoms, functional status, and disability.[5-7,70] In this study, the proportion of patients treated surgically increased from 7% in QTFC 1 (LBP only) to 84% in QTFC 6 (appropriate symptoms, physical and imaging findings of nerve root compression). The treatment decision was relatively clear at the extremes of symptoms and findings but a similar percentage of patients were treated surgically and nonsurgically in QTFC 2-4 indicating a greater degree of ambiguity in the majority of patients. In fact, the commonly held belief that nerve root compression on imaging studies is a criterion for surgery was not borne out. In this study, this finding also defined patients who were more likely to improve without surgery.

## Osteomyelitis

The single most important differential consideration to exclude when discal and adjacent marrow changes are noted is vertebral osteomyelitis. Vertebral osteomyelitis with discitis comprises 2% to 4% of all cases of osteomyelitis.[125] Despite its low incidence, the potential morbidity and mortality of vertebral osteomyelitis are great. Accurate and specific imaging is required not only for diagnosis but to also guide biopsy for a microbiologic culture. MRI provides the best combination of sensitivity and specificity. Other imaging tests such as plain films, nuclear medicine imaging, and CT may provide additional information.

In a series of 37 adult patients with vertebral osteomyelitis from the Cleveland Clinic, *Staphylococcus aureus* was the responsible organism in 68% of patients (25 of 37).[34] *Staphylococcus epidermidis*, streptococci, gram-negative aerobic bacilli, and *Mycobacterium tuberculosis* were each identified in 5% (2 of 37) of the remaining patients. In a review of the literature on pyogenic vertebral osteomyelitis by Sapico *et al.*,[129] *S. aureus* was also the dominant organism responsible for 57% of cases. Overall gram-positive bacteria accounted for 68% of cases and gram-negative bacteria (*Escherichia coli*, *Proteus* spp., and *Pseudomonas aeruginosa*) accounted for 29% of cases. Hematogenous osteomyelitis is almost always monomicrobial. The risk of spinal osteomyelitis is increased in patients with sickle cell anemia, tuberculosis, malnutrition, alcoholism, diabetes mellitus, rheumatoid arthritis, and steroid use due to compromise of host defenses.[21] The incidence of diabetes mellitus in patients with vertebral osteomyelitis (19%) is far out of proportion to that in the general population. In elderly males with genitourinary tract infections, vertebral osteomyelitis is caused most often by *E. coli* and *Proteus* spp.[129] In intravenous drug abusers, *P. aeruginosa*, other unusual gram-negative bacilli, and staphylococci cause spinal infection most frequently.[129,130] In a series of 43 adult patients, Hitchon *et al.*[60] reported that 98% presented with local spine pain of longer than 6 weeks duration and 50% presented with fever. All had elevated sedimentation rates. In a series of 150 patients with vertebral osteomyelitis, Malawski *et al.*[83] found that a lumbar vertebral body was involved in 213 instances, a thoracic vertebral body in 113 cases, and a cervical vertebral body in 19 cases. Seventy percent of cases had two vertebral bodies involved, 23% had greater than two vertebral bodies involved, and 6% had single vertebral body involvement.

Spinal epidural abscess represents a serious complication of vertebral osteomyelitis. Darouiche *et al.*[35] reported that 44% of all spinal epidural abscesses were associated with vertebral osteomyelitis. Epidural abscess, in association with vertebral osteomyelitis, tends to occur ventrally within the spinal canal, as opposed to those occurring without osteomyelitis, which tend to occur dorsally (Figure 130.17).

Colmenero *et al.*[31] retrospectively reviewed 219 cases of vertebral osteomyelitis. They compared the features of brucellar versus pyogenic versus tuberculous vertebral osteomyelitis. Brucella was present in 48% of patients, pyogenic in 33%, and tuberculosis in 19%. The mean age was 50, with no significant differences among the three groups. There was a male predominance in the pyogenic and brucellar groups. In the tuberculous group, the male to female ratio was equal. Pyogenic vertebral osteomyelitis

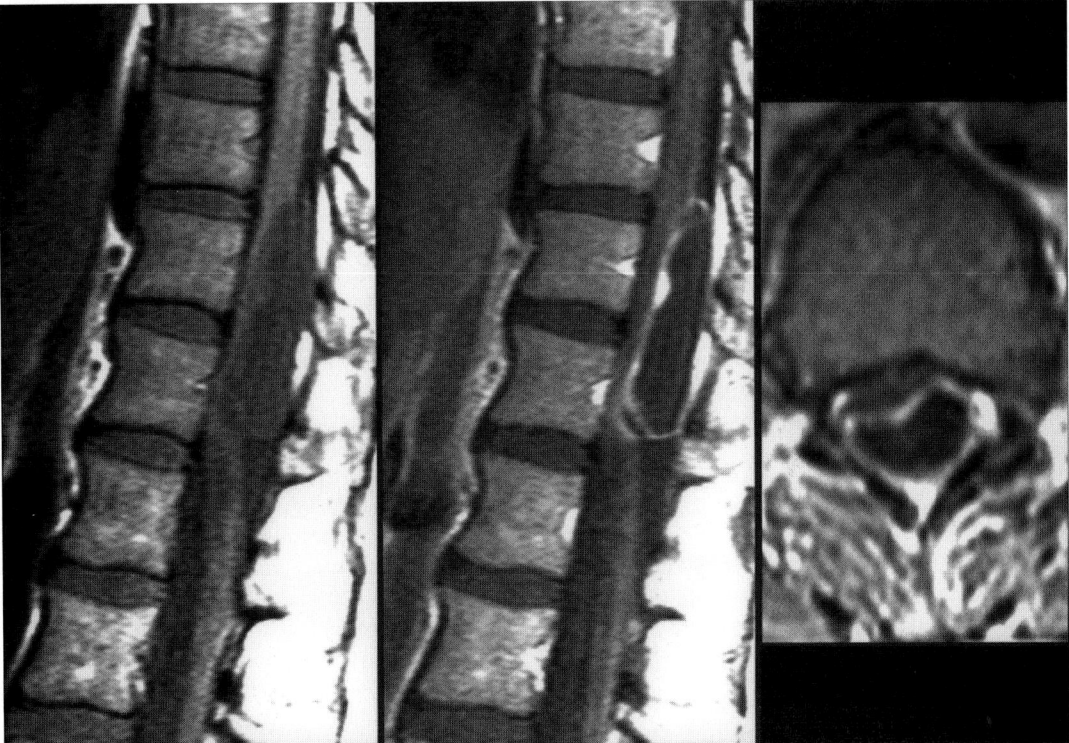

**Figure 130.17** Epidural Abscess. Sagittal T1 precontrast and postcontrast and axial postcontrast images. There is a large mass dorsally within the spinal canal, which demonstrates peripheral enhancement. At surgery, this was found to be an epidural abscess. There is no evidence of bone involvement.

was linked to diabetes, intravenous drug abuse, chronic debilitating disease or immunosuppression, prior infection, previous bacteremia, and recent surgery. Leukocytosis, neutrophilia, and elevated erythrocyte sedimentation rate (ESR) were associated with pyogenic vertebral osteomyelitis. Tuberculous vertebral osteomyelitis had a prolonged course without fever. In cases of skeletal tuberculosis, the vertebral bodies are affected in 25% to 60% of cases.[64,133] The thoracic and lumbar spine are most commonly involved, with a predilection for the thoracolumbar junction.[62,133] Usually more than one vertebral body level is involved, with 50% of cases involving two adjacent vertebral bodies.[72] Solitary and skip lesions can occur.[132-134,142] The ventral aspect of the vertebral body is most commonly involved. The dorsal elements are involved in 2% to 10% of cases.[133] Less than 2% of cases have been reported to present with only dorsal arch involvement, with sparing of the vertebral body.[116]

Brucellosis is an insidious febrile illness with nonspecific signs and symptoms. Between 25% and 34% of cases have involvement of osteoarticular structures.[4] Gottuzo et al.[53] reported a series of patients with brucellosis with skeletal involvement; 6% of these patients had vertebral osteomyelitis.

## Modes of Infection

There are three routes by which vertebral osteomyelitis can be established: (1) hematogenous, (2) iatrogenic, and (3) contiguous spread.[31]

### Hematogenous

Both the venous and arterial routes have been proposed as possible routes for the development of vertebral osteomyelitis. Batson[12] in 1940 described a valveless, low-pressure vertebral venous system. This is composed of tributaries from the vertebral body metaphyses that drain into a large channel that exits the vertebral body via the nutrient foramen into the plexus of veins lining the spinal canal in the extradural space. There are also connections through the vertebral body cortex to a plexus of veins on the ventral and lateral aspects of the spine.[12,13] Batson[12] demonstrated rich anastomoses of this vertebral venous system with the thoracic and abdominal cavities, and pelvic veins. Slight increases in pressure in the vena caval system resulted in a diversion of blood into the vertebral venous system.

Septic embolization via the arterial system has also been proposed as a route for vertebral osteomyelitis. The arterial system of the spine forms a ladder-like anastomosis on its surface. The horizontal components are segmental arteries (1 to 3mm) arising from the abdominal aorta that lie at the equator of the vertebral body, and two metaphyseal (200mm) anastomosing arteries at each vertebral metaphysis. The vertical components join the segmental arteries to the metaphyseal anastomosing arteries, the metaphyseal anastomosing arteries of adjacent vertebral arteries, as well as metaphyseal anastomosing arteries of the same vertebral body. The intraosseous arteries arise from the segmental and metaphyseal anastomosing arteries and parallel the disc surface. Children have rich anastomoses of the intraosseous arteries, which involutes by adulthood. Thus, in an adult, infection of the disc cannot occur directly via hematogenous means. It can occur via contiguous spread from an adjacent infected vertebral body. Ratcliffe[117] has proposed that septic emboli were more likely to enter the greater number of arteries at the metaphysis and the smaller caliber of the vessels allowed for the development of thrombosis with resultant infarction, which is required for osteomyelitis to develop. These two observations explain the propensity for vertebral osteomyelitis to involve the subchondral aspect of the body with relative sparing of the central portion of the vertebral body. The vertical anastomoses among the metaphyseal anastomosing arteries allowed for the spread of infection across disc spaces as well as within the same vertebral body with sparing of the central portion. The intraosseous anastomoses in children would prevent large foci of bony infarction thus resulting in smaller foci of osteomyelitis.[117]

Whereas metastatic spread from the pelvic venous system to the vertebral bodies via the vertebral venous plexus has been shown in animals,[32,94] the spread of infection via the vertebral plexus could not be demonstrated experimentally.[30] Further arguments supporting arterial spread is that vertebral osteomyelitis is usually preceded by symptomatology compatible with bacteremia (sepsis). If spread is via the venous route, extradural thrombophlebitis with meningismus should be expected to represent a prominent feature of osteomyelitis.[147] This has not proven to be the case.

### Iatrogenic or Posttraumatic

Organisms can be directly implanted secondary to surgical procedures or penetrating spinal trauma. Discitis has been reported as a complication of cervical and lumbar discography,[56,151] chemonucleolysis (chymopapain injection),[36,49] and laminectomy.[48,104] Discitis as a complication of discography is uncommon. Its incidence has been reported as 0.05% to 1.4% in various series. An aggravation or increase of neck and back pain and fever are typical presenting complaints.[56,151]

Chymopapain has been used in the nonoperative treatment of lumbar disc disease. An incidence of discitis of up to 2.5% has been reported with chemonucleolysis.[36,49] As with discography, persistent or intensification of pain is the most usual presenting symptomatology. In an experimental model, Fraser et al.[49] demonstrated that end plate erosions only occurred at infected disc levels following chemonucleolysis, whereas levels that were not infected only demonstrated disc space narrowing following chemonucleolysis. Deeb et al.[36] used the interval development of vertebral end plate irregularity and mottled-appearing vertebral bodies to suggest the diagnosis of disc space infection and to guide needle biopsy with CT scans.

The diagnosis of disc space infection following discectomy is problematic. Patients typically present 2 to 6 weeks following surgery with recurrence of pain after initially having experienced the relief of symptoms. Patients are often febrile with muscle spasm and a positive straight leg raising test.[48] The sedimentation rate is elevated. Roentgenographic findings appear several weeks after initial symptoms, with a decrease in the intervertebral disc space height and end plate erosions.

### Contiguous Spread

Vertebral osteomyelitis or disc space infection can result from contiguous spread from an adjacent infected source. It is the least common of the three mechanisms discussed here.[118] Contiguous spread requires the spread of a superlative soft tissue focus through the periosteum, cortex, and marrow of the vertebral body or through the longitudinal ligaments, annulus fibrosus, and nucleus pulposus of the disc. Contiguous spread of infection to the spine is encountered in the sacral region in association with infected decubitus ulcers, and genitourinary and intestinal processes.[118] Vertebral osteomyelitis and disc space infection have been reported as complications of colonic,[121] hypopharyngeal,[79] esophageal[11,88] perforations or instrumentation; and pelvic abscesses.[52,118] Lesions of the aorta or of an aortic graft, such as mycotic aneurysm or pseudoaneurysm, may predispose to the development of vertebral osteomyelitis.[91] A case has also been reported where an infected retroperitoneal hematoma from an abdominal aortic aneurysm resulted in vertebral osteomyelitis.[37] When considering vertebral osteomyelitis as a result of contiguous spread, the question often arises as to whether the infection was actually a result of hematogenous spread, either arterial or venous, rather than truly contiguous with direct invasion.[8,93,139] For example, the direct invasion of a vertebral body by a lung lesion is felt to be an unlikely sequence of events due to an effective barrier provided by the pleura.[8] Here it has been postulated that spread actually occurs via pleural veins communicating with Batson's plexus.

### Conventional Radiography

In general, the early findings of disc space infection on plain radiography consist of minimal disc space narrowing and erosions or indistinctness of the end plates. In addition to the bony changes, soft tissue swelling due to paraspinal phlegmon or abscess may also be evident on plain films. In the lumbar region this presents as enlargement of the psoas shadows. In the thoracic region disc space infection will appear as a paraspinal mass. In the cervical spine there will be prevertebral soft tissue swelling. As the disease progresses, the disc space narrowing worsens. The destruction of the end plates will become more obvious. In addition, sclerosis of the end plates and periosteal reaction also become evident. In general, with healing, the disc space remains markedly narrowed or will fuse, and there may be a concomitant loss of height of the vertebral body with resultant spinal deformity.

Digby et al.[42] reported the following time sequence for the radiographic changes to correlate with the pathologic changes: at 2 weeks decreased disc space height becomes evident; at 6 weeks, lytic vertebral body lesions are seen; reactive sclerosis is present at 8 weeks; and at 6 months, new bone formation and fusion are present. Malawski et al.[83] also reported the time sequence of radiographic changes in a series of 150 cases of vertebral osteomyelitis. They found that radiologic changes became apparent after

4 to 6 weeks. In their series, an early sign was also a decrease in disc space height. After several weeks, lytic vertebral body lesions and end plate disruption were evident.

Unique presentations of vertebral osteomyelitis have also been reported. McHenry et al.[90] reported a series of six patients with osteomyelitis who presented with underlying osteoporosis and compression fracture of a single vertebral body. On the initial plain radiographs, the end plates were intact. This unique presentation accounted for 13% of all hospitalized patients with vertebral osteomyelitis and 2.4% of inpatients with osteoporotic compression fractures over a 5-year period at the Cleveland Clinic.

## Nuclear Medicine

In the setting of vertebral osteomyelitis, the three-phase bone scan demonstrates increased uptake in flow and blood pool phases, and delayed images. Intense uptake in two adjacent vertebral bodies with loss of the disc space is seen on the bone scan in patients with vertebral osteomyelitis. The three-phase bone scan is sensitive for vertebral osteomyelitis. However, it lacks specificity. In the spine, it can be problematic to separate increased radionuclide uptake due to degenerative disc disease, benign compression fracture, or metastatic disease from vertebral osteomyelitis. Moreover, there have been reports of bacteriologically proven vertebral osteomyelitis that have had a negative bone scan at 2 weeks following the onset of symptoms.[44,131] In addition, the increased uptake of tracer does not differentiate active from inactive osteomyelitis, since increased uptake can persist for long periods of time following resolution of the infection.[71]

Gallium scanning also demonstrates increased uptake in the setting of vertebral osteomyelitis. It also gives information about the surrounding soft tissues. The combination of gallium scanning and three-phase bone scan may increase the specificity up nearly 100%.* The sensitivity is approximately 90%. The two tests provide complementary information.[78] It is generally accepted that the combination of bone and gallium imaging is able to identify vertebral osteomyelitis when (1) the distribution of the 2 tracers is spatially incongruent or (2) their distribution is spatially congruent and the relative uptake of gallium exceeds that of technetium.[106] The combination of the two studies is currently the nuclear medicine study of choice for vertebral osteomyelitis. Gratz et al.[54] were able to demonstrate that 67Gallium(Ga)-citrate single photon emission tomography (SPET) activity correlated with the severity of infection in a small series of patients who had been receiving antibiotic treatment for an average of 7 weeks prior to scanning The sensitivity in detecting vertebral osteomyelitis was 80% for individual foci within patients and 100% sensitive in detecting vertebral osteomyelitis in a patient. In addition, 67Ga-citrate SPET detected foci of infection outside of the spine before other imaging techniques demonstrated these.[54]

Although highly specific, indium 111 labeled white blood cells demonstrated poor sensitivity for the diagnosis of vertebral osteomyelitis. Increased or decreased activity

can be seen with indium 111 scanning in cases of bacteriologic-proven vertebral osteomyelitis. Palestro[105] reported a specificity of 98% and a sensitivity of only 39% when increased uptake was used as the criteria for vertebral osteomyelitis. Using decreased activity as the criteria for osteomyelitis, the specificity was 52% and sensitivity was 54%. In another series of patients, Whalen et al.[145] reported a specificity of 100% and sensitivity of 17% using increased uptake as a criterion. They reported that 50% of their patients with proven osteomyelitis had decreased activity on scanning. Indium 111 leukocyte imaging has little or no usefulness in detecting vertebral osteomyelitis and has been shown to be unreliable.[106] This may be due to the destruction of cells of the hematologic system that occurs with infection.[67]

With the exception of combined bone scan-gallium imaging, nuclear medicine imaging for vertebral osteomyelitis has been unsatisfactory. Promising initial results have been reported in 7 patients with vertebral osteomyelitis and fluorodeoxyglucose-positron emission tomography (FDG-PET) imaging.[67] FDG-PET imaging demonstrates the increased glucose metabolism in inflammatory cells such as leukocytes, granulocytes, and macrophages due to increased activity of activated inflammatory cells. High FDG uptake was seen in 7 patients with vertebral osteomyelitis in their series of 15 patients with osteomyelitis at various sites. Follow-up was available in 3 patients with vertebral osteomyelitis. In 1 patient, FDG-PET was of limited value in early postoperative phase due to nonspecific tracer uptake. Normal or reduced tracer uptake correlated with normalization of clinical data in 2 patients. An additional advantage is that FDG-PET is not affected by metal implants. It may be useful in evaluating patients with hardware for infection. FDG-PET has better resolution than other nuclear medicine imaging techniques and can differentiate bone from soft tissue infection. Low FDG-PET uptake has been shown in fractures and pseudoarthrosis. FDG-PET may be useful in differentiating these from vertebral osteomyelitis. However, malignancy cannot be differentiated from vertebral osteomyelitis. Both have increased uptake.[67]

## Computed Tomography

CT is also used in the diagnosis of vertebral osteomyelitis and discitis. It allows detection of bony destruction and paraspinal swelling. The addition of intrathecal contrast provides better delineation of epidural masses. CT demonstrates a decrease in the density of the affected vertebral body and disc.[69,74,118] The CT criteria for the diagnosis of pyogenic vertebral osteomyelitis includes diffuse moth-eaten or permeative bone destruction, gas within the bone or adjacent soft tissues, involvement of the intervertebral disc primarily and prevertebral soft tissue involvement[118,140] (Figure 130.18). Granulomatous vertebral osteomyelitis may present with fragmented end plates rather than as a purely lytic lesion, with paraspinal masses that extend for a greater length than the vertebral body itself, and with paraspinal masses that may demonstrate calcifications.[133] With treatment and resolution of the infection, the density of the vertebral bodies increases and associated soft tissue masses decrease in size. At the

*References 24,44,71,77,93,96,114.

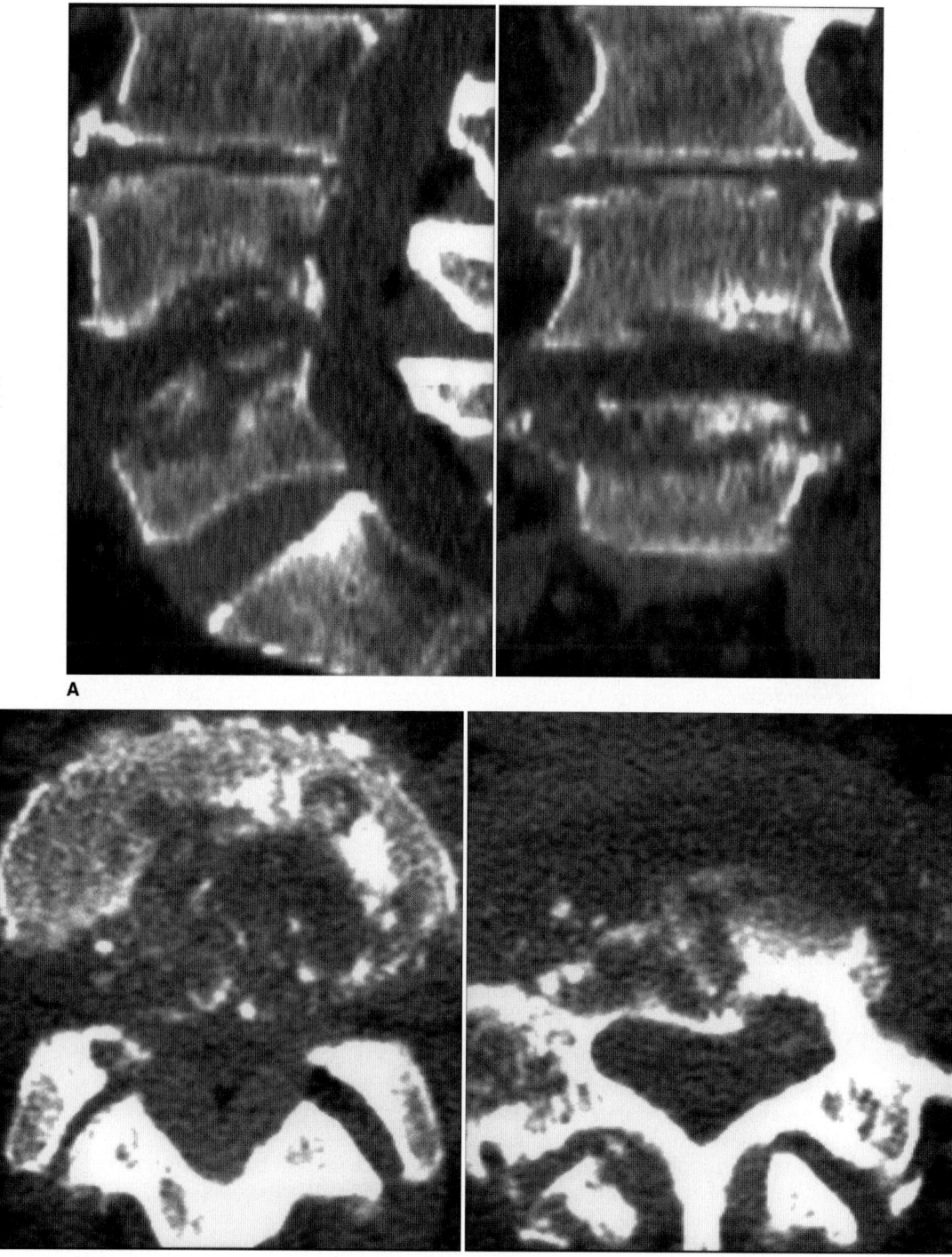

**Figure 130.18** Vertebral Osteomyelitis. **(A)** Sagittal and coronal multiplanar (MPR) CT of the L4-5 disc space. **(B)** Axial CT through the L4-5 disc. There is a permeative destructive process involving the L4-5 level centered at the disc space.

Cleveland Clinic, CT is most often used for guiding needle biopsy for definitive diagnosis and microbiologic culture, rather than as a method of diagnosis.

## Magnetic Resonance Imaging

MRI has been found to have a sensitivity of 96%, a specificity of 92%, and an accuracy of 94% in the diagnosis of vertebral osteomyelitis.[96] This is comparable to the combination of technetium 99m bone scanning and gallium scanning as discussed previously. MRI is also more sensitive and specific for the diagnosis of vertebral osteomyelitis than is plain radiography.[96] It is superior to CT regarding its contrast resolution, its demonstration of epidural disease, and in detecting the effect of the infection on the spinal cord and thecal sac. The classic MRI

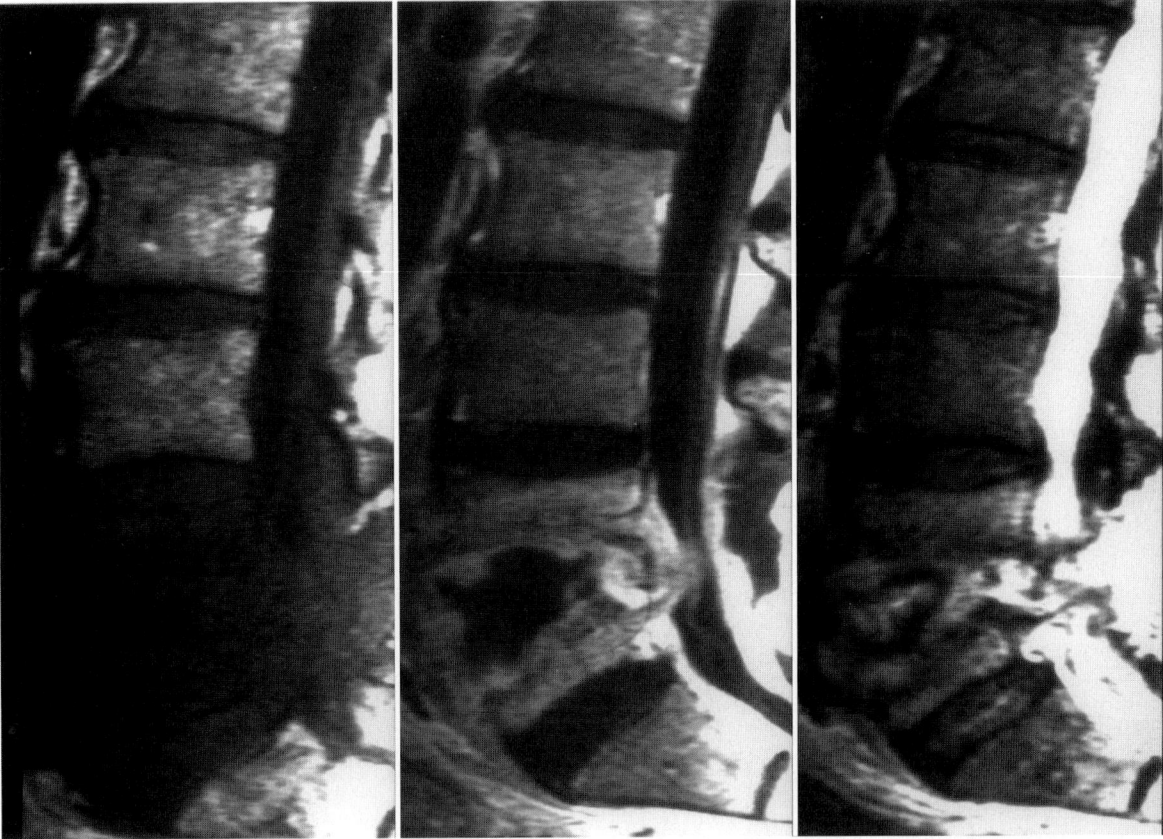

**Figure 130.19** Vertebral Osteomyelitis, Pyogenic. Sagittal T1 precontrast, T1 postcontrast, and $T_2$-weighted images. There is confluent decreased signal intensity of the intervertebral disc and adjacent vertebral bodies at the L4-5 level with the inability to discern a margin between the two on $T_1$-weighted images. There is enhancement of the involved portions of the adjacent vertebral bodies and peripheral disc enhancement. There is an increased signal intensity of vertebral bodies adjacent to the involved disc on $T_2$-weighted images and an abnormal configuration and increased signal intensity of the intervertebral disc with loss of the nuclear cleft.

appearance of vertebral osteomyelitis is as follows: a confluent decreased signal intensity of the intervertebral disc and adjacent vertebral bodies with the inability to discern a margin between the two on $T_1$-weighted images; an increased signal intensity of vertebral bodies adjacent to the involved disc on $T_2$-weighted images; and an abnormal configuration and increased signal intensity of the intervertebral disc with loss of the nuclear cleft on $T_2$-weighted images[96] (Figures 130.19 and 130.20). The addition of gadolinium enhancement to routine MRI has been found to increase the accuracy of the diagnosis of vertebral osteomyelitis and discitis in cases with equivocal MRI scans.[112] The involved portions of the adjacent vertebral body and disc typically enhance following the administration of gadolinium. Enhancement patterns of the disc may include the homogeneous enhancement of the majority of the disc, patchy nonconfluent areas of disc enhancement, or thick or thin areas of peripheral disc enhancement.[112]

Recently, the author has reevaluated the MRI findings of vertebral osteomyelitis.[34] In 37 cases of vertebral osteomyelitis with 41 disc levels of involvement, the typical T1 vertebral body, end plate, and T2 disc changes as described above were found in 95% of cases. However, only 56% demonstrated the typical T2 vertebral body changes. Atypical changes included isointense or increased signal intensity vertebral bodies and lack of end plate erosion on $T_1$-weighted images. On $T_2$-weighted images, atypical changes included vertebral bodies that were isointense or decreased in signal intensity. The absence of increased signal in the vertebral body on the $T_2$-weighted images, in the presence of other T1 and T2 signal changes consistent with vertebral osteomyelitis, should not dissuade the clinician from this diagnosis.

Post et al.[112] described abnormal enhancement of the vertebral bodies, disc and paraspinal soft tissues that progressively decreased on follow-up imaging in patients successfully treated with antibiotics. Gillams et al.[51] also followed patients on antibiotic therapy with MRI. They saw both decreasing, stable and even increasing enhancement patterns in patients who were improving clinically on medical therapy. They concluded that while decreasing spinal and soft tissue enhancement were useful signs, persistent or increasing enhancement alone did not indicate treatment failure.

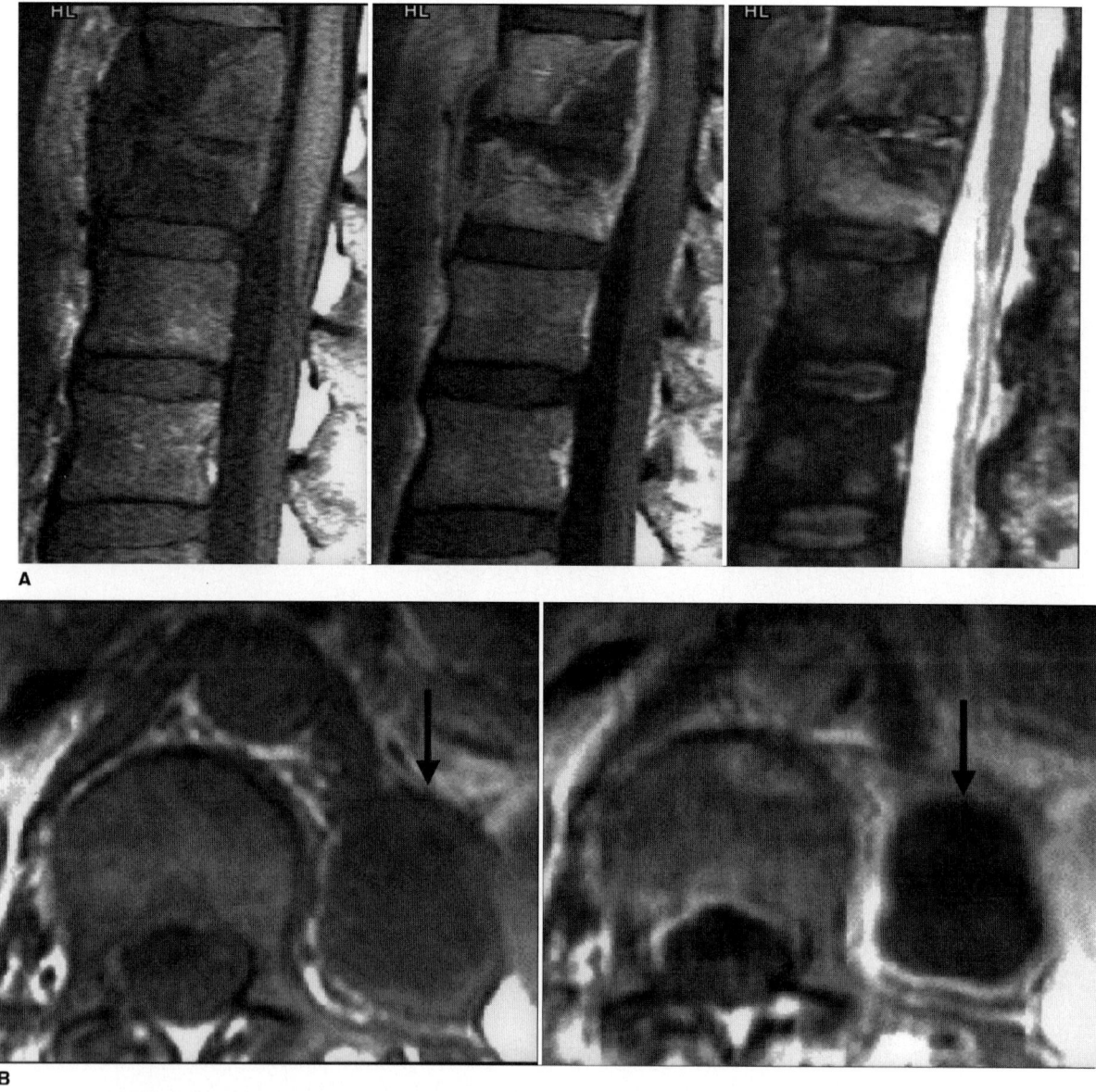

**Figure 130.20** Vertebral Osteomyelitis, Tuberculosis. **(A)** Sagittal $T_1$ precontrast, $T_1$ postcontrast and $T_2$-weighted images. **(B)** Axial $T_1$-weighted images precontrast and postcontrast through the T11-12 disc space. There is abnormal decreased signal intensity of the T11 and T12 vertebral bodies with relative sparing of the disc space and an associated paravertebral abscess *(black arrows)*.

## Specific Etiologies
### Postoperative Discitis

Differentiating postoperative discitis from normal postoperative disc space change can be difficult. Boden *et al.*[19] reported postoperative MRI changes in 15 asymptomatic patients and 7 patients with proven postoperative discitis. They found gadolinium enhancement to be useful. Four of the asymptomatic patients had MRI findings that could also be seen in patients with discitis. All 7 discitis patients and 1 asymptomatic patient had vertebral bone marrow enhancement. Five of the discitis patients and 3 of the asymptomatic patients had disc space enhancement, and all 7 discitis patients and 13 asymptomatic patients had

dorsal annulus fibrosis enhancement. The entire triad of vertebral bone marrow enhancement, disc space enhancement, and annulus fibrosis enhancement was not seen in any of the asymptomatic patients in their series. Ross *et al.*[124] evaluated 94 asymptomatic postoperative patients with MRI. Approximately 20% (19 of 94) of the patients showed intervertebral disc enhancement at the surgical level 3 months after surgery. All but one case demonstrated linear enhancement in the rostral and caudal aspects of the disc that paralleled the end-plate margins (Figure 130.21). Seven (7%) of the 94 patients had intervertebral disc enhancement and Type I marrow changes at the surgical level that also enhanced postoperatively (Figure 130.22). Type I marrow changes represent the

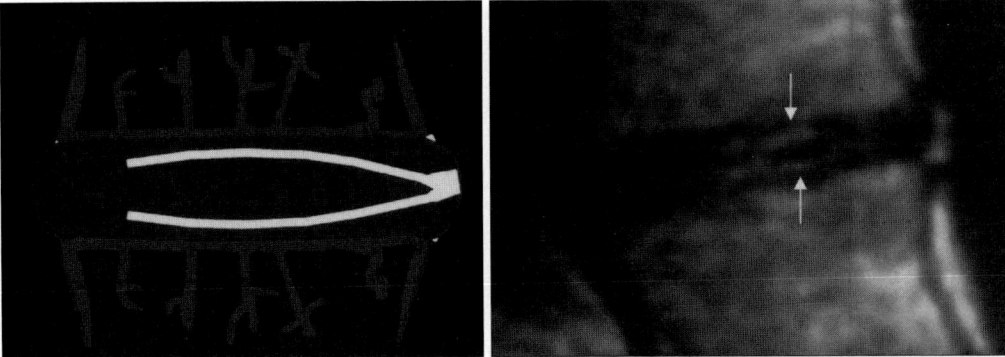

**Figure 130.21** Normal Postoperative Discal Enhancement. Sagittal diagram and T$_1$-weighted postcontrast image of the L4-5 disc. Note the linear areas of enhancement *(white arrows)*.

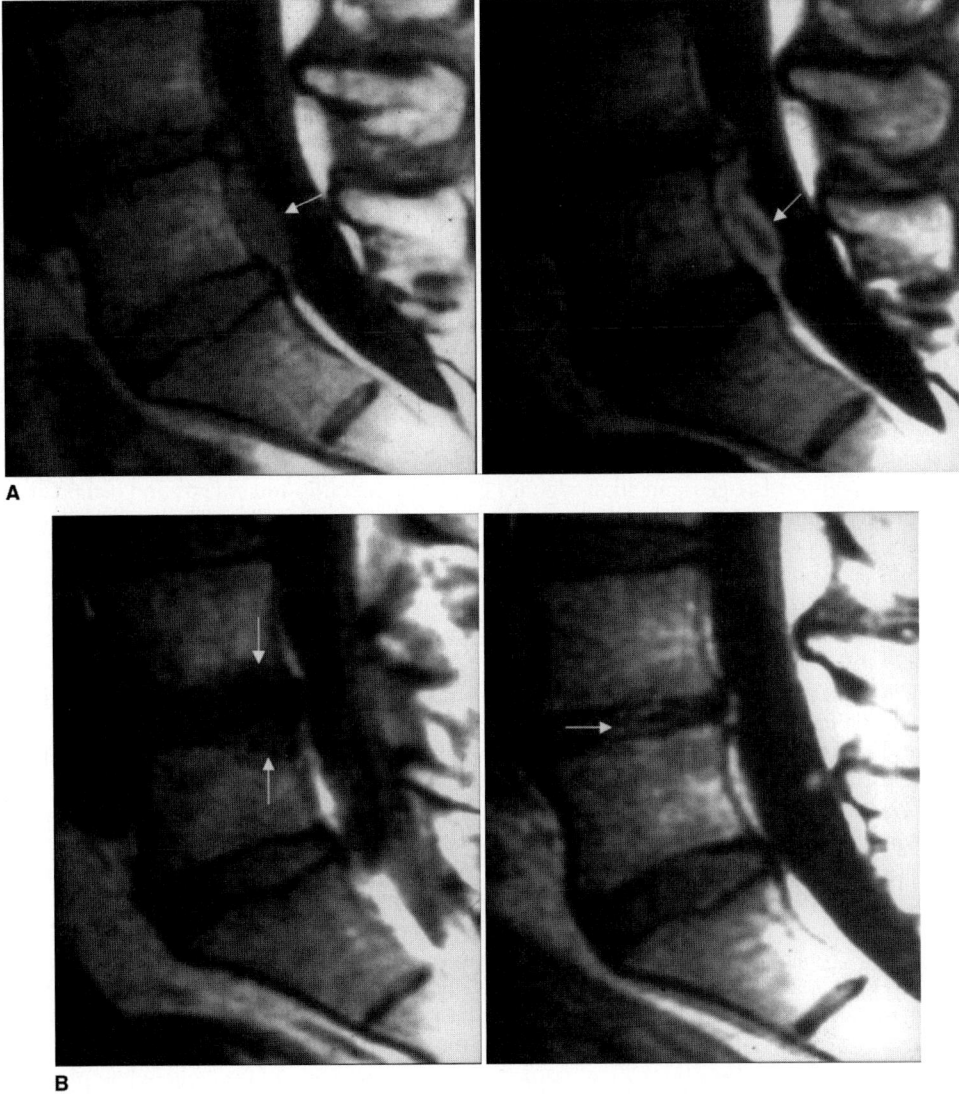

**Figure 130.22** **(A)** Sagittal T$_1$-weighted images of the lower lumbar spine precontrast and postcontrast. There is a caudally migrated free fragment from the L4-5 disc level, which lies behind the body of L5. Following contrast, there is peripheral enhancement of the disc herniation *(white arrows)*.

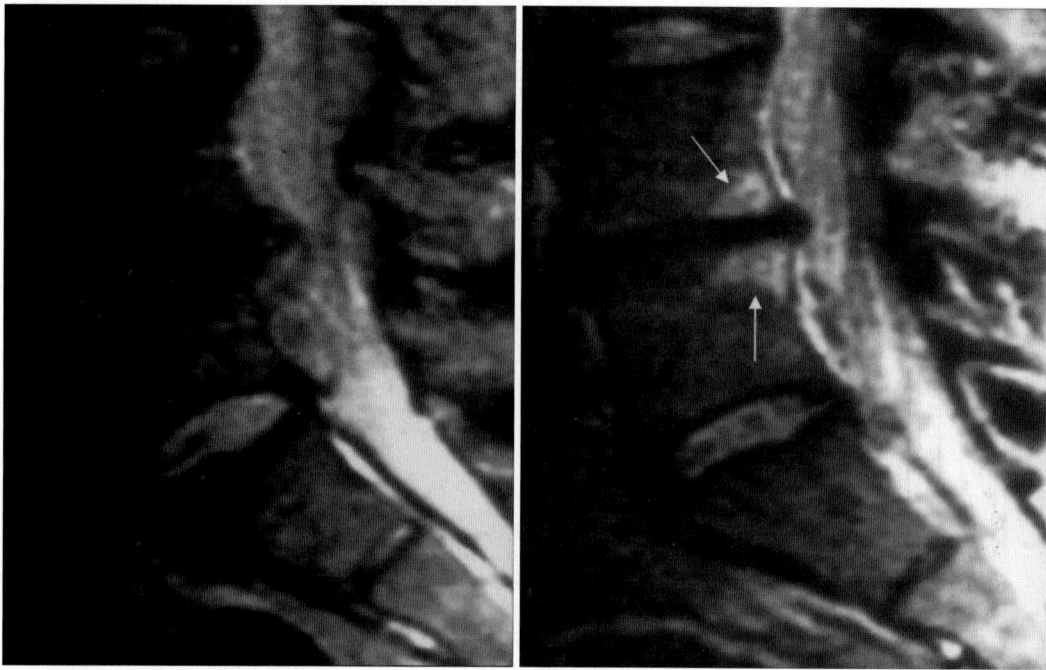

C

**Figure 130.22 *cont'd*** **(B)** Sagittal precontrast and postcontrast enhanced T$_1$-weighted images postoperatively. Note the successful removal of the disc fragment and typical Type I marrow changes of decreased signal of the posterior margins of L4 and L5 *(vertical white arrows)* and enhancement back to normal marrow signal following contrast. There is typical postoperative linear enhancement within the disc *(horizontal white arrows)*. **(C)** Sagittal T$_2$-weighted images preoperative and postoperative. Note the successful removal of the disc and typical high signal within the marrow space of Type II changes *(white arrows)*.

conversion of normal marrow to fibrovascular marrow with low signal on T$_1$-weighted images and high signal on T$_2$-weighted images.[97] Some patients showed no marrow changes between preoperative and postoperative MRI scans, while others exhibited a change to Type I enhancing marrow conversion on the postoperative scan. They emphasized the necessity of understanding normal asymptomatic postoperative changes, and that asymptomatic postoperative disc enhancement coupled with enhancing marrow changes can look similar to osteomyelitis, but can be distinguished from infection by the smooth linear bands of enhancement within the disc. They also reported increased signal from the disc at 3 months postoperatively in 7 of 19 patients who demonstrated disc enhancement; in 6 of these 19 patients there was also an associated decrease in disc space height.

### Spinal Epidural Abscess

One distinct advantage of MRI is its ability to noninvasively detect epidural disease and to demonstrate the presence or absence of a mass effect within the spinal canal. Epidural phlegmon and abscess appear as a mass on MRI. Phlegmon is defined as inflammation of soft tissues with no liquid component or pus. They are usually isointense or hypointense to the spinal cord on T$_1$-weighted images and have high signal on T$_2$-weighted images. However, their appearance can be variable, and they can have mixed signal intensities on T$_1$- and T$_2$-weighted images.[34,110,111,128]

Most of these epidural masses occur adjacent to the level of osteomyelitis and discitis and usually involve two to four vertebral segments.[9,111] Epidural abscesses can be extensive, noncontiguous, and even distant from the site of osteomyelitis. MRI offers a distinct advantage in its ability to easily and noninvasively image the entire spinal column and therefore detect the presence of such distant foci of disease.

Postcontrast MRI exhibits enhancement of the epidural mass. This provides excellent distinction between the high signal enhancing epidural process and the lower signal of the cerebrospinal fluid and spine on T$_1$-weighted images[112] (see Figure 130.17). The administration of contrast aids in differentiating between epidural phlegmon versus abscess. Dense homogeneous enhancement of the mass suggests phlegmon while peripheral or ring enhancement of the mass suggests an abscess.[2,34,128] The author has not found the unenhanced T$_1$- and T$_2$-weighted image signal characteristics to be helpful in differentiating phlegmon from abscess.[34] This distinction clinically may be important since an abscess usually requires surgical decompression and drainage while phlegmon does not.

### Tuberculous Spondylitis

Tuberculous spondylitis may be indistinguishable from pyogenic spondylitis, as discussed above. However, there are distinct imaging characteristics that, when present, should suggest the diagnosis of tuberculous rather than pyogenic spondylitis.[135] Tuberculous osteomyelitis tends to involve the ventral aspect of the vertebral body at the metaphysis. The infectious process tends to spread via the anterior longitudinal ligaments to adjacent vertebral bodies. Involvement of the intervertebral disc is relatively limited compared to the amount of vertebral body involvement (see Figure 130.20). Mycobacterium requires a well-oxygenated environment to survive. It is able to infect the well-oxygenated, well-vascularized environment of the vertebral body but has difficulty invading the intervertebral disc.[25]

### Differential Diagnosis

Many disease entities can mimic vertebral osteomyelitis radiographically. Malignancies, both primary and metastatic, can also be difficult to distinguish from infectious spondylitis.

Type I degenerative marrow changes may mimic vertebral osteomyelitis. In addition, Type I marrow signal intensity changes may enhance following the administration of gadolinium, and enhancement of the central portion of the cervical and lumbar intervertebral discs in unoperated patients does occur in the setting of degenerative disc disease.[123] In advanced disc degeneration, blood vessels once again can be seen within the disc. Usually, the signal intensity of the disc on $T_2$-weighted images helps differentiate the two entities. The disc is usually decreased in signal on $T_2$-weighted images in degenerative disc disease. On occasion in degenerative disc disease, the intervertebral discs may be increased in signal. However, the increased signal is usually linear in configuration. In infectious spondylitis, the distribution of the increased signal intensity on $T_2$-weighted images does not conform to the anatomic configuration of the disc. Clinical history and the presence or absence of ESR helps to differentiate the two entities. Only 4% of patients in a series of 474 patients with degenerative disc disease demonstrated the Type I pattern.[97]

Metastatic disease can be differentiated from vertebral osteomyelitis by its sparing of the intervertebral disc space. Disc involvement with metastatic disease is rare.[63,119] In addition, metastatic disease commonly involves the pedicles of the vertebral body, while osteomyelitic foci tend to be subchondral and do not affect the pedicle.

Primary tumors of the spine are rare compared to metastatic tumors. There are, however, primary tumors of the spine that may involve contiguous vertebral body levels and may therefore have disc involvement. Such tumors include plasmacytoma,[91,92] eosinophilic granuloma,[81] aneurysmal bone cysts,[137] giant cell tumors,[43] and chordoma.[98] Libshitz et al.[76] reported MRI findings in a series of 32 patients with multiple myeloma. On $T_1$-weighted images, the signal intensity of the vertebral body was approximately equal to that of muscle in 14 cases and intermediate between fat and muscle in 18 cases; foci of decreased signal were seen in 8 cases. On $T_2$-weighted images, the marrow signal approximated that of muscle in 17 cases and was intermediate in 15 cases; foci of increased signal were seen in 17 patients. Eosinophilic granuloma presents with lytic vertebral body lesions that can progress to near complete destruction of the vertebral

body or vertebra plana. Despite this, the adjacent intervertebral discs usually remain intact, allowing differentiation from disc space infection. Aneurysmal bone cysts and giant cell tumors of the spine can be characterized by lytic lesions that can span vertebral body levels. However, these tumors usually involve the dorsal elements. These tumors may be more difficult to distinguish from tuberculous spondylitis than from pyogenic spondylitis. Chordomas are uncommon tumors derived from notochordal elements. They can be found throughout the spinal column with a marked propensity for the clivus and sacrococcygeal regions. They are isointense or hypointense in signal on $T_1$-weighted images and increased in signal on $T_2$-weighted images. The intervertebral disc and adjacent vertebral bodies are commonly affected. A paraspinal soft tissue mass is often present.[98]

Spinal neuroarthropathy is most commonly related to tabes dorsalis, syringomyelia, or diabetes mellitus and can be difficult to differentiate from infectious spondylitis on plain films and CT. Park et al.[108] found MRI to be useful for distinguishing between the two entities. MRI in neuropathy demonstrated hypointensity in the abnormal disc and adjacent vertebral bodies on both $T_1$- and $T_2$-weighted sequences. In neuroarthropathy, the disc space and surrounding marrow were of lower signal intensity on $T_2$-weighted images than seen in spinal osteomyelitis.

Wagner et al.[141] evaluated the plain film, CT, and MRI findings in 14 patients with spinal neuroarthropathy versus 19 patients with disc space infection. They found that facet involvement with narrowing or erosions and vacuum disc were more common in spinal neuroarthropathy on imaging studies and rare in disc space infection. Vertebral body spondylolisthesis, osseous joint debris, joint disorganization, disc rim enhancement, and diffuse vertebral body enhancement were more frequent imaging findings in spinal neuroarthropathy.

Spondyloarthropathy has been described in patients undergoing long-term hemodialysis.[68,101,115] Plain film changes include disc space narrowing and irregular end plate destruction. This entity typically demonstrates decreased signal from the disc on $T_2$-weighted images and absence of an associated soft tissue mass that helps to distinguish it from vertebral osteomyelitis. Distinction between these two entities may be difficult since the sedimentation rate is typically elevated in both groups. Intervertebral disc biopsy may be required.

Patients with ankylosing spondylitis can develop pseudoarthrosis following fracture of the spine, which can mimic disc space infection.[46] It is usually seen at the thoracolumbar junction. Radiographic and CT findings of ankylosing spondylitis are difficult to differentiate from discitis. On MRI, the pseudoarthrosis exhibits an increased signal on $T_2$-weighted images. Low signal intensity bands may be seen adjacent to the high signal intensity pseudoarthrosis on $T_2$-weighted images that correlate with sclerosis seen on plain films. The remainder of the vertebral bodies are bright on $T_2$-weighted images due to marrow edema. In addition, paraspinal soft tissue swelling representing the pseudoarthrosis is also seen. Based on MRI alone, it may be difficult to differentiate pseudoarthrosis from osteomyelitis. However, if extension of the mass to the posterior elements can be demonstrated, this suggests a diagnosis of a pseudoarthrosis rather than discitis.

The diagnosis of vertebral osteomyelitis is critical due to its potential morbidity and mortality. Suspicion on the part of the physician is required in the appropriate clinical setting. Several imaging modalities are available to aid in diagnosis as well as to guide biopsy. In the correct clinical setting, these modalities and combinations of these modalities can be very specific and sensitive for the establishment of the diagnosis of vertebral osteomyelitis.

# REFERENCES

1. Ackerman SJ, Steinberg EP, Bryan RN, et al: Trends in diagnostic imaging for low back pain: has MR imaging been a substitute or add-on? *Radiology* 203:533-538, 1997.
2. Angtuaco EJC, McConnell JR, Chadduck WM, Flanigan S: MR imaging of spinal epidural abscess. *AJNR* 8:879, 1987.
3. Aoki J, Yamamoto I, Kitamura N, et al: End plate of the discovertebral joint: degenerative change in the elderly adult. *Radiology* 164:411-414, 1987.
4. Applebaum GD, Mathisen G: Spinal Brucellosis in a southern California resident. *West J Med* 166(1):61-65, 1997.
5. Atlas SJ, Deyo RA, Patrick DL, et al: The Quebec task force classification for spinal disorders and the severity, treatment, and outcomes of sciatica and lumbar spinal stenosis. *Spine* 21:2885-2892, 1996.
6. Atlas SJ, Deyo RA, Keller RB, et al: The Maine Lumbar Spine Study, part II: one year outcomes of surgical and nonsurgical management of sciatica. *Spine* 21(15): 1777-1786, 1996.
7. Atlas SJ, Deyo RA, Keller RB, et al: The Maine Lumbar Spine Study, part III: one year outcomes of surgical and nonsurgical management of lumbar spinal stenosis. *Spine* 21(15): 1787-1795, 1996.
8. Awad I, Bay JW, Petersen JM: Nocardial osteomyelitis of the spine with epidural spinal cord compression—a case report. *Neurosurgery* 15:254-256, 1984.
9. Baker AS, Ojemann RG, Swartz MN, Richardson EP: Spinal epidural abscess. *N Engl J Med* 293(10):463-468, 1975.
10. Bangert BA, Modic MT, Ross JS, et al: Hyperintense signal of the intervertebral discs on T1WSE imaging. *Radiology* 195:437-443, 1995.
11. Barr RJ, Hannon DG, Adair IV, et al: Cervical osteomyelitis after rigid oesophagoscopy: brief report. *J Bone Joint Surg Br* 70:147, 1988.
12. Batson OV: The function of the vertebral veins and their role in the spread of metastases. *Ann Surg* 112(1): 138-149, 1940.
13. Batson OV. The vertebral vein system. *AJR* 78(2):195-212, 1957.
14. Battie MC, Haynor DR, Fisher LD, et al: Determinants of lumbar disc degeneration. *Spine* 20(24):2601-2612, 1995.
15. Bell GR, Rothman RH: The conservative treatment of sciatica. *Spine* 9:54-56, 1984.
16. Berns DH, Ross JS, Kormos D, Modic MT: The spinal vacuum phenomenon: evaluation by gradient echo MR imaging. *J Comput Assist Tomogr* 15(2):233-236, 1991.
17. Bielecki DK, Sartoris D, Resnick D, et al: Intraosseous and intradiscal gas in association with spinal infection: report of three cases. *AJR Am J Roentgenol* 147:83-86, 1986.
18. Boden SD, Davis DO, Dina TS, et al: Abnormal magnetic resonance scans of the lumbar spine in asymptomatic subjects. *J Bone Joint Surg Am* 72(3):403-408, 1990.
19. Boden SD, Davis DO, Dina TS, et al: Postoperative diskitis: distinguishing early MR imaging findings from normal postoperative disk space changes. *Radiology* 184:765-771, 1992.
20. Bozzao A, Gallucci M, Masciocchi C, et al: Lumbar disc herniation: MR imaging assessment of natural history in patients treated without surgery. *Radiology* 185:135-141, 1992.
21. Broner FA: Spinal infections in the immunocompromised host. *Orthop Clin North Am* 27(1):37-47, 1996.
22. Brown TR, Quinn SF, D'Agostino AN: Deposition of calcium pyrophosphate dehydrate crystals in the ligamentum flavum: evaluation with MR imaging with CT. *Radiology* 178:871-873, 1991.
23. Bush K, Cowan N, Katz DE, et al: The natural history of sciatica associated with disc pathology: a prospective study with clinical and independent radiologic follow-up. *Spine* 17:1205-1212, 1992.
24. Cahill DW, Love LC, Rechtine GR: Pyogenic osteomyelitis of the spine in the elderly. *J Neurosurgery* 74:878-886, 1991.
25. Calderone RR. Overview and classification of spinal infections. *Orthop Clin North Am* 27(1):1-8, 1996.
26. Caragee EJ, Kim DH: A prospective analysis of magnetic resonance imaging findings in patients with sciatica and lumbar disc herniation. *Spine* 22(14):1650-1660, 1997.
27. Castillo M, Malko JA, Hoffman JC: The bright intervertebral disk: an indirect sign of abnormal spinal bone marrow on $T_1$-weighted MR images. *AJNR Am J Neuroradiol* 11:23-26, 1990.
28. Cherkin DC, Deyo RA, Street JH, Barlow W: Predicting poor outcomes for back pain seen in primary care using patients' own criteria. *Spine* 21:2900-2907, 1996.
29. Cherkin DC, Deyo RA, Wheeler K, Ciol MA: Physician variation in diagnostic testing for low back pain. *Arthritis Rheum* 37(1):15-22, 1994.
30. Collis JL: The etiology of cerebral abscess as a complication of thoracic disease. *J Thorac Surg* 13:445, 1944.
31. Colmenero JD, Jimenez-Mejias ME, Sanchez-Lora FJ, et al: Pyogenic tuberculous and brucellar vertebral osteomyelitis: a descriptive and comparative study of 219 cases. *Ann RheumDis* 56(12):709-15, 1997.
32. Coman DR, Delong RD: The role of the vertebral venous system in the metastasis of cancer to the spinal column. *Cancer* 4:610-618, 1951.
33. Cowan NC, Bush K, Katz DE, Gishen P: The natural history of sciatica: a prospective radiological study. *Clin Radiol* 46:7-12, 1992.
34. Dagirmanjian A, Schils J, McHenry M, Modic MT: Vertebral osteomyelitis revisited. *AJR Am J Roentgenol* 167(6):1539-1543, 1996.
35. Darouiche RD, Hamill RJ, Greenberg SB, et al: Bacterial spinal epidural abscess: review of 43 cases and literature survey. *Medicine* 71:369-385, 1992.

36. Deeb ZL, Schimel S, Daffner RH, *et al:* Intervertebral disk-space infection after chymopapain injection. *AJR Am J Roentgenol* 144:671-674, 1985.

37. Dehlinger KR: Salmonella osteomyelitis of the spine associated with abdominal aortic aneurysm. Report of a case. *N Engl J Med* 238:728-732, 1948.

38. Delauche-Cavallier MC, Budet C, Laredo JD, *et al:* Lumbar disc herniation. *Spine* 17(8):927-933, 1992.

39. deRoos A, Kressel H, Spritzer C, *et al:* MR imaging of marrow changes adjacent to end plates in degenerative lumbar disk disease. *AJR Am J Roentgenol* 149:531-534, 1987.

40. Deyo RA, Bigos SJ, Maravilla KR: Diagnostic imaging procedures for the lumbar spine. *Ann Intern Med* 111: 865-867, 1989.

41. Deyo RA: Magnetic resonance imaging of the lumbar spine: terrific test or tar baby? *N Engl J Med* 331:115-116, 1994.

42. Digby JM, Kersley JB: Pyogenic non-tuberculous spinal infection: an analysis of thirty cases. *J Bone Joint Surg Br* 61:47-55, 1979.

43. DiLorenzo N, Spallone A, Nolletti A, Nardi P: Giant cell tumors of the spine: a clinical study of 6 cases, with emphasis on the radiological features, treatment and follow-up. *Neurosurgery* 6:29-34, 1980.

44. Elgazzar AH, Abdel-Dayem HM, Clark JD, Maxon HR: Multimodality imaging of osteomyelitis. *Eur J Nuc Med* 22(9):1043-1063, 1995.

45. Enzmann D: On low back pain. *AJR Am J Neuroradiol* 15:109-113, 1994.

46. Eschleman DJ, Beers GJ, Naimark A, *et al:* Pseudoarthrosis in ankylosing spondylitis mimicking infectious diskitis: MR appearance. *AJNR Am J Neuroradiol* 12:1113-1114, 1991.

47. Fager CA: Identification and management of radiculopathy. *Neurosurg Clin North Am* 4:1-12, 1993.

48. Fernand R, Lee CK: Postlaminectomy disc space infection: a review of the literature and a report of 3 cases. *Clin Orthop* 209:215-218, 1986.

49. Fraser RD, Osti OL, Vernon-Roberts B: Discitis following chemonucleolysis: an experimental study. *Spine* 11(7): 679-687, 1986.

50. Gagnerie F, Tailan B, Euller-Ziegler L, Ziegler G: Intravertebral vacuum phenomenon in multiple myeloma. *Clin Rheumatol* 6(4):597-599, 1987.

51. Gillams AR, Chaddha B, Carter AP: MR appearances of the temporal evolution and resolution of infectious spondylitis. *AJR Am J Roentgenol* 166:903-907, 1996.

52. Gordon EJ: Infection of disc space secondary to fistula from pelvic abscess. *South Med J* 70:114, 1977.

53. Gotuzzo E, Alarcon GS, Bocanegra TS: Articular involvement in human brucellosis: A retrospective analysis of 304 cases. *Semin Arthritis Rheum* 12(2):245-255, 1982.

54. Gratz S: 67Ga-citrate and 99mTc-MDP for estimating the severity of vertebral osteomyelitis. *Nuclear Medicine Communications* 21(1):111-120, 2000.

55. Grenier N, Grossman RI, Schiebler ML, *et al:* Degenerative lumbar disk disease: pitfalls and usefulness of MR imaging in detection of vacuum phenomenon. *Radiology* 164:861-865, 1987.

56. Guyer RD, Collier R, Stith WJ, *et al:* Discitis after discography. *Spine* 13(12):1352-1354, 1988.

57. Hakelius A: Prognosis in sciatica: a clinical follow-up of surgical and nonsurgical treatment. *Acta Orthop Scand* 129(Suppl):5-76, 1970.

58. Henkelman RM, Watts, JF, Kucharczyk W: High signal intensity in MR images of calcified brain tissue. *Radiology* 179:199-206, 1991.

59. Hirsch C, Schajowikz F: Studies on structural changes in the lumbar annulus fibrosus. *Acta Orthop Scand* 22: 185-231, 1952.

60. Hitchon PW, Osenbach RK, Yoj WTC, Menezes AH: Spinal infections. *Clin Neurosurg* 38:373, 1992.

61. Ho PS, Yu S, Sether L, Wagner M, *et al:* Calcification of the nucleus pulposus with pathologic confirmation in a premature infant: abbreviated report. *AJNR Am J Neuroradiol* 10:201-202, 1989.

62. Hodgson AR: Infectious diseases of the spine. In Rothman RH, Simeone FA (eds): *The Spine.* Philadelphia, WB Saunders, 1975, p 567.

63. Hubbard DD, Gunn DR: Secondary carcinoma of the spine with destruction of the intervertebral disk. *Clin Orthop* 88:86-88, 1972.

64. Jaffe HL: *Metabolic, Degenerative and Inflammatory Diseases of Bone and Joints.* Philadelphia, Lea and Febiger, 1972.

65. Jensen M, Brant-Zawadzki M, Obuchowski N, *et al:* MRI of lumbar spine in people without back pain. *N Engl J Med* 331:69-73, 1994.

66. Jinkins JR, Osborn AG, Garrett D Jr, *et al:* Spinal nerve enhancement with Gd-DTPA: MR correlation with the postoperative lumbosacral spine. *AJNR Am J Neuroradiol* 14:383-394, 1993.

67. Kalicke T, Schmitz A, Risse JH, *et al:* Fluorine-18 fluorodeoxyglucose PET in infectious bone diseases: results of histologically confirmed cases. *Eur J Nuc Med* 27(5):524-528, 2000.

68. Kaplan P, Resnick D, Murphey M, *et al:* Destructive noninfectious spondyloarthropathy in hemodialysis patients: a report of four cases. *Radiology* 162:241-244, 1987.

69. Kattapuram SV, Philips WC, Boyd R: CT in pyogenic osteomyelitis of the spine. *AJR Am J Roentgenol* 140:1199, 1983.

70. Keller RB, Atlas SJ, Singer DE, *et al:* The Maine lumbar spine study, part 1: background and concepts. *Spine* 21(15):1769-1776, 1996.

71. Kern RZ, Houpt TB: Pyogenic vertebral osteomyelitis: diagnosis and management. *Can Med Assoc J* 130: 1025-1028, 1984.

72. Kricun R, Kricun M: Computed tomography. In Krichin ME: *Imaging Modalities in Spinal Disorders.* Philadelphia, WB Saunders, 1988, pp 376-467.

73. Kumpan W. Salomonowitz E, Seidl G, Wittich GR: The intravertebral vacuum phenomenon. *Skeletal Radiol* 15: 444-447, 1986.

74. Larde D, Mathieu D, Frija J, *et al:* Vertebral osteomyelitis: disk hypodensity on CT. *AJR Am J Roentgenol* 139:963, 1982.

75. Lester JW, Miller WA, Carter MP, Hemphill JM: MR of childhood calcified herniated cervical disk with spontaneous resorption. *AJNR Am J Neuroradiol* 10:S48-S50, 1989.

76. Libshitz HI, Malthouse SR, Cunningham D, *et al:* Multiple myeloma appearance at MR imaging. *Radiology* 182:833-837, 1992.

77. Lisbona R, Derbekyan V, Novales-Diaz J, et al: Gallium-67 scintigraphy in tuberculous and nontuberculous infections spondylitis. *J Nuc Med* 34:853-859, 1993.

78. Lisbona R, Rosenthall L: Observations on the sequential use of 99mTc-phophate complex and 67Gallium imaging in osteomyelitis, cellulitis, and septic arthritis. *Radiology* 123:123-129, 1977.

79. Lloyd TV, Johnson JC: Infectious cervical spondylitis following traumatic endotracheal intubation. *Spine* 5:478, 1980.

80. Long DM: Decision making in lumbar disc disease. *Clin Neurosurg* 39:36-51, 1992.

81. Madsen JR: Weekly clinicopathological exercises. *N Engl J Med* 326:1070-1076, 1992.

82. Maigne J, Rime B, Delignet B: Computed tomographic follow-up study of forty-eight cases of nonoperatively treated lumbar intervertebral disc herniation. *Spine* 27(9):1071-1074, 1992.

83. Malawski SK: Pyogenic infection of the spine. *International Orthopaedics (SICOT)* 1:125-131, 1977.

84. Maldague BE, Noel HM, Malghem JJ: The intravertebral vacuum cleft: a sign of ischemic vertebral collapse. *Radiology* 129:23-29, 1978.

85. Malter AD, Larson EB, Urban N, Deyo RA: Cost-effectiveness of lumbar discectomy for the treatment of herniated intervertebral disc. *Spine* 21(9):1048-1055, 1996.

86. Masaryk TJ, Boumphrey F, Modic MT, et al: Effects of chemonucleolysis demonstrated by MR imaging. *J Comput Assist Tomogr* 10:917-923, 1986.

87. Masaryk TJ, Ross JS, Modic MT, et al: High resolution of sequestered lumbar intervertebral disks. *AJR Am J Roentgenol* 150:1155-1167, 1988.

88. Mattingly WT, Dillon ML, Todd EP: Cervical osteomyelitis after esophageal perforation. *South Med J* 75:626, 1982.

89. McCarron RF, Wimpee MW, Hudkins PG, Laros GS: The inflammatory effect of nucleus pulposus, a possible element in the pathogenesis of low back pain. *Spine* 12:760-764, 1987.

90. McHenry MC, Duchesneau PM, Keys TF, et al: Vertebral osteomyelitis presenting as spinal compression fracture. *Arch Intern Med* 148:417-423, 1988.

91. McHenry MC, Rehm SJ, Krajewski LP, et al: Vertebral osteomyelitis and aortic lesions: case report and review. *Rev Infect Dis* 13:1184-1194, 1991.

92. Meszaros WT: The many facets of multiple myeloma. *Semin Roentgenol* 9:219-228, 1974.

93. Meyers P, Wiener S: Diagnosis of hematogenous pyogenic vertebral osteomyelitis by magnetic resonance imaging. *Arch Intern Med* 151:683-687, 1991.

94. Mitten RW: Vertebral osteomyelitis in the dog due to nocardia-like organisms. *J Small Animal Pract* 15:563-570, 1974.

95. Modic MT, et al: Morphologic alterations in patients with low back pain vs. those with radiculopathy. Submitted to the RSNA 2002 (abstract).

96. Modic MT, Feiglin DH, Piraino DW, et al: Vertebral osteomyelitis: assessment using MR. *Radiology* 157:157-166, 1985.

97. Modic MT, Masaryk TJ, Ross JS, Carter JR: Imaging of degenerative disk disease. *Radiology* 168:177-186, 1988.

98. Modic MT, Masaryk TJ, Ross JS: *Magnetic Resonance Imaging of the Spine*, ed 2. St Louis, Mosby, 1994.

99. Modic MT, Ross JR, Obuchowski N, et al: Contrast enhanced MR imaging in acute lumbar radiculopathy: a natural history study. *Radiology* 195:429-435, 1995.

100. Modic MT, Steinberg PM, Ross JS, et al: Degenerative disk disease: assessment of changes in vertebral body marrow with MR imaging. *Radiology* 166:193-199, 1988.

101. Naidich JB, Mossey RT, McHeffey-Atkinson B, et al: Spondyloarthropathy from long-term hemodialysis. *Radiology* 167:761-764, 1988.

102. Naul LG, Peet GJ, Maupin WB: Avascular necrosis of the vertebral body: MR imaging. *Radiology* 172:219-222, 1989.

103. Otake S, Matsuo M, Nishizawa S, et al: Ossification of the posterior longitudinal ligament: MR evaluation. *AJNR Am J Neuroradiol* 13:1059-1067, 1992.

104. Ozuna RM, Delamarter RB: Pyogenic vertebral osteomyelitis and post surgical disc space infections. *Orthop Clin* 27(1):87-94, 1996.

105. Palestro CJ, Kim CK, Swyer AJ, et al: Radionuclide diagnosis of vertebral osteomyelitis: indium-111-leukocyte and technetium-99m-methylene diphosphonate bone scintigraphy. *J Nucl Med* 32:1861-1865, 1991.

106. Palestro CJ, Torres MA: Radionuclide imaging in orthopedic infections. *Semin Nucl Med* 27:334-345, 1997.

107. Park WM, McCall IW, O'Brien JP, Webb JK: Fissuring of the posterior annulus fibrosus in the lumbar spine. *Br J Radiol* 52:382-387, 1979.

108. Park Y-H, Taylor JAM, Szollar SM: Imaging findings in spinal neuroarthropathy. *Spine* 19:1499-1504, 1994.

109. Pearce J, Moll JMH: Conservative treatment and natural history of acute lumbar disc lesions. *J Neurol Neurosurg Psychiatry* 30:13-17, 1967.

110. Post MJD, Bowen BC, Sze G: Magnetic resonance imaging of spinal infection. *Rheum Dis Clin North Am* 17(3):773-794, 1994.

111. Post MJD, Quencer RM, Montalvo BM, et al: Spinal infection: evaluation with MR imaging and intraoperative US. *Radiology* 169:765, 1988.

112. Post MJD, Sze G, Quencer RM, et al: Gadolinium-enhanced MR in spine infection. *J Comput Assist Tomogr* 14(5):721-729, 1990.

113. Postacchini F: Spine update: results of surgery compared with conservative management for lumbar disc herniations. *Spine* 21(11):1383-1387, 1996.

114. Quinn SF, Murray W, Clark RA, et al: MR imaging of chronic osteomyelitis. *J Comput Assist Tomogr* 12:113-117, 1988.

115. Rafto SE, Dalinka MK, Schiebler ML, et al: Spondyloarthropathy of the cervical spine in long-term hemodialysis. *Radiology* 166:201-204, 1988.

116. Raglan R, Abdelwahan IF, Braffman B, et al: Posterior spinal tuberculosis: a case report. *AJNR Am J Neuroradiol* 11:612, 1990.

117. Ratcliffe JF: Anatomic basis for the pathogenesis and radiologic features of vertebral osteomyelitis and its differentiation from childhood discitis. *Acta Radiologica Diagn (Stockh)* 26:137-143, 1985.

118. Resnick D, Niyawana G: Osteomyelitis, septic arthritis, and soft tissue infection: the axial skeleton. In Resnick D,

Niyawana G (eds): *Diagnosis of Bone and Joint Disorders,* ed 2. Philadelphia, WB Saunders, 1988, pp 2419-2447.

119. Resnick DE, Niwayama G: Intervertebral disc abnormalities associated with vertebral metastasis: observations in patients and cadavers with prostatic cancer. *Invest Radiol* 13:182-190, 1978.

120. Resnick D, Niwayama G, Guerra J, *et al:* Spinal vacuum phenomena: anatomical study and review. *Radiology* 139-341-348, 1981.

121. Romanick PC, Smith TK, Kopaniky DR, *et al:* Infection about the spine associated with low-velocity-missile injury to the abdomen. *J Bone Joint Surg Am* 67:1195, 1985.

122. Ross JS, Modic MT, Masaryk TJ: Tears of the anulus fibrosus: assessment with Gd-DTPA-enhanced MR imaging. *AJNR Am J Neuroradiol* 10:1251-1254, 1989.

123. Ross JS, Modic MT, Masaryk TJ, *et al:* Assessment of extradural degenerative disease with Gd-DTPA-enhanced MR imaging: correlation with surgical and pathological findings. *AJNR Am J Neuroradiol* 10:1243-1249, 1989.

124. Ross JS, Zepp R, Modic MT: The post-operative lumbar spine: enhanced MR evaluation of the intervertebral disk. *AJNR Am J Neuroradiol* 17:323-331, 1996.

125. Rothman ML, Zoarski GH: Imaging basis of disc space infection. *Sem US, CT, MRI* 14(6):437-445, 1993.

126. Saal JA, Saal JS: Nonoperative treatment of herniated lumbar intervertebral disc with radiculopathy: an outcome study. *Spine* 14:431-437, 1989.

127. Saal JA, Saal JS, Herzog RJ: The natural history of lumbar intervertebral disc extrusions treated nonoperatively. *Spine* 15(7):683-686, 1990.

128. Sandhu FS, Dillon WP: Spinal epidural abscess: evaluation with contrast-enhanced MR imaging. *AJNR Am J Neuroradiol* 12:1087-1093, 1991.

129. Sapico FL, Montgomerie JZ: Pyogenic vertebral osteomyelitis: report of nine cases and review of literature. *Rev Infect Dis* 1:754-776, 1979.

130. Sapico FL, Montgomerie JZ: Vertebral osteomyelitis in intravenous drug abusers: report of three cases and review of the literature. *Rev Infect Dis* 2:196-206, 1980.

131. Schlaeffer F, Mikolich DJ, Mates SM: Technetium-99m diphosphate bone scan. False normal findings in elderly patients with hematogenous vertebral osteomyelitis. *Arch Intern Med* 147:2024-2026, 1987.

132. Sharif HS, Clark DC, Aabed MY, *et al:* Granulomatous spinal infections: MR imaging. *Radiology* 177:101-107, 1990.

133. Sharif HS, Morgan JL, Alshahed MS, Al Thagafi YA: Role of CT and MR imaging in the management of tuberculous spondylitis. *Radiol Clin North Am* 33(4):787-794, 1995.

134. Smith AS, Blaser SI: Infectious and inflammatory processes of the spine. *Radiol Clin North Am* 29:809, 1991.

135. Smith AS, Weinstein MA, Mizushima A, *et al:* MR imaging characteristics of tuberculous vs vertebral osteomyelitis. *AJR Am J Roentgenol* 153:399-405, 1989.

136. Sox H, Stern S, Owens D, Abrams HL: *Assessment of Diagnostic Technology in Health Care: Rationale, Methods, Problems and Directions.* Washington DC, National Academy, 1989.

137. Stillwell WT, Fielding JW: Aneurysmal bone cyst of the cervicodorsal spine. *Clin Orthop* 187:144-146, 1984.

138. Thomas M, Grant N, Marshall J, Stevens J: Surgical treatment of low backache and sciatica. *Lancet* 2: 1437-1439, 1983.

139. Tokumoto JIN, Jacobs RA: Case report: nocardia osteomyelitis. *Am J Med Sci* 307(6):428-433, 1994.

140. Van Lom KJ, Kellerhouse LE, Pathria MN, *et al:* Infection vs tumor in the spine: criteria for distinction with CT. *Radiology* 166:851, 1988.

141. Wagner SC: Can imaging findings help differentiate spinal neuropathic arthropathy from disc space infection? *Radiology* 214(3):693-699, 2000.

142. Weaver P, Lifeso RM: The radiological diagnosis of tuberculosis in the adult spine. *Skeletal Radiol* 12:178, 1984.

143. Weber H: Lumbar disc herniation: a controlled, prospective study with ten years of observation. *Spine* 8:131-140, 1983.

144. Weber H, Holme I, Amlie E: The natural course of acute sciatica, with nerve root symptoms in a double blind placebo-controlled trial evaluating the effect of piroxicam (NSAID). *Spine* 18:1433, 1993.

145. Whalen JL, Brown ML, McLeod R, *et al:* Limitations of indium leukocyte imaging for the diagnosis of spine infections. *Spine* 16:193-197, 1991.

146. Wiesel SW, Tsourmas N, Feffer HL, *et al:* A study of computer-assisted tomography. I. The incidence of positive CT scans in an asymptomatic group of patients. 1984 Volvo Award in Clinical Sciences. *Spine* 9(6): 549-551, 1984.

147. Wiley AM, Trueta J: The vascular anatomy of the spine and its relationship to pyogenic vertebral osteomyelitis. *J Bone Joint Surg Br* 41(4):796-809, 1959.

148. Yu S, Haughton VM, Ho PSP, *et al:* Progressive and regressive changes in the nucleus pulposus. II. The adult. *Radiology* 169:93-97, 1988.

149. Yu S, Haughton VM, Sether LA, *et al:* Criteria for classifying normal and degenerative lumbar intervertebral disks. *Radiology* 170:523-526, 1989.

150. Yu S, Haughton VM, Sether LA, Wagner M: Annulus fibrosis in bulging intervertebral disks. *Radiology* 169: 761-763, 1988.

151. Zeidman SM, Thompson K, Ducker TB: Complications of cervical discography: analysis of 4400 diagnostic disc injections. *Neurosurgery* 37(3):414-417, 1995.

# CHAPTER 131

# Preoperative Imaging for Thoracic and Lumbar Spine Surgery

**Christopher B. Shields, Christopher M. Boxell, Frank J. Tomecek, and Stanley Pelofsky**

The diagnosis of most spinal disorders does not require imaging studies. The patient's history and physical examination are the clinician's most important diagnostic tools. Based on the results of the clinical evaluation, imaging studies may be obtained to confirm the suspected diagnosis. Radiographic abnormalities must never be interpreted without clinical correlation. Clinicians must avoid the trap of making decisions about the patient's therapy based on imaging studies alone; rather, they should use imaging studies as adjuncts to aid treatment.[66] For example, multiple congenital and acquired abnormalities, which are clinically irrelevant, are often noted on spine radiographs in asymptomatic persons.

Diagnostic tests (radiographic or other) should be performed only if the results will provide information that influences the patient's treatment. The indiscriminate and inappropriate use and timing of tests may lead to erroneous and dangerous intervention.

Throughout this text, great emphasis is placed on the importance of complication avoidance in spine surgery, based on radiographic imaging studies. The best method of preventing complications is careful review of all imaging studies preoperatively because they constitute the anatomic road map that helps the surgeon avoid dangerous mishaps intraoperatively.

The challenges to the clinician in today's medical arena of cost containment and managed care are (1) to be knowledgeable about the advantages and disadvantages of the available imaging studies and (2) to decide which studies will confirm the diagnosis at the lowest cost and least risk to the patient.

The person who orders the imaging tests should know about the natural history of the disease in question. For example, if a lumbar disc herniation is suspected in a patient with symptoms of less than 6 weeks' duration, it is unlikely that surgery would be performed. Consequently, it would be inappropriate to perform imaging studies because this period is considered the "do-nothing stage" with respect to imaging studies for disc herniation.[66]

Perhaps the most controversial and clinically challenging area of spine surgery is the diagnosis and treatment of low back pain, sciatica, and the failed back syndrome. This chapter focuses on preoperative imaging techniques that may be used to aid the surgeon in treating diseases of the lumbar spine in a safe and expeditious manner.

Since the 1970s, the number of effective imaging techniques for diseases of the thoracolumbar spine has increased, thereby enabling the surgeon to develop effective treatment plans for each patient. These procedures have also enabled spine surgeons to acquire precise knowledge of the spinal anatomy and its variations, as well as the information necessary to avoid intraoperative complications. The surgeon, in conjunction with the neuroradiologist, should review a variety of appropriate imaging studies before surgery, including thoracic and lumbar spine radiographs, computed tomography (CT), magnetic resonance imaging (MRI), CT-myelography, and lumbar discography. Occasionally, bone scans and spinal angiography may also be of value in planning surgical treatment.

This chapter focuses on thoracic and lumbar imaging because of the complex nature of the anatomy and the relative greater importance of imaging with respect to the preoperative decision-making process for this region.

## Plain Radiographs

Plain lumbar and thoracic spine radiographs should be part of the imaging investigation of back pain. Regrettably, they are often omitted. This is a dangerous oversight, because several bony abnormalities may be identified only by careful study of plain spine radiographs. Four views of the lumbar spine are routinely imaged in most centers: one ventrodorsal view, one lateral view, and two oblique views.[27] In a primary care setting, the frequency of confirming a diagnosis on a plain radiograph that required surgical treatment was only 0.2%.[55] In a tertiary referral practice, the probability of plain spine radiographs significantly affecting a specific diagnosis was 18%. Additional information that was not recognized by anteroposterior (AP) and lateral projections was obtained from the oblique views of the lumbar spine in only 4 of 86 pediatric patients. Thus oblique views usually are not obtained for pediatric patients.[82]

Rhea et al.[81] studied the lumbar spine radiographs of 200 adults and found that additional information was obtained from the oblique views in only 2% of the patients. Liang and Komaroff[55] recommend that only those patients who complain of low back pain and who have one of the following characteristics should have plain spine radiographs taken: (1) less than 65 years of age, (2) a history of fever and weight loss, (3) sustained significant trauma, (4) a history of substance abuse (e.g., alcohol, intravenous [IV] drugs), (5) systemic malignancy, (6) severe pain, or (7) neurologic complaints that involve the lower extremities. Plain spine radiographs can indicate the presence of osteoporosis that may be associated with compression fractures and back pain. It is unusual to observe disc calcification; however, if disc calcification is noted in the thoracic spine, it is more suggestive of a ruptured disc than if found in the cervical or lumbar areas. The presence of multiple disc calcifications in either the thoracic or the lumbar region raises the suspicion of ochronosis, pseudogout, degenerative disc disease, and infection.

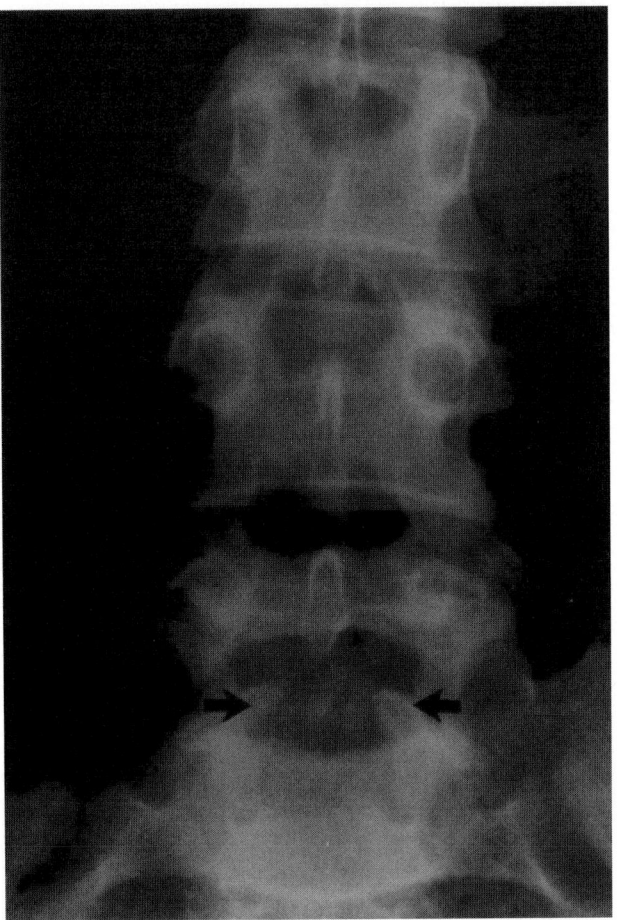

**Figure 131.1** Anteroposterior view of the lumbosacral spine with arrows on both sides of the defective lamina (spina bifida occulta). Failure to recognize this condition may result in damage to the nerve roots during the process of stripping muscle from the laminae.

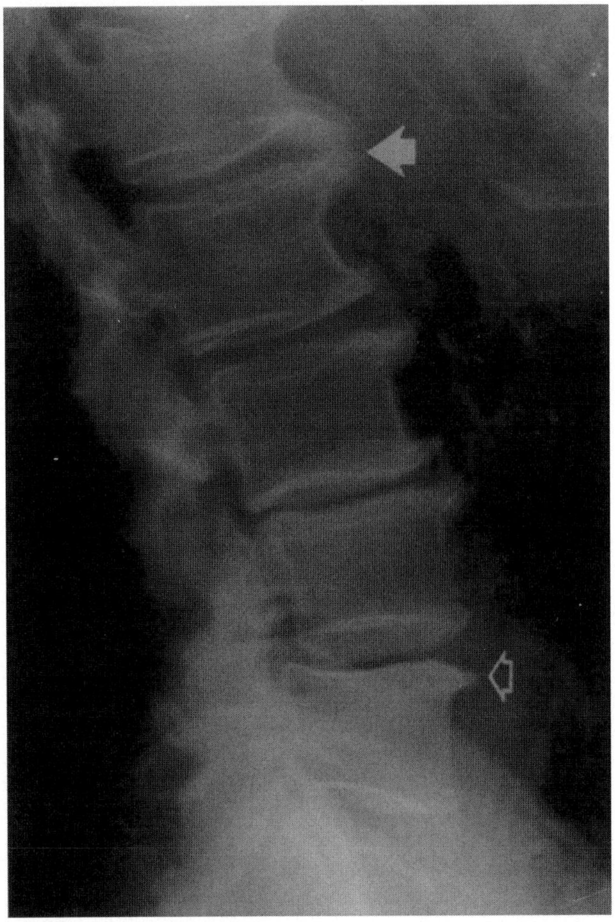

**Figure 131.2** Solid arrow points toward claw spurs on the adjacent ventral aspect of L1 and L2, and the open arrow points toward a traction spur on the anterosuperior margin of the L5 vertebral body.

Patients scheduled to undergo surgery of the thoracic or lumbar spine should always have preoperative plain radiographs taken of the level on which the surgeon is to operate. Spina bifida occulta or prior laminectomy must be recognized before proceeding with surgery (Figure 131.1). The absence of intact laminar arches must be noted to avoid the possibility of plunging a periosteal elevator through the defect in the laminar arches during surgery. This could result in a dural tear and disastrous damage to neural elements within the spinal canal.

Several types of bony spurs projecting from the lumbar vertebral bodies may be noted on lateral radiograms. Traction spurs project ventrally approximately 5mm from the vertebral end plate and usually are an indication of segmental spinal instability (SSI)[55] (Figure 131.2). These spurs arise from mechanical tensile stress at the outer annular fibers at the site of attachment to the vertebral body, from microhemorrhage, and from calcification of peripheral fibers of the annulus fibrosus.[57] Claw spurs (see Figure 131.2) occur at the level of the end plates of the vertebral body and are a result of axial loading on the annulus fibrosus. Claw spurs are considered a more benign finding than traction spurs. Calcification of the annulus fibrosus across the entire disc space results in

fusion of the adjacent vertebra, at which time the symptoms of SSI may resolve.[50]

Spinal stenosis secondary to spondylosis may result in any of the following singly or in combination: (1) narrow disc space, (2) osteoarthritic spurs, (3) narrowed interlaminar space, (4) hypertrophy of the ligamentum flavum, (5) protrusion of the annulus fibrosus, and (6) hypertrophy and subluxation of the facet joints.[93] Symptoms develop earlier in those patients with congenital lumbar spinal stenosis (i.e., a ventrodorsal diameter less than 10mm); normal is 27 to 33mm. These degenerative changes create an abnormal position for the *joint-body line,* a line coursing along the caudal surface of a vertebral body on lateral lumbar spine radiographs (Figure 131.3). Normally, this line should pass rostral to the tip of the superior articular process of the adjacent caudal vertebra. In patients with moderate to severe degenerative disc disease and changes consistent with lumbar spinal stenosis, the joint-body line passes through the facet joint.

Disc space narrowing and degenerative bone changes at multiple levels of the lumbar spine may be of little clinical significance. However, these changes are occasionally the cause of intractable low back pain, requiring surgery. Operations on one or two levels of the lumbar spine,

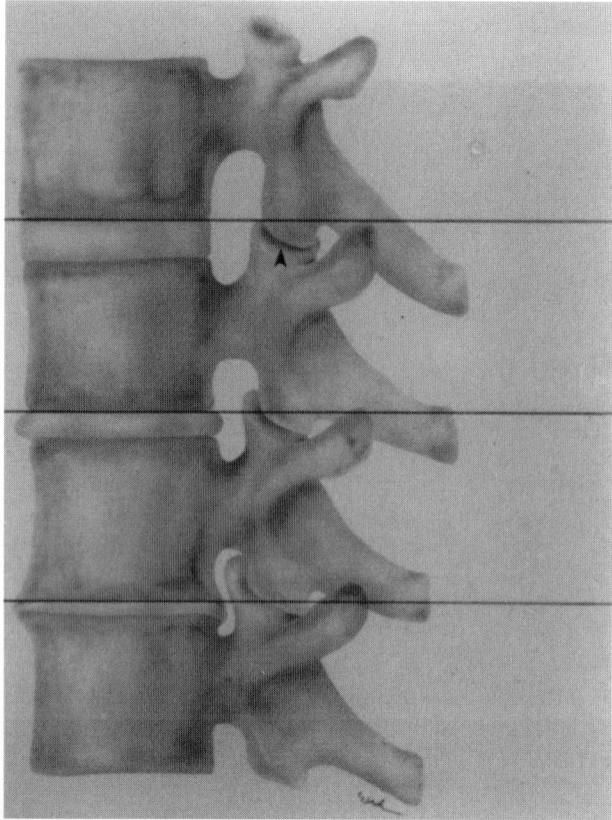

**Figure 131.3** Composite drawing of the lateral lumbar spine with a line drawn along the caudal surface of the vertebral body and continued dorsally through the dorsal articular joint (*arrowhead*). In the presence of the normal upper disc, the dorsal line passes above the articular joint. In the presence of the moderately degenerative middle disc, the line passes through the articular joint. In the presence of the severely degenerative lower disc, the line passes through the lower aspect of the articular joint.

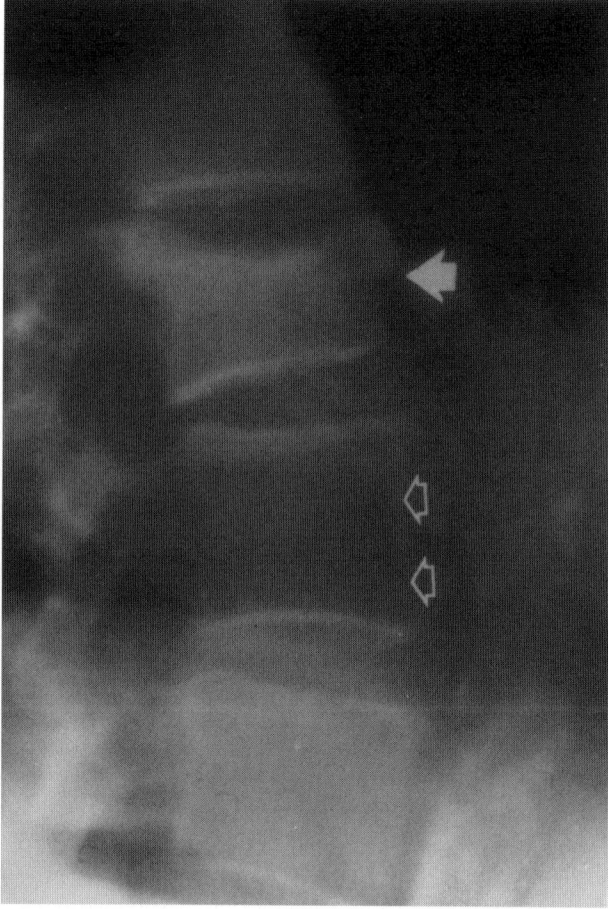

**Figure 131.4** Lateral view of the lumbar spine showing the presence of a pathologic compression fracture of L1 vertebral body (*solid arrow*) secondary to metastatic tumor. The L2 vertebral body shows osteolytic change secondary to metastatic tumor infiltration (*open arrows*).

particularly if a fusion is performed, may increase the degree of biomechanical stress on levels adjacent to the fusion. If the levels adjacent to the fusion demonstrate degenerative disc disease preoperatively, the additional biomechanical stress placed on them after surgery will likely accelerate the rate of progressive degenerative changes. Recurrent symptoms of low back pain (with or without neurologic symptoms) after lumbar spine fusion may occur several years later as adjacent levels undergo progressive degeneration.

Ventrodorsal and lateral plain radiographs are of value in determining the alignment of the vertebrae and pedicles. Plain radiographs of the lumbar spine are the optimal imaging modality for detecting spondylolisthesis,[4,103] fractures, osteolytic neoplasms (Figure 131.4), and osteoblastic neoplasms (Figure 131.5). Meyerding[65] has classified spondylolisthesis into four grades. In this classification, the ventrodorsal diameter of the vertebral body is divided into four segments. *Grade I* spondylolisthesis represents a ventral slip of the upper vertebra over the lower vertebra ranging from 0% to 25% of the ventrodorsal diameter of the vertebral body. In *grade II* spondylolisthesis, the slip ranges from 25% to 50%. In *grade III*, the slip is from 50% to 75%, and in *grade IV*, the slip is 75% to 100%. In

spondylolisthesis, the dorsocaudal margin of the upper vertebra has slipped completely over the ventral-rostral margin of the next lower vertebra.

Retrolisthesis occurs much less commonly than anterolisthesis and is characterized by the upper vertebra slipping dorsally with respect to the lower vertebra. Spondylolisthesis may occur secondary to spondylolysis. The latter is diagnosed by oblique lumbar spine radiographs that demonstrate the defect in the pars interarticularis ("Scottie dog" sign) (Figure 131.6). This defect is usually observed bilaterally.

SSI occurs when the movement between adjacent vertebrae exceeds the physiologic range. Clinically significant SSI is often recognized on lateral spine radiographs. Spinal instability may be caused by degenerative disc disease or trauma, or it can be iatrogenic in origin after a lumbar discectomy or facetectomy as part of a decompressive laminectomy. Radiographic evidence of lumbar SSI can be noted by obtaining flexion-extension radiographs (lateral view) of the lumbar spine and measuring the amount of motion between adjacent vertebrae. If there is more than 4.5mm of motion between the dorsal margins of adjacent vertebral bodies, SSI is present.[104] Use of dynamic lateral lumbar spine radiographs increases the ability to recognize

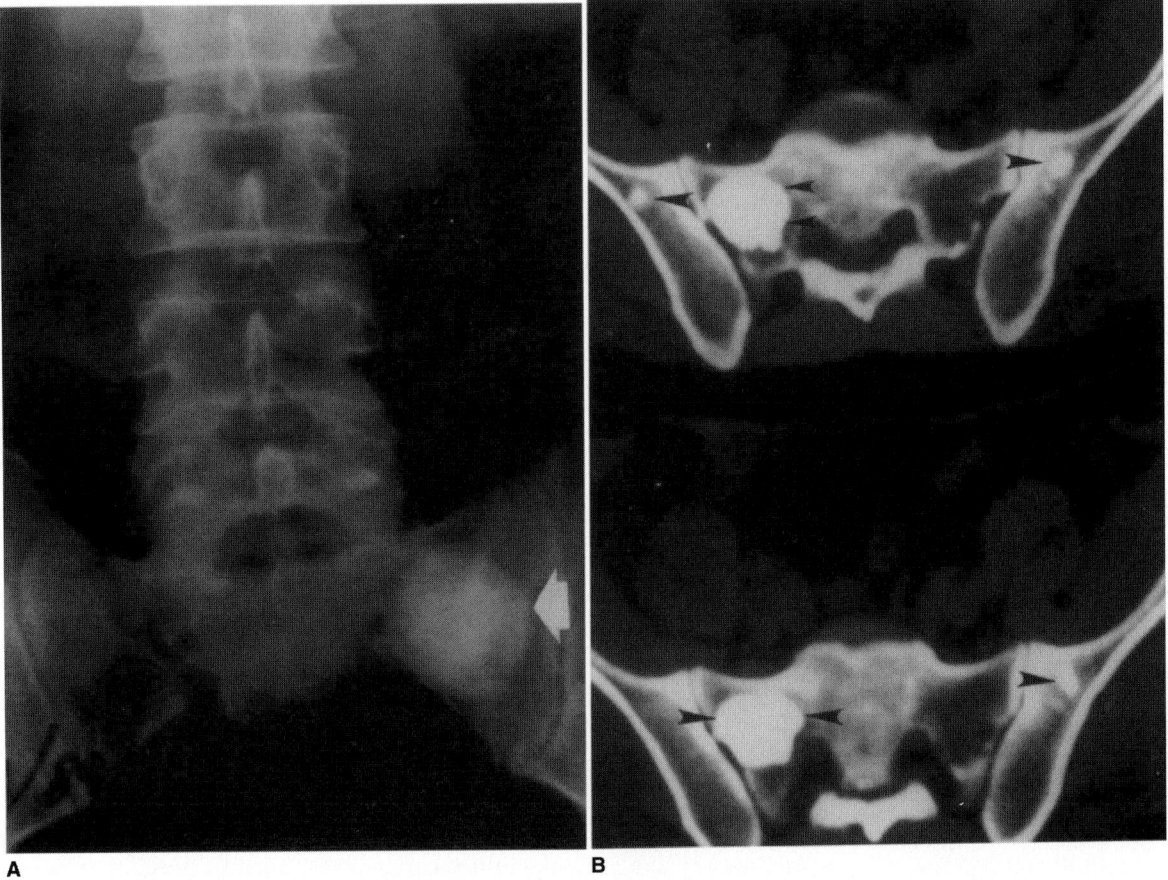

**Figure 131.5** (**A**) Anteroposterior view of the lumbar spine and pelvis showing a large osteoblastic mass in the left ala of the sacrum (*arrow*). This proved to be a metastatic deposit from a renal cell tumor. (**B**) A computed tomographic scan of the pelvis (two cuts) of the same patient showing multiple osteoblastic masses (*arrowheads*).

SSI radiographically.[51] This may be performed by having the patient sit on a low footstool and bend forward as far as possible while a lateral lumbar spine radiograph is taken. Another lateral radiograph is taken in the standing hyperextended position. The difference in vertebral body alignment between these two radiographs is a measure of the degree of SSI. The presence of excessive movement noted on dynamic flexion-extension radiographs may identify the segmental level thought to be the generator site of back pain. When intractable back pain exists, the presence of SSI often indicates the need for spine fusion across the affected segment.[109]

Ventrodorsal views of the thoracic and lumbar spines indicate the presence of scoliosis. A mild scoliotic curve (less than 15 degrees) is of little concern and may be the result of a unilateral paravertebral muscle spasm secondary to a ruptured disc. A severe degree of scoliosis in association with lateral olisthy (see Figure 53.6) and in conjunction with degenerative spondylosis presents a major technical and surgical challenge. Decompressive laminectomies at the level of lumbar spinal stenosis, without treating the scoliosis, may worsen the severity of the scoliosis by increasing the curvature, thereby exacerbating the patient's symptoms. The presence of lateral olisthy,

with or without scoliosis, noted on plain thoracic or lumbar spine radiographs, is pathognomonic of SSI. This is recognized by noting the alignment of the pedicles of the lumbar spine.

Spinal tumors alter bone structure that must be recognized for the safe surgical removal of the tumor. Vertebral body collapse (pathologic fracture), occurring after a trivial injury, may be the first indication of a neoplasm. This finding may be difficult to differentiate from a vertebral body compression fracture secondary to trauma or osteoporosis. However, radiographic evidence of bone destruction is not apparent until 30% to 50% of the trabecular bone has been destroyed. Widening of the interpedicular distance and erosion of the dorsal vertebral body (scalloping) is often noted with intradural tumors of the spine (i.e., ependymomas, neurofibromas, meningiomas). Neural foraminal erosion by the tumor, as it passes through the intervertebral foramen, is the hallmark of neurofibromas.

Osteoblastic lesions of the spinal axis suggest the presence of an osteoblastic metastatic tumor, which is usually secondary to breast or prostate cancer. Osteolytic bony changes are much more common than osteoblastic changes that suggest the presence of lymphoma, multiple myeloma, aneurysmal bone cyst, giant cell tumor, and

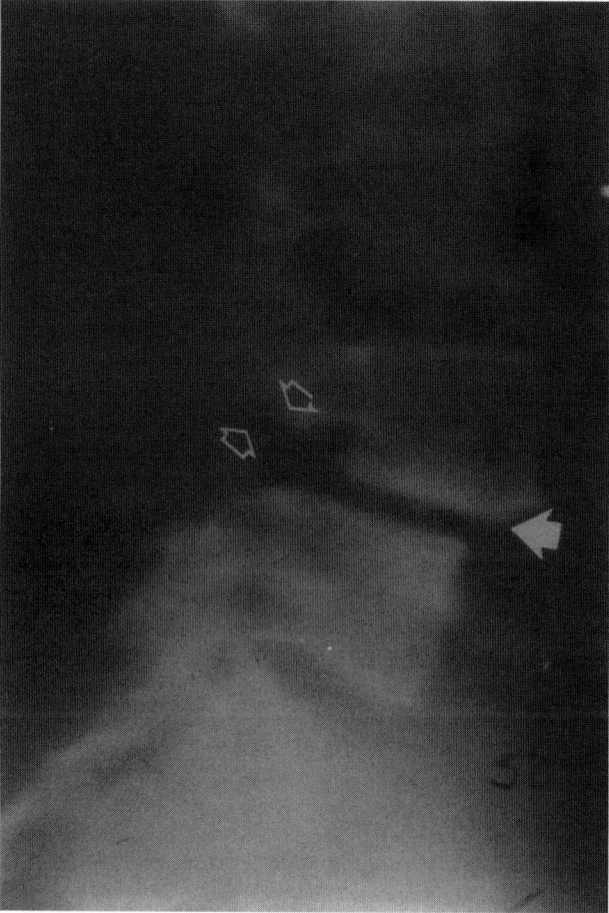

**Figure 131.6** Radiogram of a lateral view of a lumbosacral spine showing grade II spondylolisthesis of L4 on L5 *(solid arrow)*. There is a bony defect *(open arrows)* in the pars interarticularis, causing the forward slip.

metastatic carcinoma. The absence of a sharply defined cortical outline of the pedicle on the AP view of the spine is suggestive of metastatic tumor. Loss of the intact pedicle is known as the *blinking owl sign.*

Metastatic epidural tumors, located dorsal to the dural sac, often erode the laminar arch. At times, only a thin shell of outer laminar cortex remains. If the surgeon is unaware of this bony defect, forceful use of the periosteal elevator may result in plunging through the defect into the dural sac. To prevent this from occurring, the surgeon should use sharp dissection and apply minimal pressure against the bone during muscle stripping from the spinous processes and laminar arches.

Plain thoracic and lumbar spine radiographs are helpful for diagnosing fractures after trauma. Lateral spine radiographs are ideally suited for demonstrating the presence of a compression fracture of the vertebral body, as well as spinous process fractures. Often, the lateral view also demonstrates a paraspinous hematoma adjacent to the fractured vertebra. AP views of the spine are best suited for the confirmation of the presence of a fracture of the transverse processes. A fracture through the transverse process should alert the surgeon to the possibility of renal injury, because this type of fracture is usually a result of direct trauma to the dorsal lumbar area.

Although plain radiographs are ideal for the visualization of fractures of the transverse processes, CT (bone windows) is necessary for the visualization of some fractures of the facets, pedicles, and laminae. In the presence of significant interspinous ligament injury, with or without dislocation, widening of the interspinous distance is noted on lateral radiograms. Loss of the normal lumbar lordosis suggests the presence of splinting of the spine by paravertebral muscle spasm. This may be caused by a lumbar spine fracture.

Several anatomic classifications of thoracic and lumbar fractures have been described by Bedbrook,[6] Denis,[23] Holdsworth,[42] Nicholl,[70] and Whitesides and Shah.[107] CT and anatomic studies allow clinicians to divide the spine into three columns (anterior, middle, and posterior).[23,60] The *anterior column* consists of the anterior longitudinal ligament, the ventral half of the disc, the ventral half of the annulus fibrosus, the anterior longitudinal ligament, and the vertebral body. The *middle column* consists of the dorsal half of the disc, the dorsal half of the annulus fibrosus, the vertebral body, and the posterior longitudinal ligament. The *posterior column* consists of the dorsal elements of the spinal axis (facets, pedicles, and spinous processes; supraspinous and interspinous ligaments; facet joint capsules; and laminar arches). A wedge compression fracture of the vertebral body consists of destruction of the anterior column (and the posterior column); a burst fracture consists of a disruption of the anterior and middle columns; and a fracture-dislocation results from a fracture of all three columns.[23] A burst fracture often is associated with retropulsion of bone into the spinal canal. Stability or instability of a thoracolumbar fracture depends on the status of the middle column. If a fracture and failure of ligamentous integrity occurs through the middle column, the injury is considered by some to be unstable.[23] Thoracic fractures are usually stable because of the support provided by the thoracic cage. Thoracolumbar fractures (T10-L2) are often unstable as a result of large stresses applied to this area caused by the transition from the relatively nonmobile thoracic to the more mobile lumbar spine. This is important information for the surgeon to know when treating patients with spine injuries, particularly when he or she is assessing whether to mobilize the patient.

*Postinfectious discitis* is manifested by sclerosis and irregularity of the vertebral body end plates and by collapse of the disc space. Ultimately, fusion may occur across the disc space.[74] Fusion across the disc space may also be noted in patients with rheumatoid arthritis and ankylosing spondylitis.

*Venous hemangiomas* of the vertebral bodies are identified by vertical striations through them, as noted on plain radiograms. These lesions are usually of little clinical significance. However, if the end plate of a vertebra harboring a venous hemangioma is curetted during lumbar discectomy, severe hemorrhage may occur. If a vertebral body hemangioma is present on either side of a disc that is being removed, the surgeon must take care to avoid vigorous curettage through the cartilaginous end plate. Occasionally, vertebral body venous hemangiomas may be associated with an epidural soft tissue component. This may cause spinal cord or cauda equina compression with neurologic deficits.

Plain radiographs of the sacral and sacroiliac joints may reveal the presence of sacroiliitis, suggestive of early ankylosing spondylitis.[79] Additional angled pelvic radiographs, with the beam directed down the sacroiliac joint, should enable the diagnosis of sacroiliitis in 70% to 80% of patients. The presence of sacroiliitis may not be visible on plain radiographs in all patients with ankylosing spondylitis; CT scans are more helpful in detecting early sacroiliitis. A technetium bone scan is also sensitive enough to suggest this diagnosis in the early stages.

## CT-Myelography

The optimal radiographic study for imaging thoracic and lumbar intraspinal abnormalities is the CT-myelogram, using a water-soluble, absorbable, radiopaque contrast agent.[2] Although many centers use MRI or CT alone, the combination of CT and myelography provides an excellent roadmap for surgery of the thoracic and lumbar spine. For thoracic and lumbar myelograms, 10 to 16ml of iohexol (Omnipaque) (180 to 240mg/ml) is inserted at the dorsal midline L2-3 level with a 25-gauge needle.

Before performing this test, the clinician should take a careful history and should evaluate the patient's medications. If there is a history of seizures, the patient's blood level of anticonvulsant medication should be in the therapeutic range. Drugs that might lower the seizure threshold, such as monoamine oxidase inhibitors, tricyclic antidepressants, and phenothiazines, should be discontinued several days before the study. Approximately 30 minutes before injection of the contrast agent, the patient is given both phenobarbital (60mg intramuscularly) and methylprednisolone sodium succinate (Solu-Medrol) (500mg intravenously). Radiographs are taken in the ventrodorsal, lateral, and oblique projections. Water-soluble contrast agents outline the intradural nerve roots, and the dural sleeves are clearly visible. Weight-bearing radiographs may be taken with the patient in the standing position to exaggerate the appearance of the defect. This technique may be used when searching for a lumbar disc protrusion, especially at the L5-S1 interspace. Disc herniations are occasionally missed at this level on myelography, because of the large spinal canal and the relatively small dural tube. The postmyelographic CT scan increases the visualization of disc herniation. If indicated, flexion-extension myelographic radiographs may be performed. This also accentuates the abnormalities caused by lumbar spinal stenosis.[76] The presence of any radiographic abnormality may not be evident with myelography alone. By performing a thoracic or lumbar CT within 1 to 3 hours after the myelogram, the clinician can obtain additional information. Because some of the contrast agent is absorbed during this 1- to 3-hour interval, an optimal CT image is obtained. The CT is obtained with the patient in the supine position. Consequently, information about the changes that are apparent in the weight-bearing position may not be evident. Patients who undergo a routine CT-myelogram scan may be discharged from the hospital 6 hours after the procedure. Older-adult patients, those with a history of seizures, or those in whom a complete radiographic block is noted on myelography or CT should be kept in the hospital for 24 hours.

Lumbar myelography can also be performed by placing the needle into the C1-2 interspace from a dorsolateral cervical approach, with the contrast agent allowed to descend gradually to the lumbar area. This approach avoids the possibility of promoting neurologic deterioration from spinal herniation caused by alteration of spinal fluid hydrodynamics after placement of contrast agent below a complete spinal block.

The lumbar subarachnoid space usually ends between S1 and S3. Dural pouches (Tarlov's cysts) are subarachnoid cysts that extend along the extraspinal course of the lower lumbar nerve roots. Usually, these are only of anatomic interest and are of no clinical importance.[75] Occasionally, they can be extremely large, causing symptoms of adjacent nerve root compression. Dural pouches may be removed by surgical plication of the dural sheath (Figure 131.7)

Conjoined nerve roots are an anatomic variant, and they have been reported in 1.3% to 10% of studies that involved water-soluble CT-myelography and in 14% of anatomic studies.[30,38,105]

Conjoined nerve roots are the result of a nerve root that departs from the dural tube caudally; courses laterally across the disc; and exits the foramen immediately above, and often splays over, the rostral surface of the caudal pedicle.[38] This abnormality occurs most often at the L5-S1 level, with the L5 nerve root lying over the L5-S1 disc, and may be mistakenly diagnosed as a disc herniation.[78] The conjoined nerve root is fixed and therefore is vulnerable to minimal disc herniations or hypertrophy of the superior articular process. Criteria necessary to make the diagnosis from CT-myelography include the following: (1) asymmetry of the root sleeves, (2) pressure of a broad dural sheath where the roots converge from the dura, and (3) the (conjoined) nerve root taking off at a level midway between the mirror image roots.[105] It is vital to identify this abnormality preoperatively because it is necessary to surgically free up the conjoined nerve root before removing the herniated disc. A high incidence of nerve root damage has been reported after surgery in the presence of a conjoined nerve root.[105] The conjoined nerve root may be "battered" or avulsed. In addition, a portion of the nerve root that is compressed may be overlooked, leading to continued symptoms. White et al.[105] recommend pediculotomy and facetectomy to free up the nerve root before disc removal, thereby avoiding neural damage.

CT-myelogram is the most accurate and most sensitive test to use to diagnose a ruptured lumbar disc.[10] The appearance of a sharply demarcated soft tissue filling defect at the level of the disc space suggests a lumbar disc herniation (Figure 131.8). A ruptured disc may migrate in a rostral or caudal direction or into the intervertebral foramen (Figure 131.9). Such aberrant positions of the disc may raise concerns about an epidural neoplasm. A far lateral disc herniation may be located within or lateral to the intervertebral foramen. This may be missed on myelography, but the postmyelographic CT scan often displays the obliteration of the foramen by the disc tissue. At times it is difficult to differentiate between an exiting nerve root and a foraminal disc herniation, because they often have the same CT density.

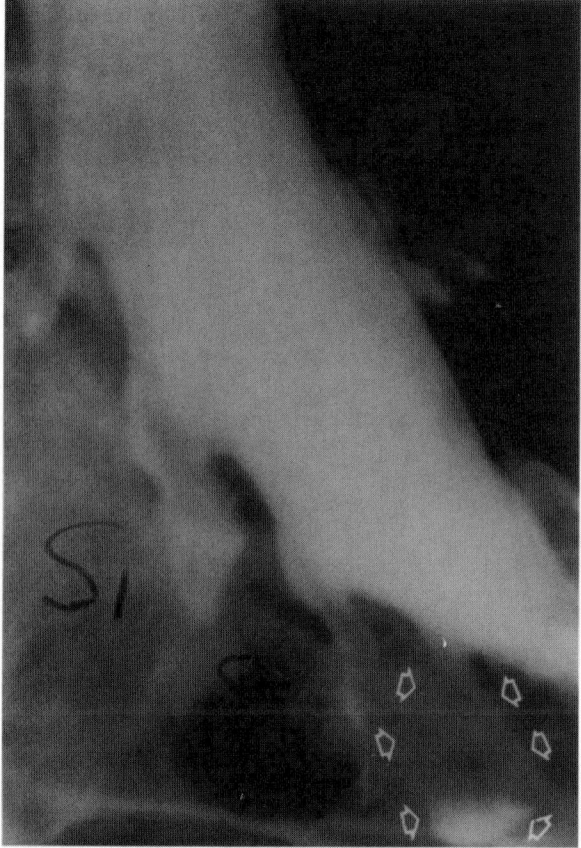

**A**

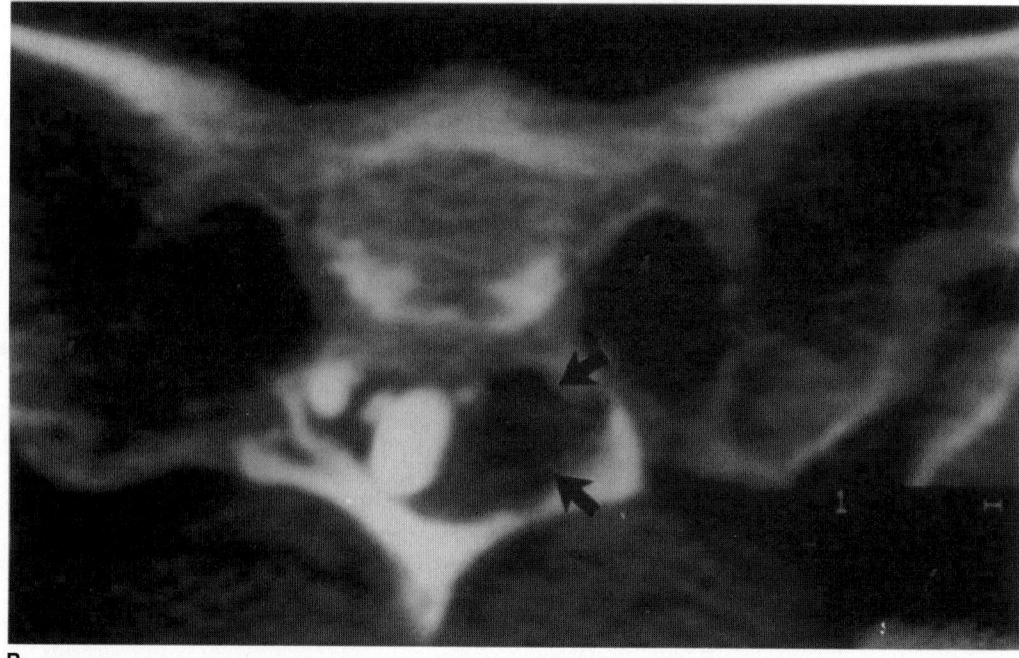

**B**

**Figure 131.7** **(A)** Lateral lumbar myelogram demonstrating contrast filling a nerve root pouch arising from the S1-2 nerve roots *(open arrows)*. **(B)** Postmyelographic computed tomographic scan demonstrating the sacral nerve root pouch *(arrows)* displacing the dural tube from right to left.

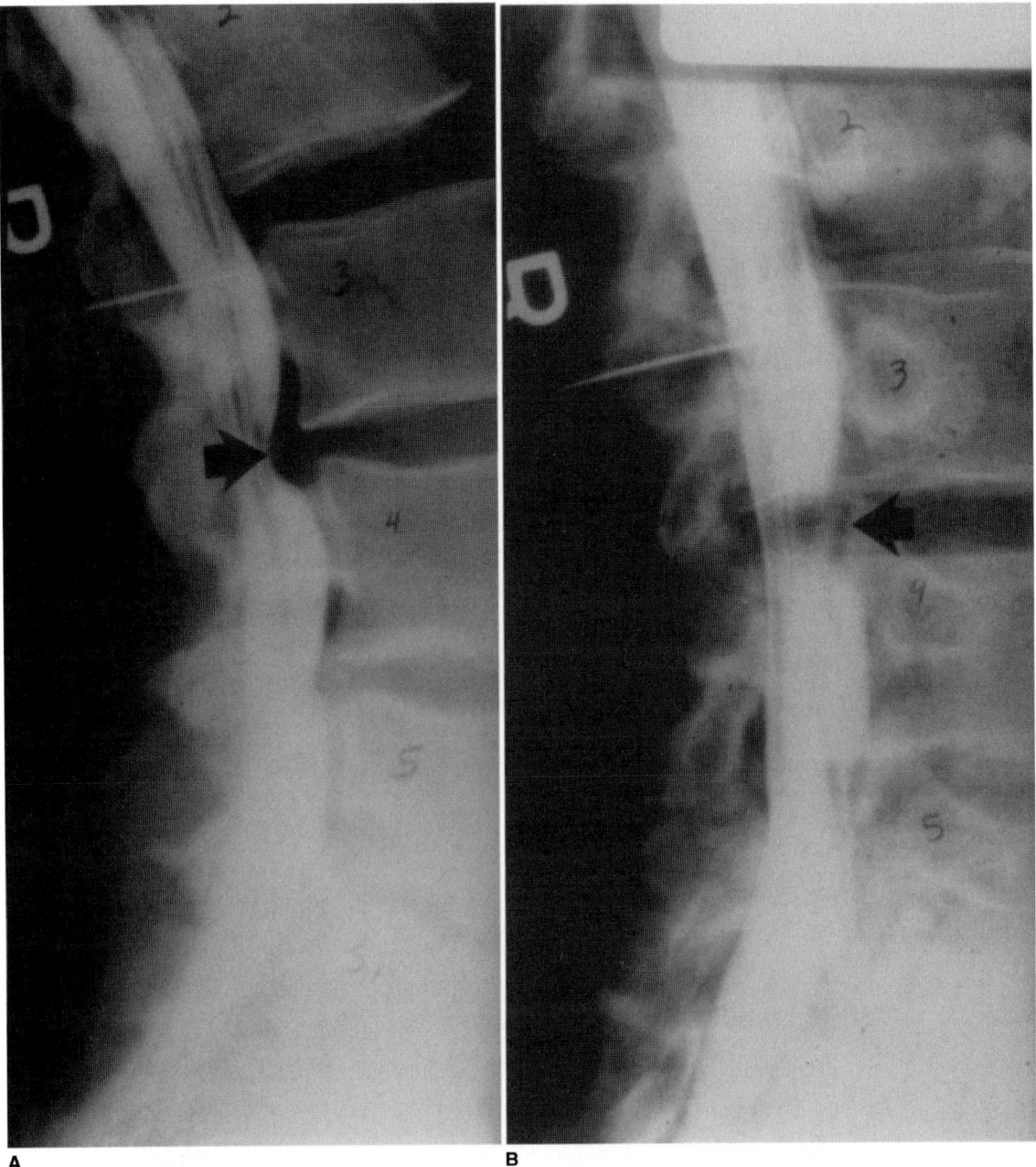

**Figure 131.8** Lateral **(A)** and oblique **(B)** myelogram images showing a disc herniation at the L3-4 interspace, predominantly on the left *(arrow)*.

*Continued*

Lumbar myelography may be technically difficult to perform in the presence of severe spinal stenosis because of narrowing of the diameter of the subarachnoid space. Severe lumbar spinal stenosis, arising secondary to spondylosis, may be associated with disc space collapse and obliteration of the interlaminar space, making insertion of the spinal needle into the lumbar subarachnoid space difficult, if not impossible.

Spinal stenosis refers to the narrowing of the normal spinal canal diameters (i.e., less than 15mm in a ventrodorsal dimension and less than 25mm in a lateral dimension). Spinal stenosis may be developmental, which causes a diffuse narrowing of the spinal canal, or it may be acquired, which usually causes focal or multifocal areas of stenosis. Developmental and acquired stenoses may coexist. This may cause symptoms at a younger age and may be clinically more severe than acquired stenosis alone.

The characteristic myelographic picture of lumbar spinal stenosis is the bilateral extradural compression of the subarachnoid space, which often assumes an hourglass deformity (Figure 131.10). Spinal stenosis may be located in the central spinal canal, causing a decrease of the ventrodorsal diameter of the spinal canal, or it may be lateral, causing a lateral recess and foraminal stenosis (Figure 131.11). On CT-myelography, there is a concentric narrowing of the spinal canal on extension and widening, with

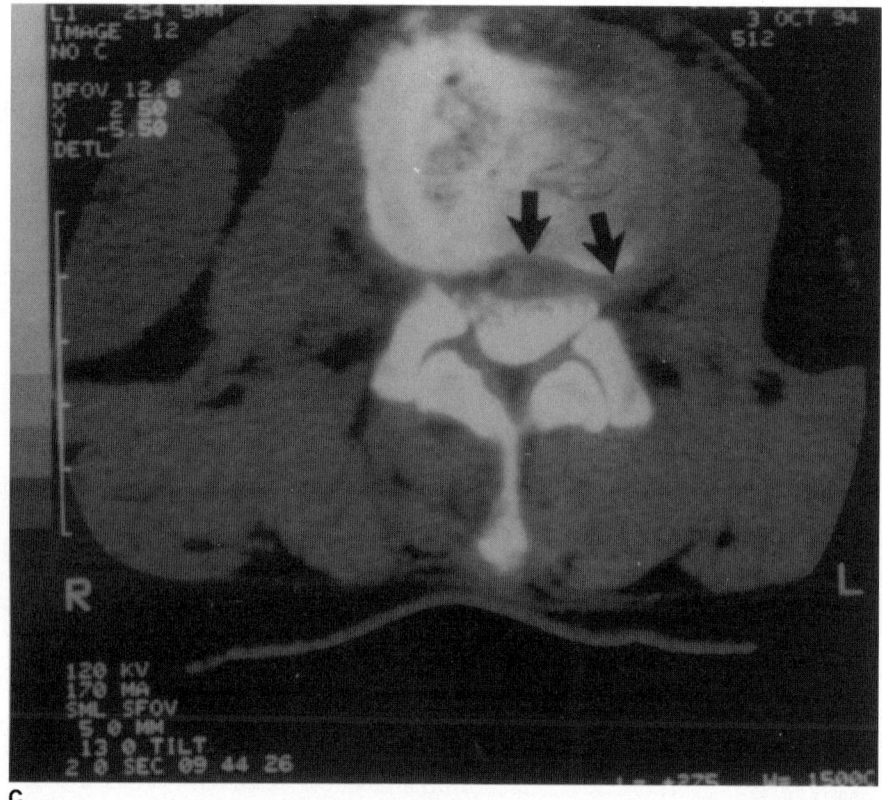

**Figure 131.8** *cont'd* (**C**) Axial computed tomography at L3-4 shows a midline and left lateral disc herniation *(arrows)*.

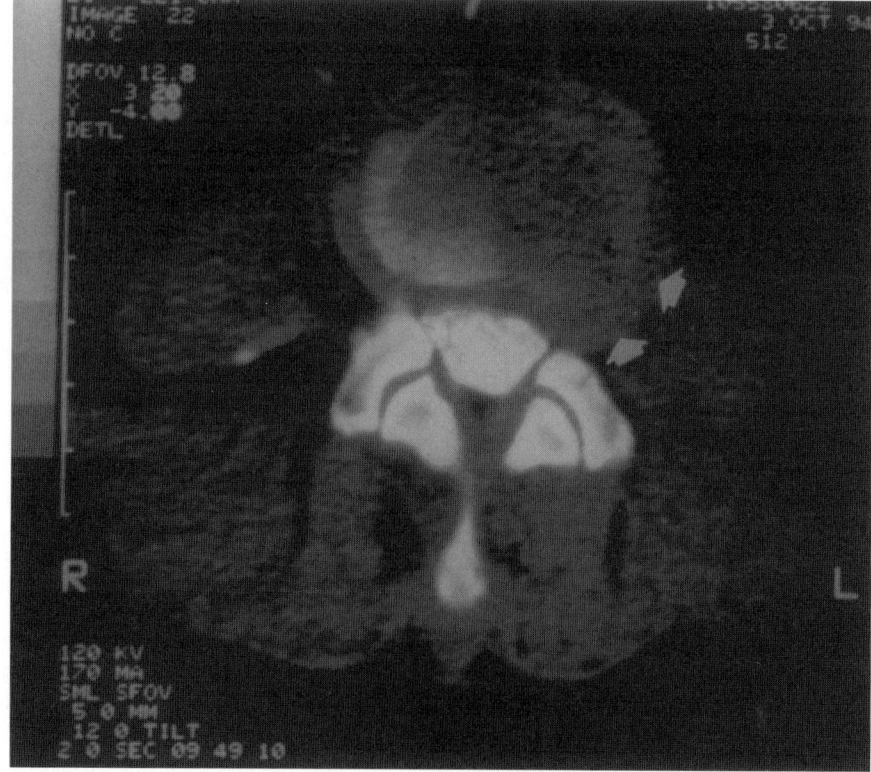

**Figure 131.9** A far lateral disc herniation is observed at the L4-5 disc space on the left *(arrows)*.

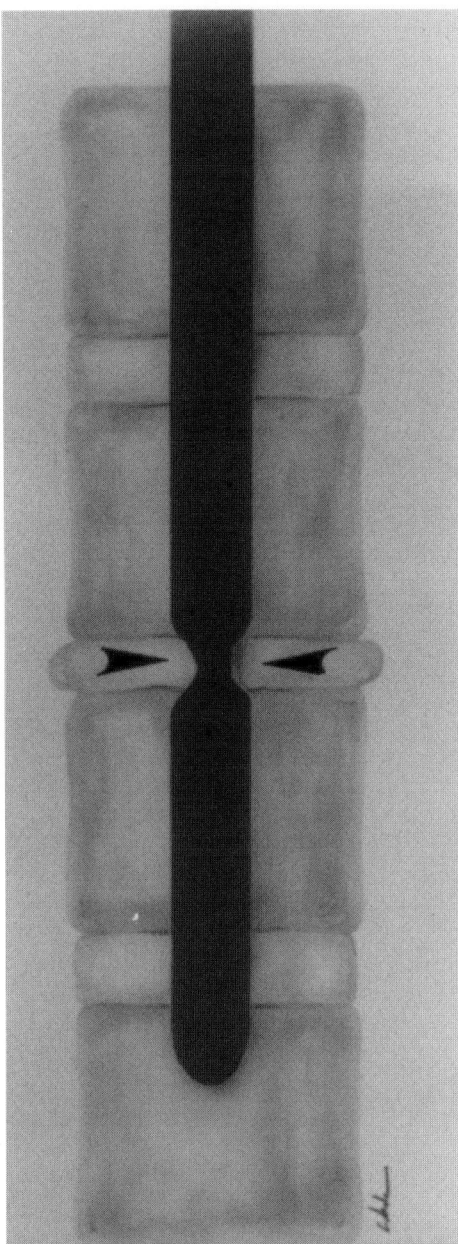

**Figure 131.10** Anteroposterior view of the lumbar spine showing concentric narrowing of the contrast column occurring at the level of a disc space (*arrowheads*).

relief of nerve root involvement, on flexion. During extension of the lumbar spine, the disc bulges toward the hypertrophic facets. This causes a pincer effect at the ventrolateral aspect of the spinal canal, with bilateral nerve root compression. These changes explain the pathophysiology of intermittent neurogenic claudication.[76]

Bilateral hypertrophic facets may be misinterpreted as a midline disc rupture (which can also produce an hourglass deformity). However, with lumbar spinal stenosis, several bony changes are often observed on CT, including (1) lateral recess stenosis, (2) foraminal encroachment, and (3) facet hypertrophy (predominantly the superior facet). These usually occur at multiple levels. There may also be a bulge of the annulus fibrosus resulting from narrowing of

the disc space. This further contributes to the degree of spinal stenosis. Severe spinal stenosis may produce a complete obstruction of the spinal canal, which may cause a paintbrush or a rat-tail appearance. This mimics a complete block that can be caused by a metastatic epidural tumor. The postmyelographic CT scan usually clarifies the differentiation between lumbar disc rupture or spondylosis and epidural tumor.

MRI may provide further information. Spinal stenosis secondary to degenerative hypertrophic facet disease usually occurs at the L3-4 and the L4-5 levels, and it is manifested by a washboard appearance (see Figure 131.11). Hypertrophic facet disease occurs less commonly at L5-S1. Hypertrophic facets cause compression of the dural sac and nerve roots from a dorsolateral direction. The clinical syndrome associated with this radiographic picture is intermittent neurogenic claudication.

Lateral recess stenosis results from hypertrophic changes of the inferior articular process, which narrows the spinal canal at the level of the facet joint (subarticular zone). The nerve root exiting the next caudal level is trapped and compressed in the lateral recess. The surgeon must be alert to the presence of lateral recess stenosis, because failure to decompress this area results in a poor outcome after surgery. Lateral recess stenosis is best identified by a postmyelographic CT scan (Figure 131.12).

Foraminal stenosis results from narrowing of the foramen through which a nerve root exits the spinal canal. This space is bounded by the rostral and caudal pedicles at the rostral and caudal boundaries of the foramen, respectively; the disc and dorsal surface of the vertebral body ventrally; and the facet joints ventrally. Foraminal encroachment may result from the following: (1) degenerative disc disease, with collapse of the disc space and dorsal bulge of the annulus fibrosus, which projects dorsally; (2) hypertrophic facets, which narrow the foramen and project ventrally; and (3) annular hypertrophy and vertebral osteophytes, which project dorsally. These sites of pathologic disease, when present together or individually, may narrow the foramen. As the degenerative disc space collapses, upward migration of the tip of the superior articular process of the lower vertebra toward the pedicle above further narrows the foramen. These mechanisms narrow the intervertebral canal and cause nerve root entrapment throughout its entire length. The entire length of the intervertebral foramen should be identified by the surgeon. This ensures that its entire length (and not just the medial aspect of the intervertebral foramen) is decompressed. It is particularly critical to decompress the lateral portion of the neural foramen. This is often neglected during foraminotomies, leading to failure to relieve the symptoms of radiculopathy.

The surgeon must be aware of the unique configuration of the L5-S1 intervertebral foramen. Some surgeons mistakenly think that the lateral margin of the superior articular facet delineates the lateral limit of the neural foramen. However, the true lateral margins of the intervertebral foramen are the lateral surfaces of the L5 pedicle, which characteristically flares laterally and caudally. The L5-S1 nerve root "canal" is not a true canal throughout its entire length. There is no dorsal wall in the lateral third of the canal (between the lateral margin of the

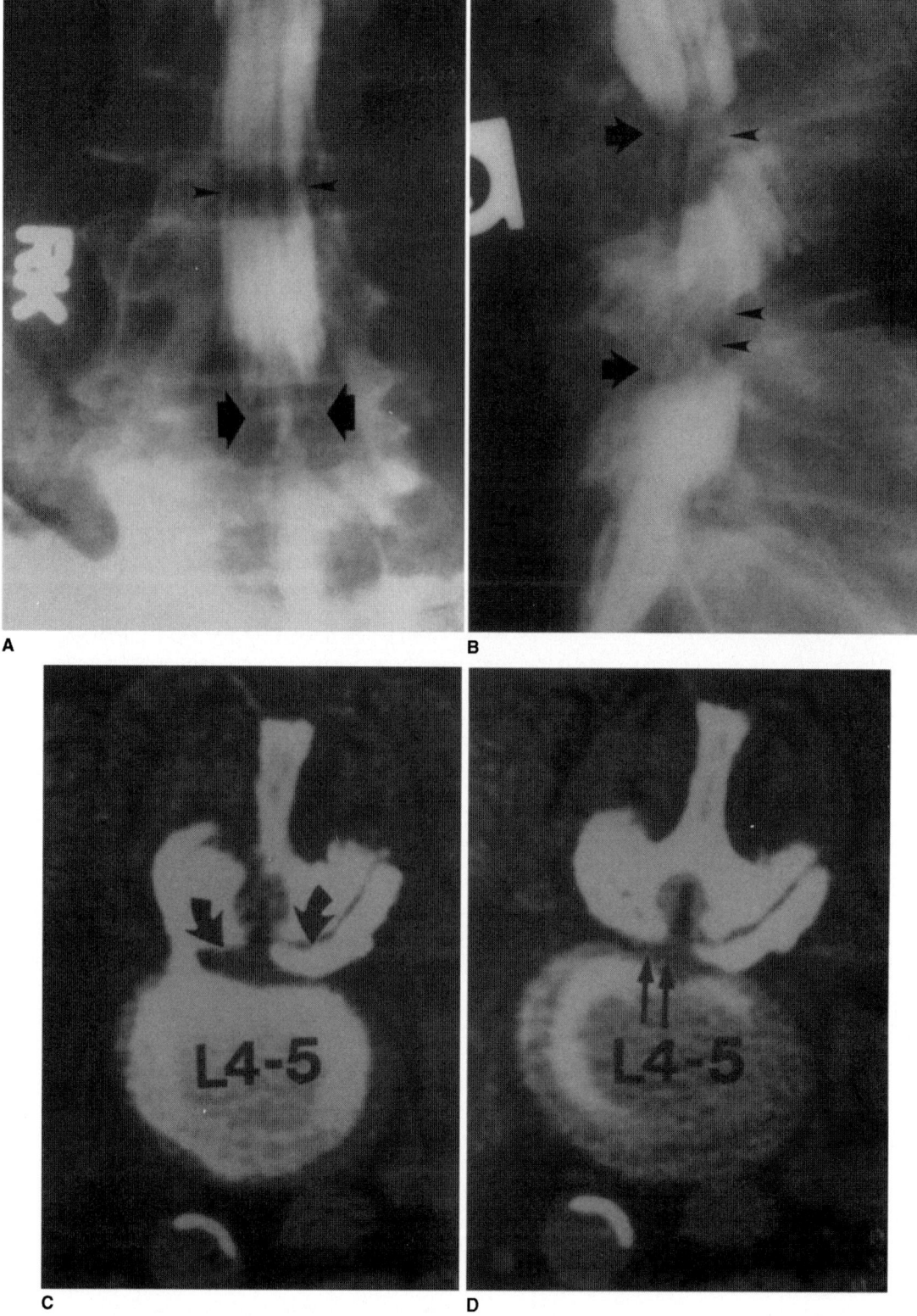

**Figure 131.11** **(A)** Anteroposterior myelogram showing high-grade stenosis of contrast column at L4-5 producing an hourglass deformity *(arrows)*. There is a lesser degree of stenosis at L3-4 *(arrowheads)*. **(B)** Lateral view of myelogram showing high-degree stenosis at L3-4 and L4-5, from dorsal facet hypertrophy *(arrows)* and ventral spondylotic spurs *(arrowheads)*. **(C)** There is marked hypertrophic facet disease *(arrows)* with narrowing of the lateral recesses and the foramina at L4-5. **(D)** A diffuse bulge of the annulus fibrosus *(arrows)* that also contributes to the severe spinal stenosis.

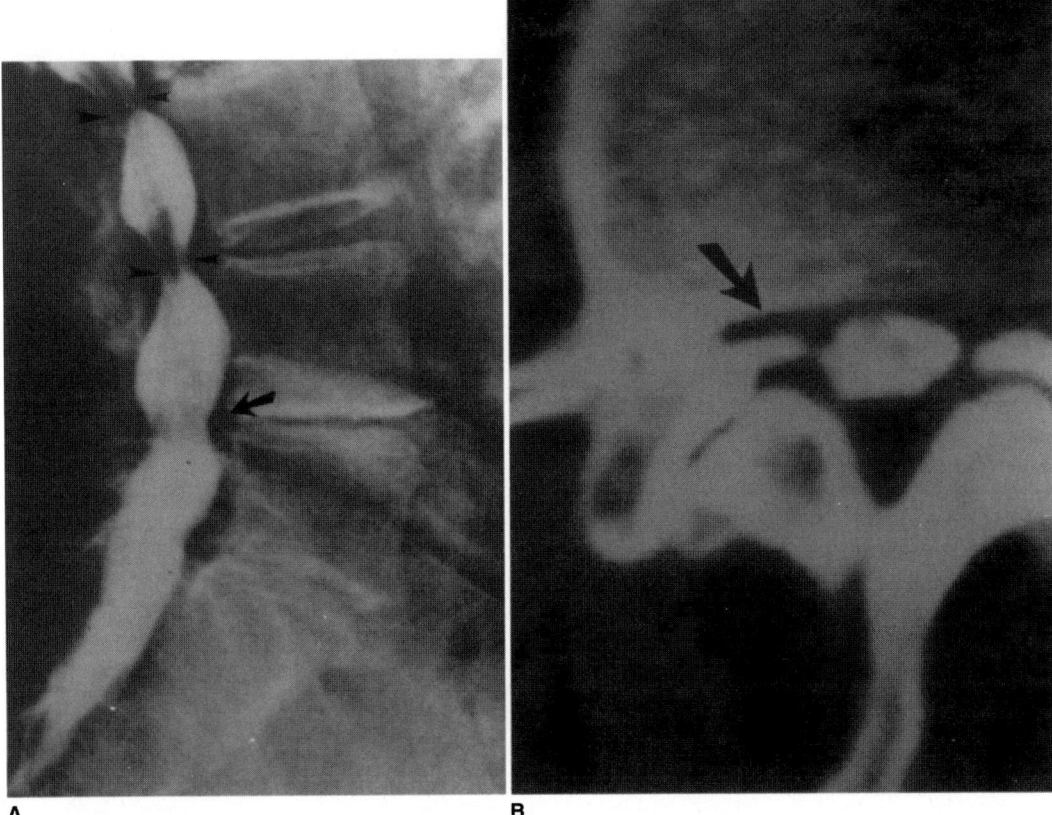

A                                          B

**Figure 131.12** (A) Lateral view of a lumbar myelogram showing collapse of the L4-5 disc space and a bulge of the annulus at that site *(arrow)*. There is also facet and disc space narrowing and associated dural sac compression at the L2-3 and L3-4 interspaces *(arrowheads)*.
(B) Postmyelographic computed tomographic scan at L4-5 demonstrates a hypertrophic superior articular facet resulting in lateral recess stenosis *(arrow)*, which causes pressure on the nerve root lying in the lateral recess.

superior articular process and the caudolateral flare of the L5 pedicle). Notably, the lateral margin of the superior articular process delineates the lateral margin of the canal at other levels. The surgeon's failure to recognize this configuration may result in incomplete decompression of the L5 nerve root, which continues to be trapped between the caudolateral margin of the L5 pedicle and the rostral margin of the end plate of S1, and of the laterally bulging L5-S1 disc.[38] Sagittal reformatted CT scans taken parallel to the caudal margin of the L5 pedicle may be required to identify this abnormality.

To prevent a greater slip after decompression, the surgeon performs lumbar spine fusion to bridge the vertebrae involved in the slip. If a severe spondylolisthesis (grade II or greater) occurs at L5-S1, the fusion with instrumentation should extend from L5 to S1 to maintain alignment.

CT-myelography is often valuable in distinguishing postoperative fibrosus from recurrent disc herniation. Hodge *et al*.[41] studied 20 patients who had recurrent symptoms after unilateral discectomy. Using a combination of CT-myelogram and CT-discography, they classified their patients into three groups. Group I consisted of 12 patients in whom the extradural mass observed on CT-myelography matched the disc fragment's size and contour noted on CT-discography. This pattern indicated the presence of recurrent disc herniation. Group II consisted of three patients in whom the extradural defect on CT-myelogram was larger than the disc fragment seen on CT-discogram. This indicated a combination of fibrosis and recurrent disc herniation. Group III consisted of five patients in whom the CT-discogram was normal, whereas the CT-myelogram demonstrated an extradural defect. Hodge *et al*.[41] interpreted this finding as an indication of the presence of epidural fibrosis without a recurrent disc rupture. MRI scans performed with and without gadolinium (Gd) enhancement have largely replaced other studies for differentiating recurrent disc herniation from epidural fibrosis. However, the results of the Gd-enhanced MRI may be equivocal if the study is performed more than 6 months postoperatively, because by then the fibrotic region has become relatively avascular and resembles the picture of a recurrent disc herniation, which is also avascular.[39] If a Gd-enhanced MRI scan is performed less than 6 months postoperatively, epidural fibrosis is highly vascular and is visible as an area of high signal, whereas a recurrent disc herniation is avascular.

Since the late 1980s, there has been a major shift away from the use of CT-myelography to Gd-enhanced MRI scans for the diagnosis of spinal tumors. One drawback to myelography is the risk of converting an incomplete to a complete neurologic deficit by altering intraspinal hydrodynamics as a result of a lumbar spinal puncture. One such event is herniation of the tumor in a caudal direction, causing greater pressure on the spinal cord or nerve roots of the cauda equina. The apparent advantages of MRI include its high anatomic resolution, noninvasiveness, and safety from neurologic deterioration.

Currently, the use of myelography alone cannot be considered a first choice; however, when used in conjunction with CT, it can be of great value for imaging the thoracic and lumbar spines (Figures 131.13 to 131.15). This is particularly important when bone compromises the spinal canal, such as in spinal stenosis secondary to spondylosis, in spondylolisthesis, in spondylolysis, or in patients with metal rods placed after a spine fusion with instrumentation. MRI has largely replaced CT-myelography for imaging spinal tumors, congenital abnormalities, and many instances of lumbar and thoracic disc disease.

## Computed Tomography

Although plain spine radiographs and CT-myelography are still used for the investigation of thoracic and lumbar pain, they have been superseded by CT and MRI in many institutions.[49] As a single test, CT with three-dimensional (3D)

slices is ideally suited for imaging bone, particularly lateral and central recess stenosis; facet hypertrophy; and disc extrusions. Multiplanar re-formations of axial, coronal, and sagittal images, as well as 3D reconstruction using software, can provide even greater imaging capabilities. Reformatted high-grade CT alone can suggest the presence of a disc herniation, but MRI may be necessary to confirm the diagnosis. At times, an IV contrast-enhanced CT facilitates the diagnosis of a disc herniation by demonstrating a line of enhancement draped over the lesion. This enhanced area may represent epidural veins or scar tissue draped over the herniated disc.[92]

CT clearly differentiates calcified disc tissue and a spondylotic spur from an acute disc rupture. The calcified disc/spondylotic spur is white and the disc herniation is a speckled gray on CT. CT clearly outlines the anatomy of apophyseal joints and demonstrates the presence of facet tropism (asymmetry of the facets), which is believed to contribute to degenerative changes in the disc and facets. Under normal circumstances, the angle of orientation of the lumbar apophyseal joints from the transverse processes is approximately 50 degrees at L3-4, 40 degrees at L4-5, and approximately 35 degrees at L5-S1.[95] It is likely that increased ventrodorsal sagittal orientation of L4 and L5 apophyseal joints contributes to the development of apophyseal joint irregularity, juxtaarticular calcification of the joint capsule, cystic changes of the facets, vacuum joint, and hypertrophic joint changes (especially the

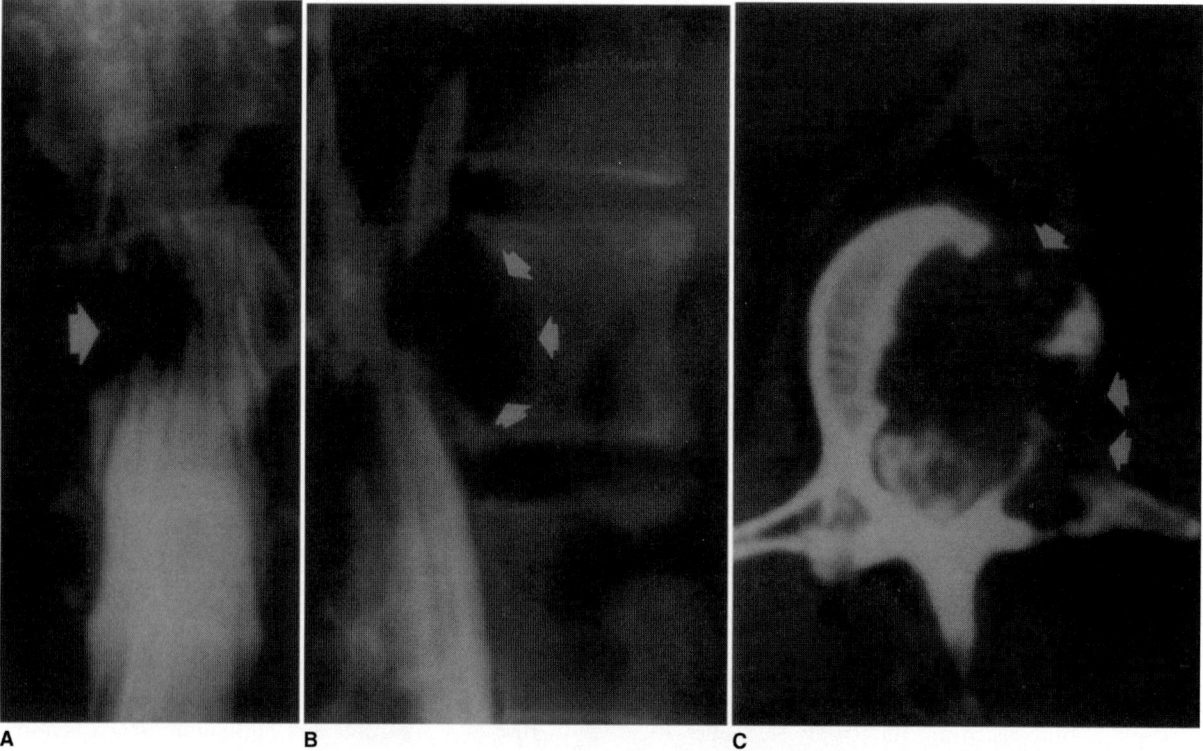

**A**    **B**    **C**

**Figure 131.13** **(A)** Anteroposterior myelogram showing filling defect on the right L3 vertebral body caused by a large osteolytic defect with dorsal epidural extension *(arrow)*. **(B)** Lateral myelogram showing destruction of the vertebral body *(arrows)*. **(C)** The postmyelographic computed tomographic scan demonstrates the extent of bone destruction of the vertebral body with involvement of the right transverse process. The border of the tumor is outlined by the arrows. This proved to be a spinal lymphoma.

superior facet). These are readily identified by bone windows of CT, and they indicate the presence of degenerative joint disease. Superior facet hypertrophy and osteophyte formation may lead to lateral recess and foraminal stenosis. This may cause compression on the descending nerve root in the lateral portion of the spinal canal, before the nerve root exits the spinal canal, caudal to the pedicle at the next lower level. The margins of the lateral recess are the inferior facet (the dorsal boundary), the dorsal surface of the vertebral body (the ventral boundary), and the pedicle (the lateral boundary). Such degenerative

changes of the apophyseal joint must be identified preoperatively for the surgeon to adequately decompress the lateral recess, ensuring a successful outcome. The presence of uncinate spurs projecting from the dorsolateral portion of the vertebral body may also trap the exiting nerve root in the foramen and, together with the adjacent hypertrophic superior articular facet, may cause major compression of the nerve root or dorsal root ganglion lying in the foramen. High-resolution parasagittal CT reconstruction of the lumbar spine and normal axial images demonstrate the narrowed foramen. Adequate ventral decompression

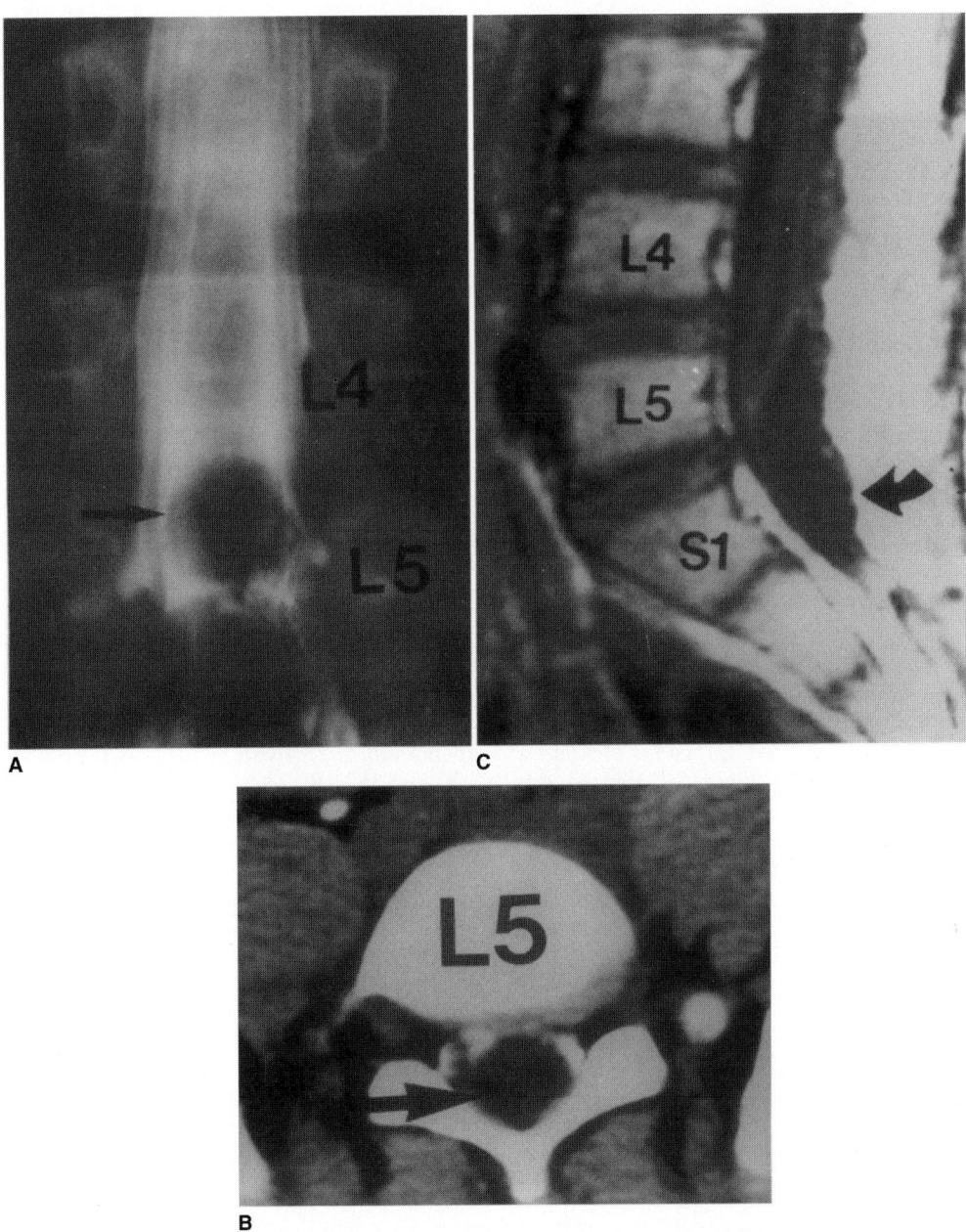

**Figure 131.14** **(A)** Anteroposterior myelogram demonstrating a spheric filling defect at L4-5 *(arrow)*, which nearly fills the dural sac at the L5 level. **(B)** The postmyelographic computed tomographic scan confirming the presence of the intradural mass *(arrow)*. **(C)** A T$_1$-weighted magnetic resonance image demonstrating an area of decreased signal behind the L5 and S1 vertebrae *(arrow)*. This proved to be an intradural lipoma arising from the filum terminale.

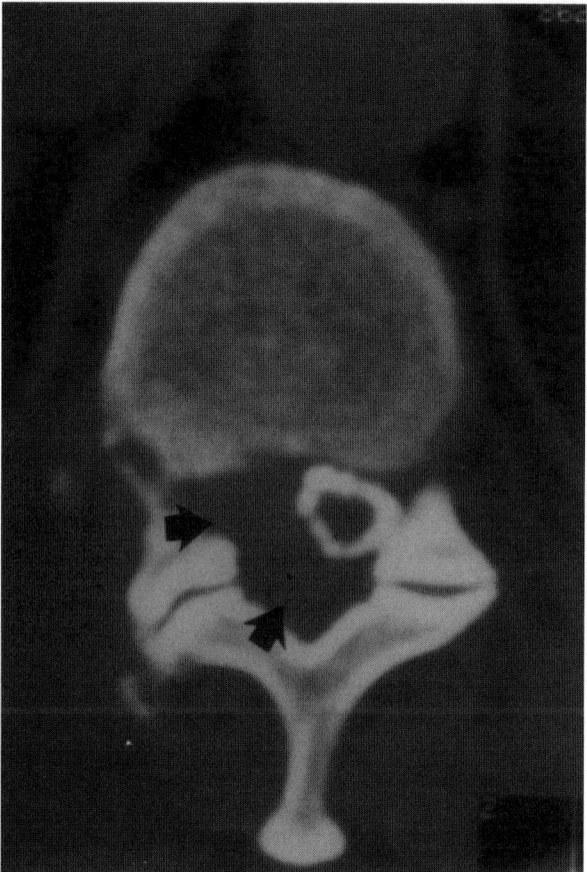

**Figure 131.15** A postmyelographic computed tomographic scan demonstrating an epidural filling defect on the left with T12 with a shift of the dural sac from left to right *(arrows)*. No bone erosion is present. This patient had metastases to the lumbar epidural space.

(of an annular bulge or disc rupture) and dorsal decompression (of a hypertrophic facet joint and osteophytes) of the foramen are necessary to provide satisfactory nerve root and dorsal root ganglion decompression. The lateral margin of the intervertebral foramen may also be narrowed by a hypertrophic ligamentum flavum.

Another drawback to performing only a lumbar CT is the possibility of missing pathologic conditions above L3-4, such as an L1-2 or L2-3 ruptured disc, because the routine CT performed to evaluate disc disease images only the L3-S1 region.

Intraspinal synovial cysts may occur in conjunction with degenerative joint disease.[11,54,59,88] These usually arise from the L4-5 level and from the ventromedial margin of the facet joint. They may contribute to nerve root compression (see Figure 53.3). The diagnosis can be made by either CT[59] or MRI.[54] Intraspinal synovial cysts are usually less than 1cm in diameter and are filled with either fluid, gas, or fat. The cyst is usually at the medial margin of the apophyseal joint and compresses the adjacent neural element. An MRI scan of the synovial fluid demonstrates low $T_1$ signal and high $T_2$ signal. High-quality CT scans may also demonstrate fluid within a synovial cyst.

CT of the sacroiliac joints is usually performed to confirm the presence of degenerative changes, which are usually suggestive of degenerative joint disease and the spondyloarthropathies. Such imaging changes may consist of subchondral sclerosis, cystic changes of bone, and juxtaarticular osteopenia.[38]

## Magnetic Resonance Imaging

MRI has contributed greatly to the successful imaging of spinal disorders. With MRI, clinicians can obtain information about the degree of disc hydration. Customarily, $T_1$-weighted MRI without Gd enhancement takes only 30 to 45 minutes. The only indications for performing Gd-enhanced MRI scans are (1) to differentiate postoperative scar tissue from recurrent disc tissue and (2) to identify the presence of a spinal tumor.

The optimal role for MRI is for the diagnosis of lumbar and thoracic disc disease (Figures 131.16 and 131.17). MRI has the advantages of being accurate, noninvasive, and relatively comfortable (except for the 1% to 3% of patients suffering from claustrophobia, who require sedation), and it does not require the use of radiation. The size, shape, and detailed locations of a herniated disc (herniated nucleus pulposus [HNP]) fragment can be identified more accurately on MRI than on a plain CT, but often not as clearly as on a CT-myelogram.

MRI is capable of imaging both intraspinal and paraspinal lesions, the foraminal diameters, and spinal cord and nerve roots. One of the major advantages of MRI is its capability to reconstruct images in multiple planes.[86] However, there are disadvantages associated with MRI scans: (1) their expense, (2) potential allergies to Gd, (3) the lack of precision in identifying abnormal areas of calcification, and (4) bone changes involving the lateral recesses and facet joints. Furthermore, MRI cannot be performed on patients with intraocular foreign bodies, cochlear implants, certain intracranial aneurysm clips, and cardiac pacemakers because of the risk of dislodging these ferromagnetic objects.

In lumbar disc disease, the disc may appear isointense, hypointense, or hyperintense on $T_1$-weighted MRI scans (Figure 131.18). The presence of a hypointense disc space is the hallmark of degenerative disc disease, which may or may not be symptomatic.[22] The incidence of some abnormality of the lumbar spine being identified by MRI may be as high as 64%,[46] but only a small fraction of these abnormal images are of significance to the point of requiring an operation.

Several variants of lumbar disc herniations can be identified by MRI. They are (1) ventral, (2) gas containing, (3) calcified, and (4) foraminal and extraforaminal disc herniation. With these images, clinicians can also differentiate between a disc herniation contained within the posterior longitudinal ligament from one that has ruptured through the posterior longitudinal ligament.

The presence of a high signal appearance of marrow in adjacent vertebral bodies on either side of the affected disc suggests the progressive bony changes secondary to degenerative disc disease. Early marrow changes noted with degenerative disc disease are secondary to vascularized granulation tissue (Type 1 change) entering the end plates of the vertebral bodies.[110] This creates a low signal

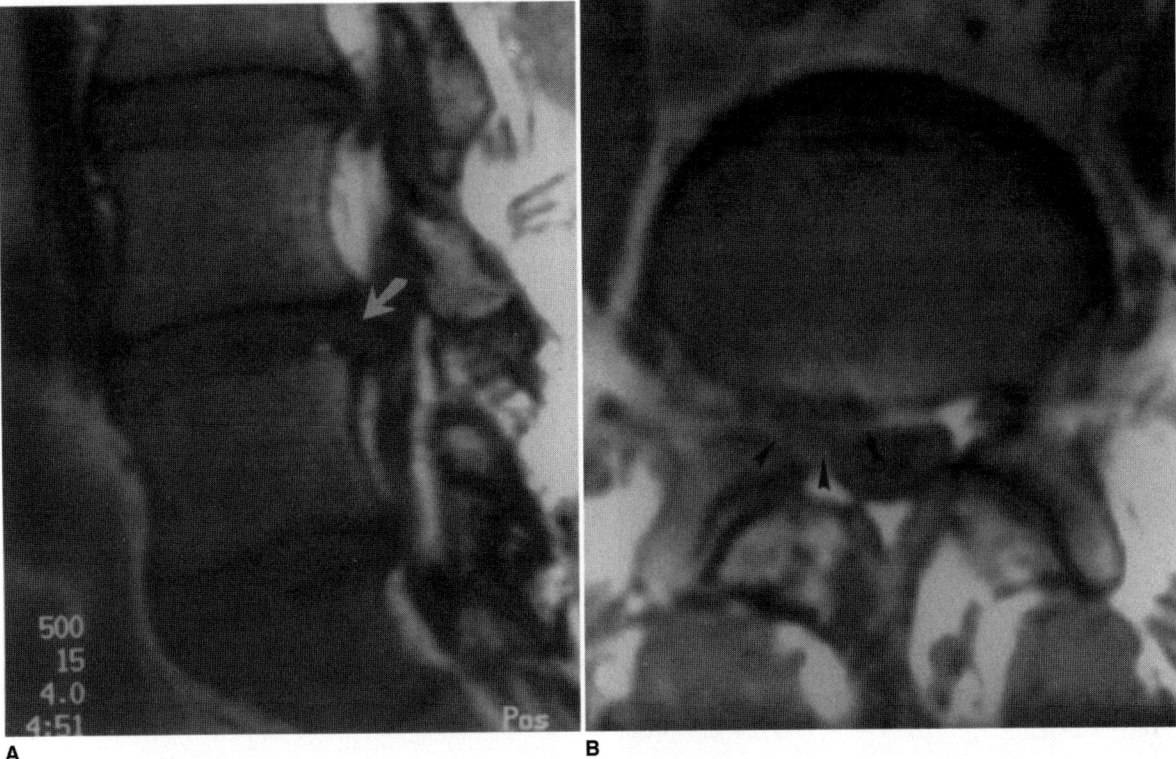

**Figure 131.16** (A) $T_1$-weighted magnetic resonance image (sagittal view) of the lumbar spine demonstrating a large disc herniation at the L4-5 level (*arrow*). (B) Axial view also demonstrates the right dorsolateral herniated disc that occludes the L4-5 intervertebral foramen (*arrowheads*).

for the marrow on either side of the affected disc on $T_1$-weighted images and a high signal on $T_2$-weighted images. As the process continues, granulation tissue becomes fibrotic and is eventually replaced by fat (Type 2 change). This is recognized by a high signal on both $T_1$- and $T_2$-weighted images. A low signal on all images is indicative of Type 3 changes, representing sclerosis or dense fibrosis.[24,67] These changes in marrow are often suggestive of SSI and may be an indication for performing a lumbar spine fusion with a lumbar discectomy.

Lumbar spondylosis may be identified on MRI that often complements the images noted on CT or CT-myelography. $T_1$-weighted MRI identifies the bony overgrowth of the facets, vertebral end plates, and lamina, whereas $T_2$-weighted MRI, which demonstrates cerebrospinal fluid within the dural sac as a white image, indicates the degree of dural compression in spinal stenosis, including central spinal canal stenosis, foraminal narrowing, and lateral recess stenosis.

Degenerative spinal stenosis causes hypertrophic facet disease, which may extend medially to the midline (causing narrowing of the lateral diameter of the spinal canal) or ventrally (leading to severe lateral recess stenosis and foraminal stenosis). The extent of stenosis caused by facet disease and disc herniation must be recognized and appreciated preoperatively if adequate decompression is to be performed. All too often, incomplete removal of the offending stenosis results in a suboptimal clinical result.

MRI is valuable for assessing the integrity of torn dorsal ligaments of the spine. Direct evidence of the presence of this injury was noted by Emery et al.[25] in 17 of 19 patients studied by MRI. These injuries are identified by the loss of integrity of the black stripes that normally represent the supraspinous ligament and the posterior longitudinal ligament. Disruption of these dorsal ligaments has occurred if any of the following are observed: (1) The black stripes are replaced by an area of increased signal; (2) there is an increased signal between the interspinous ligaments; (3) there is widening of the interspinous distance; or (4) there is subluxation of the vertebral bodies greater than 3mm, with kyphotic angulation greater than 25 degrees.

MRI is the diagnostic test of choice for spine tumors. This test does not require a lumbar puncture, as does the CT-myelogram. The latter is not only uncomfortable, but it may be dangerous because it could result in a caudal herniation of the tumor and deterioration of the patient's neurologic status. MRI (with and without Gd) has virtually replaced other tests for the diagnosis of spinal tumors. It is highly effective in differentiating intramedullary from extramedullary tumors (Figures 131.19 and 131.20). Intramedullary tumors are usually gliomas (most of which are ependymomas), which usually occur in the conus medullaris (see Figure 131.20). Astrocytomas are usually present in the cervicothoracic region. Occasionally, these tumors are associated with cysts that are easily identified via MRI. In the absence of a solid component,

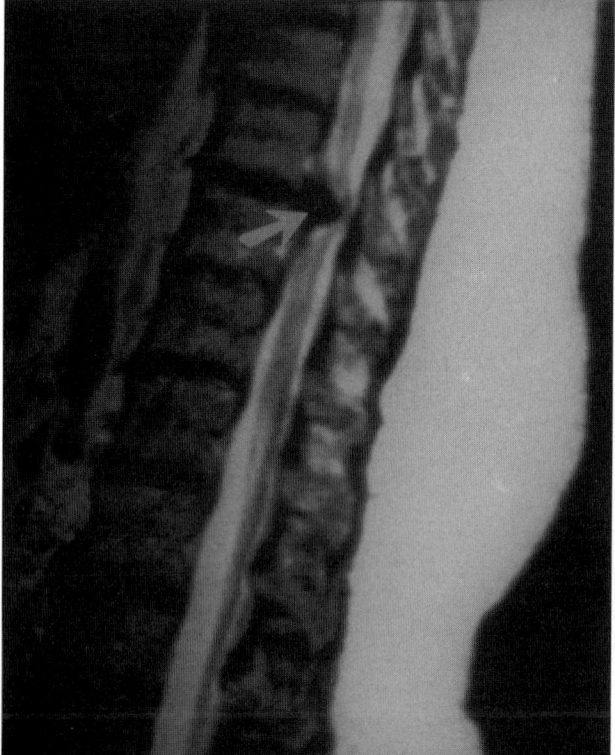

**Figure 131.17** $T_2$-weighted magnetic resonance image (sagittal view) of a thoracic spine showing a large extruded disc at the T9-10 level causing severe spinal cord displacement and compression (*arrow*).

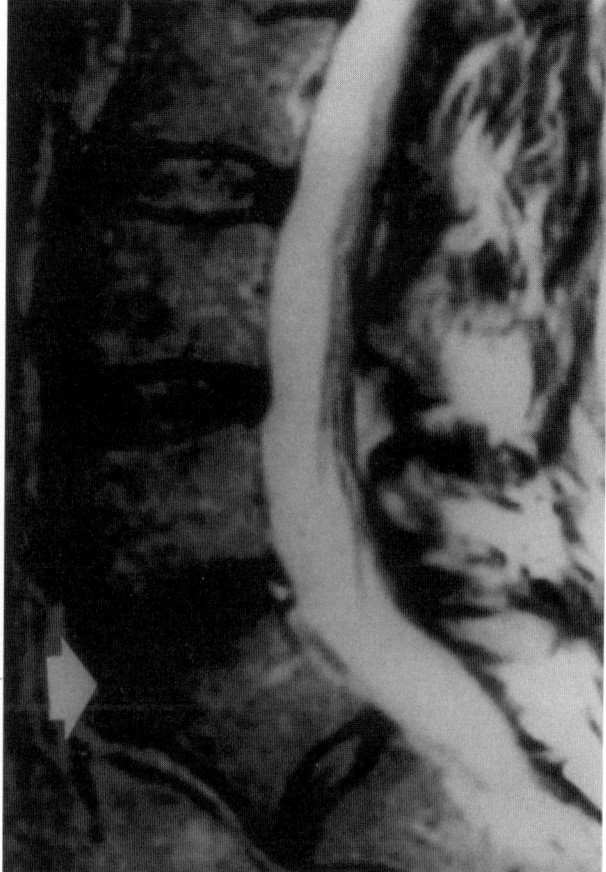

**Figure 131.18** Magnetic resonance image of a lumbar spine showing a black disc space on $T_1$-weighted scan (*arrow*). This is indicative of degenerative disc disease resulting from a decrease in the water content of the disc.

intramedullary cystic tumors may be confused with syringomyelia or a benign cystic lesion (Figure 131.21).

Benign intradural-extramedullary tumors are usually meningiomas. They constitute approximately 60% of this group of tumors. Others, in decreasing frequency, are neurilemomas and neurofibromas. Neurofibromas may have a dumbbell shape, with part of the tumor lying intraspinally and part lying extraspinally. These tumors have a variable appearance; they are isointense, hypointense, or hyperintense on $T_1$-weighted imaging. They usually show strong enhancement after Gd injection (Figure 131.22).

The diagnosis of epidural tumors is readily made with MRI. These tumors are usually of metastatic origin, most likely arising from breast,[87] prostate, lung, or kidney. Metastatic tumors often infiltrate the adjacent bony spine. MRI is highly effective in differentiating between epidural and bony spinal tumors. The high fat signal characteristic of marrow of the vertebral bodies noted on $T_2$-weighted images is often obliterated by tumor infiltration. The presence of multiple metastatic deposits may be evident throughout the entire spine, where there may be diffuse marrow infiltration[3] (Figure 131.23), and the images may also show solitary metastatic deposits to the spine (Figure 131.24).

## Discography

### Rationale

Discography has been, is, and will likely continue to be a controversial subject. Nevertheless, discography may be a useful test to evaluate patients with persistent, intractable, and disabling low back pain that is unresponsive to conservative treatment.

Discography is used in patients with low back pain to evaluate the morphology and internal structure of the disc and, more importantly, to assess the disc for pain production (provocation). A positive discogram reveals the presence of annular tears, radial fissures (Figure 131.25), protrusions, herniations, or diffuse degeneration. However, the discogram must also be supported by a report (by the patient) of precise (variously called *familiar, typical,* or *concordant*) pain reproduction to be called *positive*. Morphologic abnormalities alone, without an appropriate pain response, or with an atypical pain response denote a *negative* discogram.

Proponents of discography admit that the prevalence of radiographic findings that are interpreted as abnormal is relatively high in asymptomatic subjects. However, they emphasize that a pain-related response must be elicited during the injection of the radiopaque medium before symptoms are attributed to a clinically significant abnormality.[28] Thus just as a myelogram that is suggestive of an HNP must be corroborated with abnormal signs on physical examination (e.g., straight leg raising), proponents of discography have suggested that pain replication during the injection of the patient's typical pattern of pain

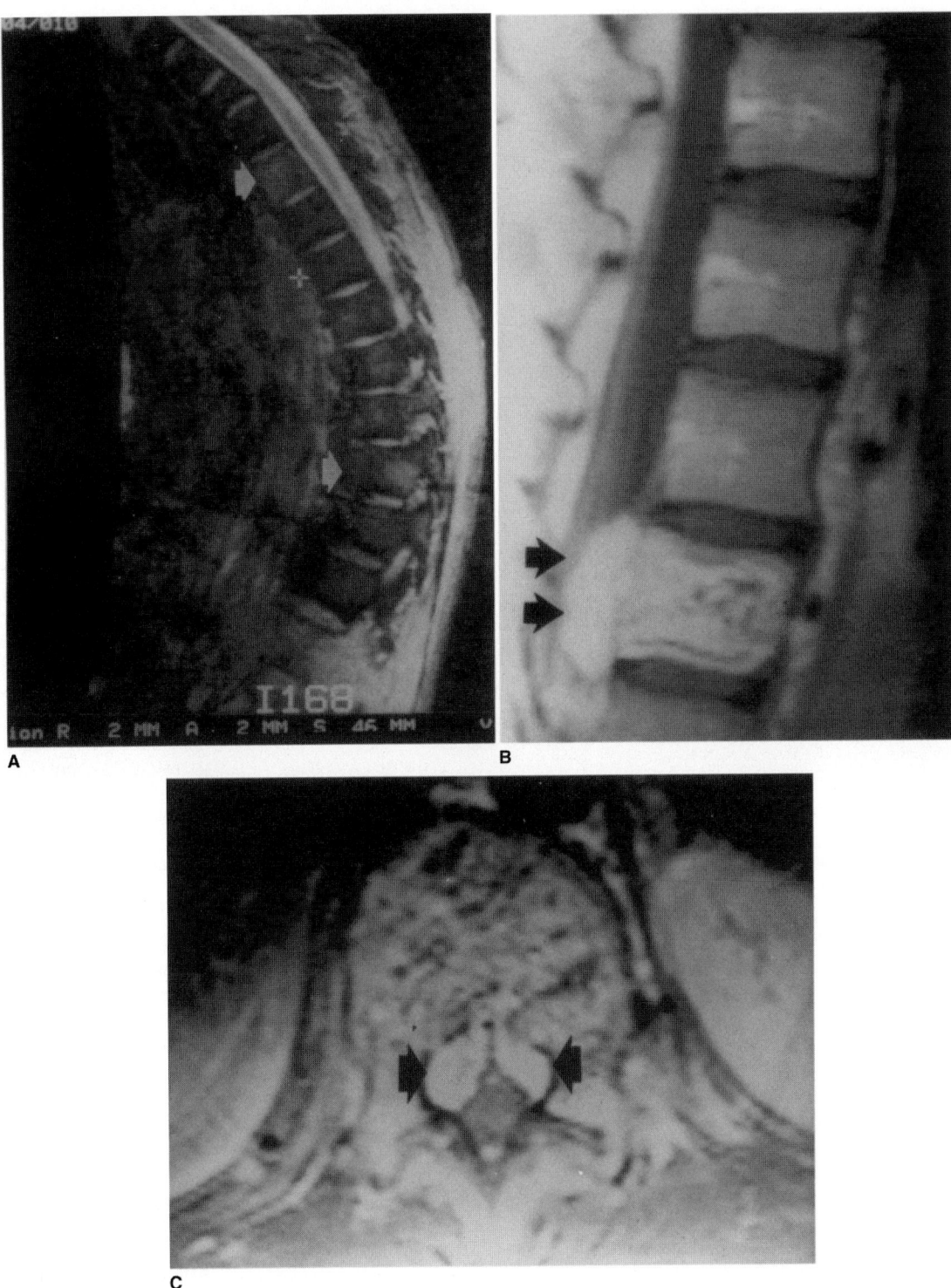

**Figure 131.19** (**A**) Lateral view of a thoracic $T_2$-weighted magnetic resonance image. The vertebral bodies of T4 and T10 have a low attenuation striated image *(arrows)* characteristic of cavernous hemangioma. Sagittal (**B**) and axial (**C**) views of gadolinium-enhanced images demonstrate the T12 soft tissue mass compressing the ventral dural sac *(arrows)*.

(provocation) must be present for a positive interpretation of a discogram.

Discography is considered by some to be particularly useful for determining the patients with degenerative disc disease and low back pain who may be candidates for surgical intervention. Degenerative morphologic changes are commonly observed on MRI, especially in older patients. Often, these studies do not expose the pain generator in patients with severe low back pain. Previously, asymptomatic disc herniations have been described in autopsy studies by McRae,[64] with myelography by Hitselberger and Whitten,[40] with CT by Johansen *et al.*,[47] and with MRI

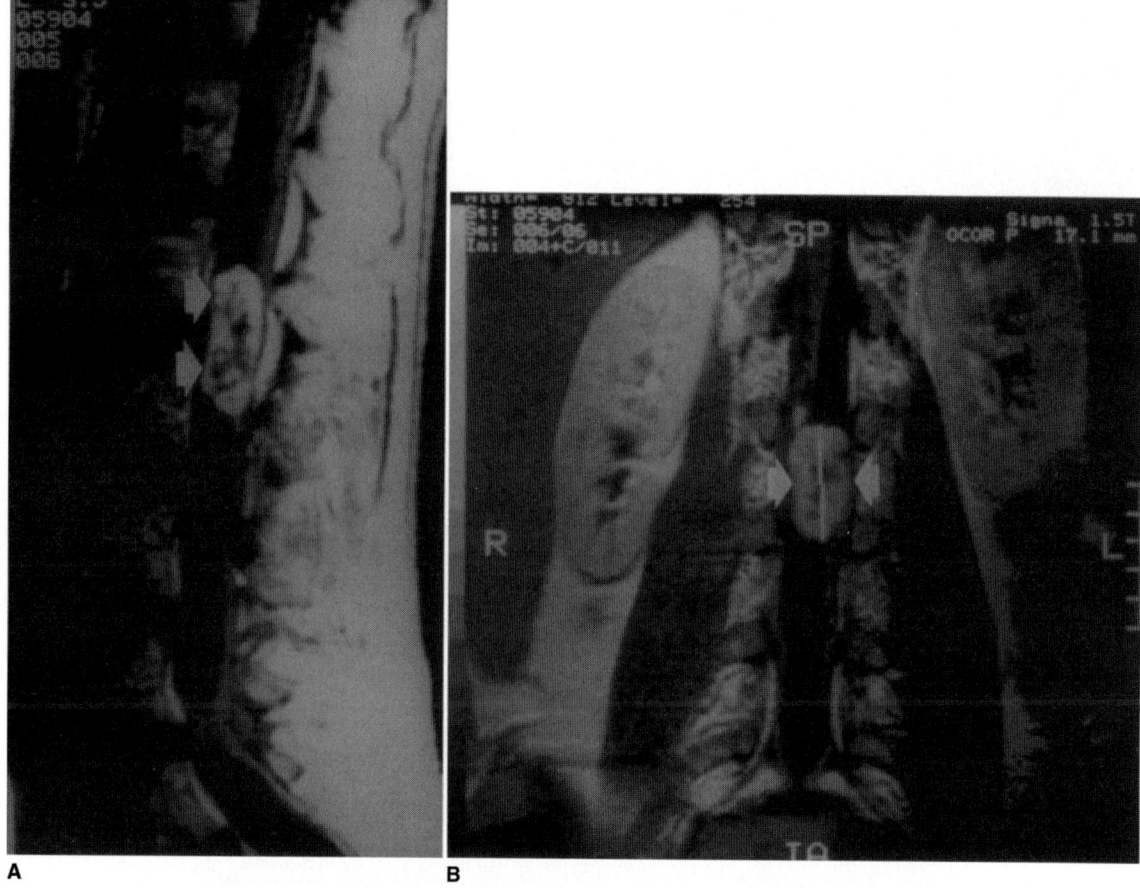

**Figure 131.20** Sagittal (**A**) and coronal (**B**) gadolinium-enhanced magnetic resonance images ($T_1$-weighted) of the upper lumbar region. An intradural ependymoma of the filum terminale/conus medullaris junction at L1-2, measuring 3 × 2cm, is depicted. A speckled, mottled appearance of the tumor is observed (*arrows*).

by Jensen *et al.*[46] and others.[26,100] Such degenerative changes should not be considered indicators for surgical intervention or for lumbar arthrodesis without corroborating symptoms or other tests.

MRI is very efficient at detecting degenerative changes in the disc. However, it is not specific at pinpointing the pain generator. Because discography is a provocative test, it can be used to supplement the radiographic information provided by MRI and, it is hoped, to identify the pain generator.

Discrepancies between MRI and discography have been documented. Simmons *et al.*[90] compared findings of awake lumbar discography with MRI in 164 consecutive patients with low back pain, with or without radicular symptoms. In all, 465 discs were injected. In 60 discs (13%) MRI showed abnormal findings, but the discograms were normal. In 34 discs (7%) the MRI showed normal findings, whereas the discograms were abnormal, with 21 (5%) recreating exact pain symptoms (provocation) and 13 (2%) causing no pain. Zucherman *et al.*[112] and Kornberg[52] were also able to show abnormal discography in patients with normal MRI.

Patients with intractable low back pain that exceeds or equals leg pain and who have documented recurrent disc herniations, spondylolisthesis,[16] gross instability, or combinations of these disorders present as relatively straightforward candidates for consideration of lumbar fusion.

However, patients with lesser degrees of abnormal radiographic abnormalities present a more difficult dilemma. Discography may help differentiate symptomatic from asymptomatic degenerative discs in these situations. A dogma against discography prevails. This dogma, in part, stems from Holt's flawed studies and conclusions reported in 1964 and 1968,[43,44] as well as other more recent studies opposing discography.[20] Holt[44] used suboptimal equipment and less than desirable asymptomatic "volunteers" in his study. The "volunteers" were prisoners without a history of low back pain. Each subject, 30 in all, was to have three levels injected, for a total of 90 discograms. However, 23% of the discs injected were judged invalid because of technical difficulties. As Walsh *et al.*[98] and Simmons *et al.*[89] point out in their critiques of Holt's study, his high rate (36%) of false-positive findings was merely a reflection of the number of discs displaying abnormal morphologic characteristics. Sixteen of the discograms were reported to show actual ruptures, and all were reported as being painful. Walsh *et al.*,[98] and even Holt,[44] conjectured that the pain response from these injections may have been a direct response to the highly irritative effects of the contrast agent (diatrizoate meglumine and diatrizoate sodium [Hypaque]) as it extravasated into the epidural space. In addition, both papers point out discrepancies between Holt's results discussed in the text and

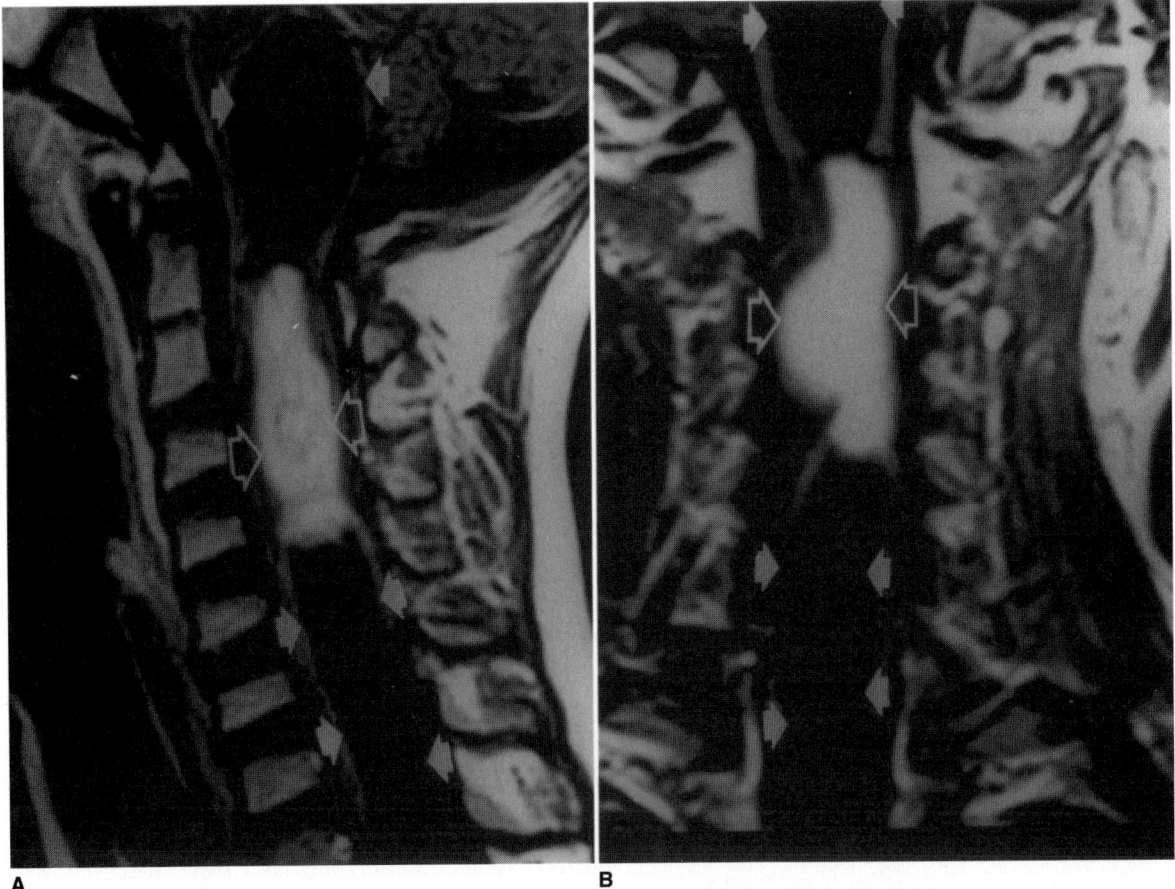

**Figure 131.21** Sagittal (**A**) and coronal (**B**) $T_1$-weighted magnetic resonance images (gadolinium-enhanced) demonstrating an intramedullary ependymoma extending from C2 to C5 (*open arrows*). An associated intramedullary cyst extends rostrally into the medulla oblongata and caudally to T1-2 (*closed arrows*).

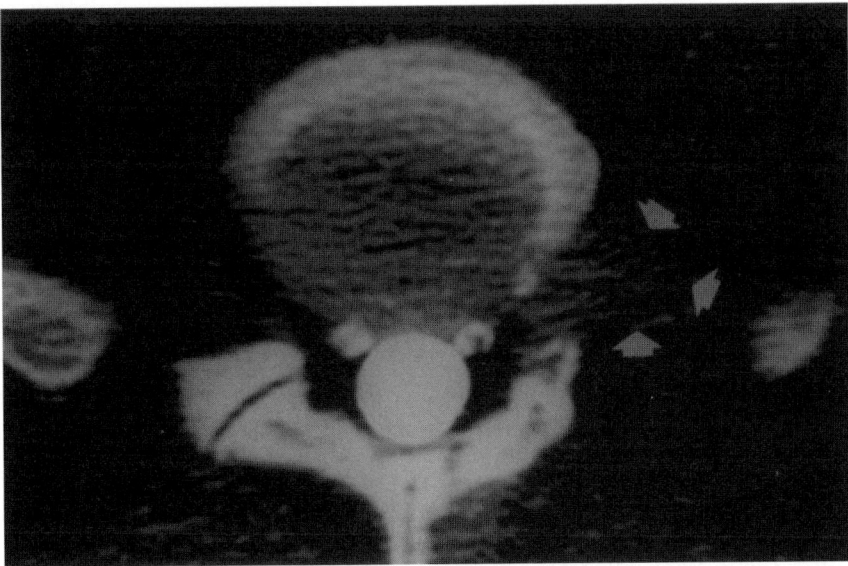

**Figure 131.22** Postmyelographic computed tomographic scan demonstrating an extraspinal neurofibroma (*arrows*) extending from the left L5-S1 foramen.

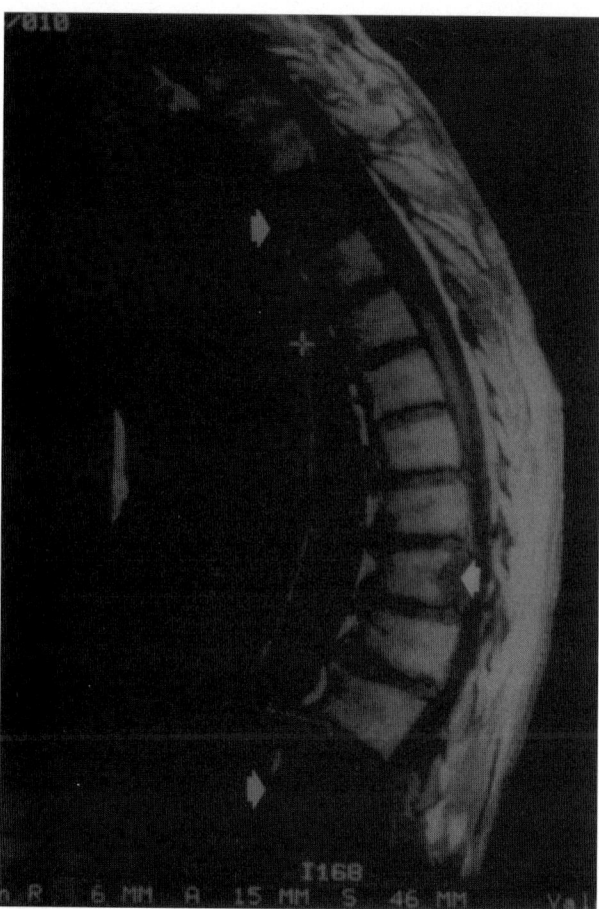

**Figure 131.23** Sagittal $T_1$-weighted magnetic resonance image demonstrating multiple metastatic deposits in the thoracic spine (*arrows*).

disc degeneration and in pinpointing truly pathologic discs.°

It is believed that the pain generated by discography occurs when annular fissures or nuclear herniations extend into the outer third of the annulus fibrosus.[68] Nerve endings from branches of the sinuvertebral nerves, the gray rami communicantes, and the lumbar ventral rami consistently innervate the outer third of the dorsal, lateral, and ventral aspect of the annulus fibrosus, respectively.[14,15,32] Histochemical studies have shown that these nerve endings contain peptides, such as calcitonin gene-related peptide, vasoactive intestinal peptide, and substance P. These are associated with nociception.[1,48,101] The typical or concordant pain response provoked by discography may relate to the stimulation of these nociceptive nerve endings by enzymes such as phospholipase $A_2$,[108] as well as nuclear degradation products in part modulated by the dorsal root ganglion. In addition, evidence shows that an autoimmune response to the nucleus pulposus and its degradation products may incite an inflammatory response in the epidural space, dura mater, and nerve roots, thereby also triggering nociceptive nerve endings.[†] Heggeness and Doherty[37] have documented end plate deflection during intradiscal injection. They postulate that such deflection may cause focal increases in the intraosseous pressure of the lumbar vertebrae.[37] Such increased intraosseous pressure has been implicated as a possible cause of low back pain.

Thus in patients without radiculopathy but with intractable, disabling low back pain, discography may be useful before recommending lumbar, and perhaps cervical,[106] and even thoracic, discectomy combined with fusion.

## Clinical Results

Approximately 70,000 lumbar spine fusions are performed annually in the United States.[111] A significant number of these are performed for the treatment of back pain secondary to degenerative disc disease; therefore it behooves the surgeon to use every possible means to identify which of the degenerated discs are painful. *The key issue regarding the use of discography is whether it can predict outcome from surgical intervention, particularly in the case of lumbar fusion.*

Colhoun et al.[21] found the results of lumbar discography to be a useful predictor of surgical outcome. Of patients with positive pain provocation at discography (with corresponding degenerative morphologic changes), 89% derived significant pain relief following surgery (93% of 195 patients underwent fusion), whereas only 52% benefited from surgery when the disc exhibited structural degenerative changes without pain provocation with discography.

Blumenthal et al.[12] investigated the role of anterior interbody fusion for discogenic pain in 34 patients and reported a 73% fusion rate, with a 74% clinical success rate.

those listed in his table. Aprill[5] points out that some of Holt's "successful" discograms, in fact, may have been annular injections.

In a controlled prospective study, Walsh et al.[98] established the specificity of lumbar discography by comparing results in 10 asymptomatic volunteers with 7 patients with chronic low back pain. In the asymptomatic individuals, the discogram was interpreted as abnormal for 17% (5) of the 30 discs injected and for 5 of the 10 asymptomatic control subjects. However, when the discogram was defined as positive when only substantial pain was associated with the injection (provocation), there were no positive interpretations for the asymptomatic individuals (a false-positive rate of 0 and a specificity of 100%). These results directly contrast with the findings in Holt's study,[44] in which discography was found to have a false-positive rate of 36%. Walsh et al.[98] attribute the following as the direct causative factors in the significantly lower rate of pain-related responses in their study: (1) advances in fluoroscopic guidance for accurate needle placement, (2) the use of CT for the evaluation of accuracy of intranuclear injection, and (3) the use of a less toxic contrast agent.

Many other studies have demonstrated the combination of discography-CT to be quite sensitive in delineating

---

°References 7,9,17-19,29,31,35,45,58,63,68,71,77,84,85,90,95,96.
†References 13,33,61,72,73,91.

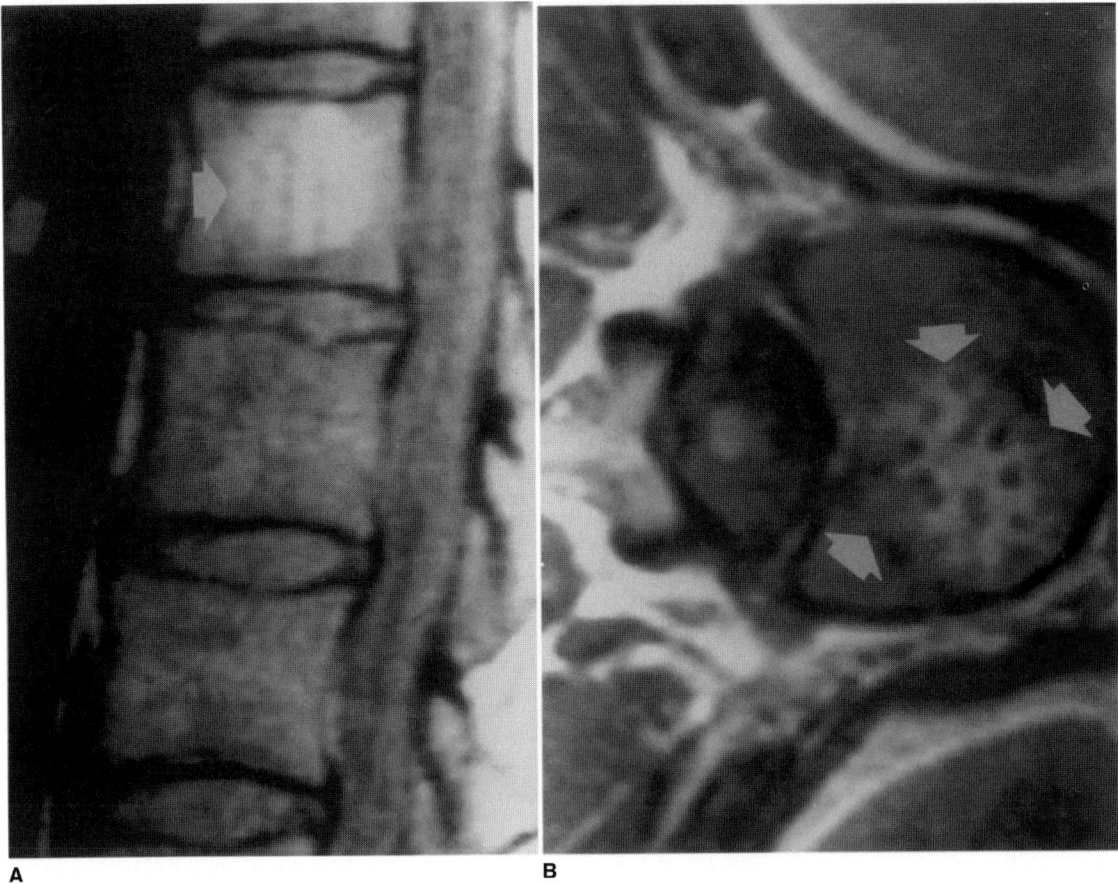

**A**                    **B**

**Figure 131.24** Sagittal (**A**) and axial (proton density) (**B**) magnetic resonance images demonstrating a metastatic prostate tumor of the T12 vertebral body (*arrows*).

Newman and Grinstead[69] achieved an 86.1% success rate in 36 patients with internal disc derangement, as diagnosed by MRI and discography with pain provocation. Their patients were treated with anterior lumbar interbody fusion, with a fusion success rate judged to be 88.9%.

In a study by Wetzel *et al.*,[102] 48 patients who (1) had been symptomatic, with a chief complaint of low back pain for a mean time of 34.4 months; (2) failed to respond to conservative treatment; and (3) displayed positive results with discography (provocation) underwent lumbar fusion. Only 23 of these 48 patients were believed to have a solid arthrodesis at final follow-up (24 to 65 months). At final follow-up, only 22 patients (46% of the total) had a satisfactory clinical outcome; however, all 22 were part of the group with solid arthrodesis. Therefore solid arthrodesis correlated with a 95.6% clinical success.

Kozak and O'Brien[53] reported their results in 27 patients with primary low back pain treated by combined ventral and dorsolateral fusion. Deranged, painful discs were identified by discography. There were 7 one-level fusions, 17 two-level fusions, and 3 three-level fusions. Fusion rate was judged at 94.6%. A good result was achieved in 74.1%. A good result was defined as 76% to 100% relief of back and leg pain, return to employment, no or slight restriction of physical activity, and no use of analgesics.

These studies and others[34,36,56] suggest that if discography reveals a painful, morphologically degenerated disc in patients with intractable low back pain, and a solid lumbar fusion can be achieved with surgery, a better than 70% good clinical result can be expected. These results compare favorably with many reports on chemonucleolysis,[62,80] microdiscectomy,[94] and even, standard discectomy for the treatment of sciatica/radiculopathy secondary to disc protrusion or herniation.

Another advantage of discography is that it can be used to assess a patient's pain threshold. The patient with a low pain threshold may be detected immediately. The surgeon may decline to operate, because such patients are unlikely to tolerate the postoperative pain associated with a lumbar fusion.

Disadvantages of discography include its invasive nature, with inherent complications such as dye allergy, nerve root injury, discitis, and exacerbation of existing low back pain. Discography may provide confusing additional information when it conflicts with results of other radiographic tests. It is uncommon for a radiographically normal disc on MRI scans to be painful at discography.[5,72] However, there are some patients who do report a pain response with injection of a normal disc. Usually, the pain reported is atypical, but sometimes it is concordant. Experience dictates that such patients will not benefit

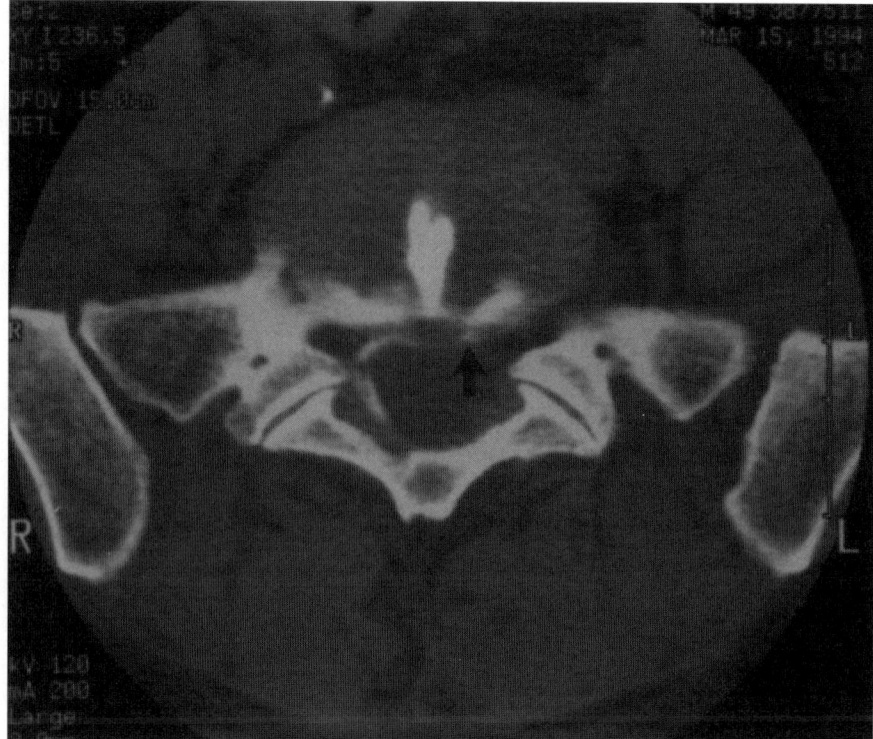

**Figure 131.25** Postdiscogram computed tomographic scan that demonstrates a large single radial tear with dorsal extravasation of the dye (*arrow*). The patient (a 49-year-old man with chronic low back pain) had concordant back pain.

from surgical treatment and thus should be directed toward other treatment avenues.

Discography may help limit the extent of surgical fusion, as in the patient with multiple degenerative discs but with only one or two painful discs[53] (Figure 131.26).

In the previously fused patient with a good outcome who develops recurrent symptoms, discography may identify a new, degenerative, painful disc above or below the fused segment.[53] Discography may also be helpful in the previously operated patient in differentiating scar from recurrent disc herniation.[5,8] Contrast from the disc injection can outline the recurrent herniation within the scar (Figures 131.27 and 131.28).

Discography can also highlight a foraminal or extraforaminal far laterally herniated disc and can aid in distinguishing such from a tumor (e.g., schwannoma, metastasis)[85] (Figure 131.29).

Last, as suggested by some,[53,99] the patient with a prior dorsolateral fusion and continued pain may still have pain emanating from the disc ventrally. Such a patient might be considered a candidate for an anterior discectomy and interbody fusion or a dorsolateral discectomy and interbody fusion in an effort to extract all nuclear material. This eliminates whatever products or process that stimulated nociceptive nerve endings within the annulus or that induced inflammatory reactions in the epidural space, nerve roots, or dura mater. This procedure should also eliminate whatever residual motion that remains ventrally at the motion segment.

## Technique of Discography

A few comments on the technique of lumbar discography are warranted. Discography should include the use of some sedation and analgesia to allay patient fear, anxiety, and pain during needle placement so that the patient is made as comfortable as possible and will not be hypersensitized before the actual disc injection. IV propofol (Diprivan) is an ideal agent for this purpose, because of its rapid onset of action and short duration. An equally effective regimen is the combination of an intramuscular narcotic and oral or IV diazepam. The effects of each can be reversed after needle placement with naloxone hydrochloride (Narcan) and flumazenil (Romazicon), respectively.

The skin is prepared with alcohol cleansing, followed by painting with povidone-iodine (Betadine) solution. It is preferable to anesthetize the skin and soft tissues down to the level of the facet joints. A single-needle (if the clinician is adept at needle placement) or a dual-needle technique is then used. With the two-needle technique, a 6-inch 18-gauge needle is placed through a lateral, oblique approach. Ventrodorsal, oblique, and lateral fluoroscopic imaging is essential for proper needle placement. The tip of the 18-gauge needle is placed in the annulus and is confirmed with radiographic imaging. This often elicits a brief pain response consisting of a report of back pain and, often, ipsilateral leg pain. This pain should resolve quickly. If it does not, the needle should be repositioned, because it may be impinging on the exiting nerve root. The needle

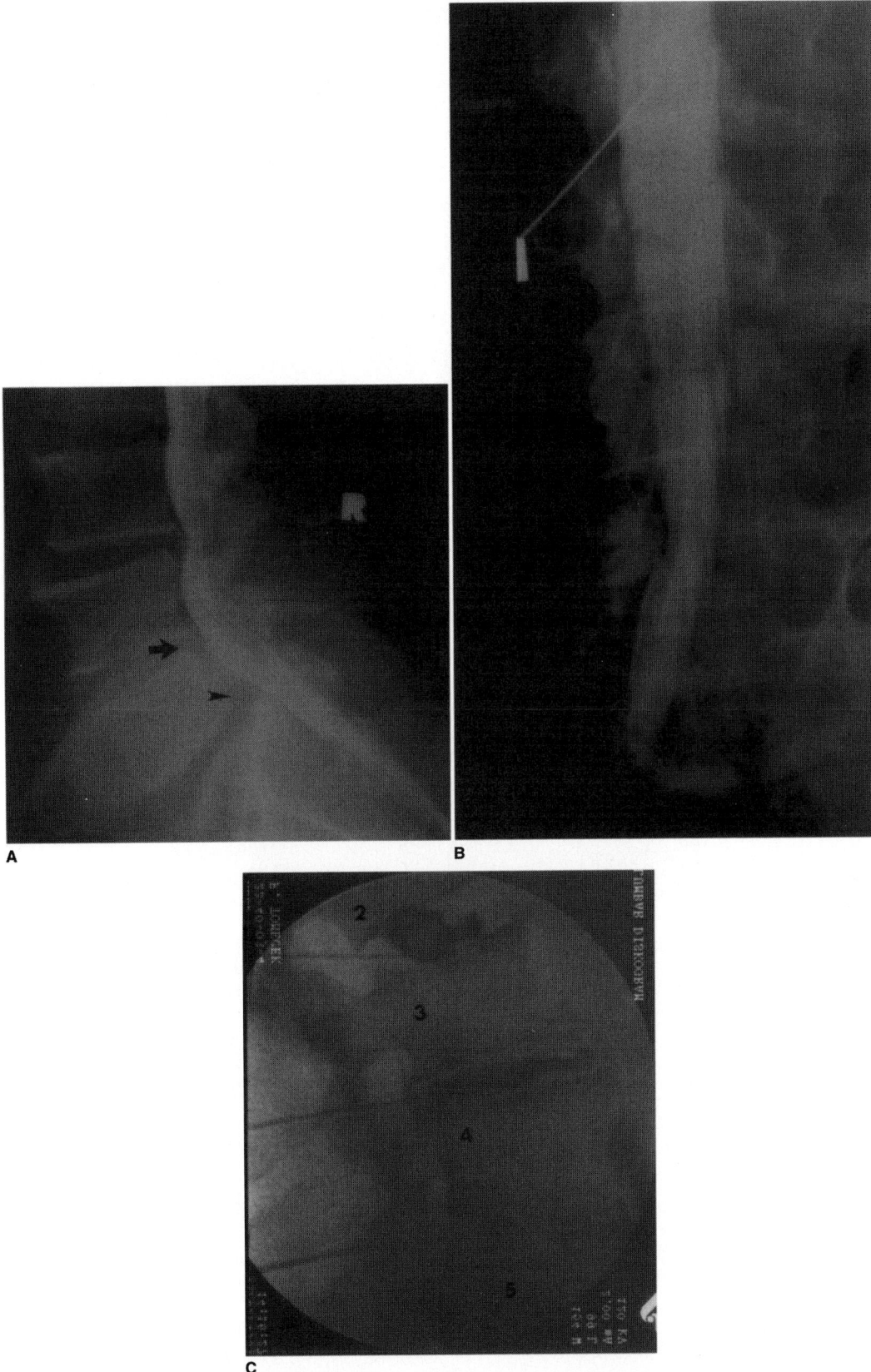

**Figure 131.26** Image of a 54-year-old man with chronic low back pain and mild right leg pain. **(A)** Lateral myelogram demonstrates multiple bulging discs and retrolisthesis of L4 on L5 *(arrow)* and grade I spondylolisthesis of L5 on S1 *(arrowhead)*. **(B)** Oblique myelogram demonstrates poor filling of right L5 and S1 nerve roots. **(C)** Lateral discogram demonstrates normal radiographic appearance at L2-3 and diffuse degenerative disc disease with concordant pain at the L3-4 and L4-5 levels.                          *Continued*

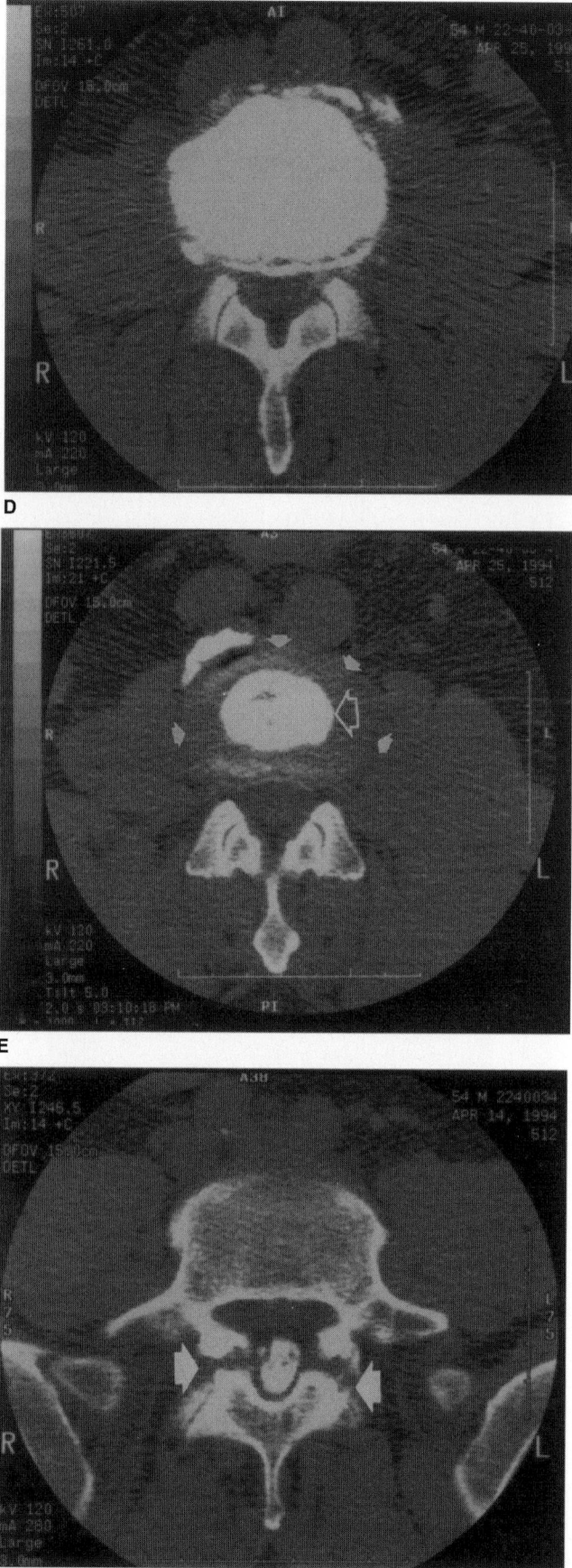

**Figure 131.26 *cont'd*** **(D)** Postdiscogram computed tomographic (CT) scan at L3-4 demonstrates an entirely incompetent annulus with contrast agent filling the entire disc space. **(E)** Postdiscogram CT scan at L2-3 demonstrates a normal disc with contrast filling the nucleus pulposus *(open arrow)*, surrounded by a normal annulus *(closed arrows)*. **(F)** Postmyelogram CT scan at L5-S1 clearly demonstrates spondylolysis and bilateral pars defects *(arrows)*.

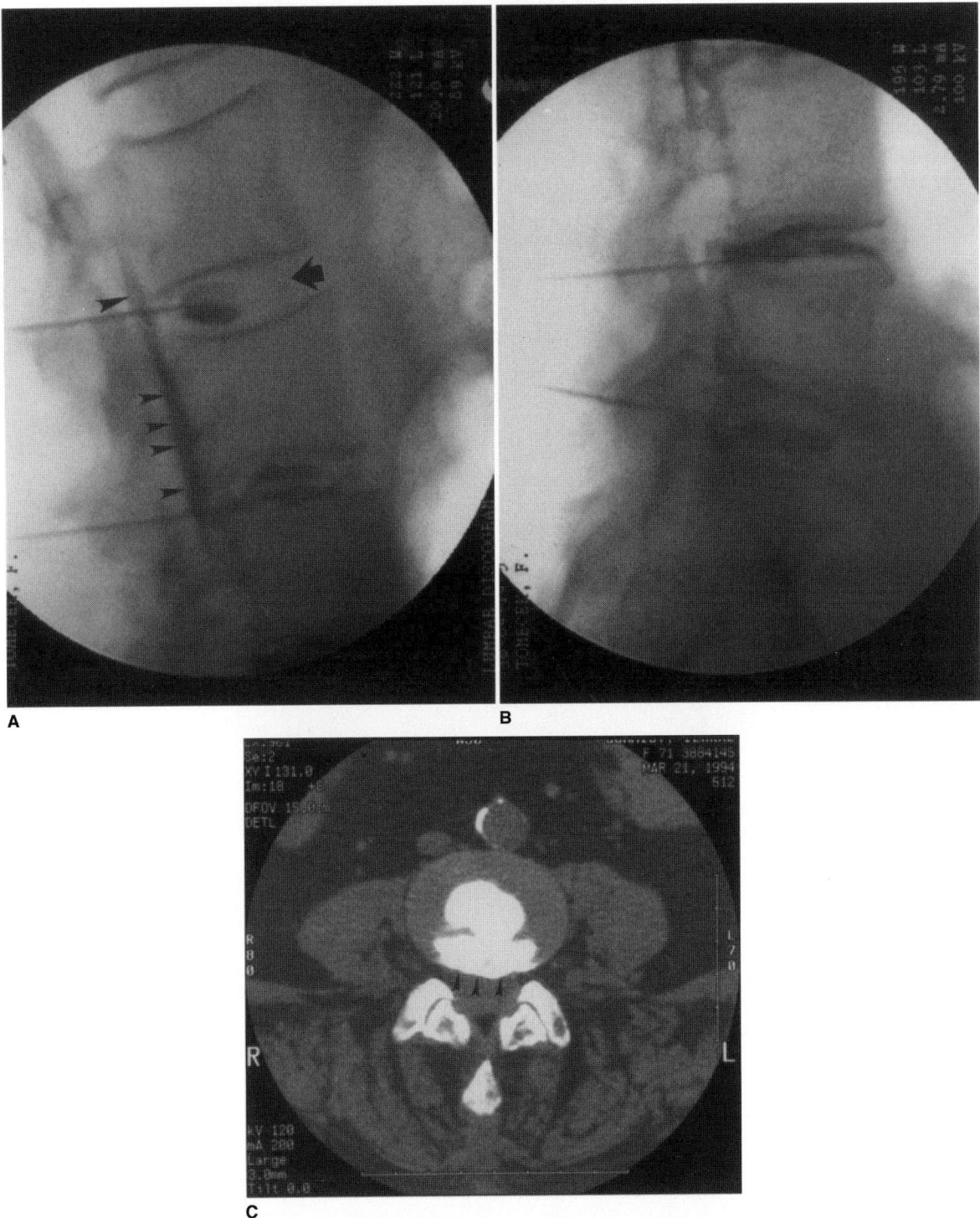

**Figure 131.27** Patient is a 71-year-old woman with chronic low back pain and left leg pain who had a history of lumbar discectomies on the left at L4-5 and L5-S1. (**A**) Lateral discogram demonstrates normal radiographic appearance at L2-3 *(arrow)*, a dorsal annular tear with concordant back pain at L3-4, and extravasation of dye into the epidural space *(arrowheads)*. (**B**) Lateral discogram at L4-5 and L5-S1 demonstrates incompetent annulus dorsally at both levels, but patient experienced concordant back and left leg pain at L4-5 and no pain at L5-S1. (**C**) Postdiscogram computed tomographic (CT) scan at L2-3 demonstrates dorsal annular tear *(arrowheads)*, but patient experienced no pain.

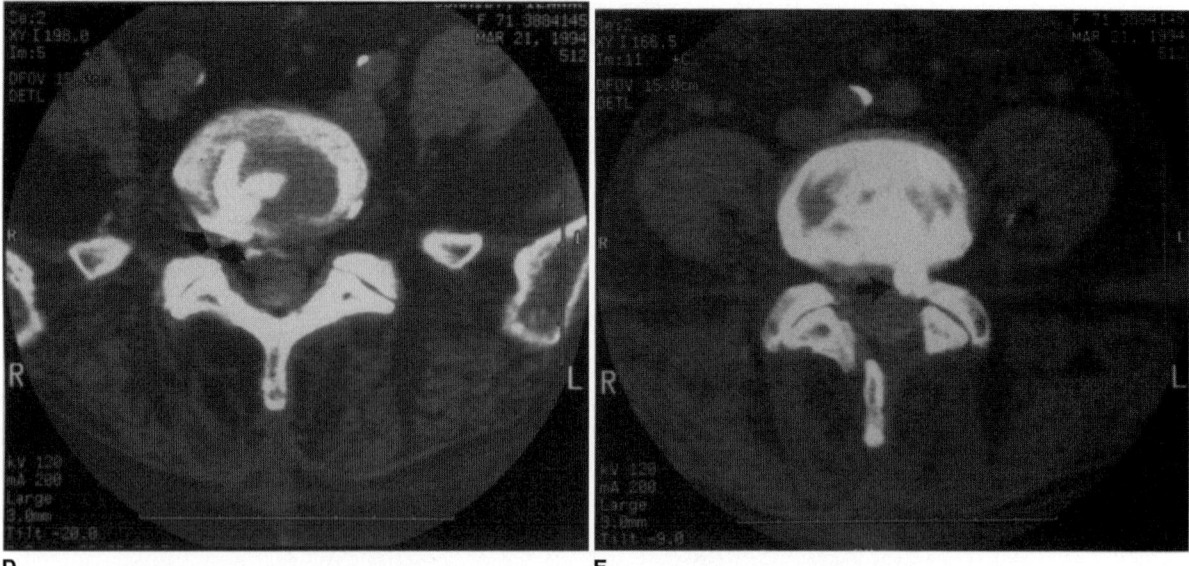

D                                    E

**Figure 131.27** *cont'd* (**D**) Postdiscogram CT scan demonstrates right-sided radial tear *(arrows)*.
(**E**) Postdiscogram CT scan demonstrates concentration of dye in a recurrent herniated disc at
the previously operated L4-5 level *(arrow)*.

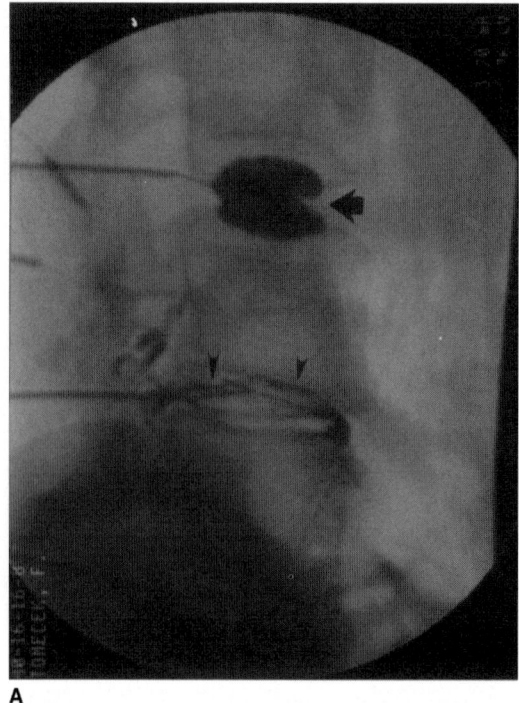

A

**Figure 131.28** Discograms of a 34-year-old woman with recurrent low back pain and left leg
pain. She had a history of an L4-5 laminectomy, discectomy, and noninstrumented fusion.
(**A**) Lateral discogram demonstrates normal radiographic appearance of L3-4 disc *(arrow)* and
diffuse annular tears and degenerative disc disease at L4-5 *(arrowheads)*. The patient exhibited
concordant back and leg pain with the L4-5 injection.

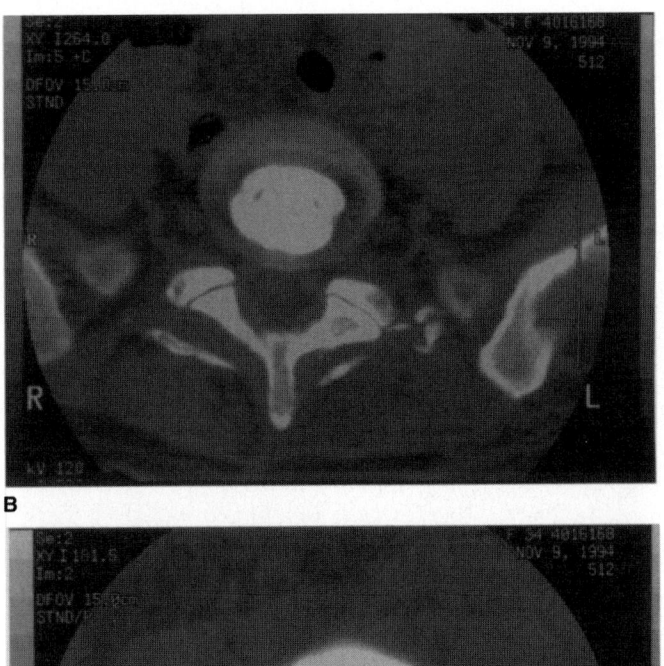

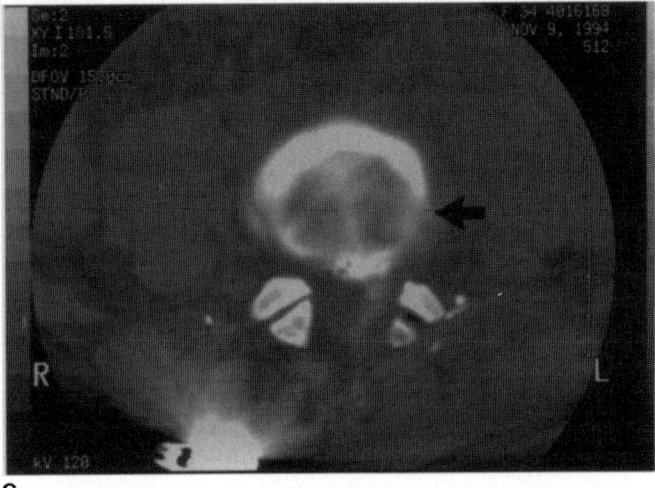

**Figure 131.28 *cont'd*** **(B)** Postdiscogram computed tomographic (CT) scan demonstrating normal L3-4 disc. **(C)** Postdiscogram CT at L4-5 demonstrates both ventral and dorsal incompetent disc and radial tear *(black arrow)* with concentration of dye in a recurrent disc fragment at the previously operated L4-5 level *(arrowhead)*.

should be inserted from the side opposite the one with the patient's most significant leg pain (if leg pain is a component of the patient's symptoms). This ensures that the exiting nerve roots on the patient's dominant side of pain are not irritated.

Once the 18-gauge needles are in place, the stylets are removed, leaving the outer sheaths undisturbed. Eight-inch 22-gauge needles with manually curved tips are then passed through the outer sheaths of the 18-gauge needles until the tips of the 22-gauge needles are as near the center of the nucleus as possible. This is confirmed with ventrodorsal and lateral radiographs. Permanent radiographs are obtained for documentation purposes.

All suspected abnormal discs, and at least one morphologically normal disc, are studied. A normal disc acts as the control for the study.

A water-soluble, nonionic contrast media such as iopamidol (Isovue) is injected into the disc. Contrast is injected slowly through a 3ml syringe. The volume of contrast used is recorded. A normal disc typically accommo-

dates 1 to 2.5ml of fluid and displays a globular or bilobular accumulation within the centrum of the disc. A firm end point is reached, and if a normal disc is injected, there is no perceived pain or the patient will note only a pressure sensation.

With an abnormal disc, various degenerative patterns are observed, a larger quantity of contrast is used, an end point may be spongy or nonexistent, and the patient may or may not report a pain response. A classification system, such as the Dallas discogram description,[84] may be used to incorporate these findings, or the findings may simply be described individually and recorded.

Clarification of the provoked pain is crucial and should be characterized as concordant or nonconcordant, typical or atypical, congruent or noncongruent, similar or dissimilar, and exact or nonexact. It is also helpful to note pain behavior and to use a visual pain scale.

Permanent radiographs should be obtained with contrast present in the discs. The patient is then transported

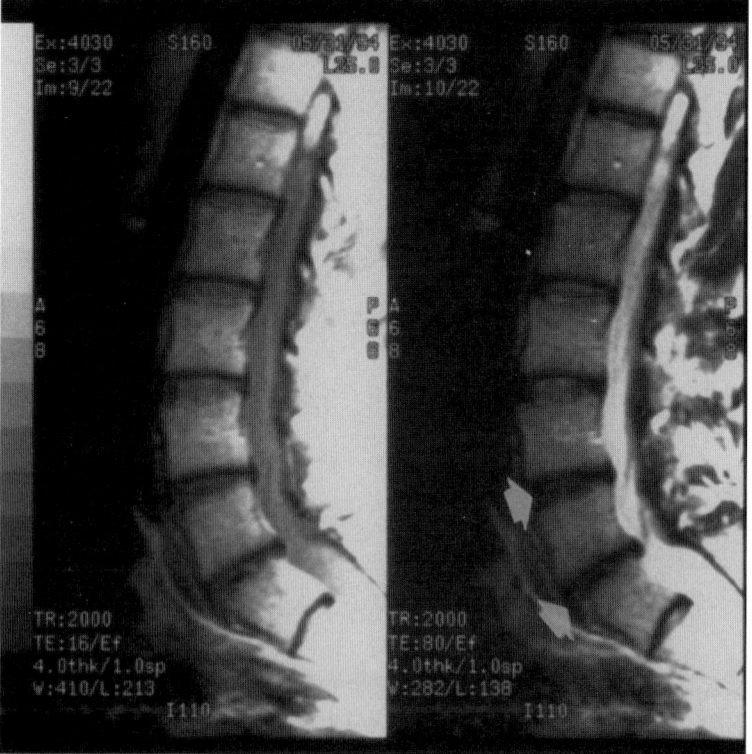

**A**

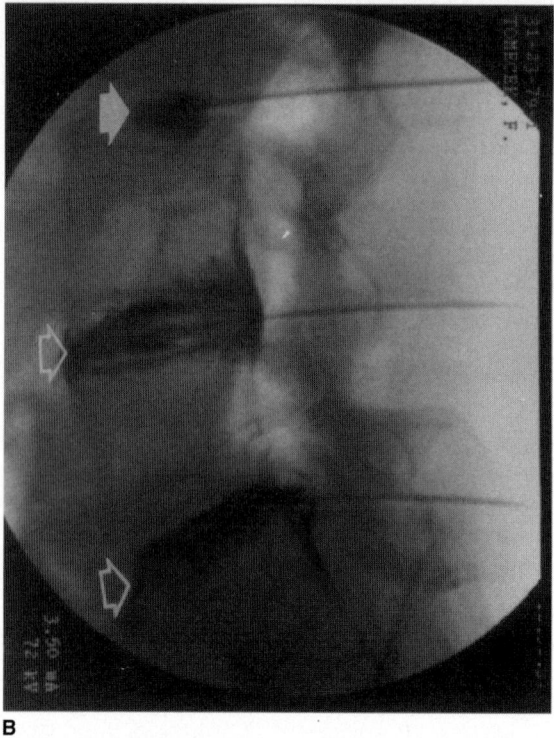

**B**

**Figure 131.29** Patient is a 45-year-old man with chronic low back pain and right leg pain. (**A**) Sagittal T$_2$-weighted magnetic resonance image demonstrates dehydrated bulging hypointense discs at L4-5 and L5-S1 (*arrows*) with loss of disc space height at those levels as well (*right*). (**B**) Lateral discogram displays normal radiographic pattern at L3-4 (*closed arrow*); multiple annular tears and dorsal extravasation of the dye is shown at L4-5 and L5-S1 (*open arrow*). The patient also displayed a concordant pain response at these lower levels.

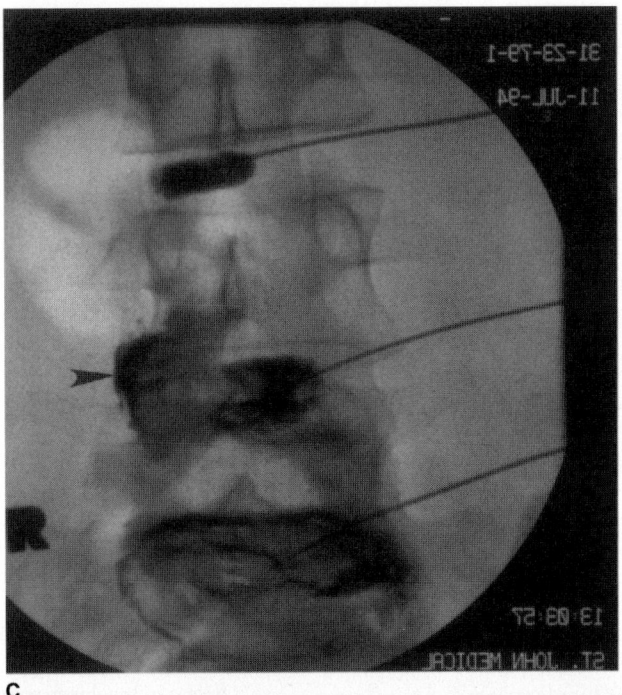

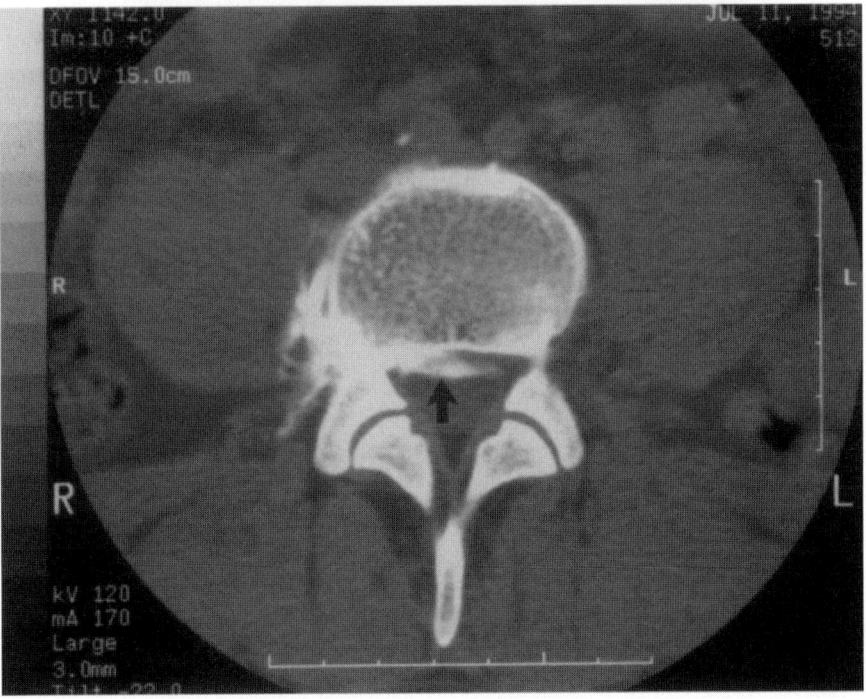

**Figure 131.29 *cont'd*** (**C**) Anteroposterior discogram displays additional finding of right-sided extravasation of the dye at L4-5 *(arrowhead)*. The patient had concordant leg pain when L4-5 was injected. Note that needles were introduced from a left-sided approach. (**D**) Postdiscogram computed tomographic scan demonstrates concentration of dye into a laterally herniated disc *(arrow)*.

to the CT unit, where high-resolution, thin-cut sections in the plane of each injected disc are obtained.

In some instances, usually involving the L5-S1 disc, a needle cannot be placed satisfactorily from the lateral approach. A more midline, transdural approach may be required, with the first needle passed to the level of the ligamentum flavum and the second needle placed transdurally between the laminae.

The test, if performed under strict conditions by a surgeon or radiologist with a good understanding of the pathophysiology of disc disease, can be of great value in determining whether the disc is generating the patient's pain. Careful correlation of the clinical findings and imaging tests (including discography) can benefit the surgeon in determining the appropriate surgical therapy.

# REFERENCES

1. Ahmed M, Bjurholm A, Kreicbergs A, Schultzberg M: Neuropeptide Y, tyrosine hydroxylase and vasoactive intestinal polypeptide-immunoreactive nerve fibers in the vertebral bodies, discs, dura mater, and spinal ligaments of the rat lumbar spine. *Spine* 18:268, 1993.
2. Albert TJ, Balderston RA, Heller JG, *et al:* Upper limb disc herniations. *J Spinal Disord* 6:351, 1993.
3. Alexander AR: Magnetic resonance imaging of the spine and spinal cord tumors. In Devlin VJ (ed): *Spine: State of the Art Reviews.* Philadelphia, Hanley & Belfus, 1998, p 499.
4. Amato M, Totty WG, Gilula LA: Spondylolysis of the lumbar spine: Demonstration of defects and laminal fragmentation. *Radiology* 153:627, 1984.
5. Aprill CN III: Diagnostic disc injection. p. 403. In Frymoyer JW (ed): *The Adult Spine: Principles and Practice,* vol 1. New York, Raven, 1991.
6. Bedbrook GM: Stability of spinal fractures and fracture dislocations. *Paraplegia* 9:23, 1971.
7. Bernard TN Jr: Lumbar discography followed by computed tomography. Refining the diagnosis of low-back pain. *Spine* 15:690, 1990.
8. Bernard TN Jr: Using computed tomography/discography and enhanced magnetic resonance imaging to distinguish between scar tissue and recurrent lumbar disc herniation. *Spine* 19:2826, 1994.
9. Birney TJ, White JJ Jr, Berens D, Kuhn G: Comparison of MRI and discography in the diagnosis of lumbar degenerative disc disease. *J Spinal Disord* 5:417, 1991.
10. Bischoff RJ, Rodriguez RP, Gupta K, *et al:* A comparison of computed tomography-myelography, magnetic resonance imaging, and myelography in the diagnosis of herniated nucleus pulposus and spinal stenosis. *J Spinal Disord* 6:289, 1993.
11. Bjorkengren AG, Kurz LT, Resnick D, *et al:* Symptomatic intraspinal synovial cysts: Opacification and treatment by percutaneous injection. *AJR Am J Roentgenol* 149:105, 1987.
12. Blumenthal SL, Baker J, Dossett A, Selby DK: The role of anterior lumbar fusion for internal disc disruption. *Spine* 13:566, 1988.
13. Bobechko WP, Hirsch C: Auto-immune response to nucleus pulposus in the rabbit. *J Bone Joint Surg* 47B:574, 1965.
14. Bogduk N: The innervation of the lumbar spine. *Spine* 8:286, 1983.
15. Bogduk N, Tynan W, Wilson AS: The nerve supply to the human lumbar intervertebral discs. *J Anat* 132:39, 1981.
16. Bridwell KH, Sedgewick TA, O'Brien MF, *et al:* The role of fusion and instrumentation in the treatment of degenerative spondylolisthesis with spinal stenosis. *J Spinal Disord* 6:461, 1993.
17. Buirski G: Magnetic resonance signal patterns of lumbar discs in patients with low back pain. A prospective study with discographic correlation. *Spine* 17:1199, 1992.
18. Buirski G, Silberstein M: The symptomatic lumbar disc in patients with low-back pain. Magnetic resonance imaging appearances in both a symptomatic and control population. *Spine* 18:1808, 1993.
19. Castro WH, Jerosch J, Hepp R, Schulitz KP: Restriction of indication for automated percutaneous lumbar discectomy based on computed tomographic discography. *Spine* 17:1239, 1992.
20. Clifford JR: Lumbar discography: An outdated procedure [Letter]. *J Neurosurg* 64:686, 1986.
21. Colhoun E, McCall IW, Williams L, Cassar-Pullicino VN: Provocation discography as a guide to planning operations on the spine. *J Bone Joint Surg* 70B:267, 1988.
22. Crock HV: Isolated lumbar disk resorption as a cause of nerve root canal stenosis. *Clin Orthop* 115:109, 1976.
23. Denis F: The three column spine and its significance in the classification of acute thoracolumbar spinal injuries. *Spine* 8:817, 1983.
24. de Roos A, Kressel H, Spritzer C, Dalinka M: MR imaging of marrow changes adjacent to end plates in degenerative lumbar disk disease. *AJR Am J Roentgenol* 149:531, 1987.
25. Emery SE, Pathria MN, Wilber RG, *et al:* Magnetic resonance imaging of posttraumatic spinal ligament injury. *J Spinal Disord* 2:229, 1989.
26. Evans W, Jobe W, Siebert C: A cross-sectional prevalence study of lumbar disc degeneration in a working population. *Spine* 14:60, 1989.
27. Frymoyer JW, Newberg A, Pope MH, *et al:* Spine radiographs in patients with low back pain. An epidemiological study in men. *J Bone Joint Surg* 66A:1048, 1984.
28. Frymoyer JW, Selby DK: Segmental instability. Rationale for treatment. *Spine* 10:280, 1985.
29. Gibson MJ, Buckley J, Mawhinney R, *et al:* Magnetic resonance imaging and discography in the diagnosis of disc degeneration. A comparative study of 50 discs. *J Bone Joint Surg* 68B:369, 1986.
30. Gomez JG, Dickey JW, Bachow TB: Conjoined lumbosacral nerve roots. *Acta Neurochir* 120:155, 1993.
31. Greenspan A, Amparo EG, Gorczyca DP, Montesano PX: Is there a role for diskography in the era of magnetic resonance imaging? Prospective correlation and quantitative analysis of computed tomography-diskography, magnetic resonance imaging and surgical findings. *J Spinal Disord* 5:26, 1992.
32. Groen GJ, Baljet B, Drukker J: Nerves and nerve plexuses of the human vertebral column. *Am J Anat* 188:282, 1990.
33. Grönblad M, Virri J, Tolonen J, *et al:* A controlled immunohistochemical study of inflammatory cells in disc herniation tissue. *Spine* 19:2744, 1994.
34. Grubb SA, Lipscomb HJ: Results of lumbosacral fusion for degenerative disc disease with and without instrumentation. Two- to five-year follow-up. *Spine* 17:349, 1992.
35. Grubb SA, Lipscomb HJ, Guilford WB: The relative value of lumbar roentgenograms, metrizamide myelography, and discography in the assessment of patients with chronic low-back syndrome. *Spine* 12:282, 1987.

36. Grubb SA, Lipscomb HJ, Suh PB: Results of surgical treatment of painful adult scoliosis. *Spine* 19:1619, 1994.

37. Heggeness MH, Doherty BJ: Discography causes end plate deflection. *Spine* 18:1050, 1993.

38. Heithoff KB, Herzog RJ: Computed tomography (CT) and enhanced CT of the spine. In Frymoyer JW (Ed): *The adult spine: Principles and practice,* vol 1. Raven, New York, 1991, p 368.

39. Herzog RJ: Magnetic resonance imaging of the spine. In Frymoyer JW (Ed): *The adult spine: Principles and practice,* vol 1. Raven, New York, 1991, p 457.

40. Hitselberger WE, Whitten RM: Abnormal myelograms in asymptomatic patients. *J Neurosurg* 28:204, 1968.

41. Hodge JC, Ghelman B, Rappoport LH, *et al:* Recurrent disk versus scar in the postoperative patient: The role of computed tomography (CT)/diskography and CT/myelography. *J Spinal Disord* 7:470, 1994.

42. Holdsworth FW: Fractures, dislocations and fracture-dislocations of the spine. *J Bone Joint Surg* 52A:1534, 1970.

43. Holt EP Jr: The fallacy of cervical discography. Report of 50 cases in normal subjects. *JAMA* 188:799, 1964.

44. Holt EP Jr: The question of lumbar discography. *J Bone Joint Surg* 50A:720, 1968.

45. Horton WC, Daftari TK: Which disc as visualized by magnetic resonance imaging is actually a source of pain? A correlation between magnetic resonance imaging and discography. *Spine* 17(Suppl 6):S164, 1992.

46. Jensen MC, Brant-Zawadzki MN, Obuchowski N, *et al:* Magnetic resonance imaging of the lumbar spine in people without back pain. *N Engl J Med* 331:69, 1994.

47. Johansen JG, Nestvold K, Sortland O: Extraspinal pathology and incidental disc herniation in patients with sciatica. *Spine* 13:437, 1988.

48. Kawakami M, Weinstein JN, Spratt KF, *et al:* Experimental lumbar radiculopathy. Immunohistochemical and quantitative demonstrations of pain induced by lumbar nerve root irritation of the rat. *Spine* 19:1780, 1994.

49. Kido DK, Wippold FJ 2nd, Wood RC Jr: The role of nonionic myelography in the diagnosis of lumbar disc herniation. *Invest Radiol* 28(Suppl 5):S62, 1993.

50. Kirkaldy-Willis WH, Farfan HF: Instability of the lumbar spine. *Clin Orthop* 165:110, 1982.

51. Knuttson F: The instability associated with disc degeneration in the lumbar spine. *Acta Radiol* 25:593, 1944.

52. Kornberg M: Discography and magnetic resonance imaging in the diagnosis of lumbar disc disruption. *Spine* 14:1368, 1989.

53. Kozak JA, O'Brien JP: Simultaneous combined anterior and posterior fusion. An independent analysis of a treatment for the disabled low-back pain patient. *Spine* 15:322, 1990.

54. Lemish W, Apsimon T, Chakera T: Lumbar intraspinal synovial cysts. Recognition and CT diagnosis. *Spine* 14:1378, 1989.

55. Liang M, Komaroff AL: Roentgenograms in primary care patients with acute low back pain: A cost-effectiveness analysis. *Arch Intern Med* 142:1108, 1982.

56. Lorenz M, Zindrick M, Schwaegler P, *et al:* A comparison of single level fusions with and without hardware. *Spine* 16(Suppl 8):455, 1991.

57. Macnab I: The traction spur. An indicator of segmental instability. *J Bone Joint Surg* 53A:663, 1971.

58. Maezawa S, Muro T: Pain provocation at lumbar discography as analyzed by computed tomography/discography. *Spine* 17:1309, 1992.

59. Maupin WB, Naul LG, Kanter SL, Chang CS: Synovial cyst presenting as a neural foraminal lesion: MR and CT appearance. *AJR Am J Roentgenol* 153:1231, 1989.

60. McAfee PC, Yuan HA, Fredrickson BE, Lubicky JP: The value of computed tomography in thoracolumbar fractures. An analysis of one hundred consecutive cases and a new classification. *J Bone Joint Surg* 65A:461, 1983.

61. McCarron RF, Wimpee MW, Hudkins PG, Laros GS: The inflammatory effect of nucleus pulposus. A possible element in the pathogenesis of low-back pain. *Spine* 12:760, 1987.

62. McCulloch JA: Alternatives to discectomy: Microsurgery and chemonucleolysis. *Semin Spine Surg* 6:243, 1994.

63. McCutcheon ME, Thompson WC III: CT scanning of lumbar discography. A useful diagnostic adjunct. *Spine* 11:257, 1986.

64. McRae DL: Asymptomatic intervertebral disc protrusions. *Acta Radiol* 46:9, 1956.

65. Meyerding HW: Spondylolisthesis. *Surg Gynecol Obstet* 54:371, 1932.

66. Modic MT, Herzog RJ: Imaging corner: Spinal imaging modalities. What's available and who should order them? *Spine* 19:1764, 1994.

67. Modic MT, Steinberg PM, Ross JS, *et al:* Degenerative disk disease: Assessment of changes in vertebral body marrow with MR imaging. *Radiology* 166:193, 1988.

68. Moneta GB, Videman T, Kaivanto K, *et al:* Reported pain during lumbar discography as a function of anular ruptures and disc degeneration. A re-analysis of 833 discograms. *Spine* 19:1968, 1994.

69. Newman MH, Grinstead GL: Anterior lumbar interbody fusion for internal disc disruption. *Spine* 17:831, 1992.

70. Nicholl EA: Fractures of the dorso-lumbar spine. *J Bone Joint Surg* 31B:376, 1949.

71. Ninomiya M, Muro T: Pathoanatomy of lumbar disc herniation as demonstrated by computed tomography/discography. *Spine* 17:1316, 1992.

72. Olmarker K, Byrod G, Cornefjord M, *et al:* Effects of methylprednisolone on nucleus pulposus-induced nerve root injury. *Spine* 19:1803, 1994.

73. Olmarker K, Rydevik B, Nordborg C: Autologous nucleus pulposus induces neurophysiologic and histologic changes in porcine cauda equina nerve roots. *Spine* 18:1425, 1993.

74. Onofrio BM: Intervertebral discitis: Incidence, diagnosis and management. *Clin Neurosurg* 27:481, 1980.

75. Paulsen RD, Call GA, Murtagh FR: Prevalence and percutaneous drainage of cysts of the sacral nerve root sheath (Tarlov cysts). *AJNR Am J Neuroradiol* 15:293, 1994.

76. Penning L, Wilmink JT: Posture-dependent bilateral compression of L4 or L5 nerve roots in facet hypertrophy. A dynamic CT-myelographic study. *Spine* 12:488, 1987.

77. Perkins PG: Lumbar discography [Letter]. *J Neurosurg* 65:882, 1986.

78. Peyster RG, Teplick JG, Haskin ME: Computed tomography of lumbosacral conjoined nerve root anomalies. Potential cause of false-positive reading for herniated nucleus pulposus. *Spine* 10:331, 1985.

79. Ramos-Remus C, Russell AS: Clinical features and management of ankylosing spondylitis. *Curr Opin Rheumatol* 5:408, 1993.

80. Revel M, Payan C, Vallee C, et al: Automated percutaneous lumbar discectomy versus chemonucleolysis in the treatment of sciatica. A randomized multicenter trial. *Spine* 18:1, 1993.

81. Rhea JT, DeLuca SA, Llewellyn HJ, Boyd RJ: The oblique view: An unnecessary component of the initial adult lumbar spine examination. *Radiology* 134:45, 1980.

82. Roberts FF, Kishore PR, Cunningham ME: Routine oblique radiography of the pediatric lumbar spine: Is it necessary? *AJR Am J Roentgenol* 131:297, 1978.

83. Rothman RH, Simeone FA: Lumbar disc disease. In Rothman RH, Simeone FA (eds): *The spine*, ed 2. WB Saunders, Philadelphia, 1982, p 508.

84. Sachs BL, Vanharanta H, Spivey MA, et al: Dallas discogram description. A new classification of CT/discography in low-back disorders. *Spine* 12:287, 1987.

85. Segnarbieux F, Van de Kelft E, Candon E, et al: Disco-computed tomography in extra-foraminal and foraminal lumbar disc herniation: influence on surgical approaches. *Neurosurgery* 34:643, 1994.

86. Shalen PR: Radiological techniques for diagnosis of lumbar disc degeneration. In Guyer RD (ed): *Spine: State of the art reviews*. Philadelphia, Hanley & Belfus, 1989.

87. Shields CB, Raque GH Jr, Gardner PK: Neurologic aspects of breast cancers. In Donegan WL, Spratt JS (eds): *Cancer of the breast*, ed 4. Philadelphia, WB Saunders, 1995, p 717.

88. Silbergleit R, Gebarski SS, Brunberg JA, et al: Lumbar synovial cysts: Correlation of myelographic, CT, MR, and pathologic findings. *Am J Neuroradiol* 11:777, 1990.

89. Simmons JW, Aprill CN, Dwyer AP, Brodsky AE: A reassessment of Holt's data on: "The question of lumbar discography." *Clin Orthop* 237:120, 1988

90. Simmons JW, Emery SF, McMillin JN, et al: Awake discography. A comparison study with magnetic resonance imaging. *Spine* 166(Suppl 6):S216, 1991.

91. Spiliopoulou I, Korovessis P, Konstantinou D, Dimitracopoulos G: IgG and IgM concentration in the prolapsed human intervertebral disc and sciatica etiology. *Spine* 19:1320, 1994.

92. Teplick JG, Haskin ME: CT and lumbar disc herniation. *Radiol Clin North Am* 21:259, 1983.

93. Tomacek FJ, Shields CB: Lumbar spondylosis: Spinal and lateral recess stenosis. In Tindall GT, Cooper PR, Barrow DL (Eds): *The practice of neurosurgery*, vol 3. Baltimore, Williams & Wilkins, 1996, pp 2489-2519.

94. Tullberg T, Isacson J, Weidenhielm L: Does microscopic removal of lumbar disc herniation lead to better results than the standard procedure? Results of a one year randomized study. *Spine* 18:24, 1993.

95. Vanharanta H, Guyer R, Ohnmeiss DD, et al: Disc deterioration in low-back syndromes. A prospective, multi-center CT/discography study. *Spine* 13:1349, 1988.

96. Vanharanta H, Sachs BL, Spivey MA, et al: The relationship of pain provocation to lumbar disc deterioration as seen by CT/discography. *Spine* 12:295, 1987.

97. van Schaik JPJ, Verbiest H, van Schaik FD: The orientation and shape of the lower lumbar facet joints. In Post MJD (ed): *Computed tomography of the spine*. Baltimore, Williams & Wilkins, 1984, pp 495-505.

98. Walsh TR, Weinstein JN, Spratt KF, et al: Lumbar discography in normal subjects. A controlled, prospective study. *J Bone Joint Surg* 72A:1081, 1990.

99. Weatherley CR, Prickett CF, O'Brien JP: Discogenic pain persisting despite solid posterior fusion. *J Bone Joint Surg* 68B:142, 1986.

100. Weinreb JC, Wolbarsht LB, Cohen JM, et al: Prevalence of lumbosacral intervertebral disk abnormalities on MR images in pregnant and asymptomatic nonpregnant women. *Radiology* 170:125, 1989.

101. Weinstein J, Claverie W, Gibson S: The pain of discography. *Spine* 13:1344, 1988.

102. Wetzel FT, LaRocca SH, Lowery GL, Aprill C: The treatment of lumbar spinal pain syndromes diagnosed by discography. *Spine* 19:792, 1994

103. Whelan MA, Chase NE: Lumbar spondylosis and spondylolisthesis. *Appl Radiol* 16:52, 1987.

104. White AA, Panjabi MM: *Clinical biomechanics of the spine*, ed 2. Philadelphia, Lippincott-Raven, 1990, p 352.

105. White JG III, Strait TA, Binkley JR, Hunter SE: Surgical treatment of 63 cases of conjoined nerve root. *J Neurosurg* 56:114, 1982.

106. Whitecloud TS, Seago RA: Cervical discogenic syndrome. Results of operative intervention in patients with positive discography. *Spine* 12:313, 1987.

107. Whitesides TE, Shah SGA: On the management of unstable fractures of the thoracolumbar spine. Rationale for use of anterior decompression and fusion and posterior stabilization. *Spine* 1:99, 1976.

108. Willburger RE, Wittenberg RH: Prostaglandin release from lumbar disc and facet joint tissue. *Spine* 19:2068, 1994.

109. Wiltse LL: Salvage of failed lumbar spinal stenosis surgery. In Hopp E (ed): *Spine: State of the art reviews*. Philadelphia, Hanley & Belfus, 1987.

110. Yu S, Haughton VM, Sether LA, *et al:* Criteria for classifying normal and degenerated lumbar intervertebral disks. *Radiology* 170:523, 1989.
111. Zdeblick TA: A prospective, randomized study of lumbar fusion. Preliminary results. *Spine* 18:83, 1993.
112. Zucherman J, Derby R, Hsu K, *et al:* Normal magnetic resonance imaging with abnormal discography. *Spine* 13:1355, 1988.

# CHAPTER 132

# Postoperative Imaging

William T. Curry, Jr., Zoher Ghogawala,
Sohrab Gollogly, and Darrel Brodke

Postoperative images of the spine are obtained for a variety of indications and, accordingly, most imaging modalities are used. Proper selection of studies and reasoned interpretation of the results depends on a thorough understanding of spinal anatomy, the mechanics of the procedure at hand and its attendant risks, and foresight regarding expected pathologic abnormalities. Postoperative spinal imaging may seek explanation of unexpected symptoms, verification of implant positioning, evaluation of fusion or healing of fractures, or extent of resection of a tumor or vascular malformation. Moreover, the structures to be viewed include muscular, bony, ligamentous, and neural elements including the spinal cord and the attached roots.

Spinal surgery for degenerative disease normally does not require postoperative imaging, except for those patients receiving hardware and awaiting bony fusion. However, should preoperative symptoms not resolve–or new ones arise–immediate imaging should be executed to define a remediable cause. The postoperative milieu differs considerably from the preoperative state, even in the absence of complications, and thus the radiographic features of the normal postoperative spine must be understood. Jinkins and Van Goethem[27] have comprehensively reviewed the imaging characteristics of the normal postoperative spine and have detailed those associated with various complications.

For most indications, magnetic resonance imaging (MRI) is the stalwart of postoperative imaging. Unless there is a specific desire to visualize metallic implants and/or bone, MRI provides the most detail, with particular regard to the spinal cord and nerves, cerebrospinal fluid (CSF), collections of fluid (abnormal and normal), and abnormal tissue. Plain films and computed tomography (CT) are best for evaluating bony abnormalities. MRI allows acquisition in several different planes and provides outstanding spatial resolution, and various sequences permit emphasis on different structures and their consistencies. For instance, $T_2$-weighted images demonstrate the water content of discs or reflect intramedullary edema. In addition, $T_2$-weighted fast spin-echo images provide superior spatial resolution and decreased motion artifact in comparison with other spin-echo sequences.[47] Gadolinium contrast administration allows delineation of inflammatory processes, vascular abnormalities, or residual tumor.

## Normal Postoperative Spine

Analysis of the postoperative image requires understanding of the anatomy involved in the surgical procedure. The first 6 to 8 weeks can be considered the acute/subacute period. The extent of bony removal at surgery greatly influences postoperative imaging appearance. The removal of bone may permit dorsal expansion of the dura mater through defects, which can resemble a pseudomeningocele. In addition, asymmetry in the paraspinal muscle-fat planes related to surgical dissection is a normal finding. Edema may obscure muscular margins. When the intervertebral disc has been violated or partially excised, distinction between epidural tissue edema and the disrupted annulus fibrosus and recurrent disc herniation or residual disc material can be complex.[27] This well-vascularized tissue usually enhances homogenously, whereas disc material typically enhances poorly or, at best, heterogeneously. Epidural fibrosis may be present in as many as 100% of patients following disc surgery. Gadolinium enhancing end plates and annulus fibrosus may also be observed and easily mistaken for early signs of infection (Figure 132.1).

Van Goethem et al.[52] prospectively studied 36 patients with excellent outcomes following lumbar discectomy and obtained MRI scans at 6 weeks and 6 months. Imaging findings in these asymptomatic patients mimicked diagnostic findings in patients with complications. That is, 20% of patients had recurrent disc herniation; nerve root enhancement was also observed in 20% of patients at 6 weeks (half of whom had recurrent discs). At 6 months, contrast enhancement was observed along the surgical tract in all patients.[52] Likewise, facet joint enhancement was also seen bilaterally and was attributed to mechanical stress during laminectomy.

The normal postoperative spinal image is far from "normal." Edema, shifting, and compression of the thecal sac; epidural fibrosis; and enhancement at almost any portion of the operative field or tract can be seen in an asymptomatic, well-treated patient.

## Unresolved or Recurrent Symptoms

The *failed back surgery syndrome* (FBSS) refers specifically to those patients who have undergone lumbar spine surgery for degenerative disease (disc herniation, foraminal stenosis, or spinal instability) who suffer severe pain in the back and legs.[51] The potential causes of FBSS are numerous and are listed elsewhere. Although not necessarily definitive regarding the cause of postoperative pain, imaging studies guide the clinician toward some diagnostic hypotheses and eliminate others. In some cases, ambiguities persist and diagnostic and therapeutic dilemmas remain unsolved. The imaging findings discussed here largely pertain to postoperative causes of radiculopathy and are not confined to the lumbar spine, nor do they cover all possible sources of postoperative pain. Complications related to spinal instrumentation and fusion are discussed elsewhere in this book.

## Recurrent Disc Herniation Versus Epidural Scar Formation

MRI with administration of gadolinium is the sine qua non for differentiating epidural scar from recurrent disc herniation. Nonenhanced MRI is approximately 85% accurate in achieving this distinction,[8] whereas enhanced MRI is 95% to 100% accurate.[25,40] Both fibrosis and disc can be hyperintense relative to bone on $T_2$-weighted images (Figure 132.2). An important technical point for these evaluations is the timing of imaging following contrast administration. Although the guiding radiologic tenet is that fibrosis enhances and discs do not, some disc frag-

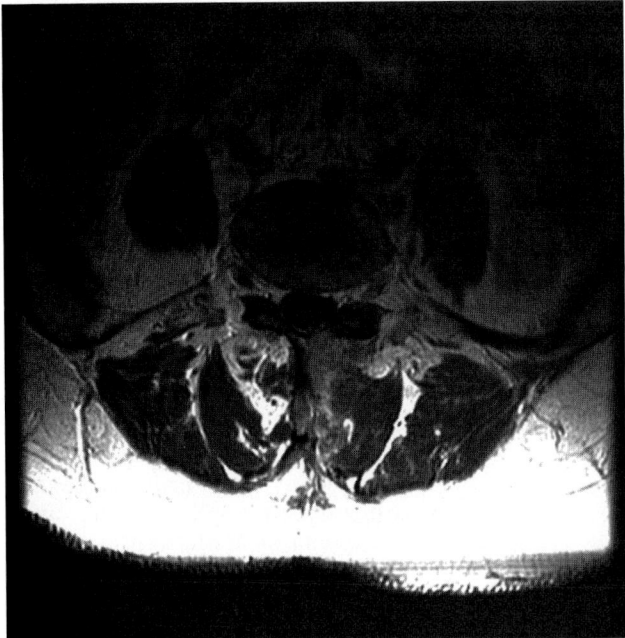

**Figure 132.1** Normal postoperative axial $T_1$-weighted magnetic resonance image with gadolinium of the lumbar spine 3 months after the patient underwent left lumbar microdiscectomy.

ments may be partially vascularized, leading to heterogeneous enhancement with a centrally nonenhancing region. In addition, as previously stated, the annulus fibrosus may enhance after disc surgery.[6] If imaging is delayed more than several minutes beyond the administration of contrast, gadolinium seeps across the disc, which is then seen to enhance more homogenously. To avoid this phenomenon and to increase the specificity for detecting fibrosis, imaging should commence within 2 minutes of gadolinium injection.

### Postoperative Hematoma

Included in the differential diagnosis for a patient who undergoes a spinal procedure and deteriorates in the early postoperative period is hematoma, usually extradural (Figure 132.3). Neurologic symptoms are rare in the lumbar spine because the canal is capacious and the roots of the cauda are mobile. However, in the cervical and thoracic spine, neural compression by a postoperative hematoma can have devastating neurologic consequences.

MRI is more sensitive for the detection of blood products in the spine than is CT,[27] and MRI usually demonstrates mixed blood breakdown products. Neural or dural compression is readily seen on sagittal and axial MRI.

### Postoperative Infection

Because of the imaging characteristics of the normal postoperative spine, diagnosis of postoperative infection can be complicated. Imaging should be complementary to the clinical scenario, including timing, symptoms, physical findings, and laboratory evaluations. Two versions of postoperative infection predominate: spondylodiscitis and paravertebral

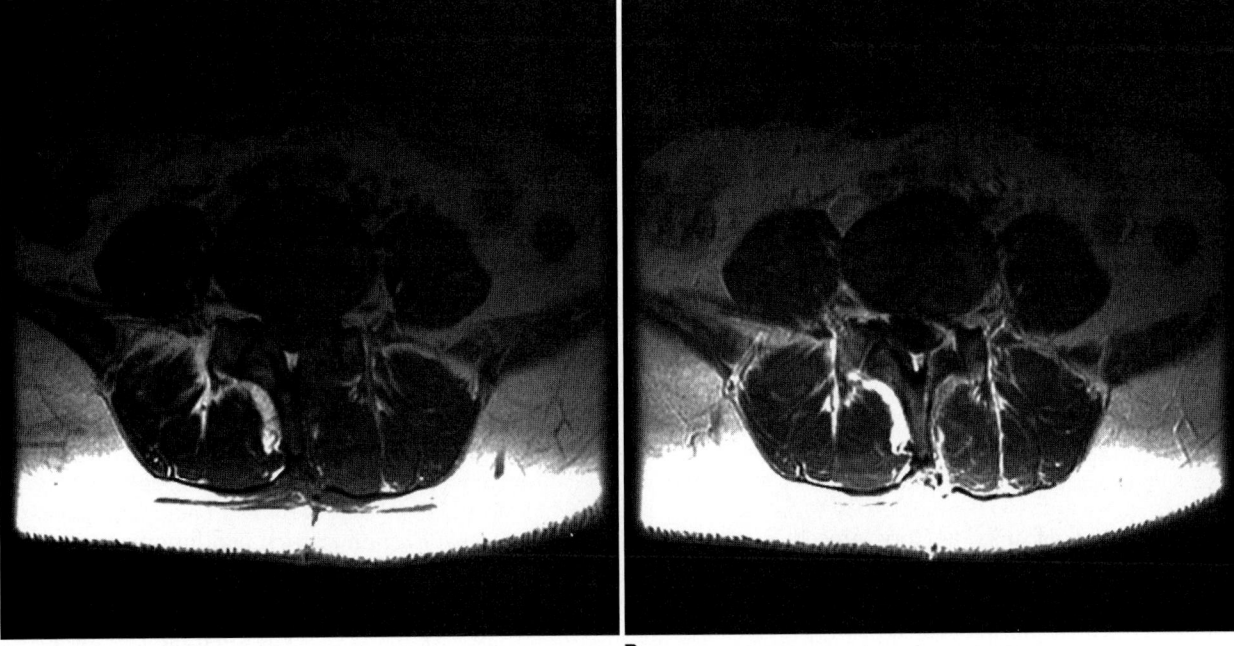

**A**  **B**

**Figure 132.2** Axial magnetic resonance images (MRIs) of a patient with a recurrent left disc herniation causing symptoms. **(A)** Axial $T_1$-weighted MRI without gadolinium. **(B)** Axial $T_1$-weighted MRI with gadolinium.

*Continued*

or epidural abscess (Figure 132.4). Spondylodiscitis may occur in up to 3% of patients.[17] Patients usually complain of pain and have muscle spasm. Fever, although occasionally present, is not always found. The wound may be tender and should be inspected for drainage. Although nonspecific and often falsely negative, adjunctive laboratory evaluations include the serum white blood cell count and the erythro-

cyte sedimentation rate. A number of reports suggest that C-reactive protein is a superior test.[23,27,45] A suspicious disc may be biopsied percutaneously and submitted for Gram stain and culture. Likewise, fluid collections may be tapped.

Radiographs and CT are not sensitive for detecting acute or subacute spondylodiscitis. MRI may be supplemented with radionuclide scintigraphy. Although it may be less sensitive than MRI, radionuclide scintigraphy also is more specific (92% vs. 100%).[38]

However, this theory is disputed in some studies.[6] Jinkins and Van Goethem[27] describe the MRI findings of postoperative spondylodiscitis:

- Vertebral end plate or marrow changes (low signal on $T_1$-weighted images and high signal on $T_2$-weighted images)
- Enhancing bone marrow adjacent to disc
- Enhancing spinal canal tissue
- Enhancing paravertebral soft tissue mass: rim (abscess) or homogenous (phlegmon) enhancement

Although some of the aforementioned signal changes can occur normally postoperatively (including disc enhancement), extensive contiguous enhancement of the disc and adjacent marrow is more consistent with infection. However, as previously stated, enhancement can be seen along the entire surgical tract in the normal postoperative spine. The issue of aseptic discitis, which is virtually indistinguishable from septic discitis on MRI,[23] further complicates the diagnostic and therapeutic issues. Cultures from the suspicious area must be obtained to ensure appropriate treatment and guide antibiotic selection, if appropriate.

Infected epidural collections enhance either homogenously, if phlegmonous, or in a rim fashion, as with

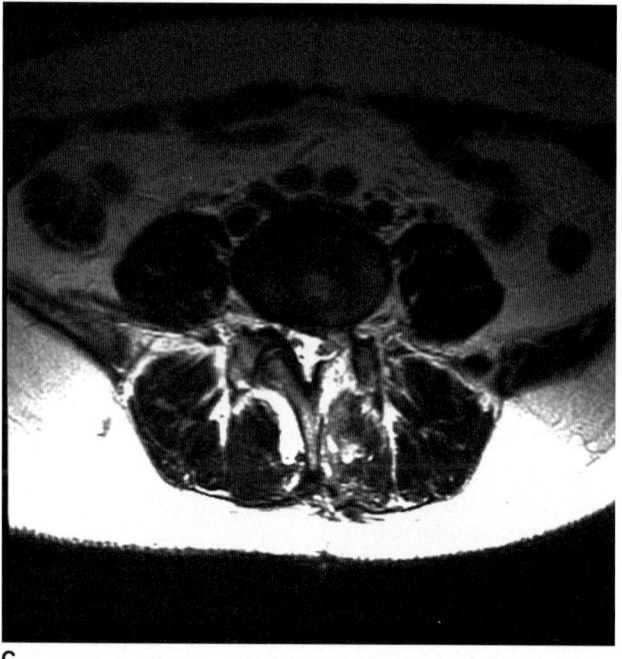

**C**

**Figure 132.2 *cont'd* (C)** Axial $T_2$-weighted MRI image.

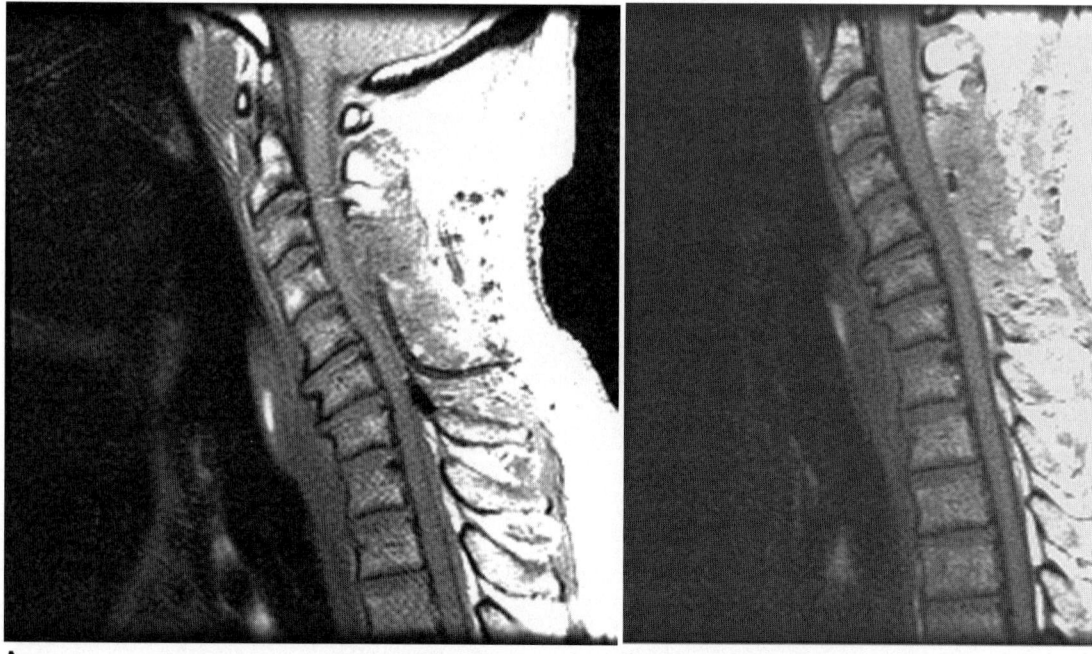

**A**                                    **B**

**Figure 132.3** Quadriparesis was observed in this patient following uneventful C3-5 laminectomies for spinal stenosis. **(A)** An isointense epidural hematoma is seen compressing the the cal sac and spinal cord. Following evacuation of the clot **(B)**, the patient's weakness improved.

abscesses. Epidural abscesses may exert mass effect on neural elements, and they should be drained emergently if symptomatic.

## Postoperative Arachnoiditis

A potential cause of FBSS that is difficult to manage is chronic arachnoiditis.[10] The potential causes of arachnoiditis are protean, but not proven. The inflammatory response may result from blood, infection, trauma, contrast, or any other intrathecally injected substance. Clinical findings of radiculopathy do not necessarily correlate with the severity of arachnoiditis as appreciated on imaging.[9]

Myelography, with and without CT, and MRI (particularly $T_2$-weighted fast spin-echo sequencing) both depict arachnoiditis with high accuracy, and classic findings on each correlate well with each other[20] (Figure 132.5). Shafaie et al.[47] summarize the three imaging patterns of arachnoiditis:

1. Matted or clumped nerve roots
2. An "empty" thecal sac caused by adhesions of the nerve roots to the walls of the thecal sac
3. An intrathecal soft tissue mass with a broad dural base that may obstruct CSF pathways

Although meninges and roots may enhance on MRI, gadolinium uptake is variable, and its absence does not provide diagnostic information. MRI can detect arachnoiditis with 92% sensitivity, 100% specificity, and 99% accuracy.[19]

## Postoperative Radiculitis

Enhancement of nerve roots is caused by disruption of the blood-nerve barrier. This can be reflective of a traumatized root or one that is undergoing repair (e.g., after chronic or severe compression from a herniated disc). The significance of an enhancing nerve root in the postoperative period changes over time and varies with circumstance. Nerve root enhancement can be seen in asymptomatic patients for 6 to 8 months postoperatively, after which it resolves.[6] Thereafter, in the chronic postoperative period, nerve root enhancement correlates well with radiculopathy.[26]

The causes of radiculitis and ongoing nerve root enhancement with radiculopathy are not fully explained,

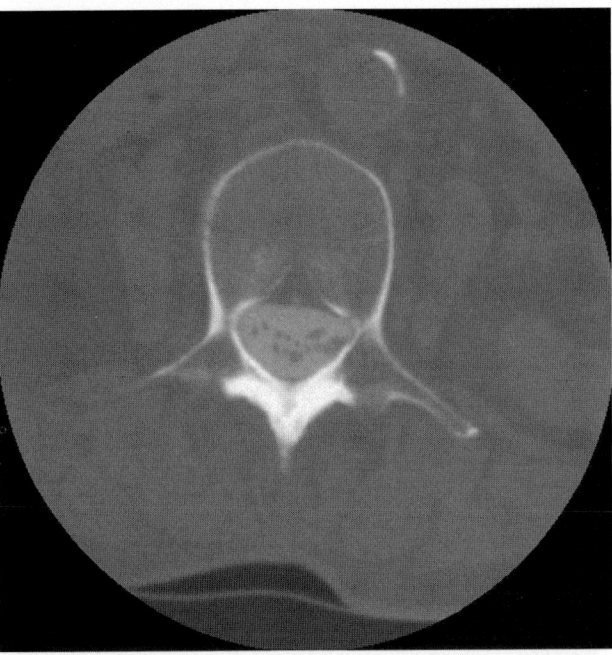

A

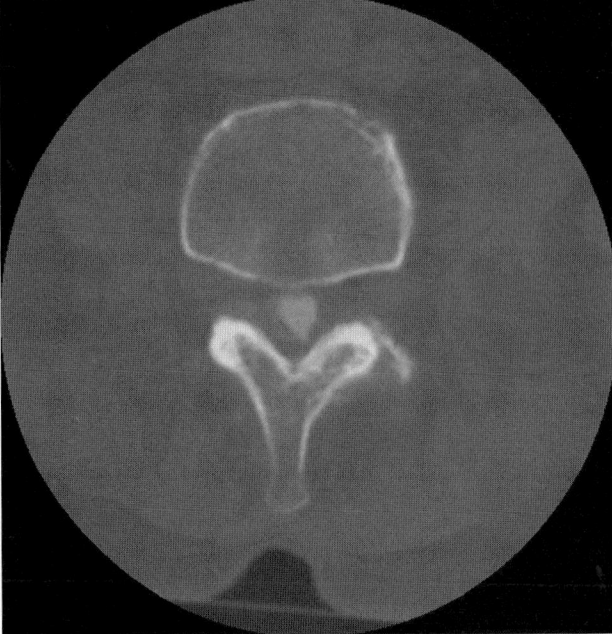

B

**Figure 132.5** Axial computed tomography myelogram image (**A**) demonstrates normal appearance of the nerve roots. (**B**) The nerve roots are clumped on one side. This is consistent with arachnoiditis.

**Figure 132.4** Postoperative epidural abscess. A rim-enhancing epidural collection is apparent dorsal to the thecal sac, opposite the L3-4 disc.

but probably relate to both trauma and ischemia from unresolved compression or to traction or constriction by postoperative epidural fibrosis and scarring. Management of the latter entity is usually frustrating, so the clinician should be compelled to exclude alternative causes of postoperative radiculopathy, including recurrent disc herniation and foraminal or lateral recess stenosis.

## Pseudomeningocele

A pseudomeningocele is a collection of CSF not lined by arachnoid or dura mater. Intraoperatively, a dural violation is either not recognized or inadequately repaired, resulting in a persistent opening. Back pain or radiculopathy can ensue. Most commonly, the imaging characteristics of CSF are identified (Figure 132.6); in the immediate postoperative period, blood products may be mixed in.

As mentioned previously, other radiographically identifiable causes of postoperative pain include foraminal or lateral recess stenosis and spinal instability. Although surgery may cause or exacerbate these features, their evaluation postoperatively and the imaging characteristics are similar to primary preoperative scenarios and, accordingly, are not discussed in detail in this chapter.

## Instrumentation

Since the introduction of the rod and hook construct by Harrington,[24] pedicle screw and plate fixation by Roy-

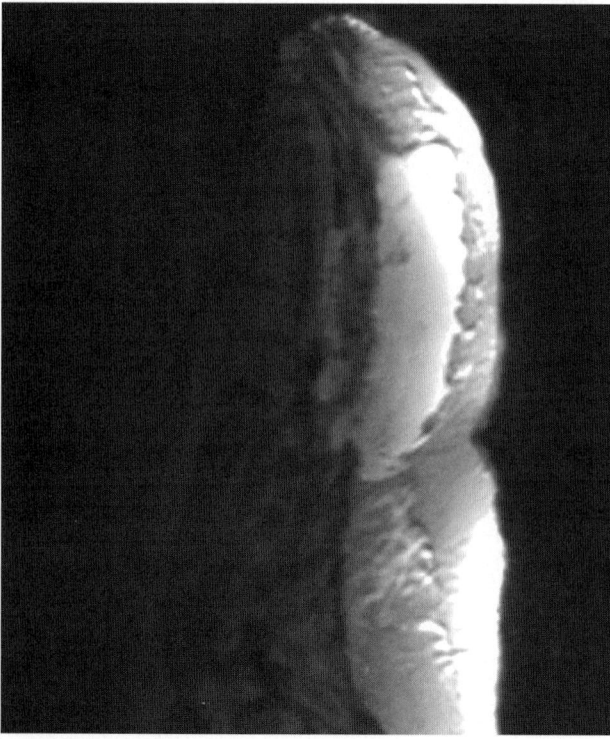

**Figure 132.6**  Pseudomeningocele. Laminectomy and successful removal of a thoracic schwannoma was complicated by formation of this massive dorsal thoracic pseudomeningocele, which is demonstrated by the dorsal hyperintensity on sagittal $T_2$-weighted magnetic resonance imaging.

Camille et al.,[42] and Caspar ventral cervical plating,[11] surgeons have attempted to bolster spinal stability with instrumentation at ever-increasing rates. Review of the indications and the imaging characteristics of each individual construct is beyond the scope of this chapter, because many options and variables exist. However, common principles of postoperative neurodiagnostic imaging can be applied to the analysis of studies obtained after spinal instrumentation of any set of spinal segments so that reasoned measures may be considered, if necessary.

To appropriately choose and interpret postoperative imaging of hardware, the clinician's goals of instrumentation should be fully understood and placed within each patient's clinical context. Spinal instrumentation is not an end unto itself, but replaces instability with rigidity, providing a permissive environment for the establishment, over time, of solid bony fusion. Almost any artificial construct will succumb to fatigue and inevitably fail if required to support the stresses of providing spinal stability without successful arthrodesis.

Selection and accurate placement of spinal instrumentation is guided, in large part, by preoperative and intraoperative imaging. Once the indication for instrumentation is established, the proper dimensions of screws, plates, hooks, or rods can be predicted by measurements of bony anatomy obtained from plain radiographs or CT, particularly in the axial plane. Important information regarding bone density also can be gleaned from plain films or CT. The equivalent mineral density—calculated from quantitative CT—has been correlated with the ability of cancellous bone to hold screws.[54] Placement of instrumentation is often guided by intraoperative biplanar fluoroscopy or by CT, and accurate understanding of instrument position is often possible in real time. Postoperative images should always be considered with respect to the preoperative films so that old pathologic findings are not confused with iatrogenic new ones.

As is the case with all postoperative spinal imaging, the evaluation of spinal implants occurs in two contexts: (1) at routine follow-up at various intervals and (2) in the assessment of unexpected signs or symptoms. Immediately postoperatively, implants are usually imaged to confirm placement at the correct level and proper positioning of screws, including depth of penetration into cancellous bone or across cortical thresholds. Routine early postoperative imaging serves the additional purpose of surgeon education, permitting appraisal and refinement of technique.

Patients who develop new pain or neurologic deficits, either immediately postoperatively or in a delayed fashion, should be expediently imaged so that the clinician can determine if there is a reversible hardware-related complication. Specific imaging of spinal implants is best achieved by plain radiography and by computed tomography with sagittal and coronal reconstructions. MRI is largely impractical for this purpose, because solid cortical bone is not well delineated, and even with the use of modern titanium implants, image artifact may obscure details.

For many purposes, conventional radiographs remain the foundation of instrumentation evaluation. The use of at least two perpendicular planes (anteroposterior [AP] and lateral) greatly enhances the ability to detect complications such as bony fracture or misplaced screws. Likewise, serial radiographs permit detection of subtle changes in implant positioning over time that may reflect screw loosening or breaking and may foreshadow complications that are more serious. Plain films are usually adequate, readily obtained, and not costly.

As titanium implants progressively replace steel and chrome and imaging artifact is diminished, the use of CT has increased. Advantages of CT over conventional radiographs include the ability to obtain axial images, permitting evaluation of the spinal canal. In addition, precise information regarding cortical bone is provided.[28] The evolution of high-speed helical CT permits image reformation and creation of sagittal, coronal, and three-dimensional reconstructions, which may offer more thorough information about implant positioning.

## Thoracolumbar Pedicle Screws

The use of routine postoperative imaging after pedicle screw fixation in the thoracolumbar spine provides an example in which to consider the relative accuracy of imaging via competing modalities and, importantly, the clinical relevance of any advantages. Consideration must be given to the rates of instrumentation (pedicle screw) misplacement in the hands of experienced spine surgeons and the consequences of such, particularly in the setting of a postoperative patient without new pain or neurologic symptom. Therefore the complications associated with pedicle screws are reviewed, followed by an attempt to frame the role of immediate postoperative imaging.

Review of the literature suggests that placement of pedicle screws in the thoracolumbar spine is safe, but that accuracy varies and that rates of misplacement reach as high as 41%, even in the hands of experienced spine surgeons using intraoperative fluoroscopic guidance.[46] Difficulties in understanding rates of misplacement arise because of discrepancies in how accuracy is measured (e.g., by plain films,[18] by CT,[55] or in cadaveric specimens[12]). Likewise, investigators vary regarding their opinion of whether or not a breach or erosion of cortical bone or screw penetration exceeding 2mm constitutes misplacement.[56] In a review of 915 procedures, Lonstein et al.[34] reported that 95% of 4800 screws had been placed "within the pedicle and vertebral body," as assessed by plain radiographs. Defining accurate placement as "within 2mm of the medial border of the pedicle," Gerstein and Robbins[21] used postoperative CT to determine a screw misplacement rate of 19%. The generally accepted rate of misplacement per patient is approximately 5%, garnered through surveys of American Back Society members compiled by Esses et al.[16]

How accurately do various modalities of postoperative imaging reflect the accuracy of pedicle screw placement? Again, variation exists, but most evidence favors the superiority of CT over plain radiographs. Using plain radiography, Weinstein et al.[53] reported that, in cadavers, the position of 21% of 124 screws was inaccurately predicted. In a similar in vitro study,[18] plain films were accurate for 73% to 83% of screws.

CT, particularly with axial cuts displaying the length of the pedicle and delineating cortical bone, is most accurate. In 42 screws placed in 4 cadavers, in vitro analysis demonstrated 10 cortical penetrations, which was 100% in concordance with CT results.[12] Somewhat contrastingly, Yoo et al.,[55] assessing screw placement in lumbar cadaveric spines, demonstrated CT sensitivity of 68% for cobalt-chrome screws and 87% for titanium, concluding that the use of "CT alone can lead to inaccuracies."[55]

Several studies suggest that many cortical penetrations identified on CT cannot be identified on roentgenograms. In a prospective study of 30 patients with lumbar pedicle screw fixation, postoperative plain films detected only 10% of cortical transgressions identified by CT.[29] Berlemann et al.[3] also note a significant difference in sensitivity, with CT detecting of 50% more misplaced screws. In contrast, comparing lateral plain films and CT, and judging pedicle screw position as "in," "out," or "questionable," Sapkas et al.[43] studied 35 patients with 220 thoracolumbar pedicle screws and noted that no statistical difference in detection existed between the two modalities (96% "in" by plain film vs. 94% by CT). Again, the literature is not definitive; however, particularly in patients with new neurologic symptoms, CT may yield more information because of its depiction of the spinal canal, wherein nerve roots course caudally before exiting through neural foramina.

The clinical significance of a misplaced pedicle screw, in an asymptomatic postoperative patient, is unclear. The most dreaded complication associated with hardware misplacement is neurologic injury. Class I evidence suggesting that instrumentation improves outcome when combined with dorsolateral fusion does not exist, although pedicle screw fixation probably decreases the rate of pseudoarthrosis.[44] Therefore the consequences of screw misplacement with regard to final outcome are, likewise, difficult to determine.

A high rate of screw malposition does not necessarily correlate with neurologic complication.[46] In a study (as determined by CT) of 50 patients undergoing 360-degree lumbar fusion, 41% of pedicle screws were outside of the pedicle to some extent: 20.9% were outside of the pedicle by less than 2mm; 11.1% were outside of the pedicle by 2 to 4mm; 6.1% were outside by 4 to 6mm; and 2.9% were outside by more than 6mm. In addition, 32% of screws were misplaced medially, potentially endangering neural elements. Of those screws that penetrated cortical bone by more than 6mm, three missed medially, and all of them were located in the lumbar spine. The four laterally missing screws were placed in the thoracic spine. "Apparent displacement of dura" was associated with each of the medially placed screws; however, only one patient (0.5%) issued neurologic complaint (S1 pain).[46] Despite a 41% pedicle screw misplacement, only one patient suffered nerve root irritation. All patients in this study "fused as expected." Similarly, in the study by Castro et al.,[12] 5 of 30 patients suffered postoperative deficits ipsilateral to the side of a misplaced screw (as determined by CT). Each of these patients had screw misplacement of 6mm or more. No symptoms were ascribed to screws penetrating cortex by less than 6mm at any level. Normal spinal anatomy dictates that there is an epidural "cushion" in the lumbar spinal canal that provides a margin for error for extrapedicular screw placement. Other anatomic studies reveal even wider epidural zones of safety.[48] Less margin for error may exist in the thoracic spine because the spinal cord is not as mobile as are the nerve roots. However, because of the anatomy of thoracic pedicles, misplaced screws tend to be lateral, where neural elements are not at risk, although vascular and visceral structures may be endangered.[56]

Although CT may be considered the "gold standard" for assessing the placement of spinal instrumentation, its advantages over less costly plain films may be of little relevance in patients enjoying smooth postoperative courses. As discussed at the beginning of this section, changes in the positioning and the integrity of hardware are important to follow longitudinally. Even micromotion can be the cause of persistent pain. However, prudence may limit the use of CT to patients with symptoms, either new or unresolved, following surgery.

Although the aforementioned discussion pertains specifically to immediate postoperative imaging after placement of thoracolumbar pedicle screws, its principles may be considered for other applications. The availability of a more precise measuring stick does not necessarily mandate its routine use, particularly if management and prognosis are unlikely to be altered by the information. As surgeons gain more expertise and confidence in surgical technique, limiting the use of postoperative CT may become feasible and, in fact, prudent.

## Fusion

Except for patients with limited life expectancy (e.g., metastatic cancer), one of the chief goals of any stabilizing spinal procedure, with or without instrumentation, is the fusion of bony elements. Although successful fusion does not necessarily lead to good outcome,[2,4,15] documentation of arthrodesis is an essential component of patient follow-up. It is well established that pseudoarthrosis, which is the leading complication associated with thoracic and lumbar spinal arthrodesis,[39] can contribute greatly to persistent postoperative pain.[49]

Successful fusion depends on the establishment of a contiguous mass of bone across a motion segment, preventing movement in any plane across that segment.[42] A spinal pseudoarthrosis is defined as "an absence of bridging bone between adjacent vertebrae."[39] In a review of thoracolumbar pseudoarthrosis, Raiszadeh *et al.*[39] define atrophic, transverse, shingle, and complex nonunions. "Atrophic" pseudoarthrosis presents as withering and resorption of the bone graft. When significant growth of bone between segments is disrupted by a horizontal band of fibrous tissue, the pseudoarthrosis is considered "transverse." In a "shingle" pseudoarthrosis, a defect in the fusion mass passes sagittally and obliquely, preventing contact of the graft with the underlying vertebra. When contact between the fusion mass and adjacent vertebrae is lost in multiple areas, the pseudoarthrosis is "complex." Radiographic detection of failed fusion can be straightforward, as in the case of progressive deformity or atrophic pseudoarthrosis, or it can be more challenging, as with transverse or shingle pseudoarthrosis. Motion demonstrated on flexion-extension radiographs strongly suggests pseudoarthrosis. The gold standard for determining instability and pseudoarthrosis is a second-look operation, at which time the fusion mass and any motion can be visualized directly.[35] A variety of radiographic methods has been used for assessing fusion.

### Radiographs

Much information regarding fusion can be garnered from plain radiographs, if the fusion mass is properly visualized. In a study of pseudoarthrosis after allograft posterior lumbar interbody fusion with pedicle screw and plate fixation, Brantigan[7] enumerates radiographic criteria by which to determine failed, uncertain, and successful fusion:

*Radiographic pseudoarthrosis:* Collapse of construct, vertebral slip, broken screws, resorption of the bone graft, or major lucency or gap visible in the fusion area
*Uncertain fusion:* Bone graft visible in the fusion area at approximately the density originally achieved surgically, or a small lucency or gap visible involving a portion of the fusion area, with at least half of the graft area showing no lucency between the graft bone and vertebral bone
*Radiographic fusion:* Bone in the fusion area radiographically more dense and more mature than originally achieved in surgery, no interface between the donor bone and the vertebral bone, mature bony trabeculae bridging the fusion area, resorption of ventral vertebral traction spurs, anterior progression of the graft within the disc space, facet joint fusion

Serially following the evolution of the fusion mass from the immediate postoperative period to the time of satisfactory radiographic fusion and patient recovery is critical for assessing changes in density and position of the graft, as well as for evaluating alterations in hardware positioning. Likewise, bony changes associated with chronic instability can be observed to regress.

The importance of proper visualization of the fusion mass and joint across which it passes is demonstrated by Dawson *et al.*[14] in their appraisal of plain radiographs for pseudoarthrosis in the lumbar spine. For patients with dorsolateral lumbar fusion, visualization of the facet joints by oblique radiographs increases the sensitivity of plain radiographs from 48% to 82% over AP and lateral views alone. Dawson *et al.*[14] and Raiszadeh *et al.*[39] note that the sensitivity of oblique films is diminished in cases of kyphosis or rotational deformity.

### Dynamic Radiography

Dynamic radiography is often used to assess spinal instability and has been applied toward the assessment of pseudoarthrosis. Flexion-extension or lateral bending films help detect gross instability but seem poorly able to demonstrate the subtler motions often associated with failed fusion. Plain radiographs with proper views are superior to dynamic radiography, with comparative sensitivities of 82% versus 23% in one study.[1]

### *Technetium Scintigraphy*

Absorption of technetium by healing bone may offer complementary information in the assessment of fusion.[39] Technetium scintigraphy seems most useful 1 year after surgery, once bony remodeling is complete. Combined planar scintigraphy and single photon emission CT scintigraphy may be more sensitive than flexion-extension radiography; however, false-positive rates are unacceptably high when scans are performed before 1 year, probably because of continued bone remodeling in immature fusion.[36,40,49]

### Tomograms

Although the use of tomograms has declined, evidence suggests great sensitivity in the detection of pseudoarthrosis. AP views yield more information than do lateral views, although the latter may be useful for patients with kyphotic deformities. Correlation between known pseudoarthrosis and detection on AP tomograms has been reported to be as high as 96%.[14]

### Computed Tomography

Some authors have reported the usefulness of CT for documenting pseudoarthrosis.[13] Historically, CT has been less useful than plain radiographs for detecting pseudoarthrosis, particularly because of inability to demonstrate transverse disruptions in the fusion mass.[31] The recent ability to obtain thin-cut CT scans and to fashion high-detail sagittal, coronal, and 3D reconstructions may increase CT sensitivity for detecting pseudoarthrosis, although such has not been rigorously studied[30] (Figure 132.7).

### Magnetic Resonance Imaging

MRI possesses great sensitivity for detecting subtle fractures in long bones, particularly because of rendering of the marrow and cancellous bone. Nevertheless, MRI has not been used routinely for the assessment of fusion, largely because of hazards and artifact from associated hardware and difficulties in viewing cortical bone. Reports have demonstrated its use in cases of suspected pseudoarthrosis, wherein plain radiographs demonstrated sclerotic zones between motion segments, typically reflective of successful fusion. MRI can demonstrate subtle gaps of intermediate signal intensity on $T_1$-weighted images and high $T_2$ signal intensity that are otherwise undetected.[22]

The radiographic diagnosis of failed fusion and pseudoarthrosis remains somewhat vexing. No single radiographic modality consistently identifies pseudoarthrosis with great sensitivity and specificity. Rendering therapeutic decisions regarding fusion or the consideration of second-look or corrective surgery requires the application of clinical judgment in the context of radiographic findings. Relative inaccuracies in commonly relied on imaging techniques are highlighted by Larsen et al.,[31] who found no statistically significant correlation between radiographic appearance on plain radiographs, flexion-extension radiographs, CT, and bone scintigraphy with intraoperative verification of pseudoarthrosis.

## Postoperative Imaging for Tumor

In most instances, postoperative imaging after spinal tumor resection is performed to confirm gross total resection or the degree of removal and to serve as a baseline for subsequent follow-up studies. In benign intradural

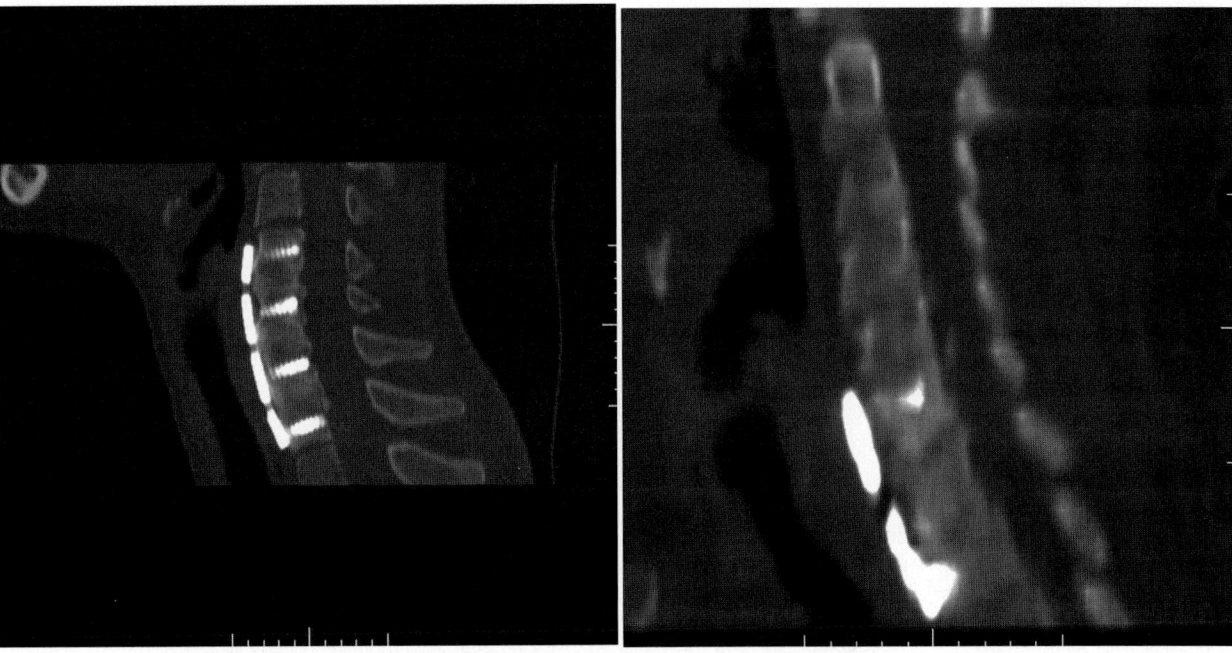

**A**                    **B**

**Figure 132.7** Computed tomographic sagittal reconstruction imaging of the cervical spine. **(A)** The image demonstrates solid fusion 3 months after surgery at three levels with ventral cervical plating. **(B)** The patient had neck pain with movement 1 year after surgery. At the upper level, there is a pseudoarthrosis, whereas at the lower level there is fusion. Flexion-extension images demonstrated movement at the level of pseudoarthrosis.

extramedullary diseases such as meningioma or schwannoma, gross total removal is usually achieved. However, yearly follow-up imaging is generally recommended to identify recurrence before the onset of symptoms. The recurrence rate for spinal meningioma is approximately 1% at 5 years and just higher than 5% at 10 years.[33,50]

Intramedullary spinal tumors can be either benign or malignant. Advances in microsurgical technique permit gross total resection in most cases of benign tumors such as ependymomas and hemangioblastomas. For ependymomas, Lee et al.[32] recommend postoperative imaging immediately after surgery, at 6 months after surgery, and then annually. Radiation treatment is recommended only in cases where gross total resection is not achieved. Intramedullary spinal lipomas are generally treated with internal decompression and can be followed clinically.

In the case of medulloblastoma, postoperative imaging is often used to stage the disease. Spinal MRI has been found to have greater accuracy than CSF cytologic analysis after surgery. Imaging performed after 2 weeks postoperatively appears to reduce false-positive results. The identification of disseminated disease on postoperative imaging is associated with poor prognosis.[37]

# REFERENCES

1. Albert TJ, Pinto M, Denis F: Management of symptomatic lumbar pseudarthrosis with anteroposterior fusion. A functional and radiographic outcome study. *Spine* 25:123, 2000.
2. Bailey SI, Bartolozzi P, Bertagnoli R, et al: The spinal fixator system. A preliminary report of a 2-year prospective, international multicenter study in a range of indications requiring surgical intervention for bone grafting and pedicle screw fixation. *Spine* 21:2006, 1996.
3. Berlemann U, Heini P, Muller U, et al: Reliability of pedicle screw assessment using plain radiographs versus CT reconstruction. *Eur Spine J* 6:406, 1997.
4. Blumenthal SL, Gill K: Can lumbar spine radiographs accurately determine fusion in postoperative patients? Correlation of routine radiographs with a second surgical look at lumbar fusions. *Spine* 18:1186, 1993.
5. Boden SD, Davis DO, Dina TS, et al: Contrast-enhanced MR imaging performed after successful lumbar disk surgery: Prospective study. *Radiology* 182:59, 1992.
6. Boden SD, Davis DO, Dina TS, et al: Postoperative diskitis: Distinguishing early MR imaging findings from normal postoperative disk space infections. *Radiology* 14:765, 1992.
7. Brantigan JW: Pseudoarthrosis rate after allograft posterior lumbar interbody fusion with pedicle screw and plate fixation. *Spine* 19:1271, 1994.
8. Bundschuh CV, Modic MT, Ross JS et al: Epidural fibrosis and recurrent disk herniation in the lumbar spine: MR imaging assessment. *AJR Am J Roentgenol* 150:923, 1988.
9. Burton CV: Lumbosacral arachnoiditis. *Spine* 3:23, 1978.
10. Burton CV, Kirkaldy-Willis WH, Yong-Hing K, et al: Causes of failure of surgery on the lumbar spine. *Clin Orthop* 157:192, 1981.
11. Caspar W, Barbier DD, Klara PM: Anterior cervical fusion and Caspar plate stabilization for cervical trauma. *Neurosurgery* 25:491, 1989.
12. Castro WH, Halm H, Jerosch J, et al: Accuracy of pedicle screw placement in lumbar vertebrae. *Spine* 24:1320, 1996.
13. Chafetz N, Cann CE, Morris JM, et al: Pseudoarthrosis following lumbar fusion: Detection by direct coronal CT scanning. *Radiology* 162:803, 1987.
14. Dawson EG, Clader TJ, Basset LW, et al: A comparison of different methods used to diagnose pseudoarthrosis following posterior spinal fusion for scoliosis. *J Bone Joint Surg* 67A:1153, 1985.
15. Dickman CA, Fessler RG, Macmillan M, et al: Transpedicular screw-rod fixation of the lumbar spine: Operative technique and outcome in 104 cases. *J Neurosurg* 77:860, 1992.
16. Esses SI, Sachs BL, Dreyzin V: Complications associated with the technique of pedicle screw fixation: A selected survey of ABS members. *Spine* 18:2231, 1993.
17. Fernand R, Lee CK: Post-laminectomy disk space infection: A review of the literature and a report of three cases. *Clin Orthop* 209:215, 1986.
18. Ferrick MR, Kowalski JM, Simmons ED: Reliability of roentgenogram evaluation of pedicle screw position. *Spine* 22:249, 1997.
19. Firooznia H, Krischeff II, Rafii M, et al: Lumbar spine after surgery: Examination with intravenous contrast-enhanced CT. *Radiology* 163:221, 1987.
20. Fitt GJ, Stevens JM: Postoperative arachnoiditis diagnosed by high resolution fast spin-echo MRI of the lumbar spine. *Neuroradiology* 37:139, 1995.
21. Gerstein SD, Robbins SE: Accuracy of pedicle screw placement in vivo. *Spine* 15:11, 1990.
22. Ghazi J, Golimbu CN, Engler GL: MRI of spinal fusion pseudarthrosis. *J Comput Assist Tomogr* 16:324, 1992.
23. Grane P, Josephson A, Seferlis A, et al: Septic and aseptic post-operative discitis in the lumbar spine: Evaluation by MR imaging. *Acta Radiol* 39:108, 1998.
24. Harrington PR: Treatment of scoliosis: Correction and internal fixation by spine instrumentation. *J Bone Joint Surg* 44A:591, 1962.
25. Hueftle MG, Modic MT, Ross JS, et al: Lumbar spine: Postoperative MR imaging with Gd-DTPA. *Radiology* 167:817, 1988.
26. Jinkins JR, Osborn AG, Gattet D, et al: Spinal nerve enhancement with Gd-DTPA: MR correlation with the postoperative lumbosacral spine. *AJNR Am J Neuroradiol* 14:383, 1993.
27. Jinkins JR, Van Goethem JWM: The postsurgical lumbosacral spine: Magnetic resonance imaging evaluation following intervertebral disk surgery, surgical decompression, intervertebral bony fusion, and spinal instrumentation. *Radiol Clin North Am* 39:1, 2001.
28. Kaech DL, Meier G: Principles, imaging, and complications of spinal instrumentation. In Jinkins JR (ed): *Posttherapeutic neurodiagnostic imaging.* Philadelphia, Lippincott-Raven, 1997, pp 267-302.
29. Laine T, Makitalo K, Schlenzka D, et al: Accuracy of pedicle screw insertion: A prospective study in 30 low back patients. *Eur Spine J* 6:402, 1997.
30. Lang P, Genant HK, Chafetz N, et al: Three-dimensional computed tomography and multiplanar reformations in the

assessment of pseudoarthrosis in posterior lumbar fusion patients. *Spine* 13:69, 1988.

31. Larsen JM, Rimoldi RL, Capen DA, *et al:* Assessment of pseudoarthrosis in pedicle screw fusion: A prospective study comparing plain radiographs, CT scanning, and bone scintigraphy with operative findings. *J Spinal Disord* 9:117, 1996.

32. Lee TT, Gromelski EB, Green BA: Surgical treatment of spinal ependymoma and post-operative radiotherapy. *Acta Neurochir* 140:309, 1998.

33. Levy WJ, Bay J, Dohn DF: Spinal cord meningioma. *J Neurosurg* 57:804, 1982.

34. Lonstein JE, Denis F, Perra JH, *et al:* Complications associated with pedicle screws. *J Bone Joint Surg* 82A:1519, 1999.

35. McMaster MJ, James JIP: Pseudarthrosis after spinal fusion for scoliosis. *J Bone Joint Surg* 58B:305, 1976.

36. McMaster MJ, Merrick MV: The scintigraphic assessment of the scoliotic spine after fusion. *J Bone Joint Surg* 62B:65, 1980.

37. Meyers SP, Wildenhain SL, Chang JK, *et al:* Postoperative evaluation for disseminated medulloblastoma involving the spine: Contrast-enhanced MR findings, CSF cytologic analysis, timing of disease occurrence, and patient outcomes. *AJNR Am J Neuroradiol* 21:1757, 2000.

38. Modic MT, Feiglin DH, Pirano DW, *et al:* Vertebral osteomyelitis: Assessment using MR. *Radiology* 157:156, 1985.

39. Raiszadeh R, Heggeness M, Esses SI: Thoracolumbar pseudoarthrosis. *Am J Orthop* 29:513, 2000.

40. Rawlins BA, Michelsen CB: Failed lumbosacral fusions: State of the art reviews. *Spine* 8:563, 1994.

41. Ross JS, Masaryk TJ, Schrader M, *et al:* MR imaging of the postoperative lumbar spine: Assessment with gadopentetate dimeglumine. *AJR Am J Roentgenol* 155:867, 1990.

42. Roy-Camille R, Saillant G, Mazel C: Plating of thoracic, thoracolumbar, and lumbar injuries with pedicle screw plates. *Orthop Clin North Am* 17:147, 1986.

43. Sapkas G, Papadakis SA, Stathakopoulos DP, *et al:* Evaluation of pedicle screw position in thoracic and lumbar spine fixation using plane radiographs and computed tomography. A prospective study of 35 patients. *Spine* 24:1926, 1999.

44. Schnee CL, Freese A, Ansell LV: Outcome analysis for adults with spondylolisthesis treated with posterolateral fusion and transpedicular screw fixation. *J Neurosurg* 86:56, 1997.

45. Schulitz KP, Assheur J: Discitis after procedures on the intervertebral disc. *Spine* 19:1172, 1994.

46. Schulze CJ, Munzinger E, Weber U: Clinical relevance of accuracy of pedicle screw placement. *Spine* 23:2215, 1998.

47. Shafaie FF, Bundschuh CV, Jinkins JR: The posttherapeutic lumbar spine. In Jinkins JR (ed): *Posttherapeutic Neurodiagnostic Imaging.* Philadelphia, Lippincott-Raven, 1997, pp 223-243.

48. Sjostrom L, Jacobsson O, Karlstrom G, *et al:* CT analysis of pedicles and screw tracts after implant removal in thoracolumbar fractures. *J Spinal Disord* 6:225, 1993.

49. Slizofski WJ, Collier BD, Flatley TJ, *et al:* Painful pseudoarthrosis following lumbar spinal fusion: Detection by combined SPECT and planar bone scintigraphy. *Skeletal Radiol* 16:136, 1987.

50. Solero CL, Fornari M, Giombini S: Spinal meningiomas: Review of 174 operated cases. *Neurosurgery* 25:153, 1989.

51. Van Goethem JWM, Parizel PM, Perdieus D, *et al:* Imaging findings in patients with failed back surgery syndrome. *J Belge Radiol* 80:81, 1997.

52. Van Goethem JWM, Van de Kelft EV, Biltjes IG, *et al:* MRI after successful lumbar discectomy. *Neuroradiology* 38:S90, 1996.

53. Weinstein JN, Spratt KF, Spengler D, *et al:* Spinal pedicle fixation: Reliability and validity of spinal roentgenogram-based assessment and surgical factors on successful screw placement. *Spine* 13:1012, 1988.

54. Wittenberg RH, Shea M, Swartz DE, *et al:* Importance of bone mineral density in instrumented spinal fusion. *Spine* 16:647, 1991.

55. Yoo JU, Ghanayem A, Petersilge C, Lewin J: Accuracy of using computed tomography to identify pedicle screw placement in cadaveric human lumbar spine. *Spine* 22:249, 1997.

56. Youkilis AS, Quint DJ, McGillicuddy JE, *et al:* Stereotactic navigation for placement of pedicle screws in the thoracic spine. *Neurosurgery* 28:771, 2001.

# CHAPTER 133

# Intraoperative Imaging of the Spine

**Iain H. Kalfas, Bruce M. McCormack, and Hansen A. Yuan**

Few surgical specialties are as dependent on intraoperative imaging as is the field of spinal surgery. Whether it involves obtaining a lateral radiograph to confirm the level of a lumbar disc herniation or using ultrasonic imaging to localize an intramedullary syrinx, intraoperative imaging provides information that can significantly affect the course of the surgery.

The most commonly used intraoperative imaging techniques are plain film radiography, fluoroscopy, and ultrasonography. These techniques each have their own advantages and disadvantages, but when used appropriately, each can provide valuable information. In addition to these standard intraoperative imaging techniques, image-guided spinal navigation (IGSN) has evolved over the past few years into a proven and versatile tool for orienting the spinal surgeon to the complex three-dimensional anatomy of the spinal column. This chapter reviews each imaging technique, as well as the indications for their use.

## Plain Film Radiography

Plain film radiography was the first imaging technique applied to spinal surgery. The segmented bony anatomy of the spinal column lends itself readily to this form of imaging. Images are easily obtained, relatively inexpensive, and generally reliable. Differential attenuation of x-rays by the various tissues provides the image contrast seen in a radiograph. Attenuation differences result from the variations in tissue density and tissue thickness and from the energy spectrum of the x-ray beam. Bone attenuates x-rays the most, followed by muscle, fat, and air, which attenuate very few x-rays. However, plain film radiography does not show soft tissue structures, such as the spinal cord, nerve roots, or intervertebral discs.

In spinal surgery, plain radiography is typically used to localize a specific spinal level. During the surgical exposure of the cervical, lumbar, or thoracic spine, a radiopaque marker (i.e., clamp, probe, spinal needle) is positioned in the surgical field. For the lumbar of cervical spine, a lateral radiograph is obtained with the lumbosacral or occipitocervical junction at one end and the inserted marker at the other end. The number of vertebral levels between the imaged junction and the marker can be determined and the appropriate spinal level easily localized. In general, the range of view from the occipitocervical junction extends caudally to the cervicothoracic junction, depending on the prominence of the patient's neck and shoulders. The range of view from the lumbosacral junction extends rostrally to the lower thoracic region.

Spinal levels in the midthoracic and upper thoracic spine can be more difficult to precisely localize because of their distance from a reliable anatomic reference point. In this case, an alternative to the conventional method of radiographic localization is to obtain two adjacent lateral images. The first film is placed to include the lumbosacral or occipitocervical junction at one end and an instrument marker attached to the spinal anatomy at the other end. A second film is then obtained that includes the first instrument marker and a second instrument marker centered in the operative field. The location of the first instrument marker can be determined on the first film by its relationship to the lumbosacral or occipitocervical junction. The location of the appropriate spinal level can be determined on the second film by determining its relationship to the first instrument marker.

Radiographic imaging of the upper thoracic spine can be difficult because the patient's shoulders may obstruct the view on a lateral radiograph. An alternative to the lateral radiograph is the anteroposterior (AP) view. This view can be obtained by positioning the patient on a radiolucent operating table. The film cassette can then be placed immediately below the table, and an AP view can be obtained. With this view, either the T1 or the T12 vertebrae and their associated ribs serve as the reference point for spinal level identification (Figure 133.1).

When intraoperative localization involves exposure of the spinal column at the level of collapsed or fractured vertebrae, the relationship of the operative field to the lumbosacral or occipitocervical junction is not as critical. A film that centers over the operative field can approximate the appropriate level. The abnormal vertebrae can usually be identified on a lateral radiograph and the appropriate exposure confirmed.

The most common error related to the use of intraoperative plain radiography is incorrectly identifying the marked spinal level. This is usually because of poor image quality that may obscure the appropriate spinal anatomy. It can also be caused by the surgeon misinterpreting either the intraoperative anatomy or the radiograph itself. Localization errors can occur by incorrectly counting the number of spinal levels from the lumbosacral or occipitocervical junction to the operative field. Therefore it is imperative that a satisfactory radiograph be obtained before continuing with the procedure. This may require repeating the film or more carefully interpreting the initial radiograph.

In addition to localization of the spinal level, plain radiography can be used during spinal surgery to assess the extent of neural decompression. This is more practical for anterior decompressive procedures than for posterior procedures. This technique is particularly helpful for transoral decompressive procedures or for anterior decompressive procedures in the setting of a kyphotic deformity. It involves placing a radiopaque contrast medium into the decompressed site immediately before obtaining a lateral radiograph. The radiograph demonstrates the extent of the decompression and can be compared with the preoperative study. If the configuration and location of the contained contrast medium does not approximate the configuration and location of the epidural compression on the preoperative studies, the operative site can be modified until a satisfactory decompression of the neural elements is achieved (Figure 133.2).

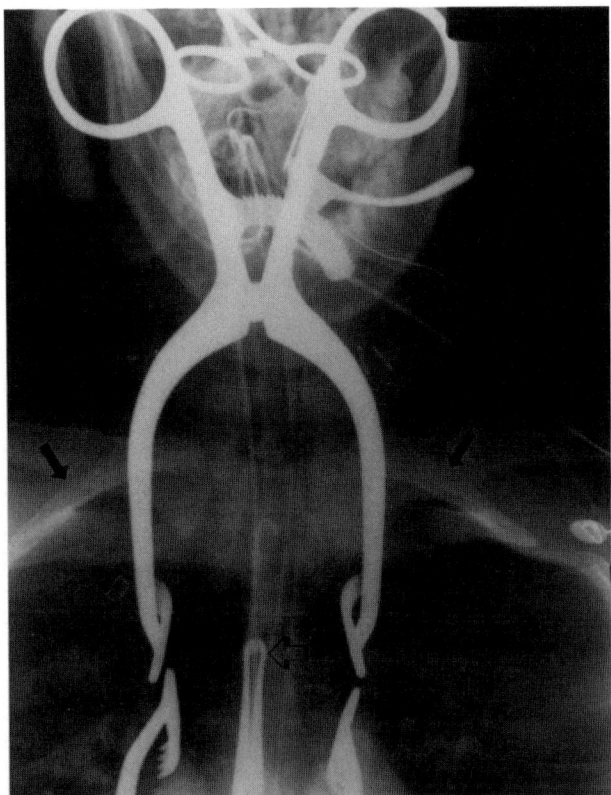

**Figure 133.1** Anteroposterior radiograph of the upper thoracic spine showing a clamp on the spinous process of T3 *(open arrow)*. The reference point for localization is the first pair of ribs *(arrows)*.

In certain instances, an intraoperative myelogram may help determine the extent of canal decompression (Figure 133.3). For example, when a posterolateral approach is used in the setting of a thoracolumbar vertebral body burst fracture with ventral epidural compression, radiopaque dye can be placed in the subarachnoid space by a small-gauge spinal needle. A lateral radiograph is taken and the relationship of the dye to the ventral spinal cord can be assessed.[23]

## Fluoroscopy

Fluoroscopy is used when "real-time" imaging of the spine is required. The x-rays are produced continuously and the film/screen combination used in radiography is replaced with an image intensifier and television monitor system. The image can be produced with a lower radiation dose compared with standard radiography. A camera records the image and displays it on a monitor. The images can be recorded on x-ray film, cinefluoradiography film, or videotape.[1]

The primary use of fluoroscopy in spinal surgery is to facilitate the optimal positioning of spinal fixation screws, interbody cages, or percutaneous methylmethacrylate injected into vertebral bodies. Each of these techniques requires a precise orientation to the unexposed spinal anatomy. Suboptimal screw placement can result in neural and/or vascular injury, as well as inadequate spinal fixation, which may lead to a pseudoarthrosis or fixation failure.[6]

Fluoroscopy provides the surgeon with real-time imaging of the spinal column in several planes depending on the positioning of the fluoroscope's C-arm. When used for the insertion of pedicle screws, the C-arm can be positioned to provide a lateral view of the spinal column. This shows the sagittal (rostral-caudal) orientation of a pedicle screw or its proposed trajectory (Figure 133.4). By rotating

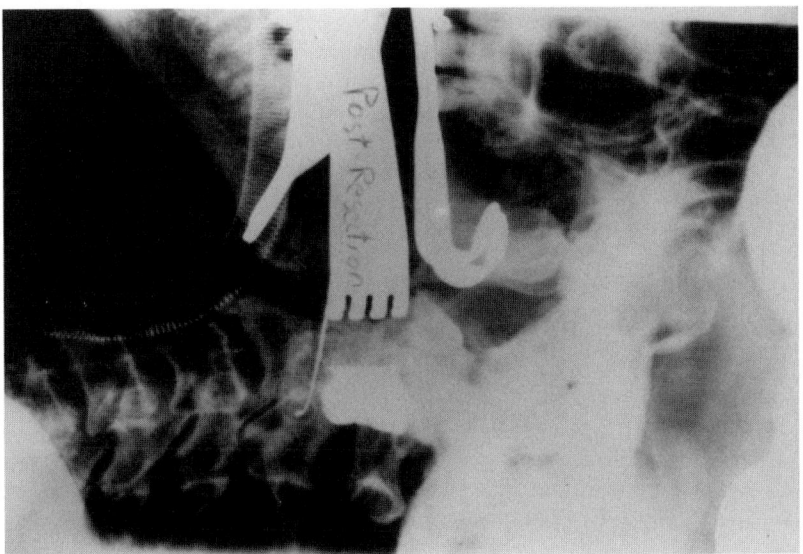

**Figure 133.2** Lateral radiograph after a transoral odontoidectomy. Radiopaque contrast media has been placed into the decompressed site. The position and configuration of the contrast media can be compared with the preoperative studies to confirm a satisfactory decompression.

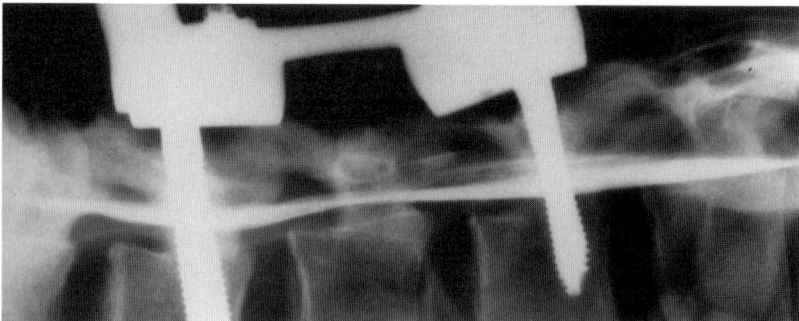

**Figure 133.3** Intraoperative lateral myelography after lumbar decompression and fixation.

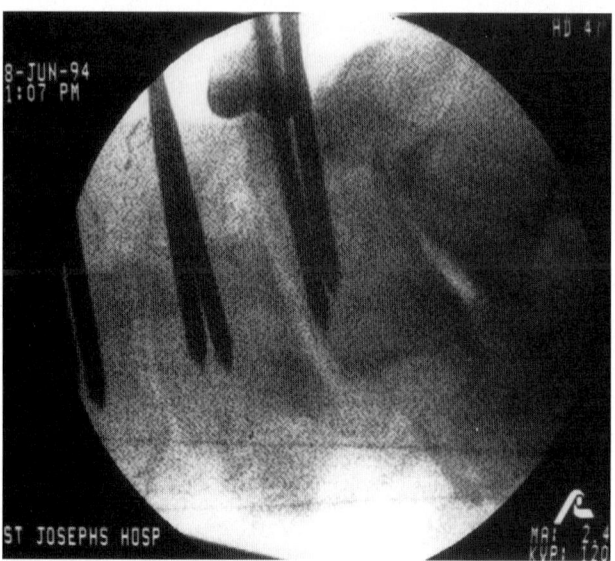

**Figure 133.4** Lateral fluoroscopic view of the lower lumbar spine showing the sagittal orientation of Steinmann pins placed within the pedicles of L3, L4, and L5.

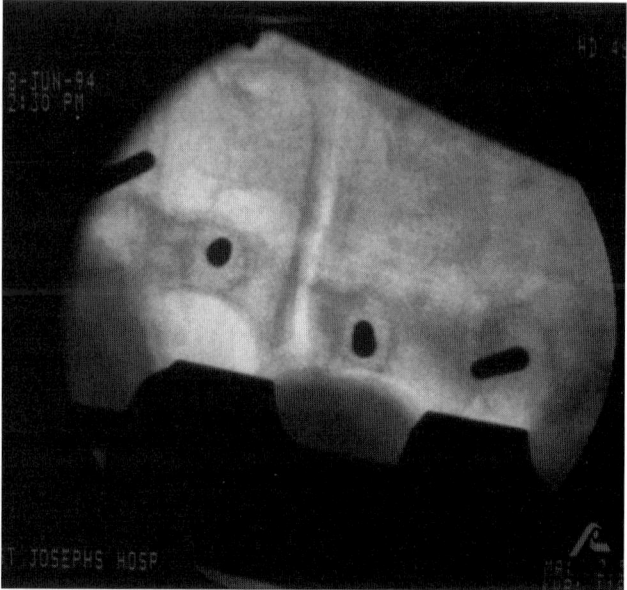

**Figure 133.5** Oblique fluoroscopic view of the lumbar spine showing the pedicles in cross section. Three Steinmann pins have been placed within the pedicles and are noted to be lying within the cortical margins of the pedicles.

the C-arm from the lateral position toward the AP position, the radiologist can obtain an oblique view of the spinal column. In the lumbosacral region, this view can show the individual pedicle in cross section.

Before screw insertion, a localizing marker (i.e., K-wire or Steinmann pin) can be placed into each pedicle to be instrumented. The oblique fluoroscopic view demonstrates these markers within the cortical margins of the individual pedicles if the entry point and screw trajectory in both the sagittal and axial planes have been properly selected (Figure 133.5). When these parameters are confirmed, the markers can then be removed and the pedicle screws inserted along the same path.[11]

When fluoroscopy is used for cervical screw fixation (i.e., anterior odontoid screw fixation), an AP and a lateral view may be required. This can be obtained by alternating the position of a single C-arm unit from the lateral to the AP position or by using two separate fluoroscopy machines with arms positioned 90 degrees with respect to each other.[10] The latter option requires careful positioning of the two fluoroscopic units so that they do not interfere with the access of both the surgeon and the anesthesia team to the patient.

Fluoroscopy has also been used for ventral cervical plate instrumentation procedures to assist in the positioning and placement of the fixation plates and screws.[2] However, the lower cervical and upper thoracic regions can often be difficult to visualize because of image obstruction by the patient's shoulders. This problem can occasionally be alleviated either by placing an interscapular roll beneath the patient and taping the shoulders down to the table or by using wrist slings to pull down on the patient's arms during imaging. With the development of ventral cervical plating systems that use unicortical instead of bicortical screw placement, fluoroscopy is now used less commonly for anterior cervical fixation surgery.

A disadvantage of fluoroscopy is that it can be difficult to manipulate and time-consuming to use. It requires the surgical team to wear lead aprons during imaging or to move away from the operative field to stand behind radiopaque barriers. Furthermore, as with all intraoperative imaging modalities, fluoroscopy provides only two-dimensional imaging of the spinal column in any one view. The surgeon must reposition the C-arm to obtain a second two-dimensional view. For example, two fluoroscopic views (lateral and oblique) are required for pedicle screw insertion because each view alone does not supply complete information regarding the screw entry point and trajectory. A lateral fluoroscopic view may show a satisfactory trajectory in the sagittal plane but does not show errors in the axial plane that involve excessive medial or lateral inclination of a screw. An oblique view is needed to provide this information, but it is often difficult to interpret.

Another problem associated with the use of fluoroscopy for spinal surgery is the difficulty in obtaining a true lateral image. This difficulty can produce a parallax effect that can result in the suboptimal positioning of fixation screws. In the cervical spine, this problem can be addressed by ensuring that the angle of one mandible viewed on the fluoroscopy screen overlaps the angle of the other mandible. In the thoracic and lumbosacral spine, the rostral and caudal cortical margins of the vertebrae can be used to ensure a true lateral image. If two cortical margins are seen at one end of a vertebral body, a true lateral image has not been obtained, and an adjustment of the C-arm is needed.

## Ultrasonography

The application of ultrasonography to spinal surgery was first reported in 1982.[3,4] Like fluoroscopy, ultrasonography provides continuous and real-time imaging. However, unlike fluoroscopy, which provides only images of the bony spinal column, ultrasonography can image the adjacent neural and soft tissue structures, as well.

Diagnostic ultrasound scanners consist of a scan head containing transducers that convert electrical energy to mechanical or sound energy. For an ultrasonographic image to be obtained, the scan head of the ultrasound probe is placed against a contact surface. A short ultrasonic pulse is generated by the transducers and is transmitted into the contact surface. This pulse travels continuously into the medium until it strikes another surface or encounters a change in acoustic impedance. Acoustic impedance is a physical property that depends not only on tissue density, but also on the actual composition and internal structure of a tissue substance.[5]

When the ultrasound pulse strikes a surface, some of the energy is reflected back to the transducer and some of the energy continues forward. Structures that reflect most or all of the ultrasound pulses striking them, specifically air and bone, prevent the imaging of structures behind them. A reflected ultrasonic pulse returns to the scan head and hits the transducer. The shape of the crystal in the transducer is changed, inducing a voltage across it. This voltage is recorded with the amplitude dependent on the strength of the reflection that contacts the transducer face. The location within the tissue from which the reflection came can be calculated easily once the speed of sound in the tissue being scanned and the interval of time between the generation of the impulse and the reception of the reflected wave are known.

The spinal canal can be imaged with ultrasonography during surgery by filling the wound with saline after a laminectomy has been performed. The tip of the transducer is immersed in the saline and manipulated in several directions to give the surgeon an orientation to the specific anatomy. By rotating the scan head 90 degrees, the images can be changed from a longitudinal to a cross-sectional image of the structure.

Anatomic structures that are dense in composition and therefore are capable of reflecting ultrasonic pulses are termed *echogenic* and appear white on the ultrasound images. These structures include the spinal cord, the vertebral body, and any solid intramedullary or extramedullary lesion. The nonechogenic black layers consist of the saline immediately beneath the transducer tip, the subarachnoid space on either side of the spinal cord, and any intramedullary syrinx or cystic lesion (Figure 133.6).

Ultrasonography can be used to localize a variety of lesions within the spinal canal. It is effective for localizing and characterizing intramedullary spinal cord tumors and intradural extramedullary tumors. Ultrasonography can be used before opening the dura to visualize the extent of the tumor and to localize specific areas of interest such as a cyst within the tumor. The images guide the opening of the dura and can often direct the surgeon to a particular location to start the myelotomy and exploration.[19] When a cystic tumor such as a hemangioma is present, ultrasonography can identify the specific mural nodule of the tumor.[20]

Edema proximal or distal to the tumor also causes widening of the cord seen on ultrasound and can create confusion in determining the absolute limits of the tumor. However, in most cases, the tumor border is well defined and the edema is less echogenic than the tumor.[21]

In the setting of syringomyelia, ultrasonography can be used to localize the maximal extent of the syrinx and to identify any small septa present[20] (see Figure 133.6). If a drainage catheter is placed into the syrinx, ultrasonography can be used to assess the degree of collapse of the cavity and to determine whether additional catheters are needed.

Ultrasonography has also been used in the setting of vertebral body fractures or dislocations to assess the spinal canal following a decompressive procedure. This is particularly useful in the thoracic and thoracolumbar areas, at which a posterolateral approach is often used to access anterior and anterolateral epidural compression. If a laminectomy is also performed, the ultrasound probe can be placed over the dorsal dura and the extent of the ventral decompression can be assessed.[16,17]

## Image-Guided Spinal Navigation

IGSN involves the use of an image-processing workstation coupled with a digitized localizer system to virtually link preoperative computed tomography (CT) images of the spine to the corresponding surgical anatomy. By providing the ability to manipulate multiplanar images through any surgical point, IGSN gives the surgeon a greater degree of orientation to the unexposed, and therefore nonvisualized, spinal anatomy. Although it is not an intraoperative imaging device, IGSN does provide the spinal surgeon with valuable intraoperative image information regarding nonvisualized spinal anatomy.

The development of image-guided technology for spinal surgery was influenced by the difficulties of intraoperative spatial orientation associated with surgery for complex spinal disorders.[15,18] The three-dimensional anatomy of the spinal column can present challenges for even the most experienced surgeon. Standard dorsal surgical approaches expose only a portion of the spinal column at a given level. Although this partial exposure is not problematic for most laminectomy or discectomy procedures, it can be limiting in the setting of complex spinal column disorders such as fractures, neoplasms, or deformities.

The increased acceptance and use of spinal instrumentation devices and the development of more complex operative exposures have expanded the options for managing complicated spinal disorders. Consequently, proper orientation to the unexposed spinal anatomy has become even more critical. In particular, the various fixation techniques that require placing bone screws into the pedicles of the thoracic, lumbar, and sacral spine; into the lateral masses of the cervical spine; and across joint spaces in the upper cervical spine require "visualization" of the unexposed spinal anatomy. Although intraoperative fluoroscopy, serial radiography, and ultrasonography have proven useful, they are all limited in that they provide only two-dimensional imaging of a complex three-dimensional structure. Consequently, the surgeon is required to extrapolate the third dimension based on an interpretation of the images and knowledge of the pertinent anatomy. This so-called "dead reckoning" of the anatomy can result in varying degrees of inaccuracy when the surgeon is placing screws into the unexposed portions of the spinal column.

Several studies have shown the unreliability of routine radiography in assessing pedicle screw placement in the lumbosacral spine. The rate of penetration of the pedicle

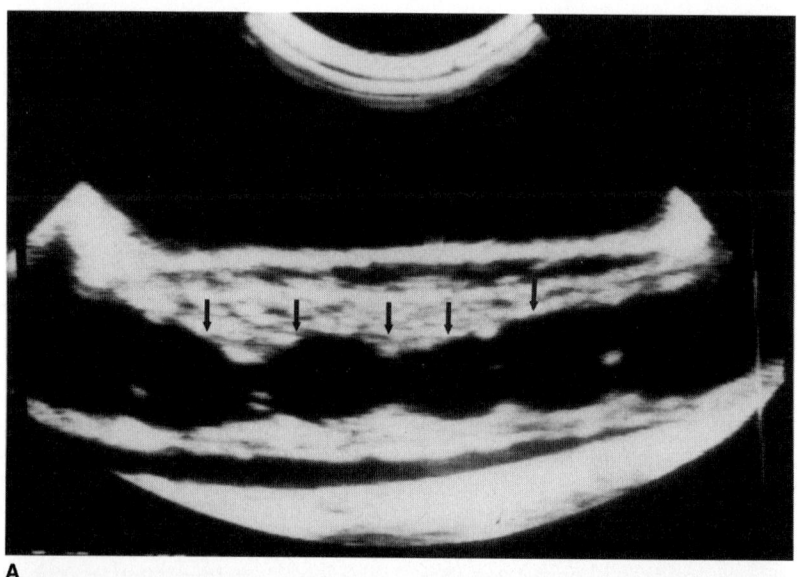

A

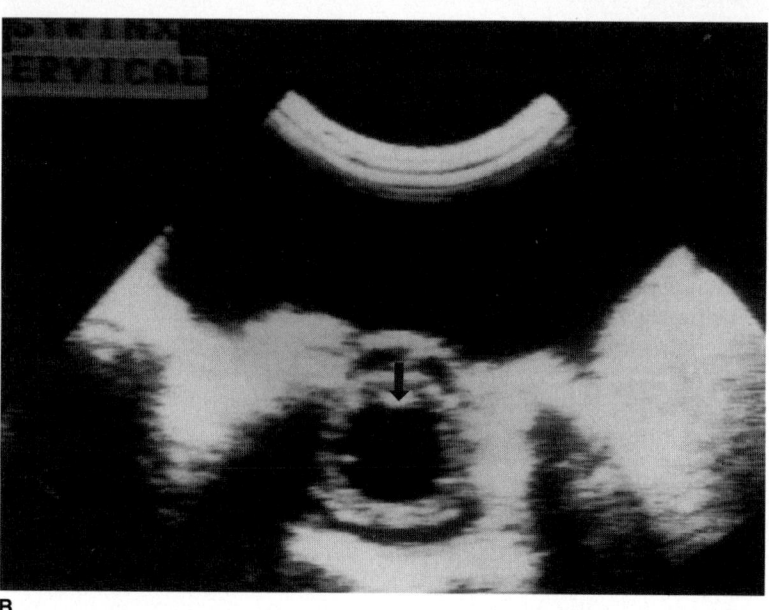

B

**Figure 133.6** **(A)** Sagittal ultrasound image of the cervical spinal cord demonstrating a large syrinx *(arrows)*. **(B)** Axial ultrasound image of the same patient demonstrating the syrinx *(arrow)*.

cortex by an inserted screw ranges from 21% to 31% in these studies.[8,9,24] However, Steinmann *et al.*,[22] using an image-based technique for pedicle screw placement that combined CT axial images of cadaver spine specimens with fluoroscopy, were able to demonstrate a reduction of this screw insertion error rate to 5.5%.

The application of image-guided navigational technology to spinal surgery provides three-dimensional and multiplanar views of image data to improve the surgeon's visualization of the spinal anatomy. These image data are provided in near real time and can be manipulated to show every aspect of the intraoperative spinal anatomy through any selected point in the surgical field.[12-15,18]

## Navigational Technique

The primary components of an image-guided navigational system include an image-processing computer workstation interfaced with a two-camera optical localizer (Figure 133.7). Customized navigational probes with three to four small reflective spheres attached in a known arrangement serve as the tools that link the surgeon to the navigational system (Figure 133.8). The optical localizer camera system emits an infrared beam toward the surgical field, where the beam is captured by the spheres on the probe and reflected back to the camera. The spatial orientation of the reflected light is passed on to the computer workstation, which can then use mathematical principles of localization by triangulation to localize and track not only the exact position of the probe's tip but also the position of any anatomic structure in the surgical field on which the probe tip rests.

Bone landmarks on the exposed surface of the spinal column provide the frame of reference necessary for image-guided navigation. Specifically, any anatomic landmark that can be identified during surgery and in the preoperative image data set can be used as a reference point. Typically, for spinal surgery, the reference points used are the tips of the spinous process and transverse processes at each spinal level to be instrumented, although other bony landmarks such as facet joints or prominent osteophytes can also be used.[12-15,18]

After surgical exposure, each selected reference point in the image data set is mapped onto its corresponding point in the exposed surgical anatomy by a process called *registration*. This process involves highlighting one of the selected reference points in the image data set while placing the navigational probe on the corresponding point in the surgical field. As the camera localizer system tracks the position of the probe, the spatial location of the probe tip is relayed to the computer workstation, and the selected anatomic point in the surgical field is linked spatially to its corresponding image data point. This paired-point registration step is then repeated for each of the three to five reference points required for accurate registration.

Alternatively, the surgeon can perform the registration process by creating a surface map of the exposed spinal anatomy. This technique involves placing the probe on multiple nondiscreet points on the exposed and débrided surface in the surgical field. The positional information of these points is transferred to the workstation, and a topographic map of the selected anatomy is created and "matched" to the patient's CT data set. This surface-mapping technique is more time-consuming and inherently less accurate than the paired-point registration technique.[14]

The registration process represents the step during image-guided navigation that can have the greatest effect on navigational accuracy. Registration accuracy depends on the surgeon carefully selecting the correct reference points or performing the contour mapping process. If properly performed, registration allows for the display of reformatted, multiplanar CT images or magnetic resonance images to assist the surgeon with orientation to the unexposed spinal anatomy.[18]

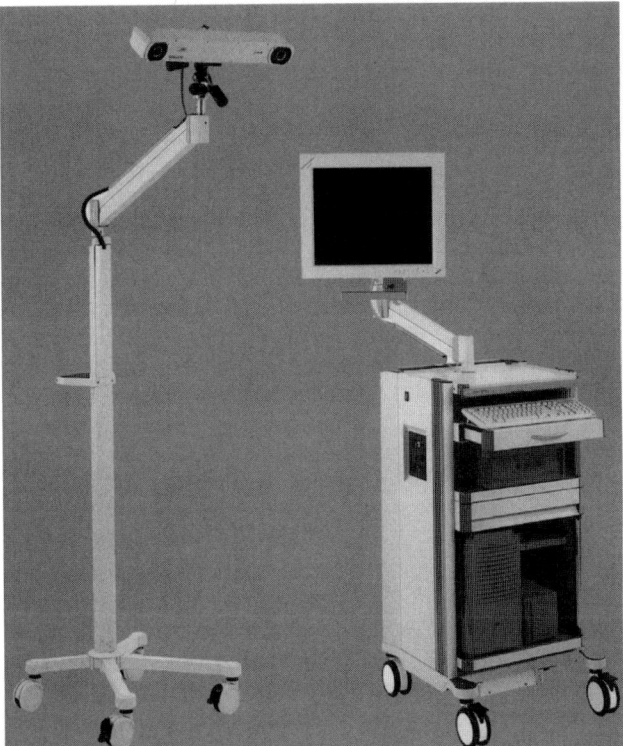

**Figure 133.7** Image-guided navigation system. Image-processing computer workstation (*right*) and an infrared camera (*left*).

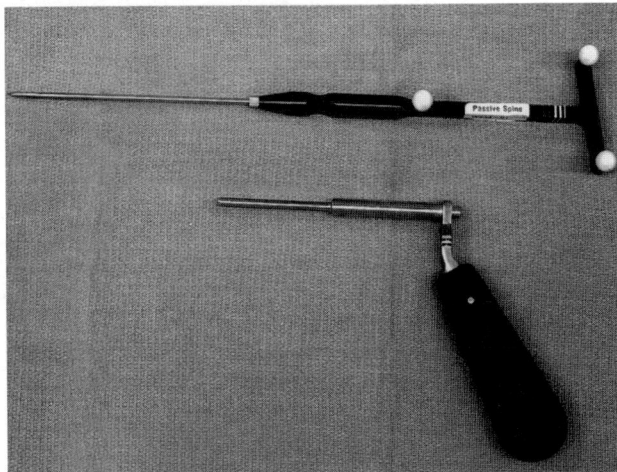

**Figure 133.8** Navigational probe (with passive reflectors) and handheld drill guide.

The registration process establishes a precise spatial relationship between the image data and the spinal anatomy. If the patient is inadvertently moved after registration, the spatial relationship is distorted and the navigational information is inaccurate. This problem can be minimized by the optional use of a spinal tracking device, which consists of a separate set of passive reflectors attached to a spinous process in the surgical field. This tracking device alerts the system if any inadvertent movement of the spine occurs and provides for the necessary correction that keeps the registration process accurate and eliminates the need to repeat the registration process. The disadvantage of such a tracking device is the added time needed for its attachment to the spine, the need to maintain a line of sight between it and the camera, and the inconvenience of having to perform the procedure with the device placed in the center of the surgical field.

Once the registration process is completed, the surgeon can place the navigational probe on any exposed point in the operative field and the workstation will automatically generate three reformatted images through the selected point. The three planar images are oriented perpendicular to one another in relationship to the long axis of the probe. For pedicle screw fixation, these three reformatted images are the corresponding axial, coronal, and sagittal images through a selected point. On each reformatted image, a cursor or trajectory line marks the position of the navigational probe in the surgical field. The diameter of the cursor and the width of the trajectory line can be adjusted in proportion to the selected screw diameter. The length of the trajectory line relative to the imaged spine is displayed in millimeters, providing for accurate screw length selection (Figure 133.9). As the surgeon moves the probe through the surgical field, each planar image updates immediately to show the probe's orientation to the spinal column and to provide the surgeon with an optimal orientation to the pertinent spinal anatomy and the precise screw entry point and trajectory.

At each level to be instrumented, the surgeon identifies standard bony landmarks used for selection of a screw's entry point and trajectory. The navigational probe is placed through a drill guide onto the selected entry point. The navigational images are generated, and the surgeon can then make subtle modifications to the selected entry point and trajectory as needed by simply changing the angle or location of the drill guide-probe assembly. When the appropriate entry point and trajectory have been determined, the navigational probe is removed from the

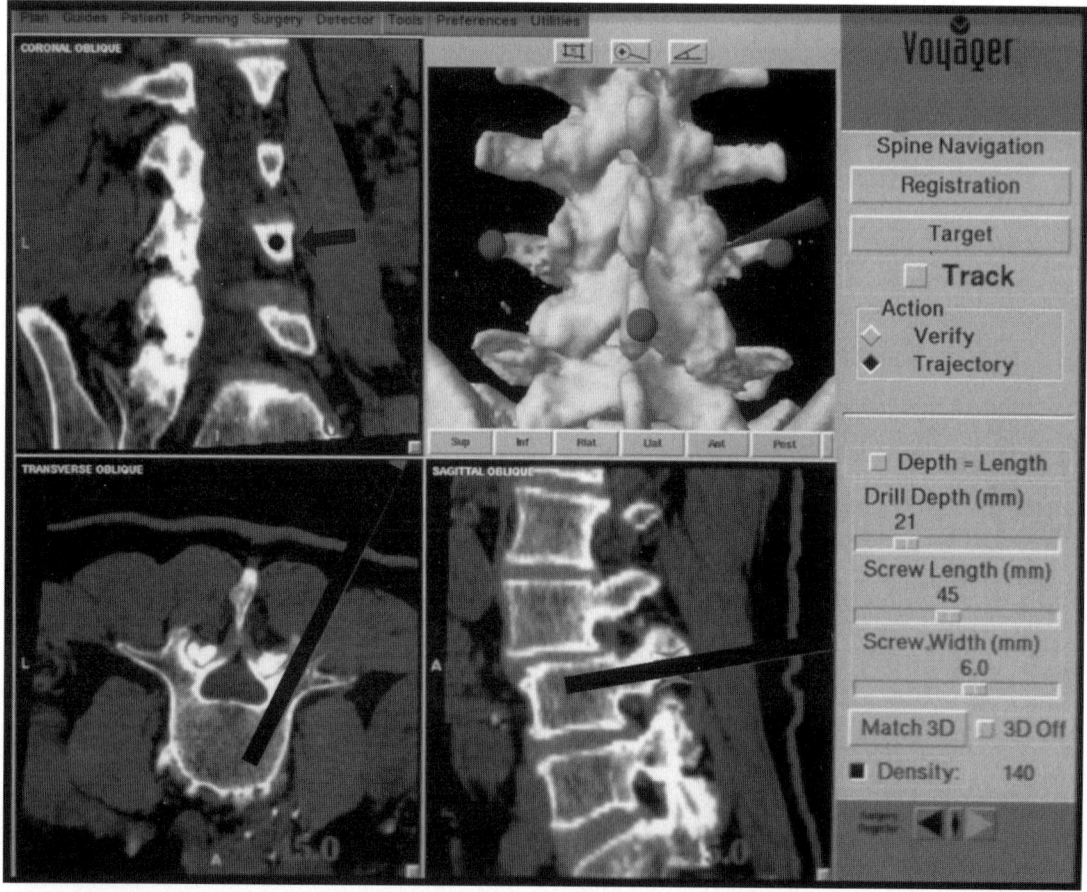

**Figure 133.9** Image-guided workstation screen demonstrating a satisfactory trajectory selection through the L4 pedicle. The upper left quadrant displays the coronal image with the computer cursor positioned within the cross section of the pedicle *(arrow)*. The left and right lower quadrants show the selected trajectory in the axial and sagittal planes, respectively. The length of the trajectory line is set at 45mm, and its diameter set at 6mm. The upper right quadrant displays a surface-rendered image of the imaged spinal anatomy.

drill guide and a 3.0mm pilot hole is drilled along the selected trajectory. The process is then repeated for the contralateral side. Each level to be instrumented undergoes a separate registration process. This segmental registration eliminates the potential error that can occur with changes of vertebral body position between the preoperative scanned position and the intraoperative position. Because each vertebra is a rigid body, the spatial relationship of registration points at a single vertebral level to the pedicles of the same vertebrae remains unchanged regardless of changes in patient positioning.

At any point during the orientation procedure, the accuracy of the system can be tested by placing the probe on a known bony landmark and confirming its location on the workstation screen. If there is any discrepancy between the position of the probe and the corresponding position of the cursor on the workstation screen, the registration process can easily be repeated.

When applied to screw fixation of the spinal column, IGSN reduces or eliminates the need for intraoperative imaging.[12,14,15,18] It can facilitate the optimal placement of screws within the spinal column. However, unlike intraoperative ultrasonography or fluoroscopy, IGSN does not provide true real-time imaging. It does not show changes in the spinal anatomy as they occur. The system functions as a confirmation tool to assist the surgeon in identifying the pedicle and relating its position and orientation to the exposed spinal anatomy. It is an alternative method to the more conventional means of interpreting two-dimensional images of the spine, relating them to the surgeon's knowledge of the pertinent anatomy, and estimating the location of the pedicle. It is not intended to function as a substitute for an understanding of the appropriate spinal anatomy and the indications and techniques for insertion of pedicle screws.

An extensive application of this technology to spinal surgery over the past decade has proven IGSN to be a practical and extremely useful alternative and adjunct to conventional intraoperative imaging. It has been used routinely for pedicle screw fixation in the lumbosacral and the thoracic spines. It is invaluable for placing transarticular screws at the C1-2 level (Figure 133.10) and for providing optimal orientation to spinal anatomy during transoral surgery and during anterior thoracolumbar surgery.[12,14,15,18]

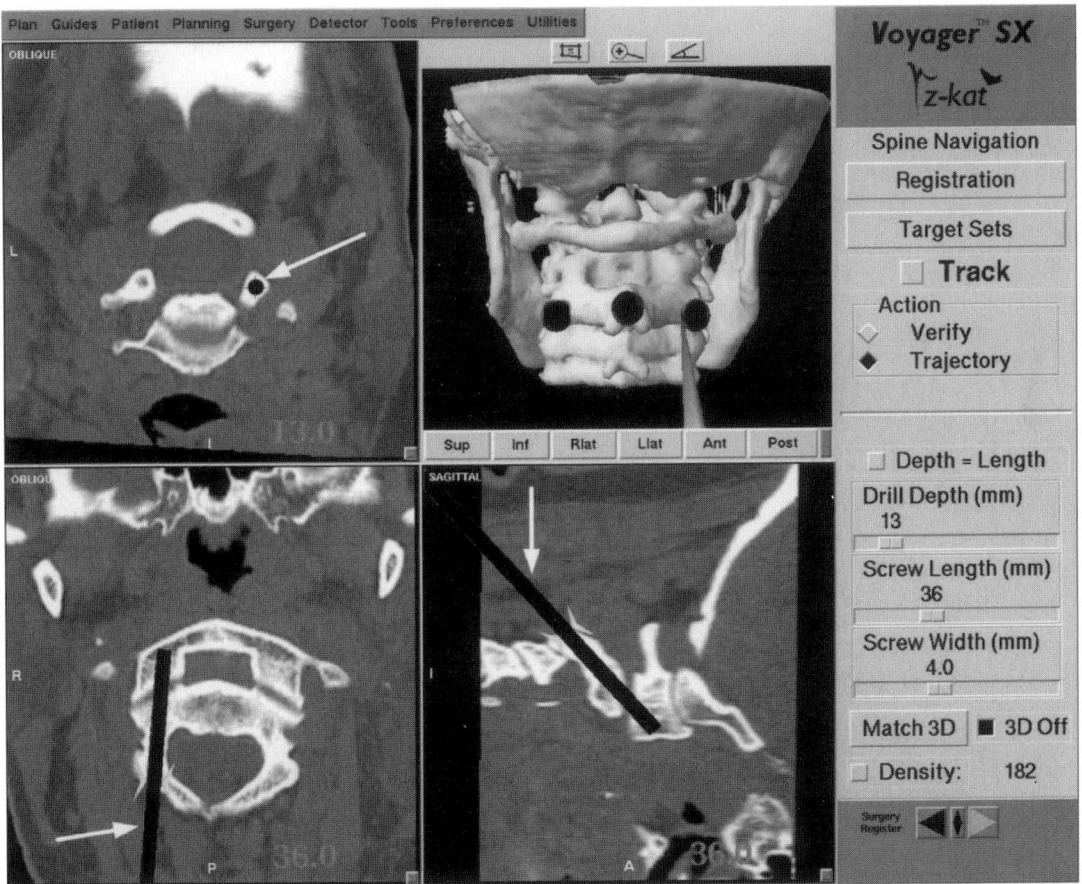

**Figure 133.10** Image-guided workstation screen demonstrating screw entry point and trajectory for C1-2 transarticular screw fixation. The upper quadrant displays the virtual position of a screw tip placed along the selected trajectory *(arrow)*. The two lower quadrants display the selected screw trajectory in the sagittal plane (right lower quadrant) and in a plane that is perpendicular to the long axis of the navigational probe (left lower quadrant). This latter view represents an oblique plane that is midway between a coronal and an axial plane. The length of the trajectory line is set at 36mm, and its diameter set to 4mm. The selected trajectories in both lower quadrants are indicated by the arrows. The right upper quadrant shows a surface-rendered image of the cervical anatomy.

In addition, it serves as a highly effective image-manipulation system, allowing the surgeon to scroll through CT images in any selected plane before and during surgery. This allows the surgeon to better conceptualize the complex three-dimensional anatomy of the spinal column as compared with the standard method of viewing multiple two-dimensional image sheets.

## Fluoroscopic Navigation

Fluoroscopic navigation is the combination of standard fluoroscopy with image-guided navigational technology. It was developed to counter the user difficulties of some earlier image-guided systems, which typically took much longer to use than standard fluoroscopy.[7] Fluoroscopic navigation uses the same computer workstation and localizer system used for IGSN; however, instead of using preoperative CT images, it uses AP and lateral fluoroscopic images acquired intraoperatively (Figure 133.11). The presumed advantages of fluoroscopic navigation are that a preoperative CT image is not required and that the navigational image can be updated at any point during the surgical procedure. The advantage over conventional fluoroscopic techniques is that the amount of intraoperative fluoroscopic time is reduced.

The disadvantage of fluoroscopic navigation is that it is still only fluoroscopy. The same difficulties experienced with standard fluoroscopy are present with fluoroscopic navigation. Specifically, only an AP and lateral images are provided. The critical plane for most spinal screw fixation procedures is the axial plane. This is the only plane that can definitively demonstrate violation of the spinal canal by a medially displaced screw. Only CT-based image-guided navigation can demonstrate this view, although current developments with standard fluoroscopy will eventually allow for axial reconstructions. Furthermore, any region of the spinal column that is difficult to image with standard fluoroscopy (i.e., upper thoracic) is difficult to image with fluoroscopic navigation.

The early goals of image-guided spinal navigation were to improve the surgeon's orientation to the intraoperative spinal anatomy in a time- and cost-efficient manner and to ultimately replace fluoroscopy. Many of these earlier CT-based image-guided systems were difficult to use and were time-consuming. Fluoroscopic navigation was an attempt to solve this problem. However, after several years of clinical experience, CT-based navigational technology has become significantly easier to use than earlier models. This improved ease of use coupled with the ability to obtain axial imaging, as well as its superior accuracy, image manipulation, and orientation capabilities, provides image-guided

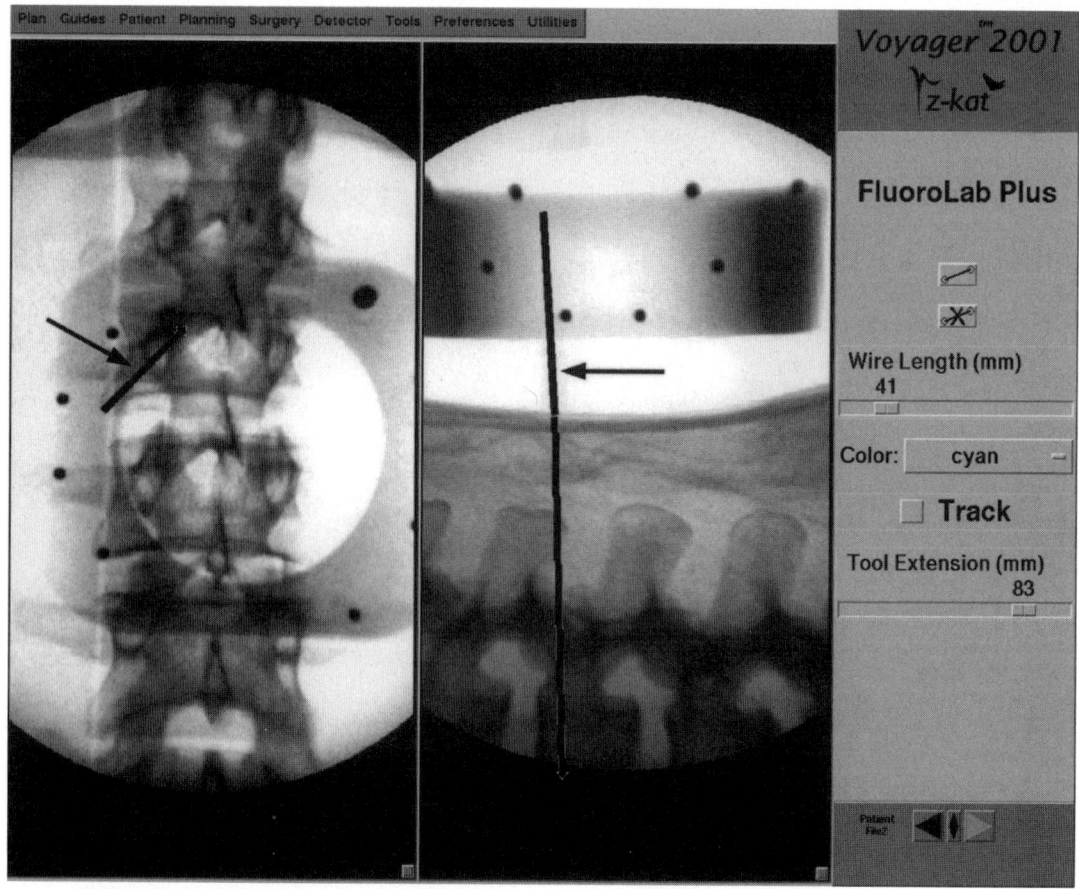

**Figure 133.11** Fluoroscopic workstation screen demonstrating selected trajectory (*arrows*) through the L2 pedicle in the sagittal and coronal planes. An image in the axial plane is not available with fluoroscopic navigation.

technology with a clear advantage over any fluoroscopic-based technology.

## Summary

Intraoperative imaging of the spinal column is an important aspect of spinal surgery. It is used not only to provide the surgeon with localization capabilities, but also to provide a greater degree of orientation to the unexposed spinal anatomy. Although several imaging options are available, they are all dependent on the careful interpretation of images obtained by the surgeon. Furthermore, they are not a substitute for a thorough knowledge of the pertinent spinal anatomy and surgical technique.

## REFERENCES

1. Brunberg JA, Gabrielsen T, Rubin J, et al: Diagnostic imaging technology. In Crockard A, Hayward R, Hoff JT (eds): *Neurosurgery: The Scientific Basis of Clinical Practice*, ed 2. Boston, Blackwell Scientific, 1992, pp 758-786.
2. Caspar W: Anterior cervical fusion and interbody stabilization with the trapezial osteosynthetic plate technique. Aesculap Scientific Information Leaflet S-039. Aesculap Instruments Corp, Burlingame, CA, 1986.
3. Chandler WF, Knake JE, McGillicuddy JE et al: Intraoperative use of real-time ultrasonography in neurosurgery. *J Neurosurg* 57:157, 1982.
4. Dohrmann GJ, Rubin JM: Intraoperative ultrasonic imaging of the spinal cord: Syringomyelia, cysts, and tumors—A preliminary report. *Surg Neurol* 18:395, 1982.
5. Dohrmann GJ, Rubin JM: Intraoperative diagnostic ultrasound. In Wilkins RH, Rengachary SS (eds): *Neurosurgery*. New York, McGraw-Hill, 1985, pp 457-463.
6. Duane SH, Myers DL: Complications of lumbar spinal fusion with transpedicular instrumentation. *Spine* 17:184, 1992.
7. Foley KT, Simon DA, Rampersaud YR: Virtual fluoroscopy: Computer-assisted fluoroscopic navigation. *Spine* 26:347, 2001.
8. George DC, Krag MH, Johnson CC, et al: Hole preparation technique for transpedicle screws: Effect on pull-out strength from human cadaveric vertebrae. *Spine* 16:181, 1991.
9. Gertzbein SD, Robbins SE: Accuracy of pedicle screw placement in vivo. *Spine* 15:11, 1990.
10. Grob D, Jeanneret B, Aebi M, Markwalder T: Atlanto-axial fusion with transarticular screw fixation. *J Bone Joint Surg* 73B:972, 1991.
11. Hernstorf JE, Gaines RW, Steffee AD: Transpedicular fixation of spinal disorders with Steffee plates. Surgical Rounds for Orthopedics, 1987.
12. Kalfas IH: Image-guided spinal navigation: Application to spinal metastasis. In Maciunas RJ (ed): *Advanced Techniques in Central Nervous System Metastasis*. AANS Publications, Park Ridge, IL, 1998, pp 245-254.
13. Kalfas IH: Image-guided spinal navigation. *Clin Neurosurg* 46:70, 1999.
14. Kalfas IH: Frameless stereotaxy assisted spinal surgery. In Rengachary SS (ed): *Neurosurgery Operative Color Atlas*. AANS Publications, Park Ridge, IL, 2000, pp 123-134.
15. Kalfas IH, Kormos DW, Murphy MA, et al: Application of frameless stereotaxy to pedicle screw fixation of the spine. *J Neurosurg* 83:641, 1995.
16. McGahan JP, Benson D, Chehrazi B, et al: Intraoperative sonographic monitoring of reduction of thoracolumbar burst fractures. *AJR Am J Radiol* 145:1229, 1985.
17. Montalvo BM, Quencer RM, Green BA, et al: Intraoperative sonography in spinal trauma. *Radiology* 153:125, 1984.
18. Murphy MA, McKenzie RL, Kormos DW, Kalfas IH: Frameless stereotaxis for the insertion of lumbar pedicle screws: A technical note. *J Clin Neurosci* 1:257, 1994.
19. Platt JM, Rubin JM, Bowerman RA, et al: Intraoperative sonographic characterization of a cystic intramedullary spinal cord lesion appearing as solid. *AJNR Am J Neuroradiol* 9:614, 1988.
20. Platt JM, Rubin JM, Chandler WF, et al: Intraoperative spinal sonography in the evaluation of intramedullary tumors. *J Ultrasound Med* 7:317, 1988.
21. Sanders WP, Ausman JI, Dujovny M, et al: Ultrasonic features of two cases of spinal cord hemangioblastoma. *Surg Neurol* 26:453, 1986.
22. Steinmann JC, Herkowitz HO, El-Kommos H, Wesolowski DP: Spinal pedicle fixation: Confirmation of an image-based technique for screw placement. *Spine* 18:1856, 1993.
23. Walker J, Gillespie R, Davis J, Dawson W: Water-soluble contrast medium for intraoperative evaluation of anterior cervical discectomy: Technical note. *J Neurosurg* 68:491, 1988.
24. Weinstein JN, Spratt KF, Spengler D, et al: Spinal pedicle fixation: Reliability and validity of roentgenogram-based assessment and surgical factors on successful screw placement. *Spine* 13:1012, 1988.

# C H A P T E R   1 3 4

# Stereotactic Radiosurgery of the Spine

**William E. McCormick, Michael P. Steinmetz, Allan J. Hamilton, Richard Crownover, Iain H. Kalfas, and Edward C. Benzel**

The term *stereotactic radiosurgery* was coined by Leksell in 1951 and describes the use of stereotactic localization to administer a large radiation dose to a precise target while exposing normal structures to safely tolerated doses.[12] This represented a significant departure from conventional radiation therapy, in which radiation is given over a large field in fractionated doses to capitalize on the differential response of normal tissue and tumor cells to radiation. The efficacy of stereotactic radiosurgery in the management of intracranial neoplasms is well known and accepted. Several neoplasms that have been successfully treated by intracranial radiosurgery are commonly found in the spine, including metastatic tumors, vascular malformations, neurofibromas, and meningiomas. Until recently, however, there were substantial obstacles to applying radiosurgery to the treatment of spinal lesions. Intracranial radiosurgery uses targets that are fixed with respect to the cranium, which is immobilized rigidly in a stereotactic frame. Accurate targeting and delivery of a radiation dose is more complex in the spine. The spine moves relative to respiration and has a large amount of surrounding soft tissue. This makes securing the spine to a frame technically difficult.[29] Frames with clamps that attach to the dorsal elements have been developed, but there are drawbacks to this method. It requires an invasive surgical procedure that increases the duration of the procedure and the risks of potential surgical complications.[29] The Cyberknife, an image-guided, frameless robotic stereotactic radiosurgery system, is used to treat intracranial lesions and possesses an overall treatment outcome that is comparable with the results of conventional frame-based radiosurgery.[1-3,6-8] More recently, the Cyberknife has been used to treat extracranial neoplasms, including lesions of the spine.[1-3,5,8]

In this chapter, the limitations of conventional radiation therapy in the management of spinal neoplasms are reviewed. Two specific spinal stereotactic radiosurgery techniques, bone screw fixation and a frameless robotic stereotactic system, the Cyberknife, are discussed, and the limited clinical data associated with these two techniques are reviewed. Finally, the potential advantages and disadvantages of the use of stereotactic radiosurgery to treat lesions in the spine are addressed.

## Neoplastic Spinal Disease

There are a number of reasons for stereotactic radiosurgery to be of potential future importance in the management of spinal lesions. One such factor is the sheer number of spinal neoplasms, particularly metastases, that occur every year. The axial skeleton is the third most common site of cancer metastases after the lung and liver, and the incidence of spinal metastases in the United States is approximately 100,000 per year.[31] Spinal cord compression is estimated to complicate the course of 5% to 10% of all patients with metastatic cancer.[22] Finally, in 50% to 70% of patients, especially those with breast and prostate cancer metastases, multiple levels of involvement are noted.[9]

The median survival for patients with metastatic spinal disease is 10 months, and death typically results from the systemic malignancy.[32] Thus spinal vertebral metastases commonly signal disseminated disease in which open surgery may not be a realistic alternative. Despite this overall grim prognosis, treatment is warranted, particularly in regards to quality of life. The goals of surgery or radiotherapy in these patients are not for cure, but rather for the preservation or restoration of ambulation and bladder control, as well as pain relief.

In a review of 18 clinical series examining the overall results of radiation therapy alone in patients with spinal cord compression from metastatic tumor, Siegal *et al.*[31] found that 28% to 50% of patients either regained or maintained ambulation at the end of treatment. Several studies that have addressed the issue of pain control in patients with spinal metastases have shown that 50% to 80% of patients receive pain relief from radiotherapy alone.[5,10] However, the success of conventional radiotherapy is limited. Only some neoplasms, such as lymphoreticular or prostate tumors, are radiosensitive. Many of the common primary tumors that metastasize to the spine are only moderately radiosensitive (breast) or are radioresistant (non–small cell lung cancer, renal cell carcinoma, melanoma, and gastrointestinal carcinomas).

The vertebral body is the region of the spine that is most commonly affected by metastases. Vertebral body metastases often invade the dorsal elements, as well as the ventral epidural space. This can complicate the dose-planning process in radiation therapy.[35] However, what limits conventional radiotherapy more than any other factor is the relative radiosensitivity of the spinal cord. Conventional radiotherapy lacks the precision to allow large doses of radiation to targets in close proximity to the radiosensitive spinal cord.

## Spinal Cord Radiosensitivity

Radiation myelopathy is a devastating complication of conventional radiation therapy of the spinal cord and has no effective treatment. Morphologically, it is characterized by demyelination and myelomalacia, as well as nonspecific vascular changes that include increased vascularity, hyaline degeneration, vasculitis, thrombosis, and frank hemorrhage.[30] Radiation myelopathy usually occurs with a latency of 6 months to 2 years after cessation of radiation therapy and may progress to total paralysis.

The most widely observed dose limit for the spinal cord is 45Gy in 22 to 25 fractions. It has been shown that the spinal cord is relatively more sensitive to large doses per fraction than most other tissues.[24] This sensitivity was discovered clinically after a number of published reports of myelopathy following schedules of 10 fractions of 4Gy.[30] Marcus and Million[13,14] have shown that 45Gy, conventionally fractionated, lies at the flat region of the dose-response curve and that lower doses result in no appreciable decrease in the incidence of myelopathy. Schultheiss et al.[30] argue that a conventionally fractionated dose that would result in a 5% incidence of radiation myelopathy is between 57 and 61Gy. They believe that such a schedule may be considered in cases in which the spinal cord is particularly threatened by tumor growth.

It has been observed that the spinal cord is also sensitive to hyperfractionation. Both rodent and primate studies show that shortening the intervals between irradiation from 24 hours to 6 to 8 hours reduces spinal cord tolerance by 10% to 15%.[30] It appears that the intervals between treatments allow less repair of radiation damage at the subcellular level.

A common problem in radiation oncology is the treatment of late recurrences or secondary tumors near a previously irradiated site. Many radiation oncologists are reluctant to retreat previously irradiated tissues, particularly if the spinal cord is involved, for fear of causing radiation myelopathy.[30] Reliably accurate delivery of radiation that minimizes exposure to normal spinal cord tissue provides a solution to such problems.

## Spinal Stereotactic Radiosurgery Techniques

Two different techniques for stereotactic radiosurgery of the spine have been described. These consist of bone screw fixation and frameless stereotaxis.

### Bone Screw Fixation

Bone screw fixation involves the use of an extracranial stereotactic frame, the Hamilton-Lulu frame. It is based on the traditional principles of rigid skeletal fixation and consists of a rigid box that is $200 \times 50$cm in length and 18cm deep, in which the patient is placed prone[35] (Figure 134.1). Fixation is achieved by clamping the exposed spinous processes above and below the target area (Figure 134.2). In the distal spine, bilateral pelvic fixation pins can replace spinous process clamps, and for cervical and high thoracic targets, a head ring can be substituted for the clamps. Once coordinates for the target are acquired from computed tomography images, the patient and frame are transferred into the linear accelerator (LINAC) treatment tube, and alignment is accomplished using LINAC guide lasers (Figure 134.3).

Clinical experience with the Hamilton-Lulu frame consists of 12 reported patients, four with renal cell carcinoma, two with adenocarcinoma of unknown origin, two with metastatic sarcoma, and two with metastatic breast carcinoma[35] (Figure 134.4). All patients had imaging-confirmed tumor recurrence or tumor progression after standard fractionated radiotherapy to the spine. All were thought to have exhausted all alternative treatment modalities. Eighteen tumors were treated in these 12 patients, and the

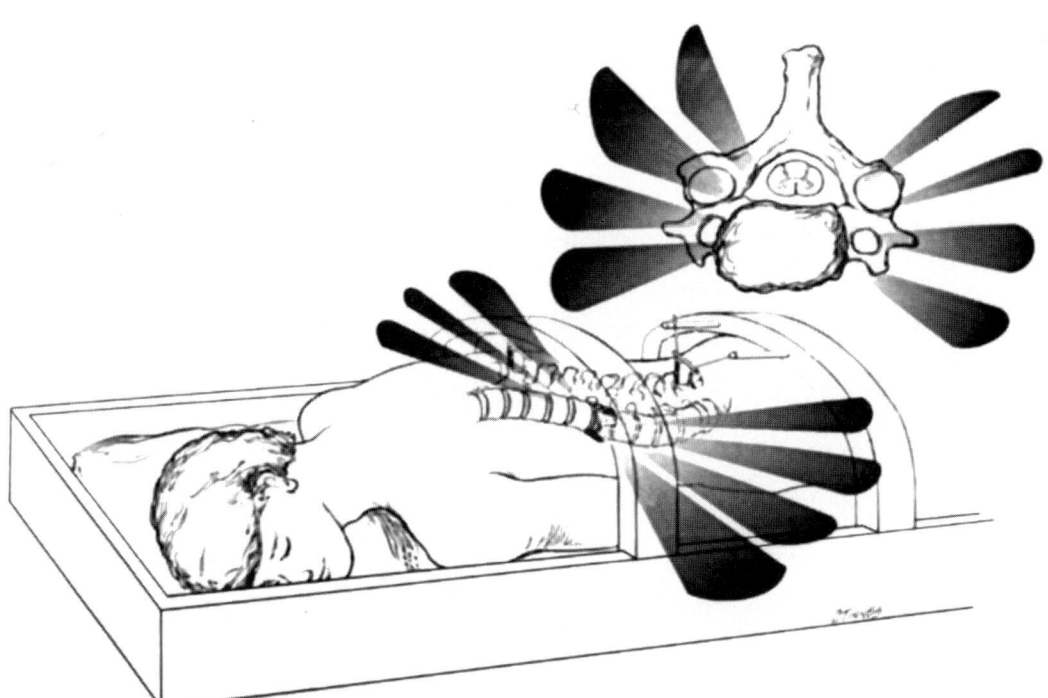

**Figure 134.1** Illustration of a spinal stereotactic radiosurgical frame that encompasses a region between the two arcades depicted. The insert in the upper right corner illustrates how beams of radiation could be aimed at a tumor to avoid inadvertent radiation injury to the adjacent spinal cord.

tumor volume ranged from 0.9 to 521.0cm³. Dose per isocenter varied from 8 to 18Gy in these patients, with the maximal calculated delivery of radiation to the thecal sac ranging from 50 to 100cGy. Median radiation exposure to the spinal cord was 4 to 68cGy. Measured stereotactic radiation treatment error using this frame has been assessed through experiments and is approximately 2mm.[35]

In the series by Takacs and Hamilton,[35] 10 of 12 patients had radiographic follow-up for 3 months or longer. Four tumors showed growth arrest, four tumors showed regression, and two tumors continued to grow. Two patients had superficial wound infections after frame fixation, and one patient had radiation-induced esophagitis. No other major complications were noted, and no instances of radiation myelopathy have occurred. Spinal

cord function indices remained stable in 73% of patients and worsened in 27% of patients. Karnofsky performance scale scores improved or remained stable in 93% of these patients.[30] These results showing 8 of 10 patients experiencing tumor regression or growth arrest are encouraging. Disadvantages with this system include the potential risks that accompany general anesthesia and the surgical procedure necessary for the skeletal fixation.

## Frameless Stereotactic Radiosurgery

The Cyberknife is an image-guided, frameless robotic stereotactic radiosurgery system. It has three main differences from conventional frame-based radiosurgery. (1) It references the position of the treatment site to internal radiographic features, such as skeletal anatomy, rather than to a frame. (2) It uses real-time x-rays to establish the position of the lesion during treatment and then brings the treatment beam into alignment with the observed position of the treatment site. (3) It aims each beam independently without a fixed isocenter. Thus changes in patient position during treatment are compensated for by adaptive beam pointing rather than attempting to control motion by rigid immobilization.[29]

The Cyberknife consists of a robot with a mounted 6-MV X-band LINAC, coupled with a real-time image guidance system (Figure 134.5). The treatment site is imaged by two x-ray fluoroscopes, and bony landmarks are referenced to the hardware components. After the location of the bony landmarks are determined relative to the robot, the target lesion position is then determined and the computer relates these coordinates to the previously acquired treatment planning images. Unlike the gantry-mounted LINAC used with rigid bone fixation, the treatment beam can be positioned and pointed nearly anywhere in space. Because treatment beams are not confined to isocentric geometry, they can be arranged in complex overlapping patterns that conform to irregular dose-volume contours. Thus, careful

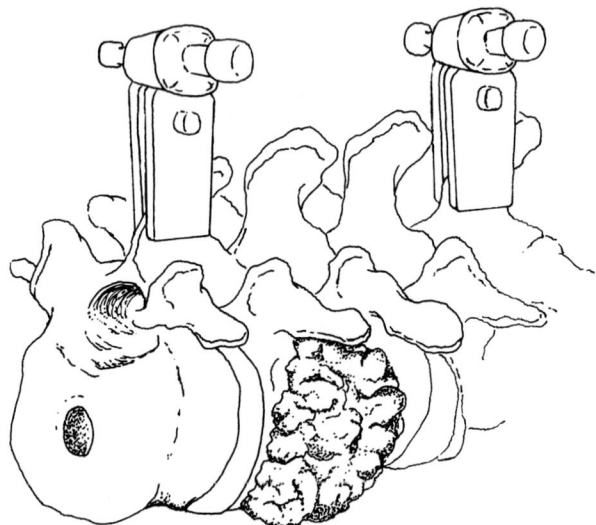

**Figure 134.2** Illustration of spinous process clamp fixation above and below the area of interest. This serves as the skeletal fixation for a stereotactic spinal frame.

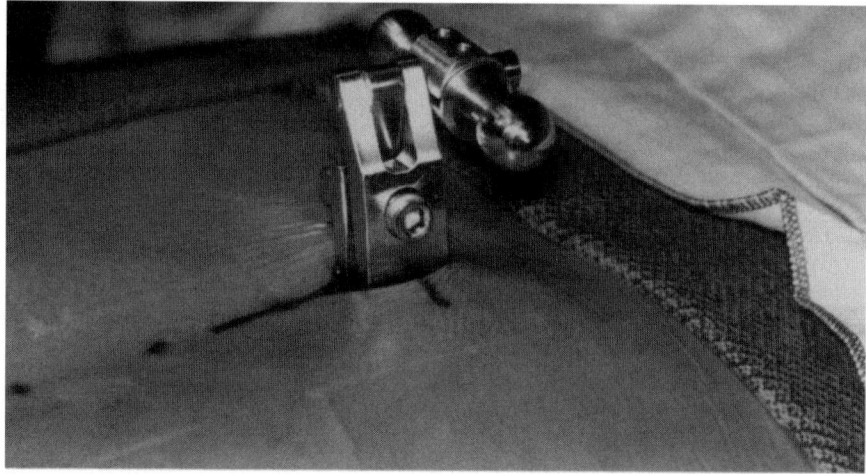

**A**

**Figure 134.3 (A)** A spinous process clamp in position on a patient. The small object that extends from the clamp with spherical attachments at either end is used to affix the patient to the spinal frame by means of a universal joint (which adapts over the end of the spherical projections).

planning can allow beam patterns that wrap around the spine, minimizing spinal cord exposure[29] (Figure 134.6).

For each fraction of radiation, the dose is separated among 100 or more beam directions called *nodes*. The robotic arm moves the LINAC sequentially through the prescribed nodes during treatment. The LINAC stops at each node, the imaging system checks the target position, and corrective changes are then made accordingly. This allows correction for patient movement during the treatment. The combined overall accuracy of the Cyberknife has been assessed by using imaging and dosimetry phantoms. The total root-mean-square targeting error was approximately 1.0 to 1.2mm.[29] Cyberknife accuracy was also tested independently by Murphy and Cox,[20,21] and the mean total radial error was found to be 1.6mm with the positioning error along each axis to be ±0.9mm. These values are equal to or better than that of frame-based systems.

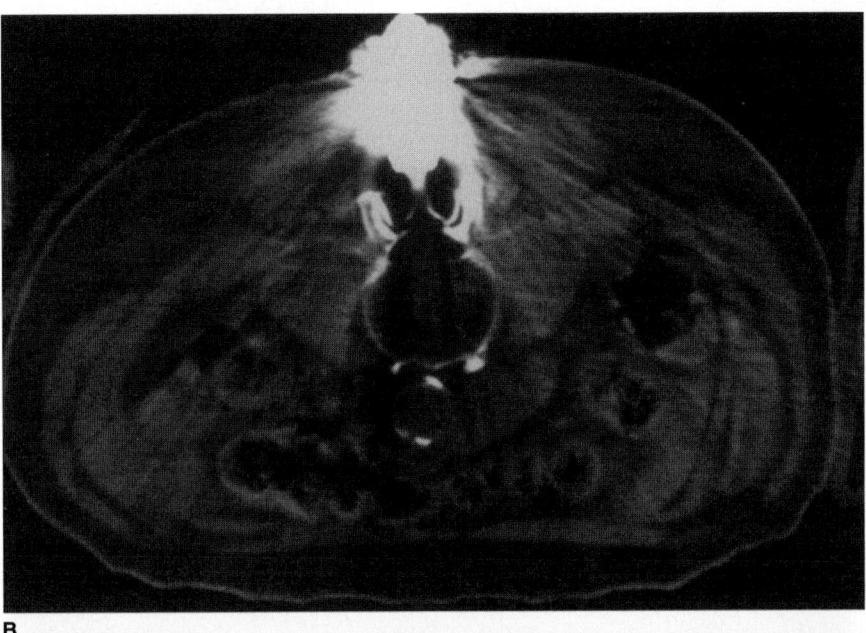

B

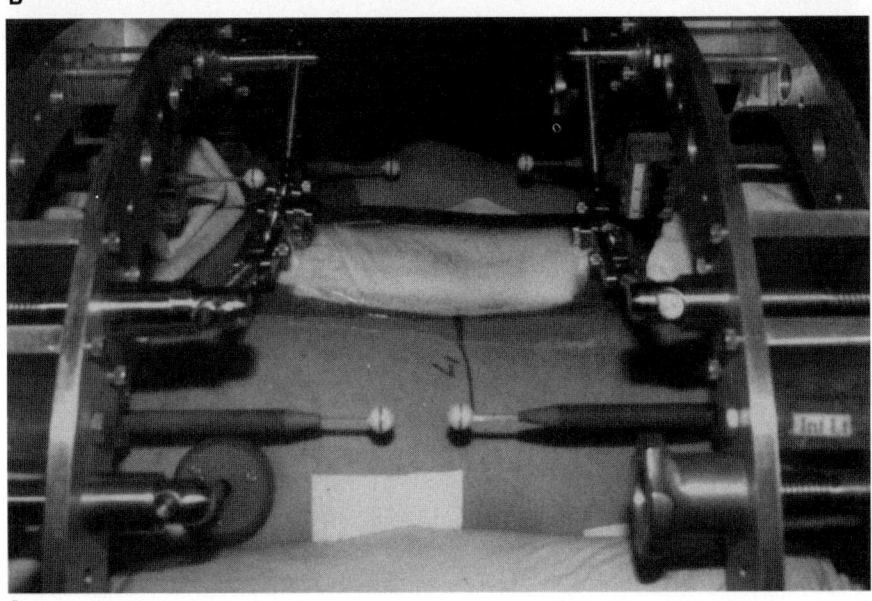

C

**Figure 134.3** *cont'd* **(B)** A computed tomographic (CT) scan that shows the spinous process clamp in position on a spinous process. The obvious advantage of such spinous process fixation is that it permits the spinal canal to be free of invasive skeletal fixation, such as might be obtained with a screw. **(C)** A patient with a tumor at the L1 vertebral body that is indicated in the lower middle portion of the photograph. Spinous process fixation has been obtained above and below the area of the lesion for the purposes of delivering stereotactic radiosurgery. The spherelike projections off the metal arcades are external calibration targets used for aligning the planes of the CT scanner and the linear accelerator; they also serve as internal checks on the computer software before delivering radiosurgery.

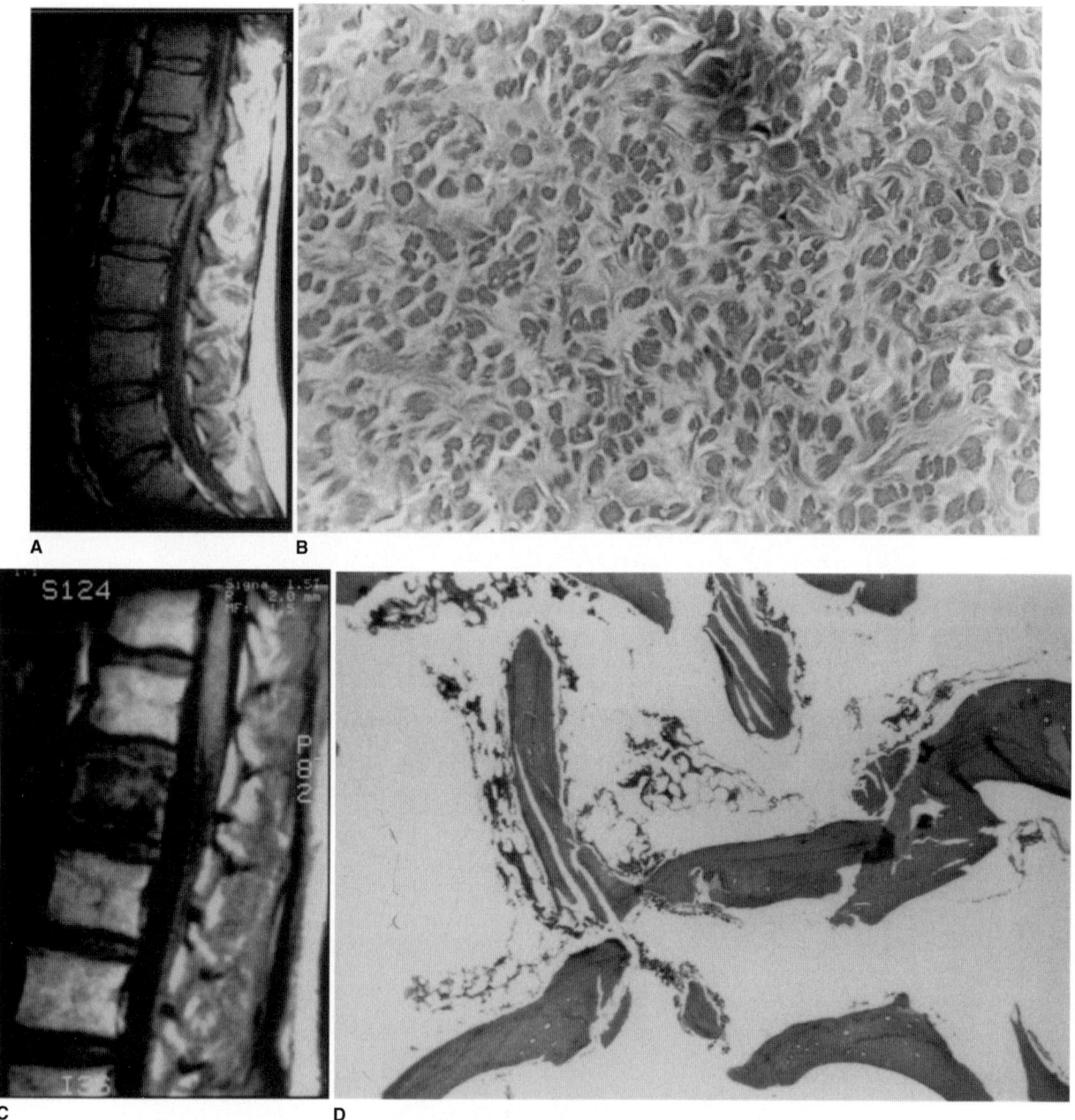

**Figure 134.4** (**A**) A sagittal magnetic resonance image that shows a metastatic osteosarcoma at L1 with obvious tumor in the epidural space. (**B**) A biopsy of this region with demonstrated infiltrating neoplasm. (**C**) The same patient 8 months after spinal stereotactic radiosurgery, with complete regression of the epidural tumor. (**D**) A biopsy of the same site (after radiosurgery) shows complete histologic regression of the tumor with new bone growth.

Ryu *et al.*[29] reported 16 patients who underwent Cyberknife treatment of spinal cord lesions. Treatment was performed between 1997 and 2000 at the Stanford University Medical Center. Spinal lesions included six spinal vascular malformations, five metastatic cancers, two schwannomas, one hemangioblastoma, one meningioma, and one chordoma. Clinical and radiographic follow-up data ranged from 3 to 48 months. Nine of the 16 patients had cervical spine lesions. Cervical vertebrae are easily imaged using the diagnostic x-ray cameras of the Cyberknife. Thus cervical spine targeting was referenced

to the vertebral bodies nearest the treatment site. It is more difficult to clearly image the specific thoracic and lumbar vertebrae because of increased opacity from the chest and abdomen. Therefore for thoracic and lumbar lesions, 2 × 6mm surgical stainless steel fiducial markers were implanted percutaneously before radiosurgery. This was performed with the patient under conscious sedation. The fiducial markers were implanted near the dorsal bony elements of the vertebral levels adjacent to the lesion being treated. No complications of fiducial placement occurred, and all patients were discharged home the same day.

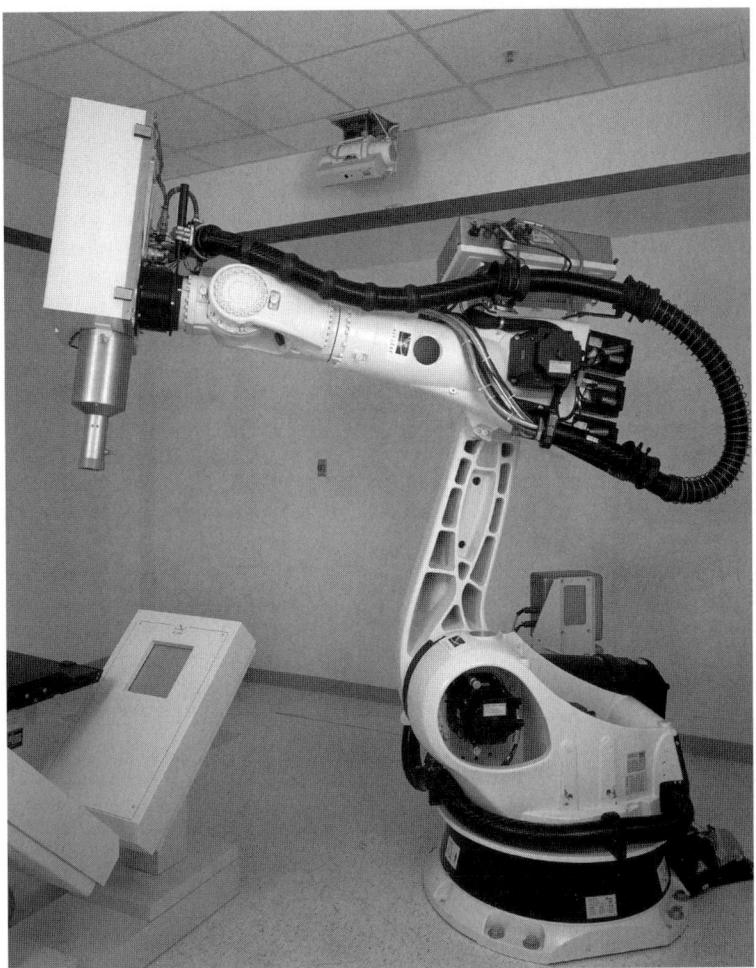

**Figure 134.5** The Cyberknife.

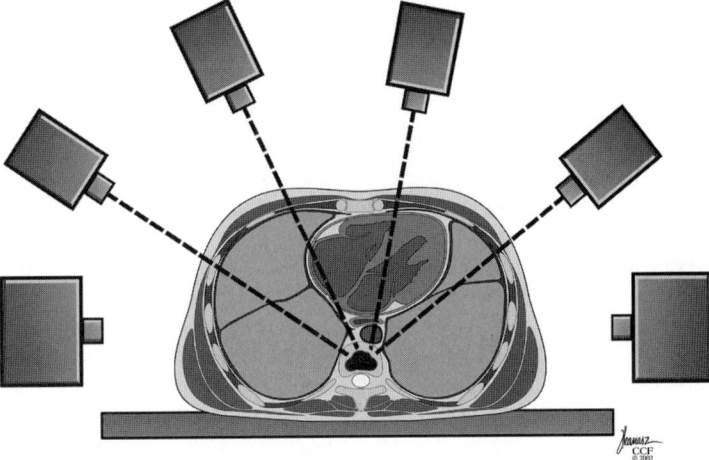

**Figure 134.6** Schematic of the Cyberknife robotic arm treating a vertebral body lesion. Treatment beams can be arranged in multiple planes to minimize spinal cord exposure. Imaging detectors on either side of the patient detect movement of the lesion or some other internal landmark and allow movement of the linear accelerator to stay targeted on the lesion. (*Copyright © 2002 Cleveland Clinic Foundation.*)

With the exception of the six patients with vascular malformations, all patients had prior surgical resection, radiotherapy, or both before radiosurgery. Patients were treated with a total dose of 100 to 2500cGy in 1 to 5 fractions. In all cases, the dose delivered to the spinal cord was less than 800cGy. No patients had neurologic changes, hemorrhage, or symptom exacerbation following therapy. Limited follow-up data are available. However, preliminary data showed that six patients had local control of tumor size on follow-up magnetic resonance imaging up to 1 year posttreatment.[29] Of the patients with spinal cord vascular malformations, only one has had follow-up angiography, because the other patients are less than 3 years posttreatment. The patient who had follow-up angiography had 80% reduction in size of the arteriovenous malformation (AVM) 3 years after initial treatment and has successfully undergone a second course of radiosurgery. Despite the use of radiosurgery for some spinal AVMs, it should be noted that the standard of treatment for spinal AVMs remains surgical with the goal of complete obliteration.

## Cost Issues

One potential advantage of stereotactic radiosurgery is cost. Comparative economic data have been examined for intracranial stereotactic radiosurgery. Sperduto and Hall[33] assessed the application of whole brain radiation therapy (WBRT) plus stereotactic radiosurgery versus WBRT plus surgical resection for patients with a solitary brain metastasis. Excluding those patients who required surgical relief from mass effect, Sperduto and Hall[33] calculate that radiosurgery would save society $175 million each year. Mehta et al.[19] assessed LINAC radiosurgery versus surgical resection for single brain metastases in a retrospective review of a single institution's data. They found that surgical resection resulted in a 1.8-fold increase in cost compared with radiosurgery. Both modalities yielded superior survival and functional independence compared with WBRT alone. Rutigliano et al.[28] performed the same analysis for intracranial Gamma Knife surgery and found stereotactic radiosurgery to be similarly more cost-effective. Although these studies involve intracranial radiosurgery, there is good reason to believe that similar cost-effectiveness may be seen in spine surgery—where surgical intervention commonly involves the additional expenses of complex instrumentation systems.

## Potential Drawbacks to Spinal Radiosurgery

One of the most obvious limitations of spinal stereotactic radiosurgery is the lack of long-term follow-up. The two clinical series using the Hamilton-Lulu frame and the Cyberknife are relatively recent, with the latter series having a median follow-up of only 6 months.[29] In the series by Takacs and Hamilton,[35] patient selection was limited to those with end-stage diseases and was purely palliative. Reserving treatment for only this patient population also limits follow-up. The safety and usefulness of stereotactic radiosurgery of the spine will not be fully determined until longer-term results are obtained.

An additional concern regarding spinal radiosurgery is its potential effect on spine stability. Postradiation spinal deformity has been well documented in children following radiotherapy for malignant disease, such as neuroblastoma, Wilms' tumor, and medulloblastoma.* Radiation affects the vertebral epiphysis and the soft tissues, resulting in fibrosis and contractures. Neuhauser et al.[23] have shown that growth disturbances of cartilage and bone pro-

duced by radiation are directly related to dose. Radiation effects on the growing axial skeleton are often manifested by scoliosis and kyphosis. Various authors have reported a 50% to 80% incidence of scoliosis in children administered radiation for Wilms' tumor and neuroblastoma.[17,18,25] Of these children, 11% to 12% had postradiation scoliosis severe enough to warrant management.

There are few data on the long-term effects of radiotherapy on the adult spine with regards to deformity. It is known that the scoliosis and kyphosis seen in children following radiation does not show progressive change until the adolescent growth spurt.[16] Therefore the degree of postradiation deformity seen in children is not anticipated in adults following radiosurgery. However, other adverse effects are possible. Matsubayashi[15] described the process by which repair takes place following the irradiation of bony spine metastases. After degeneration and necrosis of tumor cells, vascular invasion and fibrous tissue fills the space left by the lesion. Collagen fibers become mineralized, and osteoblastic activity forms woven immature bone that remodels into mature lamellar bone. Recalcification of the involved area can be seen within 3 to 4 months, and complete healing can be seen at 6 months. Takacs and Hamilton[35] point out that, should the rate of neoplastic cell death after radiosurgery be greater than the rate of osteoblastic growth, involution of the vertebral body may occur and lead to compression fractures and spinal deformity (Figure 134.7). This may ultimately lead to neural compression. As the use of spinal stereotactic radiosurgery is expanded to include patients with lesions that translate into better prognosis and thus longer follow-up periods, an increase in symptomatic spinal deformity may be observed.

## Summary

There are several potential advantages to the application of stereotactic radiosurgery to the spine. It represents a less invasive alternative to surgical intervention, which carries the morbidity of general anesthesia and long, often involved operations that require significant recovery periods. This is an important advantage in those patients with metastatic lesions, because they commonly have advanced systemic disease and often a poor prognosis.

Stereotactic radiosurgery can also avoid the problem of the relative radiosensitivity of the spinal cord. Because the dose is conformed more precisely to treatment volume, larger doses of radiation should increase the likelihood of tumor control–as has been shown by intracranial radiosurgery.[29] In fact, many of the lesions treated by Ryu et al.[29] were previously deemed untreatable as a result of their proximity to radiosensitive structures. Spinal stereotactic radiosurgery may also bypass the problem of tumor recurrence in areas that have received so-called maximal irradiation. Recurrent tumors that, in the past, were no longer treatable following radiation therapy are now potentially treatable.

Stereotactic radiosurgery of the spine also expands the range of lesions that are potentially treatable. Up to 50% or more of patients with spinal metastases have multiple sites of involvement.[9] Aggressive surgical resection of multiple lesions in some patients may be unrealistic because of advanced systemic disease and limited prognosis. Such

---

*References 4,11,17,18,23,25,27,34,36,37.

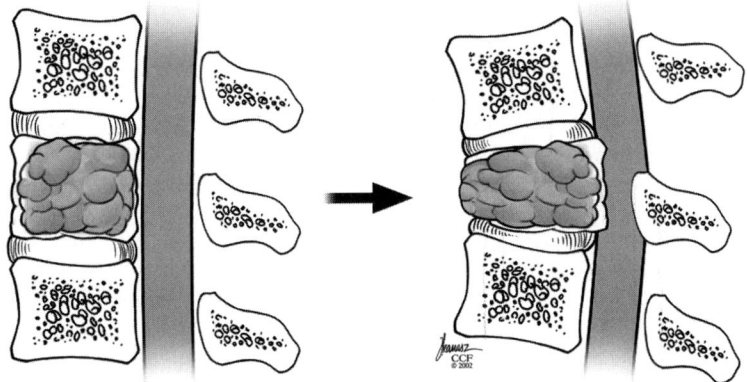

**Figure 134.7** A potential complication of radiosurgery. If the rate of neoplastic cell death after radiosurgery is greater than the rate of osteoblastic growth, compression fractures and spinal deformity may result. *(Copyright © 2002 Cleveland Clinic Foundation.)*

patients may benefit from radiosurgery, because its invasiveness can be limited to the placement of small fiducials near the spinal dorsal elements.

Several concerns exist regarding spinal stereotactic radiosurgery. More clinical studies and longer follow-up data are necessary to demonstrate its effectiveness. The effect this therapy may have on spinal stability must also be considered. If the use of spine radiosurgery is to be extended to those patients with longer survival, then long-term complications such as vertebral body collapse and progressive spinal deformity should be anticipated and considered. Stereotactic radiosurgery of the spine represents a novel form of therapy for several different spinal lesions and possesses a number of potential benefits. Ultimately, further studies and longer clinical follow-up will determine its safety and effectiveness.

## REFERENCES

1. Adler JR, Chang SD, Murphy MJ, *et al:* The Cyberknife: A frameless robotic system for radiosurgery. *Stereotact Funct Neurosurg* 69:124, 1997.

2. Adler JR, Cox R: Preliminary clinical experience with the Cyberknife: Image-guided stereotactic radiosurgery. In Alexander E, Kondziolka D, Loeffler J (eds): *Radiosurgery 1995.* Karger, Basel, New York, 1996, pp 316-326.

3. Adler JR, Murphy MJ, Chang SD, Hancock SL: Image-guided robotic radiosurgery. *Neurosurgery* 44:1299, 1999.

4. Arkin AM, Pack GT, Ransohoff NS, Simon N: Irradiation-induced scoliosis: A case report. *J Bone Joint Surg* 32A:401, 1950.

5. Byrne NT: Spinal cord compression from epidural metastases. *N Engl J Med* 327:614, 1992.

6. Chang SD, Murphy MJ, Doty J, Adler JR: Stereotactic radiosurgery: New innovations. In Fisher WS III (ed): *Perspectives in Neurological Surgery.* Baltimore, Williams & Wilkins, 1999, pp 145-153.

7. Chang SD, Murphy MJ, Martin DP, Adler JR: Frameless stereotactic radiosurgery. In Petrovich Z, Brady LW, Apuzzo MLJ, Bamberg M (eds): *Combined Modality Therapy of Central Nervous System Tumors.* New York, Springer, 2000, pp 387-396.

8. Chang SD, Murphy MJ, Martin DP, Adler JR: Image-guide robotic radiosurgery: Clinical and radiographic results with the Cyberknife. In Kondziolka D (ed): *Radiosurgery 1999.* New York, Karger, Basel, 2000, pp 23-33.

9. Heldman U, Myschetzky PS, Thomsen HS: Frequency of unexpected multifocal metastases in patients with acute spinal cord compression: Evaluation of low-field MR imaging in cancer patients. *Acta Radiol* 38:372, 1997.

10. Helwig-Larsen S: Clinical outcome in metastatic spinal cord compression: A prospective study of 153 patients. *Acta Neurol Scand* 94:269, 1996.

11. Katzman J, Waugh T, Berdon W: Skeletal changes following irradiation of childhood. *J Bone Joint Surg* 51A:825, 1969.

12. Leksell L: The stereotactic method and radiosurgery of the brain. *Acta Chir Scand* 102:316, 1951.

13. Marcus RB, Million R: The risk of radiation myelitis after treatment of the cervical spinal cord. Presented at the 31st Annual Scientific Meeting of the American Society for Therapeutic Radiology and Oncology. San Francisco, CA, 1989.

14. Marcus RB, Million R: The incidence of myelitis after irradiation of the cervical spinal cord. *Radiology* 93:3, 1990.

15. Matsubayashi T: The reparative process of metastatic bone lesions after radiation therapy. *Jpn J Clin Oncol* II(Suppl):253, 1981.

16. Mayfield JK: Postradiation spinal deformity. *Orthop Clin North Am* 10:829, 1979.

17. Mayfield JK, Riseborough EJ, Jaffe N, Nehme M: Irradiation spine deformity in children treated for neuroblastoma. In *Late Biological Effects of Ionizing Radiation, Proceedings of a Symposium,* vol 1. Vienna, Austria, International Atomic Energy Agency, 1978, pp 155-166.

18. Mayfield JK, Riseborough EJ, Jaffe N, Nehme M: Spinal deformity in children treated for neuroblastoma. *J Bone Joint Surg* 63A:183, 1981.

19. Mehta M, Noyes W, Craig B, *et al:* A cost-effectiveness and cost-utility analysis of radiosurgery vs. resection for single-brain metastases. *Int J Radiat Oncol Biol Phys* 39:445, 1997.

20. Murphy MJ: An automatic six degree of freedom image registration algorithm for image guided frameless stereotactic radiosurgery. *Med Phys* 24:857, 1997.

21. Murphy MJ, Cox RS: The accuracy of dose localization for an image guided frameless radiosurgery system. *Med Phys* 23:2043, 1996.

22. Nather A, Bose K: The results of decompression of cord or cauda equina compression from metastatic extradural tumors. *Clin Orthop* 169:103, 1982.

23. Neuhauser EBD, Wittenberg MH, Berman CZ, Cohen J: Irradiation effects of roentgen therapy on the growing spine. *Radiology* 59:637, 1952.

24. Phillips TL, Buschke F: Radiation tolerance of the thoracic spinal cord. *Brain* 105:659, 1969.

25. Riseborough EJ, Grabias SL, Burton RI, Jaffe N: Skeletal alterations following irradiation for Wilms' tumor. *J Bone Joint Surg* 58A:526, 1976.

26. Rubin P, Andrews JR, Swarm R, Gump H: Radiation induced dysplasia of bone. *AJR Am J Roentgenol* 82:206, 1959.

27. Rubin P, Duthie RB, Young LW: The significance of scoliosis in postirradiated Wilms' tumor and neuroblastoma. *Radiology* 79:539, 1962.

28. Rutigliano MJ, Lunsford LD, Kondziolka D: The cost-effectiveness of stereotactic radiosurgery vs. surgical resection in the treatment of solitary metastatic brain tumors. *Neurosurgery* 37:445, 1995.

29. Ryu SI, Chang SD, Kim DH, *et al:* Image-guided hypofractionated stereotactic radiosurgery to spinal lesions. *Neurosurgery* 49:838, 2001.

30. Schultheiss TE, Kun LE, Ang KK, Stephens LC: Radiation response of the central nervous system. *Int J Radiat Oncol Biol Phys* 31:1093, 1995.

31. Siegal T, Siegal T, Shohami E, Shapiro Y: Surgical management of malignant epidural tumors compressing the spinal cord. In Schmidek HH (ed): *Operative Neurosurgical Techniques: Indications, Methods, and Results,* ed 4. Philadelphia, WB Saunders, 2000, pp 2171-2197.

32. Sioutos PJ, Arbit E, Meshulam CF, Galicich JH: Spinal metastases from solid tumors: Analysis of factors affecting survival. *Cancer* 76:1453, 1995.

33. Sperduto PW, Hall WA: Radiosurgery, cost-effectiveness, gold standards, the scientific method, cavalier cowboys, and the cost of hope. *Int J Radiat Oncol Biol Phys* 36:511, 1996.

34. Tachdjian MD, Matson DD: Orthopaedic aspects of intraspinal tumors in infants and children. *J Bone Joint Surg* 47A:223, 1965.

35. Takacs I, Hamilton AJ: Extracranial stereotactic radiosurgery: Applications for the spine and beyond. *Neurosurg Clin North Am* 10:257, 1999.

36. Vaeth JM, Levitt SH, Jones MD, Holttreter C: Effects of radiation therapy in survivors of Wilms' tumor. *Radiology* 79:560, 1962.

37. Whitehouse WM, Lampe I: Osseous damage in irradiation of renal tumors in infancy and childhood. *AJR Am J Roentgenol* 70:721, 1953.

# CHAPTER 135

# Somatosensory Evoked Potential for Spine Surgery

**Jorge Gonzalez-Martinez, Ashwini D. Sharan, and Dileep Nair**

The prevalence of degenerative spinal conditions and deformities are such that spinal surgical procedures are common. Furthermore, evolution and understanding of spinal mechanics and physiology has allowed the introduction of many newer spinal surgical techniques. Nevertheless, a small proportion, less than 0.5%, of patients may develop a persistent neurologic deficit immediately postoperatively. Careful surgical techniques, including stabilization of the spine during surgery, have helped reduce this complication somewhat. However, it is apparent that a neurologic injury related to such an intervention can be disabling. For this reason, the monitoring of somatosensory evoked potentials (SSEPs) from peripheral nerve stimulation (posterior tibial, peroneal, or median nerves) during spinal column or spinal cord surgery is common.*

The spinal cord and nerve roots are at risk during a variety of surgical procedures performed on the spinal cord and surrounding structures. The risk varies with the underlying disease, as well as the type and location of surgery.[3,6,7,12] Patients with intramedullary tumors, syringomyelia, spinal arteriovenous malformation, thoracoabdominal aneurysms, and any other disorder associated with a baseline neurologic deficit are at greatest risk. The frequency of neurologic injury following scoliosis surgery, correction of congenital spinal deformities, and decompression (with and without spinal fusion) is low, but when damage to the spinal cord occurs, the resulting deficits are often severe, permanent, and devastating.[2,4,12] The detection of significant changes in the monitored evoked potentials (MEPs) often indicates early spinal cord dysfunction and may permit appropriate intervention to prevent spinal cord damage.

In the 1970s, the "wake-up test" was developed in an attempt to reduce the risk of spinal cord injury in patients undergoing scoliosis surgery. This technique rapidly became the standard with which other monitoring techniques were compared. Although helpful, the wake-up test disrupts the surgical procedure, can be performed only intermittently, and is associated with considerable risks (e.g., extubation, pulmonary embolism). Furthermore, it is not applicable to patients undergoing surgical procedures in which no period of major risk is defined, as in resections of spinal neoplasms.

In the 1980s, SSEP monitoring was developed as an alternative to the wake-up test. SSEP recordings provided the means to monitor spinal cord function continuously without interfering with surgery or producing additional risk. A large body of data, including clinical experience in thousands of patients, has provided significant information regarding the utility and limitation of SSEP monitoring during spinal surgery, but no prospective controlled trial of SSEP monitoring has ever been published.*

## Neuroanatomic and Functional Basis

The SSEP is dependent on the dorsal columns. Consequently, if the dorsal columns are preserved, injury to other important pathways could occur without a change in the SSEP.[10,15,27]

Specifically, SSEPs are used to assess whether the lemniscal somatosensory system is intact. Impulses generated from the median nerve at the wrist (radial aspect) are transmitted through the sensory fibers to the dorsal horn of the cervical spinal cord. Next, impulses follow the dorsal tract (*fasciculus cuneatus*) to the ipsilateral posterior tract nuclei (*nucleus cuneatus*) located in the dorsal medulla. Conduction then leaves the medullary nuclei through the medial lemniscus, which, after crossing the midline, terminates in the ventrobasal nucleus of the thalamus. From the thalamus, there are multiple radiations to the primary sensory cortex. When received at the level of the cortex, afferent volleys are processed, both in the somatosensory cortex and in the parietal association fields. Median nerve SSEPs reflect spinal cord function from C1 to C7.

In addition, SSEPs recorded from upper extremity stimulation do not reflect lower extremity abnormalities. Posterior tibial potentials must also be recorded. Stimulation at the level of the medial malleolus generates afferent volleys that are transmitted by sensory fibers to the dorsal horn at the conus medullaris and then carried by the dorsal tract (*fasciculus gracilis*) to the dorsal medullary nucleus (*nucleus gracilis*). Cortical conduction is then achieved via the medial lemniscus and thalamus.

## Methods of Monitoring

The two basic types of spinal cord monitoring currently used in surgery use noninvasive or invasive techniques.

### Noninvasive Techniques

The noninvasive techniques involve the monitoring of potentials generated by spinal, subcortical (brainstem), or cortical pathways from the skin surface or from subdermal needle electrodes. In all the noninvasive studies, peripheral nerves in the upper (median or ulnar nerve) or lower extremity (posterior tibial or peroneal nerve) are stimulated. Recordings outside the operating field (noninvasive technique) are by far the simplest and can be performed without disturbing the surgeon's attention from the surgical

---

*References 1,5,9,11,13,14,16-19,21-25,27,29-33,35,37-45.

*References 1,2,5,13,16,21,24,25,34.

field. Recordings are most commonly made from standard scalp derivations, usually CZ-FZ (International 10-20 System)[20] with leg stimulation, and C3 (C4)-FZ with arm stimulation. Other reference electrodes, such as the ears, are also used. Most of the early studies of surgical monitoring used peripheral stimulation with scalp recording, which generally gives a well-defined, although unstable, response.

The technique of monitoring potentials from a single recording site (i.e., cortical potentials) has some criticisms that must be mentioned. If the responses change or disappear during monitoring, it is difficult if not impossible to differentiate this from technical problems versus an alteration of spinal cord function. Another criticism of recording only cortical potentials is that they are very sensitive to the effects of changing levels of anesthesia and decreases in blood pressure as opposed to the subcortical or spinal cord potentials.

### Invasive Techniques

A number of methods of recording in the operating field have been developed to facilitate recording closer to the neural tissue.* These methods include subarachnoid, epidural, spinous process, and intraspinal ligament recordings. The spinal cord recording (not cortical potentials) facilitates direct evaluation of segmental changes that occur above and below the operative site. Dinner *et al.*[11] assessed 70 of 100 scoliotic patients who were monitored with interspinous electrodes and confirmed that the spinal evoked potentials were both reliable and reproducible, whereas the wires posed little risk to neurologic function. Lüders *et al.*[29] successfully used spinal evoked responses during 40 spinal procedures, 32 for scoliosis and Harrington rod placement and 8 for syrinx drainage and resection of tumors and arteriovenous malformations.

Although recordings in the surgical field can yield a much larger response, they are associated with technical problems including disturbing the surgeon's attention, adding to the risk of infection; with mechanical artifact; and with being limited to those surgical procedures in which the spine is opened to expose the dura. In general, such recordings require much technical expertise for satisfactory recordings and require that the surgeon be familiar and cooperative with the procedure. Recordings in the surgical field are most useful for spinal cord surgery (e.g., for tumors or arteriovenous malformations), in which recorded potential can localize the area of damage or record responses that are too small to record with other methods.

Spinal cord evoked potential monitoring, another method of invasive recording, can be achieved by direct, segmental spinal cord stimulation using subdural electrodes. Polyphasic action potentials produced by these subdural electrodes are larger in amplitude and less likely to deteriorate or vary with minimal adjustments in anesthetic concentrations as compared with those noted during cortical monitoring. Simultaneous ascending and descending signals are generated and can be assessed in shorter periods of time. Recordings are made over 1- to 2-minute intervals with the interspinous ligament or

spinous process devices, whereas longer 10- to 230-second intervals are required when extradural or subarachnoid thoracolumbar potentials are followed. Spinal potentials may also be used in conjunction with other monitoring modalities such as the MEP or cortical evoked responses. Limitations of this technique include intraoperative displacement of monitoring electrodes, which results in unreliable recordings and/or inadvertent neurologic injury.

### Monitoring Techniques

SSEPs are recorded from the cortex with only two of the many electrodes composing the cortical array used by the International 10-20 System.[20] One electrode is placed in the midsagittal plane (CZ1), and the second is applied more ventrally in the midline. A third ground is always added (FZ). Placing an additional cervical needle electrode (at C2) helps confirm whether cortical changes reflect true spinal cord changes, as opposed to local cortical variations that may occur in response to alterations in anesthetic administration. Such needle electrodes may also be placed over a lumbar spinous process (L5) to differentiate between similar alterations. SSEP skin and surface electrodes are noninvasive and are applied far away from the operative field, and monitoring may begin before induction and continue through closing.

The large mixed peripheral nerves (median, ulnar, peroneal, or posterior tibial nerves) receive short 200-msec pulses at rates of 3 to 5 per second. The larger-diameter peripheral sensory A alpha and A beta fast-conducting fibers are stimulated with stimulus intensities set at two or three times the motor threshold, sufficient to produce a motor twitch.[26] Two hundred recordings are then averaged and passed through band-pass filters of 10 to 500Hz for increased clarification and noise reduction. Alternate stimulation of the right and left sides allows both waveforms to be simultaneously monitored with a split-screen array. This requires 50 seconds (means of 200 recordings) for two extremities and 100 seconds for all four extremities. Findings may be reproduced by repeating stimulation of one or both sides, enabling the surgeon to be alerted to significant changes in any of the four extremities within minutes.

The most reliable SSEP recordings are produced by electrical stimulation of large mixed nerves in the limbs. Stimulation is applied to distal nerves (e.g., ulnar, median, tibial) with surface electrodes or to proximal nerves (e.g., sciatic, cauda equina, brachial plexus). Each nerve is stimulated unilaterally in a consecutive fashion so that those pathways carrying information from all potentially affected limbs are monitored. Bilateral simultaneous stimulation may miss a unilateral injury and therefore is performed only when an adequate response cannot be obtained with unilateral stimulation. Stimulation duration and intensity is adjusted (0.2 to 0.5msec, 5 to 90mA) to produce maximal stimulation of sensory axons. The rate of stimulation is kept under 5Hz to minimize rate-dependent attenuation of the SSEP, which is accentuated by anesthetics. Rates less than 2Hz are sometimes required to record cerebral potentials in children and adolescents, especially at deeper levels of anesthesia.

---

*References 8,11,22,28,29,36,39.

Stimulation rates that are even fractions of 60Hz are avoided to prevent averaging of 60-cycle interference into the recording. The number of stimuli required for averaging varies with the amount of background noise, as well as with the size and reproducibility of the SSEP. In the absence of a preoperative deficit or excessive artifact, 250 stimuli are usually necessary for recordings made from surface electrodes. The number of stimuli averaged should be kept to a minimum so that the surgeon receives feedback as rapidly as possible.

The type of electrode recording used depends on the location of recordings sites and the type of surgery. Scalp electrodes are standard and are similar to those used for SSEP recordings in the outpatient setting. They are firmly attached with collodion and filled with conductive gel to ensure stability and low impedance during long surgical procedures. Esophageal or nasopharyngeal electrodes are used to record cervical cord potentials outside the surgical field in cervical spine surgery. Needle electrodes inserted between spinous processes or over the lamina of the spine can be used to record spinal cord activity. Needle electrodes placed in the interspinous ligaments can be used within the operative field if the dorsal vertebral elements are left intact. Small cotton-tipped electrodes or platinum electrodes are used to record directly from the surface of the spinal cord or cerebral cortex.

For each of these active electrodes, an appropriate reference must be chosen. Nearby electrodes reduce noise, but distant electrodes enhance signal amplitude. In general, active and reference electrodes should be of the same material to minimize impedance mismatch, which increases noise. Recordings can be made at multiple peripheral and central sites along the sensory pathways. Adherence to this important principle minimizes the incidence of false-positive changes and makes troubleshooting for technical errors more efficient.

Signal amplification and filter settings are similar to those used for diagnostic outpatient SSEP recordings, although at times the sensitivity must be reduced or the band-pass restricted because of the amount of noise in the surgical environment. Amplification of 5 to 10uV/cm, sweep speed of 2 to 10msec/cm, low frequency filters of 30 to 100Hz, and high frequency filters of 2000 to 3000Hz are generally satisfactory. The equipment used for intraoperative SSEP recordings must be versatile and easily tailored to the specific type of procedure being monitored. The ability to record other modalities (e.g., electromyogram [EMG], MEP) concurrently with SSEP may be essential. Preamplifiers need to tolerate high current loads caused by cautery and other sources of electrical interference. Automatic cautery suppression; artifact rejection; and software for digital filtering, trend analysis, data reproduction, and storage are desirable features.

## Anesthesia

Anesthesia reduces the amplitude and increases the latency of cortical SSEP recordings. This is especially true in the presence of disease and in children and adolescents. Because the reduction of amplitude is directly related to depth of anesthesia, the level of anesthetic agents should be kept as light as possible. Anesthetic effect varies with the agent used, with halogenated anesthetics producing the greatest effects, followed by moderate changes with intravenous barbiturates and nitrous oxide, and the least with narcotics and benzodiazepines. Etomidate and ketamine have been shown to enhance the amplitude of the cortical SSEP potentials. These drugs can be used occasionally to record cortical potentials during surgery when responses are absent with standard anesthetics. Alterations in blood pressure can also reduce the amplitude of the evoked response, especially with mean blood pressures lower than 70mmHg.

To further limit perioperative morbidity, a consistent anesthesia protocol should accompany SSEP monitoring. In cervical spine surgery, the risk of spinal cord injury related to intubation led to the adoption of the awake, nasotracheal, fiberoptic intubation protocol, with patients at times immobilized in hard cervical collars. Often, when patients with severe cervical spinal cord compromise are being positioned, the neutral position is not the optimal position. SSEP changes may indicate that a greater or lesser degree of flexion or extension may be warranted. Induction of anesthesia proceeds only after the SSEPs return to baseline levels, because bolus injections of barbiturates transiently compromise the SSEP response for 5 to 10 minutes.

The anesthesia protocol uses preoperative and intraoperative medications. Premedications include hydroxyzine 1mg/kg, meperidine 1mg/kg, and atropine (0.2 to 0.4mg). Numbing of the nasopharyngeal passageways is achieved with either 4% cocaine applied with cotton swabs to the nasopharynx or 10ml of 2% lidocaine jelly applied with a 14-Fr nasotracheal catheter to the same area. Both regimens include a transtracheal injection with 5ml (100mg) of 2% Xylocaine. Next, a 7 to 8mm anode tube, placed over an adult fiberoptic bronchoscope, is introduced through the nares into the larynx and trachea, with the patient receiving midazolam 1 to 5mg as needed.

Although patients who undergo ventral surgery remain supine, those who undergo dorsal procedures may be brought to the sitting position. In this case, while the patient is still awake, a Mayfield head holder is applied using 15ml of 1% Xylocaine and 1:200,000 epinephrine to locally anesthetize the pins sites. Careful attention must be given to positioning the arms. They should be elevated, gently flexed, and padded at the elbows to reduce traction of nerve roots or the brachial plexus.

When bringing a patient to the sitting position, it may be preferable to keep him or her awake to avoid hypotension while preserving intact barometric reflexes. However, even with these precautions, some awake patients demonstrate declines in both amplitudes and latency responses. These changes are attributed to a relative drop in spinal cord perfusion despite systemic normotension (relative hypotension). This may readily be reversed by the pharmacologic induction of hypertension.

During induction, infusing a bolus of thiopental 2 to 3mg/kg or propofol (Diprivan) 1 to 2mg/kg results in a transient 5- to 10-minute decline in SSEP responses. Inhalation anesthetic concentrations are kept between 0.2% and 0.4%, and nitrous oxide is maintained below 60% to 70%.

Vecuronium is given in a loading dose of 0.1mg/kg and then administered repeatedly as required. Local anesthetic infiltrated into the operative wound may allow the anesthesiologist to use lower doses of anesthetic throughout surgery, and this may be desirable for monitoring. Patients are immediately awakened and neurologically assessed on the operating table after surgery. Only then are the patients brought to the recovery room.

## Interpretation

Animal and human studies have shown that SSEP changes can occur when there is injury to adjacent motor pathways at the spinal and brainstem level.[4,9,10,12] Assuming that appropriate stimulation and recording can be achieved, a major issue to be resolved is what constitutes a significant change and how reliably this can be detected. To further complicate matters, the primary disease often produces an SSEP abnormality that can be recognized in baseline recordings.° Recording methods may have to be modified. Despite averaging, multiple sources of artifacts may result in unstable potentials that are different for each patient. It is essential to determine the limits of SSEP amplitude and latency variation with repeated samples during the early part of the surgery. Significance criteria can be determined that are beyond the baseline limits of variability. In patients with high amplitude, well-defined potentials at peripheral, spinal, and cortical levels; a reproducible drop in amplitude of 50% or greater or an increase in latency of 2msec or greater (or more than a 5% to 10% prolongation of latency); or both is considered significant.

SSEPs rely on the recording of amplitude and latency values elicited from median and posterior tibial nerve stimulation. The responses are recorded from the postcentral sulcus (noninvasive technique). Amplitude is measured, in microvolts, from the wave's height to its trough. The amplitude reflects the integrity of a number of fibers being simultaneously stimulated to form an action potential. Amplitude varies from patient to patient according to age, height, temperature, and integrity of the system being tested. Comparison of right and left side and assessment of changes compared with the patient's preoperative baseline is important.

If baseline recordings with the patient under anesthesia show highly variable, low-amplitude cortical or spinal potentials, then all potentials recorded rostral to the area at risk might be required to disappear for the change to be considered significant. Implicit in these judgments is the understanding that effects of a change in physiologic variable, limb position, artifacts, and technical failures be identified and either corrected or accounted for before a final decision regarding the significance of a change in the SSEP is made.

Early in the procedure, an effort is made to identify and eliminate all sources of noise, especially 60-cycle interference. Care must be taken to avoid ground loops. Any conductor in contact with the patient (including intravenous lines) or electrical equipment in the room can be a source of interference. The recording system should suppress

°References 3,9,21,24,30,33,40,45.

input during cautery and reject high-amplitude artifact. EMG activity from surrounding muscle can also produce unwanted artifact if neuromuscular activity is not blocked. Especially with the patient under light anesthesia, EMG activity can obscure the SSEP. A short, constant, controlled level of short-acting neuromuscular blocking agent or intermittent doses of benzodiazepines can be used to control muscle artifact in cases that require simultaneous monitoring of SSEP and EMG.

In the upper extremities, although the entire waveform from N10 (brachial plexus), N12a/N12b (segmental ascending dorsal column), N13a/N13b (dorsal horn/cuneate nucleus), and N14 (medial lemniscus) is recorded, the final cortical median N20 proves to be the most clinically relevant. Similarly, N22/P22 (dorsal horn T10 to L1), N29 (cervical gracile nucleus), P31 (medial lemniscus), and N34 (thalamus/brainstem) are noted, but the P38/N38 and P40 constitute the most used cortical potentials.

The cortical potential recorded from median nerve stimulation shows three positive peaks before the final negative trough of N20. The first of the waves at P15 indicates the afferent volley arriving at the thalamic level, whereas P16 and P18 indicate transmission via the thalamocortical tract to the primary sensory cortex. Once at the volley arrives at the cortex, additional positive peaks up to P25 indicate additional volley transmission to the surrounding sensory cortical regions.

Cortical responses noted after tibial nerve stimulation follow a similar but more prolonged pattern. The mean latency for the posterior tibial response P40 is typically 38.8 msec. Multiple initial negative peaks may also be visualized with these responses. These varied responses reflect the different anatomic locations along the somatosensory pathway of the posterior tibial nerve to the cauda equina, lumbosacral spinal cord, gracile nucleus, thalamus, and cortex.

Somatosensory cortical evoked responses (compared with invasive spinal evoked responses) have the disadvantage of being more vulnerable to changes in anesthetic techniques and are susceptible to changes in peripheral skin conditions (i.e., temperature). Cortical responses are also smaller in amplitude, and they more readily deteriorate, particularly in the presence of excessive electroencephalographic (ECG) activity or environmental noise. Averaging 200 responses per recording enhances the response, largely by allowing random noise to be eliminated.

## Resuscitative Measures

Anesthetic and surgical resuscitative measures may be instituted as soon as significant SSEP deterioration is detected. This measure may take place either during the first 50 seconds or after findings have been reproduced at 100 seconds. The more rapid the adoption of these techniques in response to imminent tissue damage, the faster the potentials return to baseline.

Medical causes of SSEP changes include hypotension, hypothermia, increased levels of halogenated inhalation anesthetics (greater than 0.4% fluorane), and intravenous

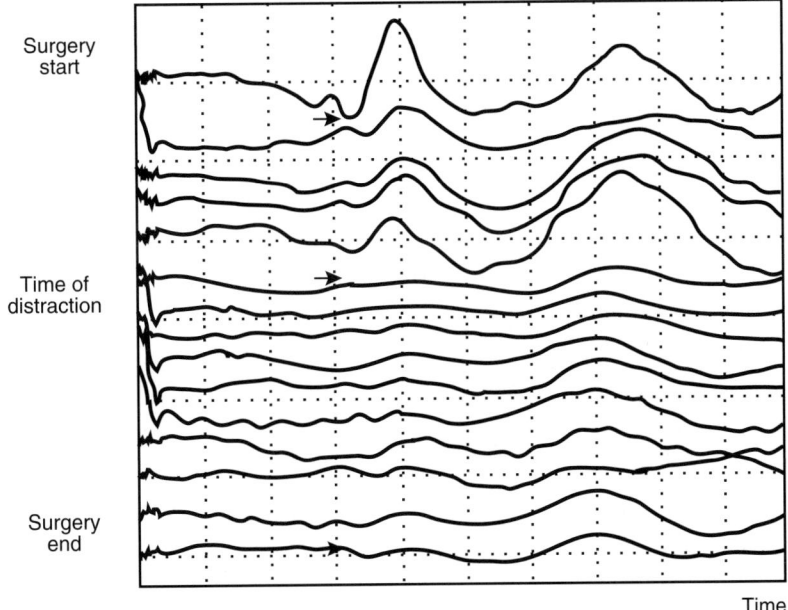

**Figure 135.1** Example of intraoperative somatosensory evoked potentials recording (tibial nerve stimuli) during spine surgery for scoliosis procedure. During the first stage of surgery, the P32 potential is clearly evidenced (*top arrow*), but soon after surgical distraction, the potential almost disappears (*middle arrow*). The surgeon was informed and the distraction was reversed. The potential returned at the end of the procedure, but with smaller amplitude (*bottom arrow*).

sedation. These may be reversed by inducing hypertension and hyperthermia artificially and by hyperoxygenating the wound with peroxide irrigation while increasing systemic oxygenation. The reduction or elimination of inhalation anesthesia by switching to a barbiturate "balanced" technique may also foster recovery. High-dose methylprednisolone may be emergently administered to limit neurologic injury signaled by persistent SSEP abnormalities.

Surgical maneuvers may require cessation of surgical manipulation, release or elimination of distraction, removal of excessively large grafts resulting in overdistraction, and removal of instrumentation. An example of cortical SSEP changes during spine surgery for scoliosis in shown in Figure 135.1. For patients with ossification of the posterior longitudinal ligament, changes in SSEP responses are common. Therefore for these individuals, distraction is avoided until the pathologic abnormality has been fully excised.

## Summary

SSEP monitoring is a relatively juvenile form of monitoring when compared with other techniques such as ECG or even blood pressure monitoring. Despite its relatively recent introduction, SSEP monitoring has already contributed much to the ability of the spine surgeon to deal with difficult problems that only a few years ago were considered too risky to even to consider. SSEP plays a valuable role during spine surgery by decreasing patient risk and improving outcome. It is essential that spine surgeons continue to improve intraoperative monitoring techniques to provide optimal care for their patients.

## REFERENCES

1. Allen A, Starr A, Nudleman K: Assessment of sensory function in the operating room utilizing cerebral evoked potentials: A study of fifty-six surgically anesthetized patients. *Clin Neurosurg* 28:457, 1981.
2. Allison T: Recovery functions of somatosensory evoked responses in man. *Electroencephalogr Clin Neurophysiol* 14:331, 1962.
3. Bennett MH: Effects of compression and ischemia on spinal cord evoked potentials. *Exp Neurol* 80: 508, 1983.
4. Brodkey JS, Richards DE, Blasingame JP, *et al:* Reversible spinal cord trauma in cats. Additive effects of direct pressure and ischemia. *J Neurosurg* 37:591, 1972.
5. Brown JC, Axelgaard J, Rowe DE: Monitoring of the human spinal cord. *Orthop Trans* 3:123, 1979 (abstract).
6. Coles JG, Wilson GJ, Sima AF, *et al:* Intraoperative detection of spinal chord ischemia using somatosensory cortical evoked potentials during thoracic aortic occlusion. *Ann Thorac Surg* 34:299, 1982.
7. Croft TJ, Brodkey JS, Nulsen FE: Reversible spinal cord trauma: A model for electrical monitoring of spinal cord function. *J Neurosurg* 36:402, 1972.
8. Cusick JF, Myklebust J, Larson SJ, Sances A Jr: Spinal evoked potentials in the primate: Neural substrate. *J Neurosurg* 49:551, 1978.
9. D'Angelo CM, VanGilder JC, Taur A: Evoked cortical potentials in experimental spinal cord trauma. *J Neurosurg* 38:332, 1973.
10. Deecke L, Tator CH: Neurophysiological assessment of afferent and efferent conduction in the injured spinal cord of monkeys. *J Neurosurg* 39:65, 1973.

11. Dinner DS, Lüders H, Lesser RP, *et al:* Intraoperative spinal somatosensory evoked potentials monitoring. *J Neurosurg* 65:807, 1986.

12. Dolan EJ, Transfeldt EE, Tator CH, *et al:* The effects of spinal distraction on regional spinal cord in cats. *J Neurosurg* 53:756, 1980.

13. Engler GL, Spielholz NI, Bernhard WN, *et al:* Somatosensory evoked potentials during Harrington instrumentation for scoliosis. *J Bone Joint Surg* 60A:528, 1978.

14. Giblin DR: Somatosensory evoked potentials in healthy subjects and in patients with lesions of the nervous system. *Ann NY Acad Sci* 112:93, 1964.

15. Griffiths IR, Trench JG, Crawford RA: Spinal cord blood flow and conduction during experimental cord compression in normotensive and hypotensive dogs. *J Neurosurg* 50:353, 1979.

16. Grundy BL: Monitoring of sensory evoked potentials during neurosurgical operations: Methods and applications. *Neurosurgery* 11:556, 1982.

17. Grundy BL, Nelson PB, Doyle E, Procopio PT: Intraoperative loss of somatosensory-evoked potentials predicts loss of spinal cord function. *Anesthesiology* 57:321, 1982.

18. Hahn JF, Lesser R, Klem G, *et al:* Simple technique for monitoring intraoperative spinal cord function. *Neurosurgery* 9:692, 1981.

19. Halliday AM, Wakefield GS: Cerebral evoked responses in patients with dissociated sensory loss. *Electroencephalogr Clin Neurophysiol* 14:786, 1962 (abstract).

20. Jasper HH: The ten-twenty electrode system of the International Federation. *Electroencephalogr Clin Neurophysiol* 10:371, 1958.

21. Jones SJ, Edgar MA, Ransford AO, *et al:* A system for electrophysiological monitoring of the spinal cord during operations for scoliosis. *J Bone Joint Surg* 65B:134, 1983.

22. Klem G, Andrish J, Gurd A et al: Spinal cord evoked potentials recorded from ligamentum interspinalis. *Electroencephalogr Clin Neurophysiol* 50:221, 1980.

23. Kobrine AI, Evans DE, Rizzoli HV: Correlation of spinal cord blood flow, sensory evoked response, and spinal cord function in subacute experimental spinal cord compression. In Cervos-Navarro J, Betz E, Ebhardt G, *et al* (eds): *Pathology of cerebrospinal microcirculation. Advances in neurology,* vol 20. New York, Raven Press, 1978, pp 389-394.

24. LaMont RL, Wasson SL, Green MA: Spinal cord monitoring during spinal surgery using somatosensory spinal evoked potentials. *J Pediatr Orthop* 3:31, 1983.

25. Larson SJ, Sances A Jr, Christenson PC: Evoked somatosensory potentials in man. *Arch Neurol* 15:88, 1966.

26. Lesser RP, Koehle R, Lueders H: Effect of stimulus intensity on short latency somatosensory evoked potentials. *Electroencephalogr Clin Neurophysiol* 47:377, 1979.

27. Lesser RP, Raudzens P, Lüders H, *et al:* Postoperative neurological deficits may occur despite unchanged intraoperative somatosensory evoked potentials. *Ann Neurol* 19:22, 1986.

28. Lüders H, Andrish J, Gurd A, *et al:* Origin of far-field subcortical potentials evoked by stimulation of the posterior tibial nerve. *Electroencephalogr Clin Neurophysiol* 52:336, 1981.

29. Lüders H, Gurd A, Hahn J, *et al:* A new technique for intraoperative monitoring of spinal cord function: Multichannel recording of spinal cord and subcortical evoked potentials. *Spine* 7:110, 1982.

30. Maccabee P, Levine DB, Kahanovitz N, *et al:* Monitoring of spinal and subcortical somatosensory evoked potentials during Harrington rod instrumentation. *Orthop Trans* 6:19, 1982 (abstract).

31. MacEwen GD, Bunnell WP, Sriram K: Acute neurological complications in the treatment of scoliosis. A report of the Scoliosis Research Society. *J Bone Joint Surg* 57A:404, 1975.

32. Macon JB, Poletti CE, Sweet WH, *et al:* Conducted somatosensory evoked potentials during spinal surgery. Part 2: Clinical applications. *J Neurosurg* 57:354, 1982.

33. McCallum JE, Bennett MH: Electrophysiologic monitoring of spinal cord function during intraspinal surgery. *Surg Forum* 26:469, 1975.

34. McNeal D, Passoff T, Swank S, *et al:* Spinal cord monitoring using epidural electrodes for stimulation and recording. *Orthop Trans* 6:19, 1982 (abstract).

35. Nash CL Jr, Lorig RA, Schatzinger LA, *et al:* Spinal cord monitoring during operative treatment of spine. *Clin Orthop* 126:100, 1977.

36. Nordwall A, Axelgaard J, Harada Y, *et al:* Spinal cord monitoring using evoked potentials recorded from feline vertebral bone. *Spine* 4:486, 1979.

37. Nuwer MR, Dawson EC: Intraoperative evoked potential monitoring of the spinal cord. A restricted filter, scalp method during Harrington instrumentation for scoliosis. *Clin Orthop* 183:42, 1984.

38. Raudzens PA: Intraoperative monitoring of evoked potentials. *Ann NY Acad Sci* 388:308, 1982.

39. Schramm J, Hashizume K, Fukushima T, *et al:* Experimental spinal cord injury produced by slow, graded compression. Alterations of cortical and spinal evoked potentials. *J Neurosurg* 50:48, 1979.

40. Spielholz NI, Benjamin MV, Engler GL, *et al:* Somatosensory evoked potentials during decompression and stabilization of the spine. Methods and findings. *Spine* 4:500, 1979.

41. Tamaki T, Tsuji H, Inoue S, *et al:* The prevention of iatrogenic spinal cord injury utilizing the evoked spinal cord potential. *Int Orthop* 4:313, 1981.

42. Tsuji S, Lüders H, Lesser RP, *et al:* Subcortical and cortical somatosensory potentials evoked by posterior tibial nerve stimulation: normative values. *Electroencephalogr Clin Neurophysiol* 59:214, 1984.

43. Tsuyama N, Tsuzuki N, Kurokawa T, *et al:* Clinical application of spinal cord action potential movement. *Int Orthop* 2:39, 1978.

44. Wilber RG, Thompson GH, Shaffer JW, *et al:* Postoperative neurological deficits in segmental spinal instrumentation. A study using spinal cord monitoring. *J Bone Joint Surg* 66A:1178, 1984.

45. Worth RM, Markand ON, DeRosa GP, *et al:* Intraoperative somatosensory evoked response monitoring during spinal cord surgery. In Courjon J, Mauguiere F, Revol M (eds): *Clinical applications of evoked potentials in neurology. Advances in neurology,* vol 22. New York, Raven Press, 1982, pp 367-373.

# CHAPTER 136

# Electronic Diagnostic Studies

Jeffrey Owen and John Regan

The increased use of pedicular instrumentation by orthopedic and neurologic surgeons has resulted in the need to develop cost-effective intraoperative procedures that are sensitive to nerve root and pedicle wall status. At the present time, no single procedure is sensitive to the status of both of these structures. However, by using a multimodality approach, it is possible to provide the surgeon with information regarding these structures. Based upon the format and methods of acquiring data, these procedures can be divided into two major categories: electrophysiologic and imaging.

Electrophysiologic procedures provide the surgeon with information regarding the functional integrity of nerve roots and the structural integrity of pedicle walls. These procedures record responses that are obtained through electromyograms (EMG) and are divided into two categories based on their method of elicitation. If the EMG response is elicited by mechanical or thermal irritation of a nerve root, the response is known as a free-run or spontaneous EMG (S-EMG). The S-EMG is directly sensitive to nerve root status, but provides only indirect information regarding pedicle wall status. If the EMG is elicited by electrical stimulation of the pedicle screw or pedicle wall, the response is known as an electrically elicited EMG (E-EMG). The E-EMG is directly sensitive to the structural integrity of pedicle walls, but provides only indirect information regarding nerve roots. Because of the differential sensitivity of S-EMG and E-EMG data, their procedures complement each other during surgery. Table 136.1 lists the acquisition parameters typically used to administer these tests.

In addition to electrophysiologic studies, it is possible to obtain information regarding the pedicle walls and screws using imaging studies. Intraoperative imaging consists of plain film radiography, fluoroscopy, and image guidance procedures.[14] The primary purposes for using these procedures are to localize a specific spinal level, provide images of the spine during placement of pedicle screws, and ensure correct orientation and placement of pedicle screws. Intraoperative imaging studies are not useful in determining the functional status of neurologic structures or the occurrence of nerve root irritation.

Comparatively, imaging studies provide direct and, in some applications, real-time (but gross) information regarding pedicle walls and the placement of pedicle screws within the pedicles. Neurophysiologic procedures provide more-detailed information regarding pedicle wall structure, as well as functional information regarding nerve roots.

The purpose of this chapter is to (1) provide a very brief review of intraoperative imaging techniques in the operating room, (2) present an overview of electrophysiologic procedures that have been used during surgeries for spinal degeneration, and (3) provide information regarding traditional and new applications of EMG procedures during surgeries that use transpedicular screw placement.

## Limitations of Intraoperative Imaging Techniques

As has been reported in numerous studies, the use of pedicle screws can result in pedicle wall breakthrough. The consequences of breakthrough include an unstable construct and the potential for nerve root or spinal cord damage. The incidence of breakthrough is directly related to the instrumentation used, surgeon experience, and variations in pedicle anatomy.[13] Incidence figures for pedicle wall breakthrough, with or without neural irritation or damage, ranges from 1.2% to 28.8%.[10,11,25]

The potential consequence of pedicle wall breakthrough to neural and other structures depends upon the location of the breakthrough. According to Halliday et al.[11] the following complications can occur as a function of site of breakthrough:

1. Rostral breach leads to penetration of the intervertebral disc and poor screw fixation.
2. A caudal breach risks injury to dura mater and nerve roots.
3. A medial breach leads to encroachment into the spinal canal and potential injury to the spinal cord and nerve roots.
4. A lateral screw breach can result in injury to segmental vessels and possible retroperitoneal penetration, along with poor screw purchase.

According to the authors, the use of intraoperative imaging (i.e., fluoroscopy) to confirm the location of the pedicle screw is commonly used. However, even with intraoperative imaging studies, the incidence of pedicle wall breakthrough remains high.

In addition to an unstable construct, pedicle wall breakthrough by pedicle screws poses a risk to adjacent neural and anatomical structures. The most common type of insult is nerve root injury due to the screw entering into the nerve root foramen. According to Esses et al.,[9] the incidence of neurologic injury during the placement of pedicular screws occurs in approximately 2.5% to 7.5% of surgeries. Damage to nonneural structures can occur, but is uncommon (i.e., dural tears occur in less than 2.5% of patients).[4]

The purpose of any intraoperative pedicle screws fixation study, whether imaging or electrophysiologic, is to ensure proper placement of the pedicle screws. If the pedicle screws are properly placed, injury to neural and other anatomic structures is avoided, and a more stable construct is achieved. However, because imaging studies are not typically performed during the use of placement hardware (i.e., pedicle finder or tap) or the actual placement of a pedicle screw, the surgeon has no information regarding the location of the hardware or screw relative to

**TABLE 136.1**

**Parameters Used to Administer Electrically Elicited Electromyograms or Spontaneous Electromyograms**

| Parameter | Elicitation method | |
|---|---|---|
| | E-EMG | S-EMG |
| Filter settings | 5-5000Hz | 5-5000Hz |
| Time base | 507ms | 1-2 sec |
| Sensitivity | 10% rejection | 10% rejection |
| Stimulus presentation rate | 2.1-3.1/sec | Not applicable |
| Stimulus intensity | 7mA or 20V | Not applicable |

*E-EMG,* Electrically elicited electromyogram; *S-EMG,* spontaneous electromyogram.

the pedicle wall or neural structures. While fluoroscopy is used to determine hardware and screw location at various times during placement, images are not usually obtained while the hardware or screw is actually being placed. For example, during the placement of a pedicle screw, the surgeon needs to advance the screw, stop and record an image, and then continue with screw placement. Because imaging data are not collected continuously, the surgeon has no feedback during times at which the nerve roots and pedicle walls are at greatest risk. An alternative approach is to use an electrophysiologic procedure during the placement of the pedicle hardware or screw.

## Overview of Electrophysiologic Procedures

Historically, two electrophysiologic procedures have been used to provide the surgeon with information regarding the pedicle wall and/or nerve roots: dermatomal somatosensory evoked potential (DSEP) and EMG.

Prior to discussing DSEPs and EMGs, it is necessary to present criteria against which the efficacy of any electrophysiologic procedure can be compared. For an electrophysiologic procedure to be effective and helpful to the surgeon, it must demonstrate the following characteristics:

1. The duration of time needed to administer the procedure must not significantly increase surgical time.
2. The procedure should be administered continuously during those periods of surgical intervention that place a structure at risk.
3. Test results should provide instantaneous and accurate information regarding the status of the structure or structures at risk.
4. The procedure must be reliable and cost-effective.

### Dermatomal Somatosensory Evoked Potentials

DSEPs were first reported for diagnostic use by Aminoff et al.[1] This initial application was further developed for operating-room use and reported by Cohen and Huizenga,[6] Herron et al,[12] and Owen et al.[20] The DSEP is elicited by electrically stimulating a peripheral dermatomal field and recording the response at sites caudal

and rostral to the level of surgery. The purposes for administering DSEP procedures are to determine level or levels of nerve root involvement and the adequacy of nerve root decompression.[20]

With regard to the criteria listed above, DSEPs can be performed nearly continuously, testing does not increase the duration of surgery, and the procedure is not expensive to administer. However, test results are not instantaneous, are less than 100% accurate to the level (or levels) or degree of nerve root involvement, and unfortunately, are unreliable.[18,21]

The limitations of DSEPs were compounded by the development of transpedicular fixation techniques and the change of the surgeon's focus away from level and degree of nerve root compression to functional and structural status of nerve roots and pedicle walls. To provide the surgeon with this type of information, monitoring techniques that record an EMG response were developed.

## Electromyographic Monitoring

Based upon their intended purpose and their method of elicitation, EMG procedures are divided into two categories: E-EMGs and S-EMGs.

### Electrically Elicited Electromyograms

The first EMG procedure intended for use with pedicular instrumentation was reported by Calancie et al.[2] In that study, EMG procedures were administered to animals in an effort to determine whether E-EMGs could determine the structural integrity of pedicle walls. The study was not intended to investigate EMG sensitivity to nerve root irritation. Procedurally, a low-intensity cathodic stimulus was applied to the walls of the pedicle and to the head of a pedicle screw. The anode electrode was placed in the surgical field. The premise of this test was that an intact pedicle wall demonstrated an adequate amount of resistance that prevented a flow of current between the cathode- and anode-stimulating electrodes. If the pedicle wall were fractured, resistance would be decreased and allow the low-intensity current to flow from the cathode to the anode electrode. This flow of current would result in stimulation of the adjacent nerve root, which would elicit an EMG response in the myotome innervated by the nerve root (Figure 136.1).

**Interpretation and Intervention.** E-EMG interpretation is based upon the threshold of the response. In their original study, Calancie et al.[3] used a stimulating procedure that consisted of presenting the stimulus at a starting intensity level (SIL) of 20V or 7mA. (Note: 4V = ~1mA.) If no response was elicited at 20V, it was assumed that the pedicle wall was intact. If a response was elicited at 20V, the stimulus intensity was decreased until the threshold of the response was determined.

Determination of EMG threshold is important because the efficacy of intervention is based on changes in this level. In a study by Darden et al.,[8] the efficacy of intervention was investigated. In that study, intervention consisted of either reorienting the pedicle hole or removing and reinserting the pedicle screw. EMG thresholds were reestablished following these maneuvers. If the EMG threshold was increased to at least the original SIL, none of the patients were found to demonstrate a surgically induced neurologic deficit. However, if no intervention was initiated, the incidence of surgically induced neurologic deficits was increased.

As with most clinical procedures, modification of the original methodology has occurred with increased use of the test. In regard to the E-EMG response, a modification

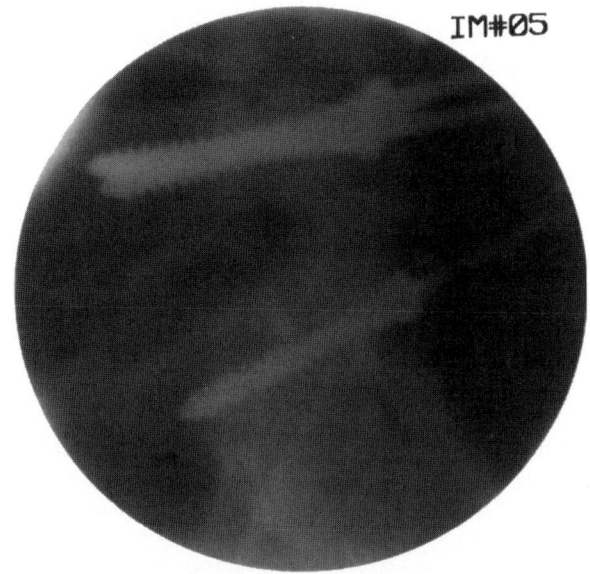

**Figure 136.1** Fluoroscopic image of pedicle screws and monopolar stimulator used to elicit the E-EMG during surgery.

of the original E-EMG procedure involves the use of cathodic stimulation of the pedicle finder, tap, or screwdriver. By stimulating these tools during their use, it is possible to obtain real-time information regarding pedicle wall status when the pedicles are at their greatest risk for breakthrough.

**Case Study 1.** A male who was 38 years of age underwent surgery for correction of spinal stenosis from L4 to S1. Preoperatively, the patient complained of pain in the lower extremities in an L5-S1 distribution. Surgery consisted of decompressing the nerve roots from L4 through S1, bilaterally, and placing pedicle instrumentation at L4, L5, and S1.

During surgery, E-EMG monitoring techniques were used. The specific methodology consisted of stimulating the pedicle holes and pedicle screws after their placement. Based on electrophysiologic measurements, an SIL of 20V was used.

Figure 136.2 depicts a composite of results recorded after placement and stimulation of the six pedicle screws. Six traces of data that represent the six myotome recording sites are shown. These traces/recording sites are as follows:

1. Trace 1: left quadriceps femoris muscle group (L4)
2. Trace 2: right quadriceps femoris muscle group (L4)
3. Trace 3: left tibialis anterior muscle (L5)
4. Trace 4: right tibialis anterior muscle (L5)
5. Trace 5: left medial gastrocnemius muscle (S1)
6. Trace 6: right medial gastrocnemius muscle (S1)

As indicated in Figure 136.2, no EMG activity was elicited when stimulating the left or right pedicle screws placed at L4 or L5, bilaterally. A large and well-formed

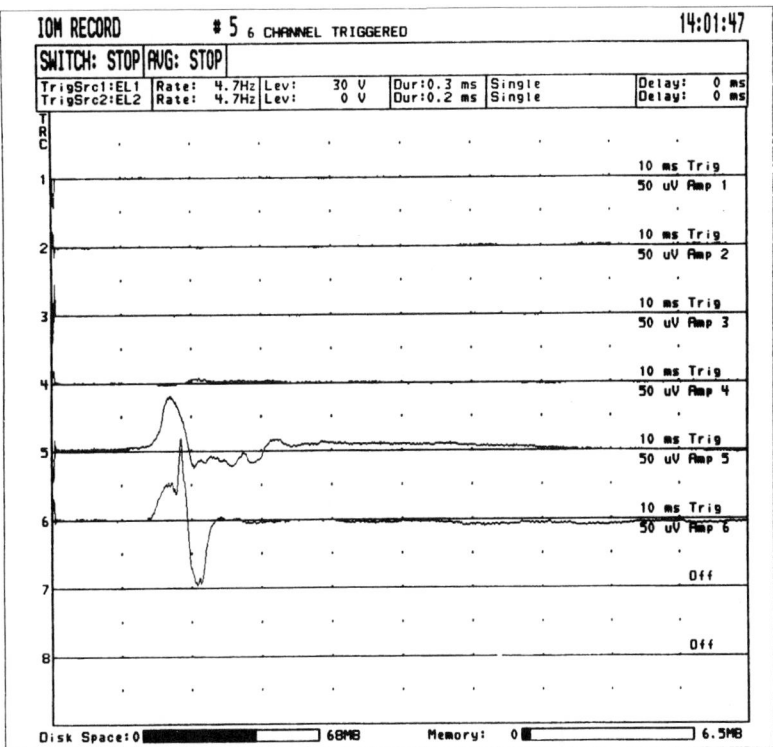

**Figure 136.2** Composite of E-EMG data recorded from Case Study 1. Note EMG activity present in traces 5 and 6.

response was elicited at a threshold of less than 20V for the left (trace 5) and right (trace 6) S1 pedicle screws. This information was relayed to the surgeon, who visually inspected the pedicle walls. In both instances, pedicle wall breakthrough had occurred. The pedicle screws that tested positive were removed, reoriented, and reinserted. After reinsertion, another test was administered, and EMG threshold was reestablished at an intensity level equal to at least the SIL. This patient did not demonstrate any new neurologic deficits after surgery.

**Accuracy.** Calancie et al.[3] investigated the ability of E-EMG to accurately determine if pedicle wall breakthrough had occurred. In this study, 102 pedicle walls and screws were stimulated using routine methods. In addition to the electrophysiologic testing, the pedicle walls were palpated and visually inspected for integrity. Based on the results from the EMGs and palpatory examination, 68% of the pedicle screws had been placed in a satisfactory manner (true-negative). In 19% of the screws, a positive EMG response and pedicle wall breakthrough were present. These were missed by initial visual inspection or palpation (true-positive). In the remaining 13% of the screws, electrophysiologic evidence indicated a breakthrough, but there was no evidence of this using visual inspection or palpation (false-positive). No patients demonstrated any postoperative morbidity associated with malpositioned screws.

**Limitations.** When Calancie et al.[2] first reported the E-EMG procedure, their purpose was to develop a method for providing the surgeon with information regarding pedicle and nerve root status. However, it is possible to obtain a positive E-EMG finding, consistent with pedicle wall breakthrough, without any concomitant change in nerve root status. This relationship between pedicle walls versus nerve root status reveals a major limitation of E-EMG. If information regarding pedicle wall status is needed during surgery, E-EMG is the electrophysiologic method of choice. However, if information regarding nerve root status is desired, alternative methods need to be considered. This limitation of E-EMG to nerve root status lead to the development of a procedure that records an S-EMG.[19]

The results from Calancie et al.[3] indicate that if pedicle wall breakthrough occurs, the E-EMG will detect its presence. However, this method also demonstrated a 13% false-positive rate. E-EMG testing demonstrated pedicle wall breakthrough, even though other methods of evaluation were negative. Patients, however, did not demonstrate a surgically induced neurologic deficit. This later finding makes an important point regarding E-EMG testing. This test only determines if pedicle wall breakthrough has occurred; it is not a direct test of nerve root function. In addition, the test only assesses pedicle wall status after the pedicle hole has been made or the pedicle screw has been placed. Consequently, it is possible to damage a nerve root during the use of transpedicular instrumentation and only detect this damage after the injury has occurred. Although these limitations exist, the E-EMG test is very sensitive to pedicle wall integrity and should be administered during the static phases of surgeries that use transpedicular

instrumentation. These phases include testing the pedicle hole after it has been made and the pedicle screw after it has been placed.

### Spontaneously Elicited Electromyograms

**Background and Elicitation.** In 1994, Owen et al.[19] reported the development of a procedure that recorded EMGs that had been elicited by mechanical irritation of a nerve root by transpedicular instrumentation. This technique was developed because of the limitations associated with the E-EMG method. As indicated earlier, the E-EMG method is administered during the static phases of surgery. However, during the dynamic stages of surgery (i.e., during the sounding of the pedicle hole or the actual placement of the pedicle screw), the nerve roots are not monitored. Consequently, a nerve root could be damaged during these surgical maneuvers, but the damage could remain undetected until the pedicle hole or screw is electrically stimulated. It also appears prudent to provide a direct measure of nerve root function rather than infer nerve root status based upon measures of pedicle wall integrity. The presence of pedicle wall breakthrough does not necessarily indicate that the nerve root has been or will be irritated. Consequently, results from the E-EMG procedure could indicate that pedicle wall breakthrough had occurred, without the development of a new postoperative radiculopathy (false-positive). To avoid these limitations, the S-EMG was developed for recording spontaneous EMG activity that had been elicited by actual mechanical stimulation of a nerve root.

To elicit the S-EMG, the nerve root must be irritated by a mechanical or thermal stimulus. The sources of mechanical irritation include, but are not limited to, the pedicle sound, pedicle tap, and pedicle screw. Thermal irritation usually occurs following the use of irrigating fluids that are too cold. Unlike the E-EMG, the S-EMG is a direct measure of nerve root irritation. Consequently, the S-EMG is recorded during the dynamic stages of surgery and will only be elicited by actual irritation of the nerve root.

To administer the S-EMG method, the monitoring instrumentation is set up to monitor muscle function continuously (e.g., free run). If a nerve root is irritated, the involved peripheral nerve will depolarize and "fire," which produces a contraction in the innervated muscle. This contraction is recorded as an EMG. The electrical activity associated with the contraction is observed on a monitor as an EMG wave and also heard on a loudspeaker as a "popping" sound. By turning up the intensity of this sound, the surgeon can hear the popping sound associated with nerve root irritation and immediately stop the maneuver producing the irritation. Therefore, any instantaneous changes to nerve root function can be immediately detected and avoided or reversed.

**Interpretation and Intervention.** Interpretation of the S-EMG consists of determining the visual and/or auditory presence of muscle contraction through the use of the elicited EMG. If a nerve root has been irritated, the nerve fiber should fire and produce a contraction of the innervated muscle. Interpretation of the response is basically "all or none." This means that no activity is consistent with no nerve root irritation, whereas the presence of activity indicates that nerve root irritation is occurring. To intervene, the surgeon must immediately stop all surgical maneuvers being performed and visually identify the source of irritation.

To determine the sensitivity and specificity of the S-EMG to nerve root irritation, Owen *et al.*[19] recorded data from 89 patients who underwent surgery for spinal degeneration and in which transpedicular instrumentation was used. During these surgeries a total of 476 nerve roots were monitored. Results indicated that 85 nerve roots (17.8%) demonstrated some type of firing during surgery. In 98.5% of the firings, the EMG activity correlated exactly with the segmental level at which the surgeon was working. In the remaining cases, EMG activity did not correlate with this level. However, it was determined that in these cases the activity was due to the temperature of the irrigating fluids (i.e., cold), which identifies one of the weaknesses of S-EMG procedures. More specifically, any type of nerve root irritation (i.e., mechanical or thermal) can elicit an S-EMG. Therefore, it is necessary to rule out the effects from these more perisurgical sources when considering the initiation of intervention.

**Case Study 2.** A male who was 64 years of age underwent surgery for correction of spinal stenosis. The patient complained of low back pain with radicular symptoms demonstrating an L4-5 pattern. Surgery consisted of decompression of the nerve roots and the use of transpedicular instrumentation.

Electrophysiologic monitoring consisted of recording S-EMGs during the dynamic stages of surgery and mixed nerve somatosensory evoked potentials (SSEPs) during the remaining periods of the surgery. SSEPs were elicited by stimulating the ulnar nerve and posterior tibial nerve and recording the responses cervically and cortically. Although SSEPs do not provide useful information regarding individual nerve root function, these data were recorded in order to protect the brachial plexus and spinal cord during surgery. The ulnar nerve SSEP was used to monitor brachial plexus function in order to ensure that the patient did not develop a plexopathy due to positioning on the operating table. Posterior tibial nerve SSEPs were recorded in order to monitor spinal cord function during surgery. Although the spinal cord was not at direct surgical risk, this proved to be an additional precaution that may be useful to the patient and surgeon and that does not increase monitoring costs.

Figures 136.3 and 136.4, six channels of EMG activity and two channels of SSEP data, depict the results obtained from this patient. In both figures, traces (channels) 1 through 6 represent EMG data recorded from the following muscle groups:

1. Traces 1 and 2: left and right quadriceps femoris muscle groups (L4)
2. Traces 3 and 4: left and right tibialis anterior muscle groups (L5)
3. Traces 5 and 6: left and right medial gastrocnemius muscle groups (S1)

Traces 7 and 8 show ulnar nerve data (see Figure 136.3) and posterior tibial nerve data (see Figure 136.4). In both figures, the same recording sites were used. Trace 7 was recorded from C5, and trace 8 was recorded from over the somatosensory cortex. All SSEP data remained within normal limits throughout surgery and are not described further.

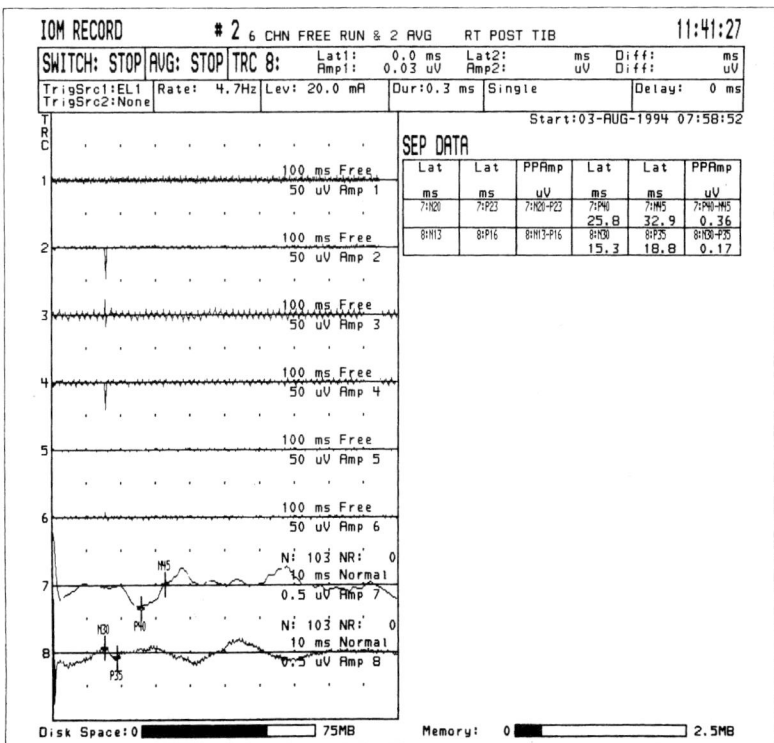

**Figure 136.3** Artifactual data (traces 2 and 4) recorded during surgery in Case Study 2.

Figure 136.3 depicts the presence of what appears to be a single downward-oriented spike of S-EMG activity on traces 2 and 4. However, closer inspection of this activity indicates that this was an artifact and not an actual EMG response from mechanical irritation. A true EMG response must demonstrate a polyphasic morphology and not consist of a single polarity spike.

Figure 136.4 demonstrates a prolonged and polyphasic discharge of EMG activity on trace 2 (right quadriceps femoris muscle group). This activity was due to mechanical irritation of the nerve root by the pedicle tap. The surgeon heard the popping sound produced by the muscle contractions and immediately stopped the use of the pedicle tap. The surgeon was also informed of the activity by the monitorist. The tap was removed and the pedicle inspected and palpated. It was found that pedicle wall breakthrough had occurred and that the nerve root was being irritated. The pedicle hole was reoriented, and no further activity was elicited. The patient did not demonstrate new surgically induced neurologic deficits after surgery.

### Limitations of Electromyographic Monitoring

As with all medical procedures, EMG testing for nerve root function demonstrates several limitations. First, chronic nerve root compression can increase the threshold of EMG activity to electrical stimulation. This accounts for the findings of Lenke *et al.*[15] and the need to stimulate the pedicle at intensities adequate to find EMG threshold. Second, cold irrigating fluids can result in the firing of a nerve root. This necessitates the use of warm irrigating fluids in order to avoid false-positive results. Finally, the efficacy of any monitoring program is influenced by the training and experience of the examiner and, if appropriate, the supervisor.[17] If these individuals are not adequately trained, the incidence of false-negative results increases.

### Advanced Applications of Electromyographic Testing

E-EMG and S-EMG procedures were originally developed for monitoring the thoracolumbar spine. Since that time, the development and use of pedicular instrumentation in the thoracic spine has occurred. This new application has put the thoracic nerve roots at risk, which has resulted in the development of EMG procedures for this surgical application.

A review of the literature pertaining to the placement of thoracic pedicle screws reveals a breach of the pedicle in 20% to 41% of the screws placed.[5,24,28] Cinotti *et al.*[5] have even suggested that the pedicles from T4 to T8 are not wide enough for the safe insertion of pedicle screws. The difficulties associated with thoracic screw placement are due to smaller pedicles compared with those of the lumbar spine and the greater degree of variability of anteromedial and cephalad angulation.[25,26] According to Vaccaro *et al.*,[25] the distance between the ventral vertebral cortex and the structures of the dorsal mediastinum are within 5mm, which makes the margin for error very small.

To record EMGs during surgeries that use thoracic pedicle screws, several procedural questions need to be

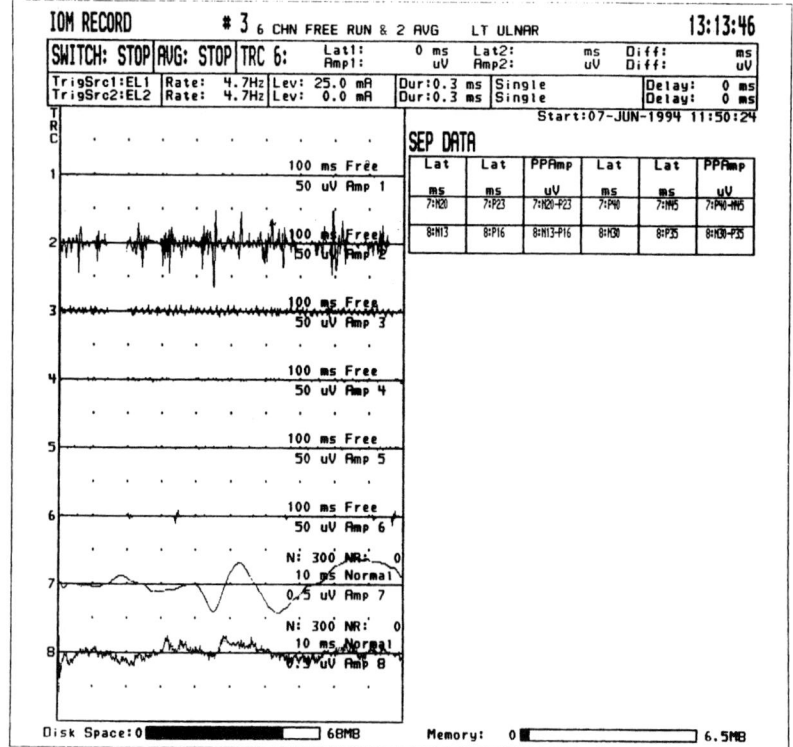

**Figure 136.4** S-EMG data recorded from right quadriceps femoris muscle groups during nerve root irritation (Case Study 2).

addressed. Because of the similarities between these levels of surgery (i.e., thoracic vs. lumbosacral), the parameters used to record the data will be identical. Additionally, the specific procedures (i.e., E-EMG and S-EMG) and the sites used to elicit the E-EMG (e.g., stimulation of the pedicle holes, screws, etc) are very similar. However, questions that need to be addressed include: Where will the EMG data be recorded? What type of stimulus should be used to elicit the data? What criteria will be used to interpret the E-EMGs?

Several studies that have been reported in the literature have addressed the questions regarding the stimulus parameters used to elicit the EMG, recording sites for this response, and the criteria to interpret the data. Danesh-Clough et al.[7] investigated E-EMGs in six sheep. In that study, EMGs were elicited by electrically stimulating the internal walls of the pedicle and the pedicle screws from T8 to L2. EMGs were recorded from the transversus abdominus muscles at three levels: the lower two intercostal spaces and the psoas. Using a constant voltage stimulus, the authors found that EMG thresholds less than 10V demonstrated a 94% sensitivity and a specificity of 90% to pedicle wall breakthrough.

In a study by Lewis et al.[16] E-EMGs were recorded from intercostal muscles from T6 to T15 in five pigs. In this study, pedicle wall status was divided into one of three categories: intact pedicle walls (group A), removal of medial pedicle wall (group B), and screws placed in contact with neural elements (group C). Results from this study indicated that there was no significant difference in mean EMG threshold as a function of animal group. What this means is that no "cut-off" threshold could be determined below which intensity levels were consistent with breakthrough.

In a recent study by Shi et al.,[24] E-EMG data were collected from 22 patients undergoing spinal surgery that included thoracic instrumentation. In this study, EMGs were recorded from intercostals or abdominal muscle groups, depending on the level or levels of screw placement. Results from 87 screws indicated that stimulation thresholds above 11mA had a 97.5% predictive value, meaning that the screws were within the pedicles.

Finally, in a study by Raynor et al.,[22] EMGs were recorded from rectus abdominus muscles in 92 patients in whom screws were placed from T6 to T12. Thresholds were divided into three categories based upon the integrity of the pedicle walls: (1) greater than 6mA and intact placement, (2) less than 6mA with intact medial pedicle wall, and (3) less than 6mA with medial wall perforation. Status of the medial wall was determined by tactile and/or visual inspection. In addition to using a fixed cut-off point of 6mA as suggesting medial pedicle wall breakthrough, the authors also compared thresholds that were less than 6mA with thresholds that were greater than 6mA. If thresholds were less than 6mA, medial wall defects were more likely to occur when the difference of the threshold at a suspected segmental level was at least 65% from all other screws in that patient. This later measure takes into consideration the "outliers" and allows the examiner to use the patient's own bone characteristics as a variable in determining whether pedicle wall breakthrough had occurred.

Overall, these results indicate that E-EMGs can be recorded in humans undergoing thoracic surgery that involve pedicle screw placement. Data can be recorded from intercostals and rectus abdominus muscles. Although no definitive information is available from this literature regarding whether a constant voltage versus a constant current stimulus should be used, it appears that a threshold greater than 6mA or 10V is consistent with an intact medial pedicle wall. To compensate for the effects from pathology on the impedance characteristics of the pedicle wall, the examiner should compare absolute thresholds with the mean overall threshold of responses obtained at greater than 6mA. If the difference is greater than 65% between these two values, a medial wall breakthrough should be suspected. This latter method of measurement is applicable regardless of whether a constant voltage or current stimulus is used and should be considered when interpreting data.

In a somewhat different application, it is possible to use E-EMGs to help determine the location of an offending screw that is irritating an individual nerve root. In a study by Rowan et al.,[23] a patient undergoing correction of idiopathic scoliosis was administered mixed nerve SSEPs and motor evoked potentials (MEPs). EMGs were not recorded during the initial surgery. Correction consisted of a posterior spinal fusion with instrumentation being placed from T2 to L3. During surgery, SSEPs and MEPs remained unchanged, but the patient demonstrated no motor function in the left quadriceps immediately postoperatively. The patient was returned to the operating room, and the conus medullaris was electrically stimulated at T12-L1 using percutaneous needle electrodes. E-EMGs were recorded from the following muscle groups: quadriceps, anterior tibialis, medial gastrocnemius, and hamstring. The purpose for this testing was to determine what was offending the nerve root or roots and at which level or levels. A variety of stimulation sites were used, rostral and caudal to the conus medullaris, in order to determine the location or locations of nerve root involvement. Based upon clinical information, it appeared that the pedicle hooks at L2 or L3 or both could have been producing degraded nerve root function and the observed postoperative motor deficit. Prior to any hook removal, no reliable EMG response was obtained from the left quadriceps, but reliable data were recorded from the other muscle groups. Following the removal of hooks at L2 and L3, on the left side a reliable response was recorded from the quadriceps. By using the E-EMGs, it was possible to determine which hook was irritating the nerve root(s) and how much correction could be placed on instrumentation without any deleterious effects on nerve root function. Following surgery, the patient demonstrated a return of function of the left quadriceps, and adequate correction of the spine was still achieved. Although this application is atypical, it does demonstrate that E-EMGs can provide useful information regarding the presence and location of nerve root irritation. Additionally, this information can be rapidly obtained, usually in less than 1 minute, which allows the surgeon to determine the efficacy of intervention without prolonging surgical time.

### Costs Versus Benefits of Electromyographic Monitoring

A question often raised about the use of intraoperative monitoring, regardless of the modality being administered or the type of surgery monitored, is its cost-benefit ratio. Whereas studies have reported the benefits of other types of monitoring, no information relative to the use of transpedicular instrumentation has been available. To answer this question, the author recently investigated the postoperative neurologic status of patients who underwent surgery using transpedicular instrumentation. Based on whether EMG monitoring was performed, the patients were divided into two groups: Group I (*n* = 185) without monitoring and Group II (*n* = 205) with E-EMG and S-EMG monitoring. The same surgeons, who were well experienced with the use of transpedicular instrumentation, performed the surgeries. There were no significant differences between the two groups of subjects relative to age, duration of symptoms, or gender. The incidence of surgically induced radiculopathies for Group I was 9.6%, whereas the incidence of the same type of pathology for Group II was less than 1%. These results indicate that EMG monitoring was effective in significantly reducing the incidence of surgically induced neurologic deficits.

The costs associated with a surgically induced deficit are difficult to estimate, but they include the need for additional surgery, radiologic studies, prolonged hospitalization, and the need for inpatient and outpatient physical therapy. In addition, lost income to the patient must be considered, as well as the costs associated with medicolegal matters. The cost of administering intraoperative EMG monitoring varies among hospitals. Typical hospital costs for monitoring a 6-hour surgery range from $500 to $600. Obviously, the costs and benefits associated with a monitoring program outweigh the costs resulting from a surgically induced neurologic deficit if the incidence of these deficits approaches the 9.6% rate observed by the author.

### Summary

Intraoperative applications of EMG procedures have been shown to be an effective method to monitor individual nerve root function during surgeries that place these structures at risk. Compared with traditional neurophysiologic techniques (i.e., DSEPs), E-EMGs and S-EMGs are more reliable, specific, and sensitive to the onset of a surgically induced neurologic deficit. When used appropriately, the use of EMG procedures should decrease the incidence of surgically induced deficits, with a concomitant decrease in the postsurgical costs resulting from these problems.

### REFERENCES

1. Aminoff JM, Goodin DS, Barbaro NM, *et al:* Dermatomal somatosensory evoked potentials in unilateral lumbosacral radiculopathy, *Ann Neurol* 17:171-176, 1985.
2. Calancie B, Lebwohol N, Madsen P, Klose KJ: Intraoperative evoked EMG monitoring in an animal model: a new technique for evaluating pedicle screw placement, *Spine* 17:1229-1235, 1992.
3. Calancie B, Madsen P, Lebwohl N: Stimulus-evoked EMG monitoring during transpedicular lumbosacral spine instrumentation: initial clinical results, *Spine* 19:278-286, 1994.
4. Chozik BS, Toselli R: Complications of spinal instrumentation. In Benzel E (ed): *Spinal Instrumentation.* Park Ridge, IL, American Association of Neurological Surgeons, 1994, pp 257-274.
5. Cinotti G, Gumina S, Riponi M, Postacchin F: Pedicle instrumentation in the thoracic spine: a morphometric and cadaveric study for placement of screws, *Spine* 24:114-119, 1999.
6. Cohen BA, Huizenga BA: Dermatomal monitoring for surgical correction of spondylolisthesis: a case report, *Spine* 13:1125-1128, 1988.
7. Dansch-Clough T, Taylor P, Hodgson B, Walton M: The use of evoked EMGs in detecting misplaced thoracolumbar pedicle screws, *Spine* 26:1313-1316, 2001.
8. Darden BV, Wood KE, Hatley M, *et al:* Evaluation of pedicle screw location monitored by intraoperative evoked electromyography, *J Spinal Disord* 9:8-16, 1996.
9. Esses S, Sachs B, Dreyzin V: Complications associated with the technique of pedicle screw fixation, *Spine* 18:2231-2239, 1993.
10. Gertzbein SD, Robbins SE: Accuracy of pedicle screw placement in vivo, *Spine* 15:11-14, 1990.
11. Halliday AL, Zileli M, Stillerman CB, Benzel EC: Doral thoracic and lumbar screw fixation and pedicle fixation techniques. In Benzel EC (ed): *Spine Surgery: Techniques, Complication Avoidance, and Management,* vol 2. New York, Churchill-Livingstone, 1999, pp 1053-1064.
12. Herron LD, Tripp AC, Gonyea M: Intraoperative use of dermatomal somatosensory evoked potentials in lumbar stenosis surgery, *Spine* 12:379-383, 1987.
13. Jacob RP, Mack C, Fessler RG: Pedicle screws: biomechanics, uses, and current assessment of outcomes, *Neurosurg Q* 4:39-50, 1994.
14. Kolfas IH, McCormack BM: Intraoperative imaging. In Benzel EC, editor: *Spine Surgery: Techniques, Complication Avoidance, and Management,* vol 2. New York, Churchill-Livingstone, 1999, pp 1221-1231.
15. Lenke LG, Padberg AM, Russo M, Bridwell KH: *Triggered EMG stimulation threshold for accuracy of pedicle screw placement: an animal model and clinical correlation.* Paper presented at the annual meeting of the Scoliosis Research Society, Portland, OR, 1994.
16. Lewis SJ, Lenke LG, Raynor B, *et al:* Triggered electromyographic threshold for accuracy of thoracic pedicle screw placement in a porcine model, *Spine* 26:2485-2490, 2001.
17. Nuwer MR, Dawson EG, Carlson LG, *et al:* Somatosensory evoked potential spinal cord monitoring reduces neurologic deficits after scoliosis surgery: results of a large multicenter survey, *Electromyogr Clin Neurophysiol* 96:6-11, 1995.
18. Owen JH, Bridwell KH, Lenke LG: Innervation pattern of dorsal roots and their effects on the specificity of dermatomal somatosensory evoked potentials, *Spine* 18:748-754, 1993.
19. Owen JH, Kostuik JP, Gornet M: The use of mechanically-elicited electromyograms to protect nerve roots during surgery for spinal degeneration, *Spine* 19:1704-1710, 1994.

20. Owen JH, Padberg AM, Holland L, *et al:* Clinical correlation between degenerative spine disease and dermatomal somatosensory evoked potentials in humans, *Spine* 16:S201-205, 1991.
21. Phillips LH II, Park TS: Electrophysiologic mapping of the segmental anatomy of the muscles of the lower extremity, *Muscle Nerve* 14:1213-1218, 1991.
22. Raynor BL, Lenke LG, Kim Y, *et al:* Can triggered electromyograph thresholds predict safe thoracic pedicle screw placement? *Spine* 27:2030-2035, 2002.
23. Rowan BA, Thomson JD, Owen JH, Hyams ES: Postoperative motor deficit despite intraoperative somatosensory and motor evoked potential monitoring: a case study, Submitted for publication.
24. Shi YB, Binette M, Martin WH, *et al:* Electrical stimulation for intraoperative evaluation of thoracic pedicle screw placement, *Spine* 28:595-601, 2003.
25. Vaccaro AR, Rizzolo SJ, Allardyc TJ, *et al:* Placement of pedicle screws in the thoracic spine: part I: morphometric analysis of the thoracic vertebra, *J Bone Joint Surg Am* 72:1193-1199, 1995.
26. Weinstein J, Rydevik B, Rauschning W: Anatomic and technical considerations of pedicle screw fixation, *Clin Orthop* 284:34-46, 1992.
27. West JL III, Oglivie JW, Bradford DS: Complications of the variable screw plate pedicle screw fixation, *Spine* 16:576-579, 1991.
28. Xu R, Ebraheim NA, Ou Y, Yeosting RA: Anatomic considerations of pedicle screw placement in the thoracic spine: Roy-Camille technique versus open lamina, *Spine* 23:1065-1068, 1998.

# CHAPTER 137

# Spine Surgery Monitoring

## William Mitchell, Abm Salah Uddin, and Edward C. Benzel

Spinal surgery is continuously evolving and becoming increasingly complex. Surgeons are routinely tackling more difficult pathology. Technical and material advancements have made this possible. Adjunctive measures such as a myriad of monitoring techniques have been present and available for some time but have varied in their usage and proven effectiveness. To understand the role of intraoperative monitoring and the technique used, the available information is presented.

## Wake-up Test

A number of methods have been developed for the intraoperative monitoring of spinal cord function. In 1973, Vauzelle et al.[49] described the intraoperative wake-up test, which is still considered the "gold standard" by some centers. This enables the surgeon to perform a brief, neurologic examination to directly evaluate the functional integrity of the neuronal structures, as opposed to an indirect evaluation by neurophysiologic monitoring. The patient is awoken from general anesthesia to undergo a neurologic examination. Therefore, the surgeon can assess significant neurologic deficits that may have occurred as a result of surgical manipulation or instrumentation. If there is a neurologic deficit, the deformity correction and/or instrumentation can be revised.

The requirements of the intraoperative wake-up test are simple. The patient must first be screened preoperatively to assess degree of tolerance. The ability to participate may be limited by the patient's premorbid personality. This assessment is not only difficult, but often an unreliable predictor of the patient's tolerance for intraoperative awakening. Nevertheless, a full explanation must ensue, describing the procedure and expected conditions upon awakening (i.e., intubation, confusion, levels of discomfort). Language barriers may be overcome by prerecording commands for examination.[31]

The technique of anesthesia is critical for patient wakefulness and degree of discomfort. Introduction of local anesthetic to the pharynx and larynx, either by transcutaneous injection or spray, is paramount for patient comfort upon awakening. An initial loading dose of a narcotic with continuous infusion is the preferred anesthetic regime, because concomitant electrophysiologic monitoring may be affected by halogenated anesthesia. However, halogenated anesthetics may be used sparingly and should be reserved for younger patients with iatrogenic hypertension. Narcotics and halogenated anesthesia, preferably fentanyl and isoflurane, are discontinued 30 minutes prior to awakening. Approximately 10 minutes prior to awakening, paralytic agents are reversed and nitrous oxide is discontinued. Strict adherence to this regimen should provide a wakeful patient who is able to follow commands in approximately 5 minutes.

Once awakened, the patient is asked to appropriately move the arms and legs. Discovered deficits require reevaluation of the patient's position, the instrumentation, or consideration of vascular compromise. Therefore, both the surgeon and anesthesia team must be prepared for re-awakening following their initial assessment.

Although current means of electrophysiologic monitoring may obviate the need for the intraoperative wake-up test, technical difficulties or potentially misleading results of the neurophysiologic monitoring may warrant a wake-up test. Therefore, although crude, the wake-up test should remain a tool in the surgeon's armamentarium. However, there are two fundamental disadvantages associated with this test: (1) It provides only momentary information about the integrity of the nervous system, and (2) the information pertains to voluntary movements only.

## Current Techniques

The use of the intraoperative wake-up test is limited by patient tolerance, additional operative time, and a limited assessment of the neurologic status during the test only. Modern neurophysiologic monitoring provides the benefit of patient comfort with the indirect continuous assessment of neurologic status during surgery.

Currently available techniques for intraoperative spinal cord monitoring include somatosensory spinal evoked potentials (SSEPs), spinal recording of spinal evoked potentials (SPSEPs), dermatomal somatosensory evoked potentials (DSEPs), motor evoked potentials (MEPs), and electromyogram (EMG). Continuous neurophysiologic monitoring is an important tool that may reduce intraoperative morbidity. The principles, advantages, and disadvantages are discussed.

### Somatosensory Spinal Evoked Potentials (SSEPs)

Somatosensory Spinal Evoked Patient (SSEP) Monitoring was first introduced in 1972. The principle of SSEP monitoring is related to the continuous real-time recording of conduit function.[10,47] The spinal cord is the conduit through which stimulation of a peripheral nerve provides an afferent signal. It is conducted through the spinal cord and recorded either at the level of the spinal cord or cerebral cortex. The majority of signals is conducted via the dorsal columns and only a fraction through the ventral tracts.[11,15] Therefore, SSEP monitoring reflects dorsal column function. Moreover, in part, because of this selectivity, false-negative and false-positive recordings have been reported. Although reported rates vary, a large series of 50,000 patients demonstrated a 0.067% false-negative rate.[12] On average, the false-negative rate is reported to be less than 2%, and the false-positive rate is less than 3%[13,16,17,19,25] (Figures 137.1 to 137.3).

While relying on neurophysiologic monitoring, one must be aware of its technical limitations and reliability to avoid misinterpretation. It is, therefore, a common practice to secure both peripheral and central recording sites for the afferent volley. This aids in the differentiation of technical failure from neurologic injury. A technical failure affects changes in the latencies or amplitude in both the peripheral and central recorded responses. Alternatively, neurologic injury affects only central responses. Moreover, one must realize that following significant surgical manipulation that may affect the spinal cord, changes in SSEP signals may be delayed for up to 30 minutes.[17] Therefore, it is imperative to continue recording for at least 30 minutes following maneuvers considered to be at substantial risk for neurologic injury. This emphasizes a major limitation in that the feedback is often significantly delayed.

SSEP may be recorded either cortically or subcortically. During surgical monitoring, there is significant reduction of muscle noise from anesthesia and muscle relaxants with the subcortical responses. Subcortical responses are more reliable than the cortical responses because they are less sensitive to changes related to anesthesia or other systemic factors, such as blood pressure or temperature. During cervical spine procedures, median nerve stimulation is appropriate for upper to mid cervical levels. However, ulnar stimulation must be instituted for lower cervical levels. For thoracic and lumbosacral pathology, the posterior tibial nerve is routinely stimulated. In

the advent of a severe peripheral neuropathy, the common peroneal nerve can be stimulated.

Currently, there are no universally accepted criteria for interpreting the significance of intraoperative changes in SSEP monitoring. However, changes in amplitude greater than 50% and/or increases in latency greater than 10% should remain a guideline for impending spinal cord injury.[1] Because of the shortened volley, latency changes become less important in subcortical recording. Moreover, although changes in velocity may be a sensitive indicator of spinal cord injury, quantification has proven to be cumbersome and therefore does not play a significant role in SSEP monitoring.

Inhalational anesthetics such as halothane, isoflurane, and enflurane all have a consistent dose–response effect regarding SSEP recording.[1,24,30,42] The effects are poorly understood yet produce a reliable prolongation of latency and reduction of amplitude. Narcotics such as morphine and synthetic narcotics such as fentanyl, alfentanyl, and sufentanyl also affect signals.[24,30] Although more commonly observed with higher doses, bolus dosing of potent narcotics has a varying effect upon signal amplitude and latency. Benzodiazepines reduce the amplitude of the cortical responses without affecting the latency significantly, but they have been shown to reduce muscle noises.[1,30]

Anesthetic regimens should not include the use of paralytic agents and rely on balanced nitrous inhalation, with a continuous infusion of narcotics (without bolus). The use of halogenated anesthetics should be kept to a minimum, especially when used during cortical recording.

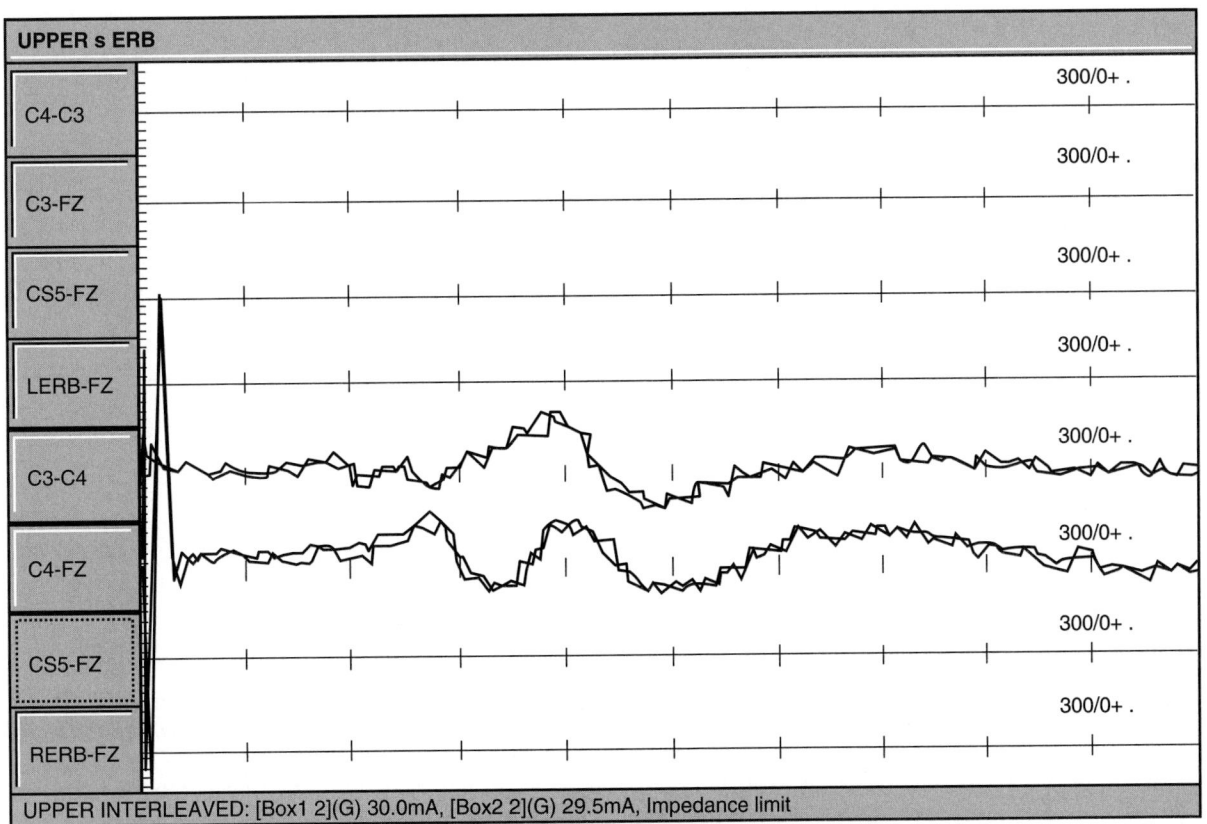

**Figure 137.1** Intraoperative monitoring during intradural left L3 tumor resection. Normal baseline in the right upper extremity SSEP.

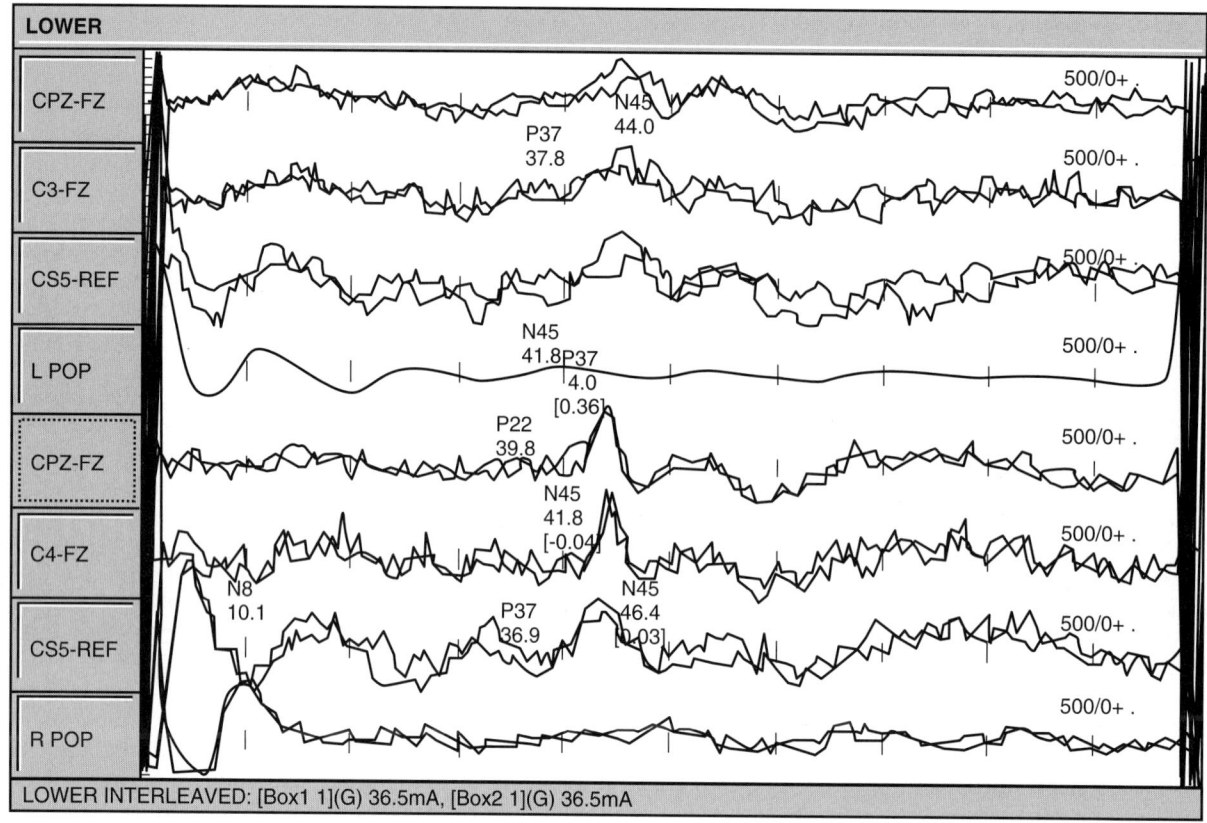

**Figure 137.2** Intraoperative monitoring during intradural left L3 tumor resection. Normal lower extremity intraoperative SSEP.

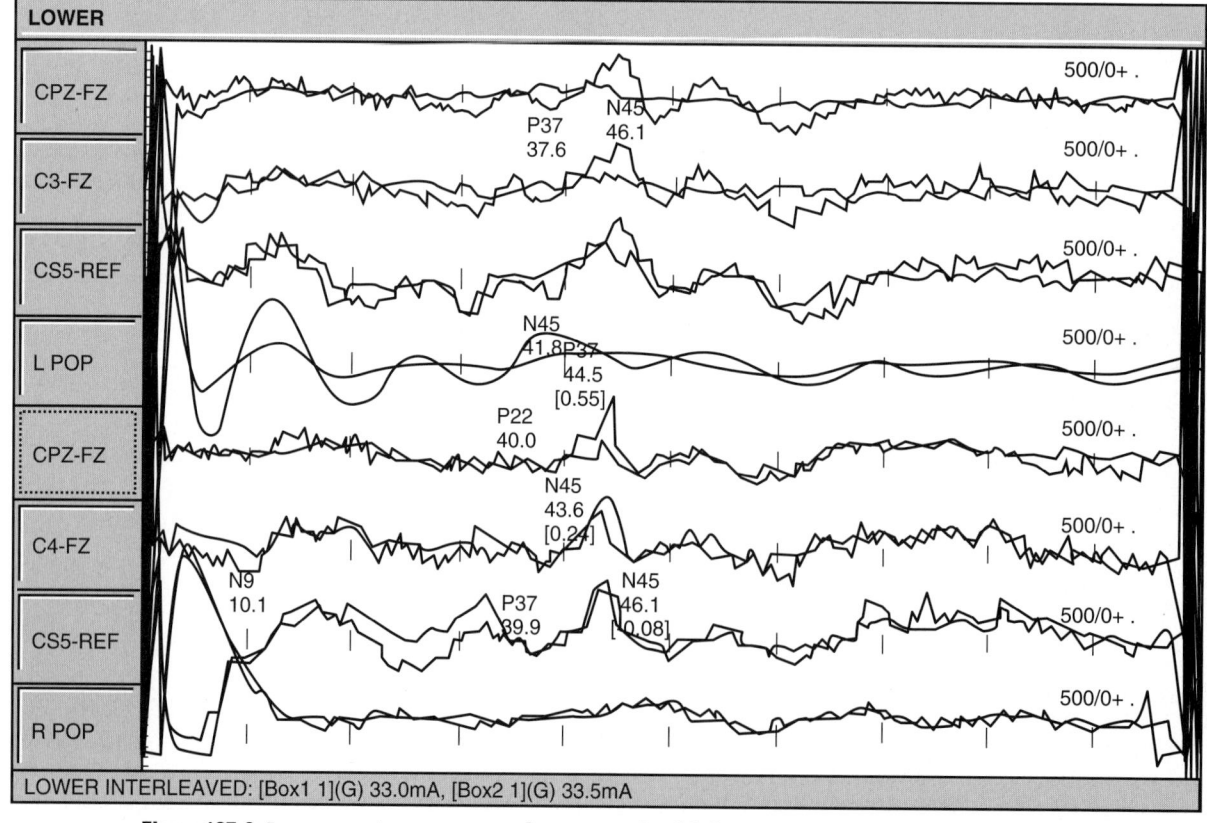

**Figure 137.3** Intraoperative monitoring during intradural left L3 tumor resection. Decreased amplitude of the left lower extremity SSEP (CPZ-FZ-CX5-REF).

The introduction and use of propofol has had a profound effect in neuroanesthesia and is a preferred regimen because it does not affect the subcortical component, such as N13, and it increases the latency of the early cortical responses by only 10% without affecting their amplitude.[42]

Factors that play a role in the sensitivity of SSEP to anesthetic depression are essentially twofold. First, recording from lower order neurons (fewer synapses) reduces the incidence of anesthetic depression. In addition, previous spinal cord injury has been shown to increase the sensitivity of neurons to anesthetic depression.[14]

Other than anesthesia, environmental and physiologic factors that play a significant role in signal recording include 60Hz noise from other operating equipment (e.g., electric drills, warming blankets Bair Hugger, headlights, etc.), hypocarbia, hypothermia, and hypotension.[23,42] Changes in amplitude and/or latency are the warning signs of possible neurologic injury. Animal studies have shown susceptibility to neurologic injury at the time of surgical manipulation during periods of hypotension via ischemia.[14] This is also evident in humans with decreases in SSEP amplitudes and prolongation of latency during periods of relative intraoperative hypotension. Although no definitive data exist, maintaining a mean arterial pressure (MAP) at 10% above the patient's baseline MAP is a practical rule in spinal decompression, instrumentation, and deformity correction surgery.

SSEP monitoring may help the surgeon during deformity surgery, as observed by Nuwer et al.[33] in their survey of 50,000 monitored spinal surgeries (60% scoliosis, 7.5% fractures, 6.5% kyphosis, and 5.5% spondylolisthesis); they found incidence of false-negative SSEP to be 0.063%. The major limitations in using SSEP for monitoring the spinal cord are the time delay between injury and manifestation of SSEP and the lack of definitive correlation with anterior column function. Motor tracts have been damaged without a change in SSEP.[6,13,36] Therefore, the surgeon must avoid developing a false sense of security based solely on SSEP. If used, they must be considered to be only one instrument in the surgeon's armamentarium. In addition, the surgeon must be prepared for the false-positive results and their ramifications. The false-positive rate ranges from 9% to 28%, depending upon the location and number of channels and recording sites.[2,27] False-positive can lead to premature termination of surgical decompression or a misguided alteration in surgical strategy. This negative aspect of electrophysiologic monitoring may alone denigrate its use.

## Spinal Recording of Spinal Evoked Potentials (SPSEPs)

The aforementioned principle of reduction in the number of synapses has significant benefits. Spinal stimulation and recording provide both a reduction in the sensitivity to anesthetic depression, as well as higher baseline amplitudes. In addition, significant peripheral nerve disease may hinder adequate recording with SSEP. This problem is avoided by the use of spinal cord stimulation and recording. Spinal evoked potentials provide a more consistent response when compared to cortical SEP.[45,48] Additionally, a more rapid acquisition of responses can be achieved because of the need for fewer repetitions, adding to overall efficiency.[45,48]

Recording and stimulation electrodes are placed in the epidural or subarachnoid space. Although invasive, reported complications remain exceedingly low via percutaneous implantation or under direct visualization.[45] The predominant technical challenge of percutaneous placement is the difficulty associated with achieving midline placement. Paramedian recording or stimulation may result in unilateral monitoring and changes in the spinal potentials.[35] Electrodes may migrate during the procedure. This may herald alarming (but clinically insignificant) changes in amplitude and latency. While reducing the number of synapses, this method contains the same limitations as SSEP.

## Dermatomal Somatosensory Evoked Potentials (DSEPs)

Dermatomal Somatosensory Evoked Potentials (DSEPs) can be used intraoperatively during procedures where specific nerve roots are at risk, as opposed to the spinal cord. It is seldom used for spine monitoring. However, recent technologic advancements warrant an overview.

A specific dermatome is stimulated. The evoked electrical activity travels through the same pathway as the SSEP. However, dermatomal stimulation yields responses of smaller amplitude and increased latency because excited nerve fibers are smaller in diameter and fewer in number. It is also more difficult to record than SSEP because of its low amplitude.

Achievement of proper cutaneous stimulation requires each electrode to be positioned in each targeted dermatome. Baseline recording should include comparative analysis of each side to allow for measurement of between-limb latencies.[21] This may be useful to monitor the C5 nerve root, which is a sensitive cervical root and has been shown to have a higher injury rate than other cervical roots with overdistraction and manipulation.[41] Additionally, it may be useful in the lumbar spine or when the pathology is at the nerve root level.

## Motor Evoked Potentials (MEPs)

The shortcomings of SSEP monitoring are that of posterior column selectivity, limitations resulting from peripheral nerve disease, time delay, and a variable false-negative rate. An undetermined fraction of monitoring error results from unrecorded injury to the anterior spinal cord.[1,42]

The need for monitoring ventral spinal cord function becomes increasingly important with deformity correction and ventral surgical decompression procedures. Deformation of the ventral spinal cord may have a limited effect on dorsal column function, thereby increasing the false-negative rate of SSEP. Furthermore, vascular compromise of the ventral spinal cord will likely spare the posterior columns and thereby not be manifested by changes in SSEP. Although used less frequently, motor evoked potentials (MEP) monitoring enables the assessment of the ventral spinal cord and is associated with a shorter delay between injury and changes.

First introduced by Levy and York[26] in 1983, intraoperative MEP has gained significant interest within the surgical community. Rostral stimulation can be achieved at the cortical, brain stem, or spinal cord level. Caudal recording sites may be located at the spinal level, peripheral nerve, or muscle. As with SSEP monitoring, similar principles of dual volley recording should be applied.

Transcranial cortical stimulation must overcome the resistance of the skull. As such, current requirements are higher and associated with a significant degree of discomfort.[37,43] A balance must be maintained between the quantity of stimulation and the anesthetic to control the normal physiologic responses to pain. Pre-induction baseline recording is therefore not possible because of the discomfort associated with MEP stimulation.

Obvious contraindications to transcranial MEP include awake procedures, as well as a previous history of seizure activity. Continued MEP stimulation may result in seizure activity that may remain unrecognized during general and/or paralytic anesthesia.

For the aforementioned reasons, magnetic current induction of the cerebral cortex is now becoming more prevalent. First introduced in 1985, transcranial magnetic stimulation achieves a compound motor action potential without the need for signal averaging.[3,4] A magnetic field (usually in the form of a skull cap) is placed over the patient's head and rotated, thereby inducing an electrical current as first described by Faraday in 1831. In addition, it is painless and provides a more rapid means of signal analysis due to the obviated need for averaging.[32,40] Although expensive and cumbersome, this technology will no doubt take the place of transcranial stimulation as the technology improves.

There are several significant restrictions regarding magnetic stimulation, including anesthesia techniques, technical difficulties with the cap, interpretations, and FDA approval.

One can electrically stimulate the spinal cord to record MEP. Electrodes may be placed in the epidural space,[28,29,44] interspinous ligaments outside the surgical field,[9] and lamina.[36] Significant amplitude changes range from 20% to 50%.[7,18,34,44,45] Fifty percent is also recommended level for MEP[22,50] (cortical) and SEP.[20]

The changes in MEP are immediate, as opposed to those of SSEP. In addition, it enables direct assessment of the motor function. It does not rely upon posterior column assessment to infer anterior column integrity.

### Electromyography (EMG)

Electromyography (EMG) has been increasingly used during lumbar pedicle screw placement. Electrodes are placed on the muscles innervated by the nerve roots in question. Bipolar recording electrodes (an active and a reference electrode) are placed over the belly of muscles, separated by 2 to 3 inches. Subdermal needle electrodes or surface electrodes may be used. Muscle relaxation must remain constant when recording (two to three twitches out of a train of four). Free run EMG is continuously monitored for mechanical responses, which are identified by an audible sound reminiscent of "popping popcorn." This is easily identified by the high-amplitude spikes, which differentiate them from background noise. The triggered EMG can aid in the evaluation of the integrity of the pedi-

cle wall. If there is no stimulation of adjacent nerve roots manifested by EMG activity, the wall of the pedicle is presumed to be intact. The stimulus can be recorded in milliamps or volts. Darden et al.[8] found (1) EMG threshold greater than 7mA or 30V indicates an intact pedicle; (2) EMG threshold less than 20V or 6mA, the pedicle is likely breached; and (3) EMG threshold greater than 20V or 6mA and less than 30V or 7mA, one should inspect the pedicle and use the appropriate intervention. The data can be confusing at times, especially with a fractured pedicle, because the clinical impact of a fractured pedicle is unknown (Figures 137.4 and 137.5).

## Summary

Intraoperative neurophysiologic monitoring is becoming increasingly available for spine surgery. Each modality has its advantages and limitations. However, combining multimodality monitoring such as SSEP, MEP, and EMG may overcome the shortcomings of each individual modality. Modern techniques allow for multimodality monitoring. When properly used, intraoperative monitoring during spine surgery may possibly help minimize neurologic deficits in selected situations.

No monitoring technique can replace meticulous operative technique and attention to detail. Specifically, the surgeon should position the patient in a neutral position and not attempt deformity correction until the decompression is completed. The MAP may be maintained 10% above the baseline preoperative MAP. Preoperative planning based upon radiologic imaging and anatomy can minimize the risks of instrumentation.

Electrophysiologic monitoring may be beneficial and therefore is appropriate in selected deformity correction surgical procedures, surgery for nerve root tumors, and possibly spinal cord tumors. With deformity correction surgery, the surgeon is unable to intraoperatively assess whether or not the deformity correction has injured the spinal cord. Therefore, intraoperative neurophysiologic monitoring can be helpful. However, SSEP is associated with a 30-minute delay and does not always correlate with motor function. Therefore, if possible, MEP may be used. It is useful to help ensure that correction has not injured the ventral spinal cord. The same principle holds true for spinal cord tumors. The myelotomy itself typically affects SSEP such that they are not helpful. In addition, the pathology typically lends itself to either a clean dissection plane or the absence of such. If there is no clean plane, the surgeon may only perform a biopsy. If there is a clean plane (e.g., ependymoma, metastasis), the surgeon will often use this plane for a complete resection. MEP may be useful in this scenario to provide feedback about the stress on the ventral cord. EMG can be useful in nerve sheath tumors to assess the viability of the nerve root in question. If there is evidence of transmission and preserved neural function, the surgeon should make every effort to dissect the tumor off of the nerve root. If there is no evidence that the root is conducting or functional, the surgeon may elect to sacrifice the nerve root without consequence.

Intraoperative neurophysiologic monitoring is an evolving tool in the spine surgeon's armamentarium. However,

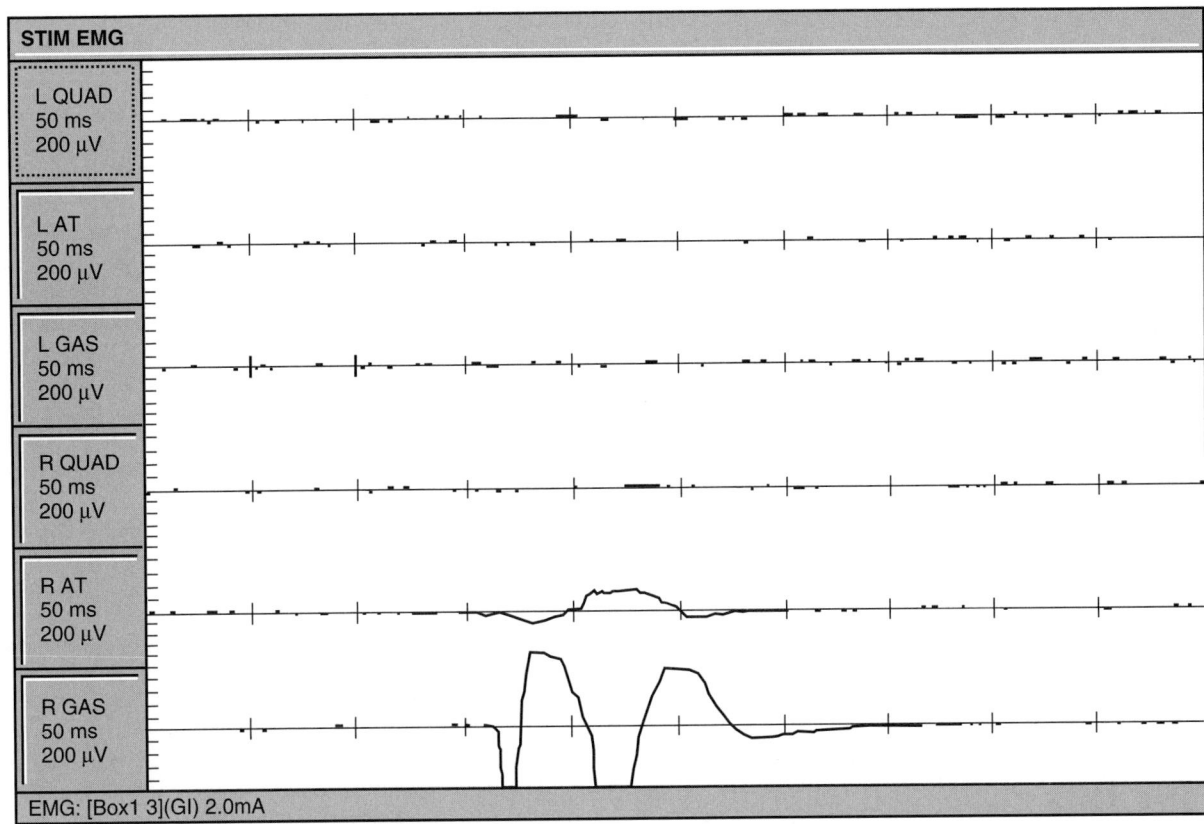

**Figure 137.4** Intraoperative monitoring during lumbar laminectomy and fusion with instrumentation from L3-S1. Direct S1 nerve root stimulation at 2mA.

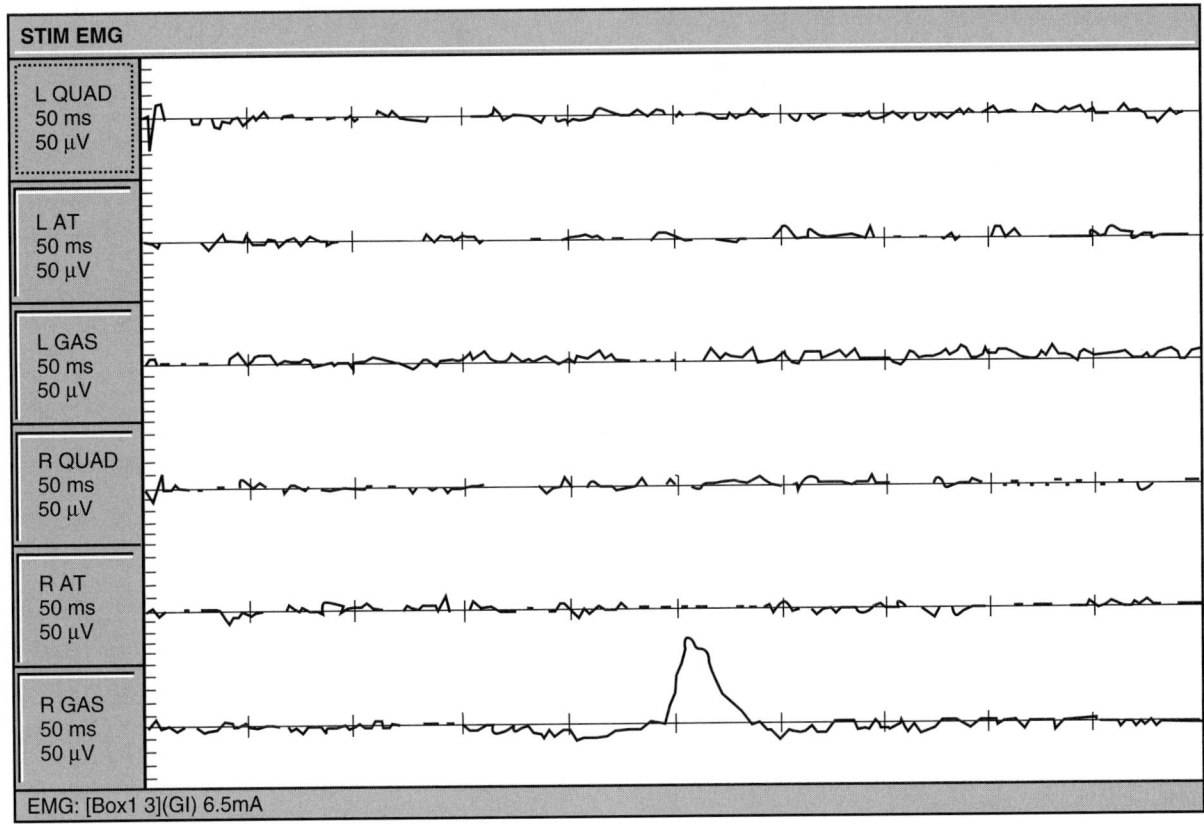

**Figure 137.5** Intraoperative monitoring during lumbar laminectomy and fusion with instrumentation from L3-S1. Right S1 pedicle screw stimulation at 6.5mA suggesting breached pedicle.

it is only one of many tools. It cannot replace surgical decision making and technique. It does add time, cost, and information (some useful, some potentially misleading) to every case. It has not conclusively shown to be a significant advantage in every case. However, it may provide the greatest advantage for spine deformity correction and for nerve sheath tumor surgery. It may also be helpful for intramedullary spinal cord tumors.

# REFERENCES

1. American Electroencephalographic Society Evoked Potentials Committee: American electroencephalographic society guidelines for intraoperative monitoring of sensory evoked potentials. *J Clin Neurophysiol* 4:397-416, 1987.
2. Ashkenaze D, Mudiyan B, Boachie-Adjei O, Gilbert C: Efficacy of spinal cord monitoring in neuromuscular scoliosis. *Spine* 18:1627-1633, 1993.
3. Barker AT, Freeston IL, Jalinous R, *et al:* Magnetic stimulation of the human brain. *J Physiol* 369:3, 1985.
4. Barker AT, Jalinous R, Freeston IL, *et al:* Noninvasive magnetic stimulation of the human cortex. *Lancet* 2:1106-1107, 1985.
5. Been HD, Kalkman CJ, Traast S, *et al:* Neurologic injury after insertion of laminar hooks during Cotrel-Dubousset instrumentation. *Spine* 19:1402, 1994.
6. Ben-David B, Haller G, Taylor P: Anterior spinal fusion complicated by paraplegia: a case report of false-negative somatosensory evoked potential. *Spine* 12:536, 1987.
7. Burke D, Hicks R, Stephen J, *et al:* Assessment of corticospinal and somatosensory conduction simultaneously during scoliosis surgery. *EEG Clin Neurophysiol* 85:388-396, 1992.
8. Calancie B, Klose J, Baier S, *et al:* Isoflurane induced attenuation of motor evoked potentials caused by electrical motor cortex stimulation during surgery. *J Neurosurg* 74:879, 1991.
9. Coe JD, Mongan PD, Chambers HG, Peterson RE: Spinal cord monitoring with neurogenic motor evoked potentials using percutaneously placed interspinous electrodes: a new technique for spinal cord stimulation. Paper presented at American Academy of Orthopaedic Surgeons 1994 Annual Meeting, Scientific Program, New Orleans, LA, February 28, 1994.
10. Croft BA, Brod JS, Nuisen FE: Reversible spinal cord trauma: a model for electrical monitoring of spinal cord function. *J Neurosurg* 36:299, 1972.
11. Cusick JF, Myklebust JF, Larson SJ, Sances A, Jr.: Spinal cord potentials in the primate: neural substrate. *J Neurosurg* 49:551, 1978.
12. Dawson EG, Carlson LG, Kanim LEA, Sherman JE: Somatosensory evoked potential spinal cord monitoring reduces neurological deficits after scoliosis surgery: results of a large multicenter survey. *EEG Clin Neurophysiol* 96:6, 1995.
13. Dinner DS, Luders H, Lesser RP, *et al:* Intraoperative spinal somatosensory evoked potential monitoring. *J Neurosurg* 65:807-814, 1986.
14. Dinner DS, Shields RW, Jr., Luders H: Intraoperative spinal cord monitoring. In Rothman RH, Simeone FA (eds): *Spine,* vol II. Philadelphia, WB Saunders, 1992, p 1801.
15. Giblin DR: Somatosensory evoked potentials in healthy subjects and in patients with lesions of the nervous system. *Ann N Y Acad Sci* 112:93, 1964.
16. Ginsburg HH, Shetter AG, Raudzens PA: Postoperative paraplegia with preserved intraoperative somatosensory evoked potentials: case report. *J Neurosurg* 63:296-300, 1985.
17. Grundy BL: Monitoring of sensory evoked potentials during neurosurgical operations: methods and applications. *Neurosurgery* 11:556-575, 1982.
18. Imai T: A clinical study on intra-operative spinal cord monitoring with spinal evoked potential for scoliosis. *J Jpn Orthop Assoc* 62:511-521, 1988.
19. Jones SJ, Carter L, Edgar MA, *et al:* Experience of epidural spinal cord monitoring in 410 cases. In Schramm J, Jones SJ (eds): *Spinal Cord Monitoring.* Berlin, Springer-Verlag, 1985, pp 215-220.
20. Jones SJ, Edger MA, Ransford AO, Thomas NP: A system for the electrophysiological monitoring of the spinal cord during operations for scoliosis. *J Bone Joint Surg Br* 65:134-139, 1983.
21. Katifi HA, Sedgwick EM: Somatosensory evoked potentials from posterior tibial nerve and lumbosacral dermatomes. *EEG Clin Neurophysiol* 65:249-259, 1986.
22. Kitagawa H, Itoh T, Takano H, *et al:* Motor evoked potential monitoring during upper cervical spine surgery. *Spine* 14:1078-1083, 1989.
23. Kochs E: Electrophysiological monitoring and mild hypothermia. *J Neurosurg Anesthesiol* 7:222-228, 1995.
24. Koht A: Anesthesia and evoked potentials: overview. *Int J Clin Monit Comput* 5:167-173, 1988.
25. Lesser RP, Raudzens P, Luders H, *et al:* Postoperative neurological deficits may occur despite unchanged intraoperative somatosensory evoked potentials. *Ann Neurol* 19:22-25, 1986.
26. Levy WJ, Jr., York DH: Evoked potentials from the motor tracts in humans. *Neurosurgery* 12:422, 1983.
27. Lubicky JB, Spadoro JA, Yuan HA, *et al:* Variability of somatosensory evoked potential monitoring during spinal surgery. *Spine* 14:790-798, 1989.
28. Machida M, Weinstein SL, Yamada T, Kimura J: Spinal cord monitoring: electrophysiological measures of sensory and motor function during spinal surgery. *Spine* 10(5):407, 1985.
29. Machida M, Weinstein SL, Yamada T, *et al:* Dissociation of muscle action potentials and spinal somatosensory evoked potentials after ischemic damage to the spinal cord. *Spine* 13:1119, 1988.
30. McMeniman WJ, Purcell GJ: Neurological monitoring during anesthesia and surgery. *Anaesth Int Care* 16:358-367, 1988.
31. Mizutani AR, Drummond JC, Karagianes TG: A less than rude awakening. *Anesthesiology* 69:287, 1989.
32. Mills KR, Murray NMF, Hess CW: Magnetic and electrical transcranial brain stimulation: physiological mechanisms and clinical applications. *Neurosurgery* 20:164-168, 1987.
33. Nuwer MR, Dawson EG, Carlson LG, *et al:* Somatosensory evoked potential spinal cord monitoring reduces neurologic deficits after scoliosis surgery: results of a large multicenter survey. *EEG Clin Neurophysiol* 96:6, 1995.
34. Ohmi Y, Tohno S, Harada S, Nakano K: Spinal cord monitoring using evoked potentials recorded from epidural

space. In Homma S, Tamaki T (eds): *Fundamentals and Clinical Application of Spinal Cord Monitoring.* Tokyo, Japan, Saikon Press, 1984, pp 203-210.

35. Owen JH: Evoked potential monitoring during spinal surgery. In Bridwell KH, Dewald RL (eds): *The Textbook of Spinal Surgery.* Philadelphia, Lippincott, 1997, pp 31-64.

36. Owen GH, Bridwell KH, Grubb R, *et al:* The clinical application of neurogenic motor evoked potentials to monitor spinal cord function during surgery. *Spine* 16:S385, 1991.

37. Owen JH, Laschinger J, Bridwell K, *et al:* Sensitivity and specificity of somatosensory and neurogenic-motor evoked potentials in animals and humans. *Spine* 13:1111, 1988.

38. Owen GH, Naito M, Bridwell KH: Relationship among level of distraction, evoked potentials, spinal cord ischemia and integrity and clinical status in animals. *Spine* 15:852, 1990a.

39. Owen GH, Naito M, Bridwell KH, Oakley DM: Relationship between duration of spinal cord ischemia and post-operative neurologic deficits in animals. *Spine* 15:618, 1990b.

40. Rothwell JC, Day BL, Thompson PD, *et al:* Some experiences of techniques for stimulation of the human cerebral motor cortex through the scalp. *Neurosurgery* 20:156-163, 1987.

41. Saunders RL: On the pathogenesis of the radiculopathy complicating multilevel corpectomy. *Neurosurgery* 37(3):408, 1995.

42. Schramm J: Spinal cord monitoring: current status and new developments. *Cent Nerv Syst Trauma* 2:207-227, 1985.

43. Shimuzu H, Shimoji K, Maruyama Y, *et al:* Human spinal cord potentials produced in lumbosacral enlargement by descending volleys. *J Neurophysiol* 48:1108, 1982.

44. Tamaki T, Noguchi T, Takano H, *et al:* Spinal cord monitoring as a clinical utilization of spinal evoked potentials. *Clin Orthop* 185:58-64, 1984.

45. Tamaki T, Tsuji H, Inoue S, Kobayashi H: The prevention of iatrogenic spinal cord injury utilizing the evoked spinal cord potential. *Int Orthop (SICOT)* 4:313-317, 1981.

46. Tomaki T: Spinal cord monitoring with spinal potentials evoked by direct stimulation of the spinal cord. In Desmedt JE (ed): *Neuromonitoring in Surgery.* Amsterdam, Elsevier, 1989, p 139.

47. Tomaki T, Yamashita T, Kobayashi H, Hiryama H: Spinal cord monitoring. *Jpn J Electroencephalogr Electromyogr* 1:196, 1972.

48. Tsuyama N, Tsuzuki N, Kurokawa T, Imai T: Clinical application of spinal cord action potential measurement. *Int Orthop (SICOT)* 2:39-46, 1978.

49. Vauzelle C, Stanara P, Jouvinroux P: Functional monitoring of spinal cord activity during spinal surgery. *Clin Orthop* 93:173, 1973.

50. Zentner J: Noninvasive motor evoked potential monitoring during neurosurgical operations on the spinal cord. *Neurosurgery* 24:709-712, 1989.

# CHAPTER 138

# Intraoperative Nonparalytic Monitoring

George W. Sypert, Richard L. Saunders, and Edward C. Benzel

Electrophysiologic monitoring techniques have been the subject of numerous publications, yet objective evidence of efficacy is sparse. True class I evidence does not exist. Its routine use, therefore, must be solely at the discretion of the surgeon. Alternative monitoring techniques, such as nonparalytic monitoring techniques, may provide an alternative approach. This chapter focuses on this strategy.

The earliest documented systematic approach to the intraoperative monitoring of spinal cord function was via the wake-up test.[3] This technique often provided an unequivocal demonstration of the integrity of long motor tract function. However, it provided this information for one point in time, and, in fact, after any potentially harmful surgical manipulation had taken place. The advent of the ability to monitor evoked potentials accurately heralded another wave of spinal cord function monitoring enthusiasm.[1,3,5,7] The popularity of this monitoring modality has increased over the years.

Many successful surgeons, however, do not use intraoperative electrophysiologic monitoring during the majority of their procedures. Indeed, there are no rigorous scientific data that prove the clinical utility of intraoperative evoked potential monitoring techniques. Furthermore, evoked potential monitoring clearly does not demonstrate accurately the intactness of vital neural pathways to the surgeon.[2,4,6,8,10] Based on an 80-plus year cumulative clinical experience that includes the surgical treatment of patients who were electrophysiologically monitored during surgery, the authors believe that the data acquired from intraoperative evoked potential monitoring are most often less helpful than the immediate surgical feedback provided by observation of unparalyzed muscles in the majority of spine surgery cases.

Immediate intraoperative feedback during nonparalytic anesthesia is a motor response to intraoperative spinal cord or nerve root manipulation. Whereas immediate intraoperative feedback monitoring requires that the patient not be pharmacologically paralyzed, intraoperative evoked potential monitoring mandates pharmacologic paralysis. Although pharmacologic paralysis eliminates the potentially critical and immediate feedback provided by the observation of the motor response to the inadvertent manipulation of neural tissue, it provides muscle relaxation and lessens the dosages of inhalation and intravenous anesthetic agents, both of which are somewhat advantageous to the surgeon and to the anesthesiologist.

The spine surgeon, therefore, must determine the relative benefits and risks associated with these alternative techniques of intraoperative monitoring. To assist in this process, a brief historic perspective is presented.

## The Origins of Intraoperative Monitoring of Neurologic Function

The wake-up test was introduced in the early 1970s as a method of monitoring spinal cord function during scoliosis surgery. It involves the elevation of the plane of anesthesia, such that the patient can move the extremity placed at risk by a prior operative intervention (e.g., the correction of a scoliotic deformity). Preoperative patient education is imperative. It is, however, associated with a multitude of drawbacks. These include anesthetic difficulties, inadequate assessment, the risks associated with excessive patient movement, and excessive operative delays. Therefore, its popularity has waned since the mid-1980s.[3]

Intraoperative electrophysiologic monitoring quickly found widespread use. Its clinical use, however, was not clearly established. Anecdotal and retrospective reports appeared in the literature.[1,3,5,10] Although some of the reports touted the "effectiveness" of monitoring regarding the prevention of neurologic injury, all were significantly flawed. Small control groups, uncontrolled series, and the use of otherwise inadequate controls contributed to the flawed nature of these reports.

## The Deficiencies of Electrophysiologic Monitoring

Electrophysiologic monitoring, by virtue of its nature, dictates that the observation of an electrophysiologic response to an intraoperative adverse neural event becomes manifest after the event occurs. Thus the event, such as surgical trauma, is followed by its documentation by electrophysiologic means. This type of monitoring is not *on-line*.

Furthermore, electrophysiologic monitoring efficacy is sensitive to anesthetic variables and technique. The potential alteration of intraoperative electrophysiologic observations by anesthetic technique further detracts from the value and validity of the technique itself. Surgical delays, hurried operations, and unnecessary intraoperative anesthetic alterations often result.

The most common type of electrophysiologic monitoring is of somatosensory evoked potentials (SSEPs). SSEPs monitor sensory function transmitted through the posterior columns of the spinal cord.[1,4,8] The majority of operations for extra-axial compressive lesions are ventral spinal decompression procedures. The posterior columns are, therefore, positioned farthest from the operative site of all spinal tracts. One must, therefore, question their validity on an anatomic basis alone. Although motor evoked potential monitoring has been used, the technique has not been perfected and is not without risk. Failure to detect injury has been reported.[2,6,7]

## The Rationale for Nonparalytic Anesthesia Intraoperative Monitoring

Sypert[9] commented on the use of the intraoperative observation of surgical manipulation evoked motor responses as a monitoring technique in 1988. He pointed out that the majority of surgical procedures during which the monitoring of neural function might be beneficial involves neural decompression.[9] The surgeon, however, is able to observe directly the neural elements during the critical components of such an operation. This "direct observation" type of monitoring is, indeed, the most useful to the surgeon. For example, the observation of the dural sac and its relationship to surrounding and confining bony and soft-tissue structures affords the skilled and alert surgeon the opportunity to monitor the extent of neural distortion and compression in an on-line manner.

Electrophysiologic mapping of the cerebral cortex and the monitoring of seventh nerve responses are well-established important adjuncts in some forms of cranial surgery. Simplistically, such methods are used for the precise localization of exquisite anatomy, not simply as a measure of surgical tolerance. Transference of these important electrophysiologic observations to refine surgery of the spinal cord may not be entirely appropriate; that is, spine surgeons are not mapping a territory or attempting to locate the spinal cord. Their requirement is an ongoing measurement of how well the spinal cord is tolerating the surgical strategy. This is not at all similar to the situation in cranial surgery.

The best electrical example of tolerance monitoring is observed in scoliosis surgery. There is, however, a difference between scoliosis surgery and decompressive surgery with regard to the nature of the surgical stresses. Whereas with scoliosis the spinal cord is threatened by the ischemia associated with stretching or tethering, the surgical hazard in decompression is distortion and concussion. Neither type of surgery is necessarily dependent on a particular spinal cord geography (as is the case in cranial surgery); the critical determination is the measurement of tolerance.

It is not insignificant that electrophysiologic monitoring approaches a standard of care in scoliosis surgery but not decompression surgery. This is primarily because spinal cord stretching is not known to provoke predictable motor response and the blinded (to the surgeon) correction of the deformity may injure neural tissue (unbeknownst to the surgeon).

Exclusive of scoliosis, the adept surgeon does not depend on the determination of spinal tolerance. The spinal cord is not distorted and not concussed intentionally in the properly performed procedure. Accordingly, because the spine surgeon knows where the spinal cord is, electrophysiologic methodology has not found a clear place in nonscoliosis spinal surgery. Indeed, because anesthetic requirements in electrical monitoring dampen surgically provoked intraoperative motor responses, the defensive boilerplate of "black box" paraphernalia is a questionable trade-off.

An inherent advantage of immediate intraoperative feedback through a motor response "felt" by the surgeon during a particular maneuver is of immense significance.

There is no delay; the patient's movement is indeed so frightening that one stops reflexively whatever endeavor evoked the response. Inherent to most electrophysiologic monitoring, however, is the requirement for waveform averaging. This, by definition, causes a delay in the surgeon's response. This is further compounded because it is the person watching the box, not the surgeon, who first appreciates the monitored change. Even if minuscule, these delays are unacceptable when compared with the immediacy of clinical monitoring of the unparalyzed patient. The second author (RLS) has systematically used intraoperative nonparalytic anesthesia monitoring in spinal cord surgery since 1987 on the basis of the foregoing rationalizations. Motor responses consistent with nerve root stimulation have been noted frequently with bipolar or unipolar coagulation on the lateral vertebral body and the posterior longitudinal ligament, presumably resulting from heat transmission. A similar motor response with instrumentation in the cervical foramina has been noted but not with the same frequency as the heat observation. Six patients have had a more global total body movement, which was believed to represent a spinal cord response. Although this has been observed with coagulation of the posterior longitudinal ligament, most of these cases were in response to inadvertent impact on or distortion of the spinal cord. Of these six patients, one had a persisting postoperative worsening of a severe myelopathy and a second had transient bilateral arm aching. The latter raises the question of a minor central cord injury. The remaining four patients were unaffected. No patient without a motor response during surgery suffered an immediate adverse myelopathic change.

One case, in particular, illustrates the value of immediate intraoperative feedback. The spinal cord was sharply indented by an area of focal ligamentous hypertrophy. Failing to appreciate this area of focal spinal cord distortion, the surgeon forcefully compounded the compression by ligamentous excision, with a resulting sudden profound total body "jump." The surgical effort was reflexively stopped. The pathology was only then recognized, and without question, injury to the spinal cord was avoided. Had the patient been under paralytic anesthesia for conventional electrical spinal cord monitoring, the spinal cord would have been substantially distorted before the surgeon was "electrically alerted." Such immediacy of motor response, which is unique to the nonparalyzed patient, is a simple but elegant means by which to detect inadvertent spinal cord stress. Until evoked response monitoring forms can provide this immediacy, they will remain a potentially dangerous embellishment rather than refinement to spinal surgery. Conventional electrophysiologic "monitoring" in spinal surgery may be a false assurance to the inexperienced or heavy-handed surgeon.

## Summary

If inadvertent neural trauma occurs from heating, compression, distraction, or trauma, a motor response in affected nonparalyzed muscles usually occurs. This, in a sense, is the equivalent of an on-line motor evoked potential. Immediate surgical feedback is, therefore, provided by two means: (1) direct observation of the relationship between the neural elements and the surrounding structures and (2) observation of the motor response to intraoperative neural manipulation. Surgical maneuvers that are potentially harmful can be immediately altered or discontinued. Immediate feedback to the surgeon allows this to be an effective method of neurologic injury prevention.

Intraoperative nonparalytic anesthesia monitoring, however, is not foolproof. Feedback, although immediate, may still be provided to the surgeon after irreversible injury has been incurred by the patient. The depth of anesthesia or pharmacologic paralysis may be excessive, thus not allowing surgical trauma-evoked motor responses. Certain motor pathways may be resistant to traumatically induced elicitation of motor responses. Finally, neural distraction often results in depression of neural transmission rather than neural hyperactivity. This latter point renders this technique less useful for the graduated correction of spinal deformity.

Electrophysiologic monitoring is perhaps clinically advantageous when direct neural element observation (visual) is not possible during operative manipulation. This may occur during such maneuvers as deformity correction.

Finally, technologic advances, such as electrophysiologic monitoring, cannot be used to replace intelligent surgeon input into the intraoperative decision-making process. Common sense will, in most clinical scenarios, outweigh electrophysiologic monitoring as an intraoperative decision-making tool.

## REFERENCES

1. Aminoff MJ: The use of somatosensory evoked potentials in the evaluation of the central nervous system. *Neurol Clin* 6:809, 1988.
2. Ben-David B, Haller G, Taylor P: Anterior spinal fusion complicated by paraplegia: a case report of false-negative somatosensory evoked potential. *Spine* 12:536, 1987.
3. Brown RH, Nash CL, Jr.: Intra-operative spinal cord monitoring. In Frymoyer JW (ed): *The Adult Spine: Principles and Practice*. Philadelphia, Lippincott-Raven, 1991, p 549.
4. Cusick JF, Mykelbust J, Larson SJ, et al: Spinal evoked potentials in the primate: neural substrate. *J Neurosurg* 49:551, 1978.
5. Engler GI, Spielholz NI, Bernhard WN, et al: Somatosensory evoked potentials during Harrington instrumentation for scoliosis. *J Bone Joint Surg* 60A:528, 1978.
6. Ginsburg HH, Shetter AG, Raudzens PA: Postoperative paraplegia with preserved intraoperative somatosensory evoked potentials: case report. *J Neurosurg* 63:296-300, 1985.
7. Lesser RP, Raudzens P, Luders H, et al: Postoperative neurological deficits may occur despite unchanged intraoperative somatosensory evoked potentials. *Ann Neurol* 19:22, 1986.
8. Powers SK, Bolger CA, Edwards MSB: Spinal cord pathways mediating somatosensory evoked potentials. *J Neurosurg* 57:472, 1982.
9. Sypert G: Stabilization procedures for thoracic and lumbar fractures. *Clin Neurosurg* 34:340, 1988.
10. Wilber RG, Thompson GH, Shaffer JW, et al: Postoperative neurological deficits in segmental spinal instrumentation: a study using spinal cord monitoring. *J Bone Joint Surg* 66A:1178, 1984.

# CHAPTER 139

# Anesthesia

## Marc L. Bertrand and Brion J. Beerle

Historically, spine surgery has played "second fiddle" to intracranial neurosurgery in the minds of many anesthesiologists. With advances in surgical technique and concomitant improvements in anesthetic management, however, surgical spine procedures are performed increasingly on elderly and medically compromised patients. Spine surgeons are able to perform procedures, once considered impossible, that provide anesthesiologists with some of their greatest challenges. This chapter acquaints spine surgeons with anesthetic concerns and with some techniques used during anesthesia for spine surgery.

## Preoperative Assessment

With preoperative evaluation, the anesthesiologist becomes familiar with the spine surgery patient's functional status, coexisting medical diseases, medications, allergies, and anesthetic concerns. It provides the opportunity to obtain informed consent for anesthesia. A thorough review of any symptoms attributable to cardiac or respiratory dysfunction is especially important during the preoperative interview because these systems contribute most to postoperative morbidity. Anesthesiologists can assess airway anatomy and cervical spine mobility to identify patients who may require specialized airway management.

## Laboratory Studies

Routine laboratory screening tests, including coagulation studies, rarely reveal abnormalities that were not apparent from the history and physical examination. It is reasonable to check a preoperative hemoglobin and hematocrit in patients with coexisting disease or a history of anemia and serum electrolytes in patients being treated with diuretics. Chronic hypokalemia, to a serum potassium of 3.0mmol/L, is not a contraindication to elective surgery in the absence of cardiac comorbidity, symptomatic arrhythmias, or digitalis therapy.[88] Symptomatic chronic hypokalemia in the perioperative period requires oral replacement on an outpatient basis because rapid intravenous supplementation may lead to an increase in morbidity and mortality.[46] Preoperative electrocardiograms and chest x-rays should be limited to elderly patients or to those with known or suspected cardiopulmonary disease.

## Considerations in Patients with Spinal Cord Injury

Preoperative considerations in spinal cord injury (SCI) patients vary with the timing of surgery in relation to the injury and the anatomic level of injury. Patients who show symptoms of neurologic deficits secondary to acute SCI are the most challenging. SCI patients must have sufficient respiratory muscle strength to oxygenate and ventilate effectively. They may have impaired coughing ability and significant ventilation perfusion mismatch.[60] Pneumonias are common in patients with acute or chronic SCIs because of the high incidence of aspiration and pulmonary dysfunction with lesions above T7.[29] Associated injuries related to trauma must be considered, such as rib fractures, pneumothoraces, closed head injuries, and pelvic fractures. Most of these patients show symptoms of varying degrees of hypotension as well as impaired myocardial contractility resulting from acute sympathetic denervation. They require volume loading and, often, vasopressors and/or inotropes to maintain organ perfusion pressure. Depolarizing muscle relaxants may result in fatal hyperkalemia. A history of autonomic hyperreflexia in the chronic SCI patient usually portends an intraoperative exacerbation.

## Considerations in Patients with Scoliosis

It is important to evaluate the degree of preoperative pulmonary compromise in the patient with scoliosis. Pulmonary function tests are quite useful in this patient population. The FVC and $FEV_1$ are the best indicators of the extent of restrictive lung disease caused by the thoracic deformity. Baseline arterial blood gas measurement or preoperative oximetry may also be helpful in guiding patient postoperative care.

## Considerations in Patients with Rheumatoid Arthritis

Patients with rheumatoid arthritis must be evaluated carefully for the extent of their systemic disease so that the risks of surgery and anesthesia may be minimized. Deformities produced by articular involvement may make intravascular catheter placement difficult and increase the risk of positioning-related injury. Cervical spine films should be obtained because up to 30% of these patients may have asymptomatic cervical instability.[77] Cervical spine instability or significant temporomandibular joint disease may require awake fiber-optic airway management and strict attention to positioning. The electrocardiogram should be examined for the presence of conduction abnormalities and an echocardiogram should be obtained if there are any history or physical examination findings compatible with valvular dysfunction. The serum blood urea nitrogen and creatinine should be checked to assess renal function in patients taking high doses of nonsteroidal anti-inflammatory drugs. Liver function tests are useful in patients taking cytotoxic drugs. Finally, stress dose steroids should be ordered for all patients with a recent history of steroid use.

## Other Disorders

A variety of other disorders impact on spine surgery patients in the preoperative period. Patients with mass lesions of the cervical spine require preoperative assessment to determine whether specialized airway management is necessary. Patients with primary vascular spinal cord tumors require preoperative preparation for massive transfusion. Those with a history of myelomeningocele,

SCI, or other disorders that require chronic catheterization may be sensitive to latex. A latex-free environment should be ensured at the time of surgery for patients with a history of latex sensitivity. Consideration should be given to preoperative prophylaxis with $H_1$- and $H_2$-receptor blockers and steroids in patients with a documented history of significant reaction to latex.

## Pharmacology

Preoperative medications serve a variety of functions, including sedation, amnesia, anxiolysis, and aspiration prophylaxis. The goal of premedication in the neurosurgical patient is to provide anxiolysis with minimal sedation at the termination of surgery. Benzodiazepines have largely supplanted barbiturates and anticholinergics for this purpose. The reliability of midazolam in the immediate preoperative period has greatly reduced the need for longer-acting premedicants. $H_2$ blockers raise the pH of gastric fluid[15] and usually decrease gastric volume in patients at risk for aspiration. However, the routine use of histamine blockers for aspiration prophylaxis in patients not at risk is difficult to justify, given their cost.

### The Ideal Agent

The ideal anesthetic agent for spine surgery provides stable hemodynamics with rapid awakening to permit prompt neurologic assessment postoperatively. In addition, it would be beneficial if such an agent conferred some neurologic protection against ischemic injury. Most anesthetic agents in current use have been studied extensively in relation to these goals for intracranial procedures. Few studies, however, have examined their effects specifically on the spinal cord. The following pharmacologic descriptions are based on studies that examined cerebral physiology and cerebral protection primarily.

### Induction

Agents used to induce anesthesia include barbiturates, narcotics, benzodiazepines, and a variety of other unclassified drugs. Since the early 1940s, the barbiturates have been used for this purpose and reliably decrease cerebral blood flow, $CMRO_2$, and ICP. Treatment with barbiturates after a global ischemic event does not appear to provide any neuronal protection. Barbiturate administration after focal or partial ischemic events, however, seems to provide some protection from neurologic injury.[37] These agents have limited use in maintaining anesthesia secondary to their prolonged effects. Most of them depress cardiac output and systemic vascular resistance, so care must be taken when they are given to a hypovolemic or traumatized patient.

### Propofol

Propofol, a sedative hypnotic agent, seems to possess all the benefits of the barbiturates with regard to reduction of cerebral blood flow and $CMRO_2$.[72] Propofol is cleared rapidly and produces prompt awakening in patients shortly after an infusion is discontinued. The autoregulatory capacity of the cerebral circulation remains intact during propofol anesthesia.[17] To date, there is little experimental evidence indicating that propofol provides any significant degree of neurologic protection in temporary focal ischemia models. The only animal study suggesting some protective benefit of propofol in burst suppressive doses failed to measure or control cerebral perfusion pressure.[89]

### Ketamine

Ketamine, a phencyclidine derivative, differs from most induction drugs because it raises cerebral metabolic rate, blood flow, and ICP.[76] It is thus less ideal for neuroanesthesia, but these are desirable properties for use in the hypovolemic patient. Ketamine preserves central circulating volume and afterload in patients with traumatic spinal cord lesions secondary to the release of endogenous catecholamines. However, in severely hypovolemic patients who have exhausted their sympathetic reserve, the bolus administration of ketamine may result in hemodynamic collapse because of its unopposed direct myocardial depressant effects.

### Inhalation Agents

Inhalation anesthetics are the agents used most commonly for the maintenance of general anesthesia. Their mode of delivery and pharmacokinetics allow for controlled, predictable action and easy reversal. They are typically mixed with inspired gases via vaporizers, which are devices that make adjustments for temperature, flow rate, and anesthetic vapor pressure so that a known quantity can be delivered over a wide range of conditions. The inhalation agents act on the brain via an unknown mechanism. Hypothesized mechanisms include membrane protein inhibition and membrane depolarization through membrane swelling or carrier protein inhibition.[45] Anesthetic potency parallels the lipid solubility of the agent. A standard known as the minimum alveolar concentration (MAC) is used as a guide to compare anesthetics of different potency. One MAC of any anesthetic is the end-tidal concentration that will render 50% of patients immobile to the surgical incision. The MAC for different anesthetic agents is additive; 0.5 MAC of nitrous oxide mixed with 1 MAC of isoflurane gives 1.5 MAC of anesthetic.

A number of factors determine the rate of increase of the partial pressure of an anesthetic in the brain, and hence its speed of onset. These factors include the concentration of the anesthetic delivered, solubility of the anesthetic in both the blood and the brain, alveolar ventilation, cardiac output, and presence of intrapulmonary or intracardiac shunts.[70] For example, nitrous oxide is a poorly soluble gas with a MAC of 105% that is routinely delivered in high concentrations (50% to 70%) and has the most rapid onset of action. Isoflurane has intermediate solubility, a MAC of 1.2%, and a slower onset.

The inhalation anesthetics currently in common use include isoflurane, desflurane, and sevoflurane. They all possess cerebral vasodilator properties and decrease blood pressure by reducing either cardiac output or systemic vascular resistance. The increased cerebral blood flow seen with isoflurane can be attenuated by hyperventilation and a reduction in $pCO_2$.[23] Desflurane and sevoflurane are both less soluble in blood than isoflurane and possess the theoretic advantage of more rapid emergence. Their effects on the cerebral vasculature parallel those of isoflurane,[34] although desflurane has been demonstrated to raise cerebrospinal fluid (CSF) pressure via its effects on CSF dynamics.[64] Nitrous oxide is the least potent and most used inhalation agent and exhibits a favorable safety profile in spine surgery. It causes a mild rise in blood pressure and ICP when used alone. It is not clear if any inhalation agent confers specific advantages in spinal cord surgery, and agent choice should be dictated by the overall anesthetic plan.

## Narcotics

Narcotics are used frequently in conjunction with other agents as part of a balanced anesthetic. They provide reliable suppression of the catecholamine response to surgical stimulation and superior analgesia without appreciable changes in spinal cord blood flow. Narcotics also provide a stable background for intraoperative neurophysiologic monitoring. The use of continuous infusion techniques for narcotic administration allows for predictable pharmacokinetics and reliable termination of action at the termination of surgery.

Remifentanil, one of our newest narcotic agents, is unique in that it does not demonstrate any significant accumulation over prolonged periods of infusion. Recovery from remifentanil is essentially dose-independent because of its rapid esterase metabolism.[19] Remifentanil is particularly useful in cases involving SSEP or MEP monitoring as well as any case requiring a total intravenous anesthetic (TIVA). Because of the rapid offset of remifentanil, which is faster than the onset of most other analgesics, care must be taken to provide supplemental analgesics prior to stopping remifentanil in cases where substantial postoperative pain is anticipated.[2]

## Muscle Relaxants

The use of muscle relaxants in spine surgery provides for optimal intubating conditions, an immobile surgical field, and reduces the risk of patient coughing and straining. Muscle relaxants may be broadly classified into two groups: depolarizing and nondepolarizing. Succinylcholine, the only depolarizing agent approved for use in the United States, has a rapid onset and short duration, qualities that make it useful when rapid intubating conditions are desired. This agent actively depolarizes the muscle at the myoneural junction until it becomes refractory to further stimulation. Typically, administration of succinylcholine produces a rise in serum potassium of 0.5mEq/L.[27] Succinylcholine also depolarizes extrajunctional acetylcholine receptors in patients with burns or denervation injuries. These receptors are more numerous and have a greater ionic permeability, leading to acute, profound hyperkalemia when stimulated.[25] The risk of hyperkalemia is greatest after 3 to 7 days post injury and may persist for several years.[59] Life-threatening succinylcholine-induced hyperkalemia has been hypothesized but not reported after immobilization or disuse atrophy in the absence of other causal factors.[5] Succinylcholine is also a triggering agent for malignant hyperthermia and is contraindicated in any patient with a family history of malignant hyperthermia or a history of degenerative muscular disease. The routine use of succinylcholine is also contraindicated in children based on several reports of post-administration hyperkalemic cardiac arrest presumed secondary to unrecognized or undiagnosed muscular dystrophy.

The nondepolarizing muscle relaxants, including pancuronium, vecuronium, atracurium, mivacurium, and rocuronium, differ from one another primarily in onset and durations of action. These agents irreversibly bind to the myoneural junction and competitively inhibit the binding of acetylcholine. The extent of neuromuscular blockade is monitored intraoperatively in a number of ways. The most reliable method is with the use of a train-of-four (TOF) monitor. This device allows for subjective or objective comparison of the ratio of the first and fourth muscle stimuli, which correlates well with the density of receptor occupation. A ratio less than 0.25 correlates with dense paralysis and a ratio greater than 0.75 correlates well with the patient's ability to maintain protective airway reflexes after extubation.[3]

Muscle relaxants provide both optimal intubating conditions during induction of anesthesia and maintenance of muscle relaxation intraoperatively. Paralysis is preferred by some spine surgeons and ensures a quiet operative field. Other surgeons prefer to avoid muscle relaxation so that any direct stimulation of peripheral nerves will be readily apparent (nonparalytic anesthetic intraoperative monitoring).

Muscle relaxation is reversed by the administration of anticholinesterase agents. These agents will reliably reverse a blockade when the effects of the nondepolarizing muscle relaxant have begun to fade. Because these compounds increase acetylcholine levels at all cholinergic receptors, they are usually given in conjunction with a muscarinic anticholinergic drug (e.g., atropine or glycopyrrolate) to prevent unwanted tachycardia, salivation, and bronchial secretions.

The most important factors that affect the ability to reverse muscle relaxation are the depth of block at the time of reversal, choice and method of administration of relaxant, and the dose of reversal agent. Other factors that may antagonize the ability to reverse a nondepolarizing blockade include hypothermia, metabolic acidosis, respiratory alkalosis, and the administration of certain antibiotics.[62] As previously mentioned, reversal is followed with the TOF monitor. The best clinical assessment of adequate reversal is the ability of the patient to sustain an unassisted head lift for at least 5 seconds. Assessment of less cooperative patients can be carried out by observing the negative inspiratory force generated during spontaneous ventilation. A negative inspiratory force of less than approximately 25cm of water correlates well with adequate reversal but not airway protection.[69]

## Monitoring

### General Monitoring

The single most important monitors in the operating room are the anesthesia providers. They are responsible for collecting and analyzing both subjective and objective data about the patient's vital organ function. The perioperative use of monitoring equipment greatly enhances their ability to perform this vital function. Routine monitoring during spine surgery includes electrocardiography, noninvasive blood pressure measurement, pulse oximetry, end tidal carbon dioxide, temperature, urine output, neuromuscular blockade, and the auscultation of breath and heart sounds. More invasive forms of hemodynamic monitoring may be indicated based on the complexity of the operative procedure or the severity of coexisting disease. Electrocardiographic monitoring is useful to detect myocardial ischemia and cardiac conduction disturbances and in the analysis of arrhythmias.

Patients with both acute and chronic cervical spine injuries may show symptoms of a variety of specific electrocardiographic abnormalities. These abnormalities have been attributed to the autonomic imbalance created by disruption of sympathetic pathways located in the cervical cord. Severe acute cervical spine injury is frequently associated with marked sinus bradycardia. It also carries an increased incidence of ventricular and supraventricular arrhythmias, as well as cardiac arrest, when compared with injury of the thoracolumbar spine.[50] Multilead ST-segment elevation has been noted in a significant percentage of patients with chronic, complete SCI. These alterations in ventricular repolarization are hypothesized to be manifestations of central sympathetic dysfunction and, indeed, resolve with low-dose isoproterenol infusion.[51]

Systemic blood pressure is used as an indirect monitor of organ perfusion. For the majority of elective spine procedures, noninvasive blood pressure monitoring is adequate and sufficient. Invasive monitoring of arterial blood pressure is recommended for patients with a history of significant cardiopulmonary disease, those with preoperative hemodynamic instability, those in whom induced hypotension is to be used, and those who may require a period of postoperative ventilatory support when frequent blood gas measurements are anticipated.

Central monitoring of venous or pulmonary artery pressure may be indicated in patients with a history of ischemic heart disease or left ventricular dysfunction, particularly in the setting of anticipated large blood loss or fluid shifts. In patients with normal cardiac function, central venous pressures provide an adequate estimate of left ventricular end-diastolic volume. A pulmonary artery catheter, however, may provide a more accurate assessment of left ventricular volume in patients with ventricular dysfunction. Acute cervical spine injury with spinal shock is associated with substantial hemodynamic lability and a high incidence of left ventricular dysfunction.[56] These patients are less tolerant of aggressive fluid replacement and more prone to develop pulmonary edema. The acutely quadriplegic patient qualified for surgery should be monitored with both an arterial line and either a central venous or pulmonary artery catheter.

In the majority of spine surgery patients, their intravascular volume status can be monitored without invasive central monitoring techniques. For those patients in whom central monitoring is necessary, two practical points should be considered. First, long-arm placement of central lines is the preferred approach to cervical spine procedures because it allows for optimal field avoidance.

Second, the absolute accuracy of central monitoring in general, and pulmonary wedge pressures in particular, is questionable in positions other than supine. This may impact the decision of whether or not central monitoring is employed.

## Neurophysiologic Monitoring
### The Awake Patient

The awake patient is the ultimate spinal cord monitor. There are several case reports describing the use of local anesthesia for spine surgery in the awake patient, although it is not a common means of neurologic monitoring. Chang[12] and Drummond et al.[21] both describe the use of anesthesia by local infiltration for dorsal cervical osteotomy. From these descriptions it appears that at least a short period of unconsciousness may be required because of significant discomfort associated with the fracturing of the anterior longitudinal ligament. Zigler et al.[90] presented a series of 34 consecutive cases of dorsal cervical stabilization and fusion in patients with unstable cervical spines and variable degrees of neurologic injury using local anesthesia in conjunction with light sedation. They encountered no untoward complications and found that the technique was well tolerated by patients, although occasionally bone graft harvesting under local anesthesia was uncomfortable.

### The Wake-Up Test

In 1973, Vauzelle et al.[84] described their use of an intraoperative "wake-up" with observation of limb movement for the assessment of spinal cord function. This simple test is an excellent monitor of gross motor function and is used most commonly during surgical procedures involving spinal column instrumentation and distraction. Its use is based on clinical evidence that neural impairment resulting from distraction is reversible when the distracting forces are modified during its early phase.[21,33] Currently, an awake patient is the only available monitoring modality to provide unequivocal intraoperative documentation of intact motor function.

An advantage of the wake-up test over more highly technical forms of neurophysiologic monitoring is that specialized equipment or ancillary monitoring personnel are unnecessary. Two limitations are that the patient can only be awakened intermittently and, therefore, the anesthesiologist and surgeon are restricted to a few spot checks of the integrity of motor pathways. It is possible that neurologic impairment may occur despite a successful wake-up test. Diaz and Lockhart[20] reported one case of unresolved paraplegia after a normal wake-up test. This test may be difficult or impossible to perform in young children, patients with cognitive difficulties, and those with significant hearing impairment. A number of complications of this technique have been described, including dislodgement of spinal hardware, displacement of intravenous lines and monitors, accidental extubation, air embolism, and the possibility of intraoperative recall. These complications appear to be uncommon in the clinical setting, although they are always a reason for concern.[33,80]

The most important factors contributing to the successful performance of an intraoperative wake-up include adequate preoperative rehearsal with the patient and good intraoperative communication between the surgeon and anesthesiologist about the timing of the wake-up. There are a wide variety of anesthetic techniques that can provide suitable conditions, namely a patient who is free of discomfort, is able to follow commands, and has amnesia for the event. A common technique is a nitrous oxide/narcotic/relaxant-based anesthetic with the addition of a low-dose volatile agent as needed. Frequently, a narcotic infusion provides better control of analgesia and timing of the wake-up. Other possibilities include the use of a nitrous oxide/narcotic/relaxant technique in conjunction with a propofol infusion or a total intravenous anesthetic using propofol and remifentanil infusions. The choice of anesthetic may be influenced and/or limited by the concurrent use of evoked potential monitoring.

The general procedure for an intraoperative wake-up is as follows. The wake-up protocol is reviewed in detail with the patient preoperatively. If a nitrous oxide/narcotic/relaxant technique is used, the narcotics, relaxant, and any background volatile agent are discontinued approximately 30 minutes before the anticipated wake-up. The muscle relaxation is monitored using a nerve stimulator and, if necessary, reversal may be given. As a rule, patients become responsive shortly after the discontinuation of the nitrous oxide. Patients are first asked to grip the anesthesiologist's hand to assess their ability to respond to commands, and then to flex and extend their feet within the direct vision of the surgical team. It is helpful to provide some gentle restraint of their head and arms in case struggling should occur. One should always be prepared to administer a bolus dose of a sedative/hypnotic agent immediately if struggling becomes problematic. The risk of air embolism may be minimized if the wound is packed and flooded with irrigating solution. Generally, the choice of anesthetic matters far less than the skill and attention with which it is administered.

### Nonparalytic Anesthesia/Intraoperative Monitoring

The provision of anesthesia without the use of muscle relaxants has become increasingly popular during spine surgery. This technique provides the surgical team with a real-time means of monitoring the effects of electrocautery and surgical manipulation on neural tissues. It also presents anesthesiologists with some of their most significant problems. Without paralysis, anesthesiologists lose their "safety net" to prevent patient movement during periods of mismatch between the level of anesthesia and the level of surgical stimulation. In other words, a greater degree of vigilance is required to maintain a quiet surgical field when muscle relaxants are not used.

### Somatosensory Spinal Evoked Potentials

Somatosensory spinal evoked potentials (SSEPs) are the electrophysiologic responses of the central nervous system to stimulation of a peripheral nerve. SSEPs may be categorized as either peripheral, spinal, subcortical, or cortical, based on the location of the recording site. Clinically, cortical SSEPs are the most commonly used, with the stimulus applied to either the posterior tibial, peroneal, and/or median nerves.

Interpretation of SSEP data is based on changes in response amplitude and latency. Amplitude is defined as the vertical dimension of the waveform and can be measured as the difference between two peaks of opposite polarity or between a specific peak and a reference point of zero potential. Latency is defined as the elapsed time between the stimulus and the response. Apel et al.[4] considered a clinically significant change in SSEPs to have occurred if latency was increased by 10% or amplitude was reduced by at least 50%. Owen,[67] however, believes that an interpretation criterion of 50% for amplitude reduction may be too sensitive and may result in unnecessary false-positive findings. He recommends that the surgeon be informed of degraded data if latency increases more than 10% or amplitude decreases more than 60% relative to baseline.

The clinical usefulness of SSEPs lies in their ability to demonstrate the functional integrity of neural pathways in an anesthetized and presumably unresponsive patient. Grundy et al.[30,31] have shown that intraoperative SSEPs are very sensitive indicators of hypoxia and ischemia associated with spine manipulation. Numerous cases have been reported in which early recognition of SSEP changes appeared to have prevented permanent neurologic damage by alerting the surgeon to the need for appropriate corrective action. There are also several case reports of false-negative SSEPs in which postoperative neurologic deficits occurred with preserved intraoperative waveforms.[6,53]

There are several reasons why SSEP monitoring may not always be reliable. Because SSEPs primarily assess posterior column function, false-negative results may occur if the neural injury is located outside the tract being monitored, that is, the anterior motor tracts. Alternatively, technical problems may result in suboptimal recordings leading to undetected changes, or a deficit may be a result of a slowly progressive structural change that began, but was not detectable, intraoperatively. As with many monitoring modalities, SSEPs appear to be reasonably reliable but not perfect.

In the operating room, baseline SSEPs should be recorded after the induction of anesthesia and skin incision. Serial intraoperative recordings are obtained and should always be interpreted relative to these baseline measurements. If significant changes are noted in the SSEPs, a review of the monitoring equipment and all temporally related surgical and anesthetic events should ensue. Physiologic alterations that may impact SSEPs include hypotension, hypothermia, anemia, hypoxemia, and changes in arterial $pCO_2$. Changes in the depth of anesthesia may have profound effects on evoked potential waveforms, and every effort should be made to avoid alterations in the inhaled gas concentration and/or bolus injection of hypnotic agents during periods of risk. If the SSEP changes persist without adequate explanation, the possibility of injury to neural tissues exists and a wake-up test should be performed.

The preferred anesthetic for SSEP monitoring is one that allows for the recording of adequate baseline waveforms and avoids rapid alterations in anesthetic depth during the course of the surgical procedure. Many techniques satisfy these requirements but the most commonly used anesthetic is a balanced $O_2/N_2O$/narcotic technique with low-dose isoflurane supplementation (no more than 1%). Although this regimen decreases the amplitude of SSEPs, most believe that it is compatible with effective monitoring. The use of a continuous narcotic infusion will have the least effect on evoked potential monitoring and provides additional hemodynamic stability to any anesthetic regimen. As noted in Table 139.1, intravenous agents generally have only modest effects on SSEPs, whereas volatile agents, such as isoflurane, attenuate the SSEP waveforms in a dose-dependent fashion. Care must be taken to maintain isoflurane concentrations at the lowest practical level.

SSEP monitoring has been associated with several unique complications. Legatt and Frost[49] reported electrocardiogram artifact produced by the triggering of the pacer enhancement circuitry in the electrocardiogram monitor by the somatosensory stimuli. Merritt et al.[61] described a case of pacemaker-mediated tachycardia induced by intraoperative SSEP stimuli. The tachycardia and associated hypotension were a result of mistaken interpretation by the programmable pacemaker of the SSEP stimulus as its own intrinsic atrial event.

### Motor Evoked Potentials

Motor evoked potentials (MEPs) are the electrical activity measured in peripheral nerves and muscles after cortical or spinal stimulation. MEPs appear to provide a useful measure of the functional integrity of motor pathways. Theoretically, when used in conjunction with SSEPs, they allow for the monitoring of both motor and sensory pathways in the anesthetized patient and may provide more complete information about neural integrity.

MEPs may be categorized as either transcranial or spinal, depending on the location of the stimulating electrode. The stimulus may be either electrical or magnetic, with electrical stimulation being the most commonly used. The same interpretation criteria used for SSEPs of 60% loss of amplitude and 10% prolongation of latency may also be used for MEPs.[68]

MEPs are extraordinarily sensitive to anesthetic agents. Transcranial MEPs are more sensitive than spinal cord MEPs. The anesthetic techniques normally used during the monitoring of SSEPs are not compatible with MEP

| TABLE 139.1 | | |
| --- | --- | --- |
| **Effects of Anesthetic Agents on Somatosensory Spinal Evoked Potentials (SSEPs)** | | |
| **Agent** | **Amplitude** | **Latency** |
| Isoflurane | Decrease | Increase |
| Nitrous oxide | Decrease | Minimal change |
| Propofol | Minimal change | Increase |
| Pentothal | Mild decrease | Increase |
| Ketamine | Increase | Increase |
| Etomidate | Marked increase | Increase |
| Fentanyl | Minimal increase | Mild increase |
| Midazolam | Decrease | Minimal increase |

monitoring. Volatile anesthetics, nitrous oxide, and sodium pentothal all cause significant depression of MEPs.[28,39,40,54] Ketamine, etomidate, propofol, and narcotic agents appear to produce less significant changes.[48] The bolus injection of any of these agents during MEP monitoring may cause a transient decrease in amplitude, suggesting that continuous infusion techniques are preferable to repeated boluses.[41] The most common anesthetic currently used at our institution to provide adequate monitoring conditions for MEPs is a total intravenous anesthetic technique using propofol and remifentanil infusions.

A controlled level of neuromuscular blockade (90% reduction in twitch), as provided by an infusion of a neuromuscular blocking agent, permits recording of compound muscle action potentials while eliminating motor activity that could interfere with surgery.[1] However, our neuromonitoring team feels that the complete avoidance of neuromuscular blockade provides the optimal conditions for monitoring motor evoked potentials.

## Anesthetic Techniques

With increasing numbers of diagnostic and therapeutic procedures performed in an outpatient setting, demands for safe, short-acting analgesia from the anesthesia care team have increased. The concepts of monitored anesthesia care and conscious sedation have developed from these needs. Many drugs or techniques may be used. The most common drugs for sedation are intravenous narcotics, benzodiazepines, or an infusion of propofol. The essential aspects of care dictate that appropriate monitors of ventilation, oxygenation, and sedation are used, and that someone skilled in airway management is given the sole task of monitoring the patient during the procedure.

### Regional Anesthesia

Regional anesthesia may be used for spine procedures, including lumbar discectomy. Advantages include an awake patient at the end of surgery, a lower incidence of postoperative nausea and vomiting, and more complete suppression of the stress response to surgery. Typically, with spinal anesthesia an intermediate-acting local anesthetic such as bupivacaine is used. The disadvantage of using spinal anesthesia for spine procedures is the discomfort some patients may experience with prolonged prone positioning. The anesthesiologist may be concerned about emergent airway management in a prone patient, should problems arise during surgery. When spine surgeons and anesthesia personnel are knowledgeable in this technique, however, they use regional anesthesia with great safety and patient satisfaction.

### Regional Analgesia

Regional analgesia is a useful adjunct for the management of postoperative pain after thoracic or lumbar spine surgery. Epidural or intrathecal morphine provides long-lasting analgesia and improved pulmonary mechanics with fewer systemic side effects than if given intravenously. Patients receiving neuraxial opioids require some sort of monitoring for respiratory depression, a rare but potentially fatal side effect.

## General Anesthesia

Given the location and positioning requirements, most procedures that involve the spine are performed under general anesthesia. After appropriate preoperative evaluation and premedication, uncomplicated patients qualified for general anesthesia are preoxygenated with 100% oxygen for several minutes before induction. This maneuver denitrogenates the patient so that if gas exchange is impaired after induction of anesthesia, more time will be available for airway management efforts before desaturation. After routine monitors are applied, the patient is given an intravenous induction agent. Usually, this is a short-acting barbiturate or propofol. Narcotics may be added to further blunt the hemodynamic response to laryngoscopy. A short-, intermediate-, or long-acting muscle relaxant is then administered and the TOF monitor is observed for desired suppression of twitch height. If the patient has a history of gastroesophageal reflux, symptomatic hiatal hernia, prior gastric surgery, gastroparesis, or recent food ingestion, a rapid sequence induction may be selected. In this case, the induction agent and rapid-onset muscle relaxant are given simultaneously without bag-mask ventilation. Endotracheal intubation can usually be accomplished within 60 seconds of patients losing their airway reflexes. Correct endotracheal tube position is then confirmed by auscultation of breath sounds and documenting the presence of end-tidal carbon dioxide in the expired gases. The endotracheal tube is secured, the eyes are protected, and the patient is positioned for surgery.

After induction, the patient is usually given an inhalation agent or continuous intravenous infusion for the maintenance of anesthesia with or without further muscle relaxation. Gas exchange, systemic perfusion, and body temperature are monitored frequently throughout the case. At the end of the procedure, the maintenance agents are discontinued, muscle relaxation is reversed, and the patient is extubated after adequate strength and responsiveness can be demonstrated. The patient is transported to the recovery room for continued monitoring of vital signs.

## Airway Management

The inability to manage a patient's airway successfully has resulted in as many as 30% of intraoperative deaths attributable to anesthesia.[11] More than 85% of all respiratory-related malpractice claims result in neurologic damage or death. Effective airway management in the patient qualified for spine surgery must account for any abnormalities in airway anatomy as well as any potential or known instability in the cervical spine.

## Preoperative Evaluation

Preoperative evaluation of the airway can be accomplished using three relatively simple tests that predict the difficulty of orotracheal intubation. The quality of visualization of the dorsal pharynx, when the patient faces the examiner in a neutral position with tongue protruded, predicts the difficulty of visualization of the airway during laryngoscopy.[16,58] In addition, if the distance between the thyroid cartilage and the end of the mandible is greater than 7cm, adequate space is usually available for ventral displacement of the tongue during visualization.[26] The third parameter is an assessment of atlantooccipital mobility. Adequate neck extension ensures that proper alignment of the oral, pharyngeal, and laryngeal axes can be obtained.

## The Difficult Intubation

The probability that a patient will be difficult, if not impossible, to intubate increases within certain disease states. The most common of these are (1) congenital facial and upper airway deformities, (2) maxillofacial trauma, (3) airway tumors and any known or suspected need for cervical spine immobility secondary to prior surgery, and (4) degenerative disease or trauma to the cervical spine. When patients appear to be difficult to intubate, it is advisable to secure additional information while they are still awake. Using topical anesthesia, one may perform gentle laryngoscopy to determine whether the laryngeal view will be adequate. If any uncertainty remains at this juncture, awake fiber-optic intubation should be used.

The American Society of Anesthesiologists has developed an algorithm that is designed to facilitate appropriate airway management during rapidly evolving clinical situations[7] (Figure 139.1). Patients who are known to be difficult to intubate are much less likely to suffer morbidity secondary to airway management because proper preparations can be made before the delivery of anesthesia. Awake fiber-optic intubation under light sedation and airway topicalization allows the anesthesiologist to definitively secure the airway while the patient is spontaneously ventilating. In addition, retrograde intubation via a guidewire fed through the cricothyroid membrane and out the upper airway may be used as a guide for intubation during spontaneous ventilation. The retrograde technique is most useful in patients with significant maxillofacial trauma in whom visualization of the airway with a fiber-optic scope may be quite difficult because of the presence of blood and secretions.

Sometimes a difficult airway is not recognized in advance and general anesthesia is induced in the usual fashion. An immediate decision for the best management strategy centers on the ability to maintain oxygenation and ventilation through a mask airway. If the patient can be ventilated with ease using a mask and positive pressure, there is obviously more time to allow for positioning and gathering of personnel and equipment to facilitate intubation. In situations when the patient cannot be ventilated with a mask or intubated, one must quickly provide oxygenation from a site below the oral aperture. This is accomplished most easily by the placement of a large-bore intravenous catheter into the trachea via the cricothyroid membrane. The catheter is then connected to a high-flow gas injection system, such as a jet ventilator. Jet ventilation provides oxygenation until the patient is intubated or a cricothyroidotomy can be performed.

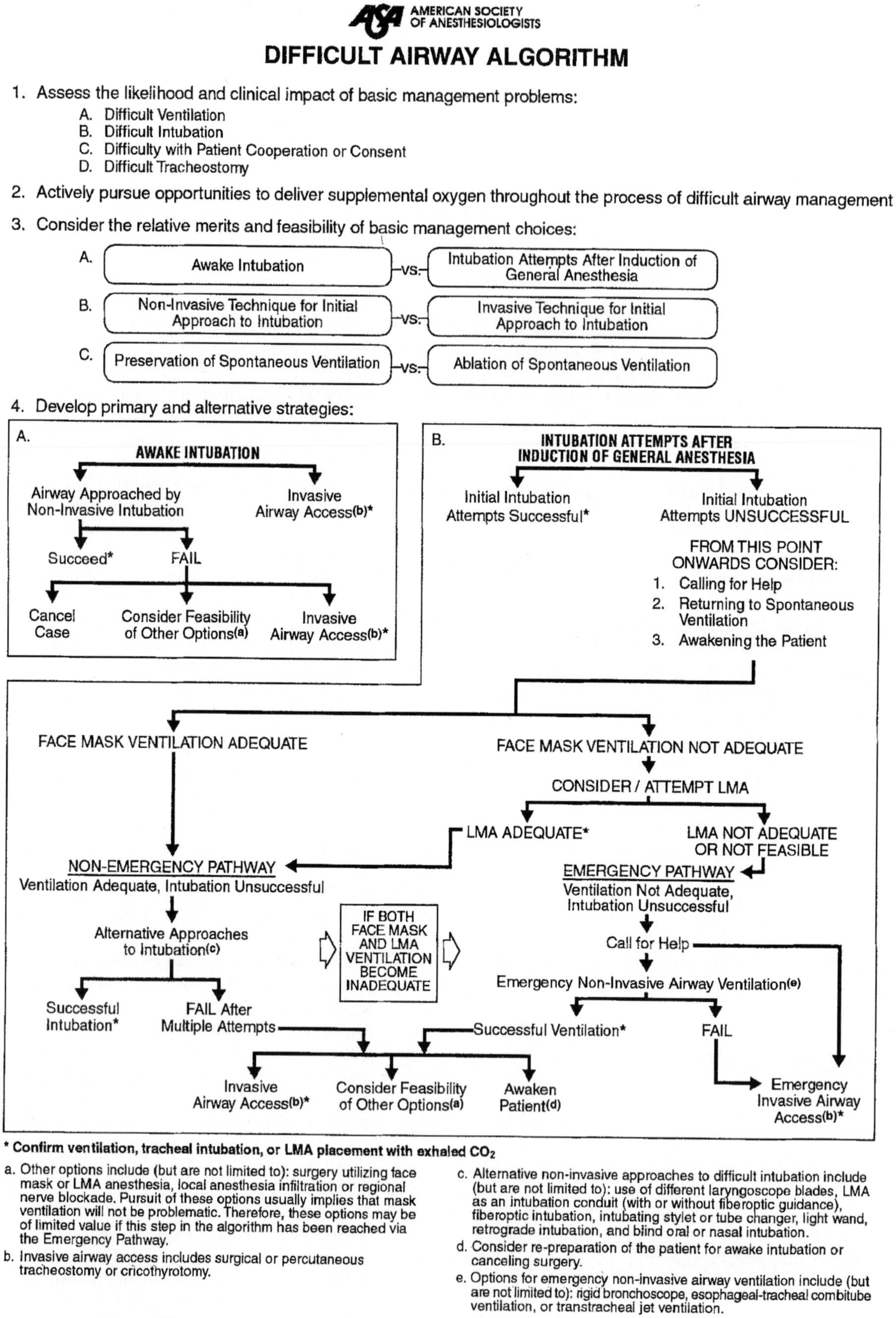

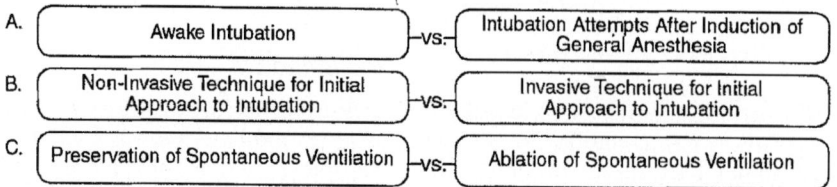

## DIFFICULT AIRWAY ALGORITHM

1. Assess the likelihood and clinical impact of basic management problems:
   - A. Difficult Ventilation
   - B. Difficult Intubation
   - C. Difficulty with Patient Cooperation or Consent
   - D. Difficult Tracheostomy

2. Actively pursue opportunities to deliver supplemental oxygen throughout the process of difficult airway management

3. Consider the relative merits and feasibility of basic management choices:

   - A. [ Awake Intubation ] -vs- [ Intubation Attempts After Induction of General Anesthesia ]
   - B. [ Non-Invasive Technique for Initial Approach to Intubation ] -vs- [ Invasive Technique for Initial Approach to Intubation ]
   - C. [ Preservation of Spontaneous Ventilation ] -vs- [ Ablation of Spontaneous Ventilation ]

4. Develop primary and alternative strategies:

**A. AWAKE INTUBATION**

Airway Approached by Non-Invasive Intubation     Invasive Airway Access(b)*

Succeed*     FAIL

Cancel Case     Consider Feasibility of Other Options(a)     Invasive Airway Access(b)*

**B. INTUBATION ATTEMPTS AFTER INDUCTION OF GENERAL ANESTHESIA**

Initial Intubation Attempts Successful*     Initial Intubation Attempts UNSUCCESSFUL

FROM THIS POINT ONWARDS CONSIDER:
1. Calling for Help
2. Returning to Spontaneous Ventilation
3. Awakening the Patient

**FACE MASK VENTILATION ADEQUATE**     **FACE MASK VENTILATION NOT ADEQUATE**

CONSIDER / ATTEMPT LMA

LMA ADEQUATE*     LMA NOT ADEQUATE OR NOT FEASIBLE

**NON-EMERGENCY PATHWAY** Ventilation Adequate, Intubation Unsuccessful

**EMERGENCY PATHWAY** Ventilation Not Adequate, Intubation Unsuccessful

Alternative Approaches to Intubation(c)

IF BOTH FACE MASK AND LMA VENTILATION BECOME INADEQUATE

Call for Help

Emergency Non-Invasive Airway Ventilation(e)

Successful Intubation*     FAIL After Multiple Attempts

Successful Ventilation*     FAIL

Invasive Airway Access(b)*     Consider Feasibility of Other Options(a)     Awaken Patient(d)

Emergency Invasive Airway Access(b)*

* Confirm ventilation, tracheal intubation, or LMA placement with exhaled $CO_2$

a. Other options include (but are not limited to): surgery utilizing face mask or LMA anesthesia, local anesthesia infiltration or regional nerve blockade. Pursuit of these options usually implies that mask ventilation will not be problematic. Therefore, these options may be of limited value if this step in the algorithm has been reached via the Emergency Pathway.

b. Invasive airway access includes surgical or percutaneous tracheostomy or cricothyrotomy.

c. Alternative non-invasive approaches to difficult intubation include (but are not limited to): use of different laryngoscope blades, LMA as an intubation conduit (with or without fiberoptic guidance), fiberoptic intubation, intubating stylet or tube changer, light wand, retrograde intubation, and blind oral or nasal intubation.

d. Consider re-preparation of the patient for awake intubation or canceling surgery.

e. Options for emergency non-invasive airway ventilation include (but are not limited to): rigid bronchoscope, esophageal-tracheal combitube ventilation, or transtracheal jet ventilation.

**Figure 139.1** American Society of Anesthesiologists' difficult airway algorithm.

## The Laryngeal Mask Airway

A relatively recent and useful adjunct to airway management is the laryngeal mask airway (LMA).[8] The LMA consists of a reusable silicon tube fused at a 30-degree angle to a soft, spoon-shaped mask that, when positioned above the airway and inflated, stents open the airway above the epiglottis (Figure 139.2). The advantage of this device as an adjunct to the management of the difficult airway is that it may be inserted blindly and rapidly into the airway, producing acceptable gas exchange in most instances. It may then be used to facilitate fiber-optic or blind endotracheal intubation. One potential disadvantage of the LMA in patients qualified for spine surgery is the need for cervical spine extension during placement, although the success rate of placement of the device with the head in a neutral position in experienced hands has been reported to be as high as 95%.[9] The LMA does not provide protection against the aspiration of stomach contents and is, therefore, contraindicated in elective airway management of the patient at risk for aspiration.

## The Patient with Cervical Spine Injury

In patients with potential or known cervical spine injury, airway management must be dictated by the acuity of the situation. Patients who require immediate intervention secondary to hemodynamic instability, acute respiratory failure, inability to protect their airway, or elevated intracranial pressure probably are best managed with bag and mask assisted ventilation followed by tracheal intubation with direct laryngoscopy. Usually, this can be safely accomplished with in-line stabilization of the neck in a neutral position. The risk of neurologic complications from direct laryngoscopy in patients with unstable cervical spines has not been quantified, but is probably quite low. Atlantoaxial extension with minimal movement of the lower cervical spine has been demon-

strated during laryngoscopy in anesthetized patients.[57] Movement of the cervical spine is also significantly reduced when in-line stabilization is performed during laryngoscopy.[36] There are several studies in the literature that showed no neurologic deterioration in patients with known cervical spine injuries after direct laryngoscopy with stabilization of the cervical spine,[13,73,78,81] and Holly[38] reported similar safety with nasotracheal intubation. Although the risk of neurologic injury secondary to direct laryngoscopy is low, it is not zero. Recent studies of different intubation strategies on cervical spine motion suggest potential advantages with the use of fiber-optic bronchoscopy as well as the Bullard laryngoscope.[14,35,86]

## The Patient with Rheumatoid Arthritis

Airway abnormalities in patients with rheumatoid arthritis deserve special mention. In addition to having atlantooccipital instability, these patients may exhibit scoliotic deformities of the larynx and trachea, making intubation difficult even with a fiber-optic bronchoscope.[42] Arthritic changes of the cricoarytenoid joint associated with this disease have been reported as a source of upper airway obstruction in these patients postextubation.[71]

## Extubation

Extubation of the patient with a difficult airway should proceed with caution. Extra care must be taken to ensure that the effects of all respiratory depressant anesthetics are removed and that the patient has fully recovered from any neuromuscular blockade. This can be assessed most effectively by examining the patient's ability to maintain a voluntary head lift for greater than 5 seconds. This maneuver correlates well with the ability to maintain protective airway reflexes postextubation and to cough effectively.[69] When there are doubts about the integrity of the airway resulting from surgical trauma, altered anatomy, hematoma formation, facial edema, or neurologic injury, prudence would dictate a period of postoperative mechanical ventilation with the patient in a head-elevated position until full recovery. Then it is possible to topicalize the trachea and extubate the patient under direct vision using the fiber-optic bronchoscope to assess airway integrity. A guidewire or intubating stylette may be left in place in the patient's airway after extubation to facilitate reintubation, if needed.[7]

There are several case reports of upper airway obstruction after multilevel cervical corpectomies.[24] The etiology of the airway compromise is unclear but may relate to severe hypopharyngeal and supraglottic swelling secondary to either disruption of lymphatic drainage during the operative dissection, inflammation, and/or venous obstruction from small blood clots. Some centers have developed guidelines to minimize postoperative airway complications in these patients. This includes 48 hours of postoperation intubation if a multilevel corpectomy is performed, or if operative time exceeds 5 hours.[10] Intermittent retractor release throughout the surgical procedure may help prevent this complication.

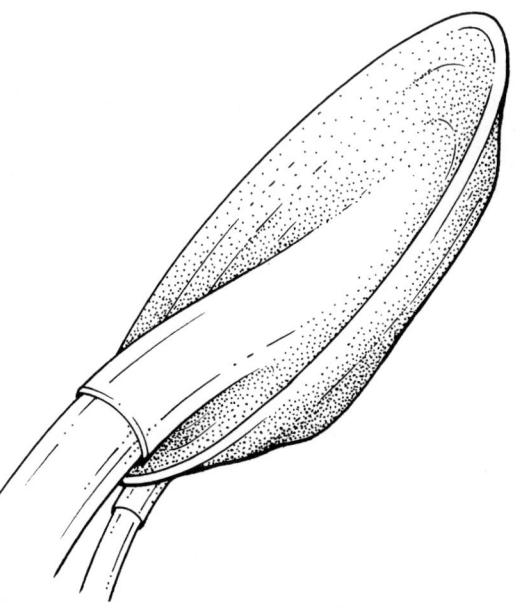

**Figure 139.2** Laryngeal mask airway.

# Positioning

Surgery on the spine may be performed with the patient in a variety of positions including, but not limited to, the lateral, prone, knee-chest, Concorde, or sitting position. Proper positioning and careful padding of the patient is of utmost importance and may occupy a significant period of time after the induction of anesthesia. When the patient is moved out of the supine position, the risk of positioning-related nerve and soft-tissue injury increases dramatically. The time spent padding and checking all pressure points is time well spent and should be a priority for all those in the operating room.

## Peripheral Nerve Injury

Brachial plexus injury accounts for the greatest number of positioning-related peripheral nerve injuries. The brachial plexus is very susceptible to both excessive compression and stretch injury. Arms should not be abducted more than 90 degrees, and care should be taken to keep supports and axillary rolls well away from the axilla. The ulnar nerve is the most common nerve injury of the upper extremity and the ulnar groove should be well padded and protected at all times. The peroneal nerve is the most common nerve injury of the lower extremity because of its vulnerable course as it wraps around the head of the fibula. Care should be taken to avoid any pressure over this area. The head should be positioned to avoid pressure on the ears, eyes, and nose. Excessive extension or torsion of the neck should also be limited. When the patient is in position, breasts and genitalia should be checked to guard against the possibility of compression or abrasion injury.

## Postoperative Visual Loss

Postoperative visual loss (POVL) after spine surgery is a relatively rare event that, unfortunately, has been reported with increasing frequency over the past 5 to 10 years.[47,79,85] Concern regarding the apparent increased reporting frequency of this event led the ASA Committee on Professional Liability to establish the ASA Postoperative Visual Loss Registry in July 1999. The Registry collects detailed information on cases of POVL in an effort to better define intraoperative risk factors and patient characteristics that may predispose a patient to this perioperative complication.[47] Anonymous reporting is encouraged and the standardized, anonymous case report form can be accessed via the internet at www.asaclosedclaims.org under the POVL Registry subheading.[47]

The precise etiology of POVL is not well understood but is most likely a multifactorial phenomenon. Suggested contributing factors include hypotension, large blood loss, high-volume fluid resuscitation, anemia, direct ocular pressure, head dependent position, long operative time, and the presence of vascular disease. Review of the POVL Registry data as of Winter 2001[47] shows that the majority of cases reported involved patients in the prone position for spine procedures (Figure 139.3). The most common type of ophthalmic lesion associated with POVL is ischemic optic neuropathy (90%) with only 6% of cases associated with central retinal artery occlusion. Based on

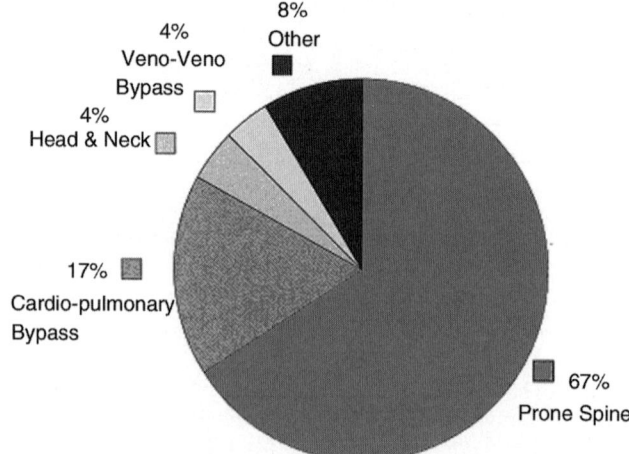

Figure 139.3  Percentage of cases in the ASA POVL Registry associated with a particular operation (n = 47). (From Lee L: ASA postoperative visual loss (POVL) registry. Anesthesia Patient Safety Foundation Newsletter 16(4):56-57, Winter 2001-2002.)

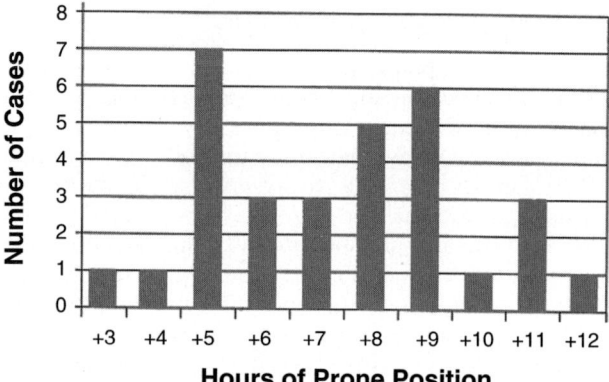

Figure 139.4  ASA POVL Registry data: number of cases of visual loss versus duration of prone position (n = 31). (From Lee L: ASA postoperative visual loss (POVL) registry. Anesthesia Patient Safety Foundation Newsletter 16(4):56-57, Winter 2001-2002.)

their data, the incidence of POVL appears to increase with increased time spent in the prone position (Figure 139.4) and occurs across all age ranges (Figure 139.5). Younger age does not appear to guarantee protection against this complication. It should be noted that the Registry does not contain denominator data of all cases of prone spine surgery; therefore, definitive conclusions regarding risk cannot be made.[47]

## The Sitting Position

The sitting position provides the anesthesiologist with some very unique challenges. It provides some distinct advantages for the surgeon but poses some risk to the patient including cardiac instability, venous air embolism, and quadriplegia. The sitting position can induce significant venous pooling, which may lead to severe hypotension. This problem may be attenuated by judicious fluid administration, the use of compressive stockings, the slow

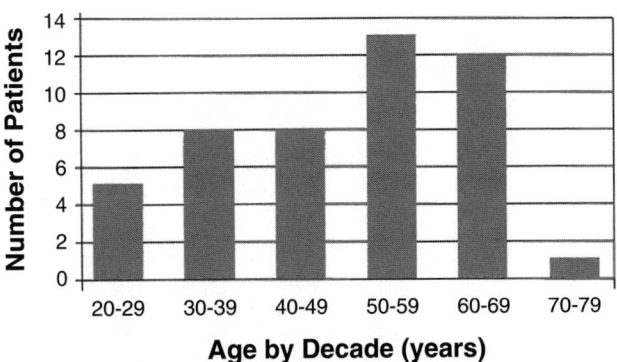

**Figure 139.5** ASA POVL Registry data: number of patients per decade of age with postoperative visual loss. *(From Lee L: ASA postoperative visual loss (POVL) registry. Anesthesia Patient Safety Foundation Newsletter 16(4):56-57, Winter 2001-2002.)*

assumption of the sitting position, and maintenance of the knees at the chest level. Contraindications to the sitting position include: (1) documented patent foramen ovale or right-to-left shunt, (2) cerebral ischemia in the upright position while awake, and (3) cardiac instability.

Venous air embolism is one of the most feared complications of the sitting position. The incidence of air embolism during spine surgery in the sitting position appears to be substantially less than that during intracranial procedures in the sitting position (7% vs. 43%).[55] The most sensitive monitors for venous air embolism include $ETCO_2$, $ETN_2$, the precordial Doppler and, most sensitive of all, the transesophageal echocardiogram. A long-arm central venous line is routinely placed for aspiration of air should an embolus occur. It may be accurately positioned just below the junction of the superior vena cava and the right atrium under electrocardiographic guidance within a matter of minutes.[18] Treatment of an air embolus involves the identification of the source, flooding the field to prevent further influx of air, aspiration of air through the central venous line, discontinuation of nitrous oxide to avoid expansion of the air bubbles, and supportive therapy with fluids and pressors.

### Spinal Cord Infarction

Cervical spinal cord infarction is a rare injury but may occur secondary to extreme flexion or inadequate spinal cord perfusion pressure. Over-aggressive flexion may also result in facial swelling and macroglossia requiring postoperative intubation for airway control. Confirmation that two fingers fit between the chin and the chest once the patient has been positioned will help to avoid these complications.

### Fluid and Blood Therapy

Goals of fluid management in anesthesia for spine surgery include the maintenance of adequate plasma volume to preserve spinal cord perfusion pressure while avoiding decreases in plasma oncotic pressure and interstitial fluid accumulation. Fluid replacement can be accomplished with isotonic crystalloid solutions, colloid preparations, or blood products to satisfy these goals. Glucose-containing solutions should be avoided in the absence of documented hypoglycemia because of their demonstrated ability to worsen neurologic outcome following temporary focal ischemia.[22] Hypertonic saline has been used with a safety record similar to isotonic fluids and provides more rapid restoration of intravascular volume after trauma.[83]

### Blood Loss and Replacement

When blood losses become greater than one blood volume, many patients develop a progressive increase in bleeding from all sites. Presumably this occurs due to dilution of circulating procoagulants and platelets. In 1984, at a National Institutes of Health (NIH) consensus conference, the group concluded that during massive transfusion, the component required most frequently when increased bleeding occurred was not fresh frozen plasma but platelets.[65] Thrombocytopenia or a qualitative platelet dysfunction is probably the most likely cause of bleeding even in the presence of elevated prothrombin and partial thromboplastin times.[63] With the exception of surgical hemostasis, disseminated intravascular coagulation is the most common unanticipated cause for major bleeding in patients without an underlying coagulopathy.

Given the worldwide concern over the risks of transfusion-related infectious disease transmission, much work and development has taken place to minimize the administration of donated blood products. Currently, only 2% to 5% of transfusions in the United States are of autologous blood. Units of blood when donated and preserved with ADSOL have a shelf life of 42 days, making preoperative anemia after donation less of a concern. The aggressive preoperative administration of adequate iron supplements and erythropoietin could reduce requirements greatly for allogeneic blood.

There is debate over the optimal hematocrit for surgical procedures,[75] and this mystical value has drifted downward over time.[87] Acute normovolemic hemodilution remains a safe and effective means of intraoperative blood conservation in those patients expected to have blood losses of 1 to 2L. Reduction in hematocrit reduces the oxygen-carrying capacity of blood, thus decreasing the "margin of safety" of effective oxygen transport. However, this reduction in hematocrit also causes a reduction in viscosity and an increase in cardiac output. A normovolemic decrease in hematocrit from 40% to 20% will induce a 50% drop in oxygen-carrying capacity, but only a 10% drop in oxygen delivery secondary to increased cardiac output. This change parallels the decrease in oxygen consumption seen with the institution of general anesthesia or mild hypothermia. This form of therapy should be reserved for moderately healthy patients without preexisting cardiac, cerebrovascular, or pulmonary disease. There is no evidence that hemodilution has adverse effects on wound healing, infection rates, or immunologic status. Conversely, hemoconcentration may have detrimental effects based on animal studies of focal ischemia.[43]

Replacement of blood losses during surgery with the patient's own shed blood is also an attractive conservation option. Most cell-saving devices currently in use mix salvaged blood with an anticoagulant, then wash and concentrate it to a hematocrit about 50%. The effluent, which contains plasma fractions, platelets, leukocytes, free hemoglobin, anticoagulant, saline, and other debris, is discarded. Induction of disseminated intravascular coagulation does not appear to be a problem with these devices.[82] Their use is contraindicated in the presence of tumor cells or bacterial contamination. Residual anticoagulation is not a problem with sufficient washing.

## Induced Hypotension

Induced hypotension may be useful to help minimize blood loss and transfusion therapy during spine surgery, although its efficacy has not been consistently demonstrated.[66] With the use of high concentrations of volatile anesthetics or direct-acting vasodilators such as nitroprusside or nicardipine, the mean arterial pressure may be dropped to the lower limits of autoregulatory control of blood flow, thereby reducing capillary venous pressure and blood loss. Obviously, this technique should be reserved for the otherwise healthy patient.

## Pharmacologic Aids

Agents that attempt to reduce bleeding pharmacologically have also been used. Desmopressin (DDAVP), an analog of the natural hormone vasopressin, induces endothelial cells to release von Willebrand factor, tissue-type plasminogen activator, and certain prostaglandins.[74] With these effects in mind, DDAVP has been used in two human trials during scoliosis surgery with variable results.[32,44] Aprotinin is a serine protease inhibitor that preserves platelet integrity and adhesiveness. It has shown promise as an agent for the prevention of blood loss during cardiac surgery in multiple studies and appears to reduce blood loss and transfusion requirements in spine fusion procedures as well.[52]

## REFERENCES

1. Adams DC, Emerson RG, Heyer EJ, et al: Monitoring of intraoperative motor-evoked potentials under conditions of controlled neuromuscular blockade. Anesth Analg 77: 913-918, 1993.
2. Albrecht S, Schuttler J, Yarmush J: Postoperative pain management after intraoperative remifentanil. Anesth Analg 89:S40-S45, 1998.
3. Ali HH, Utting JE, Kitz RJ: Evaluation of recovery from nondepolarizing neuromuscular block using a digital neuromuscular transmission analyzer. Anesth Analg 52: 740-745, 1973.
4. Apel DM, Marrero G, King J, et al: Avoiding paraplegia during anterior spinal surgery: the role of SSEP monitoring with temporary occlusion of segmental spinal arteries. Spine 16:S365-S370, 1991.
5. Azar I: The response of patients with neuromuscular disorders to muscle relaxants: a review. Anesthesiology 61:173-187, 1984.
6. Ben-David B, Haller G, Taylor P: Anterior spinal fusion complicated by paraplegia. Spine 12:536-539, 1987.
7. Benumof JL: Practice guidelines for management of the difficult airway. Anesthesiology 98:1269-1277, 2003.
8. Brain AIJ: The laryngeal mask: a new concept in airway management. Br J Anaesth 55:801-804, 1983.
9. Brimacombe J, Berry A: Laryngeal mask airway insertion: a comparison of the standard versus neutral position in normal patients with a view to its use in cervical spine instability. Anaesthesia 48:670-671, 1993.
10. Caldwell MW, O'Hara RC, Bloom MJ, et al: Postoperative airway complications in patients undergoing anterior cervical corpectomy with graft placement: a review of the Pittsburgh experience. J Neurosurg Anesthesiol 6:311, 1994.
11. Caplan RA, Posner KL, Ward RJ, Cheney FW: Adverse respiratory events in anesthesia: a closed claims analysis. Anesthesiology 72:828-833, 1990.
12. Chang J: Anaesthesia for cervical osteotomy. Can Anaesth Soc J 21:83-91, 1974.
13. Chekan R, Weber S: Intubation with or without neuromuscular blockade in trauma patients with cervical spine injury. Anesth Analg 70:S54, 1990.
14. Cohn AI, Zornow MH: Awake endotracheal intubation in patients with cervical spine disease: a comparison of the Bullard laryngoscope and the fiberoptic bronchoscope. Anesth Analg 81:1283-1286, 1995.
15. Coombs DW, Hooper D, Colton T: Acid aspiration prophylaxis by use of preoperative oral administration of cimetidine. Anesthesiology 51:352-356, 1979.
16. Cormack BS, Lehane J: Difficult tracheal intubation in obstetrics. Anaesthesia 39:1105-1111, 1984.
17. Craen RA, Gelb AW, Murkin JM, Chong KY: Human cerebral autoregulation is maintained during propofol air/O$_2$ anesthesia, abstracted. Anesthesiology 77:A220, 1992.
18. Cucchiara RF, Messick JM, Gronert GG, Michenfelder JD: Time required and success rate of percutaneous right atrial catheterization: description of a technique. Can Anaesth Soc J 27:572-573, 1980.
19. Dershwitz M, Randel GI, Rosow CE, et al: Initial clinical experience with remifentanil. Anesth Analg 81:619-623, 1995.
20. Diaz JH, Lockhart CH: Postoperative quadriplegia after spinal fusion for scoliosis with intraoperative awakening. Anesth Analg 66:1039-1042, 1987.
21. Drummond JC, Abitbol JJ, Sanford TJ, Garfin SR: Transient paraplegia during posterior cervical osteotomy. Anesthesiology 74:628-630, 1991.
22. Drummond JC, Moore SS: The influence of dextrose administration on neurologic outcome after temporary spinal cord ischemia in the rabbit. Anesthesiology 70:64-70, 1989.
23. Entrei C, Leszcniewski W, Carlsson C: Local application of 133 Xenon for measurement of cerebral blood flow during halothane, enflurane and isoflurane anesthesia in humans. Anesthesiology 63:391-399, 1985.
24. Emery SE, Smith MD, Bohlman HH: Upper-airway obstruction after multilevel cervical corpectomy for myelopathy. J Bone Joint Surg 73A:544-551, 1991.
25. Fambrough DM: Control of acetylcholine receptors in skeletal muscle. Physiol Rev 59:165-227, 1979.
26. Frerk CM: Predicting difficult intubation. Anaesthesia 46:1005-1008, 1991.

27. Fung DL, White DA, Jones BJ, Gronert GA: The onset of disuse-related potassium efflux to succinylcholine. *Anesthesiology* 55:547-549, 1991.

28. Ghaly R, Stone J, Kartha R, *et al:* Effect of neuroleptanalgesia on motor potentials evoked by transcranial magnetic stimulation in primates. *Anesthesiology* 75:A595, 1991.

29. Giffen JP: Anesthesia for patients with spinal cord injury: acute and chronic. *ASA Refresher Course Lectures* 22:152, 1991.

30. Grundy BL, Heros RC, Tung AS: Intraoperative hypoxia detected by evoked potential monitoring. *Anesth Analg* 60:437-439, 1981.

31. Grundy BL, Nash CL, Brown RH: Deliberate hypotension for spinal fusion: a prospective randomized study with evoked potential monitoring. *Can Anaesth Soc J* 29: 452-461, 1982.

32. Guay J, Reinberg C, Poitras B, *et al:* A trial of desmopressin to reduce blood loss in patients undergoing spinal fusion for idiopathic scoliosis. *Anesth Analg* 75:405-410, 1992.

33. Hall JE, Levine CR, Sudhir KG: Intraoperative awakening to monitor spinal cord function during Harrington instrumentation and spine fusion. *J Bone Joint Surg* 60A:533-536, 1978.

34. Hanson TD, Warner DS, Todd MM, Vust LJ: The role of cerebral metabolism in determining the local cerebral blood flow effects of volatile anesthetics: evidence for persistent flow-metabolism coupling. *J Cereb Blood Flow Metab* 9:323-328, 1989.

35. Hastings RH, Vigil AC, Hana R, *et al:* Cervical spine movement during laryngoscopy with the Bullard, Macintosh, and Miller laryngoscopes. *Anesthesiology* 82:859-869, 1995.

36. Hastings RH, Wood PR: Head extension and laryngeal view during laryngoscopy with cervical spine stabilization maneuvers. *Anesthesiology* 80:825-831, 1994.

37. Hayek DA, Veremakis C: Cerebral resuscitation. In Pinsky MR, Dhainault JF (eds): *Pathophysiologic Foundations of Critical Care.* Baltimore, Williams & Wilkins, 1993, pp 753-777.

38. Holly J, Jordon R: Airway management in patients with unstable cervical spine fractures. *Ann Emerg Med* 18: 1237-1239, 1989.

39. Kalkman CJ, Drummond JC, Ribberink AA: Low concentrations of isoflurane abolish motor evoked responses to transcranial electrical stimulation during $N_2O$/opioid anesthesia in humans. *Anesth Analg* 73: 410-415, 1991.

40. Kalkman CJ, Drummond JC, Ribberink AA: Effects of propofol, etomidate, midazolam and fentanyl on motor evoked responses to transcranial electrical or magnetic stimulation in humans. *Anesthesiology* 76:502-509, 1992.

41. Kalkman CJ, Ubags LH, Been HD, Porsius M: Ketamine or etomidate used as a supplement to sufentanil/$N_2O$ anesthesia does not disrupt monitoring of myogenic transcranial evoked responses. *J Neurosurg Anesthesiol* 6:322, 1994.

42. Keenan MA, Stiles CM, Kaufman RL: Acquired laryngeal deviation associated with cervical spine disease in erosive polyarticular arthritis. *Anesthesiology* 58:441-449, 1983.

43. Kiyohara Y, Fujishima M, Ishitsuka T, *et al:* Effects of hematocrit on brain metabolism in experimentally induced cerebral ischemia in spontaneously hypertensive rats. *Stroke* 16:835, 1985.

44. Kobinsky NL, Letts RM, Patel LR, *et al:* 1-Desamino-8-D-arginine vasopressin (desmopressin) decreases operative blood loss in patients having Harrington rod spinal fusion surgery. *Ann Intern Med* 107:446-450, 1987.

45. Kublin DD: Mechanisms of action. In Miller RD (ed): *Anesthesia.* New York, Churchill-Livingstone, 1993, 51-83.

46. Lawson DH: Adverse reactions to potassium chloride. *Q J Med* 43:433-440, 1974.

47. Lee L: ASA postoperative visual loss (POVL) registry. *Anesthesia Patient Safety Foundation Newsletter* 16(4): 56-57, Winter 2001-2002.

48. Lee VC: Spinal and cortical evoked potential studies in the ketamine-anesthetized rabbit: fentanyl exerts component-specific, naloxone-reversible changes dependent on stimulus intensity. *Anesth Analg* 78:280-286, 1994.

49. Legatt AD, Frost EAM: EKG artifacts during intraoperative evoked potential monitoring. *Anesthesiology* 70:559, 1989.

50. Lehmann KG, Lane JG, Piepmeier JM, Batsford WP: Cardiovascular abnormalities accompanying acute spinal cord injury in humans: incidence, time course and severity. *JACC* 10:46-52, 1987.

51. Lehmann KG, Shandling AH, Yusi AU, Froelicher VF: Altered ventricular repolarization in central sympathetic dysfunction associated with spinal cord injury. *Am J Cardiol* 63:1498-1504, 1989.

52. Lentschener C, Cottin P, Bouaziz H, *et al:* Reduction of blood loss and transfusion requirements by aprotinin in posterior lumbar spine fusion. *Anesth Analg* 89:590-597, 1999.

53. Lesser RP, Raudzens P, Luders H, *et al:* Postoperative neurological deficits may occur despite unchanged intraoperative somatosensory evoked potentials. *Ann Neurol* 19: 22-25, 1986.

54. Losasso TJ, Boudreaux JK, Muzzi DA, *et al:* The effect of anesthetic agents on transcranial magnetic motor evoked potentials in neurosurgical patients. *Anesthesiology* 75:A1032, 1991.

55. Losasso TJ, Muzzi DA, Dietz NM, Cucchiara RF: Fifty percent nitrous oxide does not increase the risk of venous air embolism in neurosurgical patients operated upon in the sitting position. *Anesthesiology* 77:21-39, 1992.

56. Mackenzie CF, Shin B, Krishnaprasad D, *et al:* Assessment of cardiac function during surgery on patients with acute quadriplegia. *J Neurosurg* 62:843-849, 1985.

57. Majernick T, Bieniek R, Houston J, Hughes H: Cervical spine movement during orotracheal intubation. *Ann Emerg Med* 15:417-420, 1986.

58. Mallampati SR, Gatt SP, Gugino LD, *et al:* A clinical sign to predict difficult tracheal intubation: a prospective study. *Can J Anaesth* 32:429-434, 1985.

59. Martyn JJ, White DA, Gronert GA, *et al:* Up and down regulation of skeletal muscle acetylcholine receptors. *Anesthesiology* 76:822-843, 1992.

60. McMichan JC, Michel L, Westbrook PR: Pulmonary dysfunction following traumatic quadriplegia. Recognition, prevention, and treatment. *JAMA* 243:528, 1980.

61. Merritt WT, Brinker JA, Beattie C: Pacemaker-mediated tachycardia induced by intraoperative somatosensory evoked potential stimuli. *Anesthesiology* 69:766-768, 1988.

62. Miller RD, Roderick LL: Acid-base balance and neostigmine antagonism of pancuronium neuromuscular blockade. *Br J Anaesth* 50:317-324, 1978.

63. Murray DJ, Olson J, Strauss R, Tinkder JH: Coagulation changes during packed red cell replacement of major blood loss. *Anesthesiology* 69:839-845, 1988.

64. Muzzi DA, Losasso TJ, Dietz NM, *et al:* The effect of desflurane on cerebrospinal fluid pressure in neurosurgical patients, abstracted. *Anesthesiology* 73:A1212, 1990.

65. NIH Consensus Conference: Fresh frozen plasma indications and risks. *JAMA* 253:551-553, 1984.

66. Nuttall GA, Horlocker TT, Santrach PJ, *et al:* Predictors of blood transfusions in spinal instrumentation and fusion surgery. *Spine* 25(5):596-601, 2000.

67. Owen JH: Update on evoked potentials during spinal surgery. *Curr Opin Orthop* 4:12-20, 1993.

68. Owen JH, Bridwell KH, Grubb R, *et al:* The clinical application of neurogenic motor evoked potentials to monitor spinal cord function during surgery. *Spine* 16: S385-S390, 1991.

69. Pavlin KG, Holle RH, Schoene RB: Recovery of airway protection compared with ventilation in humans after paralysis with curare. *Anesthesiology* 70:381-385, 1989.

70. Pharmacokinetics and pharmacodynamics of inhaled and injected drugs. In Stoelting (ed): *Pharmacology and Physiology of Anesthetic Practice.* Philadelphia, Lippincott-Raven, 1991, pp 1-32.

71. Phelps JA: Laryngeal obstruction due to cricoarytenoid arthritis. *Anesthesiology* 27:518-519, 1966.

72. Ravussin P, Guinard JP, Ralley F, Thorin D: Effect of propofol on cerebrospinal fluid pressure and cerebral fluid pressure and cerebral perfusion pressure in patients undergoing craniotomy. *Anaesthesia* 43(suppl):37-41, 1988.

73. Rhee KJ, Green W, Holcroft JW, Mangilli JA: Oral intubation in the multiply injured patient: the risk of exacerbating spinal cord injury. *Ann Emerg Med* 19: 511-514, 1990.

74. Richardson DW, Robinson AG: Desmopressin. *Ann Intern Med* 103:228-239, 1980.

75. Robertie PG, Gravlee GP: Safe limits of isovolemic hemodilution and recommendations for erythrocyte transfusion. *Int Anesthesiol Clin* 28:197-204, 1992.

76. Shapiro HM, Wyte SR, Harris AB, *et al:* Acute intraoperative intracranial hypertension in neurosurgical patients: mechanical and pharmacologic factors. *Anesthesiology* 37:399, 1972.

77. Skues MA, Welchew EA: Anaesthesia and rheumatoid arthritis. *Anaesthesia* 48:989-997, 1993.

78. Stellin GP, Barker S, Saboe L, Miller J: Etiology and clinical course of missed spine fractures. *J Trauma* 27: 980-986, 1986.

79. Stevens WR, Glazer PA, Kelley SD, *et al:* Ophthalmic complications after spine surgery. *Spine* 22:1319-1324, 1997.

80. Sudhir KG, Smith RM, Hall JE, Hansen DD: Intraoperative awakening for early recognition of possible sequelae during Harrington-rod spinal fusion. *Anesth Analg* 55:526-528, 1976.

81. Talcucci RC, Shaikh KA, Schwab CW: Rapid sequence induction with oral endotracheal intubation in the multiply injured patient. *Am Surg* 54:185-187, 1988.

82. Thurer RL, Lytle BW, Cosgrove DM: Autotransfusion following cardiac operations: a randomized, prospective study. *Ann Thorac Surg* 27:500-507, 1979.

83. Vassar MJ, Perry CA, Gannaway WL, Holcroft JW: 7.5% sodium chloride/dextran for resuscitation of trauma patients undergoing helicopter transport. *Arch Surg* 126:1065-1072, 1991.

84. Vauzelle C, Stagnara P, Jouvinoux P: Functional monitoring of the spinal cord during surgery. *Clin Orthop* 93:173-178, 1973.

85. Warner ME, Warner MA, Garrity JA, *et al:* The frequency of perioperative vision loss. *Anesth Analg* 93:1417-1421, 2000.

86. Watts AD, Gleb AW, Bach DB, Pelz DM: Comparison of the Bullard and Macintosh laryngoscopes for endotracheal intubation of patients with a potential cervical spine injury. *Anesthesiology* 87:1335-1342, 1997.

87. Woerkens ECSM, Trouwborst A, Lanschot JJB: Profound hemodilution: what is the critical level of hemodilution at which oxygen delivery-dependent oxygen consumption starts in an anesthetized human? *Anesth Analg* 75:818-821, 1992.

88. Wong KC, Schafer PG, Schultz JR: Hypokalemia and anesthetic implications. *Anesth Analg* 77:1238-1260, 1993.

89. Young Y, Menon DK, Tisavipat N, *et al:* Propofol neuroprotection in a rat model of ischaemic reperfusion injury. *Eur J Anaesthesiol* 14:320-326, 1997.

90. Zigler J, Rockowitz N, Capen D, *et al:* Posterior cervical fusion with local anesthesia: the awake patient as the ultimate spinal cord monitor. *Spine* 12:206-208, 1987.

# CHAPTER 140

# Perioperative Management

**Seth M. Zeidman, Laurence D. Rhines, and Nathan H. Lebwohl**

The spectrum of spinal surgery ranges from straightforward cervical procedures in healthy, young adults to emergent fixation of unstable thoracolumbar spinal fractures in clinically unstable patients with multiple traumatic injuries. Preoperative evaluation and postoperative care share equal importance with the surgical procedure. The continuum of care begins at the initial meeting of the surgeon and patient and continues long after surgery. The clinician should be cognizant of coexisting medical problems and their implications, commonly used anesthetic and surgical techniques, potential postoperative complications, and prophylactic measures that can minimize postoperative morbidity. This chapter provides an overview of these issues.

The purpose of preoperative evaluation is to identify problems affecting surgical risk and in so doing, to reduce perioperative morbidity and mortality. Preoperative evaluation often uncovers other health problems that need attention, regardless of whether they directly impact the proposed operation. A complete health history should be obtained, including the present illness, past illnesses, and associated diseases. One should inquire about bleeding tendencies, current medications, and allergies. Coexisting medical problems are common in spinal surgery patients and can be associated with an increased incidence of postoperative complications and a lengthy hospital stay.

## General Conditions Affecting Surgical Risk
### Age

Patients at either extreme of the life span are at risk for complications or death from operation because of their narrower margin of safety. Small errors that are well tolerated by young, healthy adults are quickly compounded in children or geriatric patients, sometimes with catastrophic results.

Infants and young children have a relatively low tolerance for infection, trauma, blood loss, and nutritional and fluid disturbances.[8] The management of these disorders in infants and children differs from their treatment in adults. Particular aspects of surgical care deserving special attention include fluid and electrolyte management, nutrition, and temperature maintenance.[8,33]

Advanced age is an independent risk factor for postoperative morbidity, and the prevalence of coexisting medical problems increases with age.[38] As a result, elderly patients who undergo spinal procedures have higher rates of postoperative complications, including excessive bleeding,

postoperative confusion, and urinary tract infections.[48] They tend to recuperate more slowly than do their younger counterparts.

It is safe to consider every patient over age 65 to be at high risk for generalized atherosclerosis and for potential limitation of myocardial and renal reserve. Elderly patients often develop cardiac failure if they are fluid overloaded. Close monitoring of vital signs, intake, output, body weight, and serum electrolytes is mandated. Elderly patients generally require smaller doses of narcotics, sedatives, and anesthetics than do younger patients. Barbiturates, sedatives, and steroids may cause confusion, and narcotics can produce respiratory depression.[5]

Osteoporosis and falls are common in the geriatric population and result in an increased incidence of spinal fractures with advancing age. Elderly patients with spinal fractures after a fall pose special problems. In addition to assessing the overall medical condition, the clinician should evaluate the cause of the fall because it may uncover an important coexisting medical condition and, in turn, help to prevent future injury. Although most falls are results of accidents or environmental factors, they can also be caused by important cardiovascular or neurologic disorders, including arrhythmia, orthostatic hypotension, or cerebral ischemia. Special consideration should also be given to alcohol and drug use as possible causes. The incidence of falls in the elderly has been correlated with use of benzodiazepines, antidepressants, and diuretics.

Finally, advanced age is an important independent risk factor for postoperative deep venous thrombosis and pulmonary embolism that are major causes of morbidity and mortality after surgical procedures.

### Obesity

Obesity increases the technical difficulty of surgery and anesthesia. Obese surgical patients have a greater incidence of serious concomitant disease and higher rates of postoperative wound breakdown, thromboembolic complications, and pulmonary disease. Early patient mobilization, aggressive pulmonary toilet, and appropriate prophylaxis against deep venous thrombosis are all necessary adjuncts to good perioperative care. Occasionally, it may be advisable to delay elective surgery until the patient loses weight by appropriate dietary measures.

### Coagulation Abnormalities

Spinal procedures may result in substantial blood loss. Excessive bleeding at the surgical site increases the chances of wound infection and impaired wound healing. Although the prevalence of underlying coagulopathies is no higher in spinal surgery patients, many regularly take nonsteroidal anti-inflammatory drugs (NSAIDs). Because NSAIDs are reversible inhibitors of platelet aggregation, their use can increase postoperative bleeding. NSAIDs should be discontinued at least 1 week before a major spinal procedure. NSAIDs have also been shown to inhibit the healing of spinal fusions. In patients undergoing spinal fusion, NSAIDs should be avoided in the postoperative period as well.[12,20]

## Malnutrition

Increasing evidence suggests that many surgical patients are moderately to severely malnourished.[6] The increased metabolic demands of patients undergoing or recovering from spinal surgery are often unmet because of insufficient caloric intake. With inadequate caloric intake, the hypercatabolic state induced by trauma or surgery results in significant visceral and skeletal protein depletion. Malnourished patients have increased rates of mortality and morbidity from sepsis, wound complications, impaired healing, and protracted rehabilitation. Although no single test demonstrates malnutrition conclusively, a variety of laboratory studies and physical measurements can help reveal nutritional inadequacies.[13] These include preoperative weight loss of more than 10 pounds, serum albumin less than 3.5g/dL, and total lymphocyte count less than 1500 to 2000 cells/mm.[29]

If malnutrition is identified, a vigorous regimen of nutritional supplementation should begin, preferably before surgery, and the patient should be monitored throughout the perioperative period.[13] Total or peripheral parenteral nutrition should be considered in patients who either cannot tolerate or cannot meet their caloric needs with enteral nutrition alone.[24,26,31,34]

## Smoking

The harmful effects of smoking tobacco on the rate of postoperative pulmonary, cardiac, and thromboembolic complications are well known. In a recent study of 875 patients undergoing orthopedic reconstructive surgery, the incidence of cardiopulmonary complications in smokers was double that of nonsmokers. In that study, smoking was identified as the single most important risk factor for the development of complications after elective hip or knee arthroplasty. Similarly increased rates of pulmonary complications were identified in a multicenter review of 400 patients undergoing abdominal surgery.[3,16,40,65]

A review of wound infections following dorsal spinal operations involving instrumentation implicated smoking as a significant risk factor for developing an infection.[61]

Wound complications in soft tissue procedures have also been reported to occur much more frequently in smokers. In a study of 425 patients undergoing reconstruction after breast cancer surgery, the risk of skin flap necrosis was nine times as high in heavy smokers than in nonsmokers. Similarly, in a review of patients undergoing face-lift, the risk of skin slough was 12.5 times as high in smokers, compared with nonsmokers.[45,55]

Stopping smoking prior to surgery has been shown to decrease the rate of postoperative complications, but only if a significant amount of time elapses between smoking cessation and surgery. A 2-week smoke-free period in a study of 60 patients prior to colorectal surgery did not decrease the rate of postoperative complications. In contrast, 4 weeks of smoking cessation significantly reduced the rate of wound infections in a randomized, controlled trial of minor dermatologic procedures. In another randomized trial of 120 patients scheduled to undergo hip or knee replacement, enrollment in a smoking cessation program at least 6 weeks prior to surgery resulted in a substantial decrease in complication rates. Wound complications

decreased from 31% to 5%, and cardiovascular complications decreased from 10% to 0%.[41,56,57]

In addition to the general postoperative problems discussed above, tobacco smoking has been associated with unique complications following spinal surgery. Smoking was identified as a significant risk factor regarding the development of postoperative airway obstruction after cervical corpectomy. In a review of 133 patients undergoing cervical corpectomy, six of seven patients who developed airway obstruction were smokers. Two of these patients died as a result of this complication. Other risk factors were myelopathy and multilevel surgery. In patients with these risk factors the authors[14] recommend delayed extubation, and careful assessment of the airway for swelling prior to extubation.

Smoking has been shown to inhibit the healing of spinal fusions in many clinical reviews. This effect has been well documented in patients undergoing spinal fusion surgery and in animal models. In a randomly selected retrospective study of 50 smokers and 50 nonsmokers undergoing uninstrumented lumbar posterolateral fusion, the pseudoarthrosis rate was 40% for smokers and 8% for nonsmokers. A corresponding diminution in resting oxygen saturation was identified. The authors[4] theorized that this relative hypoxia was responsible for the failure of the arthrodesis to heal.

Animal studies, however, have shown that the inhibition of fusion can be attributed directly to the pharmacologic effects of systemically administered nicotine, without hypoxia.[53]

Inhibition of bone graft vascularization has been shown in the animal models. Cytokine expression is decreased, suggesting that the inhibitory effects of nicotine involve more than just local vasoconstriction.[9,62]

Although the effect of hypoxia has not been studied independently, these observations suggest that the negative effects of smoking on arthrodesis cannot be avoided by switching from inhaled tobacco to oral or transdermal nicotine.

Smoking has been demonstrated to be a risk factor for nonunion following thoracic and cervical fusion surgery as well. In a review of 90 patients undergoing ventral instrumented spinal fusion for adolescent scoliosis, four of five patients who developed a nonunion were smokers.[60]

A retrospective review of 131 patients who had multilevel cervical discectomies and fusions with autogenous interbody graft without instrumentation found a pseudoarthrosis rate of 50% in smokers, compared with 24% in nonsmokers.[23]

In animal models, bone morphogenic protein was effective in reversing the inhibitory effects of nicotine on spinal fusion.[52]

In some clinical series, the use of instrumentation and electrical stimulation has been reported to help overcome the inhibitory effects of smoking on spinal fusion.[2,42]

Two studies have assessed whether the negative effects on fusion can be reversed by smoking cessation, with conflicting results. Glassman et al.[20] reported that while smokers had a nonunion rate of 26.5% following lumbar fusion surgery, those who stopped smoking for more than 6 months after surgery had a successful arthrodesis rate of 82.9%. This was not significantly different than the union rate of 85.8% in nonsmokers. However, Deguchi et al.[12] found no improvement in arthrodesis rate in their patients who stopped smoking.

## Infection

Urinary tract infections are frequent in spinal surgery patients. When associated with bacteremia, these infections are of particular concern because of the possibility of bacterial seeding of hardware. Thus, it is important to identify and treat established urinary tract infections before spinal instrumentation is applied.[11]

## Compromised Host

The capacity of a compromised host to respond to infection or trauma is significantly impaired by disease or medication. Increased susceptibility to infection and delayed wound healing are the major postoperative problems in these patients and may arise from drugs such as corticosteroids, immunosuppressive agents, or cytotoxic agents and from prolonged antibiotic therapy. Infections in these patients can be caused by either common or opportunistic organisms. Malnutrition, renal failure, diabetes mellitus, and other immunocompromising diseases, including acquired immunodeficiency syndrome, significantly increase susceptibility to infection.

## Multiple Trauma

Many spinal surgery patients are the victims of severe accidents and have sustained multiple concomitant traumatic injuries. In such cases, urgent repair of spinal injuries almost always takes precedence over assessment and treatment of chronic medical problems, because acute spinal stabilization dramatically reduces mortality, incidence of adult respiratory distress syndrome, length of hospital stay, and need for mechanical ventilation.

Patients suffering multiple trauma are often in their best state of health upon admission. Efforts to delay spinal stabilization may not be in their best interest.

After surgery, it is important to search for factors contributing to the accident, including alcohol and drug abuse, unrecognized or untreated conditions such as liver disease, withdrawal syndromes, myocardial infarction, arrhythmias, seizures, and hypoglycemia. All these conditions have postoperative implications and may require specific diagnostic and therapeutic interventions.

## Rheumatologic Conditions

Patients with rheumatoid arthritis undergo a variety of spinal procedures, particularly cervical fusion. Rheumatoid arthritis patients experience high complication rates for all surgical procedures. Wound breakdown, infection, loosening of instrumentation, and pseudoarthrosis occur more frequently in rheumatoid arthritis patients and can be attributed to poor tissue integrity, compromised vascular status, as well as the use of immunosuppressive drugs.[49,54]

Rheumatoid arthritis patients should be examined for cervical spine involvement. Dynamic flexion and extension radiographs should be obtained to exclude occult instability, before the administration of general endotracheal anesthesia. A variety of other problems including anemia, pulmonary fibrosis, and pleural effusions may be present. Chronic steroid use often results in adrenal suppression requiring administration of perioperative stress-dose steroids. Similarly, patients with systemic lupus erythematosus and other rheumatologic conditions require thorough preoperative evaluation and may prove difficult to manage.[28]

Particular attention should be paid to patients with ankylosing spondylitis. These patients warrant very different management than the typical spinal surgery patient with degenerative disease, especially with regard to positioning, traction, and orthoses.

# Nonsurgical Diseases Affecting Surgical Risk
## Cardiac Disease
### *Preoperative Evaluation*

The most common symptoms of heart disease are dyspnea, fatigue, chest pain, and palpitation. It is important to inquire about exercise tolerance, paroxysmal nocturnal dyspnea, orthopnea, peripheral edema, irregular heartbeat, and chest pain. One should document significant past illnesses such as congenital heart disease, rheumatic fever, myocardial infarction, atherosclerotic cerebrovascular and peripheral vascular disease, diabetes mellitus, hypertension, and autoimmune disease. Also, use of cardiac pacemakers, previous cardiac surgery, and past or present use of diuretics, digitalis, coronary vasodilators, antihypertensives, and antiarrhythmics should be noted. A history of angina pectoris, myocardial infarction, Adams-Stokes attacks, stroke, cerebral ischemic attacks, intermittent claudication, or previous treatment for heart disease or hypertension should alert the surgeon to the possibility of a cardiac abnormality requiring further evaluation.

Conditions contraindicating elective surgery because of increased risk are acute myocardial infarction, recent or crescendo angina pectoris, aortic stenosis, and atrioventricular block.

**Physical Examination.** The heart rate and rhythm must be recorded and any cyanosis, clubbing, petechiae, neck vein distention, and peripheral edema noted. The lungs should be auscultated for rales or wheezes. Auscultation permits evaluation of the first and second heart sounds, as well as of gallops and murmurs.

**Radiologic Examination.** Most preoperative patients require an anteroposterior chest radiograph to exclude cardiac enlargement, pulmonary vessel distention, and pulmonary infiltrates. Lateral views permit diagnosis of individual chamber enlargement.

**Electrocardiography.** An electrocardiogram (ECG) can help detect arrhythmias, conduction defects, chamber enlargement, and myocardial ischemia. Routine preoperative ECGs are obtained on all adult patients undergoing spinal surgery. The ECG is useful diagnostically and also as a baseline measurement to evaluate subsequent changes in the myocardium and conduction system. In general, a stable abnormality on the ECG, in the absence of cardiac failure or angina pectoris, is indicative of only slightly increased perioperative risk.

**Laboratory Tests.** Serum concentrations of hemoglobin, sodium, potassium, and calcium may be relevant in the assessment of cardiac function. Arterial blood gas and pH studies indicate the adequacy of oxygenation.

**Hemodynamic Studies.** Pulse rate and cuff blood pressure are useful indicators of cardiac function. Monitoring arterial pressure with an intraarterial line provides a more accurate value and permits waveform analysis. Central venous pressure (CVP) and pulmonary capillary wedge pressure (PCWP) indicate cardiac preload. PCWP reflects left ventricular filling pressure and left ventricular performance, whereas CVP reflects right ventricular function.

Elevations of CVP above 10 mmHg suggest right ventricular failure. In most patients, left heart function correlates with right heart function. CVP exceeding PCWP by greater than 5 mmHg indicates pulmonary artery hypertension; PCWP exceeding CVP by more than 5 mmHg indicates isolated left ventricular failure. However, presence of a normal CVP does not exclude left ventricular failure. PCWP below 10 mmHg may be associated with shock; and a PCWP above 25 mmHg, with pulmonary edema.

For patients with cardiac or pulmonary disease, monitoring of PCWP with a Swan-Ganz catheter provides the best indication of left ventricular preload. Cardiac output can be measured by thermodilution using a Swan-Ganz catheter. Serial measurements can guide fluid therapy, even in the presence of left ventricular failure.

Echocardiography is a noninvasive method of studying cardiac anatomy and function. Cardiac catheterization with coronary angiography remains the most definitive cardiac diagnostic study, showing the vascular supply to different areas of the myocardium. This type of study is not without inherent risks.

### Preoperative Preparation

The cardiac status of a spinal surgery patient with cardiac dysfunction should be optimized before surgery. Special attention should be paid to correction of electrolyte imbalance, fluid excess, and anemia. It is important to avoid hypotension, hypoxia, fluid overload, and undue pain or excitement.

### Cardiac Contraindications

Relative cardiac contraindications to operation are recent myocardial infarction (MI), uncontrolled congestive heart failure (CHF), unstable angina pectoris, intractable cardiac arrhythmias and conduction defects, and uncontrolled hypertension. Preoperative evaluation is directed toward detecting and treating these conditions.

Mortality after a major operation is 25% if the surgery is within 3 weeks of MI, 10% if within 3 months, and 5% if within 6 months. A patient with a healed MI has an added mortality risk of about 3%. Only emergent and urgent operations are indicated within 3 months; only

semiurgent procedures are indicated from 3 to 6 months. Elective operations should be postponed until 6 to 12 months after MI.

Treatable causes of CHF include myocardial ischemia and its sequelae, valvular disease, bacterial endocarditis, sepsis, arrhythmias, hyperthyroidism, and hypertension. Careful perioperative management of these conditions will certainly decrease morbidity. Anginal chest pain may reflect severe coronary artery disease. Symptoms and signs denoting severe angina include associated sweating and nausea, poor response to coronary vasodilators (nitroglycerin), no relief with rest, frequent attacks, prolonged pain, and ECG evidence of ischemia.

High-risk coronary artery lesions include left main coronary artery occlusion, high left anterior descending artery lesions, and lesions in multiple vessels. Elective procedures should be postponed in patients with such lesions. Nonelective procedures may necessitate preliminary or coincident coronary artery bypass surgery. Patients who need urgent or emergent procedures require intensive perioperative management.

In hypertensive patients the blood pressure should be normalized preoperatively. There is a linear correlation between preoperative blood pressure and postoperative myocardial ischemia.[23]

### Postoperative Management

Patients with significant cardiac disease require close postoperative monitoring. Monitoring typically includes treatment in an intensive care setting for the first 24 hours postoperatively.

Most postoperative MIs occur on the second or third postoperative day, and hence serial ECGs for 3 days are indicated in patients with known coronary artery disease. Chest pain is often difficult to evaluate in the postoperative period, and an MI may become apparent only because of hypotension or arrhythmia. Serial cardiac isoenzyme studies are especially useful for identifying postoperative infarcts, and should be obtained as well. Postoperative treatment for MI entails vigorous support and monitoring. Arrhythmias and cardiac failure should be treated as they arise.

Typically, cardiac failure shows symptoms of hypotension or oliguria and is most often a result of hypovolemia in the postoperative patient. If hypotension or oliguria persists after intravenous fluids are administered, the patient must undergo complete evaluation. When cardiac failure results from hypertensive crisis, blood pressure can be reduced with nitroprusside.

Cardiac failure unresponsive to other measures may respond to afterload reduction. Judicious use of drugs with a positive inotropic effect (e.g., dopamine, dobutamine, isoproterenol, and digitalis) may also prove to be beneficial. Heart performance is most efficient at a rate of 100 to 120 beats/min.

Pericardial restriction resulting from constrictive pericarditis or pericardial effusion is suggested by a decreased cardiac output with a high CVP. Typically, jugular veins are distended, and a paradoxical pulse may be present. Echocardiography may assist in making the diagnosis. Treatment consists of pericardiocentesis or pericardiotomy.

In the presence of bradycardia, one should look for anesthetic excess, hypoxia, atrioventricular block, or vagal stimulation by visceral traction, carotid sinus compression, or traction on extraocular muscles.

In the presence of falling blood pressure, one should look for anesthetic excess, myocardial ischemia, or inadequate preload caused by blood or fluid losses, obstruction of venous return, or vasodilation. In the postoperative patient, absence of blood pressure, carotid pulse, or respiration is an ominous sign. Treatment should include identification of the underlying cause and immediate correction of the abnormality (e.g., for ventricular fibrillation, electrical defibrillation should be used; for asystole, cardiac massage, vagolytic or sympathomimetic drugs, or cardiac pacing should be used). Cardiopulmonary resuscitation should be initiated immediately and continued until the underlying problem has been corrected. Four minutes without blood flow to the brain results in a fatal ischemic injury. Preexisting inadequacy of cerebral blood flow and oxygenation shortens the time available for correction. Closed chest cardiopulmonary resuscitation is the initial method of resuscitation. Open chest cardiac massage should be undertaken only as a last resort.

Treatment of the major arrhythmias is a complex problem requiring close collaboration of the internist and surgeon. If the surgeon is required to provide emergency treatment until the internist arrives, a general knowledge of cardiac arrhythmias and their treatment is important. Diagnosis of the arrhythmia is made from the ECG.

Atrial fibrillation decreases cardiac efficiency and may cause congestive failure. Treatment involves slowing the rate by adequate digitalization. Calcium channel blockers can be used in patients with no history of heart failure or cardiomyopathy. Conversion to normal sinus rhythm by quinidine or direct current (DC) countershock may be required if shock or pulmonary edema is noted.

Atrial flutter often causes congestive failure. Digitalization will slow the rate, either by increasing the degree of block or converting the flutter to sinus rhythm or atrial fibrillation. DC countershock is the treatment of choice, especially if the rhythm is poorly tolerated.

Paroxysmal supraventricular tachycardia often occurs in patients with otherwise normal hearts. In the absence of heart disease, serious effects are rare. Digitalis toxicity must be excluded as a cause. Vagal stimulation (carotid sinus massage, Valsalva) should be tried initially. If mechanical measures fail, pharmacotherapy is indicated. There is, however, no unanimity on the most effective medical therapy. Digitalis, vasopressors, procainamide, and propranolol can all be tried. Continuous ECG and blood pressure monitoring are essential. DC cardioversion may be indicated if the patient's condition deteriorates.

Ventricular tachycardia and ventricular fibrillation are usually associated with myocardial damage, especially myocardial infarction. Lidocaine is the drug of choice for emergency treatment because of its short duration of action. If the arrhythmia recurs, an IV infusion may be given or the IV injection repeated. If lidocaine has no effect, DC cardioversion is preferable to additional pharmacotherapy.

Ventricular fibrillation produces cardiac arrest and requires defibrillation and cardiopulmonary resuscitation.

DC cardioversion is often effective in converting patients back to sinus rhythm. If the initial attempt at cardioversion is unsuccessful, repetition with sequentially higher energy levels is indicated.

## Pulmonary Disease
### Preoperative Evaluation

The most common symptoms of pulmonary disease are dyspnea at rest or after minor exertion, cough, sputum production, wheezing, chest pain, and hemoptysis. It is important to document any history of tuberculosis, recent upper respiratory infection, chronic pulmonary disease, or asthma. One must determine the degree of tobacco and alcohol use as well as previous occupational exposures to coal dust, asbestos, and silica dusts. Establishment of a medication history, particularly regarding the use of corticosteroids, is especially important.

**Physical Examination.** The examiner must look for physical signs of pulmonary disease such as cyanosis or nail clubbing. It is important to observe the respiratory rate and respiratory effort as well as to percuss the chest for dullness or hyperresonance and to determine inspiratory diaphragm excursion. Auscultation of the chest allows the examiner to hear rales, rhonchi, wheezes, and decreased breath sounds.

**Radiologic Examination.** The chest radiograph may demonstrate pulmonary infiltrates, granulomas, atelectasis, hyperlucency, pneumothorax, abnormalities of pulmonary vasculature, or a mass. A normal radiograph does not exclude pulmonary disease.

**Laboratory Examination.** Yellow, green, or brown sputum suggests active infection. Sputum culture is indicated to identify specific organisms and to determine antibiotic sensitivities. Arterial blood gas measurements help evaluate pulmonary gas exchange. The arterial partial pressure ($Pa_{O_2}$) of oxygen is an indicator of oxygen uptake by the blood in its passage through the lungs. $Pa_{O_2}$ is affected by the fraction of inspired oxygen, right-to-left shunting, and diffusion capacity across the alveolocapillary membrane. Normally, $Pa_{O_2}$ is 70mmHg or greater. A $Pa_{O_2}$ of 60mmHg indicates mild respiratory failure; a $Pa_{O_2}$ of 50mmHg or less indicates severe pulmonary disease. The oxygen saturation ($Sa_{O_2}$) reflects the percentage of hemoglobin actually bound by oxygen. Normally, $Sa_{O_2}$ is 93% or more; an $Sa_{O_2}$ of 90% indicates mild respiratory failure; an $Sa_{O_2}$ of 84% or less indicates severe pulmonary disease. The arterial partial pressure of carbon dioxide reflects the adequacy of ventilation. Normally, $Pa_{CO_2}$ is 38 to 43mmHg. A $Pa_{CO_2}$ of 44 to 54mmHg indicates mild impairment of ventilation; a $Pa_{CO_2}$ of 55mmHg or greater indicates severely impaired ventilation. Arterial blood pH is affected by both metabolic and respiratory factors. Normally, the arterial blood pH is 7.38 to 7.42.

**Spirometry.** The vital capacity (VC) is the maximum volume expired after a maximum inspiration. VC is decreased in restrictive disease but is usually normal in obstructive disease. A VC that is 50% or less of predicted indicates severe disease. The forced expiratory volume is the maximum volume expired after a maximum inspiration. Forced expiratory volume equals VC in restrictive disease but is less than VC in obstructive disease.

### Preoperative Preparation

Patients without pulmonary symptoms can be expected to tolerate surgery from a respiratory standpoint. If a patient can climb two flights of stairs without shortness of breath, further evaluation of respiratory status is generally unnecessary. Factors that can predispose a patient to postoperative pulmonary complications are long-term cigarette smoking, chronic obstructive pulmonary disease, upper abdominal and thoracic procedures, acute respiratory infections, and restrictive disorders such as obesity, pulmonary fibrosis, and neuromuscular and skeletal disease. Patients with one or more of these factors require careful preoperative preparation, and most should undergo complete pulmonary evaluation. Elective procedures should be postponed until maximum pulmonary function has been achieved. All patients should stop smoking at least 2 weeks before any elective operation. Overweight patients should try to achieve ideal body weight. All patients should receive preoperative instruction in coughing, deep breathing, and use of the incentive spirometer.

Respiratory infections should be treated before elective operations. Viral infections resolve with symptomatic treatment; bacterial infections can be treated with the appropriate antibiotics. Whenever possible, preoperative preparation and treatment should be performed on an outpatient basis to avoid superinfection with hospital-acquired antibiotic-resistant organisms. Adequate hydration, humidified air, and expectorants can help liquefy sputum. Postural drainage and chest percussion can help clear these secretions. Bronchodilators are often helpful for patients with chronic obstructive pulmonary disease. In addition, patients with bronchospasm or asthma may benefit from the administration of bronchodilators either by aerosol or by intermittent positive pressure breathing. Corticosteroids may be necessary for patients with severe asthma or pulmonary fibrosis.

If aspiration is observed, endotracheal intubation, airway suctioning, and saline lavage should be performed immediately. Bronchorrhea will neutralize the acidic gastric juices within 10 minutes so lavage after this interval is of no benefit. Moreover, steroid treatment has no objective benefit. Antibiotics should be reserved to treat specific organisms and should not be used prophylactically.

No patient should be denied operation for emergent and urgent conditions because of pulmonary disease. Whenever possible, the risks should be recognized and pulmonary function optimized.

### Postoperative Management

The postoperative effects of major procedures under general anesthesia include decreases in total lung capacity, vital capacity, functional residual volume, and compliance. Aggressive postoperative care minimizes these effects. Administering low doses of analgesics at frequent intervals promotes improved respiration by controlling pain without compromising respiratory drive. Frequent change of position and early ambulation are also beneficial. Changing the volume of ventilation prevents atelectasis. Incentive spirometry promotes deep inspiration that can also help prevent atelectasis.

Oxygen administration should be used when necessary, but with judiciousness; 100% oxygen promotes atelectasis and may result in oxygen toxicity. Administering oxygen to patients with chronic hypercapnia may depress respiratory drive. The elderly and patients with acutely impaired respiratory function may require ventilatory support over the first postoperative night. Arterial blood gases and fluid therapy should be closely monitored; administration of both insufficient and excessive fluid impairs respiratory function. Patients with bronchospasm may benefit from bronchodilator therapy.

### Pulmonary Complications

Ventilatory impairment is typical after ventral thoracic and lumbar approaches to the spine. In most instances, the impairment does not prevent spontaneous breathing. However, if the operative procedures are extensive, if there has been massive trauma, if the patient is elderly, or if the patient has preexisting chronic disease or malnutrition, ventilatory impairment may be so great that a period of assisted ventilation is necessary.

The first postoperative hours are critical because this is when acute ventilatory failure most commonly occurs. The effects of muscle relaxants may not have worn off completely, and muscle weakness can cause reduced vital capacity. If a respiratory complication develops, decreased lung compliance may also contribute to inadequate ventilatory function.

Pneumothorax is an uncommon complication in elective surgical procedures, but it should be considered in any patient who develops acute respiratory distress or intraoperative deterioration. The principal cause of pneumothorax in hospitalized patients is iatrogenic lung puncture during percutaneous central venous catheter placement. It can also occur in a patient who coughs and thereby ruptures a pulmonary bleb or bulla. Diagnosis is made on the basis of decreased or absent breath sounds on the affected side, with hyperresonance to percussion. When a tension pneumothorax develops there may also be lateral shift of the trachea away from the affected side. Any patient who develops respiratory distress after insertion of a central venous catheter should be presumed to have a pneumothorax, and a chest tube should be inserted immediately and not delayed for the radiograph. If pneumothorax is suspected but the patient is comfortable, one should first obtain the chest radiograph and insert a chest tube if indicated.

Atelectasis is the most common complication in the first 2 to 3 postoperative days. It results from collapse of the most dependent portions of the lung. Clinical signs include fever, tachypnea, and tachycardia that typically develop within the first 2 postoperative days. Chest radiographs usually show linear densities in dependent segments of the lungs or frank areas of collapse. There is often radiographic evidence of volume loss in the affected lung. Treatment entails deep breathing and coughing to expand underventilated lung segments. The patient should be mobilized if there are no contraindications. Mechanical devices, including the incentive spirometer and devices to maintain positive airway pressure help achieve adequate ventilation.

If the above methods fail to reverse atelectasis, bronchoscopy may be indicated for suctioning secretions out of the atelectatic segment. This is rarely necessary and should be used only when the atelectasis is severe and involves an entire lobe, if the patient is developing respiratory distress, or if blood gas levels are deteriorating.

Acute pulmonary edema is common in elderly patients with compromised cardiac function or in patients with significant cardiac disease. Typically, it develops on the second or third postoperative day as third-space fluid is mobilized. Alternatively, it can occur with excessive administration of fluid during surgery or immediately postoperatively if cardiac or renal function is compromised. Healthy patients with normal cardiac and renal function usually tolerate fluid overload with prompt diuresis and no pulmonary symptoms.

The diagnosis of acute pulmonary edema is made by the presence of tachypnea, tachycardia, shortness of breath, and orthopnea. These symptoms are often coupled with elevated CVP, distended neck veins, and wet rales bilaterally in the basilar lung segments. These rales may extend two-thirds of the way up the lungs. In addition, the sputum is often frothy and pink. Chest radiographs show symmetric perihilar fluffy infiltrates, cardiac enlargement, prominent pulmonary vascular shadows, and lymphatic congestion in the costophrenic angles (Kerley's B lines).

Pneumonia, in the postoperative patient, usually results from inadequately treated atelectasis, airway contamination, or preexistent pulmonary disease, most commonly a consequence of cigarette smoking. Pneumonia rarely develops earlier than 4 to 5 days after operation unless an unusual event, such as aspiration, occurs. The source is almost always bacterial, and if the patient has been given prophylactic or therapeutic antibiotics from the time of surgery, one may assume that the organism causing the pneumonia is resistant to the antibiotics.

The diagnosis is made by the presence of fever, leukocytosis, increased sputum production, decreased breath sounds or rales on physical examination, and a localized or diffuse infiltrate on radiographs. Gram staining of the sputum usually reveals heavy colonization by a single organism, and a large number of polymorphonuclear leukocytes are present. If pneumonia is diagnosed, antibiotic therapy should be started immediately, on the basis of the Gram stain. Confirmatory cultures must be obtained, and the antibiotic sensitivities checked. Antibiotic therapy can then be guided by these sensitivities. Therapy should include supportive care as well as measures directed at the underlying cause of the pneumonia. Blood gases should be monitored and endotracheal intubation and ventilation carried out, if the patient's status deteriorates.

**Adult Respiratory Distress Syndrome.** In rare instances after extensive surgery or massive trauma, patients develop tachypnea, hypoxemia, diffuse pulmonary infiltrates, and decreased compliance of the lungs. Physical examination does not reveal rales, bronchospasm, or evidence of alveolar edema. In these situations, the diagnosis of adult respiratory distress syndrome (ARDS) is made. In many cases, ARDS appears to be related to pulmonary microembolism, and the findings are similar to those described for fat embolism. Evidence of intravascular coagulation is common with this syndrome, but the role of intravascular coagulation as a specific cause has not been proved. ARDS normally does not develop until 3 days postoperatively, and it is often associated with sepsis.

When the disease is mild, supportive care with oxygen administration may be sufficient. In most cases, the symptoms are severe, and hypoxemia mandates intubation and mechanical ventilation. In severe cases, positive end expiratory pressure must be used to improve oxygenation.

A pulmonary artery catheter, to monitor PCWPs, is mandatory for careful titration of fluid therapy. Because of the high mortality associated with the development of renal failure in patients with ARDS, attempts must be made to preserve renal function by adequately hydrating these patients. At the same time, one must avoid overhydration, which can increase pulmonary interstitial edema. PCWPs should be kept as low as possible, while adequate peripheral perfusion and a urine output of 0.5ml/kg/hr are maintained. Wedge pressures should not exceed 15mmHg. Steroids and diuretics have not been shown to be of benefit.

Fat embolism syndrome may occur after extensive trauma. Although the true etiology of this syndrome is poorly defined, it was initially postulated to result from embolization of marrow fat to the pulmonary capillaries, producing symptoms by mechanical obstruction and inflammation. Arguing against this mechanism are the pathologic findings of fat in pulmonary, renal, and cerebral capillaries in traumatized patients without fractures or evidence of bony injury. The symptoms are nearly indistinguishable from those of ARDS: tachypnea, hypoxemia, pulmonary infiltrates, and decreased lung compliance. The only clinical difference is a higher incidence of cerebral symptoms, including disorientation, confusion, and progressive obtundation without localizing signs.

**Pulmonary Embolism.** Dyspnea, pleuritic chest pain, and hemoptysis are the classic symptoms of pulmonary embolism. Physical examination may reveal decreased breath sounds, pleural rub, or pleural effusion. Moreover, chest radiograph may demonstrate a wedge-shaped density, and the ECG may show evidence of right ventricular strain. Ventilation-perfusion scan of the lungs often reveals areas of decreased perfusion. Pulmonary angiography, the gold standard for diagnosis, occasionally shows obstruction of large pulmonary arteries.

Pulmonary embolism accompanied by circulatory and respiratory instability mandates treatment with high-dose IV heparin. Placement of a Greenfield filter or ligation of the inferior vena cava may be required if anticoagulants are contraindicated, if bleeding complications develop in a patient receiving anticoagulants, or if pulmonary embolism recurs in a fully anticoagulated patient.

## Renal Disease
### Preoperative Evaluation

Urine frequency and volume, dysuria, nocturia, poor stream, incontinence, and hematuria must be checked for.

It is important to note any history of renal disease, calculi, diabetes mellitus, or hypertension and to establish whether there has been any use of diuretics or nephrotoxins.

A history of the use of acetaminophen, a potential nephrotoxin, is particularly revealing in patients who undergo spinal surgery. Often, patients with low back pain consume substantial quantities of acetaminophen without recognizing its potential harm. Symptoms and signs of renal disease frequently reflect the degree of renal failure; however, it is not uncommon for patients with marked impairment of renal function to be asymptomatic.

Urinary tract obstruction should be suspected in any anuric patient. Upper tract obstruction must be bilateral for azotemia to occur. A renal hippurate scan, infusion intravenous pyelogram, renal ultrasound, and retrograde ureteral catheterization are important diagnostic tests. Renal scans are very useful for detecting acute obstruction. Sonography, infusion intravenous pyelogram, and retrograde catheterization are indicated in patients with chronic obstruction. Obstruction of the lower tract is recognized by the inability to insert a Foley catheter.

**Physical Examination.** Edema or dehydration must be carefully checked for. Metabolic acidosis may result in hyperventilation, and pericardial effusions can sometimes produce a friction rub.

**Laboratory Examination.** Blood urea nitrogen (BUN) and serum creatinine measurements and routine urinalysis are adequate screening tests for renal disease. A freshly voided urine sample yields much information about renal status.

Hematuria may be secondary to glomerular disease or to a lesion in the collecting system. In addition, the finding of different types of casts in the urine may be a sign of advancing renal disease. Red cell casts are suggestive of acute glomerular dysfunction, whereas white cell casts are indicative of acute pyelonephritis. It must be kept in mind that in patients with reduced muscle mass, serum creatinine levels can remain within the normal range even though creatinine clearance is no more than 20% of normal values. BUN-to-creatinine ratios greater than 10:1 may reflect prerenal azotemia, gastrointestinal bleeding, or enhanced catabolic states or may be secondary to catabolic drug effects.

Random urine samples usually have a specific gravity of 1.012 to 1.015. A higher specific gravity reflects dehydration or the presence of solutes, such as radiograph contrast medium, glucose, or mannitol. Dilute urine (specific gravity less than 1.007) reflects overhydration, diuretic therapy, water intoxication, or diabetes insipidus. A fixed specific gravity of 1.010 to 1.014 (isosthenuria) signifies a lack of renal tubular concentrating ability and occurs in renal parenchymal disease, congenital tubular defects, and acute tubular necrosis.

The normal pH range of the urine is 4.3 to 5.0. This range can be affected by diet and other factors. Aciduria may result from metabolic or respiratory acidosis, potassium depletion, starvation, or fever. Alkaline urine results from metabolic or respiratory alkalosis, certain urinary infections, and carbonic anhydrase-B-inhibiting diuretics.

Transient proteinuria may result from fever, cold exposure, strenuous exercise, and acute stress. Persistent proteinuria may signify true renal disease. Proteinuria is the earliest sign of aminoglycoside toxicity. Glucosuria usually signifies diabetes mellitus but may result from benign renal glucosuria, renal tubular disorders, pregnancy, or glucose infusion. The presence of reducing agents in the urine may also yield significant information about the patient's status. Ketonuria occurs with diabetic ketoacidosis, excessive vomiting, starvation, cachexia, and after strenuous exercise and cold exposure. One must keep in mind that ascorbic acid, cephalosporins, salicylates, paraldehyde, and chloral hydrate can alter reactions that measure urinary reducing agents. The dipstick test for occult blood is a useful screening test. It is positive with more than 10 red blood cells per high-power field in a spun urine sediment. However, myoglobinuria and hemoglobinuria can also give a positive reaction.

BUN concentration varies with dietary nitrogen consumption, hepatic urea production, and endogenous protein catabolism. It is increased by dehydration, gastrointestinal hemorrhage, hemolysis, corticosteroid therapy, and the tissue breakdown of trauma, shock, or sepsis.

Finally, the serum creatinine concentration is an important value as it reflects glomerular filtration. Creatinine production is correlated to muscle mass and, in a given individual, remains nearly constant in the absence of muscle destruction. Creatinine clearance (CLcr) is a more exact indicator of glomerular filtration and is defined by the equation

$$Clcr = (U[cr] \times V) \, P[cr]$$

where U[cr] = urine creatinine concentration in mg/dL, P[cr] = serum creatinine concentration in mg/dL, and V = urine volume in mL/min. Normal creatinine clearance is $125 \pm 25 \, mL/min/1.73 m^2$. A minimum clearance of $10 \, mL/min/m^2$ is needed to maintain life without dialysis. Serum creatinine level may remain normal until the clearance is reduced by more than half.

### Preoperative Preparation

In the preoperative period, it is important to assess renal function carefully and correct any electrolyte abnormalities. Anephric patients, if managed carefully, tolerate operations well. Preoperative preparation should maximize renal function and is important for preventing postoperative failure. Urinary tract infection should be treated preoperatively with appropriate antibiotics as determined by urine culture and sensitivity tests.

Obstructive lesions of the urinary tract should be removed or corrected, if possible, before other major operations are planned. Dehydration, hypovolemia, and electrolyte imbalance should be corrected, and adequate urine volume should be ensured preoperatively. Metabolic acidosis, even though compensated for, should be corrected with sodium bicarbonate.

Anemia is a frequent finding in patients with renal disease and should be evaluated preoperatively. A hemoglobin level of 9gm/dL and a hematocrit of 25% are satisfactory for patients with chronic renal insufficiency. Hemodialysis patients adapt to hematocrits in the range of 20% and do not need transfusions unless there are significant losses of blood. Blood transfusion should be used cautiously to avoid cardiac decompensation.

Coagulation defects in patients with chronic renal disease should be identified and corrected. Patients with severe renal failure often have platelet dysfunction that can cause bleeding. Elective procedures should be delayed until platelet dysfunction is corrected with hemodialysis on the day before surgery. Follow-up hemodialysis, with its attendant anticoagulation and fluid shifts, can be delayed until the second or third postoperative day.

It is important to maintain all antihypertensive medications, including β-blockers and catecholamine-depleting drugs, until the night before surgery. Discontinuation of clonidine may result in paroxysmal hypertension, and abrupt withdrawal of certain β-blockers can produce cardiac dysrhythmia. Patients who take diuretics may require correction of volume contraction and hypokalemia. When possible, one should avoid nephrotoxic drugs and be on the alert for medications that accumulate because of decreased renal excretion. Use of nephrotoxic intravenous contrast media should be limited.

### Postoperative Management

The diseased kidney is unable to concentrate urine and must excrete a urine volume greater than normal to rid the body of metabolic end products. At the same time, the kidney may be unable to excrete water and electrolytes. There is a slim margin between further renal insufficiency from dehydration and CHF secondary to excess salt and water retention. Effective management requires monitoring of body weight, intake and output, serum electrolytes, pH, CVP, and pulmonary artery wedge pressure. Keeping track of urine electrolyte concentrations and of all measurable fluid losses helps guide appropriate fluid therapy. Urine output and specific gravity do not, however, in and of themselves, reliably reflect the state of hydration.

Nephrotoxic drugs must be administered carefully and in reduced doses to patients with impaired renal function. These agents include aminoglycoside antibiotics, cephaloridine, colistin, polymyxin B, and amphotericin B. Spot checks for urine protein are useful for detecting early aminoglycoside toxicity. Drugs requiring major dose modification in the renally impaired patient include allopurinol, digoxin, methotrexate, phenobarbital, procainamide, quinidine, and tolbutamide.

Postoperative urine output less than 25ml/hr requires immediate evaluation. Oliguria suggests prerenal or renal parenchymal failure. Anuria suggests vascular obstruction, cortical necrosis, or urinary tract obstruction.

**Acute Renal Failure.** The hallmark of acute renal failure is rapidly progressive azotemia, generally accompanied by oliguria (urine output less than 400 ml/24hr). Prerenal azotemia results from renal hypoperfusion caused by volume depletion (dehydration or blood loss) or decreased cardiac output from pump failure (CHF). An expeditious diagnosis of prerenal azotemia is essential because the condition is easily reversible, and persistent renal hypoperfusion will result in acute tubular necrosis.

The physician must assess the patient's volume status frequently (fullness of neck veins, skin turgor, orthostatic changes in blood pressure and heart rate, and peripheral perfusion). Examination of the heart and lungs may reveal signs of CHF.

Bladder catheterization can be helpful for obtaining urine specimens and for monitoring urine output carefully. Measurements of serum BUN, creatinine, electrolytes, and osmolality, as well as of urine electrolytes and osmolality, can also be of diagnostic value.

Following the above suggestions should help distinguish whether prerenal azotemia is secondary to hypovolemia or CHF. In patients with tenuous cardiac function, measurement of central venous or even pulmonary arterial wedge pressures may be necessary before therapy is instituted.

Hypovolemic patients should be given normal saline solution at a rate of 100 to 500ml/hr depending on the severity of volume depletion. Diuretics should not be administered before hypovolemia is corrected.

If there is no improvement in urine output after blood volume has been replenished, a bolus of furosemide or mannitol may be administered. Mannitol should be infused carefully because if oliguria persists, failure to excrete mannitol will produce volume expansion and pulmonary edema. If there is no response to these diuretics, acute tubular necrosis (ATN) or obstructive uropathy is probably present.

The clinical setting and the laboratory tests, especially the results of urinalysis, are generally sufficient to establish the diagnosis of ATN. ATN may be a consequence of ischemia, nephrotoxins, or unknown mechanisms. The course of ATN is divided into three phases: pre-ATN, oliguric, and diuretic phases. As the kidneys recover, the urine output gradually increases. Occasionally, this postoliguric diuresis is massive. The severity of renal damage varies. In mild cases, there may be high urinary output rather than oliguria (nonoliguric ATN). Anuria (urine output less than 50mL/24hr) is rare in ATN. Bilateral cortical necrosis, acute glomerulonephritis, urinary obstruction, and thrombosis of the major renal vessels are more likely to produce anuria.

The abnormalities described in chronic renal failure also occur in acute renal failure, frequently with greater severity because of the acuteness of renal dysfunction. Fluid and electrolyte abnormalities are invariably present, and profound acidosis and severe hyperkalemia are common. In ATN, infection and gastrointestinal bleeding are the major associated complications. Infection is the principal cause of death.

Treatment of ATN is supportive and is directed at preventing or treating complications until renal function returns to normal. There is no evidence that the course of established ATN is modified by the administration of furosemide or mannitol. Diuretics should not be given.

Measurable fluid losses and insensible losses should be replaced. Fluid intake, fluid output, and body weight should be meticulously assessed. In addition, sodium losses from urine or other measurable sources should be replaced. Hyponatremia developing in the course of ATN is usually indicative of fluid excess, rather than of sodium deficit, and is best treated by fluid restriction. Additionally, hyperkalemia frequently occurs in these patients. A variety of factors contribute to hyperkalemia, including acidosis and potassium release from tissues secondary to excessive catabolism, trauma, or hemolysis. The serum potassium concentration and the ECG must be monitored.

Severe hyperkalemia (serum potassium level greater than 7mEq/L) requires more urgent therapy, including administration of sodium bicarbonate or hypertonic glucose solution and an insulin drip. Life-threatening cardiac arrhythmias due to hyperkalemia should be treated by IV calcium gluconate, or calcium chloride dialysis may be required to remove excess potassium. It is advisable to restrict magnesium and check for hypocalcemia. Acidosis in ATN may be treated cautiously with sodium bicarbonate, but this may result in hypernatremia and heart failure. Acidosis associated with volume overload is best treated by dialysis.

Adequate nutrition is fundamental in the treatment of ATN. Dosages of drugs, including antibiotics, digoxin, and magnesium-containing antacids, must be modified. If a nephrotoxin may have caused the ATN it should be discontinued.

As suggested above, the indications for dialysis include uncontrollable hyperkalemia or acidosis, overhydration, and the development of uremic symptoms. Peritoneal dialysis and hemodialysis are equally effective. Early and aggressive dialysis seems to result in improved survival in patients with ATN.

ATN has an overall mortality rate of 50%. Mortality is approximately 80% in patients with burns, trauma, or surgical procedures and only 30% with medical ATN. This is presumably because there are more complications of the underlying condition in the surgical group.

**Urinary Retention.** Inability to urinate after surgery is a frequent problem and may be seen after any operation. Causes include reflex spasm of the voluntary sphincter because of pain or anxiety, medications (usually anticholinergics and narcotics), preexisting partial bladder outlet obstruction (e.g., enlarged prostate), and intraoperative overdistention.

Preoperative voiding patterns should be evaluated if a bladder outlet obstruction is suspected. Obstruction can be corrected before operation, or catheter drainage may be instituted immediately after surgery. One should avoid excessive use of narcotics and parasympatholytic drugs. Patients scheduled for lengthy operations should be catheterized preoperatively and the bladder drained throughout the procedure.

If a patient is unable to pass urine for several hours postoperatively, and there is no urge to urinate, one must explore the possibility of oliguria as a consequence of diminished volume status. Occasionally, a heavily sedated patient does not recognize the sensation of fullness and does not urinate for that reason.

A palpable bladder in the midline above the symphysis pubis is highly suggestive of acute urinary retention. Any patient who does not urinate for 6 hours after operation should be evaluated carefully. In this way, overdistention of the bladder, which may induce bladder atony and even myogenic damage to the bladder wall, can be avoided.

Urinary retention can be relieved in a variety of ways. Narcotics or sedatives may help relieve local pain.

Moreover, if the condition permits, the patient can be positioned in the standing or sitting position instead of the supine position for urination. Cholinergic drugs such as bethanechol chloride may be administered.

When all other measures fail, if the bladder is markedly distended and severe bladder contractions occur without voiding, single-pass, straight catheterization should be performed so that patients can void on their own. A preoperative history of any voiding difficulty is very important to help decide on the duration of catheter drainage. If there was minimal preoperative obstruction, the patient should be able to resume normal voiding spontaneously. Under no circumstances should the bladder be allowed to overdistend. If the patient cannot void spontaneously after two catheterizations, and there is evidence of overstretching or mild mechanical obstruction, a Foley catheter should be left in place for 2 to 3 days before testing for spontaneous voiding again. It is of note that men after middle age often have mechanical obstruction secondary to prostatic enlargement. Women are more susceptible to detrusor atony after overstretching, especially if the period of overstretching is prolonged.

## Gastrointestinal Complications
### Gastric Distention and Dilatation

The stomach frequently becomes distended with gas during anesthesia induction, and further quantities of air are swallowed in the postoperative period. Gastric juices and duodenal secretions that reflux into the stomach contribute to this distention. Marked gastric distention can result in nausea and vomiting. Moreover, the distended stomach may impair diaphragmatic excursion and cause tachypnea. Nasogastric intubation for 12 to 24 hours is usually sufficient treatment; however, intubation for longer periods is occasionally necessary.

Vomiting immediately after an operation may be the result of a direct anesthetic effect or the result of gastric distention. Regardless of the cause, the best management is nasogastric intubation and suction to maintain an empty stomach for 12 to 24 hours. Medications that suppress nausea are less effective and can have untoward side effects, including vasodilatation. Vomiting later in the postoperative period may be the result of drugs, ileus, mechanical obstruction of the gut, or other problems and should be investigated.

Gastric dilatation occurs when the stomach becomes massively distended. Hemorrhage from the gastric mucosa can develop. This uncommon surgical complication is an occult cause of shock in the first few hours after operation. If the fluid is vomited, aspiration may occur. The distended tympanitic stomach may be visible in the epigastrium or on a radiograph. Typically, nasogastric intubation yields dark bloody fluid. Fluid and electrolyte losses must be replaced. Acute gastric dilatation can be fatal if it is unrecognized, and prompt treatment usually results in dramatic improvement.

Paralytic ileus is the cessation of effective gastrointestinal motility after trauma, severe illness, or surgery. Ileus is primarily a gastric phenomenon because the remainder of the gut can usually handle fluids earlier than the stomach. Vomiting and abdominal distention are the main manifestations. Decreased bowel sounds are an unreliable finding. Abdominal radiographs show gas in the stomach, small bowel, and colon. Mechanical bowel obstruction must be excluded in such patients. Any patient with ileus should be given bowel rest (given nothing by mouth) and should have a nasogastric tube inserted and left in place until the ileus resolves.

Another potential gastrointestinal complication is constipation. There are several factors contributing to postoperative constipation. First, taking nothing by mouth eliminates gastrocolic reflexes and reduces fecal bulk. Second, dehydration encourages fluid absorption from the colonic contents, desiccating the stool. Third, ileus has a component of impaired colonic motility. Finally, incisional pain makes patients unwilling to increase intraabdominal pressure, eliminating an important force contributing to defecation. Physical inactivity removes stimuli to movement of feces through the colon. Furthermore, opiates and antacids containing calcium or aluminum exacerbate constipation. Often attempts to defecate on a bedpan are unsuccessful because the patient is semirecumbent. The normal sitting or squatting position raises abdominal pressure and helps evacuate the rectum.

Hiccups are another potential complication. Typically, they are self-limited; however, they can be sufficiently persistent and exhausting to endanger life in a severely debilitated patient. They are produced by any process that stimulates the afferent or efferent phrenic nerve pathways. Therefore, the causes are quite varied and include central nervous system, cardiopulmonary, and gastrointestinal conditions, as well as renal failure, infectious diseases, and steroid therapy.

Treatment should be directed at the cause when possible, but therapy is frequently only symptomatic. Breath holding, drinking a large glass of water, or gastric lavage with a warm 1% solution of sodium bicarbonate may be effective. Rebreathing into a paper bag or administration of 10% to 15% carbon dioxide by face mask induces hyperventilation and may interrupt the reflex. Tranquilizing drugs such as chlorpromazine hydrochloride or other phenothiazine preparations are worth trying in patients with prolonged hiccups. Barbiturate sedation may be effective.

## Disorders of Hemostasis

Patients with preexisting hemostatic disorders undergo operations more frequently than in the past. Because specific replacement therapies are available, it is essential to identify the exact defect preoperatively whenever possible. Occasionally, the first sign of a hemostatic defect is excessive bleeding at operation. This distressing situation will seldom arise from a preexisting disorder if a bleeding history and screening laboratory tests are obtained before surgery.

### Screening Procedures

Blood is the most potentially dangerous substance prescribed by most physicians. Complications are common and may be fatal. Transmission of syphilis, malaria, bacteria, and viruses is infrequent with current blood banking practices. Hepatitis, however, remains a problem.

Blood products carry a hepatitis risk proportional to the number of donors contributing to the blood pool. Recently, available assays for hepatitis have greatly reduced the potential of distributing blood from hepatitis carriers, but most cases of hepatitis that occur after transfusion in the United States are not a result of hepatitis B or other known viruses. The statistical risk of hepatitis is unknown because the majority of cases are subclinical. Blood is an allograft, and the recipient may become immunized against human leukocyte antigens, platelet antigens, and red cell antigens. Reactions to leukocyte antigens are the probable cause of many febrile responses to transfusions. Reactions to transfusions of proteins, especially IgA, are frequently severe and may be hemolytic in nature.

Administration of blood to the wrong recipient is the most common error and is usually the result of a clerical error such as incorrect specimen labeling. Such an error can cause serious immunologic complication. Massive hemolysis may occur, leading to renal failure and death. Symptoms of early hemolysis are chills, fever, back pains, circulatory collapse, and hemorrhage. Delayed hemolysis occurs from several days to 1 month after transfusion and is manifested by anemia or mild jaundice.

### Transfusion Reactions

In the case of a transfusion reaction, the transfusion should be immediately halted and the remaining blood returned to the bank for investigation of the appropriateness of the cross-match, the Rh compatibility, and the Coombs' test. The patient should be adequately hydrated. Samples of plasma and urine should be tested for hemoglobin. The presence of hemoglobin in these fluids implies hemolysis. Cultures should be obtained of the recipient's blood and the donor blood. If a severe reaction has occurred, renal function should be evaluated and protected by administration of mannitol and bicarbonate. Febrile reactions, without hemolysis, should be treated with antihistamines and acetaminophen. Isoimmunized patients who require subsequent transfusions should receive washed red cells.

Surgical patients usually receive blood transfusions for the restoration of red cell mass or blood volume. Anemic patients who are asymptomatic are able to tolerate operations of almost any magnitude if operative blood loss is minimal. If a surgical procedure commonly associated with substantial blood loss is planned, anemia should be corrected 1 to 2 days before operation so that the storage-related defects of transfused blood can be normalized. Moreover, preoperative transfusion permits preoperative detection of transfusion reactions. Red cell concentrates are preferred for correction of preoperative anemia in stable patients.

The need for transfusion to correct mild postoperative anemia is assessed by measurement of the reticulocyte count. If the count is elevated and if the patient does not have postural hypotension or dyspnea, transfusion is not indicated. If the reticulocyte count is low, the response to oral or parenteral iron should be determined before giving blood. Chronically ill patients frequently have a regenerative anemia and may require serial blood transfusions.

Banked blood lacks functioning platelets. Platelets lose their aggregability in cold storage, and preservatives do not maintain platelet viability beyond 72 hours. In addition, most banks with component programs routinely remove the platelets from donated blood. Absent or non-functioning platelets contribute to post-transfusion bleeding, and the magnitude of the problem is proportional to the number of units of blood administered. Platelet concentrates (or platelet packs) should be given to patients receiving 10 or more units of blood within 1 hour.

Whole blood is preferable for patients with exsanguinating hemorrhage because red cell concentrates cannot be rapidly administered.

## Prophylaxis
### Autologous Blood Donation

Autologous blood transfusion avoids most of the complications associated with transfusion of homologous blood, including transmission of disease, hemolytic transfusion reactions, and other immune phenomena. Despite existing medical problems, most patients are able to donate at least two units of autologous blood before surgery. This could potentially enable over 90% of patients to avoid homologous transfusion during major spinal procedures. Autologous blood can normally be stored for up to 40 days (longer storage requires an expensive and complex freezing process). One unit of autologous blood can be processed from a given patient every 3 days up to 3 days before surgery, provided the hematocrit remains at least 34%. Iron supplementation is recommended. Treatment with erythropoietin can increase the patient's hematocrit and allow more blood to be stored in advance of surgery. It can also be used without pre-donation to minimize the need for transfusion at the time of surgery.[32]

There are two forms of autotransfusion. In one type, a patient donates blood in advance of elective operation, and this blood is stored for transfusion back into the donor, should it be required. This practice permits stimulation of erythropoiesis and results in restoration of red cell mass to near normal levels by the time of operation. A further advantage is the availability of the safest possible blood, should the patient require it.

The other type of autotransfusion is useful in emergencies. Blood lost by the patient is collected into an apparatus designed for this purpose (e.g., the cell-saver), anticoagulated, and immediately returned to the circulation. This type of autotransfusion is most useful in cases of massive bleeding. It may be lifesaving when compatible blood is unavailable. Reinfusion of large amounts of blood, however, can cause coagulopathies.

### Antibiotic Prophylaxis

Prophylactic antibiotics are administered routinely to patients undergoing spinal surgery, particularly those undergoing spinal instrumentation, because of the severe consequences of infected prostheses. Short courses of antibiotics are safe and effective. Longer courses have been associated with *Clostridium difficile* colitis.

Prophylaxis for endocarditis is not necessary for clean spinal procedures because the risk of bacteremia is low.

### Prophylaxis for Thromboembolism

The most important prophylaxis issue in patients undergoing spinal surgery is the prevention of deep venous thrombosis and pulmonary embolism. The incidence of deep venous thrombosis in spinal surgery is not known. Estimates as high as 60% have been made. Prophylaxis for thromboembolism should therefore be considered in all patients undergoing major spinal procedures. Low-dose warfarin and adjusted-dose heparin have proven to be effective. Thigh-length sequential compression devices, thromboembolic stockings, and low-dose heparin may also serve as prophylaxis for deep venous thrombosis in elective spinal surgery. Initial studies suggest that low molecular weight heparin and heparinoids may be effective and safe in these patients. The benefits of prophylactic anticoagulation must be balanced against the risk. Cain[7] reported a high rate of complication due to therapeutic heparinization after pulmonary embolus in spinal surgery patients. In a poll of Scoliosis Research Society members representing more than 13,000 thoracic and lumbar fusions, he identified nine patients who were treated with heparin anticoagulation. Complications attributable to anticoagulation were reported in two-thirds of these patients.

### Anticoagulation

Anticoagulation is defined as suppression of the coagulation mechanism. The term is used loosely in clinical practice, however, and it may refer to the suppression of clotting or the inhibition of platelet aggregation.

The only absolute anticoagulant is heparin, a physiologic substance present in mast cells that suppresses thrombin formation. Oral anticoagulant agents are less effective. They block coagulation indirectly by depressing certain factors in the clotting cascade. Antiplatelet-aggregating agents interfere with the platelet contribution to coagulation.

Venous clots are composed of fibrin. As a result, anticoagulants are effective for preventing and treating venous thrombosis. Arterial clots are composed mainly of platelets. Therefore, antiplatelet-aggregating medications are useful for preventing arterial thrombosis.

Heparin can be administered either subcutaneously or intravenously. Subcutaneous heparin is used only when small amounts of heparin are required, most often for prophylaxis against clotting. Larger doses of heparin required to treat thrombotic states should be administered intravenously.

Generally, for clotting prophylaxis, sufficient heparin is administered to decrease the coagulation tendency without altering coagulation parameters. This avoids the complications inherent in systemic anticoagulation. Clotting measures such as the Lee-White clotting time, the activated partial thromboplastin time, or the prothrombin time are all used for this purpose. These tests help to quantify the effect of a given dose of anticoagulant.

A dose of heparin is metabolized in 4 to 8 hours. In the presence of bleeding complications, it may be necessary to reverse the heparin immediately by infusing protamine sulfate. Not more than 1mg of protamine should be given for every 100 units of heparin. Administration of too much protamine can produce hypotension or bleeding complications. Protamine, therefore, should be administered slowly and carefully.

Anaphylactic reactions to heparin are very rare. Hemorrhage is the primary complication. Patients at risk should have their hematocrit checked frequently (at least twice daily). Typically, bleeding occurs into wounds or into the retroperitoneum and is not serious if the problem is promptly recognized and appropriately treated. Cerebral hemorrhage is a rare but serious complication.

Depression of platelet function occurs in some patients after 3 to 4 days of heparin therapy. The risk of hemorrhage is greatest in these patients. This complication can often be anticipated, however, because it is usually preceded by a decrease in the platelet count to below 100,000.

Heparin should be given in adequate doses. The rate of heparin infusion should be adjusted to maintain a partial thromboplastin time that is 1.5 to 2 times the control value. Enoxaparin, a low molecular weight heparin, is an alternative that does not require continuous infusion or such careful monitoring and regulation of laboratory values. The usual dose for prophylaxis is 40mg given subcutaneously once daily. The dose for treatment of deep vein thrombosis is 1mg/kg body weight given subcutaneously every 12 hours. Special caution is necessary when treating the elderly, those with renal impairment, or patients weighing less than 45kg.

Coumadin is less effective than heparin but is practical for prophylaxis, especially in outpatients, because it is administered orally. The dosage required in individual patients varies considerably. The preferred regimen for initiation of oral anticoagulation is 10mg of warfarin orally each day until anticoagulation is obtained. The dose is then adjusted to maintain a prothrombin time that is 1.5 to 2 times the normal value. The average maintenance dose is 5mg/day.

The prothrombin time returns to normal within 3 to 4 days after warfarin is discontinued. Rapid reversal is obtained by administering 5 to 10mg of IV vitamin K. Immediate reversal can be obtained by the administration of fresh frozen plasma IV.

The most common complication of oral anticoagulation is hemorrhage, frequently into the retroperitoneum or into the urinary or gastrointestinal tract. The urine and stool should be monitored for the presence of blood. Abdominal pain suggests retroperitoneal hemorrhage.

Antiplatelet-aggregating agents are used to treat arterial thrombotic conditions. These agents carry less risk of hemorrhage than do anticoagulants, but they are not as effective. Aspirin, dipyridamole, and related drugs depress platelet aggregation for the life span of the platelet. Reversal of drug effect therefore depends upon generation of new platelets. The half-life of platelets is approximately 4 days; therefore, these agents are effective for 1 to 2 days.

Plasma volume expanders can also depress platelet aggregation. Low molecular weight dextran reduces viscosity, increases microcirculatory flow, and decreases the tendency toward platelet aggregation. This agent is often used postoperatively.

## Postoperative Complications
### Nonspecific Complications
#### Fever

Pulmonary atelectasis is the most common cause of fever during the first 2 days after major spinal procedures. Typically, the pulse and respiratory rates are elevated along with the temperature (the "triple response"). Pneumonia seldom develops before the third postoperative day unless pulmonary disease was present at the time of operation or unless the patient aspirates.

Wound infection caused by β-hemolytic streptococci or clostridia can develop within hours of operation. Other bacterial wound infections require several days before they progress sufficiently to cause fever.

In general, cystitis alone does not cause fever, but infection of the upper urinary tract does. Infection in the operative site (deep to the incision) can also cause fever. Examples include epidural abscess, empyema, meningitis, and graft infection. Intravenous catheters can become infected quickly unless rigid aseptic precautions are used during and after insertion.

Reactions to drugs, notably antibiotics, may cause fever. The extent to which fever is investigated by laboratory tests and radiographs depends on the interval between operation and appearance of fever, the severity of fever, and the physician's certainty about the cause on the basis of the history and physical examination. The patient must be questioned about symptoms (e.g., dysuria, unusual pain) that may be clues to the source of fever. Physical examination, including auscultation of the chest, inspection of the wound, and examination of IV sites, is essential.

Leukocyte count and urinalysis are ordered in nearly every case. Cultures of urine, sputum, blood, and drainage fluid may be indicated. Chest radiographs are not necessary for patients with a clinical diagnosis of atelectasis in the first day or two after operation. Persistent fever of suspected pulmonary origin, however, requires a chest radiograph. Radiographs of other areas (e.g., the abdomen) are obtained as indicated. The search for deep infections may require special tests such as gallium scan, liver scan, ultrasound, computed tomography (CT), or magnetic resonance imaging (MRI) scans.

Postoperative fever is treated best by correction of the underlying cause. Because high fever (temperature greater than 38.5°C) is itself debilitating, antipyretic drugs (e.g., acetaminophen or aspirin) can be given by mouth or by rectal suppository while the cause is being investigated. Application of ice packs or 70% alcohol to the skin surface or placement of the patient on a refrigerated blanket are other methods of lowering body temperature.

If the cause of fever remains undefined, IV catheters and central lines should be removed and new ones placed. Potentially fever-causing drugs should be changed or discontinued.

## Confusion and Delirium

Elderly patients and those who are acutely and severely ill may become psychotic postoperatively. Causative factors include pain, sleep deprivation, isolation, and unfamiliar surroundings. The patients may become disoriented, hallucinatory, agitated, combative, and fearful of personnel who are caring for them, particularly at night. The derangements are transient, and patients usually regain their former mental status as the recovery from the operation progresses. It is essential to determine whether a patient with these symptoms is hypoxemic. Hypoxemia is a common cause of postoperative restlessness and mental status alteration, and the administration of analgesics or sedatives to a hypoxic patient may be lethal.

Simple helpful measures include keeping a light on in the room and providing a companion. Efforts should be made to reorient confused patients as often as possible. Mechanical restraints should be avoided unless the patient is at risk of self-injury or injury to others. Tranquilizers should be used cautiously, especially in elderly patients.

## Delayed Wound Healing and Dehiscence

Many systemic factors contribute to wound healing failure by altering collagen metabolism or impairing oxygen delivery to the wound. Local and technical problems may cause impaired blood supply or inadequate resistance to mechanical forces. Infection, corticosteroid or cytotoxic drug use, malnutrition, hypovolemia, hypoxemia, increased blood viscosity, tissue irradiation, and errors in technique may all contribute to impaired wound healing.

Wounds may dehisce because tissue is devitalized by dissection or strangulated by placement of too many sutures or by tying sutures too tightly. The latter is a common technical cause of dehiscence, which is confirmed when intact sutures are found to have cut through the tissue on one side of the wound. Inadequate suture strength or number or premature suture removal may also lead to similar complications. Absorbable sutures may not maintain their tensile strength long enough for secure healing, especially in debilitated patients.

Dehiscence of the skin is apparent on inspection. Fascial dehiscence is manifested by spontaneous serosanguineous fluid drainage from the wound. One must assume that fascia has dehisced when this type of drainage appears, especially when it persists. Fluid from a seroma or hematoma is not serosanguineous, and it usually does not continue to drain.

Obvious major dehiscence of the fascia should be treated by resuture under anesthesia in the operating room. Minor disruptions of fascia may be managed without resuture; however, the extent of fascial disruption is often underestimated until the skin is opened and the wound is explored. It is best to do this under aseptic conditions in the operating room.

Bleeding from the incision is apparent within minutes to hours after the operation is completed. Bleeding vessels may be in the skin, in the cutaneous fat, or at the fascial level.

## Decubitus Ulcers

Decubitus ulcers are caused by sustained pressure on the skin, usually over bony prominences such as the sacrum, ischium, trochanter, and heel. Poor nutrition is the most important factor leading to decubitus formation. The ulcers occur in bed-ridden patients who are weak, aged, malnourished, or paralyzed and who are receiving inadequate nursing care. Soiling of the bed because of bowel or urinary incontinence frequently leads to skin irritation, which in turn increases the risk of ulcer development. Unrelieved pressure of only a few hours may be sufficient to produce a decubitus ulcer in a susceptible individual. Usually, decubiti begin as small areas of erythema and tenderness that soon break down to form indolent ulcers, unless they are protected from further pressure. In neglected cases, large defects in skin and soft tissues may result from the combined effects of pressure, infection, and poor healing capability. Osteomyelitis of underlying bone may occur.

The most important elements in prevention of decubitus ulcers are vigilant nursing care, mobilization, and nutrition. Bedridden patients should be inspected frequently for areas of skin damage that may progress to ulcer formation. Soiling of the bed by incontinent patients should be prevented as much as possible. An alternating pressure or foam rubber mattress may be used to decrease pressure on the skin. Washable sponge pads under pressure points are also protective.

It is essential to change patient position frequently and protect involved skin areas by pillows and pads. The clothing and skin must be kept clean and dry. Correction of malnutrition and anemia and control of infection are often critical to healing.

Decubitus ulcers should be kept clean and well débrided. They may be exposed to air or covered with dry sterile dressings. Topical applications have little value. Invasive local infection should be treated with drainage, saline compresses, and systemic antibiotics, as indicated.

Surgical treatment of large, resistant lesions consists of complete débridement, including removal of any bony prominences or sequestra and closure of the wound with a local myocutaneous flap. This provides an adequate pad over the bone and avoids suture lines over the critical area of pressure. The donor area may be closed frequently by direct approximation, but a split-thickness skin graft may be required.

## Postoperative Complications Specific to Spinal Surgery
### Infection

**Spinal Surgical Wound Infection.** Spangfort[58] reviewed more than 10,000 laminectomy cases and reported an operative infection rate of approximately 2.9%. More recent series indicate that preoperative antibiotic prophylaxis may lower the incidence of infection.[47,51]

In 1980, Ramirez and Thisted[44] reported an incidence of infection of 0.3% in an analysis of 28,395 patients who underwent lumbar laminectomy for radiculopathy in the United States.

The clinical and radiographic characteristics of interspace infection were described first by Milward,[39] in 1936, after the inadvertent introduction of microorganisms into a disc space during lumbar puncture. Gieseking[19] reported the first postoperative interspace infection in 1951. Typically, patients with aseptic necrosis or interspace infection are asymptomatic immediately after surgery but begin to experience excruciating spasms in the lower back, with or without radiation into the legs within 2 weeks. Typically, the white blood cell count and temperature are often normal but the sedimentation rate is elevated, often to more than 100mm/h. Lumbosacral radiographs may reveal erosion of the cartilaginous plates as the disease progresses. Needle aspirations of the interspace may reveal the offending organisms but are often negative.[43] Patients with a clear-cut syndrome should be placed on IV antibiotics.

Wound infection should be suspected when persistent temperature elevation occurs several days postoperatively. The wound should be examined for erythema, swelling, tenderness, and drainage. Management should include a Gram stain and culture, with antibiotic treatment if the clinical suspicion is strong. In the presence of probable infection or persistent infection despite antibiotic treatment, the patient should be returned to the operating room and the wound reopened, thoroughly débrided, and irrigated. Hardware should not be removed. If there is substantial tissue necrosis, the wound can be managed open, with frequent dressing changes. If the tissues look healthy and well vascularized, the wound can be closed over drains.

**Discitis.** The incidence of postoperative intervertebral disc space infection (discitis) is 0.75%. Disc space infection rates vary from 0.1% to 3.8%.[10,25,36,46,58] The higher incidence of disc space infection with microsurgery has been attributed to the presence of the microscope over the open wound.[37] Postoperative discitis produces persistent intense back pain with unremarkable associated physical findings 2 weeks to 3 months after discectomy.

Elevated erythrocyte sedimentation rates are typical. Bone scan, CT, and MRI are quite sensitive for detecting discitis and can identify changes associated with discitis earlier than can plain radiographs. CT is effective in the early diagnosis of discitis, hypodensity of the affected disc space being detected as early as 10 days postoperatively. The responsible bacteria are identified in less than 50% of cases, with *Staphylococcus* species being the most common organisms cultured.[43] Early diagnosis and immediate treatment are important for preventing chronic infection. Immobilization is often effective for pain relief, and 4 to 6 weeks of intravenous antibiotic therapy is recommended.[43] Uncomplicated discitis should not require surgery, and most patients undergo spontaneous interbody fusion. Occasionally, lumbar epidural abscesses may develop that produce paresis. Under these circumstances, immediate decompressive laminectomy is indicated.

**Postoperative Osteomyelitis.** Infection may be introduced directly into the intervertebral disc space during surgery and can spread to the adjacent vertebral bodies, producing osteomyelitis. Surgery for protruding or herniated discs is the most frequent factor in the direct introduction of infection into the intervertebral disc space.[*] This

complication occurs in less than 1% of patients who undergo disc surgery. Organisms may be inadvertently inoculated at the time of surgery, and residual hematoma, necrotic tissue, and foreign bodies provide an environment conducive to bacterial proliferation. Weeks, months, or even years may elapse before the diagnosis of a disc space infection is established. Symptoms may not be apparent immediately after operation. Often there is initial pain relief followed by recurrence several days to weeks later. Fever may be transient, intermittent, or nonexistent, and there is often no evidence of infection when symptoms develop. The degree of pain may appear to be out of proportion to the objective findings and may be attributed erroneously to hysteria, malingering, or even psychoneurosis.

The typical radiologic changes of vertebral osteomyelitis may not be apparent for months. Radionuclide bone scans are quite sensitive and often demonstrate evidence of infection before plain films of the spine show any changes. However, they are not specific; surgical edema and disc changes may yield false-positive results.[18] Furthermore, early in the course of disc space infection, the bone scan may be negative in a significant proportion of patients.[21] CT scans may show destructive changes of the vertebral bodies before these are evident on plain films. End-plate irregularities on CT scan, however, are not specific for discitis, and normal curettage changes in vertebral end plates may mimic erosions of discitis.[230] MRI may show changes of discitis long before any changes are apparent radiologically.[1] It is, however, important to note that MRI and CT studies may be negative early in the course of postoperative or post-traumatic discitis,[21] and a high index of suspicion is necessary. Any patient with increasing back pain more than 2 weeks postoperatively and an erythrocyte sedimentation rate greater than 50mm/h should be considered to have discitis until proven otherwise.[1] Percutaneous disc biopsy can be helpful in the diagnosis of postoperative discitis,[17] but this is often falsely negative.

In a study comparing MRI, plain radiographs, and radionuclide studies in the evaluation of vertebral osteomyelitis, MRI was judged to be as accurate and sensitive as combined bone and gallium scanning and more sensitive than plain radiography. The MRI appearance of pyogenic infection is characteristic, making MRI a rapid noninvasive method for the detection of vertebral osteomyelitis and its complications, including epidural abscess. On $T_1$-weighted images, infected disc material shows decreased signal intensity from the intervertebral disc space and contiguous vertebral bodies relative to the normal vertebral signal. On $T_2$-weighted images, these tissues show increased signal. MRI provides more anatomic detail than radionuclide scanning and allows differentiation of neoplasm and degenerative disease from osteomyelitis. The disc space is nearly always spared in neoplastic disease, whereas degenerative disease with nucleus desiccation produces decreased disc signal on $T_2$-weighted images. Gallium scans may show positive results earlier than MRI scans in the course of infection, and this technique is more sensitive to changes arising from treatment and decreasing inflammation.

In many patients, postoperative discitis and vertebral osteomyelitis resolve spontaneously, and a diagnosis is never made.[50] In some patients with postoperative

---

[*]References 1,15,17,27,43,59,63,64.

vertebral osteomyelitis, intermittent antibiotic therapy obscures the diagnosis and permits the illness to go undetected for years.[27,35] Kern[27] reported a patient in whom vertebral osteomyelitis and meningitis became manifest 2.5 years after lumbar spinal surgery. The ability of infections to remain dormant and recur after long periods is illustrated by a patient in whom postoperative staphylococcal lumbar vertebral osteomyelitis developed and cleared after 3 years of treatment. Thirty-four years later, after 30 years without symptoms, the patient developed a staphylococcal psoas abscess.[35]

**Epidural Abscess.** Spinal epidural abscess (SEA) is an uncommon entity, but its clinical importance overshadows its rarity. Although epidural abscess is rare, it should be considered in any patient with increasing neurologic symptoms and signs in the early postoperative period. It may be difficult to differentiate from an expanding hematoma in the absence of systemic evidence of infection.

The importance of early diagnosis of SEA was emphasized by Heusner as early as 1948. Several studies have emphasized the frequently rapid deterioration and substantial permanent morbidity associated with this infection. Despite the recognition of spinal epidural abscess as a potential neurosurgical emergency and the increased sophistication of diagnostic studies, the morbidity and mortality associated with spinal epidural abscess remains significant. Advances in imaging have made the diagnosis of spinal epidural abscess less elusive and the options for therapeutic intervention more rational.

Spinal epidural abscesses are categorized as acute lesions (gross pus in the epidural space), usually with accompanying sepsis, or chronic lesions (granulation tissue in the epidural space) that may persist for months. The clinical presentation of an acute SEA is often stereotyped, but it can be difficult to appreciate in its earliest stages. The classic triad is intense localized back pain, progressive neurologic deficit, and fever. The initial complaint is almost uniformly axial pain. Paresthesias are also very common. Fever or other symptoms of infection are present about 50% of the time. Without treatment, the progression and time course of symptoms beyond this point is astoundingly uniform. Within 3 days, patients generally note radicular symptomatology, followed within 36 hours by weakness. Rapid deterioration to paralysis occurs typically over the next 24 hours. This pattern of symptoms is so uniform that some authors[66] suggest that this establishes the diagnosis until proven otherwise.

Laboratory findings are often unhelpful. Fever and leukocytosis are useful markers when present but are absent in more than 50% of the cases. Leukocytosis is common in the acute group (average white blood cell count of less than 16,000/mm[6]). The erythrocyte sedimentation rate is almost universally elevated but is a nonspecific indicator.

Plain radiographs are typically unremarkable in the absence of concomitant osteomyelitic involvement of adjacent vertebral bodies. The vertebral end plates directly adjacent to the disc space may show erosion. This often develops as late as 4 to 6 weeks after the onset of infection. The degree of local bone destruction from associated osteomyelitis is best appreciated by CT, and this information is often essential to formulation of the optimal management strategy.

CT myelography is an excellent technique that is often diagnostic. Lateral C1-2 puncture is our preferred method. This identifies the upper limit of any epidural mass but may not define the lower edge, and a second puncture below the block is required occasionally. Myelography has the added benefit of providing a cerebrospinal fluid sample for a cell count with differential, protein and glucose levels, Gram stain, and culture. The cerebrospinal fluid profile is generally consistent with parameningeal inflammation, although up to 15% of patients have concurrent meningitis. Myelography, however, carries the risk of converting an epidural process into a subdural empyema by subarachnoid contamination from puncture of the thecal sac during traversal of an unsuspected focus of epidural infection. Because of this potential morbidity, MRI is used as a first line diagnostic imaging modality.

MRI is indispensable for diagnosing spinal epidural abscess and is extremely valuable in guiding the patient's management. MRI is considered the diagnostic test of choice, and it is diagnostic in nearly every case. MRI rapidly and accurately identifies inflammatory foci, defines the degree of spinal cord compression, and shows the predominant location of the abscess and will often dictate the surgical approach. MRI provides more information than does CT about the extent of abscess involvement and degree of cord compromise.

The traditional therapy for spinal epidural abscess has been immediate surgical spinal cord decompression. Early studies of spinal epidural abscess recommended this policy and warned of patients who had deteriorated before delayed surgical decompression could be performed. The fundamental principles of surgical management are drainage of pus, débridement of granulation tissue, copious irrigation, and postoperative drainage.

## Summary

The perioperative management of the spinal surgery patient is both straightforward and potentially complex. It is critical to evaluate patients carefully, both preoperatively, to avoid intraoperative catastrophes, and postoperatively, to eliminate development of preventable associated morbidities. Perfect surgical procedures are often negated by suboptimal perioperative care. Spine surgery should never be considered potentially less morbid than other areas of neurosurgery.

## REFERENCES

1. Bircher MD, Tasker T, Crawshaw C, Mulholland RC: Discitis following lumbar surgery. *Spine* 13:98-102, 1988.
2. Bose B: Anterior cervical instrumentation enhances fusion rates in multilevel reconstruction in smokers. *J Spinal Disord* 14:3-9, 2001.
3. Brooks-Brunn JA: Predictors of postoperative pulmonary complications following abdominal surgery. Chest 111(3):564-571, 1997.

4. Brown CW, Orme TJ, Richardson HD: The rate of pseudarthrosis (surgical nonunion) in patients who are smokers and patients who are nonsmokers: a comparison study. *Spine* 11(9):942-943, 1986.

5. Brown MD, Seltzer DG: Perioperative care in lumbar spine surgery. *Orthop Clin North Am* 22:353-358, 1991.

6. Buzby GP: Perioperative nutritional support. *JPEN J Parenter Enteral Nutr* 14(suppl5):1975-1995, 1990.

7. Cain JE, Jr., Major MR, Lauerman WC, *et al:* The morbidity of heparin therapy after development of pulmonary embolus in patients undergoing thoracolumbar or lumbar spinal fusion. *Spine* 20(14)1600-1603, 1995.

8. Coran AG: Perioperative care of the pediatric patient. *Surg Annu* 1:31-55, 1991.

9. Daftari TK, Whitesides TE, Jr., Heller JG, *et al:* Nicotine on the revascularization of bone graft: an experimental study in rabbits. *Spine* 19(8):904-911, 1994.

10. Dauch W: Infection of the intervertebral space following conventional and microsurgical operation on the herniated lumbar intervertebral disc. *Acta Neurochir* 82:43-49, 1986.

11. David TS, Vrahas MS: Perioperative lower urinary tract infections and deep sepsis in patients undergoing total joint arthroplasty. *J Am Acad Orthop Surg* 8(1):66-74, 2000.

12. Deguchi M, Rapoff AJ, Zdeblick TA: Posterolateral fusion for isthmic spondylolisthesis in adults: analysis of fusion rate and clinical results. *J Spinal Disord* 11(6):459-464, 1998.

13. Ellis LM, Copeland ED, Souba WW: Perioperative nutritional support. *Surg Clin North Am* 71:493-507, 1991.

14. Emery SE, Smith MD, Bohlman HH: Upper-airway obstruction after multilevel cervical corpectomy for myelopathy. *J Bone Joint Surg Am* 73(4):544-551, 1991.

15. Ford L, Key J: Postoperative infection of the intervertebral disc space. *South Med J* 48:1295-1303, 1955.

16. Forrest JB, Rehder K, Cahalan MK, Goldsmith CH: Multicenter study of general anesthesia. III. Predictors of severe perioperative adverse outcomes. *Anesthesiology* 76(1):3-15, 1992.

17. Fouquet B, Goupille P, Jattiot F: Discitis after lumbar disc surgery. *Spine* 17:356-358, 1992.

18. Fraser R, Ostio, Vernon-Roberts B: Discitis after discography. *J Bone Joint Surg* 69B:26-35, 1987.

19. Gieseking H: Lokalisierte spondylitis nach operiertem Bandscheibenvorfall. *Zentralbl Chir* 76:1470-1477, 1951.

20. Glassman SD, Rose SM, Dimar JR, *et al:* The effect of postoperative nonsteroidal anti-inflammatory drug administration on spinal fusion. *Spine* 23(7):834-838, 1998.

21. Guyer RD, Collier RR, Ohnmeiss DD, *et al:* Extraosseous spinal lesions mimicking disc disease. *Spine* 13:328-331, 1988.

22. Hilibrand AS, Fye MA, Emery SE, *et al:* Impact of smoking on the outcome of anterior cervical arthrodesis with interbody or strut-grafting. *J Bone Joint Surg Am* 83A(5):668-673, 2001.

23. Howell SJ, Hemming AE, Allman KG, *et al:* Predictors of postoperative myocardial ischaemia: the role of intercurrent arterial hypertension and other cardiovascular risk factors. *Anaesthesia* 52(2):107-111, 1997.

24. Hu SS, Fontaine F, Kelly B, Bradford DS: Nutritional depletion in staged spinal reconstructive surgery. The effect of total parenteral nutrition. *Spine* 23:1401-1405, 1998.

25. Hudgins W: The role of microdiscectomy. *Orthop Clin North Am* 14:589-603, 1983.

26. Jevsevar DS, Karlin LI: The relationship between preoperative nutritional status and complications after an operation for scoliosis in patients who have cerebral palsy. *J Bone Joint Surg Am* 75(8):1256, 1993.

27. Kern C: Delayed death following disc surgery. *Texas State Med J* 50:158-160, 1954.

28. Khanam T: Anaesthetic risks in rheumatoid arthritis. *Br J Hosp Med* 52:320-325, 1994.

29. Klein JD, Hey LA, Yu CS, *et al:* Perioperative nutrition and postoperative complications in patients undergoing spinal surgery. *Spine* 21:2676-2682, 1996.

30. Kopecky K, Gilmor RL, Scott JA, Edwards MK: Pitfalls of computed tomography in diagnosis of discitis. *Neuroradiology* 27:57-66, 1985.

31. Lapp MA, Bridwell KH, Lenke LG, *et al:* Prospective randomization of parenteral hyperalimentation for long fusions with spinal deformity, its effect on complications and recovery from postoperative malnutrition. *Spine* 26:809-817, 2001.

32. Lee JH, Lee SH, Oh JH: Minimal effective dosage of recombinant human erythropoietin in spinal surgery. *Clin Orthop* 412(7):71-76, 2003.

33. Mammel M, Thompson TR: Perioperative management of the pediatric patient. *Urol Clin North Am* 10:139-148, 1983.

34. Mandelbaum BR, Tolo VT, McAfee PC, Burest P: Nutritional deficiencies after staged anterior and posterior spinal reconstructive surgery. *Clin Orthop* 234(9):5-11, 1988.

35. Mansour A, Nabos J, Taddonio R: Psoas abscess: thirty-four years after pyogenic osteomyelitis of the spine. *Orthopedics* 2:262-264, 1979.

36. Mayfield F: Complications of laminectomy. *Clin Neurosurg* 23:435-439, 1976.

37. McCulloch J: *Principles of Microsurgery for Lumbar Disc Disease.* Philadelphia, Lippincott-Raven, 1989.

38. Miller RW, Coulthard SW: Anesthesia for the elderly and debilitated patient. *Otolaryngol Clin North Am* 14:715-722, 1981.

39. Milward F: Changes in the intervertebral discs following lumbar puncture. *Lancet* 2:183-185, 1936.

40. Moller AM, Pedersen T, Villebro N, Munksgaard A: Effect of smoking on early complications after elective orthopaedic surgery. *J Bone Joint Surg Br* 85(2):178-181, 2003.

41. Moller AM, Villebro N, Pedersen T, Tonnesen H: Effect of preoperative smoking intervention on postoperative complications: a randomised clinical trial. *Lancet* 359(9301):114-117, 2002.

42. Mooney V, McDermott KL, Song J: Effects of smoking and maturation on long-term maintenance of lumbar spinal fusion success. *J Spinal Disord* 12(5):380-385, 1999.

43. Pilgaard S, Aarhus N: Discitis following removal of lumbar intervertebral disc. *J Bone Joint Surg* 51A:713-716, 1969.

44. Ramirez L, Thisted R: Complication and demographic characteristics of patients undergoing lumbar discectomy in community hospitals. *Neurosurgery* 25:226-231, 1989.

45. Rees TD, Liverett DM, Guy CL: The effect of cigarette smoking on skin-flap survival in the face lift patient. *Plast Reconstr Surg* 73(6):911-915, 1984.

46. Roberts M: Complications of lumbar disc surgery. *Spinal Surg* 2:13-19, 1988.

47. Rubinstein E, Findler G, Amit P, Shaked I: Perioperative prophylactic cephazolin in spinal surgery: a double-blind placebo-controlled trial. *J Bone Joint Surg Br* 76(1):99-102, 1994.

48. Saleh KL: The elderly patient in the post anesthesia care unit. *Nurs Clin North Am* 28:507-518, 1993.

49. Sawin PD, Dickman CA, Crawford NR, *et al:* The effects of dexamethasone on bone fusion in an experimental model of posterolateral lumbar spinal arthrodesis. *J Neurosurg* 94(suppl1):76-81, 2001.

50. Scherbel A, Gardner W: Infections involving the intervertebral discs: diagnosis and management. *JAMA* 174:370-374, 1960.

51. Schnoring M, Brock M: Prophylactic antibiotics in lumbar disc surgery: analysis of 1,030 procedures. *Zentralbl Neurochir* 64(1):24-29, 2003.

52. Silcox DH, III, Boden SD, Schimandle JH, *et al:* Reversing the inhibitory effect of nicotine on spinal fusion using an osteoinductive protein extract. *Spine* 23(3):291-296, 1998.

53. Silcox DH, III, Daftari T, Boden SD, *et al:* The effect of nicotine on spinal fusion. *Spine* 20(14):1549-1553, 1995.

54. Skues MA, Welchew EA: Anaesthesia and rheumatoid arthritis. *Anaesthesia* 48:989-997, 1993.

55. Sorensen LT, Horby J, Friis E, *et al:* Smoking as a risk factor for wound healing and infection in breast cancer surgery. *Eur J Surg Oncol* 29(5):482, 2003.

56. Sorensen LT, Jorgensen T: Short-term pre-operative smoking cessation intervention does not affect postoperative complications in colorectal surgery: a randomized clinical trial. *Int J Colorectal Dis* 5(4): 347-352, 2003.

57. Sorensen LT, Karlsmark T, Gottrup F: Abstinence from smoking reduces incisional wound infection: a randomized controlled trial. *Ann Surg* 238(1):1-5, 2003.

58. Spangfort E: The lumbar disc herniation: a computer aided analysis of 2,504 operations. *Acta Orthop Scand* 142(suppl):1-95, 1972.

59. Sullivan C, Bickel W, Svien H: Infections of vertebral interspaces after operations on intervertebral discs. *JAMA* 166:1973-1977, 1958.

60. Sweet FA, Lenke LG, Bridwell KH, *et al:* Prospective radiographic and clinical outcomes and complications of single solid rod instrumented anterior spinal fusion in adolescent idiopathic scoliosis. *Spine* 26(18):1956-1965, 2001.

61. Thalgott JS, Cotler HB, Sasso RC, *et al:* Postoperative infections in spinal implants. Classification and analysis: a multicenter study. *Spine* 16(8):981-984, 1991.

62. Theiss SM, Boden SD, Hair G, *et al:* The effect of nicotine on gene expression during spine fusion. *Spine* 25(20): 2588-2594, 2000.

63. Thibodeau A: Closed space infection following removal of lumbar intervertebral disc. *J Bone Joint Surg* 50A:400-410, 1968.

64. Turnbull F: Postoperative inflammatory disease of lumbar discs. *J Neurosurg* 10:469-473, 1953.

65. Weis JC, Betz RR, Clements DH, III, Balsara RK: Prevalence of perioperative complications after anterior spinal fusion for patients with idiopathic scoliosis. *J Spinal Disord* 10(5):371-375, 1997.

66. Zeidman S, Rigamonti D: Spinal epidural abscess. *Surg Neurol* 52(2):189-196, 1999.

# CHAPTER 141

# Medical Management of the Patient with Spinal Cord Injury

**Michael J. Rosner, Andrea L. Halliday, and Perry A. Ball**

Spinal cord injury (SCI) has historically been associated with high mortality. Between 1980 and 1985 this rate was reduced by 60%, and by a further 90% since 1986.[29] The leading cause of death associated with SCI remains respiratory failure (mainly from pneumonia) in both the acute and the chronic phases of quadriplegia. Other causes are sepsis, cardiovascular problems, and renal complications.[28] Medical management is crucial to the reduction of mortality and improvement in the quality of life and is based on known postinjury pathophysiologic changes. Although some of the pathophysiology remains vague and ill-defined, several well-established phenomena provide a rational basis for management of patients with SCI.

The following are important considerations for medical management: (1) respiratory changes that are mostly secondary to interaction of the denervated intercostal and abdominal musculature with an intact diaphragm, (2) cardiovascular and gastrointestinal (GI) events that relate to generalized sympathectomy and unopposed vagal innervation; (3) the more general consequences of immobility and its interaction with skin, muscle mass, joints, lungs, and in particular, the venous system, and (4) the interaction of these changes with the patient's systemic and psychological condition.

## Respiratory Complications and Care

Pneumonia and atelectasis are the most common respiratory problems, and these occur more often in "complete" quadriplegia (in 80% to 90%) than in patients with "incomplete" lesions (15% to 20%).[66] Pleural effusion, hemopneumothorax, and pulmonary edema occur in 15% to 20% of the cases.[61]

Because most early morbidity and mortality cases result from respiratory causes, many neurosurgeons eschew early intubation of SCI patients for fear that the patient will never be ventilator free. This is not the case. Whereas the patient with complete cervical quadriplegia spends approximately 3 weeks on the ventilator, compared with only 3 to 5 days for the patient with incomplete quadriplegia, most severely injured patients are successfully weaned from the ventilator and the intensive care unit (ICU).[66,110]

For the few patients whose injury does not allow return of adequate function, home ventilatory support can be very successful.[35,100] Some of these techniques require tracheostomy, but many procedures can be employed noninvasively, with oral intermittent positive pressure ventilation being the method most frequently used. Nasal, thoracic, or abdominal devices are the next in frequency of use.[7] Standard volume ventilation can also be used successfully.[100]

Furthermore, over 6 weeks to 6 months, forced vital capacity (FVC) and forced expiratory volume improve by 30% to 100%. The degree of improvement relates poorly to the lesion level. It correlates only weakly with the degree of initial severity of the SCI[11,16,97] and can be improved with exercise.[25] Decisions about early ventilation and intubation should therefore be based on the objective assessment of respiratory function after injury and not on a guess about ultimate outcome. Furthermore, ventilation should be used aggressively before severe pulmonary dysfunction progresses.[72,110]

## Respiratory Physiology in Quadriplegia

### Muscles of Respiration

Surgeons have traditionally been taught that after SCI the diaphragm is intact, and therefore respiratory function should be relatively normal. Most SCIs occur below level C4 (the predominant nerve root level of the phrenic nerve) and leave the diaphragm intact. However, this traditional teaching has impeded the surgeon's understanding of the importance of the intercostal muscles and accessory muscles of respiration in the pathophysiologic processes involved with SCI* and respiratory failure. Normally, intercostal muscles provide little for active ventilation during periods of rest or relative inactivity. However, they play an important role in maintaining the chest wall as a relatively rigid structure, against which the diaphragm can act to generate tidal volume. An analogy is a syringe in which the diaphragm is represented by the plunger. As long as the syringe barrel is stiff and rigid, a substantial negative force, based only on movement of the plunger (diaphragm), can be generated. If the syringe barrel were to become flexible, negative forces generated within the syringe by plunger withdrawal would cause the wall to collapse and pucker. This is exactly what happens to the quadriplegic patient with paralysis of intercostal musculature. The diaphragm is intact, but the chest wall functions as in a severe flail chest injury, and the negative inspiratory forces generated are inadequate to produce the required tidal volume ($V_t$).

In middle and low cervical quadriplegia the scalene muscle (C3-8), the clavicular portion of the pectoralis major muscle (C5-7), and the laryngeal, glossopharyngeal, latissimus dorsi, and cranial portions of the serratus anterior muscles are all eventually able to augment respiratory mechanics. It is these cervically innervated muscles that allow earlier weaning of the patient with middle or low cervical quadriplegia. The patient with high quadriplegia (C0-4) may or may not lose diaphragmatic function but may lose these accessory muscles.[78]

---

*References 31,66,71,72,97,99.

Patients with low quadriplegia or high thoracic paraplegia have functionally similar respiratory characteristics. The frequency of pulmonary contusion and the high energy exerted in thoracic paraplegia often increase the latter patients' risk of pulmonary complications.[61]

## Respiratory Weaning and Intubation Parameters

The negative inspiratory force (NIF), FVC, and $V_t$ of 30 consecutive, nonintubated patients with quadriplegia or high thoracic paraplegia were measured from the time of admission until discharge from the ICU (Rosner, unpublished data). It was found that at admission, NIF averaged $-44 \pm 15$cm $H_2O$, FVC averaged 1.08L, and $V_t$ averaged approximately 300ml (Table 141.1). Table 141.2 lists parameters that are generally used as a guideline for elective intubation. The average FVC is at the level at which elective intubation would normally be considered. The NIF is also low. In general these profound respiratory abnormalities are almost exclusively the result of the functionally flail chest produced by paralysis of the intercostal muscles.[31,72,97]

The consequences of low $V_t$ are apparent immediately as wasted ventilation. Anatomic wasted ventilation is defined

### TABLE 141.1

**Selected Pulmonary Physiologic Variables in Patients With Respiratory Compromise**

| | Normal* | Respiratory Failure* | Acute Quadriplegia† |
|---|---|---|---|
| Forced vital capacity (L) | 4.5–5.25 | 1.05 | $1.08 \pm 0.4$ |
| Negative inspiratory force (cm $H_2O$) | −75 to 100 | ≥−25 | $-43 \pm 14$ |
| Compliance (nonintubated) ml/cm $H_2O$ | 100 | <20 | 24 |
| $Pao_2$ ($Fio_2 = 0.21$) (mmHg) | 80–95 | <70 | $95 \pm 32$ ($Fio_2 = 0.30$) |
| $(A-a)o_2$ ($Fio_2 = 1$) (mmHg) | 25–65 | >450 | 75 ($Fio_2 = 0.30 \pm 0.08$) |
| $Paco_2$ (mmHg) | 35–45 | >55 | $36 \pm 5$ |
| Wasted ventilation ($V_d/V_t$) (anatomic) | 0.2–0.3 | 0.55–0.6 | 0.5 |

$Pao_2$, partial arterial pressure of $O_2$; $Fio_2$, Fraction of inspired $O_2$; $(A-a)o_2$, alveolar-arterial $O_2$ gradient; $Paco_2$, partial pressure of $CO_2$; $V_d$, dead space; $V_t$, tidal volume.
*Data from Demling.[27]
†Data on newly admitted patients.

### TABLE 127.2

**Definitions of Selected Respiratory Parameters Useful for Monitoring Patients With SCI**

| | |
|---|---|
| Forced vital capacity (FVC) | The maximal volume that can be exhaled after a maximal inhalation. It is usually 65 to 75ml/kg of ideal body weight. In most males it approximates 5L. |
| Tidal volume ($V_t$) | The air moved during a typical spontaneous breath. Normally this is 5 to 7ml/kg of ideal body weight or 350 to 500ml during rest and mild activity. |
| Functional residual capacity (FRC) | The volume remaining in the lung after exhalation—high FRC reduces risk of atelectasis. |
| Negative inspiratory force (NIF) | The negative pressure that can be generated by a maximal inspiratory attempt. It is measured at the bedside. Normal individuals can generate negative pressures of −75 to −100ml $H_2O$. However, many bedside meters do not measure pressures higher than −60ml $H_2O$. |
| Pulmonary compliance ($\Delta V/\Delta P$) | The change in volume ($\Delta V$) generated by a change in pressure ($\Delta P$). PEEP must be subtracted from the peak inspiratory pressure to define the $\Delta P$ or the change in pressure. The normal value for nonintubated patients is approximately 100ml/cm $H_2O$. For intubated patients the normal value is approximately 30 to 40ml/cm $H_2O$ because of the additional force required to expand the chest wall. |
| Dead space ($V_d$) | The volume of air that does not reach the alveoli for gas exchange. It is estimated to be 2ml/kg of ideal body weight and is about 150ml for the average adult. |
| Anatomic wasted ventilation ($V_d/V_t$) | Dead space divided by $V_t$. This is the percentage of each breath that is not available for gas exchange. It is normally 20% to 30%, based only on anatomic dead space. Physiologic dead space is always greater because it includes those alveoli that are ventilated but not perfused. |
| (Alveolar-arterial) $O_2$ gradient ($[A-a]o_2$) | Estimate of relative hypoxemia and calculated as $(A-a)o_2 = Fio_2$ (760mmHg − 47mmHg $H_2O$) − ($PAco_2/0.8$) − $Pao_2$. Normally, the $Pao_2$ should approximate the $PAo_2$ (e.g., if $Fio_2 = 0.4$, $Pao_2$ should be about 235mmHg). |
| Ideal body weight (Dallas-Hall Formula*) | Male = 106lb + 6lb/in (over 60 inches)<br>Female = 100lb + 5lb/in (over 60 inches) |

PEEP, Positive end-expiratory pressure; $Fio_2$, fraction of inspired $O_2$; $PAco_2$, partial alveolar pressure of $CO_2$; $Pao_2$, partial arterial pressure of $O_2$; $PAo_2$, partial alveolar pressure of $O_2$
*From Zeman.[114]

by the ratio of the ventilatory dead space ($V_d$) to the total $V_t$ or $V_d/V_t$. Anatomic wasted ventilation exceeding 50% to 60% signals the need for elective intubation based on impending ventilatory failure. Normal $V_d$ is approximately 2ml/kg, or about 150ml for the average adult male (on the basis of ideal body weight). If the $V_t$ is only 300ml, wasted ventilation is already at 50%.

If the patient continues with low $V_t$ relative to dead space (high wasted ventilation), inadequate NIF (low NIF), and an inability to generate an effective cough or to take deep breaths (low FVC), the respiratory consequences are predictable. Diffuse microatelectasis develops and can become severe; although early on, chest radiographs may remain nearly normal. Similarly, auscultation and physical examination of the chest may be close to normal. As the process of atelectasis continues and becomes more generalized the lungs stiffen and begin to demonstrate decreased compliance.

Compliance is defined by the ratio of the change in volume to the change in pressure required to generate the change in volume. As the lungs stiffen, or compliance decreases, the pressure (NIF) required to generate a given $V_t$ increases and the work of breathing increases.[72] However, the inspiratory force of the quadriplegic patient, which is already near the lower limits of normal, generally cannot be increased significantly.

Decreasing compliance, with high wasted ventilation and an inability to generate deep breaths and cough, which adequately reexpands the lungs, potentiates the process of atelectasis. This results in a vicious cycle of decreasing $V_t$s and decreasing compliance that further decreases the $V_t$. Hypoxemia and respiratory failure ensue.

In its purest form, this process is demonstrated with serial measurements of weaning parameters. Close attention should also be paid to the respiratory rate. Although unable to generate an adequate $V_t$, patients are able to increase their respiratory rate. Progressive tachypnea is usually the first sign of impending respiratory failure. In this case patients tire and eventually are unable to support their ventilation (especially because of the high wasted ventilatory effort). The result may be acute respiratory arrest.

### Blood Gas Determinations

Blood gas determinations, when used as the primary method to assess adequacy of pulmonary function, may provide misleading results. Arterial blood gas values are the least sensitive indicators of pulmonary function, and they change only after pulmonary and cardiovascular reserves are depleted. Early in the process, tachypnea, even with high wasted ventilation, results in a normal to low partial pressure of carbon dioxide in alveoli ($PaCO_2$). Hypocapnia may be misinterpreted as evidence of perfectly adequate respiratory reserve, whereas it actually represents a response to respiratory distress. It is the result of the activation of primary pulmonary receptors that produces dyspnea (vagal afferents) and increases the ventilatory drive.[102] At this stage it has very little, if any, input from the carotid chemoreceptors and does not represent a response to hypoxemia. As this process continues the $PaCO_2$ often falls, with increasing tachypnea.

Hypoxemia begins to develop, although it tends to be mild. At this stage treatment with supplemental oxygen may mask further pulmonary impairment and neither addresses nor alters the basic pathophysiologic events. Supplemental oxygen may improve hypoxemia, but it does not address the cause. No patient in the ICU is hypoxemic from a lack of oxygen in the environment (at least at sea level). Atelectasis, ventilation-perfusion abnormalities, and failure to mobilize secretions are common underlying causes.

As the patient tires, wasted ventilation increases and microatelectasis continues to develop. These processes all interact, and the patient's respiratory rate can no longer be sustained. Effective alveolar ventilation reaches low levels, and the $PaCO_2$ begins to increase. Hypoxemia becomes profound and respiratory arrest may be imminent.

Another key to the early detection of impending ventilatory failure is the alveolar-arterial oxygen ($[A–a]O_2$) gradient. If a healthy person receives supplemental oxygen, such that the fraction of inspired oxygen ($FiO_2$) is 0.40, partial arterial pressure of $O_2$ ($PaO_2$) should be 200 to 235mmHg. This is rarely the case in quadriplegic patients. This phenomenon represents a large ($A–a)O_2$ gradient and suggests pulmonary dysfunction. If the $PaO_2$ is 70mmHg, tissue oxygenation is adequate and arterial saturation of hemoglobin is 90% or more. Nevertheless, the relatively low $PaO_2$ is a sign of pulmonary abnormality. For example, if the respiratory rate is 35, the $PaCO_2$ is 25mmHg, and the $PaO_2$ is 65 to 70mmHg with apparent dyspnea, the patient would not be optimally treated by adding nasal prongs and low-flow oxygen to the treatment regimen, even though $PaO_2$ may transiently improve. Therapy would more appropriately be directed at the underlying pathophysiology (i.e., a failure of adequate expansion of the lungs).

### Airway Secretions

Concomitant with the inability to take deep breaths and to cough is the inability to clear airway secretions. If airway secretions accumulate, there is progressive obstruction of small bronchioles and pulmonary segments distal to the obstruction. These segments become atelectatic and contribute to decreasing pulmonary compliance and hypoxemia.

Pulmonary secretions tend to be more viscous after SCI and are increased in volume,[10,58] and the airways are abnormally reactive.[101] Both problems resolve with time but require aggressive early management.

Chest auscultation may fail to identify a significant secretion problem for three reasons: (1) poor tidal volume may not move enough of the secretions to produce rhonchi, (2) an upright position will allow secretions to drain to the dependent portions of the lung, in which ventilation is minimal and which does not generate rhonchi, and (3) dehydration may harden secretions such that they become immobile and rhonchi are not generated.

Systemic hydration of the patient is mandatory for adequate mobilization of secretions; warm, humidified air also aids immensely in secretion clearance.

The early use of bronchodilators may improve both mucus secretion and ciliary action[10,99] and may also reduce airway resistance.[101] The latter will improve cough (expiratory velocity), reduce work of breathing, and help preserve lung volumes.

## Atelectasis

The use of additional oxygen to treat the mild hypoxemia associated with this early form of respiratory compromise may actually potentiate the development of atelectasis. Absorption atelectasis represents a decrease in alveolar volume as a result of the absorption of oxygen. Room air consists of approximately 80% nitrogen, which is neither well nor rapidly absorbed from the alveoli. If the patient is placed on an inspired oxygen concentration of 0.40 (almost double the oxygen concentration of room air), the volume by which the alveolus can be expected to decline or collapse doubles. The use of supplemental oxygen must be considered very carefully in patients with SCI. The process of alveolar collapse may be potentiated through the loss of volume via the absorbable gas. This is another factor that may accelerate the cycle of progressive atelectasis.

A further complication is that as the $FiO_2$ is increased, hypoxemia may improve at first and instill a false sense of security. A key observation is the improvement in $PaO_2$ followed, within hours, by a decrement in $PaO_2$ to the level before oxygen treatment. This decline is a signal to the clinician that lack of oxygen was not the cause of hypoxemia, that more oxygen will not help, and that lung volume, pulmonary shunt, and secretions ought to be managed better.

Upper lung segments are well ventilated but poorly perfused; lower segments are well perfused but poorly ventilated. In quadriplegic patients with intact accessory muscles the upper chest may expand (ventilating the upper lobes) but leave the lower thorax with paradoxical motion (but functionally flail) and relatively poor ventilation.[31,97] The ventilation-to-perfusion ratio (V/Q) mismatch potentiates basilar atelectasis, especially in the upright position.

Normally, a person increases vital capacity in the upright position; quadriplegic patients decrease their vital capacity when upright. The reasons include less effective diaphragmatic contraction in this position, increased basilar congestion (blood volume), which increases basilar atelectasis, and dependent drainage of secretions into the lung bases.[31,46,72]

## Pulmonary Trauma

One must consider the interaction of pulmonary contusion, aspiration, hemopneumothorax, and other pulmonary injuries that occur in 20% to 40% of patients with SCI. Even patients with clear chest radiographs may have aspirated or have suffered a pulmonary contusion (especially thoracic fractures). Most of the physical signs in this group of patients are normal or nearly normal, or are so masked by rhonchi, the noise of tubes and ventilators, and other ambient sounds that the presence of intrinsic pulmonary pathologic processes is not evident. The reasons may well be one or more of the following: (1) increased $(A–a)O_2$ gradient (relative hypoxemia), (2) decreased pulmonary compliance, (3) abnormalities on chest radiograph, such as fractured ribs and clavicles or other

injuries, and (4) thoracic spine fractures that are often associated with pulmonary contusion. Critical interpretation of all information obtained at admission can be very useful for establishing a plan to follow a patient serially for respiratory failure or for electively intubating the patient before the process is difficult to reverse. Serial parameters taken multiple times per day can be very helpful.

## Respiratory Failure

The consequence of neglecting changes in respiratory parameters goes beyond respiratory failure. As respiratory failure continues it becomes difficult to re-expand the lungs, even with tracheal intubation and mechanical ventilation. The lungs are often extremely stiff, with significantly decreased compliance. Thick and colonized secretions begin to accumulate, and infection may develop very rapidly.

The interaction of bronchopulmonary infection, profoundly atelectatic lungs, pulmonary contusion, or factors such as aspiration and chest injury in a patient whose immune response is already abnormal may result in rapid development of the adult respiratory distress syndrome (ARDS). Mortality from ARDS is reported to be as high as 40% in many series. Equally important is the prolonged period of ventilation required to reverse the pulmonary capillary changes. This may require 4 to 6 weeks or more of ventilatory support. The results, in terms of prolonged mechanical ventilation and ICU stay, can be devastating and extraordinarily expensive. The patient who would otherwise have become ventilator independent may be permanently ventilator dependent.

## Diagnostic Pitfalls

The chest examination, including auscultation, may be misleading in the patient with thick or dried secretions. Auscultation suggests clear chest fields. If the secretions are too thick to move as tidal ventilation occurs, rhonchi are not heard. Often the atelectatic process is so diffuse that areas of inadequate breath sounds either are not heard or are masked by ambient noise. Therefore the patient with an increased $(A–a)O_2$ gradient, but with relatively normal auscultation and chest radiograph that reveal clear lung fields, may be manifesting the pulmonary effects of dehydration or inadequate humidification of the inspired gas, with poor mobilization of secretions.

A similar pitfall of the physical examination is the ease with which expiratory wheezes are missed with continuous positive airway pressure (CPAP) or positive end-expiratory pressure (PEEP). The positive airway pressure maintains functional residual capacity (FRC) by preventing collapse of alveoli. At the same time terminal velocity of flow may be decreased, and wheezing because of bronchospasm may be missed or misinterpreted. If this process continues unchecked and unrecognized, the patient can develop severe problems from acute asthma. If bronchodilator therapy is not instituted, the patient may continue to deteriorate. This is manifested as a rising $PaCO_2$, rising peak inspiratory pressure, and hyperinflation of the lungs from air trapping. Pneumothorax or permanent bullous emphysema may result. These changes may not necessarily be reversible in all patients.[6] It is easy to ascribe the deteriorating pulmonary condition either to developing ARDS or to some concomitant pulmonary injury and change, such as aspiration pneumonia or pulmonary contusion. Although ARDS, atelectasis, and pulmonary edema are best treated with increasing PEEP and increasing mechanical ventilation, the effects of bronchospasm may be worsened by increasing PEEP or $V_t$, or with a higher respiratory rate because of air trapping. Bronchodilators should be used in most patients with ARDS.

## General Management Principles

The prevention of the respiratory failure cascade is based on maintaining the FRC, which implies maintaining lung expansion by adequate $V_t$ and by secretion clearance. This is normally accomplished by assisting the patient to cough.

Just as inspiration is ineffective against a relatively flaccid chest wall, so is the cough. The high positive pressures generated by glottic closure, and the abdominal and chest wall tension present in normal coughing, are lost in the quadriplegic patient with a flaccid chest and abdominal wall. However, in the partially injured patient, coughing can be assisted with manual compression of the epigastrium or abdominal binder. These techniques are best used in the more chronic phase of paralysis.[46,62]

Nasotracheal or oral tracheal suctioning should be used early and aggressively, before obvious pulmonary dysfunction develops. Sick patients *will* have secretions, and if the cough is not productive, the secretions must be suctioned.

Severe pulmonary failure is best diverted by a rational and careful plan directed at the following considerations: (1) maintaining FRC, (2) clearing secretions, (3) using a careful and expectant approach to intubating those patients not already intubated, and (4) recognizing that in the unintubated patient, the most objective indicators for elective intubation are not blood gas results but progressive tachypnea, inadequate or declining FRC, low $V_t$ associated with high wasted ventilation, and low and declining NIF. If the patient has a Swan-Ganz catheter, pulmonary dysfunction may be signaled at an even earlier stage by an increasing pulmonary shunt fraction.

A kinetic therapy bed has been shown to be very effective in improving pulmonary shunt fraction. Qs/Qt (15% to 20%) can thus be used as a criterion for moving patients to a kinetic therapy bed and back to a regular hospital bed.[92]

## Continuous Positive Airway Pressure

It may be clinically beneficial to use CPAP by mask or other currently available appliances to maintain FRC. In a recent study of surgical patients treated with coughing, deep breathing, and turning (vs. incentive spirometry or CPAP by mask), pulmonary complications in the group receiving CPAP by mask were essentially nonexistent, compared with the baseline rates obtained in the more traditional treatment groups. Similarly, just as the cough and deep breathing techniques have intrinsic limitations because of the pulmonary changes brought about by the SCI, so does incentive spirometry. Regardless of how great the incentive is, when FVC is less than 700ml, mechanical assistance will be required to maintain lung volume.

## Mobilization of Secretions

The mobilization of secretions is extraordinarily important. The use of mechanical techniques such as suctioning, either via endotracheal or nasotracheal routes, is mandatory in many severely injured patients with SCI. It is equally important to maintain these secretions in a fluid and liquid state so that they can be easily mobilized. Adequate humidification is the most important aspect of this process, and can most often be accomplished by a nebulizer, as either a cold or a warm mist. The former is usually adequate; however, there are times when a warm mist will produce a better result because the partial pressure of water is directly related to temperature. Molecular water can penetrate more deeply into and through the small airways and can help liquefy secretions that are located in areas that are difficult to reach. Humidified air at 37°C will not cause fever (but it does require heater lines inside the tubing to avoid blocking of the tubing from excessive condensation). Warmed air also reduces bronchospasm.

Metaproterenol (Alupent; 1mg/2.5ml; q 6 to 8 hr) and albuterol (2.5mg/3ml; q 6 to 8 hr) are sympathomimetic bronchodilators that may assist in mobilizing secretions by maintaining an open airway.[101] Ipratropium (Atrovent; 500μg/2.5ml, q 6 to 8 hr) is an anticholinergic bronchodilator that may be used to complement the sympathomimetic agents. All these agents can be started at lower doses than those given here because their systemic effects may be amplified in the quadriplegic patient. Evidence also suggests that the activity of pulmonary cilia is improved by such therapy.

Systemic steroids (e.g., methylprednisolone; 125 to 1000mg, q 6 hr) are highly effective against bronchospasm. It may be prudent to begin steroids when problematic bronchospasm is recognized. Because steroids become effective in about 6 hours, additional agents may be needed initially. When ARDS is developing, it may be prudent to treat bronchospasm and infection early.

Acetylcysteine (Mucomyst) can at times be useful to break up secretions. It should be used with great caution, however, because of the risk of bronchospasm and inflammation of the tracheal and bronchial endothelia. Endotracheal saline is very useful and safe.

Oscillating beds or frequent turning to the full lateral decubitus position may help clearance of secretions. The patient is rotated from side to side, and secretions are drained in a dependent fashion. Some beds can be programmed to vary the time and angle of elevation to either side. Keeping the more atelectatic (nondependent) lung higher for a longer period (15 to 30 seconds) than the better-inflated lung may help immensely with reinflation.

If a pulse oximeter is used to monitor $SpO_2$ continuously, it is useful to note when saturation decreases in the rotation cycle. When the more severely affected, atelectatic lung is at a lower elevation, $SpO_2$ should decrease because of an augmented V/Q abnormality. Changing the cycle to keep this lung higher for a longer time should speed reexpansion.

Bronchoscopy is useful in clearing foreign bodies from the tracheobronchial tree. However, if repeat bronchoscopy is needed for secretion management, patient ventilation should be reassessed for inadequate $V_t$, inadequate PEEP, excess $Fio_2$, or airway temperatures lower than 37°C. Inadequate or infrequent suctioning usually accompanies this situation.

## Management of Infection

Although it is imperative to treat infection at an early stage, prophylactic antibiotics are rarely indicated, because quadriplegic patients are long-term patients. Within 2 to 3 days of hospitalization an alteration of the normal flora occurs in almost all patients, even those in relatively good health. There is a shift in the standard oral flora toward a mix of nosocomial organisms. This shift is unpreventable, is usually potentiated by prophylactic antibiotics, and leads to the selection of resistant, robust organisms that can colonize the patient. The tracheobronchial tree can never be sterilized by the use of antibiotics.

Achieving sterile pulmonary secretions should not become the goal of therapy. Before an antibiotic is selected and used, the following factors should be taken into account: (1) the types of bacteria seen after a Gram stain, (2) the white blood cell (WBC) numbers (3+ or 4+), (3) the quality, quantity, and characteristics of the secretions (e.g., thick, purulent), (4) the presence of infiltrates on chest radiographs, (5) other measures of pulmonary dysfunction, (6) declining platelet and WBC counts (i.e., the clinician should define the evidence for infection vs. colonization), and (7) fever.

The criteria for success and termination of antibiotic usage should be identified at the time that therapy is instituted and should clarify the goals of therapy to avoid prolonged and questionable drug therapy.

Similarly, antibiotics should not be withheld for obvious pneumonia, sepsis, or other infection. Antibiotics should be directed at the most likely organisms, usually nosocomial, and should have a broad spectrum of activity. They should never be withheld from a deteriorating patient with progressive infection while culture results are pending.

Antibiotics should be used for specific infections, for specific periods, or with objective criteria, such as clearance observed on progressive chest radiographs. A culture report suggesting different or additional organisms should only rarely lead to a change in antibiotics if the patient has been improving. Antibiotic therapy should be discontinued if the pneumonia has cleared, as determined by chest radiography, physical examination, sputum criteria, defervescence of the patient, decreasing WBC count, or normalization of the differential WBC count.

When antibiotics are discontinued after 1 to 2 weeks, the patient often develops a new fever. It may be best to withhold treatment until a new culture is obtained and a clear source of the fever is identified. Often the fever disappears over the next 48 to 72 hours without the need for further antibiotics.

Indiscriminate antibiotic use can cause resistant organisms to develop and can suppress normal flora. Often after cessation of antibiotic therapy, the fever subsides and the problem disappears. This is not related to clearing of "drug fever" or to an antibiotic reaction, but is the result of a normal mix of flora beginning to exert itself and control pathogenic organisms.

## Weaning from Ventilator Support

When a patient is ready for ventilator weaning, serial measures of FVC, NIF, and $V_t$, augmented by blood gas determinations, physical examination, and respiratory rate evaluation, provide the objective basis to accelerate the rate of this process. Asking patients about their comfort level is a powerful but often neglected component of the process.[57]

A reliable method of weaning quadriplegic patients from ventilatory support is by gradually decreasing the synchronized intermittent mandatory ventilation (SIMV) rate. A rate of four breaths per minute with low (approximately 5cm $H_2O$) PEEP is usually well tolerated. At this level of mechanical support the patients provide most of their minute ventilation for most of the day and night. Concomitantly, the work of breathing can be diminished with the use of positive airway pressure (PEEP or pressure support) and by the reduction in dead space associated with tracheotomy. The reduction of IMV rates to 4 is usually tolerated well by most ventilator-dependent quadriplegic patients. Further reduction from this level of support is often difficult.

Two factors are important at this point. First, the progression of fibrosis or spasticity of the intercostal musculature that allows the diaphragm to be more efficient requires time—usually 4 to 16 weeks. Second, the physical strengthening of the muscle groups that are functional depends on exercising and stressing those muscles. Exercise must be combined with adequate rest.[11,66,69]

Alternating periods of very low SIMV (<4) that progress to no ventilator breaths (0 SIMV) with maintenance of a PEEP/CPAP level of about 5cm $H_2O$, alternating with SIMV of 4 can work well. The patient may initially tire after 5 to 10 minutes and must be placed back on ventilator support for 1 to 2 hours of rest. The work time can be increased until it equals the rest time; the former is increased and rest time is decreased until the patient can manage throughout the day without rest. A full night's rest is crucial to success, and elimination of nighttime ventilator support is the last stage of weaning.

For a reasonable night's rest (10 PM to 6 AM), the patient may be placed on a SIMV rate of 10 to 14 or on at least a comfortable rate. The active weaning process is reinstituted the next morning. It is imperative that sedatives be avoided. "Anxiety" during this stage may represent dyspnea and too rapid a withdrawal of support, rather than purely psychological effects, and is not incompatible with the quadriplegic patient's natural fear at the prospect of ventilator withdrawal. Dyspnea and air hunger may be expressed in the patient by the following finding: Usually the $Pao_2$ is normal with a low $Paco_2$—a finding that does not rule out too-rapid weaning. Treatment of dyspnea and anxiety is achieved by providing reassurance and by increasing ventilatory support, or by holding the weaning process at the current level. It is not treated with drugs. Too-rapid weaning can lead to pneumonia, atelectasis, and pulmonary changes that may take weeks to resolve or may permanently damage the lungs.[6]

As weaning proceeds to a CPAP of 0, a T-tube trial with 0 CPAP is a better tolerance test than 12 or 24 hours of CPAP alone. A T-piece connected to warmed, humidified air eliminates the higher resistance and increased work of breathing associated with most ventilator circuits. Therefore once the mechanical aspects of augmenting $V_t$ are no longer required, the wall humidifier is often a better alternative than continued use of the mechanical ventilator circuit. Even if CPAP is required, delivery via a Down's valve on the T-piece is very efficient.

Continuous measurement of end-tidal $CO_2$ (ET-$CO_2$) and $SpO_2$ can provide an objective assessment of "tiring." Some quadriplegic patients become extremely anxious when IMV rates are dropped to very low levels and may demand to be placed back on the ventilator, even though they may be capable of longer periods without support. Monitoring this process by continuous ET-$CO_2$ measurement can be effective. Most ET-$CO_2$ monitors have alarms to signal high and low respiratory rates, as well as high and low ET-$CO_2$. The initial response to inadequate pulmonary reserve is tachypnea. Determining a patient's baseline parameters allows weaning on the basis of changes in respiratory rate and ET-$CO_2$. Respiratory rates that increase from 15-20 to 35-40 breaths per minute will not be tolerated for long. Similarly, developing hypocapnia usually signals tiring of the patient *before* $CO_2$ retention. A rest, with return to the baseline respiratory rate and ET-$CO_2$ before the next trial, is prudent. Patients move through this stage at highly varying rates, depending on their age, level and severity of their neurologic and pulmonary disease, preexisting factors, and concomitant injuries.[61,66]

In the difficult to wean, minimal reserve patient, residual mechanical chest problems can limit ventilator weaning. Reevaluation of the chest, especially after direct trauma, can lead to improvement in respiratory function. Localized scar, atelectasis, abscess, and lung deformity after tube thoracostomy placement can be the problem.[85]

Anemia or low red blood cell (RBC) mass can reduce $O_2$-carrying capacity and can limit exercise tolerance to the point that weaning is blocked or fails. Transfusion of packed RBCs should improve $O_2$-carrying capacity, and it may mobilize extracellular water from pulmonary and other tissues. Serial measures of NIF, FVC, and $V_t$ can help evaluate the response to treatment.

Inadequate cardiac reserve can also limit weaning and may be difficult to diagnose. The problem is often a relatively high cardiac output that is ineffectively distributed. Catecholamines and pacemakers can be of assistance before the development of denervation hypersensitivity and chest wall spasticity.

If weaning is instituted early, while the chest wall is still flaccid, even low (5 to 10cm $H_2O$) CPAP or PEEP can lead to overdistension of the lungs and chest, increase the work of breathing, and slow or limit weaning. Conversely, a too low PEEP may allow progression of atelectasis and may decrease compliance, with the same result (i.e., poor weaning).

Psychological dependence on the ventilator should not be underestimated. All weaning difficulties, however, cannot be attributed to psychological factors. Recourse to behavioral explanations should occur only after objective physiologic changes have been eliminated. Patience on the part of the medical staff should lead to the most rapid ventilator weaning.

## Tracheal Extubation and Tracheotomy

If the patient has been treated with continuous endotracheal or nasotracheal intubation and does not move through weaning trials at an acceptable rate, a tracheotomy may be considered. Tracheotomy reduces anatomic dead space to half or less, thus decreasing wasted ventilation. If the patient's $V_t$ is only 200ml and the dead space with intubation is 125ml, wasted ventilation is more than 60%. If dead space can be reduced to 50 to 75ml with a tracheotomy, wasted ventilation will only be 25% to 30% (50ml/200ml), even though $V_t$ (200ml) may not have changed. This represents a substantial improvement in effective use of the weakened pulmonary and chest wall structures and may free the patient from prolonged ventilator dependency.

The consequences of premature extubation may be no worse than reintubation or as serious as respiratory arrest or death. Usually, 1 to 2 weeks are lost as a result of unsuccessful extubation. Extubation results in an increased dead space and usually leads to a decreased FRC, as a result of reduced lung expansion. Furthermore, secretions are less adequately mobilized by suctioning. All of this may allow the process of atelectasis to recur. Therefore even after extubation, the patient must be monitored for adequate FRC, including the use of the bedside adjuncts of CPAP, respiratory treatments, bronchodilators, nasotracheal suctioning, and adequate humidification.

## Cardiovascular Complications

### Hemodynamic Response to Spinal Cord Injury

Most of the unique cardiovascular responses of the quadriplegic patient can be explained by sympathectomy, in combination with intact vagal efferent and afferent nerves (Tables 141.3 and 141.4 and Box 141.1).

Approximately 25% of patients are hypotensive (systolic blood pressure less than 90mmHg) after injury and have heart rates less than 90 beats/min.[67] These vital signs are often present, even after 4000 to 6000ml of in-field fluid administration and a normal to high normal central venous pressure (9 ± 3mmHg). Therefore hypovolemia generally does not explain the hypotension.

The cardiac index (CI) of patients with acute quadriplegia averages 4.5 ± 0.9L/min/m². This CI is at or above normal in at least 50% of the patients. If CI is high and mean arterial pressure (MAP) is low, systemic vascular resistance index (SVRI) must be low. Indeed, a calculation suggests the SVRI to be less than 1600 dyne-sec-cm⁵-m² in more than half the patients. This is the result of the sympathectomy effort and the loss of the ability to vasoconstrict. This hyperdynamic state is similar to that observed with sepsis but is not associated with tachycardia.

While cardiac output is increased, systemic vascular resistance is decreased via generalized vasodilatation. The sympathetic nervous system is unable to shift vascular

**TABLE 141.3**

**Definitions of Useful Hemodynamic Variables**

| | |
|---|---|
| Cardiac index (CI) (L-min$^{-1}$–m$^2$) CI = CO/BSA | Cardiac output corrected for body surface area |
| Systemic vascular resistance index (SVRI)° SVRI = MAP − CVP × BSA CO | Vascular resistance corrected for body surface area |
| Pulmonary vascular resistance index (PVRI)° PVRI = PAP − PCWP × BSA CO | Estimate of pulmonary vasoconstriction or tone—corrected for body surface area |
| Pulmonary capillary wedge pressure (PCWP) | Also known as pulmonary artery occlusion pressure; estimates left ventricular end-diastolic pressure |
| Pulmonary shunt fraction (Qs/Qt) | Estimate of percentage of cardiac output not involved with gas exchange |

*CO, Cardiac output; BSA,* body surface area; *MAP,* mean arterial pressure; *CVP,* central venous pressure; *PAP,* positive airway pressure; *PCWP,* pulmonary capillary wedge pressure.
°Units: mmHg-L$^{-1}$ − min-m$^{-2}$ × 80 = Dyne-sec-cm$^{-5}$-m$^2$.

**TABLE 141.4**

**Hemodynamic Profile of Normal Subjects and Patients with Quadriplegia**

| Variable | Normal° | Quadriplegia |
|---|---|---|
| Heart rate (beats/min) | 60–100 | 76 ± 11 |
| CVP (mmHg) | 0–6 | 11 ± 4 |
| PCWP (mmHg) | 6–12 | 15.5 ± 4.7 |
| Cardiac index (L-min$^{-1}$-m$^{-2}$) | 2.5–4 | 4.4 ± 1 L |
| MAP (mmHg) | 80–100 | 93 ± 14 |
| SVRI (dyne—sec-cm$^{-5}$) | 1800–2500 | 1525 ± 518 |
| PVRI (dyne—sec-cm$^{-5}$) | 50–220 | 185 ± 113 |
| Qs/Qt (%) | <8 | 22 ± 6.7 |

*CVP,* Central venous pressure; *PCWP,* pulmonary capillary wedge pressure; *MAP,* mean arterial pressure; *SVRI,* systemic vascular resistance index; *PVRI,* pulmonary vascular resistance index.
°Data from Passmore JM, Byrnes TJ, Goldstein RA: Hemodynamic support of the critically ill patient.. In Dantzker DR (ed): *Cardiopulmonary Critical Care.* Orlando, FL, Grune & Stratton, 1986, pp 359-402.

**BOX 141.1**

**Some effects of sympathectomy in patients with SCI**

Hypotension with:
  Low systemic vascular resistance (index)
  High cardiac index
Failure to redistribute cardiac output with organ hypoperfusion and microcirculatory abnormalities
Bradycardia/bradyarrhythmias
Bronchospasm and pulmonary obstruction
Increased viscosity of pulmonary secretions
Gastroesophageal motility impairment
Impaired gastric emptying
Impaired small bowel peristalsis
Abnormalities of bowel mucus
Impaired colonic peristalsis
Denervation hypersensitivity to catecholamines
Autonomic dysreflexia
Abnormal thermoregulation
  Impaired sweating
  Hyperthermia

volumes from one vascular bed to another. Therefore the patient is unable to shift vascular volume from the musculoskeletal system to the splanchnic and renal beds, as may be required. This may lead to decreased organ perfusion, even with what appears to be adequate blood pressure, adequate central venous pressure, adequate pulmonary capillary wedge pressure (PCWP), and adequate intake.[3]

The hemodynamic problem after SCI is one of distribution or distributive shock on a neurogenic basis. It results primarily from loss of vasoconstrictor tone and the inability to generate a tachycardia, or to shift blood volume from a peripheral to a more central vascular distribution. Note that spinal shock *is not* synonymous with neurogenic shock. The former is hypotonia and areflexia and occurs independently of the neurogenic, distributive shock observed with the SCI patient.

Even the patient with complete motor and sensory quadriplegia may demonstrate relatively intact sympathetic and respiratory reserve when CI, SVRI, FVC, NIF, and other measures are invoked. Indeed, these measures of autonomic function may predict improvement and should be included in future definitions of complete versus incomplete quadriplegia and paraplegia.[65,67]

Approximately 50% of patients in a typical SCI series demonstrate a profound sympathectomy effect, but the remainder may demonstrate only partial effects or none, depending on the severity of the lesion. Notably, patients with high thoracic paraplegia have lost most of their sympathetic vasoconstrictor outflow. Because the cardioaccelerator fibers exit between T2 and T4, some of these patients may be able to generate a tachycardia better than patients with cervical quadriplegia.

### Hemodynamic Management
#### Fluid Management

Because overall volume status is usually adequate in the resuscitated quadriplegic patient, low urine output and mild hypotension may not be effectively or optimally treated by further fluid loading. Although these patients may require additional fluids early in their course, even before the PCWP approaches 14 to 15mmHg, great care should be exercised in infusing additional fluids.

The consequences of excess fluid administration under these circumstances are congestive heart failure, pulmonary edema, and hyponatremia. In part, this is because the PCWP relates most directly to end-diastolic load of the left ventricle and only indirectly to ventricular and systemic volume. When systemic resistance is low, as in SCI, left ventricular afterload is reduced and PCWP will be low. Administration of fluid until a normal or high PCWP is reached will result in excessive fluid retention. Even if pulmonary edema and congestive heart failure do not develop, increased lung fluid leading to decreased pulmonary compliance, may precipitate respiratory failure in patients with no reserves.

Treatment of inadequate organ perfusion in the SCI patient is most precisely managed by the early use of vasopressors. The most effective vasopressor is norepinephrine in low doses (0.05 to 0.2μg/kg/min), because it has both alpha (vasoconstrictive) and beta (chronotropic and inotropic) effects. Because much of the musculoskeletal vascular bed dilates with beta stimulation, the increase in SVRI after norepinephrine administration is much less than expected and far less than that observed with phenylephrine.

A pure alpha agent such as phenylephrine is an excellent choice for increasing vascular resistance, but it may potentiate bradycardia through stimulation of the carotid baroreceptors and increase vagal outflow. The net result can be a decrease in MAP and urine output. In occasional cases phenylephrine can precipitate bradycardia to the point of asystole.

Dopamine can be as effective as norepinephrine, but it is less reliable. Additionally, much of its hemodynamic effect is exerted via norepinephrine (dopamine is a precursor to norepinephrine), and its effect on urine output occurs through direct diuretic effects on the kidney. In some patients dopamine may decrease MAP by stimulation of further vasodilatation.

Because of the generalized sympathectomy of SCI, catecholamines and sympathomimetic drugs should be very effective at low doses. It is best to begin their infusion at a low level (approximately 20% of the normal dose) and slowly increase the dose to the needed effect. This sensitivity becomes more marked (not less so) as the SCI patient moves further from the time of injury. Some evidence suggests a sixfold to tenfold increase in sensitivity to catecholamine infusions.[5] This sensitivity may also present as an increased systemic response to inhaled bronchodilators.

Spinal cord contusion is associated with reduced spinal cord blood flow and progressive ischemia over the several hours after injury. Blood flow reduction may be as great as 60% to 80%. About two thirds of this decrement may be caused by concomitant systemic hypotension as a result of the sympathectomy effect.[80,108,112] In theory spinal cord ischemia resulting from hypotension should be preventable.

It has therefore been suggested that SCI patients require normal or higher than normal blood pressures to maximize recovery of the damaged spinal cord. This principle has not been proved in clinical practice. However, maintenance of normal blood pressure of 80 to 90mmHg (mean blood pressure) is reasonable. This MAP level should maintain adequate mental status (or at least ease

the suspicion that abnormalities in mental function are not related to mild hypotension), urine output, and organ perfusion.

Urinary outputs higher than 0.5ml/kg/hr are adequate, but higher outputs may accompany the higher MAP required for spinal cord perfusion and should be supported with appropriate fluids. A fluid intake volume of 30 to 100ml/hr more than the output should avoid net dehydration, especially if the patient is being infused with a vasoactive drug.

If signs of cardiac failure, pulmonary edema, oliguria, or peripheral edema occur, hemodynamic support may be required. The exact method of support may vary according to both local practice and the specific circumstances of a patient.

### Bradyarrhythmia Management

Although profound bradyarrhythmias (heart rate less than 40) are unusual in the young quadriplegic patient, they are common and life threatening in older patients who may have preexisting coronary artery disease. They can result in hypotension and spontaneous asystole.

Classically, treatment has been directed at the use of anticholinergic drugs, such as atropine or propantheline bromide, to block vagal efferents.[1] Although this is often life saving and very effective, use of atropine and its relatives may lead to enough drying and thickening of pulmonary secretions to exacerbate concurrent respiratory problems. These drugs may potentiate the development of ileus and may adversely impact hemodynamic and respiratory changes. Chronotropic agents such as norepinephrine or dopamine do not have these side effects. Furthermore, they produce an effect that is more easily controlled and titrated. Occasionally, the problem may be severe and of sufficient duration to require a pacemaker.

### Management of Congestive Heart Failure

Heart failure is an unusual problem in the quadriplegic patient. It tends to occur in the elderly or in those patients with preexisting heart disease. Most of these patients have cardiac outputs that are in the high to normal range. However, they may have low urine output, prerenal azotemia, and hyponatremia with low urinary sodium, thus confusing the clinical situation.

When this problem occurs, it is typically in a patient who requires mechanical ventilation. The use of mechanical ventilation, high inspiratory pressures, and even relatively low levels of CPAP or PEEP often mask the development of rales and other pulmonary findings consistent with congestive heart failure. Therefore a negative physical examination of the lungs does not rule out the presence of congestive heart failure. The use of a pulmonary artery catheter, combined with a higher index of suspicion, may be worthwhile.

Managing patients with congestive heart failure can be difficult. Use of digitalis may potentiate bradyarrhythmias. Alpha agents or even oral ephedrine can, at times, be useful when an increase in afterload is desired. However, most patients need inotropic and chronotropic drugs, and a combination of these agents, along with carefully administered diuretics, is often necessary. A pacemaker is usually beneficial because these individuals are generally not able to increase their own heart rate to improve cardiac output.

### Autonomic Dysreflexia

The sympathectomy effect after SCI also results in hypersensitivity to both endogenous and exogenous catecholamines. This denervation hypersensitivity is thought to form the basis for the symptoms and signs of autonomic dysreflexia.

The complex of diaphoresis, plethora, nasal congestion, pilomotor reflexes, headache, and severe acute hypertension with bradycardia occurs when afferent stimuli produce sympathetic discharges from the thoracoabdominal spinal cord when it is isolated from the cervical spinal cord and other inhibitory regions. The stimulus, often bladder or rectal distension, increases catecholamine levels and leads to vasoconstriction and other sympathetic effects. Intact vagal efferents produce bradycardia. The extreme autonomic effects are probably the manifestation of denervation hypersensitivity interacting with only mild catecholamine increases.[5,84,95] The treatment for autonomic dysreflexia is to drain the bladder and empty the rectum. Rarely, other stimuli may be at fault. Blocking agents, such as alpha blockers (prazosin), beta blockers (propranolol), or both, may be considered. The problem is rare in acute quadriplegia but may manifest itself after a few weeks in the ICU.

## Gastrointestinal Complications

In the patient with pure high SCI, the pathophysiology associated with GI dysfunction seems to be based on the absence of sympathetic innervation of the bowel in the presence of intact vagal efferents. This leads to an initial abdominal examination characterized by intact or even hyperactive bowel sounds. However, gastric emptying and peristalsis are not effective without sympathetic modulation, and ileus develops. This may not be apparent until 2 or 3 days after injury.

The effect includes the gastroesophageal sphincter, stomach, small bowel, large bowel, and rectum. Both laboratory and clinical evidence suggests that peristalsis is not effective in any segment of the gut after acute SCI.[34,77,82]

The results of premature feeding of even small volumes during the acute period may be acute gastric dilatation or extensive GI ileus. Often the SCI patient, with or without an endotracheal tube, spontaneously swallows large volumes of air, potentiating gastric and bowel dilatation. Gastric dilatation may precipitate reflex bradycardia, bradyarrhythmias, and asystole.

As abdominal distension progresses the diaphragm is pushed farther into the chest cavity, reducing total lung volume and FRC. The increased work of breathing tires the patient, further reducing inspiratory force; atelectasis and decreased lung compliance worsen, with respiratory failure developing because of progressive abdominal distension. As ileus develops, intestinal third space and nasogastric fluid losses via suction potentiate hypovolemia and electrolyte imbalance.

### Management

It is generally wise to delay enteral feeding until flatus is passed spontaneously and bowel movements have returned. Suppositories, enemas, and stimulants may seem to speed the process, but they are not effective in the reinstitution of peristalsis.

The large bowel is also dyssynergic, and often, ileus may take on the characteristics of an obstructive pattern on radiographs of the abdomen. Fecal impaction is frequent and may worsen the process. The unwary radiologist may suggest the presence of mechanical obstruction. Great caution should be exercised because the consequences of laparotomy include cardiovascular instability, increased ventilatory requirements, excessive fluid shifts, and prolonged ICU stay.[107]

Parenteral feeding of the SCI patient may begin if GI tolerance does not quickly follow. The most frequent error is excessive alimentation. The SCI patient may be in negative nitrogen balance for months because of paralysis. No amount of nutritional or caloric support will change this.

A limited intake of 1400 to 1600Kcal/day, or about 20Kcal/kg of ideal weight, is more than sufficient to supply quadriplegic patients' nutritional needs until they can regulate their own intake. Excess feeding may result in azotemia (with little increase in creatinine). There is also evidence that quadriplegic patients may generate more heat as a result of feeding. This can cause low-grade fever ($37.5°$ to $38°C$).[2,3]

Vomiting after tolerating enteral feeding may represent recurrent ileus, other intraabdominal catastrophic processes, or something simpler, such as the superior mesenteric artery syndrome. In patients with significant weight loss from lying supine in bed, the fourth portion of the duodenum may be trapped between the aorta and the superior mesenteric artery. Vomiting occurs soon after tube feeding or eating. Most quadriplegic patients can be treated by being rotated to the right at 30 to 60 degrees during feeding. If the problem resolves, the diagnosis is evident. It usually manifests 3 to 6 weeks after injury. Either parenteral nutrition or, occasionally, surgery may be required.[38,73,83,86]

Patients with SCI are at risk for severe GI hemorrhage. GI bleeding can be difficult to diagnose in the insensate patient with an ileus resulting from quadriplegia. Routine abdominal radiographs, physical examination, and a high index of suspicion for declining platelet and hematocrit values help. A rising blood urea nitrogen level, in the presence of a good urine output and stable creatinine, suggests blood in the GI tract.[4]

Prophylactic $H_2$ blockers may help. Ranitidine, 50mg IV q 6 hr, has been shown to significantly reduce the risk of GI hemorrhage (from 43% to 17%).[20] Others have not observed such an effect in SCI patients.[30] Steroids have not been shown to increase the risk of GI hemorrhage.[4,30,32]

When hemorrhage is suspected, endoscopy is diagnostic and may have therapeutic value. Therapeutic embolization by interventional radiology may be the next step at some institutions. Laparotomy may be lifesaving and should not be withheld. Most bleeding from the GI tract can be conservatively managed with antacids (to maintain the gastric pH at 4 to 5), $H_2$ blockers as continuous infusions, and patience. Gastric feeding can be helpful if GI function has returned. The nasogastric tube itself may cause gastric erosions and bleeding. Endoscopy can help with the latter diagnosis.

## Genitourinary Complications

The most frequent debate has revolved around the merits of early intermittent catheterization versus continuous Foley catheter drainage. In 1966 Guttman and Frankel reported reduced rates of urinary tract infection and other complications with intermittent catheterization.[51,70] As a result many physicians favor intermittent catheterization of the bladder, primarily to minimize infection. However, for intermittent catheterization to succeed, certain conditions must be met. First, adequate personnel must be available because the bladder must be emptied every 4 to 6 hours (4 to 6 times each day). Second, fluid restriction to about 1500ml/day is required so that no more than 500ml accumulates at any time. Overdistension and stretch injury to the bladder may impair the ultimate development of continence.[49]

The advantages of continuous catheter drainage are the ability to monitor urinary output and the avoidance of overdistension of the bladder. The use of vasopressors, the maintenance of normal MAP, and the use of PEEP with increased fluid requirements mandate continuous catheter drainage of the bladder.

Over the long term it is useful to switch from continuous Foley catheterization to an intermittent technique. The change can take place several weeks into the course of quadriplegia with no reduction in the success rate, in terms of ultimate continence or reduction of complications.[68] Therefore while patients are acutely ill and require critical care with support of the respiratory and hemodynamic systems, continuous bladder catheterization is indicated; this can later be followed by an intermittent catheterization protocol without fear of compromising outcome.

Over the short term, 100% of patients with new-onset quadriplegia or paraplegia develop urinary tract infection, regardless of the method of management. These methods also include suprapubic cystostomy. The long-term (more than 6 to 12 months) use of continuous catheter drainage does result in more renal and bladder calculi, bladder hyperreflexia, and other complications, but this is not relevant to the initial ICU care.[68]

Chronic, continuous catheterization is associated with a 50% to 100% increase in abnormal intravenous pyelograms (IVPs), autonomic dysreflexia, calculi, urethral lesions, leakage, and urinary tract infection relative to intermittent catheterization. However, the same guideline holds: that acute ICU care is best managed with continuous Foley catheterization and does not interfere with or delay long-term bladder rehabilitation.[75]

Treatment of urinary tract infection follows the principles used for pulmonary infection—colonization of the bladder is the rule and treatment should be reserved for infection. Large numbers of bacteria (3+ or 4+; or a colony count of more than $10^5$), WBCs (more than 50 per high-power field), and fever justify an antibiotic course.

However, one must be aware of patients who are febrile from deep vein thrombophlebitis or heterotopic ossification, with bacteria in their urine.

## Integument Complications

For reasons that are predominantly related to relative hypotension and decreased skin perfusion, the patient with SCI is extremely susceptible to the development of decubiti. If the patient is left too long on a spine board (the time may be as short as 6 to 12 hours), decubiti can develop. Manual log rolling has been a classic, traditional, and effective management scheme. However, mechanical adjuncts, such as oscillating beds, the BioDyne bed, and the KinAir bed, may play a role in the management of the insensate integument in select cases. None of these modalities eliminate the need for frequent inspection, cleanliness, and good nursing care.

Prevention of pressure sores or decubitus ulcers is a primary goal of quadriplegic patient care. Established pressure sores can cost $20,000 to $40,000 in prolonged hospitalization and surgical care and can cause more than 10% of fevers.[9,50]

The mainstay of prevention is elimination of pressure points through padding, positioning, and frequent turning of the patient. Nursing the patients on pneumatic or rotating beds can partly relieve the burden on personnel. The kinetic therapy table is effective at improving pulmonary function but is less so at improving skin care. Flotation beds may be more effective.

Beyond the recognition that frequent turning of the patient is a key to preventing ulceration is the understanding that a decubitus ulcer represents ischemic necrosis of the dermis and underlying tissue. It is caused by disturbance of the microcirculation of the skin, with decreased oxygen delivery.[74]

Quadriplegic patients are immobile, are unable to shift patterns of circulation to areas of increased need, and are unable to raise their blood pressure and, often, have been treated with dehydration. These factors adversely affect the microcirculation of all organs, including the dermis.

Although no proof is available, improved hydration and the maintenance of MAP and CI may well improve circulation to the dermis. This may be associated with fewer and less severe decubiti that heal more quickly. These techniques are used to facilitate healing of myocutaneous flaps.[93]

Bunny boots and other bootlike appliances that strap around the foot have been purported to maintain dorsiflexion of the foot and to reduce the risk of heel decubiti; however, these appliances have not been shown to be effective. The use of foam on the heels increases the area over which skin pressure is distributed only slightly, and heel decubiti may still develop. These adjuncts are harmless but may give the nursing and physician staff a false sense of security and in addition, may reduce the frequency of inspection. One of the easiest methods to achieve diminished heel pressure is simply to place a pillow under the patient's calves. This suspends the heel entirely and distributes the weight of the leg over the entire calf-pillow area.

## Deep Vein Thrombosis and Pulmonary Emboli

Deep vein thrombosis (DVT) is a common complication that is more likely to occur concomitantly with immobility, limb weakness, trauma to the legs, congestive heart failure, obesity, advancing age, and surgery. A disproportionate number of risks are present in neurosurgical patients, with an incidence of DVT of 30% to 100% estimated by radiolabeled fibrinogen scanning. Compared to general trauma patients, patients with SCI bear a nearly ninefold greater risk. Of patients with paralysis, 70% to 100% develop DVT, compared with only a small percentage in patients immobilized with, but not paralyzed by, spinal fractures.*

Regrettably, the high risk of DVT in patients with SCI parallels that of pulmonary embolism (PE). The general surgical population has a risk of 0.1% to 0.8% of a fatal PE. The SCI patient has a risk of 2% to 10% for fatal PE.[48]

Some data suggest that pneumatic compression stockings lower the risk of DVT when they are used prophylactically,[98,106] but this use does not seem to lower the risk of PE.[59,105] Similarly, prophylactic heparin and minidose heparin that reduce risk of DVT in general surgical and orthopedic patients[21,23] do not seem to be as effective after SCI.[41,105] Low molecular weight heparin is probably no more effective or safer than an equivalent dose of standard heparin.[60] Low molecular weight dextran is useful for patients undergoing general or orthopedic surgery, but it does not seem to be effective in neurosurgical patients.[21,47,105,109]

The literature suggests that at best, standard prophylactic measures for DVT may be helpful in reducing the risk of lower extremity thrombosis (but not necessarily pelvic vein thrombosis), but have little effect on reducing the rate of fatal PE. The use of prophylactic vena caval filters offers protection against large, life-threatening saddle emboli, but does not decrease the risk of pelvic or lower extremity vein thrombosis[88,111] or even small, recurrent PE.

Prophylactic heparin, minidose heparin, or pneumatic compression stockings are optional because the data to recommend them are insufficient. If these modalities are used, one should be aware of the attendant risks. Heparin induces an immunologically based thrombocytopenia in about 5% of patients, which increases the risk of thrombosis.[96,109] Low-dose heparin carries about the same risk.

Antiembolism stockings must be brought to above the knee. Often they roll and form tourniquets on the calves and thighs, thus essentially neutralizing the small benefit. One study suggested that 50% of the antiembolism stockings and pneumatic compression devices were applied incorrectly at the outset.

Thrombosis is potentiated by venous stasis. Anticoagulants and compression devices are aimed at this pathophysiology. The hypercoagulable state of trauma and SCI are less easily altered. Research on antiplatelet agents, antithrombin III, and hematologic defects, such as resistance to activated protein C and antiphospholipid syndrome, may all contribute to the hypercoagulable state, and yield to specific surveillance and treatment.[26,69,104,109]

---

*References 41,56,59,76,79,105.

The prevention of venous stasis can be aided significantly by normal hydration of the patient. Fluid restriction to prevent overdistension of the bladder causes dehydration and probably increases the risk of venous thrombosis. In a series of 157 quadriplegic and paraplegic patients managed from the outset with pulmonary artery catheters, hydration, and vasopressors, there were no cases of fatal pulmonary artery embolism. Approximately 50% of the patients were treated with pneumatic compression hose, and fewer with prophylactic heparin (Rosner, unpublished data).

Treatment of DVT or PE consists of acute anticoagulation with heparin to a partial thromboplastin time that is 1.5 to 2.5 times the normal value. Low molecular weight dextran may be helpful, but this agent is also a diuretic, and dehydration should be avoided. If heparin is not tolerated, or is contraindicated because of concomitant gastrointestinal hemorrhage, a vena caval filter should be placed.[63,88,109] This can usually be accomplished by percutaneous routes.

After acute heparinization, most patients should be placed on coumadin for 3 to 6 months. INR levels of 1.5 to 2.5 are generally recommended.[56]

The diagnosis of PE in the patient with SCI can be elusive. Patients with PE rarely have obvious thrombophlebitis in the lower extremities or may have emboli from the more proximal pelvic veins. Physical examination does not help identify the patient at risk. Furthermore, the rate of laboratory diagnosis of DVT is so high that it has no practical discriminatory value.

When PE presents in the SCI patient with acute hypotension and cardiorespiratory arrest, the diagnosis is usually straightforward. However, with smaller emboli the only signs may be acute episodes of anxiety, dyspnea, and tachypnea.[37] Blood gas values may or may not reflect an acute change, and an underlying marginal pulmonary status makes interpretation of arterial blood gas values more difficult. Continuous bedside recording and monitoring of $SpO_2$ may reveal a short-lived decrease in oxygen saturation. Tachypnea may reduce $PaCO_2$ and shift the $O_2$ saturation curve to the left, thus making $O_2$ saturation appear normal. Added $O_2$ will almost eliminate the sensitivity of the $SpO_2$ monitor as well.

If PE is suspected, a ventilation-perfusion scan, or a ventilation scan alone, may justify heparin therapy or placement of a vena caval filter. Rarely, pulmonary arteriography is required. This is a complex examination that may miss small emboli, especially if it is performed after a delay.

Recurrent or unexplained fever in the SCI patient can also be caused by PE. Patients who are being treated for sepsis on the basis of fever spikes associated with recurrent, mild decrements in systemic blood pressure (with or without tachycardia) should be evaluated carefully.[9,36,103]

## Fever

Fever is common in patients with SCI and occurs at a rate of 34 episodes per patient per month.[9] Approximately 80% of patients have identifiable single sources of fever. The most common (44%) is urinary tract infection. Soft-tissue infections account for 11% of infections. Box 141.2 lists the common sources of fever observed in the first few weeks after SCI.

Patients with SCI have the same sources of fever as do other trauma patients. However, two major points should be considered in the fever work-up. First, the patient with SCI may be anesthetic in an area of inflammation. The physical examination may be benign relative to sensate patients. Guarding, rebound tenderness, and pain during range of motion of a joint may be absent. Thus a high index of suspicion is required for diagnosis. More frequent use of diagnostic aspiration (e.g., to differentiate between traumatic and septic arthritis and effusion of a knee) may be required to firmly establish a diagnosis of infection versus sterile collection.

Second, many fevers are not caused by infection. Pulmonary emboli, thrombophlebitis, and heterotopic ossification do not respond to broad-spectrum antibiotics, and definitive therapy can be delayed. Additional sources include perforated gastric or duodenal ulcers, septic phlebitis, atelectasis, and excessive respiratory work during ventilator weaning. All these causes have primary treatment that may or may not involve antibiotics, but they will continue to cause fever if an accurate diagnosis is delayed.

A general principle is that antibiotics should be withheld until a clear diagnosis is established and an endpoint of therapy is defined—for example, resolution of fever and infiltration and clearing of purulent sputum. An exception is the hemodynamically unstable, septic patient. This patient should be administered additional fluids, and cultures or Gram stains of the sputum, urine, blood, and wounds should be performed. Antibiotics should then be administered without delay.

## Heterotopic Ossification

Heterotopic ossification (HO) occurs in approximately 20% of patients with SCI. It most typically occurs in the hip, elbow, or shoulder joints, and is an inflammatory process that may present with swelling in the thigh or arm, limitation of joint motion, and fever. Leukocytosis is often mild.

---

**BOX 141.2**

**Sources of fever in acute SCI**

Urinary tract infection
Pneumonia, bronchopneumonia
Atelectasis°
Soft-tissue infection (decubiti)
Pulmonary emboli°
Thrombophlebitis°
Epididymitis
Heterotopic ossification°
Excessive bleeding°
Line sepsis
Tracheitis

°Not related to infection.

---

The swelling is often spongy, feels warm, and frequently is mistaken for thrombophlebitis. If DVT is demonstrated by ultrasound (as it will be in 50% to 70% of patients), it may be treated with heparin. Heparin will not worsen HO but will delay other therapy. Permanent loss of joint motion is a risk of HO.[24,39,40,94]

The diagnosis is best made with a radionuclide bone scan. Plain radiographs demonstrate the process too late for optimal intervention. HO can begin as early as 1 to 2 weeks after injury. Antiinflammatory agents (nonsteroidal antiinflammatory drugs) are the mainstay of therapy but are often avoided in acute situations. Etidronate disodium (Didronel) can be used with minimal risk of GI bleeding or coagulopathy and may be given IV or PO. It works by a reduction of bone formation and resorption. Oral dosage is 20mg/kg/day for 14 days, followed by 10mg/kg/day, for a total of 12 weeks of therapy.

## Drug Therapy

Currently, drug therapy is being directed at the biochemical events surrounding SCI. Three types of pharmacologic agents are most commonly used: (1) steroids and antioxidants, (2) opiates, and (3) gangliosides.

Methylprednisolone (MPSS) in very large doses is a putative scavenger of free radicals and is thought to interrupt lipid peroxidation and to prevent further membrane damage after injury.[19,53-55] On this basis two cooperative studies—National Acute Spinal Cord Injury Study (NASCIS) I and NASCIS II—were organized. NASCIS I examined relatively low doses of MPSS after SCI (a 100mg bolus followed by 100mg/day for 10 days vs. a 1000mg bolus followed by 1000mg/day for 10 days). No effect on SCI outcome was demonstrated.[15,16]

However, because the laboratory evidence was so compelling, NASCIS II was organized. This study used higher doses of MPSS (a 30mg/kg bolus followed by 5.4mg/kg/hr for 24 hours, or approximately 10,000mg over 24 hours for most patients). It examined the outcome in patients treated within 8 hours and those treated after 8 hours of injury. Naloxone was also studied as part of the NASCIS II protocol. NASCIS II data were interpreted as demonstrating a positive, statistical effect on neurologic outcome after SCI. The effect was a 3% to 4% improvement in those receiving MPSS within 8 hours of injury.[17] Those receiving MPSS more than 8 hours after injury demonstrated no improvement and perhaps did less well than the placebo-treated patients. Naloxone was judged as showing no beneficial effect. There was no functional difference in outcome at 1 year after SCI with any of the regimens, including MPSS given within 8 hours.[12,13,18]

As a result of these studies MPSS has become standard therapy in the treatment of acute SCI. However, no current study has shown MPSS to improve the functional category postinjury, the effect being small at best. There is a suggestion that aberrations in the placebo group may have contributed to the study's findings.[14,91] Other issues, including an increased number of deaths in patients treated with MPSS, cloud its use,[89,90] and the debate continues.[113]

GM-1 ganglioside was shown to improve functional neurologic recovery in some patients with SCI in a small study.[42,43] The effect was on the long tracts, and treatment resulted in a greater number of ambulators.[44]

A class of steroids with much greater antioxidant effect is the 21 aminosteroids that are also known as "lazaroids." These agents have shown promise in the laboratory in improving the outcome after acute SCI.[8,22,33,52] However, the preliminary results of a clinical trial (NASCIS III) failed to demonstrate superiority over MPSS treatment alone. Concerns about an excessive number of deaths haunt the early results of this study as well, but these should be resolved soon.

## Emotional Reaction

A patient's emotional reaction (grief) to SCI is of major concern. A condition such as quadriplegia causes a grief reaction that parallels that of the loss of a family member or friend. Not only do patients undergo a grieving process, so do relatives and friends.

Typically, the stages of grief begin with denial of the injury. After denial the patient feels anger and hostility, depression and sadness, then resolution and acceptance. As the injury is accepted, patients begin to plan realistically and to pursue rehabilitation. A patient must experience and conclude each stage before completing the full process. There are unique manifestations of this process in acute quadriplegia.

### Denial

The denial stage is especially profound in young quadriplegic patients because they do not accept their own mortality—they *know* they will walk again. Family members express this denial when they tell medical staff that the patient is a fighter. The acute medical problems that accompany quadriplegia and paraplegia and the medical activity associated with these problems make it easy for both the family and the patient to focus on issues other than how they are to deal with their loss.

The medical staff may potentiate this distraction by their preoccupation with medical issues and problems. Often the medical staff finds that during the denial stage, patients are extremely compliant and very easy to manage. They are grateful for all the activity and attention and are not very demanding. Similarly, the family tends to be preoccupied with medical and surgical decisions and is tractable and unquestioning at this stage.

If the physicians and nurses are uncomfortable with the patient's prognosis, they often focus discussion on these immediate medical or surgical procedures. The family and patient are passively encouraged not to speak of longer-term issues. Alternatively, a poor prognosis may be mentioned once but is not reinforced. Another approach, too often designed to protect the physician, is to offer such a dismal prognosis that survival and any improvement are considered miracles.[64] Failure to deal objectively at the outset may well enhance the denial reaction.

### Anger and Hostility

As denial begins to resolve and the truth about the severity of loss becomes obvious, the family and patient may become angry and hostile. This is often expressed as frustration with the perceived unfairness of the entire situation. The anger may be directed at a third party who may be, or is perceived to be, responsible for the injury, or the hostility may be very diffuse and not directed whatsoever. The latter situation is not as benign as it may seem. The patient or family may become extremely demanding of the medical staff. They may call the nurses frequently, become angry and agitated, and be intolerant of delays in the delivery of physical therapy, occupational therapy, or dietary trays. They may focus this hostility on a particular person; however, it is rarely directed at the attending or primary physician. Failure to resolve anger and hostility not only prevents the patient and family from moving on to acceptance of the illness, but may also result in litigation.

### Depression and Sadness

As anger and hostility subside depression and sadness follow. Frequently patients become withdrawn and passive. They may complain of severe pain and may require narcotics. This pain is often ill defined and is not based on the injury. The complaint of pain often justifies the use of narcotics by the patient, as a method of dulling sadness and depression by producing emotional analgesia rather than physical analgesia. It is quite easy to promote narcotic addiction by treating every pain complaint with narcotics—the patient becomes more tractable and less demanding, the family quiets down when they see the patient as being more comfortable, and the ability of all to accomplish the tasks associated with care of the patient becomes easier. Patients who do not move through this phase effectively become drug dependent. Thus this period requires insight on the part of the physicians and nurses. A careful, detailed explanation to the patient and family may be needed about why narcotic and other sedatives are being withheld.

### Resolution and Acceptance

Resolution and acceptance of the injury are not usually observed in the acute ICU situation. This occurs most often after the patient has been transferred to a rehabilitation unit or after the patient is in the chronic phase of the rehabilitative process.[87]

### Completing the Grieving Process

Because successful adaptation to the injury depends on completion of the grieving process, the medical and nursing staff must foster and guide it, rather than delay or divert it. Generally, family requests to not tell patients of the probable permanent nature of the disability are not helpful. Although there is no ideal time to inform the patient, there is little to be gained by allowing denial, ignorance, and misinformation to prolong the period of denial. This request usually represents the inability of family members themselves to accept and deal with the injury. Often there is an associated guilt among the family members. For example, they may think that they failed to prevent the injury. This may be the case, but the guilt of the family, whether appropriate or inappropriate, is of no benefit to patients who must adjust to the circumstances.

It is important to stress that the outcome of acute quadriplegia and paraplegia is variable. Clear data are available to provide a prognosis, depending on the type of injury, its mechanism, and its location (thoracic, cervical, or lumbar), and these can provide appropriate information for the family. At the same time it is prudent to inform them that it is often difficult to prognosticate accurately. However, being unduly pessimistic (e.g., informing the family that the patient has no chance of improving [when 10% to 30% of patients may have some degree of improvement in a hypothetical case]), is neither useful nor accurate.

From an early stage the medical treatment should include a compassionate approach to patient and family education, an explanation of what the deficit is and how it was incurred, and the provision of an overall plan for management of the patient. It is likely that the family will neither understand nor remember what is said. However, these are issues that need to be brought up and faced.

## REFERENCES

1. Abd AG, Braun NM: Management of life-threatening bradycardia in spinal cord injury. *Chest* 95:701-702, 1989.
2. Aksnes AK, Brundin T, Hjeltnes N, *et al*: Meal-induced rise in resting energy expenditure in patients with complete cervical spinal cord lesions. *Paraplegia* 31: 462-472, 1993.
3. Aksnes AK, Brundin T, Hjeltnes N, *et al*: Glucose-induced thermogenesis in tetraplegic patients with low sympathoadrenal activity. *Am J Physiol* 266:E161-E170, 1994.
4. Albert TJ, Levine MJ, Balderston RA, *et al*: Gastrointestinal complications in spinal cord injury. *Spine* 16:S522-S525, 1991.
5. Arnold JM, Feng QP, Delaney GA, *et al*: Autonomic dysreflexia in tetraplegic patients: evidence for alpha-adrenoceptor hyper-responsiveness. *Clin Auton Res* 5: 267-270, 1995.
6. Bach JR: Inappropriate weaning and late onset ventilatory failure of individuals with traumatic spinal cord injury. *Paraplegia* 31:430-438, 1993.
7. Bach JR, Alba AS: Noninvasive options for ventilatory support of the traumatic high level quadriplegic patient. *Chest* 98:613-619, 1990.
8. Behrmann DL, Bresnahan JC, Beattie MS: Modeling of acute spinal cord injury in the rat: neuroprotection and enhanced recovery with methylprednisolone, U-74006F and YM-14673. *Exp Neurol* 126:61-75, 1994.
9. Beraldo PS, Neves EG, Alves CM, *et al*: Pyrexia in hospitalised spinal cord injury patients. *Paraplegia* 31: 186-191, 1993.
10. Bhaskar KR, Brown R, O'Sullivan DD, *et al*: Bronchial mucus hypersecretion in acute quadriplegia. Macromolecular yields and glycoconjugate composition. *Am Rev Respir Dis* 143:640-648, 1991.
11. Bluechardt MH, Wiens M, Thomas SG, *et al*: Repeated measurements of pulmonary function following spinal cord injury. *Paraplegia* 30:768-774, 1992.
12. Bracken MB: Treatment of acute spinal cord injury with methylprednisolone: results of a multicenter, randomized clinical trial. *J Neurotrauma* 8(Suppl 1):S47-50, 1991.
13. Bracken MB: Pharmacological treatment of acute spinal cord injury: current status and future prospects. *Paraplegia* 30:102-107, 1992.
14. Bracken MB, Holford TR: Effects of timing of methylprednisolone or naloxone administration on recovery of segmental and long-tract neurological function in NASCIS 2. *J Neurosurg* 79:500-507, 1993.
15. Bracken MB, Collins WF, Freeman DF, *et al*: Efficacy of methylprednisolone in acute spinal cord injury. *JAMA* 251:45-52, 1984.
16. Bracken MB, Shepard MJ, Hellenbrand KG, *et al*: Methylprednisolone and neurological function 1 year after spinal cord injury. Results of the National Acute Spinal Cord Injury Study. *J Neurosurg* 63:704-713, 1985.
17. Bracken MB, Shepard MJ, Collins WF, *et al*: A randomized, controlled trial of methylprednisolone or naloxone in the treatment of acute spinal-cord injury. Results of the Second National Acute Spinal Cord Injury Study [see comments]. *N Engl J Med* 322:1405-1411, 1990.
18. Bracken MB, Shepard MJ, Collins WF, *et al*: Methylprednisolone or naloxone treatment after acute spinal cord injury: 1-year follow-up data. *J Neurosurg* 76:23-31, 1992.
19. Braughler JM, Hall ED: Current application of "high-dose" steroid therapy for CNS injury. *J Neurosurg* 62: 806-810, 1985.
20. Chan K, Lai ECS, Tuen H, *et al*: Prospective double-blind placebo-controlled randomized trial on the use of ranitidine in preventing postoperative gastroduodenal complications in high-risk neurosurgical patients. *J Neurosurg* 82:413-417, 1995.
21. Clagett GP, Reisch JS: Prevention of venous thromboembolism in general surgical patients: results of meta-analysis. *Ann Surg* 208:227-240, 1988.
22. Coates JR, Sorjonen DC, Simpson ST, *et al*: Clinicopathologic effects of a 21-aminosteroid compound (U74389G) and high-dose methylprednisolone on spinal cord function after simulated spinal cord trauma. *Vet Surg* 24:128-139, 1995.
23. Collins R, Scrimgeour A, Yusuf S, *et al*: Reduction in fatal pulmonary embolism and venous thrombosis by perioperative administration of subcutaneous heparin: overview of results of randomized trials in general, orthopedic, and urologic surgery. *N Engl J Med* 318: 1162-1173, 1988.
24. Cope R: Heterotopic ossification. *South Med J* 83: 1058-1064, 1990.
25. Crane L, Klerk K, Ruhl A, *et al*: The effect of exercise training on pulmonary function in persons with quadriplegia. *Paraplegia* 32:435-441, 1994.
26. Dahlback B, Hildebrand B: Inherited resistance to activated protein C is corrected by anticoagulant cofactor activity found to be a property of factor V. *Proc Natl Acad Sci USA* 91:396-400, 1994.
27. Demling RH: Pulmonary dysfunction.. In Wilmore DW, Cheung LY, Harken AH, *et al* (eds): *Care of the Surgical Patient*, vol 1. Critical Care. New York, Scientific American, 1996, pp 1-26.

28. DeVivo MJ, Ivie CS III: Life expectancy of ventilator-dependent persons with spinal cord injuries. *Chest* 108:226-232, 1995.

29. DeVivo MJ, Black KJ, Stover SL: Causes of death during the first 12 years after spinal cord injury. *Arch Phys Med Rehabil* 74:248-254, 1993.

30. Epstein N, Hood DC, Ransohoff J: Gastrointestinal bleeding in patients with spinal cord trauma. Effects of steroids, cimetidine, and mini-dose heparin. *J Neurosurg* 54:16-20, 1981.

31. Estenne M, De Troyer A: Mechanism of the postural dependence of vital capacity in tetraplegic subjects. *Am Rev Respir Dis* 135:367-371, 1987.

32. Fadul CE, Lemann W, Thaler HT, *et al*: Perforation of the gastrointestinal tract in patients receiving steroids for neurologic disease. *Neurology* 38:348-352, 1988.

33. Farooque M, Olsson Y, Holtz A: Effect of the 21-aminosteroid U74006F and methylprednisolone on motor function recovery and oedema after spinal cord compression in rats. *Acta Neurol Scand* 89:36-41, 1994.

34. Fealey RD, Szurszewski JH, Merritt JL, *et al*: Effect of traumatic spinal cord transection on human upper gastrointestinal motility and gastric emptying. *Gastroenterology* 87:69-75, 1984.

35. Fischer DA: Long-term management of the ventilator patient in the home. *Cleve Clin Q* 52:303-306, 1985.

36. Fluter GG: Pulmonary embolism presenting as supraventricular tachycardia in paraplegia: a case report. *Arch Phys Med Rehabil* 74:1208-1210, 1993.

37. Frisbie JH, Sharma GV: Pulmonary embolism manifesting as acute disturbances of behavior in patients with spinal cord injury. *Paraplegia* 32:570-572, 1994.

38. Fromm S, Cash JM: Superior mesenteric artery syndrome: an approach to the diagnosis and management of upper gastrointestinal obstruction of unclear etiology. *S D J Med* 43:5-10, 1990.

39. Frost FS: Role of rehabilitation after spinal cord injury. *Urol Clin North Am* 20:549-559, 1993.

40. Garland DE: Clinical observations on fractures and heterotopic ossification in the spinal cord and traumatic brain injured populations. *Clin Orthop* 233:86-101, 1988.

41. Geerts WH, Code KI, Jay RM, *et al*: A prospective study of venous thromboembolism after major trauma. *N Engl J Med* 331:1601-1606, 1994.

42. Geisler FH: GM-1 ganglioside and motor recovery following human spinal cord injury. *J Emerg Med* 11 (Suppl 1):49-55, 1993.

43. Geisler FH, Dorsey FC, Coleman WP: Recovery of motor function after spinal-cord injury—a randomized, placebo-controlled trial with GM-1 ganglioside [published erratum appears in *N Engl J Med* 325:1659-1660, 1991] [see comments]. *N Engl J Med* 324:1829-1838, 1991.

44. Geisler FH, Dorsey FC, Coleman WP: GM-1 ganglioside in human spinal cord injury. *J Neurotrauma* 9(Suppl 2): S517-S530, 1992.

45. Geisler FH, Dorsey FC, Coleman WP: Past and current clinical studies with GM-1 ganglioside in acute spinal cord injury. *Ann Emerg Med* 22:1041-1047, 1993.

46. Goldman JM, Rose LS, Williams SJ, *et al*: Effect of abdominal binders on breathing in tetraplegic patients. *Thorax* 41:940-945, 1986.

47. Green D, Chen D, Chmiel JS, *et al*: Prevention of thromboembolism in spinal cord injury: role of low molecular weight heparin. *Arch Phys Med Rehabil* 75: 290-292, 1994.

48. Green D, Twardowski P, Wei R, *et al*: Fatal pulmonary embolism in spinal cord injury. *Chest* 105:853-855, 1994.

49. Grundy D, Russell J: ABC of spinal cord injury. Urological management. *Br Med J* 292:249-253, 1986.

50. Gunnewicht BR: Management of pressure sores in a spinal injuries unit. *J Wound Care* 5:36-39, 1996.

51. Guttman L, Frankel HL: The value of intermittent catheterisation in the early management of traumatic paraplegia and tetraplegia. *Paraplegia* 4:63, 1966.

52. Haghighi SS, Perez-Espejo A, Geng XZ, *et al*: Effect of 21-aminosteroid pretreatment in compression trauma to the spinal cord. *Neurol Res* 16:268-272, 1994.

53. Hall ED: The neuroprotective pharmacology of methylprednisolone. *J Neurosurg* 76:13-22, 1992.

54. Hall ED, Braughler JM, McCall JM: Antioxidant effects in brain and spinal cord injury. *J Neurotrauma* 9(Suppl 1): S165-S172, 1992.

55. Hall ED, Yonkers PA, Andrus PK, *et al*: Biochemistry and pharmacology of lipid antioxidants in acute brain and spinal cord injury. *J Neurotrauma* 9(Suppl 2):S425-S442, 1992.

56. Hamilton MG, Hull RD, Pineo GF: Venous thromboembolism in neurosurgery and neurology patients: a review. *Neurosurgery* 34:280-296, 1994.

57. Hess D, Hodgkin JE, Burton GG: Mechanical ventilation: initiation, management, and weaning. In *Anonymous Respiratory Care: A Guide to Clinical Practice.* Philadelphia, Lippincott-Raven, 1993, pp 599-624.

58. Hincman HO, Bhaskar KR, O'Sullivan DD, *et al*: Lipids in airway mucus of acute quadriplegic patients. *Exp Lung Res* 16:369-385, 1990.

59. Hull RD: Venous thromboembolism in spinal cord injury patients. *Chest* 102:658S-663S, 1992.

60. Hull RD, Raskob GE, Pineo GF, *et al*: Subcutaneous low-molecular weight heparin compared with continuous intravenous heparin in the treatment of proximal-vein thrombosis. *N Engl J Med* 326:975-982, 1992.

61. Jackson AB, Groomes TE: Incidence of respiratory complications following spinal cord injury. *Arch Phys Med Rehabil* 75:270-275, 1994.

62. Jaeger RJ, Turba RM, Yarkony GM, *et al*: Cough in spinal cord injured patients: comparison of three methods to produce cough [see comments]. *Arch Phys Med Rehabil* 74:1358-1361, 1993.

63. Jarrell BE, Posuniak E, Roberts J, *et al*: A new method of management using the Kim-Ray Greenfield filter for deep venous thrombosis and pulmonary embolism in spinal cord injury. *Surg Gynecol Obstet* 157:316-320, 1983.

64. Langer KG: Depression and denial in psychotherapy of persons with disabilities. *Am J Psychother* 48:181-194, 1994.

65. LeDoux MS, Rosner MJ: Importance of cardiopulmonary function in prognosis after spinal cord injury. *J Neurosurgery* 74:364A, 1991.

66. Lemons VR, Wagner FC Jr: Respiratory complications after cervical spinal cord injury. *Spine* 19:2315-2320, 1994.

67. Levi L, Wolf A, Belzberg H: Hemodynamic parameters in patients with acute cervical cord trauma: description,

intervention, and prediction of outcome. *Neurosurgery* 33:1007-1016, 1993.

68. Lloyd LK, Kuhlemeier KV, Fine PR, *et al*: Initial bladder management in spinal cord injury: does it make a difference? *J Urol* 135:523-527, 1986.

69. Lockshin MD: Antiphospholipid antibody syndrome. *JAMA* 91:1396-1400, 1992.

70. Luce JM: Medical management of spinal cord injury. *Crit Care Med* 13:126-131, 1985.

71. Luce JM, Culver BH: Respiratory muscle function in health and disease. *Chest* 81:82-90, 1982.

72. Mansel JK, Norman JR: Respiratory complications and management of spinal cord injuries [see comments]. *Chest* 97:1446-1452, 1990.

73. Massoud WZ: Laparoscopic management of superior mesenteric artery syndrome. *Int Surg* 80:322-327, 1995.

74. Mawson AR, Siddiqui FH, Biundo JJ Jr: Enhancing host resistance to pressure ulcers: a new approach to prevention. *Prev Med* 22:433-450, 1993.

75. McGuire EJ, Savastano J: Comparative urological outcome in women with spinal cord injury. *J Urol* 135: 730-731, 1986.

76. Merli GJ, Crabbe S, Paluzzi RG, *et al*: Etiology, incidence, and prevention of deep vein thrombosis in acute spinal cord injury. *Arch Phys Med Rehabil* 74:1199-1205, 1993.

77. Meshkinpour H, Harmon D, Thompson R, *et al*: Effects of thoracic spinal cord transection on colonic motor activity in rats. *Paraplegia* 23:272-276, 1985.

78. Morgan MDL, De Troyer A: The individuality of chest wall motion in tetraplegia. *Eur Bull Physiopathol Respir* 20:547-552, 1984.

79. Myllynen P, Kammonen M, Rokkanen P, *et al*: Deep venous thrombosis and pulmonary embolism in patients with acute spinal cord injury: a comparison with nonparalyzed patients immobilized due to spinal fractures. *J Trauma* 25:541-543, 1985.

80. Ohashi T, Morimoto T, Kawata K, *et al*: Correlation between spinal cord blood flow and arterial diameter following acute spinal cord injury in rats. *Acta Neurochir (Wien)* 138:322-329, 1996.

81. Passmore JM, Byrnes TJ, Goldstein RA: Hemodynamic support of the critically ill patient.. In Dantzker DR (ed): *Cardiopulmonary Critical Care*. Orlando, FL, Grune & Stratton, 1986, pp 359-402.

82. Pedersen E: Regulation of bladder and colon-rectum in patients with spinal lesions. *J Auton Nerv Syst* 7:329-338, 1983.

83. Pedoto MJ, O'Dell MW, Thrun M, *et al*: Superior mesenteric artery syndrome in traumatic brain injury: two cases. *Arch Phys Med Rehabil* 76:871-875, 1995.

84. Perkash I, Friedland GW: Catheter-induced hyperreflexia in spinal cord injury patients: diagnosis by sonographic voiding cystourethrography. *Radiology* 159:453-455, 1986.

85. Peterson WP, Whiteneck GG, Gerhart KA: Chest tubes, lung entrapment, and failure to wean from the ventilator. Report of three patients with quadriplegia. *Chest* 105:1292-1294, 1994.

86. Raissi B, Taylor BM, Taves DH: Recurrent superior mesenteric artery (Wilkie's) syndrome: a case report. *Can J Surg* 39:410-416, 1996.

87. Redner JE, Prigatano GP, Trieschman RB: Neuropsychological management of patients with spinal

cord injury. In Menezes AH, Sonntag VKH (eds): *Principles of Spinal Surgery*. New York, McGraw-Hill, 1996, pp 987-998.

88. Rogers FB, Shackford SR, Wilson J, *et al*: Prophylactic vena cava filter insertion in severely injured trauma patients: indications and preliminary results. *J Trauma* 35:637-641, 1993.

89. Rosner MJ: National acute spinal cord injury study of methylprednisolone or naloxone, letter. *Neurosurgery* 28:628-629, 1991.

90. Rosner MJ: Methylprednisolone for spinal cord injury, letter. *J Neurosurgery* 77:324-325, 1992.

91. Rosner MJ: Methylprednisolone and spinal cord injury, letter. *J Neurosurgery* 80:954-955, 1994.

92. Rosner MJ, Coley I, Elias Z: Oscillating therapy and pulmonary shunt fraction after severe spinal cord injury. In Green BA, Summer WR (eds): *Continuous Oscillation Therapy: Research and Practical Applications*. Coral Gables, FL, University of Miami Press, 1986, pp 31-38.

93. Rubayi S, Cousins S, Valentine WA: Myocutaneous flaps. Surgical treatment of severe pressure ulcers. *AORN J* 52:40-47, 50, 52-55, 1990.

94. Rush PJ: The rheumatic manifestations of traumatic spinal cord injury. *Semin Arthritis Rheum* 19:77-89, 1989.

95. Santajuliana D, Zukowska-Grojec Z, Osborn JW: Contribution of alpha- and beta-adrenoceptors and neuropeptide-Y to autonomic dysreflexia. *Clin Auton Res* 5:91-97, 1995.

96. Schmitt BP, Adelman B: Heparin-associated thrombocytopenia: a critical review and pooled analysis. *Am J Med Sci* 305:208-215, 1993.

97. Sharp JM, Ledsome JR: Pulmonary function in acute cervical cord injury. *Am Rev Respir Dis* 124:41-44, 1981.

98. Skillman JJ, Collins RE, Coe NP, *et al*: Prevention of deep vein thrombosis in neurosurgical patients: a controlled, randomized trial of external pneumatic compression boots. *Surgery* 83:354-358, 1978.

99. Slack RS, Shucart W: Respiratory dysfunction associated with traumatic injury to the central nervous system. *Clin Chest Med* 15:739-749, 1994.

100. Splaingard ML, Frates RCJ, Harrison GM, *et al*: Home positive-pressure ventilation. Twenty years' experience. *Chest* 84:376-382, 1983.

101. Spungen AM, Dicpinigaitis PV, Almenoff PL, *et al*: Pulmonary obstruction in individuals with cervical spinal cord lesions unmasked by bronchodilator administration. *Paraplegia* 31:404-407, 1993.

102. St John WM, Zhou D: Reductions of neural activities to upper airway muscles after elevations in static lung volume. *J Appl Physiol* 73:701-707, 1992.

103. Stallman JS, Aisen PS, Aisen ML: Pulmonary embolism presenting as fever in spinal cord injury patients: report of two cases and review of the literature. *J Am Paraplegia Soc* 16:157-159, 1993.

104. Svensson PJ, Dahlback B: Resistance to activated protein C as a basis for venous thrombosis. *N Engl J Med* 330: 517-522, 1994.

105. Swann KW, Black PM: Deep vein thrombosis and pulmonary emboli in neurosurgical patients: a review. *J Neurosurg* 61:1055-1062, 1984.

106. Turpie AG, Hirsh J, Gent M, *et al*: Prevention of deep vein thrombosis in potential neurosurgical patients: a

randomized trial comparing graduated compression stockings alone or graduated compression stockings plus intermittent pneumatic compression with control. *Arch Intern Med* 149:679-681, 1989.

107. Wade TP, Andrus CH: Cardiorespiratory effects of laparotomy in patients with spinal cord injury. *Am Surg* 59:689-691, 1993.

108. Wallace MC, Tator CH: Spinal cord blood flow measured with microspheres following spinal cord injury in the rat. *Can J Neurol Sci* 13:91-96, 1986.

109. Weinmann ER, Salzman EW: Deep-vein thrombosis, review article. *N Engl J Med* 331:1630-1641, 1994.

110. Wicks AB, Menter RR: Long-term outlook in quadriplegic patients with initial ventilator dependency. *Chest* 90:406-410, 1986.

111. Wilson JT, Rogers FB, Wald SL, *et al*: Prophylactic vena cava filter insertion in patients with traumatic spinal cord injury: preliminary results. *Neurosurgery* 35:234-239, 1994.

112. Yeo JD, Hales JR, Stabback S, *et al*: Effects of a contusion injury on spinal cord blood low in the sheep. *Spine* 9:676-680, 1984.

113. Young W, Bracken MB: The Second National Acute Spinal Cord Injury Study. *J Neurotrauma* 9(Suppl 1):S397-S405, 1992.

114. Zeman FJ: Disorders of energy balance and body weight. In Zeman FJ (ed): *Clinical Nutrition and Dietetics*, ed 2. New York, Macmillan, 1991, pp 470-516.

# CHAPTER 142

# Nutritional Care of the Spinal Cord Injured Patient

## James S. Harrop, Donna J. Rodriguez, and Edward C. Benzel

Through a better understanding of spinal biomechanics, bone fusion principles, and spinal stabilization with instrumented constructs, spine surgeons have dramatically improved the treatment of spinal fractures during the last several decades. However, the spine trauma patient typically presents with not only a spinal fracture, but also concurrent multiorgan dysfunction from a spinal cord injury (SCI) or multisystem trauma. The treating physicians in the acute and even in the chronic setting, tend to focus on direct injuries such as spinal fractures, and often overlook or minimize the nutritional requirements of these patients.

These multisystem trauma patients' hospitalizations and rehabilitation courses often involve surgical treatment and infectious complications, including sepsis. Major surgical intervention, trauma, sepsis, and SPIs have all been independently shown to elicit well-documented and well-characterized metabolic responses that include hypermetabolism and hypercatabolism. If adequate nutritional support is not instituted, these responses can result in malnutrition and loss of lean body mass. The SCI patient's nutritional status is further complicated by the neural disruption and subsequent functional losses. These initiate a chain of events that produce several additional and unique metabolic derangements, along with the concurrent multisystem trauma injuries.

The use of early and aggressive nutritional support in the critically ill patient has been increasingly recognized to reduce patient morbidity and mortality. The optimization of the metabolic milieu after trauma, surgery, sepsis, and SCI can minimize complications associated with these injuries. This chapter defines basic nutritional formulas (Table 142.1), describes the unique metabolic characteristics and nutritional support techniques for SCI patients.

## Estimating Nutritional Requirements
### Prediction of Calorie Requirements

The ability to accurately estimate nutritional requirements is a major component of the management of critically ill patients (see Appendix 142.1 at end of this chapter). Underfeeding results in muscle wasting, decreased immunocompetence, and poor wound healing. However, overfeeding is associated with fluid overload, hyper-

glycemia, elevated blood urea nitrogen (BUN), elevated triglyceride levels, abnormal hepatic enzyme levels, respiratory distress caused by increased $CO_2$ production, and ventilator weaning difficulties.[34,52] Therefore accurate and individualized nutrient supplementation is desired.

### Standard Nutritional Requirement Formulas

The estimation of calorie and protein requirements has progressed beyond a few simple calculations. Therefore the expertise of a registered dietitian or clinician is often necessary to evaluate clinical and morphometric data. These professionals are able to choose and apply the appropriate formulas from the several methods available, so that an accurate prediction of energy and nitrogen requirements can be made. The more commonly used formulas and equations are defined and listed in Table 142.1.

The energy required to fuel basic life processes in healthy, resting, fasting individuals is defined as the basal energy expenditure or BEE. Factors that directly affect the BEE are age, gender, body surface area, and fasting versus fed states.[40] The Harris-Benedict equation is the most common method used to estimate this energy requirement in which weight is measured in kilograms, height in centimeters, and age in years.[40] BEE is figured differently for men ($BEE_m$) and women ($BEE_w$), as shown in the following equations:

$$BEE_m = 66 + (13.7 \times weight) + (5 \times height) - (6.8 \times age)$$
$$BEE_w = 655 + (9.6 \times weight) + (1.7 \times height) - (4.7 \times age) \quad (1)$$

Critically ill patients require more energy than is indicated by the BEE, because of their traumatic injuries. This energy requirement is named the predicted energy expenditure (PEE) and is estimated by multiplying the BEE by an activity factor (1.2 for bedrest) and a stress/injury factor (1.6 to 1.75 for major trauma).[76,77] In the SCI patient this posttraumatic hypermetabolic and hypercatabolic state is superimposed with a state of muscle inactivity caused by paralysis. Therefore the use of the usual activity factor of 1.2 for bedrest may overestimate caloric needs and result in excessive delivery of calories.[17,27,63,76]

### Factors That May Escalate Energy Expenditure

Major injury increases metabolic rate and has been described as a "sudden stimuli to which the organism is not quantitatively or qualitatively adapted."[27] The extensive multisystem trauma and long bone fractures that commonly occur in association with SCI can augment the hypermetabolic response.[62]

Postinjury hypermetabolism is at least in part caused by the hormonal effects of increased glucagon, cortisol, and catecholamine levels. The small decrease in plasma thyroxine associated with SCI does not appear to influence the metabolic rate.[21] However, pancreatitis, a relatively common complication of SCI,[8,13] significantly increases energy expenditure.

Increases in body temperature after SCI are commonly caused by pulmonary or urinary tract infections. However,

| TABLE 142.1 | |
|---|---|
| **Definitions of Basic Nutritional Terms** | |
| **Term** | **Definition** |
| BEE (basal energy expenditure) | Energy required to fuel basic life processes in healthy, resting, fasting individuals. This is estimated most commonly using the Harris-Benedict equation.[40] |
| PEE (predicted energy expenditure) | Energy expenditure for the patient taking into account his or her additional requirements because of activity and stress or injury. This is estimated using the BEE multiplied by a referenced activity and stress factor. |
| REE (resting energy expenditure) | Energy used by the patient in a resting state measured by either direct or indirect calorimetry. This is measured most commonly with the use of indirect calorimetry (metabolic cart) and the Weir equation. |

the loss of sympathetic innervation and the inability of muscles to shiver can lead to wide ranges in basal metabolic rates.[10,20,81] The degree of impairment of temperature regulation is proportional to the extent and spinal level of the paralysis. Also, greater fluid retention and subsequent increased body weight result in falsely elevated predictions. Ventilated patients do not require as much energy because they are not performing spontaneous breathing. Critically ill patients who are sedated and relatively motionless are in a lower energy state.[88]

Although the Harris-Benedict equation does account for activity and the metabolic stress/injury response, other factors including infection, body temperature, nutritional support regimens, clinical procedures, surgical operations, and medications are not considered. Patient variability with regard to these factors can complicate the use of predictive equations for energy expenditures. Therefore the sicker the patient, the poorer the ability to predict metabolic rates based on these equations and formulas. Actual energy expenditure measurements are therefore necessary and fortunately available.

### Calorimetry: Measurement of Energy Expenditures

Calorimetry is a more sophisticated technique to determine energy expenditure than the use of predictive equations and formulas. However, it is more expensive and requires precision equipment and technical skills. Nevertheless, energy expenditures can be accurately determined by using either direct or indirect calorimetry.

Direct calorimetry measures heat production or heat loss by the body.[30] To measure it, a subject is placed in a sealed chamber with a supply of oxygen. Because the chamber is well insulated, the heat produced by the body is absorbed by a known volume of water that circulates through pipes located in the chamber. The change in water temperature reflects the heat loss and represents expended metabolic energy. Although this method is very precise, it is not practical or feasible for acutely traumatized patients.

Indirect calorimetry is a useful and accurate alternative to the direct method. This technique is used to measure energy expenditure in critically ill patients. Heat production or resting energy expenditure (REE) is determined with a metabolic cart (Critical Care Monitor, Medical Graphics Corporation, St. Paul) by measuring respiratory gas exchange between the inspired and expired samples.[30]

The basis for this is that oxygen consumption ($VO_2$) and carbon dioxide production ($VCO_2$) accurately reflect a significant portion of systemic intracellular metabolism. The REE is determined from the data obtained by the metabolic cart study and the Weir equation,[87] as explained in the following equation:

$$REE = (3.9 \times VO_2 + 1.1 \times VCO_2) \times 1.44 \qquad (2)$$

An additional feature of the metabolic cart is the ability to not only calculate the REE, but also the respiratory quotient (RQ) from the measured $VO_2$ and $VCO_2$. The respiratory quotient is the ratio of $VCO_2/VO_2$, and can be used as an indicator of substrate use.[30] Each energy source (carbohydrate, protein, and fat) is oxidized at a known RQ, ranging from 0.7 to 1 (Table 142.2). Therefore the RQ can be used occasionally to determine the predominant substrate used. For example, when the measured RQ is greater than 1, lipogenesis is assumed to occur. Substrate adjustments can be made in the nutritional support regimen based on information acquired from the metabolic cart study.

## Overview of the Metabolic Stress Response

### Major Trauma, Surgery, and Sepsis

After suffering a spinal cord injury the patient's metabolism sustains a hypermetabolic and hypercatabolic state, which is similar to that seen after trauma, major surgical interventions, and sepsis. This hypermetabolic and hypercatabolic state results in a remarkable increase in energy expenditure, total body protein catabolism, and nitrogen

| TABLE 142.2 | |
|---|---|
| **Respiratory Quotient (RQ) as per Substrate Used** | |
| **Substrate Used** | **RQ** |
| Ethanol | 0.67 |
| Fat | 0.71 |
| Protein | 0.82 |
| Mixed substrate oxidation | 0.85 |
| Carbohydrate | 1 |
| Ketone bodies | 1 |
| Lipogenesis | >1 |

excretions.* The energy requirements of the trauma patient, often in excess of 200% of BEE, are necessary to maintain lean body mass. If the nutritional requirements are not met from exogenous sources, the body will use internal sources, such as body fat and muscle reserves. For example, increased protein turnover indicates that postinjury caloric requirements are much higher than maintenance levels. This accelerated protein breakdown results in a supply of amino acids for the gluconeogenesis that is needed to fuel anaerobic glycolysis in the injured tissues.

The multitude of metabolic variables in the critically ill patient deserves close scrutiny. Maintaining close attention to the nutritional status of these patients helps prevent the detrimental consequences of depleted muscle mass, increased susceptibility to infections, and impaired wound healing. The SCI patient differs from other patients in that the neuronal disconnection of the muscles causes a decrease in muscle use and a compensatory atrophy, thus lowering the energy expenditure. In addition, there are two metabolic responses superimposed on this already complex pathophysiologic process. These two different metabolic responses to SCI can be separated into an acute and a delayed nutritional response.

## Acute Nutritional Response to Spinal Cord Injury

In the acute period after a SCI, which is defined here as less than four weeks, the patient's metabolic response is influenced by the hypermetabolism related to the traumatic injury, as well as by the decreased energy requirements related to the muscle paralysis. The degree of neuronal injury resulting in loss of muscle stimulation and atrophy has directly been correlated to REE.[†] Therefore a quadriplegic patient has a lower energy expenditure than a paraplegic patient, whose energy expenditure is less than a patient without an SCI.[64]

Actual resting energy expenditures, measured by indirect calorimetry during the first and second weeks after SCI, have demonstrated that calorie needs are overestimated when the Harris-Benedict equation for BEE (see Equation 1) is used in conjunction with injury and activity factors.[76] Kearns and associates[45] also reported that the average REE after acute SCI was lower than predicted by the Harris-Benedict BEE. They hypothesized that nonspecific changes in neurogenic stimuli and decreased oxygen consumption by flaccid muscles contributed to their findings. Their hypothesis was further supported by the observation that the REE increased by 5% as muscle tone returned.[45] Young and associates excluded the injury and activity factors used in the Harris-Benedict equation for PEE in four acute SCI patients despite their traumatic injuries.[90] This calculation, which was significantly lowered because of the loss of the activity and trauma and additional factor adjustments, was determined to be 97% of the predicted value using indirect calorimetry.[90] This emphasizes the inaccuracy and elevation of PEE using standard formulas and equations for the acute SCI patient.

These patients also have persistent negative nitrogen balance during the first 3 weeks after injury despite aggressive nutritional replacements.[33,75,76] This is an obligatory negative nitrogen balance that is not corrected with increased caloric intake.[75]

## Delayed Nutritional Response to Spinal Cord Injury

Resolution of the hypermetabolic and hypercatabolic states after spinal cord injury occurs between the third and fourth week. The patient then enters the delayed nutritional response to SCI. This change in metabolism is indicated by the resolution of a negative nitrogen balance.[43,45,49,75,76] Several investigators have reported that the delayed metabolic response to SCI is marked by a reduction in energy expenditure of up to 67% and is associated with a progressive loss in lean body mass. Agarwal et al.[1] studied 15 quadriplegic patients at a mean of 9.2 years after injury and measured energy expenditures, which were markedly reduced from calculated expenditures based on the Harris-Benedict BEE. This results of this study illustrated that the delivery of calories based on the Harris-Benedict formula leads to overfeeding. This was further demonstrated by Kearns and associates, whose five chronic quadriplegic patients showed that the Harris-Benedict equation (BEE) exceeded energy expenditure by a factor of 1.5.[44] Although the time frame of this study in relation to injury was not specified, they suggested reducing the estimated number of calories by 20% in the chronic SCI patient.[44]

The reduced caloric needs of SCI patients appears to be proportional to the spinal level of the neurologic lesion or the mass of denervated muscle.[4,17,28,63,80] By studying 22 SCI patients at more than 2 months after injury, Cox et al.[28] showed that quadriplegic patients required 22.7 kcal/kg/day, whereas paraplegic patients required 27.9 kcal/kg/day. Cox further noted that upon allowing uncontrolled diets, patients gained on average 1.7 kg per week.[28] Mollinger et al.[63] also confirmed lower caloric needs of SCI patients (than predicted by BEE) and a significant correlation of energy expenditure with the level of the spinal cord lesion. Clarke[17] concluded that metabolic data obtained from healthy subjects could not be used to predict caloric expenditures in paraplegic patients, even when allowances were made for body weight. Sedlock and Laventure[80] attributed this discrepancy to the loss of lean body mass after paralysis.

## Basic Nutritional Requirements

### Carbohydrate Requirements

Glucose is the preferred energy substrate by the central nervous system (CNS) tissue, blood cells, granulation tissue, testes, and renal medulla. A minimum of 100 to 150 g of glucose per day is required for these functions and for the prevention of excessive protein breakdown.[83] The rate at which the body oxidizes carbohydrate or glucose is approximately 2 to 4 mg/kg/min under normal conditions. During severe stress the oxidation rate of glucose is elevated to 3 to 5 mg/kg/min. In most patients the provision of more than 400 to 500 g of glucose per day exceeds the body's ability to oxidize it and use it for energy. The excess glucose is converted to fat and can be measured by calorimetry as an increased $VCO_2/VO_2$ ratio (increased

---

*References 12,28,29,34,35,38,46,47,89.

[†]References 4,17,28,43-45,56,75,80.

RQ).[12] Despite the central nervous system's need for glucose, chronic SCI patients have been shown to have glucose intolerance because of an insulin intolerance.[6]

The relationship between derangements in glucose metabolism and neural injury has been studied extensively, especially with regard to ischemia.[32,55,57,72,74] The results of these studies suggest that hyperglycemia at the time of, and immediately after, neurotrauma (including SCI) may worsen outcome. High serum glucose levels increase the substrate available for anaerobic glycolysis, and thus for the production of lactic acid.[59] This CNS acid production may have an adverse effect on the recovery from neurologic injury.[7] Control of serum glucose levels (prevention of hyperglycemia), especially during the first 2 to 8 hours postinjury, appears to be crucial for optimal recovery. However, increased glucose availability may be advantageous after 2 to 8 hours postinjury, and thus allows for early calorie supplementation.[7]

## Lipid Requirements

After glucose is stored, the body prefers lipid metabolism and breakdown rather than depleting protein stores.[60] Provision of lipid as a concentrated source of calories can facilitate protein sparing, decrease the risk of carbohydrate overfeeding, and help limit total fluid volume. Fat should generally constitute 30% of the total calorie delivery. In the acute postinjury stage large amounts of fat (greater than 30%), especially linoleic or omega-6 fatty acids, can have an immunosuppressive effect by stimulating the release of arachidonic acid.[83] This precursor leads to prostaglandin formation, and subsequently, depressed delayed cell-mediated hypersensitivity, lymphocyte proliferation, and natural killer cell function. High serum triglyceride levels also indicate fat intolerance and the need to reduce the delivered amount of intravenous lipid emulsions. A minimum of 4% of total energy needs should be provided as essential fatty acids to avoid deficiency.[83]

## Protein Requirements

Proteins are essential for tissue growth, maintenance and repair, and for the synthesis of hormones, enzymes, antibodies, and transport molecules. All amino acids serve important functions. When excess protein is ingested, it is either metabolized into energy or stored as fat. The recommended dietary allowance for healthy adults is 0.8g of protein per kilogram of ideal body weight daily (ideal body weight for males is estimated to be 106lb for the first 5 feet in height plus 6 additional pounds for every inch taller; for females, it is 100lb for the first 5 feet plus 5 pounds for every inch taller).[3] Protein requirements increase dramatically to 2g per kilogram of ideal body weight after multiple trauma, major burns, or severe sepsis. Increased levels of protein are also recommended after acute SCI.[16]

After glycogen stores are depleted in the muscles and liver through glycogenolysis, the body protein is catabolized by gluconeogenesis. As a part of this process, for every 6.25g of protein broken down 1g of nitrogen is excreted.[85]

## Micronutrients
### Calcium

Alterations in calcium metabolism after acute SCI has been well documented.[18,22,62] Bone homeostasis is a balance between bone destruction and building. After SCI the skeleton is no longer placed in a position such as to carry and support the body. This immobilization causes bone reabsorption below the level of injury that begins within 10 days of injury and occurs for at least 6 months.[23,61] This may lead to high serum and urine calcium levels. Adults are susceptible to hypercalcemia because of impaired renal function and excretion difficulties, whereas children also may have accelerated levels caused by increased bone turnover.[6,86] Although rare after SCI, symptoms of hypercalcemia include anorexia, nausea and vomiting, abdominal cramps, constipation, headache, and lethargy.

A low calcium diet does not appear to be effective in decreasing serum calcium levels.[51] Ultimately, this negative calcium balance leads to osteoporosis in all skeletal structures below the lesion. Ragnarsson and Sell[69] showed, in a retrospective study, that a greater incidence of lower-extremity fractures occurs in paraplegic patients rather than in quadriplegic patients. This is believed to be caused by greater activity levels of the former group. Most of these fractures occurred in osteoporotic bones without known trauma or after trivial injuries.[69]

### Iron

Anemia is a common complication of acute SCI, even in the absence of significant blood loss.[16,41] In the study of Huang et al.,[41] of 28 acute SCI patients, 71% were found to have normochromic, normocytic anemia, and 14% had normochromic, microcytic anemia. They speculated that iron deficiencies, immune system changes that alter bone marrow maturation, and the effects of stress were causative factors. The process of erythropoiesis was not found to be altered in SCI patients.[41]

Anemia associated with chronic disorders, such as decubitus ulcers or urinary tract infections, was the most common type discovered in the long-term SCI patients studied by Perkash and Brown.[67] Anemia has also been identified as a factor related to increased length of stay of patients admitted to rehabilitation centers.[11] Recognition of the potential causes of anemia might speed the rehabilitation process.

### Sodium

The prevalence of hyponatremia in acute SCI patients is reportedly much higher than in general surgical populations.[19,68] The strongest predictor of the development of hyponatremia is the extent of the neurologic injury. The highest risk is observed with motor and sensory complete SCI patients. Low serum sodium levels (less than 135mM/L after correction for hyperglycemia) usually occur within the first week postinjury. Possible mechanisms include increased fluid intake, intrarenal defects in water excretion, resetting of the osmostat, and excessive sodium losses.[54]

# Feeding Modalities

After admission to the intensive care unit patients are typically not fed because efforts are concentrated on other factors, such as acute life-saving interactions, and reduction and stabilization of the initial fractures. Feeding the acute spinal cord injured patient is further complicated by mechanical ventilation, traction, immobilization, and abdominal distention.[15] Cooper and associates[27] stated "it is not a rare occurrence to see a patient who is paraplegic . . . literally die of starvation, despite vigorous attempts to supply adequate nutrients." Many factors hinder adequate nutrient intake and assimilation in spine surgery, spine trauma, and SCI patients.

Frequently, gastrointestinal (GI) function in acute and chronic SCI patients is compromised as a result of a posttraumatic ileus and neuronal motility dysfunction.[50] This lack of nutritional support during a time of hypermetabolism can result in malnutrition if not addressed immediately. Although many patients with SCI present with paralytic ileus, bowel activity commonly returns within the first postinjury week.[62] SCI patients commonly experience dysphagia caused by cervical fractures, retropharyngeal hematomas, and immobilization devices, but nutritional intake can be improved with pureed or mechanical soft diets and supplemental tube feedings.[9] Also, constipation can possibly be avoided by adequate dietary intake of fiber and fluids, and an appropriate bowel regimen.

## Diet-Oral Intake

The preferred route of nutrition support in any patient is by oral intake. Paraplegic SPI patients can typically provide adequate nutrition support if they do not have multiorgan injuries. Unlike quadraplegic patients, they have full use of their hands and arms and do not often require ventilatory support. The use of oral nutritional supplements can be tailored for the individual patient to meet their needs (Table 142.3).

**TABLE 142.3**

### A Guide to Enteral Feeding Formulas

| | cal/ml | Protein g/L | Fat g/L | Carb g/L | mOsm/kg H$_2$0 | Special Features |
|---|---|---|---|---|---|---|
| **Oral Supplements** | | | | | | |
| Boost | 1 | 43 | 18 | 173 | 640 | Multiflavor |
| Boost with Fiber | 1 | 43 | 18 | 178 | 480 | Fiber |
| Boost Plus | 1.5 | 59 | 58 | 200 | 720 | High calorie |
| Boost HP | 1 | 61 | 23 | 210 | 540 | High protein |
| Choice | 1 | 39 | 43 | 101 | 380 | Diabetics |
| Ensure | 1 | 37 | 25 | 165 | 470 | Multiflavor |
| Ensure Plus | 1.5 | 55 | 47 | 210 | 690 | Multiflavor |
| Kindercal | 1.1 | 30 | 44 | 135 | 440 | Ages 1-10 |
| Resource 1.5 | 1.5 | 67 | 67 | 230 | 600 | |
| Resource Shake | 1.7 | 55 | 74 | 240 | 600 | |
| Resource 2.0 | 2 | 108 | 103 | 270 | 600 | |
| Sustacal | 1 | 61 | 22 | 132 | 650 | High protein |
| **Standard Tube Feeds** | | | | | | |
| Comply | 1.5 | 60 | 61 | 180 | 460 | Restricted fluids |
| Isocal | 1 | 34 | 44 | 135 | 270 | |
| Isosource | 1 | 51 | 35 | 142 | 240 | |
| Osmolite | 1 | 37 | 34 | 151 | 300 | Isotonic |
| Nutren 1.0 | 1 | 40 | 38 | 128 | 300 | |
| Ultracal | 1 | 45 | 39 | 142 | 360 | Moderate nitrogen |
| Kindercal TF | 1.1 | 30 | 44 | 135 | 345 | Ages 1-10 |
| **Fiber-Containing Supplements** | | | | | | |
| Ensure Fiber with FOS | 1.1 | 38 | 25 | 169 | 470 | |
| Glucerna | 1 | 42 | 59 | 96 | 355 | Diabetics |
| Jevity | 1 | 44 | 35 | 155 | 300 | |
| Jevity Plus | 1.2 | 55 | 39 | 173 | 365 | |
| Isosource Fiber | 1 | 38 | 34 | 138 | 275 | |
| Nutren 1.0 with fiber | 1 | 40 | 38 | 128 | 300 | Vanilla |
| Ultracal HN plus | 1.2 | 54 | 40 | 156 | 370 | |
| **High-Calorie Density Formulas** | | | | | | |
| Comply | 1.5 | 60 | 61 | 180 | 460 | Restricted fluids |
| Deliver 2.0 | 2 | 75 | 101 | 200 | 640 | Restricted fluids |
| Ensure Plus HN | 1.5 | 63 | 49 | 202 | 650 | |
| Isocal HNplus | 1.2 | 54 | 40 | 156 | 400 | |
| Isosource Energy | 1.6 | 57 | 62 | 200 | 390 | |

*Continued*

**TABLE 142.3**

## A Guide to Enteral Feeding Formulas *cont'd*

| | cal/ml | Protein g/L | Fat g/L | Carb g/L | mOsm/kg H₂0 | Special Features |
|---|---|---|---|---|---|---|
| **High-Calorie Density Formulas *cont'd*** | | | | | | |
| Magnacal Renal | 2 | 75 | 101 | 200 | 570 | Renal dialysis |
| Nepro | 2 | 70 | 96 | 333 | 665 | Renal dialysis |
| Nutren 1.5 | 1.5 | 60 | 68 | 170 | 430 | |
| Nutren 2.0 | 2 | 80 | 106 | 196 | 710 | |
| Probalance | 1.2 | 54 | 41 | 156 | 350 | Elderly |
| Pulmocare | 1.5 | 63 | 93 | 106 | 475 | Vent patient |
| Suplena | 2 | 30 | 96 | 255 | 600 | Renal dialysis |
| TwoCal HN | 2 | 84 | 91 | 219 | 690 | High nitrogen |
| **High-Protein Formulas** | | | | | | |
| Ensure High Protein | 1 | 50 | 25 | 130 | 470 | |
| Isocal HN | 1.1 | 44 | 45 | 124 | 270 | |
| Isosource Protein | 1.2 | 66 | 40 | 148 | 300 | |
| Osmolite HN | 1 | 44 | 45 | 144 | 300 | |
| Osmolite HN plus | 1.2 | 55 | 39 | 158 | 360 | |
| TwoCal HN | 2 | 84 | 91 | 219 | 690 | |
| Ultracal HN plus | 1.2 | 54 | 40 | 156 | 370 | |
| **Special Disease State Formulas** | | | | | | |
| ChoiceDM | 1 | 45 | 51 | 119 | 300 | Diabetics |
| Deliver 2.0 | 2 | 75 | 101 | 200 | 640 | Restricted fluids |
| Glucerna | 1 | 42 | 59 | 96 | 355 | Diabetics |
| Introlyte | 0.5 | 22 | 18 | 71 | 200 | Starting tube feeds |
| Lipisorb | 1.4 | 57 | 57 | 161 | 630 | Fat malabsorption |
| Magnacal Renal | 2 | 75 | 101 | 200 | 570 | Renal dialysis |
| Oxepa | 1.5 | 63 | 94 | 106 | 493 | Lung injured, ventilated |
| Probalance | 1.2 | 54 | 41 | 156 | 350 | Elderly |
| Protain XL | 1 | 57 | 30 | 145 | 340 | Wound healing |
| Pulmocare | 1.5 | 63 | 93 | 106 | 475 | Vent patient |
| Respalor | 1.5 | 75 | 68 | 145 | 400 | Limited resp function |
| Subdue | 1 | 50 | 34 | 130 | 450 | Impaired GI function |
| Suplena | 2 | 30 | 96 | 255 | 600 | Renal dialysis |
| Traumacal | 1.5 | 82 | 68 | 142 | 560 | Trauma |
| **Elemental Formulas** | | | | | | |
| AlitraQ | 1 | | 16 | 165 | 575 | Impaired GI tract |
| Peptamen | 1 | 40 | 39 | 127 | 260 | Ready to feed |
| Peptamen VHP | 1 | 63 | 39 | 105 | 300 | Ready to feed |
| Perative | 1.3 | 67 | 37 | 177 | 385 | |
| Subdue | 1 | 50 | 34 | 130 | 330 | Malabsorption pts |
| Subdue plus | 1.5 | 76 | 51 | 127 | 400 | Calorically dense |
| Optimental | 1 | 51 | 28 | 139 | 540 | Malabsorption pts |
| Criticare HN | 1 | 38 | 5 | 220 | 650 | Malabsorption pts |
| **Modular Supplements** | | | | | | |
| Casec powder | 3.8 | 90 | 2 | N/A | N/A | Protein powder |
| Moducal powder | 3.8 | N/A | N/A | N/A | N/A | Glucose polymers |
| Microlipid | 4.5 | N/A | 45 | N/A | 80 | Fat emulsion |
| MCT oil | 7.7 | 0 | 0 | N/A | N/A | MCT |
| Polycose powder | 2 cal/ml | N/A | N/A | N/A | N/A | Glucose polymers |
| Promod powder | 12 cal/T | 3 g/L | N/A | N/A | N/A | Protein powder |
| **Pediatric Formulas** | | | | | | |
| Isosource Jr | 1.2 | 54 | 94 | 340 | 346 | Ages 1-12 |
| Kindercal TF | 1.1 | 30 | 44 | 135 | 345 | Ages 1-10 |
| Pediasure Enteral | 1 | 30 | 48 | 110 | N/A | Ages 1-10 |
| Pediasure Enteral with fiber | 1 | 30 | 44 | 114 | N/A | Ages 1-10 |

Successful nutritional management often includes assistance in meal selection, change of meal patterns to six small meals daily, high nutrient density, commercial supplements, and nocturnal tube feedings. In Laven et al.'s[53] study of 51 acute SCI patients, 57% reported that anorexia was present 2 weeks after injury and continued until 8 weeks postinjury in 33% of the population. Depression and the sensation of early satiety are common causes of decreased appetite in these patients. Assistance by nursing staff at mealtimes may be necessary in the acute stages. Patients may become more independent by using assistive eating devices.

Chronic SCI patients require increased vitamin, mineral, and complex carbohydrate intake and decreased fat intake.[56] High levels of fat intake, low intake of dietary fiber, nominal activity levels, and a predisposition to the development of cardiovascular disease place SCI patients at an increased risk for cardiopulmonary morbidity and mortality.

## Parenteral Nutrition

### Indications

Because of the common complications of GI dysfunction and prolonged ileus after SCI, total parenteral nutrition (TPN) is essential if an optimal nutritional status cannot be maintained by the enteral route.[90] The combination of TPN (to provide nutrient needs) and small volumes of enteral feedings (to maintain gut integrity) may provide the best of both worlds in selected situations. If the GI tract is not provided with a minimum amount of nutritional support (i.e., 10 to 20ml/hr of enteral feeds), the mucosal villi will atrophy.[2] This atrophy impairs the natural immunogenic barrier and allows bacteria to translocate across the mucosa and into the blood stream.

### Administration

Specialized nutritional support techniques are available to prevent malnutrition (Figure 142.1). Either central or peripheral veins can be used for delivering TPN. Concentrated TPN formulas should only be infused through a central venous catheter to prevent thrombophlebitis of the smaller peripheral veins.[84] Central vein access is appropriate for TPN delivery needed for more than 5 to 7 days. TPN solutions with osmolarities of less than 900mOsm can be administered via peripheral vein access. However, peripheral access is difficult to maintain for more than 5 to 7 days.

Most institutions have standard TPN solutions that can be ordered from stock. Information about these TPN formulas can be obtained from the institutions' pharmacies. Patient-specific formulas can also be designed to meet individuals' calorie, protein, and fluid requirements. The energy substrates used in TPN are dextrose solutions ranging from 5% to 70% concentrations, and lipid emulsions in concentrations of 10% (1.1kcal/ml) to 20% (2kcal/ml).[84] Protein is provided by commercial crystalline L-amino acid solutions in concentrations of 3% to 15%. Electrolyte additives, multivitamins, trace element preparations, and medications can also be administered in TPN solutions according to each patient's needs.

### Complications

Complications of TPN include mineral and electrolyte imbalances, acid-base disorders, substrate intolerances (hyperglycemia, hypertriglyceridemia, elevated BUN levels), and catheter-related infections.[84] In the acute postinjury stage daily monitoring of serum electrolytes, glucose, BUN, and creatinine is necessary to detect and minimize excesses or deficiencies. Changes in sodium, potassium,

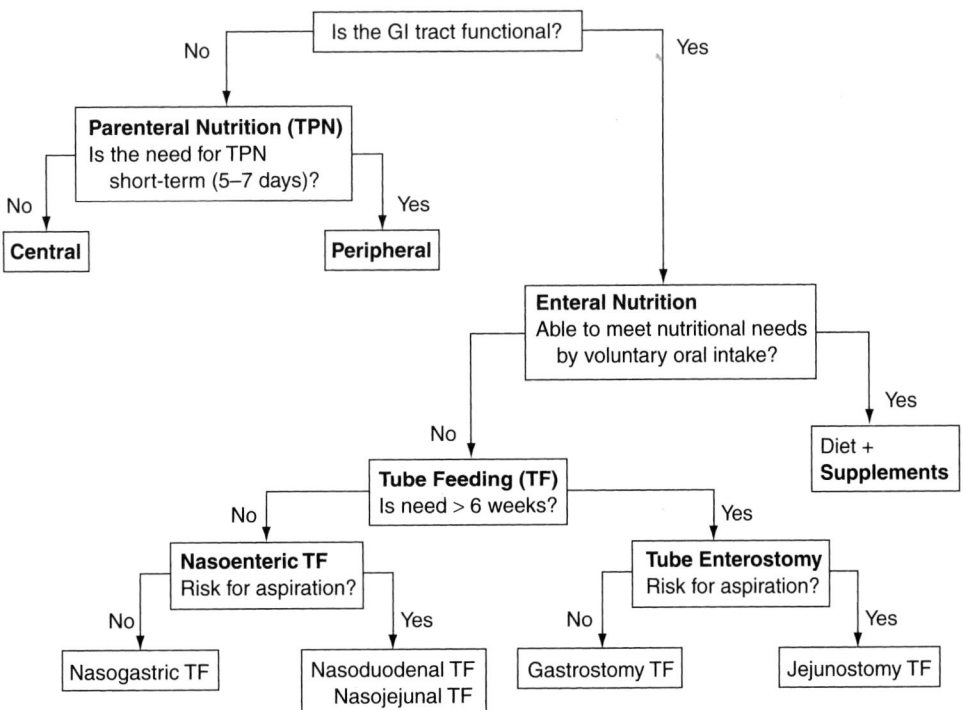

**Figure 142.1** The decision-making process for nutritional support.

magnesium, and phosphorus deliveries are frequent in critically ill patients. Careful evaluation of fluid balance by daily weights and intake and output records is necessary to prevent volume depletion or overload. Meticulous line care is essential for reducing catheter-related infections. However, parenteral nutrition has been shown to promote the bacterial translocation from the intestine to the blood stream.[2] This bacterial translocation is a result of loss of the intestinal barrier because of atrophy of the mucosa from disuse. Therefore trophic tube feeds (10 to 20ml/hr) while using parenteral nutrition, can prevent the disuse atrophy and bacterial translocation. This flow rate is minimal and well tolerated in most posttraumatic ileus states.

### Enteral Nutrition (Tube Feeding)

#### Indications

When adequate dietary intakes cannot be achieved orally, and the GI tract is functional, enteral nutrition via a tube is the preferred method for nutritional support. The enteral route for nutrient administration is always preferable to parenteral feedings. The benefits of enteral feedings include more physiologic metabolism and use of nutrients, maintenance of gut integrity, decreased risk of bacterial translocation, decreased expense of nutrient delivery, and decreased risk of catheter-related infections.[42] Use of the enteral route is contraindicated in the presence of mechanical obstruction of the GI tract, prolonged ileus, severe GI hemorrhage, severe diarrhea, intractable vomiting, and high-output GI tract fistula.

#### Administration

The decision regarding the type of enteral access depends on the anticipated duration of tube feeding and the risk of pulmonary aspiration of gastric contents (see Figure 142.1). Short-term (less than 6 weeks) enteral access is possible via the nasogastric, nasoduodenal, or nasojejunal routes. Surgical or percutaneous endoscopic gastrostomy and jejunostomy tubes can be inserted for long-term (more than 6 weeks) nutritional support.[79] Gastric feedings should not be instituted in patients without an intact gag reflex, with gastroesophageal reflux, with gastroparesis, with gastric outlet obstruction, or with gastric atony.[42] Jejunal feedings can usually be initiated immediately after injury, and potentially reduce the risk of aspiration.

A wide variety of specialized commercial formulas are available for both oral and tube feeding supplementation (see Table 142.3). These supplements differ by calorie and protein densities, fiber contents, form of nutrients, and the amount of micronutrients.[42] Selection of the appropriate formula is based on the individual's digestive and absorptive capacity, and the specific characteristics and indications of the product. Most commercial formulas provide the recommended dietary allowances for vitamins and minerals in approximately 1 to 1.5L.

Formulas can be administered by bolus, intermittent, or continuous methods. Bolus feedings involve the rapid delivery of 300 to 400ml of formula over 10 minutes several times daily. Intermittent feedings are also given several times daily, but over at least 30 minutes. The bolus and intermittent methods are especially suited for gastric feedings. Small-volume, continuous drip feedings over 10 to 24 hours are recommended for intestinal delivery of nutrients. Continuous feedings are usually better tolerated than bolus feedings in critically ill patients.[42]

The final goal amount of delivered formula depends on the product's nutrient density and the individual estimated daily calorie and protein requirements. Bolus or intermittent feedings can be initiated with 100ml of formula. The bolus volume can be advanced by 50ml every 4 hours to the goal amount if gastric residuals are not significant (less than 100ml or half the volume previously delivered) when aspirated before each feeding.[25] Initiation of continuous tube feeding can range from rates of 20 to 40ml/hr. Rates are then advanced by 10 to 25ml/hr every 6 hours to the goal amount as the patient tolerates.

#### Complications

Complications of enteral feedings interrupt adequate nutrient deliveries (Table 142.4). Diarrhea and tube obstruction are the most common problems associated with tube feedings. Recognition of the causes and solutions to these complications can improve formula tolerance and increase nutrient deliveries.[42]

## Monitoring of Nutritional Status

There is little documentation of the effectiveness of early aggressive nutritional support in terms of improved outcome or decreased incidence of complications for SCI.[43,53] However, there is a large body of evidence supporting improved outcomes in other neurologic injuries, such as head trauma.[36,39,70,90] Applying this data to the SCI population supports that hospitalized SCI patients should be maintained at optimal nutritional status. Two thirds of the SCI patients admitted to rehabilitation units are reportedly malnourished.[65] In addition, quadriplegic patients are at a higher risk for malnutrition than are paraplegic patients and should be even more aggressively supported.[66]

### Body Composition

Patients with serious injuries, such as major fractures, will often lose 10% to 25% of their body weight during recovery from the injury.[46,47] Studies regarding tissue composition show that protein accounts for 8% to 12% of the total weight loss, and fat accounts for 15% to 30%. However, in SCI patients early weight loss consists primarily of muscle rather than fat.[53]

Several studies have demonstrated that the loss of muscle tissue and body cell mass (BCM) after SCI is a progressive process that occurs over a prolonged period.[19,37,80,82] Body composition studies by Sedlock and Laventure[80] indicate that although their SCI subjects were not overweight, they had an increased proportion of body fat with a decreased lean body mass. Rasmann Nuhlicek and associates[71] also compared controls to SCI patients and showed no difference in body weight or extracellular water, but an increase in the ratio of extracellular to total body water, along with

**TABLE 142.4**

### Complications of Enteral Feeding

| Complications | Possible Causes | Suggestions for Prevention or Treatment |
|---|---|---|
| **Gastrointestinal** | | |
| Diarrhea | Formula hyperosmolarity | Initiate feeding at slow rate (10-20ml/hr); advance rate gradually as patient tolerates |
| | Bolus feedings | Change to continuous drip feedings |
| | Low-residue formulas | Use fiber-containing formulas |
| | Gut atrophy (prolonged NPO status) | Deliver peptide-based formulas or initiate slow rates of formulas and gradually advance |
| | Concurrent drug therapy | Evaluate medication regimen (antibiotics, magnesium-containing antacids, oral potassium supplements, sorbitol); adjust as possible |
| | Bacterial contamination | Limit formula hang-time to no more than 8 hours; change tube feeding bag and extension tubing every 24 hours |
| | Bacterial overgrowth | If stool culture for *C. difficile* is positive, treat with vancomycin; Lactinex granules, 1 package 3X daily |
| | Lactose intolerance | Use lactose-free formulas |
| Gastric residuals | Delayed gastric emptying | Confirm placement of feeding tube distal to the ligament of Treitz; trial metoclopramide (10mg IV every 6 hours) |
| | Bolus feedings | Change to continuous drip feedings |
| **Mechanical** | | |
| Tube obstruction | Medications given via tube | Use crushed medications or elixirs only; irrigate tube before and after each medication; use nasogastric tube (instead of nasoduodenal) for delivery of medications |
| | Irregular irrigation of tube | Irrigate tube with 30-50ml of water every 4 hours for continuous feeding or before and after each bolus feeding |
| Tube displacement | Removal by patient | Consider use of feeding tube bridle or modified nasal cannula |

an increased fat mass in higher-level injuries. Claus-Walker and Halstead[19] demonstrated that connective tissue, lipids, and water replace the atrophied muscle. Greenway and associates[37] noted no consistent trends in body composition changes in long-term SCI patients. They commented that caloric restriction compensates for reduced muscle activity, and that it can control increases in body fat. Shizgal *et al.* stated that in well-nourished quadriplegic patients, the loss of BCM is accompanied by a similar loss of extracellular mass (ECM) as body size decreases.[19,82] In malnourished SCI patients, however, body weight may actually increase as a result of expansion in the ECM, even in the presence of a corresponding loss of BCM. Therefore it was concluded that body weight is a poor predictor of nutritional status.

### Anthropometric Measurements

Anthropometric measurements are an inexpensive and easily applied tool to access and follow nutritional status in the healthy individual. These measurements consist of direct measurements of weight, height, the triceps, skinfold thickness, midarm circumference, and midarm muscle circumference. Unfortunately, SCI patients typically undergo water shifts, denervation muscle atrophy, increased percentage of body fat, and unavoidable weight and body compositional changes, which questions the accuracy and validity of these nutritional gauges.[16,63,66] The Metropolitan Life Insurance guidelines of ideal body weight for a given height and frame size for long-term SCI patients illustrates these changes.[10] Paraplegic patients are approximately 10 to 15lb (and quadriplegic patients are approximately 15 to 20lb) below the recommended guideline weights for long-term patients.[10]

### Serum Protein Markers

Serum total protein and albumin levels are not useful as nutritional assessment parameters for acute SCI patients. Albumin levels are often distorted by fluid shifts and acute blood loss. Hepatic transport proteins respond as acute-phase reactants and serum levels decline following acute stress.[27] Also, SCI patients have an extremely high elimination rate of serum albumin.[16,66] With its long half-life of 18 to 21 days, serum albumin is an insensitive marker for adequacy of nutritional support. In fact, serum albumin may be a better indicator of severity of illness than of nutritional status. Serum prealbumin is a more appropriate parameter, with its half-life of 1 to 2 days.[34]

### Creatinine-Height Index

Creatinine-height index is based on the amount of creatinine excreted in the urine over 24 hours. This index is typically compared with standard values to assess nutritional status. However, denervation muscle atrophy after spinal cord injuries causes a dramatic increase in creatinine excretion, regardless of dietary intake or nutritional status. Thus the creatinine-height index does not truly reflect the acute SCI patient's nutritional status.[10] Despite this a standard index of less than 60% has been established as an indicator of nutritional risk in SCI patients.[66]

## Nitrogen Balance and Nitrogen Turnover

Nitrogen balance (NB) occurs when nitrogen intake equals nitrogen output (NB = 0), and is also referred to as nitrogen equilibrium.[34] A positive NB or anabolic state exists when nitrogen intake exceeds nitrogen output. A net 24-hour positive NB of 2 to 4g is optimal for anabolism. When nitrogen excretion is greater than nitrogen intake, a negative NB or catabolic state exists.

NB can be calculated by subtracting the total nitrogen output from total nitrogen intake. The total nitrogen intake is determined by dividing the daily protein intake (grams) from both enteral and parenteral sources by 6.25. Nitrogen output consists primarily as urine urea nitrogen (UUN). An aliquot of a 24-hour urine collection is assayed for its urea nitrogen content by a standard enzymatic laboratory technique (Beckman Astra, Beckman Instruments, Fullerton, CA).[76] This value, plus 4 (the constant used for nitrogen losses from the skin and feces), is subtracted from the grams of nitrogen intake during the same 24-hour period to calculate the NB, as demonstrated in the following equation:

$$NB = [\text{Protein Intake (g)}/6.25] - (24 \text{ hour UUN} + 4) \quad (3)$$

The provision of inadequate calories forces the body to break down muscle mass to meet energy demands. This muscle breakdown results in nitrogenous by-products: urea, creatinine, and 3-methyl-histidine, which are excreted in the urine.[45] Endogenous protein stores are also used as an amino acid supply when insufficient exogenous protein is provided. Increasing calorie and protein deliveries, therefore, can minimize net protein losses. Glucocorticoid administration can increase the catabolism of protein. In this situation the catabolized protein fuels gluconeogenesis.[43]

After non-SCI major trauma and surgery, REE and nitrogen excretion levels are parallel. However, in SCI patients calorie needs decrease, whereas urinary nitrogen losses, primarily from muscle tissue,[26] increase in proportion to the severity of the SCI.[27] This negative NB ensues in the spinal cord–injured population, despite more than adequate caloric and protein administration.[43,76] This same phenomenon has been observed with severe cases of botulism poisoning that have resulted in muscle paralysis.[14]

Nitrogen losses after SCI are obligatory and persist for at least 7 weeks.[26,27,49,76] Peak negative NB has been previously observed in SCI patients during the third week after injury, despite adequate delivery of predicted and measured calories.[75] Cooper and Hoen[26] reported that urinary nitrogen excretion of greater than 25g/day during the first 2 postinjury weeks is a poor prognostic sign for the eventual functional return of paralyzed muscles. In some patients the administration of growth hormone has reduced nitrogen loss.[58] Growth hormone studies after SCI, however, have not been conducted.

During the first week after injury, many SCI patients have been observed to have a transiently positive NB.[76] This observation may be reflective of a delay in protein losses. Dietrick et al.[31] evaluated four conscientious objectors who were immobilized in pelvic girdles and leg casts for 6 to 7 weeks on a metabolism ward. All four subjects showed an increase in nitrogen excretion and negative NBs. This, however, took 4 to 5 days to develop. From the data presented by Dietrick et al., it is concluded that acute immobilization could contribute to the nitrogen excretion increase observed in paralyzed patients that begins approximately 1 week after injury. Rodriguez and associates[75] showed an obligatory negative NB in 11 of 12 SCI patients, despite excessive feedings, and the only patient who did not have a negative NB was an incomplete myelopathy. They concluded that relying on NB determinations to calculate nutritional requirements in SPI patients resulted in overfeeding.

## Nutritional Deficiency–Related Wound Complications

SCI patients are at increased risk of developing wound-related or skin breakdown problems. In the perioperative period SPI patients are typically insensate over the operative region. This results in prolonged pressure and decreased blood supply and nutrition in an already nutritionally compromised patient. Klein and associates showed that even without spinal cord injuries, a spine patient's preoperative nutritional status was an independent predictor of postoperative infectious complications.[48]

Decubitus ulcers can also develop acutely or in the chronic SCI, and their development is associated with prolonged focal pressure application and the completeness of the SCI.[73] Other factors include anemia, immobility, hypoproteinemia, and systemic infections. After SCI an increased degradation of integument collagen results in the excretion of hydroxyproline, hydroxylysine, and glucosyl-galactosyl hydroxylysine in the urine.[22,78] This leads to a decreased amino acid content per unit weight of skin in SCI patients, and may account for its decreased tensile strength and increased susceptibility to decubiti. Decubiti may lead to protein depletion of up to 50g/day.[53] The larger the pressure ulcer, the greater the protein loss from the wound, which further augments protein deficiencies.

Lack of weight-bearing results in collagen degradation, as does weightlessness in astronauts.[24] Poor circulation below the level of the injury can reduce nutrient and oxygen delivery to the tissues, thus further increasing the risk of decubiti formation.[78] Defective wound healing has also been reported in nondecubitus wounds below the level of the spinal lesion.[5] Notably, growth hormone levels have been observed to be elevated in SCI patients. This may be, in fact, related to an overall increase in collagen turnover.[21]

## Summary

Consideration of nutritional support is necessary for the maintenance of optimal nutritional status in critically ill and rehabilitating SCI patients. Methods for estimating caloric and nutritional needs can provide the *best guess* for initial nutritional management. Actual metabolic measurements with indirect calorimetry can then provide fine-tuning of subsequent nutrient needs. Adjustments can also be made based on the patients' clinical conditions, available feeding routes, their tolerance of substrates, and the modification of requirements as the hospital course progresses. The use of a variety of nutritional supplements and available assessment techniques should further optimize nutritional management and outcomes of SCI patients.

# REFERENCES

1. Agarwal N, Lee BY, Corcoran L, Del Guerico LRM: Energy expenditure in quadriplegic patients, abstracted. *JPEN* 8:98, 1984.

2. Alverdy JC, Aoys E, Moss GS: Total parenteral nutrition promotes bacterial translocation from the gut. *Surgery* 104(2):185-190, 1988.

3. American Diabetic Association and American Dietetic Association: *A Guide for Professionals: The Effective Application of Exchange Lists for Meal Planning.* New York, 1977, p 17.

4. Barboriak JJ, Rooney CB, El Ghatit AZ, *et al*: Nutrition in spinal cord injury patients. *J Am Paraplegia Soc* 6:32-36, 1983.

5. Basson MD, Burney RE: Defective wound healing in paraplegic patients. *Surg Forum* 32:78-80, 1981.

6. Bauman WA, Spungen AM: Carbohydrate and lipid metabolism in chronic spinal cord injury. *J Spin Cord Med* 24:266-277, 2001.

7. Benzel EC, Wild GC: Biochemical mechanisms of posttraumatic neural injury. In Barrow DL (ed): *Perspectives in Neurological Surgery.* St Louis, Quality Medical Publishing, 1991, pp 95-126.

8. Berlly MH, Wilmot CB: Acute abdominal emergencies during the first four weeks after spinal cord injury. *Arch Phys Med Rehab* 65:687-690, 1984.

9. Bildsten C, Lamid S: Nutritional management of a patient with brain damage and spinal cord injury. *Arch Phys Med Rehab* 64:382-383, 1983.

10. Blissitt PA: Nutrition in acute spinal cord injury. *Crit Care Nurs Clin North Am* 2:375-384, 1990.

11. Burr RG, Clift-Peace L, Nuseibeh I: Haemoglobin and albumin as predictors of length of stay of spinal injured patients in a rehabilitation centre. *Paraplegia* 31:473-478, 1993.

12. Bynoe RP, Kudsk KA, Fabian TC, Brown RO: Nutritional support in trauma patients. *Nutr Clin Pract* 3:137-144, 1988.

13. Carey ME, Nance FC, Kirgis HD, *et al*: Pancreatitis following spinal cord injury. *J Neurosurg* 47:917-922, 1977.

14. Cashman MD, Wightkin WT, Madden JE, Phillips RS: Massive azoturia and failure to achieve positive nitrogen balance in a botulism patient. *JPEN* 10:316-318, 1986.

15. Charney KJ, Juler GL, Comarr E: General surgery problems in patients with spinal cord injuries. *Arch Surg* 110:1083-1088, 1975.

16. Chin DE, Kearns P: Nutrition in the spinal-injured patient. *Nutr Clin Pract* 6:213-222, 1991.

17. Clarke KS: Caloric costs of activity in paraplegic persons. *Arch Phys Med Rehab* 47:427-435, 1966.

18. Claus-Walker J: Clinical implications of the disturbance in calcium and collagen metabolism in quadriplegia. *Int J Rehab Res* 3:540-541, 1980.

19. Claus-Walker J, Halstead LS: Metabolic and endocrine changes in spinal cord injury: I. The nervous system before and after transection of the spinal cord. *Arch Phys Med Rehab* 62:595-601, 1981.

20. Claus-Walker J, Halstead LS: Metabolic and endocrine changes in spinal cord injury: II (Section 1). Consequences of partial decentralization of the autonomic nervous system. *Arch Phys Med Rehab* 63:569-575, 1982.

21. Claus-Walker J, Halstead LS: Metabolic and endocrine changes in spinal cord injury. III. Less quanta of sensory input plus bedrest and illness. *Arch Phys Med Rehab* 63:628-631, 1982.

22. Claus-Walker J, Halstead LS: Metabolic and endocrine changes in spinal cord injury: IV. Compounded neurologic dysfunctions. *Arch Phys Med Rehab* 63:632-638, 1982.

23. Claus-Walker J, Halstead LS, Carter RE, *et al*: Calcium excretion in the quadriplegia. *Arch Phys Med Rehabil* 53:14-18, 1972.

24. Claus-Walker J, Singh J, Leach CS, *et al*: The urinary excretion of collagen degradation products by quadriplegic patients and during weightlessness. *J Bone Joint Surg* 59A:209-212, 1977.

25. Clevenger FW, Rodriguez DJ: Decision-making for enteral feeding administration: the why behind where and how. *Nutr Clin Pract* 10:104-113, 1995.

26. Cooper IS, Hoen TI: Metabolic disorders in paraplegics. *Neurology* 2:332-340, 1952.

27. Cooper IS, Rynearson EH, MacCarty CS, Power MH: Metabolic consequences of spinal cord injury. *J Clin Endocrinol* 10:858-870, 1950.

28. Cox SAR, Weiss SM, Posuniak EA, *et al*: Energy expenditure after spinal cord injury: an evaluation of stable rehabilitating patients. *J Trauma* 25:419-423, 1985.

29. Cruse JM, Lewis RE, Dilioglou S, *et al*: Facilitation of immune function, healing of pressure ulcers and nutritional status in spinal cord injury patients. *Exp Mol Pathol* 68:38-54, 2000.

30. Damask MC, Schwarz Y, Weissman C: Energy measurements and requirements of critically ill patients. *Crit Care Clin* 3:71-96, 1987.

31. Dietrick JE, Whedon GD, Shorr E: Effects of immobilization upon various metabolic and physiologic functions of normal men. *Ann J Med* 4:3-36, 1948.

32. Duckrow RB, Beard DC, Brennan RW: Regional cerebral blood flow decreases during hyperglycemia. *Ann Neurol* 17:267-272, 1985.

33. Frankenfield DC, Stanley Smith J, Cooney RN: Accelerated nitrogen loss after traumatic injury is not attenuated by achievement of energy balance. *JPEN* 21:324-329, 1997.

34. Fry DE, Borzotta AP: Options in nutritional support of the surgical patient. *Probl Gen Surg* 4:427-440, 1987.

35. Garfin SR, Shackford SR: Care of the multiply injured patient with cervical spine injury. *Clin Orthop* 239:19-29, 1989.

36. Grahm TW, Zadrozny DB, Harrington T: The benefits of early jejunal hyperalimentation in the head-injured patient. *J Neurosurg* 25(5):729-735, 1989.

37. Greenway RM, Houser HP, Lindan O, Weir DR: Long term changes in gross body composition of paraplegic and quadriplegic patients. *Paraplegia* 7:301-318, 1970.

38. Hadley MM: Hypermetabolism after CNS trauma. *Nutrition* 5:143, 1989.

39. Hadley MN, Grahm TW, Harrington T, *et al*: Nutritional support and neurotrauma: A critical review of early nutrition in forty-five acute head injury patients. *Neurosurgery* 19(3):367-373, 1986.

40. Harris JA, Benedict FG: A biometric study of basal metabolism in man. Carnegie Institute of Washington, Publication no 279. Philadelphia, Lippincott-Raven, 1919, pp 190-227.

41. Huang CT, DeVivo MJ, Stover SL: Anemia in acute phase of spinal cord injury. *Arch Phys Med Rehab* 71:3-7, 1990.

42. Ideno KT: Enteral nutrition. In Gottschlich MM, Matarese LE, Shronts EP (eds): *Nutrition Support Dietetics Core Curriculum.* Silver Springs, MD, American Society of Parenteral and Enteral Nutrition, 1992, pp 71-104.

43. Kaufman HH, Rowlands BJ, Stein DK, *et al*: General metabolism in patients with acute paraplegia and quadriplegia. *Neurosurgery* 16:309-313, 1985.

44. Kearns PJ, Pipp TL, Quirk M, Campolo M: Nutritional requirements in quadriplegics, abstracted. *JPEN* 6:577, 1982.

45. Kearns PJ, Thompson JD, Werner PC, *et al*: Nutritional and metabolic response to acute spinal-cord injury. *JPEN* 16:11-15, 1992.

46. Kinney JM: Calories-nitrogen-disease and injury relations. *Drug Intell Clin Pharm* 6:261-265, 1972.

47. Kinney JM, Duke JH Jr, Long CL, Long FE: Tissue fuel and weight loss after injury. *J Clin Pathol* 14:65-72, 1970.

48. Klein JD, Hey LA, Yu CS, *et al*: Perioperative nutrition and postoperative complications in patients undergoing spinal surgery. *Spine* 21(22):2676-2682, 1996.

49. Kolpek JH, Ott LG, Record KE, *et al*: Comparison of urinary urea nitrogen excretion and measured energy expenditure in spinal cord injury and nonsteroid-treated severe head trauma patients. *JPEN* 13:277-280, 1989.

50. Krogh K, Mosdal C, Laurberg S: Gastrointestinal and segmental colonic transit times in patients with acute and chronic spinal cord lesions. *Spinal Cord* 38:615-621, 2000.

51. Lagger L: Spinal cord injury: nutritional management. *J Neurol Nurs* 15:310-312, 1983.

52. Lanschot JJB, Feenstra BWA, Vermeu CG, Bruining HA: Calculation versus measurement of total energy expenditure. *Crit Care Med* 14:981-985, 1986.

53. Laven GT, Huang C-T, DeVivo MJ, *et al*: Nutritional status during the acute stage of spinal cord injury. *Arch Phys Med Rehab* 70:277-282, 1989.

54. Leehey DJ, Picache AA, Robertson GL: Hyponatremia in quadriplegic patients. *Clin Sci* 75:441-444, 1988.

55. LeMay DR, Gehua L, Zelenock GB: Insulin administration protects neurologic function in cerebral ischemia in rats. *Stroke* 19:1411-1419, 1988.

56. Levine AM, Nash MS, Green BA, *et al*: An examination of dietary intakes and nutritional status of chronic healthy spinal-cord injured individuals. *Paraplegia* 30:880-889, 1992.

57. Longstreth WT Jr, Inui TS: High blood glucose level on hospital admission and poor neurologic recovery after cardiac arrest. *Ann Neurol* 15:59-63, 1984.

58. Manson JM, Wilmore DW: Positive nitrogen balance with human growth hormone and hypocaloric intravenous feeding. *Surgery* 100:188-197, 1986.

59. Marsh WR, Anderson RE, Sundt TM: Effect of hyperglycemia on brain pH levels in areas of focal incomplete cerebral ischemia in monkeys. *J Neurosurg* 65:693-696, 1986.

60. Marvin JA: Nutritional support of the critically injured patient. *Crit Care Nurs* 11:21, 1988.

61. Maynard FM: Immobilization hypercalcium following spinal cord injury. *Arch Phys Med Rehabil* 67:41-44, 1986.

62. McCagg C: Postoperative management and acute rehabilitation of patients with spinal cord injuries. *Orthop Clin North Am* 17:171-182, 1986.

63. Mollinger LA, Spurr GB, Ghatit EL, *et al*: Daily energy expenditure and basal metabolic rates of patients with spinal cord injury. *Arch Phys Med Rehab* 66:420-426, 1985.

64. Monroe MB, Tataranni PA, Prately R, *et al*: Lower daily energy expenditure as measured by a respiratory chamber in subjects with spinal cord injury compared with control subjects. *Am J Clin Nutr* 68:1223-1227, 1998.

65. Newmark SR: Nutritional support in an inpatient rehabilitation unit. *Arch Phys Med Rehab* 62:634-637, 1981.

66. Peiffer JC, Blust P, Leyson LF: Nutritional assessment of the spinal cord injured patient. *J Am Diet Assoc* 78:501-505, 1981.

67. Perkash A, Brown M: Anemia in patients with traumatic spinal cord injury. *J Am Paraplegia Soc* 9:10-15, 1986.

68. Peruzzi WT, Shapiro BA: Hyponatremia in spinal cord injured patients. *Crit Care Med* 22:252-258, 1994.

69. Ragnarsson KT, Sell H: Lower extremity fractures after spinal cord injury: a retrospective study. *Arch Phys Med Rehab* 62:418-423, 1981.

70. Rapp RP, Young B, Twyman D, *et al*: The favorable effect of early parenteral feeding on survival in head-injured patients. *J Neurosurg* 58:906-912, 1983.

71. Rasmann Nuhlicek DN, Spurr GB, Barboriak JJ, *et al*: Body composition of patients with spinal cord injury. *Eur J Clin Nutr* 42:765-773, 1988.

72. Rawe SE, Lee WA, Perot PL: Spinal cord glucose utilization after experimental spinal cord injury. *Neurosurgery* 9:40-46, 1981.

73. Richardson RR, Meyer PR: Prevalence and incidence of pressure sores in acute spinal cord injuries. *Paraplegia* 19:235-247, 1981.

74. Robertson CS, Grossman RG: Protection against spinal cord ischemia with insulin-induced hypoglycemia. *J Neurosurg* 67:739-744, 1987.

75. Rodriguez DJ, Benzel EC, Clevenger FW: The metabolic response to spinal cord injury. *Spinal Cord* 32:599-604, 1997.

76. Rodriguez DJ, Clevenger FW, Osler TM, *et al*: Obligatory negative nitrogen balance following spinal cord injury. *JPEN* 15:319-322, 1991.

77. Rodriguez DJ, Sandoval W, Clevenger FW: Is measured energy expenditure correlated to injury severity score in major trauma patients? *J Surg Res* 59:455-459, 1995.

78. Rodriguez GP, Claus-Walker J: Biochemical changes in skin composition in spinal cord injury: a possible contribution to decubitus ulcers. *Paraplegia* 26:302-309, 1988.

79. Sangster W, Swanstrom L: Laparoscopic-guided feeding jejunostomy. *Surg Endosc* 7:308-310, 1993.

80. Sedlock DA, Laventure SJ: Body composition and resting energy expenditure in long term spinal cord injury. *Paraplegia* 28:448-454, 1990.

81. Sherrington CS: Notes on temperature after spinal transection, with some observations on shivering. *J Physiol* (Lond) 58:405-424, 1924.

82. Shizgal HM, Roza A, Leduc B, *et al*: Body composition in quadriplegic patients. *JPEN* 10:364-368, 1986.

83. Shronts EP, Lacy JA: Metabolic support. In Gottschlich MM, Matarese LE, Shronts EP (eds): *Nutrition Support Dietetics Core Curriculum.* Silver Springs, MD, American Society of Parenteral and Enteral Nutrition, 1992, pp 351-365.

84. Skipper A, Marian MJ: Parenteral nutrition. In Gottschlich MM, Matarese LE, Shronts EP (eds): *Nutrition Support*

*Dietetics Core Curriculum.* Silver Springs, MD, American Society of Parenteral and Enteral Nutrition, 1992, pp 105-123.

85. Stanek GS: Metabolic and nutritional management of the trauma patient. In Cardona VD, Hurn PD, Mason PJ, *et al* (eds): *Trauma Nursing: From Resuscitation Through Rehabilitation.* Philadelphia, WB Saunders, 1988, pp 284-315.

86. Tori JA, Hill LL: Hypercalcemia in children with spinal cord injury. *Arch Phys Med Rehabil* 59:443-447, 1978.

87. Weir JB: New methods for calculating metabolic rate with special reference to protein metabolism. *J Physiol* 109:1, 1949.

88. Williams RR, Fuenning CR: Circulatory indirect calorimetry in the critically ill. *JPEN* 15:509-512, 1991.

89. Young B, Ott L, Phillips R, McClain C: Metabolic management of the patient with head injury. *Neurosurg Clin North Am* 2:301-320, 1991.

90. Young B, Ott L, Twyman D, *et al*: The effect of nutritional support on outcome from severe head injury. *J Neurosurg* 67:668-676, 1987.

# APPENDIX 142.1

# A Nutritional Support Algorithm for Spine Trauma and SCI Patients

**OBJECTIVE:** *To assess the optimal nutrient deliveries for spine trauma and SCI patients.*

1. Determine ideal body weight (IBW) and actual percentage of IBW.

   Ideal Body Weight:

   Men: 5 feet = 106lb + 6lb for every inch taller

   Women: 5 feet = 100lb + 5lb for every inch taller

   If patient is 20% greater than ideal weight, use adjusted IBW° to calculate basal energy expenditure (BEE).

2. Determine an estimate of actual caloric needs by determining predicted energy expenditure (PEE).

   Acute Postinjury Stage:

   $$\text{PEE} = \text{BEE} \times (\text{injury and stress factor})$$
   $$(\text{range } 1.6\text{-}1.75)$$
   $$\text{Men: BEE} = 66 + (13.7 \times \text{Wt}^\dagger)$$
   $$+ (5 \times \text{Ht}^\dagger) - (6.8 \times \text{age})$$
   $$\text{Women: BEE} = 655 + (9.6 \times \text{Wt}^\dagger)$$
   $$+ (1.7 \times \text{Ht}^\dagger) - (4.7 \times \text{age})$$

   Chronic Stage:

   Quadriplegics: PEE = 22.7kcal/kg/day

   Paraplegics: PEE = 27.9kcal/kg/day

---

°Adjusted IBW: If 20% over IBW, subtract IBW from actual weight and multiply by 0.25; add the product to the IBW.
†*Wt*, Weight in kilograms; *Ht*, height in centimeters, age in years.

3. Determine estimated protein requirements.

   Protein: 2g/kg IBW (acute stage)

   1.2-1.5g/kg IBW (postacute stage)

4. Select appropriate nutritional support access route and formula for administration of nutrient needs.

   a. Formula selection is based on clinical condition and patient tolerance. Standard formulas can be modified if necessary to meet patients' needs. Enteral tube feeding formulas can be selected from Table 142.3.

   TPN formulas should be determined by the aforementioned nutritional requirements and via regional or institutional standards. Contact the hospital IV pharmacy for information on standard formulas and compositions. IV lipid emulsions are available in 10% (1kcal/cml) or 20% (2kcal/ml) concentrations.

   b. Initial goal rates of tube feedings, TPN, and IV lipids are based on the amount of formula needed to meet assessed calorie, protein, and fluid needs.

5. Serially monitor physiologic, energy, and nutritional parameters in the acute stage.

   a. Daily:
   Weights
   Fluid intake and output
   Tolerance to nutritional support regimen
   Strict calorie counts (when on oral diet)
   Electrolytes, glucose, BUN, creatinine, complete blood count with differential

   b. Weekly:
   Prealbumin (if receiving enteral nutrition)
   Liver function profile, prealbumin, triglycerides (if receiving TPN)

   c. Biweekly:
   Indirect calorimetry or metabolic cart studies (ideally when tube feeding or TPN and IV lipids are at goal rates)

6. Adjust calorie and nutrient delivery parameters on a regular basis.

   Adjustments in calorie delivery goals can be made according to indirect calorimetry measurements. Protein delivery should remain at approximately 2g protein/kg IBW during the acute stage; 1.2 to 1.5g protein/kg during the postacute stage. Tube feeding, TPN, and IV lipids can be tapered as oral diet intake improves (documented by calorie counts).

# CHAPTER 143

# Skin and Wound Care

**Ann M. Henwood, Sait Naderi,
and Edward C. Benzel**

A multidisciplinary approach to skin care can effectively minimize the unnecessary morbidity and mortality secondary to pressure ulcers (PUs). In addition to contributing to patient morbidity, PUs also result in considerable expense. It has been reported that 1.6 million PUs develop in U.S. hospitals every year. A total cost to treat PUs has been estimated to be between $2.2 billion to $3.6 billion annually. Approximately $125 to $200 is spent for each Stage I and Stage II PU that develops, and $14,000 to $23,000 is spent for each Stage III and Stage IV PU. Seventy-five percent of acute-care acquired ulcers occur in patients who have undergone a surgical procedure that lasted 3 hours or longer. This same group accounts for 30% to 40% of the total cost associated with PUs.[7]

It has been estimated that 25% of the medical costs associated with spinal cord injuries (SCIs) are incurred as a result of PUs. Overall, the average cost of treating a single PU can range from $5000 to $50,000[36,55]; 1 to 6 months of additional hospital stay is often required. Infectious complications of PUs, such as cellulitis, osteomyelitis, sepsis, and endocarditis, account for more than 60,000 deaths annually.[1,69,71]

Skin is the largest organ of the body and is composed of a sequence of layers (epidermis, dermis, and subcutaneous fat) that together provide its varied features. The outermost layers provide protection from the elements. These layers permit secretion, excretion, insulation, sensation, and thermoregulation.

A PU (also known as a pressure sore, decubitus ulcer, or bedsore) is an area of damaged skin and underlying soft tissues resulting from prolonged unrelieved pressure between a bony prominence and an external surface. In a patient, pressure ulcer injury occurs over the scapula, occiput, sacrum, and heels when placed in the supine position; the ear, shoulder, greater trochanter, medial knee, malleolus, and foot edge when laterally positioned; and the nose, forehead, chest iliac crests, foot edge, and toes when placed in the prone position.[46]

## Incidence and Prevalence

The incidence of PUs occurring in postoperative patients varies from 12% to 45%[62]; others report a 12% to 66% incidence.[32,58,62] In one study the prevalence of ulcer development within 4 days of surgery, by stage, ranged from 0.65% (unstageable) to 6.44% (Stage I). The total number of intraoperatively acquired PUs is 23% of the total number of ulcers developed in hospitals.[7]

PUs occur in 28% of SCI patients. According to the National Spinal Cord Injury Statistical Center, the incidence of PUs during the initial hospital stay is 32%.[38] Another study reported a PU rate of 30% to 85% during the first month after injury.[*] In a retrospective study of SCI the PU rate was found to be 60% and 50% in quadriplegic and paraplegic patients, respectively; also, multiple PUs developed in most quadriplegic cases.[17,37,56,64,70]

## Etiology

Although various factors are involved in the incidence of PUs, it is clear that the main cause of PUs is pressure over a bony prominence.

Historically, PUs have been blamed on poor nursing care and have been used as outcome indicators to quantify good versus poor nursing care.[22,58] In fact, PUs are acute injuries that develop rapidly when compression of tissues causes ischemia and necrosis during serious illness and trauma, including surgery.[6] The primary factor contributing to PU formation is constant pressure for extended periods. Pressure induces ischemia and causes reactive hyperemia. Because muscles and subcutaneous tissues are more susceptible than epidermis to pressure-induced injury, PUs are usually worse than they initially appear. The visible portion of a PU is not truly indicative of the extent of the problem.[57]

The mean skin capillary pressure in healthy persons is approximately 25mmHg.[34] External compression with a pressure of more than 30mmHg occludes the blood vessels, so that the surrounding tissue becomes anoxic and cell death occurs. Tissue pressure, however, depends on the patient's health. In addition, the amount of tissue damage is proportional to the magnitude and length of application of the pressure. Pressure ulcers can develop within 24 hours of the insult and take as long as 5 days to manifest themselves.[57] Kosiak[34] demonstrated that applying a constant pressure of 70mmHg to the skin caused irreversible changes in less than 2 hours. He also demonstrated an inverse relationship between time and pressure. Intense pressure for short periods was tolerated by patients as well as low pressure for long periods of time without sustaining tissue injury. Even a brief period of pressure relief can reduce the likelihood of PUs.

## Risk Factors and Their Assessments

Numerous factors that influence PU formation have been documented. The intrinsic and extrinsic factors that contribute to the risk of the development of a PU are discussed in the following paragraphs.

## Intrinsic Risk Factors

### Age

Several changes that occur in normal skin with aging may predispose older persons to PU development. These factors include decreased epidermal turnover, flattening of

---

[*]References 12,20,40,44,45,59,68.

1887

the dermoepidermal junction, and decreased number of dermal blood vessels. Bridel[15] reported gradual reduction in collagen formation between the ages of 20 and 60. A marked drop in collagen synthesis with concurrent loss of its protective mechanism occurs after the age of 60. In general the risk of PU development doubles after the age of 40 and triples after the age of 70.

### Pattern of Spinal Cord Injury

Each year 25% of SCI patients will develop a PU. Regardless of the type of treatment of these PUs, they will recur in 5% to 91% of SCI patients.[57] The pattern of SCI (completeness of neurologic deficit, level of injury [quadriplegia vs. paraplegia], and muscle tone [spastic vs. flaccid plegia]) can affect skin care and PU formation. Richardson and Meyer[59] examined variables related to PU formation in acutely injured SCI patients and found that quadriplegic patients with complete injuries were more likely to develop PUs than were those with lower level or incomplete injuries. However, Curry and Casady[20] reported that cervical injuries were not associated with an increased rate of PU formation. They reported PUs in 22.2% and 28.5% of patients with cervical and thoracolumbar injuries, respectively. Spasticity can contribute to PU development. Shearing forces in SCI are increased threefold, partly as a result of lower limb spasticity.

### Immobility

Immobility has been found to be the most significant risk factor for PU development.[11] Immobility may be caused by mental status changes, physical deficit, or neurologic deficit, or may occur during surgery.

### Malnutrition

Increased PU risk occurs in malnourished patients by the reduction of tissue tolerance.[13] Integrity of the skin and support structures is influenced by nutritional status. Low serum albumin levels have been shown to predict injury from pressure.[38] Collagen and elastin can diminish the ability of soft tissue to absorb pressure. Lack of vitamins and trace elements necessary for collagen formation and cell metabolism can predispose the patient to increased risk of pressure damage.[18]

Decreased fluid intake in the malnourished patient can lead to increased risk for dehydration. Dehydration can affect tissue perfusion, resulting in reduced pliability, and dry, flaky, or scaling skin associated with fissuring and cracking of the stratum corneum. This ultimately places the patient at an increased risk for PU formation.[57]

The patient's nutritional status has an important effect on the maintenance of tissue vitality. Wound healing can be affected by several variables, such as a negative nitrogen balance, anorexia, obesity, and repeated infections. Negative nitrogen balance and anorexia after SCI frequently contribute to weight loss and tissue wasting. Thus bony areas become more prominent, resulting in an increase in the applied force per unit area. Obesity can also contribute to the formation of PUs by decreasing mobility.

### Body Weight

The emaciated patient has little padding over bony prominences and is vulnerable to pressure injury. The obese patient may be malnourished with poor tissue perfusion, and may be difficult to move while avoiding shearing and frictional forces. Patients are at risk of pressure damage if they are less than 90%, or more than 120%, of their ideal body weight.[62]

### Cardiovascular Changes

Some cardiovascular changes secondary to SCI can diminish tolerance to pressure and pressure-induced ischemia. The loss of sympathetic innervation and unopposed parasympathetic activity contribute to vascular stasis and tissue hypoxia in SCI patients. The loss of vasomotor tone produces vasodilatation, bradycardia, and an increased cardiac index. This results in an increased stroke volume and a decreased venous return. The reduction in venous return is further accentuated by decreased muscle tone and the absence of the muscle pump. Gravity, acting mainly when the patient is in the sitting position, and a decreased negative inspiratory force, resulting from pulmonary insufficiency, may also diminish venous return. In SCI patient, soft-tissue blood flow below the level of injury is reduced to 33% of its normal value. A decrease in transcutaneous oxygen tension is observed in the SCI patient, even in the absence of pressure.[45] All of these factors contribute to the formation of PUs. In summary, poor tissue oxygenation, poor cell nutrition, and a decrease in venous return may accentuate the process of PU formation.

## Extrinsic Risk Factors

Extrinsic risk factors are those elements that may be manipulated through interventions and help to prevent pressure ulcers.

### Shearing

Shearing forces are the second key factor in the development of PUs. Shear forces are defined here as forces created by sliding adjacent structures, which cause a relative displacement of tissue and, in turn, occlusion of capillaries. Shear forces can be more significant than pressure itself in the dermis (where capillaries run perpendicular to the skin) and near the bone (where nutrient vessels pierce the fascia, also in a perpendicular manner) (Figure 143.1). Shear forces, alone or in combination with pressure, significantly compromise circulation in tissues, whereas the skin may remain stationary. The elevation of the head of the bed by more than 30 degrees may increase shearing forces.

### Friction

Another important external force that acts directly on the epidermis is friction. Friction between skin and stationary surfaces, such as bed clothes, results in the loss of stratum corneum and, in turn, causes intraepidermal blisters and superficial erosions. Lack of this protective layer leads to further breakdown.

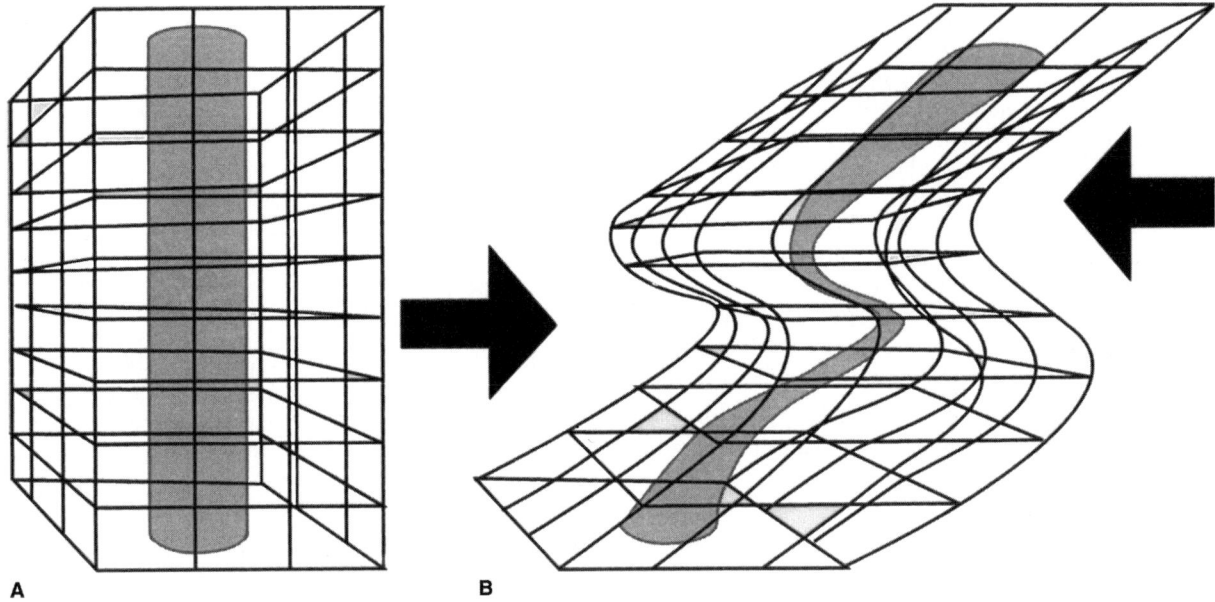

**Figure 143.1** (**A**) Appearance of the skin and relationship between a perpendicular capillary and skin. (**B**) Application of a shear force can lead to obstruction of the capillary and results in PU formation.

Frictional forces indirectly underlie shearing, and like shear forces, friction alters the critical pressure-time relationship affecting skin ischemia. Because friction contributes to PU formation, SCI patients should not be dragged across the bed; rather they should be lifted and moved, with a bed sheet used as a *drag sheet*.

### Moisture

Contact of skin with moisture, resulting from urine and stool incontinence, leads to skin maceration and edema. This makes the epidermis more susceptible to abrasion. The likelihood of further tissue breakdown thus increases. The effect of moisture on PU formation is well known. One study demonstrated that incontinence caused a 5.5-fold increase in the incidence of PUs.[41] Fecal incontinence is a greater risk factor for PU development than urinary incontinence, because stool contains bacteria and enzymes that are caustic to the skin.[57,58]

### Surgery

Preoperative factors that place patients at risk for PUs include the following comorbidities: diabetes, underlying respiratory disease, hypertension, and vascular disease. Low preoperative hemoglobin and hematocrit, as well as a preoperative serum albumin level lower than 3g/dL, also have been shown to place patients at greater risk for PU.[4,38,53]

Patients are at an increased risk because of forced immobility during surgery.[58] The amount of time on the operating room (OR) table is the most statistically significant risk factor associated with PU injury in perisurgical patients.[62] Studies have shown variable amounts of time before pressure ulcer injury occurs. Hoshowsky and Schramm[31] found that PU injury can occur in as little as

2.5 hours on the OR table. Surgery lasting more than 4 hours can triple the risk of skin changes and quadruple the risk of PU formation. Hicks[29] found that PU injury was twice as likely to occur if time on the OR table was more than 4 hours.

Not only does the amount of time on the OR table contribute to PU formation, but anesthetic agents lower blood pressure and alter tissue perfusion, which also contributes to tissue damage.[5] Surgical patients' skin may be made more susceptible to PUs because of pooled prep solution, causing skin maceration, change in skin pH, and the removal of protective oils.[58,62] In addition, one study had shown that 75% of patients placed on a hyperthermia blanket during surgery went on to develop PUs.[28,32,62]

Firm positioning devices in the OR are used to hold patients in place by exerting pressure on bony prominences, and retractors increase pressure on internal tissues while OR personnel increase pressure on external tissues by leaning on the patient.[58] All of these events can cause pressure over bony prominences, eventually leading to PU injury.

## Assessment and Staging of Pressure Sores

Routine skin inspection is customarily included in any skin care program because it provides important information regarding the formulation and evaluation of skin care plans. At least once daily the skin should be examined from head to toe, and high-risk areas should be assessed more frequently with special attention paid to bony prominences. Assessment involves the entire integument, not just the ulcer, and is the basis for a treatment plan and its evaluation. PU assessment should include location, size (length, width, and depth), the extent of sinus tract undermining or tunneling, exudate, color of wound bed, epithelialization, and staging.[58] Photographs can document PU status better than hand-drawn diagrams.

Although several different staging and classification systems have been developed for PU classification, the Agency for Healthcare Research and Quality (AHRQ) (formerly the Agency for Healthcare Policy and Research) has adopted the National Pressure Ulcer Advisory Panel's (NPUAP) pressure ulcer classification system as part of the pressure ulcer clinical practice guidelines. PUs are staged to classify the degree of observed tissue damage. The use of this classification tool permits universal assessment and consistent communication of the severity of tissue damage among health care personnel.[4]

"Stage I: An observable pressure-related alteration of intact skin when compared with adjacent skin.

Observable changes may include skin temperature (e.g., warmth, coolness), tissue consistency (e.g., firm, boggy), and skin sensation (e.g., pain, itching).
Stage II: Superficial with partial thickness skin loss that presents clinically as a blister or abrasion.
Stage III: Full thickness skin loss extending down to the fascia that presents as a deep crater.
Stage IV: Full thickness skin loss with extensive destruction or damage to muscle, bone or supporting structures." (Figure 143.2)[68]

Skin inspection should be followed by laboratory investigations, such as culture and assessment for infection markers. In the case of a chronic nonhealing PU and underlying osteomyelitis, a triad of a white blood cell count higher than 15,000, plain radiographic signs, and a

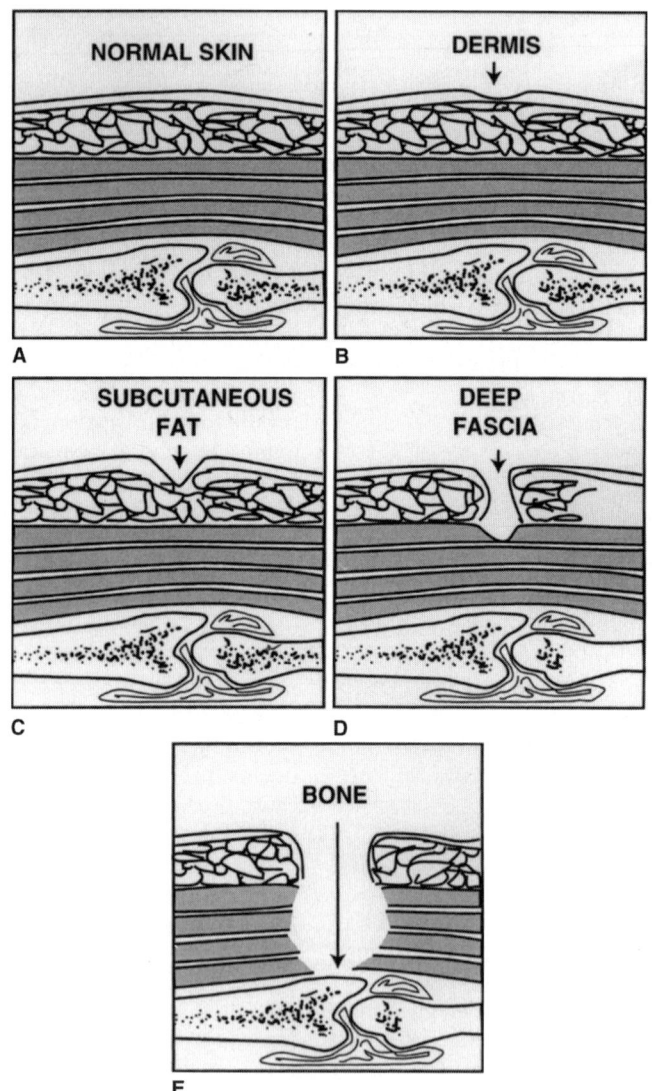

**Figure 143.2** Normal gross anatomy of the skin and its changes in the different stages of the PU. **(A)** Normal anatomy. **(B)** Stage I: An observable pressure-related alteration of intact skin when compared with adjacent skin. Observable changes may include skin temperature, tissue consistency, and skin sensation. **(C)** Stage II: Superficial with partial thickness skin loss that presents clinically as a blister or abrasion. **(D)** Stage III: Full thickness skin loss extending down to the fascia that presents as a deep crater. **(E)** Stage IV: Full thickness skin loss with extensive destruction or damage to muscle, bone or supporting structures.

high sedimentation rate (greater than 100mm/hr) provides a sensitivity and specificity of 90% for diagnostic screening of this complication.[55]

## Prevention

The foundation for the prevention of pressure ulcers is based on the elimination of risk factors. The first step in the prevention of PUs is to be knowledgeable of risk factors, specifically which ones make the patient a high risk for PU development. The second step in prevention is to be aware of the interventions that reduce the risk of pressure injury. The third step is to evaluate the effectiveness of the intervention.[57] Proper measures can minimize the PU rate by as much as 59%.[10,23,50,55,64] Prevention is a 24-hour, ongoing process. Management of PU risk includes an understanding of body positioning, turning, and mobilization of the patient in the bed and wheelchair. It also includes paying attention to hygiene, and the use of pressure reduction devices and strategies, as well as the appropriate monitoring of nutritional and hydration status.

### Mobilization and Turning Program

The primary goal of this program is to relieve pressure, which is achieved by regular turning. The patient should be placed in the full lateral decubitus position when it is safe. A patient with a very unstable spine perhaps should not be aggressively turned until the spine is surgically fixated. This restriction is uncommon.

At-risk patients should be turned every 2 hours to minimize pressure on bony prominences.[3,33,40] A written schedule for systematically turning and repositioning the

patient should be used. Norton *et al.* reported a lower incidence of PUs in at-risk patients who were turned every 2 to 3 hours.[51]

The goal of repositioning is to facilitate tissue reperfusion before the tissue becomes ischemic. Repositioning should involve a sustained relief of pressure. As skin tolerance improves the amount of time spent in one position may be increased gradually.

After the acute phase of care, when the SCI patient is able to tolerate wheelchair activities, continuation of pressure relief techniques in the wheelchair is equally important. These activities serve to relieve pressure and maintain (and increase) the strength in the upper extremities. Wheelchair push ups, lateral weight shifts to each side, and forward over-the-knees positioning are some of the effective pressure relief techniques used.[47]

Improper transport of the patient increases the incidence of PUs. When transferring patients, care should be taken to not slide or drag the skin across the bed surface.[43] The patient may also help prevent friction injuries by taking an active role and using the trapeze during turning and repositioning (if the spine is stable).

Ischial PUs are a manifestation of prolonged sitting, without focal pressure reduction. Appropriate care, patient education, and patient diligence should minimize incidence of this complication (Figure 143.3). Sacral PUs also may be caused by sitting, particularly if an inappropriate or worn-out chair is used or if the patient sits with the pelvis excessively flexed.

Uninterrupted sitting in a chair or wheelchair is a common cause of PU. When in a wheelchair, SCI patients should reposition themselves at least once every hour and shift their weight every 15 minutes. If the patient needs assistance, simply standing the patient and reseating in the chair may minimize the risk of tissue injury. Small shifts in

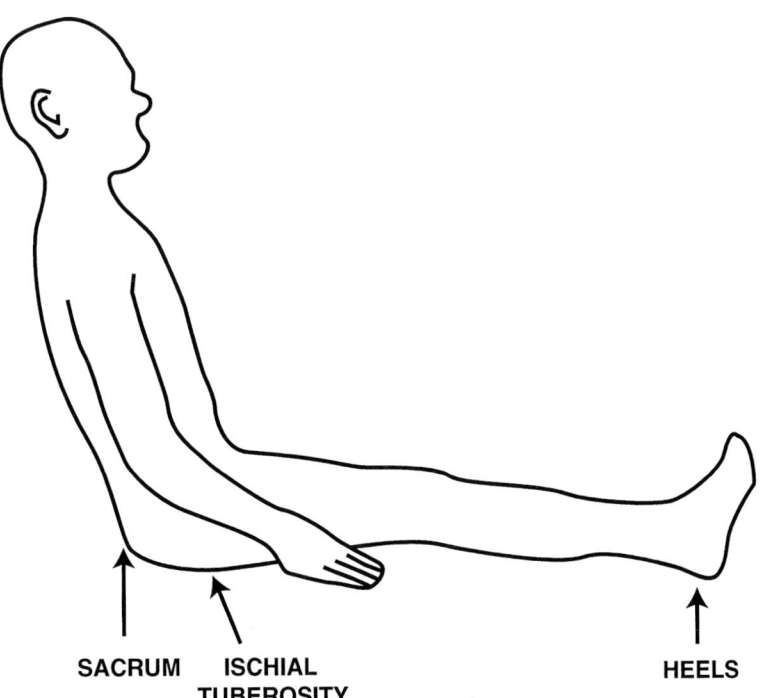

**SACRUM   ISCHIAL                                    HEELS**
**TUBEROSITY**

**Figure 143.3** Potential sites for pressure in the sitting position.

weight such as elevating the legs can help to reduce the risk of tissue injury.[57]

## General Hygiene

Proper patient hygiene can help to prevent or at least minimize the likelihood of PUs. Bathing programs should include washing with mild soap and water to avoid excessive skin drying and cracking. The skin should be kept clean and free of moisture from urinary and fecal incontinence, perspiration, and wound drainage. However, it is important to keep the skin well lubricated with a simple standard hospital skin moisturizer. Studies have shown that petrolatum is more effective than lanolin on dry skin.[25]

The type of material next to the skin may either diminish or increase moisture retention. Cotton disperses moisture, whereas nylon and plastic materials cause moisture to be retained. Clothes should fit properly without causing excessive focal pressure or friction. Tight clothes make dressing difficult and may also cause localized pressure and vasomotor changes. Similarly, the patient's shoes should be one half or one full size larger than normal.

## Nutrition

Proper nutrition is an important factor in maintaining the vitality of intact tissues. A high-protein diet, with an increased caloric intake, is initially needed to replace weight loss and to prevent protein deficiency and anemia.

Adequate fluid intake is 30 to 35ml/kg of body weight. Patients on air-fluidized beds for the prevention of PUs must have their fluid intake increased an additional 10 to 15m/kg of body weight to prevent dehydration.[14]

The nutritional state of the patient is also affected by drugs, alcohol, nicotine, and caffeine. Nicotine and caffeine are vasoconstrictive, leading to a decrease in tissue oxygenation and, in turn, affecting tissue healing. Smokers have a higher rate of extensive PUs than do nonsmokers.[9,24,35,50]

## Patient Support Surfaces

Patients with an unstable spine, who cannot tolerate frequent turning, may require a pressure support surface that can lower the surface pressure below capillary filling pressure (32mmHg). Thick foam mattresses, water mattresses, alternating-pressure air mattresses, and static multilayered air mattresses have been found useful in preventing PUs. Air-fluidized beds and low air–loss beds, which have elaborate support surfaces, probably provide the most effective surface for functionally dependent patients with large, deep, or multiple PUs.

## Beds

A variety of beds can be used to prevent PUs, with some being appropriate for patients with unstable spines. For patients with a stable spine, low-air–loss beds, oscillating low-air–loss beds, or air-fluidized beds can be used alternatively. The patient, the caregiver, and the family may develop a false sense of security with use of these beds.

Specialized beds do not prevent PUs but can minimize the likelihood of PUs. However, skin care may be difficult when using these beds.

In general, studies comparing several specialized beds show no statistical significance in the prevention or healing of PUs from one bed to another. However, studies do show that PUs heal more quickly on specialized beds when compared to foam overlays or standard hospital mattresses.[42]

## Rotating Beds

A patient with an unstable spine can be placed on a rotating bed that rocks side to side in a continuous motion, or on an oscillating support surface or kinetic treatment table to prevent PUs. These beds are often used in trauma or intensive care units but are usually not practical for rehabilitation units. A rotating bed must be adjusted properly; otherwise it slides the patient back and forth as it rocks. This sliding, in turn, subjects the skin to shear forces, causing, rather than preventing, skin breakdown.

## Air-Fluidized Beds

An air-fluidized bed is an oval space with up to 2000lb of glass beads covered by a polyester sheet. The beads are fluidized by a flow of warm, pressurized air that floats the polyester cover on which the patient is placed. Feces and body fluids are able to flow through the polyester sheet; thus the skin is kept dry. Most studies have demonstrated a rapid rate of wound healing using these beds, compared with conventional treatment.[1,2,8,23] These beds have a bactericidal effect because of sequestration and desiccation of microorganisms by the ceramic beads. Adverse effects include fluid loss, dehydration, dry skin, scaly skin, and epistaxis from the flow of the dry air. Turning and repositioning may be difficult.

## Beds

Low-air-loss beds consist of multiple inflatable fabric pillows that are attached to a modified hospital bed frame. An electric fan maintains the buoyancy of the pillows. The head and foot of the bed can be elevated. They are cooler and more portable than air-fluidized beds. However, urine and feces cannot pass through the fabric. Their use was found to be associated with a threefold increase in tissue healing.[23]

## Cushions

There are several different forms of gel- or water-filled mattresses and cushions for use with beds or wheelchairs. These mattresses and cushions may aid or inhibit patient mobility, particularly during transfer. Smooth surface cushions provide less resistance to sliding and aid in board placement during transfer. However, they do not optimally eliminate pressure. Furthermore, the patient cannot perform meticulous skin care and inspection. Cushions and mattresses may increase local tissue temperature, which, in turn, causes an additional rise in tissue metabolism and greater oxygen demand.

## Patient Positioning

Perhaps the most important anatomic and soft-tissue bony prominences in the bedridden patient are the sacrum and the heels.[26] The importance of these pressure points is diminished when the patient assumes other positions.

The sacrum is located superficially at its dorsal aspect, with very little soft tissue separating the bone from the integument. When the supine position is assumed, significant pressure is applied to this point. Although the sacrum is a common site for PU formation related to supine positioning, the scapula and occiput are also potential points of pressure (Figure 143.4). Both regions have bony prominences with minimal overlying soft tissue. The prevention of sacral, scapular, and occipital PUs is predicated on limiting the time spent in the supine position.

Evidence suggests that when the side-lying position is used, pressure on the greater trochanter should be minimized and the patient should be placed at a 30-degree laterally inclined angle rather than a 90-degree angle to avoid direct pressure on the greater trochanter.[58] Placing a patient in a position that is intermediate between the full lateral decubitus and the supine position perhaps applies significant pressure to the downside scapula, while lessening pressure on the sacrum. Dorsolateral buttock pressure is also increased. This, however, is usually tolerated well because of the significant soft tissue mass overlying this region. This position, for the reasons listed, is a reasonable alternative intermittent position. No single position should be maintained for any significant length of time. The full lateral decubitus position exposes the downside greater trochanteric region to significant focal pressure, if proper technique is not used. The anatomic arrangement of the greater trochanter and surrounding soft tissues is of great importance in this regard. One must keep in mind the dynamic relationship between the overlying soft tissues and the bony prominence (greater trochanter).[58]

In the hip flexed position the greater trochanter is more superficial (exposed) relative to both the immediately overlying soft tissue surrounding the trochanter itself. The latter is composed of the gluteus maximus and the lateral thigh muscles. When the hip is extended (leg straightened), the greater trochanter retracts relative to the surrounding soft tissue. This extended position results in a distribution of pressure over a significantly wider surface area, thereby minimizing focal trochanteric pressure (Figure 143.5). It would therefore seem prudent to straighten the downside leg in the full lateral decubitus position. This essentially eliminates the negative effects of the lateral decubitus position previously reported (Figure 143.6).[58]

Heels are at an increased risk of PU development because they have higher tissue interface pressures than other tissues covering bony prominences. Heels must be elevated off the bed surface by some protective mechanism. A common practice is to use pillows under the calves to prevent heels from bearing pressure loads, which prevents them from resting on the surface of the bed.[57]

## Treatment of Pressure Sores

When a PU occurs it can be treated either medically or surgically, depending on the chronicity, position, and size. Many of the components used in prevention of PUs are also used in the treatment, but at a more intense level of management. The extrinsic and intrinsic contributing factors of the PU formation must be identified. Eliminating the cause of pressure should improve the course of the treatment.

The stage of a PU determines its treatment. A stage I PU most often heals spontaneously, simply following relief of pressure. Depending on the source of the trauma to the skin pressure relief may be easily attained by adjusting an orthosis or, with multiple PUs, by avoiding a certain posture. A special bed may be occasionally necessary to reduce the pressure.

The treatment of an open wound (stages II, III, and IV), however, is more complex. Prevention or elimination of infection facilitates healing. Local treatment combined with systemic antibiotic and supportive therapy often heals a PU. Chronic PUs, however, are more resistant to therapy.

With respect to wound care the goal is to achieve a clean wound with a low level of bacteria that is kept moist with a nonadherent dressing until complete wound healing has occurred.[58]

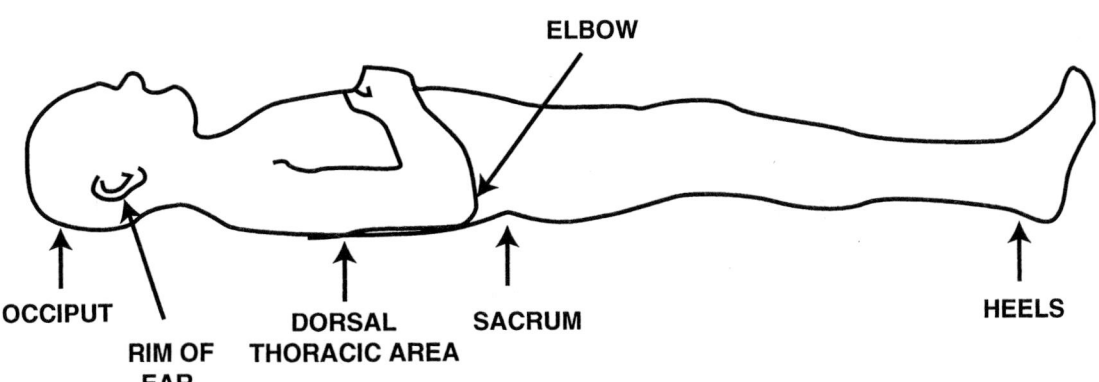

**Figure 143.4** The supine position can lead to pressure application predominantly on the sacrum, the scapula, heels, and the occiput.

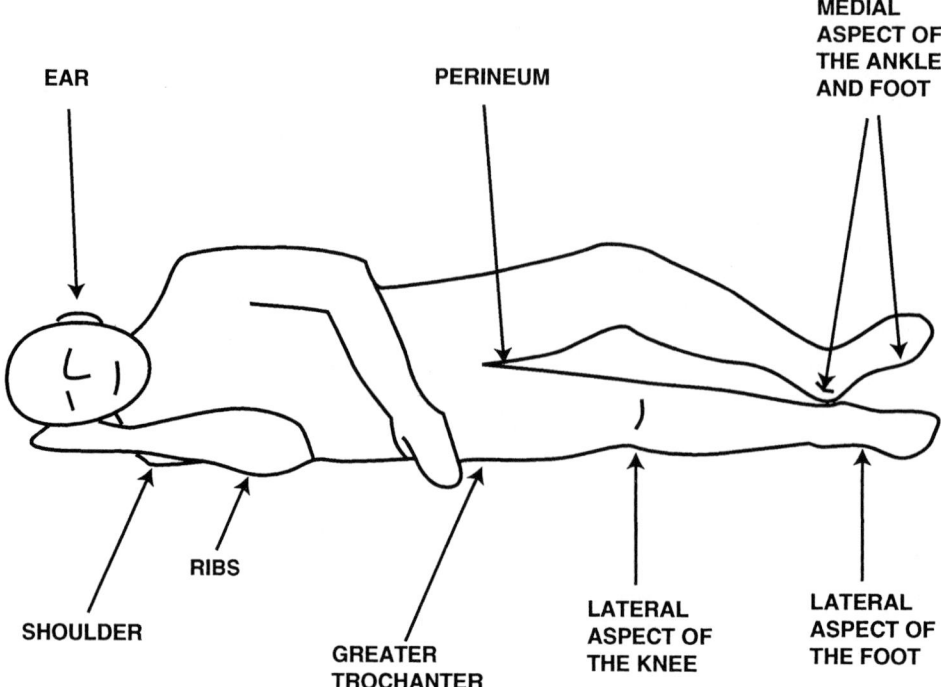

EAR    PERINEUM    MEDIAL ASPECT OF THE ANKLE AND FOOT

SHOULDER    RIBS    GREATER TROCHANTER    LATERAL ASPECT OF THE KNEE    LATERAL ASPECT OF THE FOOT

**Figure 143.5** The lateral position can lead to pressure application on the greater trochanter, ribs, shoulder, and lateral aspect of the knee and feet. Note that the perineum and lateral aspect of the foot and ankle may also be exposed to increased focal pressure.

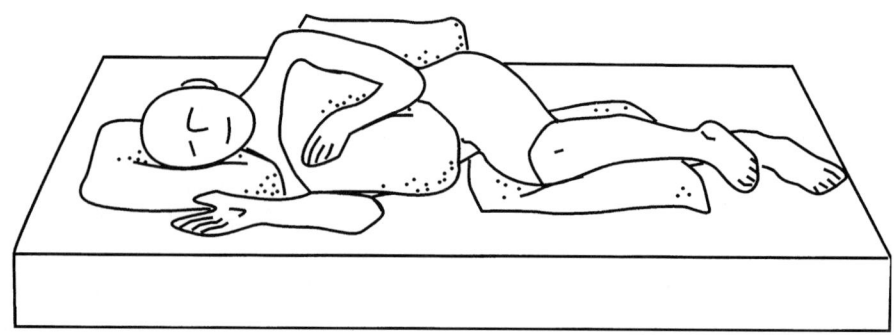

**Figure 143.6** The lateral decubitus position, using pillows, may reduce the pressure applied to the body surface, particularly the greater trochanter.

## Systemic Therapy

In some circumstances oral antibiotics and vitamin C may be indicated. Vitamin C has been found to help in chronic nonhealing PUs.[66]

With osteomyelitis, cellulitis, and sepsis, and also as prophylaxis for endocarditis, systemic antibiotic therapy may be indicated.[39] Sepsis secondary to PU infections is associated with a 50% mortality in the hospital setting (Figure 143.7). Gentamicin and clindamycin are antibiotics of choice in patients with good renal function. In older patients cefotetan disodium (Cefotan) or ticarcillin-clavulanic acid (Timentin) and fleroxacin are reasonable alternatives.[21,55] First-generation cephalosporins do not penetrate PU wounds well and should not be used.

## Topical Therapies

Topical therapies for PUs include a variety of cleaning and open-air wound care regimens, antibiotics, topical surface materials, biologic, mechanical, and chemical débridement, electrical stimulation, laser therapy, whirlpools, and hyperbaric oxygen strategies.

### Wound Dressings

Traditional wound dressings are considered to be passive products because they protect the wound from further injury while healing occurs. However, there are many new wound dressings that are interactive in that they act to alter the local wound environment. Regardless of the type of dressing selected, the main purpose is to absorb

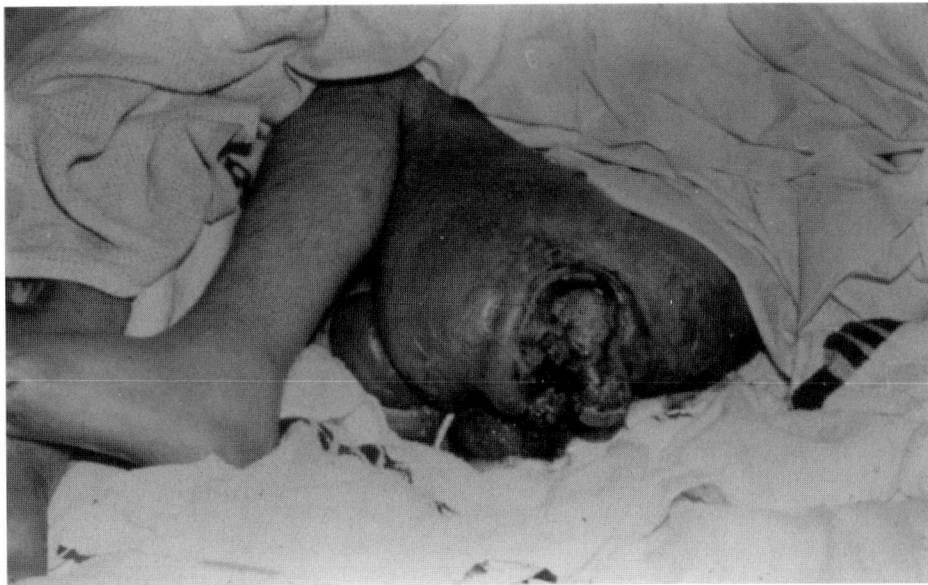

**Figure 143.7** Macroscopic appearance of a stage IV PU in a patient who developed osteomyelitis and deep soft-tissue infection. He ultimately died of these complications.

exudates, provide thermal insulation, allow gaseous exchange, protect the wound from infection, maintain a moist wound environment, and relieve pain. Interactive dressings have a varying number of properties and are currently undergoing research.[19,57]

**Gauze.** Currently most gauze dressings are inexpensive. They must be changed two or three times daily. Maintaining moistness may be difficult with gauze dressings, and if they become dry, they may adhere to the wound. Their removal may then be painful and the risk of removing healthy granulation tissue is increased. Gauze dressings must be fixed with a cover dressing or wrap.

**Films.** Semipermeable polyurethane films allow gases to pass through, but are impermeable to water. They are believed to mimic the function of the skin and may enhance healing by sequestering wound fluids. Because the films are transparent, the wound can be directly visualized with the dressing in place. Such a dressing can remain in place as long as 7 days. This type of dressing, if used, is appropriate for Stage I PUs.

**Foams.** Semipermeable polyurethane foams are transparent and waterproof. They absorb excessive wound exudate. At the same time a moist environment is maintained, and excessive autolysis or maceration is avoided. Because these foams do not adhere to the wound, they must be fixed with a cover dressing or tape, hence the direct visualization of the wound is obscured. Foams can be used for Stage I and Stage II PUs. They should not be used for deep PUs extending into the underlying muscle, sores covered by eschar, infected sores, or heavily exuding PUs.

**Hydrocolloid.** Hydrocolloids contain an adhesive material that physically interacts with wound fluid. These occlusive or semiocclusive dressings encourage wound cleansing and débridement through the process of autolysis. They promote the development of granulation tissue by stimulating angiogenesis. They may not adhere to highly exudative wounds. They can be used for Stage II and Stage III PUs.[23,72] Currently hydrocolloids are cost effective and require changing every 3 to 7 days.

**Hydrogel.** Hydrogels are three-dimensional hydrophilic polymers that interact with aqueous solutions by swelling and maintaining water in their structure. They are nonadhesive and conform to the wound surface. Hydrogels are very absorbent and dehydrate easily. They can be used in Stage IV PUs.

**Alginate Dressings.** Alginate dressings, derived from seaweed, are highly absorbent. They have been used for PUs with copious drainage. They should not be used for dry wounds and must be fixated with a cover dressing or tape.

**Amino Acid Copolymer Membrane.** Amino acid copolymer membranes are moderately permeable to water vapor and impermeable to bacteria. Early results have shown that they are helpful for tissue healing.[30]

### Cleansing Agents

AHRQ guidelines recommend cleansing PUs at each dressing change. Techniques should be chosen that use the least amount of chemical and mechanical trauma necessary to cleanse the wound adequately. For some wounds isotonic saline irrigation is a sufficient cleanser. Extremely dirty wounds may need a stronger cleanser and more mechanical force. As the wound heals and becomes cleaner less mechanical force and a gentler cleanser should be used.[52,58]

It has been shown that whirlpool therapy resulted in faster wound healing than standard treatment. Pulsatile irrigation and lavage of PUs has been shown to be more effective than whirlpool therapy.[58]

Although irrigation with saline can retard bacterial growth in open PUs, povidone-iodine, acetic acid, hydrogen peroxide, and sodium hypochlorite are cytotoxic and may impair wound healing. Some antimicrobial agents such as mupirocin ointment and silver sulfadiazine may decrease the bacterial count. In general, topically applied antibiotics do not penetrate deeply into the ulcer, and their use is not recommended. They can lead to a resistance to antibiotics, as well as cause hypersensitivity reactions, contact dermatitis, and drug toxicity from drug absorption.[60]

## Adjunctive Therapies

The role of several adjunctive therapies in PUs has been investigated. These therapies include electrotherapy, infrared therapy, ultraviolet therapy, low-energy laser irradiation therapy, ultrasound therapy, hyperbaric oxygen therapy, vacuum assisted closure, constant tension approximation, normothermia, use of miscellaneous topical agents (e.g., sugar, vitamins, elements, hormones, cytokine growth factors, skin equivalents), and systemic drugs other than antibiotics, such as vasodilators, hemorheologics, serotonin inhibitors, and fibrinolytic agents.*

### Electrical Stimulation

Low-voltage direct current and high-voltage pulsed galvanic stimulation has been used successfully in treating PUs. During treatment the negative electrode is placed directly on the wound, and the positive electrode is placed at some point distally. In a randomized, double-blind, multicenter study, electric stimulation has been shown to increase the rate of healing of PUs. The Pressure Ulcer Guideline Panel recommended the use of electrotherapy in Stage III and Stage IV PUs that have proven to be unresponsive to conventional therapy. Electrical stimulation may also be useful for recalcitrant Stage II PUs.[23,49,52]

### Hyperbaric Oxygen Therapy

Hyperbaric oxygen therapy is defined here as the use of high-pressure, pure, humidified oxygen that is applied by a portable chamber to either the entire body or to an extremity. The chamber forces 100% oxygen into superficial tissue and assists with wound healing. This modality has been found helpful in SCI patients, because they have an underlying intact arterial supply.[27,50] However, the AHRQ does not recommend this therapy, because its effectiveness has not been established.[52]

### Ultrasound

The use of ultrasound for healing of PUs has produced equivocal results, with some studies demonstrating efficacy, but more series finding it ineffective.[57,67]

### Laser

Laser therapy has been used effectively in animal models for the treatment of PUs. Studies have demonstrated healing of PUs using the helium-neon laser in one third of the cases, compared with nonlaser-treated wounds.[50] Research on the use of lasers for human PUs is still in the early stages.

### Growth Factors

Growth factors are naturally occurring proteins secreted from platelets and macrophages that direct the migration of cells into wounds and lead to the process of repair. In current experimental studies topically applied, platelet-derived growth factors and fibroblast growth factors have been used to promote healing of chronic PUs. Preliminary data suggest improved wound healing.[16,70] Other growth factors, such as TGF-beta and epidermal growth factor, have been identified as potential therapies.[54] Although these modalities hold promise, they are still investigational, and consequently, not yet recommended for routine use.

### Vacuum-Assisted Closure and Constant Tension Approximation

Both of these therapies use tension to cause cellular stretching. Because of the constant controlled forces of stretching, a mitotic response is stimulated and wound healing is assisted. Vacuum assisted closure uses an open-celled foam that can be cut to the size of the PU and placed on top of or inside of the PU. It is then secured with a transparent film. Negative pressure is applied to the wound by means of flexible tubing that is embedded in the foam and attached to a vacuum pump. Although this is a new adjunctive therapy, studies have shown this method of treatment to be quite effective. Constant tension approximation uses a device to place tension traction on the wound margins.[52]

### Normothermia

Normothermia therapy is used to encourage local blood flow and oxygen to the wound. A foam collar is placed around the wound, and a transparent film is attached to the collar and placed over the wound. A warming device controlled by a temperature control unit is placed into a pocket on the transparent film, and the environment underneath the film cover is kept at 38°C. Initial studies are showing positive results.[52]

### Débridement

Débridement, the removal of necrotic tissue, is fundamental to the healing of a PU. Wounds must be clean for healing to take place. The removal of inflammatory stimuli such as devitalized tissue, reactive chemicals, and bacteria requires débridement and cleansing.[58] Large numbers of bacteria normally reside in necrotic tissue. The presence of necrotic material dictates local débridement to decrease the bacterial cell count to 100,000 per gram of tissue. There are different methods of débridement, which on occasion may be combined to achieve the best result.

---

*References 23,45,56,64,65,67.

## Mechanical Débridement

Mechanical débridement is accomplished by local cleansing and dressing techniques. Soap and water or hydrogen peroxide and saline, used in a ratio of 1:3 or 1:2, are some of the more common agents used in cleansing the wound.

The most commonly used method of mechanical débridement is the wet-to-dry dressing technique. It has been shown that woven gauze with larger pores and coarser weave, compared to nonwoven cotton sponges, is more effective for débridement.[48] This is most effective when used on PUs with necrotic tissue in stages II, III, and IV. The wet-to-dry technique is painful and should be discontinued when the wound bed looks pink.[57]

## Sharp Débridement

Sharp débridement is performed by scissors, forceps, and/or scalpel. This is indicated in Stage II, Stage III, and Stage IV PUs. Eschars underlying necrotic tissue are best removed by sharp débridement. The sharp débridement can be facilitated by chemical débridement.

## Chemical Débridement

Autolytic débridement is less painful. When the wound is kept moist with an occlusive dressing, the wound uses its own enzymes to digest the nonviable tissue and viscous exudates.[57] To enhance autolysis, exogenous enzymes may be applied to the wound. Enzymatic preparations may be fibrinolytic or collagenolytic and cause the liquefaction of necrotic tissue and facilitate its removal by sharp or mechanical débridement. As far as possible, eschars should be removed from the wound; the remaining devitalized tissue should be scored with a scalpel before enzymatic débridement.[58] Enzymatic preparations are used in the treatment of stages II, III, and IV PUs. Although they are not able to débride hard eschars, these preparations can loosen them.

## Biologic Débridement

Biologic débridement using maggots has been recognized for centuries as an aid to wound healing. Maggots liquefy necrotic tissue but not healthy tissue. They disinfect the wound and stimulate tissue growth. Sherman et al.[63] reported that maggot therapy débrided most of the necrotic wounds within 1 week, which was more rapid than all other nonsurgical methods. They found maggot therapy to be beneficial, safe, and inexpensive.

## Surgery

Unfortunately, not all PUs respond to conservative measures. Surgical intervention, which may allow the patient to mobilize more rapidly, is required when a deep PU fails to heal. Surgical intervention may be considered in every PU larger than 10cm. Currently flap grafts and myocutaneous flaps provide useful reconstructive techniques. However, recurrence is a concern, and patients should remain vigilant about pressure-relieving measures.

## Complications

All stage I PUs should heal rapidly. If a PU does not heal or respond to appropriate therapy, the possibility of infection should be considered. Associated infectious processes include chronic local infection, cellulitis, osteomyelitis, sepsis, and death. The chronic and nonhealing PUs occasionally show neoplastic changes.[62]

One of the causes of the fever in SCI patients is localized soft-tissue infection. The infected sore can progress and lead to osteomyelitis or sepsis. Beneath the infection site one may occasionally observe an abscess. Figure 143.7 depicts an unhealed and infected PU.

In the case of persistent and recurrent drainage from a wound, osteomyelitis must be considered. Unexpected fever, unhealed PU, leucocytosis, and radiographic appearance point to this diagnosis. Wound culture, the use of systemic antibiotics, and if necessary, surgical débridement, are the treatments of choice.

## Summary

The management of PUs is complex and should be targeted towards prevention. The best, most cost-effective, and easiest treatment is prevention. Prevention necessitates education of both the patient and the treating team. Treatment of sores of the integument, "the largest organ of the body," is aided by a team approach.

## REFERENCES

1. Allmann RM, Laprade CA, Noel LB, *et al*: Pressure sores among hospitalized patients. *Ann Intern Med* 105:337-342, 1986.
2. Allmann RM: Pressure ulcers among the elderly. *N Engl J Med* 320:850-853, 1989.
3. Alterescu V, Alterescu KB: Pressure ulcers: assessment and treatment. *Orthop Nursing* 11: 37-49, 1992.
4. Armstrong D, Bortz P: An integrative review of pressure relief in surgical patients. *AORN J* 73:645,647-648, 2001.
5. Aronovitch SA: Intraoperatively acquired pressure ulcer prevalence: A national study. *J Wound Ostomy and Cont Nurs* 26:130-136, 1999.
6. Bader DL (ed): *Pressure Sores: Clinical Practice and Scientific Approach.* Basingstoke, United Kingdom Macmillan, 1990.
7. Beckrich K, Aronovich SA: Hospital acquired pressure ulcers: a comparison of costs in medical vs. surgical patients. *Nurs Econ* 17:263-271, 1999.
8. Bennett RG, Bellantoni MF, Ouslander JG: Air-fluidized-bed treatment of nursing home patients with pressure sores. *J Am Geriatr Soc* 37:235-242, 1989.
9. Bergstrom N, Braden B: A prospective study of pressure sore risk among institutionalized elderly. *J Am Geriatr Soc* 40:747-758, 1992.
10. Bergstom N: Pressure ulcer treatment. *Am Fam Physician* 51:1207-1222, 1995.
11. Berlowitz D, Wilking S: Risk factors for pressure sores: A comparison of cross-sectional and cohort-derived data. *J Am Geriatr Soc* 37:1043-1050, 1989.

12. Bliss MR: Acute pressure area care. *Lancet* 339:221-223, 1992.

13. Braden B, Bergstrom N: A conceptual scheme for the study of the aetiology of pressure sores. *Rehabil Nurs* 12:12-16, 1987.

14. Breslow RA: Nutrition and air-fluidized beds: A literature review. *Adv Wound Care* 7:57-62, 1994.

15. Bridel J: The aetiology of pressure sores. *J Wound Care* 2:230-238, 1993.

16. Brown GI, Nanney ZB, Griffey J, *et al*: Enhancement of wound healing by topical treatment with epidural growth factor. *N Engl J Med* 321:76-79, 1989.

17. Colen SR: Pressure sores. In McCarthy JG, May JW, Littler JW (eds): *Plastic Surgery*. Philadelphia, WB Saunders, 1990, pp 3797-3838.

18. Cullum N, Clark M: Intrinsic factors associated with pressure sores in elderly people. *J Adv Nurs* 17:427-431, 1992.

19. Cullum N, Nelson EA, Flemming K, Sheldon T: Systematic reviews of wound care management: (5) beds; (6) compression; (7) laser therapy, therapeutic ultrasound, electrotherapy and electromagnetic therapy. *Health Technol Assess* 5:1-221, 2001.

20. Curry K, Casady L: The relationship between extended periods of immobility and decubitus ulcer formation in the acutely spinal cord-injured individuals. *J Neurosci Nurs* 24:185-189, 1992.

21. Cutler NR, Seifert RD, Sramek JJ: Fleroxacin treatment of stage IV pressure ulcers with associated osteomyelitis. *Ann Pharmacother* 28:117, 1994.

22. Dealy C: Pressure sores: the result of bad nursing? *Br J Nursing* 1:748, 1992.

23. Evans JM, Andrews KL, Chutka DS, *et al*: Pressure ulcers: prevention and management. *Mayo Clin Proc* 70:789-799, 1995.

24. Finucane TE: Malnutrition, tube feeding and pressure sores: data are incomplete. *J Am Geriatr Soc* 43:447-451, 1995.

25. Frantz R, Gardner S: Clinical concerns: Management of dry skin. *J Geront Nurs* 20:15-18,45, 1994.

26. Graff MK, Bryant J, Beinlich N: Preventing heel breakdown. *Orthop Nurs* 19:63-69, 2000.

27. Grimi PS, Gottlich IJ, Boddie A, Batson I: Hyperbaric oxygen therapy. *JAMA* 26:2216-2220, 1990.

28. Grous CA, Reilly NJ, Gift AG: Skin integrity in patients undergoing prolonged operations. *J Wound Ostomy Continence Nurs* 24:86-91, 1997.

29. Hicks DJ: An incidence study of pressure sores following surgery. In *ANA Clinical Session: 1970 Miami*. New York, Apple-Century-Crofts, 1970, pp 49-54.

30. Honde C, Derks C, Tudor D: Local treatment of pressure sores in the elderly: Amino acid copolymer membrane versus hydrocolloid dressing. *J Am Geriatr Soc* 42:1180-1183, 1994.

31. Hoshowsky VM, Schramm CA: Intraoperative pressure sore prevention: An analysis of bedding materials. *Res Nurs Health* 17:333-339, 1994.

32. Kemp MG: Factors that contribute to pressure sores in surgical patients. *Res Nurs Health* 13: 293-301, 1990.

33. Kemp MG, Faan C, Krouskop TA: Pressure ulcers. Reducing incidence and severity by managing pressure. *J Gerontol Nurs* 20:27-34, 1994.

34. Kosiak M: Etiology and pathology of decubitus ulcers. *Arch Phys Med Rehabil* 40:62-68, 1959.

35. Lamid S, Ghatit AZ: Smoking, spasticity and pressure sores in spinal cord injured patients. *Am J Phys Med* 62:300-306, 1983.

36. Langemo D: Incidence and prediction of pressure ulcers in five patient care settings. *Decubitus* 4:25-33, 1991.

37. Leigh IH, Bennet G: Pressure ulcers: prevalence, etiology, and treatment modalities. A review. *Am J Surg* 167:25S-30S, 1994.

38. Lewicki LJ, Mion L, Splane KG, *et al*: Patient risk factors for pressure ulcer during cardiac surgery. *AORN J* 65: 933-942, 1997.

39. Lewis VL, Bailey MH, Pulawski G, *et al*: The diagnosis of osteomyelitides in patients with pressure sore. *Plast Reconstr Surg* 81:229-232, 1988.

40. Linares HA, Mawson AR, Suarez E, Biundo JJ: Association between pressure sores and immobilization in the immediate post-injury period. *Orthopaedics* 10:571-573, 1987.

41. Lowthian PT: Underpads in the prevention of decubiti. In Kennedy RM, Cowden JM, Scalesc JT (eds): *Bed Sores Biomechanics: Proceedings of a Seminar on Tissue Viability and Clinical Applications*. Baltimore, University Park Press, 1976, pp 141-145.

42. Maklebust J: An update on horizontal patient support surfaces. *Ostomy Wound Management* 45:70S-77S, 1999.

43. Maklebust J: Pressure ulcers: etiology and prevention. *Nurs Clin North Am* 22: 359-377, 1987.

44. Mawson AR, Biundo JJ Jr, *et al*: Risk factors for early occurring pressure ulcers following spinal cord injury. *Am J Phys Med Rehabil* 67:123-127, 1988.

45. Mawson AR, Siddiqui FH, Biundo JJ Jr: Enhancing host resistance to pressure ulcers: a new approach to prevention. *Prev Med* 22:433-450, 1993.

46. Mayrovitz HN: Pressure and blood flow linkages and impacts on pressure ulcer development. Paper presented at First Annual OR-Acquired Pressure Ulcer Symposium, Atlanta, March 1998.

47. Minnis RJ, Sutton RA, Duffus A, Mattison R: Underseat pressure distribution in the sitting spinal injury person. *Paraplegia* 22:297-304, 1984.

48. Mulder GD: Evaluation of three nonwoven sponges in the débridement of chronic wounds. *Ostomy Wound Management* 41:62-67, 1995.

49. Mulder GD: Treatment of open-skin wounds with electric stimulation. *Arch Phys Med Rehabil* 72:375-377, 1991.

50. Nawoczenski DA: Pressure sores: prevention and management. In Buchanan LE, Nawoczenski DA (eds): *Spinal Cord Injury. Concepts and Management Approaches*. Baltimore, Williams & Wilkins, 1994, pp 99-121.

51. Norton D, McLaren R, Exton-Smith AN: *An Investigation of Geriatric Nursing Problems in the Hospital*. London, National Corporation for the Care of Old People, Center for Policy on Aging Report, 1962.

52. Ovington LF: Dressings and adjunctive therapies: AHCPR guidelines revisited. *Ostomy Wound Management* 45: 94S-106S, 1999.

53. Papantonio CT, Wallop JM, Kolodner KB: Sacral ulcers following cardiac surgery: incidence and risk. *Adv Wound Care* 7:24-36, 1994.

54. Patterson JA, Bennet RG: Prevention and treatment of pressure sores. *Am Geriatr Soc* 43:919-927, 1995.

55. Perez ED: Pressure ulcers: updated guidelines for treatment and prevention. *Geriatrics* 48:39-44, 1993.

56. Pope R: Pressure sore formation in the operating theatre: 1. *Brit J Nurs* 8:211-214, 1999.

57. Ratliff CR: Pressure ulcer assessment and management. *Lippincott's Primary Care Practice* 3:242-258, 1999.

58. Reuler JB, Cooney TG: The pressure sore: pathophysiology and principles of management. *Ann Int Med* 94:661-666, 1981.

59. Richardson RR, Meyer PR: Prevalence and incidence of pressure sores in acute spinal cord injuries. *Paraplegia* 19:235-247, 1981.

60. Rodeheaver GT: Pressure ulcer débridement and cleansing: A review of current literature. *Ostomy Wound Management* 45:80S-85S, 1999.

61. Scott EM: Hospital acquired pressure sores as an indicator of quality: a research programme centered in the operating theatre. *Br J Theatre Nurs* 8:19-24, 1998.

62. Scott SM: Mayhew PA, Harris EA: Pressure ulcer development in the operating room: nursing implications. *AORN J* 56:242-250, 1992.

63. Sheman RA, Wyle F, Vulpe M: Maggot therapy for treating pressure ulcers in spinal cord injury patients. *J Spinal Cord Med* 18:71-74, 1996.

64. Singh RVP, Suys S, Villanueva PA: Prevention and treatment of medical complications. In Benzel EC, Tator CH (eds): *Contemporary Management of Spinal Cord Injury.* Park Ridge, IL, American Association of Neurological Surgeons, 1995, pp 195-215.

65. Stankard CE, Cruse CW, Wells KE, Karl R: Chronic pressure ulcer carcinomas. *Ann Plast Surg* 30:274-277, 1993.

66. Taylor TV, Rimmer J, Day B, *et al*: Ascorbic acid supplementation in the treatment of pressure sores. *Lancet* 2:544-546, 1974.

67. Ter Riet G, Kessels AGH, Knipchild P: Randomized clinical trial of ultrasound treatment for pressure ulcers. *BMJ* 310:1040-1041, 1995.

68. Treatment of Pressure Ulcers, Clinical Guideline No. 15, AHCPR Pub. No. 95-0652, December 1994.

69. Vidal J, Sarrias M: An analysis of the diverse factors concerned with the development of pressure sores in spinal cord injured patients. *Paraplegia* 29:261-267, 1991.

70. Wharton GW, Milani JC, Dean LC: Pressure sore profile: cost and management. *Paraplegia* 26:124, 1988.

71. Yarkony GM: Pressure ulcers: a review. *Arch Phys Med Rehabil* 75:908-917, 1994.

72. Young JS, Burns PE: Medical changes incurred by spinal cord injury patients during first six years following injury. *Sci Digest* 4:19-26, 1982.

73. Xakellis GC, Chrichilles EA: Hydrocolloid versus saline-gauze dressings in treating pressure ulcers: a cost-effectiveness analysis. *Arch Phys Med Rehabil* 73:463-469, 1992.

# CHAPTER 144

# Medical Management of Adult and Pediatric Spinal Cord Injury

Jack E. Wilberger, Mehdi Sarkarati, Edward C. Benzel, and Charles H. Tator

The three primary goals of both adult and pediatric spinal cord injury (SCI) management are to optimize neurologic outcome, provide for early mobilization, and facilitate rehabilitation. These goals are difficult to meet when medical complications supervene. Unfortunately, SCI patients are uniquely vulnerable to a variety of complications that at a minimum prolong hospitalization, increase costs, and delay entry into rehabilitation, and that at the other extreme may impair neurologic recovery.

Fortunately, mortality after SCI is relatively low (approximately 4%) and continues to decline. However, morbidity, even in children, remains significant. Thus attention to the medical management of SCI is essential, and the skills of a multidisciplinary team of neurosurgeons, critical care specialists, and physiatrists are often required.

Recently, *Guidelines for the Management of Acute Cervical Spine and Spinal Cord Injuries* were published.[33] This document provides a comprehensive overview of current practice regarding a number of issues discussed in this chapter.

## Pharmacologic Intervention

Methylprednisolone administration within 8 hours of adult SCI has been shown to improve the odds of neurologic recovery.[4] Pediatric patients were not included in this study's patient population because of Food and Drug Administration regulations. However, pathophysiologically there is no reason to believe that children would not respond similarly, and thus it is generally recommended that suspected or confirmed SCI in adults or children be treated with a 30mg/kg bolus of methylprednisolone as soon as feasible after injury. Subsequently, a 5.4mg/kg/hr infusion should be continued for the next 23 hours. Because there is a suggestion that treating with methylprednisolone more than 8 hours after SCI results in a slight decrease in neurologic recovery, it is not advisable to use the drug in such a situation.[5]

A recent methylprednisolone trial has been completed that compares the previously described regimen with 48-hour methylprednisolone dosing and the new free radical scavenger, Tirilazad.[4,5] Children were excluded from this trial also. At 6 weeks follow-up the 48-hour dosing of

methylprednisolone, if started within 3 to 8 hours of injury, resulted not only in improvement in neurologic recovery but also in improvement in functional recovery. However, also accompanying this was a significant increase in the steroid-related complications of infection and gastrointestinal (GI) hemorrhage.

Debate continues, however, over the true utility of methylprednisolone after SCI, and perhaps as important, its promulgation as a standard of care in this setting. In the recent guidelines the following conclusion is drawn: "the evidence suggesting harmful side effects is more consistent than any suggestion of clinical benefit."

Information from the GM-1 ganglioside SCI study has just become available.[32] More than 800 patients were randomized between GM-1 and placebo (with all having received the previously described steroid protocol). Although those patients receiving GM-1 recovered neurologic function at a faster rate, in the end there was no difference in recovery between groups. Thus at this juncture there is no indication of any clinical benefit in SCI.

## Spectrum of Medical Complications

Every organ system can be affected by SCI, irrespective of whether the system is primarily injured in the traumatic event. The National Acute Spinal Cord Injury Study (NASCIS) data (Figure 144.1) provides the most recent comprehensive statistics on medical complications after adult SCI. The overall decrease in medical complications, as demonstrated by NASCIS, may be attributable to coordinated care in specialized acute SCI centers. Tator *et al.* [27] recently described a reduction in hospital length of stay of almost 50% when a multidisciplinary team approach for medical management was used. Thus constant vigilance must be maintained to prevent these complications and to manage them as rapidly and comprehensively as medically feasible when they do occur.

Because the incidence of pediatric SCI is quite low (less than 1% of all new spinal cord injury cases per year), the incidence of medical complications in children is not well documented. However, with the exception of pulmonary embolism (PE), it should be anticipated that pediatric medical considerations are not dissimilar to those of adults.

## Pulmonary Considerations

The respiratory system is uniquely susceptible to SCI because primary neurologic dysfunction profoundly affects respiratory physiology directly, as well as indirectly. Although cervical injury is more commonly associated with pulmonary complications, these may also occur with a thoracic level injury. Pulmonary complications are the single most common cause of morbidity and mortality after pediatric SCI.

The muscles of respiration include the abdominal, intercostal, diaphragm, and cervical accessory muscles. The abdominal muscles are the primary muscles of active expiration and account for more than 50% of expiratory capacity. Thus thoracic SCI, with abdominal muscle

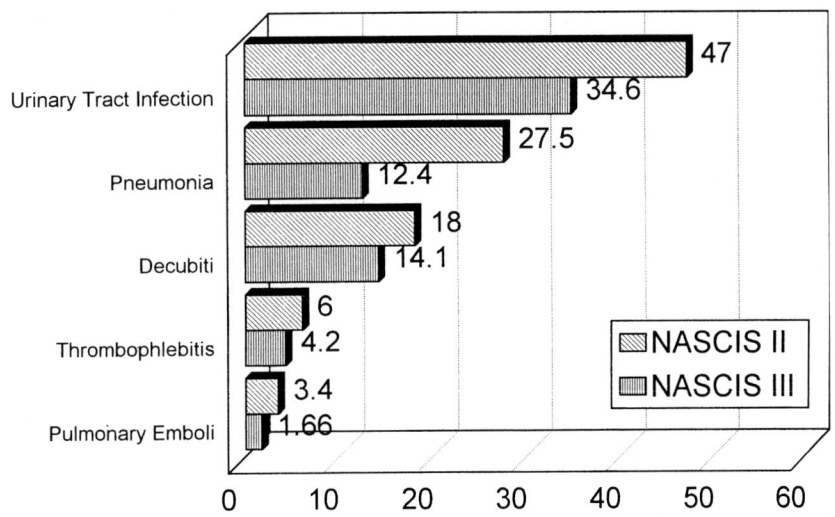

**Figure 144.1** Comparison of complication rates of National Acute Spinal Cord Injury Studies II and III.

paralysis, may lead to ineffective expiration, excessive end-tidal volumes, and subsequently, a diminished lung capacity.[16,18]

The intercostal muscles play an important role in stabilizing the chest wall during inspiration. Their paralysis results in a functionally flail chest, in which the chest wall collapses during inspiration and expands during expiration, resulting in an overall loss of tidal volume.

The diaphragm muscles account for approximately 50% to 60% of the inspiratory force generated. When the other muscles of respiration are nonfunctional, however, the diaphragm assumes 100% of the workload and may rapidly fatigue.[11]

Overall, generalized muscle weakness contributes to diminished contraction force for effective coughing and clearing of secretions. These muscle abnormalities, singly or in combination, may ultimately result in significant decreases in functional residual capacity, tidal volume, and inspiratory and expiratory volumes, while markedly increasing residual lung volumes.[21]

In the majority of instances careful monitoring via pulse oximetry or arterial blood gas measurement is an essential component of early management. Postural changes, nasotracheal suctioning, and chest physiotherapy aid in clearing secretions and minimizing atelectasis.[17]

It should be borne in mind that the vital capacity and the tidal volume of the quadriplegic patient are greater in the supine than in the upright position. In the supine position the weight of the abdominal contents helps in forcing the diaphragm rostrally, which leads to a decrease in residual volumes.[10]

Despite attention to these details, some patients may require intubation for respiratory support. The two primary indications are inability to ventilate effectively (partial pressure of carbon dioxide greater than 50mmHg) and inability to oxygenate adequately (partial arterial oxygen pressure less than 80mmHg). Intubation is also occasionally necessary to allow for more vigorous clearing of secretions by intermittent bronchoscopy.[22]

Intubation with current endotracheal tubes can be safely achieved for several weeks, although there are some proponents of early tracheotomy (with the belief that it facilitates patient care and simplifies weaning of ventilatory support). One disadvantage of early tracheotomy, however, is that it may interfere with ventral cervical surgery in those patients who require internal stabilization from such an approach.

Except for quadriplegic patients with injury at very high levels, most SCI patients can be weaned from ventilatory support during acute hospitalization.[13,30] A number of different weaning regimens have been advocated, although no regimen has a significant advantage over any other. Most patients can be successfully weaned when the vital capacity is greater than 1L, maximal negative inspiratory force exceeds 30cm $H_2O$, and minute ventilation is less than 10L.[29]

Despite attention to these details, atelectasis and subsequent bronchial pneumonia are still common in the SCI population, and thus constant vigilance is of utmost importance to rapidly diagnose and treat pneumonia. The use of prophylactic antibiotics is not encouraged, even in those patients who require prolonged intubation or tracheostomy. Routine use may increase the occurrence of antibiotic-resistant infection.[12,16]

Another potential pulmonary complication of SCI is sleep apnea. Automatic respiration is regulated by spinal cord tracts that lie in the rostral cervical spinal cord. If these pathways are significantly damaged, only voluntary respiration (which is dependent on consciousness) is possible, and breathing may cease during sleep. One should maintain a high index of suspicion of this syndrome in any patient with a high cervical SCI. An apnea monitor or pulse oximeter must be used on a continuous basis for 7 to 10 days after injury in such patients.

## Hemodynamic Considerations

The transection of sympathetic pathways after SCI, with concomitant unopposed vagal activity or hyperactivity, accounts for the majority of cardiovascular complications associated with SCI.[19] Recent monitoring with a Swan-Ganz catheter, however, has documented far-reaching hemodynamic derangements in these patients. The primary immediate concerns are generally bradycardia and neurogenic spinal shock. Whereas the majority of patients with cervical SCI will have bradycardia, only rarely does this become of significant clinical concern to warrant treatment with atropine or use of a temporary transvenous cardiac pacer. Nevertheless, it is important to continue electrocardiographic monitoring during the early phase after injury.[23]

Neurogenic spinal shock results from an inadequate circulating fluid or blood volume because of loss of vascular tone, pooling of blood in the periphery, and third spacing of fluids. Systemic vascular resistance may be less than 50% of the normal level in these patients. As a result fluid resuscitation alone may be insufficient to restore normal blood pressure, and pressor agents are often required. Alpha-adrenergic agonists and beta-adrenergic agonists, such as phenylephrine, norepinephrine, dopamine, and dobutamine, are most frequently used. On occasion, however, these agents produce a paradoxical effect by decreasing cardiac output and by secondarily decreasing tissue perfusion.

The importance of stabilizing the hemodynamic situation as soon as possible after SCI lies in its potential to impact neurologic recovery. A number of experimental models suggest improved outcomes after spinal cord blood flow is maximized by careful attention being paid to systemic resuscitation.[9,14]

A recent detailed study by Levi et al.[20] not only documented hemodynamic derangements in 50 SCI patients, but also demonstrated a correlation with neurologic prognosis. The absence of significant decrements in pulmonary vascular resistance and systemic vascular resistance, or an appropriate response to aggressive therapy, was associated with improved motor recovery.

Several recent studies have advocated an aggressive critical care protocol, with particular emphasis on hemodynamic monitoring, stabilization, and blood pressure treatment. In 1997 Vale and colleagues at the University of Alabama maintained mean arterial pressure above 85mmHg for 7 days after injury. More than 50% of patients required pressors to maintain such levels. In a nonrandomized, pilot study of 77 consecutive SCI patients these authors concluded that neurologic outcome was enhanced by early and aggressive volume resuscitation and blood pressure augmentation.[34]

Another manifestation of sympathetic denervation is orthostatic hypotension. Children seem particularly predisposed to this problem. Raising an SCI patient abruptly from the supine to the upright position may result in a significant drop in blood pressure because of an inability to regulate vascular tone. Thus the mobilization of these patients often requires progressive elevation, with the use of tilt tables or other similar maneuvers.

## Deep Venous Thrombosis and Pulmonary Embolism

Deep venous thrombosis (DVT) has been reported to occur in up to 100% of SCI patients, but the incidence of overtly symptomatic DVT is less than 15%. Paraplegic patients have a slightly higher incidence (16%), compared with quadriplegic patients (12%). Motor complete quadriplegia is associated with an incidence of 23%. In contrast, motor incomplete quadriplegic patients have an incidence of 9%.[28] Venous pooling secondary to decreased vascular resistance, combined with a lack of muscle contraction, are the primary factors in its occurrence.

The incidence of PE is approximately 5% in adults, with an equal occurrence in paraplegic and quadriplegic patients.[28] Pulmonary thromboembolism after DVT is one of the catastrophic complications of acute SCI. It results in the death of approximately 4% of acutely hospitalized patients. PE has rarely been reported after pediatric SCI. Because DVT may not be clinically overt, a high index of clinical suspicion is required, and these patients are best managed with aggressive preventive measures.

External sequential pneumatic compression stockings have become popular as an adjunctive treatment, and have been shown to lower the incidence of DVT, but not PE, in other patient populations.[2] Heparin (5000 units subcutaneously every 8 hours), administered approximately 72 hours after SCI, is the mainstay of prophylaxis. Earlier administration is not recommended because of the remote possibility of extending any areas of parenchymal spinal cord hemorrhage that are often observed after SCI.

The Guidelines recommend prophylactic treatment of thromboembolism in all patients with severe motor deficits, with the use of low molecular weight heparin, rotating beds, low dose heparin, pneumatic compression stockings, or electrical stimulation—typically in combination.

The clinical diagnosis of DVT is difficult to establish, and therefore some surgeons advocate the routine use of Doppler venography on a regular schedule. Such studies have a 90% accuracy in detecting significant venous thrombosis.

When DVT is established, full anticoagulation with heparin, followed by coumadin, is instituted, unless medically contraindicated. An increased vigilance for the possibility of PE must be maintained because signs and symptoms may be absent or misleading. Fever is often the first manifestation, because SCI patients may not be able to perceive pleuritic pain or mount a tachycardic and tachypneic response to altered pulmonary perfusion. Because of the unreliability of chest radiography and ventilation-perfusion scans in diagnosing PE, pulmonary angiography is most often necessary.

When PE occurs, even with full anticoagulation, interruption of the vena cava is indicated; this is highly effective in preventing recurrences. Some practitioners have even advocated prophylactic vena caval interruption in all SCI patients.[31]

## Gastrointestinal Considerations

GI concerns in the SCI patient vary from minimizing gastric and abdominal distension and stress ulcerations to providing nutrition and bowel retraining.

The simplest and most effective means of preventing most acute GI complications is by using nasogastric suction. Gastric atony and paralytic ileus may compromise respiratory function by further decreasing lung capacity or by leading to vomiting and aspiration.

Stress ulcerations occur at a low rate but may increase the use of high-dose steroids. The monitoring of gastric pH and the institution of treatment to maintain a pH greater than 4.5 should minimize the risk of ulceration. Antacids may be administered via a nasogastric tube, or alternatively, intravenous $H_2$ blockers may be used.

More severe and life-threatening acute abdominal complications such as splenic rupture or liver lacerations, or chronic complications such as bowel obstruction or perforation, or other similar conditions, may be obscured because of a lack of pain perception after SCI. Occasionally, vague pain may be appreciated secondary to autonomic visceral afferent branches that are conducted into the spinal cord via the splanchnic nerves. Also, if the SCI is not above the C5 level, referred pain secondary to diaphragmatic irritation may be felt in the shoulder region. Other signs of ongoing abdominal complications, such as temperature elevation, elevated white blood cell count, or associated ileus, are not reliable signs for the identification of abdominal disease in these patients. Similarly, clinical examination may be misleading because localized abdominal tenderness, muscle guarding, and rigidity are likely to be absent, even though peritonitis may be present. Thus it must be recognized that patients with SCI can develop such abdominal complications. The patient must be observed carefully for any indirect signs that may point to an ongoing acute abdominal problem.[6]

Because SCI patients are hypermetabolic and hypercatabolic acutely, nutrition should be started as soon as the gut permits or within 7 days of injury, if parenteral alimentation is required. Supplying nutrition via the GI tract is a much more physiologic means of replacing calories and providing protein substrates. A number of solutions are available for this purpose. Initial feeding rates of 20 to 30ml/hr are increased incrementally as long as there is no significant gastric retention. If there is significant gastric retention and aspirates remain high, small-bore nasoduodenal tubes may allow the patient access to nutrition. Elemental feeding formulas can help if diarrhea becomes a problem.[3]

As the SCI patient recovers the need for caloric support progressively decreases. Most patients require 30 to 40kcal/kg/day acutely, whereas subacute or chronic quadriplegics require approximately 22kcal/kg/day, and paraplegics require 27kcal/kg/day.[8]

Bowel retraining is a critical component of GI management and should be begun early after injury. The most effective bowel regimen is a daily routine of a combination of rectal suppositories and stool softeners.

## Urologic Considerations

Initial urologic management mandates the use of an indwelling Foley catheter until hemodynamic stability is assured. However, the longer the need for an indwelling catheter, the greater the risk of urinary tract infection. Renal problems account for the majority of long-term medical issues in the chronic SCI patient. The prophylactic use of antibiotics, in association with indwelling Foley catheters, has not been shown to decrease this risk.[24,26] Thus as soon as is feasible, clean, intermittent catheterization should be initiated, and bladder retraining begun.[7]

Depending on the level of the SCI, the bladder may be areflexic and flaccid, or dyssynergic and spastic. With an areflexic bladder, voiding may be accomplished by using abdominal pressure—the Crede maneuver. However, if residual urine remains high, this maneuver must be supplemented by clean, intermittent catheterization.[1] With a spastic bladder, spontaneous voiding is possible as long as the intravesicular pressure is not too high and there is no overriding sphincter spasticity. In this situation, at least in men, an external condom catheter is acceptable.[15] If the pressure is too high or if the sphincter is spastic, pharmacologic intervention may be helpful. The bladder musculature may be relaxed with anticholinergics such as propantheline or smooth muscle relaxants such as oxybutynin.

Pediatric SCI regimens for bladder management depend on the age, gender, size, and weight of the child and the type of bladder. Fluid intake and output are crucial in establishing programs and schedules. In infants and toddlers, for whom the use of diapers is appropriate, one must ensure adequate emptying of the bladder. With school age children, diapers are no longer appropriate, and their continued use may be detrimental to the child's self-esteem and self-image. Clean, intermittent catheterization is an alternative and can be instituted at any age.

## Skin Care

Development of pressure areas is an undesirable complication of SCI. Immobility and the lack of sensation predispose to pressure necrosis of the skin and subsequent skin breakdown. Thus pressure over the skin, particularly the bony prominences, must be avoided. The most common sites for the development of decubiti are the ischial, sacral, malleolar, trochanteric, and coccygeal prominences. In children who are confined to the supine position for long periods, the occiput is particularly vulnerable to the development of a pressure ulcer. Also, pressure points may be created by orthotic devices. These areas must be diligently checked, padded, and protected when found.[25]

## Psychological and Rehabilitation Issues

Not only does SCI create physical disability, but it is also a severe psychological stress on both the patient and the family members. Because this stress may not be readily appreciated initially, it is important to provide appropriate levels of psychiatric support and counseling within a few days of SCI. For some patients who become rapidly depressed from their physical limitations, the use of antidepressant medications may be appropriate.

Additionally, SCI rehabilitation aims to facilitate maximal neurologic recovery while helping the individual develop compensatory strategies for the neurologic loss that has occurred. Rehabilitation issues should be addressed early in critical care management, and the appropriate team should be assembled to address the physical disabilities.

# REFERENCES

1. Barkin M, Dolfin D, Herschorn S, *et al*: The urologic care of the spinal cord injured patient. *J Urol* 129:335-339, 1983.

2. Black PM, Baker MF, Snook CP: Experience with external calf compression in neurology and neurosurgery. *Neurosurgery* 18:440-444, 1986.

3. Blissitt PA: Nutrition and acute spinal cord injury. *Crit Care Clin North Am* 2:375-383, 1990.

4. Bracken MB, Shepard JJ, Collins WF Jr, *et al*: A randomized controlled trial of methylprednisolone or naloxone in the treatment of acute spinal cord injury. The results of the National Acute Spinal Cord Injury Trial. *N Engl J Med* 322:1459-1461, 1990.

5. Bracken MB, Shepard JJ, Collins WF Jr, *et al*: Methylprednisolone or naloxone in the treatment of acute spinal cord injury: one year follow-up results of the National Acute Spinal Cord Injury Study. *J Neurosurg* 77:324, 1992.

6. Charney KJ, Juler GL, Comarr AE: General surgery problems in patients with spinal cord injuries. *Arch Surg* 110:1083-1088, 1975.

7. Comarr AE: Intermittent catheterization for traumatic cord and bladder patients. *J Urol* 108:79-81, 1972.

8. Cox S, Weiss S, Posunick E, *et al*: Energy expenditure after spinal cord injury: an evaluation of stable rehabilitating patients. *J Trauma* 25:419-423, 1985.

9. Ducker TB, Salcman M, Perot PL, *et al*: Experimental spinal cord trauma. I: Correlation of blood flow, tissue oxygen, and neurologic status in the dog. *Surg Neurol* 10:60-62, 1978.

10. Estenne M, DeTroyer A: Mechanism of the postural dependence of vital capacity in tetraplegic subjects. *Am Rev Resp Dis* 135:367-371, 1987.

11. Estenne M, DeTroyer A: Respiratory muscle involvement in tetraplegia. *Prob Resp Care* 3:360-374, 1990.

12. Fishburn MJ, Marino RJ, DiTunno JF: Atelectasis and pneumonia in acute spinal cord injury. *Arch Phy Med Rehabil* 71:197-200, 1990.

13. Gardner BP, Watt JWH, Crishnan KR: The artificial ventilation of acute spinal cord damaged patients: A retrospective study of 44 patients. *Paraplegia* 24:208-220, 1986.

14. Guha A, Tator CH: Acute cardiovascular effects of experimental spinal cord injury. *J Trauma* 28:481-490, 1988.

15. Herschorn S, Gerridzen RG: The management of the neurogenic bladder. In Bloch RF, Basbaum M (eds): *Management of Spinal Cord Injuries*. Baltimore, Williams & Wilkins, 1986.

16. Kocan MJ: Pulmonary considerations in the critical care phase. *Crit Care Clin North Am* 2:369-374, 1990.

17. LaSala PA, Frost EAM: Intensive care management of spinal cord injury. In Alderson JD, Frost EA (eds): *Intensive Care*. London, Butterworth, 1990.

18. Ledsome JR, Sharp JM: Pulmonary function and acute cervical cord injury. *Am Rev Resp Dis* 124:41-44, 1981.

19. Lehman KG, Lane JG, Piepmeier JM: Cardiovascular abnormalities accompanying acute spinal cord injury in humans: Incidence, time course, and severity. *J Am Coll Cardiol* 10:46-56, 1987.

20. Levi L, Wolf A, Belzberg H: Hemodynamic parameters in patients with acute cervical cord trauma: A description, intervention, and prediction of outcome. *Neurosurgery* 33:1007-1013, 1993.

21. Mansel JK, Norman JR: Respiratory complications in management of spinal cord injuries. *Chest* 97:1440-1452, 1990.

22. McMichan JC, Michel L, Westbrook PR: Pulmonary dysfunction following traumatic quadriplegia. Recognition, prevention, and treatment. *JAMA* 243:528-531, 1980.

23. Meincke FW: Regulation of the cardiovascular system in patients with fresh injuries to the spinal cord. *Paraplegia* 9:109-112, 1971.

24. National Institute on Disability and Rehabilitation Research: Consensus Statement. The prevention and management of urinary tract infections among people with spinal cord injuries. *J Am Parapleg Soc* 15:194-204, 1992.

25. Nsenis JE, Sarmiento A: The pathophysiology and management of pressure sores. *Orthop Rev* 2:25-34, 1973.

26. Pearman JW: Prevention of urinary tract infection following spinal cord injury. *Paraplegia* 9:95-104, 1971.

27. Tator CH, Duncan EG, Edmons VE, *et al*: Neurological recovery, mortality, and length of stay after acute spinal cord injury associated with changes in management. *Paraplegia* 33:254-262, 1995.

28. Waring WP, Karunas RS: Acute spinal cord injuries and the incidence of clinically occurring thromboembolic disease. *Paraplegia* 28:8-15, 1991.

29. Weber RK: Respiratory management of acute cervical cord injuries. In Tator CH (ed): *Early Management of Acute Spinal Injury*. Philadelphia, Lippincott-Raven, 1982.

30. Wicks AB, Mentor RR: Long-term outlook in quadriplegic patients with initial ventilator dependency. *Chest* 90: 406-410, 1986.

31. Wilson TI, Rogers FB, Wald SL, *et al*: Prophylactic vena cava filter insertion in patients with traumatic spinal cord injury: preliminary results. *Neurosurgery* 35:234-239, 1994.

32. Geisler FH, Coleman WP, Grieco G, *et al*: The Sygen Study Group: The GM-1 ganglioside multi-center acute spinal cord injury study. *Spine* 26(24 suppl)S87-S98, 2001.

33. Guidelines for the management of acute cervical spine and spinal cord injuries. *Neurosurgery* 50(3 suppl)S1-S199, 2002.

34. Vale FL, Burns J, Jackson AB, *et al*: Combined medical and surgical treatment after spinal cord injury. Results of a prospective pilot study to assess the merits of aggressive medical resuscitation and blood pressure management. *J Neurosurg* 87:239-246, 1997.

# CHAPTER 145

# Spinal Traction

## Michael A. Morone and Perry A. Ball

Currently spinal traction is used almost exclusively for the correction of cervical spine pathology. Spinal traction results in a longitudinal pull along the spine that reduces deformity, restores normal anatomic alignment, and stabilizes the spine. The use of spinal traction for the treatment of thoracic and lumbar spine pathology is of questionable benefit because of the large forces required for significant vertebral movement.[27,30] After a review of studies involving lumbar traction, the Quebec Task Force on Spinal Disorders concluded that there was no scientific evidence to support the use of lumbar spinal traction devices.[32] Caution should be applied if lumbar traction devices are to be used, especially those that use gravity inversion, because of the potential for ocular and cardiovascular side effects.[13]

The history of spinal traction goes back 2000 years, when Hippocrates described a form of treatment for dorsal dislocations of the vertebrae in which the patient was placed in a prone position and traction was applied to both ends of the body.[18] Downward pressure was then applied over the protruding vertebrae. In 1650 Glisson used a traction sling for the treatment of rickets-induced spinal deformities.[36] Taylor, in 1929, described the use of a physician-controlled manual head halter traction device for the reduction of a fracture-dislocation of the cervical spine.[38] Cervical traction devices involving attachment to the bony calvarium were introduced in 1933 by Crutchfield, who placed sharp tongs into the parietal eminences, and then attached the tongs to a halter-type traction device.[5] Later, Crutchfield designed his own tongs (Figure 145.1) that were to be placed in the parietal regions bilaterally. This allowed the sequential addition of weights to gradually reduce a dislocation, and it provided a means of maintaining alignment until definitive stabilization could be achieved. Crutchfield's original patient was maintained in traction for 30 days.[5] These tongs had blunted tips and required skull trephinization through the outer cortical table for placement. Because of the narrow distance between the tongs (10 to 11cm) patients could be easily turned in bed, but the tongs could also just as easily become dislodged. At weights greater than 30lb, these tongs often became dislodged. Other disadvantages included the need to shave a large portion of the patient's hair, the need for an assistant during placement of tongs, and the need to use drills and other instrumentation.

Crutchfield tongs remained in use until the early 1970s. McKenzie reported the use of modified ice tongs that had a depth stop of ⅛ inch for the tong points and a mechanism for locking the points into position.[28] These points had to be driven into place with a mallet. In 1936 Hoen described a technique of cervical traction using a wire passed between two burr holes on each side of the head.[19] The

wire often cut through the calvarium and scalp, causing dural lacerations and meningitis. More than a decade later the Vinke tongs were introduced, and these were easier to apply.[39] These tongs fit over the horizontal aspect of the skull above the temporal ridge in the parietal region, rather than over the calvarial apex (Figure 145.2). In addition, an eccentric blade was attached to the diploic space between the inner and outer tables of the skull, allowing more secure fixation to the skull and more weight to be applied. However, the Vinke tongs still required the use of additional instrumentation (drills and undercutting drill blades). In 1973 Gardner introduced the tongs that have largely supplanted the Crutchfield and Vinke tongs.[14] The tips of the Gardner tongs are applied below the greatest diameter of the skull, and there is a spring-loaded pin that allows only 30lb of compressive force to be applied (Figure 145.3). The advantage of the Gardner-Wells tongs is its relative ease of use, requiring neither hair shaving nor use of other instrumentation. In addition, a small metal plate attached to each set of tongs lists the steps to be followed during tong application. In comparison to previous tongs the Gardner-Wells tongs provide the most secure traction of the various tong devices and are less likely to slip out of place. Recent modifications of the Gardner-Wells tongs include the use of graphite to allow use during magnetic resonance imaging (MRI). In 1968 Nickel and associates introduced the halo ring as a traction device.[29] The cranial halo provides a more efficient means of fixation to the skull (Figure 145.4). With the halo traction device, both the lateral and the rotatory directions of the traction force can be better controlled than with the Gardner-Wells tongs. The same halo can eventually be attached to a plastic body jacket, which allows for early ambulation.

## Head Halter Traction

### Indications

Head halter traction is noninvasive and has two primary indications. Halter traction may be used as either a type of conservative treatment (nonsurgical) or as an adjunct during cervical spine surgery. The conservative indications for cervical halter traction include its use for nuchal muscle spasm, disk herniations, and spondylosis. The nonsurgical placement can be performed on either an inpatient or, more commonly, an outpatient basis. The patient can be recumbent in bed or in a sitting position while using halter traction.[25] The direction of the traction should be that which is most comfortable for the patient (usually neutral or slightly flexed), and the maximum weight is usually no more than 10lb. Traction is often applied two to four times a day, with the patient engaging in normal activities between traction sessions. Intraoperatively, traction is usually used for spinal distraction to facilitate placement of a bone graft in a discectomy or vertebrectomy site. When traction is released, compressive forces hold the graft in place, and thus even when the patient is recumbent, some compressive forces are still applied to the bone graft. Compression of the bone graft should lead to a greater chance of bone fusion. Halter traction should not be used for stabilization or as an attempt at spinal realignment

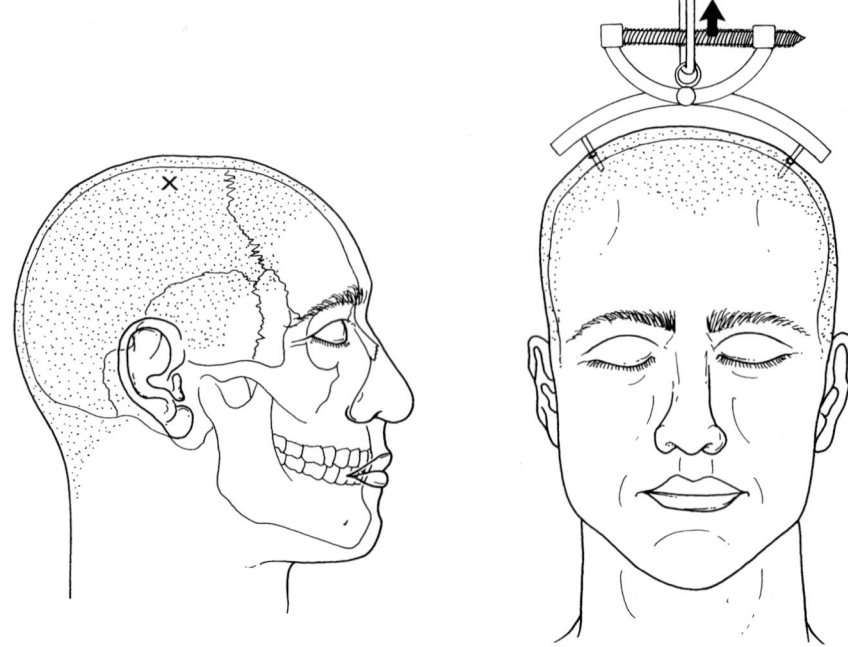

**Figure 145.1** Crutchfield tongs are applied to the crown of the skull along the plane of the external auditory meatus. The tips of the tongs should be perpendicular to the plane of the skull. *X*, Point of insertion.

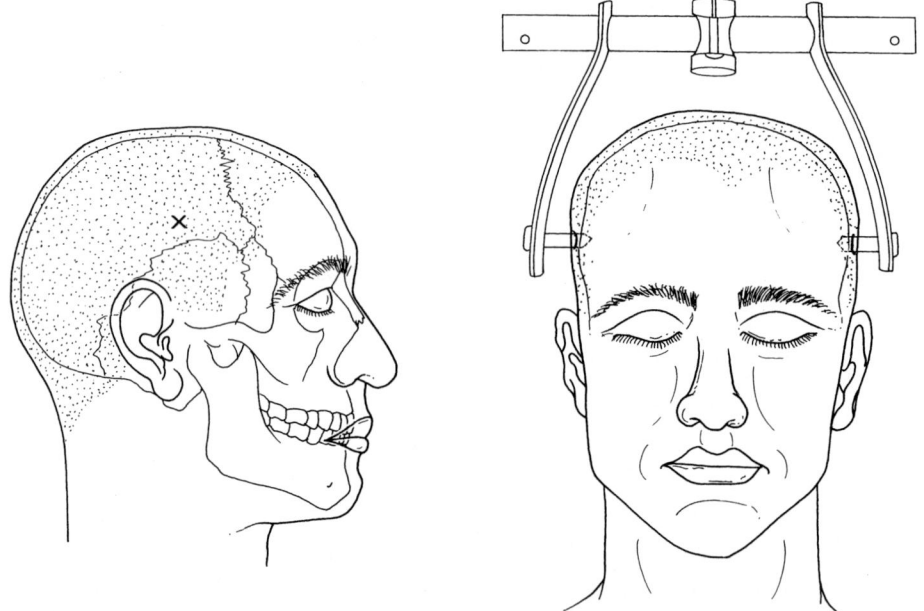

**Figure 145.2** Vinke tongs are applied to the widest portion of the skull above the ears. Special tools are provided, such as a drill with a stop to prevent penetration of the inner table of the skull and an undercutting tool to cut the bone between the outer and inner tables of the skull. The tips of the tongs are equipped with a flat eccentric metal table, which expands within the space cut between the outer and inner tables of the skull and locks the tongs to the skull. *X*, Point of insertion.

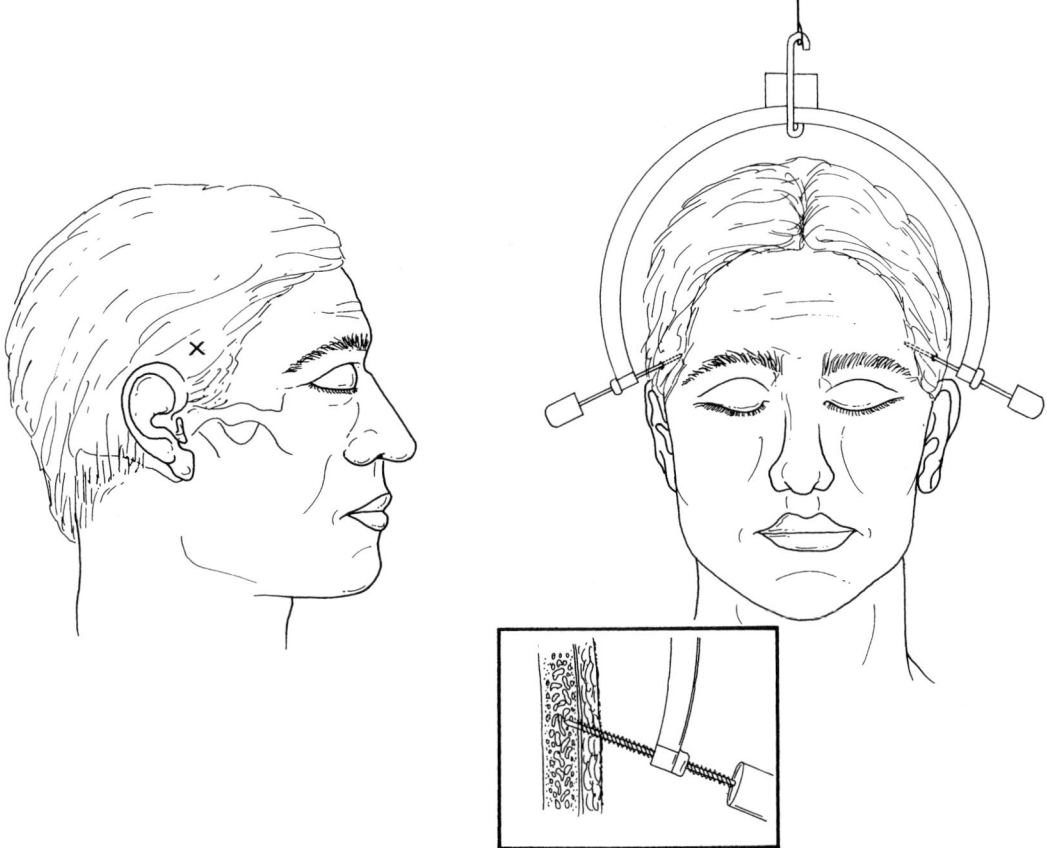

**Figure 145.3** Gardner-Wells tongs may be applied without shaving hair. The regions over the ears are thoroughly prepared with a sterilizing solution, and a local anesthetic is instilled into the skin, subcutaneous tissue, and the periosteum. Once the device is properly aligned, the screws are tightened until the pressure indicator (*inset*) appears.

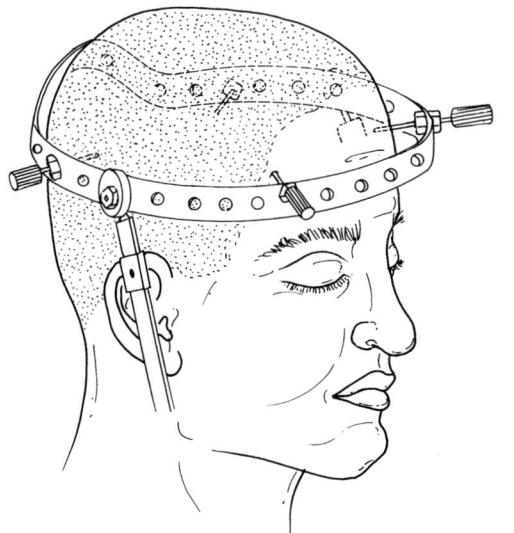

**Figure 145.4** The halo traction ring provides four-point skeletal fixation using pins that pierce the outer table of the skull. These pins are attached by threads to a circumferential steel or titanium ring. The pins are locked to the ring by hexagonal nuts.

after cervical spine injuries, such as fractures, dislocations, or fracture-dislocations.

### Application

Head halter systems are noninvasive and usually consist of two pads, one placed under the chin and the other under the occiput. The pads should be fitted so that pressure is applied evenly to both pads. A metal elbow (spreader) is often used to attach the pad straps to the traction so that the lateral soft tissues of the head and face are not compressed by the straps when traction is applied. For outpatient halter traction some surgeons prefer the type of traction that requires the patient to be recumbent rather than seated. While the patient is recumbent, the head of the bed is elevated 30 to 45 degrees, with the patient's hips and knees flexed.[25] A complaint of too much pressure on either of the pads may require neck flexion or extension by lowering or raising the head of the bed. This type of traction may be used for several sessions each day to achieve pain relief.

Intraoperatively, the halter traction is applied after the patient is endotracheally intubated. The halter is adjusted so that the pads fit easily under the chin and occiput. The chin and occiput straps are then attached to a metal spreader, which, in turn, is attached to a rope that is in about 40 degrees of flexion, so that the head is held in a neutral position. Dorsal to the shoulders, a transverse roll is placed, along with an intravenous fluid bag, behind the patient's neck to maintain the cervical lordotic curvature and also to act as a support while tapping the bone graft in place. A soft foam donut is placed behind the patient's head for support and to prevent direct pressure on the occiput. Halter traction should not be used intraoperatively in the presence of spinal instability.

### Risks

The risks are few for the patient who has been appropriately and completely instructed in the use of halter traction. Patient instruction should include a thorough demonstration of proper traction setup, followed by the patient's own demonstration of the setup and safe use of the device. Most complaints are of excessive pressure on the skin at the pad sites. This can be alleviated with extra padding or by reducing the weight to an amount that is still beneficial to the patient. If the traction increases patient discomfort, the patient should be instructed to discontinue use and request physician consultation.

Intraoperative risks of halter traction include excessive pressure on the skin associated with a prolonged operative time. The rope used for the traction should be of a length such that the weights are close to the ground; thus if the weights should come loose and traction should be lost, the spine will not be jerked violently. Such a violent movement could occur at a critical point in the operation and could potentially result in neural injury. In addition, the anesthesiologist should be familiar with the use of the traction device, and care should be taken not to pull or trip on the traction rope. The traction rope should hang freely and not get tangled with other tubes and wires, because inadvertent extubation or loss of spinal traction could occur. Recently the use of distraction posts that are placed into the vertebral bodies adjacent to the discectomy or vertebrectomy site has eliminated much of the need for cervical halter traction during ventral cervical spine surgery.

## Skeletal Traction

### Indications

Cervical skeletal traction is invasive because it requires attachment to the bony calvarium. This form of traction is appropriate for the treatment of cervical spinal injuries that have the potential for instability (fractures, dislocations, or combinations thereof). In addition, this type of traction can also be used for the reduction of deformities that have a degenerative, rheumatoid, or infectious cause. Skeletal cervical traction allows for pull along the axis of the spine while providing for alignment and maintaining the cervical spinal canal volume. This, in turn, may protect the spinal cord. The benefit of this type of traction is that it allows for the gradual and regulated realignment of the spinal column while the neurologic status of the patient is closely monitored. Skeletal traction can be continued over several

days as needed. Traction should begin at 5 to 8 lb. A lateral radiograph should be obtained. Weights can be added in 5 to 10 lb increments every 30 to 60 minutes until realignment is obtained. Crutchfield recommended a maximum weight of traction that depended on the level of the injury. This is often called the rule of fives; the weights begin with 10 lb for the head and are increased by 5 lb for each spinal level (Table 145.1).[5] For example, an injury at level C4-5 would be associated with a maximum of 30 lb of traction (C4, being the fourth level, would have 20 lb of traction; with 10 lb added for the head, the total weight is 30 lb). Greater weight would increase the risk of neurologic injury or overdistraction. After each weight increment, and before more weight is added, a radiograph should be obtained to monitor for realignment, to determine the need for more distraction, and to monitor for overdistraction. Once realignment is obtained, the amount of weight should be slightly reduced by 5 to 10 lb. Muscle relaxants and analgesics can be used as adjuncts in achieving realignment. The tongs should be checked daily and tightened only if loose. If tightening is aggressive, the pins may penetrate the inner table of the skull. Pin care should be performed twice a day by the nursing staff with diluted hydrogen peroxide, followed by bacitracin ointment.

### Types of Skeletal Cervical Traction

#### Cranial Tongs

The Gardner-Wells tongs are the most common type of cranial tongs used today (see Figure 145.3). The Vinke and Crutchfield tongs, discussed earlier, are of historical importance only. The Gardner-Wells tongs are easy to use and require no additional instrumentation. For a discussion of the application of the Crutchfield and Vinke tongs, the reader is referred to Johnson et al.[20]

**Application.** The Gardner-Wells tongs consist of a C-shaped rectangular rod with an S-shaped link welded to its center to which the traction rope is attached (see Figure 145.3). Also welded to this link are the directions for applying these tongs. At each end of the C that arches over the head are threaded bolts with sharp, pin-pointed ends. These sharp points are simply screwed into place. It is emphasized that the points must be sharp. The entire apparatus should be sterilized before use. On one pin is a spring device that protrudes 1 mm when the appropriate amount of tension is applied to penetrate the outer table of the calvarium.

**TABLE 145.1**

**Cervical Traction Weights**

| Level of Injury | Minimum Weight (lb) | Maximum Weight (lb) |
|---|---|---|
| C1 | 5 | 10 |
| C2 | 6 | 12 |
| C3 | 8 | 15 |
| C4 | 10 | 20 |
| C5 | 12 | 25 |
| C6 | 15 | 30 |
| C7 | 18 | 35 |

Before the traction is applied it is imperative that the patient's hemodynamic and pulmonary status be stabilized; this includes the placement of intravascular monitoring catheters and intubation, if indicated. In addition, a baseline neurologic examination should be performed and a lateral cervical spine radiograph should be obtained. The location of the pins will depend on whether traction is desired with the cervical spine in the neutral, flexed, or extended position. A fixation point that is on a line from the tip of the mastoid process to the top of the pinna will result in traction, with the cervical spine in neutral orientation (i.e., the traction line is parallel to the long axis of the spine). If the site selected is ventral to this point, traction will be applied in extension. Conversely, if the site selected is dorsal, the result will be traction with the neck in flexion. Alternatively, the amount of extension or flexion can also be altered by altering the angle of the traction line with respect to the long axis of the spine. This can be done by altering the height of the pulley (e.g., if the pulley is raised, flexion is obtained, and if the pulley is lowered, extension results).

For fixation in the neutral position the head and neck are stabilized by sandbags, if needed. The hair is combed and maintained vertically, or a small area is shaved. An antiseptic solution is rubbed on the area above each ear. The pin is located just below the equator of the skull and just above the ears (2 to 3cm), in line with the external auditory meatus and the mastoid process. This site places the pins in the longitudinal axis of the spine, thus balancing the extension and flexion forces. The selected pin entry sites are infiltrated with 1% lidocaine. The anesthetic should adequately infiltrate the skin, subcutaneous tissue, and periosteum. The pins are twisted into place by hand; the knurled knobs are twisted in the exact area without making any incision in the skin or drilling into the skull. The knurled handles of the pins are twisted with the fingers until the spring device pushes out 1mm; this indicates that at least 25lb of force is applied. At this point the tongs are tilted back and forth to set the pins. Nuts on the threaded pins allow the depth of the position to be precisely fixed. Traction can then be applied. Within 12 to 24 hours a slight tightening should be attempted. After this the pins should not be disturbed.

**Risks.** Complications may occur in relationship to the use of traction devices.[10] When applying the Gardner-Wells tongs care must be taken to ensure that the site of pin entry is adequately anesthetized; inadequate anesthesia may cause the patient to move excessively, resulting in movement of an unstable cervical spine. Careful attention must be paid to the spring pin. Tightening the pins beyond the recommended amount could lead to a pin penetrating the inner table of the skull. In addition, the location of the pin should be verified by a surgeon experienced in application of tongs. If the pin is above the equator of the skull, traction weight may be sufficient to dislodge the tongs, with resultant scalp laceration. Insertion of the pin greater than 3cm below the equator of the skull may lead to penetration of the pins through the thin squamous portion of the temporal bone. In this

thinner area of bone the spring pin may protrude no more than 1mm before the inner table is violated. This could lead to intracranial hemorrhage or meningitis. The pin sites must be cleaned daily and observed for loosening and infection. Infected pins should be removed and replaced at a slightly different site. As with any condition in which the patient is immobile, pressure sores should be prevented with scheduled log rolling of the patient. For cervical traction specifically, occipital pressure sores should be watched for.

### Cranial Halo Traction

The cranial halo traction device was first introduced by Perry and Nickel in 1959 for the management of severe cervical instability secondary to poliomyelitis.[31] In 1968 Nickel and associates introduced the halo ring for use as a traction device.[29] The cranial tong devices are limited because they apply traction in only the longitudinal direction. Halo traction devices allow for three-dimensional positioning of the cervical spine (see Figure 145.4). Cranial halo traction devices are supplanting the Gardner-Wells tongs in many of the centers that treat spinal disorders. If the spine surgeon plans to maintain the patient in a halo vest, either as a primary method of spinal fixation or after a surgical stabilization procedure, the initial use of cranial halo traction will obviate the need to change four Gardner-Wells tongs to cranial halo tongs during the switch from traction to the attachment of the halo to a vest. Most halo rings that are part of halo vest systems on the market can be used with traction devices. Spine surgeons should become familiar with several systems, learning the finer points of each before selecting one or two types to use. Cranial halo traction provides four-point skeletal fixation through a circumferential steel ring. This rigidly controls the head and, when attached to a body jacket with metal uprights, allows for early mobilization of the patient. The direction of the traction force, both lateral and rotatory, can be controlled better than with the Gardner-Wells tongs.

**Indications.** The indications for use of halo traction are the same as those for cranial tongs; in addition, the halo traction device can be converted for use with a plastic jacket for patient mobility (Figure 145.5). In situations in which long-term halo immobilization is desired, either as a means of postsurgical stabilization (orthosis) or for early immobilization, the spine surgeon may prefer to use the halo traction device instead of cranial tongs. This early mobilization of the patient, while still maintaining traction, is the primary advantage of the halo device. Halo traction has been used to stabilize fractures and reduce fracture-dislocations and dislocations of the upper and lower cervical spine after trauma, infection, inflammation, and tumor invasion. The halo vest provides good stabilization of the upper (C1 and C2) cervical spine. Upper cervical spine movement ranges from 4% to 30% in patients wearing halo vests.[2,21] In contrast to the upper cervical spine the subaxial cervical spine tends to be less fixated with halo vests.[2,22] Injuries that are purely ligamentous do not heal well with the use of halo traction and vests.

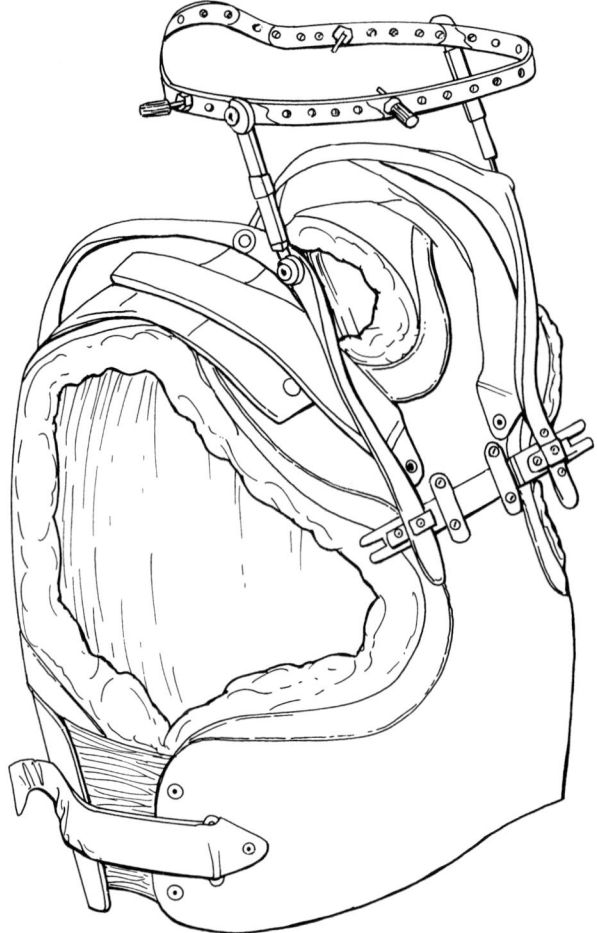

**Figure 145.5** The halo ring may be attached to a plastic vest, plaster of Paris body cast, or pins through the pelvis through rigid metal uprights. This controls the head and neck rigidly and allows the patient with an unstable spine to transfer or ambulate, speeding the course of rehabilitation and avoiding the morbidity associated with prolonged bed rest and traction.

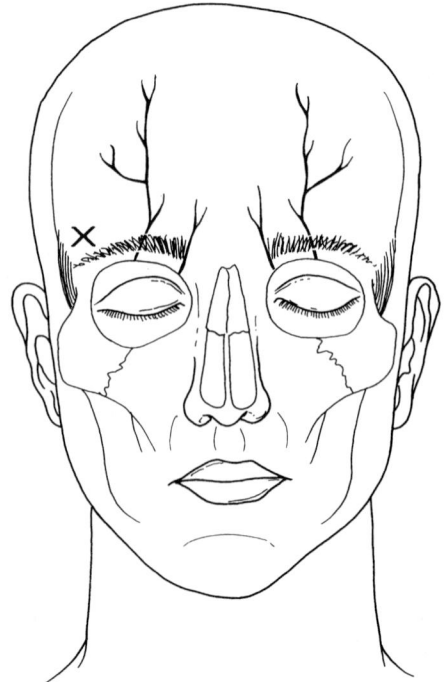

**Figure 145.6** The safe area for anterior pin placement is over the lateral eyebrow. Care must be taken to avoid the nerves and frontal sinus medially, and the thin temporal bone and the temporalis muscle laterally.

**Application.** There are a variety of halo ring traction devices on the market. Spine surgeons should become familiar with several of these before deciding which one to use in their practice. When used for cervical traction the halo ring is placed with the anticipation that it will eventually be connected to a plastic jacket that will allow patient mobility. The patient is positioned in the same manner as for placement of the Gardner-Wells tongs. To relieve the patient's anxiety and pain associated with halo application an explanation of the procedure, followed by a mild sedative and an analgesic, is helpful. Halo rings are available in different sizes; ideally a halo to skull clearance of 1 to 1.5cm should be present (see Figure 145.4). The hair is shaved at the planned sites of pin placement, and the skin is prepared with povidone-iodine (Betadine) and infiltrated with local anesthetic. The halo pins have a broad base and a narrow tip to prevent penetration beyond the outer table of the skull. Four proposed pin sites are chosen. The ventral pin sites are located approximately 1cm above the lateral third of the eyebrows. This position avoids injuring the supraorbital nerve (Figure 145.6). The dorsal pins are diagonally opposite the ventral pins in

channels approximately 1.5cm above the ears. Before the halo ring is placed, it is held in position by an assistant. Many systems have suction-tipped pins to hold the halo in position until the skull pins are placed. The use of suction-tipped pins permits one person to place the halo safely. Hexagonal lock nuts should be loosely placed on each pin outside the ring before advancing the pin. The skull pins are advanced gently until the outer layer of the dermis is penetrated. The ventral and diagonally opposite dorsal pins are simultaneously tightened by hand. The diametrically opposite pins are tightened to a maximum of 6kg, using the torque screwdriver. Alternate tightening of the skull pins prevents the displacement of the halo ring into an asymmetric position. The pins should penetrate only the outer table of the skull. The pins should be placed so that they are perpendicular to the skull. If all pins are placed properly, an excellent grip on the calvarium should be achieved. This prevents rostral migration of the halo ring when traction is applied. Once the pins are placed, the hexagonal nuts are tightened against the halo ring, securing the positions of the pins and also preventing their backing out. Plastic caps can then be placed on the ends of the pins to act as a guard against injury by the exposed metal. Twenty-four hours later the hexagonal nuts should be loosened and the skull pins tightened with the torque screwdriver to confirm 6kg of pressure; the hexagonal nuts are then retightened. No further tightening of the skull pins is necessary; otherwise, the inner table of the skull may be violated. Most systems come with a traction loop that can be attached to a rope and weights. A cervical spine radiograph should be taken to check spinal alignment. The halo ring traction device is then handled as previously described for cranial tong traction. At the appropriate time the traction device can be converted for use with a plastic body jacket.

**Risks.** As with cranial tong traction devices most complications are related to the skull pins. Most of the risks can be prevented with proper initial placement of the halo ring and pins, as well as meticulous daily care of the pin site. The potential risks are the same as those with cranial tong devices and include the risk of penetration of the inner table of the skull, with resultant intracranial hemorrhage, brain injury, or meningitis. Other risks include infection at the pin site that may be confined to the soft tissue or that may result in osteomyelitis of the bone at the pin entry site. Infections at the pin site can present as increased local pain, as drainage, or as a loose skull pin. For a pin site infection, the skull pin should be removed and a new sterile pin should be placed at a new site. Soft-tissue infections usually respond to local care and antibiotics; if there is no improvement, an osteomyelitis may be present, and this may require débridement. Pin loosening, with the potential risk of rostral migration of the halo ring, can occur with osteomyelitis at the pin site. Other complications, such as overdistraction with use of the halo ring, have been previously discussed for cranial tong traction devices.

## Management of Specific Injuries

Cervical traction can be a useful adjunct in the management of several specific injuries. For cervical spine injuries, only skeletal types of traction, not halter traction devices, should be used.

### Atlas (C1) Burst Fractures

Fractures of the atlas ring are relatively common injuries. They usually occur as a result of axial loading, with forces transmitted through the occipital condyles in the lateral masses of the atlas. The resulting fractures may be unilateral or bilateral, but often result in a widening of the ring and the space available for the spinal cord. A key consideration in the management of these injuries is the integrity of the transverse (atlantal) ligament and the stability of the relationship between the atlas and the dens. If the transverse ligament is intact, these fractures are relatively stable and should heal with immobilization in a cervical orthosis, such as a Philadelphia collar. Spence demonstrated that if on an open-mouth radiograph there is more than a 7mm offset from the edge of C1 to the lateral mass of C2, the likelihood of rupture of the transverse ligament is high.[37] Results of several recent studies, however, have shown that up to 25% of atlas fractures may be missed on plain radiographs.[6,15,16] MRI may be a better method for determining whether the transverse ligament is intact.[7] If the transverse ligament is disrupted, the fractures are unstable. The management of atlas fractures is controversial. Levine and Edwards[23] have argued that isolated C1 ring fractures, with a disrupted transverse ligament, should be managed by traction to reduce the displacement, as indicated by an open-mouth radiograph, using up to 30lb if necessary. They argue that the traction should be

maintained for 6 weeks, to prevent redisplacement, before the halo vest is applied. Because injury is caused by axial loading, traction applied in neutral orientation is biomechanically appropriate. However, Hadley et al.[16] managed five patients with greater than 7mm of displacement with a halo vest alone, and without using prolonged traction, and achieved good results.

### Hangman's Fractures

Hangman's fractures, which involve a fracture through the pars interarticularis of C2, were classified by Effendi et al.[11] into three types—a classification that has been modified by Levine and Rhyne.[24] In this classification scheme, hangman's fractures are defined in terms of both angulation and translation between the C2 and C3 vertebrae. Type I fractures are through the neural arch at the base of the pedicle and have up to 3mm of displacement and no angulation. These injuries can be treated with an orthosis, such as a Philadelphia collar. Type II fractures have more than 3mm of translation of C2 on C3. Levine and Rhyne[24] have postulated that this is a flexion-compression injury. In this situation traction, applied with mild cervical extension, can be used to reduce the amount of translation before a halo vest is applied. Levine and Rhyne used 15 to 20lb to reduce type II hangman's fractures in a series of 22 patients and were able to achieve substantial reduction of 19 of these patients. In this situation caution must be used in a subgroup of patients with type IIa fractures, as designated by Levine and Rhyne, who have substantial angulation of the body of C2.[24] In type IIa fractures the fracture line runs obliquely, ventrocaudally to dorsorostrally in the neural arch. Additionally, these fractures are identified because of their severe angulation without resultant translation. The authors noted that when these patients are placed in traction, the translation worsens, and thus the mechanism of injury is probably flexion-distraction.[24] In this situation treatment in a halo vest, with compression and extension, is appropriate. Type III fractures are unusual injuries that result from flexion-compression and involve a dislocation of C2-3 facets, either unilaterally or bilaterally. In this situation traction may be applied in extension in an attempt to reduce this dislocation. However, depending on the location of the fracture, it may not be possible to reduce these injuries with closed techniques.

### Facet Dislocations

Facet dislocations of the middle and lower spine are common injuries. Unilateral facet dislocations are thought to result from flexion and rotation. The characteristic radiographic appearance is that of subluxation of less than 50% of the width of the vertebral body. Subluxation of 50% or more of the width of the vertebral body is indicative of bilateral facet dislocation. The presumed mechanism of these injuries is that of flexion and distraction. Cervical traction has been most widely applied for reduction of facet dislocations; this is also the indication for which the use of cervical traction has aroused the most controversy.

The advantage of reducing facet dislocations is not in question because acute bilateral facet dislocations are highly unstable. The structures that resist further flexion, the interspinous ligaments and the facet capsules, have been completely disrupted in such injuries. The dislocation substantially narrows the space available for the spinal cord, and therefore most of these injuries are associated with a neurologic deficit. Reduction serves to reconstitute the spinal canal and reappose the facet surfaces to allow for healing.

The stability of unilateral facet dislocations is less clear-cut. Because the facet capsule on the side opposite the dislocation is usually intact, there is clear advantage to reduction. Approximately half of these injuries are associated with a neurologic deficit—either a radiculopathy or a myelopathy—and thus reduction probably enhances the chance for neurologic recovery. When unilateral facet dislocations are allowed to heal unreduced, there is a substantial incidence of chronic pain.

Reduction of these injuries can be achieved with axial traction or, alternatively, through open reduction from either a ventral or a dorsal approach. The results of several series of closed reduction of facet dislocations using tongs or halo traction have been published.[1,4] Notably, there has been substantial variation among these series in terms of the success rate, the amount of weight used, and the time required to achieve reduction.

A flexion mechanism is involved in facet dislocations. Therefore reduction can usually be accomplished more readily if the traction is applied with some degree of flexion. It is best to begin with a small weight, such as 10lb, and to then perform a neurologic examination and obtain a lateral radiograph. Weight is sequentially added in 10lb increments. After each addition of weight examination and radiography are repeated. The radiograph should be reviewed not only for alignment, but also for evidence of distraction. A reasonable radiographic indicator of distraction is the widening of the disk space by greater than 5mm. If this is detected, weights should be removed and attempts at closed reduction should be abandoned. The examination should focus on motor and sensory function, as well as on patient complaints, such as increasing pain. If any deterioration in neurologic function occurs, an MRI scan or myelogram should be obtained to exclude spinal cord compression by a disk fragment.

If the lateral radiograph demonstrates that normal alignment has been achieved, all but 5lb of weight can be removed to permit maintenance of the reduction. Closed reduction performed in this manner allows for rapid restoration of vertebral alignment, with the patient awake and neurologic function monitored.

Neurologic deterioration has been reported with the use of traction for reducing facet dislocations, principally because of overdistraction and disk herniation.[12,35] This has led to the two substantive areas of controversy. The first is the total amount of weight that should be used before the effort is abandoned and open reduction is undertaken. The second is whether MRI should be performed to exclude the presence of traumatic disk herniation before closed reduction is attempted. In some respects both controversies are part of the same question: do the benefits of obtaining normal vertebral alignment as rapidly as possible exceed its potential risks?

Distraction has been demonstrated to produce spinal cord dysfunction in experimental animals. How this relates to the clinical situation is not clear. Crutchfield's original recommendations were that a maximum of 5lb should be used per cervical vertebral level.[5] Several authors have argued that no more than 10lb should be used per level. Others have maintained that the use of larger amounts of weight, even up to 150lb if necessary, is safe and effective.[33] Traction tongs tolerate a large amount of weight; cadaver studies have demonstrated that stainless steel Gardner-Wells tongs pull out when traction in excess of 200lb is applied, whereas with titanium tongs, this occurs at about 75lb.[3] When the published results are compared, it is clear that the use of greater weights results in greater success in achieving reduction. It is not clear from the published results, however, whether the patients in these series have a higher rate of neurologic complications. Furthermore, the reported incidences of deterioration as a result of distraction have occurred when less than 10lb have been applied per level. Careful, sequential examination of the patient and the radiograph are most likely preferable to the arbitrary choice of a weight.

The issue of whether MRI should be performed before attempted closed reduction has generated substantial controversy. There have been reports of neurologic deterioration after attempts at closed reduction, because when these patients underwent MRI, disk herniations were observed. This has led to the recommendation that MRI should be performed before traction is applied. If disk herniation is observed, ventral discectomy and open reduction should be performed in lieu of traction. Some surgeons have refuted this by arguing that in awake and cooperative patients traction can be safely applied in a sequential manner. Rizzolo et al.[33] reported a series of more than 100 patients in whom they performed closed reduction without prior MRI. None of these patients suffered a new permanent neurologic deficit. Rizzolo et al.[33] argued that this allows normal vertebral alignment to be restored in the shortest time. To determine the optimal approach, it is necessary to understand the significance of timing of decompression and the incidence of traumatic disk herniations in the presence of facet dislocations.

The significance of timing of decompression in the presence of spinal cord injury remains unsettled. Some evidence suggests that rapid reduction and decompression may improve outcome.[8,9] In Hadley's[17] series, patients who improved neurologically were those in whom reduction was performed within 8 hours. This must be balanced by the fact that any acute intervention in spinal injury carries some risk; 11% of the patients in Hadley's series deteriorated. Similarly, Marshall et al.[26] observed a 5% rate of neurologic deterioration in patients with acute spinal cord injuries, mostly related to some type of intervention in management, including surgery and traction.

The incidence of disk herniation in the setting of facet dislocation was evaluated by MRI by Rizzolo et al.[34] These patients, however, were imaged after the dislocations had been reduced with traction. They found a 40% incidence of disk herniation in patients with unilateral facet dislocations and an 80% incidence in patients with bilateral dislocations. This high incidence of disk herniation, in comparison with the low rate of neurologic deterioration in most series, implies that in many situations closed reduction can be achieved safely in the presence of disk herniation. The more significant conclusion, however, is that restoring vertebral alignment does not necessarily mean that decompression of the neural elements has been achieved. Thus an MRI study obtained before the application of traction can provide information about whether closed reduction alone will be sufficient. With disk herniation, even if closed reduction can be performed safely, complete decompression would necessitate subsequent anterior discectomy. In such a situation it may be most expeditious to proceed with discectomy and open reduction. Finally, the issue of surgical stabilization remains. If ligamentous injuries heal poorly with nonoperative treatment, surgical stabilization is necessary. The risks and benefits of both closed reduction and subsequent surgery should be critically appraised.

# REFERENCES

1. Beatson TR: Fractures and dislocations of the cervical spine. *J Bone Joint Surg* 45B:21-35, 1963.
2. Benzel EC, Hadden TA, Saulsbery CM: A comparison of the Minerva and halo jackets for stabilization of the cervical spine. *J Neurosurg* 70: 411-414, 1989.
3. Blumberg KD, Catalano JB, Cotler JM, Balderston RA: The pullout strength of titanium alloy MRI compatible and stainless steel MRI incompatible Gardner-Wells tongs. *Spine* 18:1895-1896, 1993.
4. Braakman R, Vinken PJ: Unilateral facet interlocking in the lower cervical spine. *J Bone Joint Surg* 49B:249-257, 1967.
5. Crutchfield WG: Skeletal traction for dislocation of the cervical spine: report of a case. *South Surgeon* 2:156-159, 1933.
6. Dickman CA, Hadley MN, Browner C, et al: Neurosurgical management of acute atlas-axis combination fractures: a review of 25 cases. *J Neurosurg* 70:45-49, 1989.
7. Dickman CA, Mamourian A, Sonntag VKH et al: Magnetic resonance imaging of the transverse atlantal ligament for the evaluation of atlantoaxial instability. *J Neurosurg* 75:221-227, 1991.
8. Dolan EJ, Tator CH, Endrenyi L: The value of decompression for acute spinal cord compression injury. *J Neurosurg* 53:749-755, 1980.
9. Ducker TB, Bellagarrigue R, Salcman M, Walleck C: Timing of operative care in cervical cord injury. *Spine* 9:525-531, 1984.
10. Dunn DJ, LeClair WE: How to reduce complications in treatment of cervical spine trauma. *AAOS Instructional Course Lectures* 34:155-162, 1985.
11. Effendi B, Roy D, Cornish B, et al: Fractures of the ring of the axis: a classification based on analysis of 131 cases. *J Bone Joint Surg* 63B:319-327, 1981.
12. Eismont FG, Arena MJ, Green BA: Extrusion of intervertebral disc associated with traumatic subluxation or dislocation of cervical facets. *J Bone Joint Surg* 73A: 1555-1559, 1991.
13. Friberg TR, Weinreb RN: Ocular manifestations of gravity inversion. *JAMA* 253:1755-1757, 1985.
14. Gardner WJ: The principle of spring loaded points for cervical traction. *J Neurosurg* 39:543-544, 1973.

15. Greene KA, Marciano FF, Dickman CA, et al: Prospective evaluation of stability of traumatic axis fractures. *J Neurotrauma* 10:S220, 1993.
16. Hadley MN, Dickman CA, Browner CM, Sonntag VKH: Acute traumatic atlas fractures: management and long-term outcome. *Neurosurgery* 23:31-35, 1988.
17. Hadley MN, Fitzpatrick BC, Sonntag VKH, Browner CM: Facet dislocations injuries of the cervical spine. *Neurosurgery* 30:661-666, 1992.
18. Hippocrates: On the articulations. In Adams R (ed): *The Genuine Works of Hippocrates. Translated from Greek with a Preliminary Discourse and Annotations*, vol 2. New York, William Wood, 1986, pp 75-156.
19. Hoen TLI: A method of skeletal traction for treatment of fracture dislocation of cervical vertebrae. *Arch Neurol Psychiatry* 36:158-161, 1936.
20. Johnson RM, Murphy MJ, Southwick WO: Surgical approaches to the spine. In Rothman RH, Simeone FA (eds): *The Spine*, ed 3. Philadelphia, WB Saunders, 1992, pp 1639-1643.
21. Johnson RM, Hart DL, Simmons ET, et al: Cervical orthosis: a study comparing their effectiveness in restricting cervical motion in normal subjects. *J Bone Joint Surg* 59A:332-339, 1977.
22. Lemons VR, Wagner FC: Stabilization of subaxial cervical spinal injuries. *Surg Neurol* 39:511-518, 1993.
23. Levine AM, Edwards CC: Fractures of the atlas. *J Bone Joint Surg* 73A:680-691, 1991.
24. Levine AM, Rhyne AL: Traumatic spondylolisthesis of the axis. *Semin Spine Surg* 3:47-60, 1991.
25. Lewis RC Jr: *Handbook of Traction, Casting, and Splinting Techniques*. Philadelphia, Lippincott-Raven, 1977, pp 20-26.
26. Marshall L, Knowlton S, Garfin SR, et al: Deterioration following spinal cord injury: a multicenter study. *J Neurosurg* 66:400-404, 1987.
27. Matthew JA, Mills SB, Jenkins VM, et al: Back pain and sciatica: controlled trials of manipulative, traction, sclerosant and epidural injections. *Br J Rheum* 26:416-423, 1987.
28. McKenzie KG: Fracture, dislocation, and fracture-dislocation of the spine. *Canad Med Assoc J* 32:263-269, 1935.
29. Nickel VL, Perry J, Garrett A, et al: The halo: a spinal skeletal traction fixation device. *J Bone Joint Surg* 50A:1400-1409, 1968.
30. Pal B, Mangion P, Hossain MA, Diffey BL: A controlled trial of continuous lumbar traction in the treatment of back pain and sciatica. *Br J Rheumatol* 25:181-183, 1986.
31. Perry J, Nickel VL: Total cervical spine fusion for neck paralysis. *J Bone Joint Surg* 41A:37-60, 1959.
32. Quebec Task Force on Spinal Disorders: Scientific approach to the assessment and management of activity related spinal disorders: a monograph for clinicians. Report of the Quebec Task Force on Spinal Disorders. *Spine* 12:S1-S59, 1987.
33. Rizzolo SJ, Vaccaro AR, Cotler JM: Cervical spine trauma, review. *Spine* 19:2288-2298, 1994.
34. Rizzolo SJ, Piazza MR, Cotler JM, et al: Intervertebral disk injury complicating cervical spine trauma. *Spine* 16:S 187-189, 1991.
35. Ruflin G, Jeannerett B, Magrel F: Tetraplegia following cervical spine fusion. Cervical Spine Research Society Meeting, St. Gallen, Switzerland, 1989.

36. Schneider RC: Cervical traction, with evaluation of methods, and treatment of complications. *Int Abstr Surg* 104:521-530, 1957.

37. Spence KF Jr, Decker MS, Sell KW: Bursting atlantal fractures associated with rupture of the transverse ligament. *J Bone Joint Surg* 52A:543-549, 1970.

38. Taylor AS: Fracture dislocation of the cervical spine. *Ann Surg* 90:321-341, 1929.

39. Vincke TH: A skull traction apparatus. *J Bone Joint Surg* 30:522-524, 1948.

# CHAPTER 146

# Orthoses: Complication Prevention and Management

Eric J. Woodard, Robert J. Kowalski, and Edward C. Benzel

Spinal bracing encompasses a variety of time-honored techniques that provide external support to injured or diseased segments of the vertebral column. The practice of bracing is as old as medicine itself, having appeared throughout history in the medical and surgical writings of Hippocrates, Galen, Pare, Levacher, and Andry.[2,48,66,69] In more modern times, Frankel[23] showed that bed rest and immobilization can be effective means of achieving bony fusion. The pressures of modern day medicine, however, require early mobilization to both decrease hospital length of stay and minimize medical complications.

Although many of the basic principles the ancients used have not changed significantly, great strides have been made in understanding both the art and science of orthotics in the era of modern medicine. This mainly reflects interval advances in materials technology and development of the field of spinal biomechanics.

A spinal orthotic or brace is a unique type of spinal instrumentation, with similar principles of application and complications of use as its internally fixed counterparts. For the modern spine surgeon prescribing an appropriate orthosis, the avoidance of device-related complications requires thorough consideration of the intended purpose of the device. The biomechanics of the spinal pathology of interest, the biomechanics of the appliances available, and a variety of patient-specific factors are key elements in orthotic decision making. This chapter emphasizes the principles of spinal bracing and device classification, reviews the complications of spinal bracing, and concludes with some of the new advances and developments.

## Principles of Spinal Bracing

By definition, all orthoses are externally applied devices that apply indirect forces to the spine for correcting or preventing deformity, stabilization, unloading, and/or supportive effects (e.g., massage, warmth, psychological comfort).[56] The most common element among these goals is motion restriction.

### The Spine As a Column

The manner by which orthoses exert restrictive effects is perhaps best understood in terms of column mechanics.

Several authors have described the spine as a complex variant of an ideal column with a fixed base and free upper end.[20,48] As a theoretical structure this "ideal" column is considered a homogeneous rod of constant composition, length, and cross-sectional area. Its behavior when loaded by a balanced axial force has been described mathematically by Euler's relationship for long-segment column dynamics:

$$P \propto \frac{E(A)^2}{L^2}$$

where $P$ is the magnitude of the applied axial load, $E$ is related to the modulus of elasticity of the column material, $A$ is the cross-sectional area of the column, and $L$ is the length[72] (Figure 146.1A). As the structure is progressively loaded, it initially shortens along its longitudinal axis. Once the axial load $P$ exceeds a critical load specific for the column, failure occurs by elastic buckling.[20] Methods for stabilizing or increasing the column axial bearing load capacity involve altering one or more of three variables: (1) column elasticity ($E$), (2) cross-sectional area ($A$), or (3) length ($L$).

Prototypical spinal orthoses consist of two end-fixation elements and a connecting longitudinal member (see Figure 146.1B). An example is the chair-back, thoracolumbosacral orthosis (TLSO) that purchases the rib cage with a thoracic band and the hips with a pelvic band. Uprights interconnect the thoracic and pelvic bands.[66] Sleeve-type orthoses, such as the clamshell TLSO (see below), incorporate these elements into their circumferential design.[2] In terms of column mechanics, braces add to the relative cross-sectional area and the total modulus of elasticity of the spine, thus creating a heterogeneous composite structure that shares the axial load.

Internal segmental fixation applies direct immobilization to spinal segments while most spinal orthoses apply their forces at some distance from the spine. There is an inverse relationship between the thickness of the soft tissue separating the spine from the inner surface of the orthosis and the resulting effectiveness of immobilization. Conformation of the brace to the body helps maintain the cylindrical body shell, thereby increasing the stability of the spine.[54,55,58,71] Also, longer braces provide more stability than shorter ones, and therefore the length-to-width ratio of the orthotic significantly affects efficacy (see Figure 146.1A).

Orthoses may also apply balanced transverse forces in a three-point bending arrangement that resists bending forces and thus contributes to axial load bearing.[2,8,72] The Jewett brace utilizes the aforementioned biomechanical advantage of a three-point bending force application produced by applying dorsal forces at the sternum and pubis, in combination with a ventral force at the affected thoracic or lumbar vertebra.[58,69] The long lever arms minimize the force required to produce a sufficient bending moment. Three-point bending also effectively divides the column functionally into two portions of smaller length increasing the critical failure load of the whole column to that of each segment (see Figure 146.1C).

An underlying principle in long bone splinting is the immobilization of the fractured bone from one joint above to one joint below the site of injury. Extrapolating

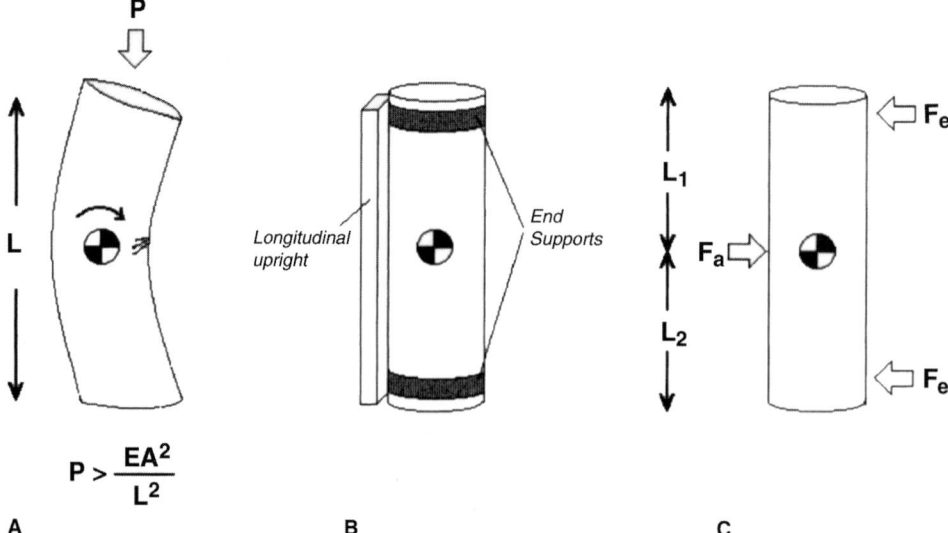

**Figure 146.1** **(A)** Elastic buckling of an ideal column of length $L$, under an axial load $P$. This column has failed by buckling because $P$ exceeds the critical load for this column as given by Euler's relationship, where $E$ is the modulus of elasticity for the column material, $A$ is the cross-sectional area of the column, and $L$ is the length. **(B)** Prototype spinal orthosis consisting of at least two end-stabilizing elements, such as circumferential bands, and an interconnecting longitudinal upright. **(C)** Three-point bending strategies of orthoses utilize two horizontal end forces, $F(e)$, which are balanced by a third oppositely directed force, $F(a)$, at or near the axis of rotation for the column. This effectively segments the column into two shorter columns, increasing their respective axial load-bearing capacities.

this concept to the axial skeleton, one may consider it to be composed of five segments, each of which may be considered a long bone (cranial, cervical, thoracic, lumbar, and sacropelvic) (see Figure 146.1A,B). Therefore one segment above and one segment below the unstable motion segment would be included in the brace.

Although the *in vivo* spine differs considerably from an ideal column in its specific composition and mechanical behavior, this model can serve as a useful paradigm for thinking about the mechanisms underlying the beneficial effects of orthoses.

### Dynamic and Passive Control

All orthoses control spinal motion by a combination of dynamic and passive mechanisms. Dynamic control describes the significant role of intrinsic musculature in actively stabilizing the spine and is the major component in the action of most orthoses. It has been demonstrated experimentally that opposing muscular forces significantly stiffen the spinal column, increasing its load-bearing capacity.[54] If isolated from its muscular support, the osseous and ligamentous spinal column holds only 2kg of axial load before failure by buckling.[48] In terms of a column, model muscular action directly affects the modulus of elasticity and relative cross-sectional area of the composite spinal column. Orthoses promote this muscular stabilization by tactile feedback that guides the patient to maintain proper positioning of the body. Pressure at the orthosis-skin contact site creates a reminder to maintain a safe position and limit unwanted gross body motion.[3,8,32,40,69] The patient therefore is able to prevent

undesirable motion of the spine by using only intrinsic muscular support guided by the orthosis. A stiffer, more securely worn appliance is more effective at limiting motion than a flexible brace because of the heightened sensation of resistance that it produces. Sypert and others have noted that the effectiveness of an appliance is directly related to the level of its discomfort.[66,69] This may, however, also contribute to higher levels of noncompliance.

Passive mechanisms for motion control are important in three-point bending mechanisms and are derived from intrinsic properties of the orthosis itself such as design, size, and material composition. The two common design elements of all orthoses are similar in principle to internal fixation constructs and include end-stabilizing elements (e.g., thoracic bands, pelvic bands) and longitudinal members or uprights that interconnect the end elements.[2] Passive mechanisms apply reactive forces to the body that oppose forces resulting from physiologic movements of the head or trunk; viscoelastic forces of ligaments, discs, and muscles; and gravitational force.[68] As summarized by White and Panjabi,[72] passive mechanical strategies form the basis for most orthotic techniques and include spinal distraction, fluid compression, balanced transverse force application, and skeletal fixation. Most appliances use a combination of techniques for spinal motion control.

### Distraction

Distracting the ends of a column is a useful means of correcting or preventing deformity. Its effectiveness depends on the efficiency of transmitting the distracting force directly to the column. Spinal distraction is a major strategy of internal fixation devices used for spinal correction and stabilization. This is best illustrated by the Harrington apparatus.[20] Distraction is also the technique used to reduce acutely unstable spine fractures with tong or halo traction. A braced column in distraction can be considered a composite of an externally applied distracting force plus the axial supporting properties of the original structure.

Distraction orthoses typically act on the head and thorax and cannot directly affect individual vertebral segments. Purchase of the head is either indirect with pads located at the mandible and the occiput (conventional orthoses) or direct by means of skull pins (halo-skeletal fixation). Thoracic purchase is obtained at the sternum and rib cage through a combination of pads, straps, or vest attachment. The effectiveness of a distraction orthosis depends on the efficiency of force transmission to the vertebral segment of interest and the mechanical rigidity of the orthosis material itself.[8] Inefficiency in transmitting external force to the spine has been termed "the transmitter problem" by White and Panjabi[72] and represents the loss of energy that occurs when force is applied to "low-stiffness, viscoelastic" structures such as overlying soft tissues, intervening normal joints, and ligaments. In the cervical area, distraction applied to the mandible is compromised by cushioning effects of soft tissue under the chin, the temporomandibular joint, cervical muscle tone, the C0-1 articulation, and each successive segmental articulation above the level at which the force is to have its effect (level of pathology). A more-rigid brace with a tighter fit improves the efficiency of transmitting force by compressing intervening soft tissue.[68] These factors paradoxically increase the risk of pressure injury to overlying soft tissues.[50] Skeletal fixation improves the effectiveness of force transmission by directly purchasing the skull, minimizing the risk of pressure injury in the head and neck region.

Point-of-contact problems also exist with thoracolumbar braces that involve the shoulder girdle, pectoral muscles, rib cage, and upper abdomen. The shoulders have a significant amount of overlying skin, fat, and muscle and are by definition highly mobile structures involved in arm movement. Orthoses relying on shoulder straps or pads to apply a counterforce cannot consistently distract the spine because of this mobility.[8] Changes in body position from sitting to supine also produce shoulder movement contributing to the difficulty of spinal distraction. Koch and Nickel[37] studied this effect in 6 patients wearing the halo apparatus by measuring the forces of distraction and compression exerted through the device with an attached strain gauge. Distraction force varied by greater than 20 lb in a halo vest and 30 lb in a halo cast when patients changed from supine to sitting positions. Similar variations in distraction with the halo device were noted during shoulder shrugging, coughing, sneezing, and deep breathing. Shoulder purchase is thus a highly variable means of anchoring the caudal end of a distraction orthosis.

Appliances with pads overlying the pectoral areas are compromised by the energy-absorbing effects of fat, muscle, and breast tissue. Movement of the chest occurs with arm motion in a similar manner to the shoulders. Although the rib cage is generally a stable structure, deep breathing, coughing, and sneezing produce significant motion that is directly transmitted by all devices purchasing the thorax. Orthoses extending below the thorax to the upper and lower abdomen are at an even greater disadvantage because of the highly elastic nature of this fluid- and air-filled region.[72]

Therefore all orthoses are limited in their ability to distract the spine because of inherent inefficiencies in force transmission at both the rostral and caudal ends of the devices and because of limitations in exerting pressure through soft tissues. Because distraction is poorly maintained by an orthosis, even when combined with halo fixation, bracing alone is generally not recommended if distraction is required to maintain reduction or to prevent dangerous instability.

### Fluid Compression

Fluid compression refers to the ability of a tight circumferential binder, such as a corset, to compress partially fluid-filled soft tissues surrounding the spine, thus creating a fluid cylinder.[56,72] Because of its mechanical incompressibility, a fluid-filled cylinder has axial load-bearing capacity. For a column model, this technique increases the aggregate cross-sectional area by converting soft tissues into load-bearing structures. Several studies have directly measured the effect of abdominal and thoracic cavity compression, noting little effect of compression on intra-abdominal pressure.[54,56,71] In Nachemson and Morris's[57] classic report, however, a 25% reduction in intradiscal pressure was observed in lumbar segments braced with an inflatable abdominal corset. The true unloading effect of fluid compression is thought to be a minor factor for orthotic thoracolumbar stabilization and is beneficial only for restricting sagittal plane motion.[56] Fluid compression is a strategy that is not applicable for the cervical spine, in which airway, vascular, and muscular tissues make up a relatively large proportion of the cross-sectional area of the neck and do not tolerate significant compression.[69]

### Transverse Loading

Balanced transverse loading describes a common and effective strategy for restricting spinal rotation and translation. Orthoses typically use a three-point bending force application arrangement with two horizontal reactive forces applied at the ends of the column in one direction and a third balancing force in the opposite direction at the fulcrum of the deformity[8,72] (see Figure 146.1C). Because the system is in equilibrium, the sum of all horizontal forces is zero. This prevents translation. Similarly, bending moments generated by the applied forces acting at the axis of rotation for the injured segment also equal zero if rotational motion is adequately controlled.[8] Keys to an effective transverse loading strategy include (1) identifying the axis of rotation at the level of injury or point of instability by using an appliance that is centered at or near this axis of rotation and (2) using an adequately long appliance that maximizes the length of the applied moment arm to control the spinal segment of interest.[8]

## Classification

Spinal orthoses are generally considered either conventional orthotics or skeletal fixators. Conventional devices are contact-type orthoses that control spinal motion through direct contact with the skin and soft tissues of the head, neck, thorax, abdomen, or pelvis. A contact orthosis may have only limited skin contact through discrete pads and straps or extensive surface area coverage (e.g., total contact orthosis). Examples of total contact devices are the Yale brace[30] and the molded clamshell TLSO (see below). Advantages of newer contact orthoses that use thermoplastic materials include ease of application, light weight, warmth, ventilation, ability to be removed for optimal hygiene, and patient acceptance.[9,53] All conventional devices provide some control of flexion and extension but are more limited in reducing lateral bending and rotation.[31] Additional drawbacks include poor patient compliance, excessive warmth causing sweating, variability of fit, and complications of skin or soft-tissue contact. All devices have limitations that must be balanced with their advantages. Each segment of the spine must be considered individually because of the variability of anatomy, mobility, and applicability of an orthosis.

Harris[28] reported the results of a consensus task force of orthotists, spine surgeons, and other health officials who set forth a common nomenclature for conventional spinal orthoses with the intent of standardizing communication among spine professionals and avoiding the plethora of eponyms describing individual appliances (Table 146.1). In this scheme, devices are classified into cervical orthoses (CO), cervicothoracic orthoses (CTO), TLSO, lumbosacral orthoses (LSO), or sacroiliac orthoses (SIO). This classification was intended to reflect the region of the spine immobilized by the device and has become the standard nomenclature of spinal orthotics since 1973. Krag[40] has recently expanded the cervical classification into four subcategories based on the specific anatomy of the region: cervical (CO), occipital-mandibular-cervical (OMC), occipital-mandibular-high thoracic (OMHT), and occipital-mandibular-low thoracic (OMLT).

### Cervical Orthoses

COs are basically soft foam or felt collars with minimal purchase of the mandible or occiput[40] (Figure 146.2A).

These collars are light, inexpensive, easy to use, and relatively comfortable to wear. Regrettably, they offer negligible resistance to cervical motion in any plane of motion, functioning only to remind patients to limit voluntary extremes of neck movement.[15,29,34] Because they are only supportive, cervical collars are inappropriate for patients with bony instability. They can provide tactile generated support of cervical musculature and psychological comfort in cases of myofascial strain or sprain or in straightforward postoperative patients without instability.[53]

### Occipital-Mandibular-Cervical Orthoses

OMC orthoses are hard plastic collars that are more rigid than foam collars and offer slightly better purchase of the mandible or occiput[40] (see Figure 146.2B). Most usage is as a prophylactic measure, in conjunction with a backboard, in acute trauma situations. They have no thoracic extension and thus, while offering an improved cranial point of fixation, they lack a true caudal one. The addition of an adjustable chin or occipital piece increases resistance to flexion or extension to a mild degree.[15] Lateral bending and rotation are poorly controlled with these braces.[31] Like the soft collars, OMC orthoses do not provide significant immobilization to the cervical spine and are not recommended for patients with instability.

### Occipital-Mandibular-High Thoracic Orthoses

When the brace is extended caudally to the shoulders and a more rigid material is used (e.g., the Philadelphia collar), movement is restricted. As with previous devices, flexion and extension are the motions most effectively limited, and there is a general trend of decreased motion at all levels with further extension of the caudal fixation point. However, this limitation of motion can produce a parallelogram effect. The ends remain fixed along the spinal axis, but motion can occur by the rostral segment translating ventrally and the caudal segment translating dorsally, or vice versa.

Examples of OMHT orthoses are the widely used Philadelphia collar, the four-poster brace, the two-poster brace (e.g., Guilford, Duke), and several newly available hard plastic collars[40] (see Figure 146.2C-F). All OMHT appliances control head movement with occipital and mandibular supports and have better upper thoracic

| **TABLE 146.1** | |
|---|---|
| **Classification of Orthoses** | |
| **Appliance Category** | **Examples** |
| Cervical orthoses (CO) | |
| Cervical collars | Foam collar |
| Occipital-mandibular-cervical | Thomas collar, Queen Anne collar |
| Occipital-mandibular-high thoracic | Philadelphia collar, Miami J collar, Guilford two-poster brace, four-poster brace |
| Cervicothoracic orthoses (CTO) | Yale brace, Minerva brace, SOMI (sternal-occipital-mandibular immobilizer) brace |
| Thoracolumbosacral orthoses (TLSO) | Clamshell thermoplastic body jacket, Jewett extension brace, Boston overlap brace |
| Lumbosacral orthoses (LSO) | Lumbosacral corset, chair-back orthosis, Knight brace |
| Sacroiliac orthoses (SIO) | Sacroiliac corset with perineal straps |
| Halo devices | Vest halo, four-pad halo, thermoplastic Minerva body jacket |

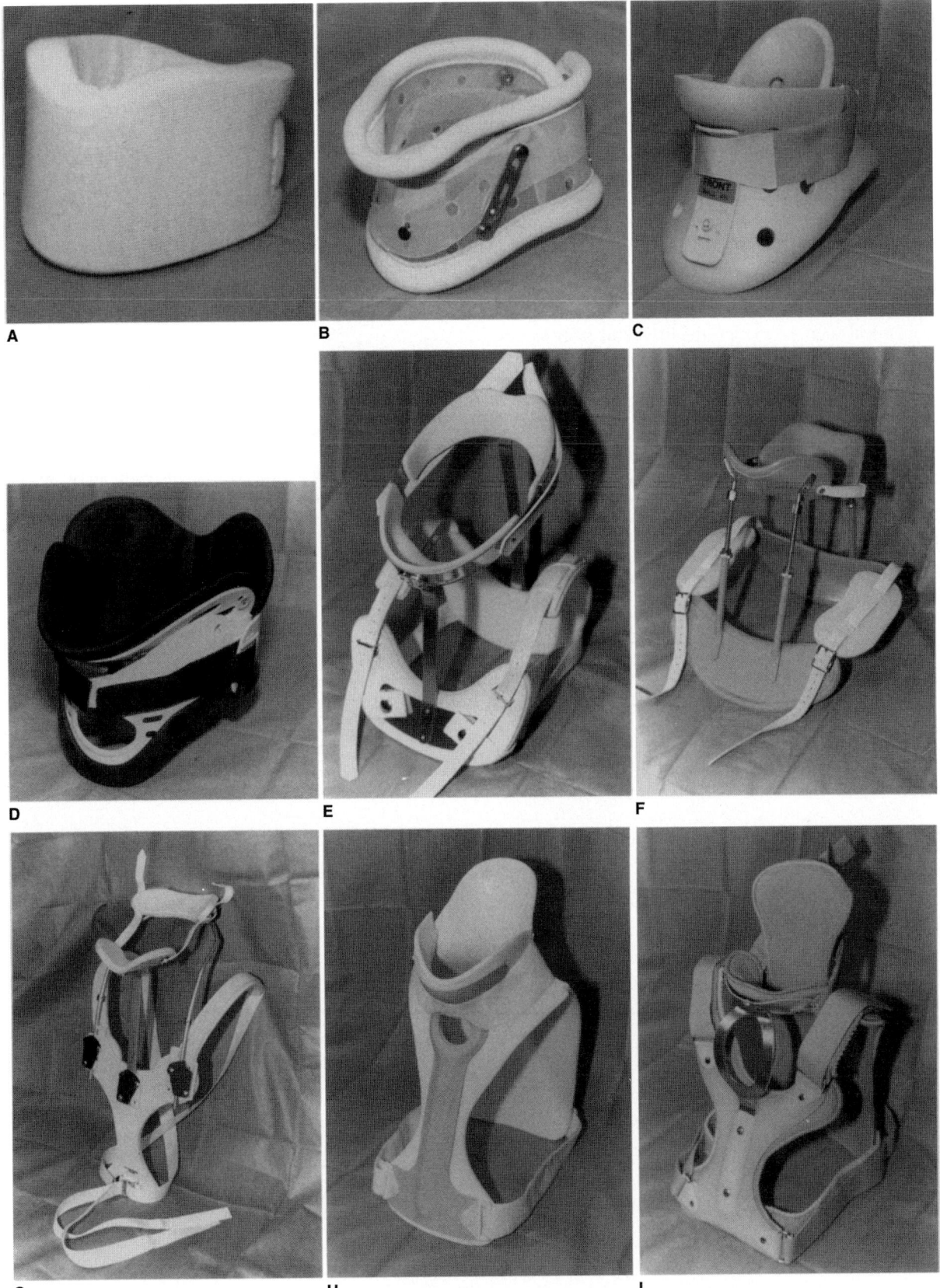

**Figure 146.2** Cervical and cervicothoracic orthoses. **(A)** Foam collar. **(B)** Thomas collar.
**(C)** Philadelphia collar. **(D)** Miami J collar. **(E)** Two-poster Guilford brace. **(F)** Four-poster brace.
**(G)** Sternal-occipital-mandibular immobilizer (SOMI). **(H)** Yale orthosis. **(I)** Minerva brace.

purchase than collars because of longer length. Like the collars, they are relatively easy to apply, are lightweight, and are relatively inexpensive.

The popular Philadelphia collar is a Plastazote foam device reinforced with hard plastic. It is available in different sizes and consists of front and back halves connected by Velcro straps.[66] Although generally well tolerated, it can be quite hot to wear, causing significant sweating and secondary skin maceration. The Plastazote material is less rigid than other OMHT appliances such as the poster orthoses.[22] Despite its limitations, Johnson *et al.*[31] found this device to be as effective in controlling upper (C0-3) flexion-extension as the rigid OMHT orthoses. It was less effective in restricting flexion-extension in the mid- and lower cervical segments (Figure 146.3) and poor in controlled rotation and lateral bending at all levels. The device is frequently used for patients with mild cervical injuries and in postoperative patients with minor instability. Polin

*et al.*[60] have recently evaluated the use of the Philadelphia collar and the halo device in odontoid fractures. Their findings indicated no significant difference in the rate of fracture healing between the two orthoses for both type II and type III fractures and suggested that the less-invasive collar may be adequate in this setting. Modifications of the Philadelphia collar have been developed that maintain cervical immobilization yet improve the comfort and convenience of a plastic removable collar. The Miami J collar is an example that is more rigid than the Philadelphia collar at all cervical levels and has the added benefit of removable chin and occipital pads for improved comfort and hygiene.

### Occipital-Mandibular-Low Thoracic Orthoses

Extending the orthotic further caudally to include the thorax adds a three-point bending moment, which provides a significant biomechanical advantage. Such devices (e.g., SOMI, four-poster, and cervico-thoracic brace) substantially restrict motion in the mid to lower cervical spine.

The OMLT orthoses are represented by the sternal-occipital-mandibular immobilizer (SOMI), the extended Philadelphia collar (Yale brace), and the Minerva brace (see Figure 146.2*G-I*). These devices are essentially longer versions of the OMHT appliances with the addition of circumferential chest straps. In general they are the most rigid of the conventional orthoses because of their increased length and better thoracic purchase[22,31] (see Figures 146.3 and 146.4). Advantages of the OMHT orthoses include best immobilization of flexion-extension and rotation of the conventional braces, noninvasiveness, and ease of application. They are, however, more cumbersome and uncomfortable to wear than the smaller appliances. With the exception of the Yale brace, they are

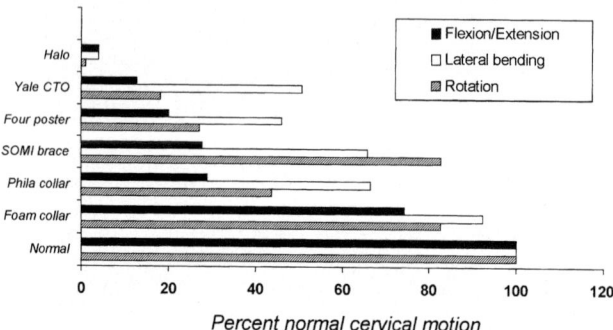

**Figure 146.3** Overall motion allowed in cervical orthoses. (*From Johnson RM, Hart DL, Simmons EF, et al: Cervical orthoses: a study comparing their effectiveness in restricting cervical motion in normal subjects.* J Bone Joint Surg 59A:332-339, 1977.)

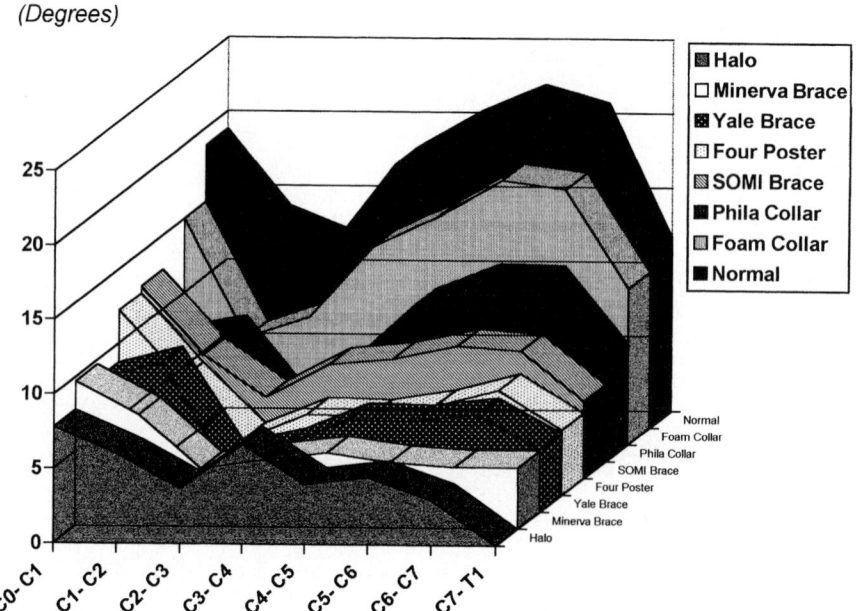

**Figure 146.4** Segmental motion allowed in cervical orthoses. (*Adapted from Johnson RM, Owen JR, Hart DL, Callahan RA: Cervical orthoses: a guide to their selection and use.* Clin Orthop Rel Res 154:34-45, 1988.)

moderately expensive and still have limited control of lateral bending.[30,31]

## Thoracolumbosacral Orthoses

Representative TLSOs include the clamshell thermoplastic body jacket and the thoracolumbar extension orthosis or Jewett brace (Figure 146.5A-C). There are a number of modifications of these two basic designs. By definition these appliances apply three-point bending forces at the upper thorax and pelvis and at the midportion of the brace across the thoracolumbar junction.[2] This class of orthotic is best suited for restricting thoracolumbar and lumbar gross-body motion[43] and poorly controls low lumbar and sacral segments.[3] Molded appliances are particularly useful for thoracolumbar junction trauma in which the total contact feature helps to control lateral bending and rotation. Velcro straps and thermoplastic materials have greatly improved the ease of wear and comfort of TLSOs in recent years, improving both compliance and effectiveness.

Jewett braces primarily control flexion-extension and are thus often used for minor flexion compression injuries such as stable compression fractures.[66] More-severe thoracolumbar injuries were recently studied by Patwardhan et al.[59] with a finite element computer model. The Jewett brace was effective at preventing deformity under physiologic flexion loading with injuries resulting in less than 50% normal spinal stiffness (single-column injuries). With injuries that reduced stiffness to between 50% and 85% (two-column injuries) and those greater than 85% (three-column injuries), the brace was ineffective for resisting spinal deformation.[59]

## Lumbosacral Orthoses

Perhaps the most frequently prescribed appliances, LSOs are also the most controversial because of their questionable effectiveness.[56] Lumbosacral corsets with or without stays, chair-back braces, and the Knight brace are representative[66] (see Figure 146.5D). LSOs stabilize the lumbar and sacral regions by encircling the upper abdomen and rib cage and the pelvis. Because of the difficulty in firmly purchasing these areas, three-point bending is probably not a major mechanism in the action of this class of orthosis. Fluid compression likely has a role, although measurements of intra-abdominal pressure while wearing the devices have been inconsistent.[54]

To quantify the effect of bracing on segmental motion, Norton and Brown[58] measured lumbar motion in volunteers by following the motion of K-wires inserted into the spinous processes. Movement at the lumbosacral junction was paradoxically greater while sitting with an LSO than without the brace. The effect was thought to be secondary to stress concentration at the caudal end of the supported segment. Waters and Morris[71] studied lumbosacral stabilization in orthoses by monitoring paraspinal muscle electromyography. Although back muscle activity during standing was reduced with an LSO, activity during fast walking was greater, possibly because of altered pelvis rotation. Lantz and Schultz[43] measured gross trunk motion and myoelectrical activity in five volunteers wearing the lumbosacral corset, a chair-back brace, and a molded TLSO during standing and sitting. Gross upper body motion was reduced up to 20% in flexion and 45% in extension, lateral bending, and rotation. The TLSO was overall the most effective device tested. Myoelectrical activity, however, varied widely, ranging from a 9% reduction to a 44% increase.[44] Axelsson et al.[3] used stereophotogrammetry in 7 patients to analyze the effects of the LSO and the molded TLSO on intersegmental lumbar spine movement. Neither device had any effect in restricting segmental translation in sagittal, vertical, or transverse planes. They concluded that the orthoses only serve as a reminder to the patient to restrict gross trunk movements.[3]

These observations substantiate clinical experience that the LSO and TLSO do not adequately stabilize segmental motion of the lower lumbar spine and lumbosacral junction. They do appear to limit gross trunk movement, which is thought to be their major mechanism of action.[43]

Consistent with the principles of long bone splinting discussed earlier, control of the pelvis may be necessary to restrict movement at the lumbosacral junction.[8,69] Fidler and Plasmans[21] have shown that including the thigh with an extension (thigh spica) reduces gross pelvis motion more significantly than a conventional LSO. Segmental translation with axial loading, however, is not affected by this device.[4] In clinical practice, patient acceptance of thigh spica orthoses is limited because of severe restriction of walking and sitting (see Figure 146.5E).

## Sacroiliac Orthoses

Rarely used today, sacroiliac orthoses were developed for pelvic instability after traumatic or postpartum pelvic disruption.[3] They are not effective at reducing motion but rather serve as a kinesthetic device to remind the patient to maintain proper pelvic posture.

## Halo Skeletal Fixation

Halo fixation is currently the most effective method of externally immobilizing the cervical spine.[40] Its basic components consist of a halo ring (or crown) for pin fixation of the skull, a plastic vest or pads secured with straps that encircle the thorax, and two or more upright connecting posts. A variety of commercial products are available that incorporate design features that reflect clinical experience and advances in metal and plastic technology[41] (Figure 146.6).

Halo bracing has several advantages over the conventional orthoses. The skin and soft tissues of the mandible and occiput are unencumbered so that it is cooler about the head and neck. The jaw is free, which allows easier eating and speaking as well as prevention of temporomandibular joint pain. Skin irritation and breakdown are avoided in the head and neck area. In difficult cases, the device may also encourage compliance both for reducing excessive activity and keeping the orthosis in place. Halo use has been credited with enabling earlier ambulation of patients with severe cervical instability, thereby allowing a more rapid entry into rehabilitation and decreasing secondary complications of immobility.

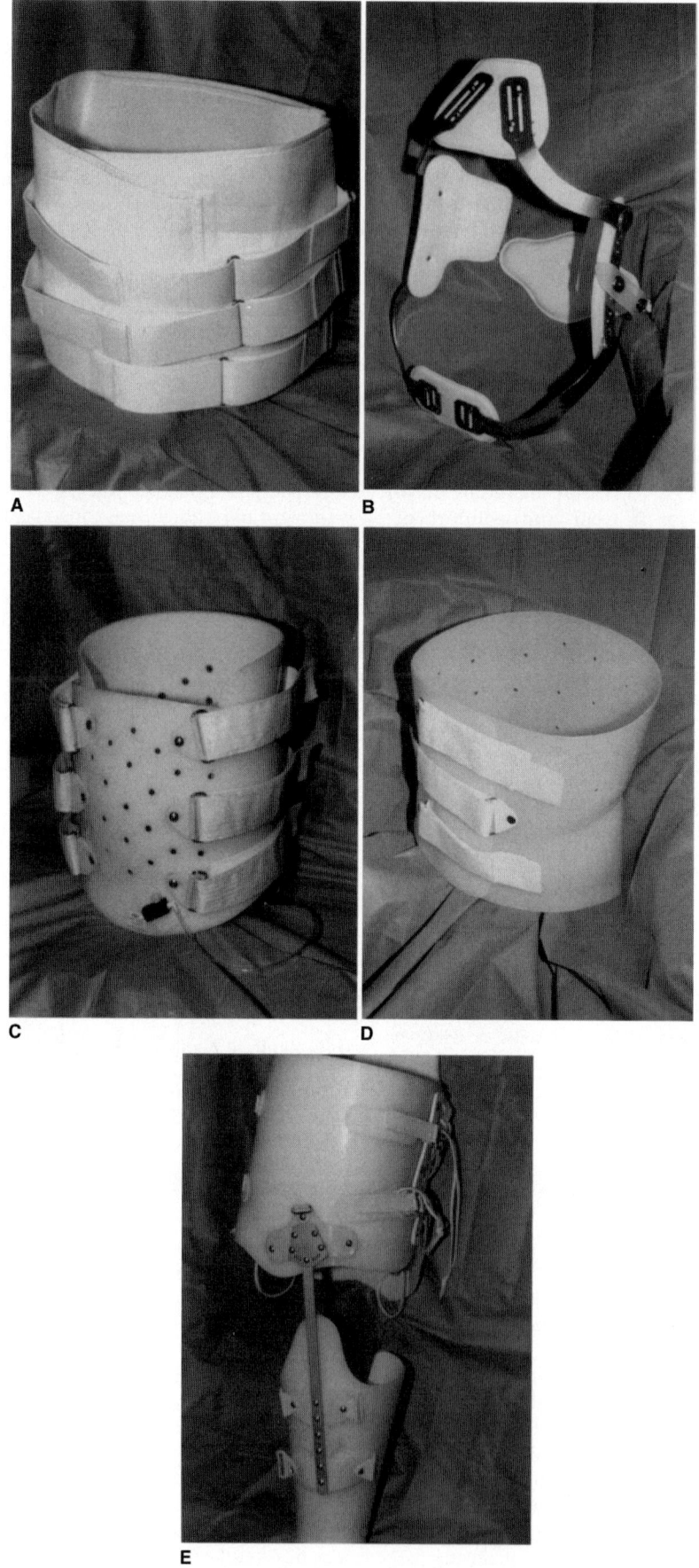

**Figure 146.5** Thoracolumbar orthoses. **(A)** Lumbosacral corset (LSO). **(B)** Jewett hyperextension brace (TLSO). **(C)** Clamshell-type molded thoracolumbosacral orthosis (TLSO). **(D)** Boston overlap brace (TLSO). **(E)** Clamshell TLSO with thigh extension (TLSO with thigh spica).

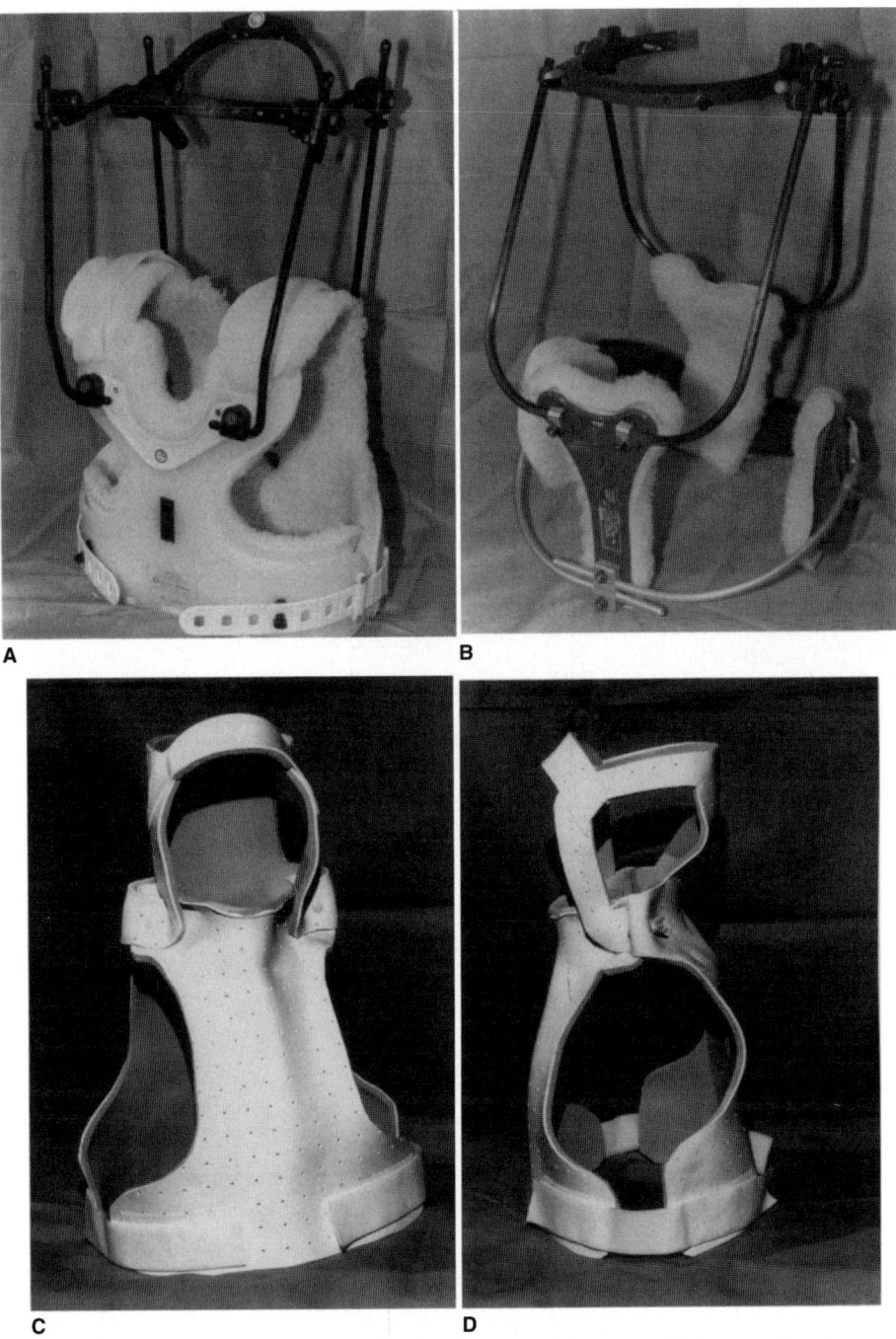

**Figure 146.6** Halo-type orthoses. **(A)** Standard halo vest. **(B)** Four-pad halo vest. **(C-D)** Thermoplastic Minerva body jacket (TMBJ).

Clearly the major advantage to the use of the halo is the degree of stabilization that can be achieved. Johnson *et al.*[31] demonstrated a reduction of lateral bending and axial rotation in 5 patients to 1% of that of normal volunteers. Whole cervical spine flexion-extension was similarly reduced to 4% of normal (see Figure 146.4). Although the halo affords a high degree of stability, persistent significant motion does occur. Koch and Nickel[37] studied halo immobilization in 6 patients with fractures, demonstrating an average of 31% normal motion for cervical spine flexion and extension at each motion segment. The greatest move-

ment occurred between C2 and C3, with the least at C7 to T1. They emphasized the importance of body position or activity such as lying, bending, or sitting in transmitting undesirable force to the cervical spine through the halo itself. Although distraction is frequently useful to maintain reduction of highly unstable spines, the ability of the halo to provide fixed distraction is limited because of this significant effect of trunk position and patient activity.[37] It should not be used as a principal distraction device.

Paradoxical spinal motion described as snaking accounts for most of the undesirable movement that occurs with the halo.[8,32] It is the segmental motion that occurs while the end points of the braced region remain relatively fixed along the spinal axis and involves simultaneous capital protraction and flexion of the upper cervical spine with extension of lower cervical segments (e.g., C0-3 flexion with C5-T1 extension on attempted neck flexion). The measured whole cervical spine movement from C0 to T1 may be minimal, yet individual midcervical segments move significantly without effective fixation[8] (Figure 146.7). Increasing the length and the conformation of a brace minimizes the parallelogram deformation of the spine and the snaking phenomenon. This also maximizes the biomechanical effect of the brace.

The thermoplastic Minerva body jacket (TMBJ)[9] is an alternative to halo bracing (see Figure 146.6). This device consists of a bivalved molded plastic shell that has contact-type purchase of the thorax like a standard halo vest and lateral extensions that incorporate a mandibular support, an occipital support, and a circumferential headband.[53] Benzel et al.[9] compared its effectiveness with the halo in 10 patients with cervical spine injuries. Each patient was tested in whole cervical spine flexion-extension with both the halo and the TMBJ. Their results indicate improved control of individual vertebral angulation at all levels except C1-C2 with the TMBJ versus the halo. There was less paradoxical movement with the molded device, indicating a higher overall level of immobilization. Eight of 10 patients reported improved comfort.[9] Maiman et al.[51]

also studied the TMBJ in 20 normal volunteers for controlling flexion-extension, lateral bending, and axial rotation. The TMBJ significantly reduced motion as compared with unrestricted controls in all planes except rotation. It was more effective than the halo in restricting flexion-extension and lateral bending when compared with the historical data of Johnson et al.[31] and Wang et al.[70] In practice, the effectiveness of the device depends on the ability to achieve an excellent fit, which requires an expert orthotist familiar with its use. The TMBJ also suffers the disadvantages of any contact orthosis such as skin irritation, mandible obstruction, discomfort, and warmth.

## Complications of Spinal Bracing

Complications of bracing can be organized into three general categories: skin and soft-tissue injuries, ineffective stabilization, and a variety of miscellaneous complications, largely related to halo skeletal fixation (Table 146.2).

### Skin and Soft-Tissue Injury

All orthoses require some degree of skin-appliance connection to apply forces indirectly to the vertebral column. Excessive pressure on the skin causes ischemia with resulting pain, breakdown, and/or frank ulceration. Pressure is defined as force per unit area and is the major cause of decubitus ulcers occurring over bony prominences in patients with poor mobility and prolonged recumbency.[68] Tissue breakdown is normally avoided because of painful exteroceptive feedback that occurs when skin pressure is prolonged. Discomfort stimulates subconscious shifting of position to unload the dependent body part. Altered sensation (Figure 146.8), consciousness, or mobility impairs normal protective mechanisms[1,8]

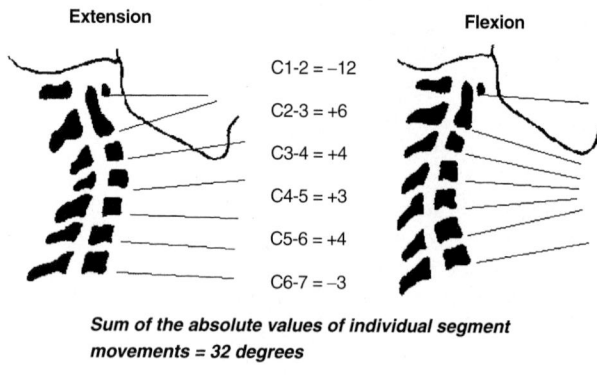

Extension     Flexion

C1-2 = –12
C2-3 = +6
C3-4 = +4
C4-5 = +3
C5-6 = +4
C6-7 = –3

*Sum of the absolute values of individual segment movements = 32 degrees*

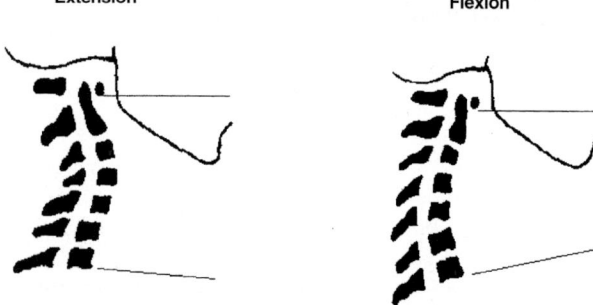

Extension     Flexion

*Total C0-T1 flexion-extension = 2 degrees*

**Figure 146.7** Paradoxical motion ("snaking") induced by the halo device. Capital flexion with simultaneous lower cervical extension produces significant absolute motion at each segment despite minimal overall motion measured between C0 and T1. *(Adapted from Benzel EC: Spinal orthotics. In Menezes AH, Sonntag VKH (eds): Principles of Spinal Surgery. New York, McGraw-Hill, 1996, 181-190.)*

| TABLE 146.2 |
| --- |
| **Complications of Orthoses** |

**Skin and Soft-Tissue Injury**
Pain
Skin/wound breakdown
Muscle atrophy, contracture formation

**Ineffective Stabilization**
Inappropriate orthotic for spinal level
Loss of reduction—halo
   Distraction, paradoxical movement ("snaking")

**Miscellaneous**
Halo pin site complications
   Overdistraction
   Dysphagia
Cardiopulmonary complications
   Pulmonary edema, reduced vital capacity
   Venous hypertension
      Varicose veins, hemorrhoids, extremity edema
   Gastrointestinal dysfunction
      Superior mesenteric artery syndrome
   Psychological dysfunction
      Secondary gain, adjustment disorders

and can lead to a variety of possible injuries, depending on the severity of the ischemic deficit[19] (Table 146.3). Careful and frequent inspection of skin contact areas beneath braces is mandatory to identify the earliest stages of injury and allow intervention before irreversible skin damage occurs.[1]

Because of their significant effect on patient management and the economic impact of treatment, decubitus ulcers have been the focus of a number of clinical and basic science investigations.[50] Important factors identified experimentally for developing pressure sores include the magnitude and duration of the applied pressure, associated shear or friction of the skin, tissue distribution, skin moisture, hydration, and general nutrition.[1,50,68] Tissue damage from pressure occurs by microvessel occlusion that impairs perfusion and leads to secondary ischemia. External pressures exceeding normal tissue capillary perfusion pressure (32mmHg)[42] will interrupt blood flow, leading to ischemia and permanent tissue death if unre-

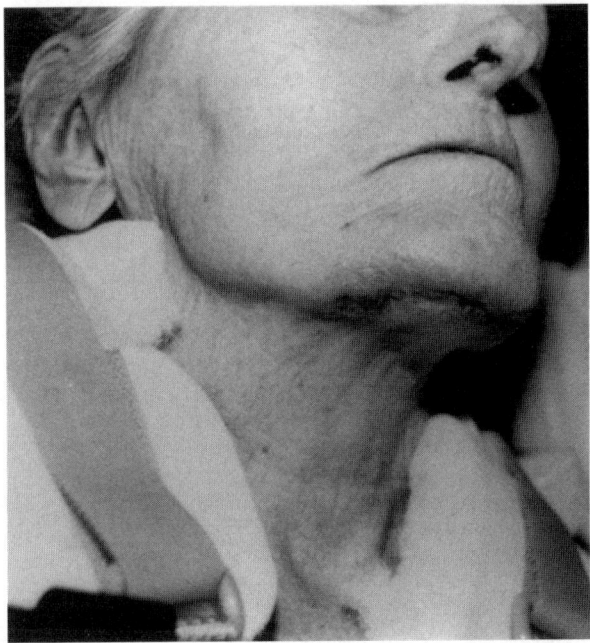

**Figure 146.8** Soft-tissue breakdown beneath the mandible in a 72-year-old woman with multiple myeloma after using the Minerva brace. Predisposing factors included pressure being applied over the prominent bony mandible, thin skin and subcutaneous tissue in this area, and poor nutrition from chronic disease.

lieved. The duration of application is inversely related to the absolute pressure.[50] Kosiak[39] has reported the relationship between duration and the risk of pressure sores in a series of studies that used a canine model. Pressures of 500mmHg applied to the skin surface for only 2 hours produced ulceration, whereas 150mmHg was tolerated for up to 12 hours. Pressure as low as 70mmHg, however, was sufficient to produce microscopic ischemic changes after only 2 hours. Thus a continuum of injury may be seen that is related to increasing pressure magnitude and duration.

Surface friction potentiates the risk of ulceration by creating shear in deeper soft tissues. Shear leads to capillary occlusion by kinking, stretching, and tearing and produces ischemia at lower absolute externally applied pressures.[1,68] A study in a porcine model compared the threshold for skin damage from a force applied with and without linear shear.[18] Ulceration occurred at less than one sixth the external pressure (45mmHg) when combined with shear than without added shearing forces (290mmHg). Surface friction also can abrade outer layers of skin, especially if the subcutaneous tissues are very firm or tightly tethered to the underlying bone.[68] Friction abrasions then further contribute to decubitus ulcer formation. Adequate systemic hydration can mitigate the effects of shear by increasing the mechanical resilience of skin.[1]

An important consequence of pressure in advanced stage injuries is the effect on muscle. Muscle is more vulnerable to ischemia than is skin, because it typically develops necrosis earlier and more extensively.[50] Pressure distribution between the skin surface and the underlying bone concentrates force at the deep bone-muscle junction because of the abrupt tissue transition from bone to muscle. Necrosis tends to be maximal at the level of the underlying bone and decreases gradually outward toward more superficial layers.[17] External skin ulceration is usually only the external manifestation of a more extensive soft-tissue injury.[1] Although vulnerable to ischemia, muscle and fat layers paradoxically are important for dissipating force through the energy-absorbing process of elastic deformation. Thus, poorly covered bony prominences such as the sacrum, greater trochanter, and heels that are without significant soft-tissue layers are particularly vulnerable to skin breakdown. Pressure dissipation plays a major role in the beneficial effects of muscle flap transfers used to cover ulcerated bony prominences.[45]

The barrier function of skin is compromised by prolonged exposure of its surface to moisture. Moisture from incontinence or sweating overhydrates the outer layer of the stratum corneum, reducing its mechanical strength

| **TABLE 146.3** | | |
|---|---|---|
| **Stages of Pressure Sore Development** | | |
| Stage I | Hyperemia | Nonblanching erythema appearing within 30 minutes of pressure that disappears within 1 hour |
| Stage II | Ischemia | Seen after 2-6 hours of continuous pressure; erythema requires 36 hours to resolve |
| Stage III | Necrosis | Skin appears blue and firm after 6 hours of pressure; skin changes do not resolve |
| Stage IV | Ulceration | Occurs 2 weeks after stage III injury appearing as ulcer formation and infection; may involve underlying bone |

(Adapted from Edberg EL, Cerny K, Stauffer ES: Prevention and treatment of pressure sores. *Phys Ther* 53: 246, 1973, with permission.)

and resistance to bacterial permeation.[1] Increased temperature caused by impaired heat convection further allows microflora to proliferate and reduce the tissue pH. These changes result in epidermal sloughing, deep layer exposure, and microbial invasion of the underlying dermis, all of which promote ulceration.

Similar conditions frequently threaten skin integrity beneath occlusive spinal orthoses. Braces that poorly dissipate pressure, impair proper hygiene, create significant shear, and allow moisture build-up are most likely to promote tissue injury. Regrettably, little data for the frequency of skin ulceration exist for conventional orthoses other than that noted in anecdotal reports. For the halo device, pressure sores have been observed in 4% to 11% of patients and usually occur over the scapulae or rib cage.[12,24,26,47] Practical means to prevent these complications include optimizing the orthotic fit, maximizing the applied surface area of the brace to dissipate pressure, and avoiding appliances with sharp or uneven edges.[68] As stated, areas over bony prominences have minimal overlying soft tissue to distribute pressure by elastic energy absorption and are most vulnerable to ischemic injury under an orthosis. Adding special padding or cutting out a hole immediately over a prominence may avoid breakdown by shifting pressure away from high-risk areas to more tolerant tissues.

Hygiene is a function of patient education and proper nursing and is greatly facilitated by modern, removable appliances.[1] Patients should be fully educated as to the risks and warning signs of early skin ulceration and should participate actively in its prevention. Special problems occur with anesthetic skin that does not produce noxious feedback to warn of excessive or prolonged pressure[8] (Figure 146.9). This can also occur in obtunded or comatose patients. Shear under an orthosis can be avoided by a properly fitted brace and by maintaining a moisture-absorbing layer between the skin and appliance at all times. A cotton undergarment that can be changed daily is useful in this regard both for hygiene and moisture reduction.

In the nutritionally depleted patient, general protein wasting may lead to tissue edema, altered tissue repair, and compromised antimicrobial mechanisms. Edema impairs tissue oxygenation, decreases elasticity, and reduces skin resistance to mechanical deformation. Marker serum proteins such as transferrin and albumin and anergy to injected antigens are common and useful indicators of nutritional status. Assessment of nutritional status and correction if inadequate may prevent or delay developing pressure sores associated with orthoses.[1]

Postoperative wounds are especially prone to skin edge maceration and secondary bacterial invasion if covered by occlusive orthoses, because of the combined negative effects of sweating, external pressure, and shearing forces[52] (Figure 146.10). Frequently changed, dry dressings over the wound reduce these effects and prevent most orthosis-associated wound infections. Alternatively, a noncontact or ventilated device may reduce this risk.

Other soft-tissue complications of spinal bracing include muscle atrophy and contracture formation.[56,69] Atrophy rapidly occurs after even brief periods of disuse because of a lack of normal motion and tone. Resulting

loss of bulk and weakness may be profound, requiring progressive weaning from the appliance and active rehabilitation after bony healing is established. Although commonly observed in this setting, atrophy associated with spinal bracing has not been thoroughly quantified. Contractures

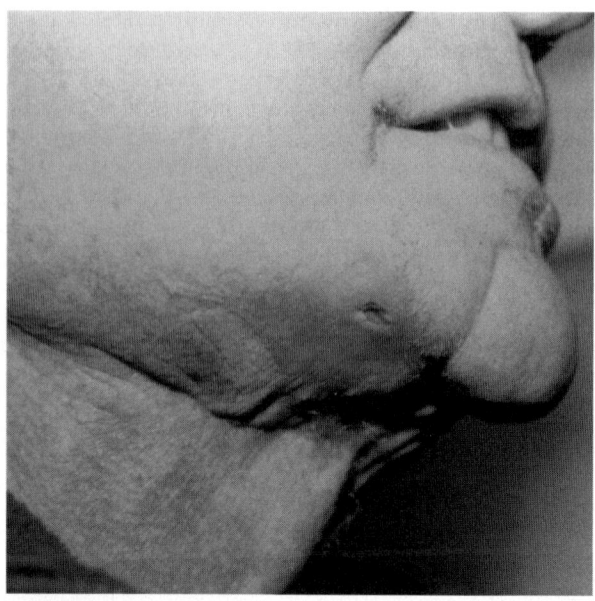

**Figure 146.9** Soft tissue ulceration beneath the mandible in a 56-year-old man using a Philadelphia collar. The skin over this area was anesthetic because of a prior radical neck dissection for laryngeal carcinoma. Anesthetic areas of skin under braces are at significant risk for breakdown, especially for patients with limited mobility.

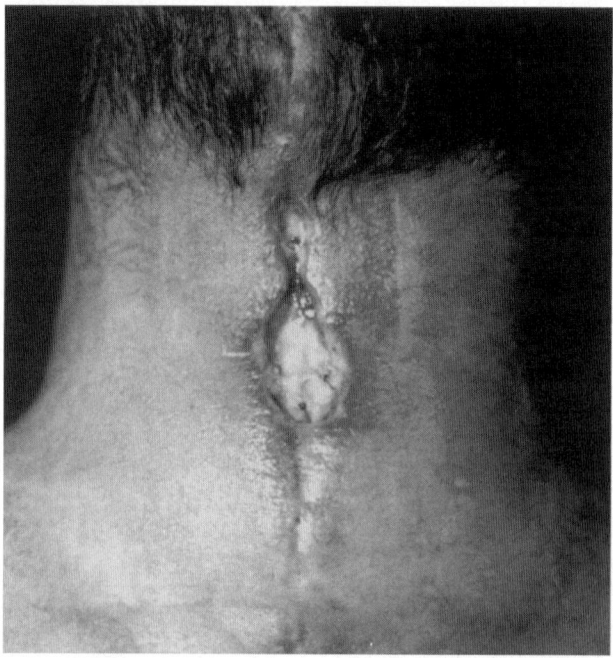

**Figure 146.10** Wound breakdown and infection in a 38-year-old man after dorsal cervical surgery, braced with a Miami J collar. External pressure and shear applied over wound edges compromise healing and risk secondary superficial infection. Orthoses that are occlusive further challenge this process by trapping moisture and heat that promote proliferation of skin microflora.

are rigid deformities of a joint caused by immobilization or unbalanced effector forces across the joint. With time, the associated muscles can become painful and permanently fibrotic. Contractures are occasionally observed with long-term cervical bracing or halo use and primarily involve limited cervical rotation. Lind et al.[47] have reported up to 80% residual neck pain and stiffness after halo bracing, which probably represents minor cervical contracture formation.

Korovessis et al.[38] recently reported an interesting soft-tissue complication associated with long-term use of a modified Boston brace in young women braced for scoliosis. The appliance uses a rigid pelvic band that covers the dorsolateral hips over the greater trochanters and is open over the lower flank region. Prolonged use (over 6 months) led to upward migration of the lateral trochanteric fat pads in 23% of 300 subjects, resulting in significant cosmetic deformity. Suction lipoplasty was required in 74% of this group. Pressure atrophy of developing fat deposits with local redistribution appears to account for this phenomenon.[38]

## Ineffective Stabilization

As previously discussed, most conventional braces poorly transmit force directly to the spine and are limited in their ability to restrict segmental motion and/or unload the vertebral column. Long conventional appliances spanning many segments across the level of interest are most effective for controlling gross body movement because of significant three-point bending.[43] Mismatch between the point of spinal instability and the optimal effective range for a particular brace (typically at its midpoint) accounts for a common cause of ineffective brace selection. Similarly, extensive instability or injuries that are only reduced by axial distraction are not usually amenable to conventional bracing. Most studies of orthotic effects involve kinematic evaluation of stability in single trials of spine motion, usually in healthy subjects. The questions of clinical effectiveness are less well answered because of limited availability of longitudinal outcome data for various devices.

Despite its limited effect on segmental motion, the TLSO may improve fusion success by restricting gross trunk motion. Johnsson et al.[33] recently studied the effect of a molded TLSO in 22 patients undergoing dorsolateral fusions. One group of 11 patients was braced for 3 months and the other for 5 months. Segmental motion was evaluated by stereophotogrammetry. Fusions became progressively more rigid beginning at 3 months in both groups. By 1 year, however, patients immobilized for 5 months showed a higher rate of fusion than the 3-month group, indicating a direct benefit of longer immobilization.[33]

Although the halo is the most rigid cervical appliance in kinematic testing, success in clinical application varies, especially with ligamentous instability. Cooper et al.[16] reviewed their experience with halo bracing of unstable injuries in 33 patients. They reported few minor complications and restored stability in 85%. In only 4 patients did therapy fail. Patients with ligamentous subluxation or angulation were most prone to lose halo reduction. Whitehill et al.[73] also reported 5 patients with unstable lig-

amentous facet dislocations or subluxations who failed to maintain reduction with the halo. Of 36 patients with facet dislocations or fracture dislocations reviewed by Beyer et al.,[11] 19 underwent halo immobilization. Only one third achieved proper alignment and one fourth achieved anatomic reduction. Half of the halo group lost reduction during bracing. They recommended open reduction and fixation of facet dislocations for better alignment and fusion results. Rockswold[62] reviewed 604 patients in five studies from the literature who were treated with halo stabilization for a variety of cervical injuries. Failed reduction and/or fusion occurred in 12% to 23% of patients. Hyperflexion ligamentous injuries had the highest failure rate. From these and other observations, it appears that the halo is an effective means for stabilizing many cervical injuries unless primary ligamentous instability exists. Paradoxical motion, or snaking, of the spine with associated midcervical angulation may account for the inadequate stability in ligamentous injuries.[8]

## Miscellaneous Complications of Spinal Bracing

### Halo Pin Site Complications

Pin site complications are among the most common limitations of halo bracing and have been studied extensively[5,12,24,47] (Table 146.4).

**Pin Loosening.** Pin loosening is seen in 36% to 60% of patients and is usually heralded by pain in the absence of associated infection.[13,47] Occasionally a fall or blunt trauma to the halo ring will result in acute loosening.[24] Current pin tip designs use a broad pin shoulder to maximize skull contact and help to limit loosening or perforation.[25] Ballock et al.[6] evaluated optimal pin site placement in a cadaver model, noting that pins inserted lower on the skull above the supraorbital ridge were more rigidly affixed than more superiorly placed pins. The lower pins were more perpendicular in orientation, which reportedly accounts for their improved rigidity. Botte et al.[13] studied the effect of pin insertion torque on subsequent pin loosening and reported improved mechanical characteristics

**TABLE 146.2**

### Complication Frequency of Halo Pin Fixation

| Complication | % |
| --- | --- |
| Loosening | 36-60[°†] |
| Pin site infection | 20-22[°†] |
| Local pain | 18[†] |
| Ring migration | 13[°†] |
| Scarring | 9-30[°†] |
| Nerve injury | 2[°] |
| Pin site bleeding | 1[°] |
| Intracranial puncture | 1[°] |

[°]Data from Garfin SR, Botte MJ, Waters RL, et al: Complications in the use of the halo fixation device. J Bone Joint Surg 68A:320-325, 1986.
[†]Data from Lind B, Sihlbom H, Nordwall A: Halo-vest treatment of unstable traumatic cervical spine injuries. Spine 13:425-432, 1988.
(Adapted from Botte MJ, Byrne TP, Abrams RA, Garfin SR: Halo skeletal fixation: techniques of application and prevention of complications. J Am Acad Orthop Surg 4:44-53, 1996, with permission.)

of the pin-bone junction at 8 inch-pounds versus 6 inch-pounds. Loosening was reduced to 7% from 36%, respectively.[13] Rizzolo et al.[61] also addressed pin insertion torque, randomizing two groups with pins inserted to torques of 8 or 6 inch-pounds. No significant difference between groups was noted, although a trend toward higher rates of loosening (26% vs. 20%) and infection (13% vs. 7%) occurred with the 8 inch-pound insertion torque. Currently, 6 to 8 inch-pounds are recommended for initial insertion torque, which is subsequently checked at 24 to 48 hours.[5] If remote loosening occurs without infection, the pins should be tightened once as long as resistance is encountered. Garfin et al.[24] found that 16% of loosened pins reloosened after tightening. Pins that were moved also loosened in 17%, suggesting that loosened pins compromise the balance of the other pins in the halo ring.[24] Repeated tightening leads to cranial perforation, because local bone erodes rapidly under pressure from the pin.

The actual force applied through the pin at the pin-skull junction appears to vary considerably for a given torque, depending on the method of insertion and the size and type of halo ring used. Whitesides et al.[74] measured force exerted through the pin for different insertion torques in several types of halo rings. They noted a wide variation in force among rings of different size and material composition. Flexibility of the ring and its effect on the coefficient of friction at the pin-ring junction reportedly accounted for the variation. Lubrication of the junction with saline significantly reduced friction between the pin and the ring. They recommended using an insertion torque specific for the type of halo used to standardize the force applied to the skull.[74] Kerwin et al.[36] also found wide variation of pin force with different ring sizes and materials. Friction between the ring and pin threads increased with ring flexibility. Addition of a locking nut paradoxically reduced pin force by either backing out the pin or altering the ring shape.

**Infection.** Skeletal fixation by definition violates the integrity of the scalp, risking local infection. Pin sites require continuous daily inspection and cleaning with hydrogen peroxide and application of a topical antibiotic such as polymyxin ointment. Despite excellent pin site care, local infection will occur in up to 22% of patients.[12] Increasing erythema and purulent drainage around the pin indicate early soft-tissue involvement and can usually be treated with a culture-specific oral antibiotic and close follow-up. Staphylococcus aureus is the most commonly involved organism. If extensive cellulitis or abscess occurs, the pin must be removed and a new pin inserted at an adjacent site. Infected pin site care follows standard principles of local wound care, including appropriate debridement and intravenous antibiotic therapy.

Brain abscess is a rare but serious result of cranial pin fixation that is typically associated with overlying soft-tissue infection and/or secondary osteomyelitis. Of five cases reviewed by Goodman and Nelson,[27] three had associated osteomyelitis, and all involved tightening a loosened pin. Rosenblum and Ehrlich[63] described a patient who presented with acute psychosis as an initial manifestation of an intracranial abscess. His halo pin had

been tightened twice because of loosening, the second time 1 week before presentation. These reports underscore the danger of repeatedly tightening loose pins. A pin that becomes loose should be retightened only once in the absence of frank scalp infection. Further loosening after initial retightening is an indication for insertion at another site.

Less frequent halo complications include frontal scarring, nerve injury, bleeding, and cranial puncture.[5] Scars from frontal pin sites are usually cosmetically acceptable for most patients. Up to 30%, however, develop severe scarring that may require further treatment.[47] Local infection, pin migration, and keloid formation may contribute to this problem. Incising the skin before insertion does not improve cosmetic outcome.[5] Garfin et al.[24] reported continuous local pain at pin sites in 17% of 180 patients treated in halos. Repeated periosteal irritation was thought to be the basis for chronic pin site pain.[24] Alternatively, pins mistakenly positioned through the temporalis muscle in the temporal fossa are also painful because of muscle trauma and continued irritation during jaw movement.[5] Paradoxically, newly developed pin site pain often indicates a loosening pin. Nerve injury with pain and paresthesias may occur with pin trauma to the supraorbital or supratrochlear nerves as they course superiorly from their foramina to innervate the frontal scalp. Pin movement is often required because of the severity of symptoms. Avoiding medial pin placement should prevent this complication.[5] By placing frontal pins into the fronto-orbital crest, obvious scars, nerve injuries, and temporalis muscle pain may be avoided. Bleeding from pin sites has been reported with patients receiving chronic anticoagulants.[24] Discontinuing anticoagulation resolves this rare and unusual complication. Intracranial puncture has been discussed in association with repeated pin tightening or frank trauma to the halo ring such as with a fall. Although rarely reported, this can lead to serious intracranial infection and loss of fixation[5] (see Table 146.1).

### Overdistraction

Because the thoracic vest of the halo transmits significant force through the device to the cranium, distraction and compression forces vary widely with different patient positions and activities.[37] Overly vigorous attempts to maintain axial traction in a halo can result in overdistraction and cause associated swallowing difficulties or neck discomfort. Dysphagia has been noted in up to 2% of patients[24] and results from impaired larynx movement required for coordinated swallowing. Avoiding excessive distraction and head extension will usually prevent this complication.

### Cardiopulmonary Complications

Cardiopulmonary complications of bracing mainly involve changes in venous pressures of the trunk, abdomen, and lower extremities. Kaplan et al.[35] described acute pulmonary edema occurring in an obese 63-year-old trauma victim after removal of a halo that had been in place for 14 weeks. Occult mitral stenosis was subsequently diagnosed. They postulated that removal of the halo vest resulted in a loss of the mechanical impediment to venous return, resulting in rapid volume loading of the heart, which was not compensated because of occult mitral stenosis. Improved ventilatory mechanics after halo removal also increased venous return, worsening pulmonary edema. Lower extremity venous hypertension is an additional concern for developing varicose veins, venous stasis with thrombosis, or hemorrhoids.[69] This is most commonly seen with the TLSO, although it has not specifically been reported or quantified.

Conventional orthoses and halo vests may compromise respiratory function by restricting expansion of the chest and abdomen. To measure this effect, Lind *et al.*[46] studied spirometry of 20 trauma patients in halos at 1 week of treatment, 3 months, and after removal of the appliance. The halo reduced vital capacity by 8% to 9%. With prolonged wearing, vital capacity increased by 10% because of adjustment of the vest, reduction in acute pain, loss of cautiousness, and respiratory training. Levels remained at all times more than adequate to support normal respiratory function.[46] Although this study demonstrates only a minimal reduction in vital capacity, the effect on patients with chronic obstructive pulmonary disease is unknown and may be more functionally significant.

### Gastrointestinal Dysfunction

Compression of the abdomen, especially combined with extension, may occasionally stretch the superior mesenteric artery across the ventral aspect of the distal duodenum, compressing it against the aorta.[8] The superior mesenteric artery syndrome or cast syndrome results in postprandial bilious emesis, epigastric pain, and distention from partial duodenal obstruction.[67] A barium study typically shows duodenal compression with delayed passage into the small bowel. Contributing factors include acute weight loss, recumbency, posturing, and spasticity.[64] Treatment is expectant with discontinued bracing, gastric decompression, parenteral alimentation, or enteral feeding through a tube passed beyond the duodenum. Refractory cases may require surgical exploration.

### Psychosocial Dysfunction

Severe psychologic problems associated with spinal bracing have been noted by a number of authors, occurring in up to 3% of patients.[14,24,56] Scoliosis bracing typically involves female adolescents with a significantly intrusive appliance that markedly affects body image. Initial adjustment disorders have been described ranging from varying degrees of depression to noncompliance and eating disorders.[7,10,65] Similar adjustment problems with other conventional devices have not been quantified, although concerns about appearance, complaints of claustrophobia, and anxiety over lost independence are commonly expressed. Orthoses are very visible symbols of infirmity, which may foster adoption of a sick role. Psychologic dependence and secondary gain is not uncommon among chronic collar users because of this change in body image and its connotation of legitimate injury.[69] Bracing should therefore be used only when indicated for specific stabilization goals having defined end points.

## New Advances and Developments

Recent developments in materials and techniques have led to many improvements in older orthoses as well as the invention of some new novel strategies. Advances have sought to both simplify their application as well as increase patient comfort, in turn delivering greater compliance. Specifically, new strap and closure configurations have made some devices easier to apply, adjust, and remove. Further front adjustments allow additional customization to follow body contour variations from the top of the torso to the waist and hips. Additional options include male and female liners, pendulous fronts, and adjustable lumbar control permitting custom curvatures from 0 degrees to 40 degrees. These advances have led some companies to claim the ability to fit 98% of the adult population (ComfAlign, The Bremer Group Company, Jacksonville, FL).

Some companies have adopted novel techniques to increase support while decreasing the incidence of skin breakdown. The Aspen cervical collar (Aspen Medical Products, Inc., Long Beach, CA) utilizes a three-layered system to achieve effective motion restriction. Two stiff inner layers of plastic provide the majority of support while an outer, more flexible layer is slotted along its edges, allowing better conformation with the patient's anatomy. The resultant better fit reduces the pressure points commonly found at the mandible, sternum, and clavicles. Studies have documented the reduced pressure from an improved fit to be significantly less than capillary closing pressure, an underlying cause of skin breakdown.[23] The advent of cleanable and replaceable liners also results in better skin care without the need for multiple collars. Large anterior and posterior openings promote better airflow, increasing patient comfort (Figure 146.11A). The Aspen CTO (Figure 146.11B), which incorporates the Aspen cervical collar, gives the practitioner the flexibility of "stepping down" the level of motion restriction as the patient progresses. The integrated system allows one to go from a four-post to a two-post and finally a stand-alone cervical collar. Other manufacturers have also developed options and attachments to increase their available applications (for example, the Jewett brace [Florida Brace Corporation, Winter Park, FL] anterior and full cervical extensions to their original hyperextension orthosis [Figure 146.12]).

The Orthotrac Pneumatic Vest (Orthofix Inc.) represents a unique, noninvasive approach to low back pain. The patient, utilizing a hand pump, activates pneumatic lifters that tie into two custom fitted belts that shift body weight from the lumbar spine onto the iliac crests (Figure 146.13). Company literature claims the vest is designed to shift up to 30% to 50% of the body weight off of the spine and distract adjoining vertebral bodies up to 1mm, which appears sufficient to off-load the spine in most cases.

Many older companies have spent much time and effort to improve their product line. Jerome Medical (Morristown, NJ), makers of the Miami J, has developed a

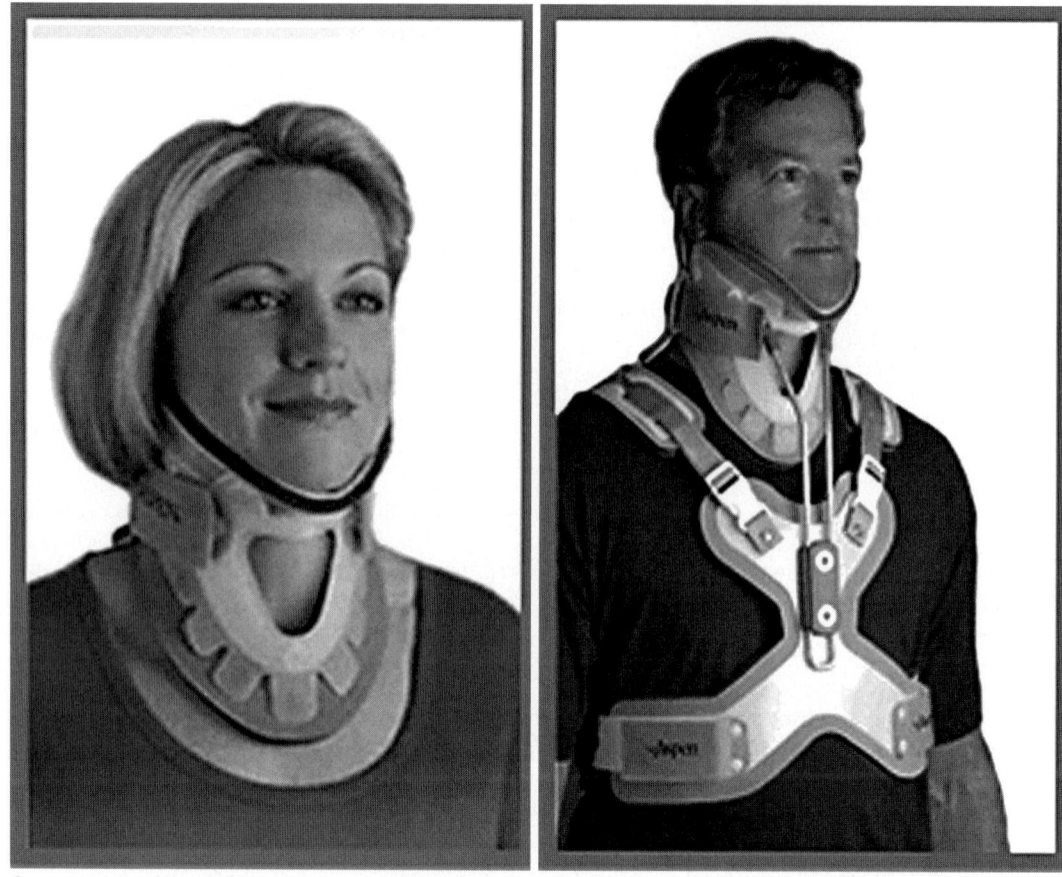

**A**                          **B**

**Figure 146.11** **(A)** The Aspen Cervical Collar (Aspen Medical Products, Long Beach, CA) incorporates large anterior and posterior openings to promote better airflow, which increases patient comfort. Their CTO incorporates the cervical collar into an integrated system, allowing the flexibility of "stepping down" from a four-post to a two-post and finally a stand-alone cervical collar **(B)**. (*From http://www.aspenmp.com.*)

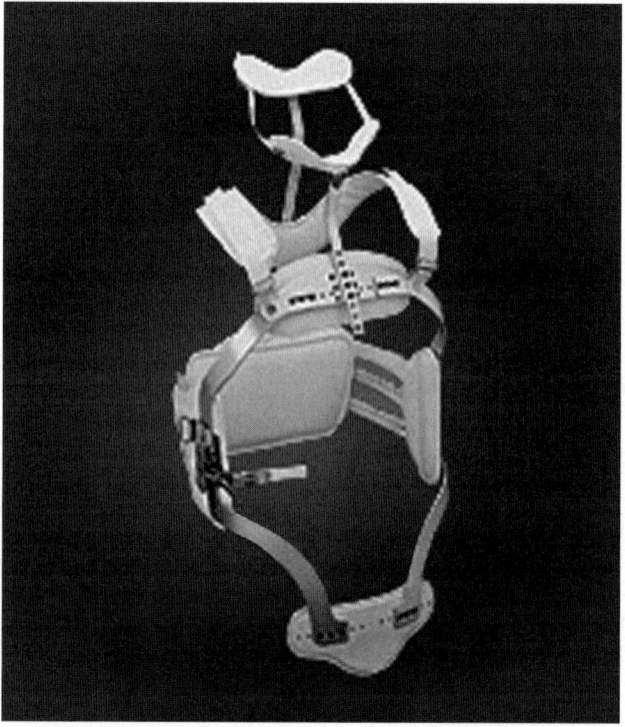

**Figure 146.12** The original Jewett® Brace (Florida Brace Corporation, Winter Park, FL) is now available with a full cervical extension. (*From http://www.flabrace.com.*)

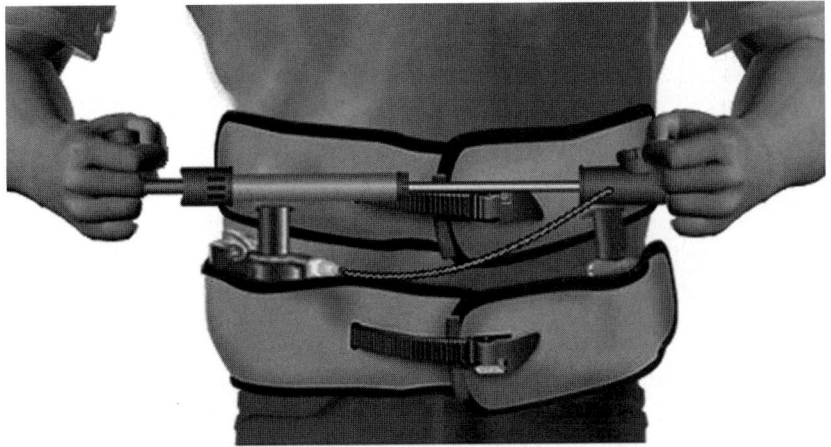

A

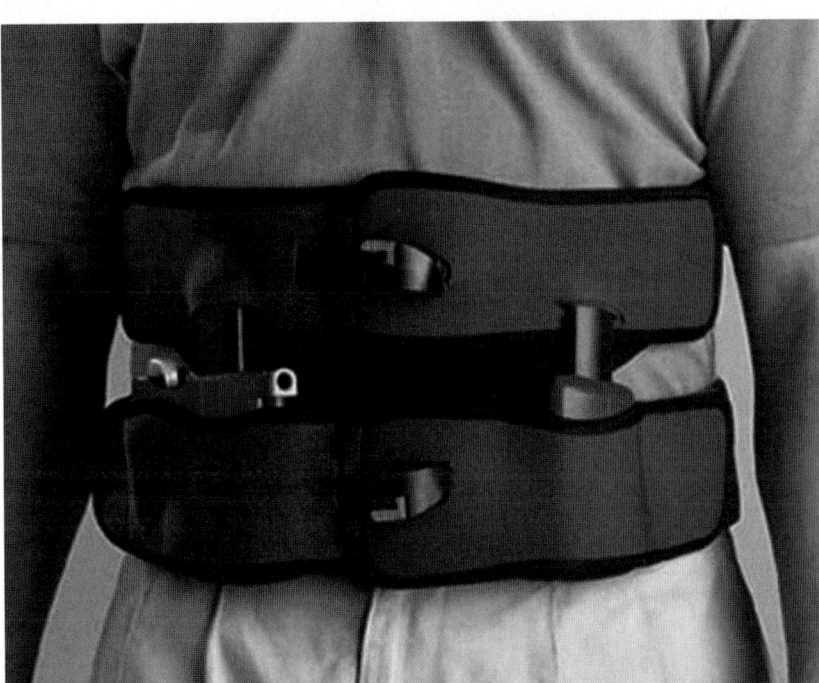

B

**Figure 146.13** The Orthotrac Pneumatic Vest (Orthofix, Inc.) utilizes a hand pump (**A**) to activate pneumatic lifters that tie into two custom-fitted belts, which shift body weight from the lumbar spine onto the iliac crests (**B**). The vest is designed to shift up to 30% to 50% of the body weight off of the spine. (*From http://www.treatmyback.com.*)

proprietary material, Sorbatek. They claim it breathes better and dries more quickly. It is also antibacterial and exhibits good thermal conductivity.

The latest model of the Halo System (PMT Corporation, Chanhassen, MN) has incorporated several changes to keep up with the times (Figure 146.14). Simply displacing the buckles yielded cleaner lateral x-rays. The use of carbon graphite and titanium materials provides clear MRI/CT scans. New nylon ball joints make assembly quicker and easier. Adjustable headblocks can now be independently adjusted three ways, allowing anterior/posterior positioning, flexion/extension, and traction/distraction.

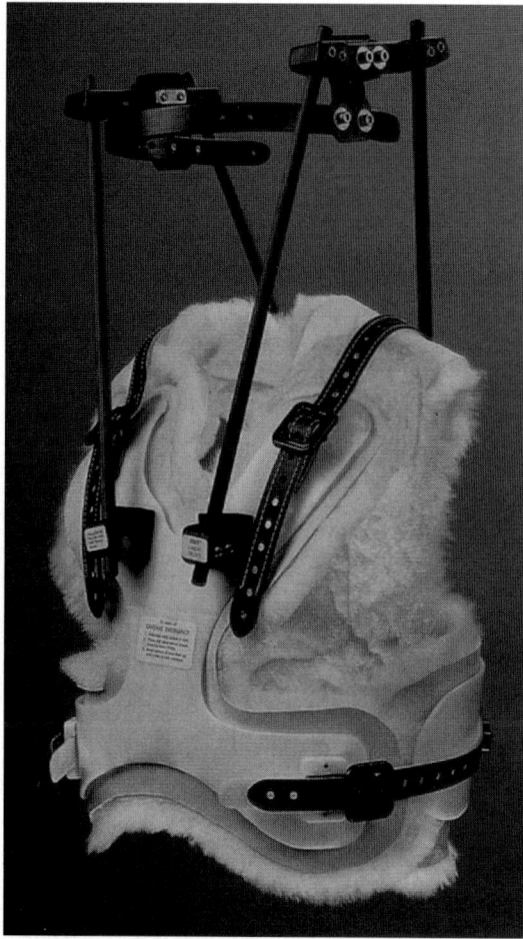

**Figure 146.14** The latest model of the Halo System (PMT Corporation, Chanhassen, MN) has incorporated several changes including displaced buckles for cleaner lateral x-rays, the use of carbon graphite and titanium materials to provide clear MRI/CT scans, new nylon ball joints to make assembly quicker and easier, and adjustable headblocks that can now be independently adjusted three ways, allowing anterior/posterior positioning, flexion/extension, and traction/distraction. *(From http://www.pmtcorp.com.)*

## REFERENCES

1. Abruzzese RS: Pressure sores: nursing aspects and prevention. In Lee BY, Ostrander LE, Cochran GVB, Shaw WW (eds): *The Spinal Cord Injured Patient: Comprehensive Management.* Philadelphia, WB Saunders, 1991, pp 210-222.

2. American Association of Orthopedic Surgeons: *Atlas of Orthoses.* St Louis, CV Mosby, 1985.

3. Axelsson P, Johnsson R, Stromqvist B: Effect of lumbar orthosis on intervertebral mobility: a roentgen stereophotogrammetric analysis. *Spine* 17:678-681, 1992.

4. Axelsson P, Johnsson R, Stromqvist B: Lumbar orthosis with unilateral hip immobilization: effect on intervertebral mobility determined by roentgen stereophotogrammetric analysis. *Spine* 18:876-879, 1993.

5. Ballock RT, Botte MJ, Garfin SR: Complications of halo immobilization. In Garfin SR (ed): *Complications of Spinal Surgery.* Baltimore, Williams & Wilkins, 1989, pp 376-388.

6. Ballock RT, Lee TQ, Triggs KJ, *et al*: The effect of pin localization on the rigidity of the halo-pin interface. *Neurosurgery* 26:238-241, 1990.

7. Bengtsson G, Fallstrom K, Jansson B, Nachemson A: A psychiatric investigation of the adjustment of female scoliosis patients. *Acta Psychiatr Scand* 50:50-59, 1974.

8. Benzel EC: Spinal orthotics. In Menezes AH, Sonntag VKH (eds): *Principles of Spinal Surgery.* New York, McGraw-Hill, 1996, pp 181-190.

9. Benzel EC, Hadden TA, Saulsbery CM: A comparison of the Minerva and halo jackets for stabilization of the cervical spine. *J Neurosurg* 70:411-414, 1989.

10. Bernstein A, Warner G: Onset of anorexia nervosa after prolonged use of the Milwaukee brace. *Psychosomatics* 24:1033-1034, 1983.

11. Beyer CA, Cabanela ME, Berquist TH: Unilateral facet dislocations and fracture-dislocations of the cervical spine. *J Bone Joint Surg* 73A:977-981, 1991.

12. Botte MJ, Byrne TP, Abrams RA, Garfin SR: Halo skeletal fixation: techniques of application and prevention of complications. *J Am Acad Orthop Surg* 4:44-53, 1996.

13. Botte MJ, Byrne TP, Garfin SJ: Application of the halo cervical immobilizer using an increased torque pressure. *J Bone Joint Surg* 69A:750-753, 1987.

14. Bunch WH, Patwardhan AG (eds): *Scoliosis: Making Clinical Decisions.* St Louis, CV Mosby, 1989, pp 237-255.

15. Colachis SC, Strohm BR, Ganter EL: Cervical spine motion in normal women: radiographic study of effect of cervical collars. *Arch Phys Med Rehabil* 54:161-169, 1973.

16. Cooper PR, Maravilla KR, Sklar FH, *et al*: Halo immobilization of cervical spine fractures. Indications and results. *J Neurosurg* 50:603-610, 1979.

17. Daniel RK, Priest DL, Wheatly DC: Etiologic factors in pressure sores: an experimental model. *Arch Phys Med Rehabil* 62:492, 1981.

18. Dinsdale SM: Decubitus ulcers: role of pressure and friction in causation. *Arch Phys Med Rehabil* 55:147-152, 1974.

19. Edberg EL, Cerny K, Stauffer ES: Prevention and treatment of pressure sores. *Phys Ther* 53:246, 1973.

20. Ferguson RL, Allen BL, Tencer AF: Biomechanical principles of spinal correction. In Cotler JM, Cotler HB (eds): *Spinal Fusion: Science and Technique.* New York, Springer-Verlag, 1990, pp 45-57.

21. Fidler MW, Plasmans CMT: The effect of four types of support on the segmental mobility of the lumbosacral spine. *J Bone Joint Surg* 65A:943-947, 1983.

22. Fisher SV, Bowar JF, Awad EA, *et al*: Cervical orthoses' effect on cervical spine motion: roentgenographic and goniometric method of study. *Arch Phys Med Rehabil* 58:109-115, 1977.

23. Frankel HL, Hancock DO, Hyslop G, *et al*: The value of postural reduction in the initial management of closed injuries of the spine with paraplegia and tetraplegia. *Paraplegia* 7(3):179-192, 1969.

24. Garfin SR, Botte MJ, Waters RL, *et al*: Complications in the use of the halo fixation device. *J Bone Joint Surg* 68A:320-325, 1986.

25. Garfin SR, Lee TO, Roux RD, *et al*: Structural behavior of the halo orthosis pin-bone interface: biomechanical evaluation of standard and newly designed stainless steel halo fixation pins. *Spine* 11:977-981, 1986.

26. Glaser JA, Whitehill R, Stamp WG, Jane JA: Complications associated with the halo vest. *J Neurosurg* 65:762-769, 1986.

27. Goodman ML, Nelson PB: Brain abscess complicating the use of a halo orthosis. *Neurosurgery* 20:27-29, 1987.

28. Harris EE: A new orthotics terminology. *Orthotics Prosthet* 27:6-9, 1973.

29. Hartman JT, Palumbo F, Hill BJ: Cineradiography of braced normal cervical spine: comparative study of five commonly used cervical orthoses. *Clin Orthop* 109:97-102, 1975.

30. Johnson RM, Hart DL, Owen JR, et al: The Yale cervical orthosis: an evaluation of its effectiveness in restricting cervical motion in normal subjects and a comparison with other cervical orthoses. *Phys Ther* 58:865, 1978.

31. Johnson RM, Hart DL, Simmons EF, et al: Cervical orthoses: a study comparing their effectiveness in restricting cervical motion in normal subjects. *J Bone Joint Surg* 59A:332-339, 1977.

32. Johnson RM, Owen JR, Hart DL, Callahan RA: Cervical orthoses: a guide to their selection and use. *Clin Orthop Rel Res* 154:34-45, 1988.

33. Johnsson R, Stromqvist B, Axelsson P, Selvik G: Influence of spinal immobilization on consolidation of posterolateral lumbosacral fusion. A roentgen stereophotogrammetric and radiographic analysis. *Spine* 17:16-21, 1992.

34. Jones MD: Cineradiographic studies of collar immobilized cervical spine. *J Neurosurg* 17:633-637, 1960.

35. Kaplan SL, Rocco TP, Tan CG, et al: Acute pulmonary edema following removal of a spinal orthosis: an unusual complication of a halo vest. *Arch Phys Med Rehabil* 71:255-257, 1990.

36. Kerwin GA, Chou KL, White DB, et al: Investigation of how different halos influence pin forces. *Spine* 19:1078-1081, 1994.

37. Koch RA, Nickel VL: The halo-vest: evaluation of motion and forces across the neck. *Spine* 3:103-107, 1978.

38. Korovessis P, Stamatakis M, Baikousis A, et al: Vertical transmission of the hip rolls due to wearing of TLSO for scoliosis. *J Spinal Disord* 9:326-333, 1996.

39. Kosiak M: Etiology of decubitus ulcers. *Arch Phys Med Rehabil* 42:19-29, 1961.

40. Krag MH: Biomechanics of the cervical spine: orthoses. In Frymoyer JW (ed): *The Adult Spine: Principles and Practice*, ed 2. Philadelphia, Lippincott-Raven, 1997, pp 1110-1117.

41. Krag MH, Begnnon BD: A new halo-vest: rationale, design and biomechanical comparison to standard halo-vest designs. *Spine* 13:228-234, 1988.

42. Landis EM: Micro-injection studies of capillary blood pressure in human skin. *Heart* 15:209-228, 1930.

43. Lantz SA, Schultz AB: Lumbar spine orthosis wearing. 1. Restriction of gross body motions. *Spine* 11:834-837, 1986.

44. Lantz SA, Schultz AB: Lumbar spine orthosis wearing. 2. Effect on trunk muscle myoelectric activity. *Spine* 11:838-842, 1986.

45. Lee BY: Plastic surgery for pressure sores. In Lee BY, Ostrander LE, Cochran GVB, Shaw WW (eds): *The Spinal Cord Injured Patient: Comprehensive Management*. Philadelphia, WB Saunders, 1991, pp 223-230.

46. Lind B, Bake B, Lundqvist C, Nordwall A: Influence of halo vest treatment on vital capacity. *Spine* 12:449-452, 1987.

47. Lind B, Sihlbom H, Nordwall A: Halo-vest treatment of unstable traumatic cervical spine injuries. *Spine* 13:425-432, 1988.

48. Lucas DB, Jacobs RR, Trautman P: Spinal orthotics for pain and instability. In Redford JB (ed): *Orthotics Etcetera*, ed 3. Baltimore, Williams & Wilkins, 1986, pp 122-152.

49. Lumsden RM, Morris JM: An in vivo study of axial rotation and immobilization at the lumbosacral joint. *J Bone Joint Surg* 50A:1591-1602, 1968.

50. Madsen BL, Barth PW, Vistnes LM: Pressure sores: overview. In Lee BY, Ostrander LE, Cochran GVB, Shaw WW (eds): *The Spinal Cord Injured Patient: Comprehensive Management*. Philadelphia, WB Saunders, 1991, pp 202-209.

51. Maiman D, Millington P, Novak S, et al: The effect of the thermoplastic minerval body jacket on cervical spine motion. *Neurosurgery* 25:363-368, 1989.

52. Massie JB, Heller JG, Abitbol JJ, et al: Post operative posterior spinal wound infections. *Clin Orthop* 284:99-108, 1992.

53. Millington PJ, Ellingsen JM, Hauswirth BE, et al: Thermoplastic Minerva body jacket: a practical alternative to current methods of cervical spine stabilization. *Phys Ther* 67:223-225, 1987.

54. Morris JM, Lucas DB, Bresler B: Role of the trunk in stability of the spine. *J Bone Joint Surg* 43A:327, 1961.

55. Morris JM: Spinal bracing. In Wilkins RH, Rengachary SS (eds): *Neurosurgery*. New York, McGraw-Hill, 1985, pp 2300-2305.

56. Nachemson AE: Orthotic treatment for injuries and diseases of the spinal column. *Phys Med Rehab* 1:11-24, 1987.

57. Nachemson AL, Morris JM: In vivo measurements of intradiscal pressure. *J Bone Joint Surg* 46A:1077-1092, 1964.

58. Norton PL, Brown T: The immobilizing efficiency of the back braces: their effect on the posture and motion of the lumbosacral spine. *J Bone Joint Surg* 39A:111-139, 1957.

59. Patwardhan AG, Li SP, Gavin T, et al: Orthotic stabilization of thoracolumbar injuries. A biomechanical analysis of the Jewett hyperextension orthosis. *Spine* 15:654-661, 1990.

60. Polin RS, Szabo T, Bogaev CA, et al: Nonoperative management of types II and III odontoid fractures: the Philadelphia collar versus the halo vest. *Neurosurgery* 38:450-456, 1996.

61. Rizzolo SJ, Piazza MR, Cotler JM, et al: The effect of torque pressure on halo pin complication rates. A randomized prospective study. *Spine* 18:2163-2166, 1993.

62. Rockswold GL: Halo management of cervical spine injuries. *Contemp Neurosurg* 13:1-6, 1991.

63. Rosenblum D, Ehrlich V: Brain abscess and psychosis as a complication of a halo orthosis. *Arch Phys Med Rehabil* 76:865-867, 1995.

64. Roth EJ, Fenton LL, Gaebler-Spira DJ, et al: Superior mesenteric artery syndrome in acute quadriplegia: case reports and review of the literature. *Arch Phys Med Rehabil* 72:417-420, 1991.

65. Schatzinger L, Nash C, Drotar D, Hall T: Emotional adjustment in scoliosis. *Clin Orthop* 125:145-150, 1977.

66. Schurr DG, Cook TM: *Prosthetics and Orthotics*. Norwalk, CT, Appleton & Lange, 1990, pp 195-215.

67. Schwartz DR, Wirka HW: The cast syndrome: a case report and discussion of the literature. *J Bone Joint Surg* 46A:1549-1552, 1964.

68. Smith EM, Juvinall RC: Mechanics of orthotics. In Redford JB (ed): *Orthotics Etcetera*, ed 3. Baltimore, Williams & Wilkins, 1986, pp 21-51.

69. Sypert GW: External spinal orthotics. *Neurosurgery* 20:642-649, 1987.

70. Wang GJ, Moskal JT, Albert T, *et al*: The effect of halo-vest length on stability of the cervical spine. *J Bone Joint Surg* 70A:357-360, 1988.

71. Waters RL, Morris JM: Effect of spinal supports on electrical activity of muscles of the trunk. *J Bone Joint Surg* 52A:51-60, 1970.

72. White AA, Panjabi MM: *Clinical Biomechanics of the Spine*. Philadelphia, Lippincott-Raven, 1978.

73. Whitehill R, Richman JA, Glaser JA: Failure of immobilization of the cervical spine by the halo vest. *J Bone Joint Surg* 68A:326-332, 1986.

74. Whitesides TE, Mehserle WL, Hutton WC: The force exerted by the halo pin: a study comparing different halo systems. *Spine* 17:S413-417, 1992.

# CHAPTER 147

# Athlete with Spinal Injury

## Julian E. Bailes, Joseph C. Maroon, and Robert C. Cantu

Injuries to the cervical spine constitute a small proportion (2% to 3%) of all sports injuries, yet their physical, emotional, and financial impact on the athlete can be devastating. Unlike the injuries usually encountered in sports medicine that cause acute discomfort, temporary loss of functional mobility, and time away from competition, trauma to the spine can result in chronic pain and functional limitation, significant disability with withdrawal from competition, and sometimes even permanent dysfunction.

When a spinal injury occurs in any sport, regardless of the type or level of competition, its treatment involves a decision-making process that goes beyond the medical to include athletic and socioeconomic concerns. Investigators of athletic injuries of the vertebral column, supporting structures, and spinal cord must first characterize the injury and provide appropriate treatment, but in addition, they must also determine the potential for future disability after such an injury and advise the athlete about whether to continue participating in sports. For athletes who have suffered neurologic compromise or significant vertebral column injury, these decisions can be relatively easy to make. However, for athletes who sustain spinal injuries with transient neurologic symptoms or radiologic evidence of an abnormal vertebral column without significant fracture or instability, the decision-making process is much less clear.

## Classification of Injuries

Athletic injuries may be categorized in two general ways. The first type occurs during recreational or unsupervised sports—such as diving, surfing, trampolining, skiing, and others—in which there are frequently no rules, training, or supervision. The lack of any structure in such activities makes it difficult to enforce safety guidelines, proper training and techniques, and manufacturing standards, which in turn limits what can be done to improve injury patterns.

The second kind of athletic injury occurs in supervised, organized sports such as football, ice hockey, wrestling, rugby, gymnastics, and others in which body contact, velocity, or torque forces; competition; and team effort are much higher. Whereas the chance for injury in such sports may be greater, the opportunity for prevention through education, regulation, rules implementation, and equipment design is also better. In our experience, injuries in

this group represent approximately 4% of total admissions to a spinal cord referral center.

## Incidence and Mechanism of Injuries

### Unorganized Sports

Water activities, such as diving and surfing, provide ample opportunity for injury to the cervical spine. In fact, the most common mechanism of spinal injury from recreational sports involves diving, usually among teenaged males during the summer months.[*] The incidence of diving accidents has been reported to comprise between 2% and 22% of all spinal injuries, with a higher incidence reported in areas with high water sports activity involving younger age groups and in times of seasonal droughts.[†] Up to 75% of recreation-related spinal cord injuries are caused by diving mishaps.[41] The true incidence of such injuries, however, is believed to be even higher, because many probably involve drowning victims.[19,53,88] Also of note is that many diving-related injuries, particularly in young men, involve alcohol consumption.[21,53,75]

Flexion, with or without axial compression, is the usual mechanism of diving injuries,[18,53] but other mechanisms such as lateral flexion or hyperextension may also produce injury.[83] In addition, the diver may occasionally enter the water in an unconventional manner, with the mechanism resembling that of a fall.[23] The most common diving injuries occur when an individual dives head first into a body of water without calculating the water's depth and strikes his head on the bottom[18,42,83,89] or, less often, when a diver strikes another swimmer or a submerged object.[19] Surfing-related cervical injuries, on the other hand, are usually the result of a variety of impact positions that the surfer assumes when propelled by a fall or tidal action, striking the head and neck.[42]

Diving injuries occur almost exclusively in the cervical spine, most frequently at the C5 level, and usually cause significant injury (complete quadriplegia).[89] The high incidence (70%) of injury at the C5 location is a result of the available range of motion at that level, in association with the relatively smaller size (1.55cm) of the spinal canal at the midcervical level.[19,24,41,83,93] Most patients with multilevel injuries also have involvement at the C5 level. The authors have identified odontoid fractures in only two patients, thus emphasizing the relative rarity of upper cervical spine diving injuries.[4]

Diving injuries are unique because the damage to the spinal cord usually occurs as an isolated event involving only hyperflexion of the neck. These patients usually have no other associated injuries. Pulmonary involvement is the major source of morbidity, owing to aspiration and near-drowning or to subsequent neurologic compromise of ventilatory mechanisms. These athletes also tend to be young and healthy and to tolerate their hospitalization well. They usually can be rapidly mobilized (e.g., by a halo brace), and physical and occupational therapy can be initiated expeditiously. Other water sports such as water skiing, high diving, skin and scuba diving, and wind surfing

---

[*]References 1,21,23,24,29,41,78.
[†]References 21,24,29,40-42,69,71.

produce a much smaller number of spinal injuries.[83] Probably no other injuries are as amenable to prevention as are diving injuries,[86] but the response to public educational programs is countered by a high rate of recidivism.

### Snow Skiing

Snow skiing mishaps comprise a less-frequent but still important source of recreational sports spinal injuries. Unfortunately, snow skiers today are probably at greater risk than in the past because of better ski equipment design, synthetic materials, and manufacturing processes that have facilitated greater skiing speeds. In his 14-year study from a major ski resort in the United States, Harris[27] found an annual incidence of two spinal cord injuries. Overall, there were 13 instances of quadriplegia, 10 of diplegia, and 3 each of paraplegia and hemiplegia. These skiers were usually young men, of expert ability, who were traveling at higher speeds than the average skier. Harris[27] noted that as the skill of an alpine skier increases, the incidence of injury may be reduced, but the severity of neurologic injury is increased. The number of such tragedies can be reduced by strong enforcement of safety guidelines for speed in all skiing activities other than competition. Helmets provide some protection against head injuries but do not prevent spinal cord injuries. Safety programs should be a part of new skier instruction to increase awareness that collisions with trees or boulders and high speeds are responsible for most snow skiing catastrophic injuries.

### Snowboarding

Snowboarding is one of the fastest growing winter sports in the world. The typical snowboarder is young and male, which is also the group known for the greatest amount of risk taking. The average age of an injured snowboarder is 20 to 21 years, approximately eight years younger than the injured skier.[8] The majority learn the sport on their own or through friends, and many have no prior skiing experience.[43] While it is estimated that snowboarders make up only a quarter of participants on the slope, some studies claim they account for nearly half of the emergency room trips from the slopes.[8] Other studies report an equal rate of injury as compared with skiing, ranging from 2 to 4 injuries per 1000 sport days.[56]

Although uncommon, spinal cord injuries do occur. Chow et al.,[8] in a study of 390 snowboarding injuries, reported that 7% were spinal. The most common spinal injury was a strain. Injuries to the spine are commonly associated with the athlete "catching air," also known as attempting an aerial maneuver. Jumping with the snowboard is a very popular activity and results in a substantial number of injuries. Shorter et al.[79] reported that at least 25% of the falls resulting in injury were the result of going over a jump.

### Bow Hunting

The most common cause of neurologic injury in bow hunting is through accidental falls from hunting tree stands. These falls have long been associated with neurologic injuries, most commonly to the back, and may result in significant long-term disability, expensive and lengthy hospitalization, and even death. A report using Oklahoma State Department of Health spinal cord injury surveillance data showed that half of the hunting-related injuries resulted in neurologic damage significant enough to cause permanent paralysis or death.[68]

### Hang Gliding

Over 30,000 people in the United States actively engage in hang gliding. Between 1973 and 1975, there were 81 known fatalities from this sport in the United States. Nonfatal injuries commonly involve the upper extremities and spine. This is in part caused by impact with the control bar. Seventeen percent of nonfatal injuries involved the spine. Cervical spine injuries are more common with the pilot flying prone, while lumbosacral injuries were more frequent in seated pilots. According to the National Spinal Cord Injury Data Research Center, the mean age of hang-gliding related spinal cord injury between 1980 and 1981 was found to be 38 years, with a range of 21 to 64 years. Seventy-five percent of injuries occurred in men. One hundred percent of the injuries occurred to an individual not participating in an organized class or team. Of those injured, 75% were considered skilled at hang gliding, and 25% resulted in quadriplegia.[9]

### Board and Body Surfing

The risk of injury in both board and body surfing is relatively low as compared with other sports. Two causes of injury predominate. The surfer can be hit by a loose board or have impact with the bottom of the ocean. The former predominates in the board surfer and carries a higher risk of head injury, while the latter is more associated with the body surfer and can lead to serious spinal injury. The majority of spinal injuries occur when the surfer is thrown into the sand at the end of a body surfing run. Cervical injuries are the most common; high thoracic and lumbodorsal injuries also are observed. Forced hyperextension of the head and neck secondary to the surfer being driven into the sand appears to be the mechanism of injury. The subarachnoid space around the cervical spine is narrowest in the C3-6 levels, making this area most vulnerable to injury. This space is decreased further with extension. Increased narrowing of this area by osteophytes and ligamentum flavum could predispose the older population with osteoarthritic changes to these injuries. Older body surfers should be aware that preexisting osteoarthrosis can increase their risk of injury.

### Weight Lifting

Neurologic injuries from weight lifting range from chronic overuse syndromes to acute quadriplegia and include spondylolysis, spondylolisthesis, intervertebral disc herniation, and various peripheral nerve injuries. Power lifting injuries have been shown to have twice as high an injury rate as bodybuilding. Injuries occur much more frequently when using free weights versus weight machines.

One of the areas of the body that is very often injured by weight lifters is the lumbar spine. These injuries are most commonly muscle strains, ligament sprains, lumbar vertebral fractures, disc injuries, and neural arch fractures. The most common serious injury to the lower back is a neural arch fracture at the pars interarticularis. Defects in the pars interarticularis of one side of the vertebrae and bilateral defects with spondylolisthesis can also occur. The Northeast Collaborative Group on Low Back Pain studied the associations between participation in several specific sports, use of free weights, and use of weight lifting equipment and herniated lumbar or cervical intervertebral discs. The study included 287 patients with lumbar disc herniation and 63 patients with cervical disc herniation. The authors found that herniated lumbar or cervical discs were not associated with the use of weight lifting machines, but a possible association was indicated between the use of free weights and cervical herniation (relative risk, 1.87%; confidence interval, 0.74 to 4.74).[58]

## Golf

Golf is an extremely popular international sport, with over 26 million participants in the United States alone. Associated joint and extremity injuries are common, but neurologic damage is infrequently encountered. In a report of 300 golfers seen in an emergency room over a 6-year period, the most common neurologic injuries were those from being hit by a club or by a ball and then the head and neck injuries that can occur from slips and falls.[103]

Most likely underreported is golf-induced stroke from vertebral artery dissection or so called "golfer's stroke."[49] Vertebral artery dissection has reportedly been caused by yoga, tennis, volleyball, judo, bow hunting and wrestling. It is no surprise, therefore, that with rapid and forceful torquing of the body while the head and neck remain fixed, such as in teeing off, vertebral artery dissection from golf is a distinct possibility.

Maroon et al.[49] recently reviewed this topic after having had a patient with major cerebellar infarction immediately following a forceful golf swing. Three additional cases were found in the medical literature. Of the 4, 1 died from stroke-related complications and the other 3 were able to return to normal activity. Compression, dissection, and occlusion of the vertebral artery occurs most frequently at the junction of C1-2, but the artery is also vulnerable at the level of C6 as it enters the transverse foramen. The presenting symptoms have included cervical pain and/or occipital headaches, dysarthria, dysmetria, ataxia, vertigo, and various neurologic deficits that may wax and wane for days to weeks.

Most neurologic deficits resolve over time without any intervention, although most are treated with heparin when diagnosed. The most likely reason for suspected underreporting of this injury is the bilateral vertebral artery supply to the brain and the usual spontaneous resolution of symptoms. Prevention of such injuries is best effected through proper stretching, conditioning, and most importantly, application of correct technique. Extremely forceful rotation of the body with the head maintained in a rigid, fixed and downward position may predispose to such injuries.

## Organized Sports
### Football

Football players are the most likely to sustain cervical trauma and constitute a group for whom reliable data regarding frequency and incidence of injury are available. Nonetheless, these data reflect wide variation, ranging from 1 quadriplegic injury per 7000 players[50] at all levels of organized football to 1 injury per 58,000 players.[57] In 1990, Cantu and Mueller[7] reported that since 1977, there was an annual incidence of fewer than 10 cases of permanent injury to the cervical spinal cord resulting from football. This is in contrast to the important work of Schneider[77] in the mid-1960s, emphasizing the relatively high incidence of such injuries. However, in the late 1970s, as the incidence of cervical spine injury among football players was declining, the number of accidents resulting in permanent quadriplegia increased. Ironically, as the design of helmets (which were intended to protect against head injury) improved, players began using their helmets as a battering weapon. The majority (83%) of cervical spinal cord injuries are sustained by the nearly 1.4 million junior and senior high school players.[7] Discrepancies in player size, age, maturity, and speed among these age groups could explain this incidence increase. Most football players are injured during the course of tackling, so that defensive backs, members of the kickoff and receiving teams, and linebackers constitute the majority of those injured.

In addition to the relevance of team position, high school players with long, slender necks appear to be most vulnerable. Almost all cervical injuries occur with high-velocity impact, usually when the player strikes his opponent with the vertex of the helmet or with the head down. This maneuver results in axial loading, often with a major or minor component of flexion. In football, impacts with the head may involve hyperflexion, hyperextension, lateral flexion, rotation, axial compression, or a combination of these. The cervical musculature, which is responsible for maintaining neck extension, is much stronger than that used in maintaining flexion. A player who lowers his head in blocking or tackling places his cervical spine in a position that is less able to absorb the opponent's energy, making him vulnerable to cervical injury via the energy forces transmitted to the spinal column. Recent laboratory and clinical evidence has shown that in almost every sport in which collisions occur, axial loading is a primary method of sustaining cervical fracture or fracture-dislocation.[72,97]

Torg et al.[94] have described a group of athletes at high risk for the development of cervical quadriplegic injury. They found that football players with (1) developmental cervical canal stenosis, (2) persistent straightening or reversal of the normal cervical spine lordotic curve, (3) evidence of preexisting posttraumatic radiographic abnormalities of the cervical spine, and (4) documentation of having previously used spear tackling techniques are predisposed to cervical spine axial injury mechanisms. This clinical entity was termed "spear tackler's spine"[94] to describe habitual users of spear tackling techniques as evidenced by radiographic documentation of prior traumatic injuries. Torg et al.[94] recommended termination of participation in contact or collision sports in individuals with this syndrome unless or until the abnormalities could be corrected.

### Rugby

Although less popular in the United States than in other countries, rugby is another organized sport that always carries a certain risk of spinal injury. The "collapsing scrum" and "crashing of the scrum" are particularly dangerous aspects of the game in which a player may have his head pushed into the ground, often with the tremendous weight of many players driving him. While in the scrum, the three front-row players join with interlocking arms and push against the opposition's front row while five additional players from each team are pushing from behind the front-row line. More than 50% of the 30 catastrophic spinal injuries in the United States since 1976 have occurred in this manner. Tackling is another common method of producing cervical injuries, comprising 55% of rugby injuries in one review.[101] Particularly dangerous are the high tackle in which the tackler wraps his arms around the opponent's neck and drags him to the ground, causing a hyperextension, often with a rotational mechanism of injury[74]; the double or "sandwich" tackle in which a player is hit by two tacklers, usually high and low[74,76]; and as in football, the head-down tackle of an opponent, producing a hyperflexion injury with or without an axial component.

### Wrestling

Neck injuries in wrestling are common, but few are catastrophic.[107] Wrestlers are usually in superior physical condition and have strong cervical soft-tissue support. Nonetheless, wrestling can place great forces on the intervertebral discs, ligaments, joints, and vertebrae as a result of rotational and horizontal shearing vectors during certain maneuvers, holds, and positions.[106,107] Also, "spearing" techniques, which drive the opponent's head into the mat, are particularly dangerous maneuvers.

Most wrestling spinal injuries are sustained by the soft tissues of the spine.[106] Takedown maneuvers in which the extensor musculature is overloaded by stress forces with hyperflexion, hyperextension, rotation, and lateral flexion cause cervical strains that frequently tear one of the musculotendinous segments of the paraspinal musculature. The acute sprain syndrome may be seen either with or without simultaneous muscle strain syndromes. In the former injuries, the ligamentous and capsular structures of the spine are involved, with pain being confined to the neck and interscapular area. Brachial plexus involvement that results in the so-called stinger or burner injury may also occur in wrestling (discussed below). Wrestlers may suffer from a traumatic herniated intervertebral disc syndrome, with the descending order of frequency being the cervical spine, the lumbar spine, and the thoracic spine. In general, although wrestling injuries are common in both the cervical and lumbar spine, catastrophic spinal cord injury is rare.[70,106] In a different, but mechanistically related, sport, judo players are also at risk of sustaining spinal injuries, most of which are minor and nonosseous. However, all athletes in the martial arts are at risk for cervical fracture-dislocation as a result of the frequent throws or violent takedowns that may occur.

### Ice Hockey

There were no reported cases of spinal injury in ice hockey players before the 1970s; however, since the establishment of an organized reporting system and with the game's increasing popularity in the United States, this sport is now recognized as having a serious risk of athletic spinal injury. Tator and associates in Canada[84,85] documented that these injuries occurred almost exclusively among young male players, with an average age of 20, during competitive, organized games and usually involved the C5 spinal level. The usual mechanism of injury is that of a player being pushed or checked from behind or falling onto the ice, causing him to strike his head with a vertex axial loading mechanism. Injury also frequently occurred when a player's head made impact against the boards around the rink, usually in a flexion posture.[17,84]

There are several additional reasons for this apparent increase in serious spinal injuries to ice hockey players. Among these are the increasing size and speed of the players; the use of helmets, which has contributed to a more aggressive style of play; lack of enforcement of rules; and poor shock absorption of the perimeter boards.[84]

### Gymnastics

The overall injury rate in gymnastics is reportedly exceeded only by football, wrestling, and softball. It is the only sport except cheerleading in which women are at high risk of catastrophic injury. Certain activities such as vaults and hyperextension cause particular impact loads that can result in repeated microtrauma injuries to the lower back. The majority of injuries happen with moves that are basic or moderately difficult and well established with the athlete.

The trampoline was the leading cause of catastrophic head and spine injuries in gymnastics. Its use, including that of the mini-trampoline, has become highly controversial. Early reports described the causes of these accidents as being related to the athlete's inexperience, fatigue, loss of concentration, carelessness, poor technique, or improper assistance.[82] More recent reports,[26,92] however, have demonstrated that neurologic injuries occur despite safety measures such as mats and spotters and were independent of both the environment and the jumper's experience.

In 1984, Torg reviewed the world literature and identified 114 quadriplegic injuries resulting from use of the trampoline and mini-trampoline.[90,92] The majority of the lesions occurred at the C4-5 and C5-6 levels and involved a highly skilled gymnast attempting to perform a forward or backward somersault. Torg concluded: "The trampoline and mini-trampoline are dangerous devices when used in the best of circumstances, and their use has no place in recreational, educational, or competitive gymnastics."[92] The best way to prevent injury on the trampoline may be to eliminate the sport altogether, or to demand only highly supervised performance of this activity. This has led to the abolition of this event as a competitive sport.

A National Registry of Gymnastic Catastrophic Injury was established in 1978.[97] Twenty gymnastic injuries of the cervical spine occurred in the first 4 years. Of those injured, 17 remained quadriplegic and 3 died secondary to the injury. Notably, most of the injuries occurred in experienced gymnasts during practice. According to the National Spinal Cord Injury Data Research Center, gymnastics accounted for 6% of all sports-related spinal cord injuries between 1973 and 1981. This represented 1% of all spinal cord injuries at the time.[56] Eighty-eight percent of the injuries occurred to an individual not participating in an organized class or team. Of those injured, 25% were considered skilled at gymnastics.[56]

The most common etiologies of back injury in this sport are repeated hyperextensions of the back, which are compounded by impact loading from tumbling and landing from height.[99] Rhythmic gymnasts, who must combine gymnastics with dance, are at particular risk for lower back injury. A study of these athletes found that 86% of the participants complained of back pain.[32] The etiologies of this pain ranged from muscle strains to complete fracture of the pars interarticularis (spondylolysis).

### Baseball/Softball

An estimated 23 million organized softball games are played in the United States per year. It has been reported that this sport causes more injuries leading to emergency room visits in the United States than any other. Between 1983 and 1989, over 2.6 million emergency room visits were documented throughout the United States.[36] Softball-related injuries can be grouped into three categories. The most common of these are injuries that occur from sliding into base. Janda[37] found base sliding to be responsible for 71% of recreational softball injuries.

Approximately 71% of softball-related injuries are caused by sliding.[80] Hosey et al.[31] studied the incidence of sliding-related injuries in seven softball and three baseball Division I collegiate teams. The overall incidence of sliding injuries was 9.51 per 1000 slides and 4.87 per 1000 game exposures, the majority of which were minor. Softball players were found to have a significantly higher incidence of sliding injuries (12.13 per 1000 slides) than did baseball players (6.01 per 1000 slides). Slides can be categorized as either feet first or head first. The head-first slide into a base seems to cause the most risk to a baseball player of catastrophic spinal cord injury. If the hands of the runner separate, the top of his head can collide with the leg of the defensive player, creating a great deal of axial load transmission to the vertebral column. While the use of breakaway bases substantially decreases the risk for occurrence of sliding-related injuries, serious injuries can still occur. The use of low-profile bases and the outlawing of sliding have also been suggested.[59] According to the National Spinal Cord Injury Data Research Center, baseball accounted for 1% of all sports-related spinal cord injuries between 1973 and 1981.[56]

### Basketball

While not considered a true collision sport, the injury rate of basketball rivals such games in many studies. Prebble

et al.[67] conducted a study of basketball injuries occurring in a rural setting. Approximately two thirds (66.4%) of those injured were males, and four fifths (78%) of injuries occurred between the ages of 10 and 19 years. Most injuries (53%) occurred during school-related activities. Actual neurologic injury accounts for only 1% to 3% of all injuries.

The most common neurologic risk in basketball is to the player's spine. According to the National Spinal Cord Injury Data Research Center, basketball accounted for 1% of all sports-related spinal cord injuries between 1973 and 1981.[56] Because the sport involves rapid changes in direction and explosive movements, repeated stress on the vertebrae of the spine can result in spondylolysis. Secondary to the athletes' rapid growth, adolescent players with these defects in the pars interarticularis are at a higher risk of vertebral slippage and spondylolisthesis.[104] Early detection of this problem in the adolescent is critical to reverse this degenerative process. If the injury is not corrected early, spinal stenosis and narrowing of the foramen can cause radiculopathy. Acute back injuries associated with basketball include lumbosacral sprains, contusions, facet joint and pars interarticularis injuries, spinal stenosis, and lumbar disc injuries or fractures.[33,34,55,60]

Disc herniation in athletes is a consequence of numerous micro-traumas of the intervertebral disc, which are further compounded by the syndrome of chronic overstraining. Basketball is a leading cause of sports-related disc disease and was the second most common cause of disc herniation among a series of 55 athletes reported by Kovac et al.[44] Facet syndrome can cause lower back pain in the basketball player. This pain radiates into the dorsal (posterior) buttocks and thigh and rarely descends below the knees. The pain is often increased with hyperextension and decreased with ambulation.[30,33] Spinal stenosis can cause chronic lower back pain and radiculopathy. It is often associated with disc disease or injury and recurrent pain while playing the game. Pars interarticularis defects can cause areas of spinal instability and low back pain in the player.[30,33,34,55] Pain from this source is greatest with hyperextension or twisting of the spine and may be unilateral. Patients with spondylolysis or spondylolisthesis with less than 50% slippage can be treated with rest. More-severe injuries require bracing of the lumbosacral spine or surgical fusion.[33,55]

Fractures of the lumbar spine are rare occurrences in basketball.[60] If a fracture does occur, timely diagnosis and treatment is essential. Compression and burst fractures are treated in a fashion similar to that in other trauma patients. Fractures of the spinous or transverse processes can be treated symptomatically. These can occur secondary to trauma or from strong muscular contraction.[33] These more commonly affect the lumbosacral area rather than the cervical spine. Overall serious injuries to the lumbar spine occur infrequently.[33,60] Cervical cord neurapraxia has been reported in basketball players. It is a transient neurologic phenomenon usually not associated with any permanent neurologic injury. No permanent morbidity has occurred in patients who returned to contact activities. Once a player experiences it, however, they have over a 50% chance of recurrence. This risk of recurrence is strongly and inversely correlated with sagittal canal diameter.[91]

### Auto Racing

Over the last two decades, auto racing safety technology has been catching up to the technology that allows cars to travel in excess of 250 mph. While speeds have increased over 20% in the last 15 years, both the injury and fatality rates have declined until there were 4 deaths in NASCAR alone in a recent 10-month period.[56] According to data collected by the professional racing organization CART, 20% of injuries sustained since 1981 have been to the axial skeleton.[98] Between 1981 and 1991, 50 Indy car drivers have incurred competition-related injuries, 3 involving the cervical spine.[98] Between 1997 and 1998, 25 spinal cord injuries related to race car driving were reported.[102] Left-sided sprains and strains are the most common injury of the cervical spine in CART drivers. These are secondary to the lateral forces endured on oval tracks, which can exceed 5.5g. Cervical spine fractures are rare. The most commonly reported vertebral fractures are spinous process avulsions or compression fractures of the cervical vertebral bodies. Rear impacts can cause whiplash and result in flexion-extension type injuries. The rollover accident carries the greatest risk of cervical spine injury. Thoracolumbar injuries are uncommon in this sport, mainly caused by the driver being so well attached in the cockpit. Studies performed by General Motors Research have found that the more reclined a driver is, the more neck load he receives during a crash.[61]

### Equestrian Sports

Horse-related injuries are recognized as a serious and common occurrence. Between 1997 and 1998, 465 spinal cord injuries related to equestrian sports were reported.[102] According to the National Spinal Cord Injury Data Research Center, equestrian sports accounted for 2% of all sports-related spinal cord injuries between 1973 and 1981. One hundred percent of injuries occurred in men, and 80% of injuries occurred in individuals considered adept at the sport. Sixty percent resulted in quadriplegia. Sixty percent of the injuries occurred to an individual not participating in an organized class or team.[9]

## Injury Patterns

### Musculotendinous Injuries

Both strains and sprains are extremely common injuries to the musculotendinous structures of the cervical, thoracic, and lumbar spine. A strain results from mechanical overloading with forces that exceed the extensor musculature capacity. The muscle responds to injury with characteristic localized pain, tenderness, and decreased or inhibited voluntary muscle contraction. Injury to the ligaments or capsular structures of the spine is termed a *sprain*, and it may occur without muscular strain. The pain is located in the neck, interscapular area, and occasionally the upper arm in cervical injuries. Lumbar ligamentous sprain is usually located in the lumbar paraspinal and midline positions. In all true sprain syndromes, the pain is nonradicular, and there is no sensory disturbance. In both strain and sprain syndromes, vertebral column and neurologic injury

must be excluded. With sprain injuries, one must be certain to exclude ligamentous damage resulting in spinal instability.

### Injuries to the Spinal Cord or Vertebral Column

Most of these kinds of athletic injuries do not involve a permanent neurologic deficit. However, for the small percentage of athletes in whom this occurs, these injuries can be devastating. Moreover, mismanagement of any unstable injury in a young athlete can sometimes lead to delayed and unnecessary neurologic involvement. It is incumbent on the personnel attending to these athletic accidents to characterize the nature of the injury, render appropriate treatment, and advise both the athlete and the family about the advisability of returning to athletic events.

### Hyperflexion

Hyperflexion was initially believed to be the primary cause of football spinal injuries. However, Torg's study in the late 1970s[95,96] identified defensive players as being three to four times more likely to suffer spinal cord injuries, with axial loading most often responsible for placing the cervical spine at risk. When an athlete improperly flexes his neck, the cervical spine can become a straight, segmented column. If loading of the straightened cervical spine is then experienced—as in a tackle—a sudden, forceful impact can cause compressive deformation of the intervertebral discs, ligaments, and vertebrae, resulting in vertebral column or in neurologic injury. In fact, axial compression with hyperflexion has also been identified as a common pathomechanical feature of most injuries common to rugby, wrestling, ice hockey, and diving.* Fracture-dislocation injury occurs in approximately 33% of all accidents, and ventral compression fractures occur in approximately 22%.[7]

Our study of 63 consecutively treated, acute athletic cervical spine injuries has enabled us to draw several conclusions about such mishaps.[3] First, for purposes of diagnosis and management, repetitive patterns of injuries have been recognized, and these are classified into three general types, as defined below. Second, the population of patients with spinal injuries resulting from competitive contact sports is young, is healthy, has few or no associated injuries, has a low incidence of complications from treatment, and can usually be discharged from the hospital after relatively short periods of stay. Last, there are a few potentially unrecognized congenital anomalies that may predispose an athlete to the risk of neurologic injury if participation in contact sports is resumed.[3]

## Types of Injuries

A classification scheme of three types of athletic spinal injuries is presented to assist the health care team with clinical evaluation and management of the injured athlete (Figure 147.1): type I, permanent spinal cord injury; type

---

*References 3,4,75,85,86,94-96.

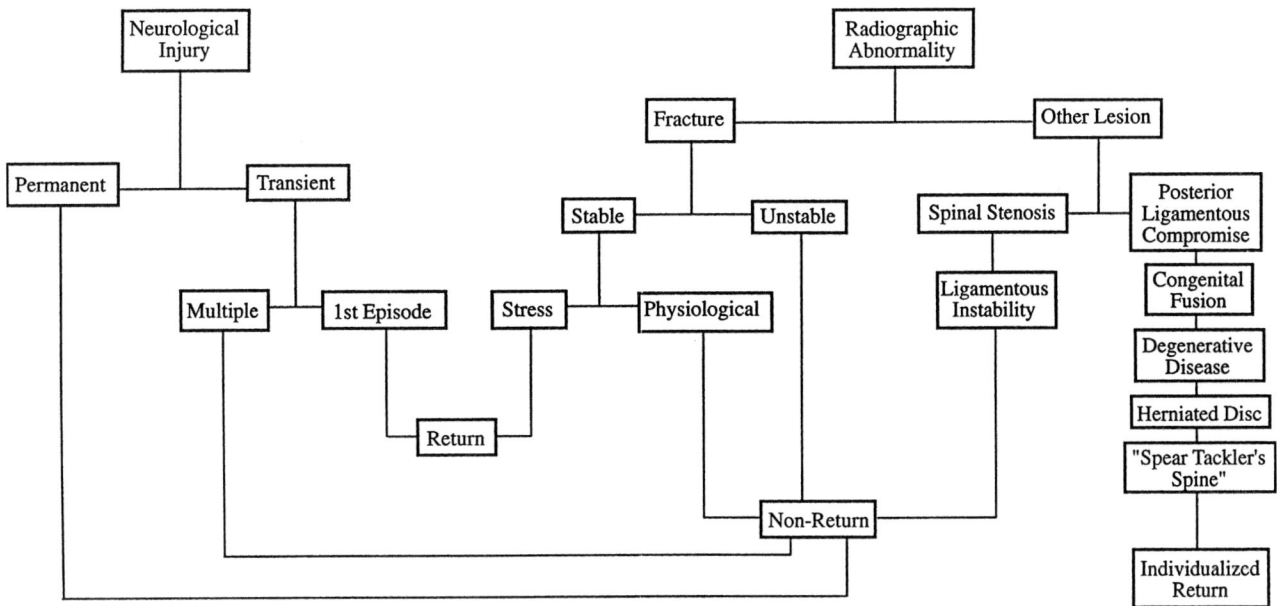

**Figure 147.1** Classification system for the types of spinal athletic injuries.

II, transient spinal cord injury; and type III, radiographic abnormality.

A type I injury causes permanent damage to the spinal cord as manifested by neurologic deficit after the injury or by symptoms that are minor or that resolve but are associated with radiographic evidence of spinal cord injury. Typically, the latter is documented by a magnetic resonance imaging (MRI) scan or by a myelogram positive for intrinsic spinal cord damage, such as swelling, hemorrhage, or contusion. For the first time, spinal cord contusion can be directly visualized on an MRI scan and is best seen on intermediate images as a high-intensity lesion within the cord. Once the spinal cord injury has been documented, either clinically or radiologically, the athlete should not be allowed to return to contact sports.

Type II injuries occur in athletes who have transient spinal cord symptoms after athletic trauma but have normal neurologic examinations and radiologic evaluations (including MRI studies). There is no vertebral fracture, spinal column instability, or intrinsic cord injury or contusion.

These transiently injured patients present a diagnostic challenge. The physician must actively seek symptoms suggestive of spinal cord involvement and follow up on them when found.[20,22] Although the prognosis for these patients is good, they must be carefully evaluated before being allowed to resume competition. Specifically, congenital or acquired spinal stenosis must be evaluated by MRI. In the absence of neurologic deficit, radiologically demonstrable injury, and congenital cervical spine anomaly, we feel that such athletes may return to full participation in contact sports. When athletes suffer from multiple episodes symptomatic of spinal cord injury, they are at a higher than normal risk for catastrophic injury, and thought should be given to prohibiting further participation.

Type III injuries are those in which the athlete has only a radiographic abnormality. An unstable fracture or fracture-dislocation requires stabilization by either a surgical procedure or external bracing. These patients should not be recommended for further participation in contact sports. In those with a bony injury that appears stable on flexion-extension radiographs, it must be determined whether this lesion is stable only during physiologic range of motion or whether it is indeed stable under the stresses to which a contact athlete would be subjected. This determination is particularly important for a fracture of an isolated lamina, spinous process, or minor portion of the vertebral body, which ordinarily would be considered to be "stress stable." A more difficult assessment involves bony injuries that have healed, are stable on physiologic range-of-motion testing (with flexion-extension radiographs), but occur in a portion of the spine that normally contributes significantly to spinal column stability.

There are few objective criteria for assessing the degree of stability of a healed fracture or ligamentous injury of the cervical spine, especially when it is placed under extreme degrees of stress. The cervical dorsal ligamentous structures contribute more to stability in flexion, whereas the ventral ligaments are more important in extension. It has been generally accepted that cervical instability exists if there is more than 3.5mm of horizontal displacement or more than 11 degrees of angular displacement between adjacent vertebrae. The contribution of the individual vertebral components to the stability of the cervical spine is unknown, especially when considering the possibility of either partial or complete ligament injuries, the healing process, the insertion of a bony graft, and the exceptional stress forces to which the athlete may be subjected. Because there are neither reliable data nor an objective way to measure stability under dynamic stress, we recommend that an athlete with any significant healed fracture of the spinal column be advised not to return to contact sports. The only exceptions to this dictum are athletes with healed, isolated fractures of the minor vertebral body, lamina, or spinous process.

## Other Radiologic Abnormalities

Type III injuries also include radiologic abnormalities other than fracture. For example, evidence of spinal motion on dynamic radiographs suggests a ligamentous injury requiring a halo brace or surgical stabilization. This individual would not be recommended for further participation in contact sports because the likelihood of injury would be significantly higher than normal. Other type III injuries include radiologic abnormalities that ordinarily would not be considered unstable but that assume a different significance in the athlete. Compromise by the dorsal ligaments would narrow the size of the cervical canal functionally, especially under high degrees of motion or stress forces and hyperextension movements. Combined with a congenitally narrow or relatively narrow cervical canal, this finding would place the athlete at a higher risk. Some surgeons believe that a bulging disc may be problematic in an athlete experiencing high-velocity collisions with a flexion component. Herniated cervical discs are relatively common in athletes and are usually treated by surgical removal that uses a ventral approach. There are no absolute guidelines regarding the decision to perform a bony fusion, but it has been suggested that healed ventral interbody fusion results in a preservation of strength in the cervical spine when tested in flexion and extension.[38,39] The authors sometimes use a dorsal surgical approach to maintain the integrity of the anterior and posterior longitudinal ligaments. This enables them to consider returning the patient to contact sports after 6 to 12 months of recuperation and after demonstration of stability on flexion-extension radiographs.

In an athlete with congenital spinal fusion, there is some increase in movement at the motion segments above and below the fused level. Unless associated with more widespread abnormalities such as Klippel-Feil syndrome, a narrowed spinal canal, multilevel fusion, motion on flexion-extension radiographs, or recurrent neurologic symptoms, this condition alone should not preclude participation in contact sports.

## Cervical Stenosis

Spinal cord injuries may be further complicated by stenosis of the cervical spinal canal, whether developmental or congenital or acquired through degeneration. In the past, spinal stenosis has most often been defined by x-ray bone measurement methods. Researchers[5,105] proposed in the 1950s that, on radiographs corrected for magnification error, canal heights of 15mm or more were normal, while spinal stenosis was felt to be present when the measurement was 12 to 13mm or less.[15,46] To eliminate the need to correct for magnification error, Torg et al.[93] in 1986 and Pavlov et al.[62] in 1987 proposed a ratio method to radiographically assess cervical spinal stenosis. The ratio method compares the height of the spinal canal from the midpoint of the posterior surface of the vertebral body to the spinolaminar line (numerator) with the height of the corresponding mid vertebral body (denominator). The authors concluded that significant spinal stenosis was present when the canal-to-vertebral body ratio was 0.80 or less.

Subsequently, serious doubts have been raised about using the ratio to diagnose cervical spinal stenosis. One problem is that x-rays do not assess the size of the neural tissue in relation to the size of the spinal canal. The size of the spinal cord has been variably reported to be between 5 and 11.5mm.[47,87] Thus, true stenosis may be present with low-normal canal measurements and a large spinal cord.

In 1990, one group[63] reported that 33% of the professional football players they studied had spinal stenosis according to the ratio. Herzog et al.[28] in 1991 reported ratios of less than 0.80 in 49% of 80 football players they studied. These authors concluded that the ratio was highly unreliable for detection of spinal stenosis and had a positive predictive value of only 12%.

Herzog et al.[28] theorized that the Torg ratio had a lot of false positives (88% of the time) because the large vertebral bodies of large athletes skewed the ratio. The cervical spinal canal heights (numerator) of all the athletes they studied were within normal limits. The athletes with abnormal Torg ratios had extremely large vertebral bodies (denominator), which brought the ratio below 0.80.

When an athlete has symptoms referable to the spinal cord such as transient quadriplegia, burning hands syndrome, bilateral motor or sensory symptoms, or nerve roots, x-rays should be a part of the initial workup. Radiographic bone measurement is still a useful screening tool; an abnormal Torg ratio should suggest the need for further workup. The physician should order an MRI after obtaining radiographs. Contrast-positive CT and myelography are useful for defining the degree of spinal stenosis; however, both techniques are invasive and usually not needed. Contrast-positive CT is more sensitive than MRI for fractures and bony abnormalities, and myelography provides a better view of spinal cord compression than MRI (Figure 147.2).

When a player has spinal cord symptoms after a sports injury and is shown to have true spinal stenosis by MRI or myelogram/contrast positive CT, return to contact sports should not be allowed.[10,13] There is a body of literature in the sports medicine, neurology, and radiology fields that indicates that spinal stenosis predisposes a patient to spinal cord injury.* Matsuura and his group,[52] for example, compared the spinal dimensions of 100 controls with those of 42 patients who had spinal cord injuries. They found that the control group had significantly larger sagittal spinal canal diameters than did the patients who had spinal cord injuries.

In the National Center for Catastrophic Sports Injury Research in Chapel Hill, NC, experience between 1989 and 2001 (Cantu RC, unpublished data, 2001) there are three cases of quadriplegia without spine fracture, and all three cases had spinal stenosis. On the other hand, there are numerous cases of quadriplegia with fracture and normal-sized canals in which complete neurologic recovery

---

*References 2,16,51,52,64,65.

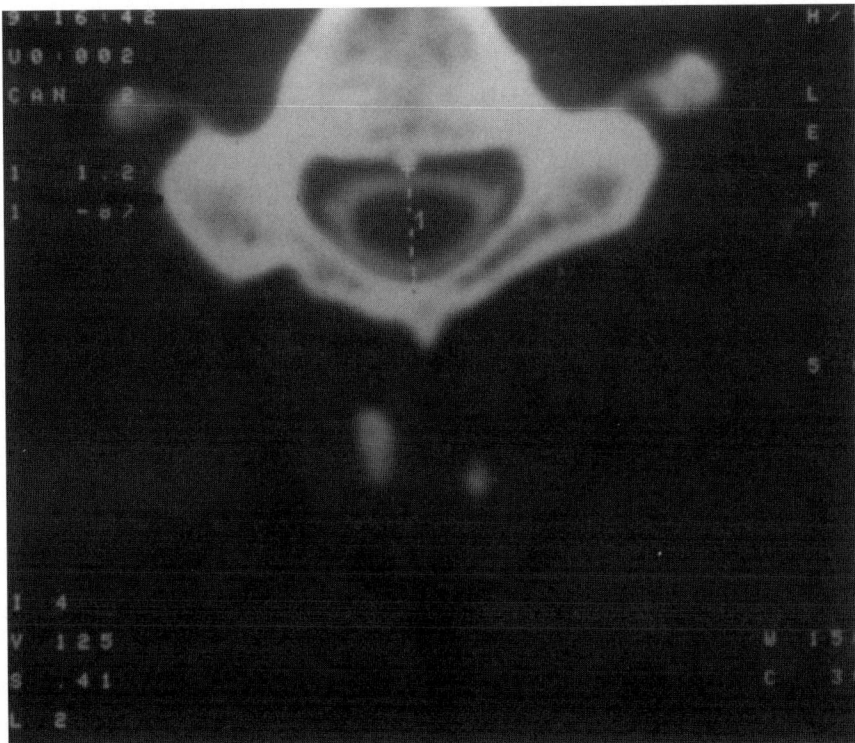

**Figure 147.2** Metrizamide cervical spine CT scan showing a 12mm canal in a professional football lineman who had repeated episodes of transient quadriplegia, resulting in his retirement from the sport.

occurred, but no cases of quadriplegia with fracture and spinal stenosis with complete, neurologic recovery.

The literature contains several articles that define spinal stenosis by the ratio method in which "stenotic" individuals were allowed to return to play collision sports.[62,93] Many didn't sustain further cervical injuries, and this fact is being used as verification that players with spinal stenosis can resume contact sports. However, the question remains: did these patients have true spinal stenosis? A 12% accuracy rate for the ratio suggests not. The consequences of this misanalysis can be devastating. Thus, when MRI does suggest spinal cord compromise, physicians can give patients clear-cut reasons for giving up contact sports[†] (Figure 147.3).

## Transient Cervical Cord Injury

Transient spinal cord injury is an uncommon but well-described phenomenon in sports having high-velocity or severe range-of-motion vectors. Symptoms include quadriplegia, quadriparesis, hemiplegia, paraplegia, and bilateral sensory loss. The incidence of transient weakness and paresthesias has been estimated at 1.3 per 10,000 participants, and the incidence of numbness and tingling at 6 per 10,000 participants.[93] Among our series of 63 athletes with

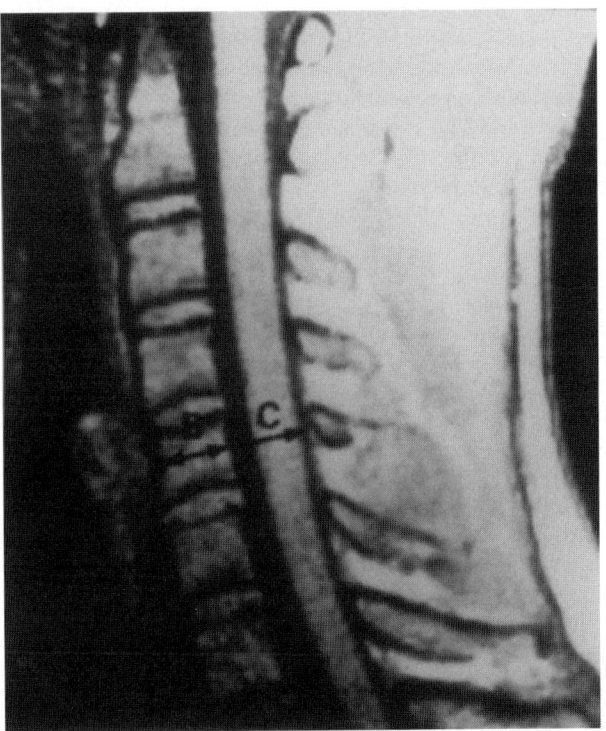

**Figure 147.3** A sagittal $T_1$-weighted MRI scan can shows the relationship between the spinal cord and spinal canal. Flexion-extension sequences give additional information concerning dynamic changes.

[†]References 2,10-13,16,51,52,64,65.

cervical spine injuries, 18 (29%) had signs and symptoms of transient neurologic cord injury and no evidence of radiographic abnormality.[3] All 18 experienced complete resolution of their symptoms. Thirteen of 18 patients were available for follow-up, and among these, 5 athletes returned to regular participation in contact sports. These 5 patients reported no recurrence of either the original or other neurologic symptoms, and all patients were neurologically intact. Each had multilevel measurements of a canal-to-cervical spinal body ratio of less than 0.80, although none had an absolute measurement of less than 14mm.

The "burning hands" syndrome described by Maroon[48] is an example of transient neurologic injury in which the athlete experiences burning dysesthesia and paresthesia, with associated weakness in both hands and arms as a result of the repeated cervical trauma experienced in contact sports. He proposed that the burning hands syndrome is a variant of central cord syndrome, without the permanent loss of function characteristic of central cord syndrome.

Distinguishing between the burner, or stinger, injury and injury with spinal cord involvement can present a diagnostic challenge. The former injury may occur in up to 50% of collegiate football players during the course of a season, and it tends to be recurrent. It is characterized by a burning, dysesthetic pain beginning in the region of the shoulder and radiating unilaterally into the arm and hand, at times associated with numbness or weakness, usually in the C5 and C6 distribution. The injury is caused by traction on the upper trunk of the brachial plexus, occurring as a force is applied that depresses the ipsilateral shoulder when the neck is laterally flexed to the contralateral side. Another mechanism involves a direct axial compression of the cervical root within the neural foramen (Figure 147.4). These injuries often resolve within several days to weeks and usually leave no residual neurologic damage. All radiologic studies are normal, and there are no findings suggestive of cord involvement such as bilaterality, lower extremity symptoms, long tract findings, sphincter distur-

bance, or sexual dysfunction. Burner and stinger injuries can often be reduced with appropriate equipment such as the high neck roll that eliminates lateral flexion and extension.[6,66,88,100]

## Lumbar Spine

A symptomatic lumbar spine in athletes can result in a significant amount of time missed from sports participation. In the skeletally immature athlete, back pain is usually of greater significance than in an adult athlete. In the young athlete, if consistent lumbar pain occurs (without radicular signs), and if this is worsened by lumbar extension, a stress reaction of the pars interarticularis is suspected. Technetium bone scans may be positive when plain radiographs are normal. It is important to detect and treat this process as early as possible to reduce the athlete's risk of developing a permanent pars defect. Treatment usually consists of curtailing sports activities and bracing in an antilordotic posture for 3 months.[45]

Spondylolysis can be associated with acquired defects in the pars interarticularis. Certain sports, such as gymnastics, have been reported to have a fourfold higher incidence of spondylolysis.[35] Female gymnasts are especially vulnerable to lumbar vertebral trauma, particularly spondylolisthesis, because excessive stresses on the low back are created by the repetitive hyperflexion-hyperextension maneuvers during flipping, vaulting, dismounting, and backbending walkovers. Football linemen also are predisposed to lumbar injury because of repetitive forceful movements in hyperextended positions. If the bone scan is indicative of an active defect, antilordotic bracing is indicated.[54] Kraus and Shapiro also recommend bracing if spondylosis occurs in conjunction with a growth spurt or if radiographs demonstrate segmental instability.[45] Treatment for spondylolisthesis depends on the amount of displacement and the skeletal maturity of the patient. If the displacement is 25% or less (grade I), all sports are allowed as long as the patient remains asymptomatic. If the injury approaches a grade II spondylolisthesis, contact sports are prohibited, and antilordotic bracing is required.[54] The authors recommend careful follow-up of the skeletally immature athlete and a conservative approach to their participation in athletics until stabilization occurs.

Fracture and fracture-dislocation of the lumbar spine are unusual with sports activities, constituting less than 5% of injuries in our experience. They are treated by using the standard guidelines for patients with such an injury. In general, the authors are impressed that an increasing number of patients may successfully heal with a thoracolumbosacral orthosis.

Although most low back pain in adult athletes is musculotendinous in nature, if the patient fails to respond to the usual local treatment or if signs or symptoms suggest nerve root involvement, a structural or degenerative etiology must be excluded. Discogenic low back pain is usually evident on the basis of the history and physical examination. Scheuermann's disease of the lumbar spine, in which disc material may herniate through the vertebral margin at the radial margin, must be considered as a cause of lumbar pain in the adolescent athlete. Certain athletes—for

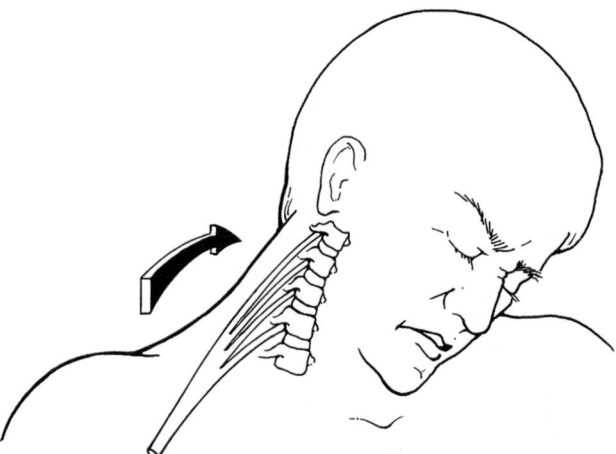

**Figure 147.4** Mechanisms that produce a "burner" or "stinger" injury by either a direct blow or ipsilateral shoulder depression with lateral neck flexion to the opposite side, causing a stretch injury to the upper trunk of the brachial plexus.

example, football offensive linemen—seem predisposed to developing degenerative disc disease, a condition probably related to their constant driving and thrusting with their legs while in a crouched position and under the load of an opposing player. The management of lumbar disc disease follows established guidelines, with our approach being as conservative as possible and relying heavily on physiotherapy. Percutaneous discectomy can be an attractive approach in the treatment of symptomatic, unresponsive herniated lumbar discs. If an athlete is not responsive to an aggressive conservative treatment regimen or if associated neurologic deficit is present, excellent results may be achieved with lumbar microdiscectomy.

## Management of Cervical Spine Injuries

Significant injury to the central nervous system as a result of participation in athletic events is an unusual occurrence. Few athletes with severe neurologic damage, however, will ever return to full activity or active competition. For those with less-serious injuries, the physician has the difficult task, in the absence of any objective criteria, of managing the return to competitive sports. This dilemma may be compounded by injured players and often their families, who may view athletics as the means to achievement, education, or financial success. For everyone involved, the consequences of the wrong decision can be devastating.

### Immediate Care

The sports medicine team present at any athletic event must first maintain a high level of on-field concentration and vigilance to recognize, prevent, or minimize potential injury to any of the players. Visualization of the exact mechanism of injury can be helpful during evaluation to confirm the presence or absence of head or neck impact. The priority when attending to any player with potential cervical injury is to achieve and maintain an adequate airway and ventilation. This task could prove difficult in a football player wearing a helmet unless special instrumentation is available to quickly remove the face mask without requiring removal of the helmet itself.

All unconscious athletes and all injured athletes who complain of numbness, weakness, paralysis, or neck pain should be handled as if they have a cervical fracture and thus potentially an unstable spine. Moving and transporting the athlete off-field should be done with sufficient personnel (usually four) so that the athlete's spinal column will not undergo motion (Figure 147.5). In particular, the caregivers should prevent flexion and extension movements that are likely to compromise the size of the cervical spinal canal. One designated person should be responsible only for immobilizing the cervical spine by cradling the shoulders and neck in his or her forearms while applying a mild traction force in the axial direction. This person should have no other role in transferring or supporting the weight of the body, and sufficient numbers of other personnel should be available or recruited so that the athlete can be easily moved without distracting the person at the head from maintaining proper cervical alignment. If necessary, the athlete's helmet can be safely removed by cutting the chin strap and pulling outward on the ear pads. This allows the helmet to be removed without movement of the neck. This maneuver is usually best accomplished once the athlete has been removed from the playing field. It is important to note that removal of a football helmet from a player wearing shoulder pads instantly forces the neck into hyperextension, and this must be avoided.

### Immediate Evaluation

The health care providers should begin their evaluation of a conscious patient by asking about extremity weakness, numbness, painful dysesthesias or paresthesias, and neck pain. A brief physical examination can determine whether there is obvious neurologic deficit and whether the athlete is unable to move all or any limbs or has gross weakness, numbness, or significant pain to palpation of the cervical region. If any of these signs or symptoms are reported by others or are present on examination or if the athlete is unconscious, he or she should be carefully transported on a spine board with the head and cervical spine in a neutral and immobilized position that is retained either manually with an external orthosis or with the use of sandbags and tape.

The initial on-field evaluation should consider the possibility of head trauma, including a brief examination of level of consciousness and cranial nerve function, with awareness that significant brain injury is possible. Although cerebral concussion is the most common head injury in football, the entire range of traumatic injuries is possible, from skull fracture to life-threatening intracranial hematomas (Figure 147.6).

Once the athlete is removed from the playing field, either to the sidelines or to the fieldhouse, the caregivers should ask in-depth questions about neurologic symptoms and should perform a more detailed examination of nervous system function, depending on the degree of suspected injury. Any persistent numbness, burning dysesthesia, or paresthesia should alert the caregiver to look closer for evidence of spinal cord injury. In examining the athlete, one should be aware that subtle degrees of weakness may be easily overlooked because these individuals are ordinarily much stronger than the average person. Any weakness should alert the examiner to the possibility of spinal or intracranial injury, just as any obvious deficit in movement, sensory disturbance, or neck pain requires that the patient be immobilized and hospitalized for a more in-depth study.

### Hospitalization

Any injured athlete who is suspected of having neurologic involvement from the history or after physical examination should undergo complete radiographic evaluation, beginning with a cervical spine radiographic series. If no abnormality is discovered, but the clinical setting suggests that the spinal column or cord is involved, further radiographic work-up is indicated, including flexion-extension radiographs for assessment of spinal stability. CT may be used to view the axial plane of the spine for fractures not discernible on routine radiographs and to analyze the relationship of bony injury to the spinal canal. The presence of

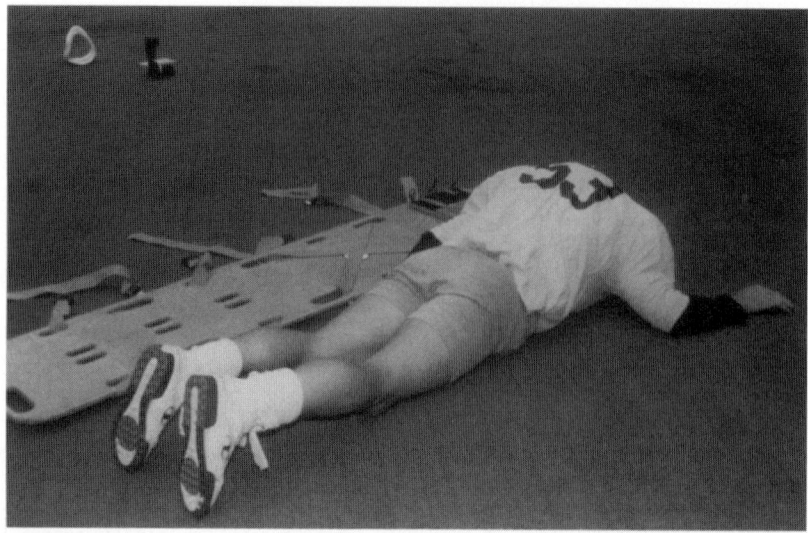

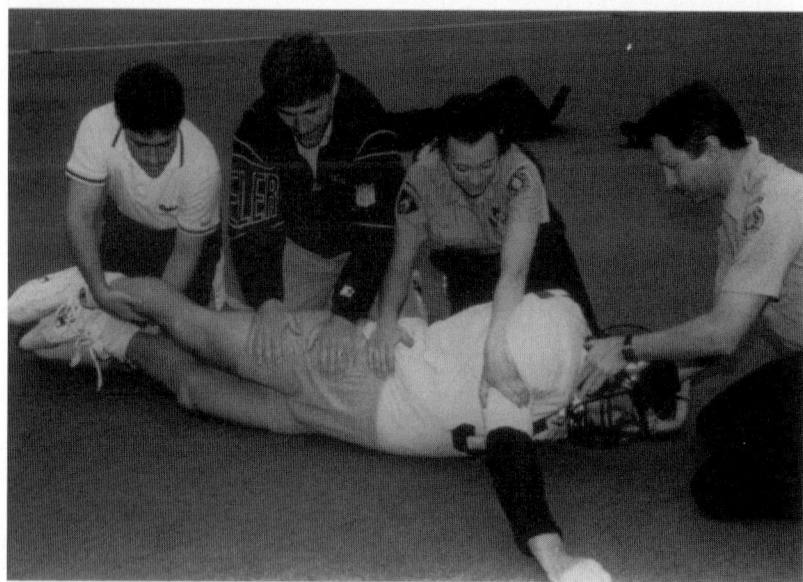

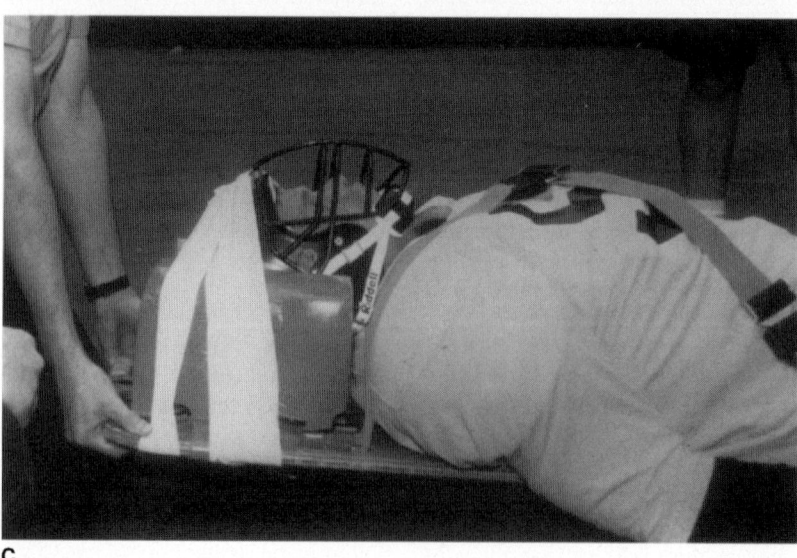

**Figure 147.5** The proper method of **(A)** transporting, **(B)** handling, and **(C)** immobilizing an injured football player.

spinal cord and canal compromise may be better appreciated with the use of metrizamide intrathecal contrast and sagittal CT reconstruction formatting. Three-dimensional CT reconstruction may provide an added advantage by delineating certain features of spinal pathology and is par-

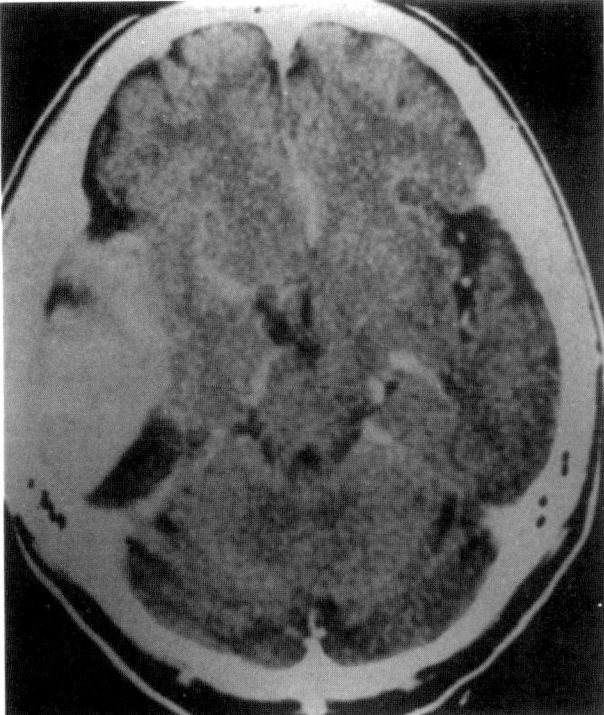

**Figure 147.6** CT scan showing a right temporal extradural hematoma that required prompt surgical evacuation. Any downed athlete must be suspected of potentially having a cervical or head injury until these can be excluded.

ticularly useful in assessing the upper cervical spine, cranioverte bral junction, and congenital anomalies in patients with concomitant injury.[25]

MRI has become increasingly popular in the diagnostic evaluation of spine-injured patients, especially when other radiologic tests fail to reveal fracture, dislocation, or instability despite persistent symptoms or signs suggestive of cord involvement (Figure 147.7). MRI can show an area of cord contusion, which is an extremely important finding, because it confirms a pathologic insult to the spinal cord (Figure 147.8), localizes the injury, and distinguishes it from a spinal nerve root or brachial plexus lesion. The latter distinction is important not only for treatment and prognosis but also in the decision-making process regarding return to contact sports participation. As mentioned, it is important for the examiner to determine whether the patient's complaints and any detectable neurologic abnormalities are caused by involvement of the nerve root, brachial plexus, or spinal cord. Nerve root symptoms usually include pain radiating into a specific dermatomal pattern and the possibility of neurologic deficits related to that sensory pattern or to the innervated muscle exists. Brachial plexus involvement is diagnosed if there is persistent pain in the entire upper extremity or in multiple sensory dermatomes or with weakness of more than one muscle. Spinal cord injury is suspected if the symptoms are bilateral and are present in the lower extremities or if long tract signs and symptoms of bladder or sexual dysfunction occur. The burning hands syndrome is distinguished by the absence of cervical pain or other signs of spinal cord injury. Root and plexus injury may often be distinguished from spinal cord involvement by electromyography, but the test usually is not positive until several weeks after the accident. Stinging and burning injuries can sometimes create

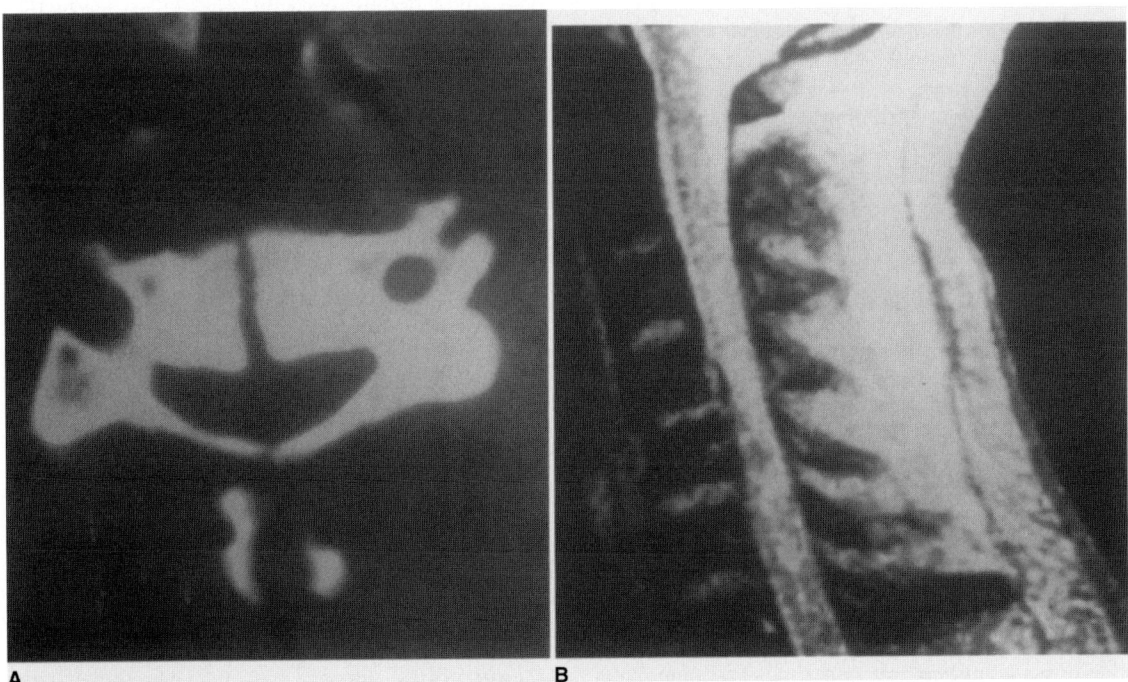

A                                        B

**Figure 147.7** CT (**A**) and MRI (**B**) scans in a 17-year-old high school football player who sustained a complete C5 quadriplegic injury while tackling an opponent.

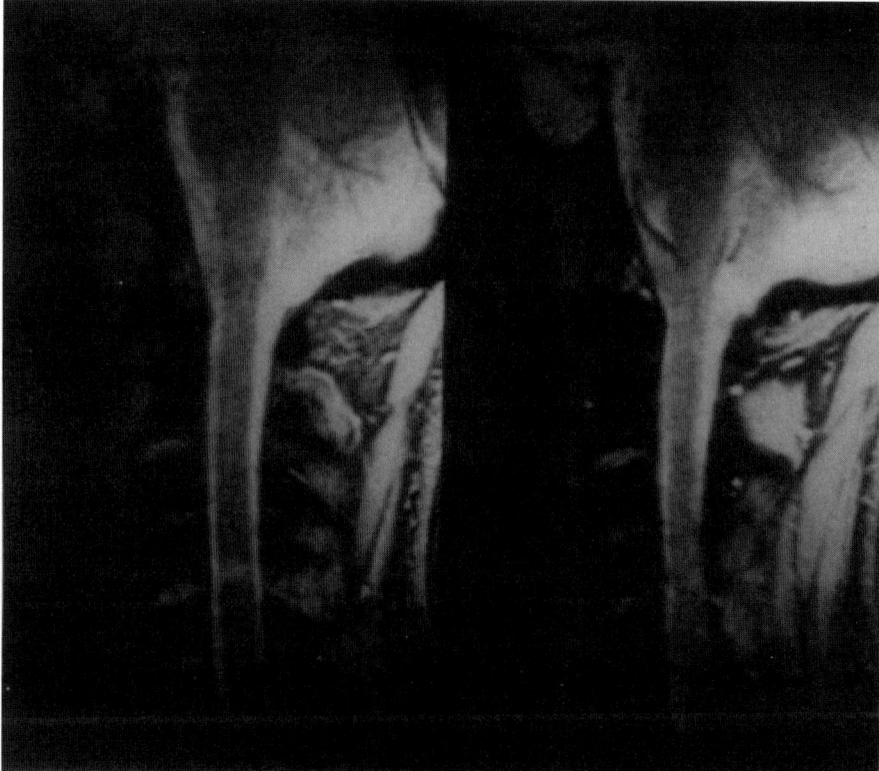

**Figure 147.8** An area of spinal cord contusion is demonstrated on an intermediate sequence MRI scan. This study documents the radiographic evidence of spinal cord injury and provides compelling evidence of definite injury in the athlete.

greater initial concern until it is determined that the injury does not involve the spinal cord.

When evidence suggests spinal cord rather than nerve root or brachial plexus injury, a thorough radiographic search must be conducted to identify any possible occult bony injury, ligamentous instability, or spinal cord contusion. Acute traumatic rupture of an intervertebral disc or traumatic hematoma must be considered as a cause of spinal cord compression and neurologic deficit. When these extremely uncommon lesions do occur in athletes, they have the ability to cause severe injury, but they are also potentially reversible.

## Treatment of Spinal Injury

When a vertebral column or spinal cord injury is documented, hospitalization becomes mandatory. With a severe injury involving vertebral column or neurologic damage, the player should be promptly transferred to a specialized care institution with adequate diagnostic and treatment facilities. Cervical traction, using a halo ring or Gardner-Wells tongs, should be instituted for adequate bony reduction and maintenance of alignment of the spine in the anatomically neutral position, as determined by radiographs and repeated physical examination of the patient. All involved health care professionals should recognize the possible respiratory and cardiovascular alterations that may occur after spinal cord injury (e.g., diminished respiratory excursion, hypotension, or brady-

cardia). An intensive care unit is usually the preferred place to treat the acute phase of such injuries.

After the patient has been evaluated and placed in cervical traction to realign the fracture-dislocation, the physician must decide whether a surgical fusion or external orthosis will be used for spinal stabilization. Nonsurgical fusion may be attempted in some cases by applying a halo vest cervical orthosis. In approximately 90% of patients thus treated, adequate bony healing occurs within 12 weeks of halo immobilization.[81] In patients with a traumatic subluxation without fracture as demonstrated by CT or tomography, adequate healing with halo immobilization has been reported in up to 82% of patients. Surgical treatment is usually still required for severe comminuted fractures of the vertebral body, fractures of the dorsal elements with extreme instability, type II odontoid fractures, and incomplete spinal cord injuries with canal or cord compromise and in patients who have neurologic deterioration with loss of higher spinal cord levels of function.

### Return to Play

The physician's decision to recommend or advise against the injured athlete's return to sports may be based on clear-cut to complex reasons. Few would argue that once there is documented evidence of spinal cord (type I) injury, either clinically or radiographically, the athlete should not be allowed to return to contact sports. This decision is based on the continuation of neurologic deficit after the injury or on the occurrence of symptoms that

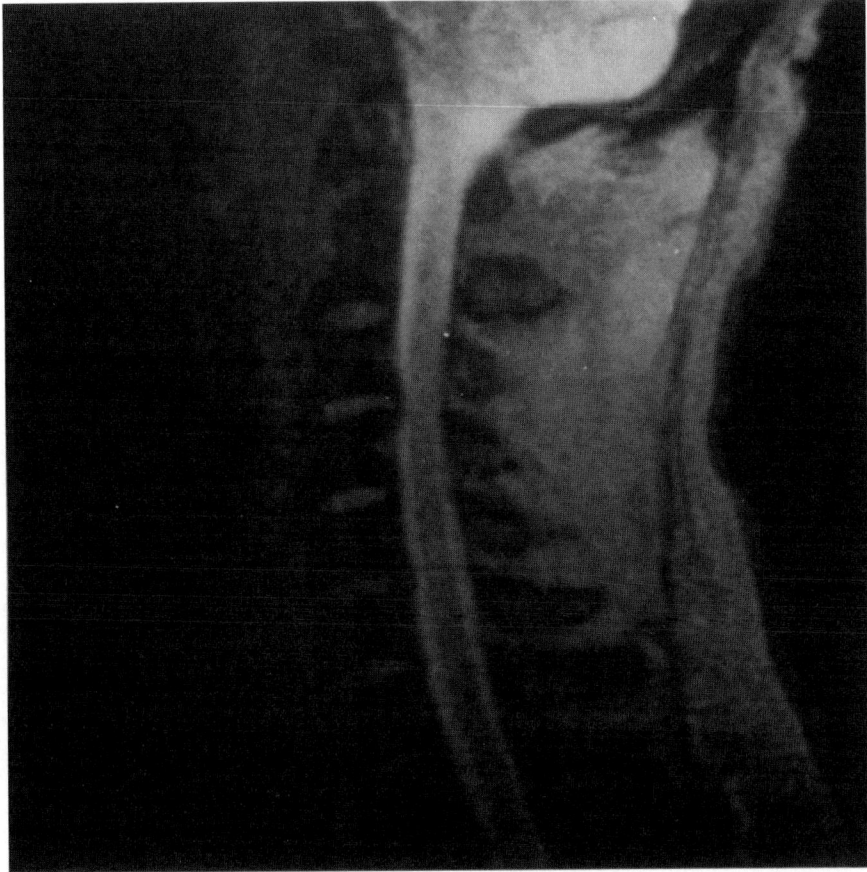

**Figure 147.9** Sagittal MRI scan showing a bulging disc at C3-4 in a professional football player. He had no symptoms referable to the spinal cord and was thus allowed to continue playing football.

are either minor or resolve but that are associated with radiologic evidence of spinal cord injury.

Transiently injured (type II) patients comprise a small but definable group of athletes who sustain repeated injuries with symptoms suggesting cervical spinal cord involvement (e.g., weakness or pain in both upper extremities). Their symptoms usually resolve rapidly, and extensive work-ups fail to disclose fracture, spinal instability, canal stenosis, or permanent neurologic deficit. Tests such as MRI and somatosensory evoked potentials should nonetheless be considered to rule out spinal cord injury either radiographically or physiologically.

Although the prognosis for these transiently injured patients is good, they must be carefully evaluated before being allowed to resume competition. In the absence of a neurologic deficit, radiologically demonstrable injury, or congenital cervical spine anomaly, we believe that they may return to full participation in contact sports. However, if repeated episodes suggestive of symptoms of spinal cord origin occur, these athletes are at a higher than normal risk for catastrophic injury and probably should not return to competitive events. As described earlier, players with the clinical and radiographic pictures of spear tackler's spine usually should be advised not to return to competition.[94] Athletes with brachial plexus trauma or burning hands syndrome may be considered healed after their symptoms resolve and after they have no abnormalities on neurologic examination.

Among type III injuries, any fracture-dislocation that requires stabilization by surgical means or external bracing precludes further participation in contact sports.[81] Patients whose fractures are determined to be stable radiographically on flexion-extension films and who do not have spinal cord injury are permitted to return to their normal daily activities. These injuries would include isolated lamina or spinous process fractures and, depending on the individual, a healed minor vertebral body fracture, which may be considered stable on the basis of flexion-extension films.

Another group of patients may have congenital spinal canal stenosis, posterior ligamentous compromise, resolved (either medically or surgically) herniated nucleus pulposus, or congenital vertebral body fusion (Figure 147.9). These patients have a heterogeneous assortment of abnormalities that, by themselves, do not require treatment yet may be associated with a higher risk of injury in contact sports. It is safe to say that in general, any patient who has had a cervical spine procedure (for example, ventral cervical discectomy, with or without fusion) will have lost some degree of inherent stability because of limited ligamentous and disc interruption and is not suitable for further contact sports. Likewise, when the MRI documents definite cervical spinal stenosis, this precludes further participation in contact sports. The disposition of those with dorsal ligamentous compromise and congenital fusion is less clear.

Within this heterogeneous group of patients, all decisions must be made on an individual basis.

## Prevention

Many sports-related accidents and collisions are either preventable or could be significantly reduced by good injury prevention techniques. The latter include adequate attention paid by everyone involved in athletic endeavors to five specific areas: (1) rules of the sport designed so as to prevent injury, (2) the use of proper equipment, (3) good preliminary training and conditioning, (4) experience of coaches, and (5) educational programs. Good education is in fact the primary way to prevent injury for individuals who engage in nonorganized, recreational sporting endeavors. For example, public education programs are today more frequently distributing information on safety in water sports, especially diving, which is particularly amenable to prevention.[86] Programs such as "Think First," sponsored by neurosurgery organizations, have dramatically reduced the incidence of diving accidents in some parts of the United States. Public service announcements and cervical spine injury prevention programs continue to be important, particularly during the summer months. Prevention should include warnings about diving in shallow water and above-ground pools, diving in places where there may be submerged objects, use of improper technique, and diving while drinking alcohol. Persons diving from deck level or higher require a water depth almost double their height to cause complete deceleration. Sadly, many "short-sighted" dives occur while the diver is intoxicated. Just as the public is cautioned about the dangers of drinking and driving, so it should be warned against drinking and diving.[3]

Organized team sports have an advantage because all five areas of injury prevention apply. Most sports have changed their rules over time in response to injury patterns. For example, the International Judo Federation Directing Committee made rule changes that severely penalize contestants who dive into the mat head first or throw a competitor head first during the execution of certain maneuvers. These rules also penalize the player if he intentionally falls backward while his opponent is clinging to his back. Injuries from amateur wrestling maneuvers are limited by rules that make it illegal to throw a wrestler to the mat "out of control" or "to spear" the opponent with the head and shoulders striking the mat. Similarly, the incidence of catastrophic spinal injuries in rugby has been reduced by instituting rules that eliminate certain dangerous techniques such as the high or late tackle.[73,76] In a 4-year period after institution of these rules, New Zealand reported no spinal cord injury during rugby events.[14] In American football, recent rule changes to avoid "spearing" contact should continue to reduce the incidence of spinal and head injuries.

Instruction on the proper techniques of sports participation is equally important to prevention. Proper positioning and techniques of blocking and tackling in football will avoid hyperflexion and initial contact with the head. Gymnastics and wrestling trainers and coaches must emphasize proper maneuvers to prevent accidents.

Particularly in football, but also in wrestling, off-season neck-strengthening exercises are a vital, and often absent, part of injury prevention programs. This type of conditioning program must be undertaken well before competition begins to allow proper neck conditioning and strengthening. Equipment designers and manufacturers have also made great strides in producing safer products for athletic competition and undoubtedly will continue to do so.

## Summary

The discussion in this chapter and the guidelines for management are based on the authors' extensive experience with a variety of sports-related vertebral column and spinal cord injuries. The scenarios involved in treating athletes with vertebral column injury, with or without central nervous system involvement, vary greatly. The physician caring for such patients must remember that they are first and foremost patients who are in need of medical treatment and advice. Spinal involvement differs from other types of sports medicine injuries in its potential for serious, devastating, and at times, life-threatening implications that supersede considerations for return to competition in contact sports. Nonetheless, in minor, healed, or transient injuries, decision making is often complex. In addition, social, personal, and parental pressures sometimes interplay. The needs and rewards of scholar-athletes and professional athletes are often difficult. The general guidelines presented in this chapter are applicable to all types of sports, levels of participation, and degrees of spinal column or spinal cord involvement. Because damage to the central nervous system is permanent, a high level of vigilance must be maintained, and decisions are made with a bias to protecting the athlete from additional, perhaps devastating injury. As always, recommendations are made on an individual basis, after consideration of all aspects of the history, physical examination, radiologic assessment, and type of athletic activity involved.

## REFERENCES

1. Albrand WO, Corkill G: Broken necks from diving accidents: a summer epidemic in young men. *Am J Sports Med* 4:107-110, 1976.
2. Alexander MD, Davis CH, Field CH: Hyperextension injuries of the cervical spine. *Arch Neurol Psychiat* 79:146-150, 1958.
3. Bailes JE, Hadley MN, Quigley MR, *et al*: Management of athletic injuries of the cervical spine and spinal cord. *Neurosurgery* 29:491-497, 1991.
4. Bailes JE, Herman JM, Quigley MR, *et al*: Diving injuries of the cervical spine. *Surg Neurol* 34:155-158, 1990.
5. Boijsen E: The cervical spinal canal in intraspinal expansive processes. *Acta Radiol* 42:101-115, 1954.
6. Cantu RC: Head and spine injuries in the young athlete. *Clin Sports Med* 7:459-472, 1988.
7. Cantu RC, Mueller FO: Catastrophic spine injuries in football. *J Spinal Disord* 3:227-231, 1990.

8. Chow TK, Corbett SW, Farstad DJ: Spectrum of injuries from snowboarding. *J Trauma* 41:321-325, 1996.

9. Clarke K: An epidemiological view. In Torg JS (ed): *Athletic Injuries to the Head, Neck and Face.* St Louis, Mosby-Yearbook, 1991, pp 19-21.

10. Cantu RC: Cervical spinal stenosis: challenging an established detection method. *Phys Sportsmed* 21:57-63, 1993.

11. Cantu RC: Functional spinal stenosis: a contraindication to participation in contact sports. *Med Sci Sports Exerc* 25(3):316-317, 1993.

12. Cantu RV, Cantu RC: Guidelines for return to contact sports after transient quadriplegia. *J Neurosurg* 80: 592-594, 1994.

13. Cantu RC: Transient quadriplegia: to play or not to play. *Sports Med Digest* 16:1-4, 1994.

14. Duda M: Reducing catastrophic injuries in rugby. *Phys Sportsmed* 16:29, 1988.

15. Epstein JA, Carras R, Hyman RA, *et al*: Cervical myelopathy caused by developmental stenosis of the spinal canal. *J Neurosurg* 51:362-367, 1979.

16. Eismont FJ, Clifford S, Goldberg M, *et al*: Cervical sagittal spinal canal size in spine injury. *Spine* 9:663-666, 1984.

17. Feriencik K: Trends in ice hockey injuries: 1965 to 1977. *Phys Sportsmed* 7:81-84, 1979.

18. Fife D, Kraus J: Anatomic location of spinal cord injury. Relationship to the cause of injury. *Spine* 11:2-5, 1986.

19. Frankel HL, Montero FA, Penny PT: Spinal cord injuries due to diving. *Paraplegia* 18:118-122, 1980.

20. Funk FJ Jr, Wells RE: Injuries of the cervical spine in football. *Clin Orthop* 109:50-58, 1975.

21. Good RP, Nickel VL: Cervical spine injuries resulting from water sports. *Spine* 5:502-506, 1980.

22. Grant TT, Puffer J: Cervical stenosis: a developmental anomaly with quadriparesis during football. *Am J Sports Med* 4:219-221, 1976.

23. Green BA, Gabrielse MA, Hall WJ, *et al*: Analysis of swimming pool accidents resulting in spinal cord injury. *Paraplegia* 18:94-100, 1980.

24. Griffiths ER: Spinal injuries from swimming and diving treated in the spinal department of Royal Perth Rehabilitation Hospital, 1956-1978. *Paraplegia* 18: 105-117, 1980.

25. Hadley MN, Sonntag VKH, Amos MR, *et al*: Three-dimensional computed tomography in the diagnosis of vertebral column pathological conditions. *Neurosurgery* 21:186-192, 1987.

26. Hammer A, Schwartzback DL, Darre E: Svaere neurologiske skader some folge af trampolinspring. *Ugeskr Laeger* 143:2970-2974, 1981.

27. Harris JB: Neurological injuries in winter sports. *Phys Sportsmed* 11:110-122, 1983.

28. Herzog RJ, Wiens JJ, Dillingham MF, *et al*: Normal cervical spine morphometry and cervical spinal stenosis in asymptomatic professional football players: plain film radiography, multi-planar computed tomography, and magnetic resonance imaging. *Spine* 16(6 suppl): S178-S186, 1991.

29. Hill SA, Miller CA, Kosnik EJ, *et al*: Pediatric neck injuries. A clinical study. *J Neurosurg* 60:700-706, 1984.

30. Hirish D, Inglemark B, Miller M: The anatomical basis of low back pain. *Acta Orthop Scand* 33:1, 1963.

31. Hosey R, Puffer J: Baseball and softball sliding injuries. Incidence and the effect of technique in collegiate baseball and softball players. *Am J Sports Med* 28:360-363, 2000.

32. Hutchinson MR: Low back pain in elite rhythmic gymnasts. *Med Sci Sports Exerc* 31:1686-1688, 1999.

33. Jackson D, Mannarino F: Lumbar spine in athletes. In Scott W (ed): *Principles of Sports Medicine.* Baltimore, Williams & Wilkins, 1984, pp 212-215.

34. Jackson D, Wiltse L: Low back pain in athletes. *Phys Sportsmed* 2: 53, 1983.

35. Jackson DW, Wiltse LL, Cirinsione RJ: Spondylolysis in the female gymnast. *Clin Orthop* 117:68-73, 1976.

36. Janda DH, Hankin FM, Wojtys EM: Softball injuries: cost, cause and prevention. *Am Fam Phys* 33:143-144, 1986.

37. Janda DH, Wojtys EM, Hankin FM, *et al*: A three-phase analysis of the prevention of recreational softball injuries. *Am J Sports Med* 18:632-635, 1990.

38. Johnson RM, Crelin ES, White AA, *et al*: Some new observations on the functional anatomy of the lower cervical spine. *Clin Orthop* 3:192-200, 1975.

39. Johnson RW, Wolf JW Jr: Stability. In Baily RW (ed): *The Cervical Spine.* Philadelphia, JB Lippincott, 1983, pp 35-53.

40. Kewalramani LS, Kraus JF: Acute spinal cord lesions from diving: epidemiological and clinical features. *West J Med* 126:353-361, 1977.

41. Kewalramani LS, Taylor RG: Injuries to the cervical spine from diving accidents. *J Trauma* 15:130-142, 1975.

42. Kiwerski J: Cervical spine injuries caused by diving into water. *Paraplegia* 18:101-106, 1980.

43. Kizer K, MacQuarrie M, Kuhn B, *et al*: Deep snow immersion deaths, a snowboarding danger. *Phys Sportsmed* 22:49-61, 1994.

44. Kovac D, Negovetic L, Vukic M, *et al*: [Surgical treatment of lumbar disc hernias in athletes]. *Reumatizam* 46:35-41, 1998 (Roman).

45. Kraus DR, Shapiro D: The symptomatic lumbar spine in the athletic. *Clin Sports Med* 8:59-69, 1989.

46. Ladd AL, Scranton PE: Congenital cervical stenosis presenting as transient quadriplegia in athletes. *J Bone Joint Surg* 68A:1371-1374, 1986.

47. Lamont AC, Zachary J, Sheldon PW: Cervical cord size in metrizamide myelography. *Clin Radiol* 32(4):409-412, 1981.

48. Maroon JC: "Burning hands" in football spinal cord injuries. *JAMA* 238:2049-2051, 1977.

49. Maroon J, Gardner P, Bejjani G, *et al*: Golf induced stroke from vertebral artery dissection: "golfer's stroke." *Neurosurgery.* Submitted for publication.

50. Maroon JC, Steele PB, Berlin R: Football head and neck injuries: an update. *Clin Neurosurg* 27:414-429, 1980.

51. Mayfield FH: Neurosurgical aspects of cervical trauma. *Clinical Neurosurgery*, vol 2. Baltimore, Williams & Wilkins, 1955.

52. Matsuura P, Waters RL, Adkins RH, *et al*: Comparison of computerized tomography parameters of the cervical spine in normal control subjects and spinal cord-injured patients. *J Bone Joint Surg (Am)* 71(2):183-188, 1989.

53. Mennen U: A survey of spinal injuries from diving. *S Afr Med J* 59:788-790, 1981.

54. Micheli LJ: Back injuries in gymnastics. *Clin Sports Med* 4:85-93, 1985.

55. Micheli L, Hall J, Miller E: Use of modified Boston brace for back injuries in athletes. *Am J Sports Med* 8:351, 1980.

56. Miele VJ, Bailes JE: Head, spine, and peripheral nerve injuries in sports and dance: an encyclopedic reference. In Bailes JE, Day AL (eds): *Neurological Sports Medicine: A Guide for Physicians and Athletic Trainers*. Rolling Meadows, IL, American Association of Neurological Surgeons, 2001, pp 181-251.

57. Mueller FO, Blythe CS: Catastrophic head and neck injuries. *Phys Sportsmed* 7:71-76, 1979.

58. Mundt DJ, Kelsey JL, Golden AL, *et al*: An epidemiologic study of sports and weight lifting as possible risk factors for herniated lumbar and cervical discs. The Northeast Collaborative Group on Low Back Pain. *Am J Sports Med* 21:854-860, 1993.

59. Nadeau MT, Brown T, Boatman J, *et al*: The prevention of softball injuries: the experience at Yokota. *Milit Med* 155:3-5, 1990.

60. NBTA Injury Reporting System: National Basketball Trainers Association. New York, National Basketball Association, 1991.

61. Olvey S: Auto racing. In Jordan B, Tsairis P, Warren R (eds): *Sports Neurology*. Philadelphia, Lippincott-Raven, 1998, pp 317-329.

62. Pavlov H, Torg JS, Robie B, *et al*: Cervical spinal stenosis: determination with vertebral body ratio method. *Radiology* 164(3):771-775, 1987.

63. Odor JM, Watkins RG, Dillin WH, *et al*: Incidence of cervical spinal stenosis in professional and rookie football players. *Am J Sports Med* 18(5):507-509, 1990.

64. Penning L: Some aspects of plain radiography of the cervical spine in chronic myelopathy. *Neurology* 12:513-519, 1962.

65. Nugent GR: Clinicopathologic correlations in cervical spondylosis. *Neurology* 9:273-281, 1959.

66. Poindexter DP, Johnson EW: Football shoulder and neck injury: a study of the "stinger." *Arch Phys Med Rehabil* 65:601-602, 1984.

67. Prebble TB, Chyou PH, Wittman L, *et al*: Basketball injuries in a rural area. *Womens Med J* 98:22-24, 1999.

68. Price C, Mallonee S: Hunting-related spinal cord injuries among Oklahoma residents. *J Okla State Med Assoc* 87:270-273, 1994.

69. Raymond CA: Summer's drought reinforces diving's dangers. *JAMA* 260:1199-1200, 1988.

70. Requa R, Garrick JG: Injuries in interscholastic wrestling. *Phys Sportsmed* 9:44-49, 1981.

71. Richards RN: Rescuing the spine-injured diver. *Phys Sportsmed* 1:63-65, 1973.

72. Roaf R: A study of the mechanics of spinal injuries. *J Bone Joint Surg* 42B:810-818, 1960.

73. Scher AT: Rugby injuries to the cervical spine and spinal cord. *S Afr Med J* 51:473-475, 1977.

74. Scher AT: The high rugby tackle: an avoidable cause of cervical spinal cord injury. *S Afr Med J* 53:1015-1018, 1978.

75. Scher AT: Diving injuries to the cervical spinal cord. *S Afr Med J* 59:603-605, 1981.

76. Scher AT: Rugby injuries of the spine and spinal cord. *Clin Sports Med* 6:87-99, 1987.

77. Schneider RC: Serious and fatal neurosurgical football injuries. *Clin Neurosurg* 12:226-236, 1966.

78. Shields CL Jr, Fox JM, Stauffer ES: Cervical cord injuries in sports. *Phys Sportsmed* 6:71-76, 1978.

79. Shorter NA, Mooney DP, Harmon BJ: Snowboarding injuries in children and adolescents. *Am J Emerg Med* 17:261-263, 1999.

80. Sliding associated injuries in college and professional baseball: 1990-1991. *MMWR Morbid Mortal Wkly Rep* 42:223,229-230, 1991.

81. Sonntag VK, Hadley MN: Nonoperative management of cervical spine injuries. *Clin Neurosurg* 34:630-649, 1988.

82. Steinbruck K, Paeslack V: Trampolinspringen-ein gefahrlicher sport? *Munchen Med Wochenschr* 120:985-988, 1978.

83. Steinbruck K, Paeslack V: Analysis of 139 spinal cord injuries due to accidents in water sports. *Paraplegia* 18:86-93, 1980.

84. Tator CH: Neck injuries in ice hockey: a recent unsolved problem with many contributing factors. *Clin Sports Med* 6:101-114, 1987.

85. Tator CH, Edmonds VE: National survey of spinal injuries in hockey players. *Can Med Assoc J* 130:875-880, 1984.

86. Tator CH, Edmonds VE, New ML: Diving: a frequent and potentially preventable cause of spinal cord injury. *Can Med Assoc J* 124:1323-1324, 1981.

87. Thijssen HO, Keyser A, Horstink MW, *et al*: Morphology of the cervical spinal cord on computed myelography. *Neuroradiology* 18(2):57-62, 1979.

88. Torg JS (ed): *Athletic Injuries to the Head, Neck, and Face*. Philadelphia, Lea & Febiger, 1982.

89. Torg JS: Epidemiology, pathomechanics, and prevention of athletic injuries to the cervical spine. *Med Sci Sports Exerc* 17:295-303, 1985.

90. Torg JS: Trampoline-induced quadriplegia. *Clin Sports Med* 6:73-85, 1987.

91. Torg JS, Corcoran TA, Thibault LE, *et al*: Cervical cord neurapraxia: classification, pathomechanics, morbidity, and management guidelines. *J Neurosurg* 87:843-850, 1997.

92. Torg JS, Das M: Trampoline-related quadriplegia: review of the literature and reflections on the American Academy of Pediatrics' position statement. *Pediatrics* 74:804-812, 1984.

93. Torg JS, Pavlov H, Genuario SE, *et al*: Neurapraxia of the cervical spinal cord with transient quadriplegia. *J Bone Joint Surg* 68A:1354-1370, 1986.

94. Torg JS, Sennett B, Pavlov H, *et al*: Spear tackler's spine. An entity precluding participation in tackle football and collision activities that expose the cervical spine to axial energy inputs. *Am J Sports Med* 21:640-649, 1993.

95. Torg JS, Truex RC Jr, Marshall J, *et al*: Spinal injury at the level of the third and fourth cervical vertebrae from football. *J Bone Joint Surg* 59A:1015-1019, 1977.

96. Torg JS, Truex RC Jr, Quedenfeld TC, *et al*: The national football head and neck injury registry. *JAMA* 241:1477-1479, 1979.

97. Torg JS, Vegso JJ, Sennett B: The National Football Head and Neck Injury Registry: 14-year report on cervical quadriplegia (1971-1984). *Clin Sports Med* 6:61-72, 1987.

98. Trammell T: Motor sports. In Watkins R (ed): *The Spine in Sports*. St Louis, CV Mosby, 1995.

99. Wadley GH, Albright JP: Women's intercollegiate gymnastics. Injury patterns and "permanent" medical disability. *Am J Sports Med* 21:314-320, 1993.

100. Watkins RG: Neck injuries in football players. *Clin Sports Med* 5:215-246, 1986.

101. Wessels LDG: Rugby injuries in South Africa. *S Afr Sports Med* 8:14-18, 1980.

102. Wilberger JE: Athletic spinal cord and spine injuries. *Clin Sports Med* 17:113, 1998.

103. Wilkes J, Jones D: Golf-related injuries seen at hospital emergency departments. *Aust J Sci Med Sport* 28:43-45, 1996.

104. Wiltse L, Widell E, Jackson D: Fatigue fracture: the basic lesion in isthmic spondylolisthesis. *J Bone Joint Surg* 57:27, 1975.

105. Wolfe BS, Khilnani M, Malis L: The sagittal diameter of the bony cervical spinal canal and its significance in cervical spondylosis. *J Mt Sinai Hosp* 23:283-292, 1956.

106. Wroble RR, Albright JP: Neck and low back injuries in wrestling. *Clin Sports Med* 9:44-49, 1981.

107. Wu WQ, Lewis RC: Injuries of the cervical spine in high school wrestling. *Surg Neurol* 23:143-147, 1985.

# CHAPTER 148

# Nonoperative Management of Neck and Back Pain

Ann M. Henwood, Mark S. Adams, George W. Sypert, and Edward C. Benzel

Low back pain (LBP) is second only to upper respiratory problems as a reason that patients visit a primary care provider (PCP).[25] Pain of spinal origin will affect 70% to 85% of the population at some point in their lives and is the most common cause of disability in patients aged younger than 45 years.[1] It accounts for a large fraction of the health care budget. LBP treatment costs increased from $4.6 billion in 1977 to $11.4 billion by 1997. Annually, $20 to $50 billion is spent on workers compensation claims, with 10% of back pain patients accounting for 85% to 90% of the costs.[1,6,17] Although most adults experience low back and neck pain, only a small percentage require surgery (approximately 1%). Therefore the nonoperative management of these complaints is of significance. The natural history of LBP suggests that the passing of time is the best treatment, as 90% of cases resolve spontaneously within 2 weeks to 3 months of onset.[1,10] LBP effects men and women equally, and the onset most often occurs between the ages of 30 and 50 years. Eighty percent of the population will experience acute LBP at least once, and 30% of this group will become chronic sufferers. The annual prevalence ranges from 14% to 45%.

Nonoperative management can be complex and time consuming because of the selection of the most appropriate management scheme for any one individual. The data on the effectiveness of the variety of management schemes are sometimes misleading. Even the establishment of the etiology of back pain is not consistent in the literature. This complicates the interpretation of outcome data. Unlike most drug treatments, it is difficult to blind clinical trials of physical treatments. Many studies have grouped pain syndromes into single treatment groups, which in turn degrade the meaningfulness of the results. A particular pain syndrome may respond well to a particular management scheme. A statistically significant result, however, may not be observed because of a grouping. Given the natural history of these pain syndromes, most patients recover rapidly; therefore it is difficult to know if the therapeutic interventions are efficacious or if the passing of time played a larger role.

## Etiology

Spine pain has been recognized as having a multifactorial etiology. The cause of LBP may originate within spinal structures such as ligaments, facet joints, vertebral perios- teum, paravertebral musculature and fascia, blood vessels, the annulus fibrosus, and spinal nerve roots.[17] Disease states or processes such as cancer, infection or musculoligamentous injuries are also causes of spinal pain, as are degenerative processes of the spine such as spinal canal stenosis, foraminal stenosis, and disc disease. No pathoanatomical diagnosis can be given to 85% of patients with isolated spine/LBP because of the poor association between symptoms and imaging results.[17] Strain and sprain are commonly used as catch-all diagnoses for generalized LBP in the absence of major red flags.

## Classification of Spinal Pain

### Mechanical

This is generally described as deep and agonizing pain. It is worsened with loading of the spine during activity and relieved or alleviated by unloading of the spine with rest. It is usually associated with degenerative conditions seen in older adults or the development of a pseudoarthrosis after a failed fusion. It may also be present with tumor.[7]

### Myofascial

This type of pain is consistent with "muscle spasm." Patients with significant trapezius "spasm" will describe tension-type headaches. Myofascial pain is usually self-limiting. This responds well to stretching exercise and muscle relaxants. Patients with underlying instability or mechanical pain will often describe associated myofascial pain. Strains and sprains of the neck or low back are catch-all terms used for nonspecific spine pain and are generally grouped within this category.[7]

## Risk Factors

Risk factors for low back and neck pain include advancing age up to 55 years, Caucasian race, living in the western United States, prolonged driving of a motor vehicle, heavy lifting and twisting, overexertion, prolonged sitting or standing, trauma, obesity, poor conditioning, and smoking.[23,32-34] In addition, there is a high prevalence of major depression in patients with chronic pain.[49]

Special attention should be given to the definite link between psychologic variables and pain of spinal origin that are exhibited in the literature. Psychologic variables emphasize the need for highlighting the multidimensional view of caring for individuals with spine pain. Psychologic distress can more than double the risk of low back pain.[47] Stress, distress, anxiety, mood, emotion, cognitive functioning, personality factors, and abuse have been shown to be variables linked to the onset of back and neck pain. Psychologic variables may not only play a role in chronic pain but also in the etiology of the onset of acute pain.[35] Resultant disability caused by LBP may be a psychologic stress-related disorder.[57] A complex pathway of how physical work demands, one's reaction to the psychosocial environment, and the unique attributes of the person may affect physical loading on the spine, increasing the risk of LBP.[39]

## Prevention

Ultimately, the practice of prevention is the reduction of risk factors. Patient education focusing on the prevention of episodes of LBP should include participation in an exercise program consisting of aerobic exercise, stretching, and strengthening exercise.[31] Exercises showed strong positive results as an effective preventive measure against back and neck pain.[36] Stretching and strengthening exercises may be done at home, thereby helping to reduce the monumental financial burden on the health care system. Smokers should be instructed to quit, because smokers have more severe symptoms that are present a greater portion of the day when compared with nonsmokers.[60] Another preventive intervention includes keeping one's weight appropriate to one's height, because obesity is positively linked to LBP.[34] Linton and van Tulder[36] reviewed 27 controlled trials regarding interventions for the prevention of back and neck pain. Their review found that back schools were not effective for prevention. Evidence showed that lumbar supports were consistently negative, and there is strong evidence that they are not effective. Ergonomic interventions as well as risk factor modification could not be considered because of a lack of quality-controlled trials and subsequent evidence.

## Current Treatment Therapies

### Points for Patient Education

First and foremost, management of spine pain should include educating the patient with regard to the probable cause of their pain, including a brief explanation of the anatomic pain generators. By understanding the cause of their pain, patients are more likely to become active participants in their treatment plan. Second, discuss the process of eliminating or reducing risk factors for future episodes of LB or neck pain and reinforce the lifetime commitment at working toward this goal. Third, reassurance should be given to the patient that with the passage of time their symptoms should abate. Fourth, the patient should be informed that because LBP has a multifactorial etiology, more than one intervention/treatment method will be necessary. Fifth, whichever treatment methods are chosen, follow-up care is essential, whether by the doctor initiating the treatment or referral to another physician/health care provider.

The following paragraphs discuss acute pain syndromes as those lasting 6 weeks or less from onset and chronic pain symptoms as lasting 12 weeks or more from onset. It is also important to recognize that patients may have acute exacerbations of a chronic pain syndrome.

### Medication Therapy

Non-steroidal anti-inflammatory drugs (NSAIDs) have been shown to be effective for short-term improvement in patients with LBP. No single type of NSAID is more effective than any other.[58] Evidence suggests analgesics are not more effective than NSAIDs.[59] Evidence has shown that muscle relaxants reduce pain intensity and that the different types are equally effective. Evidence for the use of muscle relaxants for LBP lasting longer than 3 months is lacking. However, the results show symptom relief when compared with a placebo.[59] Evidence shows more effective symptom relief when medications are used in conjunction with NSAIDs and are prescribed around the clock rather than on an as-needed basis.[17,38]

Antidepressant drug therapy may be beneficial, as one third of chronic LBP sufferers also have depression and may benefit. Antidepressants may decrease the patient's perception of pain by treating underlying depression and improving sleep.[56] Hypotheses of similarities between the physiology of pain and depression exist. Hence, there may be beneficial effects of antidepressant drug therapy on pain separate from the drug's antidepressant effects.[19] Treating patients who do not have signs and symptoms of clinical depression is controversial. However, treating non-depressed patients with tricyclic antidepressants has been shown to be effective in the treatment of neuropathic-type pain and significantly increased pain relief over placebo without a significant difference in functioning.[2,45] Antidepressants may not be effective for chronic LBP.[58]

### Exercise Therapy

Stretching and strengthening exercises have mixed results. Nearly the same number of studies show positive as negative results. Overall, evidence suggests that exercise improved pain and functional status more than other treatments for LBP. No one exercise is more beneficial than another for the treatment of LBP.[45]

### Aerobic Activity

Benefits of aerobic exercise include weight loss and psychologic effects of improved mood and lessened anxiety. The sense of well-being and accomplishment achieved from a planned aerobic exercise program creates a positive self-image and increases the level of motivation and commitment to the prescribed therapy. Objective evidence of the benefit from this treatment, however, is lacking. Nevertheless, it is commonly prescribed. Some have suggested that particular types of high-impact exercise should be avoided because of the potential for raising intradiscal pressure.[44] This stance, however, has not been backed by objective data. Patients participating in an aerobic exercise program have been shown to receive few prescriptions for pain, were given fewer physical therapy referrals, and had improved mood states and lessened depression.[52]

### Stretching Exercises

Stretching exercises help to improve the extensibility of muscles and other soft tissues, and to reestablish normal joint range of motion. Pain commonly limits mobility. Muscle spasm, or sprain, may also be present. Stretching is thought to maintain mobility and reduce spasm. Kraus[30] reported a study of the effects of stretching exercises on back pain. He found that nearly 80% of people with chronic back pain who entered the program reported improvement at the end of a 6-week training session.[40] More recent investigations have found that unless the exercises are continued, the benefit of stretching exercise may be lost.[16] Patient compliance is, again, a large determinant in the outcome.

## Isometric Exercises

Isometric exercises and exercise regimens have enjoyed significant popularity. Several studies[62,46] suggested that isometric flexion offered the best relief of pain and improved function for LBP and neck pain. With regard to LBP, the rationale was that flexion (1) widened intervertebral foramina and facet joints, reducing nerve compression; (2) stretched hip flexors and back extensors; (3) strengthened abdominal and gluteus muscles; and (4) reduced dorsal fixation of the lumbosacral junction. There has been concern over the use of flexion exercises, specifically regarding substantial increases in intradiscal pressure that may aggravate bulging or herniation of an intervertebral disc.[42] Randomized controlled trials have shown conflicting results.[14,22,29]

McKenzie more recently advocated extension exercises. These limit the risk of aggravating nerve root compression via extruding a disc fragment. This program is complicated and is individualized according to the patient's symptoms. Some investigators have suggested that it offers an advantage over the Williams method. However, there is a very high noncompliance rate.

Based on mounting evidence, weak muscles are associated with back and neck pain.[27,40,53] Therefore, strengthening exercises may reduce or eliminate back and neck pain. The supporting muscles of the spinal column provide support and prevent excessive or abnormal spinal movement. Activities that stress the spine without simultaneously strengthening muscles that support the spine (ventral and dorsal support muscles) could result in stress/muscle strength imbalance. This could result in an application of excessive stress to the spine, thus accelerating degenerative changes and worsening pain.

## Bed Rest

Bed rest for the treatment of acute episodes of LBP is controversial. Contrary to what was once recommended, bed rest is not effective in the treatment of LBP and may have harmful effects on the treatment of an acute episode of nonspecific LBP.[15,24,61,58]

There are significant disadvantages to bed rest. These include its psychologic association with a severe illness that requires many days in bed. This may lead to depression, exacerbation of pain, and a predisposition to a diminished effort in an exercise program. Deconditioning, with muscle atrophy (1% to 1.5% per day[41]), cardiopulmonary function loss (15% in 10 days),[12] and bone mineral loss occurs relatively rapidly. In addition, medical complications, including deep venous thrombosis and pneumonia, are more common with bed rest.

## Smoking Cessation

It has been shown that smokers have more severe pain present for longer periods during the day when compared with nonsmokers, and smoking may exacerbate episodes of pain.[51,60] Smokers should be encouraged to quit,

because this may reduce severity as well as duration of LBP.[32,33]

## Appropriate Weight for Height

Obesity is modestly positively associated with LBP chronicity as well as its recurrence.[34] Obese patients have been shown to have more severe pain symptoms as compared with non-obese patients.[18]

## Bracing

Bracing does diminish and may alleviate acute LBP because it lends support to the muscles of the spine. However, long-term use of bracing may lead to atrophy of these supporting muscles, ultimately resulting in a chronic pain syndrome. Wearing a brace may lead to weakening the supportive muscles of the spine.[3] Lumbar braces in the workplace have been shown to not have an effect on muscle fatigue or lifting.[37] There is a lack of evidence in the literature for the effectiveness of orthosis in the treatment of LBP.[58] Ultimately, lumbar braces probably serve best as reminder to the patient to use correct spine mechanics when performing activities such as lifting and bending.[38]

## Traction

Theoretically, the use of traction is to stretch the back and neck, distracting the vertebrae, and thereby potentially reducing protrusion of a bulging or herniated disc. Approximately 1½ times a patient's body weight is needed to develop distraction of the vertebral bodies. This may cause compliance issues, as it may be burdensome and time consuming. Conventional traction has not been shown to be efficacious for back or neck pain, acute nor chronic[4,46]; therefore, the use of traction is not recommended for the treatment of back or neck pain symptoms.

# Adjunct Therapies

The etiology of LBP is multifactorial; so is its treatment. Patients in a passive modality-intensive program have poor functional outcomes when compared with patients in an exercise-based program.[28] Therefore, adjunct therapies should be used in conjunction with conservative treatment therapies and not as a sole treatment for pain of spinal origin.

## Injection Therapy

The types of injection therapy most commonly used for LBP and radiculopathy include trigger point injections (TPIs) and nerve root, epidural, and facet joint injections (FJIs). All injection therapy should be used in conjunction with stretching and strengthening exercises to maximize the benefit of the effect of reduced pain, thereby increasing function. Multiple reviews of controlled trials show that epidural steroid injection use has conflicting evidence and probably should not be used for acute or chronic LBP.[38,46,59] Limited evidence supports trigger point therapy as a therapeutic treatment for LBP. TPI should be prescribed for muscle spasm when a patient has not responded to 4 to 6 weeks of medication and exercise therapy.[38] FJIs are not indicated during the first 4 to 6 weeks of treatment of LBP. FJI therapy is controversial, and once again, evidence is lacking for its use. When compared with placebo, no significant difference in pain relief was noted.[45] If FJI therapy is prescribed, it should be used in patients for whom surgery is not an option. FJIs may help patients who complain of LBP with walking, standing, and extension activities and have an otherwise normal neurologic exam.[38]

## Ice and Heat Therapy

Within the first 24 hours of the back or neck pain caused by a benign injury, alternating treatments of ice and heat for 20-minute periods can be effective in reducing inflammation.[10] When used in conjunction with home exercise therapy, patients may be instructed to use heat to warm the affected muscles prior to home exercise and ice packs after home exercise therapy for symptomatic relief. Insufficient data exist for the treatment of acute and chronic neck pain with thermotherapy.[46]

## Continuous Low-Level Heat Wrap Therapy

Heat wrap therapy has been shown to be effective on LBP. It has also been shown to be superior to ibuprofen or acetaminophen for relief of LBP. The heat wrap is worn around the lumbar region and secured with Velcro. It heats to 104°F for up to 8 hours.[43]

## Ultrasound

Ultrasound is used as a deep-heating modality because it reaches tissue depths that superficial heat cannot reach. Its use is not recommended for acute inflammatory conditions because it may only increase the inflammatory response.[38] Controlled research trials on its use for or against the treatment of LBP are lacking in the literature.[58] Reviews of the literature found no clinical benefit for the use of ultrasound for chronic neck pain and lacking evidence for acute neck pain.[46]

## Massage Therapy

Massage therapy improved symptoms and function and was found to be more effective when used in combination with a program for the treatment of LBP.[45] Further studies are needed to confirm these findings.[20]

## Transcutaneous Electrical Nerve Stimulation (TENS)

Several studies have shown no clinically or statistically significant effect of TENS in the treatment of acute or chronic LBP nor of acute neck pain.[45,59]

## Percutaneous Electrical Nerve Stimulation (PENS)

PENS is a combination of acupuncture and TENS therapy. This treatment has been shown to be effective in providing short-term pain relief and improved physical function in patients with long-term LBP.[21]

## Chiropractic or Manual Therapy

Modest evidence shows that chiropractic/manual therapy is more effective than a placebo but not more effective than other forms of therapies when treating patients with acute LBP.[13,58] For the treatment of chronic LBP, chiropractic/manual therapy has been shown to be more effective than traditional therapies.[58]

## Acupuncture

Limited discussion with regard to acupuncture occurs in spine literature. However, it has been shown to have positive effects on LBP and return to work.[8,50]

## Bipolar Permanent Magnet Therapy

Magnet therapy has been shown to have no effect on LBP.[11]

## Whole-Body Vibration Exercise

Vibration exercise significantly reduced pain sensation in a study group of patients experiencing LBP. This new type of exercise elicits muscular activity through stretch reflexes.[48] At one time, continuous vibration was considered a cause of LBP and now is considered to be helpful in the treatment of LBP.

## Intradiscal Electrothermal Annuloplasty (IDET)

IDET is a minimally invasive procedure that has received mixed reviews because of the relative newness of this procedure, uncertain mechanism of action, and minimal-yet-positive follow-up data; hence, this procedure is not widely accepted. IDET is recommend for use with patients who have discogenic pain, in whom other conservative treatment therapies as well as modalities have failed, and who may be candidates for lumbar fusion surgery.[26] To perform the IDET procedure, provocative discography must be performed (prior to the IDET procedure) to determine whether or not an intervertebral disc is the source of low back pain. Discography is yet another cause of controversy. Evidence for the reliable use of discography as a diagnostic method for degenerative disc disease is mixed.[5,55] In addition, there have been several reports of previously asymptomatic patients having long-term back symptoms after diagnostic provocative discography.[9,26]

Overall, patients should be encouraged to return to their normal lifestyle as quickly as possible, taking into consideration the type of work a person performs. Light multidisciplinary treatment for LBP is cost-effective treatment for LBP. This type of treatment includes evaluation by a physiotherapist, a nurse, and a psychologist if necessary. The patient is then instructed on exercise, lifestyle, and fear-avoidance of reoccurrence of pain.[54]

## Algorithm for Aggressive Nonsurgical Management of Back Pain

An ideal exercise program should be efficacious and associated with a high level of compliance. It should also be cost-effective. Similarly, it should incorporate a lifestyle alteration component (active rather than passive participation in the program). Patient motivation should be assessed by monitoring compliance with exercises.

In most cases, regardless of the type of spine-related pain present, the nonoperative management scheme is similar. What follows is a four-point management scheme. It may be individualized to patient syndromes (e.g., flexion exercise elimination from the regimen of patients with acute sciatica, to prevent further herniation of disc fragments, etc.).

Four management components (a four-point program) are integral to the nonsurgical management process associated with mechanical back pain: (1) general health promotion; (2) aerobic exercise; (3) stretching exercises; and (4) strengthening exercises (GASS). Each of these requires patient education as an integral component of the pain management process, on the part of either the surgeon or the midlevel health care providers, or more appropriately, both.

### General Health Promotion

Well-being augmentation causes the patient to simultaneously become a better surgical candidate (if surgery, indeed, is deemed appropriate) and assists in a physiologically and biomechanically improved clinical status, all by improving attitude. This process includes a program for the cessation of smoking and weight loss. Tobacco use and obesity are associated with back and neck pain. Both can and should be objectively assessed and recorded on a periodic basis. If the patient cannot demonstrate progress in these areas, his or her motivation may be insufficient to warrant surgery, or even further nonoperative care.

### Aerobic Exercise

Aerobic exercise progress can similarly be quantified (at least by patient history) and recorded. The sense of well-being and accomplishment acquired from a planned aerobic exercise program (walking, running, swimming, cycling, etc.) creates a positive internal milieu and further establishes the extent of the patient's motivation.

### Stretching Exercise

The augmentation of flexibility is an integral component of the program. The spine of a patient with mechanical instability should be thought of as being akin to a frozen joint associated with immobilization. Flexibility can be improved via stretching, and progress can be quantitatively monitored. Toe touching can be monitored by asking patients to reach for their toes with knees locked and to hold the lowest position achievable for 20 seconds. The distance from the floor is measured and recorded. Bouncing is discouraged. Documentation is mandatory. Progress is encouraged. In fact, lack of progress may very

well be a manifestation of a lack of adequate motivation. Other exercises include extension; however, they are not as easily quantified and monitored (Figure 148.1). Less-aggressive exercises may be more appropriate initially.

### Strengthening Exercise

Much of the pain of spinal origin associated with mechanical instability may often be reduced by an appropriate strengthening program. The supporting muscles of the spinal column can be thought of as such (supporting muscles). These muscles assist in activities of daily living, provide support, and prevent excessive spinal movement. If an asymmetry of muscle strength exists, excessive stresses may be placed on the spine or on its supporting muscles. In this case, strengthening the muscles that stress the spine, such as by weight lifting or by running, without strengthening the muscles that support the spine (abdominal and paraspinous muscles), could result in an excessive spinal stress application/spinal support muscle strength ratio. This may augment the dysfunctional nature of a dysfunctional motion segment.

The muscle groups to be specifically exercised include the dorsal paraspinous muscles and the abdominal muscles. Specific exercises include supine leg lifts progressing to sit-ups for abdominal muscle strengthening and prone leg lifts progressing to the airplane or rocking chair exercise for the paraspinous muscle strengthening (see Figure 148.1). Initially, less-aggressive exercises may be more appropriate. Similarly, strengthening exercises for cervical pain may be used (Figure 148.2).

It is emphasized that spine surgeons cannot divorce themselves from exercise and educational programs. Without an active participation by both the patient and the surgeon, the chance of failure of the management plan will assuredly increase.

## Patient Education

A patient education component of the program is essential. If patients understand the importance of their active participation, achieving the goal of the program is more likely. The documentation of patient progress is also imperative for longitudinal monitoring purposes. If patients cannot or refuse to participate, they have demonstrated their relative inability to succeed in a program such as outlined above. These patients should, perhaps, seek relief elsewhere.

In conclusion, due to the multi-factorial etiology of LBP and neck pain, the treatment therapies and modalities should also be multiple. The natural history of LBP shows that most patients will recover from their symptoms within a relatively short period of time; patients need reassurance of this. Early identification of risk factors and implementation of preventive measures seem to be the most effective methods to avoid future episodes of LBP and neck pain and would greatly affect the huge financial strain on the health care system. Interestingly, research has provided evidence that LBP and neck pain are manifestations of psychologic stressors. Psychologic variables cause patients to have more-severe pain. Bed rest is not

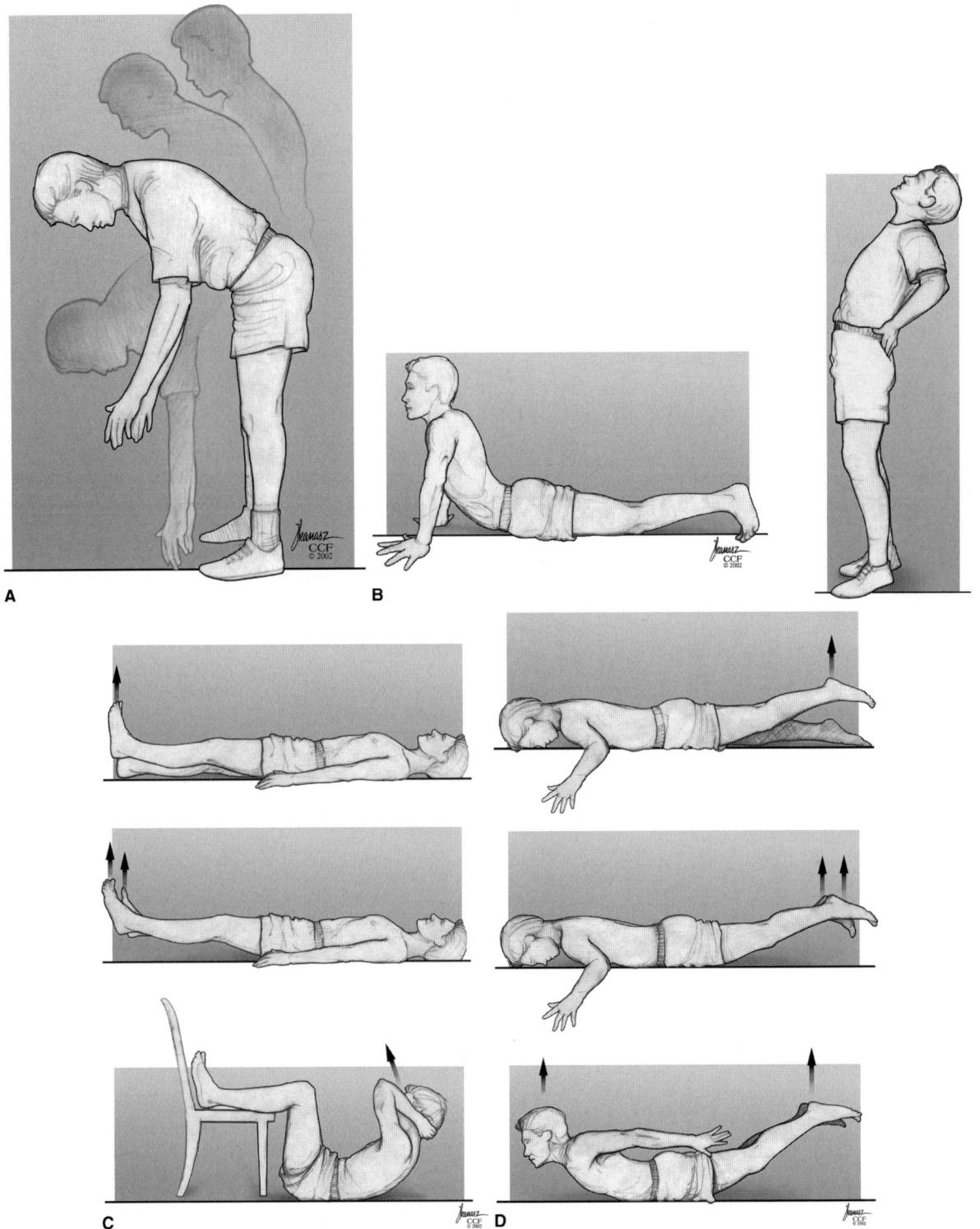

**Figure 148.1** Progressive degrees of stretching (**A** and **B**) and strengthening (**C** and **D**) exercises are depicted. For stretching exercises (**A** and **B**), the patient must hold the position for 10 to 20 seconds. For strengthening exercises, strength imbalances may increase pain. Both abdominal (**C**) and paraspinous (**D**) muscle strengthening are thus recommended. Progress may be measured in terms of duration and progression of complexity of exercises. (*Courtesy The Cleveland Clinic Foundation.*)

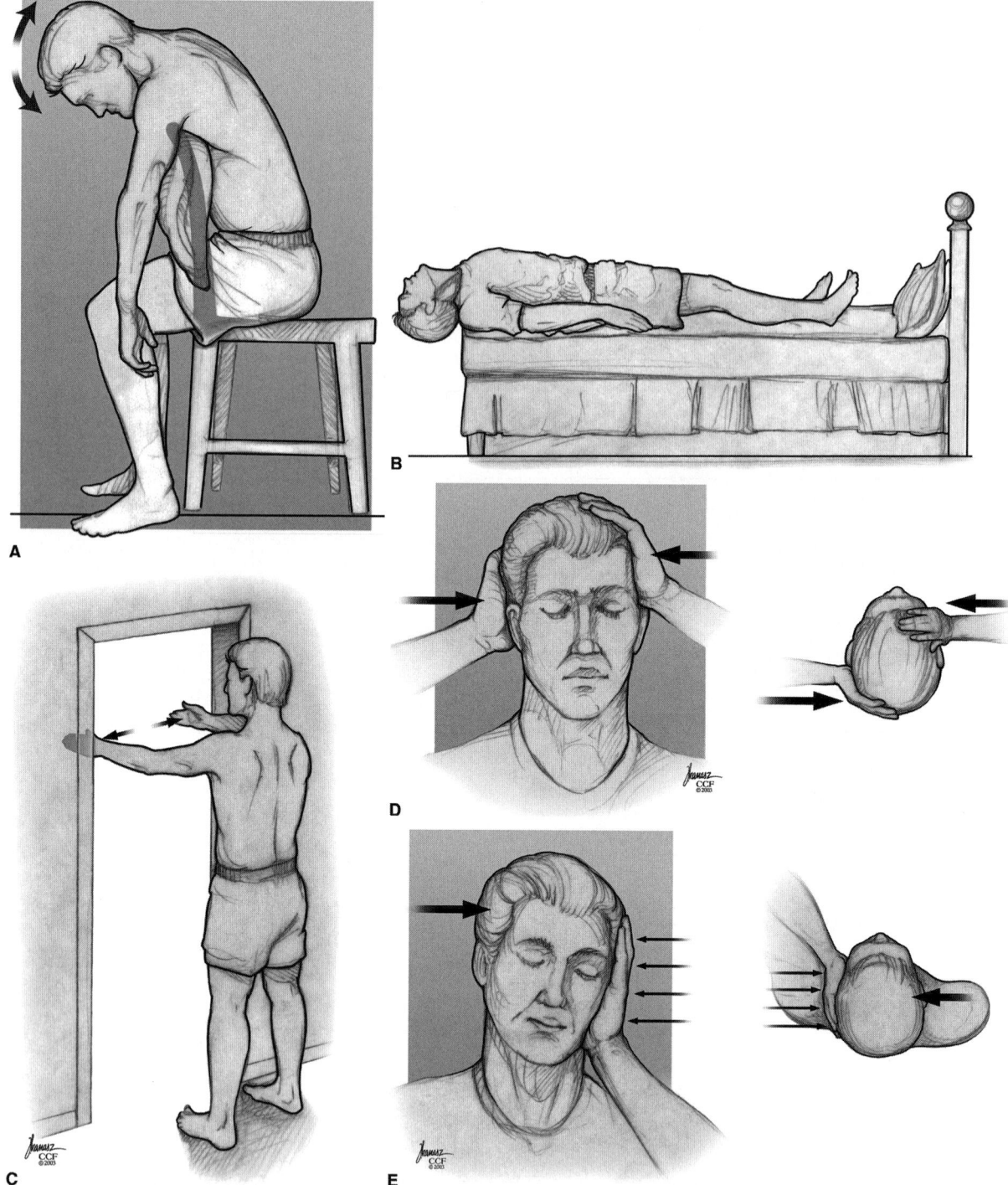

**Figure 148.2** (**A-B**) Stretching exercises; each position should be held for 10-20 seconds. (**C-E**) Resistance exercises; the goal time of each position is to hold resistance for 1 minute. (**C**) Back of arms are pushing against the door frame. (**D**) Rotational resistance (mirror and birds-eye views are depicted). (**E**) Resistance to left lateral bending; however, both right and left resistance should be practiced. (*Courtesy The Cleveland Clinic Foundation.*)

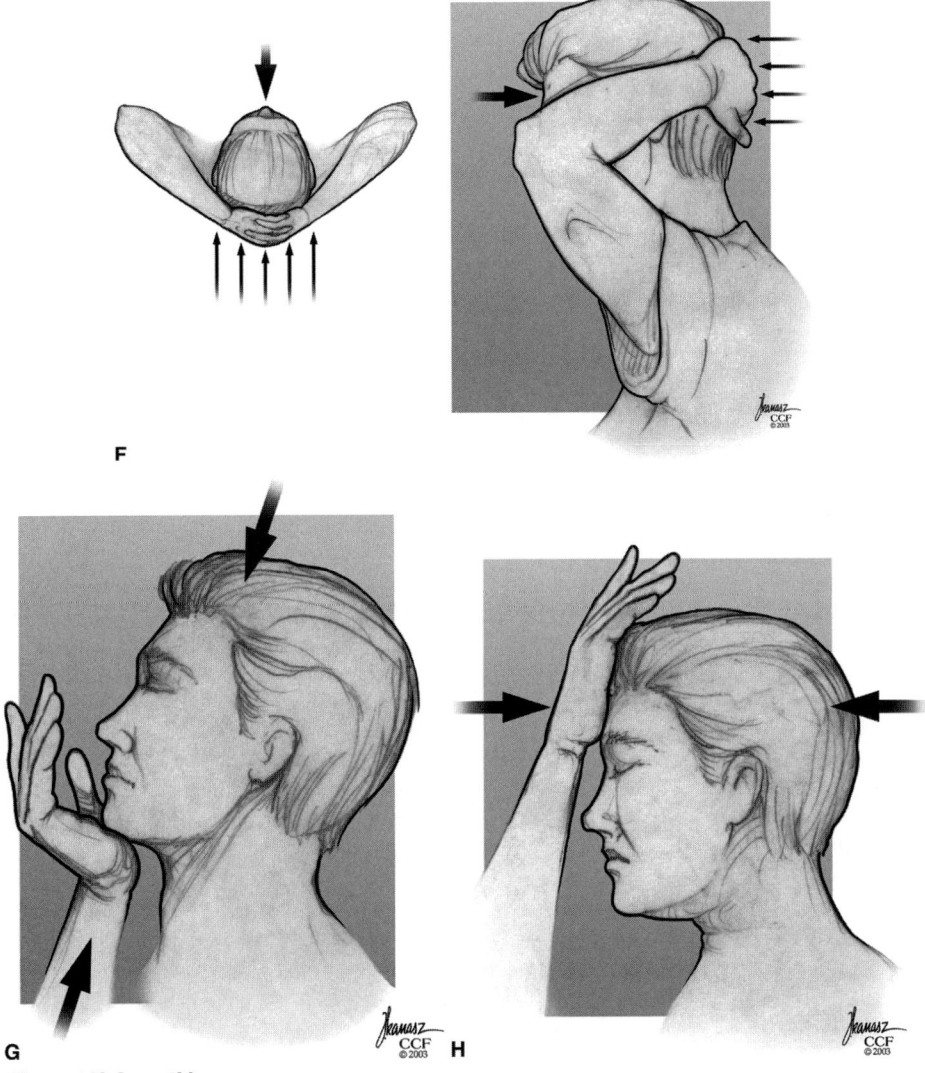

**Figure 148.2** *cont'd*

recommended for episodes of acute or chronic LBP. Return to normal daily activities is the best treatment, along with the appropriate use and management of NSAIDs for acute episodes of LBP. Isometric exercises are the best treatment for neck pain. Weight control, smoking cessation, and back exercises have been shown to reduce pain level and duration as well as aid in the treatment of chronic LBP. Many therapies and modalities in the treatment of back and neck pain exist; many have been shown to be effective and others not effective at all. However, many of the effective methods may have benefited, as the patient has, by the passing of time, and the symptoms may have improved in spite of the prescribed therapy. Larger and repeated studies are necessary to further the advancement of appropriate prevention and treatment of episodes of LBP and neck pain. Monumental patient education campaigns are needed to reduce risk factors.

## REFERENCES

1. Andersson GBJ: Epidemiologic features of chronic low-back pain. *Lancet* 354(9178):581-585, 1999.
2. Atkinson JH, Slater MA, Wahlgren DR, *et al*: Effects of noradrenergic and serotonergic antidepressants on chronic low back pain intensity. *Pain* 83(2):137-145, 1999.
3. Benzel E: Exercise, conditioning, and other non-operative strategies. In Benzel EC (ed): *Biomechanics of Spine Stabilization*. Rolling Meadows, IL, The American Association of Neurological Surgeons, 2001, pp 343-356.
4. Beurskens AJ, de Vet HC, Koke AJ, *et al*: Efficacy of traction for nonspecific low back pain. *Spine* 22(23):2756-2762, 1997.
5. Block AR, Vanharanta H, Ohnmeiss DD: Discographic pain report: influence of psychological factors. *Spine* 21:334-338, 1996.
6. Buti R: Herniated lumbar discs: diagnosis and management. *J Am Acad Nurs Prac* 10(12):547-550, 1998.

7. Byrne TN, Benzel EC, Waxman SG: Pain of spinal origin. In Byrne TN, Benzel EC, Waxman SG (eds): *Diseases of the Spine and Spinal Cord*. New York, Oxford University Press, 2000, pp 91-123.

8. Carlsson C, Sjolund B: Acupuncture for chronic low back pain: A randomized placebo-controlled study with long-term follow-up. *Clin J Pain* 17(4):296-305, 2001.

9. Carragee EJ, Chen Y, Tanner CM: Can discography cause long-term back symptoms in previously asymptomatic subjects? *Spine* 25:1803-1808, 2000.

10. Cohen RI, Chopra P, Upshur C: Low back pain, part 1: Primary care work-up of acute and chronic symptoms. *Geriatrics* 56(11):26-37, 2001.

11. Collacott EA, Zimmerman JT, White DW: Bipolar permanent magnets of the treatment of chronic low back pain: A pilot study. *JAMA* 283(10):1322-1325, 2000.

12. Convertino V, Hung J, Goldwater D: Cardiovascular responses to exercise in middle-aged men after 10 days of bed rest. *Circulation* 65:134-140, 1982.

13. Curtis P, Carey TS, Evans P: Training primary care physicians to give limited manual therapy for low back pain. *Spine* 25(22):2954-2961, 2000.

14. Davies JE, Gibson T, Tester L: The value of exercises in the treatment of low back pain. *Rheumatol Rehabil* 18:243-247, 1979.

15. Deyo RA, Diehl AK, Rosenthal M: How many days of bed rest for acute low back pain? A randomized clinical trial. *N Engl J Med* 315(17):1064-1070, 1986.

16. Deyo RA, Walsh N, Martin D, *et al*: A controlled trial of transcutaneous electronic nerve stimulation (TENS) and exercise for chronic low back pain. *N Engl J Med* 322:1627-1634, 1990.

17. Deyo RA, Weinstein JN: Low back pain. *N Engl J Med* 16(2):363-370, 2001.

18. Fanuele JC, Abdu WA, Hanscom B, *et al*: Association between obesity and functional status in patients with spine disease. *Spine* 27(3):306-312, 2002.

19. Feinmann C: Pain relief by antidepressants: Possible modes of action. *Pain* 23(1):1-8, 1985.

20. Furlan AD, Brosseau L, Imamura M, *et al*: Massage for low-back pain: A systematic review within the framework of the cochrane collaboration back review group. *Spine* 27(17):1896-1910, 2002.

21. Ghoname EA, Craig WF, White PF, *et al*: Percutaneous electrical nerve stimulation of low back pain. *JAMA* 281(9):818-823, 1999.

22. Gilbert JR, Taylor DW, Hildebrand A, *et al*: Clinical trial of common treatments for low back pain in family practice. *Br Med J* 291:7910-7914, 1985.

23. Goldberg MS, Scott SC, Mayo NE: A review of the association between cigarette smoking and the development of nonspecific back pain and related outcomes. *Spine* 23(8):995-1014, 2000.

24. Hagen KB, Hilde G, Jamtvedt G, *et al*: The Cochrane review of bed rest for acute low back pain and sciatica. *Spine* 25(22):2932-2939, 2000.

25. Hart LG, Deyo RA, Cherkin DC: Physician office visits for low back pain: frequency, clinical evaluation, and treatment patterns from a U.S. national survey. *Spine* 20:11-19, 1995.

26. Heary RF: Intradiscal electrothermal annuloplasty: the IDET procedure. *J Spinal Disord* 14:353-360, 2001.

27. Hultman G, Nordin M, Saraste H, *et al*: Body composition, endurance, strength, cross section of area and density of erector spiny muscles in men with and without low back pain. *J Spinal Disord* 6:114-123, 1993.

28. Jette DU, Fett AM: Physical therapy and health outcomes in patients with spinal impairments. *Phys Ther* 76:930-941, 1996.

29. Kendall PH, Jenkins JM: Exercises for backache: a double-blind controlled trail. *Physiotherapy* 54:154-157, 1968.

30. Kraus H, Melleby H, Gaston SR: Back pain correction and prevention. National voluntary organizational approach. *NY State J Med* 77:1335-1338, 1977.

31. Lahad A, Malter AD, Bert AO, *et al*: The effectiveness of four interventions for the prevention of low back pain. *JAMA* 272(16):1286-1291, 1994.

32. Leboeuf-Yde C: Smoking and low back pain. *Spine* 24(14):1463-1470, 1999.

33. Leboeuf-Yde C, Kyvik KO, Bruun NH: Low back pain and lifestyle: part I: smoking. *Spine* 23(20):2207-2214, 1998.

34. Leboeuf-Yde C, Kyvik KO, Bruun NH: Low back pain and lifestyle: part II: obesity. *Spine* 24(8):779-784, 1999.

35. Linton SJ: A review of psychological risk factors in back and neck pain. *Spine* 25:1148-1156, 2000.

36. Linton SJ, van Tulder MW: Preventive interventions for back and neck pain problems: What is the evidence? *Spine* 26(7):778-787, 2001.

37. Majkowksi GR, Jovag BW, Taylor BT, *et al*: The effect of back belt use on isometric lifting force and fatigue of the lumbar paraspinal muscles. *Spine* 23:2104-2109, 1998.

38. Malanga FA, Nadler SF: Nonoperative treatment of low back pain. *Mayo Clin Proc* 74:1135-1148, 1999.

39. Marras WS, Davis KG, Heaney CA, *et al*: The influence of psychosocial stress, gender and personality on mechanical loading of the lumbar spine. *Spine* 25(23):3045-3054, 2000.

40. Mayer TG, Smith SS, Keeley J, *et al*: Quantification of lumbar function. Plane trunk strength in chronic low back patients. *Spine* 10:91-103, 1985.

41. Muller EA: Influence of training and inactivity on muscle strength. *Arch Phys Med Rehabil* 51:449-462, 1970.

42. Nachemson A: The lumbar spine: an orthopaedic challenge. *Spine* 1:59-71, 1976.

43. Nadler SF, Steiner DJ, Erasala GN, *et al*: Continuous low-level heat wrap therapy provides more efficacy than ibuprofen and acetaminophen for acute low back pain. *Spine* 27(10):1012-1017, 2002.

44. Nutter P: Aerobic exercise in the treatment and prevention of low back pain. *Occ Med* 3(1):137-145, 1988.

45. Pennick V, Sinclair S: What is the optimal evidence-based management of chronic non-specific low-back pain? *Linkages: Transferring Research into Practice*. August 2002. http://www.iwh.on.ca/Pages/Publications/linkages/linkages-review.htm

46. Philadelphia Panel: *Philadelphia Panel Evidence-Based Clinical Practice Guidelines on Selected Rehabilitation Interventions for Neck Pain*. 81:1701-1717, 2001.

47. Power C, Frank J, Hertzman C, *et al*: Predictors of low back pain onset in a prospective British study. *Am J Pub Health* 91:1671-1678, 2001.

48. Rittweger J, Just K, Kautzsch K: The treatment of chronic lower back pain with lumbar extension and whole-body vibration exercise. *Spine* 27(17):1829-1834, 2002.

49. Rush AJ, Polatin P, Gatchel RJ: Depression and chronic low back pain: Establishing priorities in treatment. *Spine* 25(20):2566-2571, 2000.

50. Schmitt H, Zhao J, Brocai D: Acupuncture treatment of low back pain. *Schmerz* 15(1):33-37, 2001.

51. Scott SC, Goldbert MS, Mayo NE, *et al*: The association between cigarette smoking and back pain in adults. *Spine* 24:1090-1098, 1999.

52. Sculco AD, Paup DC, Fernhall B, Sculco MJ: Effects of aerobic exercise on low back pain patients in treatment. *The Spine Journal* 1:95-101, 2001.

53. Shirdo O, Kaneda K, Ito T: Trunk muscle strength during concentric and eccentric contraction: a comparison between healthy subjects and patients with low back pain. *J Spinal Disord* 5:175-182, 1992.

54. Skouen JS, Gradal AL, Haldorsen E, *et al*: Relative cost-effectiveness of extensive and light multidisciplinary treatment programs versus treatment as usual for patients with chronic low back pain on long-term sick leave. *Spine* 27(9):901-909, 2002.

55. Smith SE, Darden BV, Rhyne AL, *et al*: Outcomes of unoperated discogram-positive low back pain. *Spine* 330:1997-2000, 1995.

56. Stauffer JD: Antidepressants and chronic pain. *J Fam Prac* 25(2):167-170, 1987.

57. Truchon M: Determinants of chronic disability related to low back pain: towards an integrative biopsychosocial model. *Dis Rehab* 23:758-767, 2001.

58. van Tulder MW, Koes BW, Bouter LM: Conservative treatment of acute and chronic nonspecific low back pain: A systematic review of randomized controlled trials of the most common interventions. *Spine* 22(18):2128-2156, 1997.

59. van Tulder MW, Scholten RJPM, Koes BW, *et al*: Nonsteroidal anti-inflammatory drugs of low back pain. *Spine* 25(19):2501-2513, 2000.

60. Vogt MT, Hanscom B, Lauerman WC: Influence of smoking on the health status of spinal patients. *Spine* 27:313-319, 2002.

61. Waddell G, Feder G, Lewis M: Systematic reviews of bed rest and advice to stay active for acute low back pain. *Br J Gen Prac* 47(423):647-652, 1997.

62. Williams PC: *The Lumbosacral Spine, Emphasizing Conservative Management.* New York, McGraw Hill, 1965.

# CHAPTER 149

# Intradiscal Electrothermal Therapy

**Sung Min and Nagy Mekhail**

Chronic low back pain is one of the most challenging problems facing pain and spine specialists today. Low back pain is the most common cause of disability among young adults in the United States.[22] It has been estimated that approximately 80% of all adults experience disabling low back pain sometime in their lifetime, with an annual incidence of 5%.[3] Most acute low back pain episodes resolve within 12 weeks, but the rate of recurrence is high. Approximately 70% to 90% of patients have recurrences of back pain following the initial episode.[3] Low back pain becomes persistent, chronic, and disabling in 5% of patients.[34] Because of a poor correlation between patients' symptoms, physiologic changes, and imaging studies, only 10% to 20% of back pain can be attributed to a precise anatomic source.[15,19] Recently there has been growing evidence that the disc itself may be the source of pain in a significant portion of the chronic back pain population.[13] Chronic low back pain caused by degenerative disc disease is a widespread problem that accounts for approximately 40% of chronic back pain.[32,33]

Chronic discogenic low back pain continues to be a difficult condition to treat. Traditionally, the treatment options have been limited. Nonoperative treatments such as medications and physical therapy are frequently unable to significantly alleviate pain or improve the patient's functional status. Patients for whom the traditional nonoperative approach fails are often left facing the option of either a chronic pain management approach or surgical intervention, such as spinal fusion.[27,39] Results of surgical treatments such as discectomy and fusion have been less than satisfying, with failure rates as high as 40%.[34] Given the potential complications, morbidity, prolonged recovery period, and various outcomes, other treatment alternatives continue to be investigated. In 1997, a novel alternative for treating chronic discogenic pain called *intradiscal electrothermal therapy* (IDET) was proposed by Saal and Saal.[27]

IDET is a technique that utilizes a navigable thermal catheter that is placed into the dorsal wall of the annulus fibrosus of the affected disc. The disc annulus is then heated for a specified period of time with the intention of causing alteration in collagen architecture and destruction of nociceptors within the disc.

## The Intervertebral Disc

The human intervertebral disc consists of central nucleus pulposus surrounded by an outer concentric ring of the annulus fibrosus. The annulus is made up of rings of densely packed and highly organized sheets known as lamellae. The lamellae are composed of highly organized type I collagen that is maintained by fibroblast-like cells. They run perpendicular to one another and confer the tensile strength of the disc, which is similar to the tendon. The nucleus pulposus is a gelatinous structure composed of a proteoglycan aggregate and type II collagen that are maintained by chondrocyte-like cells. The disc is approximately 70% collagen in the annulus and 20% collagen in the nucleus pulposus. The end plate is a layer of cartilage that separates the disc from the adjacent vertebrae. Certain portions of the end plate are in close proximity to the marrow cavity. This facilitates the diffusion of nutrients from the vessels in the marrow space into the end plate and the intervertebral disc.

Multiple morphologic changes occur with disc degeneration. The nucleus pulposus loses its hydrostatic pressure and becomes dehydrated. The annular matrix undergoes myxomatous degeneration and loses its normal organization of collagen fibrils. These changes produce an increase in shear stress on the annular wall and focal segmental mobility, leading to delamination and fissuring of the annular wall. The end plate undergoes subchondral sclerosis with calcification and fissuring of hilar cartilage, resulting in the loss of nutrient delivery to the disc.[4,25,34]

The concept that the disc itself could be the source of back pain is not new. As far back as 1947, it was recognized that the disc is an innervated structure and therefore could be the pain generator.[2] The posterior longitudinal ligament and the outer third of the annulus fibrosus contain nerve endings that are the terminal nerve endings of the sinuvertebral nerve. They have been shown to contain nociceptive neurotransmitters (substance P, calcitonin, vasoactive intestinal peptide).[12,27]

Afferent nociceptive input is transmitted through the dorsal root ganglion. Nociceptive tissue has been shown to be sensitized, resulting in a decreased threshold after being treated with inflammatory mediators. Ingrowth of small unmyelinated nerve fibers and granulation tissue has been shown to occur in degenerative discs.[6] In one study. Freemont et al.[11] reported nerves extending into the inner third of the annulus fibrosus as well as into the nucleus pulposus in patients with chronic low back pain. In vivo studies of pain response to tissue stimulation during surgery on the lumbar spine demonstrated that the two most common pain generators were the posterior longitudinal ligament and the dorsal layer of the annulus fibrosus.[19] The exact mechanism of discogenic pain remains unclear. The basis for discogenic pain likely involves both mechanical and chemical interactions. Chronic discogenic pain is thought to be produced when distortion of the annular lamellae induces subsequent sensitization of the nociceptors, which may have been presensitized by substances such as phospholipase A2, metalloproteinase, interleukin 1, and nitrous oxide. Afferent stimuli create the release of substance P and nociception. As the disc continues to be loaded, the neuronal activity continues. The combination of mechanical and neural properties create an interplay leading to chronic discogenic pain.[27] Discogenic pain is predominantly axial but may cause referred pain in the lower extremities. This occurs because afferent input from innervated structures such as the disc converge on the same neurons in the dorsal horn as the afferent inputs from the lower extremity.[24] It is important to remember that the term *discogenic pain* does not imply disc protrusions or herniation causing nerve compression. The discogenic pain syndrome in this context is caused by an internal derangement of the disc itself.

## Intradiscal Electrothermal Therapy

IDET is a minimally invasive technique developed as an alternative treatment of chronic discogenic pain that is unresponsive to conservative treatment. The basis of this procedure stems from thermal treatments used to alter collagen fibers and to stabilize the joint capsule in other medical procedures such as arthroscopy and capsulorphy.[7] Previous studies have determined temperatures required to cause nerve death and alter collagen architecture. The hydrogen bonds in collagen start to break at 60°C, and the optimal temperature for collagen contraction is 65°C. A lesser temperature is required to cause denervation at approximately 45°C.[34] The strength of collagen fibers is derived from the conformation of the triple helix molecule, which is cross-linked with hydrogen bonds. Some of the hydrogen bonds are heat-sensitive and break as they are heated, resulting in a contracted state termed the *denatured state*.

The IDET procedure is postulated to work through multiple mechanisms. These include (1) alteration of collagen architecture within the disc, (2) denervation of annular nociceptors, (3) stimulation or induction of annular healing, (4) cauterization of vascular ingrowth, (5) and biochemical mediation of inflammation.[8,27] An in vitro study of human cadaveric disc by *Shah et al.*[34] found IDET to increase temperature in the dorsal annulus sufficient to induce collagen denaturation. Electron microscopy in this study demonstrated evidence of denaturation and contraction of collagen fibers. Some studies, however, were not able to reproduce temperatures sufficient for collagen denaturation. Recently Kleinsteuk *et al.*[17] examined the thermal distribution pattern during IDET in the cadaveric spine and reported that the temperature required for collagen denaturation and shrinkage was achieved only within 1 to 2mm of the catheter. The temperature required for denervation was found within 6mm of the catheter but was not reliably produced in clinically relevant regions such as the dorsal annulus. This suggests that other mechanisms of pain relief are present, or that catheter positioning is important to achieve improved outcome. Kleinsteuk also demonstrated that the disc temperatures did not reach steady state by the end of the IDET heating protocol. Kleinsteuk *et al.*[17] and Lee *et al.*[18] studied the stability of the lumbar spine following IDET treatment and found a small decrease (6% to 12%) and no changes in stability, respectively. It is therefore unlikely that this procedure will improve the stability of the disc itself. Theoretically, the heating of the annulus fibrosus could induce healing of the annular fissures. This, however, has not been proven through experimental studies.

Heating of collagen in the annulus fibrosus could theoretically stimulate the healing of annular tears. In vivo studies of collagen heating have shown fibroblastic activity following the treatment. If the inflammatory response does occur in response to the IDET treatment, one could expect an initial worsening of pain, followed by improvement or resolution of pain. Clinical improvement after IDET usually is seen after 2 to 3 months following the procedure.[23,27] If the disc pain is caused by nociceptors in the end plate or from high mechanical end plate loading, heating of the annulus likely will not improve the outcome.[8] The mechanism by which the IDET procedure relieves pain remains unclear and may be multifactorial.

## Technique

The procedure uses a catheter with a thermal resistive coil that is placed in the outer annulus fibrosus in the region of the annular tear under fluoroscopic guidance. The distal 5cm of the catheter is then heated gradually to 90°C over a 16- to 17-minute period and maintained at this temperature for 4 minutes[8] (Figure 149.1). A unilateral approach is usually sufficient to cover the entire dorsal annular wall. However, approximately 40% of the time, a bilateral approach is required. Intravenous antibiotic is administered prior to the procedure, in addition to an intradiscal injection of antibiotic for prophylaxis against discitis.[8]

## Selection Criteria

The selection criteria have become more stringent since the introduction of the procedure in 1997. Current widely accepted criteria include (1) unremitting low back pain of at least 6 months' duration that is unresponsive to trial aggressive conservative treatments; (2) normal neurologic

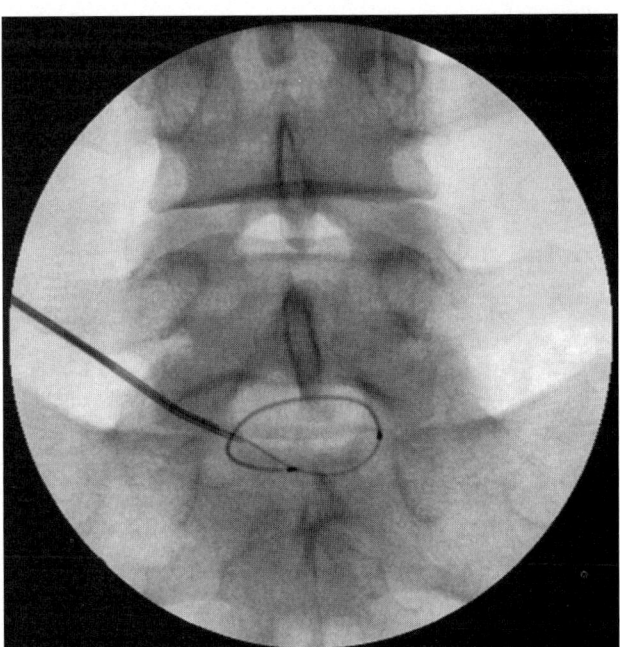

**Figure 149.1** Posteroanterior view showing how an intradiscal catheter is navigated to heat the posterior wall of the L5/S1 annulus.

examination; (3) negative straight leg raising; (4) positive discography with production of concordant pain; and (5) MRI studies that are negative for neural compressive lesions, disc protrusion less than 3mm, absence of stenosis or instability, and less than 30% decrease in disc height. A recent study by Cohen *et al.* found obesity to be a risk factor for poor outcome.

## Exclusion Criteria

Exclusion criteria include (1) inflammatory arthritis, (2) non-spinal cause of back pain, (3) medical or other condition that would preclude participation or adequate followup, (4) previous surgery at the proposed disc level, (5) greater than 50% disc height loss or instability, (6) overlying psychologic issues, and (7) extruded or sequestered disc.

## Risks and Complications

There have been relatively few reports of significant complications. Potential complications include discitis, nerve injury, and heat injury of the end plates. Several cases of cauda equina syndrome following IDET has been reported.[1,14,38] Derby *et al.*[9] reported significant disc space narrowing and disc space collapse along with biopsy evidence of end plate injury following IDET in 2 patients. Several cases of superficial skin burn have been reported as well. Vertebral osteonecrosis, as well as a case of herniated disc following the procedure, have been reported.[5,10] A recent study by Cohen *et al.*[5] found obesity to be a risk factor for poor outcome. Long-term data are still being collected, but so far, severe complications have been infrequent. Overall, IDET appears to be a relatively safe procedure when performed by an experienced physician.

## Course of Recovery

Most patients tend to experience transient worsening of pain after the procedure. The pain typically returns to baseline after 7 to 14 days. Improvement in back pain often requires 6 to 12 weeks (Figures 149.2 and 149.3).

## Postprocedure Rehabilitation

Most patients tend to experience transient worsening of pain after the procedure. They are therefore instructed on activity restrictions. Activities are gradually increased. Immediately after the procedure, bending, lifting, and prolonged sitting are not recommended. Walking and low-intensity lower extremity stretches are recommended for 4 weeks. At 4 weeks, the patients are encouraged to begin low-intensity floor stabilization exercises. At 6 months, most patients are able to begin athletic activities. See Box 149.1 regarding patient education and postprocedure instructions.

## Outcomes

The initial study by Saal *et al.*[28] reported results on 25 IDET treated patients. Eighty percent reported reduction of Visual Analog Scale (VAS) pain score of at least 2 points ($P < .0001$). Seventy-two percent reported improvement in sitting tolerance ($P < .0002$). Out of 19 patients taking analgesics, 10/19 eliminated the use of analgesics

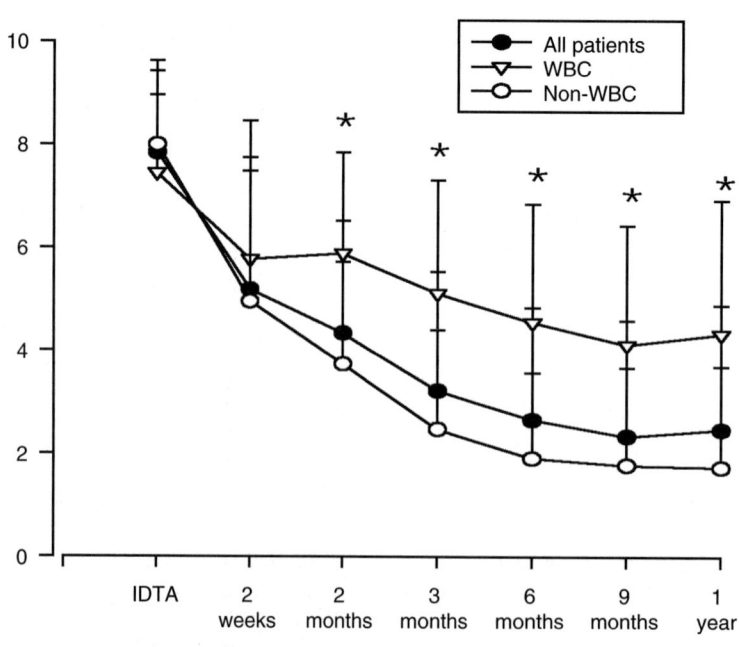

**Figure 149.2** Changes in VAS pain scores after IDET. *IDET,* Intradiscal electrothermal therapy; *IDTA,* intradiscal electrothermal anuloplasty; *VAS,* visual analog scale.

and 4/19 reduced medications by 50%. Short Form-36 (SF-36) measurement showed successful outcome (defined as change of 7 points) in 77% of patients treated at a single level and 75% treated at two or more levels. The same authors, in a subsequent study, reported the results of a 62 patient cohort with a minimum follow up of 1 year.[29] This study utilized similar inclusion and exclusion criteria as the previous study. Thirty patients underwent one-level IDET and 32 underwent multilevel treatment. VAS, SF-36, Health Status Questionnaire (Physical Function subscale), and SF-36 Bodily Pain subscale scores were assessed. This study reported a mean change of 3 in VAS ($P < .001$), a mean change in SF-36 bodily pain of 17 ($P < .001$), and a mean change of SF-36 physical function of 20 ($P < .001$). Symptomatic improvement was noted in 71% (44/62) on the SF-36 physical function subscale, 74%

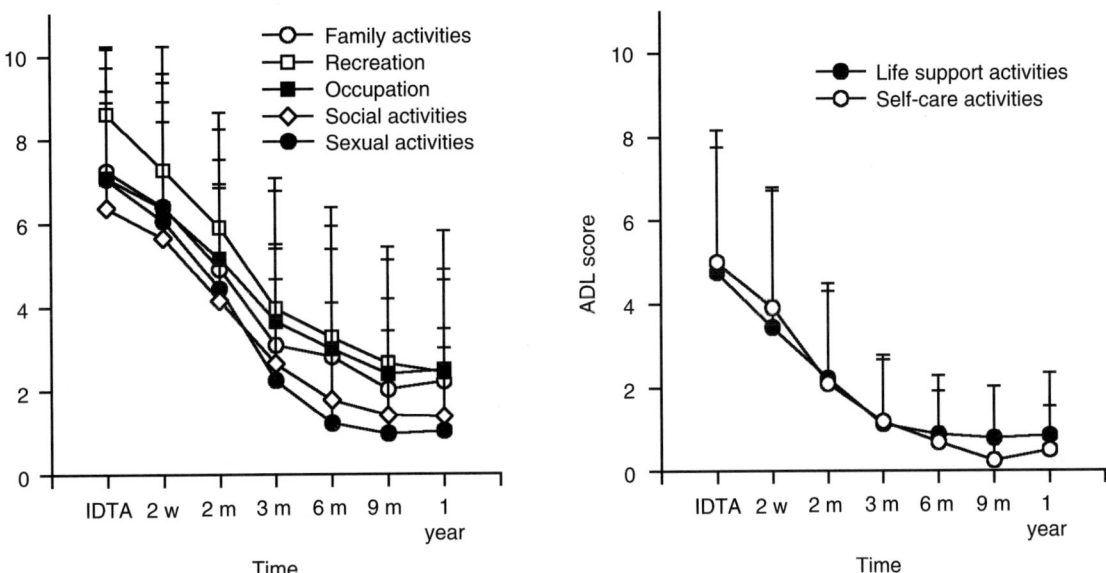

**Figure 149.3** Changes in activities of daily living after IDET. *ADL,* Activities of daily living; *IDET,* intradiscal electrothermal therapy; *IDTA,* intradiscal electrothermal anuloplasty.

---

**BOX 149.1**

## IDET postprocedure patient education and instructions

- Plan to rest for 1 to 3 days after your IDET in a comfortable position (i.e., lying down or reclining), limit sitting or walking to 10 to 20 minutes at a time.
- Return to work:
  -Sedentary work: You many return in roughly 2 weeks, however, you may still be sore after your IDET. Be aware of sitting restrictions listed below.
  -For other jobs, the decision will be made by your physician.
- Driving: None for the first 1 to 5 days, then limit your driving to 20 to 30 minutes for the first 6 weeks after your IDET. Make sure your vehicle has good lumbar support.
  -As a passenger, recline the seat and try to limit driving times to less than 45 minutes for the first 6 weeks. It is okay to recline and be driven home the day of your procedure or lie down in the back seat.
- Sitting: Limit to 30 to 45 minutes at any one time in a chair with good support for the first 6 weeks. Avoid sitting on soft couches or chairs. Use a pillow or towel to maintain your lumbar curve when sitting.
  -Standing and walking about in between sitting periods or short periods of lying down are helpful.
- Lifting: Limit 5 to 10lb for the first 6 weeks.

- No bending or twisting of the low back.
- Housework: No bending or twisting for the first 6 weeks.
- No chiropractic, manipulation, massage, inversion, or traction for the first 12 weeks.
- Exercise
  -Walk daily, beginning at the end of the first week, for approximately 20 minutes. Increase to 20 minutes twice per day, if tolerated, then progressively increase to 1 hour a day by the end of the fourth week. If back or leg symptoms increase at any point, back down on the duration of walking.
  -You may do gentle leg stretches (hamstring, piriformis) with your back flat on the floor.
  -Abdominal brace exercise can be begun at 2 to 3 weeks, with your back flat on the floor.
  -No swimming for the first 6 weeks.
  -Formal physical therapy will usually begin 6 to 8 weeks after the IDET
  -Do not use a treadmill or a StairMaster for the first 6 weeks, unless otherwise instructed.
- You will be wearing a lumbar corset, only while awake, for the first 6 weeks after your IDET.

(46/62) on SF-36 bodily pain subscale, and 71% (44/62) with VAS scores.

Saal et al.[30,31] followed the above studies with a 2-year follow-up study of 58 patients. The same inclusion and exclusion criteria were used. In this group, 27 underwent one-level IDET and 28 underwent multilevel IDET. Again, VAS and SF-36 data were collected as outcome measures. They reported mean changes in the SF-36 bodily pain subscore of 17.8 ($P < .001$) and at least a 7-point improvement in physical function subscore. In this study, no significant difference was noted in outcome between private pay and worker's compensation patients.

Karasek and Bogbuk[16] studied 35 IDET-treated patients. A total of 53 patients were considered candidates, but 17 of these patients were denied by their insurance company. This group of subjects was used by the authors as a convenient control group, and they were treated conservatively. All patients underwent discography and met the standard inclusion and exclusion criteria. VAS, return to work, Oswestry Disability Questionnaire, and opiate medication usage data were collected as outcome measures. At 3 months, only one control patient achieved significant pain relief as compared with 66% in the IDET group. They noted sustained relief at 6 and 12 months and improvement in disability, reduced drug usage, and return to work rate of 53%. The authors concluded that 60% of treated patients obtained clear benefit from the procedure and 23% obtained complete relief.

Thompson and Eckel[36,37] investigated outcome data on 211 patients obtained from 43 physicians. Significant improvement in pain (VAS and SF-36) was noted at 6 and 12 months. In this report, results were also stratified in an attempt to determine factors predictive of outcome. Treatment of multiple levels was associated with an increase in pain at all time points, but no difference in overall improvement after the procedure was observed. Smoking and gender did not predict magnitude of improvement. A trend toward decreased physical function with a lesser degree of improvement was noted in the workers' compensation group. Other earlier studies reported favorable findings in support of the procedure.[20,21,35]

Pauza et al.[26] evaluated the efficacy of IDET via a double-blinded placebo-controlled trial. To date, this is the first double-blinded placebo-controlled trial that has been reported. In this study, an average difference of 2.4 in VAS score, a 17-point improvement in the SF-36 bodily pain scale, and an 11-point improvement in the Oswestry Disability Index ($P < .05$), were reported.

Mekhail and Kapural[23] performed a prospective study to test the hypothesis that more strict patient selection criteria may improve the outcome of treatment. The additional selection criteria included disc height of at least 50%, no lumbar stenosis, no evidence of herniated nucleus pulposus, no evidence of psychologic issues, and one- or two-level degenerative disc disease. Patients were followed for 1 year. They reported improvement of VAS score of more than 6 points (on a 10-point scale) at 6 and 12 months in the non-workers compensation group. However, all the patients showed significant improvement in the activities of daily living, regardless of the type of payer (see Figures 149.2 and 149.3).

## Summary

IDET is a procedure that was introduced as a minimally invasive treatment option for treating discogenic pain unresponsive to aggressive conservative therapy. Currently, the only other reasonable interventional option for patients suffering from chronic discogenic pain is surgery such as spinal fusion. It may be a promising alternative to surgery, especially in cases where surgery is not an option. Although the procedure is not without risks, it appears to be relatively safe. Long-term data for IDET, however, is lacking. Long-term efficacy as well as the effect of thermal therapy on the disc is also unknown.

## REFERENCES

1. Ackerman III WE: Cauda equina syndrome after intradiscal electrothermal therapy. *Reg Anesth Pain Med* 27:622, 2002.
2. Bogduk: *Clinical Anatomy of the Lumbar Spine And Sacrum*, ed 3. Philadelphia, Churchill Livingstone, 2002.
3. Carey TS, Garrett JM, Jackman AM: Beyond good prognosis. Examination of an inception cohort of patients with chronic low back pain. *Spine* 25:115-120, 2000.
4. Chung SA, Khan SN, Diwan AD: The molecular basis of intervertebral disk degeneration. *Orthop Clin North Am* 34:209-219, 2003.
5. Cohen SP, Larkin T, Polly Jr DWA: Giant herniated disc following intradiscal electrothermal therapy. *J Spinal Disord Tech* 15:537-541, 2002.
6. Coppes MH, Marani E, Thomeer RTWM, et al: Innervation of "painful" lumbar discs. *Spine* 22:2342-2350, 1997.
7. Davis TT, Sra P, Fuller N, et al: Lumbar intervertebral thermal therapies. *Orthop Clin North Am* 34:255-262, 2003.
8. Debry R: *Intradiscal Electrothermal Annuloplasty (IDET)*. International Spine Injection Society Newsletter, March 2003.
9. Derby R, Bjorn E, et al: Intradiscal electrothermal annuloplasty (IDET): a novel approach for treating chronic discogenic back pain. *Int Neuromod Soc* 3(2):82-88, 2000.
10. Djurasovic M, Glassman SD, Dimar Jr JR, et al: Vertebral osteonecrosis associated with the use of intradiscal electrothermal therapy: a case report. *Spine* 27:E325-E328, 2002.
11. Freemont AJ, Peacock TE, Goupille P, et al: Nerve ingrowth into diseased intervertebral disc in chronic back pain. *Lancet* 350:178-181, 1997.
12. Freemont AJ, Watkins A, Maitre CL, et al: Nerve growth factor expression and innervation of the painful intervertebral disc. *J Pathol* 197:286-292, 2002.
13. Houp J, Conner ES, McFarland EW: Experimental study of temperature distributions and thermal transport during radiofrequency current therapy of the intervertebral disc. *Spine* 21:1808-1813, 1996.
14. Hsia AW, Isaac K, Katz JS: Cauda equina syndrome from intradiscal electrothermal therapy. *Neurology* 55:320, 2000.
15. Ito M, Incorvaia KM, Yu SF, et al: Predictive signs of discogenic lumbar pain on magnetic resonance imaging with discography correlation. *Spine* 23:1252-1260, 1998.

16. Karasek M, Bogduk N: Twelve-month follow-up of a controlled trial of intradiscal thermal annuloplasty for back pain due to internal disc disruption. *Spine* 25:2601-2607, 2000.

17. Kleinstueck FS, Diederich CJ, Nau WH, *et al*: Acute biomechanical and histologic effects of intradiscal thermal therapy on human lumbar discs. *Spine* 26:2198-2207, 2001.

18. Lee J, Lutz GE, Campbell D, *et al*: Stability of the lumbar spine after intradiscal electrothermal therapy. *Arch Phys Med Rehabil* 82:120-122, 2001.

19. Margo K: Diagnosis, treatment and prognosis in patients with low back pain. *Am Fam Physician* 49:171-179, 1994.

20. Maurer P, Squillante PC: Is IDET effective treatment for discogenic low back pain? A prospective cohort outcome study (1-2 year follow-up). Identifying successful patient selection criteria. 16th Annual Meeting, North American Spine Society, Oct 31-Nov 3, 2001.

21. Maurer P, Schlemback D, Brown M: Lumbar Intradiscal Electrothermal Annuloplasty(IDEA) for discogenic low back pain. Presented at the Intradiscal Therapy Society annual meeting. Williamsburg, VA, June 8-10, 2000.

22. McGraw JK, Silber JS, *et al*: Intradiscal electrothermal therapy for the treatment of discogenic back pain: results and follow-up. SCVIR 26th annual scientific meeting, San Antonio, TX, March 3-8, 2001.

23. Mekhail N, Kapural L: Intradiscal thermal annuloplasty for discogenic pain: an outcome study. *Pain Practice* 4(2): 84-90, 2004.

24. O'Neill CW, Kurgansky ME, Derby R, *et al*: Disc stimulation and patterns of referred pain. *Spine* 27:2276-2781, 2002.

25. Osti OL, Vernon-Roberts B, Moore R, *et al*: Annular tears and disc degeneration in the lumbar spine. A post-mortem study of 135 discs. *J Bone Joint Surg* 74-B:678-682, 1992.

26. Pauza K, Howel S, Dreyfuss P, Peloza J, *et al*: A randomized double-blinded placebo controlled trial evaluating the efficacy of intradiscal electrothermal annuloplasty for the treatment of chronic discogenic low back pain. International Spine Injection Society meeting, 2003.

27. Saal JA, Saal JS: Intradiscal electrothermal therapy for the treatment of chronic discogenic low back pain. *Clin Sports Med* 21:167-187, 2002.

28. Saal JA, Saal JS: Management of chronic discogenic low back pain with a thermal intradiscal catheter. A preliminary report. *Spine* 25:382-388, 2000.

29. Saal JA, Saal JS: Intradiscal electrothermal treatment for chronic discogenic low back pain. A prospective outcome study with minimum 1 year follow-up. *Spine* 25:2622-2627, 2000.

30. Saal JA, Saal JS: Intradiscal electrothermal treatment for chronic discogenic low back pain. *Spine* 27:966-974, 2002.

31. Saal JA, Saal JS: Intradiscal electrothermal treatment (idet) for chronic discogenic low back pain: A controlled outcome study with minimum two year follow-up. North American Spine Society 15th Annual Meeting, October 25-28, 2000, New Orleans, LA.

32. Schwarzer A, Aprill C, Derby R, *et al*: The prevalence and clinical features of internal disc disruption in patients with chronic low back pain. *Spine* 20:1878-1883, 1995.

33. Schwarzer AC, Aprill CN, Derby R, *et al*: A relative contribution of the disc and zygapophyseal joint in chronic low back pain. *Spine* 19:801-806, 1994.

34. Shah RV, Lutz GE, Lee J, *et al*: Intradiskal electrothermal therapy: a preliminary histologic study. *Arch Phys Med Rehabil* 82:1230-1237, 2001.

35. Singh V: Intradiscal electrothermal therapy: A preliminary report. *Pain Physician* 3(4):367-374, 2000.

36. Thompson KJ, Ekel TS: IDET nationwide registry preliminary results: 12 month follow up data on 211 patients. 16th Annual Meeting, North American Spine Society, Oct 31-Nov 3, 2001.

37. Wetzel FT: Cauda equina syndrome from intradiscal electrothermal therapy. *Neurology* 56:1607, 2001.

38. Wetzel FT, McNally TA, Phillips FM: Intradiscal electrothermal therapy used to manage chronic discogenic low back pain. New directions and interventions. *Spine* 27:2621-2626, 2002.

# CHAPTER 150

# Neurologic Complications

David G. Malone, Robert F. McLain,
and John R. Caruso

## Neurologic Complications of Common Spinal Operations

### Cervicomedullary Junction

Operations at the level of the cervicomedullary junction for tumor are often associated with significant risk. Three approaches are commonly used: the transoral, dorsolateral, and the lateral suboccipital. The neurologic complications associated with surgery in this area include lower cranial nerve palsy, brain stem infarction from vertebral artery damage, and direct injury to the medulla and upper cervical spinal cord. These complications may be lessened by the choice of surgical approach. Some surgeons have recommended the lateral suboccipital approach for selected lesions in this region because it provides direct visualization of the ventral surface of the brain stem and spinal cord and provides a sterile approach with ability to close the dura mater in a watertight fashion, and neither mastoidectomy nor transposition of the vertebral artery is required.[47]

### The Upper Cervical Spine

Risk factors for complications associated with upper dorsal cervical fusions are significant instability, myelopathy, prior failed fusions, and irreducible dislocations. Death has been reported from passage of a sublaminar wire at C2.[56]

### C1-2 Transarticular Fixation

Reported complications of C1-2 transarticular screw fixation include neurologic deficit including suboccipital neuralgia, hypoglossal paresis, arteriovenous fistula causing upper extremity paresis, and brainstem infarction leading to death. If brisk pulsate bleeding occurs during screw placement, arterial injury must be suspected. Screw placement can be completed on the side of the pulsatile bleeding; however, no attempt should be made to place a screw in the "normal" side.[14] A survey of the Joint Spine Section on Disorders of the Spine and Peripheral Nerves yielded important data regarding the incidence and complication rates for C1-2 transarticular screw fixation. The risk of vertebral artery injury was 2.2% per patient, and the risk of a known or suspected vertebral artery injury leading to a neurologic deficit was 3.7%. A single death was reported, for an overall morality rate of 0.1%. Intraoperative control of the

bleeding was accomplished by placing the transarticular screw, effectively tamponading the bleeding or occluding the hole with bone wax. In the survey, postoperative management of vertebral artery injury varied between observation and arteriography with balloon occlusion of the injured artery. Other data have shown that in deliberate bilateral vertebral artery occlusion, if the posterior communicating arteries are patent, the risk of vertebrobasilar insufficiency is 20%.[67] The most commonly reported complication was suboccipital numbness in 16.8% of patients.

C1-2 transarticular screws carry the potential of neurologic complications. The screw is placed in close proximity to the vertebral artery. As stated above, vertebral artery injury is reported in 3.7% of cases, with neurologic deficit occurring in a very small percentage if a single vertebral artery is injured. If vertebral artery injury occurs during screw placement, inserting the screw is often a successful method of tamponading the hemorrhage. An attempt to place a screw in the contralateral side should be avoided, since the risk of brainstem stroke greatly increases if both vertebral arteries are injured. Preoperative planning with image guidance can provide useful information to help determine if transarticular screws can even be placed at C1-2; in approximately 20% of patients the anatomy makes it unsafe to place two 3.5mm screws because of the position of the vertebral artery.[14,17,27,56,67]

### Ventral Cervical Surgery

Ventral cervical discectomy has many potential neurologic complications, but these are a rarity.[26] Injury to the cervical sympathetic chain can occur during dissection of the longus colli muscles from the ventral cervical spine.[11] The cervical sympathetic chain ascends on the lateral border of the longus colli muscles and has three ganglionic enlargements. The superior cervical ganglion is at the level of C2-3, the middle ganglion is at the level of C6, and the stellate ganglion is at the level of C7-T1. Injury to the sympathetic chain can be prevented by limiting dissection of the longus colli muscles to their medial aspect only and by careful positioning of the self-retaining retractor blades on the medial side only of the dissected muscle. The stellate ganglion may occasionally be observed during low dissection in the neck. If observed, injury may be avoided by repositioning the retractor to move this structure out of the operating field. Injury to the cervical sympathetic nerves is manifested clinically by Horner syndrome (miosis, anhydrosis, and ptosis). Injury of the cervical sympathetic chain is seldom of clinical significance, and recovery is usually spontaneous. Injury to the superior laryngeal nerve can occur during ventral cervical discectomy. This usually occurs during dissection in the deep cervical fascia because the superior laryngeal nerve is in close proximity to the superior and inferior thyroidal vessels.[8]

Injury to the recurrent laryngeal nerve may occur during ventral cervical discectomy, resulting in vocal cord paralysis.[11] The nerve is more often injured during a right-sided operative approach because of the anatomic course of the nerve. In some instances, the right recurrent laryngeal nerve does not loop around the subclavian artery and takes a more direct course, thus having a more medial position between the trachea and esophagus. However, the left nerve has a higher incidence of idiopathic palsy.[8] Vocal cord paralysis from recurrent laryngeal nerve palsy is usually the result of a stretch injury from retraction and usually resolves spontaneously within 6 months after injury. In some patients with vocal cord paralysis, the opposite vocal cord hypertrophies, allowing normal phonation. In a patient who undergoes repeat ventral surgery of the cervical spine, either the approach should be through the previously operated side or the patient should have an otolaryngologic evaluation to confirm normal vocal cord function on both sides before surgery. If vocal cord paralysis is noted, the operative approach should be on the side of the paralyzed vocal cord. Voice hoarseness is often attributable to swelling and does not reflect recurrent laryngeal nerve injury. The incidence of postoperative hoarseness has been reported to be lessened by placing a closed suction drain.[12]

Direct injury to the spinal cord and nerve roots has been reported, with an incidence of approximately 2% after ventral cervical operations for myelopathy. These can be avoided only by meticulous operating technique and proper visualization.[4,6,8]

Late postoperative complications of radiculopathy and myelopathy have been reported after ventral cervical discectomy and fusion. Five percent of patients developed myelopathy or radiculopathy an average of 5.5 years after ventral cervical discectomy and fusion, with myelography revealing pathology one level above or below the site of previous fusion. No compression was found at the previously operated site, and only 2.5% of these patients required reoperation at a second level.[6] Others have obtained different statistics. Deterioration within the first year after ventral decompression from advancing osteophytic spurring at adjacent levels occurred in 5% of cases, and deterioration in the second and third years after ventral decompressive surgery occurred in another 5% of cases because of osteophytic processes, for a total deterioration rate of 10% within 3 years of surgery.[68] Nonunion of bone graft was also noted in 7% of patients as an early cause of deterioration and in 4% of patients in the second and third years, for a combined total of 11% for deterioration caused by nonunion.[64,68] Nonunion rates may be lowered by paying meticulous attention to bone grafting and possibly by adding ventral cervical instrumentation in multilevel decompressions. Spinal cord compression from malpositioning of the bone graft occurs less often. Bilateral brachial paresis has been reported after ventral cervical surgery for spondylosis. This occurred in a delayed fashion and was associated with deformity at the surgical site, with extrusion of the bone graft.[64] Worsening of neurologic function has been reported after ventral cervical fusion from spinal cord compression by the bone graft. Neurologic function improved after removal of the offending graft.[68] Proper morticing of the graft bed is key to preventing compression of the spinal cord during graft placement. Depth measurements must be obtained at the rostral, caudal, and lateral walls as well as the length and width of the graft bed, because these measurements are not uniform. A minimum buffer of 3mm must be preserved between the decompressed spinal cord and the bone graft, with the mortices cut to provide a dorsal shelf preventing the graft from compressing the cord.

Retrospective review of complications from cervical interbody fusion found 311 neurologic complications in 36,657 cases. Horner's syndrome was reported 13 times, recurrent laryngeal nerve palsy 52 times, transient radiculopathy 14 times, intraoperative etiology of radiculopathy 124 times, worsening myelopathy in 1 case, transient mild myelopathy in 6 cases, significant permanent myelopathy in 78 cases, significant permanent radiculopathy in 22 cases, and cerebral infarction in 1 case. The overall complication rate on the basis of myelopathy was 0.1%.[22]

Neurologic deterioration after surgery for cervical myelopathy was noted to occur in 29 of 110 patients. Risk factors for deterioration were direct trauma, spinal instability, and advancing spondylosis at adjacent levels. Direct surgical trauma occurred during surgery in 1.8% of patients. Postlaminectomy instability of the spine occurred within 1 year of the procedure in 3.6% of patients and after 1 year in 1.8% of patients. Advanced spondylotic changes above and below the previously ventral operative area occurred in 3.6% of patients within 1 year of surgery and after 1 year in 2.7% of patients. Nonunion led to deterioration within 1 year in 3.6% and after 1 year in 0.9% of patients operated via a ventral approach. These complications may be lessened by including noncompressive but significantly degenerated adjacent levels in the ventral construct at the time of initial operation, and fusing the spine dorsally in the event of preoperative kyphosis or in cases where iatrogenic instability is caused during the decompressive laminectomy.[68]

## Dorsal Cervical Spine Surgery

Central cord syndrome has been reported as a delayed complication occurring several days after dorsal cervical decompressive laminectomy for cervical stenosis. The central cord syndrome often occurred after a period of hypotension and was often associated with abnormal neck position. It is recommended that laminectomy be avoided in patients with abnormal cervical posture; that hypotension be avoided, especially when the patient is mobilized for the first time postoperatively; and that a cervical collar be used in the immediate postoperative period.[36] Jackson and Simmons[29] have reported a case of cervical laminectomy in a markedly kyphotic patient who had local anesthesia, with the patient serving as his own monitor. During the operation, the patient lost neurologic function. This rapidly reversed when the dura was opened. Other reported complications of dorsal cervical surgery include death from air embolism when the sitting position was used, neurologic deterioration from poor positioning of the cervical spine during operation, and tetraplegia from epidural hematoma.[35] Neurologic worsening has been noted in myelopathic patients if a laminectomy of inadequate length or width is performed. Laminectomy should extend to the lateral margin of the thecal sac, and if more than 50% of the medial facet is resected, fusion should be considered to lessen the risk of instability. Laminectomy should extend one level higher and one level lower than the highest and lowest compressive lesions.[58] Syringomyelia has become symptomatic after cervical decompressive laminectomies for cervical stenosis in patients with an unrecognized syrinx. It is postulated that decompression changes the transmural pressures across the syrinx wall, causing an increase in syrinx size and the appearance of symptoms. This is a rare complication, and it is lessened by obtaining preoperative magnetic resonance imaging scans to differentiate between syrinx and cervical stenosis.[44]

Cervical laminectomy may cause instability if more than one half of the medial facet is removed. Other risk factors for postlaminectomy kyphosis include young age and preoperative kyphosis.[68] This may result in progressive angulation with pain and cervical spondylotic myelopathy. This complication can be lessened by restricting decompression to less than one half of the medial facet, or when more lateral decompression is needed, by performing a fusion.[7] During dorsal cervical fusion, spinal cord injury has been reported in a case in which the dorsal bone graft loosened, compressing the spinal cord and causing Brown-Séquard syndrome.[7]

Dorsal cervical foraminotomy may worsen radiculopathy.[7] Care must be taken not to place any instruments into the narrowed foramen, because this will further compress the nerve root, and the nerve root should not be retracted until the foramen is opened, thus permitting easy retraction of the nerve root.

## Thoracic Spine Surgery

Ventral approaches to the thoracic and lumbar spine can cause ischemia to the spinal cord by interrupting the blood supply to the cord. Approaches to the ventral thoracic spine at levels T4-9 are especially dangerous. The risk of causing spinal cord ischemia can be lessened by performing preoperative angiography to localize the artery of Adamkiewicz and then planning surgery to avoid this artery. In addition, temporary segmental artery occlusion with somatosensory evoked potential (SSEP) monitoring has been advocated to help identify key intersegmental arteries supplying the cord. With this approach, the segmental arteries are identified and temporarily occluded during a ventral approach to the thoracic spine while SSEP monitoring is carried out. If the SSEP waveform deteriorates, the occlusion is released and that segmental vessel is spared.[3]

Thoracic disc herniations may be treated via a variety of approaches. Neurologic complications are highest with central thoracic disc herniations approached from a dorsal laminectomy approach. In this setting, the paraplegia rate approaches 18% and is caused by excessive spinal cord retraction. Complications may be lessened by a lateral extracavitary approach, a costotransversectomy approach, or a transthoracic approach.[55] Complications may be lessened further by performing preoperative spinal angiography to avoid damage to the radiculomedullary artery of the spinal cord. Most importantly, neurologic complication rates have declined significantly with the abandonment of the standard laminectomy approach for thoracic disc herniation. Causes of the high rates of neurologic complication from standard laminectomy are thought to be related to manipulation of the spinal cord, vascular injury, and kyphotic deformity associated with laminectomy. Rates of neurologic deterioration from the variety of approaches are 22% for laminectomy, 0% for transpedular and transfacet pedicle sparing approaches, 3% for costotransversectomy, and 1% for lateral extracavitary and transthoracic.

Retained thoracic disc fragments and misidentification of the pathologic level have been identified as other reasons for neurologic deterioration. Ultrasound imaging can be extremely useful in identifying the level of pathology and confirming its removal. Radiographic imaging including preoperative marking scans, radiolucent spine frames, and intraoperative fluoroscopy or image guidance can help the correct level of operation.[41]

Spinal deformity surgery can result in neurologic injury. Risk factors for spinal cord injury in deformity surgery are instrumentation (hooks, sublaminar wires, distraction), congenital kyphosis, and diagnosis other than idiopathic scoliosis, postradiation deformity, curves greater than 100 degrees, and direct trauma.

Rates of neurologic injury in deformity surgery have decreased over the years to a rate between 0.5% and 6.4%. Injury can occur by direct surgical injury during exposure, compression by instrumentation, overdistraction of the spinal cord, and ischemia of the spinal cord. Sublaminar wires have been reported to have a higher rate of neurologic complication with a rate as high as 17%. Hooks can also cause neurologic injury by direct compression of neural elements. The rate of neurologic injury is related to the degree of curve. The higher the degree of scoliosis, the higher the risk of neurologic complications. Curves of more than 100 degrees have a 10% complication rate, compared with curves of less than 100 degrees (which have a 0.64% rate of neurologic complication).[65]

Hypotension has been implicated as a cause of neurologic deficit both intraoperatively and postoperatively. Cases have been reported in which paralysis has occurred at the level of surgery without loss of alignment or new compression in patients who have suffered hypotensive episodes. Reports also exist of restoration of function with transfusion and treatment of hypotension. Distraction of the cord to correct deformity can lessen blood flow, possibly inducing ischemia of the cord.[65]

## Vessel Ligation in Ventral Thoracic and Lumbar Surgery

A large retrospective study found almost no risk of ligating segmental vessels provided the following rules were followed. Vessel ligation is done on one side only. Vessel ligation is done on the convex side of the scoliotic curve. Vessel ligation is performed at the midvertebral body area only, not in the foramen. Vessel ligation is performed only when hypotensive anesthesia techniques are not used.[66]

SSEP monitoring and the wake-up test have been used singly and in combination to lessen the incidence of these complications. The wake-up test has proven its usefulness over the years in preventing fixed neurologic deficit. The patient is awakened during the operative procedure and neurologic function is assessed. If deficit exists, hardware is removed, correction and distraction are lessened, and compressive lesions are sought out. The wake-up test has several disadvantages in that it is not continuous (online) and is very dependent on the anesthesiologist. SSEP monitoring is helpful but is not foolproof. The false-positive rate is 1.7%, the false-negative rate is 0.2%, and in a study of 60,000 cases, there were 342 complications, with 246 of these detected by monitoring and 96 cases not detected by SSEP moniotoring.[65]

## Lumbar Spine Surgery

Injuries to the dura mater and nerve roots may occur during lumbar disc surgery. Nerve root injury may occur from laceration, thermal injury, and excessive retraction. Lacerations to the nerve root most commonly occur because of lack of identification of the nerve root or because of failure to recognize a flattened root spread over a herniated disc. Adequate illumination and magnification are extremely helpful in locating lumbar nerve roots. The annulus should never be cut until the nerve root has been positively identified. Bone and ligament should be removed until the root can be easily retracted. Further dissection of bone is often required in the lateral direction to accomplish this goal. Bipolar electrocautery is useful for providing hemostasis, but cauterization should not be attempted until the nerve root is identified to avoid electrical or thermal injury to the nerve root.[9] Dural tears may occur during lumbar surgery with an incidence of approximately 4%. Care must be taken to avoid aspirating multiple nerve roots into the suction device and thereby causing neurologic deficit. The dural tear should be covered with a cottonoid, a smaller-diameter suction device should be inserted into the field, and exposure should be improved until the dural tear is fully exposed and then closed, if possible, in a watertight fashion.[9]

Lumbar discectomy in patients with cauda equina syndrome requires rapid evaluation and treatment. Some authors have found that persistent urinary incontinence is common in patients operated on after 48 hours of presentation of symptoms but is uncommon in those operated on within 48 hours.[34] Kostuik et al.[34] found two separate modes of presentation in patients with cauda equina syndrome: (1) an acute mode with rapid onset, more severe symptoms, and a poorer prognosis after decompression; (2) a mode with more gradual onset of symptoms. In both groups of patients, those with complete saddle anesthesia tend to have permanent bladder paralysis. Kostuik et al.[34] also found no correlation between timing of surgery and extent of recovery. Despite this lack of correlation, they recommend early surgery for patients with the cauda equina syndrome.

Acute postdiscectomy cauda equina syndrome occurs at a rate of approximately 0.2%.[4] The majority of these patients develop symptoms of saddle numbness, urinary retention, motor weakness, and multidermatomal numbness in the recovery room. Stenosis of the lumbar spinal canal at the operative level with anteroposterior dimension of 13mm or less was the most common factor found in postdiscectomy cauda equina syndrome, with swelling, hematoma, retained disc fragments, and Gelfoam contributing to the compression. A large epidural fat graft has also been a reported cause of the cauda equina syndrome after lumbar discectomy.[48] In this case, a large fat graft herniated into the spinal canal on the first postoperative day, causing cauda equina syndrome. These complications may be avoided by limiting the size of the fat graft to between 5 and 8mm and by suturing the graft to adjacent paraspinous muscle tissue, by measuring the lumbar canal preoperatively, and if stenosis is present by avoiding use of keyhole laminotomy to provide the approach to the disc space. Additionally, hemostasis should be obtained to avoid hematoma formation.[43] The operation for lumbar disc herniation causing cauda equina syndrome differs from the usual lumbar discectomy in that a much wider bony exposure is required. Complete hemilaminectomy is recommended to provide space to remove the disc herniation while lessening retraction that could cause permanent deficit. Microdiscectomy should be avoided in such patients because it provides less bony exposure.[53]

The cauda equina syndrome has also been reported after surgery for lumbar spinal stenosis. Compressive hematoma has been implicated as a cause of cauda equina syndrome after decompressive laminectomy. The cauda equina syndrome has been reported to occur after application of large epidural fat grafts in lumbar decompressive laminectomies.[40] This may occur by the fat graft acting to seal a hematoma against the thecal sac or by compression of the large fat graft by the paraspinal muscles. This complication may be prevented by limiting the size of the fat graft to a thickness of 0.5 to 1.0cm and to a height less than the height of the spinous processes.[40] Several cases of cauda equina syndrome have resulted after decompressive laminectomies in which a higher lesion such as a herniated disc was later identified. To minimize these complications, the following steps should be taken. Hemostasis should be obtained before closure, or a closed suction drain should be placed if hemostasis cannot be obtained. The entire lumbar spine and thoracolumbar junction should be visualized by magnetic resonance imaging (MRI) or myelography preoperatively so that pathology in the upper portions of the spinal canal is not overlooked. Lumbar decompression should have sufficient length to include all compressed elements. The cauda equina syndrome may also occur on a vascular basis as the artery of Adamkiewicz may enter at the upper lumbar segments and may be damaged during operation at the thoracolumbar junction. Preoperative spinal arteriography should be considered carefully to verify the presence or absence of vascular supply to the spinal cord in the area of the proposed operation if the operation is to be performed in the regions from T4 to L2. In postoperative cauda equina syndrome, mechanical causes must be ruled out, and if present, removed in an urgent fashion. Only after all mechanical causes have been included should a vascular etiology be diagnosed.[4]

Automated percutaneous discectomy carries risk. The most severe reported complication is one of cauda equina syndrome caused by improper placement of the nucleotome probe in the thecal sac. In animal tests, the device could pierce dura, amputate nerve roots, and make holes in intravascular structures. Complications with the nucleotome probe can be minimized by the following procedures. The nucleotome should never be placed outside the disc space; once properly positioned, the device cannot incise the annulus, and thus it cannot exit the disc space. The thecal sac is outlined by the line of the dorsal vertebral bodies ventrally, the line of the junction of the lamina and spinous processes dorsally, and the medial borders of the pedicles laterally; therefore, the probe should be placed under radiographic guidance with these landmarks to avoid the thecal sac. The device should be used only by an operator trained in its proper usage. The procedure should only be performed under local anesthesia as patient discomfort will alert the operator to any potential injury.[38,45,57]

Surgery for lumbosacral spondylolisthesis may also cause cauda equina syndrome, even with no attempt at reduction of deformity.[52] Paresis of proximal nerve roots after reduction of lumbosacral spondylolisthesis has also been reported and is caused by stretching of proximal nerve roots after reduction of the spine.[45] The L5 nerve root is the most often damaged during reduction of lumbosacral spondylolisthesis, followed in frequency by the S1 and S2 nerve roots.[5,63] To lessen these complications, SSEP monitoring and prereduction decompression of the nerve roots should be performed. When the patient awakens from surgery, a thorough neurologic examination should be performed, and if new deficit is found, the patient should be returned to the operating room for decompression of the involved root.[52]

### Trauma

Cervical fractures with malalignment may have associated disc herniation. Neurologic deterioration has been reported at a rate of 6 per 68 cases for patients with cervical dislocation undergoing reduction. The preferred management of reduction of cervical dislocation remains controversial. One school of thought advocates closed reduction with emergent ventral cervical discectomy if the patient worsens from disc herniation. Another group recommends MRI to rule out cervical disc herniation before closed reduction to eliminate the risk of neurologic deterioration from herniated disc fragments.[19]

Gunshot wounds to the spinal cord are the third most common cause of spinal cord injury. Complication of these injuries includes osteomyelitis, meningitis, spinal instability, cerebrospinal fluid leak, and delayed paraspinal infection. Neurologic recovery is less than 1% in injuries above the T10 level, but as many as 47% of patients with injury to the terminal spinal cord or cauda equina enjoy some degree of recovery with surgical management. Complications may be minimized in patients with transperitoneal gunshot wounds to the spine by vigorous irrigation of the spinal missile track during laparotomy and with timely closure of bowel perforations. Débridement and laminectomy are advocated as soon as the patient is stable. This provides dural closure, debridement of bone and missile fragments, and the cleansing of latent infection.[16,31]

### Neoplastic Disease

Five percent of cancer patients develop neurologic deficits because of spinal metastases.[54] The majority of metastases occur in the lower thoracic and upper lumbar spine, and 80% of metastases occur ventral to the thecal sac.[51] Treatment of these lesions with laminectomy alone often causes instability with resultant paraplegia, especially when there is vertebral body involvement.[46] Vertebral body collapse is a particularly ominous finding.[21] Treatment in these cases should involve either a ventral approach or a dorsal approach with transpedicular decompression of the ventral thecal sac, reconstruction of the vertebral body with a ventral strut, instrument, or methylmethacrylate and dorsal instrumentation.[21,23,46,51,54]

### Vertebroplasty

Vertebroplasty (and kyphoplasty) has proven to be useful in treating osteoporotic compression fractures and in some cases of neoplastic disease of the spine. Contraindications include destruction of the dorsal wall of the vertebra, compression of the spinal canal, complete loss of vertebral body height, spinal instability, and presence of an osteoblastic metastatic lesion. Percutaneous approaches include the transpedicular and paramedian (beneath the transverse process). Complications include radiculopathy that is usually transient and neural compression from extravasation of acrylic. Complications are lessened by fluoroscopic control of methylmethacrylate injection, by monitoring dorsal extravasation. Acrylic may leak out of the desired area in up to 60% of cases, but is rarely of clinical significance. Direct open surgical intervention may be required in cases of acrylic extravasation.[15,39,49,61,62]

## Neurologic Complications Caused by Spinal Instrumentation

Spinal instrumentation may cause neurologic injury, either at the time of implant placement because of neural trauma, ischemia, or hemorrhage or even years after placement from compression by fibrosis or implant loosening. Harrington rods can cause nerve and thecal sac compression in a delayed fashion. Hooks placed on the L5 lamina and attached to Harrington rods have been reported over time to cut through the lamina, causing thecal sac compression. In such reported cases, the problems resolved after removal of the hardware.[28,32]

Overdistraction of the spine with spinal fixation systems can cause spinal cord injury from ischemia because distraction stretches the segmental and intrinsic vessels feeding the spinal cord, thus decreasing the cross-sectional area. Intraoperative SSEP monitoring has been useful but not infallible in detecting overdistraction.[24] If SSEP waveforms degrade during distraction, the implant should be loosened or removed. If a postoperative neurologic deficit is noted, even if SSEP waveforms are preserved, consideration should be given to removing the distraction system.[18,23] Care must be taken at sites at which the spine is predisposed to injury during distraction. Distraction over a fixed mass, during systolic hypotension, in multicolumn spinal injury, and in a kyphotic spine, increases the chance for spinal cord injury.[2,24,30]

Malpositioning of pedicle screws can cause radiculopathy, with a reported incidence as high as 7%.[10,33,42] Damage to the nerve root may be caused by the screw itself or by bone fragments from fracture of the pedicle wall. The nerve root travels along the medial border of the pedicle and exits around the caudal border of the pedicle. During placement of pedicle screws the nerve root is at risk if the medial or inferior border is violated. After the pedicle is localized and the center of the pedicle is dissected into the vertebral body, the channel should be probed to detect any breaches into the medial or lateral wall of the pedicle. If no wall defects are found, the channel may be tapped and probed after tapping to determine whether any breaches occurred during the tapping of the channel. If a defect in the wall is detected, a decision must be made as to whether the channel can be redirected in the same pedicle to avoid the breach or whether an alternative site of fixation must be used. Screw depth should be chosen to penetrate 50% to 75% of the vertebral body, and no attempt should be made to gain bicortical purchase, because neurologic injury to the sympathetic chain in the sacrum and to the presacral plexus at L5 may result. Intraoperative and preoperative imaging with plain radiographic or fluoroscopy is extremely useful for placing pedicle screws. Online EMG monitoring is very effective in evaluating cortical disruption when placing pedicle screws.[37] Imaging guidance via computer assistance is another useful method for increasing safety of insertion of spinal instrumentation.[13]

If radiculopathy is noted postoperatively in a patient who has undergone pedicle screw placement at the level of the radiculopathy, radiologic studies should be immediately performed to evaluate screw position. If malpositioning is found, the offending screw should be removed.

### Lumbar Fusion Cages

Lumbar fusion cages as used in the posterior lumbar interbody fusion (PLIF) operation can be associated with complications. The complications can be related to insertion or from loss of fixation. Significant retraction is required during cage placement to permit insertion of a properly sized cage. Too small a diameter can cause loss of fixation and retropulsion of the cage into the spinal canal, causing either radiculopathy of lumbar stenosis symptoms. Too large a diameter requires more retraction and is associated with an increased risk of nerve root injury and incidental durotomy. A durotomy rate as high as 15% has been reported.[18] Complications can be lessened by obtaining distraction of the disc space, either with interbody spacers on one side before placing a cage on the contralateral side or by the use of a distractor such as the inge sublaminar retractor to increase distraction prior to cage placement.[50,60]

### Cervical Plates

Ventral cervical fixation devices rarely cause hardware complications that result in neurologic injury. The most common theoretical complication causing neurologic injury is excessive screw length in a ventral cervical plate that compresses or impales the spinal cord. This complication may be avoided by using intraoperative fluoroscopy or plain radiographs while placing the screws. The proper length of screw may be estimated by measuring the adjacent disc space. The screw should be measured by the surgeon personally before implantation. Dorsal cervical fixation devices can lead to hardware complications that cause neurologic injury. Dorsal spinous wiring for traumatic injuries to the cervical spine has been associated with worsening of neurologic function by causing retropulsion of herniated disc fragments into the spinal canal.[1,19] Nerve root injuries during placement of lateral mass plates are possible and can be avoided by using the technique of placing the screw, beginning 1mm medial to the center of the facet and at an angle of 20 degrees superiorly and 20 degrees laterally to avoid the nerve root and vertebral artery.[20] The holes should be palpated with a probe and measured for depth. Palpation of a bottom of the hole lessens the risk of damage to neural structures. Fluoroscopy

and image guidance may improve accuracy of placement of instrumentation in the cervical spine.

### Sublaminar Wires

Sublaminar wiring techniques for segmental fixation have a 1% to 17% incidence of neurologic injury.[10] Nerve root injuries occur more frequently than do spinal cord injuries with this technique. Acute injuries caused by excessive depth of passage, attempt at passage in an acquired or congenitally narrow spinal canal, and by epidural hemorrhage are the most common causes of defects after segmental fixation. Placement of sublaminar wires through the sacral foramina has been noted to cause sacral radiculopathy. Passage of wires medially instead of laterally, thinning of the lamina to lessen length of passage, immediately crimping the wires around the lamina after passage to prevent dislodgment into the canal, and using smaller gauge double-twisted wires or cables all decrease the incidence of neurologic injury with sublaminar wiring techniques.[64] Removal of sublaminar wires may also cause neurologic injury. The wire should be cut as close to the lamina as possible to minimize the radius of arc the wire will travel during removal. Single wires and double-independent wires should be removed individually in a direction parallel to the thecal sac. Double-twisted wires should be removed with the aid of a wire extractor guide.[10]

### Complications Caused by Reduction of Spinal Malalignment

Neurologic complications caused by reducing malalignment of the spine in cases of scoliosis and spondylolisthesis are numerous. Cases of L5 radiculopathy have occurred during reduction of L5-S1 spondylolisthesis.[5] This complication may be avoided by decompression before reduction or by fusion *in situ*. There are, however, even reports of neurologic injury with *in situ* fusion for spondylolisthesis.[52]

## Neurologic Complications Caused by Surgical Technique

Neurologic complications may be caused by poor surgical technique. Unipolar electrocautery, if used improperly, can cause neurologic damage and should never be used in the vicinity of neural tissue without extreme caution being exercised. Spinal cord damage has been reported from use of unipolar cautery on the posterior longitudinal ligament.[25] Dissection of dorsal structures with electrocautery may result in dissection through the ligamentum flavum and dura mater with spinal cord or nerve root injury. Care must be used to ensure that dissection is undertaken over bone and not over the disc interspace.

Air drills have also been implicated in neurologic injury in spinal surgery.[25] Drills should never be used around unprotected neural structures. Appropriate bit selection is important. A diamond-tipped drill is less likely to wrap up adjacent tissue than is a fluted bit. The drill should begin near the region of its intended use, and a spinning drill bit should never be moved into or out of the operating field.

Neurologic damage has also been reported by incorrect identification of anatomic structures. Section of the hypoglossal nerve has been reported in ventral cervical surgery in which the nerve was mistakenly identified as the superior laryngeal artery.[25]

# REFERENCES

1. Abei M, Zuber K, Marchesi D: Treatment of cervical spine injuries with ventral plating. *Spine* 16(Suppl 3):S38-S45, 1991.

2. Allen BL, Ferguson RL: Neurologic injuries with the Galveston technique of L-rod instrumentation for scoliosis. *Spine* 11:14-17, 1986.

3. Apel DM, Marrero G, King J, *et al*: Avoiding paraplegia during ventral spinal surgery. *Spine* 16(suppl):S365-S370, 1991.

4. Boccanera L, Laus M: Cauda equina syndrome following lumbar spinal stenosis surgery. *Spine* 12:712-715, 1987.

5. Bradford DS, Boachie-Adjei O: Treatment of severe spondylolisthesis by ventral and posterior reduction and stabilization. *J Bone Joint Surg* 72:1060-1066, 1990.

6. Brandt L, Karlossin M, Holmsted L, *et al*: Myelography in the late postoperative period in patients subjected to ventral cervical decompression and fusion. *Acta Neurochir* 122:97-101, 1993.

7. Callahan RA, Johnson RM, Margolis JA, *et al*: Cervical face fusion for control of instability following laminectomy. *J Bone Joint Surg* 59A:991-1002, 1977.

8. Carrau RL, Rivera Cintron F, Astor F: Transcervical approaches to the prevertebral spine. *Arch Otolaryngol* 116:1070-1073, 1990.

9. Carrol SE, Wiesel SW: Neurologic complications and lumbar laminectomy. *Clin Orthop* 284:14-23, 1992.

10. Choi WW, Green BA, Levi AD: Computer-assisted fluoroscopic targeting system for pedicle screw insertion. *Neurosurgery* 47(4):872-878, 2000.

11. Chozick BS, Toselli R: Complications of spinal instrumentation. In: *Spinal Instrumentation*. AANS, 1994.

12. Cloward RB: Complications of ventral cervical disc operation and their treatment. *Surgery* 69:175-182, 1971.

13. Cloward RB: History of the ventral cervical fusion technique. *J Neurosurg* 63:817-818, 1985.

14. Coric D, Branch CL, Wilson JA, Robinson JC: Arteriovenous fistula as a complication of C1-2 transarticular screw fixation. *J Neurosurg* 85:340-343, 1996.

15. Cotton A, Dewatre F, Cortet B, *et al*: Percutaneous vertebroplasty of osteolytic metastasis and myeloma. *Radiology* 200:525-530, 1996.

16. Cybulski GR, Stone JL, Kant R: Outcome of laminectomy for civilian gunshot injuries of the terminal spinal cord and cauda equina: review of 88 cases. *Neurosurgery* 24:392-397, 1989.

17. Dickman CA, Sonntag VK: Posterior C1-C2 transarticular screw fixation for atlantoaxial arthordiesis. *Neurosurgery* 43:275-280, 1998.

18. Elias WJ, Simmons NE, Kapitan GJ, *et al*: Complications of posterior lumbar interbody fusion when using a titanium threaded cage device. *J Neurosurg (Spine)* 93:45-52, 2000.

19. Eisemont FJ, Arena MJ, Green BA: Extrusion of an intervertebral disc associated with traumatic subluxation or dislocation of cervical facets. *J Bone Joint Surg* 73A: 1557-1560, 1991.

20. Fehlings MG, Cooper PR, Errico TJ: Posterior plates in the management of cervical instability: long term results in 44 patients. *J Neurosurg* 81:341-349, 1994.

21. Findlay GF: The role of vertebral body collapse in the management of malignant spinal cord compression. *J Neurol Neurosurg Psychiatry* 50:151-154, 1987.

22. Flynn TB: Neurologic complications of anterior cervical interbody fusion. *Spine* 796:536-539, 1982.

23. Galasko CS: Spinal instability secondary to metastatic cancer. *J Bone Joint Surg* 73B:104-108, 1991.

24. Ginsburg HH, Shetter Ag, Raudzens PA: Postoperative paraplegia with preserved intraoperative somatosensory evoked potentials. *J Neurosurg* 63:296-300, 1985.

25. Graham JJ: Complications of cervical spine surgery. *Spine* 14:1046-1050, 1989.

26. Grisoli F, Grasiani N, Fabrizi AP, *et al*: Anterior discectomy without fusion for treatment of cervical lateral soft disc extrusion: a follow-up of 120 cases. *Neurosurgery* 24: 853-859, 1989.

27. Haid RW, Subach BR, McLaughlin MR, *et al*: C1-C2 transarticular screw fixation for atlantoaxial instability: a 6-year experience. *Neurosurgery* 49(1):65-68, 2001.

28. Hales DD, Dawson EG, Delamarter R, *et al*: Late neurological complications of Harrington rod instrumentation. *J Bone Joint Surg* 71A:1053-1057, 1989.

29. Jackson RP, Simmons EH: Dural compression as a cause of paraplegia during operative correction of cervical kyphosis in ankylosing spondylitis. *Spine* 16:846-848, 1991.

30. Johnston CE, Happel LT, Norris R, *et al*: Delayed paraplegia complication sublaminar segmental spinal instrumentation. *J Bone Joint Surg* 68A:556-563, 1986.

31. Kihtir T, Ivatury RR, Simon R, *et al*: Management of transperitoneal gunshot wounds to the spine. *J Trauma* 31:1579-1583, 1991.

32. Kornberg M, Herndon WA, Rechtine GR: Lumbar nerve root compression at the site of hook insertion. *Spine* 10:853-855, 1985.

33. Kosay C, Akcali O, Berk RH, *et al*: A new method for detecting pedicular wall perforation during pedicle screw insertion. *Spine* 26:1477-1481, 2001.

34. Kostuik JP, Harrington I, Alexander D, *et al*: Cauda equina syndrome and lumbar disc herniation. *J Bone Joint Surg* 68B:386-391, 1986.

35. Lesion F, Bouasakao N, Clarisse J, *et al*: Results of surgical treatment of radiculomyelopathy caused by cervical arthrosis based on 1000 operations. *Surg Neurol* 23: 350-355, 1985.

36. Levy WJ, Dohn DF, Hardy RW: Central cord syndrome as a delayed postoperative complication of decompressive laminectomy. *Neurosurgery* 11:491-495, 1982.

37. Maguire J, Wallace S, Madiga R, *et al*: Evaluation of intrapedicular screw position using intraoperative evoked electromyography. *Spine* 20(9):1068-1074, 1995.

38. Maroon JC, Onik G, Sternau L: Percutaneous automated discectomy. *Clin Orthop* 238:64-70, 1989.

39. Martin JB, Jean B, Sigui K, *et al*: Vertebroplasty: Clinical experience and follow-up results. *Bone* 25(Suppl 2): 11S-15S, 1999.

40. Mayer PJ, Jacobson FS: Cauda equina syndrome after surgical treatment of lumbar spinal stenosis with application of free autologous fat graft. *J Bone Joint Surg* 71A: 1090-1093, 1989.

41. McCormick WE, Will SF, Benzel EC: Surgery for thoracic disc disease: Complication avoidance, overview and management. *Neurosurg Focus* 9(4): Article 13, 2000.

42. McGuire RA, Amundson GM: The use of primary internal fixation in spondylolisthesis. *Spine* 18:1662-1672, 1993.

43. Mclaren AC, Bailey SI: Cauda equina syndrome: a complication of lumbar discectomy. *Clin Orthop* 204: 143-149, 1986.

44. Middleton TH, Al-Mefty O, Harkey LH, *et al*: Syringomyelia after decompressive laminectomy for cervical spondylosis. *Surg Neurol* 28:458-462, 1987.

45. Onik G, Maroon JC, Jackson R: Cauda equina syndrome secondary to an improperly placed nucleotome probe. *Neurosurgery* 30:412-415, 1992.

46. Onimus M, Schraub S, Bertin D, *et al*: Surgical treatment of vertebral metastasis. *Spine* 11:883-891, 1986.

47. Pritz MB: Evaluation and treatment of intradural tumors located ventral to the cervicomedullary junction by a lateral suboccipital approach. *Acta Neurochirurgie* 113:74-81, 1991.

48. Prusick VR, Lint DS, Bruder WJ: Cauda equina syndrome as a complication of free epidural fat grafting. *J Bone Joint Surg* 70A:1256-1258, 1988.

49. Ratliff J, Nguygen T, Heiss J: Root and spinal cord compression from methylmethacrylate vertebroplasty. *Spine* 26:E300-E302, 2001.

50. Ray CD: Threaded titanium cages for lumbar interbody fusion. *Spine* 22:667-679, 1997.

51. Rompe JD, Eysel P, Hopf C, *et al*: Decompression/ stabilization of the metastatic spine. *Acta Orthop Scand* 64:3-8, 1993.

52. Schoenecker PL, Cole HO, Herring JA, *et al*: Cauda equina syndrome after in situ arthrodesis for severe spondylolisthesis at the lumbosacral junction. *J Bone Joint Surg* 72A:370-377, 1990.

53. Shapiro S: Cauda equina syndrome secondary to lumbar disc herniation. *Neurosurgery* 32:743-747, 1993.

54. Siegal T, Tiqva P, Siegal T: Vertebral body resection for epidural compression by malignant tumors. *J Bone Joint Surg* 67A:375-381, 1985.

55. Skubic JW, Kostuik JP: Thoracic pain syndromes and thoracic disc herniation. In: *The Adult Spine*. Philadelphia, Lippincott-Raven, 1991.

56. Smith MD, Phillips WA, Hensinger RN: Complications of fusion to the upper cervical spine. *Spine* 116(7):702-705, 1991.

57. Stern MB: Early experience with percutaneous lateral discectomy. *Clin Orthop* 238:50-55, 1989.

58. Stoops WI, King RB: Neural complications of cervical spondylosis and their response to laminectomy and foramenotomy. *J Neurosurg* 19:986-999, 1962.

59. Transfeldt EE, Dendrinos GK, Bradford DS: Paresis of proximal lumbar roots after reduction of L5-S1 spondylolisthesis. *Spine* 14:884-887, 1989.

60. Uzi EA, Dadbby D, Tolessa E, Finkelstein JA: Early retropulsion of titanium threaded cages after posterior lumbar interbody fusion. *Spine* 26(9):1073-1075, 2001.

61. Watts NB, Harris ST, Genant HK: Treatment of painful osteoporotic vertebral fractures with percutaneous vertebroplasty or kyphoplasty. *Osteoporosis* 12:429-437, 2001.

62. Weill A, Chiras J, Simon JM, *et al*: Spinal metastasis: Indications for and results of percutaneous injection of acrylic surgical cement. *Radiology* 199:241-247, 1996.

63. West CG: Bilateral brachial paresis following ventral decompression for cervical spondylosis. *Spine* 11:176-178, 1985.

64. Wiberg J: Effects of surgery on cervical spondylotic myelopathy. *Acta Neurochir* 81:113-117, 1986.

65. Winter RB: Spine update: Neurologic safety in spinal deformity surgery. *Spine* 22:1527-1533, 1997.

66. Winter RB, Lonstein JE, Denis F, *et al*: Paraplegia resulting from vessel ligation. *Spine* 21:1232-1234, 1996.

67. Wright NM, Lauryssen C: Vertebral artery injury in C1-C2 transarticular screw fixation: reports of a survey of the AANS/CNS Joint section on Disorders of the Spine and Peripheral Nerves. *J Neurosurg* 88:634-640, 1998.

68. Yonenobu K, Okada K, Fuji T, *et al*: Causes of neurologic deterioration following surgical treatment of cervical myelopathy. *Spine* 11:818-823, 1986.

# CHAPTER 151

# Vascular and Soft Tissue Complications

## Donald A. Smith and David W. Cahill

The spine is functionally divisible into occipitoatlantoaxial, subaxial, thoracic, thoracolumbar, lumbar, and lumbosacral segments. Characteristic anatomic features within each of these spinal regions specify in part the pathologic anatomy that is encountered therein (e.g., the prevalence of degenerative disc disease in the subaxial and lumbar spine, the clustering of burst fractures at the thoracolumbar junction). The epicenter of many of these processes is in the ventral spine. For ventral approaches to the spine, it is the extraspinal anatomy, in particular that of the overlying vascular structures, that largely delimits the surgical options described elsewhere in this text. Strictly posterior approaches are less encumbered by these constraints, although the resective and reconstructive options are correspondingly restricted.

As ventral exposures to the spine have become ever more routine, spine surgeons are often assuming primary responsibility for these approaches. In general, vascular and soft tissue complications are uncommon, but when they occur they may demand reparative techniques that are not a routine part of spinal surgery training. This chapter focuses on complications related to the vascular and soft tissue anatomy ventral to the spine. Part of good preoperative planning is to foresee potential problems and to coordinate with colleagues from otolaryngology, general and vascular surgery, and urology when need of their expertise can be anticipated. Many of the complications to be described are so rare that only anecdotal experience is acquired in their management.

## Complications at the Craniovertebral Junction

The simplest and most direct ventral access to the craniovertebral junction is the transoral/transpharyngeal approach. Many different variations of this operation have been described, including combined resection of the hard palate, median labiomandibular glossotomy, maxillectomy, and LeFort osteotomies to expand the exposure from the midclivus to the C3 level. The main limitation of these procedures is the inevitable contamination of the wound by mouth flora. By reserving these approaches for extradural pathologic conditions and by using perioperative antibiotics, many of the septic complications initially encountered with this operation have been overcome.

Airway management in transoral procedures demands special attention. Significant tongue swelling is often encountered, and this can easily lead to obstruction of the oropharynx. In cases of major resections or those in which the patient has any preoperative difficulty with swallowing or aspiration, a tracheotomy is routinely performed. In more limited operations at the C1-2 level and without concurrent lower cranial neuropathy, the patient may be left intubated for 48 to 72 hours postoperatively or until glossal swelling has abated. Periodic relaxation of the intraoral retractors during surgery may mitigate the problem. Steroids are often invoked as well, but they are no substitute for controlled extubation in an intensive care unit setting by someone skilled in airway management. Close observation with a bedside tracheostomy set up is mandatory.

Although intradural procedures and bone grafting can be successfully performed through this route, these maneuvers carry a heightened risk and can be the source of significant morbidity. A layered, tensionless reapproximation of the dorsal pharyngeal musculature and mucosa with resorbable sutures is important, especially if the dura mater has been violated. In this case, reinforcement of the dural repair with a fascial graft and fibrin glue and placement of a spinal drain postoperatively are advised. If bone grafts or reconstructive cages have been inserted, they should have a low profile, without protrusion into the pharynx and resultant compromise of the soft tissue closure. Because the retropharyngeal soft tissues are well vascularized, surgeons tend to use electrocautery to divide and reflect these structures off the bone. This can result in significant retraction of the wound margins, which becomes most apparent at the time of closure. Infiltration of the retropharyngeal tissues with a dilute epinephrine solution before sharp incision and blunt reflection with the use of bipolar cautery for direct hemostasis minimizes this problem. If a primary closure cannot be obtained (or if one should subsequently break down), satisfactory repair can usually be achieved with either a pharyngeal or a septal flap reconstruction. When the soft palate has been divided, a similar degree of attention should be devoted to the tensionless anatomic reapproximation of its edges, so that a cleft or fistula does not result.

## Complications in the Subaxial Spine

The ventrolateral approach to the subaxial spine as popularized by Robinson and Smith[29] is among the most commonly performed spinal surgeries. The esophagus, larynx, and trachea are mobilized medially as a unit, and the carotid sheath is retracted laterally. The incidence of clinically significant injuries to these structures is low during primary surgeries. When an injury does occur, sharp-toothed retractors are often implicated. Handheld blunt retractors are used exclusively until the musculus longus colli have been reflected off the vertebral bodies ventrolaterally to create two soft tissue leaves into which a self-retaining retractor system can be anchored. Great care is taken with the initial placement of retractors, because this permits safe, stable, and sustained exposure that sets the stage for the remainder of the case. Toothed blades are inserted accurately under the musculus longus colli under direct vision. Proper engagement of the muscles usually requires the use of asymmetric blade lengths, with the medial blade being a bit longer.

The cervical sympathetic chain overlies the musculus longus colli more laterally. Occasionally, a Horner's syndrome ensues after reflection of these muscles or because of heat transmission from electrocautery. This is usually transient and is not functionally disabling. Other structures at potential risk are the recurrent laryngeal nerve and the vertebral arteries. Injuries to the thoracic duct are occasionally incurred in left-sided approaches at the C6-7 and C7-T1; these are reviewed separately below.

## Recurrent Laryngeal Nerve Injury

Vocal cord paresis is a complication in anterior cervical surgery that is probably underappreciated. In patients who have undergone anterior cervical dissecting and fusion, who are routinely evaluated with direct laryngoscopy postoperatively, the incidence approaches 10%.[13] Most of these are blunt injuries, believed to result from retractor pressure against the recurrent laryngeal nerve within the tracheoesophageal groove. The left recurrent laryngeal nerve has a longer course, swinging around the aortic arch before ascending in the relatively protected cleft between the trachea and esophagus, whereas the right recurrent laryngeal nerve loops around the subclavian artery and thus has a correspondingly shorter course. The extra length of nerve available on the left allegedly renders it less vulnerable to stretch injury than its counterpart on the right, but the evidence for this is scant. As a rule, functional recovery occurs over a period of weeks to months.

## Esophageal Injury

Transient swallowing disorders are commonly recorded after even uncomplicated primary anterior cervical surgeries. Symptoms usually resolve within a few weeks but may persist in up to 10% of patients, although only rarely at a level that is functionally disabling.[35] Refractory cases are investigated with manometry and swallowing studies.[7] Selected individuals can benefit from cricopharyngeal myotomy or dilation.

Esophageal perforation is a problem that is much more serious. It is in the context of reoperative surgery or surgery performed for infection, tumor, or after irradiation that most of these injuries occur. Tissues are fibrotic and sometimes friable, and tissue planes are often scarred, distorted, and unyielding. Blunt mobilization of the esophagus off the prevertebral fascia may not be successful, and sharp dissection can be equally hazardous. Passage of a nasogastric tube that can be palpated within the esophageal lumen serves as a further point of orientation and as an aid to dissection. A combination of blunt and sharp techniques may be useful for dissecting the junction between the ventral aspect of the vertebral bodies and the overlying soft tissue structures as precisely as possible. If normal planes of dissection are inapparent, exposure is extended rostrally and caudally in search of recognizable anatomy in more virginal tissues. This may enable definition of the lateral margin of the vertebral corpus concealed beneath swollen musculus longus colli. The prevertebral fascia can then be incised in a paramedian plane down to bone and the fascia and overlying laryngotracheal esophageal bundle mobilized as an undissected unit. Depending on the quality of the tissue planes that are developed in this fashion, the use of any form of toothed retractor may be eschewed. In reoperative cases, some of these difficulties may be averted altogether simply by approaching from the side opposite the initial procedure. *In this case, direct laryngoscopy should be performed preoperatively or at intubation to confirm preserved vocal cord function on the initially operated side, thereby precluding the catastrophic outcome of bilateral vocal cord paralysis at the second procedure.*

Esophageal perforation is also encountered as a delayed complication associated with ventral graft extrusion and hardware failure. This occurs most commonly because of infection, poor carpentry, a technical error in the method of instrumentation, or application of instrumentation in softened osteoporotic bone. When screws are observed to back out in follow-up radiographs, their elective removal should be considered. There are now abundant reports of esophageal injury secondary to screw migration.* Screw heads should be flush with the plate to minimize their profile and allow their locking mechanism to function properly to prevent backout. If the system is designed for bicortical fixation, it is mandatory that bicortical fixation be achieved. Plate length must be selected carefully so that there is no overhang over adjacent disc spaces, and unfused segments should not be instrumented, because these circumstances promote hardware loosening. If the quality of the bone stock is poor, bicortical screw fixation should be used. If this is not feasible, internal fixation is either best abandoned in favor of a halo orthosis or supplemented by such a device. Alternatively, dorsal fixation should be added.

## Esophageal Repair

Esophageal perforation may be apparent intraoperatively, but more often it presents postoperatively with deep wound infection, severe dysphagia, and mediastinitis.[11,21] Perforation related to hardware failure may not occur until years after the operative procedure.[9] Intraoperative tears may be either partial or full thickness. A partial-thickness injury to the esophagus is readily repaired with resorbable sutures and should not cause modification of the primary procedure. To ensure that a transmural injury has not occurred, the surgeon may instill indigo carmine dye into the hypopharynx and monitor for dye egress within the wound.

Transmural injuries are repaired primarily, again with the surgeon observing the principles of a layered, tensionless closure using resorbable sutures. The wound is irrigated copiously with antibiotic-containing solution, and systemic antibiotic coverage is broadened to include anaerobic organisms. Assuming an absence of gross contamination and a satisfactory repair, the surgeon can proceed with the intended decompression and fusion in most instances. In these circumstances, any form of spinal instrumentation should be used with caution. The patient is fed through a silastic feeding tube during the first postoperative week. Intravenous antibiotics are continued for 2 to 6 weeks postoperatively. A further course of oral antibiotics thereafter is discretionary.

---

*References 5,9,11,12,21,33.

More complicated injuries with longer segments of tissue loss that no longer allow for tensionless reapproximation require longitudinal mobilization of the mid-esophagus and a reinforced repair backed by a pedicled sternocleidomastoid muscle flap. Extensive injuries that do not lend themselves to repair in this fashion should be diverted proximally and distally to the skin surface and then reconstructed later. Primary reanastomosis may still be achievable after mobilization of the esophagus at the diaphragmatic hiatus to gain additional length. Although lacking in intrinsic coordinated propulsive activity, colonic and jejunal interpositions are yet other reconstruction options.

Delayed perforation may present with similar although less fulminant symptoms or with spinal osteomyelitis. In most cases, the original site of injury will have sealed over, although this should be evaluated with a swallowing study using a water-soluble contrast agent. Subsequent procedures depend on several factors. Any sign of contrast extravasation mandates operative repair; any deep abscess requires drainage. Grossly infected or collapsed bone grafts or vertebrae should be thoroughly débrided and regrafted after a vigorous washout. Long-term (6 weeks), organism-specific intravenous antibiotics should be administered. In less fulminant infections with good anatomic and neurologic preservation, a more conservative approach with drainage of superficial pus and administration of systemic antibiotics may be elected initially. Close clinical and radiographic follow-up is extremely important. If the patient is without signs of deep infection, nonoperative management may be a viable option, even in the presence of spinal instrumentation. The erythrocyte sedimentation rate and C-reactive protein level are useful laboratory parameters to monitor. Clinical or radiographic progression would then mandate operative management.

### Laryngotracheal Injuries

Sore throat and hoarseness are common and mostly transient complaints after anterior cervical surgery. Some have sought to relate this phenomenon to increased pressure exerted on the laryngotracheal lumen by the endotracheal tube cuff following insertion of deep retractors. Venting enough air from the cuff to create a small air leak around the endotracheal tube may alleviate at least some of this problem.[27]

Fortunately, serious injury to the trachea is rare. Minor lacerations observed intraoperatively are repaired primarily, leaving the patient intubated for 48 to 72 hours to allow the wound to seal. More severe injuries and those detected in a delayed fashion because of pneumomediastinum or neck emphysema may be more appropriately managed with primary repair and tracheostomy.

Occasionally, the parietal pleura is violated during low anterior or upper thoracic discectomy. This requires no specific treatment, as long as the visceral pleura has not been violated to cause a persistent air leak. This possibility can be assessed by flooding the wound with saline and observing for a bubble stream during positive-pressure ventilation. This bubble stream implies an ongoing air leak and indicates tube thoracostomy.

### Carotid and Vertebral Artery Injury

Carotid artery injury is unusual in the midcervical spine if care is taken during placement of toothed retractor blades. At this level, the artery is sufficiently removed from its tether points at the skull base and the aortic arch that the required degree of lateral mobilization is easily achieved. If the carotid sheath is scarred by previous radiation or operation, it should be freed longitudinally until the vessel can be displaced laterally without undue force or distortion.

Direct suture repair of carotid injuries is straightforward in virginal cases, because good proximal and distal control is readily achieved and the arterial wall willingly accepts suture. Unfortunately, this complication is most likely to occur in the reoperative and irradiated wound. Exposure is more difficult, the vessels can be very friable, and the repair is challenging.

The vertebral artery is not encountered in routine anterior cervical approaches. It may be imperiled by very lateral exploration of the neural foramen in pursuit of uncovertebral joint osteophytes. This type of injury is usually minor and is controlled with small amounts of hemostatic packing. A postoperative angiogram is obtained to rule out significant stenosis, pseudoaneurysm, or arteriovenous (AV) fistula.

More significant injury to the vertebral artery can result during cervical corpectomy if the decompression is taken too far laterally.[25] These injuries are usually incurred by overly aggressive drilling. They can be avoided if all dissection is performed under magnification and if the drill is not permitted to penetrate the deep bony cortex. The vertebra is "eggshelled out" with the drill, leaving only a thin bony cortex to be avulsed with a fine curette or thin-footed Kerrison rongeur. The ventral aspect of the transverse processes of C3-6 is also marked by a small bony tubercle that alerts the operator to the laterality of the exposure. More often, however, the point of injury occurs on the medial side of the artery, where the drill has broken through the vertebral cortex.

Bleeding can be ruinous and may not be controllable with simple packing measures. In this circumstance, the surgeon must enlarge the exposure, including deliberate resection of the ventral lip of the transverse process to uncover more of the artery proximally and distally as localized pressure is applied over a cottonoid at the point of hemorrhage. The surgeon must then weigh the options of vertebral ligation versus repair. Most patients, especially youths, tolerate unilateral vertebral ligation well.[25] However, a small number of patients will have an isolated vertebral artery terminating in the posterior inferior cerebellar artery or a compromised contralateral vertebral artery. Ligation of a vertebral artery in these circumstances could result in cerebellar or brainstem infarction. Because the status of the vertebral artery anatomy may not be known preoperatively, significant effort should be made to preserve vascular patency whenever possible.

## Complications at the Cervicothoracic Junction and in the Thoracic Spine

Ventral exposure of the cervicothoracic junction remains problematic. The standard ventrolateral cervical exposure can be extended through division of the sternocleidomastoid and anterior scalene muscles, but working angles within the narrowing confines of the thoracic inlet, along with convergence of the common carotid arteries toward the innominate artery and aortic arch, often make this an awkward endeavor. The potential for esophageal injury is probably heightened somewhat by the difficulty in applying conventional self-retaining retractor systems stably at this depth and orientation. An increased risk for pneumothorax and recurrent laryngeal nerve injury also exists at the thoracic inlet. A deliberate effort to identify the recurrent laryngeal nerve at the base of the neck before its ascent into the tracheoesophageal groove may help avert a stretch injury through injudicious placement of the retractor blades.

Between T1 and T4, transsternal approaches yield favorable working angles to the ventral spine through enlargement of the thoracic inlet. Ventral access caudal to T4 remains limited by the aortic arch and the innominate artery, which cannot be readily mobilized. Excessive spreading of the sternal retractor can cause a brachial plexus injury. Transaxillary thoracotomy centered on the third rib provides an alternative access route to this region. This yields a lateral view up to the T1-2 level, working behind and to the side of the subclavian and innominate arteries. A left-sided thoracotomy is attended with a lower frequency of recurrent laryngeal nerve palsy, but the aortic knob is rather prominent in the field at this level. Because of this prominence as well as to lessen the risk of thoracic duct injury, transaxillary thoracotomy is usually performed from the right side.

## Thoracic Duct Injuries

Although the thoracic duct is highly vulnerable to injury during operations at the level of the thoracic inlet, it is not a source of lingering morbidity. The thoracic duct ascends as an indistinct plexus behind the esophagus to join the left jugular and subclavian veins. The anatomy of the thoracic duct is variable, and ramifying branches and a right-sided confluence with the veins are not uncommon. The duct may be made visible if the patient ingests Federal Food, Drug and Cosmetic Act (FD&C) No. 6 dye preoperatively. This dye is taken up by lymphatics into the chyle, thereby aiding in the duct's intraoperative detection. If the duct is injured, the damaged segment is securely oversewn, and a low fat disc is implemented postoperatively. Thoracic duct injuries that go unrecognized intraoperatively may result in chylous effusions in the wound or chest cavity. These injuries usually resolve without treatment, but large effusions may be a source of discomfort, wound irritation, respiratory embarrassment, and significant caloric loss. Simple aspiration is usually successful as an interim measure while the point of leakage scars over. Uncontrolled leaks are reexplored (after ingestion of FD&C No. 6 dye) to assist with the intraoperative delineation of the ductal system. If the precise point of leakage can be defined, it is simply ligated. Often, only a region of leakage can be identified. In this case, multiple "stick-tie" sutures are used to imbricate the suspect tissues. This can then be backed with a buttress of fascia or muscle and a film of fibrin glue.

## Vascular Injuries

One of the principal concerns during the conduct of any transthoracic procedure is the avoidance of injury to major arterial and venous structures. The aortic arch is usually located at the T4 level. Rostral to this, the esophagus and the trachea lie immediately ventral to the spine; however, they are tethered by the brachiocephalic trunk and cannot be readily mobilized. Below the level of the arch, the descending aorta lies closely applied to the lateral aspect of the thoracic vertebrae on the left side. The thoracic duct swings dorsal to the esophagus to lie nearly in the midline, interposed between the esophagus and spine. Paired azygous veins flank the spine and anastomose extensively with each other and with the vena cava. Crossing transversely at each midvertebral body level are paired segmental arteries and veins. These are branches of the aorta and azygous systems, respectively, and they divide into an intercostal vessel and a radiculomedullary branch at the level of the neural foramen.

Vascular complications are best avoided through careful preoperative planning and exacting surgical technique. Selection of the most appropriate side for surgical approach is fundamental for a safe and effective procedure. Sometimes the lesion itself dictates this choice, as in the case of a lung tumor with direct spinal extension. However, concurrent pathologic abnormalities in the access route, such as pleural scarring from prior surgery, may sometimes indicate a contralateral approach. All else being equal, a left-sided exposure of the spine below the T6 level is preferred. Although the aorta presents ventrolaterally on the left side of the spine, it is a robust and thick-walled vessel that lends itself to mobilization; if injured, the aorta readily accepts suture for direct repair. The heart can be easily reflected ventrally out of the way, although the surgeon must be alert to altered hemodynamics because this maneuver occasionally interferes with venous return to the right and left atria, a problem that is compounded by hypovolemia. The advantage of the left-sided thoracotomy increases in the lower thoracic spine where the right hemidiaphragm is elevated into the line of sight by the underlying liver. The liver does not easily lend itself to caudal displacement, because it is tethered by the hepatic ligament and the inferior vena cava. The esophagus, which is applied to the ventral aspect of the thoracic spine, is relatively less vulnerable during transthoracic approaches, because it is flanked on either side by major vascular structures.

In primary transthoracic or thoracoscopic procedures, injury to the great vessels is usually avoidable using sound surgical technique. Segmental vessels crossing the involved vertebra are secured at the level of the midbody. Interruption at this level may enhance the probability of continued patency of the radiculomedullary branches to the spinal cord through retrograde flow from the intercostal artery. A wide flap of mediastinal pleura is then developed, one leaf of which is reflected laterally toward the pedicles and foramina, and the opposite leaf is reflected medially. Dissection proceeds in a strictly subperiosteal plane, with all instruments kept firmly applied to bone lest the aorta be inadvertently entered as the flap is developed medially. Once the edge of the anterior longitudinal ligament is reached, malleable self-retaining retractors are inserted to maintain exposure and to protect the aorta. Division of the segmental arteries and veins untethers the great vessels and permits mobilization of the mediastinal contents to the midline. Taking the segmental vessels adjacent to the rostral and caudal disc spaces to be resected assists in this mobilization and is required in any event in those patients who undergo ventral instrumentation.

Major vascular injury appears to be exceedingly uncommon during primary ventral thoracic spine operations. Oskouian and Johnson[23] recently reviewed an institutional experience of 207 patients who underwent anterior reconstructive procedures in the thoracic and lumbar spine. Direct vascular injuries were identified in seven patients, including one thoracic aortic dissection ascribed to retraction, one torn intercostal artery, and five venous injuries. Injuries recognized intraoperatively obviously mandate immediate repair. The exact technique required depends on the size and anatomy of the injury. Branch avulsions are simply ligated. Small tears in the aorta proper or the vena cava are oversewn directly with fine vascular suture technique. Larger and more complex tears require placement of vascular clamps proximally and distally to isolate the injured segment for repair. Intraoperative consultation with an experienced cardiothoracic or vascular surgeon is appropriately sought. In cases of reoperation, prior infection, or irradiation, the possibility of scarification or friability of tissues in the mediastinum may be anticipated. These dissections *can be* tedious, and occasionally, it may be advisable to place umbilical tapes about the aorta preemptively or to prepare sites for cross-clamping in those cases deemed high risk.

## Pulmonary Complications

Atelectasis and pulmonary contusion with attendant potential for AV shunting and hypoxemia are minimized by periodic reexpansion of the lung and by accurate positioning and padding of any retractors. The opportunity to reinspect the lung parenchyma at these intervals discloses evolving surface contusions that may prompt alteration in retractor placement or technique. If a rib has been removed, sharp edges should be smoothed and waxed to avoid lung impalement. Pneumothorax is an inevitable consequence of thoracotomy, and a chest tube is always placed at the time of closure to encourage lung reexpansion, to control any air leak, and to evacuate blood from the wound. Thin opalescent drainage postoperatively is suggestive of a chyle leak. Persistent or increasing volumes of chylous output may require operative reexploration as described previously.

## Thoracolumbar Junction and Lumbar Spine

The thoracolumbar junction and lumbar spine are usually approached from the left side. On the right side, access is impeded by the liver and inferior vena cava, which can be difficult to mobilize. The bifurcation of the great vessels and the width of the psoas muscles make lateral exposure through the retroperitoneum awkward below L4. The peritoneal envelope containing the stomach and spleen in

the left upper quadrant is reflected ventrally and caudally, together with the retroperitoneal structures including the kidney and ureter. Although standard operative descriptions of this approach always caution about potential injury to abdominal viscera, in practice, injuries of a clinically significant magnitude appear to be extremely uncommon.

## Splenic and Vascular Injury

Splenic injury has rarely been reported in the literature and should not present a problem as long as it is recognized promptly.[14] Recent abdominal trauma, splenomegaly, and venous hypertension may be predisposing factors. Presumably, these injuries are most often caused by overzealous mobilization or retraction. General surgical self-retaining retractor systems provide a significant advantage over handheld instruments. The smooth blades used with these systems can be placed accurately and maintained without the trauma of repeated readjustments that are the inevitable outgrowth of the fatigue of prolonged manual retraction. A large moistened laparotomy pad is placed under the retractor to minimize the risk of injury. If a splenic injury occurs, consultation with a general surgeon should be sought. Brisk bleeding from the hilum necessitates splenectomy. However, in many cases of lesser injury, the spleen can be salvaged. When it is feasible, splenorrhaphy is preferable to splenectomy because of the increased incidence of overwhelming sepsis in patients who have been splenectomized. Surgeons should bear in mind the possibility of an occult splenic injury in cases of otherwise unexplained hypotension intraoperatively or postoperatively.

The aorta lies almost directly ventral to the spine in the lumbar region. Anatomy is inconstant, but the bifurcation into the common iliac arteries usually occurs at the level of the caudal L4 body. Aortic mobilization and methods to address aortic injury have been discussed previously. The inferior vena cava lies right of the midline. It is thin walled and has an extensive and variable network of tributaries and anastomoses that are easily torn and that are less readily repaired than are arterial structures. The level of confluence of the common iliac veins to form the vena cava is variable but typically occurs opposite the L4-5 disc space, just dorsal to the proximal portion of the right common iliac artery.

## Ureteral Injury

The ureters lie in loose areolar tissue on the psoas muscles. They cross ventrally over the iliac arteries to descend into the pelvis. They can be distinguished by observing peristalsis after a momentary pinch with an atraumatic forceps. The risk of ureteral injury in primary surgeries is exceedingly small. However, if normal tissue planes have been obscured by previous surgery, retroperitoneal fibrosis, tumor, or irradiation, dissection must proceed with utmost caution. During reoperations, sponge and Kittner dissection is advantageous. Intraoperative identification of the ureter may be facilitated by retrograde placement of a stent at the outset of the procedure. If a ureteral injury is incurred, immediate repair is undertaken. The exact nature of the repair is dictated by the type of injury. Clean lacerations may be simply reanastomosed end to end, whereas a segmental injury, as may be caused by a drill or rongeur, requires segmental resection and reanastomosis with ureteral mobilization to allow for a tensionless repair. In either case, the reconstruction should be accomplished over a stent that can be subsequently retrieved cystoscopically. Injuries over segments too lengthy to permit primary repair are uncommon; however, they demand more sophisticated reconstructive techniques such as appendiceal interposition or ureteroureteral anastomosis. Obviously, the input of a urologic surgeon should be sought.

Not all ureteral injuries are recognized during surgery. The postoperative development of hydronephrosis, a urinoma, or a retroperitoneal abscess should prompt investigation of the upper urinary tract by sonography, computed tomography (CT), intravenous pyelography, or retrograde pyelography. Two instances of delayed ureteral obstruction attributed to retroperitoneal fibrosis after scoliosis surgery with Dwyer instrumentation have been reported.[6,31]

## Bowel Injury

Because the bowel is mobilized ventrally within the peritoneal envelope during a retroperitoneal approach, the possibility of an iatrogenic perforation exists. Obviously, such an event is a cause for grave concern because of the high potential for wound contamination. If a surgeon recognizes a bowel perforation intraoperatively, it is advisable that he or she establish barrier isolation of the spinal exposure to minimize the risk of further wound contamination. The perforation should be repaired primarily, and the prophylactic antibiotic coverage should be expanded to include anaerobic organisms. Once the repair is complete, the wound is thoroughly irrigated with an antibiotic-containing solution. The decision of proceeding with decompression, fusion, and instrumentation is individualized according to the phase of the procedure at which soilage occurred, its magnitude, and the relative penalty for not proceeding with a definitive procedure as planned. In most cases, the surgeon should be most reluctant to instrument a wound that he or she knows is contaminated. An extended course of antibiotics is advised postoperatively.

## Transabdominal Approaches to the Lumbosacral Spine

Ventral exposure from the L4-5 level to the sacrum can be a surgical challenge. Retroperitoneal approaches through the flank to this level are limited by the caudolaterally coursing iliac veins, by the large mass of the psoas muscles, and by the obliquity of the working angle caused by the iliac crest. The latter two difficulties can be circumvented by midline transperitoneal or retroperitoneal approaches through the hypogastrium. The overlying great vessels are still a considerable impediment to this exposure and are the major source of morbidity. Foreknowledge of advanced atherosclerotic occlusive disease or of the presence of an abdominal aortic aneurysm may temper enthusiasm for a ventral operation. Dedicated vascular studies are not routinely obtained preoperatively unless clinical circumstances warrant concern. Excellent information about the condition of the aorta and its bifurcation can usually be gleaned from the preoperative spinal imaging studies or sonography.

## Vascular Injury

Arterial anatomy is more consistent than is venous anatomy. The level of the aortic bifurcation can be anticipated at L4, and thus a direct ventral approach to the lumbosacral junction necessitates dissection within the limbs of the bifurcation. Typically, the right iliac artery has to be mobilized to uncover the L4-5 disc, and great care must be taken with insertion and removal of interbody retractors to minimize the possibility for blunt or sharp vascular injury. It is wise to confirm the presence of the femoral and pedal pulses periodically throughout the surgery. Loss of pulses should prompt an intraoperative angiogram and any indicated repair.

The venous anatomy is the more problematic aspect of these exposures. The level of confluence of the iliac veins to form the vena cava is at the L4-5 disc level in approximately 70% to 80% of patients. A more caudally situated confluence is often associated with unusually large common iliac veins. They may then directly overlie the L5 body or the L5-S1 disc space, sometimes precluding ventral access at this level entirely. These anatomic variations may be discerned in close inspection of the preoperative magnetic resonance imaging (MRI) or CT examinations.[16]

In patients who are more typical, the left common iliac vein requires the greatest mobilization. Depending on the scope and level of the surgery, this vein may have to be retracted medially, laterally, or in both directions. In inflammatory or degenerative conditions, the left common iliac vein can easily become scarred down in the soft tissues immediately ventral to the disc. Successful collapse and mediolateral retraction are possible in this case only if the vein is carefully dissected longitudinally along its axis. The middle sacral vessels originate from either the common or the internal iliac vessels, and they overlie the L5-S1 disc space. They often can be retracted with ease, although no harm attends their sacrifice. The surgeon should take care to clearly identify all major vascular structures in the field before incising the disc space. The use of monopolar cautery over the disc space should be minimized to spare the hypogastric (sympathetic) plexus. Bipolar cautery is used to secure smaller vessels, and clips or ligatures are used to occlude larger vessels.

Injuries to the common iliac veins or the vena cava are encountered in 5% to 15% of transabdominal approaches to the lumbosacral junction.[2,15,36] It is unclear whether "minimally invasive" laparoscopic procedures are more or less prone to this complication than are open techniques.* If a major vein is injured, renorrhaphy is preferred over ligation, if at all possible. Hemorrhage is initially controlled by direct pressure at the point of injury until the vessel can be isolated proximally and distally. Particularly challenging are "backside" repairs brought on through avulsion of unseen tributaries into the dorsal wall of the common iliac veins or vena cava during blunt dissection. The largest and anatomically most consistent of these tributaries are the lateral

---

*References 2,3,15,19,28,36.

lumbar veins and the iliolumbar vein. Because the inferior vena cava lies slightly to the right of midline, the most efficient strategy is to mobilize it farther rightward if it is in the way. Special effort must be taken to clearly identify, doubly ligate, and divide the lumbar and iliolumbar veins on the left side before retracting the inferior vena cava in this manner, in case the veins are avulsed or the vena cava is ruptured. Regrettably, efforts to graft veins using either autologous or prosthetic materials have been fraught with a high incidence of occlusion.

## Complications of Posterior Lumbar Discectomy

Lumbar discectomy is among the most commonly performed spine operations. Complications are few and usually relate to infection, instability, cerebrospinal fluid leak, and neurologic events. Although vascular injuries are uncommon, the potential for bowel, ureteral, and catastrophic vascular injury is now well documented. The shared mechanism of these injuries is violation of the annulus ventrally with some type of biting instrument. A recent review of the English literature since 1965 identified 98 cases of vascular injury associated with posterior lumbar discectomy and estimated an incidence of 1 to 5 events per 10,000 procedures.[24] It is likely that these complications are considerably more common than is generally appreciated.

### Vascular Injury

Vascular injury may take several forms. The most dramatic are lacerations or partial wall avulsions in large-caliber retroperitoneal arteries or veins that result in massive, acute retroperitoneal hemorrhage. Bleeding is manifest through the disc space itself in less than half of these cases. Often, the injury is first suspected because of unexplained hypotension and tachycardia, either in the operating room or during postanesthetic recovery.[4,24,26] Lesser injuries may tamponade themselves in a contained retroperitoneal hematoma, later giving rise to a pseudoaneurysm, which can present with delayed rupture or distal embolization.

Venous injuries are probably more common, but their diagnosis is less obvious. They may be a source of retroperitoneal hemorrhage, venous thrombosis, leg swelling, and pulmonary embolism. The presence of an expanding lower abdominal mass, unexplained anemia, an unexpected degree of back or leg pain, and lower extremity swelling or thromboembolism should prompt consideration of a vascular injury.

If an artery and a vein are injured in proximity to each other, the potential for the development of an AV fistula exists.[4,24] These fistulas are recognized by the presence of a thrill, symptoms of limb claudication, and cardiac overload secondary to a left-to-right shunt. Although AV fistulas may present in the first days postoperatively, full symptomatic maturation is more typically delayed by weeks to months.

Violation of the ventral annulus with curettes and rongeurs may be a much more common occurrence than is generally realized. Three of 25 patients undergoing follow-up lumbar discography were shown to have new, but asymptomatic, ventral annular defects at operated levels.[34] The L4-5 and L5-S1 levels have been implicated with equal frequency. The anatomy of the aortic bifurcation and the more variable confluence of the common iliac veins have been reviewed. Because the aorta usually terminates opposite the L4 vertebra, aortic injury per se is rare. The common iliac veins usually join at the level of the L4-5 disc space to the right of midline to form the inferior vena cava. Injuries on the lateral aspect of the disc on the right side are expected to involve the terminal inferior vena cava (at L4-5) or the proximal right common iliac vein. In paramedian injuries, the right common iliac artery and the right or left common iliac veins are vulnerable. With left lateral injuries, the left common iliac artery is at risk. With rostral bifurcation of the common iliac arteries, occasional instances of isolated internal iliac injury have been reported during L5-S1 discectomy.

The likelihood of breach of the ventral annulus is increased by the vigor with which disc space evacuation is pursued. Observing a few simple measures helps minimize this risk. The diameter of the targeted disc space along the projected axis of the discectomy can be accurately measured from preoperative MRI or CT studies acquired in axial planes oriented parallel to the disc space. Ordinarily, this varies from 37 to 48mm from L3 to the sacrum and is somewhat larger in men than in women.[1] The shafts of instruments that are to be introduced into the disc space may then be appropriately marked with a small adhesive strip as a caution against overly deep insertion. The disc rongeur should enter the disc space with the jaws in a closed position to discourage engagement of the thecal sac or a nerve root; however, once within the disc space, the jaws are opened while the rongeur is advanced to its working depth. This distributes any applied forces over two contact points and makes unintended breach of the ventral annulus more difficult.

The management of vascular complications is context specific. In the face of acute hemodynamic instability, the prone patient must be quickly returned to the supine position to aid resuscitation and enable exploratory laparotomy. Swift diagnosis and appropriate action are of paramount importance if a catastrophic outcome is to be avoided. Skin edges can be swiftly reapproximated with a whip stitch closure or staples while the anesthetic is lightened and volume resuscitation is begun. The assistance of a general or vascular surgeon should be sought immediately. The area of injury will lie beneath a bulging retroperitoneal hematoma. Exsanguinating arterial hemorrhage may be controlled with manual compression of the distal aorta until desired personnel and equipment can be mobilized. The retroperitoneal hematoma must be explored carefully to delineate the site of injury precisely and to obtain proximal and distal control. It may then be repaired primarily or grafted according to circumstances. Although retroperitoneal hematoma remains an uncommon complication of lumbar discectomy, mortality approaches 50%, in part because of delayed diagnosis. Only through early recognition of such injuries and prompt institution of corrective action can these patients be salvaged.

Less calamitous vascular injuries present in a delayed fashion in hemodynamically stable individuals.[4] Typically, such injuries are initially evaluated by an abdominal CT scan. If a retroperitoneal mass is defined adjacent to a discectomy site, it should be further evaluated angiographically. In some institutions, magnetic resonance angiography and

CT angiography can obviate the need for invasive examination in select settings. Color flow Doppler studies may also be appropriate in patients with significant lower limb swelling suggestive of proximal venous injury or thrombosis. Arterial injuries such as AV fistulas or pseudoaneurysms are repaired or reconstructed as open procedures, usually on an elective basis. Evolving reconstructive endovascular techniques may soon allow for percutaneous management of some of these conditions. Partial or complete thrombosis of an iliac vein or inferior vena cava may require either systemic anticoagulation or placement of an infrarenal caval filter, depending on the circumstances.

## Other Visceral Injury

Ureteral injury after lumbar discectomy appears to be an even rarer complication than vascular injury.[17] The ureters are located more laterally in the retroperitoneum than are the great vessels, lying in the cleft between the psoas muscles and the spine, within a bed of periureteral fat. Therefore they are somewhat more mobile than the great vessels and are less vulnerable to injury. In cases in which the ureter is not recognized as part of the operative specimen, diagnosis is usually delayed by several weeks and is announced by abdominal pain, distension, hematuria, and urinary or systemic sepsis. A urinoma may be visualized sonographically or on abdominal CT, but an intravenous or retrograde pyelogram still provides the most accurate delineation of the injury site. It is postulated that an aberrantly medial course of the ureters or a thin body habitus allowing compression of the retroperitoneal structures against the spine in the prone position are factors that contribute to this unusual complication. Treatment includes proximal diversion by nephrostomy followed by a definitive urologic reconstruction according to principles already discussed.[22] The possibility of concomitant vascular injury must be excluded by vascular imaging studies and through thorough intraoperative assessment.

Another rare but serious complication resulting from ventral penetration of the disc space is bowel perforation.[30] A 1991 review noted 13 cases in the literature.[32] Most were injuries to the ileum after L5-S1 discectomy. The mesenteric root attaches to the retroperitoneum obliquely, crossing the midline at the L5-S1 interspace as it courses toward the right sacroiliac joint. Because the great vessels bifurcate above this level, it is postulated that a narrow window is thereby created in the midline through which instruments may be passed into the mesentery. It has also been postulated that air-filled loops of bowel tend to float upward and apply themselves ventrally against the spine in the prone position. Intraoperative diagnosis is obvious if intestinal mucosa is retrieved with the rongeur. Otherwise, in the early postoperative period, patients have an acute abdomen or, in a delayed fashion, chronic wound infections attributable to intestinal flora. Treatment is usually surgical, especially when a walled-off abscess is suspected.

## Instrumentation Complications

The use of instrumentation has introduced a new level of complexity and complications to spinal surgery. Apart from issues related to biomechanical failure, the various forms of dorsal instrumentation, including assorted types of pedicle screws, claws, hooks, and sublaminar wires, mainly pose a threat of neurologic injury or cerebrospinal fluid leak. Placement of transarticular C1-2 screws must be technically exact to avoid vertebral artery injury. If an initial C1-2 screw placement results in arterial injury, a pars screw may be a preferable option on the contralateral side, rather than risking bilateral vertebral artery occlusion. It is conceivable that overly long pedicle screws could penetrate far enough through the vertebral cortex ventrally to transfix the esophagus or great vessels.

Bicortical screw fixation at the S1 level raises concern for internal iliac vein or lumbosacral trunk injury. Both of these structures lie in close apposition to the sacrum just medial to the sacroiliac joint. Based on anatomic studies in cadavers, the potential for injury to these structures seems to be increased with screws placed laterally.[20] Screws directed medially through the S2 pedicles to engage the ventral sacral cortex have only a remote chance of causing visceral injury. Major vascular structures are located more laterally, and the sigmoid colon is still attached on a short mesentery at this level. It is possible that the preparatory drilling, probing, and tapping the pilot holes are more likely to produce injury than is the placement of the screw itself. These maneuvers must be performed with extreme caution to minimize the risk of overdrilling or overtapping of the holes, which could easily puncture a vessel or viscus. Clinically relevant injuries appear to be extremely uncommon thus far, but continued strict attention to the technical details of instrumentation insertion is mandatory if these untoward events are to be avoided. Presumably, the expanding use of image-guidance technologies will add an extra margin of safety to these endeavors.

Ventral thoracic and thoracolumbar spinal instrumentation has demonstrated its potential to cause serious vascular complications. The Dunn device was withdrawn from clinical use after it was associated with the development of abdominal aneurysms in three cases. Whether this was caused by the device's design or by the method of its application in these particular individuals remains unclear. Contemporary ventral fixation systems for use in the thoracic and lumbar spine, using rod or plate constructs, have been free of vascular complications thus far. This is attributed to design parameters that emphasize a low profile and that demand an exactly lateral application on the vertebral bodies with an orthogonal screw trajectory dorsal to all major vessels. If care is taken to apply the instrumentation as intended, with screws of appropriate length, the potential for significant vascular or soft tissue injury should be exceedingly small. There is one report of aortic injury at the T6 level resultant from screw penetration during ventral spinal fixation.[18] A case of delayed aortic rupture has been attributed to erosion by a mesh cage placed for ventral reconstruction in the thoracic spine.[10] Complications such as these underscore the need for careful correlation of the field as viewed intraoperatively with preoperative and intraoperative imaging to reconfirm that spinal instrumentation is applied as intended.

Such cross-checking is especially advisable in cases of deformity correction, in which normal anatomic relations can be highly distorted. The use of screws with a blunt tip and a tapered run out to the threads may mitigate against engagement of a major vessel. Above all, surgeons must adhere to proper operative technique and pay close attention to screw length and trajectory. The width of the vertebral body and the exact location of the great vessels relative to the projected screw path can be ascertained through inspection of the axial CT or MRI scans at the levels to be instrumented.

## Summary

Contemporary surgical techniques enable both ventral and dorsal exposure of the entire spine from occiput to sacrum. This allows any pathologic condition to be addressed in an anatomically appropriate fashion. As a group, the ventral approaches are more demanding procedures because of the need to reflect overlying vascular and soft tissue structures. This inevitably subjects the patient to heightened risks of exposure-related complications compared with the simpler midline dorsal approaches.[8] This risk is justified only if it is kept acceptably low and if patient outcomes are significantly improved in relation to the natural history of the disease and to safer but possibly less definitive procedures. Sound case selection and excellent surgical technique are the keys to avoiding or minimizing these complications.

## REFERENCES

1. Anda S, Aakhus S, Skaanes KO, et al: Anterior perforations in lumbar discectomies: A report of four cases of vascular complications and a CT study of the prevertebral lumbar anatomy. Spine 16:54, 1991.
2. Baker JK, Reardon PR, Reardon MJ, Heggeness MH: Vascular injury in anterior lumbar surgery. Spine 18:2227, 1993.
3. Boos N, Kalberer F, Schoeb O: Retroperitoneal endoscopically assisted minilaparotomy for anterior lumbar interbody fusion: Technical feasibility and complications. Spine 26:E1, 2001.
4. Brewster DC, May AR, Darling RC, et al: Variable manifestations of vascular injury during lumbar disk surgery. Arch Surg 114:1026, 1979.
5. Burger R, Tonn JC, Vince GH, et al: Median corpectomy in cervical spondylotic multisegmental stenosis. Zentralbl Neurochir 57:62, 1996.
6. Cleveland RH, Gilsanz V, Lebowitz RL, Wilkinson RH: Hydronephrosis from retroperitoneal fibrosis after anterior spine fusion. J Bone Joint Surg 60A:996, 1978.
7. Daniels SK, Mahoney MC, Lyons GD: Persistent dysphagia and dysphonia following cervical spine surgery. Ear Nose Throat J 77:473, 1998.
8. Faciszewski T, Winter RB, Lonstein JE, et al: The surgical and medical perioperative complication of anterior spinal fusion surgery in the thoracic and lumbar spine in adults. A review of 1223 procedures. Spine 20:1592, 1995.
9. Finiels PJ, Hernandez G, Sabatier P, Frerebeau P: Delayed esophageal perforation after cervical osteosynthesis. Case illustration. J Neurosurg 92(1 Suppl):123, 2000.
10. Floch NR, Harvey JC, Beattie EJ Jr: Aortoesophageal fistula after reconstruction of the thoracic spine. Ann Thorac Surg 60:191, 1995.
11. Gaudinez RF, English GM, Gebhard JS, et al: Esophageal perforations after anterior cervical surgery. J Spinal Disord 13:77, 2000.
12. Geyer TE, Foy MA: Oral extrusion of a screw after anterior cervical spine plating. Spine 15:1814, 2001.
13. Heeneman H: Vocal cord paralysis following anterior approaches to the anterior cervical spine. Laryngoscope 83:17, 1973.
14. Hodge A, DeWald RL: Splenic injury complicating the anterior thoracoabdominal surgical approach for scoliosis. J Bone Joint Surg 65A:396, 1983.
15. Kaiser MG, Haid RW Jr, Subach BR, et al: Comparison of the mini-open versus laparoscopic approach for anterior lumbar interbody fusion: A retrospective review. Neurosurgery 51: 97, 2002.
16. Kleeman TJ, Michael Ahn U, Clutterbuck WB, et al: Laparoscopic anterior lumbar interbody fusion at L4-5: An anatomic evaluation and approach classification. Spine 27: 1390, 2002.
17. Krone A, Heller V, Osterhage HR: Ureteral injury in lumbar disc surgery. Acta Neurochir (Wien) 78:108, 1985.
18. Matsuzaki H, Tokuhashi Y, Wakabayashi K, Kitamura S: Penetration of a screw into the thoracic aorta in anterior spinal instrumentation. Spine 18:2327, 1993.
19. Mayer HM: A new microsurgical technique for minimally invasive anterior lumbar interbody fusion. Spine 22:691, 1997.
20. Mirkovic S, Abitol JJ, Steinman J, et al: Anatomic consideration for sacral screw placement. Spine 16(Suppl):S289, 1991.
21. Newhouse KE, Lindsey RW, Clark CR, et al: Esophageal perforation following anterior cervical spine surgery. Spine 14:1051, 1989.
22. Noyes DT, Morrisseau PM: Ureteral transection secondary to lumbar disc surgery. Urology 19:651, 1982.
23. Oskouian RJ Jr, Johnson JP: Vascular complications in anterior thoracolumbar spinal reconstruction. J Neurosurg 96(1 Suppl):1, 2002.
24. Papadoulas S, Konstantinou D, Kourea HP, et al: Vascular injury complicating lumbar disc surgery. A systematic review. Eur J Vasc Indovasc Surg 24:189, 2002.
25. Pfeifer BA, Freidberg SR, Jewell ER: Repair of injured vertebral artery in anterior cervical procedures. Spine 19:1471, 1994.
26. Raptis S, Quigley F, Barker S: Vascular complication of elective lower lumbar disc surgery. Aust N Z J Surg 64:216, 1994.
27. Ratnaraj J, Todorov A, McHugh T, et al: Effects of decreasing endotracheal tube cuff pressures during neck retraction for anterior cervical spine surgery. J Neurosurg 97(2 Suppl):176, 2002.
28. Regan JJ, McAfee PC, Guyer RD, Aronoff RJ: Laparoscopic fusion of the lumbar spine in a multicenter series of the first 34 consecutive patients. Surg Laparosc Endosc 6:459, 1996.
29. Robinson RA, Smith G: Anterolateral cervical disc removal and interbody fusion for cervical disk syndrome. Bull Johns Hopkins Hosp 96:223, 1955.

30. Shaw ED, Scarborough JT, Beals RK: Bowel injury as a complication of lumbar discectomy. *J Bone Joint Surg* 63A:478, 1981.

31. Silber I, McMaster W: Retroperitoneal fibrosis with hydronephrosis as a complication of the Dwyer procedure. *J Pediatr Surg* 12:255, 1977.

32. Smith EB, DeBord JR: Intestinal injury after lumbar discectomy. *Surg Gynecol Obstet* 173:22, 1991.

33. Smith MD, Bolesta MJ: Esophageal perforation after anterior cervical plate fixation: A report of two cases. *J Spinal Disord* 5:357, 1992.

34. Solonen KA: Perforation of the anterior annulus fibrosus during operation for prolapsed disc. *Ann Chir Gynaecol Fenn* 61:385, 1975.

35. Stewart M, Johnston RA, Wilson JA: Swallowing performance following anterior cervical spine surgery. *Br J Neurosurg* 9:605, 1995.

36. Zdeblick TA, David SM: A prospective comparison of surgical approach for anterior L4-L5 fusion: Laparoscopic versus mini anterior lumbar interbody fusion. *Spine* 25:2682, 2000.

# C H A P T E R   1 5 2

# Postoperative Spinal Deformities

## Scott T. Dull and Richard M. Toselli

Postoperative spinal deformity should be considered an iatrogenic disease. Although there are circumstances that seem to be beyond a surgeon's control, in most cases postoperative spinal deformity can be prevented. The surgeon must evaluate many factors that may be present or that arise during the initial evaluation, the preoperative planning, or the procedure, and even in the postoperative course, that directly affect the risk of a postoperative spinal deformity. However, this complication often occurs because of a disregard for or a lack of understanding of the biomechanical principles governing the surgical alteration of the spine and consequent spinal stability. Several reasons account for this.

At times, surgeons may deviate from accepted biomechanical principles because doing so may have proved successful in the past. In addition, practices that may lead to successful outcomes when performed by an experienced surgeon may not produce similar outcomes in the hands of a younger, inexperienced surgeon. Finally, many surgeons may simply lack the knowledge of these principles because spinal biomechanics is a rapidly evolving field that, until recently, has not been emphasized during surgical training.

On the other hand, an established biomechanical principle does not underlie every situation or every decision in spinal surgery. In addition, because there is no pure physiologic model for the study of spinal biomechanics, there will not always be a direct correlation between laboratory results and available clinical experience. The field of spinal biomechanics was born partly out of the necessity to establish a scientific foundation for the findings from clinical experience. In turn, its study should be used to help guide changes in the practice of spinal surgery that will improve outcome and reduce morbidity.

There is a strong relationship between the biomechanics of the spine and the clinical outcome in spinal surgery. It is especially important for the surgeon to consider this relationship when discussing postoperative spinal deformity, because so often this undesirable outcome can be prevented by adhering to basic biomechanical principles that have been established in the laboratory and that have been supported in clinical settings. The pertinent biomechanical principles related to the development of postoperative deformity are reviewed in the first part of this chapter. Next, specific types of postoperative deformity are discussed, including their incidences, causes, and treatments. An emphasis is placed on prevention, because the management of these complications is accompanied by its own potential morbidity.

## Biomechanical Considerations

Spinal deformity results from a persistent imbalance or maldistribution of the physiologic forces sustained by the spine. In general, ventral spinal elements bear compressive forces, whereas dorsal elements bear tensile stresses. Disequilibrium of these forces can be created iatrogenically during surgery in which the spinal column may be altered. This alteration (e.g., laminectomy, facetectomy, corpectomy) may be sufficient to transfer the once-shared load to the remaining spinal elements, causing either immediate instability or delayed progressive deformity. When this happens, there is an increased risk of spinal cord and nerve root injury and debilitating pain. Anticipation and prevention of postoperative deformity should be a primary concern, because treatment of this condition is often difficult and conveys its own morbidity. To prevent postoperative deformity, the surgeon must understand some biomechanical principles.

The spine has four normal curves in the sagittal plane. The cervical and lumbar regions are lordotic, whereas the thoracic and sacral regions have kyphotic curvatures. The cervical and lumbar regions are much more mobile than the relatively rigid thoracic spine. The normal thoracic curvature is 20 to 50 degrees. For the normal lumbar curvature, the range is 20 to 70 degrees. These spinal curvatures are normally balanced so that erect posture can be maintained. Spinal surgery can alter this balance, and if great enough, the alteration will result in deformity. Postoperative deformity typically occurs as an abnormal kyphosis or a listhesis.

### Cervical Spine

When postoperative deformity occurs in the cervical spine, it usually takes the form of a kyphosis or a ventral subluxation. A kyphotic deformity in this region refers to a reversal of 5 degrees or more of the natural cervical lordosis. Laminectomy is the most common surgical procedure that may lead to kyphosis. During a laminectomy, the musculus erector spinae are partially denervated and weakened. Spinous processes and laminae are removed, disrupting muscular attachments. The nuchal ligament, the supraspinous and interspinous ligaments, and the yellow ligaments are also removed. The center of gravity of the head is usually slightly in front of the cervical spinal axis. Therefore the tensile force applied by the dorsal elements must be great enough to counteract the large flexion moment created by the weight of the head. Weakening the dorsal muscles relative to the ventral cervical musculature results in an imbalance of forces. The disrupted muscular attachments reattach to scar tissue that is closer to the spine's instantaneous axis of rotation (IAR) in the sagittal plane, thus reducing the extension moment that ordinarily counteracts the flexion moment. The disrupted dorsal elements reduce the passive tensile force (tension band). Together, these alterations of dorsal elements favor the development of a kyphotic deformity. In children, the potential for kyphotic deformity is greater because of the relatively greater viscoelasticity of the immature spine and because the epiphyses in the growing spine respond to asymmetric forces by causing a ventral wedging of the vertebral bodies. Furthermore, the orientation of the cervical facet joint in the young spine is more horizontal than the 45-degree angle of the mature spine, thus creating less resistance to forward-bending moments.[85]

Despite this theory of its development, postlaminectomy kyphosis appears to be less common in adults, and the exact incidence is not well established. The contribution of the cervical musculature to spinal stability has been questioned by investigators who found that paralysis of the cervical muscles alone did not result in vertebral dislocation. In addition, experimental work by Panjabi et al.[59] suggested that the cervical spine should be stable if all of the ventral elements and at least one of the dorsal elements were intact. In the case of a simple decompressive cervical laminectomy, the remaining dorsal element would be the facets and their capsular ligaments (normally left intact). However, the risk of kyphotic deformity increases if either the C2 or the C7 spinolaminar elements are removed as part of the laminectomy. In addition, the likelihood of developing kyphosis may be higher in a postlaminectomy patient if the ventral elements are not intact at the levels of the laminectomy. For example, an adult who undergoes a C3-6 laminectomy and has an incompetent C4-5 disc is more likely to develop a kyphotic deformity than he or she would be if that disc were normal.

Although laminectomy can be complicated by a postoperative kyphotic deformity, dorsal foraminotomies or partial facetectomies have been implicated as the cause of translational deformity or subluxation. The facets clearly play a role in limiting rotation, distraction, and flexion and thus prevent translation. An abundance of biomechanical literature has evaluated the extent of instability after resection of the facet joints.

Raynor et al.[65] concluded that bilateral resection of more than 50% of the facet joint significantly compromises the shear strength of a cervical spine motion segment and that stabilization should be considered. Zdeblick et al.[98] concluded that segmental hypermobility occurred if more than 50% bilateral facetectomies were performed. Cusick et al.[15] reported that, even after unilateral facetectomy, the strength of the functional spinal unit decreased by 31% and that the potential for deformity was increased during subsequent exposure to repetitive compression-flexion loads. In a more recent study in which a multilevel cervical laminectomy and facetectomy model was used, Nowinski et al.[57] concluded that concurrent arthrodesis should be performed if more than 25% bilateral facetectomy is performed in conjunction with a multilevel laminectomy.

Despite some controversial clinical evidence that cervical laminoplasty may be beneficial in preventing the deformity that can follow a simple cervical laminectomy, no biomechanical studies are available to support the contention.

Failed ventral cervical procedures may also result in postoperative deformity. Ventral cervical discectomy or corpectomy usually requires a spacer or strut to replace and maintain the strength of the ventral spinal column. Failure of this strut results in an acute-angle kyphosis.

Several types of bone grafting techniques are available for use as a strut in ventral spinal surgery. Common autograft or allograft donor sites include ilium, fibula, and rib. These strut grafts must be able to withstand significant axial loads and to provide immediate ventral column stability. The further caudal in the spine the graft is placed, the greater the load it must withstand.

The ilium has the greatest versatility as a bone graft source. An experimental study of relative compression strengths of different iliac graft configurations revealed that the strongest was the Smith-Robinson graft, followed by the modified Bailey-Badgley graft, and then the Cloward graft.[83] All of these grafts withstood loads that were two and one-half times the average body weight. However, graft-vertebral construction, dynamic loading, joint and muscle forces, and the creeping substitution phase of bone healing were not taken into account. These conditions probably require a bone graft of greater strength than that required for isolated compression loads. Under these conditions, relative strengths of the grafts are very important.

The keystone-shaped graft, an ilial graft configuration described by Simmons and Bhalla,[74] was much stronger than the Cloward graft in flexion, extension, and lateral-bending loads. In addition, the keystone graft had 30% more surface contact with the adjacent vertebral surfaces than did the Cloward graft in a one-level procedure and 70% more surface contact in a two-level procedure. The Simmons-Bhalla graft was not compared with the other two ilial graft configurations. Other wedge-shaped grafts that are not "keystoned" into the adjacent vertebral end plates have the propensity, under compressive loads, to extrude ventrally or dorsally, depending on the direction of the wedge.

The fibula provides the strongest strut graft for resisting compression loads because of its relatively greater content of cortical bone. The slower reabsorption phase of bone graft healing with fibula implies that it can withstand compressive loads for longer periods. However, the time to achieve a solid fusion is greater because of the lower content of cancellous bone.

The rib graft can be used as a strut graft at all levels of the spine but is most convenient during ventral thoracic procedures because the rib is locally available. The rib graft has moderate strength in compression. The gentle bend of the rib allows it to conform to the natural curvatures of the spine.

Wittenberg et al.[91] suggest that in the immediate postoperative period, allograft is comparable with autograft in compressive strength, and that the ethylene oxide sterilization process of the allograft has no deleterious effects on compressive strength. Pelker and Friedlaender[61] reviewed studies of the biomechanical properties of allograft and concluded that frozen-thawed bone is better than freeze-dried bone for withstanding high torsional or bending loads, but freeze-dried bone is just as good under predominantly compressive or tensile loads. The elaborate study of Wolfinbarger et al.[92] concurs with that of Pelker and Friedlaender[61]; however, the authors state that the structural properties of freeze-dried bone can be improved to that of autograft by rehydrating with physiologic saline in vacuo for 1 hour. Microfractures in allograft formed during the rapid freezing and rehydration processes have been implicated in the reduced strength of these grafts. There is no clear consensus in the biomechanics literature regarding the relative strengths of allografts and autografts.

Adjuvant therapy seems to differentially alter the mechanical properties of bone graft. After radiation doses less than 3 megarads, the compressive strength of autograft or allograft is not significantly lowered. However, the 35% reduction in torsional strength of autograft after a 6-megarad dose of radiation is similar to that obtained with a freeze-dried allograft after only a 3-megarad dose.[61] In addition to taking into account the mechanical considerations, surgeons must consider other factors such as the biologic aspects of bone healing and the potential complications of graft harvesting when deciding between allograft and autograft for a given situation.

Positioning of the bone graft is an important consideration for postoperative mobility of the spine. Two concepts should be understood in this regard.[85] First, placement of a graft at the maximal distance from the IAR is most desirable for restricting motion about this axis. In the sagittal plane, the IAR of a motion segment is in the middle to dorsal portion of the disc. Therefore the optimal graft position for preventing rotation around the IAR is in the spinous processes dorsally rather than a ventral interbody position. Second, the placement of a bone graft dorsally allows for considerable motion at the disc space ventrally when axial loads are administered, because of the elastic properties of bone.[69] A ventral interbody graft provides the greatest weight-bearing ability.

The positioning of an interbody strut graft influences the potential for graft extrusion. Simmons and Bhalla[74] state that to prevent graft extrusion, it is ideal to place an interbody strut graft as close as possible to the "line of zero velocity," which was determined to pass through the origin of the nerve roots. A strut in this position would have nei-ther compressive nor tensile forces applied to it. Clinically, this implies that the strut graft should be placed toward the dorsal aspect of the adjacent vertebral bodies. However, when a ventral strut is required for replacement of ventral spinal elements (to prevent a kyphotic deformity or to maintain correction of a deformity), a position at a maximal distance from the IAR is best. Therefore a more ventral location is preferable.[86]

The length of a strut graft also has implications relating to its potential for failure. According to equations describing the maximal axial load before a buckling failure, the buckling load is proportional to the inverse square of the length of the loaded object.[85] Thus the longer the strut, the less the load required for it to fail by buckling. This principle becomes critical during placement of a ventral strut for the treatment of a kyphotic deformity.

The juncture between a strut graft and the adjacent vertebral body is an important consideration for the integrity of the graft. Just as graft positioning has an influence on graft extrusion, so does the graft-vertebral body juncture. First, it is important that there is maximal surface contact to achieve an even load distribution and to provide maximal area for bone fusion. Second, the graft should be under compression to aid in fusion and to help prevent extrusion. Third, the shape of the juncture can prejudice the potential for extrusion. The graft-vertebral body juncture is analogous to the various joints affecting the strength of woodwork. Joints in decreasing order of strength are the dovetail, mortise-and-tenon, dado, rabbet, and butt joints (Figure 152.1). The keystone graft, as described earlier, is somewhat analogous to a dovetail joint. The Smith-Robinson graft has a juncture like that of

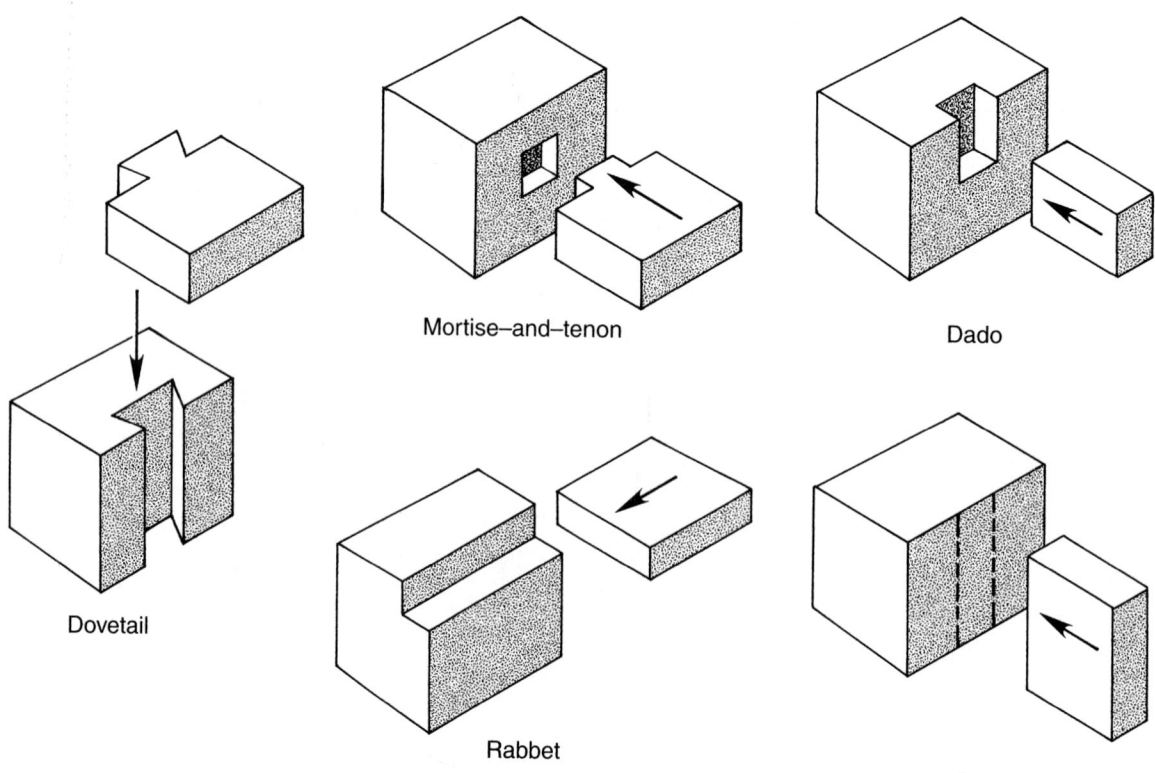

Dovetail

Mortise–and–tenon

Dado

Rabbet

Butt

**Figure 152.1** Schematic illustrations of several types of joints commonly used in carpentry.

a butt joint. The "joiners" preferred and often used by the authors for strength and practicality in ventral strut graft procedures are a shallow, slotted mortise-and-tenon joint for the rostral graft juncture and a modified, stopped dado joint for the caudal graft juncture (Figure 152.2).

## Thoracic Spine

Many of the basic biomechanical principles discussed previously can also be applied to the lower spinal regions. However, because of regional differences in the anatomy and in the physiologic forces applied, a direct correlation cannot be assumed.

Postoperative deformity of the thoracic spine most commonly occurs in the form of a kyphosis. Because of its natural kyphosis, the thoracic spine is more prone to instability during flexion or compression loads. Kyphosis in the thoracic spine can be considered abnormal if the curvature approaches 50 degrees or greater and there are symptoms associated with the curvature. The deformity can result from ventral decompressive surgery or from the more common dorsal procedures. Anatomically, the ventral elements (i.e., anterior longitudinal ligament and posterior longitudinal ligament) are more substantial than in the cervical spine. Some of the dorsal thoracic ligaments (i.e., capsular, supraspinous, and interspinous ligaments) are relatively weak. However, the ligamentum flavum is thicker and provides much of the tensile strength in the thoracic spine. The osseous and fibrous capsular components of the thoracic facets and their orientation provide the greatest resistance to flexion loads and translatory motion. The rib cage adds stability to the thoracic spine in all load situations.

In one of the only biomechanical studies using a multiple functional spinal unit (FSU) model to evaluate the effects of thoracic laminectomy, Yoganandan et al.[95] demonstrated that a two-level laminectomy decreases the load-carrying capacity of the thoracic column (by 39%), as well as the thoracic column's overall structural stiffness and energy-absorption characteristics. Because the stabilizing rib cage was not a part of this spinal model, it is difficult to gauge the absolute clinical effect of thoracic laminectomy. It is clear that the laminectomized thoracic spine's ability to resist compressive loads is diminished. Another study using thoracic single FSU models showed significant increases in motion during flexion, extension, and axial-rotation loads.[84] In addition, the results of a study involving serial sectioning of dorsal thoracic elements demonstrated that with all dorsal elements incised, the FSU remains stable until the costovertebral articulation is divided.[35] Thus although dorsal element removal alone may not result in the clinical development of a kyphosis, an accompanying abnormality (e.g., osteoporosis, tumor, infection, fracture) of the vertebral bodies at the same levels of the laminectomy may lead to kyphosis.

## Lumbar Spine

The lumbar spine is subject to the highest loads of any region of the spine. The lumbar spine is also a relatively mobile region, especially in flexion and extension. The anterior longitudinal ligament and the annulus fibrosus are the major ventral lumbar elements responsible for stability. Dorsally, the facets, their capsules, and the supraspinous ligament are the major contributors to stability, whereas the interspinous ligaments and the ligamentum flavum may be less important. In a sequential surgical alteration study of lumbar FSUs using a dynamic flexion-compression loading device, Pintar et al.[62] demonstrated that high physiologic load levels produce significant increases in the overall deflection of the FSU between bilateral facetectomy and bilateral facetectomy with posterior ligament

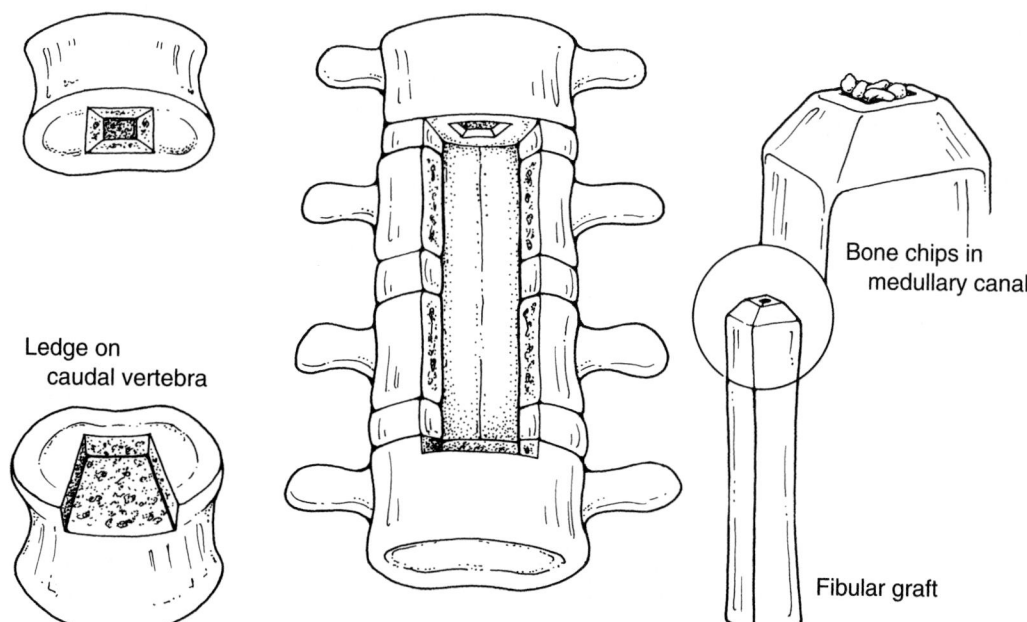

**Figure 152.2** Ventral view of a two-level corpectomy site with the rostral graft-vertebral juncture resembling a shallow mortise-and-tenon joint. The caudal juncture resembles a stopped dado joint. The fibula is filled with corticocancellous paste collected during the corpectomy.

(i.e., supraspinous and interspinous) transection but not between unilateral and bilateral facetectomy. This study emphasizes the importance of the contribution of dorsal ligaments to resisting forward-bending loads. Posner et al.[63] showed that when all dorsal elements or all ventral elements are removed, the lumbar FSU is likely to be unstable. Using another graded injury model in lumbar FSUs, Kuniyoshi et al.[42] showed the following: (1) Division of the dorsal ligaments alone did not create a significant increase in range of motion (ROM) during any of the six pure moments delivered. (2) No significant change in ROM occurred with subsequent unilateral medial and bilateral medial facetectomies for any of the moments except flexion. (3) There were significant changes in ROM during flexion and axial rotation moments after unilateral total and bilateral total facetectomies, even with intact dorsal ligaments. From these results, the authors concluded that total facetectomy, even if created unilaterally and with preservation of the dorsal ligaments, may make the lumbar FSU unstable in some spinal motion directions. They suggested that if stability is jeopardized in even one direction, supplementation with fusion is necessary.

Postoperative lumbar spine deformity manifests by either a relative kyphosis or a spondylolisthesis. A kyphosis in the lumbar spine may more appropriately be referred to as a loss of the natural lumbar lordosis, commonly known as *flat back*. Certainly, any reversal of the lordosis in this region is abnormal. This type of deformity typically occurs as a result of neglect in reestablishing the normal lordosis of the lumbar spine during instrumentation surgery. Alternatively, in the case of ventral decompression surgery, failure to place an adequate strut construct may reduce or reverse the natural lordosis. A spondylolisthesis is an abnormal translatory motion of one vertebra over another in the sagittal plane. Because of the major role the facet joints play in the stability of the lumbar spine, significant disruption during lumbar surgery places the spine at increased risk of deformity, especially under flexion and rotatory loads.

A unique abnormality of the lumbar spine is spondylolysis, in which there is a defect in the pars interarticularis.[17] This defect eliminates the contribution of dorsal spinal elements to spinal stability. A resultant progressive ventral listhesis can develop. The cause of spondylolysis has been thought to be congenital, degenerative, or traumatic. The exact mechanism(s) by which the condition develops has not been established. The surgical destruction of the pars interarticularis during a laminectomy may also result in the development of a postoperative spondylolisthesis.

## Clinical Considerations of Postoperative Spinal Deformity

Despite the significant advances made in understanding spinal instability and subsequent deformity through the use of elaborate biomechanical models, the processes are so complex and multifactorial that these models, in many cases, have not approximated the clinical conditions. Therefore actual clinical experience based on well-planned, controlled, and unbiased clinical trials should complement and support many of the basic biomechanical principles. Regrettably, few sound clinical studies are available. Therefore the available clinical experience is only an approximate guide to the "right" way to approach or manage a spinal deformity. Clinical decisions must be based on personal experience, inherited dictum, and the available literature. This section discusses the pertinent clinical aspects of postoperative deformity and provides recommendations for preventing and managing postoperative deformity.

## Postlaminectomy or Postfacetectomy Deformity
### Cervical Spine

Multisegmental cervical laminectomy is the most common procedure for cervical spondylotic myelopathy. It is also used for other conditions (e.g., for approaching intradural spinal pathologic conditions). In children, it is used most commonly for approaching spinal cord tumors. Trauma is a waning indication for laminectomy. In addition to the lack of improvement in outcome after laminectomy in traumatic spinal cord injury, laminectomy may actually contribute to deterioration because of the common concomitant multicolumn vertebral injury and resultant instability. In addition, the denervation of supporting spinal structures that accompany spinal cord injury can contribute to gradual or late deformity.

The incidence of postoperative deformity after laminectomy in adults is not well established, partly because the definition of deformity is inconsistent. The studies available vary with respect to the type and significance of deformity. For example, Mikawa et al.[52] divide postlaminectomy deformity into straight, kyphotic, and meandering types. Ishida et al.[32] classify deformity into more categories. Others consider a deformity to be present only if there are symptoms referable to that deformity. In addition, the literature does not always clarify whether the laminectomy cases reported also involved some degree of facetectomy. Another reason for the lack of clear-cut incidence data is that the length of follow-up in many studies is shorter than the time required to develop a gradually progressive postlaminectomy deformity. Nevertheless, the overall incidence of adult postlaminectomy (without facetectomy) deformity appears to be between 6% and 52%.* However, these patients rarely (0% to 3%) have symptoms directly referable to their deformity. Katsumi et al.[38] identified five risk factors that significantly increased the likelihood of cervical instability after laminectomy for spinal cord tumor in adult patients. These factors were (1) younger age, (2) preoperative abnormal cervical curvature, (3) four or more laminae removed, (4) inclusion of C2 in the laminectomy, and (5) destruction of the facet joints. The contributions of the third and fourth factors to cervical instability have not been fully supported in other studies. Callahan et al.[12] recommend dorsal cervical stabilization in the form of facet fusion after laminectomy to prevent postoperative deformity and instability in the following high-risk groups: (1) patients younger than 25 years of age; (2) patients with concomitant vertebral fracture or ligamentous traumatic injury at the levels of laminectomy; (3) patients with extensive

---

*References 27,32,34,38,52,53,72,76,96.

foraminotomies; and (4) patients with degenerative spondylosis in which laminectomy may contribute to increased motion, resulting in the progression of degenerative osteophyte formation at the laminectomized motion segments. The number of laminectomy levels did not influence the incidence of postoperative instability in this series. Most likely, the extent of the laminectomy at any level is a more important factor than the number of levels. In addition, patients with laminectomies superimposed on spinal segments with pathologic abnormalities (e.g., tumor, infection) affecting the anterior column are more at risk for deformity.

Many series have reported the incidence of cervical postlaminectomy deformity in children. The incidence ranges from 33% to 100%, with an average of 69%.[7] There seems to be a higher incidence in the subgroup of patients with spinal cord tumors, presumably because of increased spinal cord dysfunction and the effects of radiation therapy on the growing spine. That incidence may be artificially low, because many patients die of their disease before a late deformity occurs. Bell et al.[7] reported a 53% incidence of childhood cervical postlaminectomy deformity after excluding patients with primary or metastatic bone tumors, patients with neurofibromatosis, patients who underwent partial or total facetectomy, and patients who required postoperative spinal irradiation. Bell et al.[7] considered these factors to confound the true incidence of postlaminectomy deformity in children, because these factors can contribute intrinsically to deformity. Of the patients in this study group, 81% had Chiari's malformation, syringomyelia, or both. Of these deformities, 72% were kyphoses and the rest were hyperlordoses. There was a strong correlation of hyperlordosis with a peak age of 4.2 years and a weak correlation of kyphosis with a peak age of 10.5 years.

The contribution of facetectomy to postoperative deformity is significant, as evidenced in the biomechanical literature reviewed earlier. In his report comparing treatments of multilevel spondylotic radiculopathy, Herkowitz[27] noted a 75% incidence of deformity within 2 years of surgery in the subgroup of patients who underwent laminectomy with bilateral partial foraminotomies. The extent of the foraminotomy had a variable effect on the adequacy of nerve root decompression, as judged by the surgeon, and therefore was not reported in this study. Many series have demonstrated no postoperative deformity resulting from laminectomy with "limited" foraminotomies (medial facetectomies).* The term *limited* usually implies less than a 50% facet resection. This corresponds to approximately 5mm of the nerve root distal to the axilla being exposed, and it allows adequate decompression in most cases of foraminal stenosis resulting from spondylosis, especially when an undercutting of the facet is used. Even when only a unilateral (more than 50%) facetectomy is performed, there may be sufficient torsional instability to create a deformity under physiologic loads. Some laboratory evidence of this has been provided by Raynor et al.[65]

Cusick et al.[15] illustrated the importance of the dorsal (interspinous and supraspinous) ligaments for maintaining stability in the presence of bilateral cervical facetectomies.

When bilateral dorsal cervical foraminotomies are indicated, but a central decompression with laminectomy is not necessary, it may be wise to leave the dorsal ligaments intact. However, the use of stabilization techniques after bilateral (50% or less) facetectomies should not be precluded.

Cervical laminoplasty has been used since the 1970s to avoid the potential instability and to improve the clinical outcomes of laminectomies. Laminoplasty is similar to a laminectomy in that it expands the space available for the spinal cord. However, it differs in that the dorsal elements are altered, augmented, or replaced by a variety of techniques, thus providing a base for the reattachment of dorsal musculature and ligaments, as well as allowing the dorsal bony elements to fuse back to the spine.[26,28,33,43,70] Most of the described clinical reports of laminoplasties have been for the treatment of cervical spinal stenosis and ossification of the posterior longitudinal ligament. Because there is such a low incidence of symptomatic adult postlaminectomy kyphosis (except in the setting of trauma and spinal cord tumor), the efficacy of laminoplasty is difficult to determine. There is no convincing evidence in the literature to support the superiority of laminoplasty over laminectomy for preventing postoperative deformity or for improving neurologic outcome in adult patients.[30,32,55,81] Sufficient long-term data are lacking to determine whether laminoplasty may be of benefit in preventing a late deformity or whether it may provide enough stabilization of the spine to prevent the development of progressive spondylosis at the laminectomized motion segments, as has been suggested to occur after laminectomy by some authors.

The concept of laminoplasty or laminotomy in infants and children is more intriguing, because the incidence of postlaminectomy kyphosis is much greater in children than in the adult population. Only a handful of case series report results of laminoplasty in children.[60,64,73] For example, Raimondi et al.[64] illustrated a few cases of laminotomies performed with success at various regions of the spine in children. In his small series, Paraicz[60] was successful in preventing postoperative deformity in 100% of pediatric cervicothoracic laminotomy cases. Shikata et al.[73] were able to achieve good alignment, with no instability, in all 10 patients (aged 2 to 26 years) who underwent cervicothoracic laminoplasty and dorsolateral fusion, as widest from an average 3.5 year follow-up.

Although additional study is necessary to lend further support to these impressive results, using the laminotomy technique in young children would be reasonable, because the technique is relatively simple and safe. If its preventative use is ultimately established, there is no doubt that laminotomy will be preferable to later correction of a postoperative kyphotic deformity that may require both ventral and dorsal surgery.

### Thoracic and Lumbar Spine

Few clinical studies detail thoracic laminectomy deformity. Yasuoka et al.[94] reported a 0% incidence of postoperative deformity in the group of adults who did not require concomitant facetectomy and in whom surgery was not performed for trauma. Because of the support afforded by the rib cage, the occurrence of deformity after

---

*References 2,3,11,21,68,77.

an isolated thoracic laminectomy is not as common as it is in the cervical spine. However, if laminectomy is accompanied by facetectomy or if any of the ventral elements are involved with the pathologic process (e.g., an incompetent disc annulus, an osteoporotic or fractured vertebral body), the propensity for deformity increases significantly.

In the lumbar spine, an isolated laminectomy procedure ordinarily does not lead to deformity. Most of the load on the lumbar spine is borne by the vertebral bodies in the form of compressive loads, and the resistance to translation during flexion loads comes from the disc annulus and the medial aspect of the facet joint; therefore the removal of only the interspinous ligaments and the laminae is unlikely to create instability or deformity in the absence of coexisting abnormality in the anterior column and the facet complex. In the study by Yasuoka et al.,[94] no adult or child who underwent an isolated lumbar laminectomy developed postlaminectomy deformity.

Despite these results and because of a theoretical advantage of reestablishing the dorsal elements to which the extensor muscles can reattach and thereby maximize the likelihood of achieving normal spinal development, Abbott et al.[1] reported a series of 180 cases of pediatric osteoplastic lumbar laminotomies in which there were no cases of spinal deformity and in which there was at least partial osseous bridging of the laminar roof in all cases. Procedures similar to cervical laminotomy procedures in the pediatric population can be performed in the lumbar spine easily, safely, without significant additional operative time, and without instrumentation or bone graft. In the absence of any significant risk and because of a reasonably sound theoretical advantage, lumbar laminotomy is recommended in pediatric patients until or unless further study discredits it.

More commonly, a lumbar laminectomy is accompanied by some degree of facetectomy. This is especially true when the procedure is performed for acquired spinal stenosis or degenerative spondylolisthesis resulting from the hypertrophy of the facets that is inherent in the degenerative process. Because the medial aspect of the facet (as well as the disc annulus) plays a major role in preventing translational motion in the lumbar spine, the surgeon can expect an increased likelihood of the patient developing spondylolisthesis (or worsening of thereof) after laminectomy with facetectomy. In fact, the most common site of spinal stenosis and postoperative spondylolisthesis is at the L4 level. This may result in part from the stabilizing effects of the ileotransverse ligaments on the L5 vertebra and the pelvis. The incidence for worsening spondylolisthesis after decompressive laminectomy and facetectomy for degenerative spondylolisthesis is between 40% and 100%.[36,45,79,90] For acquired spinal stenosis without preoperative spondylolisthesis, the incidence is 3.7% to 20%.[36,45,71,79,82] Most patients in these studies also had discectomy performed to some extent. The effect of concomitant discectomy or age on the postoperative occurrence of spondylolisthesis is controversial. Multilevel surgery seems to portend an increased risk of postoperative slippage.[71] Although there is no definite correlation between postoperative spondylolisthesis and the clinical outcome, the long-term effects on future spinal stability and the development of low back pain, especially in patients undergoing

lumbar laminectomy with facetectomy at a relatively young age, remain unclear.

A microsurgical lumbar laminotomy is an alternative to a standard laminectomy. Microsurgical lumbar laminotomy is usually considered to involve a limited resection of the lamina rostral and caudal to the interlaminar space, the underlying ligamentum flavum, and the medial aspect of the superior facet.[5] This procedure is most often reserved for limited unilateral disease involving one or two contiguous levels. With this technique, most of the facet joint and the interspinous ligaments are preserved, thereby reducing the chances for postoperative instability. Surgeons must realize that no matter how stable they leave the spine postoperatively, the patient is not benefited unless adequate decompression is accomplished. The laminoplasty procedure can be and has been used in the thoracic and lumbar spine. However, it has not been demonstrated to be superior to laminectomy in the adult spine. As is the case in the cervical region, there may be an advantage to using laminotomy at these lower levels in children.

Similar to that in the cervical and thoracic spine, dorsal decompression in the presence of associated ventral pathologic abnormalities may result in deformity. Natelson[56] reported the occurrence of postoperative deformity that required additional surgery in several cases after lumbar laminectomy and facetectomy were performed in the presence of unrecognized or ignored anterior column abnormalities. The importance of addressing both the anterior and posterior spinal columns during surgical planning cannot be overemphasized and is therefore a recurrent theme in this chapter.

### Flat Back

Since 1973, loss of lumbar lordosis, known as *flat back*, has been considered a complication of scoliosis surgery after Harrington distraction rod instrumentation.[18] However, the application of any dorsal instrumentation system that has the capability of dorsally distracting the thoracolumbar and lumbar spine is subject to this type of deformity. The incidence is highly variable, but ranges from 5% to 49% depending on the selected patient population.[14,40,80] In a long-term follow-up study by Lagrone et al.,[44] 100% of the patients in their series had some form of distraction instrumentation extending to the lower lumbar spine or sacrum, contributing to this deformity. Other factors implicated were (1) the presence of a thoracolumbar kyphosis (usually greater than 60 degrees) caused by a lumbar curve fused to the apex of this kyphosis or by a lumbar fusion that ended at the thoracolumbar junction (in 60%), (2) pseudarthrosis associated with a loss of curvature correction (in 20%), (3) collapse of a lumbar vertebral body (in 7%), (4) fixed thoracic kyphosis of more than 40 degrees (in 5%), and (5) hip-flexion contractures (in 4%).

The two most common symptoms of flat back syndrome (symptomatic flat back) are (1) inability to stand erect and (2) back pain. The pain is typically in the upper and middle portion of the back and is worse with prolonged upright activities. Neck, thigh, and knee pain also occur because of the abnormal postures taken to compensate for the deformity. A radiographic diagnosis can be difficult because there is a wide normal range for thoracic and lumbar curvatures. However, by identifying those curvatures that have an increased distance from the sacrum to a plumb line from the seventh cervical vertebra on a standing lateral spine radiograph, the clinician can determine which symptomatic patients have a sagittal imbalance.

Treatment of this condition is often surgical, although every effort should be made at conservative management initially. During surgical correction of this deformity, the distraction hardware is removed, and multiple dorsal extension osteotomies are performed, followed by internal stabilization with a compression instrumentation system and bone graft. The rods in these systems can be contoured to re-create a more natural curvature in the thoracolumbar and lumbar regions. When there is collapse of the ventral column contributing to the deformity, ventral surgery to restore column height may be included as a staged procedure. Bracing is used during the mobilization phase of the patient's postoperative care.

According to Lagrone et al.,[44] 95% of the patients followed reported having benefitted from the corrective surgery. However, nearly 50% still had complaints of leaning forward, and 36% reported moderate or severe back pain at follow-up. There was a 60% complication rate associated with this corrective surgery. The early complications included dural tear, neuropraxia, urinary tract infection, myocardial infarction, and deep wound infection. Late complications included pseudarthrosis, hardware failure, and chronic neuralgia. Kostuik and Hall[41] reported better results and fewer complications with a single-stage ventral and dorsal procedure.

Because flat back syndrome is often more difficult to manage than the patient's original problem, making every effort to prevent this deformity from occurring is clearly advantageous. The surgeon should keep the following preventive measures in mind when performing a lower spine fusion procedure: (1) Address anterior column abnormalities that may later result in a loss of column height. (2) Position the prone patient with hips extended to maximize lumbar lordosis during surgery. (3) Avoid dorsal distraction instrumentation in the lumbar spine. (4) Contour the construct to mimic the natural curvature of the spine. (5) Avoid ending the rostral aspect of the construct at the apex of a kyphosis.

## Dorsal Surgery in the Presence of Ventral Spinal Instability

Up to half of the patients who undergo a decompressive laminectomy for spine trauma develop symptomatic kyphotic deformity. Whereas decompressive laminectomy alone is rarely indicated for spine trauma, dorsal surgical stabilization is often performed. Common indications for dorsal stabilization in the cervical spine include, for example, unilateral or bilateral facet fracture or dislocation and severe dorsal ligamentous injury in the absence of fracture. Many biomechanically sound interspinous, interlaminar, and interfacetal constructs can be used to stabilize the cervical spine dorsally when a ventral decompressive surgery is not necessary. However, any of these may fail to prevent a kyphotic deformity without sufficient anterior column support. For instance, a C5 burst fracture that exhibits no significant ventral spinal cord compression may

be managed with a dorsal stabilizing procedure. However, if there is enough ventral ligamentous and discal injury, a loss of anterior column height may occur (acutely or over time after a dorsal stabilization procedure), creating a kyphotic deformity. To avert such a problem, the surgeon may use a longer dorsal fusion construct incorporating more motion segments above and below the level of injury. Although this increased leverage may prevent an eventual kyphosis, it severely restricts mobility of the spine. Of course, the immobility would be more debilitating in the cervical or lumbar spine than in the thoracic spine. An alternative approach is to correct the ventral pathologic condition with a strut graft to restore anterior column height and alignment and to follow this with either ventral instrumentation across the affected segment or a shorter dorsal fusion construct.

## Deformity After Ventral Spinal Procedures

The most common ventral spinal procedures include discectomy and vertebrectomy for decompression at one or more levels. These procedures are often accompanied by a grafting procedure to provide support to the ventral spinal column and to establish a lattice for osteogenesis across the defect. Adjuncts such as instrumentation or external orthoses may also be used to enhance interim stability until fusion occurs. When deformity occurs after ventral spinal surgery, it typically manifests as a kyphosis that is often acutely angulated at its apex, in contrast to the round kyphosis usually observed after a multilevel laminectomy. However, if concurrent posterior column instability exists, a subluxation may also ensue. Coronal plane deformation (scoliosis) may occur as a result of asymmetric load sharing after a unilaterally focused surgical procedure. In general, deformity results from inadequate anterior column support after decompression, graft failure, pseudarthrosis, and nonunion or from unrecognized or poorly managed posterior column instability.

### Lack of Anterior Column Support

Because the primary force on the spine is axial loading and because the ventral spinal column bears the major load, removing a segment of this column and not replacing it with another supporting construct would not make sense. Failure to provide anterior column support after ventral spinal decompression may contribute to a kyphotic deformity (either immediate or delayed). Even after simple ventral discectomy, a strut should be considered, at least to preserve the load-sharing responsibilities of the anterior column and to preserve normal spinal alignment.

### Graft Failure

Graft failure can occur in the form of fracture, collapse, extrusion, and resorption. The integrity of a graft construct depends on the type, source, shape, and length of the graft; the graft juncture with adjacent vertebral bodies; the graft's intended purpose; the coexistence of posterior column instability; and the adequacy of construct immobilization (i.e., either an external orthosis, concomitant instrumentation, or no additional support) until fusion takes place.

Except for situations in which the patient is not expected to survive until fusion takes place, an osseous strut graft should be used where a spacer is necessary. Nonosseous constructs (e.g., methylmethacrylate) are doomed to eventual mechanical failure, leading to instability and deformity. Constructs that use inert lattices (e.g., titanium cages, bioabsorbable composites) to provide strength, in which interstices are filled with and incorporate bone, may become a useful alternative to a standard corticocancellous strut graft.

An osseous strut graft can be crafted from autologous or allogenic bone. The strength of either may vary depending on the condition of the donor and on the harvesting and processing methods. For example, choosing an autograft from osteoporotic bone is unwise. An iliac crest autograft that is harvested with an oscillating saw is stronger under axial compression loads than is an autograft harvested with an osteotome.[37] An allograft specimen must be carefully selected, because the strength can vary depending on the inherent quality of the donor bone and on the processing and sterilization methods. Zdeblick and Ducker[97] reported a 30% graft collapse rate with freeze-dried allograft compared with a 5% collapse rate with autograft for ventral cervical fusions. The biomechanics literature is controversial regarding any differences in the immediate strength of autograft versus allograft. The choice should probably be based more on graft availability, graft incorporation times, potential infection and immune-reaction risks, and possible donor site complications rather than on differences in immediate postoperative strength.

Common and acceptable autograft donor sites include rib, iliac crest, and fibula. Allograft is available from these sites, as well as from tibia and femur.[10,50,51,99] Each type of graft has been used in certain areas of the spine, depending on the clinical situation.

The rib is a convenient autograft source during ventral thoracic procedures,[22] but its use should be limited to short-segment struts in the thoracic region because of its relative weakness compared with the other sources. Numerous reports attest to the rib graft's propensity to fracture, collapse, or resorb.[6,35,39,78] However, multiple parallel rib grafts may be used to enhance the strength of the construct. The rib's gentle curve also conforms to the natural thoracic kyphosis.

The iliac crest is the most common source of ventral intervertebral graft for use in the cervical spine. It is also used in the thoracic and lumbar regions over short segments. The iliac crest graft's strength is maximal when it is fashioned as a tricortical strut (e.g., a Smith-Robinson graft). The tricortical graft is preferable to the dowel graft because the tricortical graft is less likely to collapse. The dowel-shaped iliac crest graft, popularized by Cloward,[13] has the greatest propensity to collapse, the incidence being 60% in one series.[29] This collapse results in kyphotic angulation, especially if multilevel interbody fusions are performed. The potential for collapse is minimized by fashioning a tricortical graft and countersinking the graft 2mm below the ventral cortex of the adjacent end plates.[9] The incidence of iliac crest graft extrusion was 2% in several series.[19,66,87] If the extrusion is minimal, fusion may still take place without surgical intervention, although it may be delayed. Only if extrusion is complete, impinges on

adjacent vital structures, or causes a deformity is reoperation necessary. Often, iliac crest graft may be limited to constructs up to three cervical segments in length because of the curvature of the iliac crest and the strength limitations imposed by these lengths.

The fibula has often been used as a strut graft in the cervical spine. The advantages of fibula grafts are that they are stronger in compression and are available in greater lengths. The main disadvantages of fibula grafts are the longer incorporation times (up to 12 to 24 months) and the high incidence (19%) of donor site complications when autologous fibula is used. Fibula graft extrusion rates have been less than 2% in several series.[20,23,25] An additional concern is the potential for the fibula graft to telescope into the adjacent vertebral body. This phenomenon is probably caused by a combination of the dissimilarity in bone density between the fibula and the vertebral body and the manner in which the graft junction is prepared. For example, older patients with osteoporotic vertebrae are especially prone to telescoping struts because the grafts tend to be harvested from younger donors with bone of higher density. When a given axial load is applied across a graft-vertebral interface, presuming the surface areas are similar, the two surfaces should exert equal and opposite forces on each other. If the load is increased, the bone surface with the lower density will fail first. This situation is also encountered when overaggressive preparation of the vertebral body results in removal of not only the cartilaginous end plate but also of the entire dense bone surface, such that the graft is resting solely on the less dense cancellous bone.

### Fusion Rates of Ventral Constructs

Iliac crest graft fusion rates are directly related to the number of ventral interbody fusion levels. Using autograft, Robinson et al.[67] achieved 94% union for one-level fusions, 73% for two-level fusions, and 50% for three-level fusions. Others have demonstrated similar results with autograft.[4,16,66,87,97] The iliac crest donor site complication rate is 2% to 20%.[88,97] Zdeblick and Ducker[97] reported the use of freeze-dried iliac crest allograft for this purpose and found a union rate of 95% for single-level fusions but a rate of only 38% for two-level fusions. Despite a respectable one-level fusion rate for freeze-dried iliac crest allograft, several reports indicate a higher graft collapse rate compared with autograft. Although graft collapse that results in a mild kyphosis ultimately may not affect the clinical outcome in this situation, it defeats the purpose of reestablishing normal anatomic disc and foraminal height, as well as anatomic alignment.

Therefore autologous bone is preferred by many surgeons for interbody fusion. Unless the disease is limited strictly to the area immediately at or adjacent to the disc spaces in a multilevel process, corpectomies with a single bridging strut graft may be preferable. If three or more vertebral levels are spanned, a fibula allograft (rather than iliac crest autograft) becomes increasingly appealing.

A modification of the Smith-Robinson technique involves using a shallow, slotted mortise-and-tenon joint rostrally and a modified, stopped dado joint caudally to seat the graft (see Figure 152.1). The cartilaginous end plates are burred to enhance fusion. Care is taken to not create too deep a trough to minimize the risk of the graft's gradual settling into the cancellous portion of the adjacent vertebral bodies. The prepared host sites are ordinarily centered on the ends of the vertebrae. In cases in which the strut graft is used to treat an existing kyphosis, the graft is placed more ventrally to obtain a greater mechanical advantage in resisting progressive deformity.

When freeze-dried fibula allograft is used in multilevel ventral cervical discectomy and interbody fusion, a partial or complete union rate of 92% within 6 months has been reported. Of the fusions, 100% were stable on flexion-extension radiographs at 8 weeks.[25] In a retrospective review of a comparison between allograft and autograft notched fibula struts for multilevel corpectomy cases, Fernyhough et al.[23] found a 27% nonunion rate for the autograft and a 41% rate for the allograft. A direct correlation existed between the fusion length and the nonunion rate, regardless of whether allograft or autograft was used. In addition, the rostral junction was more likely to develop nonunion (69%) than was the caudal junction (39%). Although the procedure is much more tedious and time-consuming, free vascularized fibula autografts have been used with ventral cervical procedures and have achieved 100% fusion rates, with union occurring within 2.5 to 5 months.[20]

Because of the relatively high donor site complication rate from fibula harvest and because of the readily available supply of allograft, fibula allograft is most commonly used for ventral cervical struts that span three or more vertebral levels. Fibula allograft is also used periodically in the cervical, thoracic, and lumbar regions for the management of kyphosis. The graft-vertebral junction is fashioned in a manner similar to that of iliac crest graft constructs. The hollow central portion of the fibula is filled with corticocancellous paste that is collected and saved during the corpectomy. Because there is no convincing evidence that instrumentation makes a significant difference in the union rate, ventral plating is not universally necessary unless the graft fit is imperfect, making the risk of extrusion unacceptable. If graft extrusion occurs, it tends to do so within 72 hours. Therefore the patient may be observed closely for that period and is then sent home with instructions to wear a firm cervical collar until follow-up radiographs reveal that bone union has occurred.

## Ventral Surgery in the Presence of Dorsal Spinal Instability

Loss of correction of alignment after a ventral decompression and grafting procedure is often secondary to graft failure. However, despite a well-constructed and well-placed strut graft, a deformity may still develop if the surgical plan did not account for posterior column instability. This is most evident in the management of trauma. In spinal trauma, injuries to both the anterior and the posterior column are often present. Ventral surgery is common in the management of spine trauma, especially for decompressing vertebral fracture fragments and traumatic disc herniations. Strut grafts are placed at the site of decompression for reestablishing alignment and providing stability. However, the incidence of postoperative deformity after ventral decompression and grafting in the setting of

trauma is as much as five times greater than in the same surgery performed for degenerative disease.[13] Of the early studies warning of this complication,[8,48,75] the one by Bell and Bailey[8] reports a 58% mechanical complication rate that included graft extrusion, spinal redislocation, and nonunion resulting in kyphosis (average of 21 degrees). Dorsal instability was present in 92% of the cases that had a mechanical complication.

This example clearly demonstrates that when ventral spinal surgery is undertaken, concomitant dorsal instability must be anticipated, recognized, and appropriately managed to avoid a likely postoperative deformity. Additional measures may include supplemental ventral instrumentation or a subsequent dorsal procedure to address the dorsal instability directly. From a biomechanical standpoint, the latter approach is the most logical. However, the extra time, potential morbidity, and cost of a second surgical procedure have prompted some surgeons to rely solely on supplemental ventral instrumentation in lieu of additional dorsal surgery. Clinical experience with ventral cervical plating in this situation has given this approach some merit.

## Deformity after Instrumentation Failure

Although it is not the scope of this chapter to review the specific implications of failure of individual instrumentation systems, general concepts regarding implant failure and its consequences deserve mention here.

There is no biomechanical model for testing instrumentation fatigue that approximates the actual conditions the implants experience in vivo. Therefore the possibility and timing of implant failure cannot be predicted. However, a widely known and long-held dictum is that all spinal instrumentation eventually fails. This seems to be true in the absence of fusion across the instrumented motion segments. The consequences of this failure depend on the intended purpose of the implant and on the timing of the failure with respect to the timing of fusion. For example, the "rod long–fuse short" concept may obligate the surgeon to remove the hardware at a point after the intended short segment has fused but before the longer segmental instrumentation has failed. Ideally, the fusion occurs before the instrumentation fails; otherwise, deformity may occur across the site of the intended fusion.

Failure of instrumentation may be a reflection of a surgeon's skill or judgment. It is vital for surgeons to be completely familiar with the instrumentation they plan to use. This implies not only technical skill in placing the implant, but more importantly, an understanding of the situations in which the implant should or should not be used. Placing unreasonable demands on the implant serves only to hasten eventual failure. For example, to expect rigid purchase of an implant in severely osteoporotic bone is imprudent.

To encourage implant fusion when instrumentation is used, surgeons should take as much care in preparing the bone graft and host site as they spend on placing the implant. When an implant succumbs before the onset of a solid fusion, the result is mechanical pain, spinal deformity, or a combination of both. If deformity occurs, neurologic deficits may ensue. The deformity is usually the same as that which the original surgery was designed to prevent or treat. In any case, the management of failed instrumentation is usually surgical.

Although a failed implant without obvious deformity is usually a telltale sign of a pseudarthrosis or nonunion, occasionally there is no radiographic evidence of a malunion. In this situation, if a patient is symptomatic, the clinician should presume that a pseudarthrosis exists. Symptomatic improvement with a trial of external bracing may help confirm this suspicion. If this is so, a decision must be made regarding a reoperation, because conservative management rarely leads to eventual fusion of an existing pseudarthrosis. In the presence of a solid fusion and in the absence of symptoms, failed instrumentation can be either left in place or removed, depending on the propensity for any of the loose components to erode through the skin or surrounding vital structures or to impinge on the spinal cord or nerve roots.

## Postfusion Degenerative Changes and Hypermobility of Adjacent Motion Segments

The literature comprises remarkably few reports describing changes that may occur in motion segments adjacent to a fusion in the cervical spine. From a biomechanical perspective, hypermobility might be expected to develop in these segments, because stress is shifted to adjacent motion segments after fusion of a segment. The increased motion theoretically translates into accelerated degenerative changes at the adjacent levels, compared with nonadjacent levels. Hunter et al.[31] followed nine patients for 7 to 15 years and found that eight of these patients had radiographic evidence of increased degenerative disease at adjacent levels (primarily in segments below the fusion) compared with nonadjacent levels. The clinical significance of these degenerative changes was not discussed. It is also not known whether these changes were in response to the altered mechanical forces on the joints adjacent to the fused segment or whether they were part of the natural progression of the degenerative disease process.

The only other study on this subject in the cervical spine[49] found that in 60 patients (101 adjacent motion segments and 134 nonadjacent segments), 10% of the adjacent motion segments and 4% of the nonadjacent motion segments developed degenerative changes during an average 3.9-year follow-up. Compared with historical controls, nonfused segments in these patients were affected by degenerative disease at a rate approximately equal to that in the general population. In addition, no hypermobility was found in any nonfused segment after evaluation with flexion-extension radiographs.

Degenerative changes in adjacent segments after lumbar fusion have received more attention in the literature. Biomechanical studies reveal that lumbar fusion induces increased stress at the adjacent segment.[47,93] The incidence of adjacent lumbar segment degeneration requiring surgical intervention is approximately 2%.[24] After lumbar fusion, the incidence of adjacent segment hypertrophic facet disease is 89%; of spinal stenosis, 44%; of severe disc degeneration, 28%; of degenerative spondylolisthesis, 11%; and of disc herniation, 0%.[46] The average time from initial fusion to onset of symptoms relating to adjacent segment abnormalities is 8.5 years.

In their review of patients who underwent operative management of the degenerated segment adjacent to a lumbar fusion, Whitecloud et al.[89] found the average interval between first fusion and operative treatment of the adjacent segment to be 11.5 years. All these patients failed conservative management and underwent spinal decompression and fusion. A pseudarthrosis rate of 80% was found in patients whose operative treatment of the adjacent segment included fusion without instrumentation versus a 17% rate when instrumentation was used. The overall rate of good results was 36% and of fair or poor results, was 64%. Poor prognostic factors included advanced osteoporosis and a short symptom-free period (less than 3 years) after the initial fusion.

Although there appears to be a high incidence of radiographic changes at adjacent segments in a lumbar fusion, the percentage of symptomatic patients who fail conservative treatment and ultimately require an operation is low. The operative treatment is met with significant complications and poor results. When an operation is necessary, decompression followed by fusion with instrumentation is best.

## Prevention of Postoperative Spinal Deformity

Prevention of a postoperative spinal deformity should be one of the primary objectives of a spine surgeon when he or she is seeking to avoid complications and to optimize outcome. As discussed in previous sections, knowledge and practice of sound biomechanical and clinical principles of spine surgery provide the framework for these goals. However, the keys to successful prevention of a postoperative spinal deformity are thorough preoperative evaluation and operative planning. Emphasis should be placed on each of the following considerations: (1) necessity versus risk for the operation, (2) appropriate and adequate neural decompression, (3) necessity of operative stabilization with bone graft or instrumentation, (4) selection of bone graft material, (5) choice of instrumentation, (6) choice of postoperative orthosis, and (7) adequate clinical and radiographic follow-up.

One of the most important challenges surgeons face is to identify patients who will benefit maximally from an operation while incurring minimum risk. This requires surgeons to be realistic and honest in their expectations and to be able to convey this clearly to the patient. Such advance communication helps ameliorate the dismay of a patient who indeed develops a kyphotic deformity after a seemingly good operation.

Most spinal operations require some degree of bone removal for purposes of exposure or decompression of the neural elements. Concern regarding the destabilization of the spine resulting from this bone removal should not overshadow the importance of achieving adequate exposure or adequate decompression of the neural elements. As long as the surgeon recognizes that the threshold for spinal stability and potential deformity has been crossed in the course of the operation and as long as appropriate contingency plans have been made, postoperative deformity can be avoided.

It is imperative for the surgeon to anticipate the need for intraoperative spinal stabilization and to preoperatively choose the appropriate graft materials and instrumentation for that particular situation. Lack of such advance planning may prompt the surgeon to use immediately available but less appropriate materials for the operation, thereby potentially exposing the patient to an increased risk for deformity.

In addition, part of the preoperative planning is the decision to use external bracing postoperatively. There are many circumstances in which bracing is a useful adjunct for enhancing immediate postoperative stability. Knowledge of the variety of orthoses available is essential so that the advantages of a particular orthotic device can be matched to the needs of the postoperative patient. Access to an orthotist is beneficial when a customized brace is needed or when the fit of a commercial orthosis needs to be adjusted.

The purpose of using external orthoses postoperatively is twofold: (1) to provide comfort and support for the spine in a normal posture while soft tissue is healing (e.g., while the paraspinal musculature is recovering and returning to its supportive role) and (2) to aid in spinal immobilization while any graft material placed during surgery is beginning to incorporate new bone and to acquire subsequent intrinsic stability. Even when these end points are achieved and the brace is removed, deformity can develop later in the postoperative course. External bracing is not a substitute for internal spinal stabilization when gross instability exists or when significant deformity is likely after a given surgical procedure. Although spinal orthoses are used as corrective devices for many types of scoliotic and kyphotic deformities, they have not been overwhelmingly successful in correcting postoperative deformity.

Care of spine surgery patients does not end when they leave the hospital with an orthosis. Diligent postoperative follow-up for an appropriate period is mandatory for several reasons. In addition to observing the progress of the patient's symptoms, neurologic status, wound healing, and the fusion process, the surgeon must watch for signs or symptoms of a progressive deformity. Early recognition of a developing postoperative deformity is the next best course of action after prevention of one. Clearly, the consequences of managing a deformity early in its progression are fewer than if intervention is accomplished in the later stages.

## Management of Postoperative Spinal Deformity

The most vigilant preoperative measures cannot ensure that all postoperative deformities will be prevented; therefore it is necessary to recognize and manage these deformities on a timely basis when they occur. Once a deformity is identified, the question is not whether to intervene, but how to intervene. A conservative approach or a more aggressive surgical approach may be indicated.

Conservative intervention for postoperative spinal deformity is appropriate only for situations in which the deformity is recognized early and is mild and the symptoms are minimal. In these cases, a trial of external bracing, physical therapy, and mild analgesics may be beneficial. The development of postlaminectomy kyphosis in children is an example of a situation in which early recognition, followed immediately by postoperative bracing, may prevent progression of the deformity. Some clinical and biomechanical evidence indicates that using a cervicothoracolumbosacral orthosis or a thoracolumbosacral orthosis to treat thoracic kyphosis in young patients will correct the deformity.[54] The biomechanical effect of this bracing technique is continuous axial spine distraction concurrent with three-point sagittal plane bending at the apex and the extremes of the kyphosis. This corrects the abnormal curvature through biomechanical adaptation of the growing spine. However, this mixed patient population includes those with traumatic and congenital kyphosis. Therefore similar results may not be exhibited by patients with postoperative deformity. Nevertheless, when progression of the deformity has been documented during conservative therapy, operative intervention is required to arrest and correct the postoperative spinal deformity.

Flat back syndrome is another condition for which conservative therapy is initially preferred. Its surgical management is fraught with such poor outcomes and such significant complications that every effort is made initially to treat this condition conservatively. Unlike progressive deformities, flat back syndrome is typically a "static" deformity, and operative intervention can be delayed until a full trial of conservative treatment has been exhausted.

Whereas nonoperative management of postoperative spinal deformities ideally serves to arrest the progression of deformity, only operative intervention has the potential for reversing or correcting the deformity. If the deformity is significant enough to have caused symptomatic neural compression, operative decompression is the only alternative. Other operative indications for postoperative spinal deformity include impairment of vital functions (namely, pulmonary or cardiac functions), jeopardy of spinal stability and balance, intractable pain, and functional debilitation. Once the decision is made to treat a postoperative deformity surgically, the surgeon must decide how it will be approached.

The decision to approach a deformity ventrally, dorsally, or from both directions depends on the region of the spine involved, the type of deformity, the need for neural decompression, the need for osteotomies to release a fixed curvature, and the appropriate graft/instrumentation construct for the type of deformity present. Of course, a unidirectional approach that addresses all of these issues is preferable.

As stated previously, except in the lumbar spine, the most common type of postoperative deformity is a kyphosis. Iatrogenic spondylolisthesis and flat back may be more common in the lumbar spine. Management of symptomatic lumbar iatrogenic spondylolisthesis requires dorsal neural decompression and dorsolateral fusion with autologous bone graft and short-segment pedicle fixation followed with a postoperative lumbosacral orthosis. Operative management of flat back syndrome has been discussed briefly in a previous section.

The same basic principles of surgical correction of kyphotic deformity can be used in the cervical, thoracic, and lumbar regions. Regardless of the approach, the more severe the deformity, the less likely the successful correction of the deformity. This reflects the need to intervene early. In general, a mild kyphosis may be approached dorsally alone. A more severe kyphosis requires ventral surgery, either alone or in combination with dorsal surgery.

One of the first surgical goals is to achieve neural decompression. The compression is usually located ventrally and is typically caused by an acute kyphotic angulation of the vertebral bodies over which the spinal cord is stretched. One or more corpectomies at the apex of the kyphosis aid in spinal cord decompression. Distraction of the spinal cord (e.g., by using excessive spinal traction or by attempting to correct the deformity, especially with distraction instrumentation) over a ventrally compressive lesion (i.e., acute-angle kyphosis) will likely lead to worsening neurologic deficits. Therefore the spinal cord must be decompressed before the deformity is corrected.

The next step is to reestablish spinal balance by correcting the abnormal curvature to the maximal degree possible. This may be as simple as placing a ventral strut graft across a distracted vertebrectomy site or as complex as requiring both ventral release (e.g., sectioning of the ventral longitudinal ligament or ventral discectomy) and dorsal osteotomy, followed by grafting and instrumentation to maintain the correction until fusion occurs. Again, the more severe and longstanding the kyphosis, the more radical the surgery needed to achieve correction.

Despite the feasibility of correcting a kyphotic deformity, correction may not be realistic in a patient who cannot withstand the rigorous surgery. In addition, severe complications of a radical correction of deformity, including aortic rupture and superior mesenteric artery syndrome, are not rare. In these cases, it is desirable at least to arrest the progression of the deformity by stabilizing across the deformity with bone graft and instrumentation.

When correcting a kyphosis, the surgeon must reduce the bending moment of the kyphosis by creating an axial distractive force across the involved segments in concert with three-point sagittal loading. Again, before distractive forces are applied, neural decompression must first be completed. Desired correctional forces can be achieved by manual application; traction devices; or instrumentation such as the combined use of Harrington compression and distraction rods, Schanz screws, and other devices that can take advantage of the "hinge principle," as described by O'Brien,[58] for correction of tuberculous kyphosis. The dorsal bony elements, dorsal ligaments, or anterior longitudinal ligament may serve as the hinge about which correction of the kyphosis occurs. The biomechanical effects are the same as those described earlier regarding the function of certain external braces (e.g., cervicothoracolumbosacral orthosis, Milwaukee brace). Ventral releases or dorsal osteotomies may be necessary before correctional bending moments are created.

To maintain the correction achieved with these maneuvers, surgeons must achieve ventral or dorsal stabilization with graft and instrumentation. When ventral releases or ventral decompressions are used, ventral strut grafts are commonly placed as spacers or bridges. The appropriate placement of these struts is important. To counteract the sagittal plane flexion bending moment (axial rotation) in a kyphotic deformity, the strut graft must be positioned as far ventral to the IAR or neutral axis as possible. To repair a short, angulated kyphosis, a single one-level strut graft at the ventral aspect of vertebral bodies at the apex may be sufficient. When the kyphosis is severe and involves many motion segments, two struts may be placed, one being longer and at a greater distance from the neutral axis than the other. Two struts are used, because despite the greater leverage of the longer, more distant strut, it has a greater likelihood of buckling and of interfering with vital structures, and it has a lower fusion rate. With biomechanical adaptation, the two struts share equal loads. In certain situations, a ventral plating system may be used to add additional immediate postoperative spinal stability and perhaps to obviate the need for additional dorsal surgery.

When correction of a kyphotic deformity is being maintained from a dorsal approach, the whole length of the kyphosis must be incorporated in the grafting and instrumentation. If not, the spine tends to lose correction over time because of the return of the flexion bending moment. This happens because of the relatively short length of the graft instrumentation, which lacks the leverage to counteract the bending moment.

No single surgical approach for kyphotic deformity has been shown to have a clear advantage. However, for moderate to severe cases, there is a trend toward using a combined ventral and dorsal approach, either at the same or at separate settings. The maintenance of the correction and the fusion rates may be better with this 360-degree approach.

## Summary

As the field of spinal biomechanics matures, as instrumentation and biomaterial technology advances, as the biology of bone healing becomes more completely understood, and as clinical experience is gained, there will undoubtedly be revisions of the strategies a spine surgeon should follow when confronted with a postoperative deformity. All spine surgeons, even the most talented, will encounter postoperative deformity as a surgical complication, and therefore postoperative deformity must be recognized and managed early in its course. Because the outcome of deformity correction is usually less than satisfactory, the most prudent surgeons are those who plan the treatment of a spinal disorder such that avoidance of complications is one of their foremost and fundamental objectives.

## REFERENCES

1. Abbott R, Feldstein N, Wisoff JH, Epstein FJ: Osteoplastic laminotomy in children. *Pediatr Neurosurg* 18:153, 1992.
2. Aboulker J, Metzger J, David M, *et al:* Les myelopathies cervicales d'origine rachidienne. *Neurochirurgie* 11:88, 1965.
3. Alsharif H, Ezzat SH, Hay A, *et al:* The results of surgical treatment of spondylotic radiculomyelopathy with complete cervical laminectomy and posterior foramen magnum decompression. *Acta Neurochir (Wien)* 48:83, 1979.
4. Aronson N, Filtzer DL, Bagan M: Anterior cervical fusion by the Smith-Robinson approach. *J Neurosurg* 29:397, 1968.
5. Aryanpur J, Ducker T: Multilevel lumbar laminotomies: An alternative to laminectomy in the treatment of lumbar stenosis. *Neurosurgery* 26:429, 1990.
6. Bailey HL, Gabriel M, Hodgson AR, Shin JS: Tuberculosis of the spine in children. *J Bone Joint Surg* 54A:1633, 1972.

7. Bell DF, Walder JL, O'Connor G, Tibshirani R: Spinal deformity after multi-level cervical laminectomy in children. *Spine* 19:406, 1994.

8. Bell GD, Bailey SI: Anterior cervical fusion for trauma. *Clin Orthop* 128:155, 1977.

9. Berchuck M, Garfin SR, Bauman T, Abitbol JJ: Complications of anterior intervertebral grafting. *Clin Orthop* 284:54, 1992.

10. Binazzi R, Po F: Sequestration of tibial cortical graft 25 years after posterior spine fusion using the Albee technique. *Spine* 11:61, 1986.

11. Bishara SN: The posterior operation in the treatment of cervical spondylosis with myelopathy: A long term followup study. *J Neurol Neurosurg Psychiatr* 13:393, 1971.

12. Callahan RA, Johnson RM, Margolis RN, et al: Cervical facet fusion for control of instability following laminectomy. *J Bone Joint Surg* 59A:991, 1977.

13. Cloward RB: Treatment of acute fractures and fracture dislocations of the cervical spine by vertebral body fusion. *J Neurosurg* 18:201, 1961.

14. Cummine JL, Lonstein JE, Moe JH, et al: Reconstructive surgery in the adult for failed scoliosis fusion. *J Bone Joint Surg* 61A:1151, 1979.

15. Cusick JF, Yoganandan N, Pintar F, et al: Biomechanics of cervical spine facetectomy and fixation techniques. *Spine* 13:808, 1988.

16. DePalma AF, Rothman RH, Lewinnek GE, Canale ST: Anterior interbody fusion for severe disc degeneration. *Surg Gynecol Obstet* 134:755, 1972.

17. Detrich M, Kurowski P: The importance of mechanical factors in the etiology of spondylolisthesis. *Spine* 10:532, 1985.

18. Doherty JH: Complications of fusion in lumbar scoliosis. Proceedings of the Scoliosis Research Society. *J Bone Joint Surg* 55A:438, 1973.

19. Dohn DF: Anterior interbody fusion for treatment of cervical disc condition. *JAMA* 179:897, 1966.

20. Doi K, Kawai S, Sumiura S, Sakai K: Anterior cervical fusion using the free vascularized fibular graft. *Spine* 13:1239, 1988.

21. Epstein JA, Janin Y, Carras R, Lavine LS: A comparative study of the treatment of cervical spondylotic myeloradiculopathy: Experience with 50 cases treated by means of extensive laminectomy, foraminotomy and excision of osteophytes during the past 10 years. *Acta Neurochir (Wien)* 61:89, 1982.

22. Fang HSY, Ong GB, Hodgson AR: Anterior spinal fusion: The operative approaches. *Clin Orthop* 35:16, 1964.

23. Fernyhough JC, White JI, LaRocca H: Fusion rates in multilevel cervical spondylosis comparing allograft fibula with autograft fibula in 126 patients. *Spine* 16(Suppl):561, 1991.

24. Frymoyer JW, Hanley E, Howe J, et al: Disc excision and spine fusion in the management of lumbar disc disease: A minimum ten-year follow-up. *Spine* 3:1, 1978.

25. Grossman W, Peppelman WC, Baum JA, Kraus DR: The use of freeze-dried fibular allograft in anterior cervical fusion. *Spine* 17:565, 1992.

26. Hattori S: Cervical myelopathy. *J Jpn Orthop Assoc* 52:581, 1978.

27. Herkowitz HN: A comparison of anterior cervical fusion, cervical laminectomy, and cervical laminoplasty for the surgical management of multiple level spondylotic radiculopathy. *Spine* 13:774, 1988.

28. Hirabayashi K, Watanabe K, Wakano K, et al: Expansive open-door laminoplasty for cervical spinal stenotic myelopathy. *Spine* 8:693, 1983.

29. Horwitz WH, Rizzoli HV: *Postoperative Complications in Neurosurgical Practice.* Baltimore, Williams & Wilkins, 1967.

30. Hukuda S, Ogata M, Mochizuki T, Shichikawa K: Laminectomy versus laminoplasty for cervical myelopathy. Brief report. *J Bone Joint Surg* 70B:325, 1988.

31. Hunter LY, Braunstein EM, Bailey RW: Radiographic changes following anterior cervical fusion. *Spine* 5:399, 1980.

32. Ishida Y, Suzuki K, Ohmori K, et al: Critical analysis of extensive cervical laminectomy. *Neurosurgery* 24:215, 1989.

33. Itoh T, Tsuji H: Technical improvements and results of laminoplasty for compressive myelopathy in the cervical spine. *Spine* 10:729, 1985.

34. Jenkins DHR: Extensive cervical laminectomy: Long-term results. *Br J Surg* 60:652, 1973.

35. Jenkins DHR, Hodgson AR, Yau ACM, et al: Stabilization of the spine in surgical treatment of severe spinal tuberculosis in children. *Clin Orthop* 110:69, 1975.

36. Johnsson KE, Willner S, Johnsson K: Postoperative instability after decompression for lumbar spinal stenosis. *Spine* 11:107, 1986.

37. Jones AAM, Dougherty PJ, Sharkey NA, Benson DR: Iliac crest bone graft: Osteotome versus saw. *Spine* 18:2048, 1993.

38. Katsumi Y, Honma T, Nakamura T: Analysis of cervical instability resulting from laminectomies for removal of spinal cord tumor. *Spine* 14:1171, 1989.

39. Kemp HBS, Jackson JW, Jeremiah JD, Cook J: Anterior fusion of the spine for infective lesions in adults. *J Bone Joint Surg* 55B:715, 1973.

40. Kostuik JP, Errico TJ, Gleason TF: Techniques of internal fixation for degenerative conditions of the lumbar spine. *Clin Orthop* 203:219, 1986.

41. Kostuik JP, Hall BB: Spinal fusions to the sacrum in adults with scoliosis. *Spine* 8:489, 1983.

42. Kuniyoshi A, Panjabi MM, Kramer KM: Biomechanical evaluation of lumbar spinal stability after graded facetectomies. *Spine* 15:1142, 1990.

43. Kurokawa T, Tsuyama N, Tanaka H, et al: Enlargement of spinal canal by sagittal splitting of spinous process. *Bessatsu Seikeigeka (Jpn)* 2:234, 1982.

44. Lagrone MO, Bradford DS, Moe JH, et al: Treatment of symptomatic flatback after spinal fusion. *J Bone Joint Surg* 70A:569, 1988.

45. Lee CK: Lumbar spinal instability (olisthesis) after extensive posterior spinal decompression. *Spine* 8:429, 1983.

46. Lee CK: Accelerated degeneration of the segment adjacent to a lumbar fusion. *Spine* 13:375, 1988.

47. Lee CK, Langrana NA: Lumbosacral spinal fusion: A biomechanical study. *Spine* 9:574, 1984.

48. MacNab I: Complications of anterior cervical fusion. *Orthop Rev* 1:29, 1973.

49. Mahring M: Segment changes in the cervical spine following cervical spondylodeses of unstable injuries. *Unfallchirurgie* 14:247, 1988.

50. Malinin TI, Rosomoff HL, Sutton CH: Human cadaver femoral head homografts for anterior cervical spine fusions. *Surg Neurol* 7:249, 1977.

51. McBride GG, Bradford DS: Vertebral body replacement with femoral neck allograft and vascularized rib strut graft. *Spine* 8:406, 1983.

52. Mikawa Y, Shikata J, Yamamuro T: Spinal deformity and instability after multilevel cervical laminectomy. *Spine* 12:6, 1987.

53. Miyazaki K, Tada K, Matsuda Y: Posterior extensive simultaneous multisegment decompression with posterolateral fusion for cervical myelopathy with cervical instability and kyphotic and/or S-shaped deformities. *Spine* 14:1160, 1989.

54. Nachemson AL: Orthotic treatment for injuries and disease of the spinal column. In *Physical Medicine and Rehabilitation: State-of-the-Art Reviews*, vol 1. Philadelphia, Hanley & Belfus, 1987, p 11.

55. Nakano N, Nakano T, Nakano K: Comparison of the results of laminectomy and open door laminoplasty for cervical spondylotic myeloradiculopathy and ossification of the posterior longitudinal ligament. *Spine* 13:792, 1988.

56. Natelson SE: The injudicious laminectomy. *Spine* 11:966, 1986.

57. Nowinski GP, Visarius H, Nolte LP, *et al:* A biomechanical comparison of cervical laminaplasty and cervical laminectomy with progressive facetectomy. *Spine* 18:1995, 1993.

58. O'Brien JP: The halo-pelvic apparatus. A clinical, bio-engineering and anatomical study. *Acta Orthop Scand Suppl* 163:1, 1975.

59. Panjabi MM, White AA III, Johnson RM: Cervical spine mechanics as a function of transection of its components. *J Biomech* 8:327, 1975.

60. Paraicz E: Laminectomy or laminotomy? *Zentralbl Neurochir* 48:327, 1987.

61. Pelker RR, Friedlaender GE: Biomechanical aspects of bone autografts and allografts. *Orthop Clin North Am* 18:235, 1987.

62. Pintar FA, Cusick JF, Yoganandan N, *et al:* Biomechanics of lumbar facetectomy under compression-flexion. *Spine* 17:805, 1992.

63. Posner I, White AA III, Edwards WT, Hayes WC: A biomechanical analysis of clinical stability of the lumbar and lumbo-sacral spine. *Spine* 7:374, 1982.

64. Raimondi AJ, Gutierrez FA, Di Rocco C: Laminotomy and total reconstruction of the posterior spinal arch for spinal canal surgery in childhood. *J Neurosurg* 45:555, 1976.

65. Raynor RB, Pugh J, Shapiro I: Cervical facetectomy and its effect on spine strength. *J Neurosurg* 63:278, 1985.

66. Riley LH, Robinson RA, Johnson KA, Walker AE: The results of anterior interbody fusion of the cervical spine: Review of 93 consecutive cases. *J Neurosurg* 30:127, 1969.

67. Robinson RA, Walker AE, Ferlie DC, *et al:* The results of anterior interbody fusion of the cervical spine. *J Bone Joint Surg* 44A:1569, 1962.

68. Rogers L: The surgical treatment of cervical spondylotic myelopathy: Mobilization of the complete cervical cord into an enlarged canal. *J Bone Joint Surg* 43B:3, 1961.

69. Rolander SD: Motion of the lumbar spine with special reference to stabilizing effect of posterior fusion. *Acta Orthop Scand* 90(Suppl):1, 1966.

70. Roy-Camille R, Benazet JP: *Atlas of Orthopaedic Surgery.* Paris, Masson, 1989.

71. Shenkin HA, Hash CJ: Spondylolisthesis after multiple bilateral laminectomies and facetectomies for lumbar spondylosis: Follow-up review. *J Neurosurg* 50:45, 1979.

72. Shields CL, Stauffer ES: Late instability in cervical spine fractures secondary to laminectomy. *Clin Orthop* 119:144, 1976.

73. Shikata J, Yamamuro T, Shimizu K, Saito T: Combined laminoplasty and posterolateral fusion for spinal canal surgery in children and adolescents. *Clin Orthop* 259:92, 1990.

74. Simmons EH, Bhalla SK: Anterior cervical discectomy and fusion: A clinical and biomechanical study with eight-year followup. *J Bone Joint Surg* 51B:225, 1969.

75. Stauffer ES, Kelly EG: Fracture dislocations of the cervical spine. *J Bone Joint Surg* 59A:45, 1977.

76. Stauffer ES, Wood RW, Kelly EG: Gunshot wounds of the spine: The effects of laminectomy. *J Bone Joint Surg* 61A:389, 1979.

77. Stoops WL, King RB: Chronic myelopathy associated with cervical spondylosis. *JAMA* 192:281, 1965.

78. Streitz W, Brown JC, Bonnett CA: Anterior fibular strut grafting in the treatment of kyphosis. *Clin Orthop* 128:140, 1977.

79. Surin V, Hedelin E, Smith L: Degenerative lumbar spinal stenosis. *Acta Orthop Scand* 53:79, 1982.

80. Swank S, Lonstein JE, Moe JH, *et al:* Surgical treatment of adult scoliosis: A review of 222 cases. *J Bone Joint Surg* 63A:268, 1981.

81. Tomita K, Nomura S, Umeda S, Baba H: Cervical laminoplasty to enlarge the spinal canal in multilevel ossification of the posterior longitudinal ligament with myelopathy. *Arch Orthop Trauma Surg* 107:148, 1988.

82. Tsou PM: Progressive symptomatic lumbar spondylolisthesis after decompressive laminectomy for acquired degenerative stenosis. Presented at the annual meeting of American Academy of Orthopaedic Surgeons, Las Vegas, January, 1985.

83. White AA III, Hirsch C: An experimental study of the immediate load bearing capacity of some commonly used iliac bone grafts. *Acta Orthop Scand* 42:482, 1971.

84. White AA III, Hirsch C: The significance of the vertebral posterior elements in the mechanics of the thoracic spine. *Clin Orthop* 81:2, 1971.

85. White AA III, Panjabi MM: *Clinical Biomechanics of the Spine,* ed 2. Philadelphia, Lippincott-Raven, 1990.

86. White AA III, Panjabi MM, Thomas CL: The clinical biomechanics of kyphotic deformities. *Clin Orthop* 128:8, 1977.

87. White AA III, Southwick WO, Duponte RJ *et al:* Relief of pain by anterior cervical fusion for spondylosis: Report of sixty-five patients. *J Bone Joint Surg* 55A:525, 1973.

88. Whitecloud TS III: Complications of anterior cervical fusion. *Instr Course Lect* 27:223, 1976.

89. Whitecloud TS III, Davis JM, Olive PM: Operative treatment of the degenerated segment adjacent to a lumbar fusion. *Spine* 19:531, 1994.

90. Wiltse LL, Kirkaldy-Willis WH, McIvor GWD: The treatment of spinal stenosis. *Clin Orthop* 115:83, 1976.

91. Wittenberg RH, Moeller J, Shea M, *et al:* Compressive strength of autologous and allogenous bone grafts for

thoracolumbar and cervical spine fusion. *Spine* 15:1073, 1990.

92. Wolfinbarger L, Zhang Y, Adam BT, *et al:* A comprehensive study of physical parameters, biomechanical properties, and statistical correlations of iliac crest bone wedges used in spinal fusion surgery. II. Mechanical properties and correlation with physical parameters. *Spine* 19:284, 1994.

93. Yang SW, Langrana NA, Lee CK: Biomechanics of lumbosacral spinal fusion in combined compression-torsion loads. *Spine* 11:937, 1986.

94. Yasuoka S, Peterson HA, MacCarty CS: Incidence of spinal column deformity after multilevel laminectomy in children and adults. *J Neurosurg* 57:441, 1982.

95. Yoganandan N, Maiman DJ, Pintar FA, *et al:* Biomechanical effects of laminectomy on thoracic spine stability. *Neurosurgery* 32:604, 1993.

96. Yonenobu K, Okada K, Fuji T, *et al:* Causes of neurologic deterioration following surgical treatment of cervical myelopathy. *Spine* 11:818, 1986.

97. Zdeblick TA, Ducker TB: The use of freeze-dried allograft bone for anterior cervical fusions. *Spine* 16:726, 1991.

98. Zdeblick TA, Zou D, Warden KE *et al:* Cervical stability after foraminotomy: A biomechanical in vitro analysis. *J Bone Joint Surg* 74A:22, 1992.

99. Zeller RD, Ghanem I, Miladi L, Dubousset J: Posterior spinal fusion in neuromuscular scoliosis using a tibial strut graft: Results of a long-term follow-up. *Spine* 19:1628, 1994.

# CHAPTER 153

# Arachnoiditis

Robert F. Heary, Bruce E. Northrup,
and Giancarlo Barolat

Spinal arachnoiditis is a nonspecific inflammatory process; it affects the arachnoid layer of the leptomeninges surrounding the spinal cord or cauda equina. The precise cause of arachnoiditis is not clear. Often, multiple conditions coexist to lead to the syndrome of arachnoiditis. The clinical result varies widely, from patients who are mildly debilitated to those who are bed bound and devastated by this process. No uniformly successful treatment, either surgical or nonsurgical, exists for patients with arachnoiditis.

## Pathogenesis

The arachnoid is an avascular membrane that lies between two vascular membranes, the pia mater and the dura mater. A chronic infection or irritation can cause the arachnoid membrane to become thickened and adherent to both the dura mater and the pia mater.[26] The pia-arachnoid carries the blood vessels to the spinal cord, and this layer contains mesenchymal cells. In 1951, Smolik and Nash[34] recognized that when the outer arachnoid layer is injured, both the blood vessels and mesenchymal cells lend themselves to extensive proliferation. The ensuing reaction between the pia-arachnoid and the dura mater leads to obliterative arachnoiditis.[34] Arachnoiditis may affect the spinal cord or the cauda equina.

The pathogenesis of arachnoiditis is similar to the response of other serous membranes such as the peritoneum and pericardium. After the arachnoid layer is exposed to an insult, an inflammatory response that is characterized by a fibrinous exudate with a negligible inflammatory cellular exudate occurs together with neovascularization, leading to fibrosis.[7,27] When this process occurs at the level of the spinal cord, vascular occlusive changes occur that reduce the blood supply to the spinal cord.[19,21,26,32] The small perforating blood vessels that supply the outer portions of the white matter may be obliterated and result in necrosis and cavitation of the spinal cord parenchyma.[19,32] Furthermore, obliteration of the venous drainage of the spinal cord may occur.[32] Ransford and Harries[26] postulated that in addition to causing the embarrassment of the blood supply of the spinal cord, arachnoiditis may cause secondary changes as a result of frank mechanical compression of neural tissue or diminished cerebrospinal fluid (CSF) circulation.

In the first half of the twentieth century, arachnoiditis was most often attributed to infectious causes. This led to changes throughout the neuraxis. More recently, lumbar arachnoiditis of noninfectious origin has become more prevalent than arachnoiditis at the spinal cord level. Lumbar arachnoiditis affects the nerve roots at the level of the cauda equina. Therefore the majority of recent experimental studies on arachnoiditis have focused on the cauda equina region.

In a classic description of lumbosacral arachnoiditis, Burton[3] described three stages in its pathogenesis. The first stage, *radiculitis,* consists of an inflamed pia-arachnoid with associated hyperemia and swelling of the nerve roots of the cauda equina. In the second stage, *arachnoiditis,* a progression of fibroblast proliferation and collagen deposition occurs. During this stage, nerve root swelling decreases, and the nerve roots adhere to each other and to the pia-arachnoid. In the third and final stage, *adhesive arachnoiditis,* marked proliferation of the pia-arachnoid occurs, with dense collagen deposition within the thecal sac. There is complete nerve root encapsulation, as well as hypoxemia of the nerve roots and progressive nerve root atrophy.[3]

Yamagami et al.[36] induced experimental arachnoiditis at the level of the cauda equina in 105 rats. They found that the development of arachnoiditis and neural degeneration directly corresponded to the magnitude of extradural inflammation and wound healing processes that occurred after laminectomy with or without retained foreign bodies. These investigators postulated that a diminished nutritional supply may be responsible for the pathologic changes in arachnoiditis. Adhesions of the arachnoid cause the nerve roots of the cauda equina to lump together, and in so doing, these nerve roots are isolated from contact with the CSF, which results in both circulatory and nutritional disturbances in the nerve roots.[36] In another study, McLaurin et al.[21] induced experimental arachnoiditis in dogs. The adhesive arachnoiditis produced a nearly solid ring of dense collagenous tissue that extended from the pia to the dura. The vessels of the subarachnoid space were embedded in this fibrous tissue and appeared to be constricted by it.[21]

The end stage of arachnoiditis, adhesive arachnoiditis, is the stage most associated with significant clinical morbidity. In this stage, the nerve roots are completely covered with collagen and become an integral part of the dural membrane. The thecal sac can appear to be an empty tube devoid of identifiable nerve fibers.[4] Many of the nerve roots passing through these sclerotic meninges degenerate and become atrophic.[19] At this stage of arachnoiditis, a lumbar puncture or surgical opening of the dura mater may lead to sectioning of the atrophic nerve fibers.[4]

## Causes

The precise cause of spinal arachnoiditis is not known; nor are the incidence and prevalence of spinal arachnoiditis in the general population. There is a great discrepancy between the incidence of radiographic arachnoiditis and the much smaller incidence of clinical arachnoiditis. In this section, the various causes of clinical arachnoiditis are reviewed.

In 1978, Burton[3] noted that back pain may be the medical problem that has the greatest socioeconomic impact in the United States. He stated that the long-term failure rate of lumbar surgery is between 10% and 40%. In patients with intractable pain and functional incapacitation secondary to failed back surgery syndrome, arachnoiditis of some degree appeared to be a common finding.[3]

As stated previously, arachnoiditis was mainly of infectious origin in the first half of the twentieth century. The more common infections included syphilis, tuberculosis, and those caused by pyogenic bacteria.[4,9] Less common infectious causes include parasitic diseases[14] and viral meningitis.[16] These infectious causes are particularly important to differentiate from the noninfectious causes of arachnoiditis because, with the exception of viral meningitis, effective treatment is available for the arachnoiditis of infectious origin. However, despite adequate treatment of the causative infection, scarring of the arachnoid membrane may lead to permanent damage and arachnoiditis beyond the period when the infection has been "successfully" treated.

There are many noninfectious causes of spinal arachnoiditis. The two most commonly implicated causes in clinical studies include postsurgical arachnoiditis and post-myelographic arachnoiditis secondary to oil-based contrast medium. These two causes have been studied extensively and have fostered considerable scientific debate.

Iophendylate (Myodil, Pantopaque) is an oil-based contrast medium used in diagnostic myelograms. Iophendylate was first used in the United States in 1944, and its usage continued for 40 years. In Sweden, iophendylate was banned from clinical use in 1948 secondary to animal studies that identified it as a causative agent for arachnoiditis.[4] Because of medicolegal concerns in the United States, at the conclusion of a myelogram, the iophendylate (Pantopaque) is removed from the intrathecal space by aspiration. Often, this removal process is not entirely successful, and in fact, may produce further trauma and cause bleeding into the CSF.[26] Despite these shortcomings, iophendylate (Pantopaque) myelography was performed on approximately 400,000 patients per year in the United States from 1944 until the 1980s.[4] In the United States, iophendylate myelography was abandoned in the 1980s in favor of myelography using water-soluble (ionic and nonionic) contrast agents. These agents were believed to result in a lower incidence of arachnoiditis as a delayed complication. Recently, two separate long-term outcome studies on patients who received iophendylate (Myodil) ventriculograms shed some doubt on the iophendylate issue. In each of these studies, there was no increased incidence of chronic symptomatic lumbar arachnoiditis after instilling iophendylate into the ventricular system and subsequently into the lumbosacral thecal sac.[13,15] This raises the possibility that the true cause of arachnoiditis after iophendylate myelography may be the combination of iophendylate and a traumatic lumbar puncture at the time of myelography. Guyer et al.[10] list the following factors as influencing the development of arachnoiditis after myelography: the type of contrast agent used (the risk is greater with oil-based than with water-soluble medium and greater with ionic than with nonionic medium), dosage of contrast medium, and the observation time after myelography.

There is general agreement that a history of spinal surgery is a risk factor for the development of spinal arachnoiditis.* In particular, some investigators have specifically stated that surgery for a herniated intervertebral disc may lead to arachnoiditis.[9,10,27,34] Furthermore, the incidence of arachnoiditis increases in patients who have had multiple spinal surgery procedures.

Carroll and Wiesel[5] showed that a postoperative pain-free interval lasting between 1 and 6 months, followed by the gradual onset of leg pain, increases the likelihood that some form of scar tissue is responsible for the symptoms. This may be either arachnoiditis or perineural fibrosis. Smolik and Nash[34] showed that simple dural retraction for the visualization of a ruptured intervertebral disc may initiate the process of arachnoiditis. The operative appearance of arachnoiditis was described by Ransford and Harries in 1972.[26] They noted that the thecal sac was opacified and, after opening of the theca, that the arachnoid was thickened and opaque and formed a circumscribed 2- to 3-mm cuff. The roots of the cauda equina were pink, swollen, and matted together with fine adhesions throughout. In addition, globules of contrast medium were trapped in the interstices of this fine adhesion meshwork.[26] Smith and Blaser[33] postulated that arachnoiditis represents an exuberant reaction to a meningeal injury as part of the normal reparative process.

In an innovative experimental study to determine the causes of focal arachnoiditis, Haughton et al.[12] studied a controlled model using monkeys in which the final observers were blinded to the treatment modality. They found that the nucleus pulposus of an intervertebral disc caused a focal arachnoiditis, whereas synovial fluid, lactic acid (produced by anaerobic glycolysis in the disc), and chondroitin sulfate (a glycosaminoglycan component of the nucleus pulposus) produced no more inflammation than did controls.[12] This study supports the view of some investigators that arachnoiditis is more likely to occur secondary to a herniated intervertebral disc.

Additional noninfectious causes of arachnoiditis have been recognized. The use of intrathecal medications, either steroids or anesthetic agents, is a risk factor for the development of arachnoiditis.† Intrathecal steroids were previously used to treat multiple sclerosis and were also explored for treatment of spinal arachnoiditis. Intrathecal steroids were subsequently proven to be ineffective for these purposes and, in fact, were proven to have caused an arachnoiditis that was localized at the unusual site of the seventh thoracic vertebra.[22] Gravity and the supine position are the reason the thoracic region may be most affected when arachnoiditis is secondary to a chemical insult.[26] Epidural injections of either anesthetic agents or steroids have also been associated with the subsequent development of arachnoiditis.[9,16,22,32] Arachnoiditis occurring after epidural injections may be secondary to accidental subarachnoid injection of the materials or to chemical damage from the preservatives used in the medications.[32]

Additional infrequent noninfectious causes of arachnoiditis include neoplasms,[10,14,18] carcinomatous meningitis,[18] arthritis (particularly ankylosing spondylitis),[14] spinal stenosis,[16] intrathecal hemorrhage,[7,16] foreign materials,[7,36] and any other type of trauma to the spine or spinal cord

---

*References 5,7,9,10,14,16,26,27,34.
†References 7,10,11,14,16,22,26.

| TABLE 153.1 | |
|---|---|
| **Causes of Spinal Arachnoiditis** | |
| **Infectious** | **Noninfectious** |
| Tuberculosis | Trauma |
| Bacterial infections | Postsurgery |
| Syphilis | Myelographic contrast medium (oil-based > water-soluble; water-soluble ionic > water-soluble nonionic) |
| Parasitic diseases | Intrathecal medications |
| Viral meningitis | Steroids |
| | Anesthesia |
| | Epidural injections |
| | Steroids |
| | Anesthesia |
| | Neoplasms |
| | Arthritis (especially ankylosing spondylitis) |
| | Spinal stenosis |
| | Herniated intervertebral disc |
| | Intrathecal hemorrhage |
| | Foreign materials |

(Table 153.1). After a spinal cord injury with the development of posttraumatic syringomyelia, arachnoiditis is not uncommon as a delayed finding.

## Clinical Course

The diagnosis of arachnoiditis requires a detailed medical history and physical examination, as well as a review of confirmatory radiographic imaging studies. Commonly, a patient will complain of more than one of the etiologic factors previously discussed. Typically, a patient has undergone multiple spinal surgeries and multiple myelograms and has been given the diagnosis of "arachnoiditis."

### History

In obtaining a medical history from a patient with arachnoiditis, the clinician should seek three major characteristics of the pain. Pain of arachnoiditis is typically described as a burning pain that is constant and worsened by activity.[3,4,9,10,33] This constant burning pain suggests an element of causalgia.[4] The pain of arachnoiditis may be located in the back or the lower limbs or both.[2,4,9,10] In a long-term follow-up study of 51 patients with arachnoiditis, Guyer et al.[10] found no consistent pattern of back pain or leg pain being more severe than the other. They found both low back and leg pain to be present in more than 90% of patients, and leg spasms and leg cramps were also common. During the follow-up period of between 10 and 21 years, these investigators found that 20% of patients developed sphincter dysfunction. The most common complaints were urinary frequency, urgency, and occasional incontinence. They did not detect any cases of fecal incontinence.[10]

The symptoms of arachnoiditis can vary from nonspecific back pain to radiculopathy and myelopathy.[33] In many patients, arachnoiditis is asymptomatic, and it is discovered as an incidental radiographic finding.[9] Intractable pain that

occurs secondary to arachnoiditis has a poorly localized paleospinothalamic pain pattern that is diffuse. This is quite unlike neospinothalamic pain, which is sharp and well localized. Because of its constancy, the pain of arachnoiditis is more depressing and more debilitating to patients than a more intense pain that is short lived.[3]

### Physical Examination

The physical examination findings in patients with arachnoiditis have been reviewed in two large clinical series. Burton[3] followed 100 patients with arachnoiditis and found little motor weakness to be present. In addition, these patients commonly had a positive straight leg raising sign, a tender sciatic notch, limited range of motion of the trunk, and paravertebral muscle spasms.[3] Guyer et al.[10] followed 51 patients with arachnoiditis for more than 10 years each and found that a decreased range of trunk motion was the most common finding. Furthermore, sensory deficits, diminished or absent deep tendon reflexes, and motor weakness were each independently present in most of their patients.[10] These two studies characterize the classic findings in lumbosacral arachnoiditis.

Occasionally, a syrinx may develop as a late complication of adhesive arachnoiditis.[2] When a syrinx develops, the typical physical examination findings of syringomyelia, including a dissociative sensory loss and variable long tract signs, may be seen. In 1939, Mackay[19] stated that cavitation of the spinal cord may occur as a result of chronic arachnoiditis. His description undoubtedly refers to the development of a syrinx after arachnoiditis.[19] Spinal arachnoiditis may cause arachnoidal adhesions to form a subarachnoid block that creates an intermittent pressure differential across the block, which may lead to an extension of its syrinx.[30] Although experimental models have demonstrated enlargement with arachnoiditis, formation of the initial syrinx cavity because of arachnoiditis has not been demonstrated in experimental studies.[6]

### Imaging Studies

Radiographic imaging studies are used to confirm the clinical impression of arachnoiditis after a history and physical examination. Plain radiographs are not useful for diagnosing arachnoiditis. The "gold standard" imaging study for diagnosing arachnoiditis is myelography[11,13,17] (Figure 153.1). As previously stated, technologic advances have led to the development of water-soluble contrast agents for myelography that have replaced the use of oil-based contrast agents (iophendylate).[3] In the United States, water-soluble myelography, with or without postmyelography computed tomography (CT), remains the examination of choice[11] (Figure 153.2).

In 1975, Jorgensen et al.[17] described the classic myelographic imaging findings in arachnoiditis. They differentiated two distinct patterns of radiographic arachnoiditis. In type I arachnoiditis, there is pure adhesion of the nerve roots to the inside of the meninges in the lower dural sac with a homogeneous contrast pattern. No nerve root shadows are seen, and there is a rounded shortening of the nerve root pocket. In type II arachnoiditis, some proliferation is added inside the dural sac that may be localized or

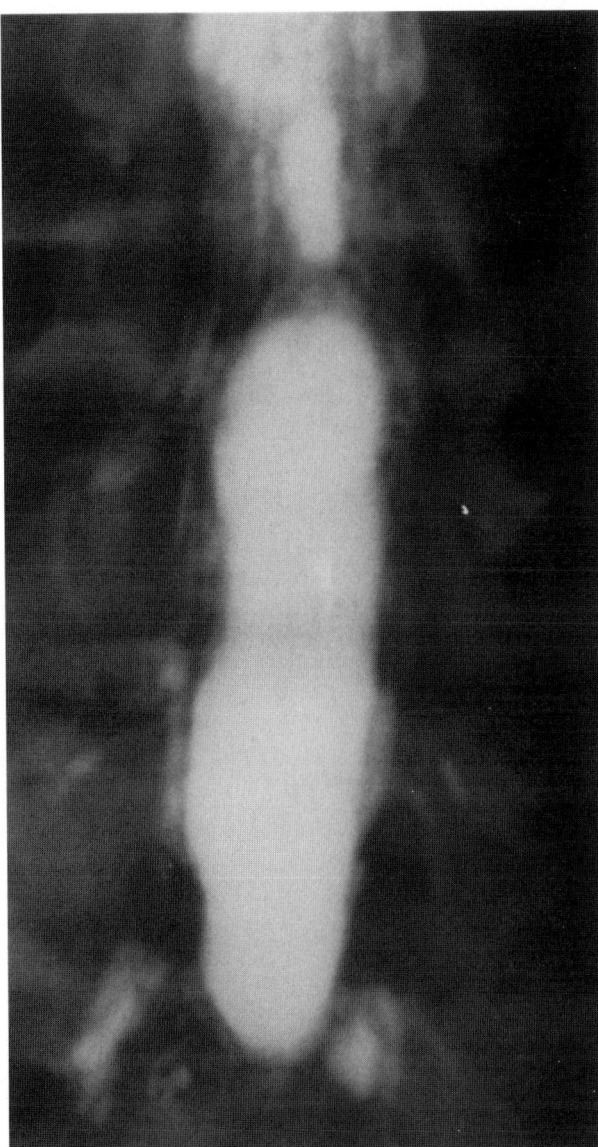

**Figure 153.1** Myelogram (anteroposterior view, oil-based contrast medium [Pantopaque]) of severe adhesive arachnoiditis. This myelogram demonstrates marked lack of filling of the nerve roots throughout the lumbar spine with blunting of the thecal sac.

sis, lymphoma, spinal arteriovenous malformation, hypertrophic interstitial polyneuritis, and neurofibroma.[18] Ransford and Harries[26] recommended, as a technical consideration, that even a hint of blood in the CSF during a lumbar puncture before myelography should preclude injection of contrast medium. This recommendation arose from their impression that the combination of intrathecal blood and contrast medium is significant in leading to the development of subsequent arachnoiditis.[26]

Magnetic resonance imaging (MRI) was developed in the 1980s. This modality has advantages over myelography because MRI is noninvasive and does not expose the patient to the dangers of ionizing radiation. In 1988, gadopentetate dimeglumine was approved by the U.S. Food and Drug Administration for human use in MRI.[35] Gadopentetate dimeglumine, commonly referred to as *gadolinium-DTPA (GAD)*, is a paramagnetic contrast agent that is injected intravenously and that results in the enhancement of edematous structures on T1-weighted images.[5] MRI with GAD is extremely useful in differentiating between scar tissue and recurrent disc herniation.[8,29] After administration of GAD, scar consistently and intensely enhances immediately. Conversely, disc material does not enhance centrally with GAD. In addition, the margins of a herniated disc are often smooth or polypoid, whereas scar usually has irregular and indistinct margins. Two distinct limitations of MRI with GAD are present. The first limitation is that the post-GAD images must be obtained in less than 30 minutes after injection or the avascular disc material may enhance, leading to an inaccurate diagnosis. The second limitation is that the MRI evaluation of a postoperative patient is unable to distinguish scar tissue within the first 2 months postoperatively. Clinicians must keep these limitations in mind when using this imaging modality in postoperative patients.[8]

Ross *et al.*[28] described three distinct groups of arachnoiditis patients with pathomorphic changes on MRI. The first group showed large conglomerations of nerve roots residing centrally within the thecal sac. In the second group, the nerve roots were clumped and attached peripherally to the meninges. No subarachnoid roots were observed, and this appearance was similar to the empty sac appearance observed on myelography (Figure 153.3). In the third group, an increased soft tissue signal was present within the thecal sac, which centrally obliterated the major portion of the subarachnoid space. When using these criteria, MRI is able to accurately diagnose moderate to severe arachnoiditis. There is an excellent correlation of MRI findings with plain film myelography or with postmyelogram CT scans.[7] Another limitation of using MRI in diagnosing arachnoiditis is that the clinician must have a thorough familiarity with the normal appearance at each level of the lumbar spine. Ross *et al.*[28] have stressed that the normal MRI appearance of the thecal sac at the L2 or L3 level could potentially be mistaken for arachnoiditis. Therefore a thorough knowledge of normal MRI characteristics is necessary before interpreting these studies. In their experienced hands, when the MRI appearance of arachnoiditis was compared with plain film myelography and postmyelogram CT, Ross *et al.*[28] found that the sensitivity was 92%, the accuracy was 99%, and the specificity was 100%.[28] This degree of diagnostic accuracy with

diffuse. The filling defects, narrowing, shortening, or occlusion of the spinal canal are also seen in this type of arachnoiditis.[17] Early arachnoiditis typically shows central nerve root clumping and thickening.[16] As the arachnoiditis progresses, the nerve roots become adherent peripherally to the thecal sac, and the terminal thecal sac appears "sleeveless" where the nerve roots do not fill out.[33] This latter finding can cause the thecal sac to appear empty.[16] Unfortunately, the myelographic pattern does not always correlate with the clinical presentation of arachnoiditis. Guyer *et al.*[10] found that the myelographic pattern of arachnoiditis did not correlate with the long-term outcome of clinical arachnoiditis in a long-term follow-up study. When nerve roots are noted to be thickened either in a nodular or a diffuse pattern on myelography, the differential diagnosis must include meningeal carcinomato-

MRI may lead to this modality replacing myelography as the procedure of choice in diagnosing patients with arachnoiditis.

## Treatment

At present, there is no proven treatment modality, either surgical or nonsurgical, that can eliminate or "cure" arachnoiditis. Arachnoiditis is a permanent problem, and therapy relates to symptomatic care.[4] The goal of treatment should be to return the patient to a functional role in society.[10] Neurologic surgeons and orthopedic surgeons may be classified into three groups, based on their outlook toward the use of surgery for treating arachnoiditis: (1) those who believe that surgery has no role, (2) those who believe that surgery has a limited role, and (3) those who believe that surgery has a significant role.

Surgical procedures used to treat arachnoiditis include spinal fusion procedures, decompressive spinal procedures without fusion, neuroablative procedures, and implantation of spinal cord stimulators. Nonsurgical modalities include the use of epidural steroid injections, intrathecal steroid injections, physical therapy programs, and pain programs relying heavily on psychologic counseling. In addition, experimental protocols using

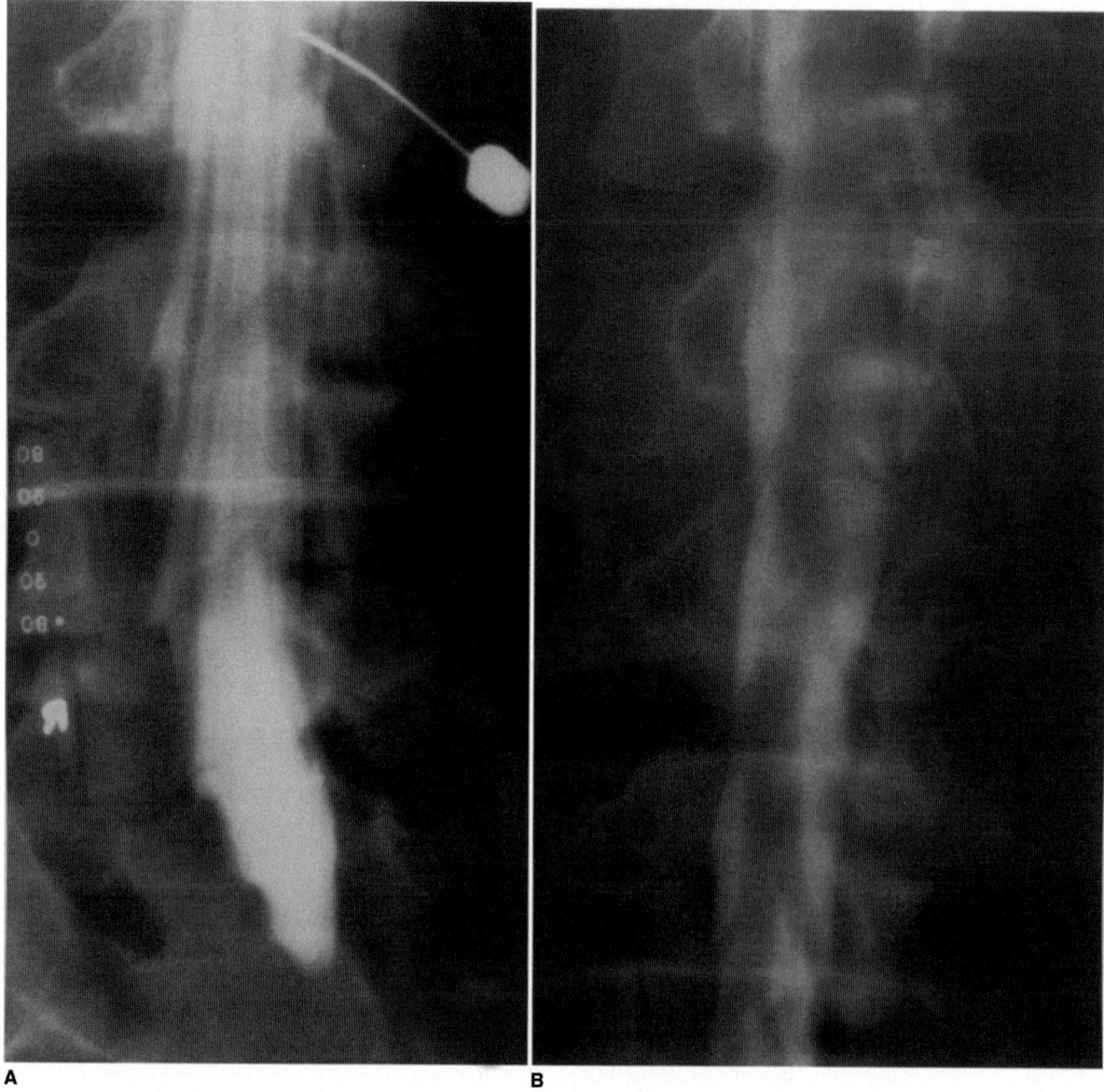

**A**                    **B**

**Figure 153.2 (A)** Myelogram (oblique view, water-soluble contrast medium [metrizamide (Amipaque)]) demonstrates normal nerve root filling throughout the cauda equina region. **(B)** Myelogram (oblique view, water-soluble contrast medium [iohexol (Omnipaque)]) of the same patient 7 years later. Clear evidence of arachnoiditis is shown by the thickened, "clumped" nerve roots that no longer show the normal filling of the nerve root sleeves.

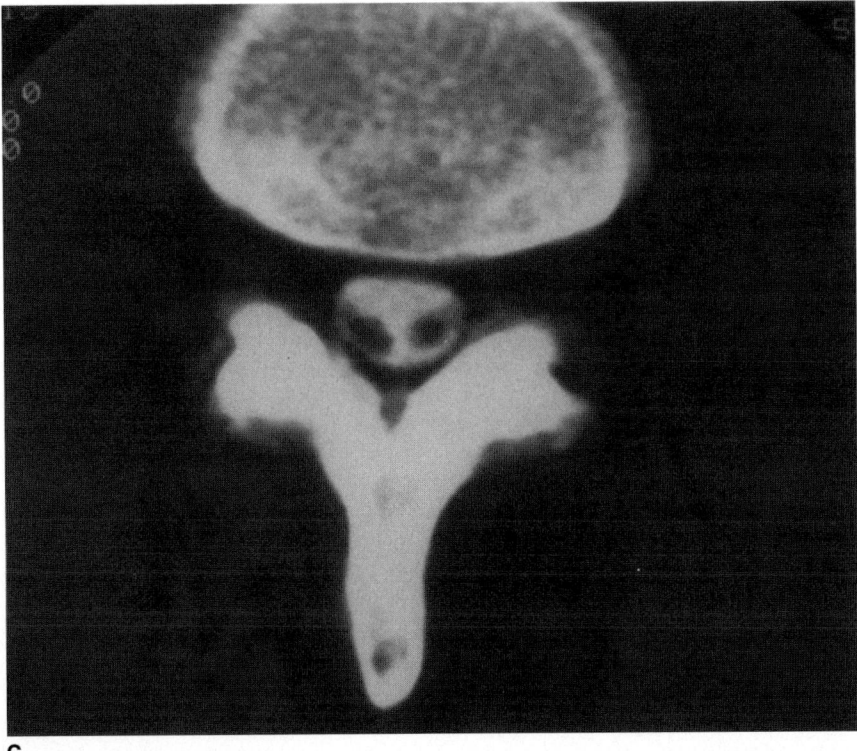

C

**Figure 153.2 *cont'd* (C)** Computed tomography scan after water-soluble myelogram demonstrates the clumping of nerve roots in the thecal sac. This study was performed in the same patient immediately after the myelogram in **(B)**.

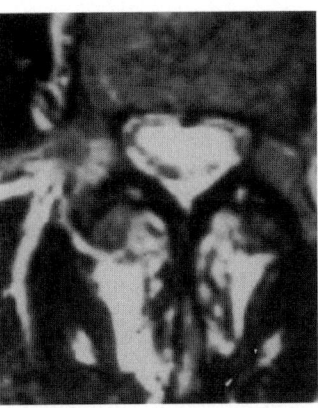

**Figure 153.3** $T_2$-weighted magnetic resonance image (MRI) demonstrates peripheral location of nerve roots in a patient with arachnoiditis. No nerve roots are seen in the central region of the thecal sac. This MRI scan is the correlate to the classic "empty sac" appearance seen on standard myelography.

both animal experiments and human clinical trials are under way.

A substantial body of literature exists that suggests that open surgical procedures are not useful in the treatment of arachnoiditis.[3,5,9,23] Carroll and Wiesel[5] observed that no surgical techniques have proven successful in either eliminating the pathologic scar tissue or significantly reducing the pain of arachnoiditis. Furthermore, if surgery is attempted, the patient's clinical condition is usually worsened.[5] Burton[4] indicated that there is no convincing evidence that neuroablative procedures for patients with adhesive arachnoiditis can provide meaningful long-term benefits when compared with the liability incurred. Grahame et al.[9] found that open surgical procedures had little or no effect on the long-term course of arachnoiditis.

A limited role for surgical procedures in the treatment of arachnoiditis has been explored by numerous investigators.[10,19,26] Mackay[19] believed that surgical intervention was of value in the early stages of arachnoiditis when only localized arachnoid cysts were present. He stated that surgery may be harmful in advanced stages of arachnoiditis when diffuse adhesions are present.[19] Other investigators have noted that although symptoms may be initially relieved after surgery, there is a high rate of relapse of symptoms at long-term follow-up.[10,26]

A more aggressive surgical approach has been recommended by a group of orthopedic surgeons in Japan. Shikata et al.[31] compared their results with microlysis for arachnoiditis with and without spinal fusion. They found that when a spondylodesis was included along with a microlysis, the clinical results were significantly improved. They suggested that spinal mobility has a detrimental effect on the development of symptoms of arachnoiditis, and therefore they believe it is better to perform a fusion in most cases of arachnoiditis.[31] The success of this type of surgical fusion procedure has not yet been duplicated in the United States.

Lesser surgical procedures include the implantation of spinal cord stimulators for long-term pain management in arachnoiditis. Initially, these procedures required an open laminectomy for the placement of an intraspinal monopolar or bipolar electrode.[25] Numerous investigators have stated that electrical stimulation of the spinal cord provides the greatest benefits in the treatment of chronic arachnoiditis.[3,9,24,25] Improved technology has led to the development of multichannel spinal cord stimulation devices that have replaced the single-channel systems. These newer devices have required further electrode positioning significantly less often and have achieved better long-term relief of pain than was obtained with the previous single-channel devices.[25] Recently, North et al.[23-25] published multiple studies detailing the importance of proper patient selection for the implantation of spinal cord stimulators, as well as specific guidelines for the technique involved. This group places an emphasis on careful psychologic screening and drug detoxification before any surgical intervention.[24] In addition, these investigators use "disinterested" third party interviewers to assess the success of spinal cord stimulation in pain management. They stress that this method is needed for any clinical studies on pain control procedures.[25]

The success of spinal cord stimulation is evaluated by the following factors: the patient's subjective estimate of pain relief, the patient's satisfaction with outcome, the use of prescription analgesics, the performance of everyday activities, the ability to return to work, and the use of the device as a sole method of pain management.[24] North et al.[23-25] used temporary percutaneous electrodes as a screening technique to demonstrate satisfactory relief of pain before implantation of a permanent spinal cord stimulation system. A minimum of 50% pain relief with temporary electrodes over a 2- to 3-day course, as well as evidence of improved activity level and stable or decreased use of analgesics, is considered satisfactory pain relief. In addition, these investigators require a superimposition of stimulation paresthesias on the topography of a patient's pain. This is necessary if a spinal cord stimulator is to achieve effective long-term pain relief.[25] Using these techniques, North et al.[23-25] found no loss of neurologic function as evaluated by both the patient and the treating staff after stimulator implantation. At a mean follow-up of 7 years after implantation of a spinal cord stimulator for failed back surgery syndrome, 52% of North et al.'s patients achieved and maintained a greater than 50% reduction in pain. Currently, these results at long-term follow-up of patients with arachnoiditis treated by spinal cord stimulation represent the best clinical control of pain in the published medical literature.[24]

Nonsurgical modalities have been used to attempt to provide symptomatic relief of arachnoiditis.[5] Because activity usually increases the pain of arachnoiditis, the benefits of physical therapy for this disease are debatable.[10] Steroids have been injected both epidurally and intrathecally in an attempt to control the pain of arachnoiditis. Nelson[22] stated that the clinical use of epidural steroid therapy is unproven and that epidural injections of any medications may be risky. Likewise, the intrathecal use of steroid medications in an attempt to treat arachnoiditis has been abandoned. Multiple investigators have shown no increased benefit with intrathecal steroids, and these injections may actually exacerbate arachnoiditis.[1,22] The use of pain-management programs relying heavily on psychologic counseling is currently ongoing; however, long-term results of this modality are not yet available.

Experimental surgical and nonsurgical trials are also under way in an attempt to improve the results of patients with arachnoiditis. MacMillan and Stauffer[20] placed vascularized omental grafts over the laminectomized spines of dogs in an experimental study. They demonstrated absorption of CSF by the omental graft and suggested that the graft may directly revascularize the nerve roots affected by arachnoiditis.[20] Reigel et al.[27] performed an experimental study in rabbits using Poloxamer 407 in an attempt to reduce arachnoidal adhesions and nerve root scarring. Poloxamer 407 is a synthetic nonionic surfactant copolymer that has been shown to reduce peritoneal adhesion formation in rats and hamsters. This compound is physically stable and chemically inert, and when placed over nerve roots and the spinal cord, it reduced the postoperative adhesions of the arachnoid. In addition, Poloxamer 407 did not alter the neurologic function or structure of the spinal cord or peripheral nerves.[27] Grahame et al.[9] performed a placebo-based, controlled 6-month crossover study of d-penicillamine in patients with chronic arachnoiditis. d-Penicillamine is a potent inhibitor of fibroblast activity and therefore of collagen synthesis. Because collagen synthesis is a major component in arachnoiditis, the theoretical benefit of d-penicillamine was tested. Unfortunately, no clear evidence of efficacy was demonstrable; however, a small subgroup of patients did show objective improvement.[9] These experimental studies all lend hope for the future management of arachnoiditis.

## Outcome

The long-term prognosis of patients with chronic arachnoiditis remains bleak. In the long-term follow-up study by Guyer et al.[10] of 51 patients with a minimum 10-year follow-up, patients compared their subjective impression of their status at follow-up with their status at the time of diagnosis. Of the patients, 7% were improved, 59% remained the same, and 33% worsened. In addition, life expectancy was shortened by 12 years when compared with age-matched controls. In this determination of life expectancy, two patients who committed suicide were excluded from the data.[10] The documentation of a minimum of 50% relief of pain in most of North et al.'s patients treated with implanted spinal cord stimulators compares favorably with treatment alternatives available for the chronic intractable pain of arachnoiditis.[24]

## Summary

Arachnoiditis is a chronic, incurable condition that must be avoided, because its management remains suboptimal. The following guidelines may help prevent arachnoiditis. Rough handling of the neural elements during surgery on intervertebral disc herniations should be avoided at all costs.[5,34] In addition, dural substitutes that remain in the body as permanent foreign bodies have the potential to induce chronic inflammation and subsequent adhesions and should be avoided. Autologous tissue is favored when a dural graft is needed.[27,36] Epidural injections of steroids have not proven effective in any long-term, prospective, well-controlled, randomized studies and therefore should be avoided in patients suspected of arachnoiditis.[22] Similarly, intrathecal steroid injections should not be used.[1,22]

With respect to radiographic imaging studies, iophendylate (Myodil, Pantopaque) should no longer be used as a contrast medium for myelography. Because of its numerous benefits and high diagnostic accuracy, MRI should be considered the diagnostic imaging modality of choice when possible. If the results of MRI are inconclusive, or if this study cannot be performed, myelography with water-soluble contrast agents should be used.

Adherence to these guidelines may help lessen the incidence of arachnoiditis; however, when arachnoiditis occurs, the following management guidelines may be used. A careful evaluation of drug habituation behavior should be obtained, and a detailed psychologic evaluation of all patients with arachnoiditis should be undertaken. After a review of the history, physical examination, and radiographic imaging studies, surgery should be reserved for radiographically confirmed mass lesions (i.e., herniated intervertebral discs), with extreme care taken to manipulate the nerve roots as little as possible. If proven spinal instability can be demonstrated on dynamic imaging studies, consideration for a spinal fusion procedure may be entertained. Currently, fusion procedures for arachnoiditis are rarely indicated. In the absence of a documented mass lesion or documented instability, implantation of a spinal cord stimulator appears to be the treatment of choice for chronic arachnoiditis. The strict guidelines proposed by North et al.[23-25] with regard to patient selection and implantation techniques should be followed carefully. As newer experimental modalities are developed, they will need to be closely monitored and subjected to the rigors of scientific proof.

In conclusion, there is a great need for a randomized, prospective, placebo-controlled, double-blind study on the management of arachnoiditis to determine the optimal method for treating this devastating problem.

# REFERENCES

1. Bernat JL, Sadowsky CH, Vincent FM, et al: Sclerosing spinal pachymeningitis. *J Neurol Neurosurg Psychiatry* 39:1124, 1976.
2. Brammah TB, Jayson MIV: Syringomyelia as a complication of spinal arachnoiditis. *Spine* 19:2603, 1994.
3. Burton CV: Lumbosacral arachnoiditis. *Spine* 3:24, 1978.
4. Burton CV: Adhesive arachnoiditis. In Youmans JR (ed): *Neurological surgery*, ed 3. Philadelphia, WB Saunders, 1990, pp 2856-2863.
5. Carroll SE, Wiesel SW: Neurologic complications and lumbar laminectomy: A standardized approach to the multiply-operated lumbar spine. *Clin Orthop* 284:14, 1992.
6. Cho KH, Iwasaki Y, Imamura H, et al: Experimental model of posttraumatic syringomyelia: The role of adhesive arachnoiditis in syrinx formation. *J Neurosurg* 80:133, 1994.
7. Delamarter RB, Ross JS, Masaryk TJ, et al: Diagnosis of lumbar arachnoiditis by magnetic resonance imaging. *Spine* 15:304, 1990.
8. Duda JJ Jr, Ross JS: The postoperative lumbar spine: Imaging considerations. *Semin Ultrasound CT MR* 14:425, 1993.
9. Grahame R, Clark B, Watson M, Polkey C: Toward a rational therapeutic strategy for arachnoiditis: A possible role for d-penicillamine. *Spine* 16:172, 1991.
10. Guyer DW, Wiltse LL, Eskay ML, Guyer BH: The long-range prognosis of arachnoiditis. *Spine* 14:1332, 1989.
11. Hardjasudarma M, Davis DR II: Neuroimaging of arachnoiditis induced by spinal anesthesia. *South Med J* 86:1293, 1993.
12. Haughton VM, Nguyen CM, Ho K-C: The etiology of focal spinal arachnoiditis: An experimental study. *Spine* 18:1193, 1993.
13. Hill CAR, Hunter JV, Moseley IF, Kendall BE: Does Myodil introduced for ventriculography lead to symptomatic lumbar arachnoiditis? *Br J Radiol* 65:1105, 1992.
14. Hoffman GS: Spinal arachnoiditis: What is the clinical spectrum? *Spine* 8:538, 1983.
15. Hughes DG, Isherwood I: How frequent is chronic lumbar arachnoiditis following intrathecal Myodil? *Br J Radiol* 65:758, 1992.
16. Jackson A, Isherwood I: Does degenerative disease of the lumbar spine cause arachnoiditis? A magnetic resonance study and review of the literature. *Br J Radiol* 67:840, 1994.
17. Jorgensen J, Hansen PH, Steenskov V, Ovesen N: A clinical and radiological study of chronic lower spinal arachnoiditis. *Neuroradiology* 9:139, 1975.
18. Kumar A, Montanera W, Willinsky R, et al: MR features of tuberculous arachnoiditis: Case report. *J Comput Assist Tomogr* 17:127, 1993.
19. Mackay RP: Chronic adhesive spinal arachnoiditis. *JAMA* 112:802, 1939.
20. MacMillan M, Stauffer ES: The effect of omental pedicle graft transfer on spinal microcirculation and laminectomy membrane formation. *Spine* 16:176, 1991.
21. McLaurin RL, Bailey OT, Schurr PH, Ingraham FD: Myelomalacia and multiple cavitations of spinal cord secondary to adhesive arachnoiditis. *Arch Pathol* 57:138, 1954.
22. Nelson DA: Intraspinal therapy using methylprednisolone acetate: Twenty-three years of clinical controversy. *Spine* 18:278, 1993.
23. North RB, Campbell JN, James CS, et al: Failed back surgery syndrome: 5-year follow-up in 102 patients undergoing repeated operation. *Neurosurgery* 28:685, 1991.
24. North RB, Ewend MG, Lawton MT, et al: Failed back surgery syndrome: 5-year follow-up after spinal cord stimulator implantation. *Neurosurgery* 28:692, 1991.
25. North RB, Kidd DH, Zahurak M, et al: Spinal cord stimulation for chronic, intractable pain: Experience over two decades. *Neurosurgery* 32:384, 1993.
26. Ransford AO, Harries BJ: Localised arachnoiditis complicating lumbar disc lesions. *J Bone Joint Surg* 54B:656, 1972.
27. Reigel DH, Bazmi G, Shih S-R, Marquardt MD: A pilot investigation of poloxamer 407 for the prevention of leptomeningeal adhesions in the rabbit. *Pediatr Neurosurg* 19:250, 1993.
28. Ross JS, Masaryk TJ, Modic MT, et al: MR imaging of lumbar arachnoiditis. *AJR Am J Roentgenol* 149:1025, 1987.

29. Ross JS, Masaryk TJ, Schrader M, *et al:* MR imaging of the postoperative lumbar spine: Assessment with gadopentetate dimeglumine. *AJNR Am J Neuroradiol* 11:771, 1990.

30. Sgouras S, Williams B: A critical appraisal of drainage in syringomyelia. *J Neurosurg* 82:1, 1995.

31. Shikata J, Yamamuro T, Iida H, Sugimoto M: Surgical treatment for symptomatic spinal adhesive arachnoiditis. *Spine* 14:870, 1989.

32. Sklar EML, Quencer RM, Green BA, *et al:* Complications of epidural anesthesia: MR appearance of abnormalities. *Radiology* 181:549, 1991.

33. Smith AS, Blaser SI: Infectious and inflammatory processes of the spine. *Radiol Clin North Am* 29:809, 1991.

34. Smolik EA, Nash FP: Lumbar spinal arachnoiditis: A complication of the intervertebral disc operation. *Ann Surg* 133:490, 1951.

35. Wolf GL: Current status of MR imaging contrast agents: Special report. *Radiology* 172:709, 1989.

36. Yamagami T, Matsui H, Tsuji H, *et al:* Effects of laminectomy and retained extradural foreign body on cauda equina adhesion. *Spine* 18:1774, 1993.

# CHAPTER 154

# Infectious Complications of Spine Surgery

**Seth M. Zeidman and Thomas B. Ducker**

Spine infections are not uncommon and certainly not rare. Hence, avoidance and treatment of spine infections should be of paramount concern to spine surgeons.

## Postoperative and Iatrogenic Spinal Infections

Infectious complications after spinal surgery and spinal diagnostic procedures include discitis, osteomyelitis, and spinal epidural abscess (SEA). The rate of infectious complications after lumbar spine surgery is reported to be between 0.5% and 5%. Spangfort[50] reviewed more than 10,000 laminectomies and reported an operative infection rate of approximately 2.9%. In an analysis of 28,395 patients who underwent lumbar laminectomy for radiculopathy in the United States in 1980, Ramirez and Thisted[44] reported an incidence of infection of 0.3%.

The clinical and radiographic characteristics of interspace infection were first described by Milward and Grout[36] in 1936 after the inadvertent introduction of microorganisms into a disc space during a lumbar puncture. Gieseking[17] reported the first postoperative interspace infection in 1951.

Patients with aseptic necrosis or interspace infections are typically asymptomatic immediately after surgery; however, within 2 weeks they begin to experience excruciating spasms in the lower back, with or without radiation to the legs. The white blood cell count and temperature are often normal, but the sedimentation rate is typically elevated, often to more than 100mm/hr. Lumbosacral radiographs may reveal erosion of the cartilage plates as the disease progresses. Needle aspiration of the interspace may reveal the offending organisms, but such aspirations are often negative.[39] Patients with a clear-cut infection syndrome should be placed on intravenous (IV) antibiotics.

Wound infection should be suspected if persistent temperature elevation occurs several days postoperatively. The wound should be examined for erythema, swelling, tenderness, and drainage. Management should include a Gram stain and culture, with antibiotic treatment if the clinical suspicion is wrong. In the presence of probable infection or persistent infection despite antibiotic treatment, the patient should be returned to the operating room and the wound should be reopened, thoroughly débrided, and irrigated.

The incidence of wound infection rises sharply when the duration of the procedure extends beyond 3 hours. Air conditioning reduces the incidence of wound contamination. However, local application of antibiotics to the wound has not been demonstrated to alter the incidence of infection.

## Postoperative Discitis

Disc space infection or discitis, an infection of the intervertebral disc with contiguous subchondral vertebral osteomyelitis, most commonly follows prior intervertebral disc surgery or arises by hematogenous dissemination.

The incidence of discitis after intervertebral disc surgery is approximately 0.7%. Bongartz et al.[8] performed 3127 open lumbar intervertebral disc operations and had 15 cases of postoperative discitis (0.5%). The higher incidence of disc space infection with microsurgery has been attributed to the presence of the microscope over the open wound.

Most cases of discitis are located in the lumbosacral spine. Discitis typically produces back pain from 2 weeks to 3 months postoperatively. The severity of the pain is often intense and has been described as being similar to an intraabdominal crisis (e.g., rupture of an abdominal aortic aneurysm). Because discitis is rare in any individual patient, postoperative back pain may initially be attributed to a poor operative result.

Clinical findings include localized spinal pain and fever. The physical findings are often unremarkable. They include extreme discomfort with tenderness to palpation, guarding against movement, and positive straight leg raising in some cases. The diagnosis may be suggested by radiologic studies such as plain radiographs, bone scan, computed tomography (CT), and magnetic resonance imaging (MRI) and is confirmed by culturing blood or material obtained from the involved disc space.

The spinal radiographs and the white blood cell count with differential are often within normal limits. The erythrocyte sedimentation rate (ESR) is one of the most sensitive tests, and it may be elevated when all other studies are normal. Postoperative discitis should be kept in mind when severe backache or muscle spasm occurs postoperatively, particularly when the ESR is elevated. Bone scan, CT, and MRI are quite sensitive for detecting discitis and can identify changes associated with discitis earlier than plain radiographs can. CT is effective in the early diagnosis of discitis. Hypodensity of the affected disc space can be detected as early as 10 days postoperatively. Both bone scan and MRI are sensitive but may be falsely positive in the postoperative patient. Aspirations of the disc space are often sterile. When an organism is identified, the most common infecting one is *Staphylococcus*.

The cause of postoperative discitis remains somewhat unclear. It has been thought to represent either an aseptic (autoimmune) inflammatory response or a low-grade bacterial infection. However, many cases respond to antibiotics, which should be continued until the ESR has returned to normal. Animal models of discitis have all required bacteria to produce the radiographic changes characteristic of discitis.[15] These findings favor a bacterial cause for postoperative discitis.

The late radiographic changes include disc interspace narrowing, end plate erosion, and the development of marginal osteophytes. Spontaneous fusion occurs in most cases.

The management of discitis is somewhat controversial. Pilgaard and Aarhus[39] noted the absence of an organism in many cases and successfully treated their patients without antibiotics. However, the organism may be elusive, and a 4- to 6-week course of IV antibiotics is advocated by many spine surgeons.

Treatment consists of IV antimicrobial therapy, spinal immobilization, and surgical intervention in selected circumstances. Early diagnosis and prompt treatment are important to prevent chronic infection. Immobilization is often successful in relieving pain and may be supplemented by a total-contact orthosis as patients become ambulatory. Uncomplicated discitis rarely requires surgery. This is in contradistinction to frank osteomyelitis, which usually requires surgical intervention. Notably, Bongartz et al.[8] reoperated on the infected intervertebral disc space to acquire material for bacteriologic culture and to remove loose fragments. They contended that reoperation facilitated early patient mobilization.

Most patients with a disc interspace infection progress to spontaneous interbody fusion over a period of 6 to 12 months. Discitis is associated with a good prognosis, but residual back pain, limited spinal mobility, and neurologic deficit may occur.

Occasionally, an epidural abscess may develop, producing paresis. Under these circumstances, immediate decompressive laminectomy is indicated.

## Postoperative Osteomyelitis

Infection may be introduced directly into the intervertebral disc space during closed-procedure surgery.[15,58] This infection can spread to the adjacent vertebral bodies, producing osteomyelitis. The most common cause of infection in the intervertebral disc space is surgery for herniated disc.* This complication occurs in less than 1% of patients undergoing disc surgery. Organisms may be inadvertently inoculated during surgery. Residual hematoma, necrotic tissue, and foreign bodies provide an environment conducive to bacterial proliferation. Weeks, months, or even years may elapse before the diagnosis of osteomyelitis is established. Symptoms may not be apparent immediately after the initial operation. Often, there is initial pain relief followed by recurrent back pain several days to weeks later. Fever may be transient, intermittent, or nonexistent, and there is often no evidence of infection when symptoms develop. The degree of pain may appear to be out of proportion to the objective findings and may be erroneously attributed to hysteria, malingering, or even psychoneurosis.

Postoperative osteomyelitis may initially present much like a severe discitis. However, the subsequent clinical manifestations are more likely to be characterized by increasing symptoms. Systemic symptoms may also be more prominent, and the ESR is usually elevated. The problem may be suspected by greater bony involvement

observed on initial imaging studies. However, postoperative osteomyelitis is often discovered only by serial radiographs that demonstrate vertebral body collapse, if the anterior and middle columns are involved. In these patients, an organism can usually be cultured. In the rare instance of posterior column involvement, the wound may demonstrate the more typical signs of infection. The typical radiologic changes of vertebral osteomyelitis may not be apparent for several months. Radionuclide bone scans are quite sensitive and often demonstrate evidence of infection before plain radiographs of the spine show any changes.

However, plain radiographs are not specific. Surgical edema and disc changes may yield false-positive results.[16] Furthermore, early in the course of disc space infection, the bone may test negative in a significant percentage of patients.[19] CT may show destructive changes of the vertebral bodies before they are evident on plain radiographs. However, end plate irregularities on CT scan are not specific for discitis, and normal curettage changes in vertebral end plates may mimic erosions of discitis.[24] MRI may show changes of discitis long before any changes are apparent radiologically. It is important to note that MRI and CT may be negative early in the course of postoperative discitis, and therefore a high index of suspicion is necessary.

Increasing back pain more than 2 weeks postoperatively and an ESR of greater than 50mm/hr should be considered to be caused by discitis until proven otherwise. Percutaneous disc biopsy is helpful in postoperative discitis diagnosis but is often falsely negative.

In a study comparing MRI, plain radiographs, and radionuclide studies for evaluation of vertebral osteomyelitis, MRI was judged to be as accurate and sensitive as a combination bone and gallium scanning and to be more sensitive than plain radiographs. The MRI appearance of pyogenic infection is characteristic, making MRI a rapid, noninvasive method for the detection of vertebral osteomyelitis and its complications, including epidural abscess. On $T_1$-weighted images, infected disc material shows decreased signal intensity from the intervertebral disc space and contiguous vertebral bodies relative to the normal vertebral signal. On $T_2$-weighted images, these tissues show increased signal. MRI provides more anatomic detail than radionuclide scanning does and allows differentiation of neoplasm and degenerative disease from osteomyelitis. The disc space is usually spared in neoplastic disease, whereas degenerative disease with nucleus desiccation produces decreased disc signal on $T_2$-weighted images. Gallium scanning may be positive earlier than MRI in the course of infection and is more sensitive to changes resulting from treatment and decreasing inflammation.

Many patients with postoperative discitis and vertebral osteomyelitis have spontaneous resolution. Therefore a diagnosis is never made.[48] In some patients with postoperative vertebral osteomyelitis, intermittent antibiotic therapy obscures the diagnosis and permits the illness to go undetected for years.

Kern[21] reported a patient in whom vertebral osteomyelitis and meningitis manifested 2½ years after lumbar spine surgery. The ability of infections to remain dormant and to recur after long periods is illustrated by a patient in whom postoperative lumbar staphylococcal vertebral osteomyelitis

---

*References 6,10,13,14,20,21,33,39,51,53,54.

developed and cleared after 3 years of treatment. Some 34 years later, after 30 years without symptoms, the patient developed a staphylococcal psoas abscess.[31]

Therapeutic decision making is based on the organism, the response to antibiotics, evidence of continuing vertebral body collapse, and signs of new neurologic involvement. The principles of treatment are identical to the management of acute hematogenous vertebral body osteomyelitis. Antibiotic treatment alone, with appropriate immobilization, may be adequate. If there is progressive neurologic deterioration or vertebral body collapse, ventral débridement and bone grafting are appropriate. If the infection is dorsal, débridement alone with antibiotic management is usually preferred.

## Postoperative Spinal Epidural Abscess

SEA after spinal decompression is rare. This condition should be suspected when the patient has increasing neurologic symptoms and signs in the early postoperative period. SEA may be difficult to separate from an expanding hematoma in the absence of systemic evidence of infection. The clinical presentation of acute SEA is often stereotyped but can be difficult to appreciate in its earliest stages. The classic triad is exquisite localized back pain, progressive neurologic deficit, and fever.[45] The initial complaint almost uniformly is axial pain. Paresthesias are also common. Fever is present in most cases.

Laboratory findings are often unhelpful. Fever and leukocytosis are useful when present, but they are absent in more than half of the cases. Leukocytosis is common in the acute group. Although nonspecific, the ESR is commonly elevated. The diagnostic test of choice is MRI.

MRI can localize the site of infection and is the diagnostic test of choice, providing more information than CT regarding the extent of abscess involvement and the degree of cord compromise. It also avoids potential subarachnoid contamination by puncture of the thecal sac when traversing an unsuspected focus of epidural infection.

Without treatment, the progression and time course of symptoms is astoundingly uniform.[46] Within 3 days, patients generally note radicular symptoms, followed within 36 hours by weakness. Rapid deterioration to paralysis typically occurs over the next 24 hours. This pattern of symptoms is so uniform that some authors have suggested that this unequivocally establishes the clinical diagnosis.

Decompression and antibiotic management are the cornerstones of therapy. Epidural abscess often arises in association with vertebral osteomyelitis and is an indication for early decompression.

## Spontaneous Spinal Infections
### Pyogenic Vertebral Osteomyelitis

Pyogenic vertebral osteomyelitis can result from spinal trauma, from infections in adjacent structures, or from hematogenous spread of bacteria to the spine. Hematogenous pyogenic vertebral osteomyelitis can have catastrophic consequences if unrecognized and untreated. The overall incidence is less than 1 per 100,000 people.[49] The rarity of this condition and its often insidious onset with vague and nonspecific signs and symptoms may delay diagnosis and subsequent treatment, often for more than 3 months from initial clinical manifestations. Pyogenic vertebral osteomyelitis has a male predominance.

Diabetes mellitus, advanced age, extended steroid therapy, and IV drug use are recognized as predisposing factors. Presumably, an infective nidus spreads bacteria to the vertebrae through the bloodstream. Bacteria initially infect the richly vascularized vertebral end plates and then spread locally.

More than 95% of pyogenic spinal infections involve the vertebral body. Less than 5% involve the dorsal elements. This likely reflects the dramatic amount of both arterial and venous blood circulation to the vertebral body.

*Staphylococcus aureus* is the most common organism found in hematogenous pyogenic vertebral osteomyelitis. Other bacterial species are common within certain subpopulations (e.g., *Pseudomonas* osteomyelitis in IV drug abusers, gram-negative osteomyelitis in patients with underlying genitourinary infections or gastrointestinal disorders).

Patients typically have a history of several weeks or months of progressive neck or back pain. Less than half of the patients are febrile at presentation. Neurologic defects most commonly result from bony collapse or associated SEA. Only 10% of patients have an acute presentation, and most have a chronic or subacute clinical picture.

The ESR is typically dramatically elevated, often over 75 mm/hr. The clinical scenarios of progressive back or neck pain with an elevated ESR should prompt a search for infection. Leukocytosis is often absent or minimally elevated in patients with a chronic pyogenic osteomyelitis, and most patients have positive blood cultures.

Findings on plain radiographs include rarefaction, loss of bony trabeculation adjacent to the cartilaginous end plate, and irregular narrowing of the intervertebral space. Vertebral body collapse is common, as is evidence of bony regeneration. Findings on CT include fragmentation of involved bone and gas formation within the involved vertebrae.

MRI is perhaps the most sensitive and specific test for detection of vertebral osteomyelitis. $T_1$-weighted images show low-density changes in the bone and intervertebral disc. The signal alterations reflect the early inflammatory response characterized by infiltration of polymorphonuclear leukocytes and fibrin deposition in the adjacent end plates. Bony destruction secondary to lytic enzymes, and the associated increased water content, is reflected by the increased signal intensity on $T_2$-weighted images. The signal alterations often precede the destructive changes. Enhancement with gadolinium demonstrates the involved structures, if present.

The goal in treating patients with vertebral osteomyelitis is preservation of neurologic function and restoration of any impaired functions. The overall plan must be individualized for each patient and must address the patient's overall medical condition, as well as the treatment of any focal abscesses.

More than three fourths of vertebral osteomyelitis cases can be treated with IV antibiotics alone. However, this requires identification of the offending organism.

Blood cultures and percutaneous biopsy overwhelmingly reveal the organism in most cases. However, if they fail to yield the diagnosis, open drainage and culture often will.

Antibiotics can be given for variable periods of time, although it appears that a 4- to 8-week course of IV antibiotics is effective for most infections. Periodic assessment of the ESR is essential to gauge the response to therapy. The presence of a persistently high ESR may reflect an untreated or partially treated infectious process.

Although most patients with pyogenic vertebral osteomyelitis respond to this therapy, some may not—particularly those with osseous involvement, neurologic deficit, septic course with clinical toxicity, failure of needle biopsy, and failure of IV antibiotics to eradicate the infection.

Once appropriate antibiotic therapy is initiated, the clinical symptoms often improve significantly. However, the MRI findings do not reflect the actual healing of vertebral osteomyelitis.

## Spinal Epidural Abscess

SEA is an uncommon entity, but its clinical importance overshadows its rarity. The overall incidence has been reported to range from 0.2 to 1.2 cases per 10,000 hospital admissions.[3] However, recent evidence suggests the incidence may be increasing. There has been a progressive increase in the incidence of SEA over the past 20 years.[45] Whether this represents a true increase or is a result of increased vigilance and the increased sensitivity of diagnostic imaging techniques is unclear. The population at risk for the development of SEA appears to be enlarging as a consequence of increasing IV drug use and a growing number of patients with human immunodeficiency virus (HIV). Advances in imaging have made the diagnosis of SEA less elusive and the options for therapeutic intervention more rational. Despite the recognition of SEA as a potential neurosurgical emergency and despite the increased sophistication of diagnostic studies, the morbidity and mortality associated with SEA remain significant.

Most cases of SEA occur in adults. Occurrence in children younger than 12 years of age is unusual. The male/female ratio is approximately 1:1, although some recent series report a male predominance. Thoracic lesions are the most common, followed by lumbar and cervical lesions. In one large series, 82% of lesions were dorsal to the spinal cord, and the rest were ventral. Patients with SEA often deteriorate rapidly, emphasizing the importance of early diagnosis.

Hematogenous spread is the source in up to 50% of cases. A primary source of infection can be identified in nearly all cases. Spread occurs either to the epidural space or in the vertebrae, with secondary extension into the epidural space. The most commonly reported foci include skin infections with furuncles, parenteral injections, bacterial endocarditis, urinary infections, respiratory infections, and pharyngeal or dental abscesses. Major risk factors for the development of SEA include IV drug use, diabetes mellitus, HIV infection, pregnancy, and prior spinal surgery. Recent spinal trauma, epidural anesthesia, malignancy, discography, and alcohol abuse have all been implicated as predisposing factors. In addition, there can be direct spread from decubitus ulcers, psoas abscesses, abdominal wounds, mediastinitis, and pyelonephritis.

SEAs are (1) acute (gross pus in the epidural space), usually with accompanying sepsis, and (2) chronic (granulation tissue in the epidural space), which may persist for months.

Despite the typically straightforward clinical presentation of SEA, in many large series, less than 20% of patients were correctly diagnosed at the time of initial presentation. This figure has particular importance, because the overall prognosis is directly proportional to the speed of diagnosis and the application of appropriate therapy. Difficulty in correctly diagnosing SEA often leads to a delay of initiation of appropriate, definitive therapy. Clinical suspicion and judicious use of radiologic imaging are the keys to timely diagnosis.

Plain radiographs are typically unremarkable in the absence of concomitant osteomyelitic involvement of adjacent vertebral bodies. The vertebral end plates directly adjacent to the disc space may show erosion. This often develops as late as 4 to 6 weeks after the onset of infection. The degree of local bone destruction from associated osteomyelitis is best appreciated on CT. This information is often essential to formulation of the optimal management strategy.

CT-myelography is an excellent technique, which is often diagnostic. Lateral C1-2 puncture is the preferred method. This identifies the upper limit of any epidural mass but may not define the lower edge. A second puncture below the block is occasionally required. Myelography has the added benefit of providing a cerebrospinal fluid (CSF) sample for cell count with differential, protein, glucose, Gram stain, and culture. The CSF profile is generally consistent with parameningeal inflammation, although up to 15% of patients have concurrent meningitis. However, myelography carries the risk of converting an epidural process into a subdural empyema. Because of this potential morbidity, MRI is favored as the first line of diagnostic imaging.

MRI provides rapid and accurate identification of inflammatory foci, defines the degree of spinal cord compression, shows the predominant location of the abscess, and often dictates the surgical approach. The MRI characteristics of SEA are distinctive. The epidural mass may be isointense or hypointense on $T_1$-weighted images and is hyperintense on $T_2$-weighted images. Occasionally, the abscess is very extensive, spanning the entire spine. It is possible to confuse the lesion with the normal spine. Noncontrast MRI allows quantitation of the degree of subarachnoid space encasement. Gadolinium-enhanced MRI often demonstrates a linear enhancement surrounding nonenhancing purulent matter. The underlying pathophysiology creating this enhancement is poorly defined. Cellulitis and granulation around the purulence, or vascular stasis in the epidural venous plexus resulting from an obstructive process in the spinal canal, may be responsible.

MRI likewise confirms achievement of adequate postoperative decompression. Follow-up studies often demonstrate a decrease in abscess size and better visualization of the subarachnoid space in conjunction with clinical improvement. The principal shortcoming of MRI is its tendency to overestimate bone involvement. In most cases, the enhancement disappears as the abscess heals.

Radionuclide scans are of limited value. Because of a lack of specificity, SEA should be considered in the differential diagnosis of any patient experiencing unexplained, rapidly increasing spinal pain, especially in the setting of fever, altered mental status, or sepsis. Three conditions to especially consider in the differential diagnosis of an epidural abscess are epidural metastasis, acute transverse myelitis, and subdural abscess.

It is particularly important to make the appropriate diagnosis in the case of epidural metastasis, because the treatment of the two disorders is distinctly different. Epidural metastases warrant radiotherapy and, occasionally, surgical intervention.

Acute transverse myelitis is more common than epidural abscess but may initially be indistinguishable. Factors favoring acute transverse myelitis include rapid evolution of neurologic deficits, a lack of significant pain, myelographic block caused by a swollen spinal cord, or recent viral infections. Subdural abscesses are rare and typically have far less associated spinal tenderness. CT-myelography or MRI demonstrates the characteristic intradural extramedullary filling defect, often with concomitant complete spinal block.

Other diagnostic possibilities include meningitis, osteomyelitis, discitis, intramedullary abscesses, epidural hematoma, intraspinal tumors, vascular lesions, disc herniation, and spinal subarachnoid hemorrhage.

The bacterial life seen in epidural abscesses includes gram-positive cocci in nearly 80% of cases. *S. aureus* is the most common organism. The remaining organisms are predominantly gram-negative rods or anaerobes. A diligent search usually identifies cutaneous, respiratory, or genitourinary sources of the infection and provides a clue to the offending organism. Other causes include *Escherichia coli, Pseudomonas aeruginosa, Diplococcus pneumoniae, Serratia marcescens, Enterobacter*, chronic infections, tuberculosis, cryptococcosis, aspergillosis, brucellosis, and *Echinococcus*. Multiple organisms or mixed flora are common and occur in as many as 10% of cases. Anaerobes can be cultured from the wound in approximately 8% of cases if proper techniques and culture media are used.

Antibiotic treatment should be initiated as soon as the diagnosis is made. Fungal and mycobacterial cultures should be obtained in view of the wide spectrum of organisms implicated in epidural abscess. Positive blood cultures may be used as strong, suggestive evidence of the causative infectious agent, although it is preferable to obtain a culture directly from the abscess before the initiation of antibiotics. Initiation of antibiotic therapy before biopsy occasionally results in failure to isolate a bacterial agent. However, there is a 48- to 72-hour window before the cultures are compromised.

The initial choice of antibiotics should provide broad-spectrum coverage and good blood-brain barrier penetration. Because *S. aureus* is the most common organism, a synthetic penicillin (e.g., nafcillin), plus an aminoglycoside (e.g., gentamicin) to provide gram-negative coverage, is a good initial regimen. Modification of the antibiotic regimen should be based on definitive culture data or identification of the source. The duration of therapy must be individualized but should not be less than 6 weeks when

there is concomitant osteomyelitis. Shorter courses (3 to 4 weeks) may be adequate for infections confined to the epidural space. Infectious disease consultation is recommended when available.

There have been sporadic reports of nonsurgical treatment of SEA. Nonoperative management of SEA has been successful in a number of cases.[56] Reported reasons for the use of nonoperative management include minor or absent neurologic deficit, poor surgical risk caused by underlying medical conditions, extensive spinal involvement, irreversible paraplegia, and refusal of surgery. When minimal or no neurologic dysfunction is present, the abscess is clearly defined by MRI, the etiologic organism is identified, and relative contraindications to surgery exist, nonoperative management of SEA represents a valid therapeutic option. Surgery may be avoided without untoward effects in selected cases, and patients with no initial neurologic deficit can be successfully managed with antibiotics alone. However, it is necessary to monitor the patient's clinical status closely, with frequent neurologic evaluations, serial MRI, and ESR measurements. Residual contrast enhancement is not, in and of itself, an indication for continuing antibiotic therapy. However, medical observation of the patient for several weeks after completion of the antibiotic treatment, as well as follow-up imaging, is indicated. ESR is a sensitive indicator of epidural abscess, and serial ESR measurements provide a helpful guide in determining the appropriate duration of antibiotic therapy. Only strict adherence to defined criteria allows nonoperative therapy to occur without devastating and potentially catastrophic consequences.

The traditional therapy for SEA has been immediate surgical spinal cord decompression. Early studies of SEA supported this philosophy, recording patients who deteriorated before delayed surgical decompression. The fundamental principles of surgical management are drainage of pus, débridement of granulation tissue, copious irrigation, and occasionally, postoperative drainage.

The location of the abscess and the presence or absence of associated osteomyelitis and vertebral body destruction dictate the approach in patients requiring surgery. Most SEAs are dorsal to the thecal sac. Extensive laminectomy is used, with closure using monofilament nylon sutures and optional postoperative drainage.

Ventral decompression with débridement and primary grafting is used for SEA ventral to the thecal sac, in conjunction with discitis/osteomyelitis. Vertebral body collapse is a strong indication for the ventral approach.

Grafts are typically stable and do not require additional stabilization with a plating system. In the presence of coexisting instability, a plating system or orthosis for several weeks can optimize fusion. Plates can be used in patients with osteomyelitis without significant added risk. Wounds either may be closed primarily with or without drainage or may be allowed to heal by secondary intention.

### The Cervical Spine

Cervical SEAs have a propensity to develop more rapid and severe neurologic deficits.[57] This propensity may reflect the smaller epidural space available in the cervical region in comparison with other spinal segments.

Likewise, the prognosis for patients with cervical epidural abscesses is generally worse than for those patients with thoracic or lumbar abscesses. Patients with cervical epidural abscesses have a correspondingly higher mortality rate. The overall mortality rate for SEA is 18%. The rate for cervical SEA is as high as 38%, despite aggressive treatment.

Cervical epidural abscesses tend to occur ventrally, whereas dorsal lesions are more common in the thoracic and lumbar spine. The increased incidence of vertebral osteomyelitis or discitis associated with cervical epidural abscess may explain this observation. A ventral approach permits direct decompression, resection of involved disc and bone, spinal reconstruction, and stabilization. Abscesses typically extend two to four vertebral levels but occasionally span the entire spinal canal. Dorsal cervical procedures are reserved for dorsal abscesses, in the absence of any ventral abnormality, such as discitis or osteomyelitis. Cervical abscesses occur more often in IV drug users (probably resulting from lymphatic spread from foci of infection in the upper extremities and neck).

### The Thoracic Spine

Thoracic epidural abscesses are especially challenging because of the common presentation with severe neurologic deficit and the technical complexity of operative decompression and stabilization. Either ventral or dorsal approaches to SEAs can be used. The initial approach depends on the location of the pathologic disease. Patients who undergo a ventral approach with corpectomy should undergo stabilization using either autologous rib or iliac crest bone graft. A construct using tobramycin-impregnated methylmethacrylate and a metal rod has been used when the operative field is very purulent. The means of spinal reconstruction after ventral débridement varies according to residual spinal stability. Packed autologous bone will incorporate after thorough débridement of infected and necrotic bone. Postoperative bracing is used. If the kyphotic deformity is likely to progress because (1) the dorsal elements are destroyed, (2) more than 50% of the vertebral body is resected, or (3) preoperative kyphosis exceeds 10 degrees despite 4 to 6 weeks of postoperative recumbency, the clinician should supplement the graft with either internal fixation or another adjunct such as antibiotic-impregnated methylmethacrylate. Short-segment dorsal fusion is performed later in patients with no initial ventral bone graft.

### The Lumbosacral Spine

The clinical course of acute and chronic epidural abscesses in the lumbar spine is usually less devastating than that for abscesses in other locations. The presence of a generous subarachnoid space, with nerve roots instead of spinal cord, is the main reason for such a difference. The threshold for surgical intervention is consequently higher than with cervical and thoracic lesions. It is important that the surgeon not perform too wide a laminectomy, because this destabilizes the spine and could result in postoperative spondylolisthesis.

Patients with associated ventral infection, and especially those with osteomyelitis, may benefit from ventral débridement and decompression. However, ventral procedures on patients with osteomyelitis affecting the lower lumbar vertebrae carry substantial morbidity.

The potentially rapid deterioration and persistent high morbidity of SEA have been stressed by several authors. Treatment of symptomatic epidural abscesses is generally an emergency. In patients with any neurologic deficit, decompression should be considered, because further neurologic progression compromises the patient's potential for recovery.

Neurologic recovery is inversely proportional to the severity and duration of paralysis. Incomplete spinal cord lesions, manifested by sensory sparing, indicate some probability of recovery. In these authors' experience, among patients treated more than 36 hours after the onset of paralysis, none recovered useful function. As stated previously, the overall mortality rate for SEA is 18%, and the rate for cervical epidural abscess is as high as 38% despite aggressive treatment.[45]

The presenting neurologic status is the most important determinant of ultimate outcome. The two other major factors in determining outcome are the interval from clinical presentation to diagnosis and the location of the abscess. Even when patients have severe neurologic deficits, good results can be attained if decompression is performed less than 24 hours from the initial manifestation of the motor deficit. Poor outcomes usually result from failing to maintain a high index of suspicion when faced with a patient complaining of severe back pain and from mistaking these disorders for more common entities until neurologic damage is irreversible. The initial reversible nature of the neurologic deficits suggests that they result more from neural compression than from ischemia.

### Spinal Subdural Empyema

Spinal subdural abscesses are rare. The available literature is largely based on case reports.[5,47] The mechanism of spread is similar to that with SEA when the abscess arises from a dermal sinus tract. The most common organism is *S. aureus*. Purulent material spreads in the subarachnoid space, inflaming the intramedullary and extramedullary blood vessels, resulting in thrombosis, occlusion, and ultimately, hemorrhagic infarction.

Clinical manifestations and the progression of neurologic deficits are also similar to those seen in SEA. The clinical presentation is likewise similar to that of an epidural abscess, except that spinal rigidity is less commonly associated with an SEA. Nuchal rigidity and meningitis may or may not be present. Plain radiographs typically do not demonstrate changes in the adjacent vertebrae. Myelography may reveal a defect that is often difficult to differentiate from an epidural lesion.[23,52] MRI is capable of defining the extent of infection and in most cases can differentiate a subdural from an epidural lesion.[28]

Operative management of spinal subdural abscesses includes laminectomy with exploration of the subdural space and débridement of suppurative material.[32]

Intraoperative ultrasound is often helpful for defining the extent of the lesion, permitting complete drainage.[41] If an associated dermal sinus is identified, it should be excised. Appropriate IV antibiotics should be administered for at least 6 weeks.[47]

The prognosis for subdural empyema is similar to that for SEA. Two thirds of the patients make a complete or good recovery after surgical treatment, in association with antibiotic therapy.[30] In a study by Probst and Wicki,[42] six patients were cured, five patients improved, and four patients died.

## Intramedullary Pyogenic Spinal Cord Abscess

Primary intramedullary abscesses of the spinal cord are rare, with only one being found in every 40,000 autopsies. The peak incidence is in the first and third decades, and males are more commonly affected than females. Approximately 25% of cases occur in children younger than 5 years of age. The thoracic spinal cord is most commonly involved. Approximately 80% of abscesses are solitary, and the rest are multiple. *Staphylococcus* and *Streptococcus* are the most commonly cultured organisms.[9] One fourth of patients have sterile intraspinal pus.

Intramedullary abscesses are most common in immunocompromised patients, including HIV-positive patients and IV drug abusers. Antecedent infections of the respiratory tract, spine, heart valves, genitourinary tract, and soft tissues, as well as midline spinal skin defects such as dermoid sinus, are found in 80% of patients. No apparent infective focus has been identified in the remaining patients.

Bacteria reach the spinal cord through (1) direct implantation secondary to trauma including lumbar puncture; (2) hematogenous spread; or (3) the lymphatics from the retropharyngeal space, mediastinum, or abdominal cavity. Lymphatics course along spinal nerves and communicate with the spinal subarachnoid space and Virchow-Robin spaces. Acute intramedullary abscesses are similar to other central nervous system abscesses, but they lack the widespread venous infarction noted with epidural abscesses. This may account for their often-favorable prognosis.

Clinically, an intramedullary abscess can have an acute, subacute, or chronic course. Neurologic symptoms and signs vary according to abscess location. Acute cases classically present with fever, transverse myelitis, and rapid deterioration of neurologic function. Pain in the neck or back may be present. Other findings include pain, urinary incontinence, dysesthesias, and monoparesis that progresses to paraparesis or quadriparesis. Patients with chronic intramedullary abscesses have a variable course simulating a spinal tumor.

CSF examination is generally unrewarding and may be misleading (e.g., pleocytosis suggesting meningitis). Myelography may show spinal cord enlargement, which is often associated with a spinal block. Postmyelography CT confirms the spinal cord enlargement but is nonspecific. On MRI, most infections demonstrate focal mass effect with decreased signal intensity on $T_1$-weighted images and increased signal intensity on $T_2$-weighted images.

Contrast-enhanced scans demonstrate nodular areas of enhancement or ring enhancement on $T_1$-weighted images. Contrast-enhanced scans allow for differentiation of the abscess from surrounding edema. The enhancement pattern on MRI is similar to that of tumor.

Operative therapy consists of laminectomy plus incision and drainage of the abscess. Occasionally, an intraspinal abscess masquerades as arachnoiditis. Henceforth, the surgeon must ensure that a cord abscess is not missed. As with all abscesses, broad-spectrum antibiotics should be begun as soon as infection is recognized. When obtained, the pus should be tested with a Gram stain and should be cultured for aerobic and anaerobic organisms and mycobacteria, as well as for fungi. Once the causative organism has been identified and its microbial sensitivities determined, specific antimicrobial therapy is initiated. Therapeutic efficacy depends on prompt diagnosis and abscess drainage. Postoperatively, patients should be followed closely for an extended period because of the high recurrence rate. Appropriate therapy results in restoration of neurologic function in more than half of treated patients. Less than 25% of treated patients experience substantial neurologic deficit.[7,34]

Patients with spinal cord abscesses caused by *Pseudomonas cepacia, Toxoplasma,* and *Mycobacterium tuberculosis* have been reported.

## Tuberculous Spondylitis

Tuberculosis may involve the vertebral column, the epidural space, the dura mater, the arachnoid, or the spinal cord itself. Tuberculous spinal infection most commonly involves the vertebral body. However, in up to 10% of patients, the neural arch, transverse processes, or spinous processes may be affected. Tuberculous spondylitis, with subsequent spinal cord compression, continues to be a major public health problem throughout much of the world.

Tuberculous spondylitis most commonly involves the lower thoracic and upper lumbar vertebrae and most commonly affects the vertebral body. It is usually confined to a single level.

Neurologic complications occur in 10% to 25% of cases, particularly if the thoracic spine is involved. Neurologic impairment may be caused by direct spinal cord compression or may be secondary to collapse of infected vertebrae, with subsequent spinal cord compression.

There are two categories of Pott's paraplegia: (1) early onset, in which the neurologic dysfunction begins within 2 years of the tuberculous spondylitis, and (2) late onset, in which neurologic deficits begins after 2 years. Early cases of Pott's paraplegia occur when the disease is active, whereas late cases are associated with a recurrence of infection.

No distinctive pattern of neurologic signs or symptoms exists with Pott's paraplegia. However, pain and local spine tenderness occur in an overwhelming number of patients. Radicular pain is common.

Radiographically, early vertebral body decalcification is observed about the disc, with slight diminution of the height of the disc space. Later, frank vertebral erosion and collapse occur, and paravertebral or psoas abscesses may appear. Sclerotic changes also may be present because of concomitant bone regeneration and fusion of vertebral bodies. Caseation beneath the anterior longitudinal ligament causes scalloping of the ventral vertebral border.

CT shows the expected vertebral body involvement. However, CT can also depict paraspinal abscess and an epidural tuberculous collection. Contrast enhancement may be useful for further delineation.

Spinal tuberculosis can be treated either medically or surgically. Treatment objectives include (1) healing the disease, (2) preventing or minimizing neurologic dysfunction, and (3) preventing any further gibbus deformity. Treatment with pharmacologic agents has been shown to be successful in multiple series.

The treatment regimen of choice for spinal tuberculosis is a combination of isoniazid, rifampin, and pyrazinamide for 2 months, followed by a 4-month or longer regimen of isoniazid and rifampin.

When the spine is stable and neurologic signs are absent or minimal, initial therapy should be pharmacologic rather than surgical. More than 85% of patients with Pott's paraplegia make an excellent recovery with pharmacotherapy. However, a patient with deteriorating neurologic function or a progressive gibbus deformity often requires ventral decompression and stabilization. Ventral procedures in the thoracic spine are extensive and are often dangerous, fraught with the potential for catastrophe. In addition, any deformity correction obtained with surgery may subsequently recede with time.

## Brucellar Spondylitis

The causative agents in brucellosis are small, nonmotile, non—spore forming, aerobic gram-negative coccobacillus organisms that are commonly found in domestic animals, including *Brucella melitensis* (goats), *Brucella abortus* (cattle), *Brucella canis* (dogs), and *Brucella suis* (swine). The organism is usually transmitted to humans by ingestion of contaminated products, skin wound contamination from infected animal tissues, and inhalation of aerosols. The disease affects approximately 500,000 people per year worldwide.[11] Increasing use of milk pasteurization has resulted in a decreasing incidence of brucellosis in the United States. Likewise, brucellosis is also uncommon in other developed countries because of milk pasteurization.

*Brucella* infections are often asymptomatic. Initial infection leads to immunity in more than 90% of cases. After an incubation period of 10 days to 3 weeks, the patient typically develops a low-grade fever, malaise, lymphadenopathy, hepatosplenomegaly, and diffuse arthralgias. The infection spreads through the lymphatic system, resulting in acute systemic infection and chronic relapsing disease (undulant fever). However, a classic undulant fever rarely occurs in patients.[43]

Failure to provide adequate treatment at this stage can result in involvement of almost any organ system. After the initial illness, which may last for several days to weeks, relapse occurs in approximately 5% of patients. Relapses seldom occur in appropriately treated patients and often are the result of focal suppurative lesions. Musculoskeletal involvement is the most common complication of brucellosis. The spine is most commonly affected. Brucellar spondylitis typically develops secondary to chronic brucellosis and occurs in 10% to 50% of patients with brucellosis.[55] Brucellosis is one of the major causes of spondylitis in the Mediterranean Basin. Of those patients with spinal brucellosis, approximately 12% will have some degree of spinal cord compromise.

Brucellar spondylitis should be part of the differential diagnosis of any patient with back and radicular pain in a region where brucellosis is endemic. Lumbar involvement is most common. Localized back pain is the most common symptom. It may be present even at rest. In most cases, radiating pelvic and girdle pains are often noted, along with restriction of movement, muscle spasms, tenderness, and signs of nerve root involvement. Neurologic deficits occur in approximately 20% of patients. Formation of a paraspinal or epidural abscess is uncommon but can occur with severe infections.[37]

Pathologic studies suggest the infection originates within the body of the vertebra, particularly in the more vascularized ventral portion, and only later extends to the intervertebral disc. The infected disc then may become necrotic and subsequently degenerate. As it bulges, the disc may press on adjacent neural structures. Usually, only one or two vertebrae are involved in brucellar infections. Infective organisms can be recovered from the infected disc or bony material in approximately 20% of cases. Serologic tests may be required to diagnose a brucellar spine infection.

Involvement of the spine can be either focal or diffuse, with a predilection to the lumbar region. Hallmarks of focal brucellar spondylitis include vertebral end plate erosion and sclerosis, inflammatory changes, and intact discs. Features of diffuse brucellar spondylitis include osteomyelitis of neighboring vertebrae, involvement of the intervening disc, and epidural extension.[1] Radiographic changes occur relatively late in the course of the disease and are similar to but less severe than those observed with tuberculosis. Plain radiographs demonstrate disc space involvement with erosion of the adjacent cortical bone, preservation of relatively intact vertebral architecture despite the amount of infection present, and absence of gibbus formations. Plain radiographs demonstrate a thinning of the disc space and erosion of the vertebral body adjacent to the involved disc. This epiphysitis usually occurs in the ventral-rostral angle and may be the main sign of bone destruction. Osteophytic bridging occurs across infected disc interspace. CT demonstrates destruction of both cortical and cancellous bone. MRI and CT findings are similar for tuberculosis and brucellosis, except that tuberculosis produces more kyphosis and paraspinal abscess formation.

The mainstay of treatment for brucellosis is antibiotic therapy. Brucellar spondylitis is typically responsive to a number of antibiotics, including tetracycline, streptomycin, doxycycline, or trimethoprim-sulfamethoxazole, which should be administered for at least 6 weeks. The current World Health Organization recommendation is doxycycline at 200mg/day and rifampin at 600 to 900mg/day for at least 12 weeks. Antibiotic therapy should continue for at least 6 weeks, or until the sedimentation rate falls to normal.[35]

Although surgery is rarely necessary, the indications for surgery for brucellar spondylitis are similar to those for tuberculosis. The role of stabilization of the spine, or decompression of the spinal cord with stabilization, is determined by the clinical condition. Surgical intervention usually is not necessary and should be reserved for tissue diagnosis. Disc excision may be required for an infected, bulging disc causing neurologic symptoms, and laminectomy may be indicated for an epidural infection producing neural decompensation. If there is spinal involvement, but surgical intervention is not warranted, the spine should be protected until healing is complete using recumbency followed by cast application or brace wear.

Brucellosis is a completely curable infection. The primary pitfall is a delay of more than 1 month in diagnosis and treatment, which can lead to multisystem involvement and severe sequelae. Many patients with brucellar spondylitis recover spontaneously, which differentiates this entity from spinal tuberculosis (which is progressive).

## Actinomycosis

The actinomycetes are a heterogeneous group whose morphology suggests fungus; however, they are classified as bacteria because of their small size, primitive nuclear organization, and cell wall composition. The usual infective organism for most cases of actinomycosis is *Actinomyces israelii*. Once known as *ray fungus, A. israelii* is now recognized as a gram-positive, non–acid-fast anaerobic Eubacterium that is intermediate between classic bacteria and higher fungi. The bacteria are present in the oral cavity, both on carious teeth and on tonsillar crypts. Endogenous organisms gain entry to the body via breaks in mucous membranes.

Actinomycosis is a noncontagious, suppurative, bacterial infection characterized by chronic inflammatory induration, sinus tract formation, fever, and leukocytosis. The pathologic reaction of the body to actinomycetes is typically suppuration. Acute and chronic inflammatory tissue is reminiscent of staphylococcal infections. Areas of infection are most characteristic for their gross appearance of sulfur granules, which are actually collections of foamy macrophages.

The common sites of involvement are the face, the thorax, and the abdomen. Involvement of the spine is rare (less than 1% of all patients with actinomycosis) and is usually the result of contiguous spread from nearby structures (e.g., thoracic infection). Early in the disease, there may be vertebral body destruction with new bone formation leading to a honeycomb appearance that may involve the pedicles, transverse processes, and ribs. After treatment, increasing sclerosis occurs, along with bone bridging and fusion between involved vertebrae. Unlike tuberculosis, from which this infection must be differentiated, actinomycosis rarely destroys the intervertebral disc.

Involvement of the central nervous system occurs by hematogenous spread from a pulmonary focus or by direct spread from lesions involving the skull, face, and throat, possibly via the lymphatics. Diagnosis is generally made by percutaneous needle biopsy and culture.

Approximately 75 cases of spinal actinomycosis have been reported since 1891. Most patients can be treated nonoperatively with antibiotics and spinal immobilization. Before the advent of penicillin, approximately 75% of cases were diagnosed postmortem. The disease involves the vertebrae and ribs in less than 1% of patients who have actinomycosis. Isolated vertebral body infections can be adequately treated nonoperatively with bed rest and aggressive antibiotic therapy. The authors' standard antibiotic regimen consists of 6 weeks of IV penicillin followed by 6 months of oral antibiotics. Clindamycin may also be used. Indications for operative intervention (i.e., open débridement) include epidural infection with spinal cord compression, large abscesses, and progressive spinal deformity.

Mortality is high in untreated or improperly treated cases. Thus it is important to distinguish actinomycosis from other vertebral infections, such as pyogenic osteomyelitis or tuberculosis. Even today, an accurate diagnosis often is not made until a late stage. Therefore assiduous efforts must be made to obtain bacterial specimens from the infected site.

## Nocardiosis

*Nocardia asteroides* is the most common human pathogen in this family of aerobic, weakly gram-positive bacteria. It is a natural soil saprophyte, often found in decaying organic matter. Infection most often occurs through the respiratory tract, although other modes of infection may occur. The infection is most commonly observed in immunocompromised hosts.

Nocardiosis may imitate a chronic granulomatous response, but more commonly, the histologic features are suppurative necrosis and abscess formation, which are typical of pyogenic infections.

The most common primary site is the pulmonary system, but dissemination to nearly any organ occurs in 45% of cases. Dissemination to the brain, meninges, and spinal cord occurs in 23% of patients, but hematogenous involvement of the vertebrae is uncommon. Epidural spinal cord compression from vertebral osteomyelitis has been reported.

If there is no spinal cord compression or large abscess, medical therapy alone is often sufficient. Sulfonamides, in conjunction with appropriate surgery, have been the mainstay of treatment since the 1940s. Many other antibiotics have been used, either alone or in combination. The optimal duration of therapy is uncertain, but because of the possibility of relapse, treatment is often continued for many months after apparent cure. A poor response to treatment may be related to the presence of a second pathogen.

## Fungal Infections

Fungal infections of the spine are rare and generally occur in debilitated, diabetic, or immunocompromised patients. Patients with acute leukemia, patients with lymphoma, recipients of organ transplants, and those receiving chemotherapy are particularly susceptible.[40] Accurate diagnosis is often delayed because other medical conditions mask the diagnosis and because fungal spondylitides are often indolent in nature. Notably, sporadic cases of fungal osteomyelitis have been reported in immunocompetent patients.[12]

Although certain radiographic features are characteristic for each type of infection, the diagnosis ultimately depends on a tissue specimen. Evaluation of specimens with fungal stains and cultures is mandated, because the latter may be negative or may take several weeks before identification is possible. Percutaneous biopsy is positive in less than 50% of cases, whereas open biopsy is positive in most cases.

The management of the different fungal infections is similar. The cornerstone of treatment is correction of those host factors that compromise wound healing or immune defense mechanisms. Antifungal agents are the mainstays of treatment, but surgery is occasionally necessary.

Surgery is generally reserved for patients with neurologic deterioration secondary to instability or progressive deformity. The selected operative approach should address the specific pathologic features encountered. Dorsal segmental instrumentation and fusion may be necessary in the face of spinal instability. However, in general, ventral débridement with stabilization is preferred.

The prognosis for patients with fungal osteomyelitis depends on the organism involved, as well as on the host. As with bacterial infections, patients with diabetes mellitus or neurologic deficits have a worse prognosis. Mortality rates following fungal infection are often high, reflecting both the severity of the fungal infection and the patient's underlying disease.

### Aspergillosis

*Aspergillus* is a saprophytic mold that is ubiquitous in the environment. It causes infection only, with rare exception, in immunocompromised hosts. Although *Aspergillus* involvement of the central nervous system does occasionally occur in otherwise healthy individuals, it is more commonly associated with IV drug abusers and severely immunocompromised patients.

Infection typically is acquired by inhaling small spores (conidia). Although uncommon, spine involvement nearly always results from hematogenous spread from the lungs. However, postoperative *Aspergillus* discitis has been reported after lumbar discectomy.[2] Vertebral involvement can also result from contiguous spread from the lung to the vertebral bodies. Vascular invasion is common in immunocompromised patients, and it leads to tissue necrosis with abundant hyphal proliferation.[38] In patients with chronic granulomatous disease, vascular invasion is uncommon and hyphae are sparse.

The radiographic findings of aspergillosis are similar to those of tuberculous spondylitis. Destruction of adjacent disc plates with subsequent collapse leads to severe pain and neurologic deficits. Disc space narrowing, involvement of adjacent vertebrae, and the presence of paraspinal abscesses are common. Dense new bone formation with small lytic lesions without sequestration may be observed. Spinal CT scans are extremely useful in delineating the extent of spinal involvement, but the radiographic picture is not specific for *Aspergillus*.

Clinically, sinus tract formation is characteristic. The incidence of epidural abscess formation, in association with neurologic deficits, is high. Diagnosis is established by percutaneous biopsy. Treatment is typically prolonged administration of amphotericin B, although ketoconazole is effective for some cases.[22]

If surgery is indicated, the principles of treatment outlined for all fungal spondylitides should be followed.[25] In cases of acute *Aspergillus* discitis, early surgery with vigorous surgical débridement, along with antifungal treatment, yields a good outcome in most cases.[2,27]

The prognosis of patients with *Aspergillus* spondylitis is guarded. Surgery has been used in most cases. The outcomes with surgical treatment have been relatively dismal.[29] There have been several reports of successful treatment with antifungal agents alone.[22]

### Coccidioidomycosis

Coccidioidomycosis is caused by *Coccidioides immitis*, a fungus that is endemic to the southwestern United States, Central America, South America, and central California, where it is often referred to as *San Joaquin Valley fever.*

The primary focus of disease is the lungs, but the disease becomes disseminated in 0.5% of cases.[4] The organism enters the body through the lungs and disseminates hematogenously. Osseous lesions are found in 20% of those with disseminated disease. Vertebral lesions are most common in the thoracic and lumbar spine. Multicentric disease is common. Radiographic studies usually reveal that the intervertebral disc is relatively uninvolved compared with the vertebral body, pedicles, and transverse processes. Contiguous rib involvement is also common. Paraspinal abscesses and skin tracts are common.

### Blastomycosis

Blastomycosis is caused by *Blastomyces dermatitidis,* a dimorphic fungus that is endemic to the southwestern and midwestern United States. Primary infection in humans occurs by inhalation of conidia, which then convert to the yeast phase in the lung. The inflammatory response resembles coccidioidomycosis, with clusters of neutrophils and noncaseating granulomas. The incubation period for acute pulmonary infection is 30 to 45 days. The symptoms are nonspecific, and acute pulmonary infection may be undetected. The organism spreads hematogenously from the lungs to the spine.[13] Men are affected nine times more commonly than women, particularly those with a history of alcohol abuse.

Thoracic and lumbar lesions are more common than cervical lesions. The radiographic findings resemble those of tuberculous spondylitis, with disc space narrowing, ventral vertebral body involvement, and the development of large paraspinal abscesses. Unlike lesions in tuberculosis, thoracic and lumbar lesions often invade adjacent ribs, involve the dorsal elements, and produce draining sinuses. Collapse and gibbus deformity are more common with blastomycosis than with any of the other fungal diseases. Diagnosis usually requires biopsy, unless blastomycosis has been reliably detected elsewhere in the body. Blastomycosis coexists with tuberculosis in nearly 10% of cases.

Skin testing is of limited value because of cross-reactivity with other fungi and a high false-negative rate. Serum complement-fixation tests are neither sensitive nor specific. An immunodiffusion test is more sensitive, more specific, and is more likely to be positive in patients with disseminated disease. A radioimmunoassay and an enzyme immunoassay are available and are quite sensitive but lack specificity. None of these tests is available for routine clinical use.

Before the availability of effective antimicrobial therapy, the mortality rate exceeded 60%.[26] At present, the recommended therapeutic agent for uncomplicated spinal blastomycosis is ketoconazole. Ketoconazole can be administered in a single daily dose of 400mg. The dose can be escalated in 200mg increments to a maximum of 800mg/day if the response to treatment is suboptimal. Amphotericin B is reserved for life-threatening disease. Amphotericin B is particularly useful in those patients with central nervous system lesions, because ketoconazole cannot cross the blood-brain barrier. Therapeutic guidelines are similar to those for aspergillosis. The role of surgery is the same as in other spinal infections.

### Cryptococcosis

Cryptococcosis is a subacute or chronic infection caused by a yeastlike fungus surrounded by a gelatinous capsule, *Cryptococcus neoformans*. Infection is acquired by inhalation of the aerosolized organism. Because many cases of cryptococcal osteomyelitis occur in normal hosts, it should be considered in the differential diagnosis even in a normal host.[18] Osseous involvement occurs in less than 5% of all cases and resembles cold abscesses. Sinus tracts and abscess formation are rare.

The onset of cryptococcosis is insidious. The bone infection typically has an indolent course. Both serum and CSF agglutination tests are available, but they are limited by their suboptimal sensitivity. Before invasive diagnostic procedures are used, cryptococcal antigen in the serum should be determined.[18] Radiographic studies show lucent lesions of the vertebral bodies with sharply scalloped margins and little, if any, reactive sclerosis or periosteal new bone formation. Radiographically, the lesions resemble those of coccidioidomycosis. The disc spaces are typically unaffected.

Treatment for cryptococcosis consists of a 6-week combined regimen of amphotericin B and flucytosine. A high relapse rate is common, particularly in patients with acquired immunodeficiency syndrome, whose disease is controlled rather than cured.

### Cysticercosis

Cysticercosis is caused by the pork tapeworm, *Taenia solium*. This disease is rare in developed areas such as the United States and Western Europe. However, it remains a significant problem for many economically deprived regions, such as Mexico, Central and South America, Africa, India, and Asia. This disease should be considered when treating patients who have recently emigrated from these areas.

Humans usually become infected by ingesting infected undercooked pork. For disseminated disease to occur, gravid proglottids or eggs must be digested by gastric juices before they hatch and liberate oncospheres, which penetrate the intestinal wall and spread widely.

Spinal cysticercosis occurs in 2% to 5% of all neurocysticercosis cases, usually as a result of intracranial parasites migrating caudally into the subarachnoid space, where they may settle at any level within the spinal canal. The presentation is variable. Backache, radiculopathy, and slowly progressive paraparesis are all possible.

Cysticercosis is suggested by a history of infection with an adult worm, multiple subcutaneous nodules, typical symptoms, previous residence in highly endemic regions where undercooked pork may have been eaten, and eosinophilia. Indirect hemagglutination tests may be positive in the blood or spinal fluid. However, a negative result does not rule out cysticercosis.

MRI is superior to CT for recognition of the subarachnoid cyst, the contained lesion, and adjacent spinal cord edema. Intramedullary inflammatory changes associated with those cysts may also be demonstrated.

Praziquantel is an effective treatment of both cerebral and spinal cysticercosis. Because of the central nervous system's inflammatory reaction to dying parasites, concomitant administration of steroids to minimize this inflammatory reaction has been recommended. Excision of the cyst has produced significant improvement in patients with neurologic deficits secondary to neural compression.

### Echinococcosis

Echinococcosis is a rare disease in developed countries. It is caused by either *Echinococcus granulosus* or *Echinococcus multilocularis*. It is more commonly seen in the sheep-rearing areas of South America, the southern and central parts of the former Soviet Union, Australia, and parts of Africa. Humans become infected after the ingestion of raw meat containing viable parasites. Under the action of gastric juices, the oncosphere is released and penetrates the intestinal wall, where it is transported to the liver and other organs. The skeleton is affected in approximately 2.4% of patients with echinococcosis. Of those cases, approximately 50% involve the spine.

Once the oncosphere reaches the vertebral body, it develops into its larval stage, commonly known as the *hydatid cyst*. The organism grows within the intratrabecular space, destroying the bone like a tumor. Unlike other organisms, it does not elicit a large inflammatory response. Adjacent bones such as ribs or the ilium may also be invaded. The organism spreads beneath the periosteum and ligaments. Spinal cord compression occurs once the bony center has been perforated.

The clinical manifestations and duration of symptoms vary considerably. Back and radicular pain are common. Paraparesis or paraplegia is a common symptom.

Plain radiographs demonstrate an expansile lytic mass that is poorly delineated and that appears multiloculated. A complete blockage of flow is a common finding with myelography. Radiologically, the disease is usually confined to a single vertebra with predilection to the thoracic spine. The cyst appears as a well-defined area in the vertebral body, which may be apparent only on tomography. The articular cartilage and the intervertebral disc are usually resistant to the cyst. However, in untreated and advanced cases, the articular surfaces and discs may be destroyed, vertebral collapse may occur, and the cyst may spread into the paravertebral tissues or beneath the psoas sheath, simulating Pott's abscess. In an endemic area, the findings suggestive of hydatid disease are ring-shaped calcification in the cyst wall, eosinophilia, and a positive Casoni's intradermal test. CT of hydatid disease reveals more specific findings than does conventional radiography. It may show cysts within the paraspinal muscles. In addition to bone destruction, the presence of daughter cysts is pathognomonic. Arachnoiditis may be demonstrated on CT or myelography. Immunologic testing may be useful, not only for diagnosis but also for following the course of the disease and the success of treatment.

Recent studies have observed an improved prognosis for what was once thought to be a uniformly fatal disease. Introduction of effective anthelminthic agents and improved surgical technique have reduced the mortality rate to less than 10% and the recurrence rate to less than 30% in most recent series.

All patients should undergo surgical débridement, with complete excision of the affected bone and stabilization, as needed. To prevent cyst recurrence, a hyperosmolar saline solution washout is recommended intraoperatively. Although its value remains to be established, presumably, the hypertonic saline solution disrupts any residual cysts osmotically.

## Schistosomiasis

Schistosomiasis is an important infectious disease in many underdeveloped countries of the world. It is caused by the human blood fluke *Schistosoma*. Central nervous system involvement is reported in less than 3% of all cases, and spinal cord involvement is even more rare.

Spinal cord disease usually takes the form of an intramedullary granuloma or a meningeal granuloma, particularly in the conus medullaris, which is involved in most cases. Transverse myelitis has been reported as the most common presentation.

Medical treatment with the antischistosomal drugs praziquantel or oxamniquine has been reported to be effective and curative in most patients. Corticosteroids have also been reported to be useful in reducing any inflammatory reaction. Laminectomy and spinal cord decompression are important adjuncts in patients who develop acute paraplegia and who deteriorate despite medical treatment.

## Syphilis

Syphilitic spinal involvement was common at the beginning of this century. The spirochete *Treponema pallidum* is responsible for syphilis. Syphilis is often referred to as *the great imitator*, because it can present and resemble many other diseases. Spinal involvement typically occurs with tertiary syphilis and presents as either Charcot's arthropathy or intraosseous gumma formation.

Neuropathic (Charcot's) arthropathy of the axial skeleton occurs in approximately 10% to 20% of patients with tabes dorsalis. Charcot's arthropathy is a neuropathic disorder producing spinal degenerative changes. Rather than reflecting a primary bone lesion, Charcot's arthropathy reflects posterior column degeneration with consequent loss of protective sensation. Degeneration of the dorsal columns results in loss of proprioceptive impulses (i.e., the afferent impulses arising in muscles and tendons, carrying the sensation of posture and joint position).

Consequently, there is subluxation and traumatization of the intervertebral joints, destruction of the discs, and fragmentation of the articular cartilage and the subchondral bone. This produces excessive bone formation within and around the joint, as well as reactive bony sclerosis and spinal deformity. These changes occur most commonly in the lumbar and thoracic spine and are identifiable on plain radiographs. Charcot's arthropathy may be detected coincidentally or may produce low back pain or nerve root involvement if destruction and hypertrophic changes are severe. Characteristically, the radiographic changes are out of proportion to the severity of the patient's complaints.

Charcot's arthropathy affecting the spine is notoriously difficult to treat. Treatment includes an orthosis to limit excessive movement and to minimize further injury. The role of fusion is undetermined.

The syphilitic gumma lesion is composed of microorganisms and the local tissue reaction to the organism and its products. Gummas are rare, destructive, and usually symptomatic, causing collapse and neurologic deficits. The clinical features of spinal gumma are often difficult to distinguish from those of coincident neuropathy, which is often present, and biopsy is necessary for the diagnosis of spinal gumma. The indications for surgically treating syphilitic gummas are similar to those for treating tuberculous spondylitis.

The treatment of choice for syphilis is penicillin. Effective alternatives include tetracycline, chloramphenicol, ceftriaxone, and other cephalosporins.

### Differential Diagnosis

The differential diagnosis should include bacterial infections, sarcoidosis, and neuropathic spine disease. Sarcoidosis rarely involves the spine but may produce paraspinal masses and circumscribed lytic spine lesions with or without a sclerotic rim. Purely sclerotic lesions occur less commonly. Neuropathic disease of the spine is limited to one to three contiguous vertebrae and is characterized by marked reactive sclerosis or destruction. Sclerosis associated with neuropathic disease of the spine parallels the base of the vertebral body and commonly involves the dorsal arch. Such sclerotic changes are associated with paraspinal debris but not with masses.

## REFERENCES

1. al-Shahed M, Sharif HS, Haddad MC, *et al:* Imaging features of musculoskeletal brucellosis. *Radiographics* 14:333, 1994.

2. Assaad W, Nuchikat PS, Cohen L, *et al: Aspergillus* discitis with acute disc abscess. *Spine* 19:2226, 1994.

3. Baker AS, Ojemann JRG, Swartz MN, *et al:* Spinal epidural abscess. *N Engl J Med* 293:463, 1975.

4. Banuelos AF, Williams PL, Johnson RH, et al: Central nervous system abscesses due to Coccidioides species. Clin Infect Dis 22:240, 1996.

5. Bartels RH, de Jong TR, Grotenhuis JA: Spinal subdural abscess. Case report. J Neurosurg 76:307, 1992.

6. Bircher M, Tasker T, Crawshaw C, Mulholland R: Discitis following lumbar surgery. Spine 13:98, 1988.

7. Blacklock JB, Hood TW, Maxwell RE: Intramedullary spinal cord abscess. J Neurosurg 57:270, 1982.

8. Bongartz EB, Ulrich P, Fidler M, Bernucci C: Reoperation in the management of post-operative disc space infection. Zentralbl Neurochir 55:120, 1994.

9. Carey ME: Infections of the spine and spinal cord. In Youmans JR (ed): Neurological surgery, ed 4. Philadelphia, WB Saunders, 1996, pp 3759-3781.

10. Dauch W: Infection of the intervertebral space following conventional and microsurgical operation on the herniated lumbar intervertebral disc. Acta Neurochir 82:43, 1986.

11. Faria F, Viegas F: Spinal brucellosis: A personal experience of nine patients and a review of the literature. Paraplegia 33:294, 1995.

12. Ferra C, Doebbeling BN, Hollis RJ, et al: Candida tropicalis vertebral osteomyelitis: A late sequela of fungemia. Clin Infect Dis 19:697, 1994.

13. Ford L, Key J: Postoperative infection of the intervertebral disc space. South Med J 48:1295, 1955.

14. Fouquet B, Goupille P, Jattiot F: Discitis after lumbar disc surgery. Spine 17:356, 1992.

15. Fraser RD, Osti O, Vernon-Roberts B: Discitis following chemonucleolysis: An experimental study. Spine 11:679, 1986.

16. Fraser R, Osti O, Vernon-Roberts B: Discitis after discography. J Bone Joint Surg 69B:26, 1987.

17. Gieseking H: Lokalisierte spondylitis nach operiertem bandscheibenvorfall. Zentralbl Chir 76:1470, 1951.

18. Gurevitz O, Goldschmied-Reuven A, Block C, et al: Cryptococcus neoformans vertebral osteomyelitis. J Med Vet Mycol 32:315, 1994.

19. Guyer RD, Collier RR, Ohnmeiss DD, et al: Extraosseous spinal lesions mimicking disc disease. Spine 13:328, 1988.

20. Hudgins W: The role of microdiscectomy. Orthop Clin North Am 14:589, 1983.

21. Kern C: Delayed death following disk surgery. Texas State Med J 50:158, 1954.

22. Kline MW, Bocobo FC, Paul ME, et al: Successful medical therapy of Aspergillus osteomyelitis of the spine in an 11-year-old boy with chronic granulomatous disease. Pediatrics 93:830, 1994.

23. Knudsen LL, Voldby B, Stagaard M: Computed tomographic myelography in spinal subdural empyema. Neuroradiology 29:99, 1987.

24. Kopecky K, Gilmor R, Scott J, Edwards M: Pitfalls of computed tomography in diagnosis of discitis. Neuroradiology 27:57, 1985.

25. Korovessis P, Repanti M, Katsardis T, Stamatakis M: Anterior decompression and fusion for Aspergillus osteomyelitis of the lumbar spine associated with paraparesis. Spine 19:2715, 1994.

26. Lagging LM, Breland CM, Kennedy DJ, et al: Delayed treatment of pulmonary blastomycosis causing vertebral osteomyelitis, paraspinal abscess, and spinal cord compression. Scand J Infect Dis 26:111, 1994.

27. Lang EW, Pitts LH: Intervertebral disc space infection caused by Aspergillus fumigatus. Eur Spine J 5:207, 1996.

28. Levy ML, Wieder BH, Schneider J, et al: Subdural empyema of the cervical spine: Clinicopathological correlates and magnetic resonance imaging. Report of three cases. J Neurosurg 79:929, 1993.

29. Liu Z, Hou T, Shen Q, et al: Osteomyelitis of sacral spine caused by Aspergillus versicolor with neurologic deficits. Chin Med J 108:472, 1995.

30. Lownie SP, Ferguson GG: Spinal subdural empyema complicating cervical discography. Spine 14:1415, 1989.

31. Mansour A, Nabos J, Taddonio R: Psoas abscess: Thirty-four years after pyogenic osteomyelitis of the spine. Orthopedics 2:262, 1979.

32. Martin RJ, Yuan HA: Neurosurgical care of spinal epidural, subdural, and intramedullary abscesses and arachnoiditis. Orthop Clin North Am 27:125, 1996.

33. Mayfield F: Complications of laminectomy. Clin Neurosurg 23:435, 1976.

34. Menezes JAH, Graf CJ, Perrett GE: Spinal cord abscesses: A review. Surg Neurol 8:461, 1977.

35. Mikolich DJ, Bsyca JM: Brucella species. In Mandell GL, Douglas RG, Bennett JE (eds): Principles and practice of infectious disease, ed 3. New York, Churchill Livingstone, 1990, pp 1735-1742.

36. Milward F, Grout J: Changes in intervertebral discs following lumbar puncture. Lancet 2:183, 1936.

37. Paz JF, Alvarez FJ, Roda JM, et al: Spinal epidural abscess caused by Brucella: Case report. J Neurosurg Sci 38:245, 1994.

38. Pfausler B, Kampfl A, Berek K, et al: Syndrome of the anterior spinal artery as the primary manifestation of aspergillosis. Infection 23:240, 1995.

39. Pilgaard S, Aarhus N: Diskitis following removal of lumbar intervertebral disc. J Bone Joint Surg 51A:713, 1969.

40. Porter SD, Noble MA, Rennie R: A single strain of Candida albicans associated with separate episodes of fungemia and meningitis. J Clin Microbiol 34:1813, 1996.

41. Price DB, Gottesman MH, Adelman R, Schneider SJ: Spinal subdural empyema: Appearance on intraoperative sonography. J Ultrasound Med 12:493, 1993.

42. Probst CH, Wicki G. Spinale subdurale empyema und abszesse. Schweiz Arch Neurol Neurochir Psychiatr 134:53, 1984.

43. Rajapakse CN: Bacterial infections: Osteoarticular brucellosis. Baillieres Clin Rheumatol 9:161, 1995.

44. Ramirez L, Thisted R: Complications and demographic characteristics of patients undergoing lumbar discectomy in community hospitals. Neurosurgery 25:226, 1989.

45. Rigamonti D, Liem L, Sampath P, et al: Spinal epidural abscess: contemporary trends in etiology, evaluation, and management. Surg Neurol 52(2):189-196, 1999.

46. Rigamonti D, Sampath P, Liem L, et al: Spinal epidural abscess: A report of seventy-five patients and review of their evaluation and management. J Spinal Disord (in press).

47. Sathi S, Schwartz M, Cortez S, Rossitch EJ: Spinal subdural abscess: Successful treatment with limited drainage and antibiotics in a patient with AIDS. Surg Neurol 42:424, 1994.

48. Scherbel A, Gardner W: Infections involving the intervertebral disks. Diagnosis and management. JAMA 174:370, 1960.

49. Silverthorn KG, Gillespie WJ: Pyogenic spinal osteomyelitis: A review of 61 cases. *NZ Med J* 99:62, 1986.

50. Spangfort E: The lumbar disc herniation. A computer aided analysis of 2,504 operations. *Acta Orthop Scand Suppl* 142:1, 1972.

51. Sullivan C, Bickel W, Svien H: Infections of vertebral interspaces after operations on intervertebral disks. *JAMA* 166:1973, 1958.

52. Theodotou B, Woosley RE, Whaley RA: Spinal subdural empyema: Diagnosis by spinal computed tomography. *Surg Neurol* 21:610, 1984.

53. Thibodeau A: Closed space infection following removal of lumbar intervertebral disc. *J Bone Joint Surg* 50A:400, 1968.

54. Turnbull F: Postoperative inflammatory disease of lumbar discs. *J Neurosurg* 10:469, 1953.

55. Zaks N, Sukenik S, Alkan M, *et al:* Musculoskeletal manifestations of brucellosis: A study of 90 cases in Israel. *Semin Arthritis Rheum* 25:97, 1995.

56. Zeidman SM, Leon L, Sampath P, Rigamonti D: Non-operative management of spinal epidural abscess: Review of 22 cases (in preparation).

57. Zeidman SM, Raycroft J, Ducker TB: Trends and complications in cervical spine surgery. *J Spinal Disord* 10(6):523-526, 1997.

58. Zeidman SM, Thompson K, Ducker TB: Complications of cervical discography: Analysis of 4400 diagnostic disc injections. *Neurosurgery* 37:414, 1995.

# CHAPTER 155

# Medical Complications

## Mark E. Shaffrey and Adam S. Kanter

Major morbidity and mortality can result from medical complications associated with complex spinal surgery. Although the relative risks are higher in patients suffering from acute trauma or multiple preexisting medical problems, the young and healthy are not immune to these difficulties. It is imperative that a sound rationale for the prevention of common medical problems be clearly defined and included in the critical pathways for spinal cord injury (SCI) and complex spinal surgeries. Despite the most comprehensive preventive measures, medical complications can occur, and clinicians must be prepared to diagnose and treat these complications expeditiously. It is only through appropriate preventive strategies, prompt recognition, and aggressive treatment of medical complications that the treatment of patients with complex spinal injuries remains safe and cost-effective.

## Thromboembolic Disease
### Incidence

Thromboembolic disease is a significant potential complication after spinal surgery, with the rates of acute deep venous thrombosis (DVT) ranging up to 15%.[30] The incidence of DVT is significantly higher in the population with SCI. Thromboembolism is reported to occur in as many as 70% of patients with complete motor paralysis. Pulmonary embolism (PE) has been reported in up to 8% of patients after spinal operations, with mortality rates as high as 0.5%.[18] Both DVT and PE are important predictors of a reduced probability of survival when compared with controls matched for gender and age.[39] Furthermore, mortality rates from PE have not changed in more than 30 years, emphasizing the need for more effective preventive measures.[39]

### Risk Factors

Risk factors for venous thrombosis are often related to Virchow's triad of venous stasis, endothelial injury, and hypercoagulability. Specific clinical risk factors that predispose to DVT include myocardial infarction, stroke, malignancy, congestive heart failure, previous DVT, previous PE, trauma, advanced age, smoking, and concurrent use of estrogen.[12,45] Spine surgery patients have an abundance of additional risk factors for developing DVT after surgical treatment. Protracted bed rest often occurs in the perioperative period. These patients often experience limitations in lower extremity movement because of neurologic deficits or pain. Complex spinal cases often demand lengthy operative times. Complex spinal surgery, with the addition of anterior and lateral approaches, often necessitates manipulation of the great vessels and thereby increases the likelihood of endothelial disruption and thromboembolic events.[12] Certain frames may compress the femoral venous system, and spinal distraction can result in compression of the left iliac vein.[18] An understanding of risk factors is critical in the development of preventive strategies for DVT.

### Prophylaxis

Recommendations for DVT prophylaxis for patients undergoing spinal procedures are varied and inconsistent. Modalities available for prophylaxis include use of gradient pressure stockings or intermittent pneumatic compression devices; administration of mini-dose unfractionated heparin, low—molecular-weight heparin, or low-dose warfarin; or placement of an inferior caval filter.

Prophylactic anticoagulation carries appropriate concerns with respect to excessive intraoperative blood loss and postoperative hematoma formation. Several studies have demonstrated effective DVT prophylaxis using mini-dose heparin in neurosurgical patients without significant bleeding complications.[4,9,14,19] However, most studies of neurosurgical patients have concentrated on gradient pressure stockings or intermittent pneumatic compression devices. Gradient pressure stockings and intermittent pneumatic compression devices appear to be clinically equivalent in reducing the risk of DVT in neurosurgical populations.[24,42] Combinations of these two modalities have not shown significant synergy.[24] Use of a prophylactic regimen reduces the risk of DVT formation in spinal injuries from 27.3% to 10.3%. Pneumatic compression devices have demonstrated efficacy similar to that of mini-dose heparin instituted on the first postoperative day.[14]

The authors adjust the prophylactic regimen according to the ambulatory status and neurologic condition of the patient. Preoperatively, hospitalized patients on bed rest or patients with neurologic deficits of the lower extremities are treated with pneumatic compression sleeves. Intraoperatively, all patients receive continuous treatment with pneumatic compression devices. It is also customary during prolonged ventral approaches to provide periodic release of retraction to decrease tension of the great vessels.[33] Postoperatively, compression devices alone are used if the patient will be ambulatory within the first 24 hours. If there are significant neurologic deficits or pain control issues that will prevent ambulation within the first 24 hours, both mini-dose heparin and pneumatic compression sleeves are used. If pneumatic compression devices cannot be tolerated because of injuries to the lower extremities, mini-dose heparin is administered perioperatively. For long-term prophylaxis, particularly in the outpatient or rehabilitation setting, low-molecular-weight heparin is used, a higher cost being traded for improvement of patient compliance and reduction in the need for laboratory monitoring. The authors advocate the use of proton pump inhibitors in lieu of $H_2$ blockers for treatment of gastric reflux and for the prophylaxis of stress ulcerations, because thrombocytopenia, a known side effect of $H_2$ blockers, may increase the incidence of thromboembolic complications.

## Diagnosis

Perhaps only 50% of patients exhibit clinical evidence of DVT, because physical examination is inaccurate in the diagnosis of this condition. Conversely, DVT is confirmed in only 20% to 30% of patients in whom it is suspected clinically.[45] Lower extremity pain and tenderness, leg edema, and low-grade fevers can be nonspecific symptoms and signs that accompany DVT. Clearly, rates of detection for DVT increase significantly as more sensitive and objective tests are used. Clinical suspicion remains an important first step in the initiation of more accurate diagnostic testing, because routine screening of asymptomatic patients after major reconstructive spinal surgery does not appear to be cost-justified.[37]

Contrast venography continues to be the "gold standard" diagnostic test for DVT. No other modality is as sensitive and specific for both proximal and distal DVT. However, high cost, limited availability, patient discomfort, and contrast reactions often encourage the use of less invasive tests.[45] By using a pressurized cuff, impedance plethysmography measures the change in electrical impedance of the lower extremity in response to occlusion of the deep venous system. The sensitivity and specificity for proximal DVT is high, but distal DVT is often missed on single examinations. Serial examinations using this modality can increase the sensitivity for detecting distal thromboses. This approach is feasible because of the low cost, wide availability, and high degree of patient compliance. B-mode ultrasonography is as sensitive as impedance plethysmography for diagnosing proximal DVT and is probably more sensitive for diagnosing distal DVT. Ultrasonography depends on radiologic interpretation and is typically more expensive than impedance plethysmography, but ultrasonography is now often considered the initial noninvasive test of choice. Venous Doppler flow analysis is seldom used as a sole diagnostic test because of its time-consuming, operator-dependent nature. However, Doppler flow analysis has proven more useful when used in conjunction with ultrasonography. In fact, duplex ultrasonography has demonstrated sensitivity rates in detecting proximal thrombi from 92% to 95%, with specificity ranging from 91% to 100%.[21] Iodine-125–labeled fibrinogen uptake scans measure the uptake of radioactive fibrinogen into forming thrombi. Although primarily a research tool, this modality may have advantages in diagnosis of distal DVT in patients with markedly abnormal venous anatomy as a result of previous DVT.[45]

## Treatment

Once the diagnosis of DVT is confirmed, the goals of treatment are thrombus resolution and prevention of embolization. General management includes bed rest, elevation of edematous extremities, and administration of appropriate analgesics (non–platelet-active agents). Definitive management of acute, proximal DVT requires a decision regarding risk of anticoagulation to the patient.

If the risk for systemic anticoagulation is acceptable, treatment of established DVT is usually initiated with a course of continuous intravenous (IV) heparin. The need for an initial course of heparin has been demonstrated in a double-blind, randomized trial with a threefold reduction in recurrent venous thromboembolic events compared with oral anticoagulants alone.[6] Most patients reach steady-state heparin levels 6 to 8 hours after an initial bolus and with continuous infusion. The therapeutic range for the activated partial thromboplastin time is 1.5 to 2.0 times control levels.[26] Both subcutaneous and intermittent IV routes have been studied as alternative routes of administration in the initial treatment of DVT, but clinical outcomes are variable.[39] The duration of heparin treatment before initiation of oral anticoagulants has been gradually reduced without significant change in bleeding or thrombotic complications.[20,25] The initiation of oral anticoagulation within the first 24 hours of heparin therapy is common. Because of variations in the half-lives of the vitamin K–dependent clotting factors, heparin should be discontinued only after the international normalized ratio is therapeutic on two measurements at least 24 hours apart, with a minimum of a 4-day overlap of heparin and warfarin. Treatment with oral anticoagulation for 3 to 4 months is standard.

The aforementioned regimen remains the authors' preferred means of managing thromboembolism. It does, however, carry risks of morbidity. The medical and surgical literature contains numerous reports of complications related to heparin therapy. These complications include thrombocytopenia and thrombotic disorders, skin necrosis, priapism, spontaneous hemorrhage, gastrointestinal bleeding, and epidural hematoma formation.[10,13,27] Decortication of the spine and the large potential dead space created during exposure predisposes the spine patient to an even higher risk of hemorrhagic complications and hematoma formation.[7] Furthermore, following decompressive surgery, hematomas are often in direct continuity with the thecal sac, placing neural structures at risk of injury, thus necessitating further surgical intervention and its additional risks.

If the risks of systemic anticoagulation are prohibitive, alternative interventions include surgical thrombectomy and caval filters. It is doubtful that surgical thrombectomy is of significant benefit if anticoagulants cannot be used to prevent rethrombosis after the procedure. In general, in patients who are at a high risk for bleeding, specifically including many patients following complex spinal surgery, caval filters should be considered.[38] These filters have been found to prevent PE in more than 98% of patients with known DVT.[5] The risk of major morbidity appears to be acceptably low, although the procedure may be complicated by extension of thrombosis into the caval system.

Management of patients with isolated calf DVT remains a topic of controversy. It is well documented that calf vein thrombi have the potential to propagate proximally.[30] Current evidence suggests that patients with calf vein thromboses must either be treated with anticoagulants or be followed closely with serial noninvasive testing. Three months of anticoagulation in patients at relatively low risk for bleeding complications, with serial, noninvasive testing being reserved for patients with significant risk for anticoagulation, is appropriate.

## Pulmonary Embolus

The diagnosis and treatment of DVT and PE are often discussed separately, but there is increasing evidence that these two entities should be considered the same disease process. Common clinical manifestations include tachypnea, dyspnea, and pleuritic chest pain. The initial evaluation for clinical suspicion of PE includes chest radiograph, arterial blood gas measurements, and electrocardiogram. The arterial blood gas measurement is useful to demonstrate alterations of oxygen transfer that accompany the ventilation of lungs that have a reduction of pulmonary vascular inflow (ventilation/perfusion mismatch). Arterial blood gases typically reveal respiratory alkalosis, variable reduction in partial arterial oxygen pressure, and widening of the alveolar-arterial oxygen pressure gradient. Chest radiographs and electrocardiograms are more important and are used to rule out other diagnoses, such as pneumonia, pneumothorax, myocardial infarction, or pulmonary edema. Occasionally, the electrocardiogram may reveal right axis deviation or a right bundle branch block that may aid in the diagnosis of PE. Most commonly, chest radiographs reveal nonspecific findings such as pleural effusion, infiltrate, atelectasis, or elevation of the hemidiaphragm. If suspicion remains high for PE after initial evaluation, either a ventilation/perfusion scan in a hemodynamically stable patient or a pulmonary arteriogram in an unstable patient is appropriate. In general, clinicians should not order initial, noninvasive studies for DVT because of the inability to completely exclude DVT with a negative test, particularly for a pelvic source of thrombus.

The treatment of PE is often determined by the patient's hemodynamic status and institutional resources. Massive PE with significant hemodynamic compromise requires urgent intervention with acute thrombolysis, surgical embolectomy, or more recently, percutaneous transvenous fragmentation or removal of emboli. For stable patients with submassive PE who can tolerate anticoagulation, the protocol of IV heparin and oral anticoagulation outlined earlier for management of DVT is appropriate. Caval filters are preferred with patients who have contraindications to systemic anticoagulation.

## Other Pulmonary Complications

Pneumonias, respiratory failure, and prolonged intubation are all common in patients undergoing major spinal procedures, especially those with SCI. Immobility, particularly when combined with neurologic injury, can lead to atelectasis, stasis of respiratory secretions, and pneumonia. In patients with an SCI above C4, phrenic nerve function is lost, and therefore diaphragmatic function is typically absent. These patients require mechanical ventilation. With injury at C4 and C5, the patient has compromise of diaphragm function and may require short-term ventilatory support (long-term support if there is preexisting pulmonary disease). At lower cervical and thoracic levels, the loss of innervation to the accessory muscles of respiration and to the intercostals can impair respiratory function. Because of the recumbent position in postoperative patients and patients with unstable spines, the respiratory capacity is decreased.

To decrease the complications associated with these factors, clinicians should immediately institute aggressive pulmonary toilet including aerosol treatments, chest physiotherapy, and frequent turning (either by logrolling or preferably by using Roto-Rest beds). Shifting the body

position prevents any portion of the lung from remaining chronically dependent. In mechanically ventilated patients, frequent suctioning is essential. Instillation of normal saline (5ml) or acetylcysteine often helps mobilize viscous secretions. Bronchoscopy may become necessary for refractory atelectasis or mucous plugging, especially in quadriplegic patients who are unable to cough and clear their own secretions. In patients who are not intubated, incentive spirometry should be encouraged hourly while they are awake. In patients with SCI, stabilization of the spinal column should be carried out as soon as the patient's medical condition permits. Early mobilization is important. Postoperatively, patients should be mobilized as soon as their condition permits, and early, aggressive physical and occupational therapy should be initiated.

## Cardiac and Vascular Complications

Neurogenic shock can occur in patients with SCI at T6 or above because of the loss of thoracic sympathetic outflow. This results in decreased venous tone, causing pooling of the blood volume in the extremities and hypotension. The decreased sympathetic tone to the heart may result in bradycardia, exacerbating hypotension. Peripheral vasculature dilation results in core hypothermia, although the skin temperature remains warm. Hypotension should be treated with pressor agents such as dopamine (which also increases the heart rate at higher doses); if there is a component of hypovolemic shock, fluid resuscitation is also necessary, but hypervolemia should be avoided.

Patients with underlying heart disease or those with multiple causes for shock may need Swan-Ganz monitoring. Bradycardia may need to be treated with atropine, but atropine dries mucous membranes, thickens secretions, and may exacerbate respiratory dysfunction. Hypothermia should be treated with a warming blanket. A heated air warmer, as opposed to a water-filled warming blanket, lessens the risk of decubiti and makes nursing care easier. The sympathetic tone begins to return in 3 to 7 days. This can result in volume overload and may produce significant diuresis.

The lumbar sympathetic chain is located on the lateral aspect of the vertebral bodies. Ventral approaches commonly damage this chain, which has generated numerous reports of sensory dysesthesias on the contralateral side.[33] This is likely a result of the affected side having lost its sympathetic vasoconstriction capabilities, thus its feeling of warmth imparts a "false" sensation of coolness in its counterpart. Most of these dysesthesias are believed to resolve in time, because few patients report long-term sequelae.[33]

## Gastrointestinal Complications
### Stress Ulcerations

The stress resulting from a complicated surgery, traumatic injury, and mechanical ventilation can predispose a patient to ulcer formation. Stress ulcerations appear to be related to ischemia of gastric capillary beds, resulting in diminished resistance of the gastric lining to the digestive secretions of the stomach.[23] There has been a gradual reduction in the incidence of severe bleeding from stress ulcerations. This is thought to result from a combination of routine prophylaxis (antacids, $H_2$ blockers, proton pump inhibitors, or sucralfate) and improved attention to tissue oxygenation.[34] The primary goal of antacids and $H_2$ blockers is to elevate gastric pH. Sucralfate is thought to enhance protective gastric mucous secretions and to increase mucosal blood flow and local prostaglandin synthesis without changing gastric pH. There have been reported concerns that elevations in gastric pH may lead to bacterial colonization of the stomach, resulting in increased risk of nosocomial pneumonias.[16] Sucralfate and continuous infusion cimetidine have been found to be less commonly associated with nosocomial pneumonias.[28,41] With cost concerns and controversies surrounding nosocomial pneumonias, sucralfate or continuous infusion cimetidine may be preferable to traditional bolus $H_2$ blocker therapy. Because of the aforementioned risks associated with $H_2$ blockade and the potential for thrombocytopenia, proton pump inhibitors have been gaining more widespread use following more complex spinal procedures.

## Adynamic Ileus

Adynamic ileus is a well-known complication of spinal surgery, and it often occurs in patients with acute, complete SCI. In SCI, this is a result of mechanical effects or of the loss of autonomic neural function. Ileus is characterized by abdominal distension and absent bowel sounds. Nausea and vomiting, respiratory distress, a feeling of constipation, or abdominal tenderness may be present. Copious gas is diffusely distributed through the intestine and colon, often with fluid levels. The diaphragm may be elevated and have diminished motion. If the clinical picture and plain radiography provide an inconclusive diagnosis, contrast medium can be given orally. In adynamic ileus, some contrast medium should reach the cecum in 4 hours; a stationary column for 3 to 4 hours indicates complete obstruction.

Treatment includes restriction of oral intake and administration of bowel stimulants, enemas, or laxatives. In some cases, nasogastric (NG) suction and replacement of electrolytes may be required. In SCI, patients rapidly become catabolic, and parenteral nutrition should begin early, often with total parenteral nutrition within 24 to 48 hours of admission. Ulcer prophylaxis should also begin. Metoclopramide, a dopamine antagonist, can increase intestinal motility without inducing spasm and can be used for postoperative ileus. In rare instances, adynamic ileus does not respond to conservative treatment, and operative intervention is needed. If no mechanical obstruction is found, a long NG suction tube is fed into the small bowel, and tube cecostomy may be indicated. This initially exacerbates the ileus. However, the bowel can now be adequately decompressed.[21]

## Ogilvie's Syndrome

Ogilvie's syndrome, or pseudoobstruction of the colon, is characterized by massive abdominal distension with a cecal diameter greater than 9cm. Nausea and vomiting, constipation, diarrhea, and pain are all more common in Ogilvie's syndrome than in adynamic ileus. The diagnosis is made by the clinical findings, including high-pitched bowel sounds, and radiographic findings of marked distension of the proximal colon with distal cutoff of colonic gas. The radiographic findings may be difficult to distinguish from cecal volvulus.

Colonic pseudoobstruction is a major contributor to morbidity and lengthened hospital stays, occurring in as many as 12% of all spinal surgery patients.[8] Delayed diagnosis can result in serious complications, including spontaneous perforation in up to 3% with an attendant mortality rate of 50%.[35] Patients at increased risk are those who have had previous abdominal surgeries, more extensive dissections, retroperitoneal hematomas, major intraoperative fluid shifts, and excessive narcotic use.[33] Ogilvie's syndrome has further been acclaimed as a harbinger for further complications instigating a down-spiral of worsening prognoses; thus prompt recognition and treatment is of paramount importance for patient well-being and for health care expenditure.[11]

Initial treatment for Ogilvie's syndrome includes NG suction, insertion of rectal tubes, cessation of oral intake, and cessation of narcotics. Patients who fail to respond to these measures may undergo pharmacologic interventions, if they are not contraindicated, before the clinician considers colonoscopic decompression. Numerous studies have reported the use of the acetylcholinesterase inhibitor neostigmine for treatment of refractory postoperative spinal surgery ileus.[1,2,31,32] The obstruction is thought to result from an imbalance in the autonomic motor system via excess parasympathetic suppression. Thus neostigmine acts to increase parasympathetic stimulation, thereby normalizing autonomic stability. Cure rates have been reported to range from 86% to 94% following a single 2mg IV bolus infusion in appropriately selected patients.[1,2,31,32] Side effects following infusion have been reported to occur in less than 5% of patients; however, it is essential to note the contraindications to using parasympathetic agents, which includes patients with bradyarrhythmias and bronchospasm. Patients must be monitored by experienced personnel and with telemetry during neostigmine infusion, and atropine must be readily available at the bedside. The total cost of neostigmine administration is approximately $50, whereas conservative observation and treatment with NG suction alone have accumulated hospital stay costs estimated in excess of $4000 per patient.[1]

If pharmacologic means fail or are contraindicated, endoscopic decompression may be performed, although undoubtedly under suboptimal conditions in an unprepared and distended colon, further complicating and increasing the morbidity and mortality of the procedure.[44] Endoscopic decompression is reported to be successful in approximately 70% of cases, although approximately one third of patients require multiple endoscopic procedures for complete resolution.[36] Failure of colonoscopic decompression requires surgical laparotomy and tube cecostomy with a concomitant mortality rate reported as high as 26%.[43] Additional factors associated with morbidity include cecal diameter, patient age, delay in decompression, and ischemia or perforation of the colon.[43]

Preventive measures for both adynamic ileus and Ogilvie's syndrome include minimizing bed rest, returning to ambulation as rapidly as possible, and limiting the use of narcotics. Early recognition and treatment of these conditions are essential to reducing morbidity and mortality.

## Genitourinary Complications

Urinary complications related to elevated bladder pressures, infections, and calculi continue to be significant sources of morbidity after all types of SCI. Acute spinal injury usually results in a period of spinal shock. During this time, patients generally demonstrate absence of detrusor motor function and bladder sensation, as well as compromise of sphincteric activity. Uninhibited reflex activity of detrusor and sphincteric activity gradually returns over 6 to 8 weeks, and a pattern of chronic dysfunction is established. After this, the clinician must investigate changes in voiding patterns to rule out causes of progressive neurologic damage, such as instability of previous fracture sites or syringomyelia.

Distension of the bladder or bowel can lead to autonomic dysreflexia in the patient with an SCI above T6 who has returning spinal cord reflexes. Symptoms include hypertension (blood pressure up to 300/180mmHg); headache; sweating; pupillary dilation; and bradycardia resulting from increased stimulation into the afferent limb of the spinal reflex, which stimulates an overreaction of the sympathetic nervous system. The initial treatment and prevention are to ensure that the bladder and bowel are not distended. This may include more frequent bladder catheterization and more aggressive bowel programs including manual disimpaction. If these measures are ineffective, medications such as amyl nitrate or nitroglycerin may be necessary. In severe cases, spinal anesthesia has been necessary.[3]

Spinal injury in the lower thoracic spinal cord generally results in impairment of bladder sensation, detrusor hyperreflexia, and sphincteric dyssynergia. Incomplete emptying of the bladder is common, and elevated bladder pressures may result. This can lead to renal damage from hydroureteronephrosis or vesicoureteral reflux if an appropriate bladder routine is not followed.

Other than in the setting of SCI, genitourinary complications are rare and are usually related to indwelling Foley catheters.[22,29] In the setting of SCI, the most common source of morbidity is sepsis related to urinary tract infection. Urine cultures are obtained with any fever (even low-grade fever) or hematuria, and the urine is kept sterile until the indwelling Foley catheter is removed. Prophylactic antibiotics are not recommended. However, any infection is treated promptly. If voluntary control of urination is not established at the time the Foley catheter is removed, intermittent clean catheterization is instituted every 4 hours, with the goal of keeping the bladder volume to less than 500ml.[15,22]

Sexual dysfunction has become increasingly recognized as a complication following complex spine surgery as ventral approaches gain in popularity. The reported incidence varies by author but has been found to occur in as many as 20% of spinal surgery–related complications. Retrograde ejaculation in particular has been reported by numerous studies, with an incidence ranging from 9% to 24% following anterior lumbar interbody fusion procedures.[33]

This is conceivably the result of injury to the superior hypogastric plexus of the sympathetic chain located anterior to the L5-S1 vertebrae.[40] Similarly, with regard to complications related to great vessel manipulation and DVT formation secondary to retraction injuries, periodic release of pressure cannot be overemphasized to help minimize the incidence of neural injury.

## REFERENCES

1. Althausen PL, Gupta MC, Benson DR, Jones DA: The use of neostigmine to treat postoperative ileus in orthopedic spinal patients. *J Spinal Disord* 14:541, 2001.
2. Amaro R, Rogers AI: Neostigmine infusion: New standard of care for acute colonic pseudo-obstruction? *Am J Gastroenterol* 95:304, 2000.
3. Apple DF: Spinal cord injury rehabilitation. In Rothman RH, Simeone FA (eds): *The Spine.* Philadelphia, WB Saunders, 1992, p 1238.
4. Barnett HG, Clifford JR, Llewellyn RC: Safety of mini-dose heparin administration for neurosurgical patients. *J Neurosurg* 47:27, 1977.
5. Becker DM, Philbrick JT, Selby B: Inferior vena cava filters. *Arch Intern Med* 152:1985, 1992.
6. Brandjes DPM, Heijboer H, Buller HR, *et al*: Acenocoumarol and heparin compared with acenocoumarol alone in the initial treatment of proximal-vein thrombosis. *N Engl J Med* 327:1485, 1992.
7. Cain JE, Major MR, Lauerman WC, *et al*: The morbidity of heparin therapy after development of pulmonary embolism in patients undergoing thoracolumbar or lumbar spinal fusion. *Spine* 20:1600, 1995.
8. Caner H, Bavbek M, Albayrak A, Altinors TC: Ogilvie's syndrome as a rare complication of lumbar disc surgery. *Can J Neurol Sci* 27:77, 2000.
9. Cerrato D, Ariano C, Fiacchino F: Deep venous thrombosis and low-dose heparin prophylaxis in neurosurgical patients. *J Neurosurg* 49:378, 1978.
10. Clark SK, Tremann JA, Donaldson JA: Priapism: An unusual complication of heparin therapy for sudden deafness. *Am J Otolaryngol* 2:69, 1981.
11. Clarke HD, Berry DJ, Larson DR: Acute pseudo-obstruction of the colon as a postoperative complication of total hip arthroplasty. *J Bone Joint Surg* 79A:1642, 1997.
12. Dearborn JT, Hu SS, Tribus CB, Bradford DS: Thromboembolic complications after major thoracolumbar spine surgery. *Spine* 24:1471, 1999.
13. Demasi R, Bode AP: Heparin induced thrombocytopenia. *Am Surg* 60:26, 1994.
14. Dennis JW, Menawat S, Von Thron J, *et al*: Efficacy of deep venous thrombosis prophylaxis in trauma patients and identification of high-risk groups. *J Trauma* 35:132, 1993.
15. Dickman CA, Sonntag VKH: The intensive care management of spinal cord injury. In Andrews BT (ed): *Neurosurgical Intensive Care.* New York, McGraw-Hill, 1993, p 248.
16. Driks MR, Craven DE, Celli BR, *et al*: Nosocomial pneumonia in intubated patients given sucralfate as compared with antacids or histamine type 2 blockers. *N Engl J Med* 317:1376, 1987.

17. Feldman RA, Karl RC: Diagnosis and treatment of Ogilvie's syndrome after lumbar spinal surgery. Report of three cases. *J Neurosurg* 76:1012, 1992.

18. Ferree BA: Deep venous thrombosis following lumbar laminectomy. *Orthopedics* 17:35, 1994.

19. Frim DM, Barker FG, Poletti CE, Hamilton AJ: Postoperative low-dose heparin decreases thromboembolic complications in neurosurgical patients. *Neurosurgery* 30:830, 1992.

20. Gallus A, Jackaman J, Tillet J, *et al:* Safety and efficacy of warfarin started early after submassive venous thrombosis or pulmonary embolism. *Lancet* 2:1293, 1986.

21. Grady-Benson JC, Oishi CS, Hanson PB, *et al:* Routine postoperative duplex ultrasonography screening and monitoring of deep vein thrombosis. *Clin Orthop* 307:130, 1994.

22. Green BA, David C, Falcone S, *et al:* Spinal cord injuries in adults. In Youmans JR (ed): *Neurological surgery.* Philadelphia, WB Saunders, 1996, pp 1987-1988.

23. Hanan IM: Gastrointestinal hemorrhage. In Hall JB, Schmidt GA, Wood LDH (eds): *Principles of Critical Care.* New York, McGraw-Hill, 1992, pp 2001-2013.

24. Huisman MV, Nurmohamed M, ten Cate JW: Mechanical prophylaxis of deep venous thrombosis. *Semin Thromb Hemost* 17(Suppl 3):269, 1991.

25. Hull RD, Raskob GE, Rosenbloom D, *et al:* Heparin for 5 days as compared with 10 days in the initial treatment of proximal-vein thrombosis. *N Engl J Med* 322:1260, 1990.

26. Hyers TM, Hull RD, Weg JG: Antithrombotic therapy for venous thromboembolic disease. *Chest* 95(Suppl 2):37S, 1989.

27. Mant MJ, O'Brien BD: Hemorrhagic complications of heparin therapy. *Lancet* 1:1133, 1977.

28. Martin LF, Booth FV, Karlstadt RG, *et al:* Continuous intravenous cimetidine decreases upper gastrointestinal hemorrhage without promoting pneumonia. *Crit Care Med* 21:19, 1993.

29. McDonnell MF, Glassman SD, Dimar JR, *et al:* Perioperative complications of anterior procedures on the spine. *J Bone Joint Surg* 78A:839, 1996.

30. Oda T, Fuji T, Kato Y, *et al:* Deep venous thrombosis after posterior spinal surgery. *Spine* 25:2962, 2000.

31. Paran H, Silverberg D, Mayo A, *et al:* Treatment of acute colonic pseudo-obstruction with neostigmine. *J Am Coll Surg* 190:315, 2000.

32. Ponec RJ, Saunders MD, Kimmey MB: Neostigmine for the treatment of acute colonic pseudo-obstruction. *N Engl J Med* 341:137, 1999.

33. Rajaraman V, Vingan R, Roth P, *et al:* Visceral and vascular complications resulting from anterior lumbar interbody fusion. *J Neurosurg* 91:60, 1999.

34. Reusser P, Gyr K, Schedegger D, *et al:* Prospective endoscopic study of stress erosions and ulcers in critically ill neurosurgical patients. *Crit Care Med* 18:270, 1990.

35. Rex DK: Acute colonic pseudo-obstruction (Ogilvie's syndrome). *Gastroenterologist* 2:223, 1994.

36. Rex DK: Colonoscopy and acute colonic pseudo-obstruction. *Gastrointest Endosc Clin N Am* 7:499, 1997.

37. Rokito SE, Schwartz MC, Neuwirth MG: Deep vein thrombosis after major reconstructive spinal surgery. *Spine* 21:853, 1996.

38. Spanier DE, Stambough JL: Delayed postoperative epidural hematoma formations after heparinization in lumbar spine surgery. A case report. *J Spinal Disord* 13:46, 2000.

39. ten Cate JW, Koopman MMW, Prins MH, Buller HR: Treatment of venous thromboembolism. *Thromb Haemost* 74:197, 1995.

40. Tiusanen H, Seitsalo S, Osterman K, Soini J: Retrograde ejaculation after anterior lumbar interbody fusion. *Eur Spine J* 4:339, 1995.

41. Tryba M: Sucralfate versus antacids or H2 antagonists for stress ulcer prophylaxis: Meta-analysis on efficacy and pneumonia rate. *Crit Care Med* 19:942, 1991.

42. Turpie AG, Hirsh J, Gent M, *et al:* Prevention of deep vein thrombosis in potential neurosurgical patients. *Arch Intern Med* 149:679, 1989.

43. Vanek VW, Al-Salti M: Acute pseudo-obstruction of the colon (Ogilvie's syndrome). An analysis of 400 cases. *Dis Colon Rectum* 29:203, 1986.

44. Vantrappen G: Acute colonic pseudo-obstruction. *Lancet* 341:152, 1993.

45. Zamorski MA, Opdycke RAC: Advances in the prevention, diagnosis and treatment of deep venous thrombosis. *Am Fam Physician* 47:457, 1993.

# CHAPTER 156

# Cerebrospinal Fluid Fistula and Pseudomeningocele After Spine Surgery

**Bruce M. McCormack, Barry M. Zide, and Iain H. Kalfas**

Cerebrospinal fluid (CSF) fistulas and pseudomeningoceles are uncommon complications of spinal surgery.[16] Most injuries heal uneventfully if the dura mater is repaired. If dural closure is not possible, CSF may drain through the surgical tract to form a cutaneous CSF fistula. Immediate measures must be taken to stop the leakage, because the fistula track is a conduit for infection.[6,12,18,28] CSF may collect in paraspinal tissues or pseudomeningocele. Pseudomeningocele may cause chronic back pain, persistent headache, and less commonly, nerve root entrapment.[9,14,17,29] Perioperative morbidity is increased, hospitalization is prolonged, and additional surgery may be needed to stop the leakage.

CSF leakage can be managed by nonoperative methods, but occasionally, operative alternatives must be used. Therefore treatment must be individualized because a single therapeutic approach is not always suitable. The appropriate treatment depends on the timing, size, symptoms, and location of the leak. Small, well-contained leaks may resolve without sequelae, with only simple measures, such as temporary CSF diversion or, perhaps, an epidural blood patch. Operative repair is performed if the fistula fails to stop following these measures. Primary dural repair may be more appropriate for select patients. Surgery is also indicated for symptomatic pseudomeningoceles that do not resolve, and the patient must be aware that all the symptoms rarely resolve.

## Incidence

In a study of 3038 operations the incidence of dural tears during the course of bone removal or during dural sac or root retraction was 5.9%.[20] The majority of dural tears heal spontaneously, and only a small percentage of patients develop symptoms. In Mayfield's review of 1408 laminectomies performed between 1971 and 1975, the incidence of CSF fistula requiring reoperation was 0.3%, and the incidence of pseudomeningocele was 0.8%.[16] The exact incidence of postlaminectomy pseudomeningocele is unknown because many cases are asymptomatic. Swanson and Fincher reported a 0.068% incidence of pseudomeningocele in a review of 1700 exploratory laminectomies.[29] Schumacher et al. reported the

incidence of pseudomeningoceles to be less than 0.1% in 3000 patients who had undergone a lumbar discectomy.[27] Teplick et al.[30] reported a 2% incidence of pseudomeningocele in a series of 400 symptomatic postlaminectomy patients examined with computed tomography (CT). In the latter series none of the patients with pseudomeningocele were treated with reoperation.

The low reported incidence of CSF wound complications is because the majority of patients underwent uncomplicated laminectomy for discectomy.[16,20,27,29,30] The incidence is much higher and has not been well reported in patients with laminectomy for spinal dysraphism or in patients with a history of prior spinal irradiation or surgery. In one report 43% of patients with intramedullary spinal cord neoplasms previously treated with radiation developed a CSF fistula or pseudomeningocele after surgery.[36] The same authors reported a high incidence of pseudomeningocele (43%) and CSF fistula (13%) in patients after surgical correction of the tethered spinal cord.[35]

The largest retrospective study of CSF fistula after spinal surgery included 39 patients.[28] Sixteen leaks occurred after intradural procedures, despite a primary closure or dural patch graft. Of the remaining 23 cases, 19 occurred in lumbar surgeries. In six out of 19 lumbar cases (33%), a dural tear was identified and repaired at the time of surgery. In 13 out of 19 lumbar cases (66%), no tear or leak was identified at the time of surgery. A myelogram was performed the day before surgery in five out of these 13 cases (38%). Three cases occurred after cervical spine surgery.

## Pathophysiology

A dural breach, either occult or recognized, is the primary event that leads to postoperative CSF cutaneous fistula and pseudomeningocele.[19] With extradural surgery it may result from excessive traction on the nerve roots, direct trauma, or laceration at the time of operation. Myelography needle puncture performed before laminectomy is another cause of postoperative CSF leaks.[28] If the dural breach is recognized, CSF leakage may still result from improper suturing of dural defects, particularly ventral and lateral rents that are difficult to repair. Resection of dura-based tumors may result in dural defects that are impossible to close in a watertight manner.

Cutaneous CSF fistulas occur in the immediate postoperative period (1 to 7 days) from egress of CSF through the wound or drain track. Pseudomeningoceles are caused either by herniation of the arachnoid through a dural tear, which forms an arachnoid-lined sac filled with CSF,[17] or by direct extravasation of CSF into the soft tissues, with eventual development of a fibrous capsule.[17,30] Once outside the confines of the dural sac, CSF pulsations force CSF into the muscular and superficial subcutaneous tissues. The size, shape, and location of the sac depend on the nature of the soft tissue into which the fluid is forced. In rare cases the capsule may ossify.[31] Entrapment of nerve roots in the pseudomeningocele may be a barrier to dural healing.[9,14]

The majority of dural breeches heal uneventfully. This suggests that there are other important pathophysiologic factors that may lead to formation of a cutaneous CSF fistula or pseudomeningocele. These include factors that delay or prevent healing of the dura mater and overlying soft tissue and that result in prolonged drainage of spinal fluid at the dural breech.[19]

Dural healing may be compromised by scar tissue, irradiation, localized infection, or foreign body reaction. These factors may also compromise healing of overlying soft tissues, which otherwise can absorb CSF, and act as a second barrier to promote eventual sealing of the dural breach. Systemic factors that impair healing include nutritional deficits, endocrine disorders (e.g., diabetes), chronic disease, and steroid administration. Spontaneous closure of large defects in the dura mater is unlikely. Similarly, patients with a paucity of soft-tissue coverage over the spine are at higher risk for wound complications. Congenital fascial defects and attenuation of myofascial coverage occur in patients with spinal dysraphism and spinal deformity, respectively. In these patients, wound closure by simple reapproximation of tissues causes undue tension on the suture lines that are not watertight, and may therefore be hazardous.

Seepage of CSF at a dural breach may be precipitated by elevated CSF pressure. For example, cutaneous CSF fistula after myelomeningocele repair is often caused by hydrocephalus (CSF pressure, 350 to 450mm $H_2O$), and it is promptly treated with ventricular shunting, which corrects the abnormal CSF dynamics. Straining can transiently elevate CSF pressure (to greater than 400mm $H_2O$) and should be avoided in the perioperative period.[26] Lumbar intradural pressure is markedly elevated with an erect posture (350 to 450mm $H_2O$), compared with supine recordings (70 to 170mm $H_2O$).[32,33] Hence patients are kept flat in bed for 3 to 4 days after intradural spinal surgery. Less commonly, CSF seepage at a dural breach is promoted by lowering of paraspinal tissue pressure by suction or by passive drains placed in proximity to dura.

## DIAGNOSIS

The diagnosis of a cutaneous CSF fistula is most often established by inspection of the patient's wound. A watery discharge is assumed to be CSF, particularly if leakage is augmented by upright posture or Valsalva maneuver, or is associated with postural headaches. Postural headaches are more severe with an erect posture and are relieved in a recumbent position. Headaches are secondary to the reduction of the CSF volume when the CSF loss through the fistula exceeds its production. The lowered intracranial pressure induces traction on pain-sensitive structures, such as meninges and blood vessels. When the patient lies down, this traction is reduced, and pain is relieved.[7] Fever or evidence of meningismus suggests bacterial meningitis. When leakage is profuse and clear at the incision site, the diagnosis is unmistakable. Small and intermittent leaks may be overlooked or misinterpreted, especially if they are mixed with blood. If the secretions produce a clear halo that surrounds a central pink stain on an absorbent surface (e.g., sheets or cotton gauze), the fluid is assumed to be CSF. Determining the presence of glucose in drainage fluid from the incision is not a reliable diagnostic test for the presence of CSF.[4]

A more specific test to identify a fluid sample as CSF is by immunofixation of B2 transferrin.[25] A high proportion of transferrin in CSF exists as a carbohydrate-free isoform (B2 transferrin) that is not present in sweat or serous fluid. Detection of B2 transferrin in such fluids is indicative of CSF leakage. Only a small sample is required (less than 1ml), and no special handling or refrigeration is required.

Pseudomeningoceles present clinically with localized back pain and postural headaches.* Localized nerve root entrapment or adhesions of roots to the dural edges of the pseudomeningocele can produce radicular symptoms.[9] Symptoms may occur several weeks to months after surgery. The clinical syndrome in the lumbar region may mimic the symptoms of lumbar disk herniation. Cervical and thoracic pseudomeningoceles may be palpable as a boggy mass. Lumbar pseudomeningoceles are usually not palpable on physical examination, but occasionally the collections track into the subcutaneous tissues.

## Imaging Studies

Magnetic resonance imaging (MRI) and CT will adequately localize the CSF fistula tract or pseudomeningocele.[14] MRI is the study of choice because of its superior imaging of soft tissue compared with CT. To best define the fistula tract for operative planning, iopamidol is injected into the subarachnoid space (Figure 156.1), followed by CT scanning. Suspected pleural CSF fistula[10,11,13]

---

*References 14,17,19,27,29,30.

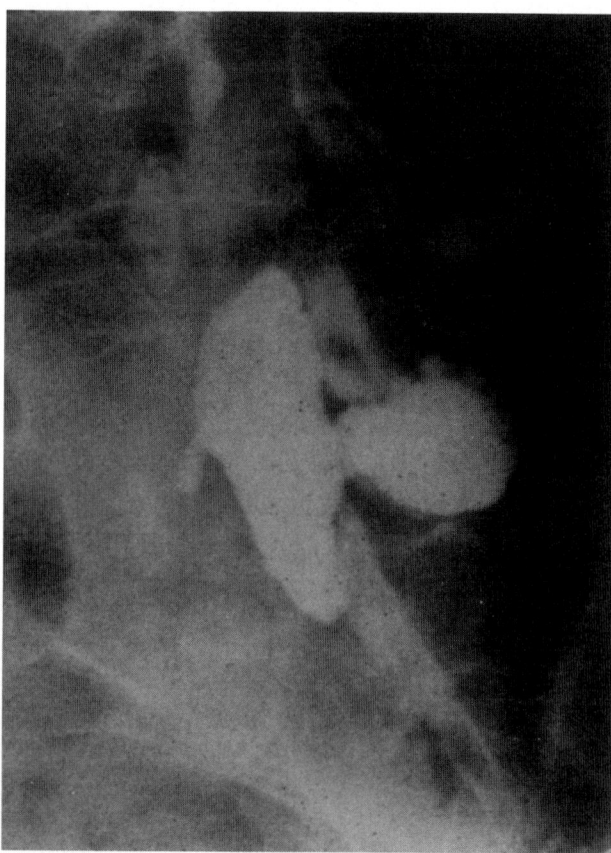

**Figure 156.1** Lumbar myelogram best demonstrates the fistulous tract of the pseudomeningocele.

or slow and intermittent leaks, such as those occurring after a lumbar puncture, are often best evaluated with radionuclide myelography.[10,24]

## Conservative Management
### Cerebrospinal Fluid Fistula

The initial treatment of postoperative CSF fistula is controversial. Successful treatment has been reported with simple measures, including bedrest, oversewing of the wound,[33] closed subarachnoid drainage,[3,6,12,18,28] and percutaneous injection of an epidural blood patch.[15] Others have recommended reoperation for repair of the dura mater as an initial treatment.[4] The authors of this chapter believe a trial of closed spinal drainage is warranted for the majority of patients and that only select patients should have immediate reoperation for dural repair.

A trial of CSF diversion predictably stops CSF cutaneous fistulas that occur after primary surgical procedures, from small dural breeches. A lumbar catheter is inserted, and CSF is drained (120 to 360ml/day) for 3 to 5 days. Spinal headaches occur in approximately 60% of patients,[12,16,28] and treatment consists of intravenous (IV) hydration, adjustment of the rate of drainage, and medication. The risk of infection is approximately 10% and includes meningitis (2.5%), discitis (5%), and wound infection (2.5%).[28] Transient lumbar nerve root irritation occurs in 24% of patients and resolves after drain removal. Catheter blockage has been reported in up to 10% of patients,[6] but this is less common with newer Teflon or silicone catheters.[28] CSF diversion stops the cutaneous fistula in 90% to 100% of cases.[12,18,28]

A percutaneous blood patch, commonly used for postlumbar puncture headache,[8] has also been reported to be effective in treating postoperative CSF fistula[15]; however, there are only a few reports in the literature. Advocates for the procedure cite a theoretically smaller risk of infection and earlier mobilization, compared with a trial of CSF diversion. Approximately 10 to 25ml of fresh autologous blood is injected into the epidural space near the dural puncture or laminectomy site.[15] Injected blood stops the leak by forming an occlusive clot over the dural breach and increasing extradural tissue pressure.

The use of prophylactic antibiotics for patients with cutaneous fistula is controversial. The majority of the literature on the use of prophylactic antibiotics for CSF fistula pertains to rhinorrhea and otorrhea. The evidence does not appear to favor their administration.[5] If antibiotics are administered, a broad-spectrum antibiotic is recommended.[23] Extrapolation of this data to postoperative leaks after spinal surgery should be interpreted cautiously.

### Pseudomeningocele

Symptomatic pseudomeningoceles that occur early after surgery for spinal dysraphism can often be dealt with effectively, using compression. Liposuction garments or abdominal binders may be used in adults. Children and infants can be fitted for Jobst garments.[34-36] Suboccipital pseudomeningocele can be treated with a compression dressing and by drainage of the collected fluid.

Early symptomatic pseudomeningoceles that occur after lumbar laminectomy and that are often associated with a CSF fistula can be treated with a trial of spinal drainage, as outlined previously.

## Surgical Management
### Indications

Surgical dural repair should be the primary treatment for patients who have accessible dural defects with profuse leakage of CSF. These fistulas are unlikely to resolve with a trial of CSF diversion. Surgery is also indicated for fistulas and symptomatic pseudomeningoceles that occur after surgery and that do not resolve with a trial of CSF diversion. Symptomatic pseudomeningoceles, diagnosed weeks to months after laminectomy, are treated with surgical dural repair.

In patients with impaired CSF absorption, a shunt should first be inserted, because direct operative repair of a fistula will fail in the presence of elevated CSF pressures. Shunts have also been successfully used to treat leaks in which wound exploration and dural repair may be complicated (e.g., pleural fistulas)[11] and fistulas at the occipitocervical junction.[3] Others have successfully treated patients with postlaminectomy cutaneous fistula with lumboperitoneal shunts in preference to a trial of temporary CSF diversion.[1] They argue that lumboperitoneal shunting minimizes the risk of infection and does not require prolonged bed rest. The authors of this book believe that these problems do not warrant a permanent shunt system.

### Surgical Principles

Novel wound closure techniques have been developed from experience with wound complications after resection of intramedullary spinal cord neoplasms in patients with multiple surgeries and irradiation.[36] Because of this experience, and a high incidence of wound complications in children after tethered spinal cord surgery,[35] a plastic surgeon is often called on to develop innovative closure techniques.[34-36] Wound complications may then be reduced to a minimum. In the majority of patients the dura mater was nearly never closed in a watertight manner. One or more myofascial layers are mobilized to provide a tension-free watertight closure. The skin is closed in three layers and a drain is placed from a distant (greater than 6cm) stab wound, and the drain tract is obliterated after removal.

### Dural Closure

Dura mater is repaired with a running 4-0 Neurolon or Prolene suture, often with loupe magnification. Occasionally a patch of fascia or cadaver dura mater is used whenever the dural defect is very large. This allows direct closure without compression of the neural elements. Such grafts or implants, however, are almost never watertight. The dural suture line may be tested by observing for CSF seepage while the anesthesiologist performs a Valsalva maneuver to increase intrathecal pressure. Alternatively, saline can be injected into the lumbar thecal sac through a small-gauge needle. Sites of leakage are sutured. If available, autologous fibrin glue may be applied to the dura and other surrounding tissues.[22] Although use of a vascularized, pedicled flap to close a thoracic dural defect has been reported,[2] such maneuvers are rarely required in our experience.

## Pseudomeningocele

The wall of the pseudomeningocele is entered. Any nerve roots herniated into the cavity are gently dissected free and reduced into the thecal sac. It is not necessary to remove the walls of the pseudomeningocele. The fistulous tract is identified at the dural surface, and the surrounding dura mater is widely exposed by widening the laminectomy defect, if necessary. The fistula is excised and the dura closed with 4-0 Neurolon. A patch graft is used, if needed.

## Myofascial Anatomy and Closure Techniques

It is useful to subdivide the back into three zones because the tissues available to the surgeon for closure are different in each of these zones (Figure 156.2). The upper and lower zones are the most difficult to close.

### Zone 1: Cervical Myofascia

One myofascial layer is mobilized for closure in the cervical region because the muscles tend to be overlapping and confluent. Skin and fat are first elevated off the underlying trapezius fascia for 3cm. Useless scar tissue is trimmed

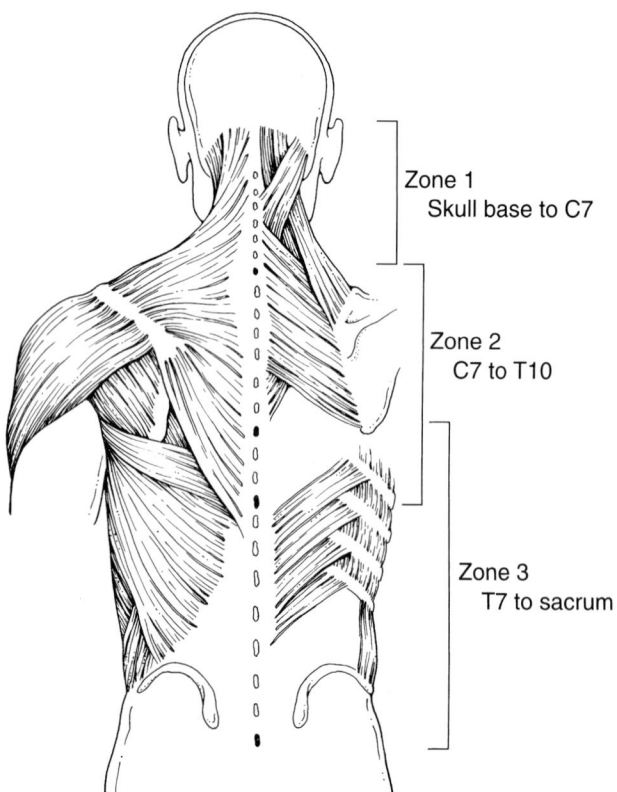

Zone 1
Skull base to C7

Zone 2
C7 to T10

Zone 3
T7 to sacrum

**Figure 156.2** The back is separated into three zones because the tissues available to the surgeon for closure differ in each of these regions.

from the muscle edges. The trapezius fascia alone is too thin in the upper neck to provide a secure closure, and therefore the underlying semispinalis capitis muscle (rostrally) and splenius capitis muscle (caudally) are used to add bulk to this layer. The heavy semispinalis capitis muscle is a vertically oriented midline muscle with fibers arising between the superior and inferior nuchal lines and running just below the upper fascia. This muscle fuses at C3-6 with the obliquely oriented splenius capitis muscle. These muscles lie just below the upper trapezius fascia. No attempt should be made to separate them, particularly if there has been previous surgery. In this case the nuchal muscle layers are fused by scar. Attempts at separation may result in multiple ribbons of poor material for suture. Rather, a sheet of conjoined muscle and fascia and associated muscle is advanced and closed. A cutting cautery is used to undermine these muscles above the vertebral laminae, leaving the overlying trapezius fascia and associated muscles for advancement and closure. If necessary, the fascia is scored in a vertical direction, 3 to 4cm from the wound edge. Traction on the medial wound edge forces the incised fascia to gape after release. The thin paraspinous muscles can be helpful in providing more bulk to this layer caudally. They are not, however, a critical layer. The craniovertebral junction region is difficult to close because it is also difficult to obtain a leak-proof closure of muscle against bone. This is especially true if a suboccipital craniectomy has been performed and the surrounding bone has been denuded. CSF may leak from the area adjacent to the bone or from the holes in the bone used for muscle traction sutures. The surgeon must release the lateral nuchal muscle insertions on the skull. These muscles are then mobilized to the midline by undermining below this muscular plane. Drill holes are then made along the calvarial edge for traction sutures. Novofil 2-0 sutures are placed through the drill holes to approximate the muscle to the skull (Figure 156.3). If sufficient soft tissue is available along the skull base, it should be used in preference to drill holes.

### Zone 2: Thoracic Myofascia

The trapezius muscle and its overlying fascia form the key anatomic structure used to obtain a "watertight" closure in this region. The skin and underlying fat are elevated from the trapezius fascia laterally for 3 to 5cm, using cutting cautery. The fascia must be clean but not violated. Excess fat can be scraped off with an elevator, and prominent spinous processes are leveled. The skin incision may be extended to allow wide exposure of the fascia. From T1 to T3 the trapezius muscle is widely elevated from the paraspinous muscles as a single layer. From T4 to T8 the rhomboid muscles are attached to the underside of the trapezius muscle. No attempt should be made to separate these muscles; rather they are elevated as a unit from the paraspinous muscles. A distinct areolar plane facilitates this maneuver, after a transverse incision into the wound edge allows the surgeon to define the separation between the paraspinous and the trapezius and rhomboid muscles. By placing an index finger into this plane, the surgeon can use the cutting cautery or scissors to separate the layer for the full length of the incision. This technique leaves a good edge of the trapezius-rhomboid layer for suturing. From T7 to T10 the fascia of the latissimus dorsi muscle adds some bulk to the trapezius fascia. The trapezius and associated muscles are mobilized medially for the entire length of the incision by undermining below this muscular plane. If necessary, the fascia is scored in a vertical direction, 3 to 4cm from the wound edge (see Figure 156.3).

The paraspinous muscles are mobilized medially. Skin hooks or wide, sharp rakes are used to hold up the medial edge of the paraspinous muscles, and the tendinous attachments are severed directly from bone to release these muscles. Protruding spinous processes at each end of the wound are rongeured off such that the paraspinal

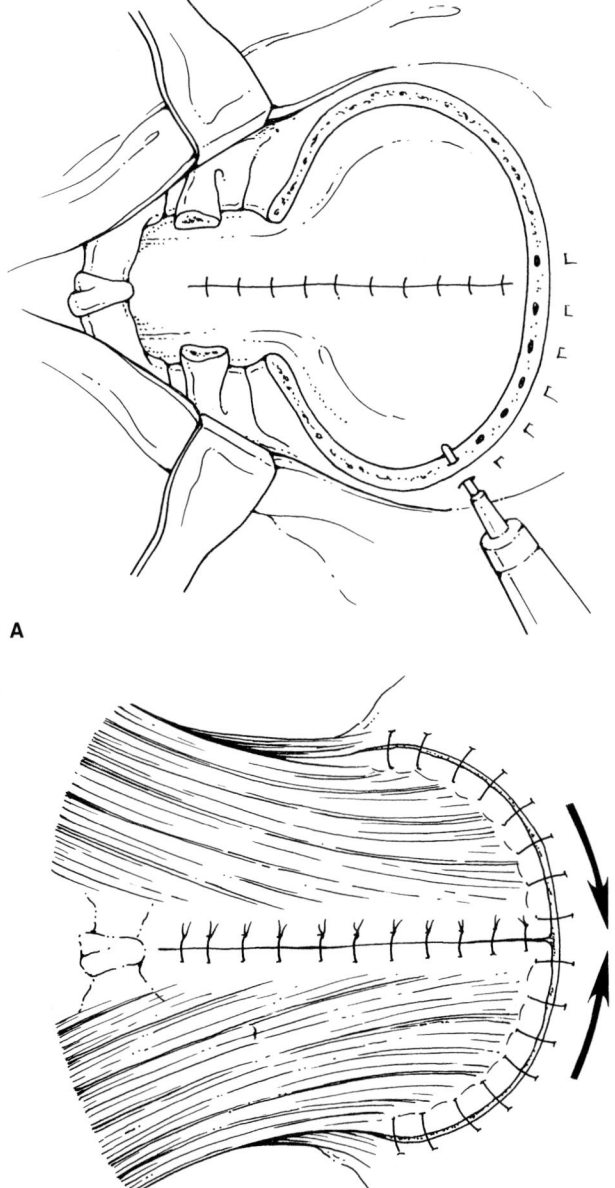

**A**

**B**

**Figure 156.3** Cervical wound closure after suboccipital craniectomy. **(A)** Drill holes are made along the calvarial edge for fixation of sutures. **(B)** These sutures are then used to pull the locally released muscle up to the bone. If sufficient soft tissue is available along the skull base, it should be used in preference to drill holes.

muscles are closed over bone, not around it. In some patients the costovertebral junctions may be prominent. Mobilization of the paraspinous muscles provides access to these bone elevations that are removed with a rongeur. Bony prominences may cause a postoperative pressure sore if they are not removed.

### Zone 3: Lumbosacral Myofascia

The fat and skin are elevated off the fascia in the thoracolumbar junction. Rostrally, the lower trapezius muscle and fascia fuse with the fascia of the latissimus dorsi muscle. No attempt should be made to separate these layers; rather the conjoined fascial layers are separated from the paraspinous muscles. As the surgeon progresses caudally the fascial insertions of the latissimus dorsi muscle become confluent with the lumbodorsal fascia. At approximately T10, the surgeon must change levels to obtain a layer thick enough for closure. When the latissimus fascia thins, the surgeon should incise a deeper layer, leaving the latissimus fascia confluent with the lumbodorsal fascia. This fascia is then separated from the paraspinous muscles below. In this manner the fascia remains thick enough to suture. Use of the thin fascial extension of the latissimus dorsi muscles, alone, for closure, will result in failure. The paraspinous muscle layer is isolated next and released from the transverse processes.

At the sacral levels the lumbodorsal fascia is nonyielding and difficult to mobilize. This may be a problem when the surgeon has to correct large defects in the lumbosacral region associated with tethered cord or myelomeningocele. In these instances relaxing incisions are made in the fascia about 3cm lateral to each medial wound edge. Relaxing incisions penetrate the fascia but not the muscle; otherwise CSF will leak through the "relaxing incision." The lumbodorsal fascia is released from the dorsal iliac bone from below with care taken not to perforate the overlying tissue plane (Figure 156.4). The gluteus muscle covers the insertion of the lumbodorsal fascia into the dorsal ilium. When this fascia is released, the gluteus muscle or fascia and the latissimus or lumbodorsal fascia can be mobilized medially.

### Tissue Expanders

Tissue expanders are useful when spinal soft-tissue coverage is severely compromised from previous surgeries or irradiation, making simple skin tissue approximation hazardous.[21] The Silastic tissue expander can augment the amount of local tissue available for closure. The deflated Silastic tissue expander is inserted below the trapezius or latissimus dorsi muscle through a small incision several weeks before the anticipated spinal surgery. Periodic expansion is performed by injections of sterile saline into the expander reservoir. The expanders, removed at the time of definitive spinal surgery, provide sufficient midline soft-tissue coverage, without undue tension.

### Closure of Layered Muscle

Evenly spaced, interrupted figure-of-eight 2-0 Novofil or Prolene sutures are used to close the myofascial

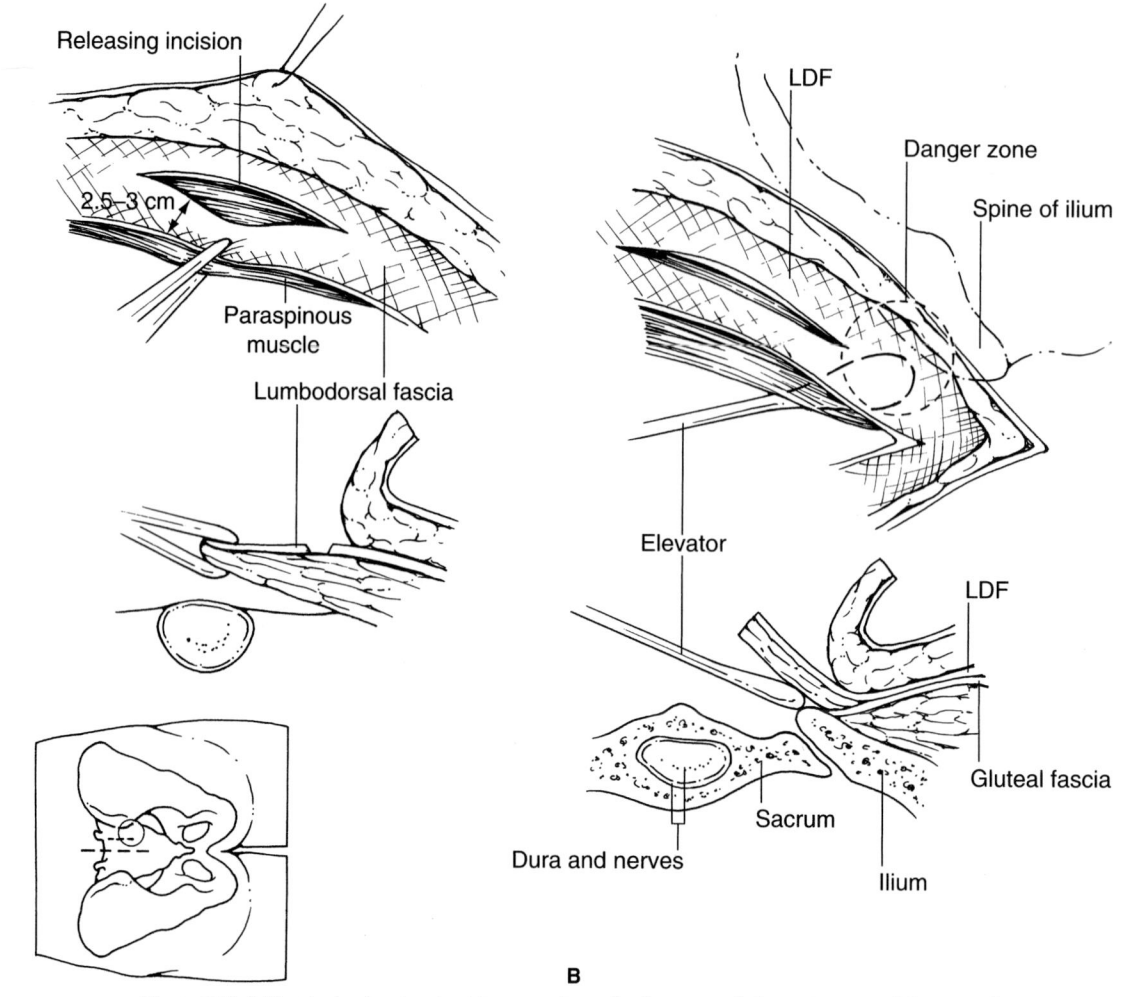

**Figure 156.4** Vertical releasing incisions made to facilitate medial movement of fascia and muscle. **(A)** Cutting through fascia only provides sufficient release. If the surgeon cuts too deeply, the operation may fail because CSF may leak through the release incision. **(B)** Proper release in the "danger zone" will usually provide sufficient laxity for closure. Extreme care must be taken to avoid cutting too deeply. *LDF,* Lumbodorsal fascia.

layer(s). The suture crosses deep and is tied tightly on the fascial surface, starting with a double granny knot. This nonabsorbable suture material provides permanent tissue approximation to prevent delayed dehiscence. Irradiated, scarred fascia is weak. Therefore permanent suture is particularly suited for this application. Because these sutures are blue, the distinctive color provides surgical midline direction if reoperation is required. Occasionally, sufficient laxity exists such that the surgeon may overlap the muscle in a "vest-over-pants" type of closure.

Just before placing the final musculofascial sutures, a large angiocatheter is passed through the muscle and fascia to lie over the dural or paraspinous muscle closure (Figure 156.5). Saline is injected through the catheter until the muscle bulges to ensure that the overlying closure is watertight. After testing, the catheter is removed and a small figure-of-eight or purse-string suture is used to tie off the stab site used for catheter insertion. Alternatively, the

end of the forceps is used to check for suture tightness along the full length of the musculofascial closure.

### Drain Placement

A suction drain is inserted subcutaneously through a distant stab incision. The drain is not placed below the myofascia because deep drainage increases pressure gradients across the dural breach and promotes CSF leakage. The stab site should be made several inches from the wound in a nonirradiated area. The farther from the wound the drain stab incision is made, the longer it can be left in. The Hemovac trocar, or long, thin clamp, is left in place along the drain tract while sutures of 0 Prolene are lightly placed with postmortem needles around the trocar or clamp. These sutures are left unknotted, to be tied later after removal of the drain (Figure 156.6). A separate purse-string suture is positioned at the drain hole.

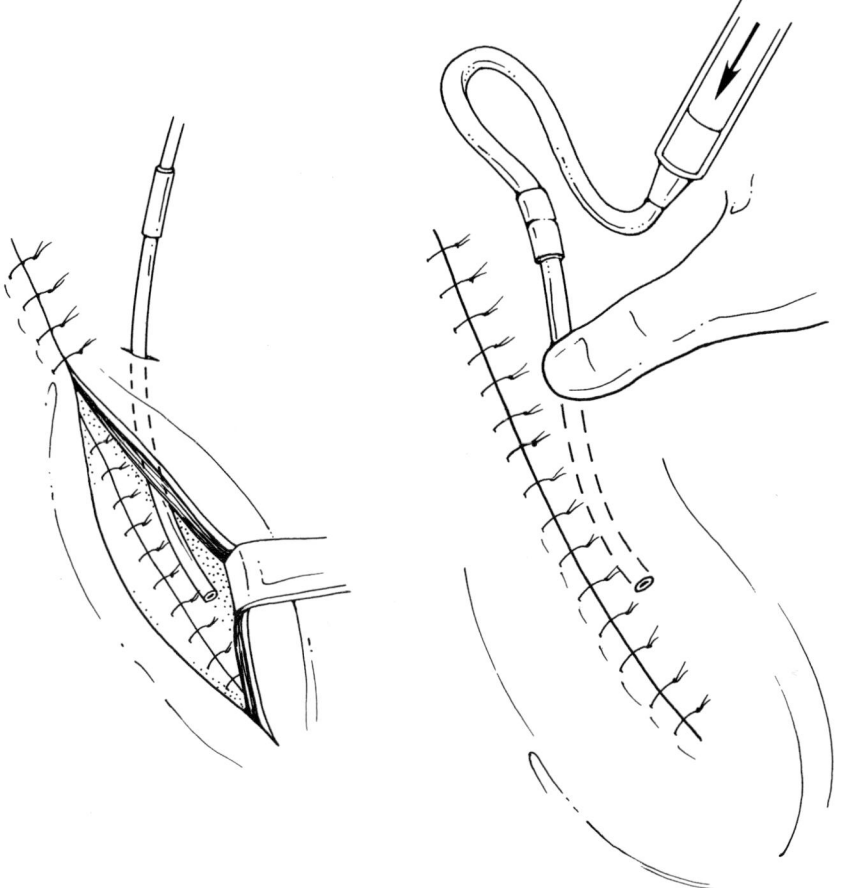

**Figure 156.5** A large catheter is passed below the myofascial layer to test its ability to prevent CSF leakage. The surgeon places a finger over the ingress site while injecting saline. Sites of leakage are oversewn. After removal of the catheter, this site is tightly closed.

## Skin Closure

Skin flap closure is performed in three layers as a contingency for leakage (Figure 156.7). The first layer is in the subcutaneous fat and everts the skin. The second layer is inverted and is in the deep dermis. Absorbable 2-0 Maxon or PDS sutures (3-0 sutures for children or infants) are used for these layers. This technique everts the wound edge, thus the incision appears humped up. The skin is then closed with interrupted or continuous tightly tied 3-0 nylon sutures.

## Postoperative Care

Adult patients are kept at bedrest for 3 days. The drainage tubes are routinely removed by the fourth or fifth postoperative day or when drainage is about 20ml/24hr. The everted skin closure flattens out rapidly after suture removal at 3 to 4 weeks.

A Jobst compression garment in children, or a liposuction garment in adults, can be fitted preoperatively to provide pressure to the wound in the perioperative period. Compression garments minimize the incidence of pseudomeningoceles. They are especially helpful in the lumbosacral region, in which binders tend to slip and seromas tend to occur.

## Summary

CSF cutaneous fistulas and pseudomeningoceles are uncommon complications of spinal surgery that increase patient morbidity, hospitalization, and cost of care. Although violation of the dura mater is the primary event leading to these wound complications, factors that adversely affect wound healing and prolong drainage of spinal fluid are contributory. Diagnosis of cutaneous fistula is made by inspection of the patient's wound, and diagnosis of pseudomeningocele is made with MRI or CT. CT myelography may help in operative planning. In the majority of uncomplicated cases, patients can be acutely treated with CSF diversion, or perhaps with a percutaneous blood patch. Surgical dural repair is indicated for select patients. If operative repair is indicated, dural and myofascial closure techniques discussed in this chapter can help minimize the incidence of wound complications in complex laminectomies. In rare instances a shunt is indicated for

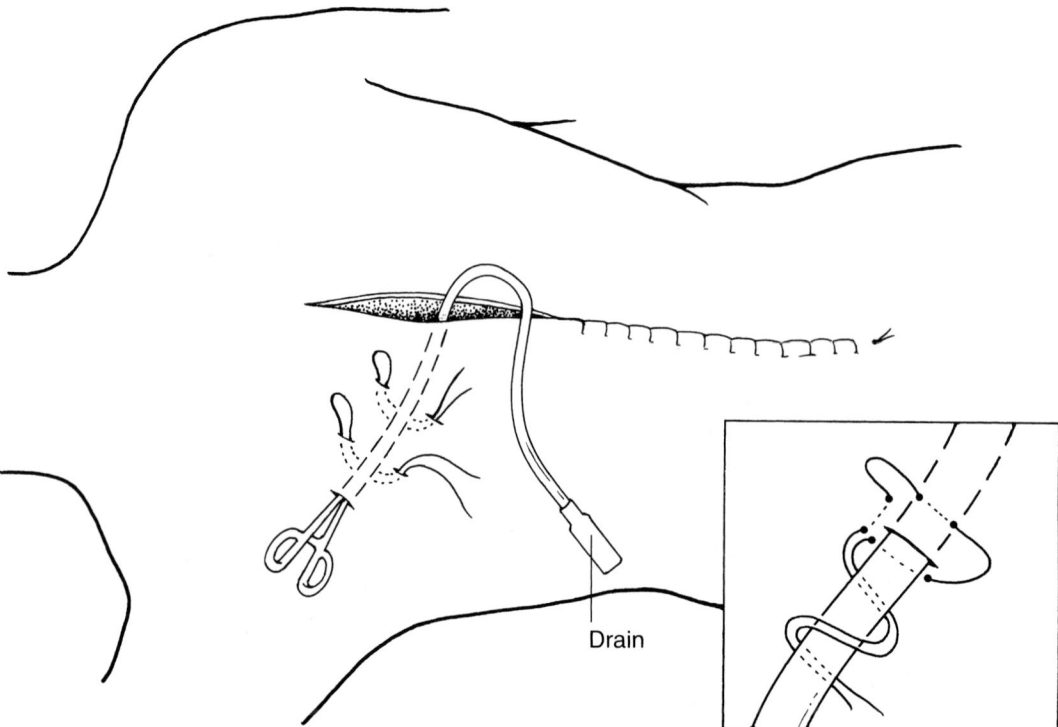

**Figure 156.6** A long, thin clamp, or Hemovac trocar, is left in situ while passing a large polypropylene (Prolene) suture around it. These sutures are left unknotted, to be tied after removal of the drain. These sutures close the drain channel.

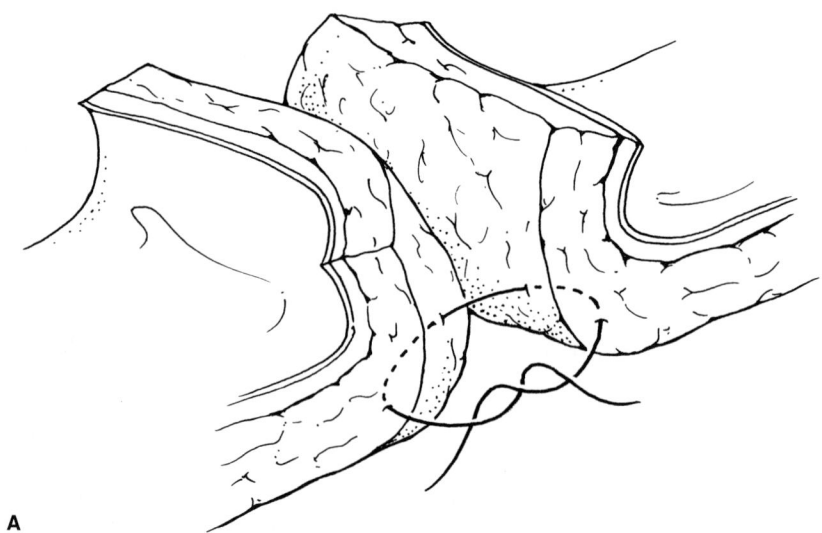

A

**Figure 156.7** **(A-C)** Diagram of the three-layer hypereverted skin closure used for maximal leak prevention, if CSF should escape into the subcutaneous space.

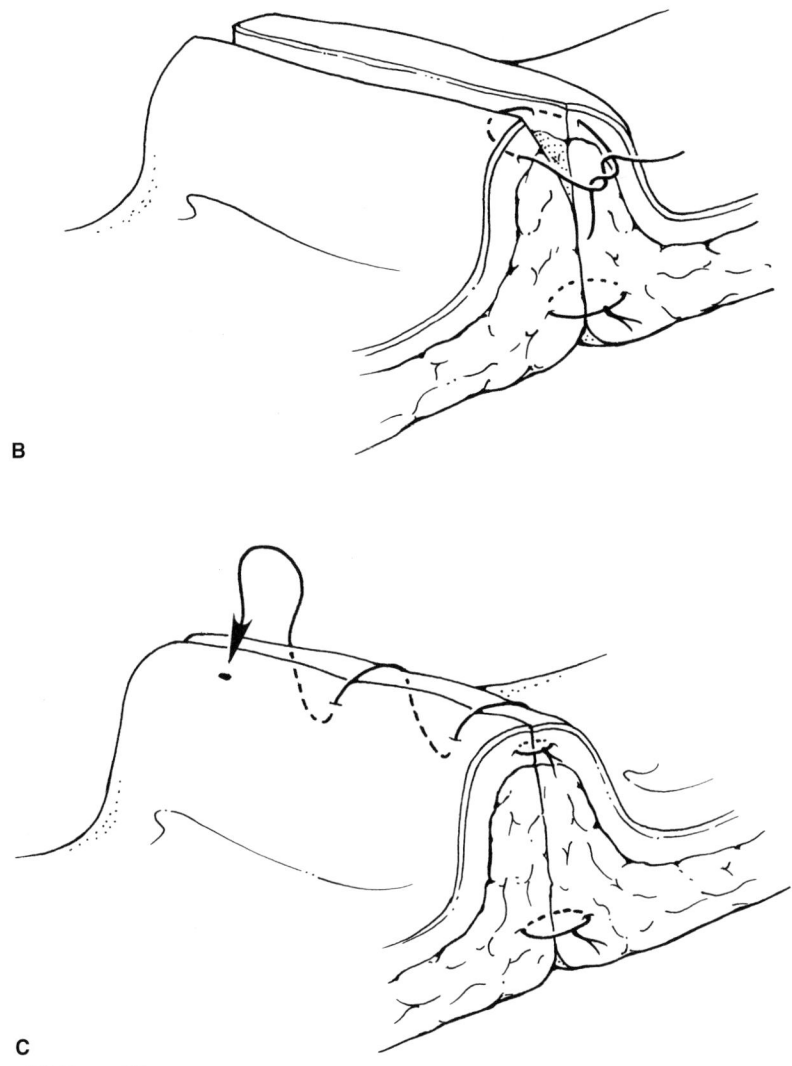

B

C

**Figure 156.7** *cont'd*

correction of abnormal CSF dynamics or for complicated wound exploration.

## REFERENCES

1. Aoki N: Correspondence: Closed continuous drainage of cerebrospinal fluid via lumbar subarachnoid catheter for treatment or prevention of cranial/spinal cerebrospinal fluid fistula. *Neurosurgery* 31:381, 1992.
2. Azizkhan RG, Roberson JB, Powers SK: Successful use of a vascularized intercostal muscle flap to seal a persistent intrapleural cerebrospinal fluid leak in a child. *J Pediatr Surg* 26:744-746, 1991.
3. Chumas PD, Kulkarni AV, Drake JM, *et al*: Lumboperitoneal shunting: a retrospective study in the pediatric population. *Neurosurgery* 32:376-382, 1993.
4. Eismont FJ, Wiesel SW, Rothman RH: Treatment of dural tears associated with spinal surgery. *J Bone Joint Surg* 63A:1132-1136, 1981.
5. Eljamel MS: Antibiotic prophylaxis in unrepaired CSF fistulae. *Br J Neurosurg* 7:501-505, 1993.
6. Findler G, Sahar A, Beller A: Continuous lumbar drainage of cerebrospinal fluid in neurosurgical patients. *Surg Neurol* 8:455-457, 1977.
7. Gass H, Goldstein AS, Ruskin R, Leopold NA: Chronic postmyelogram headache. *Arch Neurol* 25:168, 1971.
8. Gormley JB: Treatment of postspinal headache. *Anesthesiology* 21:565-566, 1960.
9. Hadani M, Findler G, Knoler N, *et al*: Entrapped lumbar nerve root in pseudomeningocele after laminectomy: report of three cases. *Neurosurgery* 19:405-407, 1986.
10. Hofstetter KR, Bjelland JC, Patton DD, *et al*: Detection of bronchopleural-subarachnoid fistula by radionuclide myelography, case report. *J Nucl Med* 18:981, 1977.
11. Katz SS, Savitz MH, Osei C, Harris L: Successful treatment by lumboperitoneal shunting of a spinal subclavicular fistula following thoracotomy. *Neurosurgery* 11:795-796, 1982.
12. Kitchel S, Eismont F, Green B: Closed subarachnoid drainage for management of cerebrospinal fluid leakage after an operation on the spine. *J Bone Joint Surg* 71A: 984-987, 1989.
13. Larson AM, Graham MM: Demonstration of pleural cerebrospinal fluid leak by In-111 DTPA

radionuclide myelography. *Clin Nuclear Med* 17:754-755, 1992.

14. Lee KS, Hardy I: Postlaminectomy lumbar pseudomeningocele: report of four cases. *Neurosurgery* 30:111-114, 1992.

15. Maycock NF, Van Essen J, Pfitzner J: Post-laminectomy cerebrospinal fluid fistula treated with epidural blood patch. *Spine* 19:2223-2225, 1994.

16. Mayfield FH: Complications of laminectomy. *Clin Neurosurg* 42:434-439, 1975.

17. Miller PR, Elder FW: Meningeal pseudocysts (meningocele spurious) following laminectomy. Report of ten cases. *J Bone Joint Surg* 50:268-276, 1968.

18. McCallum J, Maroon J, Jannetta P: Treatment of postoperative cerebrospinal fluid fistulas by subarachnoid drainage. *J Neurosurg* 42:434-437, 1975.

19. Nash CL, Kaufman B, Frankel VH: Postsurgical meningeal pseudocysts of the lumbar spine. *Clin Orthop* 75:167-177, 1971.

20. Oppel F, Schramm J, Schirmer M, *et al*: Results and complicated course after surgery for lumbar disc herniation. *Adv Neurosurg* 4:36-46, 1977.

21. Paonessa KJ, Zide B, Errico T, Engler GL: Using tissue expanders in spinal surgery for deficient soft tissue or post-irradiation cases. *Spine* 16(suppl):S324-S327, 1991.

22. Pomeranz S, Constantini S, Umansky F: The use of fibrin sealant in cerebrospinal fluid leakage. *Neurochirurgie* 34:166-169, 1991.

23. Price DJ, Sleigh JD: Control of infection due to *Klebsiella aerogenes* in a neurosurgical unit by withdrawal of all antibiotics. *Lancet* 2:1213-1215, 1970.

24. Primeau M, Carrier L, Milette PC, *et al*: Spinal cerebrospinal fluid leak demonstrated by radioisotopic cisternography. *Clin Nucl Med* 13:701-703, 1988.

25. Ryall RG, Peacock MK, Simpson DA: Usefulness of B2-transferrin assay in the detection of cerebrospinal fluid leaks following head injury. *J Neurosurg* 77:737-739, 1992.

26. Sakikawa Y, Kobayashi H, Nomura Y: Changes in cerebrospinal fluid pressure in daily life. *Ann Otol Rhinol Laryngol* 103:959-963, 1994.

27. Schumacher H-W, Wassman H, Podlinski C: Pseudomeningocele of the lumbar spine. *Surg Neurol* 29:77-78, 1988.

28. Shapiro SA, Scully T: Closed continuous drainage of cerebrospinal fluid via a lumbar subarachnoid catheter for treatment or prevention of cranial/spinal cerebrospinal fluid fistula. *Neurosurgery* 30:241-245, 1992.

29. Swanson HS, Fincher EF: Extradural arachnoidal cysts of traumatic origin. *J Neurosurg* 4:530-538, 1947.

30. Teplick JG, Peyster RG, Teplick SK, *et al*: CT identification of postlaminectomy pseudomeningocele. *Am J Roentgenol* 4:179-182, 1983.

31. Tsuji H, Handa N, Handa O, *et al*: Postlaminectomy ossified extradural pseudocyts. *J Neurosurg* 73:785-787, 1990.

32. Von Storch TJC, Carmichael EA, Banks TE: Factors producing lumbar cerebrospinal fluid pressure in man in the erect posture. *Arch Neurol Psychiatry* 38:1158, 1937.

33. Waisman M, Schweppe Y: Postoperative cerebrospinal fluid leakage after lumbar spine operations: conservative treatment. *Spine* 16:52-53, 1991.

34. Zide BM: How to reduce the morbidity of wound closure following extensive and complicated laminectomy and tethered cord surgery. *Pediatr Neurosurg* 18:157-166, 1992.

35. Zide BM, Epstein FJ, Wisoff J: Optimal wound closure after tethered cord corrections. *J Neurosurg* 74:673-676, 1991.

36. Zide BM, Wisoff JH, Epstein FJ: Closure of extensive and complicated laminectomy wounds. *J Neurosurg* 67:59-64, 1987.

# CHAPTER 157

# Nonunion

**Vinay Deshmukh, Arnold B. Vardiman, and Howard W. Morgan, Jr.**

Recent advances and refinements in internal spinal fixation devices have greatly expanded the capacity of surgeons to successfully treat complicated problems over the entire length of the spine. These systems may aid the reestablishment of normal or near-normal alignment, may apply complex multidirectional force vectors, and may allow immediate immobilization over multiple spinal segments. As important as the meticulous and thoughtful use of this instrumentation is, careful consideration must be given to the material that will, for a lifetime, bear the stresses that instrumentation supports only temporarily. Solid bony union alone provides enduring spinal stability, and failure to achieve this goal can have consequences ranging from a benign radiographic finding to persistent pain or catastrophic construct failure with permanent neurologic injury. The nonunion rate is quoted as 10% to 15% for spinal fusions.[77] A *pseudarthrosis* is defined as a documented failure of solid fusion (nonunion) 1 year after the operation with concomitant symptoms and signs.[137] As surgical frontiers broaden and patients become more medically fragile and aged, the surgeon's ability to optimize conditions that promote bony fusion and avoid nonunion/pseudarthroses becomes increasingly important.

This chapter reviews the basic principles of bony fusion, clinically relevant factors influencing fusion, and specific principles designed to minimize the incidence of nonunion. As in every other surgical arena, an understanding of basic principles, coupled with common sense, best equips surgeons to deal with the variety of problems they encounter.

## Biology of Bone Healing

Bone is a dynamic living tissue that undergoes constant remodeling; yet, it is strong and compares favorably with modern building materials.[59] It is unique in its capacity to repair and regenerate after disruption.[136] The amazing qualities of bone are derived from its unique composite structure of organic and inorganic materials. The organic component, chiefly a strongly cross-linked (type 1) collagen, gives bone plasticity that allows substantial deformation without fracture.[140] The inorganic component, chiefly in the form of hydroxyapatite, precipitates around the collagen fibers in a process of nucleation and maturation of mineral crystals.[106] The inorganic-mineral component of bone gives the tissue tremendous strength in compression and bending.[25]

The cellular components of bone include osteoblasts, osteocytes, and osteoclasts, connected through an intricate and well-organized system of canals.[120] Osteoblasts develop from mesenchymal cells and secrete the organic component of bone that occasionally is entrapped within the mineralizing bone matrix to become osteocytes. Osteoclasts are derived from monocytes and are multinucleated cells capable of enzymatically mediated resorption of bone under tight hormonal and cellular control. Osteoclasts may lie in Howship's lacunae, to occupy the space from which bone was removed. Other cellular elements of bone include the hematopoietic elements of the bone marrow and mesenchymal stem cells.

Adult bone is chiefly a cortical or cancellous bone. Cortical, compact, or lamellar bone is sheathed in a two-layered periosteum. The outer fibrous periosteal layer covers an inner cambial layer containing osteoblasts that can survive transplant and form callus.[113] An endosteum lines the trabeculae of medullary bone. The functional unit of cortical bone is the osteon or the haversian system. These cylindrical units are arranged parallel to the cortical direction and surround the haversian canal that contains the nutrient vessels, lymphatic channels, and nerves, and include the surrounding lamellar (mature) bone.[82] Volkmann's canals connect adjacent haversian canals. They provide a conduit for systemic arteries to penetrate the cortical bone, gaining access to both the haversian canals and the marrow. Osteocytes, which are osteoblasts that are entrapped in lacunae within concentric lamellar bone, have thin, filopodial processes within canaliculi and communicate with other osteocytes via gap junctions.[115]

Cancellous, trabecular, and spongy bone, as well as marrow, has a honeycombed arrangement with thin, bony trabeculae that are chiefly oriented perpendicular to the dominant external forces.[67,146] Woven bone is the initial tissue laid down during fracture repair. It forms the embryonic skeleton.[20,43] Woven bone is more rapidly deposited and resorbed and has a relatively high concentration of osteocytes; however, it has an irregular arrangement of collagen and mineralization that makes it relatively weak.[22] In nonpathologic states woven bone is generally replaced by cortical or cancellous bone.

The process of bone healing after injury is an indistinct continuous sequence of inflammation, repair, and remodeling.[21,82] The inflammatory response to injury includes vascular dilatation with exudate and edema, as well as inflammatory cell (polymorphonuclear lymphocytes, macrophages, and lymphocytes) infiltration. A variety of hormones, cytokines, growth factors, and matrix proteins (e.g., bone morphogenic protein [BMP]) are involved throughout the healing process. Nonsteroidal antiinflammatory drugs, steroids, or chemotherapeutic agents given during the first week of healing may blunt the inflammatory response and impair bone healing.[43] As the debris of the inflammatory phase is removed, fibroblasts begin laying down new matrix in the early phases of the repair. Initially a fracture callus that is composed of fibrous tissue, cartilage, and woven bone may form to bridge the bony defect. This is then replaced by woven bone and ultimately, by mature cortical or cancellous bone. This process may take 3 to 6 months or longer, depending on age and other factors.[23,43] Although the general sequence of inflammation, repair, and remodeling that occurs in long bone fracture healing also occurs with bone graft repair, there are some distinct differences. Autograft bone used in spinal fusion is initially deprived of blood supply, although a robust nonspecific inflammatory response occurs as a result of preparation of the graft recipient bed. The collection of coagulated blood around the graft is somewhat analogous to the hematoma of an acute fracture, with the complex processes of inflammation ongoing within this milieu. Although some of the periosteum, endosteum, mesenchymal cells, and osteocytes within 0.2 to 0.3mm of the borders survive transplant, most of the transplanted bone cells, separated from their blood supply, die.[140] The cancellous portion of the bone graft may be revascularized within 2 weeks, and cortical bone is revascularized within 1 to 2 months. Cancellous bone is more rapidly remodeled and is initially strengthened during the remodeling phase, because osteoblasts are first laid down over the trabeculae.[24]

Cortical bone is initially weakened during remodeling and is remodeled more slowly than cancellous bone. Bone graft is gradually replaced with new bone in a process called "creeping substitution."[104] Osteoclasts that act as cutting cones bore into the graft from the margins of host bone, followed by osteoblasts that lay down new bone. This process of healing and remodeling may leave as much as 50% to 90% of the original matrix, even after many years.[50,141] The strength of cortical autograft is halved during the first 6 months after fusion but is gradually restored over 1 to 2 years. Autograft bone provides some living bone cells with the ability to make bone (i.e., osteogenic properties). It contains some BMP, which is capable of inducing cellular differentiation (i.e., it has osteoinductive properties), and provides a scaffolding for bone growth (i.e., osteoconductive properties).[35]

## Harvesting and Handling of the Bone Graft

An effort to maximize the advantages of autograft bone as graft material begins with a plan to harvest sufficient quantity of bone for the planned application. Preoperative discussions with the patient about the potential need for multiple bone harvest sites helps avoid the problem of insufficient graft in most situations. Routinely preparing and draping both iliac crests allows ready access to alternative graft material when needed. On occasion, harvesting ventral iliac crest for a dorsal application may be performed before turning the patient into the prone position. In a situation with a high risk for nonunion, or with failed prior fusion, a sufficient quantity of autogenous bone is desired. Occasionally, unconventional graft sources should be considered and planned for in advance. Reliance on a single source for graft material, with a less than anticipated volume yield of harvested bone, may increase morbidity at that harvest site, as a result of overzealous harvest and extension of the harvest beyond safe and reasonable boundaries.

Surgical exposure of the donor site should be performed to maximize the viability of the graft. Heating of bone with the electric cautery, although frequently unavoidable, has the potential of destroying those surface osteocytes most capable of surviving via diffusion of nutrients. A sharp periosteum elevator can be used to open the subperiosteal plane in a remarkably atraumatic fashion, with minimal blood loss. For tricortical bone grafts placed in compression, harvesting with an oscillating saw provides a graft that is better at resisting compressive loads than a graft harvested with an osteotome.[46,68] The clinical significance of this is unknown. For bone used purely for onlay, one should bear in mind that 5mm is the maximal thickness that can be nourished by diffusion of nutrients.[118,119] If possible, the bone graft should be harvested within 30 minutes of planned use. The graft should be kept moist in a saline- or blood-soaked sponge before use. The graft should not be allowed to dry or make contact with toxic chemicals (e.g., antibiotic solutions).[116]

## Preparation of Recipient Bed

Because few graft osteoblasts and osteocytes survive the transplant, it is imperative that preparation of the recipient bed be undertaken with utmost care and that the bed protect the viability of the tissues that will serve as the primary source of the cellular components required for bony fusion. This process begins with meticulous subperiosteal dissection of the donor site, with complete removal of all soft tissue capable of interposition between planned fusion sites. Soft tissue should be removed to minimize thermal injury, and the use of the bipolar cautery should be emphasized when possible. Areas of planned fusion should be decorticated, allowing contact of graft with cancellous bone, while avoiding weakening the structure of the recipient bed with overzealous destruction of the cortical bone. Drilling and burring should perhaps be performed with a self-irrigating drill or with aggressive irrigation from an assistant to avoid thermal injury to the recipient bed. Bone wax should not be used in the recipient bed.

Grafts should be well fitted into the recipient site. Meticulous crafting of the graft to the recipient site cannot be overemphasized, because direct bone-to-bone contact facilitates union. In some situations cancellous bone can be packed into gaps when a perfect fit is simply not possible. The sequence of preparation of the recipient bed, decortication, and application of the bone graft must be considered relative to application of instrumentation, because access to the recipient bed may be compromised by the implant. This is particularly the case with pedicle screw fixation in which complete assembly of all of the components limits access to the transverse processes and lateral aspects of the articular surfaces. Thorough irrigation of the recipient site before placement of the graft avoids inadvertent loss of onlay graft material.

## Selection of Graft Material

There are multiple classifications of grafts. Autografts are obtained from one site in the body to be deposited in another. An allograft is bone that is transferred between two people of the same species. Xenografts are shared between members of different species. An implant is any nonviable tissue placed in the patient.[14] A transplant, in contrast, is viable tissue. The term *graft* refers to either a viable or nonviable agent.

Ideally, graft material should have the capacity to become bone (i.e., osteogenic properties), induce undifferentiated mesenchymal cells to mature into osteoblasts (i.e., osteoinductive properties), serve as scaffolding for bone healing (i.e., osteoconductive properties), harbor no risk of infection, and be genetically identical to the patient. It should also be mechanically strong, durable, potentially viable, nonreactive to the host tissue, sterile, anatomic, and cost effective.[36] Currently the only material satisfying these requirements is the patient's own (autograft) bone. Choices for autograft include iliac crest, local bone, or rib. The disadvantages of autograft include the potential for inadequate bone graft volume, poor quality of bone graft, pain at the graft site, risk of wound hernia, risk of pelvic fracture for iliac crest grafts, blood loss, instability, and nerve injury. Incidence of major complications with autograft harvesting can be as high as 10%.[36] Sawin et al.[130] reports that for dorsal cervical fusions, rib bone grafts compare favorably with iliac crest bone grafts in terms of fusion rates and donor site complications.

Allograft bone, transplanted from genetically dissimilar members of the same species, has the advantage of ready availability in multiple structural forms and without donor site morbidity. Allograft has some osteoinductive and osteoconductive, but no osteogenic, properties. Vascular ingrowth and new bone formation are delayed with allografts.[49,82,115,142] The mode of preparation of allograft may impact its success as a graft material. Allograft bone may be treated with freezing, freeze drying, or ethylene oxide to reduce its immunogenicity; but because it is genetically dissimilar to the patient, an inflammatory response similar to graft rejection noted in other tissue transplants may occur.[16,48] Fresh frozen allograft appears to have a superior fusion rate to freeze-dried graft, with ethylene oxide-sterilized grafts demonstrating uniformly poor results.[27] With careful screening the risk of human immunodeficiency virus (HIV) transmission from the allograft transplant is calculated to be less than one in a million.[20]

The use of allograft bone for single-level ventral or cervical discectomy and fusion appears to yield results that are roughly equivalent to use of autograft bone.* For multilevel ventral procedures, autograft appears to be superior.[34,54,123,155] For bone struts used over multiple segments, pseudarthrosis rates with allograft are higher (41%) than with autograft (27%).[54] When supplemented with dorsal fusion, the pseudarthrosis rate falls to 26%.[152] A separate study using notched fibular struts and a halo orthosis demonstrated delayed fusion, but seven out of eight patients had good or excellent results.[18] In fusions unsupplemented with dorsal instrumentation or a halo orthosis, autograft bone appears to be the favored graft material. For dorsal fusions, autograft bone appears to be superior.[117,136] Unlike the cervical spine the use of allograft versus autograft bone has been well studied for scoliosis.† In uninstrumented cases, autograft performed superiorly. Instrumented dorsal fusions supplemented with allograft bone performed comparably in a pediatric population (although it took a long time to achieve fusion). Ventral allograft struts supplemented with autologous bone

(packed into the hollowed marrow space of the allograft), in conjunction with dorsal fusion and segmental instrumentation, yielded better results than allograft fusion without ventral graft supplementation.[82] In the lumbar spine allograft bone plays a limited role with dorsolateral fusion; although its use as a ventral interbody strut (particularly femoral shaft allograft packed with cancellous autograft) when used with dorsal segmental instrumentation has been substantiated.‡

Each situation demands that care be taken to match the graft type to the job. With an increased ability to provide allografts with osteogenic properties, through either an autograft supplement or use of nonautograft osteogenic substances (e.g., bone morphogenic protein), the capacities of allograft will clearly be expanded. It may be prudent to reserve the use of onlay and, often, interbody allograft bone graft application for those circumstances in which the patient's bone is judged to be insufficient for the planned application. When the use of allograft is unavoidable, supplementation should be performed with autologous elements (packing autograft cancellous bone into hollowed allograft femur or supplementing morselized autograft bone with allograft) whenever possible.

Methylmethacrylate is advantageous in its ability to provide immediate stability when secured to bone. However, methylmethacrylate does not support bone healing and is not osteoconductive, osteoinductive, or osteogenic. It resists compression well but is weak when placed under tension. Methylmethacrylate can provide immediate stability when secured to bone, allowing immediate resumption of activity after surgery. Regrettably, this polymer can work loose from its bony moorings, with a resultant loss of integrity of the construct and the potential for overt spinal instability. This compound perhaps should be reserved for those patients with a life expectancy of less than 6 months.[31,43,66,95] It can, however, be a useful adjunct with autograft/allograft in patients with osteoporosis. Demineralized bone matrix facilitates bone fusion through osteoinduction and, to a lesser degree, through osteoconductive properties. The demineralization of allograft reduces its antigenicity and may uncover osteoinductive factors, including BMP. Encouraging early results have been reported using demineralized bone matrix.[90,128] Despite its promise, a recent prospective clinical trial comparing allograft and demineralized bone matrix with autograft in ventral cervical fusion demonstrated only a higher rate of graft collapse and pseudarthrosis in the allograft group.[2]

Ceramics and titanium cages have emerged as alternatives to autografts and allografts. The most commonly used ceramics are calcium phosphates (e.g., hydroxyapatite, tricalcium phosphate). The advantages of ceramics include their high degree of biocompatibility with the host. However, ceramics are exclusively osteoconductive and intact ceramics can be brittle with low impact and fracture resistance. They have 50% of the tensile strength of autograft. There is a suggestion that ceramics may also retard normal bone healing and remodeling.[126] The newest use of ceramic compounds is as carrier agents for BMP.

---

*References 18,32,33,60,63,92,123,127,131,152,153.
†References 10,44,51,83,94,96,101,105.

---

‡References 26,32,41,73,85,113,134.

While tricortical iliac crest autografts have been the gold standard for intervertebral fusion and strut graft reconstruction after corpectomy, problems with graft donor site pain have been reported to be as high as 30%.[91] Allografts remain plagued by a higher incidence of pseudarthrosis, graft collapse, and extrusion. The use of a cylindrical titanium mesh cage packed with bone salvaged from the corpectomy may avoid the need for harvesting a separate graft. Fusion rates using this method of reconstruction have been reported to be greater than 90%.[73,91] The primary disadvantages to using the cage packed with bone are the financial expense and the lack of long-term follow-up.

## Electromagnetic Factors

Direct current stimulation was first proposed in 1972 as a modality for improving fusion.[1,9] Application of pulsed electromagnetic fields for nonunion in long bone fractures appears to have no hazardous side effects.[9] Although areas of tension are associated with a net positive charge, compressive stresses are associated with a net negative charge (10 to 100mV) and osteogenesis.[9] Electromagnetic stimulation is believed to promote osteogenesis as a result of more rapid angiogenesis and decreased osteoclastic activity.[79] The effect of improved osteogenesis may be mediated by growth factors.[56] More recent evidence also suggests the activation of a second messenger system involved in bone remodeling.[110] There are three broad types of electromagnetic fields used: implantable DC current, pulsing electromagnetic fields, and capacitively coupled electrical energy.[110] Pulsing electromagnetic fields (PEMFs) and capacitively coupled electrical energy are examples of external electromagnetic fields. These are delivered via external electrodes attached to a corset. Implantable DC current requires surgical placement of the electrodes and has been shown to be the most effective.[110] Direct current may be more effective than external electrodes secondary to its increased precision in the distribution of current.[76] The cost of these devices is not insignificant. Although some investigators have noted no significant benefit of electrical stimulation for canine spinal fusions,[80,88] one randomized blinded study in 195 patients demonstrated a significant difference in fusion rates between stimulated (92%) and unstimulated (65%) groups.[102] In a study of 59 patients who underwent reoperation for failed lumbar fusions there was an 81% fusion rate in stimulated patients, versus a 54% fusion rate in unstimulated patients.[81] Another contemporary series found a 96% fusion rate with implanted stimulators versus 85% in unstimulated cases.[124] Clinical trials have been faulted for having a high degree of variation in electrical stimulation protocols, surgical intervention, and disease treated and patient populations.[110] Comprehensive, prospective, double-blinded studies regarding the effects of electrical stimulation on long-term fusion rates are yet to be published. Despite the absence of a consensus regarding the use of electrical stimulation devices to enhance spinal fusion, their thoughtful application in situations of previous nonunion or in patients judged to be at high risk for nonunion seems justified.

## Bone Morphogenetic Protein

BMP is a low-molecular–weight oligosaccharide glycoprotein and a member of the transforming growth factor beta superfamily.[69] It was initially discovered by Urist in the 1970s as an osteogenic substance present within bone matrix. It exists in the intercellular matrix and perilacunar walls. There are multiple types of BMPs, but four have been specifically shown to promote bone growth in an ectopic site.[142] BMP plays an important role in the growth and development of multiple tissues, including bone, brain, and spinal cord. It seems to be involved in regulation of cellular proliferation, survival, differentiation, apoptosis, and lineage commitment. When specific BMPs are delivered via biologic matrices, they have the capacity to induce bone, cartilage, and ligament and tendon growth in both heterotopic and orthotopic sites.[69] BMPs have been shown to be effective in animal studies; human clinical trials are under way.[13-15,89] BMPs will play a major role in the future treatment of spinal and craniofacial bony disorders.[108] Carriers for BMP include resorbable collagen sponge and porous ceramics. Porous ceramics are a more promising delivery vehicle when the graft is required to bear weight, because of the ceramic device's ability to resist compressive forces and its osteoconductive properties.[12]

## Factors Affecting Bone Healing
### Smoking

Smoking and the use of smokeless tobacco products are prevalent in the United States. Ninety percent of all initiation to tobacco begins at younger than 18 years, and despite the known health risks of smoking, tobacco use in this age group continues to grow.[6] The deleterious effects of smoking include an increased risk of pulmonary disease, cancer, and coronary artery disease. There is also a threefold to fourfold increase in the occurrence of nonunion of spinal fusions in smokers over that in nonsmokers.[11,19,64] Smoking interferes with osteoblastic function,[42] leads to increased bone resorption at fracture sites,[87] and interferes with normal bone metabolism.[71] Smoking has also been associated with bone mineral loss in several studies.[97,107,114,135] The burning of tobacco produces about 4000 compounds that can be separated into a gaseous and a particulate phase. The gaseous phase includes carbon monoxide, carbon dioxide, nitrogen oxides, ammonia, volatile nitrosamines, hydrogen cyanide, nitriles, and other compounds. The particulate phase contains nicotine and tar (which consists primarily of polycyclic aromatic hydrocarbons). It is believed that the components most likely to contribute to health hazards are carbon monoxide, nicotine, and tar.[78] Nicotine probably is the chemical most responsible for physical dependency. Animal studies have focused on its deleterious effects on revascularization of bone graft and spinal fusion.[39] Nicotine inhibits revascularization of bone graft implanted in the anterior chamber of the eye of rabbits. A follow-up study demonstrated decreased intertransverse fusion rates in rabbits receiving systemic nicotine and also suggested that the bone formed during nicotine use has inferior biomechanical properties.[132] These studies strongly indicate that the use of nicotine patches or gums, in an effort to curb patients' smoking perioperatively and during bone healing, may be ill advised. It is likely, however, that other components of cigarette smoke also have a deleterious effect on fusion, although this is less documented. Even the pulmonary compromise associated with smoking, as reflected in a decreased arterial partial oxygen pressure, has been suggested as a potential explanation for increased nonunion rates in smokers.[34]

Although there is consensus that smoking inhibits bony fusion, there is considerable disagreement over the management of the smoker facing spinal fusion. Many surgeons consider the dismal success rates of even aggressive smoking cessation programs as indication of the futility of a policy of outright refusal to perform fusions in patients who continue to smoke.[148] Others predicate decisions regarding elective spinal fusion on the patient's absolute smoking abstinence.

An intermediate approach should be used in an attempt to avoid an excessively fatalistic or autocratic view. In the nonelective settings of trauma or neurologic disability one should not predicate treatment on smoking status, although patients should be counseled for abstinence because noncompliance will place them at potential risk for nonunion. In more elective situations counseling and treatment programs should be made available. These discussions should emphasize the serious risks of smoking, as well as the potential for increased surgical complications and nonunion. The goal of smoking abstinence should be emphasized. Decisions regarding elective surgery in those patients unable to successfully abstain should be based on the patient's symptoms, coexisting risk factors for nonunion, and the planned operative procedure. For example, an otherwise healthy smoker, 35 years of age, with excruciating arm pain as the result of a C7 radiculopathy that is refractory to conservative therapy, perhaps should not be denied anterior cervical discectomy and autograft fusion, even if he or she is unable to refrain from smoking. Alternatively, a 60-year-old obese patient with adult onset (type 2) diabetes, who is unable to refrain from smoking and suffers mechanical back pain as the result of a degenerative grade II lumbar spondylolisthesis, is perhaps best managed *nonoperatively*. Although admittedly arbitrary, this policy stresses the desirability of abstaining from smoking to avoid the general health risks of smoking, including its effects on bone healing, while realizing that in some clinical situations, flatly withholding surgical intervention on the basis of smoking is unreasonable at best and punitive at worst.

## Radiation Therapy

Radiation therapy plays an important role in the treatment of many primary and metastatic tumors of the spine. Frequently the spine surgeon must consider the potential need for adjunctive postoperative radiation therapy or is consulted only after radiation has failed as the primary mode of treatment.

Radiation impairs bone healing,° inhibiting cell proliferation and producing a vasculitis that limits vascular ingrowth. Radiation delivered before long bone fracture in animals results in delayed fracture healing[47]; however, in a canine model of ventral strut grafting there was no significant difference in the biomechanical data at 3 months between controls and animals irradiated preoperatively, or at 21 days postoperatively.[55] In the same canine study radiation therapy begun on the third postoperative day resulted in the poorest bone healing, revascularization, and new bone formation. The total radiation dose, delivered preoperatively or postoperatively, has been shown to correlate well with reduction in strength of healing bone in an animal model.[93] A total radiation dose exceeding 4000cg has been proposed as a risk factor for nonfusion in patients undergoing perioperative radiation for neoplasm.

Delaying radiation, at least until after the first postoperative week, appears well founded because the untoward effects of radiation seem maximal during that interval. The total dose of radiation should be customized to the indication (tumor type and radiosensitivity), with thought given to delivering an effective but not excessive dose of radiation. In patients with a life expectancy of less than 6 months, consideration should be given to the use of polymethylmethacrylate (PMMA) as a graft material.

## Nutrition

Malnutrition has a negative impact on fracture healing,[75,121] blunts the immune response, and impairs wound healing. Whereas the ravages of advanced malnutrition are easily recognized, more subtle subclinical malnutrition may be missed on physical examination, but may be readily detected using accepted measures of nutritional assessment. A nutritional support team can provide vital preoperative evaluation and education to optimize nutritional status preoperatively and postoperatively.

## Rheumatoid Arthritis

Rheumatoid arthritis affects 1% of the world's population, with a 2:1 female-to-male predominance. The exact pathophysiology is unknown, but the disease process results in an inflammatory synovitis that can lead to the slow destruction of the joints. Although the primary joints involved are in the hands and wrists, 60% to 70% of patients with the disease eventually suffer cervical spine symptoms.[150] Cervical spine instability, a consequence of the destructive synovitis, tends to occur in three forms: atlantoaxial instability, rostral migration of the odontoid (cranial settling), and subaxial subluxation (most common at C5-6).[125] In those patients requiring fusion, bone healing is often compromised by osteoporotic bone,[125] and the direct immunosuppressive effects of the disease itself (coupled with the effects of steroid medications).[129] Furthermore, this can result in osteomyelitis.[98] Despite these factors, the use of contemporary instrumentation and arthrodesis techniques have resulted in fusion rates of 90% or higher in multiple centers.° It is prudent for the rheumatologist to taper cytotoxic medications (methotrexate) and steroids as much as possible before surgery and for as long postoperatively as is safe.

---

°References 29,40,43,47,48,55,93,149,151.

°References 30,31,53,70,86,127,143,156.

Beyond close attention being paid to instrumentation and arthrodesis, a meticulous wound closure and postoperative skin care (including care taken to ensure proper fit and padding of postoperative orthoses) is essential to successful wound healing and fusion.

The seronegative spondyloarthropathies are a group of disorders characterized by involvement of the sacroiliac joints and peripheral inflammatory arthropathy.[37] Ankylosing spondylitis is one of the best known of this group of disorders, which includes psoriatic arthropathy, Reiter's syndrome, Crohn's disease, ulcerative colitis, juvenile chronic arthropathy, and Whipple's disease. The seronegative spondyloarthropathies are occasionally referred to as "enthesopathic" disorders, because they are characterized by inflammation at the site of ligamentous insertion onto bone (the enthesis). This is distinguished from rheumatoid arthritis, which involves inflammation of the synovium. This difference is critical because the progressive destruction of the joint in rheumatoid arthritis may result in joint laxity and instability, whereas in enthesopathic disorders bony fusion usually occurs in joints adjacent to involved ligamentous insertions.[28,57] Familiarity with the enthesopathic disorders is imperative. Bony union can occur in patients with ankylosing spondylitis after surgery, and fusion rates exceeding 95% have been reported after the correction of spinal deformity.[99,133]

## Age

Surprisingly, considering that the population is increasingly mature, the issue of age as it relates to spinal fusion has been poorly addressed in the literature. Generally, skeletally immature patients have the greatest healing potential and heal more quickly.[23] It is hypothesized that children may have a greater number of undifferentiated mesenchymal cells, and that these cells may be capable of more rapid differentiation when necessary.[23,139] Bone mass changes with age in three phases: growth, consolidation, and involution. Involutional bone loss begins between the ages of 35 and 40 with cortical and trabecular bone and increases with age in both sexes. Initially the rate of cortical bone loss is 0.3% to 0.5% annually in both men and women, but this rate increases after menopause for women, with an annual rate of 2% to 3% per year, before it reverts to a lower rate 10 years later. Approximately 35% to 50% of trabecular bone mass and 25% to 30% of cortical bone mass is lost in aging women, in contrast to 15% to 45% of trabecular bone and 5% to 15% of cortical bone in aging men.[58,122] Beyond having a generally poorer bone stock, the elderly frequently suffer more medical problems than does a younger population.[111] Generally, fusion is not required, particularly with lumbar stenosis.[151] Medical clearance is obtained in most patients with coexisting disease, particularly those with coronary artery disease or pulmonary or metabolic derangements.

## Osteoporosis

Osteoporosis is the most prevalent metabolic bone disease in the United States. It is characterized by a reduction in bone mass with a preserved ratio of mineral-to-organic matrix. Although the pathophysiology of the disease is not completely understood, the development of the disorder appears to depend on the peak adult bone mass attained, and the rate at which that bone mass is lost as a result of skeletal remodeling.[65] The consequence of osteoporosis is fracture. The load-bearing axial skeleton and a relatively high percentage of trabecular bone within vertebrae make vertebral body fractures a common initial presentation of the disease. The onset of acute back pain in a postmenopausal woman with radiographic evidence of a compression fracture is a common presentation of osteoporosis. Most osteoporotic compression fractures can be conservatively managed. The pain from these injuries is usually minimal by 6 to 8 weeks. Rarely is surgical treatment of patients with osteoporotic compression fractures required. Patients with neurologic deficit present a serious challenge. One must carefully consider the biomechanics of the construct in the setting of weak bone that may readily fail at points of juncture with the hardware. Even with careful planning, scrupulous postoperative care, and orthotic support, failure of successful bony fusion in these cases can result in catastrophic failure of the construct, leaving few therapeutic alternatives. The dilemma posed by a failed construct in this setting often prompts overbuilding of these constructs by attempting to share the load over many segments. Not infrequently, this includes a ventral reconstruction, in addition to dorsal stabilization.

Ultimately, optimized peak adult bone mass (ensured by adequate calcium and vitamin D intake, with efforts to minimize the loss of bone mass, particularly in postmenopausal women) remains the focus of attempts to minimize the morbidity and mortality from this common and problematic disease. Improved medical therapies, including the bisphosphonates and potent inhibitors of osteoclast activity, hold promise for building bone mass and decreasing rates of vertebral and hip fractures.[100,144]

## Diagnosis of Nonunion

The diagnosis of pseudarthrosis remains a challenging endeavor. It has typically been based on the clinical triad of pain, radiographic evidence of instability, and loss of correction/fixation. Solid fusion of plain radiographs is demonstrated by a continuous trabecular pattern traversing the grafted segments. Roentgenographic criteria for failure of fusion are the following: lack of trabecular bone continuity from one end of the fusion to the other, collapse of the graft height with a gap present between the vertebral end-plates and the graft, a shift in the position of the graft after expected healing was to have occurred, and loss of fixation through movement of hardware. Plain static radiographs are only 80% sensitive in revealing pseudarthrosis.[137] Functional imaging (dynamic films) may reveal abnormal motion at a purportedly fused segment. Four millimeters of horizontal motion, or 10 degrees or more of angular motion on flexion/extension films, represents abnormal motion. Computed tomography (CT) has greater than 90% sensitivity in detecting nonunion. It may show defects in bridging fusion masses. Failure of fusion can often be better demonstrated on sagittal reconstructions. $T_1$-weighted magnetic resonance imaging (MRI) is not often used in verifying nonunion secondary to poor bony imaging and the length of time required for changes to be detectable on MRI. However, $T_1$-weighted MRI is useful in delineating subchondral bands adjacent to the vertebral end-plates, which suggests stable fusions. Single photon emission computed tomography (SPECT) scans have a sensitivity and a specificity around 50%, and therefore cannot be used reliably for the diagnosis of pseudarthrosis.[5] The use of ultrasound in detecting pseudarthroses has been explored. In a series by Jacobsen and Garfin, ultrasound was used to evaluate pseudarthrosis after posterolateral spinal fusion. There was a reported sensitivity of 100%, but the specificity was only 60%.[84] No single modality has been shown a high degree of accuracy. Surgical exploration, aggressive curettage, and intraoperative stress testing remain the most accurate means of diagnosing nonunion.

## Technical Aspects

Ultimately an understanding of the basic principles of bone fusion must be coupled with technical execution in the operating room. Although a well-crafted arthrodesis does not guarantee success, a poorly performed one can virtually ensure failure. Also, before any treatment of spinal pseudarthroses, one should proceed with identification of the factors that lead to failure (e.g., segmental motion or shear stresses, underlying metabolic/medical causes).

### Cervical Spine

Ventral cervical interbody fusion, using the Smith-Robinson technique, is one of the most common procedures performed by spine surgeons. Although this technique provides a high rate of solid arthrodesis, attention to some details of technique can optimize the likelihood of solid arthrodesis. Meticulous preparation of the recipient site, including the complete removal of the cartilaginous end-plates, is required. Widening the exposure to the width of the uncovertebral joints helps provide a broad surface for fusion. Very often it is helpful to remove the overhanging ventral caudal lip of the rostral vertebral body. Performed early in the decompression, this phase allows for a better view of the dorsal interspace, while also allowing for a smooth fit of the interbody graft. The final preparation of the recipient surfaces involves smoothing any irregular contours that may leave gaps in the interface between the graft and the recipient site. After the recipient site is prepared, the graft may be precisely contoured to just exceed the height of the recipient site. The graft should be impacted into the interspace, with great care taken to avoid driving it into the spinal canal. Controlled cervical traction, applied by the anesthesiologist, or an interspace spreader can provide the additional interspace height that is required to allow gentle tamping of the bone graft into position with only moderate force. Excess force, poor fit of the graft, or use of a small impactor may result in fragmentation of the graft, necessitating replacement. The graft should seat securely in the interspace, and the surgeon should be able to feel it settling solidly into position. Grafts that freely spin or move within the interspace after the release of cervical traction, or grafts that splinter, crack, or fray are suboptimal and should be replaced. Long interbody grafts require special consideration. A variety of strategies have been used that are largely based on the preference of the surgeon.[*]

Symptomatic nonunion after ventral procedures can be managed in many ways. One option, when there is no overt ventral instrumentation failure and no symptomatic ventral compressive pathology, is simply a dorsal fusion, usually employing instrumentation. A dorsal fusion that incorporates all levels included by the ventral procedure avoids reoperating through distorted anatomy. Dorsal lateral mass fusions offer particular appeal in those situations in which every effort has been made to use autograft bone and instrumentation ventrally.

If overt hardware failure or residual ventral pathology demands reoperation, one may proceed from the side opposite the initial procedure. The decision to operate through a previous exposure is largely one of personal preference, unless a recurrent laryngeal nerve injury was sustained with the initial surgery (as documented by laryngoscopy). Although the procedure is generally straightforward, a few points deserve mention with regard to ventral cervical operations.[38] First, on exposure of the ventral spine it may be difficult to precisely localize the level of suspected pseudarthrosis on gross inspection. Identifying adjacent disk space levels provides some guidance, as does an aggressive mobilization of the longus colli musculature, which provides lateral bony exposure that may reveal some preserved interspace laterally at the operated level. Second, the actual removal of graft from a previously operated level may be challenging. Usually a high-speed pneumatic drill is used to remove the previous graft. When ventral instrumentation is planned, particular care must be taken to avoid overzealous vertebral body resection adjacent to the graft site. Excessive straying into an adjacent vertebral body can quickly result in the loss of a suitable anchor point for the implant, necessitating inclusion of another level in the construct. Fluoroscopy can provide a helpful gauge of depth during drilling. One may drill down the old graft just slightly beyond the rostral and caudal margins of the graft, staying near the midline. This provides exposure of the posterior longitudinal ligament remote from previous surgical exposure. In this fashion the surgeon can easily broaden the dural exposure and extend it rostrally and caudally, beginning on tissue remote from the initial surgery. The technique of beginning far laterally and drilling on either side of the graft should be used with caution, because as the exposure deepens one may inadvertently encounter a nerve root with little warning from normal anatomic landmarks.

Dorsal cervical fusions include the occipitocervical spine, the C1-2 level, and the subaxial cervical spine. Occipitocervical fusions provide a challenge because of the complex multiplanar relationships of the skull base to the upper cervical spine. A C1 laminectomy, or a suboccipital craniectomy, magnifies this difficulty, diminishing the bony surface available for fusion. A broad exposure to the lateral aspects of the articular masses, with exposure of every available surface of the subocciput, is critical. Care must be taken to avoid damage to the vertebral artery as it courses

---

[*]References 8,17,62,74,138,147,154.

over the rostrolateral aspect of the ring of C1. A robust venous plexus around the vertebral artery can make dissection in the interval between C1 and the skull base difficult, although use of the bipolar cautery and the judicious use of Surgicel can usually control this bleeding. The laminae of C2 can be followed laterally. The rostral surface of the laminae is then followed to the pars interarticularis and down onto the superior articular surface of C2. The C1-2 articular surfaces are disrupted with a small, angled curette. Cancellous bone may then be packed into the joint space, with care taken to avoid encroachment onto the dural sac. At all levels included in the fusion, the articular surfaces are similarly disrupted and packed with cancellous bone. All available surfaces are then decorticated, and the instrumentation is positioned. The bone graft is placed and tamped firmly into place. Occasionally when sufficient graft is available, a corticocancellous sheet of bone is secured. At every phase of the arthrodesis an attempt is made to provide a contiguous sheet of bone to optimize union. Remarkably, despite the complexity of occipitocervical fusions, a high fusion rate (97%) has been reported.[7]

Many surgeons use transarticular screw fixation with all C1-2 fusions, when allowed by the patient's anatomy.[112] Revision of failed C1-2 fusions, when the anatomy will not safely allow the use of transarticular screws, is rare. Usually placement of at least a unilateral screw is possible. When a revision without screws is performed, meticulous attention must be given to preparation of the caudal aspect of the ring of C1, the usual point of failure.

The key to successful subaxial dorsal fusions is an adequate exposure of the lateral articular masses. Independent of whether a dorsal or interspinous technique or lateral mass plates are used, the articulations of the fused levels are disrupted with a small, angled curette, decorticated with a drill, and packed with cancellous bone that is tamped firmly into position.

Failure of an odontoid screw in treatment of an odontoid fracture usually occurs as a result of either screw breakage or screw cutout of the body of C2.[45] Screw removal should be followed by a dorsal C1-2 fusion with instrumentation.[112]

### Thoracic Spine

The rigidity of the thoracic spine, afforded by the articulation of the ribs, enhances the integrity of most midthoracic constructs.[3] The tremendous loads concentrated at both ends of the thoracic spine, by virtue of the leverage of the craniocervical and lumbosacral lever arms, stress constructs at these locations. This is noteworthy when one considers that surgical exposures at the extremes of the ventral thoracic spine are not straightforward. Although the surgeon with a focused practice in complex spine surgery may be intimately familiar with these approaches, those less experienced may benefit from the assistance of a thoracic surgeon during these exposures.

Failed dorsal instrumentation constructs are frequently the result of suboptimal placement of hardware. This is particularly true when lateral mass plates are used across the cervicothoracic junction. The use of lateral mass plates at these levels of transitional anatomy occasionally requires a screw to be placed into the thoracic pedicle to provide sufficient bony purchase. Some recently developed hybrid systems incorporate the strengths of lateral mass plates in the cervical spine and hook systems in the thoracic spine and allow solid dorsal stabilization across the cervicothoracic junction, without placement of pedicle screws in the thoracic spine. Dorsal thoracolumbar constructs must be carefully designed to provide sufficient strength to resist the massive forces present at this location. The addition of ventral load-bearing struts, with or without instrumentation, can be aided by thoracoabdominal or extracavitary approaches. Despite the belief that the vertebral end plate must be maintained to prevent graft subsidence, recent investigations suggest that this technical feature is of less importance than previously suspected.[72]

### Lumbar Spine

The management of failed lumbar fusions remains a source of much controversy. Every effort should be made to optimize the chance for successful fusion by analyzing the mechanism of previous nonunion and thoughtfully tailoring the planned procedure to the patient's individual situation. For example, failure of a noninstrumented dorsolateral fusion may lead to the use of spinal instrumentation to augment the dorsolateral fusion. Failure of a dorsally instrumented fusion may require not only revision of the dorsal construct, but also the addition of a ventral interbody construct.[4,61,145] Whereas ventral fusions can be safely performed,[52] most surgeons do not routinely use a combined ventral and dorsal procedure for degenerative pathologies in previously unoperated patients, as is advocated by some authors.[109] New technologies, including interbody cages that can be placed through ventral and dorsal exposures, may provide additional options in the management of symptomatic lumbar nonunion.

## Summary

Successful bony fusion requires consideration of the patient's general preoperative physiologic state, with attention paid to metabolic derangements, coexisting diseases, or habits likely to impact negatively on bone healing. An attempt must be made to modify those factors. The basic principles of biomechanics, as they apply to the patient's situation, should be used in the surgery plan. Meticulous attention is essential to the technical details of the procedure, in particular, the arthrodesis. An appropriate, well-fitted orthosis and scrupulous postoperative wound and general medical care are required. Even with the best efforts of an excellent surgeon and a compliant patient, successful bony union is occasionally not attained. In those situations in which there are persistent symptoms related to nonunion, or in which persistent motion threatens neural structures, another attempt to provide successful fusion may be made. In these circumstances every possible effort must be made to optimize the chance for successful bony union, beginning with a critical review of the previous failure. Every phase of the procedure, from preoperative and postoperative features to the planned procedure itself, must be thoughtfully optimized.

Surgical planning is critical, and simple reproduction of a previously failed procedure should be avoided. Some component of the first procedure should be altered, such as addition of hardware to a previously uninstrumented case, the addition of a dorsal construct to a ventral failure or vice versa, or the addition of a substantive postoperative orthosis. As in every other surgical arena, an understanding of the basic principles, coupled with common sense, best equips the surgeon to deal with a variety of problems.

# REFERENCES

1. Aaron RK, Coimbor DM: Electrical stimulation of bone induction and grafting. In Habal MB, Reddi AH (ed): *Bone Grafts and Bone Substitutes*. Philadelphia, WB Saunders, 1992, p. 173.

2. An HS, Simpson JM, Glover JM, Stephany J: Comparison between allograft plus demineralized bone matrix versus autograft in anterior cervical fusion. A prospective multicenter study. *Spine* 20:2211, 1995.

3. Andriachhi TP, Schultz AB, Belytseka TB: A model for studies of mechanical interactions between the human spine and rib cage. *J Biomech* 7:497, 1974.

4. Albert TJ, Pinto M, Denis F: Management of symptomatic lumbar pseudarthrosis with anteroposterior fusion. *Spine* 25:123-130, 2000.

5. Albert TJ, Pinto M, Smith MD, *et al*: Accuracy of SPECT scanning in diagnosing pseudoarthrosis: A prospective study. *J Spinal Disord* 11:197-199, 1998.

6. Anonymous: Tobacco use and usual source of cigarettes among high school students in the United States 1995. *MMWR* 45:413, 1996.

7. Apostolides PJ, Dickman CA, Golfinos JG, *et al*: Threaded Steinmann pin fusion of the craniovertebral junction. *Spine* 21:1630, 1996.

8. Awatshi D, Voorhies RM: Anterior cervical vertebrectomy and interbody fusion. Technical note. *J Neurosurg* 76:159, 1992.

9. Bassett CAL: The role of pulsed electromagnetic fields in bone grafting. In Habal MB, Reddi AH (ed): *Bone Grafts and Bone Substitutes*. Philadelphia, WB Saunders, 1992, p. 173.

10. Bridwell KH, O'Brien MF, Lenke LG, *et al*: Posterior spinal fusion supplemented with only allograft bone in paralytic scoliosis. Does it work? *Spine* 19:2658, 1994.

11. Blumenthal S, Baker J, Dossett A, Selby DK: The role of anterior lumbar fusion for internal disc disruption. *Spine* 13:566, 1986.

12. Boden SD: Biology of lumbar spine fusion and use of bone graft substitutes: Present, future, and next generation. *Tissue Eng* 6:383-399, 2000.

13. Boden SD: Evaluation of carriers of bone morphogenetic protein for spinal fusion. *Spine* 26:850, 2001.

14. Boden SD, Hair GA, Viggeswarapu M, *et al*: Gene therapy for spinal fusion. *Clinical Orthop* 379S:225-233, 2000.

15. Boden SD, Martin GJ, Morone MA, *et al*: Posterolateral lumbar intertransverse process spine arthrodesis with recombinant human bone morphogenetic protein 2/hydrodoxyapatite-tricalcium phosphate after

16. laminectomy in the nonhuman primate. *Spine* 24:1179-1185, 1999.

16. Bonfiglio M, Jeter WS, Smith CL: The immune concept: its relation to bone transplantation. *Ann NY Acad Sci* 59:417, 1955.

17. Boni M: Stabilization of the cervical spine: problems and techniques. *J Neurosurg Sci* 28:167, 1984.

18. Brown MD, Malinan TI, Davis PB: A roentgenographic evaluation of frozen allografts versus autografts in anterior cervical spine fusions. *Clin Orthop* 119:231, 1976.

19. Brown CW, Orme TJ, Richardson HD: The rate of pseudoarthrosis (surgical nonunion) in patients who are smokers and patients who are nonsmokers: a comparison study. *Spine* 8:942, 1983.

20. Buck BE, Malinin TI, Brown MD: Bone transplantation and the human immunodeficiency virus. An estimate of risk of acquired immunodeficiency syndrome (AIDS). *Clin Orthop* 240:129, 1989.

21. Buckwalter JA, Einhorn TA, Bolander ME, Cruess RL: Healing of the musculoskeletal tissues. In Rockwood A, Green DP, Bucholz RW, Heckman JD (eds): *Rockwood and Green's Fractures in Adults*, ed 4, vol 1. Philadelphia, Lippincott-Raven, 1996, p. 261

22. Buckwalter JA, Cooper RR: Bone structure and function. *Instr Course Lect* 36:27, 1987.

23. Buckwalter JA, Woo SL-Y, Goldberg VM, *et al*: Soft tissue aging and musculoskeletal function. *J Bone Joint Surg* 75A:1533, 1993.

24. Burchardt H: The biology of bone graft repair. *Clin Orthop* 174:28, 1983.

25. Burstein AH, Zika JM, Heiple KG, Klein L: Contribution of collagen and mineral to the elastic plastic properties of bone. *J Bone Joint Surg* 57A:956, 1975.

26. Butterman GR, Glazer PA, Hu SS, Bradford DS: Results of interbody allografts in revision of failed lumbar fusions. Tenth Annual Meeting of the North American Spine Society, Washington DC, October 18-21, 1995.

27. Buttermann GR, Glazer PA, Bradford DS: The use of bone allografts in the spine. *Clin Orthop* 324:75, 1996.

28. Calin A: The spondyloarthropathies. In Rubinstein E, Federman DD (eds): *Scientific American*, sec 3. New York, Scientific American, 1982, p 1.

29. Carlson HC, Williams MMD, Childs DS Jr, *et al*: Microangiography of bones in the study of radiation changes. *Radiology* 74:113, 1960.

30. Chan DP, Ngian KS, Cohen L: Posterior upper cervical fusion in rheumatoid arthritis. *Spine* 17:268, 1992.

31. Clark CR, Whitehill R: Two views of the use of methylmethacrylate for stabilization of the cervical spine. *Orthopaedics* 12:589, 1989.

32. Cloward RB: The treatment of ruptured lumbar intervertebral disc by vertebral body fusion: method of use of banked bone. *Ann Surg* 136:987, 1952.

33. Cloward RB: The anterior approach for removal of ruptured cervical disc. *J Neurosurg* 15:602, 1958.

34. Cloward RB: Gas sterilized cadaver bone grafts for spinal fusion operations: a simplified bone bank. *Spine* 5:4, 1980.

35. Cohen DB, Chotivichit A, Fujita T, *et al*: Pseudarthrosis repair: Autogenous iliac crest versus femoral ring allograft. *Clin Orthop* 371:46-55, 2000.

36. Cook SD, Whitecloud TS: Use of osteoinductive implants to facilitate spine fusions. In Bridwell KH, DeWald RL

(eds): *The Textbook of Spinal Surgery*, ed 2. Philadelphia, Lippincott-Raven, 1997, p. 2379.

37. Condemi JJ: The autoimmune diseases. *JAMA* 268:2882, 1992.

38. Coric D, Branch CL, Jenkins JD: Revision of anterior cervical pseudarthrosis with anterior allograft fusion and plating. *J Neurosurg* 86:969-974, 1997.

39. Daftari TK, Whitesides TE Jr, Heller JG, et al: Nicotine on the revascularization of bone graft. An experimental study in rabbits. *Spine* 19:904, 1994.

40. Datta R, Saha S: Quantitative determination of tolerance doses for preoperative and postoperative radiotherapy of bones. *Med Phys* 10:243, 1983.

41. Dennis S, Watkins R, Landaker S, et al: Comparison of disc space heights after anterior lumbar interbody fusion. *Spine* 14:876, 1989.

42. DeVernejoul MC, Bielakoff J, Herve M, et al: Evidence for defective osteoblastic function. A role for alcohol and tobacco consumption in middle age men. *Clin Orthop* 179:107, 1983.

43. Dickman CA, Maric Z: The biology of bone healing and techniques of spinal fusion. *BNI Quarterly* 10:2, 1994.

44. Dodd CA, Fergusson CM, Freedman L, et al: Allograft versus autograft bone in scoliosis surgery. *J Bone Joint Surg* 70:431, 1988.

45. Doherty BJ, Heggenes MH, Essess SI: A biomechanical study of odontoid fractures and fracture fixation. *Spine* 18:178, 1993.

46. Dougherty PJ, Jones AAM, Sharkey N, Benson DR: Iliac crest bone graft: Osteotome versus saw (abstract). Rosemont, IL, Cervical Spine Research Society, December 1992, p 148.

47. Emery SE, Brazinski M, Benusan J, et al: Effects of irradiation on the biological and biomechanical properties of anterior spine fusion in a canine model (abstract). Orthopaedic Research Society, 38th Annual Meeting, Washington DC, February 1992.

48. Emery SE, Hughes SS, Junglas WA, et al: The fate of anterior vertebral bone grafts in patients irradiated for neoplasm. *Clin Orthop* 300:207, 1994.

49. Enneking WF: Histologic investigations of bone transplants in immunologically prepared animals. *J Bone Joint Surg* 39A:597, 1957.

50. Enneking WF, Mindell ER: Observations on massive retrieved human allografts. *J Bone Joint Surg* 73A:1123, 1991.

51. Fabry G: Allograft versus autograft bone in idiopathic scoliosis surgery: a multivariate statistical analysis. *J Pediatr Orthop* 11:465, 1991.

52. Faciszewski T, Winter RB, Lonstein JE, et al: The surgical and medical perioperative complications of anterior spinal fusion surgery in the thoracic and lumbar spine in adults. A review of 1223 procedures. *Spine* 20:1592, 1995.

53. Fehring TK, Brooks AL: Upper cervical instability in rheumatoid arthritis. *Clin Orthop* 221:137, 1987.

54. Fernyhough JC, White JL, LaRocca H: Fusion rates in multilevel cervical spondylosis comparing allograft fibula and autograft in 126 patients. *Spine* 16:S563, 1991.

55. Finston RA, Woodard HQ, Laughlin JS: Effects of external radiation on mineral metabolism in the bones of adult dogs. *Clin Orthop* 46:183, 1966.

56. Fitzsimmons RJ, Strong D, Mohan S, et al: Low amplitude, low frequency electric field-stimulated bone cell proliferation may in part be mediated by IGF II release. *J Cell Physiol* 150:84, 1992.

57. Fox MW, Onofrio BM: Ankylosing spondylitis. In Menenzes AH, Sonntag VKH (eds): *Principles of Spinal Surgery*, vol 1. New York, McGraw Hill, 1996, p. 735.

58. Francis RM: The pathogenesis of osteoporosis. In Francis RM (ed): *Osteoporosis, Pathogenesis, and Management*. Lancaster, Kluwer, 1990, p. 51.

59. Frost HM: Tetracycline-based histologic analysis of bone remodeling. *Calcif Tissue Res* 3:211, 1969.

60. Grossman WC, Peppelman WC, Baum JA, Kraus DR: The use of freeze-dried fibular allograft in anterior cervical fusion. *Spine* 17:565, 1992.

61. Gertzbein SD, Hollopeter MR, Hall S: Pseudarthrosis of the lumbar spine-outcome after circumferential fusion. *Spine* 23:2352-2357, 1998.

62. Hanai K, Fujiyoshi F, Kamei K: Subtotal vertebrectomy and spinal fusions for cervical spondylotic myelopathy. *Spine* 11:310, 1986.

63. Hanley EN Jr, Harvell JC Jr, Shapiro DE, Kraus DR: Use of allograft bone in cervical spine surgery. *Semin Spine Surg* 1:262, 1989.

64. Hanley E, Levy J: Surgical treatment of isthmic lumbosacral spondylolisthesis, analysis of variables influencing results. *Spine* 14:48, 1989.

65. Harper KD: Osteoporosis. In Wilkins RE, Rengachary SS (eds): *Neurosurgery*, ed 2, vol 3. New York, McGraw Hill, 1996, p. 3761.

66. Harrington KD: The use of methylmethacrylate for vertebral-body replacement and anterior stabilization of pathological fracture dislocations of the spine due to metastatic malignant disease. *J Bone Joint Surg* 63A:36, 1981.

67. Hayes WC: Biomechanics of cortical and trabecular bone: implication for assessment of fracture risk. In Mow VC, Hayes WC (eds): *Basic Orthopaedic Biomechanics*. Philadelphia, Lippincott-Raven, 1991, p. 93.

68. Heggeness MH, Esses SI: Classification of pseudarthroses of the lumbar spine. *Spine* 16:449-454, 1991.

69. Helm GA, Alden TD, Sheehan JP, Kallmes D: Bone morphogenetic proteins and bone morphogenetic protein gene therapy in neurological surgery: A review. *Neurosurgery* 46:1213-1221, 2000.

70. Hey LA: Rheumatoid arthritis of the cervical spine. In Wilkins RE, Rengachary SS (eds): *Neurosurgery*, ed 2, vol 3. New York, McGraw Hill 1996, p. 3789.

71. Hollo I, Gergely I, Boross M: Smoking results in calcitonin resistance. *JAMA* 237:2470, 1977.

72. Hollowell JP, Vollmer DG, Wilson CR, et al: Biomechanical analysis of thoracolumbar interbody constructs: how important is the endplate? *Spine* 21:1032, 1996.

73. Holte DC, O'Brien JP, Renton P: Anterior lumbar fusion using a hybrid interbody graft. *Eur Spine J* 3:32, 1994.

74. Jamjoom A, Williams C, Cummins B: The treatment of spondylotic cervical myelopathy by multiple subtotal vertebrectomy and fusion. *Br J Neurosurg* 5:249, 1991.

75. Jeejeebhoy KM, Kaminski MV Jr: Nutritional assessment and intravenous support: indications for parenteral nutrition. Physician's monograph. Chicago, Medical Directions, 1978.

76. Jenis LG, An HS, Stein R, Young B: Prospective comparison of the effect of direct current electrical stimulation and pulsed electromagnetic fields on instrumented posterolateral lumbar arthrodesis 12: 290-296, 2000.

77. Jenkins LT, Jones AL, Harms JJ: Prognostic factors in lumbar spinal fusion. *Contemporary Ortho* 29:173-179, 1994.

78. Jerome JH: Drug addiction and drug abuse. In Gilman AF, Goodman LS, Rall TW, Murad F (eds): *The Pharmacological Basis of Thearapeutics*, ed 7. New York, Macmillan, 1985, p. 532.

79. Kahanovitz N: The use of adjunctive electrical stimulation to enhance healing of spine fusions. *Spine* 21:2523, 1996.

80. Kahanovitz N, Arnoczky SP, Hulse D, Shires PK: The effect of postoperative electromagnetic pulsing on canine posterior spinal fusions. *Spine* 9:273, 1984.

81. Kane WJ: Direct current electrical bone growth stimulation for spinal fusion. *Spine* 13:363, 1988.

82. Kaufman HH, Jones E: The principles of bony spinal fusion. *Neurosurgery* 24:264, 1989.

83. Knapp DR Jr, Jones ET: Use of cortical cancellous allograft for posterior spinal fusion. *Clin Orthop* 229:99, 1988.

84. Kostuik JP: Failures after spinal fusion. In Frymoyer JW (ed): *The Adult Spine: Principles and Practice*. Philadelphia, Lippincott-Raven, 1997, p. 2277.

85. Kozak JA, Heilman AE, O'Brien JP: Anterior lumbar fusion options: technique and graft materials. *Clin Orthop* 300:45, 1994.

86. Kraus DR, Peppelman WC, Agarwal AK, *et al*: Incidence of subaxial subluxation in patients with generalized rheumatoid arthritis who have had previous occipitocervical fusions. *Spine* (Suppl 10):S486, 1991.

87. Lau GC, Luck JV Jr, Marshall GJ, Griffith G: The effect of cigarette smoking on fracture healing: an animal model. *Clin Res* 37:A132, 1989.

88. Lindsey RW, Grobman J, Leggon RE, *et al*: Effects of bone graft and electrical stimulation on the strength of healing bony defects in dogs. *Clin Orthop* 222:275, 1987.

89. Lou E: Bone morphogenetic proteins: An overview of therapeutic applications. *Ortho* 24:504-508, 2001.

90. Lowery GL, Maxwell KM, Karasick D, *et al*: Comparison of autograft and composite grafts of demineralized bone matrix and autologous bone in posterolateral fusions: an interim report. *Innovation Technol Biol Med* 16:1, 1995.

91. Majd ME, Vadhva M, Holt RT: Anterior cervical reconstruction using titanium cages with anterior plating. *Spine* 24:1604-1610, 1999.

92. Malinan TI, Rosomoff HL, Sutton CH: Human cadaveric femoral head homografts for anterior cervical spine fusions. *Surg Neurol* 7:249, 1977.

93. Markbreiter LA, Pelker RR, Friedlander GE, *et al*: The effect of radiation on the fracture repair process: a biomechanical evaluation of a closed fracture in a rat model. *J Orthop Res* 7:178, 1989.

94. May VR, Mauck WR: Exploration of the spine for pseudoarthrosis following spinal fusions in the treatment of scoliosis. *Clin Orthop* 53:115, 1967.

95. McAfee PC, Bohlman HH, Ducker T, Eismont FJ: Failure of stabilization of the spine with

methylmethacrylate. A retrospective analysis of twenty-four cases. *J Bone Joint Surg* 68A:1145, 1986.

96. McCarthy RE, Peek RD, Morrissy RJ, Hough AJ: Allograft bone in spinal fusions for paralytic scoliosis. *J Bone Joint Surg* 68A:370, 1986.

97. McDermott MT, Witte MC: Bone mineral content in smokers. *South Med J* 81:477, 1988.

98. McGrath H Jr, McCormick C, Carey ME: Pyogenic cervical osteomyelitis presenting as a massive prevertebral abscess in a patient with rheumatoid arthritis. *Am J Med* 84:363, 1988.

99. McMaster MJ: A technique for lumbar spinal osteotomy in ankylosing spondylitis. *J Bone Joint Surg* 67B:204, 1985.

100. Miller PD: Critical drug appraisal: etidronate intermittent cyclic therapy for postmenopausal osteoporosis. *Br J Clin Pract* 50:23, 1996.

101. Montgomery DM, Aronson DD, Lee CL, Lamont RL: Posterior spinal fusions: allograft versus autograft bone. *J Spinal Disord* 3:370, 1990.

102. Mooney V: A randomized double blind prospective study of the efficacy of pulsed electromagnetic fields for interbody lumbar fusions. *Spine* 15:708, 1990.

103. Moskovich R, Frenkel S: Biologic materials to facilitate spinal fusions. In Bridwell KH, Dewald RL (eds): *The Textbook of Spinal Surgery*, ed 2. Philadelphia, Lippincott-Raven, 1997, p. 2385.

104. Muschler GF, Lane JM, Dawson EG: The biology of spinal fusion. In Cotler JM, Cotler HP (eds): *Spinal Fusion Science and Techniques*. Berlin, Springer-Verlag, 1990, p 9.

105. Nasca RJ, Whelchel JD: Use of cryopreserved bone in spinal surgery. *Spine* 12:222, 1987.

106. Neuman WF: Bone materials and calcification mechanisms. In Urist MR (ed): *Fundamental and Clinical Bone Physiology*. Philadelphia, Lippincott-Raven, 1980, p 83.

107. Nicita-Mauro V: Smoking, calcium, calcium antagonists, and aging. *Exp Gerontol* 25:393, 1990.

108. Oakes DA, Lieberman JR: Osteoinductive applications of regional gene therapy. *Clin Orthop* 379S:101-112, 2000.

109. O'Brien JP, Dawson MH, Heard CW, *et al*: Simultaneous combined anterior and posterior fusion. A surgical solution for failed spinal surgery with a brief review of the first 150 patients. *Clin Orthop* 203:191, 1986.

110. Oishi M, Onesti ST: Electrical bone graft stimulation for spinal fusion: A review. *Neurosurgery* 47:1041-1056, 2000.

111. Pappas CTE, Sonntag VKH: Degenerative disorders of the spine: lumbar stenosis. In Sonntag VKH, Menenzes AH (eds): *Principles of Spinal Surgery*, vol 2. New York, McGraw Hill, 1996, p. 631.

112. Paramore CG, Dickman CA, Sonntag VKH: The anatomic suitability of the C1-2 complex for transarticular screw fixation. *J Neurosurg* 85:221, 1996.

113. Pettine KA, Salib RM: Femoral diaphyseal allograft for anterior lumbar interbody fusion: long-term follow-up. *Orthop Trans* 17:12, 1993.

114. Pocock NA, Eisman JA, Kelly PJ, *et al*: Effects of tobacco on axial and appendicular bone mineral density. *Bone* 10:329, 1989.

115. Prolo DJ: Biology of bone fusion. *Clin Neurosurg* 36:135, 1988.

116. Prolo DJ: Morphology and metabolism of fusion of the lumbar spine. In Youmans JR (ed): *Neurological Surgery*, ed 4, vol 3. Philadelphia, WB Saunders, 1996, p. 2449.

117. Rao S, Yadav A, Galvan R: Posterior cervical spine stabilization under local anesthesia. *J Spinal Disord* 3:250, 1990.

118. Ray RD: Bone grafting: transplants and implants. *Instr Course Lect* 13:177, 1956.

119. Ray RD, Sabet T: Cellular survival versus induction: an experimental study in mice. *J Bone Joint Surg* 45A:337, 1963.

120. Recker RR: Embryology, anatomy, and microstructure of bone. In Coe FL, Favus MJ (eds): *Disorders of Bone and Mineral Metabolism*. Philadelphia, Lippincott-Raven, 1992, p. 219.

121. Rhoades JE, Kasinkas W: Influence of hypoproteinemia on the formation of callus in experimental fracture. *Surgery* 11:38, 1942.

122. Riggs BL, Melton LJ III: Involutional osteoporosis. *N Engl J Med* 314:1676, 1986.

123. Rish BL, McFadden JT, Penix JO: Anterior cervical fusion using homologous bone grafts: a comparative study. *Surg Neurol* 5:119, 1976.

124. Rogozinski A, Rogozinski C: Efficacy of implanted bone growth stimulation in instrumented lumbar fusion. *Spine* 21:2479, 1996.

125. Sandelin J, Santavirta S, Laasonen E, *et al*: Spontaneous fracture of atlas of cervical spine affected by rheumatoid arthritis. *Scand J Rheumatol* 14:167, 1985.

126. Sandhu HS, Boden SD: Biologic enhancement of spinal fusion. *Orthop Clin North Am* 29:621-631, 1998.

127. Santavirta S, Konttinen YT, Laasonen E, *et al*: Ten-year results of operations for rheumatoid cervical spine disorders. *J Bone Joint Surg* 73B:116, 1991.

128. Sassard WR, Eidman DK, Gray MP: Analysis of spine fusion utilizing demineralized bone matrix. Presentation. Western Orthopaedic Association Annual Meeting, August 13-17, 1994.

129. Sawin PD, Dickman CA, Crawford NR, *et al*: The effects of dexamethasone on bone fusion in an experimental model of posterolateral lumbar spinal arthrodesis. *J Neurosurg* (Spine 1) 94:76-81, 2001.

130. Sawin PD, Traynelis VC, Menezes AH: A comparative analysis of fusion rates and donor site morbidity for autogeneic rib and iliac crest bone grafts in posterior cervical fusions. *J Neurosurgery* 88:255-65, 1998.

131. Schneider JR, Bright RW: Anterior cervical fusion using preserved bone allografts. *Transplant Proc* 8S:73, 1976.

132. Silcox DH III, Dafteri T, *et al*: The effect of nicotine on spinal fusion. *Spine* 20:1549, 1995.

133. Simmons EH: Surgical treatment of ankylosing spondylitis: surgical considerations. In Rothman RH, Simeone FA (eds): *The Spine*, ed 3, vol 2. Philadelphia, WB Saunders, 1992, p. 1447.

134. Slosar PJ, Reynolds JB, Schofferman J, *et al*: Combined anterior and posterolateral lumbar fusions: primary and revision procedures. Ninth Annual Meeting of the North American Spine Society, Minneapolis, October 19-22, 1994.

135. Sparrow D, Rosner B, *et al*: The influence of cigarette smoking and age on bone loss in men. *Arch Environ Health* 37:246, 1982.

136. Stabler CL, Eismont FJ, Brown MD, *et al*: Failure of posterior cervical fusion using cadaveric bone graft in children. *J Bone Joint Surg* 67A:370, 1985.

137. Steinmann JC, Herkowitz HN: Pseudarthrosis of the spine. *Clin Orthop* 284:80-90, 1992.

138. Sypert GW, Sypert EJA: Indications for corpectomy in the cervical spine. In Menenzes AH, Sonntag VKH (eds): *Principles of Spinal Surgery*, vol 1. New York, McGraw Hill, 1996, p. 1147.

139. Tonna EA, Cronkite EP: The periosteum: autoradiographic studies on cellular proliferation and transformation utilizing tritiated thymidine. *Clin Orthop* 30:218, 1963.

140. Triffitt JT: The organic matrix of bone tissue. In Urist MR (ed): *Fundamental and Clinical Bone Physiology*. Philadelphia, Lippincott-Raven, 1980, p. 45.

141. Urist MR: Bone transplants and implants. In Urist MR (ed): *Fundamental and Clinical Bone Physiology*. Philadelphia, JB Lippincott, 1980, p. 331.

142. Urist MR, DeLange RJ, Finerman GAM: Bone cell differentiation and growth factors. *Science* 220:680, 1983.

143. Vanden Berhe A, Ackerman C, Veys E, *et al*: Occipito-cervical fusions in rheumatoid arthritis. *Acta Orthop Belg* (suppl)1:94, 1991.

144. Watts NB, Harris ST, Genant HK, *et al*: Intermittent cyclical etidronate therapy of postmenopausal osteoporosis. *N Engl J Med* 323:73, 1990.

145. Weiss LE, Vaccaro AR, Scuderi G, *et al*: Pseudarthrosis after postoperative wound infection in the lumbar spine. *J Spinal Disord* 10:482-487, 1997.

146. White AA III, Panjabi MM: *Clinical Biomechanics of the Spine*. Philadelphia, Lippincott-Raven, 1990.

147. Whitecloud TI, Larocca S: Fibular strut graft in the reconstructive surgery of the cervical spine. *Spine* 1:33, 1976.

148. Whitesides TE Jr, Hanley EN Jr, Fellrath RF Jr: Smoking abstinence. Is it necessary before spinal fusion? *Spine* 19:2012, 1994.

149. Widmann RF, Pelker RR, Friedlander GE, *et al*: Effects of prefracture irradiation on the biomechanical parameters of fracture healing. *J Orthop Res* 11:422, 1993.

150. Winfield J, Young A, William P, *et al*: Prospective study of the radiologic changes in the hands, feet and cervical spine in adult rheumatoid disease. *Ann Rheum Dis* 42:613, 1983.

151. Woodard HQ: Some effects of X-rays on bone. *Clin Orthop* 9:118, 1957.

152. Young WF, Rosenwasser RH: An early comparative analysis of the use of fibular allograft versus autologous iliac crest graft for interbody fusion after anterior cervical discectomy. *Spine* 18:1123, 1993.

153. Zdeblick TA, Ducker TB: The use of freeze-dried allograft for anterior cervical fusions. *Spine* 16:726, 1991.

154. Zdeblick TA, Bohlman HH: Cervical kyphosis and myelopathy: treatment by anterior corpectomy and strut grafting. *J Bone Joint Surg* 71A:170, 1989.

155. Zhang ZH, Yin H, Yang K, *et al*: Anterior intervertebral disc excision and bone grafting in cervical spondylotic myelopathy. *Spine* 8:16, 1983.

156. Zoma A, Sturrock RD, Fisher WD, *et al*: Surgical stabilization of the rheumatoid cervical spine. A review of indications and results. *J Bone Joint Surg* 69B:8, 1987.

# Controversies

# CHAPTER 158

# Ventral Cervical Decompression and Fusion: To Plate or Not to Plate

## Not to Plate

**Richard L. Saunders**

The multivertebral trough that is unique to decompression via central corpectomy in itself does not destabilize the spine, at least as an acute phenomenon.[30] The surgeon electing the strategy of a three-level corpectomy must consider the means by which graft complications, not stability, can be best addressed, and herein lies the argument about instrumentation. In the otherwise stable noninstrumented, three-level corpectomy, there are several common graft complications— graft displacement, graft fracture, spine-graft deformity, pseudarthrosis, and so-called subsidence or pistoning.

### Graft Displacement

The most common rationalization for the use of spinal instrumentation is the immediate fixation of the graft, especially for the surgeon not entirely comfortable with long ventral strut grafts. To avoid graft displacement, 6 weeks of bedrest, aggressive orthosis, and internal instrumentation have been advocated. Anxiety with regard to this problem is certainly appropriate. In the author's initial corpectomy experience, 12.5% of patients required immediate graft revision as a result of displacement and/or graft fracture. With experience, however, this complication has been nearly eliminated. Through practice there comes an elementary appreciation of the technical factors critical to the retention of the keystone graft. A learning curve was inevitable, because the literature available in 1984, when we first undertook cervical corpectomy, lacked detail regarding the nuances of securing a strut graft. Because there was no experience with cervical plating at that time, an attitude of presumed bone grafting competence prevailed in the orthopedic literature. Inevitably, one learns by his or her mistakes, and the frequency of graft displacement dropped. We found, for example, that the critical test of the secure graft is its resistance to displacement by flexion and extension stress under direct vision before wound closure. It is rare that a graft so tested will be displaced or fractured in the immediate postoperative convalescence period.

Perhaps the most important observation in the matter of graft displacement (and its prevention by instrumentation), is that virtually all uninstrumented grafts that dis-lodge do so in the first 2 postoperative days. The inference being, in keeping with the intraoperative flexion/extension stress test, that the displaced graft is the result of a technical error, and not simply the inherent precariousness of an uninstrumented graft. Viewed from this perspective, one could question the risk:benefit ratio of instrumentation, if it is to address poor technique and a short period of risk. A similar observation could be made on the utility of the halo vest. In the otherwise stable patient the author has not found the halo vest to be useful, even in the five-motion segment corpectomy.[4] Hardware simply for acute graft protection is overkill and ignores the added hazard of esophageal injury. Long after the "benefits" of instrumentation are forgotten an esophageal injury can remain a torment. In the instrumented cervical spine series by Newhouse[3] there was an alarming incidence of esophageal injuries.

### Graft Fracture

The second problem associated with uninstrumented grafts is that of acute graft fracture, almost unique to autogenous iliac crest constructs. This occurs most commonly, like graft displacement, immediately after surgery. The fracture is probably caused by faulty graft harvesting or preparation technique. Iliac crest graft that has been harvested with osteotomes is weakened by cortical microfractures. The graft's collapse with flexion leads to its displacement. This risk is probably greater in the osteoporotic patient. The use of instrumentation to avoid this problem may be inappropriate, because the screw-holding power in fractured or osteoporotic bone (Figure 158.1) is problematic.

Delayed bone graft fracture can occur many months after graft incorporation consequent to relatively minor stress. This is unrelated to gender or age and probably marks the weakest period in graft maturation. Whether or not this rare complication would be prevented or, conversely, compounded by spinal instrumentation, to this author's knowledge has enjoyed no commentary in the literature on graft complications.

Until recently this author has made no deliberate attempt to correct kyphotic curvatures in the course of ventral decompression and grafting, having felt that the properly performed decompression eliminates the detrimental spinal cord draping inherent to a kyphotic curve. The postoperative radiograph of a restored lordosis is unquestionably gratifying; however, without outcome data on the impact of the decompressed, but persistent kyphosis compared to that successfully reduced, the importance of deformity corrections must be kept in perspective.[2] The important aspect of this matter may lie in the spine's deterioration, which results from biomechanical alterations and the loss of cervical balance. A lengthy ventral lever arm on the instantaneous axis of rotation (IAR) inherent to the kyphotic curve invites progressive degenerative changes at the remaining motion segments.

### Spine and Graft Deformation

The critical shortcoming of the uninstrumented graft pertains to the progressive angulation of the graft with its

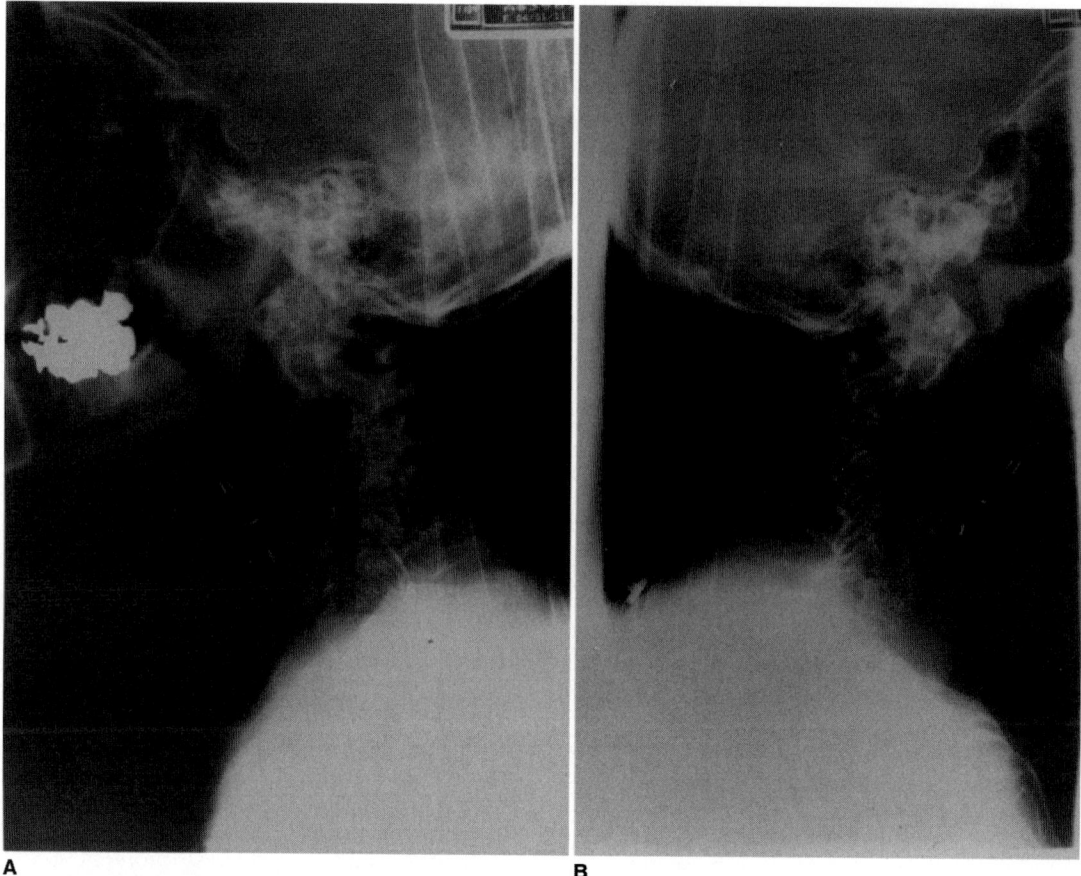

A                                                    B

**Figure 158.1** Immediate postoperative radiograph of a markedly osteoporotic iliac crest bone graft placed in an interbody position (**A**). Fracture of graft occurred soon after surgery (**B**). Hardware probably would have compounded this complication.

upper mortise (Figure 158.2). The frequency of this ordinarily asymptomatic radiographic evolution indicts the surgical method and inadequacies of current orthoses, and perhaps, supports the argument for hardware.[3] It is likely that instrumentation would prevent this complication in most cases. An untested presumption is that there is a misfit between the shape of the rostral graft tip and its mortise in such cases. More likely explanations, however, are dorsal ligamentous laxity or the biomechanical impact of the lengthened ventral moment arm acting on the IAR in spondylosis. In the uninstrumented graft this can be countered by a more ventral placement of the rostral end of the graft, using the so-called dovetailed construct to balance the biomechanical forces responsible for the kyphotic progression. Figure 158.3 illustrates this strategy, taken with graft revision 1 month after a two-level strut that had shown progressive angulation. The correction had been maintained for 2 months in a Philadelphia collar at the time of this x-ray.

A similar situation in which instrumentation is not unreasonable is that of the nonlocalizing myelopathy associated with congenital stenosis and multisegmental kyphosis. A current approach for such cases is the so-called 360-degree approach with anterior and posterior instrumentation. A simpler alternative strategy is that used in the case illustrated in Figure 158.4: this man presented with a severe asymmetrical bilateral C5 radiculopathy and minimally symptomatic myelopathy. His preoperative magnetic reso-

nance imaging (MRI) scan (see Figure 158.4A) shows congenital stenosis and broad reversal of lordosis. Progression of this imbalance was expected. There was a remote history of neck strain, but no present axial symptoms. The pathologic biomechanics were balanced by placing the cephalad end of the four-level corpectomy strut into the anterior vertebral cortex, using a dovetailed construct under moderate distraction. Figure 158.4*B* shows an MRI 4 months after surgery, at which time shoulder pain had resolved, both deltoid muscles had improved to antigravity, the myelopathic signs were unchanged, and there were no myelopathic symptoms.

## Pseudarthrosis

The final and most specific concern in noninstrumented bone grafts is that of pseudarthrosis. Hardware that is rationalized on the basis of enhanced bone graft incorporation is theoretically incontestable, especially if allograft is used. If this were not true, hardware would not be used with complex long bone fractures. The fundamental question, however, is not whether hardware will enhance bone graft incorporation or whether radiographic nonunion is a common finding absent hardware, but whether the incidence of nonunion is a significant clinical problem. The corpectomy patient with bitter complaints of neck pain 1 year after surgery is not common in this author's experience.

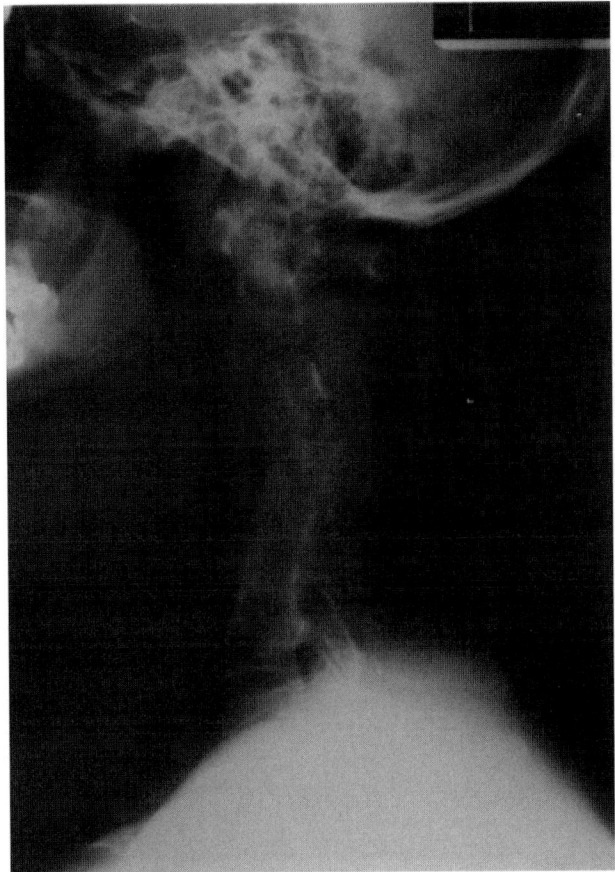

**Figure 158.2** A healed iliac crest interbody graft angled at the upper mortise. This was most likely caused by prior laminectomy, overly posterior graft placement, and inadequate orthosis. Hardware probably would have prevented this angulation.

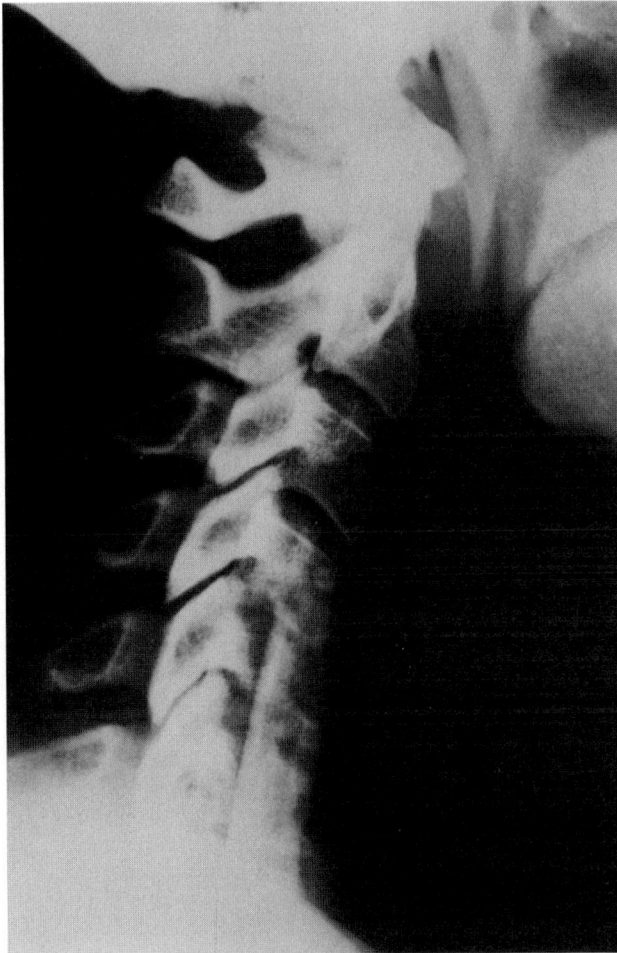

**Figure 158.3** Radiograph 2 months after two-level strut revision for progressive postoperative kyphosis. Note anterior placement of the cephalad end of graft.

The reported incidence of pseudarthrosis without instrumentation ranges widely. In the author's experience with cervical corpectomy since 1984, the incidence of radiographic nonunion with associated neck pain that was relieved by successful refusion is very small—less than 4% of cases. Neck pain without radiographic explanation is as common as symptomatic nonunion.

There is an acknowledged commonality of interobserver disagreement on radiographic interpretation of pseudarthrosis, with and without hardware. Separation of the tips of spinous processes of as much as 2mm from flexion to extension may be seen with the most assured fusion by plain films. The only absolute test of graft incorporation is open exploration. And indeed, this may be offered the patient with unexplained severe neck pain after corpectomy, regardless of radiographic assurances. A spinous process wiring will heal a radiographically evident anterior nonunion.

It is safe to say that the incidence of radiographic nonunion is generally much higher than most accept. The practical importance of this is not yet fully known; however, the frequency of this radiographic disappointment is lessened by the use of hardware, either anteriorly or posteriorly placed. Some spine surgeons report that their pseudarthrosis incidence with instrumented bone grafts is nil.[1] The fact that new iterations of cervical hardware continue to appear, along with a unique jargon, tends to sug-

gest that the last word on this enthusiasm has not been written. Such should make the thoughtful spine surgeon critical in his or her risk-benefit analyses. Perhaps not every case requires hardware.

## Subsidence

A final problem, subsidence, or pistoning of the fibula strut into a caudal mortise, has challenged instrumentation. In this author's experience with ventral surgery, subsidence has been of concern only when the pistoning followed a trajectory out of the axis of the penetrated vertebra, with the threat of fracturing off its anterior cortex. This is very rare. Ordinarily, subsidence in the unplated graft is inevitable to some degree, and not symptomatic. Figure 158.5 illustrates such a case.

## Developing a Rational Approach

Generally speaking, hardware is most logically considered in those cases where bone graft complications are likely. There are always counterbalancing considerations, however.

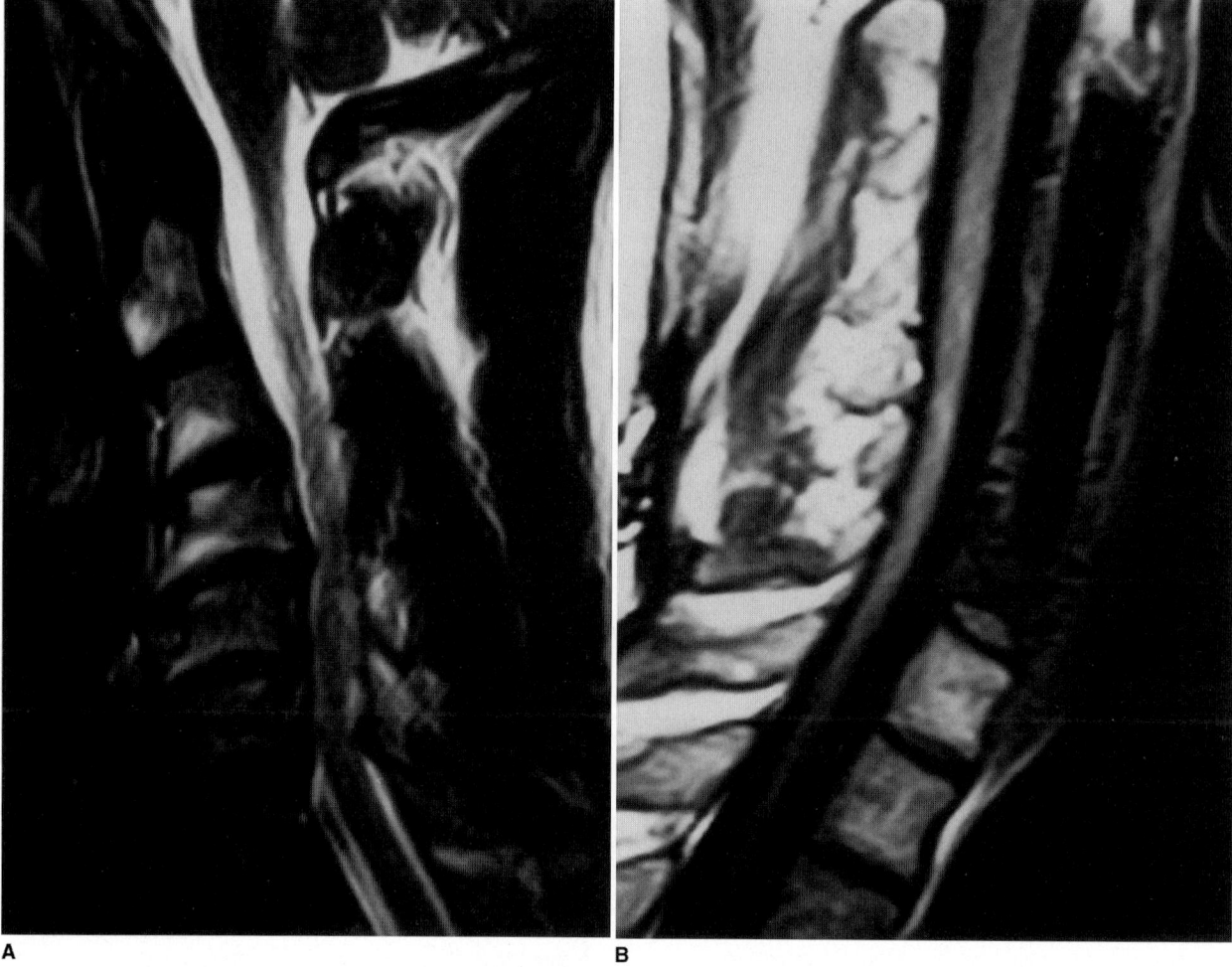

**Figure 158.4 (A)** Preoperative MRI in 40-year-old male with radiculomyelopathy. Note congenital canal stenosis and reversal of lordosis. **(B)** MRI performed 4 months after a four-level, uninstrumented corpectomy wherein the cephalad mortise/strut interface is a dovetailed construct into the anterior vertebral cortex, thus balancing the kyphotic forces of the long anterior moment arm on the IAR. Note the correction of the kyphotic attitude and capacious canal.

Instability aside, the worrisome corpectomy candidate is best characterized as one who is noncompliant, a smoker, osteoporotic, and requires a long graft. Unfortunately, this patient is not necessarily less threatening with instrumentation than without; the uncertainty of instrumenting osteoporotic bone and the unlikely benefit of plating long struts into C7 remain perplexing issues. With long struts, if internal orthosis is elected, it is probably safer to stabilize posteriorly, as well as anteriorly. Perversely, that "best case" for ventral instrumentation, the noncompliant smoker requiring a short strut, will do equally well with a simple autograft as with a plated allograft.

In the long run the complex challenges will probably have a troublingly high inherent axial morbidity. The challenge will not be to eliminate it, but how to avoid compounding its consequence. As a case in point, in a small personal series of C2 to C7 grafts without hardware, there were three immediate graft complications (6.2%).[4] Two of the three immediately displaced; one by complex fracture of severely osteoporotic iliac crest autograft, a poor choice in hindsight; and the second a proximal mortise fracture from undue extension and distraction, a significant techni-cal error. The third immediate complication occurred in a patient with an S-shaped cervical curve, who showed such subsidence in a nonaxial trajectory that fracturing off the anterior cortex of the distal vertebra was feared. He was treated in tong traction, and revision was avoided. The other two patients were revised uneventfully. Had any of these three patients been instrumented in their primary procedure, it is doubtful that the complication would have been avoided and, indeed, it is likely that the displacements would have been more complex and damaging. The management of corpectomy graft morbidity absent instrumentation, though perhaps more frequent, is relatively inconsequential; the same cannot be said about that with hardware.

Accordingly, the unequivocal argument for instrumentation is a radiographic instability pattern or evidence of spinal weakening, such as prior laminectomy, wherein the ideal would be an authoritative, but simple external orthosis, which does not exist. Similarly, the easy graft challenge, one or two levels, having risk factors such as poor compliance or health, should have excellent risk/benefit ratios favoring internal orthosis.

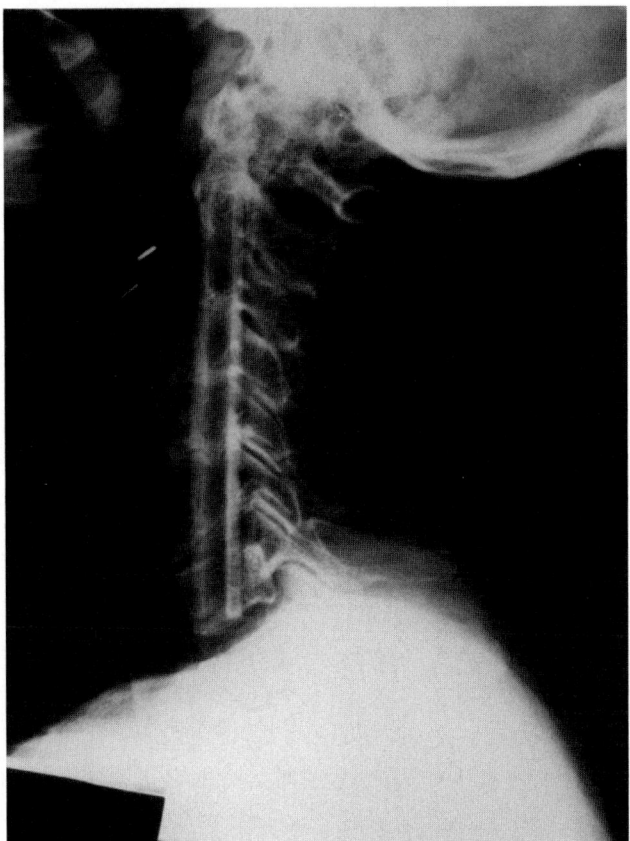

**Figure 158.5** Plain radiograph taken 2 years after four-level corpectomy and allograft fibula strut. Note extent of subsidence is actually into the next motion segment. The patient was symptom free, had had complete resolution of his preoperative myelopathy, no widening of spinous process interval with flexion from extension, and no neck pain. Note also that although the lordotic curve is straightened, there is no kyphosis in spite of subsidence.

## Summary

Whereas there is a place for ventral plating in cervical corpectomy, this ordinarily may be the exception, not the rule. That patient most prone to compromised outcome after relatively short strut placement, whether from issues of compliance, health, or stability, is a case in point. However, to derive from that patient that the standard of care in cervical corpectomy generally requires the use of anterior hardware is to overstate the case. Hardware use to forgive poor technique, or viewed as the only means to prevent progressive loss of lordosis, ignores the fact that it is an additional undertaking with attendant unique morbidities.[2]

## REFERENCES

1. Eleraky M, Llanos C, Sonntag V: Cervical corpectomy: report of 185 cases and review of the literature. *J Neurosurg (Spine 1)* 90:35, 1999.
2. Herman JM, Sonntag VH: Cervical corpectomy and plate fixation for post-laminectomy kyphosis. *J Neurosurg* 80:963, 1994.
3. Newhouse KE, Lindsey RW, Clerk CR, *et al*: Esophageal perforation following anterior cervical surgery. *Spine* 14:1051, 1989.
4. Saunders R, Pikus H, Ball P: Four-level cervical corpectomy. *Spine* 23:2455, 1999.

## To Plate

### Sait Naderi and Nevan G. Baldwin

Since its popularization the ventral approach for cervical spine surgery has been used for numerous conditions of the cervical spine, including traumatic lesions, degenerative lesions, neoplastic lesions, and infectious lesions. The ventral approach is particularly useful for the treatment of cervical spondylotic myelopathy caused by ventral compression of the spinal cord. Single- or multiple-level cervical corpectomy can be used to decompress the spinal cord and nerve roots. After a corpectomy, an appropriate bone graft (autogenous or allograft) can be placed in the defect to restore structural integrity and to maintain the cervical lordosis. A review of the literature shows that the likelihood of complications after ventral cervical surgery varies with the number of levels fused, the type of bone graft, and whether the ventral grafting is supplemented with instrumentation.* Although the reported results of single-level corpectomies with strut graft are uniformly good, the rates of pseudarthrosis formation

---

*References 1-3,6,8,9,12-15,18-21.

and graft migration are higher in multilevel corpectomy cases.[8,19-21]

After multilevel corpectomy, the addition of instrumentation to the construct has offered significant advantages.[4,7,10,11] In most series reporting on treatment without instrumentation, there is a higher incidence of graft-related problems, including pseudarthrosis, graft resorption, and graft migration.[6,9,19-21] All of these complications can lead to serious neurologic and biomechanical problems (Figure 158.6). These problems may necessitate the use of additional methods for stabilization and immobilization of the cervical spine.

External orthotic support is commonly used after cervical corpectomy procedures, including both those in which ventral plating is included and those done without instrumentation. Devices used for external immobilization include the cervical collar (multiple types), the Minerva vest, and the halo device. The halo device causes pin site scarring and discomfort. The device is also bulky and pro-

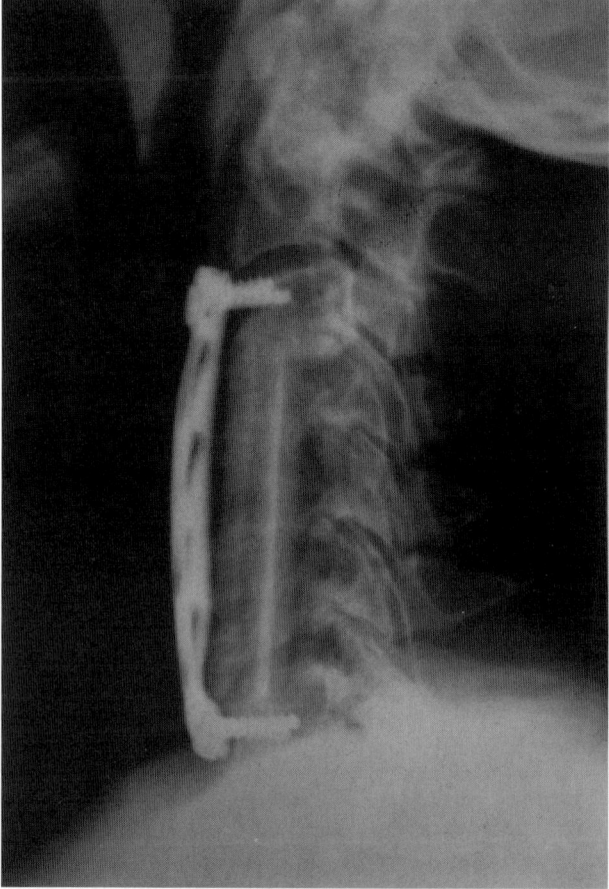

**Figure 158.6** Lateral radiograph of a 67-year-old male after three-level corpectomy, fusion with a fibular strut allograft, and ventral cervical plating. In an earlier procedure a narrow corpectomy was performed and an autograft strut was trimmed to fit the corpectomy site. This resulted in an inadequate decompression and spinal cord injury to the patient. A revision procedure with wide decompression was undertaken by a different surgeon. After the decompression the autograft strut did not fit well and was structurally inadequate. The allograft strut was therefore used.

vides only a moderate degree of immobilization. Neural injury can occur despite the halo.

Numerous studies have shown the biomechanical advantages of ventral cervical plate fixation.[5,16,18] Therefore in a case of multilevel corpectomy, to prevent postoperative graft-related problems, instrumentation should be added to the construct. The advantages of adding the internal fixation in cases of multilevel corpectomy include biomechanical improvements, improved immediate stability, improved fusion rates with acceleration of the fusion process, prevention of graft migration, and in some instances obviation of the need for external fixation.

## Biomechanical Aspects

A corpectomy effectively diminishes the structural support of the ventral and middle columns of the spine. A ventral cervical fusion without internal fixation may result in tenuous bone graft stability. A bone graft alone, used in the cervical spine, will be subjected to rotational and translational forces in three dimensions. When multiple levels are fused, the strut graft creates a lengthy moment arm that is manipulated during spinal movements.[6] This results in motion across the graft-vertebral body junction, which is a hindrance to successful fusion. Ventral cervical instrumentation helps to restrict motion at those junctions[4,10,11,17] and therefore, theoretically, promotes fusion.

When bony cortex dorsal to the plate is held in contact under load, the plate becomes part of the load-bearing, cross-sectional area.[18] Therefore after plating, the operated segment will more effectively approximate the elastic modulus (Young's modulus) of the plate, which is more than the elastic modulus of the graft alone.

Dryer et al.[5] compared the effect of the strut graft alone, strut graft plus plate, and plate alone in an experimental C5 corpectomy model of the human cadaver. They reported that the most rigid construct was the plate construct with tricortical iliac crest strut graft. The least rigid construct was the ventral strut graft alone. This study also showed that the plate alone can provide more rigid fixation than graft alone after C5 corpectomy. They concluded that the ventral plate and bone graft construct acts as reverse tension band, putting the posterior elements under tension.[5] The biomechanical effectiveness of plating after three-level corpectomy has also been shown by DiAngelo et al.,[4] Foley et al.,[7] and Kirkpatrick et al.[11] According to Kirkpatrick et al.,[11] the application of plates to the cervical spine as an adjunct to bone graft may improve the surgeon's ability to stabilize the spine after multilevel corpectomy.

## Immediate Stability

An optimal environment for fracture healing necessitates anatomic alignment, absolute immobilization, bone-to-bone contact, and compression of fracture segments. By means of a rigid internal fixation, immediate stability is improved without external bracing.[18]

## Improvement of the Rate of Fusion

The incidence of successful incorporation of a strut graft depends on the type of graft used. An iliac strut graft has a higher union rate than a fibular strut graft. The reported rates of union after single-level corpectomy are similar in cases fused with allograft or autologous graft. However, the rate of nonunion has been reported to range from 0% to 70% after multilevel corpectomy without plating. Nonunion rates tend to be especially high in cases undergoing fusion with allograft.* Yonenobu et al.,[20] using autograft, reported nonunion rates of 5% and 45% after one-level and three-level corpectomies, respectively. Fernyhough et al.[6] reported a total autograft nonunion rate of 27%, and a total allograft nonunion rate of 41% for ventral cervical fusion in cases with cervical spondylosis. In Fernyhough's series the rate of nonunion was 25% and 18% after two-motion segment fusion, 22% and 43% after three-motion segment fusion, and as high as 41% and 70% after four-motion segment fusion using autograft and allograft, respectively. Using allograft, Zdeblick and Ducker[21] reported 5% and 63% percent nonunion after one- and two-level fusion, respectively. The rate of successful fusion in most published series of patients fused with graft plus plate, however, is greater than 90%.[1-3,12-15,18,19]

Further support for the use of ventral cervical plating was reported by Lowery et al.[13] In a series of 86 patients, Lowery reported 92% and 90% rates of fusion after autograft and allograft, respectively. They concluded that plating made allograft fusion rates comparable with those of autograft.[13]

Connolly et al.[3] compared their results in ventral cervical fusions with and without ventral cervical plating. They reported that the overall graft complication rate (pseudarthrosis, delayed union, and graft collapse) was decreased with anterior cervical plate fixation. The rate of nonunion was significantly less in plated cases versus nonplated cases in the study of Yablon et al.[19] as well. They reported nonunion in nine of 60 cases undergoing fusion alone, whereas nonunion was seen in two of 111 cases undergoing fusion plus plating. Furthermore, they reported complete relief of symptoms in 39% of the nonfixation group and in 63% of the fixation group.[19]

## Acceleration of the Fusion Process

The rate of delayed union is higher in cases undergoing fusion alone. The use of plating can decrease the time of fusion. Caspar[2] reported that fusion occurred, on average, in half or less of the time in instrumented cases, compared with nonplated fixation. The rate of delayed fusion has been reported to be as high as 75% in cases undergoing fusion alone.[21]

## Prevention of Graft Migration and Collapse

The rate of graft collapse has been reported to be as high as 30%.[21] Connolly et al.[3] reported graft collapse in one of

18 cases operated without plating, and in none of 25 cases operated with plating. Yablon[19] reported graft collapse in eight of 60 cases operated without plating. Isaza et al.[9] reported 100% fusion and no graft collapse after fusion and plating. The other serious complication following grafting without plating is graft migration. Graft intrusion and extrusion can be observed despite external immobilization. Yablon et al.[19] reported graft migration in seven of 60 cases (five extrusion and two intrusion). They further reported 20% and 1% reoperation rates after grafting without and with plating, respectively.

## Obviation of External Bracing Need

Using internal fixation, additional immediate stability is provided. The use of a rigid cervical collar is usually adequate for postoperative immobilization. External fixation with a halo device, however, is usually required after multilevel corpectomy performed without plating.

## Summary

Spine stabilization with hardware is biomechanically advantageous and relatively safe. The spinal surgery literature supports the view that instrumentation is helpful to restore the stability destroyed by corpectomy. Ventral cervical plating is biomechanically sound, accelerates fusion, and lessens the incidence of graft-related complications. It also appears to improve rates of successful fusion, thereby reducing the potential need for reoperation. This is a valuable addition to the armamentarium of the spinal surgeon.

## REFERENCES

1. Apfelbaum RI: Ventral and upper cervical spine fixation techniques. In Benzel EC (ed): *Spinal Instrumentation. Neurosurgical Topics*. Park Ridge, IL: American Association of Neurological Surgeons, 1994, pp 63-96.
2. Caspar W: Anterior stabilization with trapezoid osteosynthetic plate technique in cervical spine injuries. In Kehr P, Weidner A (eds): *Cervical Spine*. I. New York, Springer-Verlag, 1987, pp 198-202.
3. Connolly PJ, Esses SI, Kostuik JP: Anterior cervical fusion: Outcome analysis of patients fused with and without anterior cervical plates. *J Spinal Disord* 9:202-206, 1996.
4. DiAngelo DJ, Foley KT, Vossel KA, et al: Anterior cervical plating reverses load transfer through multilevel strut-grafts. *Spine* 25:783-795, 2000.
5. Dryer J, Nucci R, Gorup J, et al: Two-level cervical discectomy and fusion with anterior and posterior plating: A biomechanical study. Presented at 9th Annual Meeting of North American Spine Surgery, Minneapolis, Oct 19-22, 1994.
6. Fernyhough JC, White JI, LaRocca H: Fusion rates in multilevel spondylosis comparing allograft fibula with autograft fibula in 126 patients. *Spine* 15(Suppl 10): S561-564, 1991.

*References 3,6,8,12,17,19-21.

7. Foley KT, DiAngelo DJ, Rampersaud R, *et al*: The In Vitro effects of instrumentation on multilevel cervical strut-graft mechanics. *Spine* 24: 2366-2376, 1999.

8. Herkowitz HN: Internal fixation for degenerative cervical spine disorders. *Semin Spine Surg* 7(1):57-60, 1995.

9. Isaza J, Munn BG, Williams JI, Whitecloud TS: Instrumented anterior cervical fusion in the degenerative cervical spine. Presented at 12th annual meeting of Cervical Spine Research Society, European section, Nice, France, June 5-7, 1996.

10. Isomi T, Panjabi MM, Wang JL, *et al*: Stabilizing potential of anterior cervical plates in multilevel corpectomies. *Spine* 24:2219-2223, 1999.

11. Kirkpatrick JS, Levy JA, Carillo J, Moeini SR: Reconstruction after multilevel corpectomy in the cervical spine. A sagittal plane biomechanical study. *Spine* 24: 1186-1191, 1999.

12. Law MD, Bernhardt M, White AA: Cervical spondylotic myelopathy: A review of surgical indications and decision making. *Yale J Biol Med* 66:165-177, 1993.

13. Lowery GL, Reuter MW, Sutterlin CE: Anterior cervical interbody arthrodesis with plate stabilization for degenerative disc disease. Presented at 20th annual meeting for Cervical Spine Research Society, Palm Desert, CA, 1992.

14. O'Shea JF, Sundaresan N: Use of instrumentation in degenerative disease of the cervical spine. *Mount Sinai J Med* 61:248-256, 1994.

15. Seifert V, Stolke D: Multisegmental cervical spondylosis: treatment by spondylectomy, microsurgical decompression, and osteosynthesis. *Neurosurgery* 29: 498-503, 1991.

16. Smith SA, Lindsey RW, Doherty BJ, *et al*: An in-vitro biomechanical comparison of the orosco and AO locking plates for anterior cervical spine fixation. *J Spinal Disord* 8:220-223, 1995.

17. Smith G, Goldwhite N, White A, *et al*: Complications of anterior cervical fusion. Presented at 9th Annual Meeting of North American Spine Surgery, Minneapolis, Oct 19-22, 1994.

18. Tippets RH, Apfelbaum RI: Anterior cervical fusion with the Caspar instrumentation system. *Neurosurgery* 22: 1008-1013, 1988.

19. Yablon IG, Spatz E, Ordia J, *et al*: Cervical spine fusion with and without internal fixation. Presented at 23rd Annual Meeting of Cervical Spine Research Society, Santa Fe, NM, Nov 30-Dec 2, 1995.

20. Yonenobu K, Fuji T, Ono K, *et al*: Choice of surgical treatment for multisegmental cervical spondylotic myelopathy. *Spine* 10:710-716, 1985.

21. Zdeblick TA, Ducker TB: The use of freeze-dried allograft bone for anterior cervical fusions. Spine 16:726-729, 1991.

# CHAPTER 159

# Cervical Spondylosis with Minimal Myelopathy: To Decompress or Not to Decompress

## To Decompress

**Christopher G. Paramore
and Volker K.H. Sonntag**

Decompression of the spinal cord for cervical spondylotic myelopathy (CSM) is a widely accepted treatment. However, no prospectively randomized, blinded study supports this procedure in either the neurosurgical or neurologic literature. The reason is not difficult to fathom. First, the opinion that a documented compressive lesion of the spinal cord in a patient with myelopathic signs is best addressed by surgical decompression is almost universal. This position seems logical and is supported by anecdotal experience and many retrospective clinical studies.[2,4] However, anecdotal experience is not a scientific basis for decision making, and the literature favoring cervical decompression over conservative management is plagued by nonuniform testing methods, small patient populations, and retrospective designs.

Second, and just as frustrating, is the great difficulty in organizing a randomized, prospective trial. Such a trial would no doubt require many institutions to alter their patient management strategies in the name of standardization. In the almost 7 years that have elapsed since the first edition of this book was written, only one study comparing surgical and nonsurgical management has been performed.[5] The results of this study showed no benefit in outcome for the group treated with surgery and, in fact, suggested that conservative treatment might have better outcomes. Although this trial was prospective and randomized, it is unclear that the symptoms and disability purportedly measured were actually caused by CSM and not another problem (i.e., osteoarthritis). No details of the patients' physical examinations were given. Until a better trial is performed, decisions regarding optimal treatment strategies must be made on an individual basis. These decisions depend on the skill, training, and experience of the physician. The authors' experience has led to the belief that decompression is a viable option in patients with mild myelopathy from cervical spondylosis.

## Definition of Minimal Myelopathy

Some comment on what constitutes "minimal myelopathy" is appropriate. Cervical spondylosis presumably causes a combination of upper and lower motor neuron symptoms and signs. These manifestations give rise to a recognizable clinical syndrome, cervical spondylotic myelopathy, characterized in maturity by long tract signs in the lower extremities and by weakness and wasting in the upper extremities, particularly in the intrinsic muscles of the hand. Sensory changes usually accompany these findings and assist in excluding motor neuron disease from the differential diagnosis. Typically, symptoms that arise early in the course of this disease are related either to problems of gait or to "numb, clumsy" hands.[11] Pain is an inconsistent symptom in patients with cervical myelopathy and may be a dominant symptom in patients with few neurologic complaints. Therefore an appropriate working definition of *minimal myelopathy* is "a condition in which the symptomatology outweighs the signs obtainable on physical examination, but in which the clinical pattern is clearly consistent with myelopathy." A patient so afflicted might be expected to present with complaints of decreased sensation in the hands, loss of ability to perform rigorous physical activities, or diminished dexterity. Complaints of pain may or may not be present. On examination the patient might have normal strength, and simultaneously exhibit increased muscle tone, hyperreflexia, clumsiness, difficulty with tandem gait and, perhaps, L'hermitte's sign. What then are the criteria for surgery for such a patient?

## Natural History of Cervical Spondylotic Myelopathy

The natural history of CSM is unknown. As noted by Rowland,[7] no modern study has followed patients with this disease for any significant period. Because one of the major reasons for performing surgery is to prevent the progression of the disease, it would be comforting to know that the assumption that the disease inexorably progresses is valid. This contention, however, has not been proved in a randomized, blinded fashion, although several retrospective series support the notion. Decompression in the presence of spinal cord atrophy is likely to be associated with poor results.[1] Other data suggest that the recovery rate after surgical decompression for cervical spondylotic myelopathy is inversely related to the cross-sectional area of the spinal cord at the time of clinical presentation.[6] Since the advent of magnetic resonance imaging (MRI) scans, it has been appreciated that signal changes within the spinal cord indicate a more advanced stage of CSM.[9] Obviously, to fit the definition of *minimal myelopathy*, a patient would not be expected to exhibit signal change within the cord. However, because some authors have suggested that T2 signal change worsens the prognosis of recovery after decompression,[12] it would be logical to suggest that decompression of CSM before the development of T2 signal change would be advantageous to the patient. Although it is a leap of faith to conclude that all patients with cervical spondylosis will deteriorate if left untreated, the specter of missing the "window of opportunity" to help a patient is a driving force regarding the decision to operate on the mildly symptomatic patient.

## Efficacy of Surgical Decompression

Despite its weaknesses, the existing literature touting cervical decompression for spondylotic myelopathy indicates that 60% to 80% of patients improve to some degree after surgery. The remaining patients either stabilize or worsen, the exact percentage of which depends on the individual series.[2,4,9] What is clear is that many of the "failures" reported in the literature result from either incomplete decompression of the spinal cord at surgery[3,8] or an improper surgical approach. This is particularly true of the older literature, in which laminectomy was used almost exclusively, even in the presence of ventral compression or kyphotic deformity. Although there remains an enigmatic population of myelopathic patients with documented spinal cord compression who do not respond to technically adequate surgery, their relative percentage is decreasing as both radiographic and surgical techniques become more refined. Despite the acknowledged need for a randomized, controlled study of operative versus nonoperative treatment of CSM, the more frequently asked question seems not to be "Is cervical decompression efficacious?" but "Why does cervical decompression fail?" This line of reasoning, coupled with evidence that (1) better results are achieved if decompression is performed early in the course of the disease, and (2) the fear that a trivial traumatic event may lead to catastrophic neurologic consequences, has led many to recommend aggressive treatment for the mildly myelopathic patient with documented spinal cord compression.[10] However, care and clinical judgment must be exercised if the patient's primary complaint is not neurologic dysfunction, but rather pain, because there is no guarantee that decompression of the spinal cord or fusion of the spine will result in relief of pain symptoms.

## Establishing the Diagnosis of Cervical Spondylotic Myelopathy

If the decision is made to operate early on these patients, a major caveat should be considered. The diagnosis of cervical myelopathy as the cause of the patient's symptoms must be verified. Given the prevalence of spondylotic changes in the cervical spines of the population at large, many, if not most of whom are asymptomatic, the surgeon must rule out other causes of myelopathy. These include amyotrophic lateral sclerosis, multiple sclerosis, and other spinal or intracranial lesions. Because the symptoms and signs detected are, by definition, "early," the likelihood of making an erroneous diagnosis is amplified. Nonetheless, the radiologic and bioelectrical armamentarium now available should provide adequate resources in establishing the correct diagnoses.

## Summary

The treatment of the patient with cervical spondylosis and minimal myelopathy remains controversial. In all likelihood, a subpopulation of these patients is best managed conservatively. However, our current level of knowledge does not allow us to identify the members of this group. Our best estimate is that most patients with CSM will progress, and that better surgical results are obtained in patients with less compromise of the spinal canal and shorter duration of symptomatology. Thus the authors of this book recommend early surgery for the mildly myelopathic patient. It is not clear at present if academic, market, and governmental forces will encourage or compel physicians and surgeons to resolve this issue in a scientific manner.

## REFERENCES

1. Batzdorf U, Flannigan BD: Surgical decompressive procedures for cervical spondylotic myelopathy. A study using magnetic resonance imaging. *Spine* 16:123, 1991.
2. Chiles B III, Leonard M, Choudhri H, *et al*: Cervical spondylotic myelopathy: patterns of neurological deficit and recovery after anterior cervical decompression. *Neurosurgery* 44(4):762-770, 1999.
3. Fessler R, Steck J, Giovanini M: Anterior cervical corpectomy for cervical spondylotic myelopathy. *Neurosurgery* 43(2):257-265, 1998.
4. Goto S, Mochizuki M, Watanabe T, *et al*: Long-term follow-up study of anterior surgery for cervical spondylotic myelopathy with special reference to the magnetic resonance imaging findings in 52 cases. *Clin Orthop* 291:142, 1993.
5. Kadanka Z, Bednarik J, Vohanka S, *et al*: Conservative treatment versus surgery in spondylotic cervical myelopathy: a prospective randomised study. *Eur Spine J* 9:538-544, 2000.
6. Koyanagi T, Hirabayashi K, Satomi K, *et al*: Predictability of operative results of cervical compression myelopathy based on preoperative computed tomographic myelography. *Spine* 18:1958, 1993.
7. Rowland LP: Surgical treatment of cervical spondylotic myelopathy: time for a controlled trial. *Neurology* 42:5, 1992.
8. Shinomiya K, Okamoto A, Kamikozuru M, *et al*: An analysis of failures in primary cervical anterior spinal cord decompression and fusion. *J Spinal Disord* 6:277, 1993.
9. Singh A, Crockard HA, Platts A, *et al*: Clinical and radiological correlates of severity and surgery related outcome in cervical spondylosis. *J Neurosurg* (Spine 2)94:189-198, 2001.
10. Snow RB, Weiner H: Cervical laminectomy and foraminotomy as surgical treatment of cervical spondylosis: a follow-up study with analysis of failures. *J Spinal Disord* 6:245, 1993.
11. Voskuhl RR, Hinton RC: Sensory impairment in the hands secondary to spondylotic compression of the cervical spinal cord. *Arch Neurol* 47:309, 1990.
12. Wada E, Yonenobu K, Suzuki S, *et al*: Can intramedullary signal change on magnetic resonance imaging predict surgical outcome in cervical spondylotic myelopathy? *Spine* 24(5)455-462, 1999.

# Not to Decompress

## Edward C. Benzel

## The Definition of Cervical Spondylosis and its Clinical Course

Cervical spondylosis is a relatively straightforward disease process involving: (1) the degeneration of the disk interspace, with dorsal annular bulging, followed by osteophyte formation; (2) degeneration of the facet joints with hypertrophy, resulting in a dorsolateral impingement on the dural sac; (3) soft-tissue and ligamentous hypertrophy, resulting in a dorsal impingement on the dural sac; and finally, (4) spinal deformity (most commonly kyphosis). Cervical spondylosis is an anatomic and pathophysiologic process. It, in and of itself, does not define or mandate the concurrence of neurologic symptoms. When long tract neurologic symptoms accompany the well-described anatomic and pathologic changes, as previously outlined, the process is termed cervical spondylotic myelopathy (CSM). This clinical entity has only recently been relatively well delineated.[1]

CSM is, nevertheless, still relatively poorly defined clinically, in that the diagnosis is often nebulous. Furthermore, it is often confused with other diagnoses (e.g., amyotrophic lateral sclerosis, multiple sclerosis). This is particularly true in its early phases.

The clinical course, as observed by Rowland,[1] is clearly one of a waxing and waning nature. Patients may exhibit neurologic deterioration and then enjoy neurologic improvement, without obvious reason. Furthermore, CSM may be stagnant for years. This may result either in a "missed diagnosis" (resulting from "diagnostic haste") or in a diminished indication for surgical intervention (secondary to the stable or minimal extent of the patient's symptomatology). One should not recommend a surgical procedure to a patient in whom minimal, if any, disability is present, and in whom progression of the disability is unlikely.

## Surgery for Cervical Spondylotic Myelopathy

Surgery for CSM is clearly not a benign intervention. The options include dorsal surgical approaches (with their attendant stability risks) and a ventral surgical approach (with its associated complications that often accompany spinal instrumentation and fusion, particularly in osteoporotic patients). Furthermore, nonneurologic or structural spine-related morbidity may not be insignificant, particularly in the elderly subset of patients.

The natural history of CSM, as previously mentioned, is poorly characterized. Although the symptomatology may vary from time to time in many patients, little is known about the true progression of the disease process itself. Many patients stabilize, thus demonstrating no neurologic decline over a significant time frame. Although the spondylotic process usually advances with time, it also stiffens the spine. This stiffening of the spine, in turn, usually slows the progression of degenerative changes. Furthermore, because surgery is potentially dangerous, intervention at an early stage (in a group of patients who may not progress neurologically) may be unwise.

There is no evidence that eliminating neurologic compression early in the course of the disease alters the ultimate outcome (compared to those who may have an operation during a later stage of the disease). Therefore it would seem logical that the clinical decision-making process, specifically regarding surgical intervention, should be tempered by time. If a patient progresses neurologically and indeed becomes symptomatic, the risks of surgery are potentially outweighed by the benefits of surgical intervention. Surgery in this case should obviously be entertained. If the patient does not progress neurologically, surgery has been successfully avoided, as has its attendant potential for morbidity and mortality. One can always *do* surgery. However, one cannot *undo* surgery.

## REFERENCE

1. Rowland LP: Surgical treatment of cervical spondylotic myelopathy: time for a controlled trial. *Neurology* 42:5, 1992.

# CHAPTER 160

# Bilateral Locked Cervical Facets with Incomplete Myelopathy: Open Versus Closed Reduction

## Open Reduction

**Sanford J. Larson**

Several factors deserve consideration regarding the management of a patient with bilateral locked facets at level C6-7, with some preservation of neurologic function below the level of injury. This is a flexion distraction injury in which complete circumferential disruption is usually present. Consequently, overdistraction via skeletal traction can occur. The patient whose films are shown in Figure 160.1 had abrupt and permanent increase in neurologic deficit during the course of closed reduction by skeletal traction. Displacement of intervertebral disk into the spinal canal can occur during either open or closed reduction and may produce an increase in neurologic deficit. This can be prevented by resection of the disk before reduction. Because the injury is ligamentous, satisfactory healing may not occur.[1] Dorsal fusion provides prompt stabilization and offers the best opportunity for solid healing. If an open surgical fusion is to be performed, there is little advantage provided by preoperative closed reduction.

Early reduction versus delayed reduction remains controversial. However, advocacy of early reduction is based on intuition rather than observation. Spinal cord dysfunction is produced by energy transfer at the moment of impact, and by persistent deformity of the spinal cord. Nothing can be done about the damage produced by energy transfer, and deformity of the spinal cord should not increase in a properly immobilized patient.

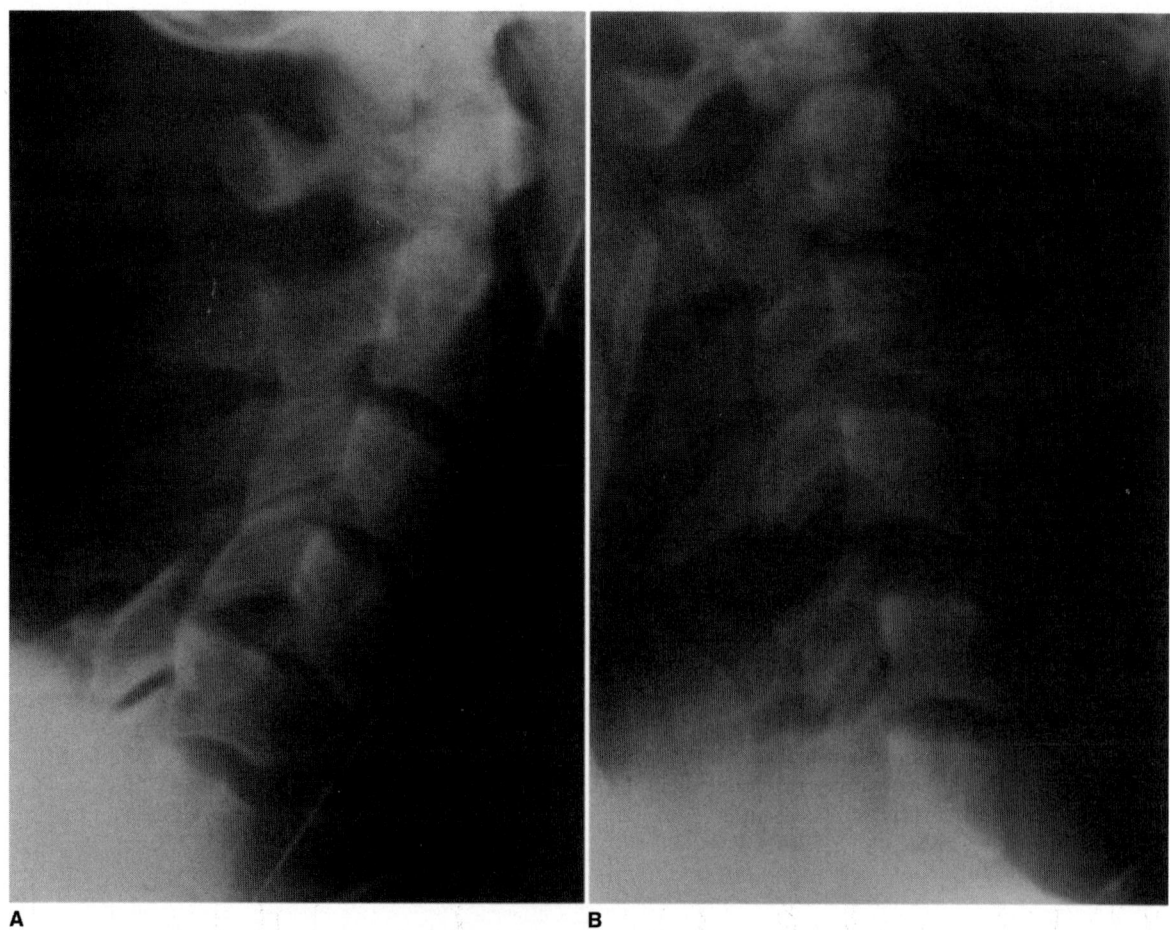

A     B

**Figure 160.1** (A) Film taken before application of skeletal traction. The patient was quadriplegic, but was ventilating without assistance. (B) Film taken during closed reduction with skeletal traction, after the patient became abruptly and permanently ventilator dependent.

Magnetic resonance imaging (MRI) for patients with bilateral locked facet is of little value before reduction. Although a postreduction scan may show displacement of disk into the spinal canal, further damage to the spinal cord may have already occurred. In the patient with residual spinal cord function a ventral approach for discectomy should be performed. This should be immediately followed by a dorsal approach for open reduction and fusion. To obtain reduction without distraction, the tips of the C7 superior articular process can be removed. Autologous iliac crest graft wired to the spinous processes and laminae gives excellent resistance to flexion and distraction. If neurologic function does not improve, MRI can be done to make sure that the spinal cord is no longer deformed.

The advantages of surgical treatment are reduction without distraction, prevention of disk prolapse, prompt and secure stabilization, and more certain healing.

## REFERENCE

1. O'Brien PJ, Schweigel JF, Thompson WJ: Dislocations of the lower cervical spine. *J Trauma* 22:710-714, 1982.

# Closed Reduction

## Patrick W. Hitchon

The patient with cervical trauma that results in C6-7 dislocation, with locked facets and an incomplete motor and sensory neurologic deficit, is presented in Figure 160.2. By virtue of its ventral subluxation, angular deformity, bilateral facet dislocation, and neurologic deficit, such a spinal injury is considered unstable.[1,3,14] These fractures of the lower cervical spine have been analyzed extensively, both clinically and in the laboratory, using cadaveric spines. The mechanism of injury is considered to be flexion distraction with resultant partial or total disruption of the interspinous ligament, bilateral capsular ligaments, posterior longitudinal ligament, and the annulus and disk.[1,3,7,11,12] Biomechanical studies were conducted on human cadaveric spines by Bauze and Ardran, and Beatson.[2,3] These studies further confirmed that for a facet dislocation to occur, the above ligaments must be injured or severed. Owing to this mechanism with primarily ligamentous injury and minor bony fractures, if any, the treatment of facet dislocations has been controversial. Whereas some experts have favored nonoperative treatment,[4,8-10,13] others have chosen operative intervention without necessarily expending time and effort into preoperative reduction.[1,5-7,12]

The argument in favor of surgery has been that ligamentous injury often heals poorly in spite of reduction and prolonged immobilization. Indeed the failure rate of immobilization in traction and halo has varied from 6%, according to some, to as high as 40% in the experience of others.[4,6,9,10,12] These results have swayed some to prefer early operative intervention to expedite rehabilitation. This enthusiasm for surgery must be tempered by the morbidity and mortality of surgical intervention, which has been estimated at greater than 10%.[11] In addition to the morbidity of operative intervention, one should also consider the failure rate of open reduction and fixation, the exorbitant cost of the implants, and the fact that some of these patients are still immobilized in a halo postoperatively.

The patient in Figure 160.2 presented with a radiculopathy and incomplete spinal cord injury secondary to a fracture dislocation at C6-7 with perched facets. Before the application of traction, an MRI is obtained to assess the spinal cord, and to rule out the presence of surgical pathology, such as a herniated disk or epidural hematoma. Generally, as in the case illustrated, the posttraumatic neurologic deficit arises from spinal cord injury and compression rather than disk herniation or a blood clot. The patient was treated with skeletal traction (70lb). The dislocation was reduced, and the patient showed some, but not total, neurologic recovery. Traction with fracture reduction and relief of spinal cord compression, followed by halo immobilization, can constitute the sole treatment necessary. Traction can be the only treatment used in patients with associated multiple injuries, such as pulmonary and cardiac contusions, visceral lacerations, long bone fractures, and occasionally, head injury. These patients often require prolonged ventilatory support and traction and immobilization for their extremity fractures.

Once reduction is achieved and the patient's condition improves, gradual mobilization with sequential radiographs in a halo commences. A postreduction MRI is indicated to confirm the adequacy of the decompression achieved by traction. This regimen of treatment is successful in at least 90% of cases.[9,10] In fact, the neurologic deficit of those treated nonoperatively has been similar to that of those treated with open reduction and internal fixation. Should the patient experience failure of the halo device, and redislocate or develop unacceptable angulation, surgical intervention may then be undertaken. Such failure is not inconsequential. As stated, it can vary from 6% to 10%, according to some,[4] and up to 40%, according to others.[6] Operative intervention with open reduction and internal fixation can then be undertaken.[1,5-7,12] Traction is time proven and controlled, with the patient generally awake and interactive. When traction fails to reduce a dislocation, or the patient redislocates in a halo, surgery can be undertaken at that time.

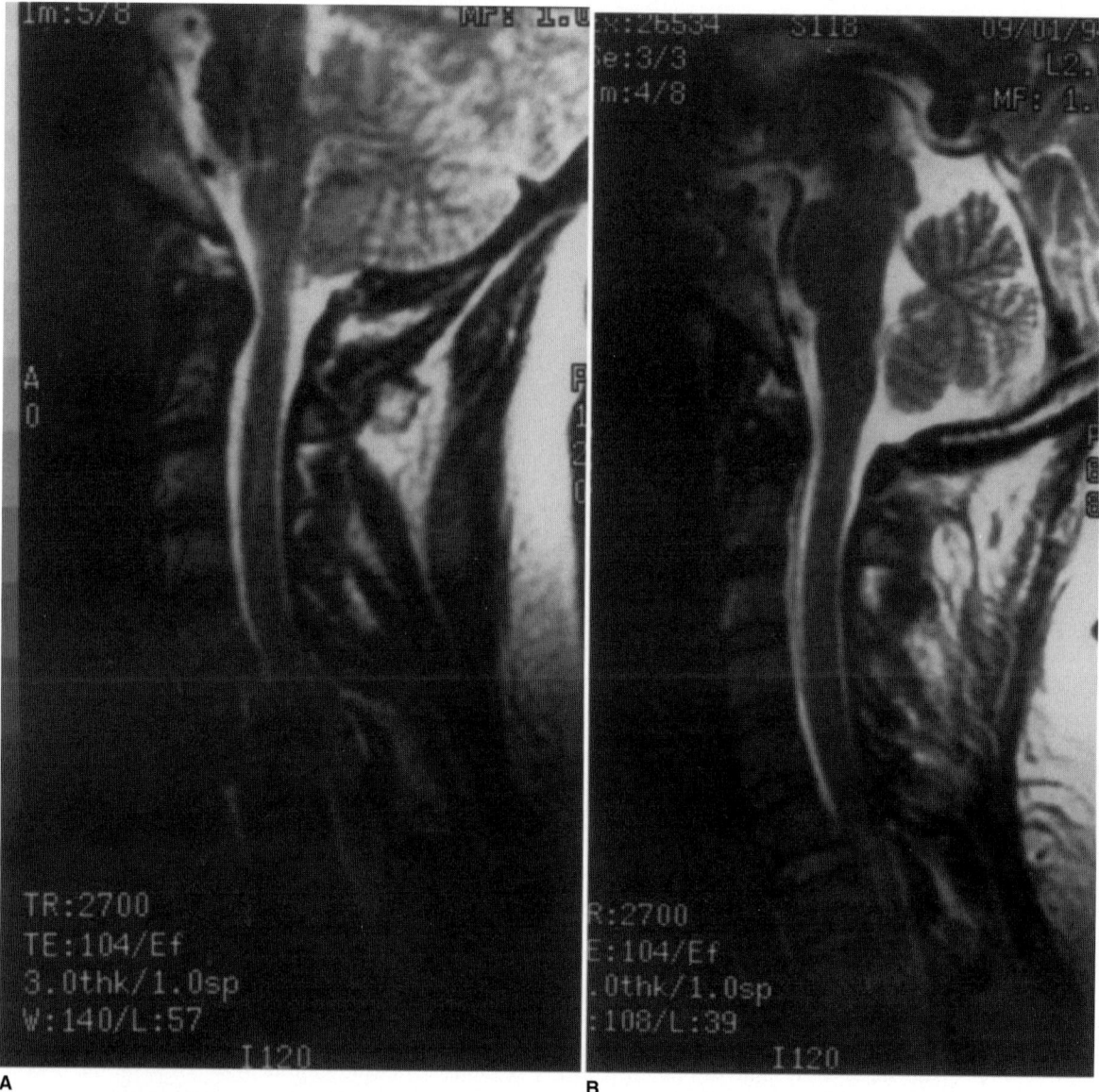

**Figure 160.2** Fracture dislocation at C6-7 in a 31-year-old woman involved in a motor vehicle accident. She presented with an incomplete C7 radiculopathy and long track signs (**A**). She was placed in traction by means of a halo; after traction with up to 70lb, reduction and correction of her alignment was achieved (**B**).

# REFERENCES

1. Allen BL, Ferguson RL, Lehmann TR, O'Brien RP: A mechanistic classification of closed, indirect fractures and dislocations of the lower cervical spine. *Spine* 7:1-27, 1982.
2. Bauze RJ, Ardran GM: Experimental production of forward dislocation in the human cervical spine. *J Bone Joint Surg* 60B:239-245, 1978.
3. Beatson TR: Fractures and dislocations of the cervical spine. *J Bone Joint Surg* 45B:21-35, 1963.
4. Bedbrook GM: Spinal injuries with tetraplegia and paraplegia. *J Bone Joint Surg* 61B:267-284, 1979.
5. Bohlman HH: Acute fractures and dislocations of the cervical spine: an analysis of three hundred hospitalized patients and review of the literature. *J Bone Joint Surg* 61A:1119-1142, 1979.
6. Bucholz RD, Cheung KC: Halo vest versus spinal fusion for cervical injury: evidence from an outcome study. *J Neurosurg* 70:884-892, 1989.
7. Cooper PR: Stabilization of fractures and subluxation of the lower cervical spine. In Cooper PR (ed): *Management of Posttraumatic Spinal Instability, Neurosurgical Topics*. Park Ridge, IL, AANS Publications Committee, 1990, pp 111-133.
8. Donovan WH, Kopaniky D, Stolzmann E, Carter RE: The neurological and skeletal outcome in patients with closed cervical spinal cord injury. *J Neurosurg* 66:690-694, 1987.

9. Dorr LD, Harvey JP Jr, Nickel VL: Clinical review of the early stability of spine injuries. *Spine* 7:545-550, 1982.

10. Lind B, Sihlbom H, Nordwall A: Halo-vest treatment of unstable traumatic cervical spine injuries. *Spine* 13:425-432, 1988.

11. Maiman DJ, Barolat G, Larson SJ: Management of bilateral locked facets of the cervical spine. *Neurosurgery* 18:542-547, 1986.

12. O'Brien PJ, Schweigel JF, Thompson WJ: Dislocations of the lower cervical spine. *J Trauma* 22:710-714, 1982.

13. Tator CH, Duncan EG, Edmonds VE, *et al*: Comparison of surgical and conservative management in 208 patients with acute spinal cord injury. *Can J Neurol Sci* 14:60-69, 1987.

14. White AA, Panjabi MM: The problem of clinical instability in the human spine: a systematic approach. In White AA, Panjabi MM (eds): *Clinical Biomechanics of the Spine*, ed 2. Philadelphia, Lippincott-Raven, 1990.

# CHAPTER 161

# Cervical Spine Fusion: Allograft Versus Autograft

## Argument for Allograft

**Bernardo Jose Ordonez**

Ventral approaches to the cervical spine were first introduced in the 1950s by Robinson and Smith,[20] Cloward,[4] and Bailey and Bagley.[2] Early surgical techniques used autologous bone grafts. The longevity of these procedures is a testament to their efficacy. However, the use of autologous bone graft is unavoidably coupled with donor site morbidity. In an attempt to eliminate donor site morbidity, the use of allograft was proposed as early as the late 1950s. Since that time, allograft has been used in spinal fusions and has met with varying degrees of success. Allograft provides a comparable means by which to obtain spinal fusion while eliminating donor site morbidity.

Review of the literature reveals that for single-level interbody cervical fusions, allograft provides similar fusion rates and clinical outcomes to that obtained by using autograft.* Multi-level interbody fusions are associated with increased nonunion rates and graft complication with both autograft and allograft.[1,3,7,23] Nonunion rates and graft complications have been shown to increase with the number of motion segments fused with both autograft and allograft.[1,3,7,23]

Various modifications in surgical technique and the use of rigid external fixation, dorsal cervical instrumentation—and most recently, ventral cervical instrumentation—have been used in an attempt to improve fusion rates for multilevel interbody cervical fusions. The use of ventral cervical instrumentation as an adjunct to multilevel interbody cervical fusions has been shown to increase fusion rates, improve clinical outcomes and reduce graft complication.[5,8,13,19] For multi-level interbody cervical fusions, the combination of allograft supplemented with ventral cervical instrumentation has been shown to provide similar fusion rates and clinical outcomes to that obtained with autograft and ventral cervical instrumentation.[5,6,8,19]

Single- or multi-level corpectomies are used for the treatment of degenerative, congenital, traumatic, infectious, and neoplastic disorders of the cervical spine. Stabilization of decompressed segments presents spine surgeons with a formidable challenge. Numerous surgical techniques with various types of grafts have been proposed and used with varying degrees of success. As with multi-level interbody cervical fusions, single- or multi-level corpectomies have an increasing rate of nonunion and graft complications with increasing number of motion segments fused for both autograft and allograft.[3,7] The literature is inconclusive regarding the ideal graft for single- or multi-level corpectomies. Some authors find autograft to be significantly superior to allograft, with increased fusion rates and decreased graft complications.[3,7,22] While other authors find no difference between allograft and autograft, they observed an increased time to incorporation of the graft.[9,11,14]

In an attempt to improve fusion rates in single or multi-level corpectomies, modifications in surgical techniques and the use of rigid external fixation, dorsal cervical instrumentation, and most recently ventral cervical instrumentation have been used. The addition of ventral cervical instrumentation provides immediate cervical spine stability, improves fusion rates, and limits graft complications.*

Various authors have found no difference in fusion rates, clinical outcome, and graft complications when comparing allograft and autograft supplemented with ventral cervical instrumentation for single- and multi-level corpectomies.[6,12,15] Most recently, an article by Mahr *et al.*[15] revealed radiographic stability in 99.2% of patients who underwent cervical corpectomies with fibular allograft reconstruction and ventral cervical instrumentation.

Allograft eliminates harvest site morbidity. Donor site morbidity has been reported to vary from 9% to 29%.† Harvest site complications include wound hematomas, osteomyelitis, wound infections, lateral femoral cutaneous nerve neuropraxia, fractures of the anterior superior iliac spine, and bowel perforations.[9,16,18] In a study by Depalma, 36% of patients had persistent donor site pain at 1 year after graft harvest. Rawlinson reported that in 45% of the patients in his study, "donor site pain had delayed their mobilization."[16] Thirty-one percent of patients in his study felt that they could have gone home sooner if not for donor site pain.[16] Other advantages of allograft include decreased operative time and blood loss.[5,9,14,15,19]

Allograft carries the potential for transmission of infectious diseases. The risk of acquiring HIV infection from allograft has been estimated to be between 1 in 1 million and one in 1.6 million.[9,19] Strict regulations regarding the testing, harvesting, treatment, handling, and storage of allograft should serve to minimize the risk of acquiring infectious disease via the implantation of allograft.

Last, the cost of bone graft harvest has been shown to be similar to the cost of purchasing allograft and ventral cervical instrumentation.[10]

The use of allograft with or without adjunctive internal ventral cervical instrumentation for fusion following cervical decompression provides an acceptable alternative to autologous bone graft. Allograft offers comparable fusion rates, similar clinical results, decreased operative time and blood loss, and eliminates donor site morbidity.

---

*References 1,3,9,17,18,21,23.

*References 5,6,8,12,13,19.
†References 1,5,7,9,14,18,19.

# REFERENCES

1. An HS, Simpson JM, Glover JM, Stephany J: Comparison between allograft plus demineralized bone matrix versus autograft in anterior cervical fusion. *Spine* 20:2211-2216, 1995.

2. Bailey R, Badgley C: Stabilization of the cervical spine by anterior fusion. *J Bone Joint Surg (Am)* 42:565-594, 1960.

3. Butterman GR, Glazer PA, Bradford DS: The use of bone allograft in the spine. *Clin Orthop Rel Res* 324:75-85, 1989.

4. Cloward R: The anterior approach for removal of ruptured cervical disks. *J Neurosurg* 15:602-617, 1958.

5. Coric D, Brunch CL Jr, Jenkins JD: Revision of anterior cervical pseudoarthrosis with anterior allograft fusion and plating. *J Neurosurg* 86:969-974, 1997.

6. Eleraky MA, Llanos C, Sonntag VK: Cervical corpectomy: report of 185 cases and review of the literature. *J Neurosurg* 90:35-41, 1999.

7. Fernyhough JC, White JI, LaRocca H: Fusion rates in multi-level spondylosis comparing allograft fibula with autograft fibula in 126 patients. *Spine* 16:726-729, 1991.

8. Geisler FH, Caspar W, Pitzen T, Johnson TA: Reoperation in patients after anterior cervical plate stabilization in degenerative disease. *Spine* 23(8):911-920, 1998.

9. Grossman W, Peppleman WC, Baun JA, Kraus DR: The use of freeze-dried fibular allograft in anterior cervical fusion. *Spine* 17:565-569, 1992.

10. Hadley MN: Banked fibula and anterior cervical locking plate [letter]. *J Neurosurg* 85:736-773, 1996.

11. Harsh GR 4th, Sypert GW, Weinstein PR, *et al*: Cervical spine stenosis secondary to ossification of the posterior longitudinal ligament. *J Neurosurg* 67:849-857, 1987.

12. Hermann JM, Sonntag VKH: Cervical corpectomy and plate fixation for postlaminectomy kyphosis. *J Neurosurg* 80:963-970, 1994.

13. Johnston FG, Crockard HA: One-stage internal fixation and anterior fusion in complex cervical spinal disorders. *J Neurosurg* 82:234-238, 1995.

14. MacDonald RL, Fehlings MF, Tater CH, *et al*: Multilevel anterior cervical corpectomy and ficular allograft fusion for cervical myelopathy. *J Neurosurg* 86:990-997, 1997.

15. Mayr MT, Subach B, Comey CH, Rodts GE, Haid RW Jr: Cervical spinal stenosis: outcome after anterior corpectomy, allograft reconstruction, and instrumentation. *J Neurosurg (Spine)* 96:10-16, 2002.

16. Rawlinson JN: Morbidity after anterior cervical decompression and fusion. The influence of the donor site in recovery and the result of a trial of surgical bone compared to autologous bone. *Acta Neurochir* 131:106-118, 1994.

17. Rish BL, McFadden JT, Penix JO: Anterior cervical fusion using homologous bone grafts: A comparative study. *Surg Neurol* 76:119-121, 1976.

18. Savolainen S, Vsenius JP, Hernesnicmi J: Iliac crest versus artifical bone graft in 250 cervical fusions. *Acta Neurochir* 131:54-57, 1994.

19. Shapiro S: Banked fibula and locking anterior cervical plate in anterior cervical fusions following cervical discectomy. *J Neurosurg* 84:161-165, 1996.

20. Smith G, Robinson R: The treatment of certain cervical-spine disorders by anterior removal of the intervertebral disc and interbody fusion. *J Bone Joint Surg (Am)* 40:607, 1957.

21. Young WF, Rosenwasser RH: An early comparative analysis of the use of fibular allograft versus autologous iliac crest graft for interbody fusion after anterior cervical discectomy. *Spine* 18(9): 1123-1124, 1993.

22. Zdeblick TA, Bohlman HH: Cervical kyphosis and myelopathy. Treatment by anterior corpectomy and strut-grafting. *J Bone Joint Surg Am* 71:170-182, 1989.

23. Zdeblick TA, Ducker TB: The use of freeze-dried allograft for anterior cervical fusion. *Spine* 16:726-729, 1991.

# Argument for Autograft

## Alexander R. Vaccaro, Jared P. Salinsky, and Bruce E. Northrup

Bone grafting is used frequently in spinal reconstruction to provide structural integrity as well as a stimulus for bony ingrowth.[12,24,29,30] Bone grafts may be classified in a variety of ways: (1) source (autograft, allograft, xenograft); (2) tissue composition (cortical, corticocancellous, cancellous); (3) anatomic origin (iliac crest, fibula, rib); (4) blood supply (nonvascularized, vascularized); and (5) preservation method (fresh, frozen, freeze-dried, irradiated).

The ideal bone graft has the strength of cortical bone and the healing properties of cancellous bone.[15] For successful healing, the graft ideally should possess osteogenic, osteoinductive, and osteoconductive properties.[17,22] *Osteogenesis* refers to the formation of new bone as derived from viable osteoprogenitor cells and osteoblasts. *Osteoinduction* refers to stimulation of osteogenic cells to produce bone through various messengers such as graft-derived growth factors (i.e., bone morphogenetic protein [BMP]). Osteoconduction refers to the physical properties of a graft as it relates to its affinity for vascular invasion and ingrowth of host bone. Osteoconductive materials may include collagen, coralline hydroxyapatite, ceramic, and tricalcium phosphate. Autologous bone graft contains both determined and inducible osteogenic precursor cells, noncollagenous bone matrix proteins including growth factors, and bone mineral and collagen.[13,15,28]

Structural autografts, such as a fibula or tricortical iliac crest bone graft, when used in an intervertebral body fusion, have the capacity to bear the mechanical compressive loads applied to the anterior column of the spine.[29] These grafts derive their strength from their cortical bone composition and may be fashioned as tricortical or bicortical struts or dowels. Autografts that are used in nonloaded or tension environments, such as the posterior and posterolateral spine, do not require cortical integrity. They can be fashioned as corticocancellous strips or morcelized fragments.[29] Autologous cancellous bone contains greater osteogenic potential than autologous cortical bone because of the large number of surviving cells within its marrow. It is physically favorable to vascular ingrowth and exposure to inductive proteins because of its large trabecular surface area and interconnected spaces.[28] Morcellization of autograft may in fact enhance osteogenesis by increasing its surface area and access to its osteoinductive and osteogenic factors.[29]

Regardless of the grafting source, the host plays a vital role in the ultimate success of a fusion. Nonsteroidal anti-inflammatory drugs, chemotherapeutic agents, tobacco, steroids, malnutrition, and systemic illness may negatively affect bone healing. Local infection, malignancy, osteopenia, and insufficient immobilization have also been implicated as negative influencing factors in bone fusion healing.[28]

Traditionally, in a patient who is in need of a three-level or greater corpectomy and fusion, the optimal grafting source is either an autologous fibular bone graft or a fibula allograft filled with local autologous or iliac crest bone graft. Autologous bone graft is often best taken from the ilium for one- or two-level cervical corpectomies or interbody fusions. The ilium provides the biomechanical strength of cortical bone as well as the osteoconductive properties of cancellous bone. The fibula is often the preferred source for more extensive bony deficits and therefore is considered the gold standard for comparison of bony healing when other sources are considered. An autologous fibular graft, besides sufficing for reconstruction of long bony deficits, also may be harvested with its vascular pedicle, unlike its allogeneic counterpart, to provide an immediate blood supply.

Vascularized cortico-cancellous autograft provides a useful grafting alternative in host fusion beds hostile to local bone ingrowth. This is frequently seen in cases of revision anterior fusion procedures, deformity in the setting of osteomyelitis, or in patients with metastatic disease who have undergone previous radiation. With a vascularized graft, ingrowth of vascular buds from the host bed with slow junctional ingrowth of host bone is no longer the primary mode of graft incorporation as with traditional nonvascularized autologous bone graft. In successfully anastomosed grafts, greater than 90% of osteocytes survive the transplantation procedure following a transient period of intraoperative ischemia. Vascularized grafts are remodeled in response to the same local mechanical stimuli (i.e., Wolff's law) as normal skeletal bone.[33,40]

The disadvantage of choosing an allogenic graft includes delayed vascular penetration, slower bone formation, fibrous tissue encapsulation, delayed or incomplete incorporation, and graft rejection.[15] Allografts are immunogenic and evoke, to various degrees, an immunologic response.[3] In addition, there is a remote potential for the spread of transmissible agents, such as the HIV virus.[6] Regardless of the source, an autograft provides unchallenged histocompatibility, the lack of transmissible agents and fresh viable tissue. In cases of significant thoracolumbar osteopenia, especially in the elderly, an autologous bone source, preferably the iliac crest, is an ideal graft source because of its similar modulus of elasticity. This is useful in reconstructive surgery following tumor excision or deformity procedures caused by osteoporosis to avoid graft telescoping or migration.

Much discussion is centered on the use of autograft versus allograft for anterior cervical reconstructive fusions. Many reports have found no significant difference between the two techniques for short segment or single-level fusions,

while other reports have found allograft to be less effective than autograft.[*] Fusions performed with autologous bone graft are consistently graded histologically superior to fusions utilizing allograft bone.[33-35] Allograft bone also has a higher reported incidence of delayed union as well as nonunion in multilevel fusion constructs.[†] In multilevel anterior cervical fusions, autograft bone has clearly been shown to be superior over allograft bone in terms of ultimate fusion success.[5,16,19,38-40] The nonunion rate for noninstrumented multilevel autogenous cervical fusions has been reported in the range of 27% to 35% as compared with a 65% to 70% nonunion rate for allograft bone.[2,16,31,38-40]

In conclusion, autologous bone graft is the preferred source of grafting material for multilevel cervical reconstructive procedures and in posterolateral fusions of the thoracolumbar spine. The literature clearly cites an improved fusion rate with autologous bone sources in virtually all spinal applications except single-level anterior cervical interbody fusion procedures. Autologous bone avoids the risk of host-versus-graft reactions or the spread of transmissible disease. When possible, an autologous bone source is the preferable form of grafting material. This should be carefully weighed against the morbidity of its harvesting procedure and the quantity necessary to complete the fusion procedure.

---

*References 5,11,16,19,21,27,37,39,40.
†References 7,8,15,16,27,31,38-40.

# REFERENCES

1. Bailey RW, Badgley CE: Stabilization of the cervical spine by anterior fusion. *J Bone Joint Surg* 42A:565-624, 1960.
2. Bohlman HH, Emery SE, Goodfellow DB, Jones PK: Robinson anterior cervical discectomy and arthrodesis for cervical radiculopathy. *J Bone Joint Surg* 75A:1298-1307, 1993.
3. Bos GD, Goldberg VM, Powell AE, Heiple KG: The effect of histocompatibility matching on canine frozen bone allografts. *J Bone Joint Surg* 65A:89-96, 1983.
4. Brown JA, Havel P, Ebraheim N, Greenblatt SH, Jackson WT: Cervical plate stabilization and bone fusion. *Spine* 13:236-240, 1988.
5. Brown MD, Malinin TI, Davis PB: A roentgenographic evaluation of frozen allografts versus autografts in anterior cervical spine fusions. *Clin Orthop* 119:231-236, 1976.
6. Buck BE, Malinin TI, Brown MD: Bone transplantation and human immunodeficiency virus: An estimate of risk of acquired immunodeficiency syndrome (AIDS). *Clin Orthop* 240:129-136, 1989.
7. Burchardt H: Biology of bone transplantation. *Orthop Clin North Am* 18:187-196, 1987.
8. Burchardt H, Enneking WF: Transplantation of bone. *Surg Clin North Am* 58:403-427, 1978.
9. Cabanela ME, Ebersold MJ: Anterior plate stabilization for bursting teardrop fractures of the cervical spine. *Spine* 13:888-891, 1988.
10. Caspar W, Barbier D, Klara PM: Anterior cervical fusion and Caspar plate stabilization for cervical spine trauma. *Neurosurg* 25:491-502, 1989.

11. Cloward RB: Gas-sterilized cadaver bone graft for spinal fusion operations: A simplified bone bank. *Spine* 5:4-10, 1980.

12. Cloward RD: Treatment of acute fractures and fracture-dislocations of the cervical spine by vertebral body fusion. A report of 11 cases. *J Neurosurg* 18:209, 1961.

13. Cotler JM, Cotler HP (eds): *Spinal Fusion Science and Technique.* Berlin, Springer-Verlag, 1990.

14. deOliveira JC: Anterior plate fixation of traumatic lesions of the lower cervical spine. *Spine* 12:324-329, 1987.

15. Dickman CA, Maric Z: The biology of bone healing and techniques of spinal fusion. *BNI Q* 10:2-12, 1994.

16. Fernyhough JC, White JI, LaRocca H: Fusion rates in multilevel cervical spondylosis comparing allograft fibula with autograft fibula. *Spine* 16:8561-8564, 1992.

17. Friedlaender GE: Bone grafts. *J Bone Joint Surg* 69A: 786-790, 1987.

18. Garvey TA, Eismont FJ, Roberti LJ: Anterior decompression, structural bone grafting and Caspar plate stabilization for unstable cervical spine fractures and/or dislocations. *Spine* 17:S431-S435, 1992.

19. Grossman W, Peppelmen WC, Baum JA, Kraus DR: The use of freeze-dried fibular allograft in anterior cervical fusion. *Spine* 17:565-569, 1992.

20. Kaufman HH, Jones E: The principles of bony spinal fusion. *Neurosurgery* 24:264-270, 1989.

21. Malinin TI, Rosomoff HL, Sutton CH: Human cadaver femoral head homografts for anterior cervical spine fusions. *Surg Neurol* 7:249-251, 1977.

22. Prolo DJ: Biology of bone fusion. *Clin Neurosurg* 36: 135-146, 1988.

23. Ripa DR, Kowall MG, Meyer PR, Rusin JJ: Series of ninety-two traumatic cervical spine injuries stabilized with anterior ASIF plate fusion technique. *Spine* 16:S46-S55, 1991.

24. Rish BL, McFadden JT, Peniz JO: Anterior cervical fusion using homologous bone grafts. A comparative study. *Surg Neurol* 5:119-121, 1976.

25. Robinson RA, Smith GW: Anterolateral cervical disk removing and interbody fusion for cervical disk syndrome. *Bull Johns Hopkins Hosp* 96:223-224, 1955.

26. Rushton SA, Albert TJ: Cervical degenerative disease: Rationale for selecting the appropriate fusion technique (anterior, posterior, and 360 degree). *Orthop Clin North Am* 29(4):755-777, 1998.

27. Sach B, Brennan W: Comparison of freeze-dried allograft versus autograft in anterior cervical spine fusions [abstract]. *Cervical Spine Res Soc* 20:140-141, 1992.

28. Sandhu HS, Boden SD: Biologic enhancement of spinal fusion. *Orthop Clin North Am* 29(4):621-631, 1998.

29. Sandhu HS, Grewal HS, Parvantaneni H: Bone grafting for spinal fusion. *Orthop Clin North Am* 31(4):685-698, 1999.

30. Schulte K, Clark CR, Goel VK: Kinematics of the cervical spine following discectomy and stabilization. *Spine* 14: 1116-1121, 1989.

31. Stabler CL, Eismont FJ, Brown MD, et al: Failure of posterior cervical fusions using bone graft in children. *J Bone Joint Surg* 67A:370-375, 1985.

32. Smith GW, Robinson RA: The treatment of certain cervical spine disorders by anterior removal of the intervertebral disc and interbody fusion. *J Bone Joint Surg* 40A:607-624, 1958.

33. Stevenson S: Biology of bone grafts. *Orthop Clin North Am* 30(4):543-552, 1999.

34. Verbiest H: Anterolateral operation for fractures and dislocations in the middle and lower parts of the cervical spine. *J Bone Joint Surg* 51A:1489-1530, 1969.

35. Wetzel FT, Phillips FM: Management of metastatic disease of the spine. *Orthop Clin North Am* 31(4):611-621, 2000.

36. Wittenberg RH, Moeller J, Shea M, et al: Compressive strength of autologous and allogenous bone grafts for thoracolumbar and cervical spine fusions. *Spine* 15: 1073-1078, 1990.

37. Young WF, Rosenwasser RH: An early comparative analysis of the use of fibular allograft vs. autologous iliac crest graft for interbody fusion after anterior cervical discectomy. *Spine* 18:1123-1124, 1993.

38. Zdeblick TA, Cooke ME, Wilson D, et al: Anterior cervical discectomy and plating: A comparative animal study. *Spine* 18:1974-1983, 1993.

39. Zdeblick TA, Ducker TB: The use of freeze-dried allograft bone for anterior cervical fusions. *Spine* 16: 726-729, 1991.

40. Zdeblick TA, Wikson D, Cooke ME, et al: Anterior cervical discectomy and fusion: Comparison of techniques in an animal model. *Spine* 17:S418-S426, 1992.

# CHAPTER 162

# Thoracic and Thoracolumbar Spine Fractures with Ventral Mass Lesion: Ventral Versus Dorsal Operation

## Ventral Decompression and Stabilization

**Meic H. Schmidt and Philip R. Weinstein**

The management of thoracic and thoracolumbar fractures remains controversial. Non-operative management has been shown to be effective if there is minimal spinal canal compromise, intact dorsal elements, and no neurologic deficit.[6] Fractures with greater than 50% loss of vertebral body height, greater than 50% spinal canal stenosis, major kyphotic deformity, neurologic deficit, intractable pain, and instability despite bracing are considered for surgery.

The role of ventral approaches for decompression and stabilization in the treatment of thoracic and thoracolumbar fractures has significantly advanced over the last two decades.[2,7-10,14] This is primarily caused by refinement of surgical approaches, improved imaging that allows for more detailed analysis of fractures and better ventral thoracolumbar instrumentation. The goals of ventral surgery are decompression of the neural elements under direct vision as well as the restoration of spinal alignment and stability without immobilizing intact motion segments.

Biomechanical studies indicate that ventral instrumentation systems, in combination with a ventral strut graft, restore spinal stability after vertebral body resection. In a porcine corpectomy model, ventral strut grafting with instrumentation was 15% stiffer during axial loading as compared with the intact spine.[5] In comparison, dorsal instrumentation alone was 76% less stiff than the intact spine. Gurr *et al.*[4] studied the ventral Kaneda device and compared it with pedicle screw systems in a bovine model. Equivalent biomechanical stiffness after corpectomy and reconstruction with the Kaneda system over three spinal segments was achieved only if dorsal instrumentation spanned at least five levels.

Dorsal decompression and stabilization techniques are still the most commonly used procedures for thoracic and thoracolumbar fractures. Although ventral decompression and stabilization can be accomplished with dorsal approaches combined with transpedicular, costotransver-sectomy, and lateral extracavitary resections, visualization of the ventral surface of the neural elements is limited, application of ventral instrumentation is difficult, and additional long construct dorsal instrumentation is frequently necessary. The complication rate with lateral extracavitary approaches, which allows the most extensive ventral canal decompression, can be significant even for experienced surgeons.[13] Indirect decompression with distraction applied via pedicle screws or hook/rod constructs can result in satisfactory ventral decompression (ligamentotaxis). However, canal clearance of retropulsed bone fragments can be incomplete, anterior and middle column reconstruction is limited, and load-bearing capacity of the injured vertebral body may not be sufficient.[1]

Ventral approaches for decompression and stabilization have always been appealing to spine surgeons because the majority of thoracic and thoracolumbar spine fractures have significant anterior and middle column pathology, and most frequently, the location of epidural compression is ventral to the dura mater.[14] However, because of the lack of ventral instrumentation, difficult, unfamiliar ventral exposures and the need for dorsal instrumentation made the direct ventral route undesirable. Recent advances in spinal instrumentation and refinement of ventral surgical approaches have changed this. The indications for a one-stage ventral decompression and stabilization continue to expand. Several clinical studies show excellent results.[3,8] The largest series by Kaneda *et al.*[8] included 150 patients treated with ventral decompression and stabilization for patients with thoracolumbar burst fracture. The mean follow-up was 8 years (range 5 to 12 years), and all patients had neurologic deficits following their injury. The fusion rate was 93%. Ten patients experienced nonunion, which was managed with dorsal instrumentation. Postoperative spinal canal stenosis measured with computer tomography ranged from 0% to 8%, with a mean of 2%. Neurologic function improved by at least 1 Frankel grade in 95% of patients. Bladder dysfunction completely recovered in 72% of patients. In addition, 86% of patients returned to work without restrictions. This study demonstrated that ventral approaches can yield excellent results for restoration of neurologic function and spinal stability. Further developments in the use of endoscopy for ventral approaches and image guidance may make the ventral route even more appealing.[11,12] These minimally invasive procedures offer the possibility of reducing postoperative pain and complications of ventral surgical approaches, especially in multiple-injury trauma patients.

## REFERENCES

1. Bradford DS, McBride GG: Surgical management of thoracolumbar spine fractures with incomplete neurologic deficits. *Clin Orthop* May:201-216, 1987.
2. Dunn HK: Anterior spine stabilization and decompression for thoracolumbar injuries. *Orthop Clin North Am* 17: 113-119, 1986.
3. Ghanayem AJ, Zdeblick TA: Anterior instrumentation in the management of thoracolumbar burst fractures. *Clin Orthop* Feb:89-100, 1997.

4. Gurr KR, McAfee PC, Shih CM: Biomechanical analysis of anterior and posterior instrumentation systems after corpectomy. A calf-spine model. *J Bone Joint Surg Am* 70:1182-1191, 1988.

5. Gurwitz GS, Dawson JM, McNamara MJ, et al: Biomechanical analysis of three surgical approaches for lumbar burst fractures using short-segment instrumentation. *Spine* 18:977-982, 1993.

6. Hitchon PW, Torner JC: Recumbency in thoracolumbar fractures. *Neurosurg Clin North Am* 8:509-517, 1997.

7. Kalfas IH: Anterior thoracolumbar stabilization. *Neurosurg Clin North Am* 8:487-498, 1997.

8. Kaneda K, Taneichi H, Abumi K, et al: Anterior decompression and stabilization with the Kaneda device for thoracolumbar burst fractures associated with neurological deficits. *J Bone Joint Surg Am* 79:69-83, 1997.

9. Kostuik JP: Anterior fixation for fractures of the thoracic and lumbar spine with or without neurologic involvement. *Clin Orthop* Oct:103-115, 1984.

10. Kostuik JP: Anterior spinal cord decompression for lesions of the thoracic and lumbar spine, techniques, new methods of internal fixation results. *Spine* 8:512-531, 1983.

11. Ohmori K, Kawaguchi Y, Kanamori M, et al: Image-guided anterior thoracolumbar corpectomy: a report of three cases. *Spine* 26:1197-1201, 2001.

12. Potulski M, Beisse R, Buhren V: [Thoracoscopy-guided management of the "anterior column". Methods and results]. *Orthopade* 28:723-730, 1999.

13. Resnick DK, Benzel EC: Lateral extracavitary approach for thoracic and thoracolumbar spine trauma: operative complications. *Neurosurgery* 43:796-802; discussion 802-793, 1998.

14. Shaffrey CI, Shaffrey ME, Whitehill R, et al: Surgical treatment of thoracolumbar fractures. *Neurosurg Clin North Am* 8:519-540, 1997.

# Dorsal Decompression and Stabilization

**Patrick W. Hitchon**

Currently there are no randomized studies regarding the role of surgery to treat spinal injuries, let alone regarding the comparison of ventral-versus-dorsal approaches to such surgery. There have been a few retrospective studies that compare ventral-versus-dorsal approaches for thoracolumbar spinal fractures.[2,7] These studies, however, were not randomized, and as the authors recognized, were subject to selection bias. With the advent of instrumentation to treat scoliosis by Harrington in 1958, similar dorsal implants were used to manage thoracolumbar fractures. Dorsal instrumentation with rods, hooks, sublaminar wires, or pedicle screws has been used with favorable results. Retrospective studies have demonstrated neurologic improvement, correction of angulation, restoration of vertebral body height and spinal canal, as well as rapid mobilization.[3-6,9] Similar results have been achieved with ventral decompression and stabilization.[10,11] These stud-

ies were nonrandomized, retrospective, and selected for a particular approach. In the author's prospective review of thoracolumbar (T11-L5) burst fractures, 58 were treated with a dorsal midline or costotransversectomy approach and 39 with a ventral or flank approach. Neurologic improvement occurred in both. Angular correction was better achieved and maintained, however, with ventral surgery.

Biomechanical studies have compared ventral and dorsal implants.[1,8,12] Such studies have not universally been in agreement. Nevertheless, ventral implants such as the Kaneda and Zielke device have been found to be comparable to the dorsal Cotrel-Dubousset and Steffe systems.

The advantage of the dorsal approach to the thoracolumbar spine is the familiarity of the spine surgeon with this access route. In case of a fracture-dislocation, with or without locked facets, the dorsal approach facilitates facet reduction and reconstitution of the spinal canal. Because of its simplicity and ability to provide stabilization and rapid mobilization, the dorsal approach is also suited in cases of total paralysis when no recovery of function is anticipated. In case of a burst fracture with retropulsed bone in the canal, adequate decompression of the spinal canal can be performed by using the transpedicular or transarticular approach. This can be performed unilaterally or bilaterally. After removal of the medial facet joint and pedicle with an air drill, retropulsed bone fragments can be removed and the spinal canal decompressed by using the air drill and reversed curettes. The adequacy of decompression can be confirmed by using the intraoperative ultrasound, which is a useful device to evaluate spinal canal morphology. Multisegmental spinal stabilization, generally (but not necessarily) two levels above and below the fracture, is thereafter accomplished by using pedicle screws solely, or in conjunction with hooks when the pedicles are small (i.e., in the upper half of the thoracic spine) (Figure 162.1). Unfortunately, in the presence of severe wedging and collapse of the vertebral body, dorsal instrumentation may fail in the absence of ventral load sharing. Thus, long multisegmental rostrocaudal fixation may be necessary to prevent construct failure. Long constructs, however, may result in stiffness and discomfort.

Although a ventral approach provides excellent visualization of the spine canal and facilitates decompression and ventral strut grafting, many spine surgeons are not optimally familiar with this approach or the anatomy. Hence, reliance on a vascular or general surgeon is customary. The ventral route to lesions above T12 often requires placement of a chest tube. The ventral approach harbors limitation regarding its failure to gain access to the facets, in cases in which dislocation and locked facets may be present. In the presence of a three-column injury, a retroperitoneal approach can prove inadequate, necessitating both ventral and dorsal stabilization. In Figure 162.1, the patient is a male aged 24 years with a burst fracture at L2 with a conus injury. The preoperative computed tomography (CT) scan shows severe spinal canal compromise from the retropulsed bone. Operative intervention through a dorsal approach facilitated adequate reconstruction of the canal and stabilization with transpedicular screws and

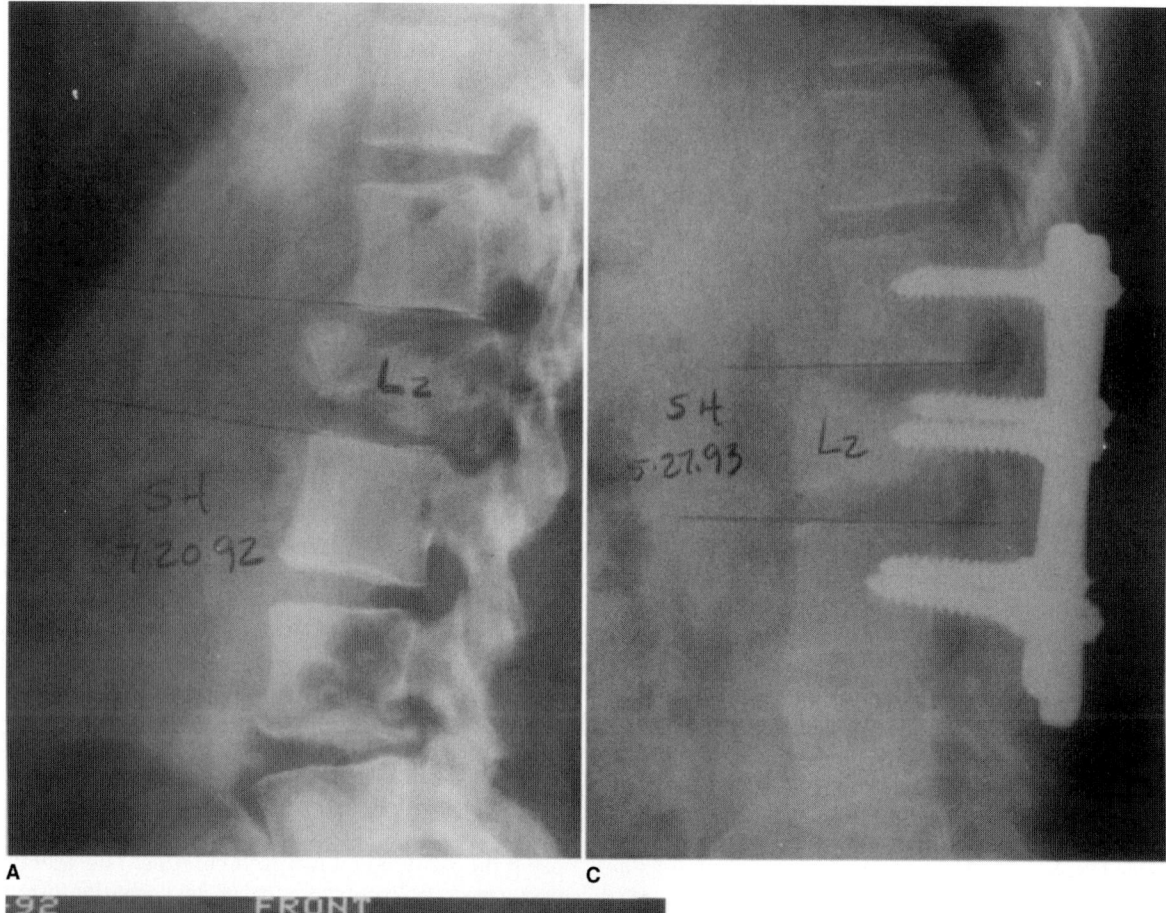

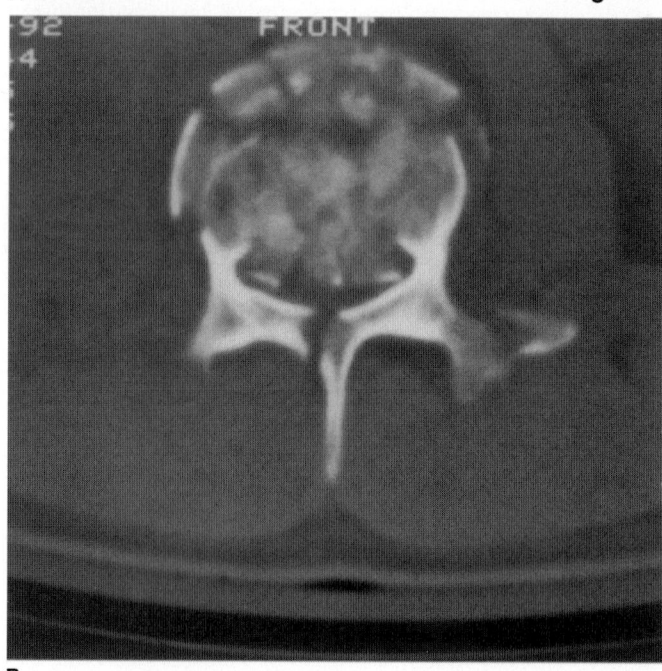

**Figure 162.1** A 24-year-old man involved in a motor vehicle accident sustained a burst fracture of L2 with conus contusion. (**A**) Lateral radiograph shows the loss in height and wedging of L2 resulting from the burst fracture. (**B**) Computed axial tomogram shows the burst fracture of L2 associated with significant compromise of the spinal canal and laminar fracture on the right side. (**C**) Radiograph obtained 10 months later shows improved alignment and restoration of vertebral body height of L2 with the pedicle screws and plates in place. The patient was now employed, but still had sphincter disturbance.

plates. The postoperative image studies demonstrate the effectiveness of this approach in well-selected patients.

# REFERENCES

1. Abumi K, Panjabi MM, Duranceau J: Biomechanical evaluation of spinal fixation devices: part III stability provided by six spinal fixation devices and interbody bone graft. *Spine* 14:1249-1255, 1989.
2. Bradford DS, McBride GG: Surgical management of thoracolumbar spine fractures with incomplete neurologic deficits. *Clin Orthop* 218:201-216, 1987.
3. Carl AL, Tromanhauser SG, Roger DJ: Pedicle screw instrumentation for thoracolumbar burst fractures and fracture-dislocations. *Spine* 17:S317-S324, 1992.
4. Crutcher JP Jr, Anderson PA, King HA, Montesano PX: Indirect spinal canal decompression in patients with thoracolumbar burst fractures treated by posterior distraction rods. *J Spinal Disord* 4:39-48, 1991.
5. Dickson JH, Harrington PR, Erwin WD: Results of reduction and stabilization of the severely fractured thoracic and lumbar spine. *J Bone Joint Surg* 60A:799-805, 1978.
6. Flesch JR, Leider LL, Erickson DL, *et al*: Harrington instrumentation and spine fusion for unstable fracture and fracture-dislocations of the thoracic and lumbar spine. *J Bone Joint Surg* 59A:143-153, 1977.
7. Gertzbein SD, Court-Brown CM, Marks P, *et al*: The neurological outcome following surgery for spinal fractures. *Spine* 13:641-644, 1988.
8. Gurr KR, McAfee PC, Shih C: Biomechanical analysis of anterior and posterior instrumentation systems after corpectomy. *J Bone Joint Surg* 70A:1182-1191, 1988.
9. Hardaker WT Jr, Cook WA Jr, Friedman AH, Fitch RD: Bilateral transpedicular decompression and Harrington rod stabilization in the management of severe thoracolumbar burst fractures. *Spine* 17:162-171, 1992.
10. Kaneda K, Abumi K, Fujiya M: Burst fractures with neurologic deficits of the thoracolumbar-lumbar spine. Results of anterior decompression and stabilization with anterior instrumentation. *Spine* 9:788-795, 1984.
11. McAfee PC, Bohlman HH, Yuan HA: Anterior decompression of traumatic thoracolumbar fractures with incomplete neurological deficit using a retroperitoneal approach. *J Bone Joint Surg* 67A:89-104, 1985.
12. Shono Y, Kaneda K, Yamamoto I: A biomechanical analysis of Zielke, Kaneda, and Cotrel-Dubousset instrumentations in thoracolumbar scoliosis: a calf spine model. *Spine* 16:1305-1311, 1991.

# Reoperation for Failed Spinal Fusion: Augmentation of Fusion with Spinal Stimulation

## Argument Against Spinal Stimulation

Jeffrey D. Gross

Failed dorsal lumbar spinal fusions create more headaches, heartaches, and backaches for patients and surgeons than most problems associated with spinal surgery. Treatments for these pseudarthroses are more complex and difficult than are many primary spinal procedures, and they themselves have a high failure rate. The need to reduce the spinal fusion failure and pseudarthrosis rates have fostered the development of augmentative therapies such as spinal stimulation. However, the clinical use of such electrical stimulating devices in the spine have remained controversial. Although supported by laboratory and animal model evidence, the application of stimulating devices for the treatment of failed spinal fusion has not been proven clinically. Furthermore, the biology of failed fusion does not parallel that of a primary fusion or of a long bone fracture or nonunion.[13,16,18] The extrapolation of our understanding of the use of such devices to the treatment of spinal disorders is incomplete.

A variety of electrical stimulators are available. They may be implanted surgically or semi-invasively with an external generator or applied completely noninvasively, with pulsed electromagnetic fields (PEMF), capacitively coupled electrical stimulation, or combined magnetic fields. These variables, combined with variations in fusion approaches and techniques for the multiple indications in differing patient populations, make comparison of relevant studies impractical.* Hence, there are few well-controlled patient studies clearly demonstrating the clinical utility of implantable or external electrical stimulating devices for pseudarthrosis in the spinal column.

## Experimental Evidence

The biochemical basis of the cellular response to electrical fields has been elucidated and nicely summarized by Brighton.[6] Cultured bone cell DNA production increased

---

*References 1,4,8,9,18,21,22,27-30.

in response to capacitive coupling, inductive coupling, or combined electromagnetic fields. These electrical fields tend to increase intracellular calcium concentrations, which increases cytoskeletal calmodulin activation and ultimately cellular proliferation. This growth and division of bone cells are the desired effects in spinal fusion.

Much of the initial work in evaluating the use of external stimulation for the augmentation of a failing arthrodesis was performed on long bone models. The relative success of these models was the impetus for the transfer of such technologies to the use in the different arena of failed spinal fusions. Initial studies of spinal stimulation for lumbar fusions, however, were performed on non-weight-bearing (i.e., quadruped) models undergoing primary spinal fusions, usually without instrumentation. There were no controls for these variables.

Nerubay et al.[24] studied implanted "direct current stimulation" (DCS) of primary dorsal spinal fusions in 30 pigs and reported a customized nonparametric score improvement of radiographic and histologic criteria 2 months after the operation. Conversely, Kahanovitz et al.[14] investigated the use of DCS in primary lumbar spinal fusions in dogs. They found no advantage for electrical stimulation in the radiologic or histologic indices for fusion until 12 weeks after the operation when using an internal control. However, each facet joint involved was considered a statistical sample, and considering the animals separately, there were no statistical differences at any time for fusion success. This same group reported the use of PEMF on a similar canine model.[16] They were unable to demonstrate radiologic or histologic differences between experimental and control groups at 6 and 12 weeks after operation. In another report, this group reported that by 12 and 15 weeks after surgery, there were no histologic or radiologic differences in dogs receiving primary spinal fusions when using instrumentation and PEMF.[15]

France et al.[10] showed the dose-dependent efficacy of subcutaneous DCS for primary, non-instrumented lumbar intertransverse process fusions in a controlled rabbit model. In a similar model, DCS increased fusion rates in a dose-dependent manner while employed with coralline hydroxyapatite as a bone graft substitute, as compared with non-stimulated rabbits with autologous bone.[5] DCS was also studied in randomized, controlled, and blinded (for outcome measure) sheep experiments while employed with titanium interbody fusion cages packed with autograft.[31] A dose-dependent rate of fusion was also observed in this study.

The use of various electrical stimulating devices for spinal fusion in animal models has met with mixed results. However, no animal studies have addressed the situation of failed fusion. Furthermore, the spinal biomechanics of quadrupeds are not identical to those in upright primates, whose weight bearing has direct influence on the fusion success.[3] Neither invasive nor external spinal stimulation has been adequately studied in an appropriate upright animal model for failed fusion of the lumbosacral spine. The use of instrumentation is a complicating factor for which there are no controlled studies with electrical stimulation in animals. Furthermore, the application of animal data to human use is controversial, since spinal fusion rates differ among species.[5] Thus there is not sufficient experimental evidence in animal studies to support the use of augmentative electrical stimulation for reoperation for failed spinal fusion.[15]

## Clinical Evidence

The results of published patient series of electrical stimulation for spinal fusion are displayed in Table 163.1. Some of the data presented have been extracted from these series to demonstrate only patients who have had implanted or external stimulation for failed lumbosacral spinal fusions. There are no studies on reoperation for failed lumbar spinal fusion that prospectively control for the type of surgery, construct variety, instrumentation, and patient status (e.g., weight, smoking status, steroid therapy.[21,23,29] Only one of these studies indicates a statistically significant improvement in the fusion rate for failed spinal fusion with electrical stimulation.[27] These 33 patients were instrumented and were not completely randomized versus controls for other factors. None of the other studies demonstrated an improvement in the fusion rate or time to fusion in the subpopulation of failed dorsal spinal fusions. In fact, one author reported that electrical stimulation had an adverse effect on the time to fusion and stated that[18] it "is not advocated for use in any type of spine fusion." Thus the clinical evidence in favor of electrical stimulation for the augmentation of failed dorsal spinal fusions is meager and requires further controlled investigation.[13]

Only recently, clinical reports have indicated the efficacy of external capacitively coupled electrical stimulation (CCES) in primary spinal fusions.[11] In this study of 179 patients (reduced from 337 for withdrawals and noncompliance), control for variables, such as a concomitant disease (i.e., diabetes), institution, bone graft materials used for fusion, and internal fixation strategies was not possible. There was no statistical significance for CCES efficacy in the smoking or previous surgery cohorts for this study. There is no parallel study for failed spinal fusions. Conversely, Jenis et al.[12] determined that neither DCS nor PEMF was able to statistically improve the fusion rate or clinical outcome of instrumented posterolateral arthrodeses.

A retrospectively random review of patients to analyze the efficacy of PEMF to augment primary spinal fusions was undertaken to measure clinical and radiologic outcome.[20] A statistically significant difference was found with 97.6% fusion success for the stimulated group and only a 52.6% fusion rate for the control group. However, there was a bias toward using PEMF on smokers, on multi-level fusions, and in conjunction with allograft use. Surgical approaches included ventral interbody, dorsolateral, and both, thereby adding further variables to the analysis of these results. The number of patients (61) was likely too small to make meaningful conclusions from the clinical outcomes. With regard to reoperation for failed spinal fusion, "...the low number of patients undergoing repeat fusion precluded specific conclusions or recommendations..." for the use of PEMF.

Recently a prospective well-designed study was published for the analysis of combined magnetic fields on primary spinal fusions.[19] This multi-center randomized, double-blind, placebo-controlled trial of 201 non-instrumented fusions demonstrated a statistically significant increase in the fusion rate at 9 months after surgery with use of a non-invasive device. When stratified by sex, this significant difference remained only for women. Also, there were only 28 patients who smoked in the entire starting population of 243, so no conclusions can be drawn for this subgroup. Furthermore, no conclusions could be drawn with regard to reoperation for failed spinal fusion.

Thus although there is increasing but incomplete evidence supporting the use of electromagnetic fields for the support of primary lumbar fusions, the study of recalcitrant subgroups such as patients with pseudarthroses has not been performed adequately, and meaningful conclusions with regard to augmentative spinal stimulation for this group cannot be made.

## Discussion

The lack of upright animal models underscores the importance for understanding the biomechanics involved in bone fusion.[16] The weight-bearing forces acting on spinal fusions in the upright position are not equivalent to those in other positions. Additionally, the pathology, fusion type, and use of instrumentation will affect the biomechanics of the construct.[1,3,16,27] Fixation alone has been shown to enhance spinal fusion.[16,18,27] These variables were not consistently controlled in the animal and patient studies published on the use of electrical stimulation for spinal fusion.[4,13,18] Furthermore, the experimental and clinical evidence supporting stimulation for bone fusion for pseudarthrosis is based on long bone data. This appendicular physiology exhibits completely different biomechanical dynamics and differs from the situation of spinal fusion where the bones are not "normally" physiologically fused bones. In other words, it is still necessary to fuse a fracture of a long bone that has failed to heal, whereas spinal segments were not meant to be linked in an immobile fashion.

Many factors affect the spinal fusion success rate, despite the method of fusion surgery. These include patient health, primary pathology, weight, weight-bearing status, steroid and NSAID use, PEMF compliance, and smoking.[18] None of the literature studies concerning electrical stimulation for failed spinal fusions were designed with complete control for these parameters, although multivariate analyses were performed in some.[21,22,27] Many authors agree that there is a paucity of appropriate controlled patient studies for electrical stimulation in spinal fusion and that further well-controlled prospective studies are warranted.* However, there is improvement in the availability of clinical studies for the use of spinal stimulation for primary lumbar fusions. The reader should be careful not to automatically extrapolate those conclusions to the case of pseudarthrosis, a more difficult and recalcitrant physiologic problem.

Furthermore, high-risk patients for fusion failure may be destined for failure despite the best surgical techniques, with or without electricomagnetic augmentation.[22] These patients' pseudarthroses are hypovascular and

---

*References 4,13,17,18,21,25.

**TABLE 163.1**

**Published Patient Series of Electrical Stimulation for Spinal Fusion**

| Year | Lead Author | Pts* | Instrumentation | Fusion Type | Stimulation | Study Type | Controls | Fusion Results | Significance |
|---|---|---|---|---|---|---|---|---|---|
| 2002 | Linovitz[19] | 201 | None | Primary posterolateral | Noninvasive combined magnetic fields | Prospective, randomized, placebo controlled, double-blinded, multicenter | Stimulation vs. placebo | 64% stim vs. 43% placebo at 9 months, although the device was worn for a minimum of 2 months | $P = .003$ overall, and .001 for female subgroup. |
| 2000 | Marks[20] | 61 | Some | Primary and revision "lumbar fusions" | PEMF | Retrospective, but random | Retrospective group | 97.6% stim vs. 52.6% control | $P < .001$, but not controlled for primary or repeat surgery. |
| 2000 | Jenis[12] | 61 | All had the same pedicle screw and rod system | Primary Posterolateral | Implanted DCS and external PEMF groups | Prospective, randomized, multi-armed | DCS and PEMF arms vs. no stimulation | Measured by fusion mass density grade | None Note: No fusion rate reported, but trend towards poor fusion grade with risk factors such as re-operation. |
| 1999 | Goodwin[11] | 179 | Some (not controlled) except interbody fusion cages. | Primary lumbar fusions: anterior and posterior interbody, posterolateral | CCES | Prospective, double-blind, randomized, placebo-controlled, multicenter | Stimulation vs. Placebo. Cohorts for age, sex, height, weight, smoking status matched | 84.7% stim vs. 64.9% placebo | Yates corrected chi-square test ($P = .0043$) overall. Stratification for posterolateral fusion over other types ($P = .006$) and internal fixation over none ($P = .013$). |
| 1996 | Rogozinski[27] | 33† | All-pedicle screws and rods | Posterolateral fusion | DCS | Prospective, semi-random | Only for stimulation | 19/19 stim vs. 11/14 control | $P = .02$ |
| 1996 | Tejano[30] | 10 | None | Posterior facet or posterolateral | DCS | Prospective | Other studies | 80%† | None |
| 1994 | Meril[21] | 24 | Some (not controlled) | PLIF or ALIF | DCS | Prospective | Retrospective, not for all factors | 92% stim vs. 73% control | $P = .3$ |
| 1990 | Mooney[22] | 2 | Some | PLIF or ALIF | PEMF | Randomized, double-blind, prospective | Not for all factors | 0/1 stim vs. 1/1 control | None |

**TABLE 163.1**

**Published Patient Series of Electrical Stimulation for Spinal Fusion** *cont'd*

| Year | Lead Author | Pts[†] | Instrumentation | Fusion Type | Stimulation | Study Type | Controls | Fusion Results | Significance |
|---|---|---|---|---|---|---|---|---|---|
| 1990 | Savini[28] | 5 | Some | Posterolateral | PEMF | Retrospective | Not controlled | All fused by 5 months | Unknown |
| 1988 | Kane[17] | 21 | None | "Standard lumbosacral fusion" | DCS | Prospective, randomized | Not for all factors | 9/11 stim vs. 4/10 control | Not reported |
| 1986 | Kornblatt[18] | 22 | All (various) | Posterolateral | DCS? | Retrospective | Retrospective | "No improvement... in fusion rate"[§] | None |
| 1985 | Simmons[29] | 13 | None | PLIF | PEMF | Prospective | None | 85% had increased bone formation | Statistics not published |
| 1974 | Dwyer[8,9] | 0 | None | Posterolateral | DCS | Prospective | None | No data on failed fusion | None |

*Subtotal of patients with failed lumbosacral fusions, if discernable.
[†]These patients represent "previous back surgery" including laminectomies, decompressions, and failed fusions.
[‡]All patients received electrical stimulation.
[§]Time to fusion was prolonged in the treatment group.

fibrotic, leading to a trend toward less-successful subsequent reoperation. This positive feedback cycle has not been borne out in the present literature analysis. Also, time to fusion was not measured in all studies, and the natural history of spinal fusion may be different in various patient populations for which the aforementioned study variables were not completely controlled.[21,29] These interrelated factors must be evaluated independently along with electrical stimulation to provide adequate evidence for their effective use as an augmentative device for failed spinal fusion. One author astutely reported that "good surgical technique remains the most important influence on surgical outcome."[27]

In addition to the paucity of animal and patient evidence in favor of utilizing electrical stimulation to augment spinal fusion for pseudarthrosis, there are numerous disadvantages and potential complications. The additional time of surgery for implantation of invasive electrical stimulators is significant and increases perioperative morbidity. Surgical use of internal stimulators provides an additional foreign body, which may increase the incidence of postoperative infection, particularly in high-risk pseudarthrosis patients such as smokers and steroid users. The invasive stimulators would thus potentially require removal, adding further surgical risks and costs to the patient's burdens.[22] Implanted leads have been shown to break and corrode on occasion.[7,8] Additionally, patients undergoing recurrent spinal surgery typically require frequent radiologic evaluations. Broken stimulator leads have been shown to abnormally heat local tissue during MRI scanning (as much as 14° C), making MRI a contraindication for those patients.[7] Also, electrical stimulators can cause significant distortion on MRI. Furthermore, there have been cases of over-stimulation, which can be deleterious to bone formation.[2] Finally, optimal electrical stimulation profiles for electrical units used in the spine are not fully elucidated.[1,14,26,29]

This analysis would not be complete without a description of the costs for the hardware and additional surgery required for stimulator implantation in the case of DCS. One supplier of electrical stimulators estimates an additional $5578 to the cost of reoperation for failed spinal fusion, which is a significant increase in health care expenditures for an unproven use. This does not take into account the additional costs related to increased operation time, potential complications, and hospital "mark-up."

## Summary

Based on animal and patient studies, the author finds no compelling evidence to advocate the use of invasive electrical stimulation to augment a failed dorsal lumbosacral fusion. Since it appears that there is no harm in using non-invasive devices after reoperation for failed spinal fusion (despite the lack of current scientific proof), these devices may be considered for application. Alternatives to fusion augmentation may include (1) attempting a more biomechanically sound fusion, with or without instrumentation; (2) having patients avoid steroids and NSAIDs; and (3) counseling patients to limit tobacco use. Further well-controlled, randomized patient studies

for the evaluation of electrical stimulation for failed fusion are indicated.

## REFERENCES

1. Bassett CA: Why are the principles of physics and anatomy important in treating osteoporosis [editorial]? *Calcified Tissue Int* 56:515-516, 1995.
2. Bassett CA, Pawluk RJ, Pilla AA: Acceleration of fracture repair by electromagnetic fields. A surgically noninvasive method. *Ann NY Acad Sci* 238:242-262, 1974.
3. Benzel EC: Spinal fusion, In Benzel EC (ed): *Biomechanics of Spine Stabilization: Principles and Practice*, New York, McGraw-Hill, 1994, pp 103-110.
4. Boden SC, Schimandle JH: Biologic enhancement of spinal fusion. *Spine* 20(suppl):113S-123S, 1995.
5. Bozic KJ, Glazer PA, Zurakowski D, et al: In vivo evaluation of coralline hydroxyapatite and direct current electrical stimulation in lumbar spinal fusion. *Spine* 24:2127-2133, 1999.
6. Brighton CT, Wang W, Seldes R, et al: Signal transduction in electrically stimulated bone cells. *J Bone Joint Surg [Am]* 83:1514-1523, 2001.
7. Chou CK, McDougall JA, Chan KW: RF heating of implanted spinal fusion stimulator during magnetic resonance imaging. *IEEE Trans Biomed Engin* 44:367-373, 1997.
8. Dwyer AF, Wickham GG: Direct current stimulation in spinal fusion. *Med J Austr* 1:73-75, 1974.
9. Dwyer AF, Yau AC, Jeffcoat KW: Use of direct current in spine fusion. *J Bone Joint Surg [Am]* 56:442, 1974.
10. France JC, Norman TL, Santrock RD, et al: The efficacy of direct current stimulation for lumbar intertransverse process fusions in and animal model. *Spine* 26:1002-1008, 2001.
11. Goodwin CB, Brighton CT, Guyer RD, et al: A double-blind study of capacitively coupled electrical stimulation as an adjunct to lumbar spinal fusions. *Spine* 24:1349-1357, 1999.
12. Jenis LG, An HS, Stein R, Young B: Prospective comparison of the effect of direct current electrical stimulation and pulsed electromagnetic fields on instrumented posterolateral lumbar arthrodesis. *J Spinal Disord* 4:290-296, 2000.
13. Kahanovitz N: Spine update. The use of adjunctive electrical stimulation to enhance the healing of spine fusions. *Spine* 21:2523-2525, 1996.
14. Kahanovitz N, Arnoczky SP: The efficacy of direct current electrical stimulation to enhance canine spinal fusion. *Clin Orthop* 251:295-299, 1990.
15. Kahanovitz N, Arnoczky SP, Julse D, Shires PK: The effect of postoperative electromagnetic pulsing on canine posterior spinal fusions. *Spine* 9:273-278, 1984.
16. Kahanovitz N, Arnoczky SP, Nemzek J, Shores A: The effect of electromagnetic pulsing on posterior lumbar spinal fusions in dogs. *Spine* 19:705-709, 1994.
17. Kane WJ: Direct current electrical bone growth stimulation for spinal fusion. *Spine* 13:363-365, 1988.
18. Kornblatt MD, Casey MP, Jacobs RR: Internal fixation in lumbosacral spine fusion. A biomechanical and clinical study. *Clin Orthop Rel Res* 203:141-150, 1986.

19. Linovitz RJ, Pathria M, Bernhardt M, et al: Combined magnetic fields accelerate and increase spine fusion. *Spine* 27:1383-1389, 2002.

20. Marks RA: Spine fusion for discogenic back pain: outcomes in patients treated with or without pulsed electromagnetic field stimulation. *Adv Ther* 17:57-67, 2000.

21. Meril AJ: Direct current stimulation of allograft in anterior and posterior lumbar interbody fusions. *Spine* 19:2393-2398, 1994.

22. Mooney V: A randomized double-blind prospective study of the efficacy of pulsed electromagnetic fields for interbody lumbar fusion. *Spine* 15:708-712, 1990.

23. Nerubay J, Katznelson A: Clinical evaluation of an electrical current stimulator in spinal fusions. *Int Orthop* 7:239-242, 1984.

24. Nerubay J, Marganit B, Bubis JJ, et al: Stimulation of bone formation by electrical current on spinal fusion. *Spine* 11:167-169, 1986.

25. Paterson D: Treatment of nonunion with a constant direct current: a totally implantable system. *Orthop Clin North Am* 15:47-59, 1984.

26. Paterson DC, Carter RF, Tilbury RF, et al: The effects of varying current levels of electrical stimulation. *Clin Orthop Rel Res* 169:303-312, 1982.

27. Rogozinski A, Rogozinski C: Efficacy of implanted bone growth stimulation in instrumented lumbosacral spinal fusion. *Spine* 21:2479-2483, 1996.

28. Savini R, DeSilvestre M, Garguilo G, Bettini N: The use of pulsing electromagnetic fields in posterolateral lumbosacral spinal fusion. *J Bioelect* 9:9-17, 1990.

29. Simmons JW: Treatment of failed posterior lumbar interbody fusion (PLIF) of the spine with pulsing electromagnetic fields. *Clin Orthop Rel Res* 193:127-132, 1985.

30. Tejano NA, Puno R, Ignacio JM: The use of implantable direct current stimulation in multilevel spinal fusion without instrumentation. A prospective clinical and radiographic evaluation with long-term follow-up. *Spine* 21:1904-1908, 1996.

31. Toth JM, Seim HB, Schwardt JD, Humphrey WB, Wallskog JA, Turner AS: Direct current electrical stimulation increases the fusion rate of spinal fusion cages. *Spine* 25:2580-2587, 2000.

# Argument for Spinal Stimulation

**Alexander R. Vaccaro, Jared P. Salinsky, and Bruce E. Northrup**

The scientific understanding of the basic principles of electricity and magnetism is about two centuries old. Electrical stimulation of human tissue has been used by medical care providers for the diagnosis and management of neuromuscular disease, stroke, spinal cord injury, and fusion metabolism. Initial experiments relating the use of electricity to bone were performed in Japan by Yasuda, who concluded that electronegativity on the concave surface of bone was the cause of new bone formation during the remodeling process.[1,2,8] Later, Bassett,[4] in North America, demonstrated abundant bone formation around the negative electrode of an implanted sterilized battery pack in the bones of dogs. The observation that a small amount of electrical current stimulates osteogenesis has been confirmed experimentally and clinically by many other researchers. Contemporary clinical applications of electrical stimulation in regards to modification of bone physiology include the management of acute bony fractures, spinal pseudarthrosis, osteoporosis, osteoarthritis, and avascular necrosis of the femoral head.

## Basic Science

The clinical application of electrical stimulation may be delivered in three distinct forms. The most direct and invasive method of applying an electric current to human tissue is through surgically implanted electrodes into the targeted tissue. The electric current is produced by an implantable generator. Another method delivers an electric current externally in the form of pulsing electromagnetic fields (PEMF). The final form generates an electric current through capacitively coupled electric (CCE) energy. PEMFs are generated by a time-varying current applied to metallic coils at a certain duration and intensity. In capacitive coupling, two charged metal plates or equivalent structures are attached to a voltage source to produce an electric field. PEMFs and capacitively coupled electric fields may be delivered through external electrodes or a corset-like or orthotic type apparatus.[36]

Research to date has demonstrated significant intracellular and extracellular events that are coupled with the active application of an electromagnetic field on cells responsible for osteogenesis. Lohmann et al.[31] found that enhanced cellular differentiation was the end result of PEMF on osteoblast metabolism, as evidenced by increased alkaline phosphatase activity, osteocalcin synthesis, and collagen production. PEMF appears to promote the production of matrix vesicles at 4 days as evidenced by increased levels of alkaline phosphatase in exposed cells as compared with controls. This is similar to the degree of osteogenic differentiation seen in response to transforming growth factor beta–one (TGF-$\beta$1). Bodamyali et al.[12] found that where bone tissue is in direct contact with a titanium cathode, the faradic products hydrogen peroxide ($H_2O_2$) and hydroxyl ion were generated, causing osteoclastic resorption. This in turn causes a release of calcium, which increases the pH. An increase in pH inhibits osteoclastic resorption and stimulates osteoblasts to lay down new bone.[12] Finally, Lorich et al.[31] found that the signal transduction mechanism that mediates the proliferation response of culture bone cells involves transmembrane calcium translocation via voltage-gated calcium channels and activation of calmodulin when stimulated by a capacitively coupled electrical field. Because calmodulin is activated by an increase in cytosolic calcium, there must be an increase in cytosolic calcium as part of the signal transduction mediating the proliferation response to an electrical field.[31,47]

Pulsed electromagnetic fields (PEMF) have been shown to be clinically effective in promoting the healing of fracture nonunions and may enhance calcification of the extracellular matrix.[3,9-11] In vitro and in vivo studies have suggested that PEMF may also modify the extracellular matrix by promoting synthesis of matrix molecules and stimulation of endochondral ossification.[3,7,9-11] Brighton et al.,[14] using direct current stimulation, explored the relationship between charge, current density, and new bone formation in the medullary canal of intact rabbit tibias. Their results indicated that the amount of new bone formed in the vicinity of a cathode is directly related to both the current density and charge. The amount of bone formed with pulsed fields approached the amount formed with constant current only when the total charge delivered by the pulsed fields neared that of the constant direct current. At the cellular level, tissue cultures exposed to electrostatic and electrodynamic fields produced a 15% to 300% increase in collagen production. Varying the electrical pulses has been shown to change the rate of calcium uptake in tissue cultured cells.[6]

## Clinical Application

Pulsed electromagnetic fields were first used in humans for the treatment of congenital pseudarthrosis of the tibia.[14,15] The use of electrical stimulation to promote healing of difficult nonunions dates back over 150 years.* Success rates as high as 95% and shortened healing time have been reported when using PEMF in conjunction with open reduction, internal fixation, and bone grafting in isolated scaphoid fractures.[27] Recently a double-blind study with PEMF in the treatment of tibial delayed unions employed the use of long leg casting and no weight bearing with either an active or control (sham) PEMF unit. Success rates of 45% were observed in the PEMF-treated patients as compared with 12% among the control patients.[30]

Electrical stimulation is also used in the management of femoral head osteonecrosis. PEMF stimulation seems to retard the radiographic progression of necrosis and improve clinical outcome after core decompression and grafting when compared with decompression and grafting alone.[33] The role of PEMF in the prevention of osteoporosis lacks an adequate clinical model, but preliminary animal studies show promise for this type of technology in a problem so prevalent in our aging society.[35] Research is actively underway to determine the effects of PEMF on the natural history of osteoarthrosis.

Electrical stimulation is now a common and popular adjunct to bone grafting in spinal fusion procedures, especially for those patients at high risk for nonunion. Surgeons are in a never-ending search for strategies that may lessen the eventuality of a symptomatic failed fusion. In this setting, an attempted revision procedure now has to be performed in a partially devascularized fusion bed because of scarring in a biologic environment that has already proven unfavorable to the promise of a successful fusion. The proven success of PEMF in bony healing in the appendicular skeleton led initially to its application in revision lumbar spinal fusions. Kahanovitz et al.[38] in 1984 demonstrated

accelerated facet fusion in a canine model with noninvasive PEMF technology. The researchers noted an early accelerated osteogenic response at 6 weeks in the stimulated group as compared with controls. However, at 12 weeks, both study groups were healed with no obvious radiographic or histologic differences in fusion mass quality. Conversely, in an identical experiment with the application of direct current stimulation, Kahanovitz and colleagues[40] found this form of electrical stimulation to significantly enhance fusion success both radiographically and histologically as compared with the control specimens.

## Electrical Stimulation and the Spine: Animal Studies

Although there is still controversy over which method is most effective, clinical evidence supports the use of direct current electrical stimulation, PEMF, and capacitive coupled electrical stimulation in increasing fusion rates in either a posterolateral or interbody lumbar spinal fusion. Additionally, all three techniques have demonstrated improved fusion healing potential in instrumented and noninstrumented fusions. Various animal studies have contributed to our current understanding of electrical stimulation as a supplement to spinal fusion.[16] Bozic et al.[49] evaluated various current densities supplied with direct current stimulation combined with an osteoconductive bone graft substitute (coralline hydroxyapatite) in a rabbit model. They found that increasing current up to 100uA improved the quality and success rate of posterolateral fusion results over lower current values. Toth et al.[49] demonstrated that direct stimulation could be used to increase the histologic and biomechanical fusion success rate of interbody fusion in sheep. Recently France et al.[20] demonstrated a trend of increasing radiographic fusion success in a rabbit posterolateral fusion model as the current density was incrementally increased (sham, 20uA, 60uA). Statistically significant differences were shown in peak load to failure ratios and stiffness; however, the most striking difference between the sham and high-current groups was observed in the host tissue response to autograft bone. Reparative granulation tissue and osteoid surrounded the autograft bone in the high current spines, whereas necrotic fibrous tissue surrounded the autograft bone in the sham group.[20]

## Electrical Stimulation and the Spine: Human Investigations

Clinical trials of electrical stimulation in humans have typically produced higher spinal fusion success rates in controlled and noncontrolled human trials. Dwyer[41] reported on its first use of direct current electrical stimulation in humans in 1974, in which all but 1 patient had a solid radiographic fusion mass. Simmons[42] used PEMF to treat established lumbar pseudarthrosis after posterior lumbar interbody fusions and achieved bony consolidation in 77% of his patients. A large multicenter nonrandomized study with a historic control, followed by a randomized prospective study, showed significantly higher fusion success rates

---

*References 5,14,17,19,23,25,26.

among the direct-current stimulated patients as compared with nonstimulated controls. This was conducted concurrently with an open investigation utilizing direct current stimulation in which the fusion success was 93%.[43,45] A randomized double-blind trial using PEMF in the setting of an anterior or posterior interbody fusion reported a radiographic fusion determined success rate of 92%, as compared with 65% for controls.[46]

## Direct Current Stimulation

Implanted direct current devices are unobtrusive, do not encumber patients in their postoperative rehabilitation, and offer no issues of patient compliance. Typically, the direct current is via two titanium leads placed paraspinally. In 1988 Kane,[27] after three separate studies, concluded direct current electrical stimulation is a useful supplement to a lumbosacral fusion or pseudarthrosis repair. Meril[34] reported statistically significant increases in fusion success in smokers, patients with no internal fixation, and patients undergoing a L4-5 fusion with direct current electrical stimulation. Seventy-seven percent of patients reported improvement in their quality of life, while 96% were noted to have successful fusion radiographically. Grottkau and Lipson[22] showed direct stimulation to increase the rate at which graft consolidation occurs in lumbar spine fusions; there was a trend toward increased fusion mass over time. Rogozinski et al.[39] found that direct current electrical stimulation combined with instrumentation in lumbosacral fusions improved fusion success rates over noninstrumented fusions. Kucharzyk[28] found, using the Modified Webster Smiley Criteria, that clinical success was greater in patients with instrumentation and direct current stimulation than in patients without electrical stimulation. He also concluded that the combination of electrical stimulation and instrumentation was significantly more cost effective than using bone grafting with electrical stimulation, instrumentation alone, or a simple in-situ noninstrumented fusion.

### Pulsing Electromagnetic Field (PEMF)

The use of external electrical stimulation such as PEMF depends primarily on patient compliance. Simmons et al.[42] found that an external orthosis containing a coil delivering a pulsed electromagnetic current centered over a failed fusion site worn 8 to 10 hours per day for 12 months could provide an effective alternative to the surgical management of failed anterior and posterior lumbar interbody fusions. Lee,[29] like Kane, argued the benefits of PEMF, reporting a 67% success rate when treating pseudarthrosis. Mooney,[36] in a double-blind prospective randomized study, reported increased fusion success rates for a PEMF-stimulated group over controls in high-risk surgical groups, including smokers (89% vs. 60%) and multilevel fusions (89% vs. 54%).

### Capacitively Coupled Electrical Stimulation (CCE)

CCE stimulation, like PEMF, is again largely dependent on patient compliance. The first successful use of CCE stimulation used to augment a lumbar spinal fusion was reported by Goodwin et al.[21] in 1999. This study found that CCE stimulation was an effective adjunct to primary posterolateral fusion and those with internal fixation. In human trials the stimulator is programmed to deliver a sinusoidal waveform pulsed at 60kHz with an amplitude of 5V peak to peak and a current of 7.1 to 10.5mA root mean square. Statistically significant fusion success rates (clinical and radiographic) have been demonstrated clinically with this form of electrical stimulation.

## Summary

Animal studies and multiple clinical trials have reported promising success rates when electrical stimulation is used in the setting of a primary or revision lumbosacral fusion. The use of this technology in clinical investigations has so far been insolated to the lumbosacral spine. Although studies are currently underway evaluating its efficacy in the cervical region, no definitive studies have conclusively supported its role in this spinal region.[24] There are no apparent adverse effects associated with direct implantable or external electrical stimulation, and the benefits of this form of technology have clearly been demonstrated. Strong consideration for the use of adjunctive electrical stimulation should be given to specific patient populations at high risk for spinal pseudarthrosis. This includes patients undergoing revision fusion procedures, active smokers, obese patients, and possibly patients with significant osteoporosis.

## REFERENCES

1. Bassett CAL: Pulsing electromagnetic fields: a new method to modify cell behavior in calcified and noncalcified tissues. *Calcif Tissue Int* 34:1-8, 1982.
2. Bassett CAL, Becker RO: Generation of electric potentials by bone in response to mechanical stress. *Science* 137: 1063-1064, 1962.
3. Bassett CAL, Caulo N, Kort J: Congenital pseudarthrosis of the tibia: treatment with pulsing electromagnetic fields. *Clin Orthop* 154:136-149, 1981.
4. Bassett CAL, Choski H, Hernandez E, et al: The effect of pulsing electromagnetic fields on cellular calcium and calcification of nonunions. In Brighton CT, Black J, Pollack S (eds): *Electrical Properties of Bone and Cartilage*. New York, Grune & Stratton, 1979, pp 427-442.
5. Bassett CAL, Mitchell SN, Gaston SR: Treatment of ununited tibial diaphyseal fractures with pulsing electromagnetic fields. *J Bone Joint Surg* 63A:511-523, 1981.
6. Bassett CAL, Mitchell SN, Gaston SR: Pulsing electromagnetic field treatment in ununited fractures and failed arthrodeses. *J Am Med Assoc* 247:623-628, 1982.
7. Bassett CAL, Mitchell SN, Schink MM: Treatment of therapeutically resistant nonunions with bone grafts and pulsing electromagnetic fields. *J Bone Joint Surg* 64A: 1214-1220, 1982.
8. Bassett CAL, Pawluk RJ, Becker RO: Effects of electric currents on bone formation in vivo. *Nature* 204:652-654, 1964.
9. Bassett CAL, Pawluk RJ, Pilla AA: Augmentation of bone repair by inductively coupled electromagnetic fields. *Ann NY Acad Sci* 238:242-262, 1974.

10. Bassett CAL, Pilla AA, Pawluk RJ: A nonoperative salvage of resistant pseudarthroses and nonunions by pulsing electromagnetic fields. A preliminary report. *Clin Orthop* 124:128-143, 1977.

11. Bassett CAL, Vades M, Hernandez E: Modification of fracture repair with selected pulsing electromagnetic fields. *J Bone Joint Surg* 64:888-895, 1982.

12. Bodamyali T, Kanczler JM, Simon B, *et al:* Effect of faradic products on direct current-stimulated calvarial organ culture calcium levels. *Biochem Biophys Res Commun* 264:657-661, 1999.

13. Bozic KJ, Glazer PA, Zurakowski D, *et al:* In vivo evaluation of coralline hydroxyapatite and direct current electrical stimulation in lumbar spinal fusion. *Spine* 24(20): 2127-2133, 1999.

14. Brighton CT, Black J, Friedenberg ZB, *et al*: A multicenter study of the treatment of non-union with constant direct current. *J Bone Joint Surg* 63A:2-13, 1981.

15. Brighton CT, Black J, Pollack SR: *Electrical Properties of Bone and Cartilage.* New York, Grune & Stratton, 1979.

16. Bush JL, Vaccaro AR: Electrical stimulation in lumbar spinal fusion. *Orthopedics* 23(7):737-743, 2000.

17. Colacicco G, Pilla A: Electromagnetic modulation of biological processes: influence of culture media and significance of methodology on calcium uptake by embryonal chick tibia in vitro. *Calcif Tissue Int* 36:167-174, 1984.

18. Dejardin LM, Kahanovitz N, Arnoczky SP, Simon BJ. The effect of varied electrical current densities on lumbar spinal fusions in dogs. *Spine J* 1(5):341-347, 2001.

19. Dwyer AF: The use of electrical current stimulation in spinal fusion. *Clin Orthop* 6:265-279, 1975.

20. France JC, Norman TL, Santrock RD, *et al:* The efficacy of direct current stimulation for lumbar intertransverse process fusions in an animal model. *Spine* 26(9):1002-1008, 2000.

21. Goodwin CB, Brighton BT, Guyer RD, *et al:* A double blind study of capacitively coupled electrical stimulation as an adjunct to lumbar spinal fusions. *Spine* 24(13): 1349-1357, 1999.

22. Grottkau B, Lipson SJ: *A Controlled Pilot Study to Determine the Effect of Direct Current (DC) Stimulation on Fusion Mass in Lumbar Spinal Fusion Patients.* Presented at the Annual Meeting of the North American Spine Society, 1995, Washington, DC.

23. Hartshorne E: Monograph on "The Causes and Treatment of Pseudarthrosis." *Am J Med Sci* 1:143, 1841.

24. Huckell CB: Clinical outcomes after cervical spine fusion. *Orthop Clin North Am* 29(4):787-799, 1998.

25. Kahanovitz N, Arnoczky SP: The efficacy of direct current electrical stimulation to enhance canine spinal fusion. *Clin Orthop* 251:295-299, 1990.

26. Kahanovitz N, Arnoczky SP, Hulse D, Shires PK: The effect of postoperative electromagnetic pulsing on canine posterior spinal fusions. *Spine* 9:273-278, 1984.

27. Kane WJ: Direct current electrical bone growth stimulation for spinal fusions. *Spine* 13:363-365, 1988.

28. Kucharzyk DW. A controlled prospective outcome study of implantable electrical stimulation with spinal instrumentation in a high risk spinal fusion population. *Spine* 24(5):465-469, 1999.

29. Lee K: *Clinical investigation of the spinal stem system, open trial phase, pseudoarthrosis stratum.* Presented at the Annual Meeting of the AAOS, Las Vegas, Nevada, 1989.

30. Lohmann CH, Schwartz Z, Liu Y, *et al:* Pulsed electrical field stimulation on MG63 osteoblast like cells affects differentiation and local factor production. *J Orthop Res* 18(4):637-646, 2000.

31. Lorich DG, Brighton CT, Gupta R, *et al:* Biochemical pathway mediating the response of bone cells to capacitive coupling. *Clin Orthop Rel Res* 350:246-256, 1998.

32. Matsunaga S, Sakou T, Ijiri K: Osteogenesis by pulsing electromagnetic fields (PEMFs): Optimum stimulation setting. *In Vivo* 10(3):351-356, 1996.

33. Melone CP, Pess GM: Treatment of scaphoid pseudarthrosis with bone grafting and pulsing electromagnetic fields. AAOS Handout, 1986.

34. Meril AJ. Direct current stimulation of allograft in anterior and posterior lumbar interbody fusions. *Spine* 19: 2393-2398, 1994.

35. Mooney V: A randomized double-blind prospective study of the efficacy of pulsed electromagnetic fields for interbody lumbar fusions. *Spine* 15:708-712, 1990.

36. Oishi M, Onesti ST. Electrical bone graft stimulation for spinal fusion: A review. *Neurosurgery* 47(5):1041-1056, 2000.

37. Paterson DC, Lewis GN, Cass CA: Treatment of delayed union and nonunion with an implanted direct current stimulator. *Clin Orthop* 148:117-128, 1980.

38. Reddi AH: Cell biology and biochemistry of endochondral bone development. *Collagen Res* 1:209-226, 1981.

39. Rogozinski A, Rogozinski C. Efficacy of implanted bone growth stimulation in instrumented lumbosacral spinal fusion. *Spine* 21:2479-2483, 1996.

40. Rubin CT, Mcleod KJ, Lanyon LE: Prevention of osteoporosis by pulsed electromagnetic fields. *J Bone Joint Surg* 71A:411-417, 1989.

41. Sharrard WJW: A double-blind trial of pulsed electromagnetic fields for delayed union of tibial fractures. *J Bone Joint Surg* 3:347-355, 1990.

42. Simmons JW: Treatment of failed posterior lumbar interbody fusions of the spine with pulsating electromagnetic fields. *Clin Orthop* 193:127-132, 1985.

43. Steinberg ME, Brighton CT, Corces A, *et al*: Osteonecrosis of the femoral head. *Clin Orthop* 249: 199-208, 1989.

44. Toth JM, Seim HB, Schwardt JD, *et al:* Direct current electrical stimulation increases the fusion rate of spinal fusion cages. *Spine* 25(2):2580-2587, 2000.

45. Uhl RL: The use of electricity in bone healing. *Orthop Rev* 18:1045-1050, 1989.

46. Yasuda I, Noguchi K, Sata T: Dynamic callus and electrical callus. *J Bone Joint Surg* 37A:1292, 1955.

47. Zhuang Z, Wang W, Seldes RM, *et al:* Electrical stimulation induces the level of TGF-β1 mrna in osteoblastic cells by a mechanism involving calcium/calmoduling pathway. *Biochem Biophys Res Commun* 237:225-229, 1997.

# CHAPTER 164

# Management of a Patient with Thoracolumbar Fracture with Complete Myelopathy and a 40-Degree Kyphotic Deformity: Operative or Recumbent Management

## Operative Management

### Sanford J. Larson

The management of a patient with thoracolumbar fracture with complete myelopathy and a 40-degree kyphotic deformity depends on whether the fracture is stable or unstable. Because myelopathy is complete, the major indication for surgery is early mobilization of the patient without the prospect of progressive deformity. If the dorsal ligamentous complex and related bony elements are intact, then the fracture is stable, and progression of deformity under the physiologic loads will not occur. By itself, a 40-degree kyphosis is not an absolute indication for an operation or for prolonged recumbency to improve alignment. If the dorsal elements have been disrupted, however, as suggested by the 40-degree deformity, surgical treatment allows the patient to be out of bed within a few days of the operation without progression of deformity. It may also allow at least partial correction of alignment. With postural management, prolonged recumbency is required, usually about 10 to 12 weeks.[1] This interferes with early, active rehabilitation treatment and introduces the possibility of recumbency-related complications. Even if it can be shown that complications are not significantly different between surgical and recumbent management, mobilization in a wheelchair is preferable to bed rest for 3 months.

The 40-degree kyphotic deformity suggests that this patient has sustained a flexion compression injury with wedging of the vertebral body. Because myelopathy is complete, reconstruction of the spinal canal is not necessary, and only a dorsal approach need be used for instru-

mentation. Correction of the deformity can be achieved by tightening sublaminar wires around Luque rods bent to the desired configuration for the vertebral column[3] or with Harrington rods[2] with more secure fixation supplied by sublaminar wiring. Alternatively, after reduction has been achieved, the Harrington rods can be replaced by segmental instrumentation, which could be with laminar hooks, transverse process pedicle hooks, or pedicle screws. To prevent substantial loss of correction, fixation should extend at least two levels above and two levels below the region of the injury. Even with this arrangement, some loss of correction can be anticipated but should not be significant. The patient can be out of bed in most instances within a few days of surgery.

The major advantages of surgical treatment for this patient are early mobilization without progressive deformity of the vertebral column and more effective rehabilitation.

### REFERENCES

1. Frankel HL, Hancock DO, Hyslop G, et al: The value of postural reduction in the initial management of closed injuries of the spine with paraplegia. Part I. *Paraplegia* 7: 179-192, 1969.
2. Kahn A: Current concepts of internal fixation. In Dunsker SB. Kahn A, Schmidek H, Frymoyer J (eds): *The Unstable Spine*. New York, Grune & Stratton, 1986, pp 45-83.
3. Larson SJ: The thoracolumbar junction. In Dunsker SB, Kahn A, Schmidek H, Frymoyer J (eds): *The Unstable Spine*. New York, Grune & Stratton, 1986, pp 127-152.

## Recumbent Management

### Patrick W. Hitchon

A fracture of the lower half of the thoracic spine or lumbar spine with an angulation of 40 degrees and a complete myelopathy is inherently unstable. Such an angular deformity with compromise of the spinal canal is associated with some disruption of the vertebral bodies and the neural arch. Based on biomechanical and clinical data,[5,12] criteria for instability in this case are satisfied, and appropriate management may therefore consist of either surgical intervention or recumbency until bony fusion occurs. Indeed, recently there has occurred an explosion of spinal implants advocated for the achievement of immediate stability.[6] The intent of such an approach has been early mobilization of the patient, a shorter hospital stay, and the achievement of neural decompression, reduction, and stabilization. Though these goals have often been achieved, the complications of surgical intervention are by no means negligible. Complications arising from surgery include hardware failure and deep vein thrombosis. These in general have exceeded those encountered in recumbency.[5,11,13] This has led to the adoption of a recumbency algorithm in patients who are intact, or those with a total lesion of the spinal cord, in which the chances of improvement are nil. Such a conservative approach in the management of thoracolumbar fractures is by no means new and dates to the 1940s with Ludwig Guttman[4] at the Stoke Mandeville Hospital and E.A. Nicoll[10] at the Mansfield General Hospital. This tradition was subsequently changed by Frankel[3] and Bedbrook[1] in patients with paralysis.

Although neurologic improvement has been found by some to be more commonly associated with surgical management,[8,9] others have reported improvement with both treatment modalities,[6,7,11,13,14] and in some cases more so in patients treated conservatively.[2] No consistent improvement has been reported in complete spinal cord injury with either surgical or recumbency treatment. It has been shown that angular deformity in recumbency patients is of greater magnitude than those treated with open reduction and fixation.[2,8,13] Nevertheless, deformity progresses with the passage of time, irrespective of treatment.[6,7] Angulation in itself, though cosmetically disconcerting, is not necessarily a harbinger of a poor outcome or intractable pain.[1,10,13] In fact, gibbous deformities of up to 40 degrees did not prohibit patients from achieving in some cases satisfactory outcomes and gainful employment in the coal mines.[1,10]

Early surgical intervention for the management of thoracic and lumbar fractures has generally been associated with a shorter hospital stay and rehabilitation times.[2,8,13,14] Although this disparity in hospital times with treatment has been quite marked, according to some, it has amounted to only 5 to 7 days according to others.[6,7,11] Indeed, the longevity of hospitalization and rehabilitation are of great concern in this age of skyrocketing medical costs. Nevertheless, the cost of surgical intervention, the use of the operating room, anesthesia, expendables, implants, and surgeon's fees are by no means negligible. In fact, a comparative analysis of hospital costs was conducted between 36 patients treated operatively and 32 treated nonoperatively.[7] This showed an overall cost of $63,000 for the former compared with $27,000 for the latter. An important consideration in this analysis, however, is the proximity and the ease with which a patient can be referred to rehabilitation subsequent to surgery. It would appear that there is no significant relationship between the incidence of pain and employability and the modality of treatment.[7,13]

In a patient with a complete lesion secondary to a thoracolumbar fracture associated with a 40-degree kyphotic deformity, surgical intervention may be contraindicated. These patients may have visceral injuries, pulmonary contusions, hemopneumothorax, and respiratory insufficiency. In addition to head injury, these patients may require prolonged ventilatory support. Their stay in the intensive care unit may further be complicated by pneumonia, sepsis, and oftentimes posttraumatic pancreatitis. These conditions militate against surgical intervention of any type, let alone a lengthy procedure of spinal stabilization with the potential for significant blood loss. Under those circumstances,

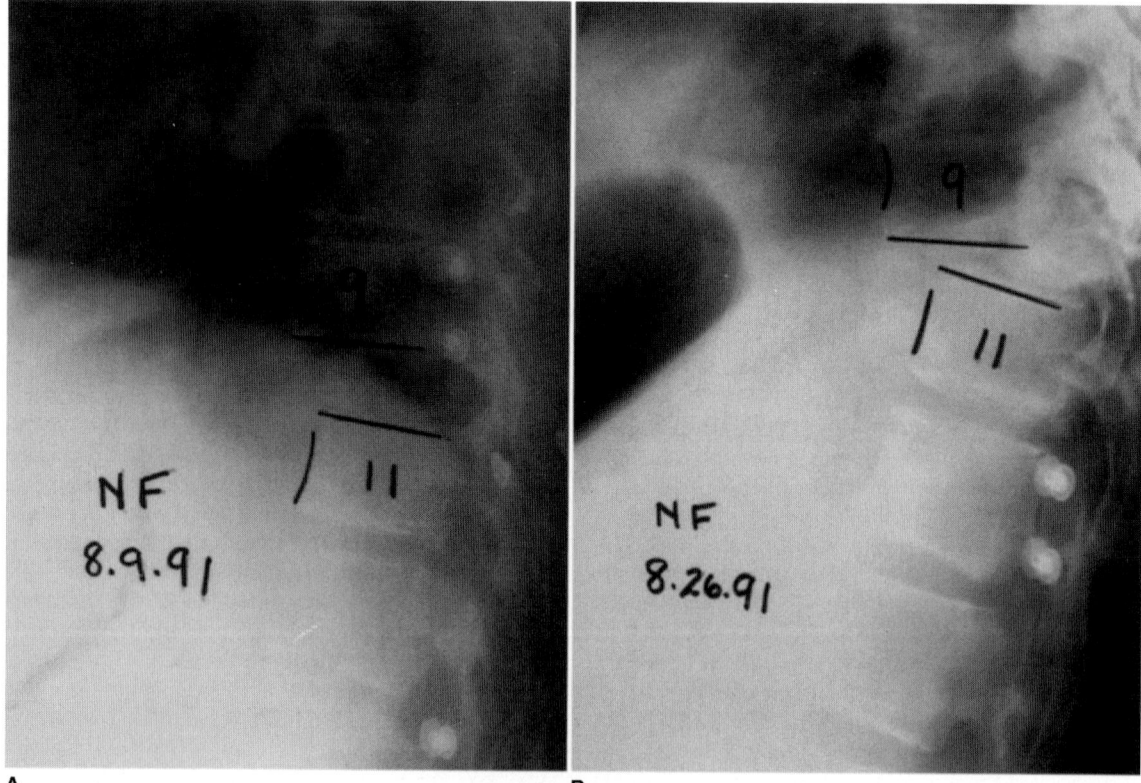

**A**    **B**

**Figure 164.1** Surgery for the unstable T10 fracture in this male aged 36 years with complete myelopathy was contraindicated owing to alcoholic hepatitis, coagulopathy, and respiratory failure. Lateral radiograph (**A**) was obtained 2 months after his injury, showing the burst fracture of T10 and ventrolisthesis of T9 on T11. After mobilization in thoracolumbar orthosis (**B**), further listhesis and angulation is noted that was associated with discomfort. With this attempt having failed, surgical intervention was undertaken in the face of a mild coagulopathy.

recumbency may often be the only treatment that can be offered to such patients. After 4 to 6 weeks of bed rest on oral, parenteral, or nasogastric feeding, bony healing is well under way. Patients can then be mobilized gradually in a customized plastic thoracolumbar orthosis. Radiographs are usually obtained sequentially at 45 and 90 degrees to confirm stability and the absence of progressive kyphosis. In the absence of instability, rehabilitation can proceed rapidly thereafter. The clamshell thoracolumbar orthosis is worn whenever the patient is sitting up for a total of 3 to 5 months, depending on the extent of dislocation or angulation. Upright films are usually obtained at 3, 6, and 12 months. In the presence of increasing pain, or progressive angulation noted on radiographs, surgical stabilization may be undertaken at that time, as was the case in the patient shown in Figure 164-1.

# REFERENCES

1. Bedbrook GM, Ohn WA: Treatment of thoracolumbar dislocation and fractures with paraplegia. *Clin Orthop Rel Res* 112:27-43, 1975.

2. Davies WE, Morris JH, Hill V: An analysis of conservative (non-surgical) management of thoracolumbar fractures and fracture-dislocations with neural damage. *J Bone Joint Surg* 62A:1324-1328, 1980.

3. Frankel HL, Hancock DO, Hyslop G, *et al*: The value of postural reduction in the initial management of closed injuries of the spine with paraplegia and tetraplegia. Part I. *Paraplegia* 7:179-192, 1969.

4. Guttmann L: Surgical aspects of the treatment of traumatic paraplegia. *J Bone Joint Surg* 31B:399-403, 1949.

5. Hitchon PW: Instability of the thoracic and lumbar spine. In Hitchon PW, Traynelis VT, Rengachary S (eds): *Techniques in Spinal Fusion and Stabilization*. Thieme, 1995, pp 51-58.

6. Hitchon PW, Torner JC, Haddad SS, Follett KF: Thoracic lumbar fractures: management analysis. In Hitchon PW, Traynelis VT, Rengachary S (eds): *Techniques in Spinal Fusion and Stabilization*. Thieme, 1995, pp 338-344.

7. Hitchon PW, Torner JC, Haddad SS, Follett KF: Management options in thoracolumbar burst fractures. *Surg Neurol* 49:619-27, 1998.

8. Jacobs RR, Asher MA, Snider RK: Thoracolumbar spinal injuries: a comparative study of recumbent and operative treatment in 100 patients. *Spine* 5:463-477, 1980.

9. McEvoy RD, Bradford DS: The management of burst fractures of the thoracic and lumbar spine: experience in 53 patients. *Spine* 10:631-637, 1985.

10. Nicoll EA: Fracture of the dorso-lumbar spine. *J Bone Joint Surg* 31B:376-394, 1949.

11. Tator CH, Duncan EG, Edmonds VE, *et al*: Comparison of surgical and conservative management in 208 patients with acute spinal cord injury. *Can J Neurol Sci* 14:60-69, 1987.

12. White AA, III, Panjabi MM: The problem of clinical instability in the human spine: a systematic approach. In White AA, III Panjabi MM (eds): *Clinical Biomechanics of the Spine*, ed 2. New York, Lippincott-Raven, 1990, pp 277-378.

13. Willén J, Lindahl S, Nordwall A: Unstable thoracolumbar fractures: a comparative clinical study of conservative treatment and Harrington instrumentation. *Spine* 10: 111-122, 1985.

14. Wilmot CB, Hall KM: Evaluation of acute surgical intervention in traumatic paraplegia. *Paraplegia* 24:71-76, 1986.

# CHAPTER 165

# Management of Symptomatic Osteoporotic Vertebral Compression

## Vertebroplasty

### John A. Carrino and Alexander R. Vaccaro

Percutaneous vertebroplasty (PV) is an imaging guided procedure that reinforces a compromised vertebra with polymethyl methacrylate (PMMA), alleviating pain and improving mobility of patients. Initially described in 1987 by two French radiologists[1] as a treatment for painful hemangiomas of the spine and subsequently reported by several groups in Europe, PV was introduced to the United States in the mid-1990s by radiologists at the University of Virginia. The most common indications for this procedure are osteoporotic compression fractures or neoplasm involving the vertebrae (typically metastatic disease or hemangiomas). Overall, the patients with osteoporosis do quite well early on with respect to pain management, and this therapeutic phenomenon has led to the popularity of this procedure.

## Background and Indications

Presently, treatments of vertebral body fractures are less than adequate, therefore there is a need for interventions that decrease the likelihood of occurrence of these fractures and improve the treatment options once they have occurred.[2] One broad category of intervention entails the augmentation of the vertebral bodies. The fundamental indications for PV are persistently painful compression fractures (typically osteoporosis related) despite correct medical (non-surgical) treatment and benign or malignant osteolytic neoplasms (aggressive hemangioma, metastasis, and myeloma). In the setting of osteoporosis, PV is primarily done for pain management and secondarily for prevention of further collapse. For neoplasm, the indications are somewhat broader, and the procedure may be done for pain management and/or stabilization. PV is not an ablative procedure per se. Reinforcement may produce analgesia or allow other therapies such as radiotherapy or surgical resection and fixation to ensue while minimizing the risk of further collapse or fracture.

The specific indications for PV are (1) osteoporotic compression fractures refractory to non-surgical therapy, typically associated with inability to perform activities of daily living; (2) Kummell's disease (osteonecrosis); (3) multiple compression deformities such that if additional collapse would occur it would result in respiratory or gastrointestinal compromise or would change the center of gravity, increasing fall risk; (4) unstable compression fractures showing movement at the wedge deformity; and (5) osteolysis related to malignant or benign neoplasms with fracture or impending risk of fracture. The indications have also been expanded to include nonunions of chronic traumatic fractures that show a pseudarthrosis with a fluid-filled cleft or cystic findings. Categorically, precise patient selection is essential to the therapeutic success of PV. Patients with prior unsuccessful spinal surgery generally do not seem to respond as well to PV.

The absolute contraindications to PV in osteoporotic patients are (1) an asymptomatic stable fracture, (2) a patient showing substantial symptomatic improvement with time, and (3) prophylactic vertebral augmentation in the setting of osteoporosis without an acute compression fracture in a patient not undergoing reconstructive spinal surgery. The absolute contraindications to PV for either osteoporotic or neoplastic conditions are (1) infection (osteomyelitis and discitis), (2) uncorrectable coagulopathy, and (3) allergy to any component required for the procedure. Acute traumatic fracture of a non-osteoporotic vertebra is also considered a contraindication.

The relative contraindications are (1) a compression fracture with a minor degree of axial pain with or without radicular pain, caused by a compressive lesion unrelated to the vertebral body collapse (if a spinal destabilization procedure will be performed then preoperative vertebroplasty may be indicated); (2) retropulsion of fracture fragment(s) causing substantial spinal canal compromise (e.g., a burst-type fracture); (3) neoplasm extending into the epidural space with substantial spinal canal compromise; (4) severe vertebral collapse such that it would be technically challenging to place a needle; (5) chronic stable fracture without pain; and (6) treatment of more than three levels performed at one time.

## Selection Process

The selection process nominally includes (1) preevaluation imaging, (2) concordant pain evaluation (for osteoporotic compression fractures), (3) candidate assessment, (4) anesthesia considerations, and (5) informed consent.

Preevaluation imaging entails demonstrating an "active" fracture by magnetic resonance (MR) imaging (i.e., bone marrow edema) or nuclear medicine scintigram ("bone scan") and excluding unknown or unsuspected malignancy or degenerative disease (e.g., herniated discs). This usually entails obtaining recent MR imaging within 7 to 10 days of consultation. A specific protocol is employed with sagittal T1-weighted CSE (conventional spin echo), sagittal $T_2$-weighted FSE (fast spin echo) or TSE (turbo spin echo) with fat saturation and axial T2 FSE through areas of abnormality. If fat suppression is not available for the $T_2$-weighted images (either in a magnet with poor homogeneity or in a low field strength system), then a STIR (short tau inversion recovery) sequence should be substituted. The fluid-sensitive sequences (T2 with fat suppression or STIR images) are necessary for the determination of the level of an "active" compression fracture. While the causes of bone marrow edema are legion, in the context of compression fractures and appropriate clinical symptoms, it often indicates a persistent pain generator. The age of the compression fracture is less important then the presence of bone marrow edema on MR imaging. This becomes relevant for people who have had symptoms for months or years. Radiography is useful for showing the degree of collapse. With complete or near complete vertebral collapse, successful PV is unlikely in most cases.

Concordant pain evaluation is also a critical aspect for determining patients with benign compression fractures that will respond to PV. A physical examination under fluoroscopy may be performed to determine whether the patient's symptoms are concordant with the level of the active compression fracture on MRI. Under fluoroscopy, the back is percussed and palpated over the spinous processes, marking the areas of tenderness. The patient also assumes any position that triggers the pain and marks the painful site. If the pain corresponds to the fractured level (usually within 1 level above or below), then the symptoms are likely to be amenable to PV at that vertebral level.

Candidate assessment consists of synthesizing the history, imaging, and fluoroscopy examination. In addition, this requires an evaluation of the patient's physical, physiologic, emotional and mental status. If the patient is a candidate, he or she will require a further work-up. In addition, there are several special situations encountered. Patients on Coumadin need to have this discontinued prior to procedure and potentially be switched to heparin for the periprocedural period. Patients with a fever, leukocytosis, or an elevated erythrocyte sedimentation rate need to wait until the cause is diagnosed and treated (presumably an infection). For patients on steroids, one will need to work closely with the primary care provider to manage the dose during the periprocedural period. If the patient is not deemed a candidate, he or she often needs referrals to other spine pain specialists.

The informed consent process is usually a comprehensive discussion of the risks, benefits, and alternatives to PV. Risks include bleeding, infection, allergic reaction to the PMMA, fracture (pedicle or rib), and PMMA extravasation. Pneumothorax is also a potential risk for thoracic levels. In the authors' opinion, informed consent also consists of an explanation of the purpose (e.g., pain management, preventing further deformity, stabilization for radiotherapy), theoretical background (stabilization by internal "casting"), technical aspects (needle procedure versus open surgery), and clinical data regarding PV. This often includes answering questions regarding the nature of osteoporosis and the status of PV as "standard of care" versus an "experimental procedure" including the off label use of the cement (PMMA) and the modification of PMMA by additional sterile barium to increase opacification (thus allowing early detection of extravasation). The need for possible emergent spinal decompression should be addressed. In the United States, informed consent must be obtained in compliance with state law.

Anesthesia considerations revolve around the patient's physiologic status. However, PV may be accomplished with neuroleptic anesthesia (conscious sedation), MAC, or general anesthesia. Advantages to using intravenous conscious sedation (IVCS) are that the patient is able to relate if there is an immediate complication and thus minimize any further damage by allowing the operator to immediately halt the injection. It also facilitates PV as a same day outpatient procedure with quicker recovery period. For these reasons, IVCS is considered the preferred mode of sedation when possible. Intravenous antibiotic (cefazolin or clindamycin if penicillin allergy) is typically given as infection prophylaxis.

## Technical Aspects (Figures 165-1 to 165-5)

The technique for PV entails penetration of the involved vertebra(e) via a transpedicular or posterolateral (parapedicular) approach followed by injection of polymethyl methacrylate (PMMA) into the vertebral body. The posterolateral (parapedicular) approach is accomplished by entering just lateral to where the pedicle joins the vertebral body (this is most typically done under CT guidance). The traditional mode has been to perform bilateral injections with a two-needle technique. However, unipedicular injections also result in substantial vertebral reinforcement when adequate volumes of cement are injected that cross the midline of the vertebral body and result in a similar distribution to bipedicular injections.[3] The ability to produce this is enhanced by using a modified transpedicular approach, which is an oblique (versus parasagittal) targeting of the pedicle while visualizing a "Scotty Dog" projection. However, to avoid the tendency for accepting suboptimal flow, some practitioners have routinely placed two needles into the body to be treated.

The modalities used are either fluoroscopy or computed tomography (CT) imaging. PV can adequately be accomplished with either single or bi-plane fluoroscopy. Bi-plane fluoroscopy is considered ideal because one can expedite viewing orthogonal projections without tube rotation. Poor quality C-arms should be avoided. The procedure time will be increased with a single-plane unit. Intermittent fluoroscopy allows the real-time or near real-time viewing of the injection, and last image hold is valuable to detect subtle differences in PMMA spread. CT is more asynchronous because of repositioning the gantry between needle manipulations, imaging and, injection. Because of the intermittent nature of table positioning, useful injection time is consumed. Some configurations have a combination of a CT and C-arm fluoroscopy, placing the needles under CT and injecting under fluoroscopy.[4] Yet another modality is CT-fluoroscopy, which allows the user to generate real-time CT sections while performing procedures. The concerns with CT-fluoroscopy revolve around the increased radiation dose delivered to the operator in the room during the procedure.

The needles used are standard bone marrow biopsy type needles that have a Luer-lock connection. Both beveled or pointed tips can be effectively used, and which to use is based largely on operator preference and experience. Initial cortical puncture and purchase should be obtained by hand,

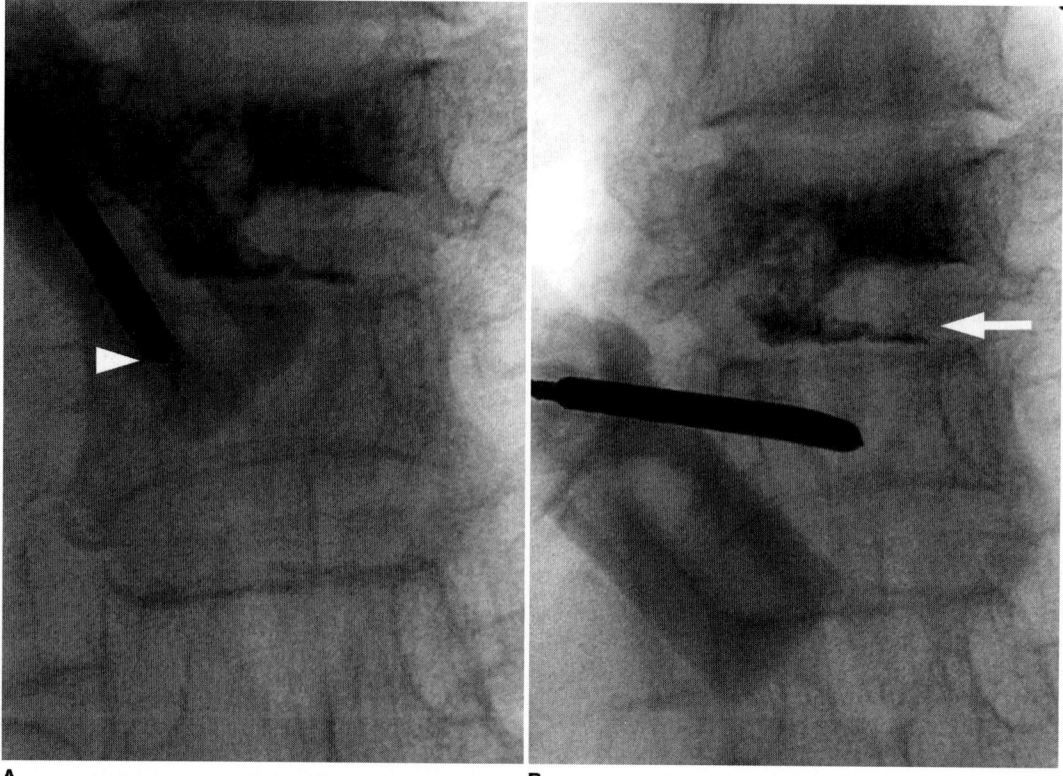

**A**                                         **B**

**Figure 165.1** Parasagittal approach. Anteroposterior projection fluoroscopic image shows typical position for the parasagittal transpedicular puncture. **(A)** Note that the initial puncture site is with the needle tip located in the superolateral corner of the ring shadow of the pedicle *(arrowhead)*. **(B)** The needle has been advanced to the anterior one third of the vertebral body and the tip is somewhat centrally located but still ipsilateral. Note the intradiscal cement from injection of the level above *(arrow)*.

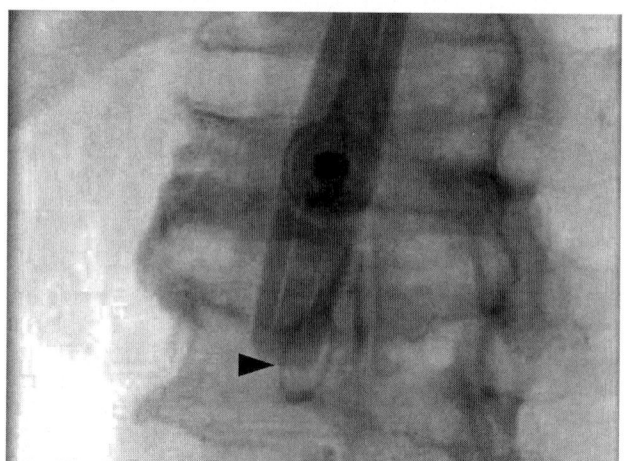

**Figure 165.2** "Scotty dog" approach. Oblique projection fluoroscopic image shows typical position for transpedicular puncture when using the "Scotty dog" approach. Note that the target is the ring shadow of the pedicle in an approximately 45-degree obliquity *(arrowhead points to the pedicle below the punctured level for reference)*. This trajectory places the needle tip centrally and facilitates filling of both sides from a unilateral injection.

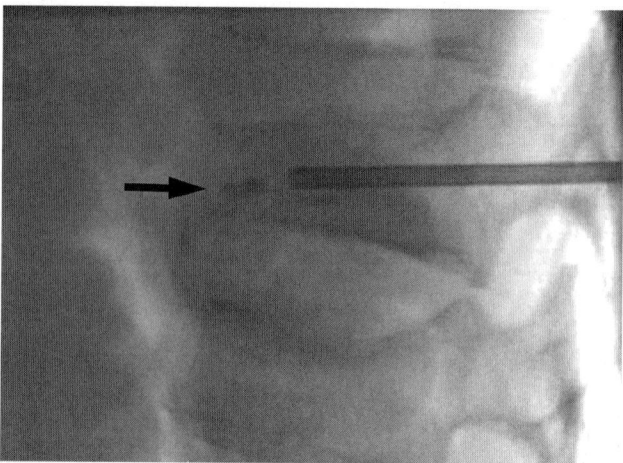

**Figure 165.3** Needle tip position. Sagittal projection fluoroscopic image shows appropriate needle tip position within the anterior one quarter to one third of the vertebral body. Note the small amount of cement injected that has begun to fill the fracture line *(arrow)*.

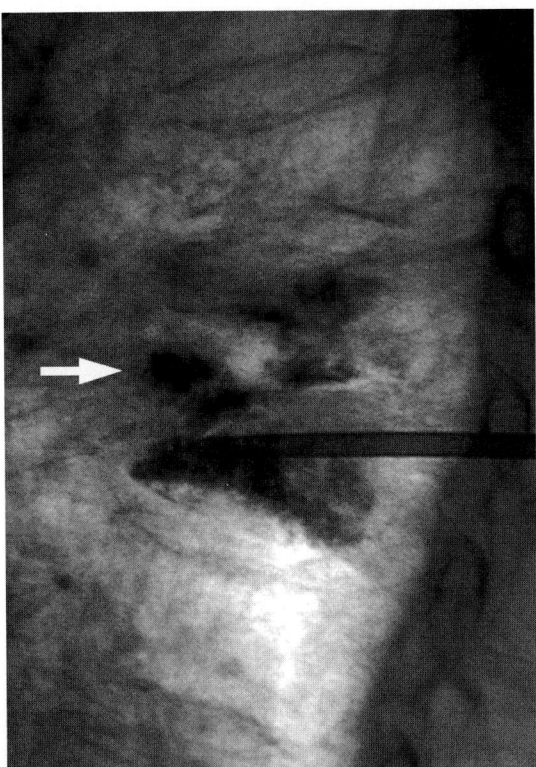

**Figure 165.4** Cement extravasation. Sagittal projection fluoroscopic image shows a small amount of cement that has extravasated anteriorly *(arrow)* outside of the vertebral body into the retroperitoneum. Extravasation in this location is usually not clinically significant.

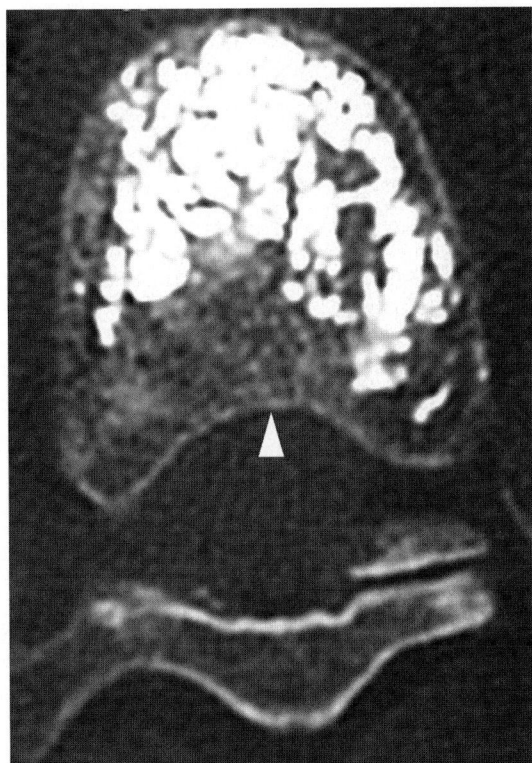

**Figure 165.5** Cement distribution. Axial CT image shows hyperattenuating cement in the anterior and mid portions of the vertebral body. Note that the posterior vertebral margin is concave *(arrowhead)*. This forms the posterior vertebral line on lateral radiography or fluoroscopy and is also the location where the basivertebral venous plexus perforates the cortex (not shown). Therefore cement should not be injected in an attempt to fill the entire posterior aspect of vertebral body under fluoroscopy.

and then needle advancement may be by hand or with the assistance of a mallet. For lumbar levels, 10-11 gauge needles are used, but for the thoracic levels, the authors prefer 13- to 14-gauge needles. The needle tips should be place in the anterior one fourth to one third of the vertebral body. This is to facilitate filling of the fracture area, which is typically anterosuperior, and to avoid injection into the larger vascular sinusoids of the basivertebral plexus, which may allow preferential flow into the epidural space.

Some practitioners perform pretreatment venography (i.e., a vertebrogram). The original rationale was to identify if the needle tip was in a major basivertebral vein branch. In this case, one might reposition the needle or change polymerization time. Experience has shown that if you do see venous opacification, PMMA does not necessarily follow suit because of the difference in viscosity. Other anecdotes describe persistent contrast in vertebra or discs that is hard to flush out even with multiple saline injections. When this occurs it might be difficult to assess cement distribution because it is obscured by the contrast (even with masking and digital subtraction imaging it can difficult because of patient motion over 10 to 15 minutes). Many practitioners did not substantially alter the injection pattern, and thus the trend has been to abandon the vertebrogram.

The cement flow needs to be carefully monitored, and the injection should cease if there is resistance or cement approaches the posterior vertebral margin. If any extraosseous cement is identified, the injection should be terminated immediately. Multiple levels, up to three, can be done in a single session. Most commonly, only one or two levels are done at a time. The risk of doing numerous levels simultaneously is that the PMMA can cause significant fat emboli because of the marrow displacement.

Post-procedure care includes keeping the patient in bed without head elevation for at least 1 hour followed by bed rest with head of bed elevated less than 45 degrees. This additional recovery period consists of 1 to 3 hours of observation depending on the patient's status. The operator or other qualified staff member should supervise initial ambulation of the patient. If any new severe pain or new neurologic symptoms develop, a CT scan should be done immediately to evaluate the distribution of cement.

The discharge plan should include post-procedure pain management in conjunction with the referring provider. Written discharge instructions are given to the patient with a plan for pain management, especially for the first few days, related to the morbidity from the needle placement. The goal is to start tapering narcotic usage at 1 to 2 weeks after the procedure. A decrease in analgesic use is encouraged on an "as needed" basis so that assessment of pain reduction can be made. For patients who have been at bed rest for a long time, a gradual increase in activity is recommended. Patients are encouraged to have a gradual return to activity with or without a short course of physical therapy. Short-term bracing may also be useful. All patients should be in a medical therapy program for treating underlying osteoporosis. Careful coordination and communication should be maintained with the referring provider regarding the patient status and expectation of benefit. Discharge follow-up involves either a phone call 24 to 48 hours after the procedure or more commonly an office visit to assess the clinical progress of the patient.

## Cement Issues

There are many issues related to the cement used in PV. These include (1) what to inject, (2) how to inject it, and (3) how much to inject. The bone cement presently used for PV is most commonly some form of polymethyl methacrylate (PMMA). The U.S. FDA (Food and Drug Administration) treats bone cement as a device, and there is currently no PMMA specifically approved for PV. The most salient considerations for choice of an agent include ability to increase vertebral strength and stiffness, visibility under fluoroscopy, ease of cement flow, and simplicity of use.

The two most popular preparations used for PV are Cranioplastic Type I Slow Set (Codman, Johnson & Johnson) and Simplex P (Stryker-Howmedica-Osteonics). Simplex P is approved by the FDA as a structural device for use in pathologic fractures in bones throughout the body, but the approval does not specify PV per se. Simplex P was the original PMMA used for the first PV by Deramond in 1984 and has remained popular for this application in Europe and the United States. In a comparison of three types of PMMA in cadavers (Cranioplastic, Osteobond, Simplex P), vertebrae were significantly stronger after cement injection, regardless of cement type. However, Simplex P restored stiffness to initial values, whereas vertebra injected with Cranioplastic were significantly less stiff than in their initial state.[5]

These preparations (mixed according to the package insert) produce cement that is difficult to inject and poorly visualized by fluoroscopy (although quite suitable for radiography). Thus the addition of an opaque agent (sterile barium, tantalum, or tungsten) is required. Sterile barium preparations are available from Parallax (Mountainview, CA) or Bryan Corporation (Woburn, MA). It has been determined that PMMA mixtures containing approximately 25% to 30% by weight of barium sulfate will provide opacification sufficient for the performance of fluoroscopically guided PV.[5,6]

Another challenge has been to obtain suitable working times for injection. This goal is accomplished by prolonging the polymerization phase. Some operators add the liquid monomer to a modified powder (PMMA with barium) until it reaches a certain consistency. However, without a specific formula or recipe, alterations in the monomer-to-polymer ratio are variable, leaving the biomechanical properties uncertain. There are descriptions of various recipes, which likely change the cement's material properties; however, it is unknown whether there is a difference in clinical therapeutic efficacy.[7] Some advocate that rather than altering the monomer to copolymer ratio, one may manipulate thermal factors (i.e., temperature) to control the work time of the cement. This is accomplished by refrigerating all the cement components (monomer, polymer, barium) for 24 hours prior to use. It is brought out just prior to mixing. In addition, the reservoir holding the PMMA mixture may be chilled with a sterile saline pack or sterile cold-water bath. Cement should not be injected in a completely liquid state (prior to beginning polymerization), as this increases the risk of leak into communicating vascular elements. As cement begins to polymerize, it remains workable after it is no longer injectable with a syringe. Reinserting the trocar and slowly emptying the cannula can introduce the residual cement (approximately 0.7ml) in this otherwise "dead space." These techniques allow one to get a very acceptable working time from the bone cement. No matter what type of cement is used, it should be mixed only after all needle placements have been completed.

There are several types of mixing and delivery systems already available (Cook, Parallax, and Stryker-Howmedica-Osteonics), and this is an avid area of development. Popular approaches have been to use high-pressure (angioplasty type) small volume (1 to 3ml) syringes and more recently reservoir-type injectors that are connected via a Luer-lock mechanism to a bone marrow biopsy type needle. Cement is loaded into the delivery system for injection only when needed (i.e., after all needles have been placed), and this keeps the cement that is not being injected chilled and prolongs its useful work time. In addition, some delivery systems use a sealed vacuum container for mixing the polymer and monomer to reduce exposure to fumes. However, at least one study has shown that for typical PV working conditions, the methyl methacrylate vapor concentrations measured are well below the recommended maximum exposure.[8]

Injection is done into one needle at a time. This is prudent for two main reasons. First, this ensures that the second needle stays clean and does not plug prematurely with polymerizing cement should an unanticipated delay occur. If the cement mixed polymerizes too rapidly and the first injection is inadequate, then a new batch can be mixed for the second injection through an unused needle. Second, there may be suitable filling from the first needle and obviate the need to inject through the second needle.

With respect to how much cement mixture to inject, there has been an *in vitro* assessment demonstrating that initial vertebral body strength is restored with as little as 2ml of cement, but significantly greater stiffness requires 4 to 8ml, depending on vertebral level and type of cement.[9] These types of data provide guidance on the cement volumes needed to restore biomechanical integrity and parallel the clinical experience that many patients do well without the need to fill an entire vertebral body. Therefore one trend has been to use less cement, thus minimizing the risk of complications from extravasation.

Because of the limitations of current PMMA and opacification agent recipes described previously, there is an interest in developing dedicated substances for use in PV. New biomaterials such as nanoparticles and Orthocomp (a glass-ceramic-reinforced BisGMA/BisEMA/TEGDMA matrix composite) are being actively pursued, and it is likely that there will be specific formulations available for PV shortly.[10]

## Neoplasm

The application of PV in the setting of neoplasm is somewhat different than in the treatment of painful osteoporotic compression fractures. The techniques are similar, but the goals and results are slightly different. PV is not an ablative procedure, and the goal is not to aim for the lesion (i.e., not targeting the center or the periphery of the tumor). In the tumor cases the primary goal is to provide structural support, and the secondary goal is pain relief. This is vice versa in osteoporosis. The amount of PMMA used may be greater because there is a trend in osteoporosis to minimize injectant volume to the location of the fracture region (i.e., filling the fracture line). The mechanism of effect is most likely related to increased strength and stiffness and not a thermal ablative phenomenon.[11]

The neoplasms most commonly treated are hemangiomas and metastases (typically from adenocarcinomas). Hemangiomas are vascular neoplasms composed of endothelial cells and have been likened to a "blood-filled sponge." While they have a benign histology, they may exhibit an aggressive growth pattern and come to clinical attention (hence the term "aggressive hemangioma"). PV consolidates the vertebral body and reduces the risk of hemorrhage. Subsequent surgery may then be focused on decompression and epidural extension resection.[12] In this fashion, PV is another adjuvant treatment akin to intralesional sclerosis or embolotherapy preoperatively. PV is also efficacious in treating osseous vertebral metastases that result in pain or instability, providing immediate and long-term pain relief, and contributes to spinal stabilization.[13] Preprocedural MR imaging in this context is used to evaluate the soft tissue extent of the tumor (e.g., spinal canal involvement, neuroforaminal encroachment, and status of the PLL).

Specific technical considerations include needle placement, cement volume, and adjuvant therapy. Needle placement is similar to that in osteoporosis cases (transpedicular or parapedicular approach) and not necessarily altered based on lesion location. Placement of the tip is into the midline of the anterior portion of the vertebral body. The goal in the PMMA application is to obtain craniocaudal filling (attempting to get superior to inferior end plate filling) that crosses the midline transversely providing a strut. The cement may fill part of the tumor. However, attempting to fill the whole tumor is not advised. This may be difficult or impossible to accomplish, and there is a risk that the neoplastic tissue would be displaced into the canal, causing a symptomatic stenosis, which may make surgical debulking more difficult. In addition, it is still controversial as to whether the PMMA is in itself toxic to the tumor, and it is generally felt that the tumor is killed within 2mm of the cement from the exothermic reaction. Thus, filling of the tumor is not the critical aspect of the procedure. However, it is vital that adjuvant therapy (surgery, chemotherapy, or radiotherapy) be performed (or at least considered) in addition to the PV so that tumor kill can be achieved. For cases involving malignant neoplasm, there is the possibility of vascular tumor seeding as the PMMA enters areas of hypervascularity and neovascularity displacing tumor into the vascular system. While there is no literature regarding this issue, it is felt to be a non-trivial risk. In addition, patients may also need to be admitted overnight (23-hour stay) for pain control and the potential for tumor necrosis factor syndrome.

## Complications

Fortunately, major complications are uncommon. The most common complication will be radicular pain caused by migration of cement into the epidural venous plexus. Paralysis has been reported, but is exceptional and less likely to occur if the procedure is performed in a controlled image-guided fashion (by using a bi-plane real time fluoroscopy suite). Also noted have been rib, pedicle, or transverse process fractures. In most patients, intradiscal and paravertebral leaks of cement have no clinical importance.[14] However, there certainly have been case reports of severe neurologic complications, which underscores the need for appropriate safeguards as outlined previously.[15] There has also been a case report of a pulmonary embolism caused by acrylic cement. This rare complication was felt to occur because periverterbral venous migration was not recognized.[16] The anticipated complication rate is higher for treating neoplasms (10%) than for osteoporotic compression fractures (1% to 3%).

## Clinical Experience

The early clinical results for PV are very promising. Overall, there is a high technical success rate reported for accomplishing PV with minimal complications by experienced operators. Several retrospective studies have been performed and uniformly report good pain relief and reduced requirements for analgesics following PV.[17-21] In one series of 26 patients treated for osteoporotic compression fracture, 90% reported significant pain relief immediately after treatment.[17] In this study, the clinical results were not correlated to the extent of vertebral body filling. The patients with osteoporosis who seem to respond best to vertebroplasty are ones that have only one or two new fractures that are not severely compressed (vertebra plana is a relative contraindication), and have had a fracture for less than 12 months. Patients who are likely to benefit have fracture(s) that demonstrate bone marrow edema on MRI or radiotracer uptake on a nuclear medicine bone scintigram. The patient should be in significant pain and the pain from the fracture should alter their lifestyle. PV is also been shown to be beneficial as part of the treatment for osteolytic metastases and multiple myeloma lesions.[18] PV cannot correct curvature (kyphosis) of the spine caused by osteoporosis but may help to prevent worsening deformity and the ensuing thoracoabdominal complications. There are no data to support the use of PV to prophylactically stabilize osteoporotic vertebral bodies at risk for fracture. Nevertheless, while the principle of vertebral body augmentation remains encouraging, data to support widespread use have been primarily retrospective, and the indications are yet to be firmly established. Prospective clinical trials and randomized control trials are underway.

## Summary

The decision to perform PV should be made by a multidisciplinary team, because the choice between vertebroplasty, kyphoplasty, surgery, radiation therapy, medical treatment, or a combination thereof depends on a number of factors. Vertebroplasty should be viewed as only one component of a comprehensive program to manage osteoporosis and its complications. Of course, medical evaluation and treatment are paramount. The augmentation of vertebral bodies that have already fractured is likely to prove useful by reducing pain, improving function, and preventing further collapse and deformity. However, meticulous attention to techniques makes PV a safe and successful procedure.

## ACR Standard

The ACR (American College of Radiology) has a standard for the performance of PV, which was developed a by a consensus panel consisting of neuroradiologists, musculoskeletal radiologists, neurologic surgeons, and orthopedic surgeons. This document is available from the ACR website (www.acr.org) as a PDF (portable document file).

## REFERENCES

1. Galibert P, Deramond H, Rosat P, Le Gars D: [Preliminary note on the treatment of vertebral angioma by percutaneous acrylic vertebroplasty]. *Neurochirurgie* 33:166-168, 1987.
2. Bostrom MP, Lane JM: Future directions. Augmentation of osteoporotic vertebral bodies. *Spine* 22(24 suppl):39S-42S, 1997.
3. Tohmeh AG, Mathis JM, Fenton DC, *et al:* Biomechanical efficacy of unipedicular versus bipedicular vertebroplasty for the management of osteoporotic compression fractures. *Spine* 24:1772-1776, 1999.
4. Gangi A, Kastler BA, Dietemann JL: Percutaneous vertebroplasty guided by a combination of CT and fluoroscopy. *AJNR Am J Neuroradiol* 15(1):83-86, 1994.
5. Belkoff SM, Maroney M, Fenton DC, Mathis JM: An in vitro biomechanical evaluation of bone cements used in percutaneous vertebroplasty. *Bone* 25:23S-26S, 1999.
6. Jasper L, Deramond H, Mathis JM, Belkoff SM: Evaluation of PMMA cements altered for use in vertebroplasty. Presented at the 10th Interdisciplinary Research Conference on Injectable Biomaterials, Amiens (France), March 14-15, 2000.
7. Jasper LE, Deramond H, Mathis JM, Belkoff SM: The effect of monomer-to-powder ratio on the material properties of cranioplastic. *Bone* 25:27S-29S, 1999.
8. Cloft HJ, Easton DN, Jensen ME, *et al:* Exposure of medical personnel to methylmethacrylate vapor during percutaneous vertebroplasty. *AJNR Am J Neuroradiol* 20(2):352-353, 1999.
9. Belkoff SM, Mathis JM, Jasper LE, Deramond H: The biomechanics of vertebroplasty the effect of cement volume on mechanical behavior. *Spine* 26(14):1537-1541, 2001.
10. Belkoff SM, Mathis JM, Erbe EM, Fenton DC: Biomechanical evaluation of a new bone cement for use in vertebroplasty. *Spine* 25(9):1061-1064, 2000.
11. Deramond H, Wright NT, Belkoff SM: Temperature elevation caused by bone cement polymerization during vertebroplasty. *Bone* 25(2 Suppl):17S-21S, 1999.
12. Ide C, Gangi A, Rimmelin A, *et al:* Vertebral haemangiomas with spinal cord compression: the place of preoperative percutaneous vertebroplasty with methyl methacrylate. *Neuroradiology* 38(6):585-589, 1996.
13. Weill A, Chiras J, Simon JM, *et al:* Spinal metastases: indications for and results of percutaneous injection of acrylic surgical cement. *Radiology* 199(1):241-247, 1996.
14. Cotten A, Dewatre F, Cortet B, *et al:* Percutaneous vertebroplasty for osteolytic metastases and myeloma: effects of the percentage of lesion filling and the leakage of methyl methacrylate at clinical follow-up. *Radiology* 200(2):525-530, 1996.
15. Harrington KD: Major neurological complications following percutaneous vertebroplasty with polymethylmethacrylate: A case report. *J Bone Joint Surg* 83:1070-1073, 2001.
16. Padovani B, Kasriel O, Brunner P, Peretti-Viton P: Pulmonary embolism caused by acrylic cement: a rare complication of percutaneous vertebroplasty. *AJNR Am J Neuroradiol* 20(3):375-377, 1999.
17. Jensen ME, Evans AJ, Mathis JM, *et al:* Percutaneous polymethylmethacrylate vertebroplasty in the treatment of osteoporotic vertebral body compression fractures: technical aspects. *AJNR Am J Neuroradiol* 10:1897-1904, 1997.
18. Cortet B, Cotten A, Boutry N, *et al:* Percutaneous vertebroplasty in patients with osteolytic metastases or multiple myeloma. *Rev Rhum Engl Ed* 64(3):177-1783, 1997.
19. Cyteval C, Sarrabere MP, Roux JO, *et al:* Acute osteoporotic vertebral collapse: open study on percutaneous injection of acrylic surgical cement in 20 patients. *AJR* 173:1685-1690, 1999.
20. Barr JD, Barr MS, Lemley TJ, McCann RM: Percutaneous vertebroplasty for pain relief and spine stablization. *Spine* 25(8):923-928, 2000.
21. Cortet B, Cotten A, Boutry N, *et al:* Percutaneous vertebroplasty in the treatment of osteoporotic vertebral compression fractures: an open prospective study. *J Rheumatol* 26:2222-2228, 1999.

# Kyphoplasty

## Daisuke Togawa and Isador H. Lieberman

Osteoporotic vertebral compression fractures are the most common of fragility fractures. Over 700,000 new cases are diagnosed each year in the United States alone.[20] It is estimated that the fractures in 200,000 of these patients become chronically painful.[3] In addition to the pain and disability associated with vertebral compression fractures, indirect consequences cause an enormous health care burden.[20] Additionally, the vertebrae adjacent to a fracture are subject to excessive stresses caused by kyphotic posturing and altered biomechanics, resulting in a fivefold increase in the risk of collapse.[12]

The first premise of orthopedics is to restore anatomy and stabilize the skeleton, to allow bone healing so that individuals with fractures may eventually resume normal function. In the face of vertebral compression fractures (VCFs) up to now, the spine community has been content to ignore these physiologic and biomechanical principles because it has not had a reliable method to address these fractures in a physiologically vulnerable geriatric population.

Methyl methacrylate vertebral augmentation (vertebroplasty or kyphoplasty) now affords patients a minimally invasive, safe, and effective method of vertebral body stabilization, rapid pain relief, and in the case of kyphoplasty, restoration of spinal alignment in the treatment of their painful progressive VCFs. There is still, however, much to learn about the biomechanics, the source of pain, and bone physiology within the osteoporotic or osteomalacic vertebral body and the effects of methyl methacrylate on the surrounding bone.

## Surgical Indication

Kyphoplasty is currently indicated for progressive, painful osteoporotic or osteolytic vertebral body wedge compression fractures. Similar to any other fragility fracture, the goals are to restore stability, anatomic alignment, and function as soon as safely possible. The current indications for vertebral augmentation include any progressive painful VCF. Even though the quoted natural history of vertebral compression fractures is for two thirds of the patients to eventually become pain free, one must appreciate that the affected vertebral bodies rarely regain normal height and that there is a five-fold increase in further fractures at adjacent or remote levels within one year.[17,23] If one subscribes to the philosophies of traditional spinal biomechanics and appreciates that "kyphosis begets kyphosis," especially in the face of low bone density, it only makes sense to intervene before the fracture progresses significantly. This minimizes the effects of sagittal imbalance on the spine. Pain relief then becomes the secondary indication and protection of sagittal spinal alignment becomes the primary indication. This is synonymous with the rationale to reduce a distal radius fracture back to its anatomic alignment to allow normal function of the distal radioulnar joint. Like hip fracture surgery, the results of vertebral augmentation are most predictable with immediate intervention.

The contraindications to kyphoplasty include local active osteomyelitis or any systemic pathology such as sepsis, prolonged bleeding times, or other cardiopulmonary pathology that precludes the safe completion of the procedure under either conscious sedation or general anesthesia. Other relative contraindications include non-osteolytic infiltrative spinal metastases, vertebral bodies with deficient dorsal vertebral body cortices, or patients presenting with neurologic signs or symptoms. Certain burst or vertebra plana fracture configurations may be technically difficult and are relative contraindications. The use of an inflatable bone tamp should be assessed on a case by case basis. Sagittal and axial CT and MRI are particularly important to plan the trajectory for the percutaneous procedure.

There exists a significant debate regarding the number of levels to augment and the indication for prophylaxis in the setting of vertebral compression fractures. Vertebroplasty proponents are more liberal in recommending multiple levels at any one time. One must, however, consider the volume of cement and the potential for monomer toxicity. It is well established that cement monomer is arrhythmogenic and cardiotoxic at the volumes used for a total hip or knee replacement. The risk appears to be somewhere in the neighborhood of 1 in 3000 to 1 in 5000.[2,6] Taking into account the volume of cement (6ml per level) and the proximity to the spine, and then assuming one is willing to accept the same degree of risk, it seems most appropriate to limit vertebroplasty or kyphoplasty to one or two levels at any surgical setting. Kyphoplasty does have a built in advantage over vertebroplasty in that the technique dictates that a thicker partially cured cement be poured into the cavity in a controlled fashion rather than a highly liquid cement forced into the closed space of the collapsed vertebral body. The liquid cement of vertebroplasty has more free monomer available to enter the circulation, and the liquid cement will obey the laws of fluid dynamics, seeking out the path of least resistance. Therefore the cement readily enters the venous sinuses or exits through vertebral body fissures and cracks, resulting in cement leaks.

## Technique

The kyphoplasty procedure may be performed under intravenous sedation with local anesthetic or under general anesthesia. The patients are positioned prone on a radiolucent table. Two C-arms are positioned to achieve AP and lateral radiographs of the affected vertebra. The vertebral body is cannulated percutaneously through a 3mm stab incision either transpedicularly or extrapedicularly, depending on what the anatomy and fracture configuration dictates. Through the working cannula, the inflatable bone tamps are positioned under the end plates in the center of the vertebral body. The bone tamps are then inflated to achieve reduction of the fracture and create a cavity to be filled with cement. The inflation is continued until anatomic height restoration is achieved, the bone tamp comes to within 1mm of any cortical or end plate surface, or the maximum pressure or volume of the balloon is achieved. Inflation of the bone tamp pushes bone from the center to the periphery of the vertebral body, thus effectively bone grafting the side walls and end plates and sealing off any cracks, fissures, or venous sinuses.[14,24] Once the cavity is created, the inflatable bone tamp is removed, the cement is mixed, and the cavity is filled in a slow and controlled fashion under fluoroscopic guidance only when the cement has thickened considerably. By virtue of the cavity, and the thick partially cured cement instilled, the risk of cement extravasation is minimal. Once the cement has hardened, the cannulae are removed and the stab incisions are closed with a single stitch. The patients are typically discharged from hospital the same day, or in physiologically compromised patients, watched over night. All patients are encouraged to resume all of their normal activities of daily living as soon as possible with no restrictions.

## Clinical Results

In the author's ongoing Institutional Review Board-approved study,[5,9,16] over 900 consecutive kyphoplasty procedures were performed in over 300 patients between April 1999 and August 2003. The mean age was 69 years (range 35 to 89). The mean duration of symptoms was 7 months. Outcome data were obtained by administering the Short Form 36 health survey (SF-36) and visual analog scale (VAS) for pain rating; additionally, the patients underwent detailed neurologic and radiographic examinations pre- and postoperatively. Perioperative and clinical follow-up revealed that the procedure was well tolerated, with improvement in pain and early mobilization. The levels treated ranged from T3 to L5, with 47% of the vertebrae located at thoracolumbar junction. Length of stay ranged from 0.5 day to 9 days (mean 1.1 day). There were no clinically significant cement leaks and no perioperative complications attributable to the inflatable bone tamp or tools. SF-36 data (preoperative and postoperative) are available on over 200 patients (67%), with follow-up ranging from 1 week to 38 months (mean 7.5 months). SF-36 scores improved in every category, statistically significant in all but the General Health modality. Physical function improved from 22.0 to 36.4 ($P \le .0001$). Role physical improved from 5.0 to 21.7 ($P \le .0001$). Bodily pain improved from 22.5 to 41.2 ($P \le .0001$). Vitality improved from 31.8 to 40.8 ($P \le .0001$). Social function improved from 37.7 to 59.6 ($P \le .0001$). Role emotional improved from 51.1 to 61.4 ($P = .021$). Mental health improved from 62.7 to 69.4 ($P \le .0001$). General health was unchanged from 51.1 to 51.1 ($P = .047$). The VAS scores improved from a preoperative level of 7 to an initial postoperative level of 3.2 ($P < .0001$). At the last follow-up examination, the value remained unchanged at 3.4 ($P < .0001$).

Ledlie et al.[15] reported functional and radiographic outcomes in the first 96 kyphoplasty patients with 133 fractures. Their follow-up period was a minimum of 12 months, and the mean patient age at the time of surgery was 76 years (51 to 93). With regard to pain as rated by the patient when using a 10-point VAS, the mean score was decreased to 1.4 at the 1-year follow-up, while the mean preoperative VAS score was 8.6. Ambulatory status was also improved postoperatively. Over 90% of the patients (27/29, 50 patients lost to follow-up) were ambulatory at 1 year, while only 35% of the patients (28/79) were ambulatory preoperatively.

Phillips et al.[19] also recently reported their early radiographic and clinical results of kyphoplasty. In this study, 29 patients with 61 fractures between T6 to L5 were evaluated. The mean age of these 29 patients was 70 years. Their clinical information including pain relief, improvement in activity, and satisfaction with the surgical procedure, as well as their sagittal spinal alignment on the standing radiographs, were assessed and followed up to 1 year. Average pain scores were significantly decreased to 2.6 and 0.6, at 1-week and 1-year, respectively, while average pain score was 8.6 preoperatively.

## Complications

In the author's series of patients,[5,16] cement extravasation was observed in less than 10% of cases. No problems were identified clinically as a result of these extravasations immediately after surgery or at final follow-up. In one patient, a myocardial infarction occurred as a result of fluid overload during the procedure. In a separate prospective multi-center series, there were 6 major complications out of 600 cases associated with the kyphoplasty procedure. Four of these were neurologic complications (0.75%). These were directly attributable to surgeon error and breach of technique. To date, no reports of primary or secondary infection of the cement mantle have been published. In this series of over 300 patients, we had no primary infections. One hematogenous infection 2 years after kyphoplasty in a patient receiving multiple blood and platelet transfusions for Waldenstroms macroglobulinemia was observed. Ledlie et al.[15] reported that asymptomatic cement leaks were noted in 9% of vertebral bodies treated, but no device- or procedure-related complications were reported. Phillips et al.[19] reported that asymptomatic cement leaks were observed in 6 of 61 vertebral fractures (9.8%). In this series as well, there were no clinical consequences attributable to the bone tamp or cement deposition.

## Kyphoplasty Versus Vertebroplasty

Although both percutaneous vertebroplasty (PVP) and kyphoplasty provide excellent pain relief,* kyphoplasty has the potential to improve spine biomechanics and decrease the risk of cement extravasation. PVP usually does not expand the vertebral body or regain normal spine alignment.

Preliminary data indicate that kyphoplasty may restore the vertebral body toward its original vertebral height, preventing kyphosis that leads to respiratory and digestive problems. In Ledlie's paper, height restoration was reported from radiographically measured anterior and midline points of the fractured vertebrae when using the two nearest normal vertebrae as reference points.[15] At 1 year, the ventral vertebral height was 85% of the predicted height and midline height was 89%, while their preoperative heights were 66% and 65%, respectively. In Phillips' paper, regarding the measurement of local sagittal alignment in the region of the fracture, the alignment was improved by a mean of 8.8 degrees for all fractures and 14.2 degrees in fractures considered reducible by kyphoplasty (that experienced at least 5 degrees of correction).[19]

Restoration of height and sagittal alignment may also work to protect vulnerable vertebral levels above or below the sites treated by minimizing force transfer. One

---

*References 1,4,5,7-9,13,16.

vertebroplasty study reported a 52% rate of remote or adjacent level fractures after vertebroplasty.[10] On the other hand, Harrop et al.[11] demonstrated that the incidence of post-kyphoplasty vertebral compression fracture in the primary osteoporotic patients was 11.25%, while the incidence in the steroid-induced osteoporotic patients was 48.6% (17 fractures/35 patients). This result suggests that the intervention, kyphoplasty, in primary osteoporotic patients does not increase the rate of remote or adjacent level fractures as compared with the published natural history reports.[17,21,22] Phillips reported that 3 out of 29 patients experienced new vertebral fractures adjacent to previously treated levels, and 2 patients experienced new fractures at levels that were remote (not adjacent) levels.[19]

PVP is much more prone to cement leaks,[13] since the PMMA is injected in a liquid state and takes the path of least resistance through cracks in surrounding bone. In performing vertebroplasty, the surgeon injects the liquid cement,[18] typically pausing or stopping once a leak becomes evident. On the other hand, the expanded kyphoplasty balloon creates a cavity that instills a partially cured cement to the point at which the cement bolus reaches and interdigitates with the bony margins. The initial kyphoplasty findings show lower rates of cement extravasation, as compared with published PVP series, supporting the hypothesis that deposition of partially cured cement into a previously formed cavity may be an improvement over the injection of liquid cement into the unreduced vertebral body.

## Summary

Kyphoplasty is a well-tolerated procedure that is indicated for the treatment of painful VCFs. Kyphoplasty is associated with early clinical improvement of pain and function, as well as restoration of vertebral body height. Favorable outcomes in early trials appear to permit early mobilization, which has the potential to decrease mortality. Considering the greater mortality that is associated with osteoporotic compression fractures, early mobilization in these patients is of prime importance.

## REFERENCES

1. Barr JD, Barr MS, Lemley TJ, McCann RM: Percutaneous vertebroplasty for pain relief and spinal stabilization. *Spine* 25:923-928, 2000.
2. Charnley J: Systemic effects of monomer. In *Acrylic Cement In Orthopaedic Surgery*. Edinburgh and London, E & S Livingstone, 1970, pp 72-78.
3. Cooper C, Atkinson EJ, O'Fallon WM, Melton LJ 3rd: Incidence of clinically diagnosed vertebral fractures: a population-based study in Rochester, Minnesota, 1985-1989. *J Bone Miner Res* 7:221-227, 1993.
4. Cortet B, Cotten A, Boutry N, *et al:* Percutaneous vertebroplasty in the treatment of osteoporotic vertebral compression fractures: an open prospective study. *J Rheumatol* 26:2222-2228, 1999.
5. Coumans JV, Reinhardt MK, Lieberman IH: Kyphoplasty for vertebral compression fractures: 1-year clinical outcomes from a prospective study. *J Neurosurg* 99:44-50, 2003.
6. Coventry MB, BeckenBaugh RD, Nolan DR, Ilstrup DM: 2,012 Total hip arthroplasties: A study of postoperative course and early complications. *J Bone Joint Surg Am* 56:273-284, 1974.
7. Cyteval C, Sarrabere MP, Roux JO, *et al:* Acute osteoporotic vertebral collapse: open study on percutaneous injection of acrylic surgical cement in 20 patients. *AJR Am J Roentgenol* 173:1685-1690, 1999.
8. Deramond H, Depriester C, Galibert P, Le Gars D: Percutaneous vertebroplasty with polymethylmethacrylate. Technique, indications, and results. *Radiol Clin North Am* 36:533-546, 1998.
9. Dudeney S, Lieberman IH, Reinhardt MK, Hussein M: Kyphoplasty in the treatment of osteolytic vertebral compression fractures as a result of multiple myeloma. *J Clin Oncol* 20:2382-2387, 2002.
10. Grados F, Depriester C, Cayrolle G, *et al:* Long-term observations of vertebral osteoporotic fractures treated by percutaneous vertebroplasty. *Rheumatology (Oxford)* 39:1410-1414, 2000.
11. Harrop JS, Prpa B, Reinhardt MK, Lieberman IH: Incidence of remote and adjacent vertebral compression fractures after kyphoplasty. *Spine* (In press)
12. Heaney RP: The natural history of vertebral osteoporosis. Is low bone mass an epiphenomenon? *Bone* 13(suppl 2):S23-S26, 1992.
13. Jensen ME, Evans AJ, Mathis JM, *et al:* Percutaneous polymethylmethacrylate vertebroplasty in the treatment of osteoporotic vertebral body compression fractures: technical aspects. *AJNR Am J Neuroradiol* 18:1897-1904, 1997.
14. Kovacic J, Lieberman IH, Togawa D, *et al:* The behavior of polymethylmethacrylate during kyphoplasty and vertebroplasty in the primate spine: A gross and histologic analysis. *Spine* 3:79S, 2003.
15. Ledlie JT, Renfro M: Balloon kyphoplasty: One-year outcomes in vertebral body height restoration, chronic pain, and activity levels. *J Neurosurg* 98:36-42, 2003.
16. Lieberman IH, Dudeney S, Reinhardt MK, Bell G: Initial outcome and efficacy of "kyphoplasty" in the treatment of painful osteoporotic vertebral compression fractures. *Spine* 26:1631-1638, 2001.
17. Lindsay R, Silverman SL, Cooper C, *et al:* Risk of new vertebral fracture in the year following a fracture. *JAMA* 285: 320-323, 2001.
18. Martin JB, Jean B, Sugiu K, *et al:* Vertebroplasty: Clinical experience and follow-up results. *Bone* 25:11S-15S, 1999.
19. Phillips FM, Ho E, Campbell-Hupp M, *et al:* Early radiographic and clinical results of balloon kyphoplasty for the treatment of osteoporotic vertebral compression fractures. *Spine* 28:2260-2265, 2003.
20. Riggs BL, Melton LJ 3rd: The worldwide problem of osteoporosis: insights afforded by epidemiology. *Bone* 17:505S-511S, 1995.
21. Ross PD, Davis JW, Epstein RS, Wasnich RD: Pre-existing fractures and bone mass predict vertebral fracture incidence in women. *Ann Intern Med* 114:919-923, 1994.
22. Ross PD, Ettinger B, Davis JW, *et al:* Evaluation of adverse health outcomes associated with vertebral fractures. *Osteoporos Int* 1:134-140, 1991.

23. Silverman SL: The clinical consequences of vertebral compression fracture. *Bone* 13(suppl 2):S27-S31, 1992.

24. Togawa D, Bauer TW, Lieberman IH, Takikawa S: Histological evaluation of human vertebral bodies after vertebral augmentation with polymethyl methacrylate. *Spine* 28:1521-1527, 2003.

# CHAPTER 166

# Management of Ossification of Posterior Longitudinal Ligament

## Cervical Laminoplasty: Open Door

**Elizabeth Vitarbo and Allan D. Levi**

Cervical spondylotic myelopathy (CSM) represents a heterogenous group of disorders first recognized in the 1950s.[6] Since that time, there has been a growing body of evidence supporting its diverse clinical symptomatology and attendant pathophysiologic changes. A clear understanding of pathology, prognosis and the role of surgical intervention is critical for all neurosurgeons, as it is one of the most frequently encountered disorders requiring neurosurgical care.

## Pathophysiology

CSM is a heterogenous group of disorders resulting from variable combinations of congenital canal stenosis (sagittal anteroposterior [AP] diameter <12mm), degenerative osteophyte formation, hypertrophy of uncovertebral and facet joint complexes, ligamentous hypertrophy, and instability. Ossification of the posterior longitudinal ligament (OPLL) and ligamentum flavum may alter the biomechanics, with resultant management implications that are addressed in the "Management" section in the next few pages. The final common denominator of these changes is a reduction in spinal canal area, ultimately leading to spinal cord compression.

While the majority of patients (70% to 85%) greater than 65 years old have radiographic evidence of multisegmental cervical spondylosis, only a small percentage become symptomatic.[19] To explain this phenomenon, Hayashi et al.[22] introduced the concept of static and dynamic forces acting in concert to influence the clinical presentation.[12] Essentially, instability and ligamentous changes represent dynamic forces, the effect of which are dependent on head and neck movement. Whereas the former may be associated with flexion and/or extension, the latter is classically implicated in hyperextension of the neck. In contrast, the remainder of the pathophysiologic changes listed above may be considered static forces, the effects of which are exacerbated by dynamic forces.

The precise contributions of static and dynamic forces to disease progression remains controversial, thus confounding attempts to define a natural history and prognosticate. However, it has become clear that the most important determinants of disease development and outcome are the degree and duration of spinal cord compression. In an autopsy series, Ono et al.[56] found that myelopathy was associated with both gray and white matter pathology that was not limited to the focal area of compression, and correlated significantly with the "AP compression ratio" (AP/lateral cord diameter).[12] Subsequent cadaveric studies confirmed these findings, with the degree of spinal cord deformity on CT (computed tomography) myelogram correlating with premortem symptom severity.[12,77] Experimentally, the importance of dynamic forces in disease progression is supported by the finding that the severity of histopathologic changes is proportional to the incidence of pathophysiologic stresses (hyperflexion, hyperextension, instability) at the site of spinal cord compression.[12,31] Additionally, clinical evidence exists that those exhibiting radiographic evidence of instability who were treated conservatively did worse than those without gross instability.[4,12]

While it is essentially impossible to accurately determine the duration of pathologic spinal cord compression, it is critical to ascertain the duration of clinical symptomatology, as this has significant implications regarding prognosis. Retrospective studies have shown that conservative management is associated with clinical improvement in 36% of patients, at best,[14] with other studies revealing essentially uniform disease progression over variable periods of time.[8,12,57,69] Importantly, clinical improvement is noted to be rare in patients with symptoms longer than 2 years.[59] While more conservative estimates contend that symptom duration less than 6 months to 1 year is critical for good outcome, the salient point is that the best outcomes are typically associated with expeditious treatment following the onset of symptoms.* This does not suggest that patients are to be operated on as soon as subtle symptoms or signs are identified, but it does dictate that a high index of suspicion be maintained for CSM in patients exhibiting signs and symptoms appropriate for the diagnosis, and, in the presence of appropriate supportive evidence, that trials of conservative management not be prolonged.

## Clinical Presentation

Although a thorough discussion of this topic is beyond the scope of this text, the following represent some of the more typical findings associated with CSM. Variable combinations of motor, sensory, and reflex changes are invariably present, and a finding of one in the absence of the others should call the diagnosis into question.

Gait changes are often the earliest and most subtle symptom. Tripping and mild unsteadiness are common, as are complaints of lower extremity spasticity and subjective

---

*References 1,18,21,41,42,52,76,78.

weakness. "Gradual gait deterioration often ensues, with a broad based, hesitant gait resulting."[12,20]

Upper extremity complaints often develop subsequent to gait changes. The so-called myelopathy hand[56] represents variable combinations of numbness and loss of fine motor function, typically in a nondermatomal distribution, resulting in significant functional limitation. Loss of power is noted, occasionally with concomitant atrophy of hand muscles. Interestingly, a significant subset of patients are noted to have unilateral or bilateral deltoid weakness as well.[12,14,59]

Sensory manifestations are logically dependent on the location of cord compression. Given that compressive factors are often concentric and diffuse, any combination of sensory alterations may manifest. However, some degree of posterior column involvement is the most consistent finding. Therefore, impairment of position and vibratory sense in both upper and lower extremities is common in CSM. On the other hand, given the dual pathways available for the transmission of touch sensation, this modality is rarely compromised unless a bilateral transverse lesion exists.[10] Finally, while it has been argued that spinal cord and nerve root compression are rarely symptomatic at the same time, it is important to consider that similar pathophysiologic changes are often at play in both disorders, and the presence of radiculopathy does not exclude the diagnosis of or mitigate the clinical importance of CSM.

Bowel and/or bladder dysfunction associated with CSM is reported in approximately 20% of cases,[15,30] although an incidence as high as 50% has been noted.[12,46] Bowel and bladder dysfunction is rarely the presenting manifestation of CSM.

In addition to the aforementioned, upper motor neuron inhibition commonly results in hyperactive reflexes. "Pathologically" hyperactive reflexes are common below the level of compression, with variable presence of a Hoffman's and/or Babinski reflex and clonus. Importantly, however, hyporeflexia may be noted in the upper extremities, depending on the level of involvement. Finally, a Lhermitte's sign may be elicited or reported, but this finding is rare.

## Management

While acute deterioration has been reported with CSM, the disease is often relatively chronic in nature, and progressive. Deterioration is most commonly stepwise, with episodic acute exacerbations superimposed on established symptoms or deficits, leading to progressive disability. A significant subset of patients exhibits slow, steady progression, devoid of "quiescent" periods. Again, although Epstein has reported a 36% rate of clinical improvement and a 38% rate of disease stabilization with conservative management,[12,14] Clark et al.,[8] found disease regression and neurologic improvement to be rare.[12] Though conflicting evidence exists, the majority of available evidence suggests that CSM is largely a surgical disease in the presence of symptoms, appropriate radiographic evidence and supportive studies.

Conservative management of CSM is largely empiric. There exist no well-designed clinical studies systematically evaluating the efficacy of common treatment modalities. The mainstay of conservative therapy is immobilization, together with antiinflammatory medications, in an attempt to address modifiable sources of static and dynamic cord compression. Theoretically, immobilization of the grossly or microscopically unstable spine may facilitate resorption of degenerative osteophytes, in addition to preventing ongoing dynamic compression.

Once surgical intervention is decided upon, the principal decision regarding surgical management is whether a ventral or dorsal approach should be employed. A ventral decompressive procedure and fusion is the most appropriate surgical procedure in the presence of ventral compressive factors limited to one or two vertebral body levels.[9,11] This procedure most directly addresses the pathology, and facilitates fusion with the use of bone graft, with or without the addition of instrumentation. "Good-excellent" clinical results have been achieved in as many as 92% of patients undergoing this procedure.[23] However, concerns regarding appropriate graft material and its stability carry significant clinical implications with longer gaps. The risk of adjacent level disease may be as high as 25% in studies that have looked at the long term results of anterior fusion surgery.[26]

Sir Victor Horsely is the first neurosurgeon credited for decompressing the cervical spine of a patient with progressive cervical spondylotic myelopathy using a dorsal approach.[71] Until the description of ventral approaches, management of CSM has traditionally consisted of a decompressive laminectomy. While this procedure effectively enlarges the functional spinal canal area, thus allowing the spinal cord to move away from compressive elements and expand, it does so at the expense of dorsal stabilizing structures. Depending on the preoperative spinal alignment, the levels of decompression and the period of time passed since surgery, development of spinal instability and gradual kyphotic deformity may be observed. Given these concerns, together with the considerable population suffering from multilevel compressive pathology necessitating dorsal decompression, Asian surgeons developed the laminoplasty procedure in the late 1970s,[58,75] with numerous modifications since that time.* This procedure, by leaving the dorsal stabilizing structures in situ, is believed to mitigate the development of kyphosis, and, with subsequent bone fusion, stabilize the cervical spine with improved outcome. While evidence exists to both support and refute these claims, it is now acknowledged that patients with preoperative kyphotic alignment are unlikely to do well with either procedure, and are best managed with a ventral surgery.

## Surgical Technique

While in the supine position with the neck minimally extended, endotracheal intubation is performed after administration of a general anesthetic. In selected cases, the surgeon may be especially concerned about the risk for

---

*References 27,34,42,43,53,73.

spinal cord injury with any extension of the cervical spine because of the severity of the stenosis and spinal cord compression. A fiberoptic intubation while the patient is awake with the aid of a bronchoscope can then be performed to reduce the risk of hyperextension of the neck and permit the surgeon to repeat the neurologic examination after placement of the endotracheal tube. In very selected cases, one may prefer to also turn the patient in the prone position awake, as this represents yet another instance in which inadvertent movements of the neck may occur and result in neurologic deterioration. Some neurosurgeons have advocated the routine use of methylprednisolone prophylaxis as a neuroprotective agent prior to the start of surgery. The rational being that provision of this drug in the setting of a potential spinal cord injury situation may reduce the severity of injury. As no data has been presented to suggest that it is effective as a neuroprotective agent in cervical decompressive surgery, its routine use cannot be recommended.

Neurophysiologic monitoring options include somatosensory evoked potentials (SSEPs), motor evoked potentials (MEPs) and electromyograms (EMGs). The value of the routine use of such monitoring is often questioned as it has been difficult to demonstrate that the information provided can actually change what the surgeon does during the surgery, which will make it safer. However, some retrospective studies have demonstrated the positive predictive value of such tests in determining outcome.[5,7] The stimulating and recording electrodes are placed and secured and baseline recordings are obtained prior to turning the patient. A number of options exist for holding the head during surgery in the prone position. The authors use the Mayfield three-pin headrest, which allows the surgeon to easily control the degree of flexion and extension of the cervical spine as well as reducing the possibility of pressure on the patient's eyes. The patient is then transferred onto the operating table in the prone position, with the head secured in a slightly flexed position. Tape can be applied to the superior and dorsolateral aspects of both shoulders, and secured to the caudal region of the operating table to assist with intraoperative radiographic visualization of the lower cervical levels as required. After the operative field is prepped and draped, the midline is infiltrated with commercially available 1% lidocaine with epinephrine to minimize skin bleeding. A midline incision is made and monopolar or bipolar electrocautery are used to control soft tissue bleeding. Midline fascia is then incised with monopolar electrocautery. Subperiosteal dissection is used to reflect the soft tissue structures off the spinous processes, lamina and mesial portions of the facets bilaterally, taking care to preserve the facet capsules.

## Open Door Expansile Cervical Laminoplasty

Cervical laminoplasty is usually recommended in patients who have multilevel cervical spondylosis and stenosis typically extending over three to four levels. Patients generally have a normal cervical lordosis and/or a relatively straight cervical spine. A dorsal decompressive procedure is avoided in the presence of significant kyphosis. The majority of patients are recommended to undergo decom-

pression from an open door cervical laminoplasty from C3 to C7 with partial laminectomies of C2 and T1 and fusion with rib allograft at C3, C5 and C7 supplemented by vertebral autograft. The decompression extends somewhat rostral and caudal to the maximum levels of compression so that the spinal cord does not migrate back and become entrapped or kinked at the rostral or caudal levels (lamina) of the decompression.

The initial portion of this procedure is identical to that described above. Soft tissue dissection and retraction of the extensor cervical muscle groups, exposure of the cervical lamina and mesial facets is obtained from the caudal portion of C2 to the rostral limit of T1. The caudal one third of the C2 lamina and the rostral one third of the T1 lamina are removed using a combination of a high-speed air drill and a 2mm Kerrison punch to visualize the underlying dura at this level. The authors also remove the spinous processes of C3 to C7 inclusively with a Horsely and morselize the bone for subsequent autografting.

The next segment of the procedure involves doing osteotomies of cervical lamina three to seven. In so doing, one creates a "open" side and a "hinged" side of the above lamina (Figure 166.1). In general the side with the greatest compression and/or the most clinically symptomatic is the open side. If one is planning to do foraminotomies in addition to the laminoplasty, the open side is best placed on the side of the intended foraminotomies. A high-speed air drill with a small bit is used to create troughs at the level of the lamina-facet junction from C3 to C7. Drilling proceeds through the outer and inner cortical margins of the lamina on the side to be "opened." On the hinge side, drilling proceeds through the outer cortical margin and cancellous bone, however, the inner cortex is not violated. After the drilling is complete, bone allografts are prepared for purposes of stabilizing canal expansion. We prefer to use rib allografts for this purpose. Again using the drill, three separate grafts are cut, each approximately 8 to16mm in length. Grooves are then made transversely along the cut surfaces of the rib grafts, approximating the thickness of the cut laminae. After the grafts have been prepared, attention is turned to "opening the door." Initially, two small curettes are introduced into the open gap produced by drilling the laminae, and advanced just deep to the outer cortex. By pulling the curettes upwards, the laminar facet gap on the open side is slowly enlarged and thus results in a green-stick fracture along the previously created trough on the hinge side. Minimal advances are made before moving to other laminae, in an effort to open all the involved laminae as a functional unit. The goal is to expand the AP diameter of the canal by approximately 4mm. Great care must be taken in order to achieve this goal without fracturing the inner cortex of the hinge side. Once this is accomplished, the rib allografts are placed in the gap that has been created at the C3, C5, and C7 levels, with the cut edges of the lamina resting in the cut groove of the rib (Figure 166.2). If done properly, the grafts should fit snugly in the gap, there should be slight "closing" force securing the graft position, and the inner cortex of the hinge side should be intact. We then use the morselized spinous process autograft and place it over the decorticated bone surfaces of the facet and

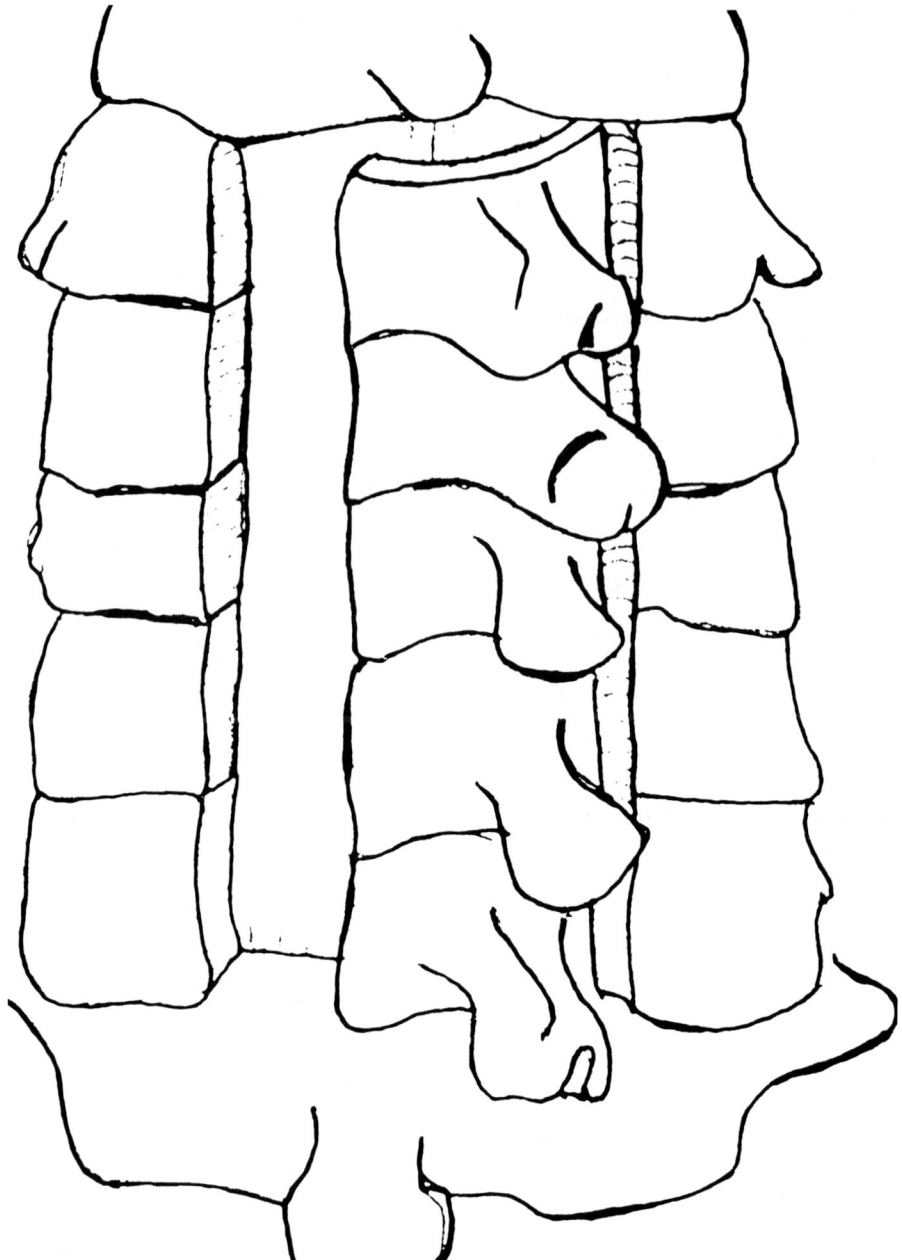

**Figure 166.1** Left open-door cervical laminoplasty. Note that on the right hinge side, drilling spares the inner cancellous bone, while the osteotomies on the left open door side involve all layers. Elevation of the posterior arches increases the lamina-facet gap on the left, and produces a green-stick fracture on the hinge side.

lamina on the hinge side to provide some "stiffness" to the construct.

Should the patient suffer from radiculopathy as well as myelopathy, one can add one or several foraminotomies to the laminoplasty procedure. Typically the foraminotomy is initiated once the lamina has been elevated and the ligamentum flavum excised. The mesial one third to one half of the facet over the exiting nerve root is drilled with a high-speed drill. The opening can be widened with 1 or 2mm angled Kerrison punches.

Should rigid stabilization be required, the addition of facet cables with or without rib allograft can be inserted. Lateral mass screws attached to a plate or a rod can also be

applied. It is sometimes difficult to position the rib allografts to hold open the lamina once additional hardware is placed but it can be done. Other variations of the approach include: Spinous process autograft instead of the rib allograft is used to hold open the lamina. Some surgeons prefer to stabilize the rib allograft with miniplates to the adjacent lamina and facet on the open side[55] or sutures. The lamina can be split in the midline with a T-handled "Gigli-like" saw and the allograft spacers positioned between the green-stick fractured hemilamina.[13]

In the authors' experience, an open door expansile cervical laminoplasty (without additional stabilization procedures) takes approximately 90 minutes to complete, with

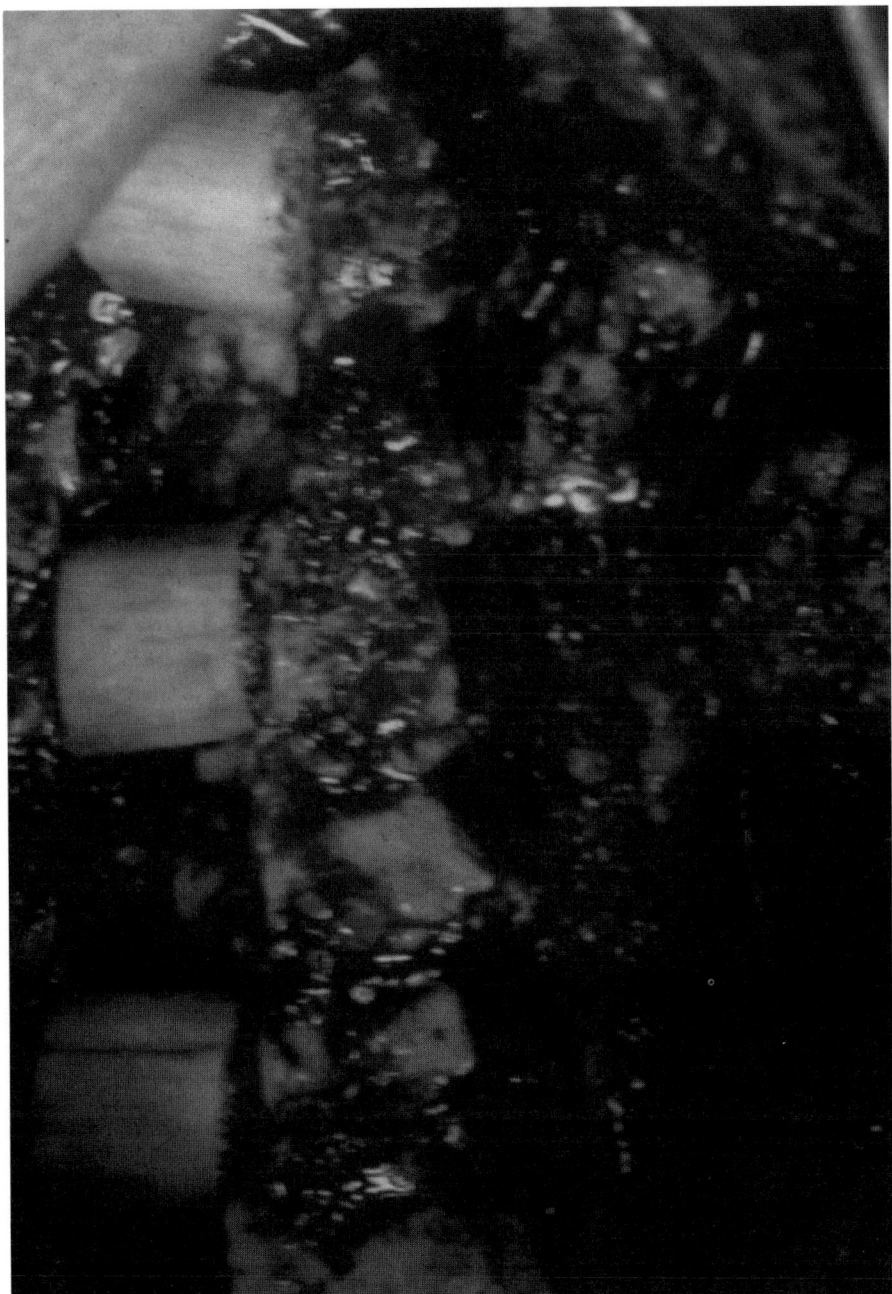

**Figure 166.2** Intraoperative photograph following left open-door cervical laminoplasty. Rib allografts are placed in the gap that has been created at the C3, C5, and C7 levels, with the cut edges of the lamina resting in the cut groove of the rib. If done properly, the grafts should fit snugly in the gap, there should be slight closing force securing the graft position, and the inner cortex of the hinge side should be intact. We then use the morselized spinous process autograft and place it over the decorticated bone surfaces of the facet and lamina on the hinge side to provide some stiffness to the construct.

an average blood loss of 200ml. The complication rate is low (see the next section), particularly when compared to decompressive operations, which attempt to achieve the same number of levels of decompression and stabilization when tackled from the front.[47] It is ideally suited for the elderly myelopathic, osteoporotic patient with multiple levels of stenosis and little or minimal neck pain. In the young patient, particularly if there is significant axial neck pain, a ventral procedure may be better suited. In

patients with acute traumatic central cord syndrome without evidence of radiographic instability, an expansile laminoplasty, again is a surgical option.[75]

## Complications

The complication rate for dorsal decompressive procedures is low[45] and includes but is not limited to infection, cerebrospinal fluid (CSF) leak, hemorrhage, spinal cord injury, nerve root injury, and the risk of the general anesthetic. Specific complications historically associated with the laminoplasty procedure itself include "sinkage" of the "open door." With the addition of stabilizing structures this risk is minimal. Delayed C5 nerve root weakness occurs at a reported rate of 4.6% to 13.3%[25,27,63] Although it is transient in most cases, recovery may require up to 6 years.[63] Axial neck and shoulder girdle pain can be problematic and usually responds to an aggressive course of physical therapy. However, axial neck pain and malalignment have little impact on ultimate outcome and Japanese Orthopaedic Association (JOA) scores,[17,25,49,62] unless associated with a decreased cervical curve index of greater than 10.[39,63]

An additional concern regarding laminectomy is the development of the "post-laminectomy membrane."[50] This entity has been implicated in arachnoiditis and restenosis, and may theoretically result in clinical deterioration.[55] These findings have not been reported following laminoplasty.

Numerous studies have demonstrated that postlaminectomy kyphotic deformity and instability can be problematic particularly in the younger patient.[24,33,48] Incidence rates as high as 43% have been reported.[27,55,66] It may occasionally develop following cervical laminoplasty,[32,70] though this is felt to be rarer.

## Outcomes

Overall, recovery rates of approximately 50% are consistently reported following laminoplasty,[*] though improvement is observed in as many as 75% of patients.[44] With respect to spondylotic radiculopathy, a retrospective study found outcomes were best following ventral decompression (92%), and only slightly worse (86%) following laminoplasty.[23] Laminectomy was associated with the poorest outcome (66%).[23]

## Summary

While management decisions must take into account a number of factors and are highly individualized, the following represents some general guidelines and our interpretation of critical literature.

Dorsal decompression is typically indicated when multisegment pathology needs to be addressed, and when predominantly dorsal pathology exists. Additionally, in the case of OPLL, significant adhesion between the posterior longitudinal ligament (PLL) and the underlying dura results in additional risk of dural laceration when approached ventrally.[76] Laminectomy has traditionally been used for decompression, and continues to be the procedure of choice for many clinicians in North America. Decompression does occur, but at the expense of the dorsal stabilizing structures. Loss of cervical lordosis or development of kyphosis are seen in as many as 43% of patients[27,55]; however, clinically signifi-

cant malalignment and instability are less common.[30,35,61,73] The crucial implication of ensuing kyphosis is its potential role in subsequent clinical deterioration, as kyphotic alignment of the spinal cord results in secondary cord compression and is associated with poorer outcome.[38] While this risk may be relatively insignificant in a patient who is otherwise debilitated with limited life expectancy, it is a very significant risk in a younger patient requiring earlier treatment due to underlying congenital canal stenosis (Figure 166.3).

Given the relatively high incidence of multilevel OPLL presenting in a younger patient population than CSM, Asian surgeons were long ago faced with the concerns of delayed kyphosis, instability, and postlaminectomy membrane following multilevel laminectomy, and the clinical implications of such. Additionally, as noted previously, dural adhesions make ventral approaches more difficult.[76] Expansile laminoplasty was developed to address these concerns. Theoretically, by minimizing "violation" of dorsal structures one can successfully enlarge the spinal canal while largely preserving dorsal stabilizing structures, thus reducing postoperative deformity or instability, and alleviating the need to perform additional fusion. While the procedure was first described by Oyama,[58,78] it did not become popularized until several years later. Initial procedures were cumbersome and lengthy, requiring complex reconstruction of the posterior arch.[58] Numerous modifications since that time have resulted in simplified, faster procedures with improved stability.[*] The importance of preserving spinoligamentous complexes in order to mitigate kyphosis has been recognized, and has resulted in tissue-sparing techniques.[†] However, such preservation is also recognized to significantly increase the closing force on the elevated laminae.[74]

In order to combat the problem of delayed closure, a variety of techniques have been employed. These primarily involve the use of spacers to buttress the created gap or the use of sutures to attach the remaining spinous process to the facet or soft tissue structures of the hinge side. We prefer the former, utilizing fibular allograft, with the closing forces maintaining firm positioning of the graft and facilitating fusion. Further stability may be obtained, in addition to or in lieu of the techniques discussed here, using onlay bone grafting at the hinge site(s).[66]

Animal studies have supported the presumed benefits of laminoplasty over laminectomy. In one study, laminectomies or laminoplasties were performed from C3 to C5 in goats, with monthly radiographic follow-up for a 6-month period. Results were compared with controls, confirming that, radiographically, laminoplasties were biomechanically superior in maintaining alignment.[3] An additional study in rabbits found that, while postoperative range of motion (ROM) was similar between groups, laminectomy was associated with increased angle deformity and poorer outcome.[16]

Clinically, studies have shown that clinical improvement directly correlates to degree of canal expansion. However, excessive expansion as well as irregular canal area[40] may be associated with additional problems. It appears that optimal canal expansion approximates 4mm

---

*References 25,32,42,49,63,65.

*References 27,42,43,53,55,72,73.
†References 18,25,28,29,36,39,43,54,62.

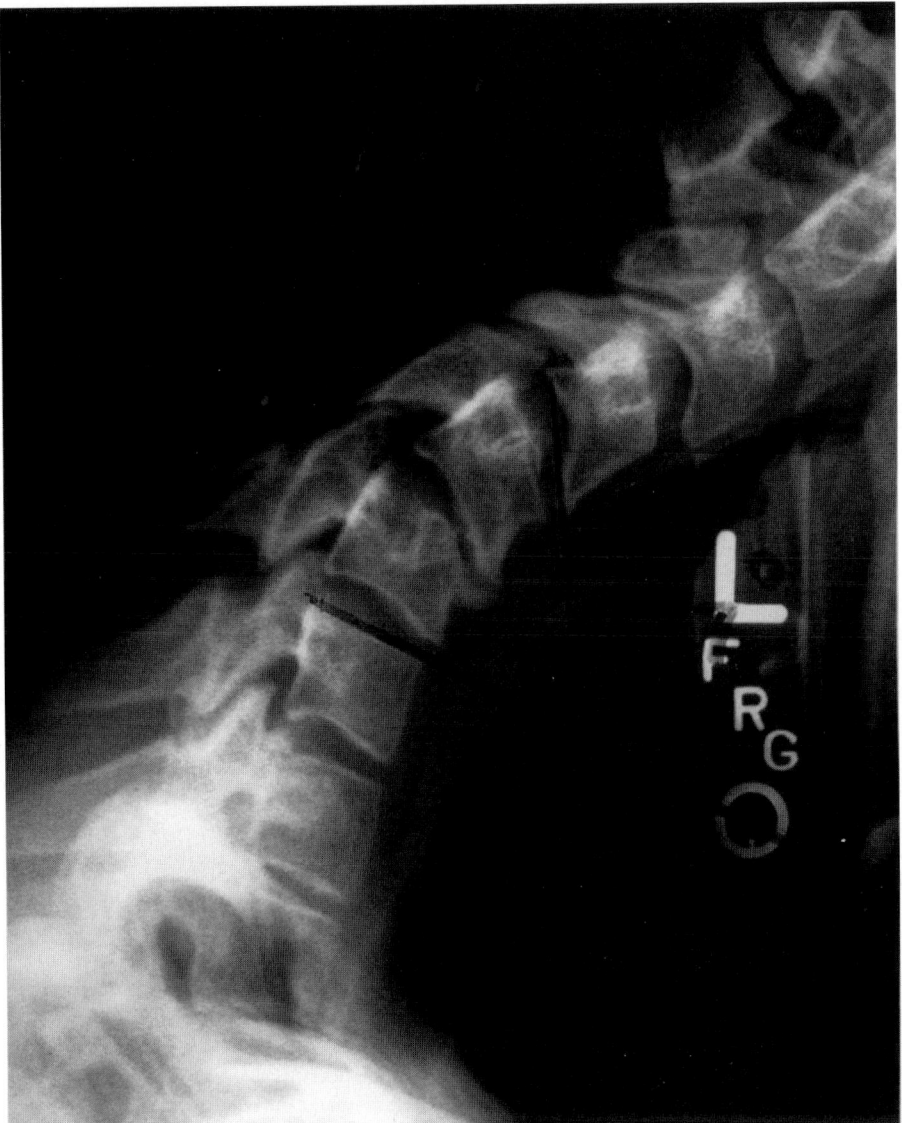

**Figure 166.3** Postoperative cervical kyphosis measuring 57 degrees in a 19-year-old female. The kyphosis was diagnosed 3 years after undergoing a cervical laminectomy from C3 to C5 for a C3-4 disc herniation.

to 5 mm in the sagittal AP diameter,[27] correlating to approximately 50% increase canal area,[2,65] and facilitating 3mm dorsal shift of the spinal cord.[68] However, decreased lordosis correlates with decreased volume expansion following laminoplasty, as well as decreased dorsal migration of the cord.[2] While improvement certainly occurs with less substantial enlargement, more aggressive enlargement is not advisable. Retrospective studies indicate increased canal diameters (beyond the ones just discussed) are associated with an increased incidence of postoperative complications, specifically C5 to C6 paresis. Presumably, this is due to traction on the nerve roots, as the C5 level frequently represents the apex of the lordotic curve, and exhibits the most significant migration. While numerous studies suggest this is a transient phenomenon in most cases, it is obviously distressing for the patient, and may take as long as 6 years to recover sufficiently.[63] Far more critical than canal expansion is subsequent cord expansion,

with studies showing a direct correlation between JOA scores and spinal cord area.[51]

Both clinically and radiographically, limited ROM is frequently observed following laminoplasty. Studies suggest that approximately 50% ROM is lost following laminoplasty, particularly extension.° This correlates well with radiographic evidence of spontaneous bony fusion.[64,66] It has been proposed that this is actually beneficial, in that it ameliorates ongoing mechanical stress or injury without being rigid and inducing stress and degeneration of adjacent levels. While numerous studies have shown no correlation between limited ROM and recovery rates or outcome, this may represent a biomechanical etiology for the postoperative axial pain, which is problematic. However, it is important to remember that the majority of

---

°References 13,27,33,37,41,64.

literature pertains to patients undergoing decompression for OPLL, which itself is associated with increased rigidity and thus may overestimate the restricted ROM attributable to the laminoplasty procedure.

In summary, while the laminoplasty procedure was designed to address some of the concerns of multilevel decompressive laminectomy, it is not without its own complications. Historically, sinkage of the open door was a concern, but this is now rare with the addition of stabilizing structures. However, axial neck pain, shoulder girdle/C5 to C6 weakness, and decreased ROM continue to be particularly problematic. Additionally, while numerous studies suggest malalignment and instability are more common following laminectomy,[33,48] both may develop following laminoplasty, occasionally at rates comparable to those seen with laminectomy.[32,70] Overall, recovery rates of approximately 50% are consistently reported following laminoplasty, with axial pain and malalignment having little impact on ultimate outcome and JOA scores,[17,25,49,62] unless associated with a decreased cervical curve index of >10.[39,63] Outcomes are comparable to,[30,53] if not better than[23] those associated with laminectomy. Laminoplasty may, however, be preferable in patients with poor bone quality, as well as younger patients with multilevel compression in the setting of lordotic alignment, as these patients are most at risk to develop delayed malalignment or instability.

# REFERENCES

1. Aita I, Hayashi K, Wadano Y, Yabuki T: Posterior movement and enlargement of the spinal cord after cervical laminoplasty. *J Bone Joint Surg Br* 80:33-37, 1998.
2. Baba H, Uchida K, Maezawa Y, et al: Three-dimensional computed tomography for evaluation of cervical spinal canal enlargement after en bloc open-door laminoplasty. *Spinal Cord* 35:674-679, 1997.
3. Baisden J, Voo LM, Cusick JF, et al: Evaluation of cervical laminectomy and laminoplasty. A longitudinal study in the goat model. *Spine* 24:1283-1288; discussion 1288-1289, 1999.
4. Barnes MP, Saunders M: The effect of cervical mobility on the natural history of cervical spondylotic myelopathy. *J Neurol Neurosurg Psychiatry* 47:17-20, 1984.
5. Bouchard JA, Bohlman HH, Biro C: Intraoperative improvements of somatosensory evoked potentials: correlation to clinical outcome in surgery for cervical spondylitic myelopathy. *Spine* 21:589-594, 1996.
6. Brain WR, Northfield DW, Wilkinson M: The neurologic manifestations of cervical spondylosis. *Brain* 75:187-225, 1952.
7. Calancie B, Harris W, Broton JG, et al: "Threshold-level" multipulse transcranial electrical stimulation of motor cortex for intraoperative monitoring of spinal motor tracts: description of method and comparison to somatosensory evoked potential monitoring. *J Neurosurg* 88:457-470, 1998.
8. Clark E, Robinson PK: Cervical myelopathy: a complication of cervical spondylosis. *Brain* 79:483, 1956.
9. Connolly ES, Seymour RJ, Adams JE: Clinical evaluation of anterior cervical fusion for degenerative cervical disc disease. *J Neurosurg* 23:431-437, 1965.
10. Daube JR, Reagan TJ, Sandok BA, Westmoreland BF: The sensory system. In Daube JR (ed): *Medical Neurosciences*, ed 2. Boston, Little Brown, 1986, pp 115-136.
11. DePalma AF, Rothman RH, Lewinnek GE, Canale ST: Anterior interbody fusion for severe cervical disc degeneration. *Surg Gynecol Obstet* 134:755-758, 1972.
12. Dillin WH, Watkins RG: Clinical syndromes in cervical myelopathy. In Rothman RH, FA Simeone FA (eds): *The Spine*, ed 3. Philadelphia, WB Saunders, 1992, pp 560-570.
13. Edwards CC 2nd, Heller JG, Silcox DH 3rd: T-Saw laminoplasty for the management of cervical spondylotic myelopathy: clinical and radiographic outcome. *Spine* 25:1788-1794, 2000.
14. Epstein JA, Epstein WE: The surgical management of cervical spinal stenosis, spondylosis and myeloradiculopathy by means of the posterior approach. In The Cervical Spine Research Society. Editorial Committee: *The Cervical Spine*, ed 2. Philadelphia, Lippincott, 1989, pp 625-643.
15. Epstein N, Epstein J, Carras R: Cervical spondylostenosis and related disorders in patients over 65: current management and diagnostic techniques. *Orthotransactions* 11, 1987.
16. Fields MJ, Hoshijima K, Feng AH, Richardson WJ, Myers BS: A biomechanical, radiologic, and clinical comparison of outcome after multilevel cervical laminectomy or laminoplasty in the rabbit. *Spine* 25:2925-2931, 2000.
17. Fujimura Y, Nishi Y: Atrophy of the nuchal muscle and change in cervical curvature after expansive open-door laminoplasty. *Arch Orthop Trauma Surg* 115:203-205, 1996.
18. Fujimura Y, Nishi Y, Chiba K, et al: Multiple regression analysis of the factors influencing the results of expansive open-door laminoplasty for cervical myelopathy due to ossification of the posterior longitudinal ligament. *Arch Orthop Trauma Surg* 117:471-474, 1998.
19. Gokaslan ZL, Cooper PR: Treatment of disc and ligamentous diseases of the cervical spine by the anterior approach. In Youmans JR (ed): *Youmans Neurological Surgery*, ed 4. Philadelphia, WB Saunders, 1996, pp 2253-2261.
20. Gorter K: Influence of laminectomy on the course of cervical myelopathy. *Acta Neurochir* 33:265-281, 1976.
21. Grob D: Surgery in the degenerative cervical spine. *Spine* 23:2674-2683, 1998.
22. Hayashi H, Okada K, Hashimoto J, et al: Cervical spondylotic myelopathy in the aged patient. A radiographic evaluation of the aging changes in the cervical spine and etiologic factors of myelopathy. *Spine* 13:618-625, 1988.
23. Herkowitz HN: A comparison of anterior cervical fusion, cervical laminectomy, and cervical laminoplasty for the surgical management of multiple level spondylotic radiculopathy. *Spine* 13:774-780, 1988.
24. Herman JM, Sonntag VK: Cervical corpectomy and plate fixation for postlaminectomy kyphosis. *J Neurosurg* 80:963-970, 1994.
25. Hidai Y, Ebara S, Kamimura M, et al: Treatment of cervical compressive myelopathy with a new dorsolateral decompressive procedure. *J Neurosurg* 90:178-85, 1999.
26. Hilibrand AS, Carlson GD, Palumbo MA, et al: Radiculopathy and myelopathy at segments adjacent to the site of a previous anterior cervical arthrodesis. *J Bone Joint Surg Am* 81:519-528, 1999.

27. Hirabayashi K, Watanabe K, Wakano K, et al: Expansive open-door laminoplasty for cervical spinal stenotic myelopathy. *Spine* 8:693-699, 1983.

28. Hirabayashi K, Toyama Y, Chiba K: Expansive laminoplasty for myelopathy in ossification of the longitudinal ligament. Review. *Clin Orthop* 359:35-48, 1999.

29. Hoshino Y, Kurokawa T, Machida H: Long term results of the double door laminoplasty by longitudinal splitting of spinous process. *Rinshou Seikeigeka* 27:257-262, 1992.

30. Hukuda S, Mochizuki T, Ogata M, et al: Operations for cervical spondylotic myelopathy. A comparison of the results of anterior and posterior procedures. *J Bone Joint Surg Br* 67:609-615, 1985.

31. Hukuda S, Ogata M, Katsuura A: Experimental study on acute aggravating factors of cervical spondylotic myelopathy. *Spine* 13:15-20, 1988.

32. Hukuda S, Ogata M, Mochizuki T, Shichikawa K: Laminectomy versus laminoplasty for cervical myelopathy: brief report. *J Bone Joint Surg Br* 70:325-326, 1988.

33. Inoue A, Ikata T, Katoh S: Spinal deformity following surgery for spinal cord tumors and tumorous lesions: analysis based on an assessment of the spinal functional curve. *Spinal Cord* 34:536-542, 1996.

34. Itoh T, Tsuji H: Technical improvements and results of laminoplasty for compressive myelopathy in the cervical spine. *Spine* 10:729-736, 1985

35. Jenkins DH: Extensive cervical laminectomy. Long-term results. *Br J Surg* 60:852-854, 1973.

36. Kamioka Y, Yamamoto H, Tani T, et al: Postoperative instability of cervical OPLL and cervical radiculomyelopathy. Spine 14:1177-1183, 1989.

37. Kawaguchi Y, Matsui H, Ishihara H, et al: Axial symptoms after en bloc cervical laminoplasty. *J Spinal Disord* 12: 392-395, 1999.

38. Kawakami M, Tamaki T, Iwasaki H, et al: A comparative study of surgical approaches for cervical compressive myelopathy. *Clin Orthop* 381:129-136, 2000.

39. Kimura I, Shingu H, Nasu Y: Long-term follow-up of cervical spondylotic myelopathy treated by canal-expansive laminoplasty. *J Bone Joint Surg Br* 77:956-961, 1995.

40. Kimura S, Homma T, Uchiyama S, et al: Posterior migration of cervical spinal cord between split laminae as a complication of laminoplasty. *Spine* 20:1284-1288, 1995.

41. Kohno K, Kumon Y, Oka Y, et al: Evaluation of prognostic factors following expansive laminoplasty for cervical spinal stenotic myelopathy. *Surg Neurol* 48:237-245, 1997.

42. Kokubun S, Sato T, Ishii Y, Tanaka Y: Cervical myelopathy in the Japanese. *Clin Orthop* 323:129-138, 1996.

43. Kurokawa T: Enlargement of the spinal canal by sagittal splitting of spinal processes. *Bessatsu Seikeigeka* 2:234-240, 1982.

44. Lee TT, Manzano GR, Green BA: Modified open-door cervical expansive laminoplasty for spondylotic myelopathy: operative technique, outcome, and predictors for gait improvement. *J Neurosurg* 86:64-68, 1997.

45. Lee TT, Green BA, Gromelski EB: Safety and stability of open-door cervical expansive laminoplasty. *J Spinal Disord* 11:12-15, 1998.

46. Lunsford LD, Bissonette DJ, Zorub DS: Anterior surgery for cervical disc disease. Part 2: treatment of cervical spondylotic myelopathy in 32 cases. *J Neurosurg* 53:12-9, 1980.

47. Macdonald RL, Fehlings MG, Tator CH, et al: Multilevel anterior cervical corpectomy and fibular allograft fusion for cervical myelopathy. *J Neurosurg* 86:990-997, 1997.

48. Matsunaga S, Sakou T, Nakanisi K: Analysis of the cervical spine alignment following laminoplasty and laminectomy. *Spinal Cord* 37:20-24, 1999.

49. Mochida J, Nomura T, Chiba M, et al: Modified expansive open-door laminoplasty in cervical myelopathy. *J Spinal Disord* 12:386-391, 1999.

50. Morimoto T, Okuno S, Nakase H, Kawaguchi S, Sakaki T: Cervical myelopathy due to dynamic compression by the laminectomy membrane: dynamic MR imaging study. *J Spinal Disord* 12:172-173, 1999.

51. Morio Y, Yamamoto K, Teshima R, et al: Clinicoradiologic study of cervical laminoplasty with posterolateral fusion or bone graft. *Spine* 25:190-196, 2000.

52. Nagata K, Ohashi T, Abe J, et al: Cervical myelopathy in elderly patients: clinical results and MRI findings before and after decompression surgery. *Spinal Cord* 34:220-226, 1996.

53. Nakano N, Nakano T, Nakano K: Comparison of the results of laminectomy and open-door laminoplasty for cervical spondylotic myeloradiculopathy and ossification of the posterior longitudinal ligament. *Spine* 13:792-794, 1988.

54. Nolan JP, Jr., Sherk HH: Biomechanical evaluation of the extensor musculature of the cervical spine. *Spine* 13:9-11, 1988.

55. O'Brien MF, Peterson D, Casey AT, Crockard HA: A novel technique for laminoplasty augmentation of spinal canal area using titanium miniplate stabilization. A computerized morphometric analysis. *Spine* 21:474-483; discussion 484, 1996.

56. Ono K, Ebara S, Fuji T, et al: Myelopathy hand. New clinical signs of cervical cord damage. *J Bone Joint Surg Br* 69:215-219, 1987.

57. Orr RD, Zdeblick TA: Cervical spondylotic myelopathy. Approaches to surgical treatment. *Clin Orthop* 359:58-66, 1999.

58. Oyama M, Hattori S, Moriwaki N, et al: A new method of posterior decompression. *Centr Jpn J Orthop Traumatic Surg* 16:792-794, 1973.

59. Phillips DG: Surgical treatment of myelopathy with cervical spondylosis. *J Neurol Neurosurg Psychiatry* 36:879-884, 1973.

60. Robinson R, Walker A, Ferlic D: The results of anterior interbody fusion of the cervical spine. *J Bone Joint Surg Am* 44:1569-1587, 1962.

61. Rogers L: The surgical treatment of cervical spondylotic myelopathy. Mobilization of the complete cervical cord into an enlarged canal. *J Bone Joint Surg Br* 43, 1961.

62. Sasai K, Saito T, Akagi S, et al: Cervical curvature after laminoplasty for spondylotic myelopathy—involvement of yellow ligament, semispinalis cervicis muscle, and nuchal ligament. *J Spinal Disord* 13:26-30, 2000.

63. Satomi K, Nishu Y, Kohno T, Hirabayashi K: Long-term follow-up studies of open-door expansive laminoplasty for cervical stenotic myelopathy. *Spine* 19:507-510, 1994.

64. Seichi A, Takeshita K, Ohishi I, et al: Long-term results of double-door laminoplasty for cervical stenotic myelopathy. *Spine* 26:479-487, 2001.

65. Shaffrey CI, Wiggins GC, Piccirilli CB, et al: Modified open-door laminoplasty for treatment of neurological

deficits in younger patients with congenital spinal stenosis: analysis of clinical and radiographic data. *J Neurosurg* 90:170-177, 1999.

66. Shikata J, Yamamuro T, Shimizu K, Saito T: Combined laminoplasty and posterolateral fusion for spinal canal surgery in children and adolescents. *Clin Orthop* 259:92-99, 1990.

67. Simmons EH, Bhalla SK: Anterior cervical discectomy and fusion. A clinical and biomechanical study with eight-year follow-up. *J Bone Joint Surg Br* 51:225-237, 1969.

68. Sodeyama T, Goto S, Mochizuki M, *et al*: Effect of decompression enlargement laminoplasty for posterior shifting of the spinal cord. *Spine* 24:1527-1531; discussion 1531-1532, 1999.

69. Symon L, Lavender P: The surgical treatment of cervical spondylotic myelopathy. *Neurology* 17:117-127, 1967.

70. Tanaka J, Seki N, Tokimura F, *et al*: Operative results of canal-expansive laminoplasty for cervical spondylotic myelopathy in elderly patients. *Spine* 24:2308-2312, 1999.

71. Theodore N, Sonntag VK: Spinal surgery: the past century and the next. *Neurosurgery* 46:767-777, 2000.

72. Tomita K, Nomura S, Umeda S, Baba H: Cervical laminoplasty to enlarge the spinal canal in multilevel ossification of the posterior longitudinal ligament with myelopathy. *Arch Orthop Trauma Surg* 107:148-153, 1988.

73. Tsuji H: Laminoplasty for patients with compressive myelopathy due to so-called spinal canal stenosis in cervical and thoracic regions. *Spine* 7:28-34, 1982.

74. Tsuzuki N: A novel technique for laminoplasty augmentation of spinal canal area using titanium miniplate stabilization: a computerized morphometric analysis. *Spine* 22:926-967, 1997.

75. Uribe J, Vanni S, Jagid J, *et al*: Acute traumatic central cord syndrome: Experience using early surgical decompression with open door expansile cervical laminoplasty. In *Joint Section on Disorders of the Spine and Peripheral Nerves (AANS/CNS)—17th Annual Meeting*. Phoenix, Arizona, 2001.

76. White AA 3rd, Panjabi MM: Biomechanical considerations in the surgical management of cervical spondylotic myelopathy. *Spine* 13:856-860, 1988.

77. Yu YL, du Boulay GH, Stevens JM, Kendall BE: Computer-assisted myelography in cervical spondylotic myelopathy and radiculopathy. Clinical correlations and pathogenetic mechanisms. *Brain* 109:259-278, 1986.

78. Yue WM, Tan CT, Tan SB, *et al*: Results of cervical laminoplasty and a comparison between single and double trap-door techniques. *J Spinal Disord* 13:329-335, 2000.

# Laminoplasty: French Door

## Anthony A. Virella and Edward C. Benzel

The purpose of a laminoplasty is to decompress the contents of the spinal canal while maintaining stability and preserving the dorsal bony ligamentous complex, which provides protection for neural elements.

Cervical spondylotic myelopathy (CSM) results from mechanical compression of the spinal cord. Laminectomy and laminoplasty are two commonly utilized surgical options to treat affected patients. Since laminectomy can produce less than optimal results (e.g., development of postsurgical kyphosis), laminoplasty has gained acceptance as an effective surgical option. Over the last two decades many laminoplasty techniques have been employed. Two common procedures, the open door laminoplasty (ODL) and the French door laminoplasty (FDL), differ regarding the reconstruction technique employed. The specific aim of this section is to distinguish the differences between the FDL and the ODL techniques.

Cervical laminoplasty has become the choice of treatment for CSM in many regions. This procedure has been recommended for CSM and OPLL. The philosophy of laminoplasty is related to its ability to prevent kyphosis and instability, postlaminectomy membrane formation, arachnoiditis, and restenosis.[3] The main goal of laminoplasty is to enlarge the spinal canal and, in turn, to increase the cross-sectional area of the spinal cord, while maintaining stability. In 1972, Hattori introduced Z-plasty, which has not been widely accepted because of the technical difficulties of the operation.[8] Open door laminoplasty was first described in 1978.[1] Laminoplasty via splitting the spinous processes (French door) was described in 1982.[4]

Today, three fundamental laminoplasty procedures are commonly used: Z-plasty; hemilateral open-door laminoplasty; and bilateral open-door laminoplasty (middorsal laminoplasty or French door laminoplasty). To date, several additional modifications have been reported. In one study comparing three modification of laminoplasty, no outcome difference between modifications was demonstrated.[5]

This section describe laminoplasty by midline enlargement, also termed Kurokawa's method or French door laminoplasty. Kurokawa *et al.*[4] reported their experience in 19 patients with cervical myelopathy. The clinical results were assessed as very effective in 6 patients, effective in 9, improved in 2, and unchanged in 2; none were worse. Kyphotic changes were found in 6 patients in whom interlaminar fusion was not performed.

## Procedure

The patient is placed in the prone position and the head is secured in the Mayfield headholder. The procedure of exposing the spinous processes and laminae is the same as for a standard laminectomy. When the tips of the spinous processes are used for bone grafting, they are removed and preserved a midline osteotomy of the laminae is then performed. The spinous processes are drilled down with a high-speed drill after removing the interspinous ligament. The drilling should be done with a small burr, usually 1.5 to 2.0mm in diameter. Drilling is taken down to the be inner cortex of the dorsal lamina.

While approaching the lamina through the spinous process, broader drilling is performed. This corresponds to the shape of the lamina and preserves the inner cortex of the lamina. The inner cortex of the lamina is then cut with a diamond burr. In each spinous process a hole is made on the side for wiring and later fixation.

Two gutters are drilled at both junctions between the lamina and the facet joints, leaving the inner cortex of the lamina elastic, so that it will provide a hinge when each half of the lamina is lifted. Both halves of the lamina are lifted as if opening a saloon door, and the center of the laminae and ligamentum flavum are cut with Metzenbaum scissors, being careful to not cause bleeding from the epidural vessels. The pulsation of the dura mater should be observed.

When the tip of the spinous process is used as a bone graft, the bone should be shaped to fit the spinous process. Enlargement of the spinal canal is determined by the size of bone. The bone graft is usually 10mm in width for use at C3 to C5, where the spinous processes are long. The length of the bone is dependent on whether or not interlaminar fusion is needed. When interlaminar fusion is planned, it is necessary for the bone to be of suitable length. A wiring hole is made in the grafted bone, and each spinous process is wired.

## Discussion

Many types of laminoplasty have been described. Each has its own advantages and disadvantages, and there is no consensus regarding on preferred method. Follow-up studies are required to determine the efficacy of each method. The one major advantage of Kurokawa's method is not only its suitability for enlarging the spinal canal, but also its utility in dealing with segmental instability by providing interlaminar fusion.

In the presence of an effective lordosis, cervical laminoplasty may be indicated in multilevel OPLL, congenital spinal canal stenosis, multilevel cervical stenosis, dorsal ligamentous hypertrophy, and as part of a staged ventral/dorsal spinal canal expansion procedure.[7] Most of the studies on CSM and OPLL have reported postoperative enlargement of the spinal canal and an improved neurologic outcome. However, several recent studies suggest that there may be no significant postoperative difference between laminectomy and laminoplasty regarding decompression, neurologic recovery, kyphosis, and instability.[2,6] Laminoplasty was found to provide increased stability, with less translation, tilting, and ROM, compared with laminectomy.[12] Comparing the results of 28 cases (10 laminectomy and 18 laminoplasty with 5-year follow-up), Hukuda et al.[2] did not find superiority of laminoplasty over laminectomy in CSM for functional recovery and enlargement of the epidural space. There was no difference in the occurrence of kyphosis or instability. They reported a reduction in neck extension in those patients who underwent laminoplasty. Naito et al.[5] compared the results of hemilateral, bilateral open door laminoplasty, and Z-plasty and found no difference among these three modifications. Yoshida et al.[11] reported 50% limitation in flexion and extension of the neck following laminoplasty. On the other hand, Tsuzuki et al.[10] reported radiculopathies following laminoplasty procedures. They hypothesized that this was caused by an extradural nerve root tethering. Although all laminoplasty techniques have been used for the prevention of kyphosis and instability, several authors reported a rate of kyphosis development of up to 28%.[2] Henceforth, and in view of the aforementioned, French-door laminoplasty as a treatment for cervical stenosis remains controversial.

## REFERENCES

1. Hirabayashi H, Satomi K: Expansive open-door laminoplasty. In Denaro V (ed): *Stenosis of the Cervical Spine. Causes, Diagnosis and Treatment.* Berlin, Springer-Verlag, 1991, pp 264-278. [Reference unverified]
2. Hukuda S, Ogata M, Mochizuki T, et al: Laminectomy versus laminoplasty for cervical myelopathy: brief report. *J Bone Joint Surg Br* 70:325-326, 1988.
3. Koshu K, Tominaga T, Yoshimoto T: Spinous process-splitting laminoplasty with an extended foraminotomy for cervical myelopathy. *Neurosurgery* 17:430-435, 1995.
4. Kurokawa T, Tsuyama N, Tanaka H, et al: [Enlargement of the spinal canal by sagittal splitting of the spinous processes.] *Bessatsu Seikeigeka* 2:234-240, 1982. [Article in Japanese] [Reference unverified]
5. Naito M, Ogata K, Kurose S, et al: Canal-expansive laminoplasty in 83 patients with cervical myelopathy. A comparative study of three different procedures. *Int Orthop* 18:347-351, 1994.
6. Nakano N, Nakano T, Nakano K: Comparison of the results of laminectomy and open-door laminoplasty for cervical spondylotic myeloradiculopathy and ossification of the posterior longitudinal ligament. *Spine* 13:792-794, 1988.
7. O'Brien MF, Peterson D, Casey ATH, et al: A novel technique for laminoplasty augmentation of spinal canal area using titanium miniplate stabilization. A computerized morphometric analysis. *Spine* 21:474-484, 1996.
8. Raynor RB, Pugh J, Shapiro I: Cervical facetectomy and its effect on spine strength. *J Neurosurg* 63:278-282, 1985.
9. Sunago K, Kawai S: [Evaluation of the enlargement of the spinal canal for cervical myelopathy.] *Seikeigeka* 37: 1171-1178, 1981. [Reference unverified] [Article in Japanese]
10. Tsuzuki N, Abe R, Saiki K, et al: Extradural tethering effect as one mechanism of radiculopathy complicating posterior decompression of the cervical spinal cord. *Spine* 21:203-211, 1996.
11. Yoshida M, Otani K, Shibasaki K, et al: Expansive laminoplasty with reattachment of spinous process and extensor musculature for cervical myelopathy. *Spine* 17:491-497, 1992.
12. Zdeblick TA, Abitbol JJ, Kunz DN, et al: Cervical stability after sequential capsule resection. *Spine* 18:2005-2008, 1993.

# Ossification of the Posterior Longitudinal Ligament: Laminectomy

**Michael P. Steinmetz, Ajit A. Krishnaney, and Edward C. Benzel**

Tsukimoto first reported OPLL in 1960.[9] The disease process begins as calcification followed by OPLL beginning rostrally and extending caudally.[4] The disease extends across vertebral bodies, spanning the intervening disc spaces.[6,12]

Initially there is a proliferation of cartilaginous cells in the periosteum.[10] Rostral and caudal expansion occurs and incorporates bony maturation and PLL vascular fibrosis. A coalescence of calcified foci occurs and the ossification process further matures with the production of active marrow.[10,12]

OPLL occurs most often in the cervical spine. Beginning around C3 and extending caudally. Eventually, the spinal canal becomes narrowed and clinical symptoms, such as myelopathy, may occur.

OPLL has been classified according to imaging characteristics.[5] The classifications include *continuous, segmental, mixed,* and *other.* Continuous OPLL includes those cases in which the process extends across intervening vertebral bodies across and including the disc spaces. Segmental OPLL includes those cases in which the process in solely behind the involved vertebral body(s) and does not extend across the intervertebral disc. Mixed includes elements of both continuous and segmental. At times, the disease process is located dorsal to the disc space, similar to a calcified herniated disc. These may be classified into the "other" category.

Initially patients may be asymptomatic. As the disease progresses, myelopathy and/or radiculopathy develop. Myelopathy is seen much more often compared to radiculopathy. Furthermore, sphincter disturbances are rarely seen.[11,12] It is rare for a patient to present with only cervical pain.

Patients that are asymptomatic or with mild symptoms and nonprogressive disease may be initially managed conservatively. Those with myelopathy, myeloradiculopathy, and/or progressive disease should be treated with surgery. Better results have been observed in those patients operated on at a younger age and in those with a better myelopathy score.[9] In general, surgical options include ventral cervical corpectomy, ventral cervical discectomy, laminectomy with or without fusion, and the multiple variants of laminoplasty. Each operation has its own relative indications, contraindications, and complications.

## Laminectomy

### Indications

The indications for laminectomy are relative and may be surgeon specific. Most important is the preoperative spinal alignment. Laminectomy is indicated for those patients with an effective cervical lordosis. Furthermore, it may be used cautiously for those with a straightened spine. (see the following section). Patients with multisegment involvement, that is, three or more levels, may be more effectively managed with laminectomy compared to a ventral approach.[12] Older patients, or those with medical comorbidities may benefit from laminectomy compared to an extensive ventral procedure. This is related to less operative time and morbidity of laminectomy compared with extensive ventral corpectomy. Lastly, in patients with severe spinal stenosis accompanying their OPLL, laminectomy may be indicated prior to performing ventral surgery.[7]

### Defining Cervical Alignment

As previously mentioned, the most important (in the authors' opinion) consideration for laminectomy is spinal alignment. Those with an effective cervical lordosis should undergo laminectomy; those with an effective cervical kyphosis should undergo ventral corpectomy or discectomy; while those with a straightened spine may be decompressed with either laminectomy or a ventral decompressive procedure. A midline lateral cervical radiograph or sagittal magnetic resonance image (MRI) may be utilized to determine spinal alignment.[1] A vertical line is drawn from the dorsocaudal aspect of the C2 vertebral body to the dorsocaudal aspect of C7. A horizontal line is then drawn at the midpoint of the vertical line. The width of this horizontal line depends on the surgeon's preferences and biases. The lines that have been drawn appear similar to a kite and will be referred to as such. If the dorsal aspect of the cervical vertebral bodies lies ventral to the "kite" then the spine is in effective cervical lordosis. If the dorsal aspect of the cervical vertebral bodies lies dorsal to the "kite," the spine is in an effective cervical kyphosis. A grey zone exists when the dorsal aspect of the cervical vertebral bodies lie within the "kite." In this circumstance, the spine is straight, and either a ventral or dorsal procedure may be performed (Figure 166.4).

## Procedure

Laminectomy is performed as previously described in Chapter 32. A few specifics to OPLL should be mentioned. Ossification frequently spreads, it was seen in 70% of cases in the series reported by Kato *et al.*[9] In their series, deterioration was seen in pauci-level laminectomies resulting from spread of ossification (that is, laminectomy of three or fewer levels). Therefore, extensive laminectomy is recommended in the management of OPLL, even when the disease is somewhat limited. The decompression should usually include C3 to C7 or at a minimum of 1 to 1.5 segments above and below the radiographic abnormal segments. Because of the risk of postlaminectomy kyphosis, lateral resection should not include greater than the medial 25% of the facets on either side.[15]

Sectioning of the dentate ligaments has been advocated by some[13] and not by others.[3] The benefit of sectioning the dentate ligaments is unclear and necessitates opening the dura mater, which exposes the patient to the inherent risks of opening the dura, such as CSF leak and/or spinal cord injury. Therefore, the author's do not recommend this procedure.

## Outcome

Outcome is adversely affected by age and severe myelopathy at the time of decompression.[9] Therefore, the authors recommend earlier surgery for patients with OPLL.

Miyazaki *et al.*[13] performed laminectomy and had at least one year follow-up on 155 patients with OPLL. Three patients developed quadriplegia following the procedure, while 6 demonstrated only transient quadriplegia during the first 24 hours following surgery. Functional outcome was evaluated using the JOA evaluation. Overall 81.9% of patients showed some improvement. Specifically, 36.8% were rated as excellent, 18.1% good, 27.1% fair, 7.1% unchanged, and 11% poor. Seventeen percent of patients demonstrated postoperative kyphosis

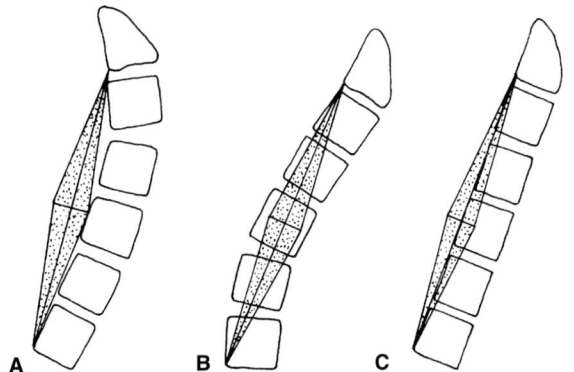

**Figure 166.4** A midline lateral cervical radiographic or sagittal MRI may be utilized to determine spinal alignment. A vertical line has been drawn from the dorsocaudal aspect of the C2 vertebral body to the dorsocaudal aspect of C7. A horizontal line is then drawn at the midpoint of the vertical line. The width of this horizontal line depends on the surgeon's preferences and biases *(see text)*. The lines that have been drawn appear similar to a kite and will be referred to as such. **(A)** If the dorsal aspect of the cervical vertebral bodies lie ventral to the "kite" then the spine is in effective cervical lordosis. Laminectomy is optimal for decompression in this situation. **(B)** If the dorsal aspect of the cervical vertebral bodies lie dorsal to the "kite," the spine is in an effective cervical kyphosis and a ventral decompressive strategy should be chosen. **(C)** A grey zone exists when the dorsal aspect of the cervical vertebral bodies lie within the "kite." In this circumstance, the spine is straight, and either a ventral or dorsal procedure may be performed. *(From Benzel EC:* Biomechanics of Spine Stabilization. *Rolling Meadows, IL, American Association of Neurological Surgeons, 2001.)*

or a worsening of their kyphotic deformity. It was not reported if the new or worsened spinal alignment negatively affected their neurologic status.

Similar results were reported by Nakano *et al.*[14] The authors performed laminectomy on 14 patients with OPLL and their outcomes were measured using the JOA score. Overall, 81.1% of patients demonstrated some improvement.

### Complications

Spinal cord injury may be seen in up to 10% of cases, while nerve root injury has been seen in up to 12.8% of cases.[2,16,17] Spinal cord injury is most often directly related to surgery and should be minimized by meticulous attention to detail. First and foremost, perioperative and intraoperative hypotension should be avoided. This may result is cord ischemia and quadriplegia. The spinal cord may also be injured during surgical decompression, that is, placing instruments under the laminae. Again, this may lessened by a careful choice and usage of instruments. The C5 nerve root may be injured during extensive cervical laminectomies, which is required for decompression of OPLL. This is most likely due to tethering of the root during dorsal migration of the spinal cord following decompression.[2,16] This deficit is usually temporary.

Postlaminectomy scar formation and kyphosis may develop following laminectomy. For these reasons, laminoplasty has been developed and widely used. The exact incidence of postlaminectomy kyphosis is unknown but may be as high as 21%.[8] Miyazaki *et al.*[13] noted that 17% of their patients either developed postoperative kyphosis or a worsening of their existing deformity. Although kyphosis and scar formation have been demonstrated following laminectomy their clinical sequelae are unknown and often do not have a negative effect on the patient's neurologic status.

In the author's opinion, patient selection and surgical technique minimizes the potential complication of postoperative kyphosis. For example, a facet-sparing laminectomy in a patient with preoperative lordosis should minimize postoperative deformity.

### Summary

Laminectomy is a highly effective surgical strategy for the management of OPLL. The procedure provides simultaneous multisegment decompression. The technique is familiar and the morbidity is low. It obviates the risk of neurologic injury and CSF leak that may be seen following a ventral procedure. Furthermore, a simultaneous fusion is avoided.

Laminoplasty has been advocated as an alternative to laminectomy. The incidence of postoperative cervical deformity and scar formation have been said to be less as compared with laminectomy. Despite these statements, there are some downsides to laminoplasty worth mentioning. Adequate decompression may be not performed on the "hinged side" of the laminoplasty. Furthermore, the hinged laminae may fracture through the inner cortex actually worsen the compression.[3] Although kyphotic worsening may be seen followed laminectomy it does not appear that this phenomenon has a negative impact on patients' neurologic status. Nakano *et al.*[14] compared laminectomy to laminoplasty for the management of OPLL and found that the outcome as measured on the JOA scale was no different between both groups.

Laminectomy should be viewed as the procedure of choice for those patients with a preoperative effective cervical lordosis and multisegment disease. Outcomes are favorable compared with the other procedures with less risk of CSF leak and neurologic injury.

### REFERENCES

1. Benzel EC: *Biomechanics of Spine Stabilization*, ed 2. Rolling Meadows, IL, American Association of Neurological Surgeons, 2001, pp 45-60.
2. Dai L, Ni B, Yuan W, Jia L: Radiculopathy after laminectomy for cervical compression myelopathy. *J Bone Joint Surg Br* 80:846-849, 1998.
3. Epstein N: Posterior approaches in the management of cervical spondylosis and ossification of the posterior longitudinal ligament. *Surg Neurol* 58:194-208, 2002.

4. Epstein N: Ossification of the posterior longitudinal ligament. In Benzel EC: *Spine Surgery: Techniques, Complication Avoidance, and Management.* New York, Churchill Livingstone, 1999, pp 489-502.

5. Hirabayashi K, Watanabe K, Wakano K, *et al:* Extensive open-door laminoplasty for cervical spinal stenotic myelopathy. *Spine* 8:693, 1983.

6. Hiramatsu Y, Nobechi T: Calcification of the posterior longitudinal ligament of the spine among Japanese. *Diag Radiol* 100:307, 1971.

7. Itoh T, Tsuji H: Technical improvements and results of laminoplasty for compressive myelopathy in the cervical spine. *Spine* 10:729, 1985.

8. Kaptain GJ, Simmons N, Replogle RE, *et al:* Incidence and outcome of kyphotic deformity following laminectomy for cervical spondylotic myelopathy. *J Neurosurg (Spine 2)* 93:199-204, 2000.

9. Kato Y, Iwasaki M, Fuji T, *et al:* Long-term follow-up results of laminectomy for cervical myelopathy caused by ossification of the posterior longitudinal ligament. *J Neurosurg* 89:217-223, 1998.

10. Kojima T, Waga S, Kubo Y, *et al:* Anterior cervical vertebrectomy and interbody fusion for multi-level spondylosis and ossification of the posterior longitudinal ligament. *Neurosurgery* 24:864, 1989.

11. Lee T, Chacha PB, Khoo J: Ossification of posterior longitudinal ligament of the cervical spine in non-Japanese Asians. *Surg Neurol* 35:44, 1991.

12. McAfee PC, Regan JJ, Bohlman HH: Cervical cord compression from ossification of the posterior longitudinal ligament in non-Orientals. *J Bone Joint Surg Br* 69:569-575, 1987.

13. Miyazaki K, Kirita Y: Extensive simultaneous multisegment laminectomy for myelopathy due to ossification of the posterior longitudinal ligament in the cervical region. *Spine* 11:31-42, 1986.

14. Nakano N, Nakano T, Nakano K: Comparison of the results of laminectomy and open-door laminoplasty for cervical spondylotic myeloradiculopathy and ossification of the posterior longitudinal ligament. *Spine* 13:92-94, 1988.

15. Raynor RB, Pugh J, Shapiro L: Cervical facetectomy and its effect on spine strength. *J Neurosurg* 63:278-282, 1985.

16. Saunders RL, Pikus HJ, Ball P: Four-level cervical corpectomy. *Spine* 23:2455-2461, 1998.

17. Yonenobu K, Hosono N, Iwasaki M, *et al:* Neurologic complications of surgery for cervical compression myelopathy. *Spine* 16:1277-1282, 1991.

# Smith-Robinson Technique

## Maxwell Boakye and Gerald E. Rodts, Jr.

Originally described by Smith and Robinson[8,9] four decades ago and subsequently modified by others,[2,4] the Smith-Robinson technique has proved to be a very successful technique for achieving arthrodesis in the cervical spine following discectomy. Ventral cervical discectomy was first performed by Smith and Robinson[8,9] and Cloward.[5] Whereas Cloward utilized a cylindrical bone dowel to replace the disc, Smith and Robinson described their approach to treatment of cervical disc disease using tricortical iliac crest bone graft. Despite the recent expanding availability of alternative graft options such as fibula allograft, premachined allografts, and polyethylether ketone (PEEK) grafts, the Smith-Robinson technique of bone grafting described next remains popular and is an excellent way to achieve satisfactory outcomes following cervical discectomy.

## Technique

Following general anesthesia and the acquisition of intravenous access, the patient is positioned for ventral cervical discectomy. The ventral cervical spine and disc spaces of interest are approached in a fashion as described in the subchapter by Boakye and Haid in Chapter 168 (Ventral Cervical Discectomy and Fusion with Allograft and Plating). Typically, the incision extends from the midline to the ventral border of the sternocleidomastoid muscle at the level of interest. Dissection is carried through the platysma muscle and through the superficial plane along the medial border of the sternocleidomastoid muscle, facilitating palpation of the carotid pulse. The carotid artery is retracted laterally as the spine is bluntly dissected. The prevertebral fascia is swept off with a Kittner (Sheavor) and the disc space of interest is confirmed by a lateral radiograph. Further exposure is obtained by release and retraction of the longus colli muscles. Vertebral body "gardening," discectomy and end plate preparation and further details of the operative approach can be obtained from the subchapter by Boakye and Haid in Chapter 168.

Following end plate preparation, a bone graft of appropriate size is placed in the disc space. The various techniques differ regarding the nature and geometry of the chosen graft. In the standard Smith-Robinson technique, a tapered horseshoe shaped tricortical iliac crest bone graft is placed in the disc space. The graft can be obtained from the ventral iliac crest using standard techniques. The graft is countersunk with the cortex facing ventrally. The ideal graft size is guided by preoperative disc height and on average is shaped to be approximately 2mm larger than the preoperative disc space height.[1] Graft size typically ranges between 6 and 10mm. Intervertebral body distraction pins are used to distract the disc space prior to graft placement. Most surgeons routinely perform osteophytectomies and removal of the PLL prior to graft placement. Smith and Robinson made no attempt to remove osteophytes, since it was their belief that bony spurs would resorb during the bone remodeling process following fusion. After discectomy and graft placement, a cervical plate can be placed at the discretion of the surgeon.

There have been some modifications of the standard Smith-Robinson technique. These include burring of the end plates to expose subchondral bone prior to graft placement (described by Emery *et al.*[6]) and reversal of the graft placement with the cortex facing dorsally (described by Bloom and Raney[2]). Reversing the bone graft is designed to lead to greater foraminal distraction, better middle column support, and lower graft extrusion rates. However, this strategy increases the chance of kyphosis due to the fact that weaker cancellous bone is placed ventrally. Excellent results have been reported using the standard Smith-Robinson as well as the modified Smith-Robinson techniques.[3,4,7] However, there is no Class I evidence supporting one approach over another. In a prospective study of 63 patients, Jenis and An[7] found no difference in clinical outcome using either the standard or the reversed Smith-Robinson technique. Both techniques can be used to achieve excellent arthrodesis and outcomes following ventral cervical discectomy. Regardless of the technique used, attention should be paid to proper vertebral body "gardening" and good end plate and graft "carpentry."

## REFERENCES

1. An HS, Evanich CJ, Nowicki BH, et al: Ideal thickness of Smith-Robinson graft for anterior cervical fusion. A cadaveric study with computed tomographic correlation. *Spine* 18:2043-2047, 1993.
2. Bloom MH, Raney FL Jr: Anterior intervertebral fusion of the cervical spine. A technical note. *J Bone Joint Surg Am* 63:842, 1981.
3. Bohlman HH, Emery SE, Goodfellow DB, et al: Robinson anterior cervical discectomy and arthrodesis for cervical radiculopathy. Long-term follow-up of one hundred and twenty-two patients. *J Bone Joint Surg Am* 75:1298-1307, 1993.
4. Brodke DS, Zdeblick TA: Modified Smith-Robinson procedure for anterior cervical discectomy and fusion. *Spine* 17:S427-S430, 1992.
5. Cloward RB: The anterior approach for the removal of ruptured cervical discs. *J Neurosurg* 15:602-615, 1958.
6. Emery SE, Bolesta MJ, Banks MA, et al: Robinson anterior cervical fusion comparison of the standard and modified techniques. *Spine* 19:660-663, 1994.
7. Jenis LG, An HS, Simpson JM: A prospective comparison of the standard and reverse Robinson cervical grafting techniques: radiographic and clinical analyses. *J Spinal Disord* 13:369-373, 2000.
8. Robinson R, Smith G: Anterior lateral disc removal and interbody fusion for cervical disc syndrome. *Bull Johns Hopkins Hosp* 69:223-224, 1955.
9. Smith G, Robinson R: The treatment of cervical spine disorders by anterior removal of the intervertebral disc and interbody fusion. *J Bone Joint Surg Am* 40A:607-624, 1958.

# Ventral Approach: Open-Window Corpectomy

## A. Fahir Özer

Compressive myelopathy is the most clinically significant problem associated with OPLL and advanced cervical spondylosis. There remains a lack of agreement about the most appropriate method of treatment of such cases. Extensive cervical laminectomy is a frequently used treatment. However, there is a continuing search for better techniques since many complications, like spinal instability, progression of spondylotic changes, spinal deformities, and constriction of the dura are frequently reported.[°] Researchers, particularly the Japanese, have developed laminoplasty techniques to prevent these complications.[†] However, in fact, such dorsal approaches are often inadequate. This is due to many factors, including the compression (usually from the ventral side), anchoring effects of the dentate ligaments and calcification or immobilization of the dura by attachment to the ossified PLL. Therefore, it has been suggested that a ventral approach may be preferable.[‡]

The technique described here is termed an open-window corpectomy because the technique leaves the ventral and the lateral portions of the vertebral body intact, and removes only the dorsal wall (i.e., a window). This provides an effective decompression through a window with minimal bone removal. This, in turn, results in minimal alterations in cervical spine biomechanics. Outcomes of the technique, based on a review of the current literature, are discussed.

## Surgical Technique

Patients are operated under general anesthesia in the supine position. Using a ventral approach, the PLL is reached following ventral discectomies. A variety of retractors may be used. The retractor used by the authors is practical and useful alternative to the existing self-retaining retractors especially for this operation,[28] particularly for Smith Robinson fusions.[33]

A high-speed drill is used upward from the connection of the PLL and the caudal surface of vertebral corpus, under a surgical microscope. The hole is broadened with the help of the drill, and the OPLL is removed (Figure 166.5). The same method is then applied to the upper discectomized intervertebral space in the downward direction (Figure 166.6). Generally, the removal of the dorsal half of the vertebral body corpus is sufficient to achieve an effective decompression. As a result, a space is formed at the dorsal aspect of the intervertebral discs and vertebral body that broadens the spinal canal (to approximately 15mm) (see Figure 166.6). The removal of the intervertebral discs and the cartilage end plates and creating a mortise for graft material, on both rostral and caudal surfaces of the vertebral body corpus, results in diminished vertebral body height. However, this shortening of the vertebral body height does not influence graft placement. After obtaining an effective decompression, a Smith-Robinson fusion is applied to the intervertebral spaces (Figure 166.7). In the surgical technique presented here, allograft fibula was used as a graft material. It is also possible to use autogenous iliac crest bone as a graft material. To minimize the incidence of graft dislodgment, the grafts are placed following distraction of the vertebral bodies, thus graft compression is achieved upon relaxation of the distraction. Additionally, the grafts are shaped since the

°References 1,2,9,12,23,24.
†References 13,17,18,21,25,26,30,31.
‡References 4,8,10,14,15,16,19,20,22,32,34.

ventral height of the graft is a few millimeter (1 to 3mm) greater than the height of dorsal surface. This minimizes dorsal dislodgement. Ventral spinal fixation is routinely used to increase the fusion rate.

This open-window corpectomy technique is particularly useful for moderate advanced cervical spondylosis or OPLL (Figure 166.8). In general, excellent results are obtained with this technique.[29]

## Rationale

Cervical spondylosis and OPLL cause progressive cervical stenosis and compressive myelopathy. Its surgical treatment is designed to decompress the spinal cord and widen the spinal canal.

Laminectomy has been accepted as the most appropriate surgical approach to achieve these goals. However,

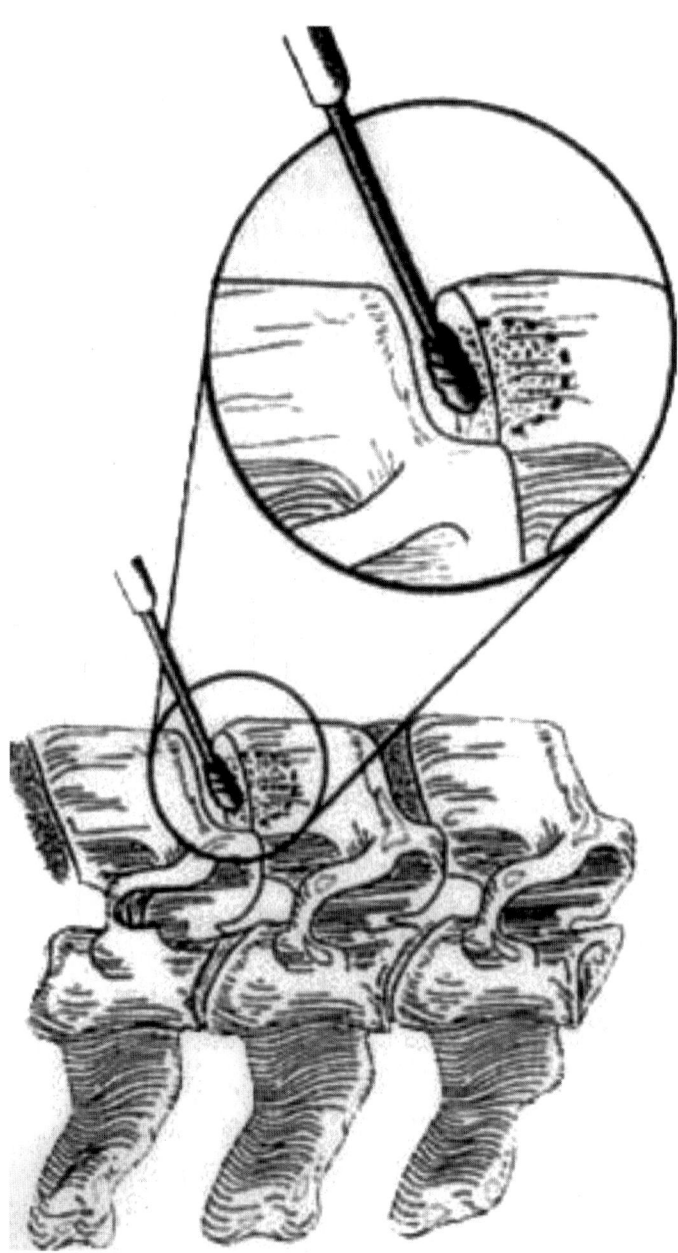

**Figure 166.5** Following removal of caudal and dorsal surface of the body, the rostral surface of the corpus in drilled towards the predrilled side.

instability and the constriction of the dura mater following laminectomy are common complications.[1,2,9,12,23,24]

Compression is generally from the ventral aspect of spinal cord in advanced spondylosis and OPLL, except for patients with a congenitally narrow spinal canal. The dura and the PLL are attached and even ossified in severe cases. The dentate ligaments, that connect the spinal cord to the ventral side of the spinal canal, and the nerve roots that bind the dura and the spinal cord

ventrally, limit dorsal spinal cord movement. For these reasons, dorsal approaches are usually insufficient to relieve the compression from the ventral side of the spinal column.*

Total OPLL extirpation is currently one of the best surgical techniques to achieve satisfactory outcome while avoiding the complications secondary to a dorsal approach.

---

*References 4,10,14-16,19,20,22,32,34.

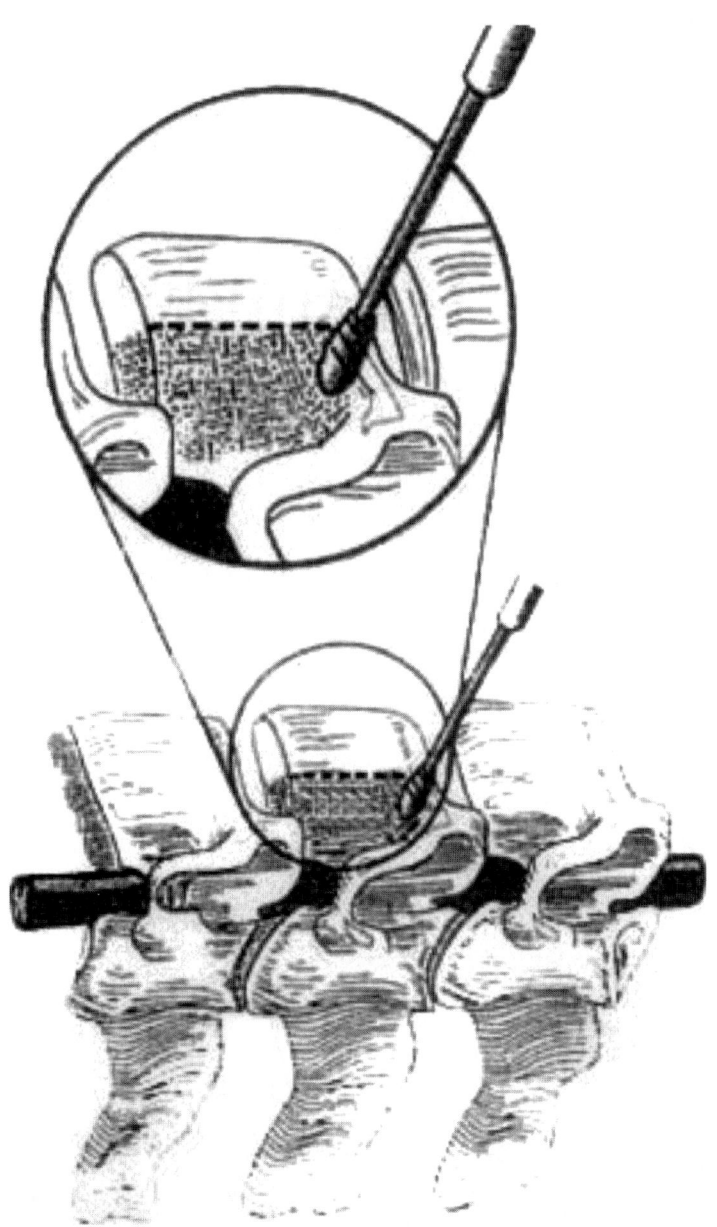

**Figure 166.6** The edges of the drilled sides are connected to each other and a window is made along with the posterior surface of the vertebra. The spinal canal is enlarged without performing total corpectomy.

With this surgical technique, the ossified annulus, the ossified cartilaginous end plates, and OPLL are totally extirpated following anterior corpectomy.°

The ventral floating technique is another commonly used surgical approach for such cases. This technique frees the OPLL over the dura after corpectomy. Incisions are made to the level of the OPLL at the upper and lower aspects of the affected levels. Thus, the expanded dura pushes the attached OPLL segment inward to the removed vertebral corpus.[19,22,33]

Both of these techniques are associated with pseudarthrosis, instability, and dislodgment due to the use of anterior strut grafts, especially when three or more disc spaces are included in the operation.[19,33,35]

## Biomechanics

The technique described here removes only the dorsal aspect of the vertebral corpus after performing appropriate ventral microdiscectomies. This provides a wide exposure of the spinal canal, along with the OPLL. After

°References 4,10,14-16,20.

removal of the OPLL, the spinal cord is decompressed. This technique allows the ventral aspect and both lateral portions of the vertebral corpus to remain intact (Figure 166.9). The importance of this is obvious with regard to the biomechanics of the spine. Biomechanically, the extent and the location of ventral spinal decompression significantly affects spinal instability.[4] The ventral vertebral body cortex provides a significant advantage regarding a buttressing effect. It bears axial loads much more effectively than the softer cancellous bone. The open-window corpectomy technique allows the bone graft to contact the three cortical margins of the vertebral body (two lateral and ventral cortical margins).

## Graft Placement

Other advantages of this technique include the ease of appropriate bone graft placement. The location of the ventral interbody bone graft significantly affects the biomechanical efficacy of the construct. Biomechanically, the optimal location of interbody bone graft placement is in-line or slightly ventral to the instantaneous axis of rotation (IAR) if the dorsal elements of the spine are intact.[5] The IAR is generally located at the junction of the anterior and

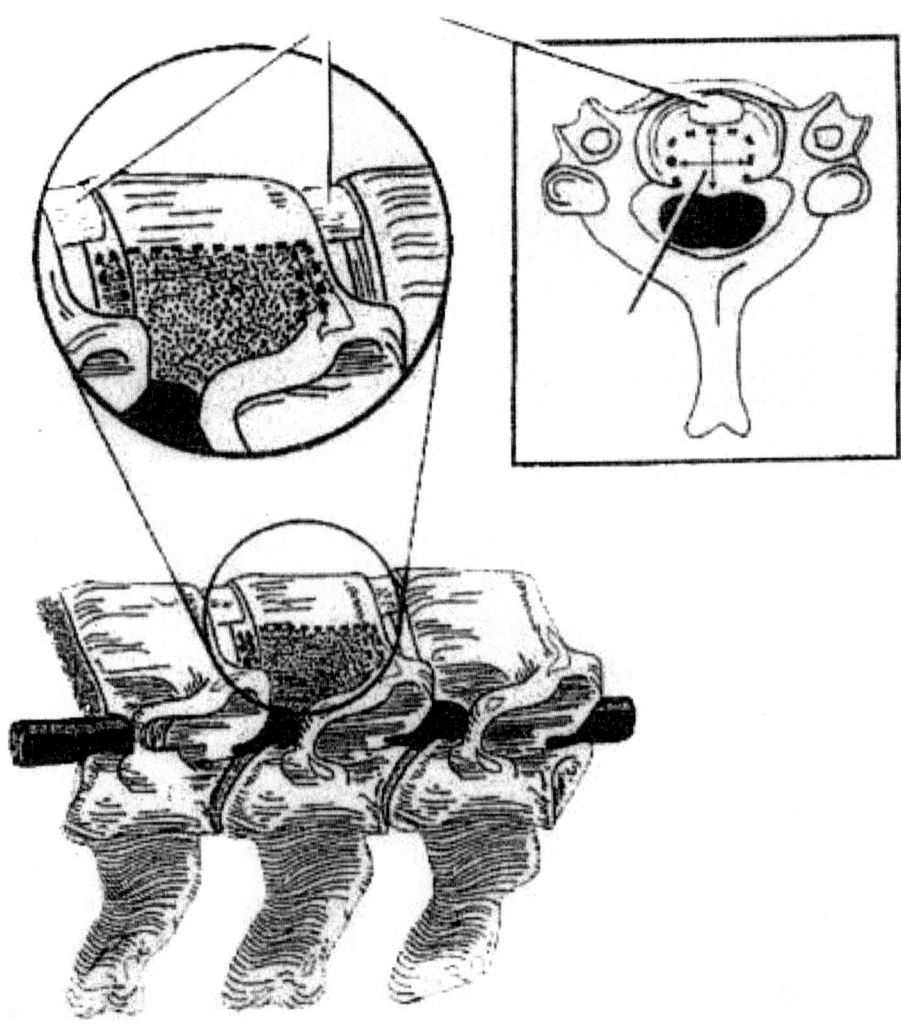

**Figure 166.7** Schematic illustration of placement of Smith-Robinson type fusions.

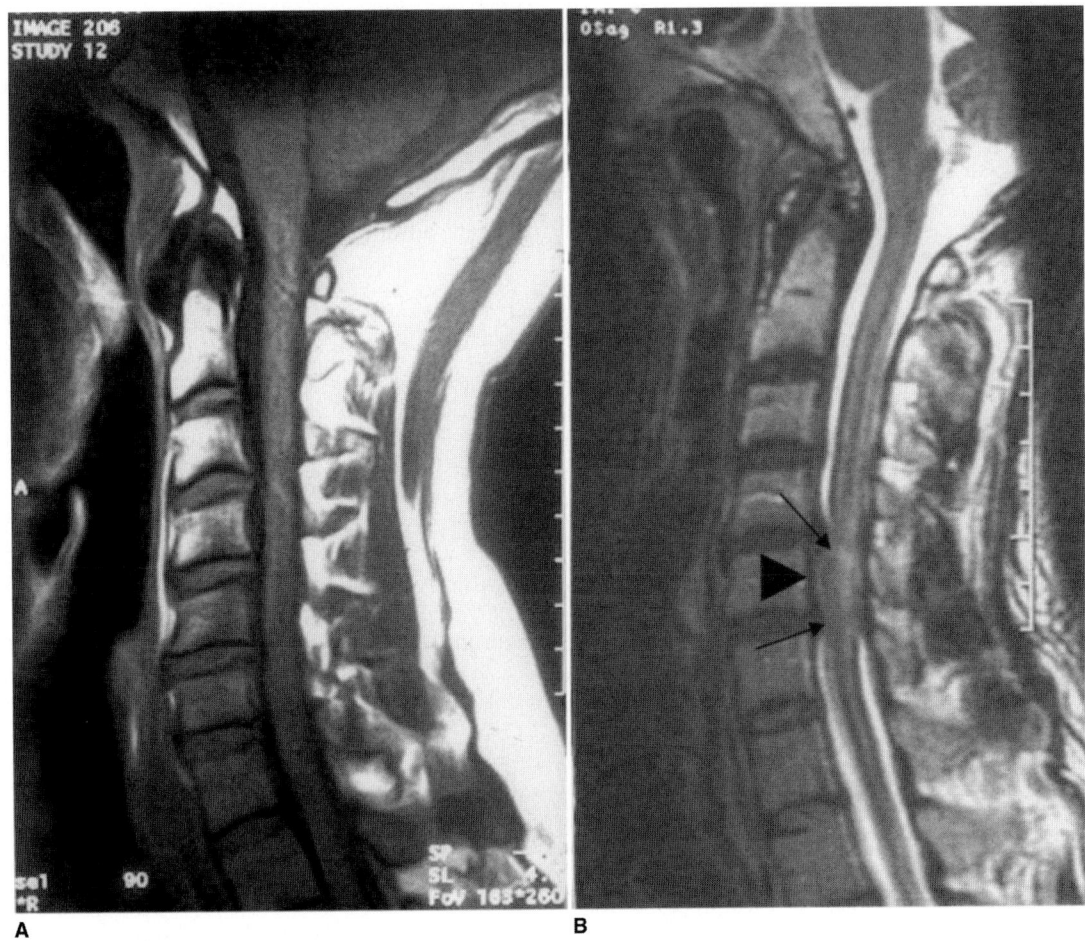

**Figure 166.8** (**A**) Case 1, (**B**) Case 2. Multiple level cervical spondylosis. Arrows depict the myelopathic areas at the effected levels. Notice loss of subarachnoid space (*arrowhead*) in posterior border of C5 corpus, compare with upper and lower levels.

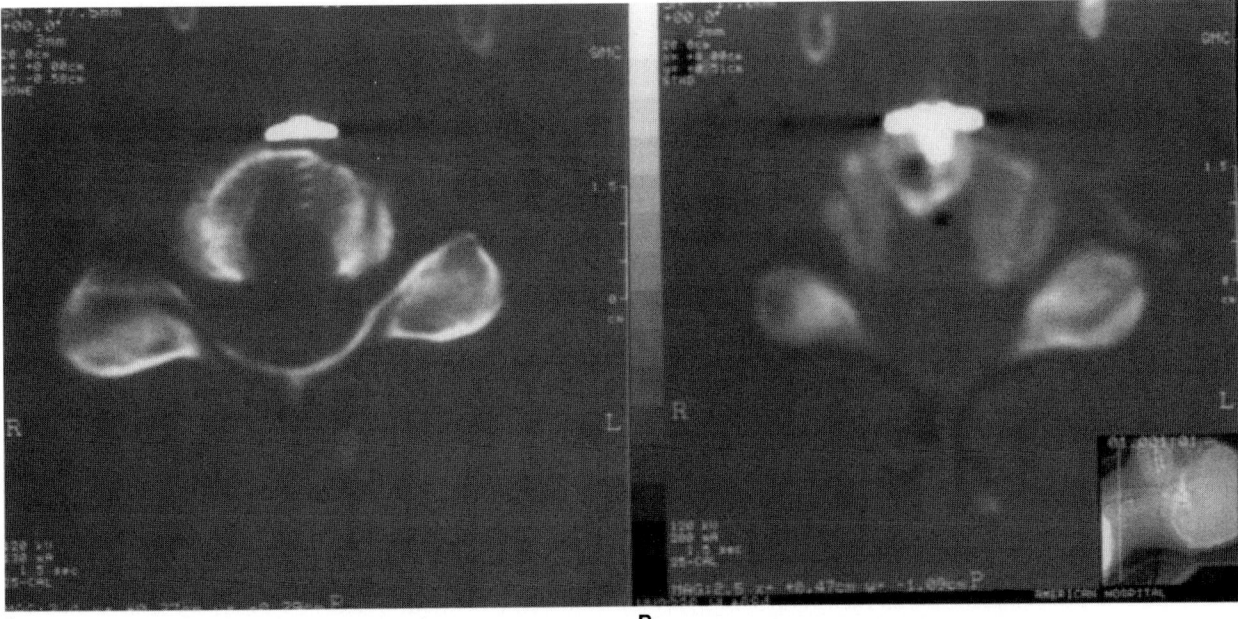

**Figure 166.9** (**A**) Case 1, (**B**) Case 2. Drilled the dorsal aspect of the vertebra. Note that the intact ventral vertebral body, sufficient decompression, and screw in the healthy corpus.

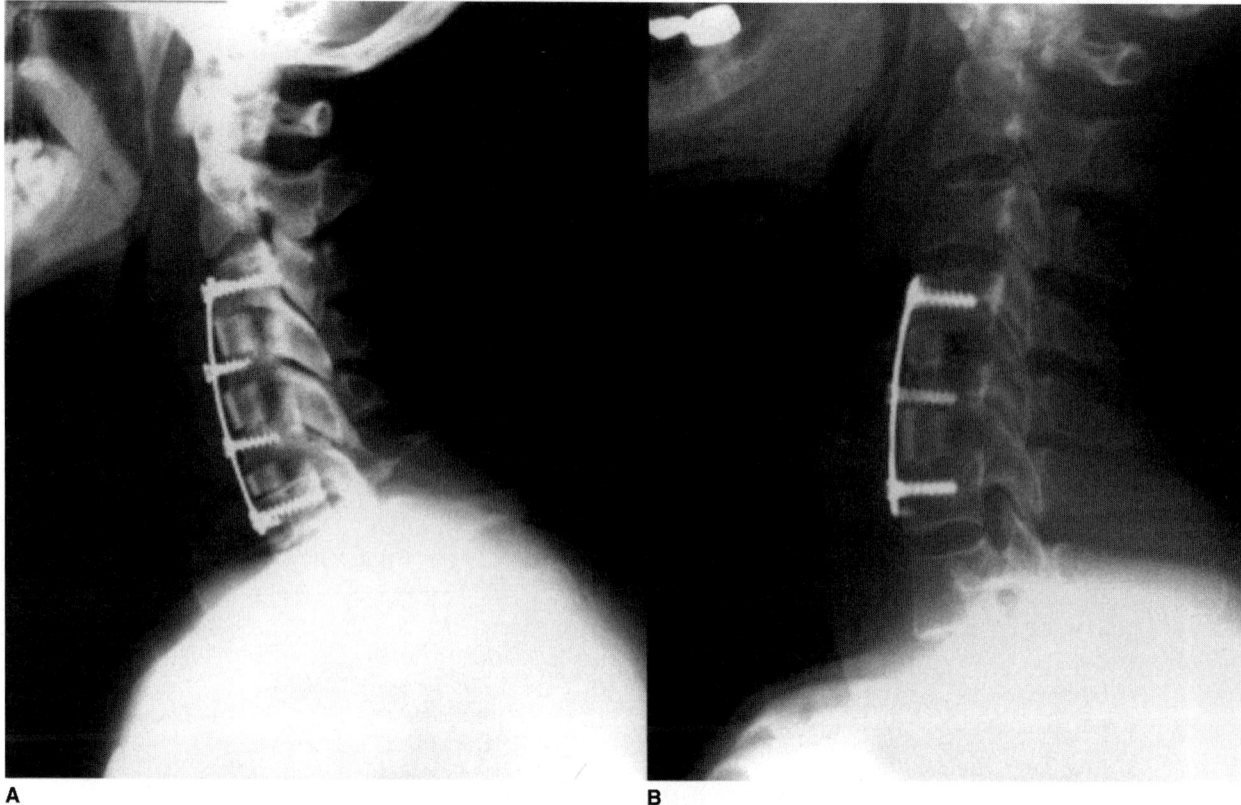

**A**                                                   **B**

**Figure 166.10** (**A**) Case 1, (**B**) Case 2. Plain lateral radiographs of the patient following the surgery. Note that the multiple fixation of the construct.

middle columns of Denis in the nonpathologic spine. The open-window corpectomy technique thus allows the placement of the interbody bone graft in an optimal location. Obviously, this should result in a substantial increase in axial-load-bearing ability.

## Multilevel Fixation

Finally, in cases where a ventral cervical fixation constructs are applied, this technique provides the option of multi-level fixation (Figure 166.10). Removal of only the dorsal aspect of the vertebral corpus permits the surgeon to place screws ventrally (Figure 166.11; see also Figure 166.9). Multilevel fixation provides the distribution of the fixation forces over multiple segmental levels. In other words, mul-tilevel fixation applies the "load-sharing" principle.[7] Although it is not yet proven experimentally, on a theoreti-cal basis, the distribution of forces decreases the stresses applied to the metal-bone interface at each segmental level. As a result, this minimizes the incidence of construct failure.[6]) Additionally, a rigid ventral construct can act as a fixed moment arm cantilever. In such an application, where two screws are used at each termini of the implant (Figure 166.12A), the construct bears axial loads relatively well. It, however, does not resist translational forces well. The addi-tion of intermediate points of fixation (Figure 166.12B) allows the implant to resist these translational forces with the utilization of three-point bending forces. Therefore, the additional fixation points not only allow axial loads to be borne more effectively by adding additional points of fixa-tion, but also allows for the resistance of translational forces as well. Moreover, a more stable construct is expected to provide a high fusion rate. In the author's paper,[29] a con-strained construct with cancellous bone screws was used. This is due to the fact that this was the only available implant during this timeframe. However, the author believes that use of a dynamic construct may be more appropriate, because it permits settling.

## Controversies

The use of multiple small grafts instead of a long strut graft is controversial. It is well known that the increase in the number of fusion sites decreases the fusion rates.[35,36] It has been also reported that placing an internal fixation implant significantly increases the fusion rate.[3,11,27] However, there is no existing data that compares plated multilevel, multi-graft fusion rates with plated multilevel, single-graft rates. The open-window corpectomy and similar techniques pro-vide improved load sharing between the implant and the vertebral bodies, and a more stable construct (by utilizing three-point bending fixation). Therefore, multiple grafts may be expected to be associated with a high union rate. As a result, problems such as dislodgment, pseudarthrosis, and construct failure may be infrequent with this method. The open-window corpectomy technique provides a wide decompression (see Figure 166.11) in a biomechanically sound manner.

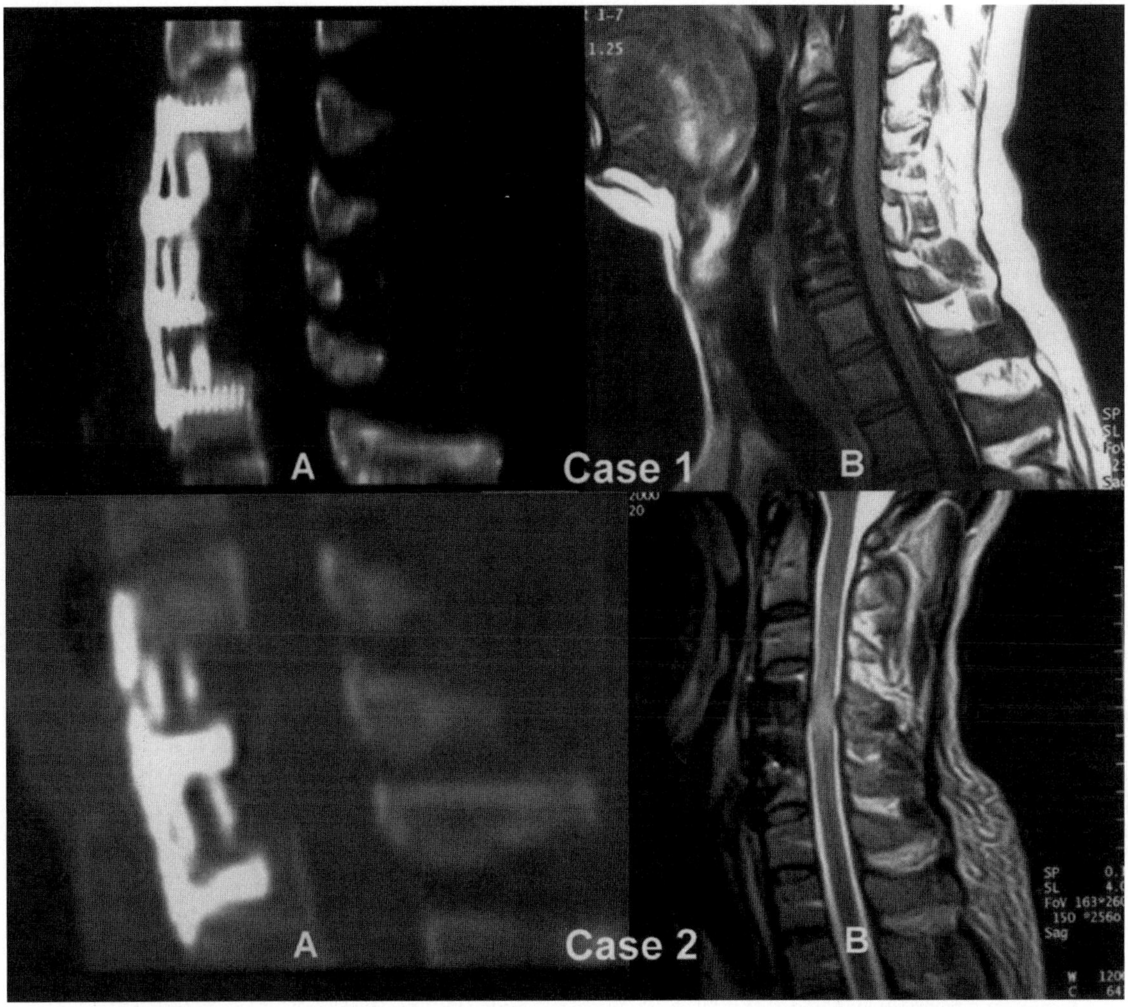

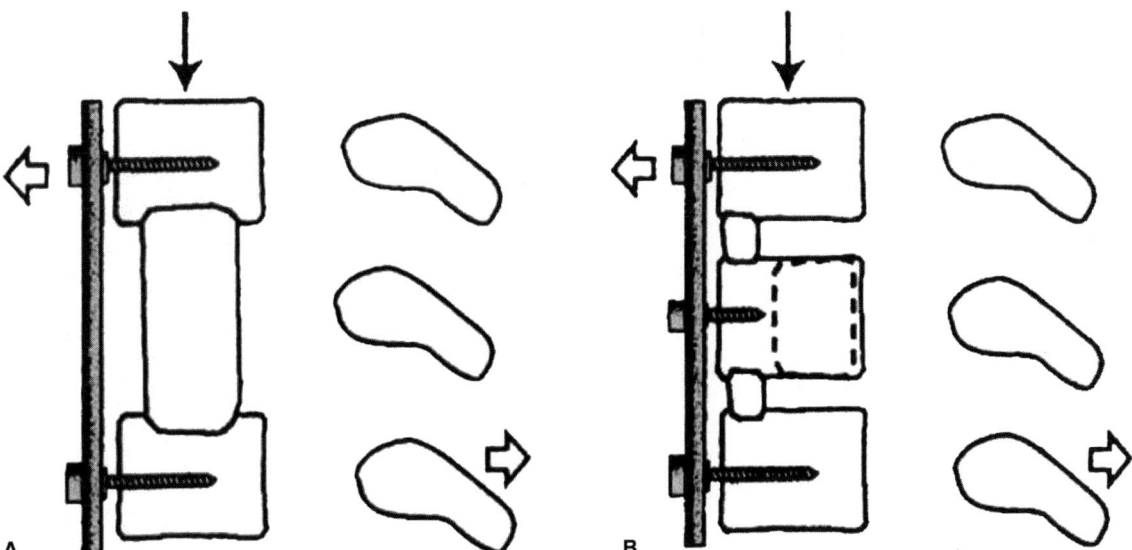

**Figure 166.11** Case 1 and 2, *A:* sagittal CT reconstruction study shows enlarged spinal canal after performing open-window corpectomy. Bony grafts are seen between vertebral bodies. The advantage of this technique is there is no necessity of the usage of long strut grafts for fusion. Note the use of multiple fixation. Case 1 and 2, *B:* Postoperative sagittal MRI study shows the satisfactory decompression of the spinal cord.

**Figure 166.12** **(A)** Illustration of multilevel long strut graft with anterior plate. Note that this construct acts like a fixed moment arm cantilever construct (*solid arrow* depicts axial force, *open arrows* depict translational forces). **(B)** Illustration of multilevel multigraft with anterior plate. Note that this construct applies three-point bending forces; thus offering better resistance to translational forces (*solid arrow* depicts axial force, *open arrows* depict translational forces).

# REFERENCES

1. Adams CB, Logue V: Studies in cervical spondylotic myelopathy. Functional effects of operation for cervical spondylotic myelopathy. *Brain* 94(3):587-596, 1971.
2. Alvisi C, Borromei A, Cerisoli M, Giulioni M: Long-term evaluation of cervical spine disorders following laminectomy. *J Neurosurg Sci* 32(3):109-112, 1988
3. Apfelbaum RI: Ventral and upper cervical spine fixation techniques. In Benzel EC (ed): *Spinal Instrumentation. Neurosurgical Topics.* Rolling Meadows, IL, American Association of Neurological Surgeons, 1994, pp 63-96.
4. Baba H, Furusawa N, Tanaka Y, *et al:* Anterior decompression and fusion for cervical myeloradiculopathy secondary to ossification of posterior ligament. *Int Orthop* 18(4):204-209, 1994.
5. Benzel EC: *Biomechanics of Spine Stabilization.* New York, McGraw-Hill,1995, pp 97-102.
6. Benzel EC: *Biomechanics of Spine Stabilization.* New York, McGraw-Hill, 1995, pp 103-108.
7. Benzel EC: *Biomechanics of Spine Stabilization.* New York, McGraw-Hill, 1995, pp 135-150.
8. Born JD. Evaluation and treatment of cervical spondylotic myelopathy by subtotal corpectomy without grafting. *Bull Mem Acad R Med Belg* 155 (3-4):171-179, 2000.
9. Butler JC, Whitecloud TS 3rd: Postlaminectomy kyphosis: causes and surgical management. *Orthop Clin North Am* 23(3):505-511, 1992.
10. Cheng WC, Chang CN, Lui TN, *et al:* Surgical treatment for ossification of the posterior longitudinal ligament of the cervical spine. *Surg Neurol* 41(2):90-97, 1994.
11. Connolly PJ, Esses SI, Kostuik JP: Anterior cervical fusion: outcome analysis of patients fused with and without anterior cervical plates. *J Spinal Disord* 9:202-206, 1996.
12. Cybulski GR, D'Angelo CM: Neurological deterioration after laminectomy for spondylotic cervical myoradiculopathy: the putative role of spinal cord ischaemia. *J Neurol Neurosurg Psychiatry* 51(5):717-718, 1988.
13. Edwards CC, Holler JG, Silcox DH: The saw laminoplasty for the management of cervical spondylotic myelopathy clinical and radiographic outcome. *Spine* 25(14):1788-1794, 2000.
14. Epstein N: The Surgical management of ossification of the posterior longitudinal ligament in 51 patients. *J Spinal Disord* 6(5):432-455, 1993.
15. Hanai K, Fujiyoski F, Kamei K: Subtotal vertebrectomy and spinal fusion for cervical spondylotic myelopathy. *Spine* 11(4):310-315, 1986.
16. Herkowitz HN: A comparison of anterior cervical fusion, cervical laminectomy and cervical laminoplasty for the surgical management of multiple level spondylotic radiculopathy. *Spine* 13(7):774-780, 1988.
17. Hirabayashi K, Satomi K: Operative procedure and results of expansive open door laminoplasty. *Spine* 13(7):870-876, 1988.
18. Hirabayashi K, Watanabe K, Wakano K, *et al:* Expansive open door laminoplasty for cervical spinal stenotic myelopathy. *Spine* 8(7):693-699, 1983.
19. Kamikozuru M: [Significance of the anterior floating method for cervical myelopathy due to the ossification of the posterior longitudinal ligament] *Nippon Seikeigeka Gakkai Zesshi (Jpn Orthop Assoc)* 65(8):431-440, 1991. [Article in Japanese]
20. Kojima T, Waga S, Kubo Y, *et al:* Anterior cervical vertebrectomy and interbody fusion for multi-level spondylosis and ossification of the posterior longitudinal ligament. *Neurosurgery* 24(6):864-872, 1989.
21. Koyama T, Handa J: Cervical laminoplasty using apatite beads as implants. Experience in 31 patients with compressive myelopathy due to developmental canal stenosis. *Surg Neurol* 24(6):663-667, 1985.
22. McAfee PC, Regan JJ, Bohlman HH: Cervical cord compression from ossification of the posterior longitudinal ligament in non-Orientals. *J Bone Joint Surg Br* 69(4):569-575, 1987.
23. Mikawa Y, Shikata J, Yamamuro T: Spinal deformity and instability after multilevel cervical laminectomy. *Spine* 12(1):6-11, 1987.
24. Miyazaki K, Kirita Y: Extensive simultaneous multisegment laminectomy for myelopathy due to the ossification of the posterior longitudinal ligament in the cervical region. *Spine* 11(6):531-542, 1986.
25. Nakano K, Harata S, Suetsuna F, *et al:* Spinous process-splitting laminoplasty using hydroxyapatite spinous process spacer. *Spine* 17(3S):41-43, 1992.
26. O'Brien MF, Peterson D, Casey AT, Crockard HA: A novel technique for laminoplasty augmentation of spinal canal area using titanium miniplate stabilization. A computerized morphometric analysis. *Spine* 21(4):474-484, 1996.
27. O'Shea JF, Sunderasan N: Use of instrumentation in degenerative disease of the cervical spine. *Mt Sinai J Med* 61:248-256, 1994.
28. Ozer AF. A novel retractor for the anterior approach to the cervical spine. *Neurol Res* 21:43-44,1999.
29. Ozer AF, Oktenoglu T, Sarioglu AC: A new surgical technique: open window corpectomy in the treatment of ossification of the posterior longitudinal ligament and advanced cervical spondylosis. Technical note. *Neurosurgery* 45(6):1481-1486, 1999.
30. Ranawat CS, O'Leary P, Pellicci P, *et al:* Cervical spine fusion in rheumatoid arthritis. *J Bone Joint Surg Am* 61-A(7):1003-1010, 1979.
31. Saruhashi Y, Hukuda S, Katsuura A, *et al:* A long term follow-up study of cervical spondylotic myelopathy treated "French Window" laminoplasty. *J Spinal Disord* 12(2):99-101, 1999.
32. Seichi A, Takeshita K, Ohishi I, *et al:* Long-term results of double-door laminoplasty for cervical stenotic myelopathy. *Spine* 1:26(5):479-87, 2001.
33. Shinomiya K, Okamoto A, Kamikozuru M, *et al:* An analysis of failures in primary cervical anterior spinal cord decompression and fusion. *J Spinal Disord* 6(4):277-288, 1993.
34. Smith GW, Robinson RA: The treatment of certain cervical spine disorders by anterior removal of the intervertebral disc and interbody fusion. *J Bone Surg Am* 40:607-624, 1958.
35. Yamaura I: [Anterior decompression for cervical myelopathy caused by ossification of the posterior longitudinal ligament: anterior floating method of OPLL] *Nippon Seikeigeka Gakkai (J of the Japanese Orthopaedic Assn)* 70(5):296-310, 1996. [Article in Japanese]

36. Yonenobu K, Fuji T, Ono K, *et al:* Choice of surgical treatment for multisegmental cervical spondylotic myelopathy. *Spine* 10:710-716, 1985.

37. Zdeblick TA, Ducker TB: The use of freeze-dried allograft bone for anterior cervical fusions. *Spine* 16: 726-729, 1991.

# CHAPTER 167

# Spondylotic Myelopathy with Cervical Kyphotic Deformity

## Ventral Approach

**Michael P. Steinmetz, Christopher D. Kager, and Edward C. Benzel**

The development of cervical spine deformity may be secondary to advanced degenerative disease, trauma, neoplastic disease, or postsurgical instability.[11] It may also occur in patients with systemic arthritides, such as ankylosing spondylitis and rheumatoid arthritis.

The most common cause of cervical kyphosis is iatrogenic (postsurgical).[2] This most commonly occurs after laminectomy. The surgical procedure involves disruption of the dorsal tension band. The incidence of clinically significant kyphosis in this situation may be as high as 21%.[12] Kyphosis may also occur following ventral cervical surgery. This may be due to pseudoarthrosis or failure to restore the anatomic cervical lordosis during surgery.[6,8]

Whatever the cause, the development of cervical deformity should be avoided and corrected when appropriate. Axial loading tends to further the kyphosis, thus creating a vicious cycle and progression of the deformity.[3] The deformity tends to cause neck pain, which is mechanical in nature.[13] The pain is due to a biomechanical disadvantage placed on the cervical musculature, and degeneration of the adjacent cervical discs. In advanced cases, forward gaze, swallowing, and respiration may be adversely affected.

## Ventral versus Dorsal Approach

Sagittal plane deformity in the cervical spine may be corrected ventrally,[4,7,10,17] dorsally,[1,5] or a combination of both.[1,9,14,15] The ventral approach is an approach that is familiar to most spine surgeons and may be performed with minimal morbidity.

Many patients with cervical kyphosis have had a prior cervical operation, often a laminectomy (Figure 167.1). A dorsal revision strategy is associated with increased morbidity regarding wound complications, pain, and the risk of neurologic injury. A ventral approach is advantageous in that "virgin" surgical territory is entered. If a prior ventral approach had been performed, the same approach may be used without difficulty, or the opposite side of the neck may be entered for the revision. These factors decrease the morbidity associated with revision cervical surgery.

In the majority of cases of cervical kyphosis there exists ventral compression of the spinal cord along with the deformity. This ventral compression must be addressed prior to deformity correction. A ventral decompression may not be adequately performed from a dorsal approach; therefore, a ventral decompression should be included with dorsal instrumentation, which increases the morbidity of the operation. A ventral approach alone permits adequate spinal cord decompression via multiple intervertebral discectomies or corpectomies. The authors favor leaving intermediate vertebral bodies and not performing multiple adjacent level corpectomies (i.e., C5, C6, and C7). A safe intermediate vertebral body is one in which there is CSF signal dorsal to the body on a $T_2$-weighted magnetic resonance image (MRI). Adequate ventral decompression may be performed with this strategy and the intervening body will be used as an intermediate point of fixation (see following discussion).

Utilizing a dorsal alone approach strategy, one is most often unable to significantly correct cervical kyphosis. Only if the deformity is "flexible" and is able to be corrected with cervical traction, may a dorsal alone approach strategy be utilized. This is not at all common. More often, a ventral release procedure is required prior to the dorsal deformity correction procedure. A dorsal deformity correction procedure, with or without a ventral release, may not fully correct the deformity. Abumi et al.,[1] even with the use of cervical pedicle screws, were only able to correct cervical deformity from 28.4 to 5.1 degrees of kyphosis with all patients achieving a solid arthrodesis. A ventral strategy provides a "better surgical leverage" for deformity correction while providing very solid fixation points if intermediate points of fixation are employed.[3]

As mentioned above, utilizing multiple points of intermediate fixation is optimal with ventral deformity correction strategies. This is accomplished by leaving intermediate vertebral bodies in place, instead of performing multiple adjacent corpectomies. These intermediate bodies provide solid fixation points for intermediate points of screw fixation. These intermediate points facilitate the "bringing of the spine" to a contoured implant to achieve further lordotic correction. They also provide three or four point bending forces to prevent deformity progression and construct failure.[3] These intermediate fixation points may also be provided with dorsal lateral mass fixation, but entail the addition of a dorsal procedure, in addition to a ventral decompression procedure.

Axially dynamic cervical implants further add to the success of a ventral deformity correction procedure. These constructs are able to provide for the placement of multiple intermediate points of fixation. The dynamic aspect of the implant is able to off load stresses at the screw/implant interface. This aids in the prevention of nonunion and construct failure, and also provides solid fixation for the prevention of cervical deformity progression.

## Recent Clinical Experience

Steinmetz et al.[16] reported their experience with the ventral correction of postsurgical cervical kyphosis. A dynamic implant was utilized in most patients. The average magni-

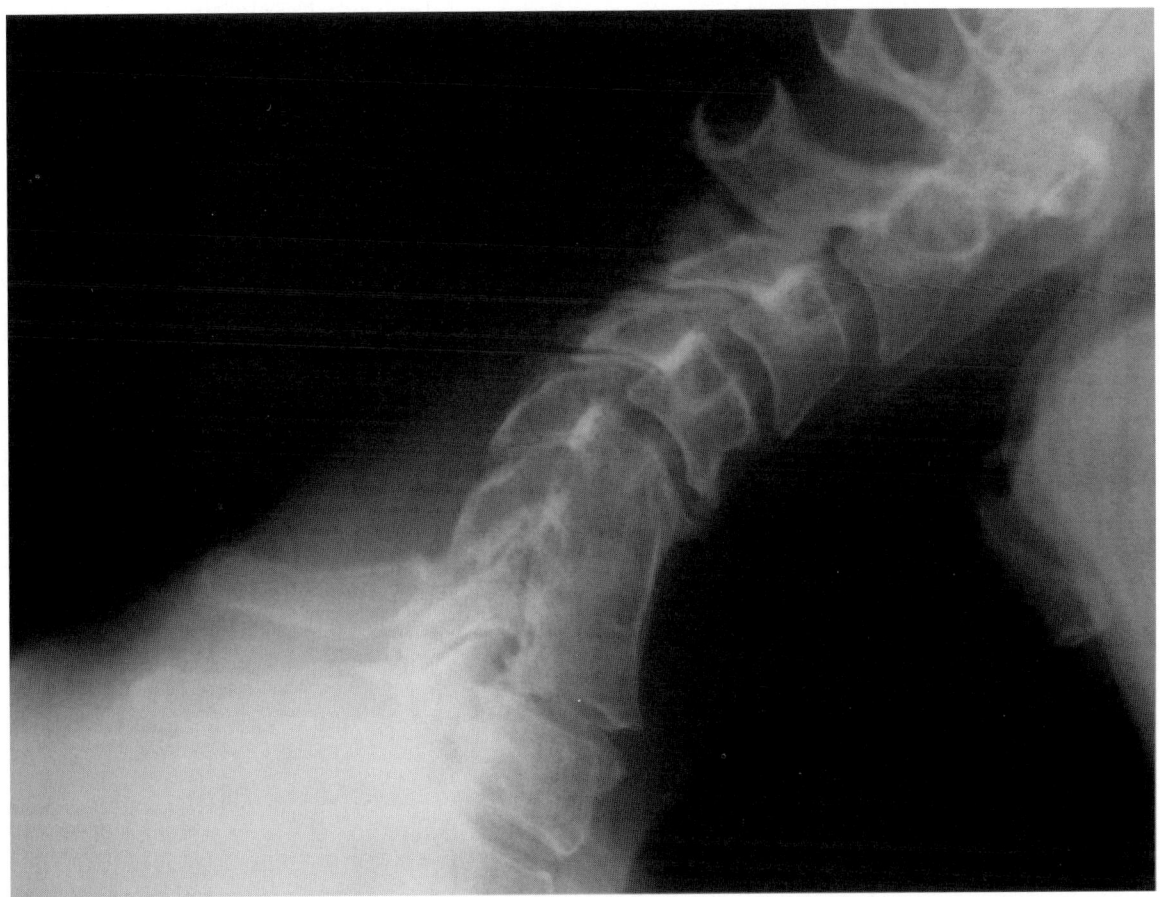

**Figure 167.1** Lateral Cervical Radiograph. The patient has a prior cervical laminectomy and also has a solid fusion mass at C4-7. The radiograph demonstrates significant kyphosis.

tude of deformity correction was 20 degrees of lordosis (Figure 167.2). The average sagittal angle following surgery was 5 degrees of lordosis. This angle was maintained effectively in the follow-up period (average 9 months), with an average change in the sagittal angle of 2 degrees of lordosis.

## Summary

It is rare that a dorsal strategy may be used alone for cervical kyphosis correction. A combined ventral/dorsal approach is used for adequate decompression and deformity correction. This strategy is associated with an increased morbidity compared with a ventral alone approach strategy. A ventral approach is familiar to spine surgeons. It permits decompression and correction via a single surgical approach. The ventral correction provides a better "surgical leverage" compared with a dorsal procedure. The correction attained is effectively maintained with strut grafting and ventral instrumentation, especially if an axially dynamic ventral construct, using intermediate points of fixation, is utilized.

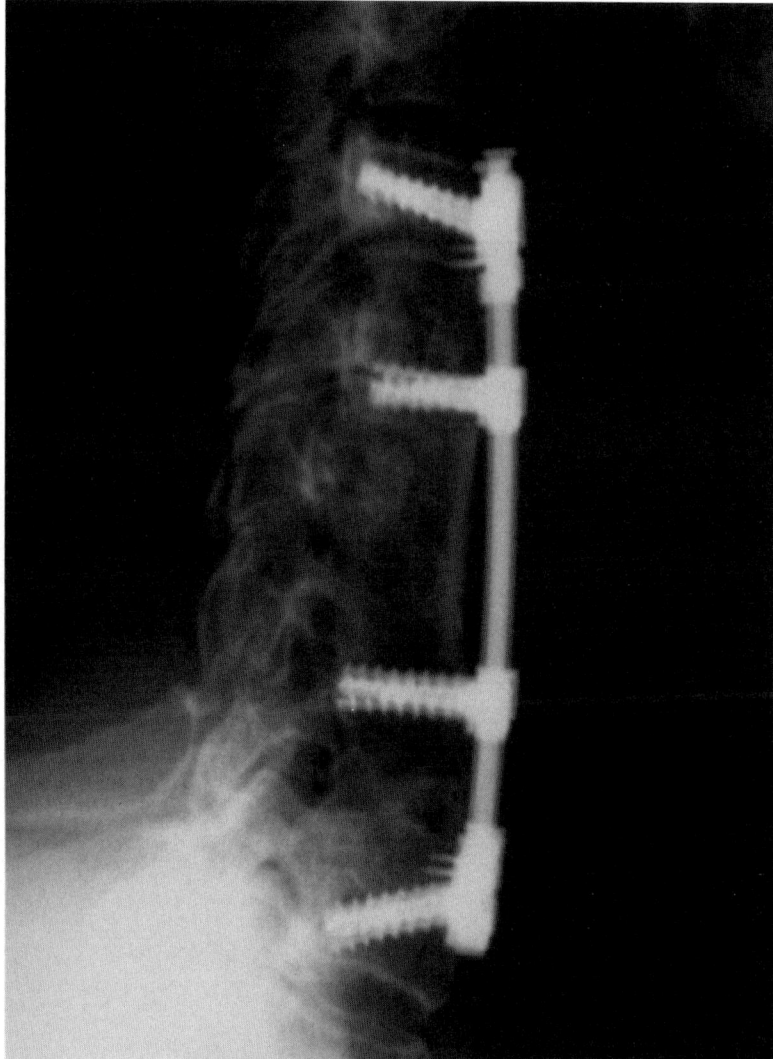

**Figure 167.2** Lateral Cervical Radiograph Following Surgery. A ventral alone strategy utilizing multiple intermediate points of fixation was used. The kyphosis is effectively reduced. (Same patient as in Figure 167.1.)

## REFERENCES

1. Abumi K, Shono Y, Taneichi H: Correction of cervical kyphosis using pedicle screw fixation systems. *Spine* 24:2389-2396, 1999.

2. Albert TJ, Vacarro A: Postlaminectomy kyphosis. *Spine* 23:2738-2745, 1998.

3. Benzel EC: *Biomechanics of Spine Stabilization*. Rolling Meadows, IL, American Association of Neurological Surgeons, 2001.

4. Buttler JC, Whitecloud III TS: Postlaminectomy kyphosis: causes and surgical management. *Clin Orthop North Am* 23:505-511, 1992.

5. Callahan RA, Johnson RM, Margolis RN: Cervical facet fusion for control of instability following laminectomy. *J Bone Joint Surg Am* 59:991-1002, 1977.

6. Caspar W, Pitzen T: Anterior cervical fusion and trapezoidal plate stabilization for re-do surgery. *Surg Neurol* 52: 345-352, 1999.

7. Cattrell HS, Clark GJ Jr: Cervical kyphosis and instability following multiple laminectomies in children. *J Bone Joint Surg Am* 49:713-720, 1967.

8. Geisler FH, Caspar W, Pitzen T, *et al*: Reoperation in patients after anterior cervical plate stabilization in degenerative disease. *Spine* 23:911-920, 1998.

9. Heller JG, Silcox III DH, Sutterlin CE III: Complications of posterior cervical plating. *Spine* 20: 2442-2448, 1995.

10. Herman JM, Sonntag VK: Cervical corpectomy and plate fixation for post-laminectomy kyphosis. *J Neurosurg* 80: 963-970, 1994.

11. Johnston FG, Crockard HA: One stage internal fixation and anterior fusion in complex cervical spinal disorders. *J Neurosurg* 82:234-238, 1995.

12. Kaptain GJ, Simmons N, Replogle RE, *et al*: Incidence and outcome of kyphotic deformity following laminectomy for cervical spondylotic myelopathy. *J Neurosurg (Spine 2)* 93:199-204, 2000.

13. Katsuura A, Hukuda S, Imanaka T, *et al:* Anterior cervical plate used in degenerative disease can maintain cervical lordosis. *J Spinal Disord* 9:470-476, 1996.

14. McAfee PC, Bohlman HH, Ducker TB: One stage anterior cervical decompression and posterior stabilization. A study of one hundred patients with a minimum of two years of follow-up. *J Bone Joint Surg Am* 77:1791-1800, 1995.

15. Savini R, Parisini P, Cervellati S: The surgical treatment of late instability of flexion-rotation injuries in the lower cervical spine. *Spine* 12:178-182, 1987.

16. Steinmetz MP, Kager C, Benzel EC: Anterior correction of postsurgical cervical kyphosis. *J Neurosurg (Spine 2)* 97:277-280, 2002.

17. Zdeblick TA, Bohlman HH: Cervical kyphosis and myelopathy: treatment by anterior corpectomy and strut-grafting. *J Bone Joint Surg Am* 71:170-182, 1989.

# Dorsal Approach

## Kuniyoshi Abumi, Manabu Ito, and Kota Suda

Expansive laminoplasty has been adopted to treat cervical myelopathy secondary to multisegmental stenotic lesions such as multisegmental spondylosis, developmental spinal canal stenosis, or continuous or mixed-type ossification of the posterior longitudinal ligament (OPLL).[12,22] Since open-door expansive laminoplasty was first designed by Hirabayashi, many modified techniques have been reported. As compared with laminectomy, laminoplasty is able to preserve spinal stability and lessen the potential hazard of postoperative kyphosis. Narrowing of the cervical spinal canal in cervical spondylosis is caused by degenerative changes of ventral and dorsal elements of the cervical spine. Therefore, both of ventral and dorsal procedures yield decompressive effects on the cervical spinal cord.

The decompressive effects of laminoplasty consist of two distinct mechanisms. One is a direct dorsal decompression, and the other is an indirect ventral decompression that is obtained by the dorsal shift of the spinal cord from the ventral compressive lesions of bony spur and bulging disc. Regarding the latter effect, cervical kyphosis may lead to poor surgical outcomes, because it may interfere with dorsal shift of the spinal cord. Baba et al.[7] showed that neurologic improvement is associated with dorsal cord shift on MRI. They reported that postoperative neurologic improvement in their study was highly correlated with the volume of the enlarged bony canal, which could be observed in patients with lordotic alignment. Sodeyama et al.[24] reported that a dorsal shift of the spinal cord of more than 3mm leads a good recovery of myelopathic symptoms. For this total decompression effect, lordotic alignment of the cervical spine is indispensable in order to facilitate dorsal spinal cord shift.

## Spinal Cord Compression in Cervical Spondylosis with Kyphosis

Several previous reports have mentioned that patients with cervical kyphosis do not gain favorable clinical results. Kimura et al.[16] reported that laminoplasty did not provide good clinical results in presence of kyphotic or S-shaped malalignment because the spinal cord was compressed at the apex of the kyphosis, disturbing dorsal shift of the spinal cord. Yamazaki et al.[26] demonstrated that morphologic limitations of dorsal decompression for cervical myelopathy were lordosis less than 10 degrees and OPLL exceeding 7mm in thickness. Suda et al.[25] reported that laminoplasty did not provide satisfactory results in patients with local cervical kyphosis exceeding 13 degrees. Masini and Maranhao[18] showed that mechanical stress on the ventral aspect of the spinal cord increases with a progression of kyphosis. Breig et al.[8,9] demonstrated that filling defects of arteries to the spinal cord occurs in cervical flexion, which leads to reduction of blood supply to the spinal cord. If the kyphotic deformity continues, myelomalacia and spinal cord atrophy will be in progress. Furthermore, flexible kyphotic deformity of cervical spondylosis may damage the spinal cord at the apex of the curvature under cervical dynamic motions.

## Correction Procedures of Spondylotic Myelopathy with Kyphosis

One of the solutions of poor outcomes of dorsal decompression procedures for cervical spondylotic myelopathy with kyphosis is direct ventral decompression. Although ventral decompression for the patients with kyphosis for short segmental compression is effective, and can be performed without serious complications,[27] a long strut graft or multilevel grafts are often required for multisegmental lesions. Moreover, multisegmental ventral decompression and fusion occasionally results in high rates of complications such as pseudoarthrosis, dislocation, or subsidence of grafted bone.[6,28] For patients with severe kyphosis, ventral decompression and a deformity correction procedure has been used as one of the solutions to restore lordotic alignment. However, the deformity correction rate for cervical kyphosis has not been shown to be sufficient, even with the support of ventral plating.[11] Alternative procedures to solve these problems are dorsal correction of kyphosis or combined ventral and dorsal procedures.[3,5,19] When the laminae cannot be used for stabilizing anchors after dorsal decompression, lateral mass screw-plate fixation or pedicle screw fixation still can be used to correct kyphosis and stabilize the segments.[3,5,10] On the basis of previous reports on cervical fixation procedures, pedicle screw fixation has been observed to provide advantages over lateral screw-plate fixation in terms of stability and pullout strength, correction rate, fusion rate, and clinical results.[5,13,17] Pedicle screw systems provide other benefits in that they can restore cervical lordosis through a single dorsal approach with simultaneous dorsal decompression, and they can maintain the correction until completion of solid bony fusion occurs.[3,5]

# Dorsal Procedure Using Pedicle Screw Fixation Systems

As for the cervical pedicle, screw insertion has been considered too risky for the neurovascular structures, except at the C2 and C7 levels.[21] However, this procedure allows rigid fixation that facilitates deformity correction and the restoration of physiologic sagittal alignment. In addition, pedicle screw fixation procedures, which do not require use of the lamina as a stabilizing anchor, are quite valuable in patients who undergo one-stage dorsal cervical decompression and stabilization and in patients who undergo dorsal reconstruction after previous cervical laminectomy. On the other hand, the risks of neurovascular complications caused by suboptimal screw placement into the cervical pedicle cannot be completely obviated.[1,4] Although, the incidence of neurovascular complications caused by dislodged screws is low, a thorough knowledge of local anatomy and the use of established surgical techniques are essential for this procedure to be optimally effective.[2]

## Preoperative Considerations

The pedicles in some patient are too small in diameter to permit screw insertion.[14,20] Preoperative oblique projection plain radiographs can be used for evaluation of pedicle size. With oblique projection plain films, the contralateral pedicle is visualized as an oval projected onto the vertebral body, showing the outer and inner diameter of the pedicle (Figure 167.3, A). Computed tomography (CT) (adjusted to bone windows) is essential to assess the pedicle morphometry and determine pedicle size, length, and direction in the coronal plane. Reconstructed CT in the oblique plane provides useful information regarding the size of the narrowed intervertebral foramina by spondylosis. The preoperative evaluation of the morphology of the vertebral artery by CT and MRI is important in preventing serious complications. The incidence of ischemic brain complication caused by

unilateral obstruction of the vertebral artery is low.[23] However, if the dominant vertebral artery is injured, serious neurologic complications can occur. Magnetic resonance angiograph (MRA) should be considered for the patients with evidence of the abnormalities or in whom these abnormalities are suspected (see Figure 167.3B-C). Preoperative lateral flexion and extension radiographs are useful to estimate the extent of correction. Correction of kyphosis can be expected to be beyond that observed on maximum extension position. If patients have a rigid kyphosis without segmental motion, a ventral release of the intervertebral discs may also be required.

## Instruments

Screws with 3.5, 4.0, and 4.5mm diameters are recommended for cervical pedicle screw fixation. Screw length is 20 or 22mm for C3-7. Twenty-four millimeter screws are required to penetrate the ventral cortex of the vertebral body at C2. Constrained type of locking mechanism is essential connecting the screws and plates/rods to obtain rigid stabilizing effect and sufficient correction capability of kyphosis.

## Surgical Technique
### Pedicle Screw Placement in the Cervical Spine

**C3-7.** The points of screw penetration for the C3 through C7 pedicles are slightly lateral to the center of the articular mass and close to the caudal margin of the inferior articular process of the cranially adjacent vertebra. The insertion angle of the pedicle screw from C3 to C7 is intended to be 25 to 45 degrees medial to the midline in the transverse plane. The lateral margin of the articular mass of the cervical spine has a notch approximately at the level of the pedicle. The pedicles are located approximately below the lateral vertebral notch at C2, at C3-6, and at or slightly above the notch at C7[15] (Figure 167.4).

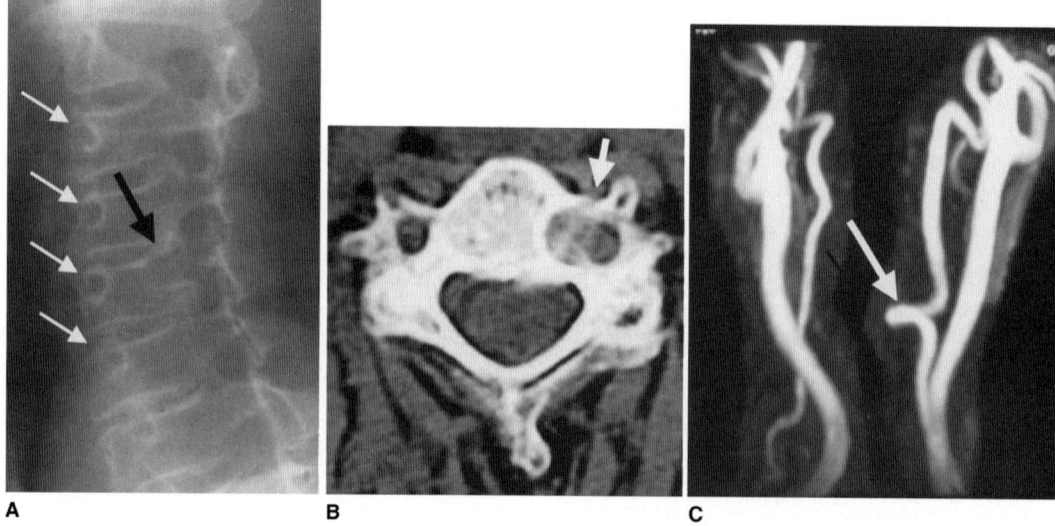

**Figure 167.3** Preoperative oblique radiographs, CT, and MRA. **(A)** In oblique projection plain films, contralateral pedicles are visualized as an oval projected onto the vertebral body *(white arrows)*. **(B)** Right vertebral artery is expanding into the vertebral body *(black arrow* in **A** and *white arrow* in **B**). **(C)** MRA demonstrates loop formation of the vertebral artery.

A          B          C

**C2.** The craniad margin of the lamina of C2 is the landmark for the point of screw penetration for C2. To confirm the screw insertion points in C2, a slightly curved, small spatula can be inserted into the spinal canal along the cranial margin of the C2 lamina to the superomedial surface of the pedicle of C2. The angle for the C2 pedicle should be 15 to 25 degrees medial to the midline in the transverse plane.

## Screw Insertion

The cortex at the point of insertion is penetrated with a high-speed burr. The surgeon can see the pedicle cavity directly in many cases by enlargement of the insertion hole with a curette. After creating the insertion hole, a small pedicle probe, tap, and screws are inserted into the pedicle with help of the lateral image intensifier to confirm the direction and insertion depth (Figure 167.5). The cortex of the cervical pedicles is always thinnest laterally toward the vertebral artery.[14,20] Therefore, the surgeon should keep this in mind during probing and tapping of the pedicle and while placing the screws. The neurocentral junction in the cervical spine, which is near the base of the pedicle in the vertebral body, is occasionally difficult to pass with the pedicle probe.[2,3] In such cases, the junction can be perforated with a Kirschner wire to establish the path for the pedicle probe into the vertebral body. A drill bit must never be used to penetrate the cortex of the lateral mass or to make a hole for screw advancement. The intended angle of screw insertion in the sagittal plane is parallel to the rostral end plate for the pedicles of C5 through C7, and in a slightly rostral direction in C2 through C4.

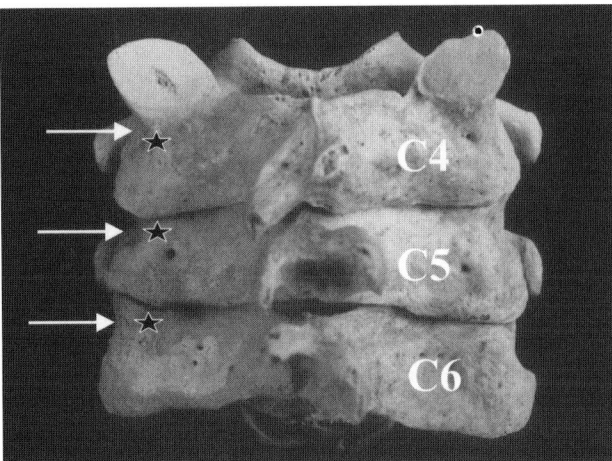

**Figure 167.4** Screw Insertion Point. The points of screw penetration for the C3 through C7 pedicles are slightly lateral to the center of the articular mass and close to the caudal margin of the inferior articular process of the cranially adjacent vertebra (*asterisks*). The lateral margin of the articular mass of the cervical spine has a notch approximately at the level of the pedicle (*white arrows*). The pedicles are located approximately below the lateral vertebral notch at C2, at C3-6, at or slightly above the notch at C7.

## Plate/Rod Application and Correction of Kyphosis

The neural foramina in patients with spondylosis are often stenotic. Therefore, a risk of iatrogenic nerve root lesion due to foraminal stenosis caused by correction of kyphosis or reduction of ventral translation exists.[1,4,10] The use of a washer under the plate/rod for the rostral vertebral screws is helpful in situations in which excessive reduction could occur during screw tightening. During the correction of kyphosis, the surgeons must also avoid applying the excessive compression force at the spinal segment with neural foraminal stenosis due to degenerative changes. The nerve root compression by foraminal stenosis can be managed with foraminotomy, without removal of the screws. The foraminotomy must be performed until the outlet of the foramen along the nerve root is reached. A prophylactic foraminotomy is recommended for the patients with marked stenosis of the neural foramen.

Prior to plate or rod application, dorsal decompression by laminoplasty or laminectomy should be performed, considering neurologic deterioration by changing of vertebral alignment after longitudinal connection of the screws. The cortex of the lateral masses and laminae must be decorticated and bone chips obtained from spinous processes and laminae are placed. In the final stage of instrumentation, inserted screws are connected to the plate or rod. Plate fixation is preferred for two-segment fixation. However, direction of the inserted screws in the coronal plane may be varied randomly in multilevel fixation. Therefore, rod fixation, with its large freedom of

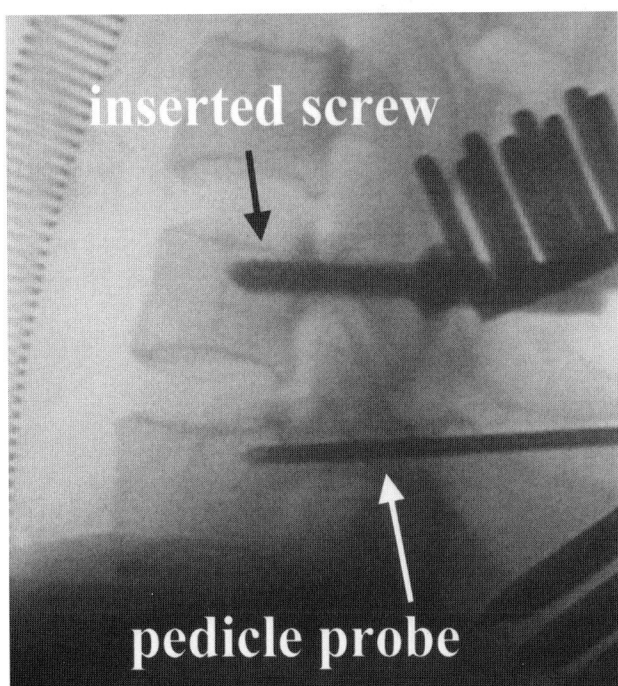

**Figure 167.5** Intraoperative Lateral Image Intensifier. After creating the insertion hole, small pedicle probe, tap, and screws are inserted into the pedicle with help of lateral image intensifier to confirm the direction and insertion depth.

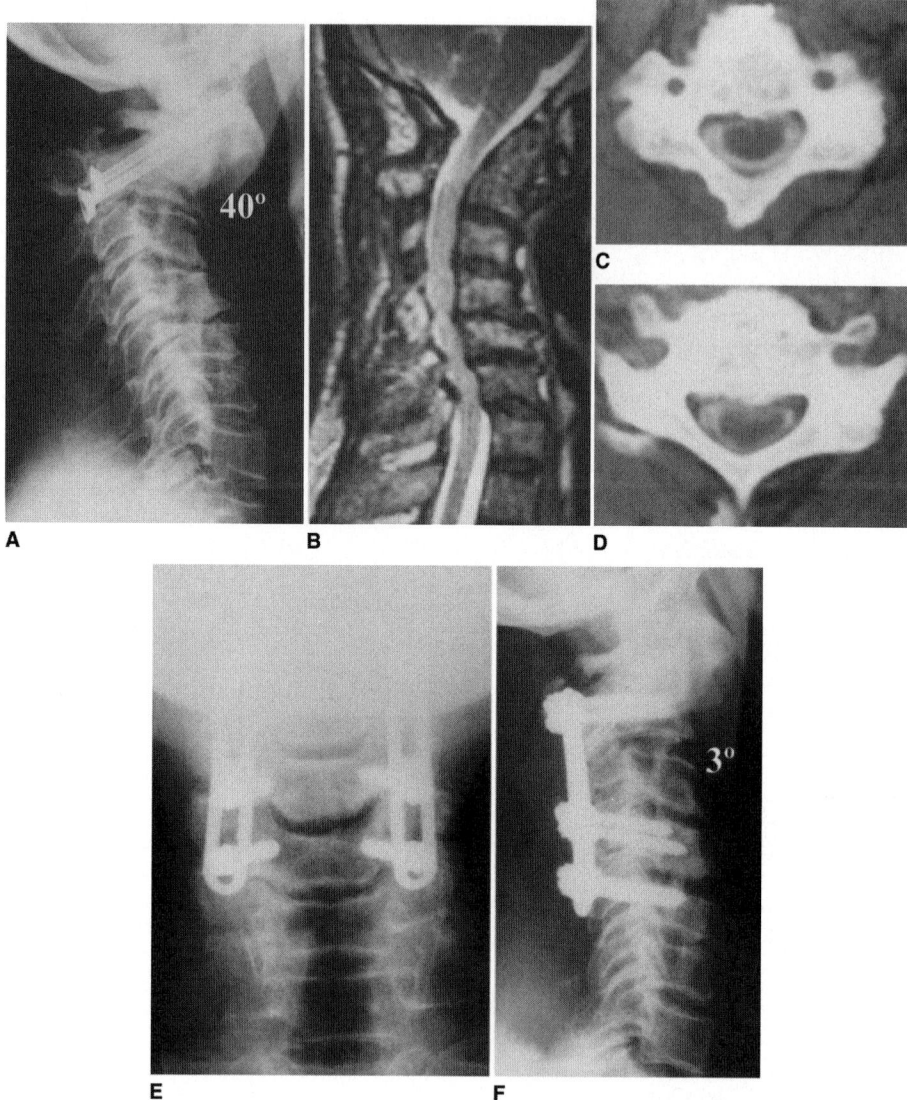

**Figure 167.6** Correction of Kyphosis Using Pedicle Screw/Plate System. The patients with cervical spondylotic myelopathy with kyphosis had undergone atlantoaxial transarticular screw fixation for odontoid fracture. (**A-D**) Cervical kyphosis and myelopathy progressed. (**E** and **F**) Simultaneous decompression by C3-7 open door laminoplasty and correction of kyphosis using cervical pedicle screw-plate was conducted. Forty degrees of preoperative kyphosis was decreased to 3 degrees. Neurologic recovery was satisfactory.

connection with the screw (rather than plate fixation) is recommended in these circumstances.

After pedicle screw insertion, rods or plates are contoured to form a physiologic lordosis. Plates are connected directly to the screws, and rods are attached to the screws using connectors. Correction of the kyphosis is performed by tightening the nuts (Figure 167.6) or by rotation of the rods using rod holders (Figure 167.7). As a consequence, the dorsal part of the cervical spine is shortened. Excessive shortening should be avoided.[1,4]

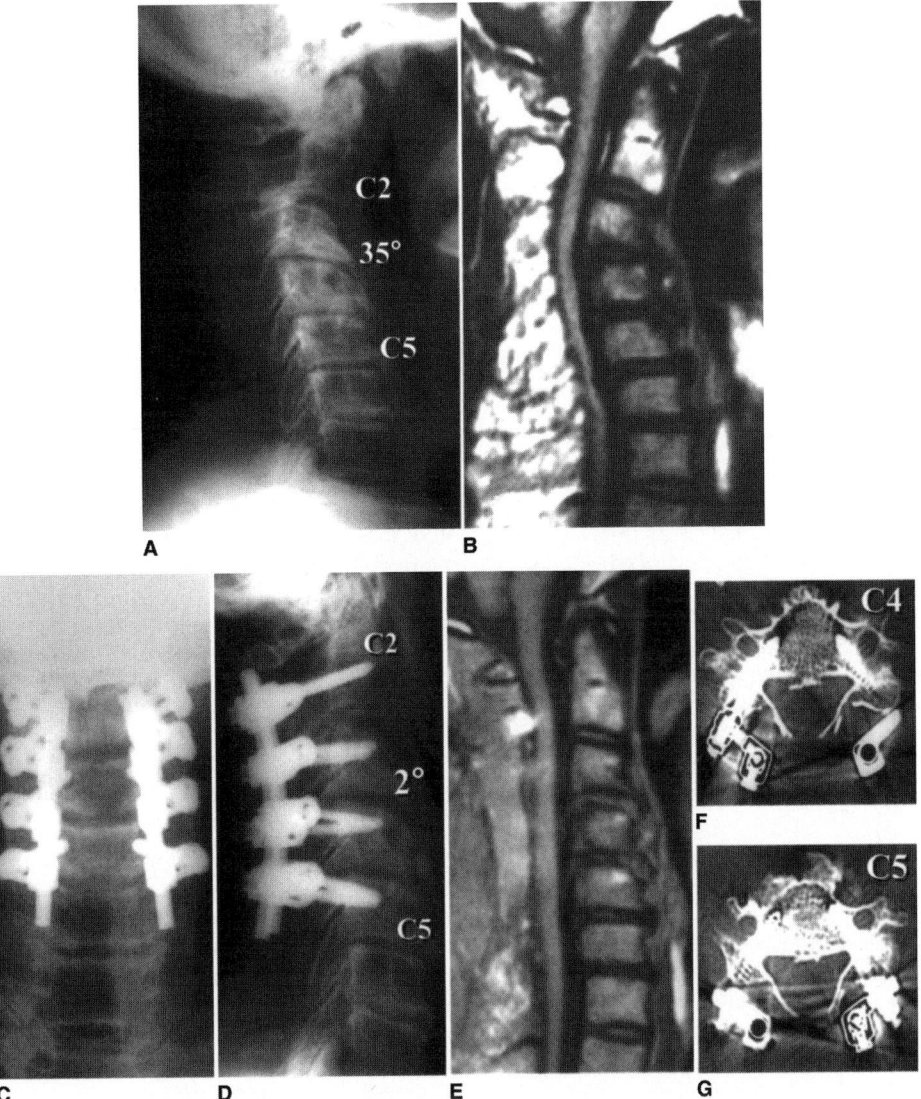

**Figure 167.7** Correction of Kyphosis Using Pedicle Screw/Rod System. (**A** and **B**) The patient sustained cervical spondylotic myelopathy with 35 degrees of kyphosis. (**C** and **D**) Open door laminoplasty from C3 to 6 and correction of kyphosis were performed by dorsal approach alone. The kyphosis improved to 2 degrees. (**E**) Postoperative MRI shows sufficient spinal cord decompression.

# REFERENCES

1. Abumi K, Ito M, Kotani Y: Complications of cervical pedicle screw placement. *Sem Spine Surg* 14:112-124, 2002.

2. Abumi K, Ito M, Kotani Y: Cervical pedicle screw fixation. In Herkowitz HN (ed): *The Cervical Spine Surgery Atlas*, ed 2. New York, Lippincott Williams & Wilkins, 2004, pp 411-422.

3. Abumi K, Kaneda K, Shono Y, *et al:* One-stage posterior decompression and reconstruction of the cervical spine by using pedicle screw fixation systems. *J Neurosurg (Spine 1)* 90:19-26, 1999.

4. Abumi K, Shono Y, Ito M, *et al:* Complication of pedicle screw fixation in reconstructive surgery of the cervical spine. *Spine* 25:962-969, 2000.

5. Abumi K, Shono Y, Taneichi H, *et al:* Correction of cervical kyphosis using pedicle screw fixation systems. *Spine* 24:2389-2396, 1999.

6. Albert TJ, Vaccaro A: Postlaminectomy kyphosis. *Spine* 23:2738-2745. 1998.

7. Baba H, Uchida K, Maezawa Y, *et al:* Lordotic alignment and posterior migration of the spinal cord following en bloc open-door laminoplasty for cervical myelopathy: a magnetic resonance imaging study. *J Neurol* 85:626-632, 1996.

8. Breig A, el-Nadi AF: Biomechanics of the cervical spinal cord: relief of contact pressure on and overstretching of the spinal cord. *Acta Radiol Diagn*: 4:602-624, 1966.

9. Breig A, Turnbull I, Hassler O: Effects of mechanical stresses on the spinal cord in cervical spondylosis: a study on fresh cadaver material. *J Neurosurg* 25:45-56, 1966.

10. Heller JG, Silcox DH III, Sutterlin CE III: Complications of posterior cervical plating. *Spine* 20:2442-2448, 1995.

11. Herman JM, Sonntag VK: Cervical corpectomy and plate fixation for postlaminectomy kyphosis. *J Neurosurg* 80: 963-970, 1994.

12. Hirabayashi K, Satomi K: Operative procedure and results of expansive open-door laminoplasty. *Spine* 13:870-876, 1988.

13. Jones EL, Heller JG, Silcox DH, *et al:* Cervical pedicle screws versus lateral mass screws: anatomic feasibility and biomechanical comparison. *Spine* 22:977-982, 1997.

14. Karaikovic EE, Daubs MD, Madsen RW, *et al:* Morphologic characteristics of human cervical pedicles. *Spine* 22:493-550, 1997.

15. Karaikovic EE, Kunakornsawat S, Daubs MD, *et al:* Surgical anatomy of the cervical pedicles: landmarks for posterior cervical pedicle entrance localization. *J Spinal Disord* 13:63-72, 2000.

16. Kimura I, Shingu H, Nasu Y: Long-term follow-up of cervical spondylotic myelopathy treated by canal-expansive laminoplasty. *J Bone Joint Surg Br* 77:956-961, 1995.

17. Kotani Y, Cunningham BW, Abumi K, *et al:* Biomechanical analysis of cervical stabilization systems: an assessment of transpedicular screw fixation in the cervical spine. *Spine* 19:2529-2539, 1994.

18. Masini M, Maranhao V: Experimental determination of the effect of progressive sharp-angle spinal deformity on the spinal cord. *Eur Spine J* 6:89-92, 1997.

19. McAfee PC, Bohlman HH, Ducker TB, *et al:* One-stage anterior cervical decompression and posterior stabilization: a study of one hundred patients with a minimum of two years of follow-up. *J Bone Joint Surg Am* 77:1791-1800, 1995.

20. Panjabi MM, Shin EK, Chen NC, *et al:* Internal morphology of human cervical pedicle. *Spine* 25:1197-1205, 2000.

21. Roy-Camille R, Salient G, Mazel C: Internal fixation of the unstable cervical spine by a posterior osteosynthesis with plates and screws. In The Cervical Spine Research Society. Editorial Committee. *The Cervical Spine,* ed 2. Philadelphia, Lippincott, 1989, pp 390-403.

22. Satomi K, Nishu Y, Kohno T, *et al:* Long-term follow-up studies of open-door expansive laminoplasty for cervical stenotic myelopathy. *Spine* 19:507-510, 1994.

23. Smith MD, Emery SE, Dudley A, *et al:* Vertebral artery injury during anterior decompression of the cervical spine. *J Bone Joint Surg Br* 75:410-415, 1993.

24. Sodeyama T, Goto S, Mochizuki M, *et al:* Effect of decompression enlargement laminoplasty for posterior shifting of the spinal cord. *Spine* 24:1527-1531, 1999.

25. Suda K, Abumi K, Ito M, *et al:* Local kyphosis reduces surgical outcomes of expansive open door laminoplasty for cervical spondylotic myelopathy. *Spine* 28:1258-1262, 2003.

26. Yamazaki A, Homma T, Uchiyama S, *et al:* Morphologic limitation of posterior decompression by midsagittal splitting method for myelopathy caused by ossification of the posterior longitudinal ligament in the cervical spine. *Spine* 24:32-34, 1999.

27. Zdeblick TA, Bohlman HH: Cervical kyphosis and myelopathy: treatment by anterior corpectomy and strut-grafting. *J Bone Joint Surg Am* 71:170-82, 1989.

28. Zdeblick TA, Hughes SS, Riew KD, *et al:* Failed anterior cervical discectomy and arthrodesis: analysis and treatment of thirty-five patients. *J Bone Joint Surg Am* 79:523-532, 1997.

# Combined Ventral and Dorsal Approach

Ajit A. Krishnaney, Michael P. Steinmetz, and Edward C. Benzel

Cervical kyphosis may be the result of a variety of pathologies, including trauma, postsurgical instability, advanced degenerative disease, or systemic inflammatory diseases such as rheumatoid arthritis or ankylosing spondylitis.[10] The most common cause of cervical deformity, however, is iatrogenic.[3] Such may be secondary to either ventral or dorsal operations, but is most commonly observed after multilevel dorsal decompression with rates of clinically significant kyphosis as high as 21%.[7,9,13]

If a kyphotic deformity is present, a flexion moment is created with the head pitched forward relative to the normal alignment of the cervical spine.[2,3,4] The abnormal posture shifts the normally neutral axial force of the head ventrally to the instantaneous axis of rotation (IAR); thus creating a flexion bending moment.[4] The ventral portions of the already compromised cervical vertebral bodies are therefore preferentially loaded and are prone to further kyphosis.[3,4] Thus a vicious cycle of abnormal forces and progressive deformity is created.[2,3,4,16] If the kyphosis becomes severe the spinal cord may be come stretched over the apex of the deformity with a resultant myelopathy.[3,15] Moreover, kyphosis places the dorsal cervical musculature at a relative mechanical disadvantage, which along with continued disc degeneration can result in mechanical neck pain.[3,14] Cervical kyphotic deformities should, therefore, be avoided. If a kyphotic deformity does develop, however, surgical intervention can be used to correct the deformity, stabilize the spine, and decompress the neural elements.

## Dorsal versus Ventral versus Combined Approaches

Once a cervical deformity is present, and the decision is made for surgical intervention, three fundamental approaches are possible: dorsal,[2,6] ventral,[5,8,11,21,22] or combined dorsal and ventral.[2,10,17,18] A number of surgical procedures utilizing the dorsal approach have been described in the literature including simple laminectomy, various derivations of laminoplasty, and laminectomy augmented with dorsal fusion (with or without instrumentation).[2,6] The advantages of the dorsal approach include familiarity, ease of decompression of multiple levels, and the ability to extend the fusion and/or fixation rostrally to the occiput and/or caudally to the thoracic spine. The major disadvantage of laminectomy and laminoplasty is the obligatory disruption of the dorsal tension band, resulting in a high rate of postlaminectomy kyphosis.[4,13] This complication has led some authors to caution against use of these procedures in patients with preexisting cervical kyphosis or even in the relative kyphosis of the "straightened" cervical spine.[3,4,15,20] Moreover, ventral compression cannot be addressed from the dorsal approach. In some cases, the use of dorsal cervical fixation, in combination with dorsal decompression, may be used to correct a mild degenerative kyphosis.[1] However, this technique requires the presence of a flexible deformity to facilitate correction of the kyphosis, without the aid of a ventral release.[2] Needless to say, this situation is a rare occurrence in the degenerative spine. Furthermore, the degree of deformity correction achieved via an isolated dorsal strategy may be limited.[2]

A number of authors have advocated the use of a ventral approach for dealing with cervical myelopathy associated with kyphosis.[5,8,11,22] This approach affords the spine surgeon the ability to both address ventral compression, as well as a ventral release via corpectomy or multiple discectomies, prior to the actual correction of the cervical deformity. Moreover, since the majority of cervical kyphotic deformities are idiopathic and the result of prior dorsal procedures, use of a ventral strategy has the added benefit of avoiding much of the morbidity associated with revision surgery.[7,9,13] Although, this strategy has been shown to be highly effective for patients with short segment stenosis and kyphosis, historically high rates of pseudarthrosis, bone graft subsidence, and graft dislocation have been seen with long segment or multisegment constructs.[3,22] These complications are largely a manifestation of the often suboptimal bony fixation sites, the poor mechanical advantage, and the reliance upon screw fixation as the only available method of bony fixation afforded by the ventral approach.[4] Some of these factors may be mitigated by the use of intermediate points of fixation and by the introduction of dynamic implants, although their true effectiveness in this regard has yet to be proven.[4] A purely ventral approach, much like the purely dorsal approach, does not permit access for dorsal decompression of the spinal cord, nor does it afford the surgeon the ability to recreate the dorsal tension band in patients who exhibit incompetent dorsal elements.

The use of a combined dorsal and ventral strategy affords all of the aforementioned advantages of each and limits the disadvantages of both approaches used alone. The surgeon is able to perform a 360-degree decompression and thereby address both dorsal and ventral neural compression. Optimal correction of sagittal plane cervical deformities can be achieved by making use of the mechanical advantage of dorsal constructs and osteotomies, in conjunction with ventral releases and reconstruction of the ventral load bearing column via interbody fusion techniques.[4,17,19] This affords the spine surgeon the ability to both lengthen the ventral column and shorten the dorsal column to achieve an optimal correction. Moreover, in the ankylosed spine with a fixed deformity, it facilitates the releases of both dorsal and ventral elements necessary for deformity correction.[17,19] Furthermore, the addition of dorsal fixation to a ventral construct may help to further minimize the risk of pseudarthrosis by loading the construct via a compressive moment and provide further translational and torsional resistance.[4] This may optimize fusion rates via Wolff's law and may be especially useful in patients with poor bone quality, comorbidities, or with prior failed surgeries. Lastly, a combined ventral and dorsal fusion strategy may obviate the need for external orthoses in many cases.[17] The chief disadvantage of the combined approach has been the relative morbidity when compared with either purely dorsal or ventral strategies. Both Schultz et al.[19] and McAfee et al.,[17] however, have reported acceptably low rates of complications and long term morbidity (5% and 11% respectively).

## Summary

Kyphotic deformities of the cervical spine may be approached dorsally, ventrally, or via a combined strategy. While both the dorsal and ventral approaches have many advantages and many patients can be successfully treated by these strategies, a subset of patients may only be optimally managed via a combined approach. This subset may include patients with severe multilevel degenerative disease and a fixed deformity, patients with both dorsal and ventral neural compression, patients with poor bone quality, patients with comorbidities that may inhibit bony fusion and wound healing, and any patient that has failed a prior attempt at deformity correction.

## REFERENCES

1. Abumi K, Kaneda K, Shono Y, et al: One-stage posterior decompression and reconstruction of the cervical spine by using pedicle screw fixation systems. J Neurosurg 90:19-26, 1999.
2. Abumi K, Shono Y, Taneichi H: Correction of cervical kyphosis using pedicle screw fixation systems. Spine 24:2389-2396, 1999.
3. Albert TJ, Vacarro A: Postlaminectomy kyphosis. Spine 23:2738-2745, 1998.
4. Benzel EC: Biomechanics of Spine Stabilization. Rolling Meadows, IL, American Association of Neurological Surgeons, 2001.
5. Buttler JC, Whitecloud III TS: Postlaminectomy kyphosis: causes and surgical management. Clin Orthop North Am 23:505-511, 1992.
6. Callahan RA, Johnson RM, Margolis RN: Cervical facet fusion for control of instability following laminectomy. J Bone Joint Surg Am 59:991-1002, 1977.
7. Caspar W, Pitzen T: Anterior cervical fusion and trapezoidal plate stabilization for re-do surgery. Surg Neurol 52:345-352, 1999.
8. Cattrell HS, Clark GJ Jr: Cervical kyphosis and instability following multiple laminectomies in children. J Bone Joint Surg Am 49:713-720, 1967.
9. Geisler FH, Caspar W, Pitzen T, et al: Reoperation in patients after anterior cervical plate stabilization in degenerative disease. Spine 23:911-920, 1998.
10. Heller JG, Silcox III DH, Sutterlin CE III: Complications of posterior cervical plating. Spine 20:2442-2448, 1995.
11. Herman JM, Sonntag VK: Cervical corpectomy and plate fixation for post-laminectomy kyphosis. J Neurosurg 80:963-970, 1994.
12. Johnston FG, Crockard HA: One stage internal fixation and anterior fusion in complex cervical spinal disorders. J Neurosurg 82:234-238, 1995.
13. Kaptain GJ, Simmons N, Replogle RE, et al: Incidence and outcome of kyphotic deformity following laminectomy for

cervical spondylotic myelopathy. *J Neurosurg (Spine 2)* 93:199-204, 2000.

14. Katsuura A, Hukuda S, Imanaka T, *et al:* Anterior cervical plate used in degenerative disease can maintain cervical lordosis. *J Spinal Disord* 9:470-476, 1996.

15. Kimura I, Shingu H, Nasu Y: Long-term follow-up of cervical spondylotic myelopathy treated by canal expansive laminoplasty. *J Bone Joint Surg Br* 77:956-961, 1995.

16. Masini M, Maranho V: Experimental determination of the effect of progressive sharp-angle spinal deformity on spinal cord. *Eur Spine J* 6:89-92, 1997.

17. McAfee PC, Bohlman HH, Ducker TB: One stage anterior cervical decompression and posterior stabilization. A study of one hundred patients with a minimum of two years of follow-up. *J Bone Joint Surg Am* 77:1791-1800, 1995.

18. Savini R, Parisini P, Cervellati S: The surgical treatment of late instability of flexion-rotation injuries in the lower cervical spine. *Spine* 12:178-182, 1987.

19. Schultz KD, McLaughlin MR, Haid RW, *et al:* Single-stage anterior-posterior decompression and stabilization for complex cervical spine disorders. *J Neurosurg (Spine 2)* 93:214-221, 2000.

20. Suda K, Abumi K, Ito M, *et al:* Local kyphosis reduces surgical outcomes of expansive open door laminoplasty for cervical spondylotic myelopathy. *Spine* 28:1258-1262, 2003.

21. Zdeblick TA, Bohlman HH: Cervical kyphosis and myelopathy: treatment by anterior corpectomy and strut-grafting. *J Bone Joint Surg Am* 71:170-182, 1989.

22. Zdeblick TA, Hughes SS, Riew KD, *et al:* Failed anterior cervical discectomy and arthrodesis: analysis and treatment of thirty-five patients. *J Bone Joint Surg Am* 79:523-532, 1997.

# CHAPTER 168

# Management of Cervical Disc Herniation

## Dorsal Laminoforaminotomy Plus Discectomy

**Jaime H. Nieto**

Treatment of cervical radiculopathy has been a subject of controversy for the past five decades. Spurling and Scoville in 1944 described lateral disc herniation.[26] Cloward,[4] as well as Smith and Robinson,[25] popularized the ventral cervical approach in the 1950s. In 1951, Scoville[22] reported the first 115 cases operated via a dorsal laminotomy and foraminotomy for cervical disc herniation. Since then, multiple studies have proven the efficacy of laminotomy and foraminotomy to treat lateral herniation of cervical disc and foraminal stenosis.

Laminoforaminotomy, with or without discectomy, is indicated for lateral disc herniation and foraminal stenosis that is not responsive to conservative treatment. This approach groups the serious potential complications such as recurrent laryngeal nerve (RLN), esophageal, and vascular injuries, as well as graft and fusion problems that are associated with the ventral discectomy.[5] The patients do not need cervical immobilization and more than one nerve root can be decompressed without the need for discectomies and or fusion.

## Biomechanics

In order to perform an adequate discectomy and foraminotomy to decompress the nerve root, part of the cervical facet must be removed. Zdeblick performed an in vitro study testing axial load, flexion, extension, and torsional movements in the human cadaveric cervical spine. He performed a C5 laminectomy and progressive (25%, 50%, 75%, and 100%) facetectomy. The study demonstrated no change in axial stiffness in the different groups. However, it showed increased segmental hypermobility when more than 50% of the facet joint was removed.[29] Raynor also reported similar results, indicating that if more than 50% of the facet joint is resected, stability is compromised.[21] Cusick also tested single-level cadaveric specimens and showed that unilateral facetectomy decreased the strength of the spine by 31% and bilateral facetectomy by 53%.[7] With dorsal foraminolaminotomy adequate decompression is achieved with removal of only one third of the facet.

## Clinical Diagnosis

Patients present with symptoms related to nerve root compression from foraminal stenosis or laterally herniated discs. It is important to rule out other causes of neck and arm pain such as primary or metastatic cancer, infection, cervical spine instability, spinal cord tumors, syringomyelia, and brachial plexopathy. Cervical disc herniation and foraminal stenosis commonly causes pain that radiates from the neck to the shoulder arm and into the hand. The dermatomal distribution of the pain and paresthesias in the arm or hand associated with motor loss, usually makes the localization of the nerve root syndrome easily recognizable. The upper cervical nerve roots usually produce pain in their dermatomal innervation. However, they may be difficult to recognize since there is no motor deficit. The most common roots involved are C6 and C7.[9,23] C3 and C4 root compression are seen only rarely. C5 nerve root compression usually presents with deltoid, supraspinatus, and infraspinatus weakness and shoulder pain. C6 symptoms include biceps weakness with numbness and paresthesias of the thumb and index finger as well as depressed biceps reflex. C7 root compression may present with triceps, wrist and finger extension weakness, and a decreased triceps reflex. C8 root syndromes include weakness of the intrinsic muscles of the hand and sensory loss in the ulnar nerve distribution. It is important to keep in mind that the syndromes are not always completely clear and isolated. There may be a significant amount of variation and overlap of innervation, or less commonly, multilevel involvement.

Clinical diagnosis should always be confirmed with the imaging findings. The work-up should begin with plain anteroposterior (AP), lateral, and oblique views as well as flexion-extension roentgenograms. Myelography, postmyelogram computed tomography (CT) and magnetic resonance imaging (MRI) are the definitive diagnostic tests. MRI and CT myelogram are the preferred studies. For spinal cord and soft tissue pathology the MRI is superior to CT myelography or myelography alone.[10] CT myelography is better when evaluating osseous pathology, foraminal spurs, and arachnoiditis.[10,13,24,27] Despite the attributes of CT myelography, MRI remains the study of choice because of its noninvasiveness, availability, and relative high specificity.[11,27] If there is a question of foraminal, or bony abnormalities or degree of stenosis on MRI, a plain CT or a CT myelogram can often supply the information needed for surgical decision-making.[21,25]

Electromyelography and nerve conduction studies should be used with caution. However, they can be helpful when the clinical picture is confusing or to evaluate potential peripheral nerve involvement, such as brachial plexus pathology.

## Surgical Technique

The surgical technique for dorsal laminotomies and foraminotomies has evolved over the last 70 years. Initially, the operation was performed with multilevel laminectomy and foraminotomies in the sitting position.[22] As microsurgical techniques have evolved, the procedure has been modified as well, from the keyhole foraminotomy[6] to recent reports that describe microendoscopic laminoforamino-tomies using minimally invasive techniques.[1,3]

## Prone Position

The patients are placed under general anesthesia. For most cases, a Foley catheter is not needed. The patient's head is placed in a three-point head frame and the patient is turned into the prone position. The Jackson frame or chest bolsters are used. All the joints are padded to avoid compression neuropathy. The neck is kept in the neutral position or slightly flexed position to open the laminae and foramina. The arms are tacked to the side and the legs are flexed at the knee. The table is placed in reversed Trendelenburg position at about 20 to 30 degrees. Flexing the knees provides support for the body when the table is in the reverse Trendelenburg position. The neck is shaved and prepped and draped in a sterile manner. A localizing lateral radiograph or C-arm fluoroscopic image is taken for localization and to minimize skin incision length. The skin incision is 2 to 3cm long and placed in the midline. An avascular plane is followed down to the spinous process. Subperiostial dissection is performed to the level of the facet joint exposing both and the superior and inferior laminae. A second localizing radiograph is taken before the laminotomy or foraminotomy is begun. With very small incisions, the operating microscope is used. However, if the incision is slightly larger then magnifying loops are used. A burr is used to perform the foraminotomy. The keyhole foraminotomy begins at the junction of the lateral aspect of the lamina and the medial margin of the facet joint. Only the medial one third to one half of the facet is drilled. The laminotomy is enlarged using the burr or small punches to remove the lateral margin of the adjacent lamina. In order to gain access to the disc space or disc fragments, the ligamentum flavum is removed carefully and the nerve root identified. The foramen is localized with a blunt nerve hook or with a Woodson instrument by feeling the pedicles above and below. The vascular cuff overlying the nerve root is coagulated and moved away, thus exposing the nerve root. The root is carefully retracted rostrally to access to the disc space or the disc fragment that is usually located under the axilla of the nerve root. The nerve root is moved caudally to look for any fragments on the rostral aspect of the root. If no disc fragment is found the posterior longitudinal ligament (PLL) is open sharply over the bulging disc to deliver the fragment.

If only a foraminotomy is to be performed, there is no need to open the ligamentum flavum but the vascular cuff overlying the nerve root is coagulated and moved away, exposing the root. One and two millimeter rongeurs are use to finish the foraminotomy laterally. The Woodson instrument should be passed easily through the foramen to assess nerve root decompression. The osteophytes are usually not removed since the foraminotomy alone achieves nerve root decompression. The wound is closed in layers. There is no need for any cervical spine orthosis postoperatively.

## Sitting Position

Scoville described the dorsal keyhole foraminotomy approach in the sitting position in the early 1950s.[22] The position is more challenging to the anesthesiologist because of the potential risks involved and the additional monitoring needed. The monitoring is directed to detection and rapid treatment of venous air embolism. The reported incidence of venous air emboli in the sitting position in the anesthesiology literature varies with the monitoring devises used. For the precordial Doppler, the incidence is between 25% and 50%.[18] The transesophageal echocardiography is a more sensitive monitor with reported incidence of venous air embolism detection of 76% for posterior fossa surgery and 7% to 25% for cervical laminectomies.[12,17]

Under general anesthesia, the patient is placed in the three-pin head holder. Thigh high stockings and an abdominal binder are applied. The back is flexed and the table is placed in the Trendelenburg position. This allows bending of the knees and avoids keeping the legs in a dependent position.

A Doppler monitor is placed over the chest. An end tidal carbon dioxide monitor is also used. A long line or central venous pressure catheter is inserted and the tip placed at the junction of the superior vena cava and the right atrium. If there is evidence of air emboli, the wound is packed with wet sponges and the air is aspirated through the central venous catheter. Once the patient is positioned, the operation is performed as described.

## Results

There have been multiple publications confirming the success rate of this operation. When patient selection is appropriately performed, there is as much as 96% resolution of the preoperative symptoms. Murphey et al.[14,15] reported their first 250 cases in 1966 followed by a larger series in 1973. Their largest series included 648 operated cases from 1939 to 1972 with 380 of these patients having a follow-up from 1 to 28 years. The most common affected nerve roots were C6 and C7, comprising 87% of all cases. They reported no deaths and 13 complications, including increased weakness of the hand and arm in 1 patient, reflex sympathetic dystrophy in 6 patients, 3 immediate recurrences treated by reexploration and removal of a residual fragment, and 3 late recurrences. Ninety percent of the patients returned to the same job. Three hundred and sixty-eight patients (96%) had between 70% and 100% improvement in symptoms.

Scoville et al.[23] reported the late results of cervical disc surgery in 383 patients with 296 having follow-up for 1 to 33 years. In this series, 83% represented lateral soft disc herniation, 13% central spondylotic type, and 4% centrally herniated soft discs. The most common levels involved were C5-6 and C6-7 in 89 % of the patients. In their series, the lateral dorsal approach was successful in over 95% on the cases, with 97% of the patients returning to their former occupations. In 1983, Henderson et al.[9] reported a retrospective study of 846 operations in 736 patients treated by cervical dorsal lateral foraminotomy from 1963 to 1980. The preoperative diagnosis was C5-6 or C6-7 in 98.7% of the cases. The long-term outcome was graded as "good or excellent" in 91.5% of the patients, "fair-poor-failure" in 8.5%. Recurrent symptoms were present in 20.3% (172 cases) and 13.9% (103 patients) eventually required a second operation for symptoms at same or new level. The complication rate was 1.5% (13 cases). There were 10 wound infections (no antibiotic prophylaxis was used in this series) and 3 cases of wound dehiscence. There were no deaths reported. Similar outcomes have been reported more recently in smaller series.[2,8,21,30]

## Summary

The dorsal foraminotomy and microlaminectomy, with or without discectomy, remains an elegant and safe method to treat lateral herniated discs or foraminal stenosis. The success is high with careful patient selection. The likelihood of potential injury to the trachea, esophagus, RLN, and major vessels are essentially nil. The limited amount of facet removal does not affect the stability of the cervical spine. There is no need for immobilization of the spine, even if several roots are decompressed. Laterally herniated discs with no myelopathic signs and minimal neck pain are excellent candidates for this operation.

## REFERENCES

1. Adamson TE: Microendoscopic posterior cervical laminoforaminotomy for unilateral radiculopathy: results of a new technique in 100 cases. *J Neurosurg* 95(1 Suppl): 51-57, 2001.

2. Aldrich F: Posterolateral microdiscectomy for cervical monoradiculopathy caused by posterolateral soft cervical disc sequestration. [See comments.] *J Neurosurg* 72(3): 370-377, 1990.

3. Burke TG, Caputy A: Microendoscopic posterior cervical foraminotomy: a cadaveric model and clinical application for cervical radiculopathy. *J Neurosurg* 93(1 Suppl): 126-129, 2000.

4. Cloward RB: The anterior approach for the removal of ruptured cervical discs. *J Neurosurg* 15:602-617, 1958.

5. Cloward RB: Complications of anterior cervical disc operation and their treatment. *Surgery* 69(2):175-182, 1971.

6. Collias JC, Roberts MP: Posterior surgical approaches for cervical disc herniation and spondylotic myelopathy. In Schmidek HH, Sweet WH (eds): *Operative Neurosurgical Techniques: Indications, Methods, and Results*, ed 4, vol 2. Philadelphia, Saunders, 1995, pp 2016-2028.

7. Cusick JF, Yoganandan N, Pintar F, et al: oganandan N, Pintar F, Myklebust J, Hussain H: Biomechanics of cervical spine facetectomy and fixation techniques. *Spine* 13(7): 808-812, 1988.

8. Davis RA: A long-term outcome study of 170 surgically treated patients with compressive cervical radiculopathy. *Surg Neurol* 1996. 46(6):523-530;discussion 530-533, 1996.

9. Henderson, CM, Hennessy RG, Shuey HM Jr, Shackelford EG: Posterior-lateral foraminotomy as an exclusive operative technique for cervical radiculopathy: a review of 846 consecutively operated cases. *Neurosurgery* 13(5): 504-512, 1983.

10. Karnaze MG, Gado MH, Sartor KJ, Hodges FJ 3rd: Comparison of MR and CT myelography in imaging the cervical and thoracic spine. *AJR Am J Roentgenol* 150(2):397-403, 1988.

11. Kuroki T, Kumano K, Hirabayashi S: Usefulness of MRI in the preoperative diagnosis of cervical disk herniation. *Arch Orthop Trauma Surg* 112(4):180-184, 1993.

12. Losasso, TJ, Black S, Muzzi DA, et al: Detection and hemodynamic consequences of venous air embolism. Does nitrous oxide make a difference? *Anesthesiology* 77(1): 148-152, 1992.

13. Modic, MT, Masaryk T, Paushter D: Magnetic resonance imaging of the spine. *Radiol Clin North Am* 24(2):229-245, 1986.

14. Murphey F, Simmons JC: Ruptured cervical disc. Experience with 250 cases. *Am Surg* 32(2):83-88, 1966.

15. Murphey F, Simmons JC, Brunson B: Surgical treatment of laterally ruptured cervical disc. Review of 648 cases, 1939 to 1972. *J Neurosurg* 38(6):679-683, 1973.

16. Murphey F, Simmons JC, Brunson B: Chapter 2. Ruptured cervical discs, 1939 to 1972. *Clin Neurosurg* 20: 9-17, 1973.

17. Papadopoulos G, Kuhly P, Brock M, et al: Venous and paradoxical air embolism in the sitting position. A prospective study with transoesophageal echocardiography. *Acta Neurochir (Wien)* 126(2-4):140-143, 1994.

18. Porter JM, Pidgeon C, Cunningham AJ: The sitting position in neurosurgery: a critical appraisal. *Br J Anaesth* 82(1):117-128, 1999.

19. Raynor RB, Pugh J, Shapiro I: Cervical facetectomy and its effect on spine strength. *J Neurosurg* 63(2):278-282, 1985.

20. Reul J, Weis J, Jung A, et al: Central nervous system lesions and cervical disc herniations in amateur divers. *Lancet* 345(8962):1403-1405, 1995.

21. Rodrigues MA, Hanel RA, Prevedello DM, et al: Posterior approach for soft cervical disc herniation: a neglected technique? *Surg Neurol* 55(1):17-22;discussion 22, 2001.

22. Scoville W, Whitcomb B, McLuarin R, The cervical ruptured disk: report of 115 operative cases. In *Transactions of the American Neurology Association*, 76th annual meeting, 1951, p 222.

23. Scoville WB, Dohrmann GJ, Corkill G: Late results of cervical disc surgery. *J Neurosurg* 45(2):203-210, 1976.

24. Shafaie FF, Wippold FJ 2nd, Gado M, et al: Comparison of computed tomography myelography and magnetic resonance imaging in the evaluation of cervical spondylotic myelopathy and radiculopathy. *Spine* 24(17):1781-1785, 1999.

25. Smith GW, Robinson RA: The treatment of certain cervical-spine disorders by anterior removal of the intervertebral disc and interbody fusion. *J Bone Joint Surg Am* 40(3): 607-624, 1958.

26. Spurling R, Scoville W: Lateral rapture of the cervical intervertebral discs. A common cause of shoulder and arm pain. *Surg Gynecol Obstet* 78:350-358, 1944.

27. Van de Kelft E, van Vyve M: Diagnostic imaging algorithm for cervical soft disc herniation. *Acta Chir Belg* 95(3): 152-156, 1995.

28. Whitecloud TS, Dunsker SB: *Anterior Cervical Spine Surgery. Principles and Techniques in Spine Surgery*. New York, Raven Press, 1993, pp xiii, 145.

29. Zdeblick TA, Zou D, Warden KE, et al: Cervical stability after foraminotomy. A biomechanical in vitro analysis. *J Bone Joint Surg Am* 74(1):22-27, 1992.

30. Zeidman SM, Ducker TB: Posterior cervical laminoforaminotomy for radiculopathy: review of 172 cases. *Neurosurgery* 33(3):356-362, 1993.

# Ventral Cervical Discectomy without Fusion

## Robert M. Galler, Nicholas Theodore, and Volker K.H. Sonntag

The surgical treatment for cervical disc herniation represents a topic of constant debate. The operative approaches for spondylosis are as numerous and variable as its clinical presentations. It seems that the more operations there are for the therapy of a particular disease, the probability exists that no single option is clearly superior. In terms of ventral approaches to single-level disc disease, the question remains: to fuse or not to fuse? Although ventral cervical discectomy without fusion is no longer the senior author's (Sonntag) preferred choice, this chapter recounts his experience with the technique and reviews the current literature to provide data for making clinical decisions about the treatment of cervical disc herniations using ventral cervical discectomy without arthrodesis.

## Clinical Features

The clinical presentation of patients with cervical disc disease varies and depends on many factors such as the level of pathology, the size and morphology of the herniated nucleus pulposus, the degree of degeneration, the curvature of the spine, and the duration of symptoms. Patients may become symptomatic with myelopathy or radiculopathy, ranging from mild to severe.

The clinical manifestations of radiculopathy can vary. Patients may complain of neck, shoulder, and arm pain and of numbness. The distribution may be myotomal or dermatomal. The pain may be described as sharp or as a dull ache. Commonly, the arm pain predominates over the neck or shoulder discomfort. Patients may not fully recognize a neurologic deficit because of pain. Instead, they may describe clumsiness or early fatigue.

Central herniation is less likely to present with an acute onset. Neck pain may predominate in these patients. A large central herniation may be associated with myelopathy, which may develop insidiously. Sensory changes may precede motor defects. The symptoms may be subtle, such as tingling of the hands or clumsiness and incoordination. Gait difficulty may appear later. Patients may become disabled progressively, or they may suffer from an acute episode associated with acute injury to the spinal cord.

## Radiographic Features

The cervical spine can be imaged with plain radiography (with or without dynamic views), CT, CT myelography, and MRI. Each modality may provide useful information regarding the involved pathology.

Plain radiography allows the overall morphology of the spinal curvature and alignment to be assessed. Bony osteophytes and subluxations are readily visualized. Plain radiographs are also useful for visualizing vertebral body fractures, for assessing the height of a disc space, and for determining the patency of the neural foramina.

CT and CT myelography are extremely useful for the same reasons as plain radiography. CT also can be used to assess the diameter of the spinal canal and the bony architecture of osteophytes in more than one plane. Reconstructions enable full visualization of the spinal architecture. CT is useful for the evaluation of patients with osteophytic spondylosis or "hard disc disease" because bony structures are well depicted by this modality. Intradural structures can be evaluated with contrast myelography.

MRI is the diagnostic imaging tool that provides the most information about the spinal cord, cervical discs, and other soft-tissue structures. The degree of spinal canal compromise and spinal cord compression is readily seen on MRI. Sequestered herniated disc fragments in almost any location are well visualized on MRI. The combination of axial, sagittal, and coronal views permits optimal surgical planning. When neoplastic disease is part of a differential diagnosis, contrast-enhanced MRI is also useful for the diagnosis of tumor.

The combination of all three imaging techniques provides valuable information about all aspects of the pathoanatomy of patients with spinal disease.

## Selection of Operative Approach

The choice of surgical approach in a patient with cervical radiculopathy, myelopathy, or both is the next major consideration. We favor the most direct operative option that provides the best exposure of the offending pathology and that is associated with a high rate of success and minimal patient morbidity. Although each patient is considered individually, most cervical disc herniations are located ventrally. Osteophytes tend to form at the posterior end plate. The ventral approach allows direct visualization for decompression of the neural elements and excision of offending pathology.[11]

To fuse or not to fuse—the controversy continues. Whether arthrodesis should be performed after a herniated cervical disc is removed is still debated. Arthrodesis should be performed when instability exists or potentially exists because an acute ruptured disc is associated with fractures of a cervical vertebral body, with extensive resection of a vertebral body, or with a previous laminectomy. Fusion should be considered when a patient is a candidate for potential laminectomy, for example, a patient with cervical stenosis who exhibits abnormal cervical alignment or loss of normal cervical lordosis. If these factors are not present, anterior cervical discectomy without arthrodesis is an excellent alternative (Box 168.1). The procedure has significantly reduced operative time, blood loss, length of stay, and complications.

Ventral cervical discectomy without fusion is usually associated with longer periods of postoperative neck and interscapular pain. During long-term follow-up (mean, 6 years), however, low-level neck and arm pain is associated with anterior cervical discectomies at the same rate, with or without fusion.[25]

## 168.1

### Radiographic features that suggest interbody fusion should accompany interspace decompression and discectomy

Cervical spine instability or subluxation
Traumatic disc herniation
Prior cervical laminectomy
Congenital fusion of segments above or below the level
   being treated
Loss of cervical lordosis
Osteophytic disease of the PLL

*PLL,* Posterior longitudinal ligament.

Donor site problems or potential allograft problems are not associated with anterior cervical discectomy without fusion. Arthrodesis after discectomy is deemed necessary when a traumatic disc rupture is present, an extensive partial corpectomy is required, a previous laminectomy or gross instability is present, normal cervical lordosis has been lost, or cervical alignment is abnormal.

## Surgical Technique

### Preoperative Preparation and Anesthesia

Careful preoperative planning helps to promote a successful procedure and to minimize intraoperative difficulties. Neurophysiologic monitoring, fluoroscopy, or image guidance should be readily available. Preoperative imaging should include CT, MRI, and a vascular examination to determine the course of the vertebral artery. Knowledge of this anatomy can prevent catastrophic complications from occurring during discectomy and decompression.

The patient is transferred to the operating table while awake and wearing antiembolic stockings. Prophylactic antibiotics are administered about 30 minutes before the skin is incised. Steroids are administered if the patient is myelopathic. However, steroids should be avoided if possible because they discourage bone fusion.[23] If a disc osteophyte is compressing the cervical spinal cord, fiberoptic intubation via either the orotracheal or nasotracheal route may be needed with the patient awake. The amount of movement and trauma should be minimized. Baseline motor evoked potentials (MEPs) and somatosensory evoked potentials (SSEPs) may be recorded to document any abnormalities before intubation (author's opinion).

### Positioning and Approach

After the appropriate vascular access is achieved and baseline SSEPs are established, the patient is placed supine with all bony prominences well padded. The head is placed in the midline position in slight extension to expose the anterior surface of the neck. Typically, the patient is placed in a Caspar headholder with a chinstrap. An interscapular bolster is then placed to immobilize the head and to provide posterior support for further exposure of the area of interest. Fluoroscopy is used from the beginning of the procedure and is available during the entire operation.

The operative approach is directed toward the side that the surgeon finds most comfortable. A right-handed surgeon may perform the operation from the right but must appreciate that the course of the RLN may be variable and the nerve is therefore susceptible to injury. Some surgeons may elect to operate from the left where the RLN may course deeper in the tracheoesophageal groove. In patients undergoing a reoperation, we gain operative exposure from the ipsilateral side to avoid the possibility of bilateral vocal cord paralysis. In such cases operative access may be extremely challenging because postoperative scarring may distort the anatomic planes.

The cervical level can be estimated using external landmarks; however, fluoroscopy is helpful for accurate placement of the skin incision. The rostral and caudal extremes of the surgical site also can be viewed to determine the orientation of the incision. Typically, a horizontal incision in a skin crease is used for a one-level procedure.

After the patient had been prepared and draped, the skin is incised down to the platysma muscle. Careful dissection and broad undermining of tissues improve mobilization of the cervical structures and full surgical exposure. The sternocleidomastoid (SCM) muscle is identified, and the fascial plane between the SCM and tracheoesophageal bundle is developed. The carotid artery should be palpated so that the dissection can be directed medially. The carotid sheath is retracted laterally with the trachea and esophagus medially. The prevertebral fascia may be pushed away to expose the anterior longitudinal ligament (ALL) covering the ventral spine. The longus colli muscles are visible bilaterally. Fluoroscopy is then used to confirm the vertebral level. The ventral spine is cleared of soft tissues, and the longus colli muscles are dissected using electrocauterization. Radiolucent self-retaining retractors can be inserted under the longus colli and in the cephalocaudal position to provide full exposure.

Distraction posts may be placed at the rostral and caudal vertebral bodies. Distraction is not performed until the annulus has been incised. Care must be taken to avoid overdistraction, which can injure the facet or ligament. At this point the operating microscope is used to provide magnification and optimal illumination of the interspace. Using a series of curettes, the disc material is removed and the end plates are exposed. The disc material is removed down to the level of the PLL and laterally to the uncovertebral joints. In cases of soft disc herniation, the PLL is opened and disc fragments that may be compressing neural structures medially or laterally in the foramen are removed. In patients who have osteophytes in addition to a herniated disc, a high-speed drill is used to accomplish the necessary bony decompression.

Figure 168.1 shows an example of decompression of the affected nerve root in a case of herniated cervical disc at C6-7.

## Potential Complications

Like all operations, ventral cervical discectomy has inherent risks. The risks related to this approach are injury to the cervical viscera (i.e., trachea and esophagus), vascular injury to the carotid or vertebral arteries, and RLN palsy. Other immediate potential problems include cerebrospinal

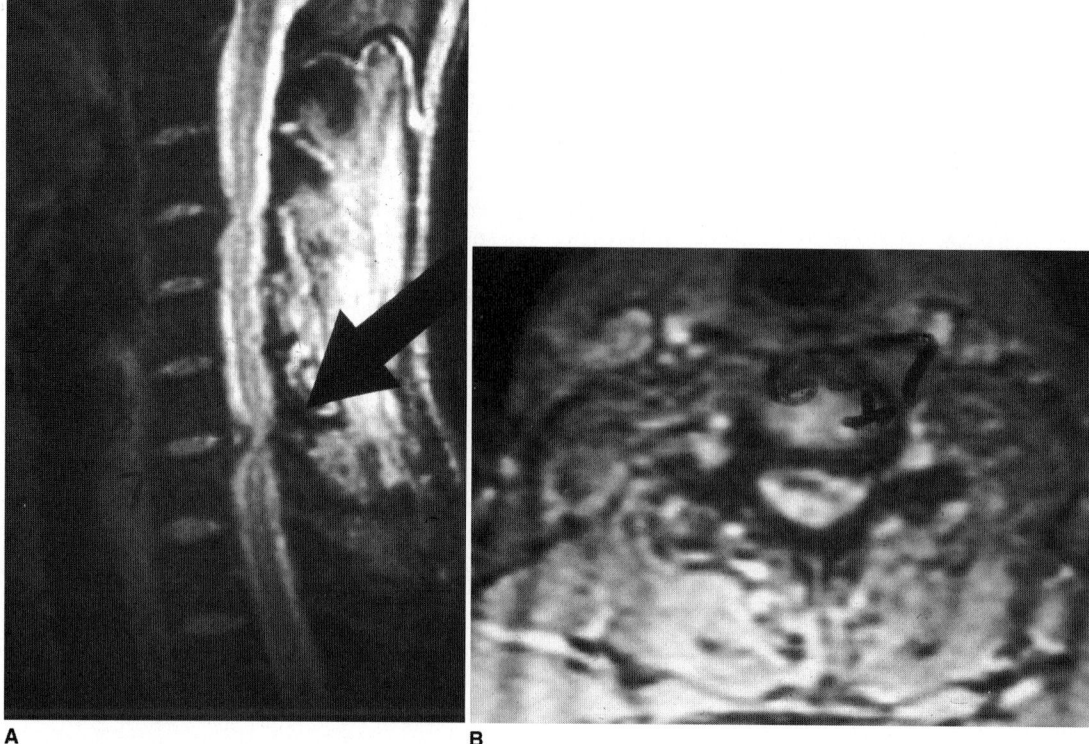

**Figure 168.1** Preoperative (**A**) sagittal and (**B**) axial magnetic resonance imaging (MRI) showing the herniated cervical disc *(arrow)* at C6-7. The disc material is paraventral to the left.

leakage, neurologic injury, infection, and postoperative hematoma. The most common postoperative problem is a persistent neurologic deficit, often the result of inadequate decompression of the involved neural element. The complications associated with graft harvest are avoided by not performing arthrodesis or by using allograft bone.

## Discussion

The ventral approach to discectomy has been used successfully for more than 35 years. As described by Bailey and Smith, the earliest reports of anterior discectomy used an approach similar to operations performed today. These descriptions record a reliable method of arthrodesis to treat trauma and degenerative disease. Soon thereafter, Cloward published his technique and described the innovative instrumentation associated with it. The ventral approach allows complete removal of disc material and is the most effective method for direct decompression of the neural elements. Its popularity has grown because of the technologic advances in operative magnification and lighting as well as the general success associated with the procedure. The literature contains many reports that describe the technique, indications, results, and complications associated with anterior cervical fusion, and many patient series have compared various surgical techniques. Still, questions have been raised about the optimal method of approach, the amount and type of decompression, and now the method of reconstruction.[10,11,17,22,24]

In the 1960s Hirsch[13,14] published a series of patients who underwent simple anterior cervical discectomy with opening of the PLL for the treatment of cervical radiculopathy. As a result, surgeons expanded this technique to include a more radical discectomy and osteophytectomy for the treatment of spondylosis. A separate literature developed exploring the indications, results, and complications of anterior cervical discectomy. The reports reviewed for this chapter included 2048 cases with 28 reoperations.*

In a consecutive series of 128 patients (with myelopathy, radiculopathy, or both), the senior author has performed ventral cervical discectomy without fusion.[10] These patients had no instability, subluxation, misalignment, or loss of cervical lordosis. The mean follow-up was 9 months. One level was decompressed in 60% of the patients, two levels in 3%, and three levels in 3%. An excellent to good outcome was achieved in 74% of these patients, 16% improved, and 10% remained unchanged. Seven patients required a reoperation, of whom only 2 had postdiscectomy collapse. Thereafter, an additional 98 patients were treated over a 4-year period with similar numerical outcomes (Tables 168.1 and 168.2).[11]

Vise[27] treated 187 patients who underwent ventral cervical discectomy without interbody fusion. In these cases the PLL was always opened for complete discectomy and

---

*References 1,2,4-7,10-14,16-18,24,29.

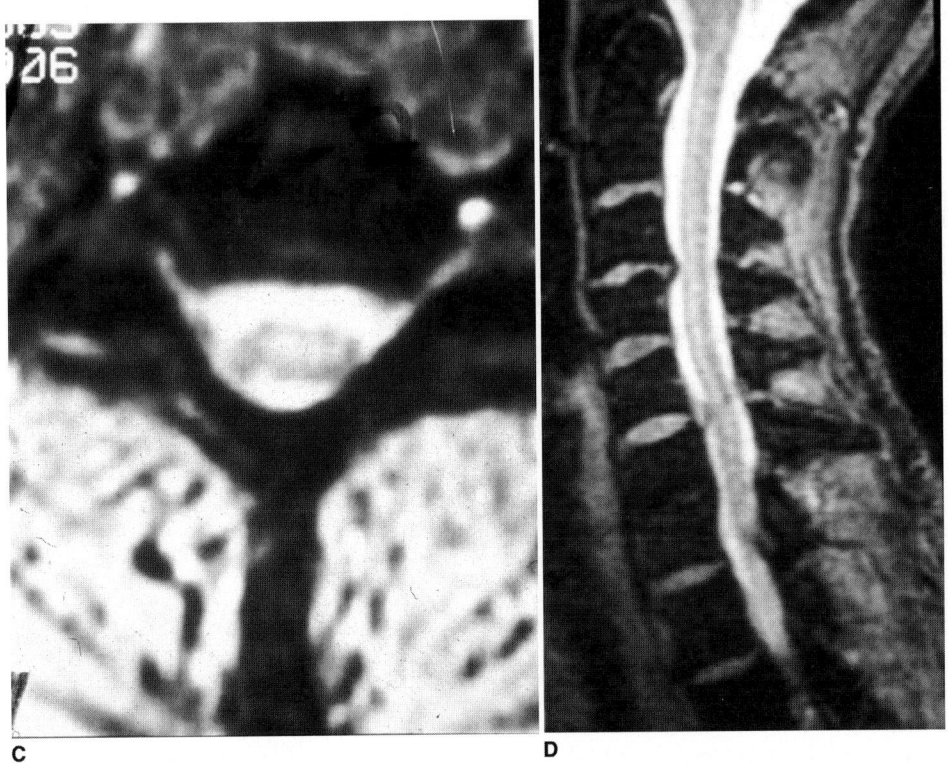

C　　　　　　　　　　　　　　D

**Figure 168.1 *cont'd*** Postoperative (**C**) axial and (**D**) sagittal MRI showing complete decompression of the affected nerve root and the absence of the herniated fragment at C6-7. Note the interbody autofusion at the operated level.

**TABLE 168.1**

**Sonntag-Hadley Series of Anterior Cervical Discectomy without Fusion**

| Author | Time of Series | No. of Patients | Mean Follow-up (months) | One-Level (%) | Two-Level (%) | Three-Level (%) | Fusion |
|---|---|---|---|---|---|---|---|
| Hadley and Sonntag[10] | Jan. 1988-Dec. 1991 | 128 | 15 | 60 | 37 | 3 | None |
| Hadley and Sonntag[11] | Aug. 1988-Aug. 1992 | 98 | 12 | 63 | 35 | 2 | None |

**TABLE 168.2**

**Outcome after Anterior Cervical Discectomy without Fusion**

| Author | No. of Patients | Excellent (%) | Good (%) | Improved (%) | Failed (%) | Failed Patients Who Improved with Reoperation and Fusion |
|---|---|---|---|---|---|---|
| Hadley and Sonntag[10] | 128 | 51 | 44 | 21 | 12 | 7 |
| Hadley and Sonntag[11] | 98 | 45 | 32 | 13 | 8 | 5 |

exploration of the epidural space. In this series 93% of the patients had good to excellent outcomes; 66% developed an autofusion at the surgical level. No patient developed instability and there were no reoperations. Table 168.3 shows data that Vise reported in his article.

Watters and Levinthal[28] reported 128 patients with cervical radiculopathy, 62 of whom underwent anterior cervical discectomy and 64 of whom underwent anterior cervical discectomy with fusion. Compared to the fusion group, the patients undergoing anterior cervical discectomy alone had significantly reduced mean operative times, blood loss, and hospitalization. Sixteen complications were associated with anterior cervical discectomy with fusion, 15 of which were related to the graft and to complications associated with anterior cervical discec-tomy. The main difference in outcome was in the early postoperative period. Patients who underwent anterior cervical discectomy alone had more neck and shoulder pain in the immediate postoperative period than those who also underwent fusion. In terms of cost, the use of a

## TABLE 168.3

### Anterior Cervical Discectomy without Bone Grafting*

| Reference | No. of Cases | Opened PLL | Results or Major Complications | No. of Levels in Reoperations | Fusion (%) | Instability | Hospital Stay (Days) |
|---|---|---|---|---|---|---|---|
| Benini et al.[1] | 25 | no | 88% good/improved | | | none | 5 |
| Bertalanffy, Eggert[2] | 164 | yes | 82% good/excellent | | 75% | 1 | 6 |
| Bertalanffy, Eggert[3] | 286 | yes | 17 worsened myelopathy 5 epidural hematomas | 5 | | 1% | 6 |
| Cuatico[4] | 81 | no | 95% good/excellent | – | | none | – |
| de Tribolet, Zander[5] | 17 | yes | 76% good/excellent | – | – | – | – |
| Dunsker[6] | 11 | yes | 100% good/excellent | – | – | – | – |
| Giombini, Solero[7] | 100 | sometimes | 80% good/excellent 3 deaths, 3 quadriparesis | 3 | 45% | none | 5 |
| Granata et al.[8] | 24 | no | 88% good/excellent | – | 63% | – | 7 |
| Grisoli et al.[9] | 120 | yes | 87% good/improved | – | 70% | none | 3 |
| Hankinson, Wilson[12] | 52 | sometimes | 89% good/excellent | – | – | 2% | 8 |
| †Hirsch et al.[14] | 45 | no | 83% good/improved | – | – | none | 4 |
| Husag, Probst[15] | 60 | yes | 82% good/excellent | – | 70% | none | 7 |
| Lunsford et al.[16] | 135 | – | 69% good/excellent | 4 | – | – | 7 |
| Martins[17] | 26 | yes | 65% good/excellent | – | – | 4% | – |
| †Murphy[18] | 26 | no | 92% good/improved | 1 | 72% | none | – |
| O'Laoire, Thomas[19] | sometimes | 96% recovery from myelopathies | | – | – | – | |
| Robertson, Johnson[21] | 135 | sometimes | 52% good/excellent-hard discs; 85% good/excellent-soft discs | | 88% | – | – |
| Rosenørn et al.[22] | 32 | – | 87% good/excellent | – | – | – | 6 |
| Tew, Mayfield[26] | 50 | – | – | – | 100% | – | – |
| †Wilson, Campbell[29] | 71 | no | 78%-95% good/improved | – | 28% | none | 5 |
| Vise[27] | 187 | always | 93% good/excellent | – | 66% | none | 1.9 (34 outpatients) |
| Total series 23 | Total patients 1822 | half opened the PLL | 52%-100% good/excellent results | 16 reoperations | about 70% fusion | excellent stability | average, about 6 days |

*Table reviews publications in the English medical literature. Different methods were used to report outcomes and types of cases selected for treatment; most were soft or soft/hard disc herniations. Most authors reverted to bone grafting for spondylosis. In some instances, outcome or fusion percentages had to be derived from the information available. Authors who did not use the outcome classification proposed by Rosenørn et al.[22] or Odom[20] (excellent, good, fair, poor) are indicated by the † symbol. The series reported by O'Laoire and Thomas[19] represented a group of patients treated for myelopathy. There were differences among authors in reporting fusion; most listed the incidence of complete radiographic fusion; this had no bearing on outcome. Several authors opened the PLL, but few resected most of it and included foraminotomies. Martin[17] defined a radical discectomy, but he did not mention foraminotomies. Bertalanffy and Eggert[2] radically excised the PLL in many patients and described an anterior foraminotomy; their most recent report of 450 cases is an addition of 286 to their earlier series of 164. Information not commented on or that could not be derived from reported data is indicated by a dash.
From Vise MW: Anterior discectomy without fusion for soft cervical disc herniation. In Al-Mefty O (ed): *Controversies in Neurosurgery*. New York: Thieme, 1995, pp 228-232, with permission.
*PLL*, Posterior longitudinal ligament

graft and plate is more expensive than a discectomy alone.

## Inconsistencies in the Literature

Many retrospective patient series have been reported, but no consistent treatment paradigm has been used. The technical preference of the surgeon often dictates the methodology used in the published reports. Therefore, comparisons must be based on many inconsistencies that cannot be completely disregarded. Some of the major differences in the technique of ventral cervical discectomy without arthrodesis involve the resection of the PLL and osteophytes and the number of levels decompressed. No prospective data based on a consistent method of diagnostic evaluation, treatment, and follow-up are available. Most reports are retrospective reviews or personal series. Without comparisons to controls or normal patients, there is no way to validate outcomes.

In terms of surgical series, each report of ventral discectomy without fusion involves different techniques. In earlier reports, discectomy was performed down to the level of the PLL but not beyond it. This simple discectomy may be used to decompress soft disc fragments, but it cannot address osteophytic disease or subligamentous disc herniation. In contrast, radical discectomy involves a complete excision of the disc, wide resection of the ALL and PLL, removal of pathologic bone and disc material posterior to the PLL, and foraminal resection of the uncovertebral joints. This approach facilitates access to free fragments that may have migrated into the neural foramen as well as to osteophytes that may be compressing the spinal cord or nerve roots. The use of simple or radical discectomies may partially account for the differences in outcomes reported in the literature. Fewer than half of the authors have reported opening the PLL as part of the procedure. Overall, outcomes have been good, ranging from 52% to 100% good or excellent results.

The success of anterior cervical discectomy with or without fusion depends on several factors. Patient selection is the most important consideration. Patients who have localized soft disc herniations ventral or ventrolateral to the spinal cord and nerve roots with minimal osteophytic bony disease are excellent candidates for an anterior cervical discectomy without arthrodesis.

## Summary

The senior author's preference is to perform ventral cervical discectomy with arthrodesis and internal fixation for single and multilevel procedures. This procedure is well tolerated and associated with early pain relief and mobilization. The use of allograft bone for arthrodesis eliminates complications related to the graft site. The placement of an internal fixation plate obviates the need for patients to wear a hard collar after surgery and permits a patient's early return to work and activity. Discectomy without fusion, however, remains an excellent alternative.

## REFERENCES

1. Benini A, Krayenbühl H, Brüderl R: Anterior cervical discectomy without fusion. Microsurgical technique. *Acta Neurochir (Wien)* 61:105-110, 1982.
2. Bertalanffy H, Eggert HR: Clinical long-term results of anterior discectomy without fusion for treatment of cervical radiculopathy and myelopathy. A follow-up of 164 cases. *Acta Neurochir (Wien)* 90:127-35, 1988.
3. Bertalanffy H, Eggert HR: Complications of anterior cervical discectomy without fusion in 450 consecutive patients. *Acta Neurochir (Wien)* 99:41-50, 1989.
4. Cuatico W: Anterior cervical discectomy without interbody fusion. An analysis of 81 cases. *Acta Neurochir (Wien)* 57:269-274, 1981.
5. de Tribolet N, Zander E: Anterior discectomy without fusion for the treatment of ruptured cervical discs. *J Neurosurg Sci* 25:217-220, 1981.
6. Dunsker SB: Anterior cervical discectomy with and without fusion. *Clin Neurosurg* 24:516-521, 1977.
7. Giombini S, Solero CL: Considerations on 100 anterior cervical discectomies without fusion. In Grote W, Brock M, Clar HE (eds): *Advances in Neurosurgery*. New York, Springer, 1980, pp 302-307.
8. Granata F, Taglialatela G, Graziussi G, et al: Management of cervical disc protrusions by anterior discectomy without fusion. Personal contribution. *J Neurosurg Sci* 25:231-234, 1981.
9. Grisoli F, Graziani N, Fabrizi AP, et al: Anterior discectomy without fusion for treatment of cervical lateral soft disc extrusion: a follow-up of 120 cases. *Neurosurgery* 24:853-859, 1989.
10. Hadley MN, Sonntag VKH: Cervical disc herniations. The anterior approach to symptomatic interspace pathology. *Neurosurg Clin North Am* 4:45-452, 1993.
11. Hadley MN, Sonntag VKH: Cervical disc herniations: the anterior operative approach without interbody fusion. In Menenzes AH, Sonntag VKH (eds): *Principles of Spinal Surgery*. New York, McGraw-Hill, 1995, pp 531-538.
12. Hankinson HL, Wilson CB: Use the operating microscope in anterior cervical discectomy without fusion. *J Neurosurg* 43:452-456, 1975.
13. Hirsch C: Cervical disc rupture. Diagnosis and therapy. *Acta Orthop Scand* 30:172-186, 1960.
14. Hirsch C, Wickbom II, Lidström A, Rosengren K: Cervical-disc resection. A follow-up of myelographic and surgical procedure. *J Bone Joint Surg Am* 46:1811-1821, 1964.
15. Husag L, Probst CH: Microsurgical anterior approach to cervical discs. Review of 60 consecutive cases of discectomy without fusion. *Acta Neurochir (Wien)* 73:229-242, 1984.
16. Lunsford LD, Bissonette DJ, Jannetta PJ, et al: Anterior surgery for cervical disc disease. Part 1: treatment of lateral cervical disc herniation in 253 cases. *J Neurosurg* 53:1-11, 1980.
17. Martins AN: Anterior cervical discectomy with and without interbody bone graft. *J Neurosurg* 44:290-295, 1976.
18. Murphy MG, Gado M: Anterior cervical discectomy without interbody bone graft. *J Neurosurg* 37:71-74, 1972.

19. O'Laoire SA, Thomas DGT: Spinal cord compression due to prolapse of cervical intervertebral disc (herniation of nucleus pulposus). Treatment of 26 cases by discectomy without interbody bone graft. *J Neurosurg* 59:847-853, 1983.

20. Odom GL, Finney W, Woodhall B: Cervical disc lesions. *JAMA* 166:23-28, 1958.

21. Robertson JT, Johnson SD: Anterior cervical discectomy without fusion: long-term results. *Clin Neurosurg* 27:440-449, 1980.

22. Rosenørn J, Hansen EB, Rosenørn MA: Anterior cervical discectomy with and without fusion. A prospective study. *J Neurosurg* 59:252-255, 1983.

23. Sawin PD, Dickman CA, Crawford NR, *et al:* The effects of dexamethasone on bone fusion in an experimental model of posterolateral lumbar spinal arthrodesis. *J Neurosurg* 94:76-81, 2001.

24. Simeone FA, Vise WM, Grob D, Henderson F: Treatment of soft cervical disc herniation. In Al-Mefty O, Origitano TC, Harkey HL 3rd (eds): *Controversies in Neurosurgery.* New York, Thieme, 1996, pp 226-238.

25. Sonntag VKH, Klara P: Controversy in spine care. Is fusion necessary after anterior cervical discectomy? *Spine* 21:1111-1113, 1996.

26. Tew JM Jr, Mayfield FH: Proceedings: anterior cervical discectomy—a microsurgical approach (abstract). *J Neurol Neurosurg Psychiatry* 38:413, 1975.

27. Vise MW: Anterior discectomy without fusion for soft cervical disc herniation. In Al-Mefty O (ed): *Controversies in Neurosurgery.* New York, Thieme, 1995, pp 228-232.

28. Watters WC 3rd, Levinthal R: Anterior cervical discectomy with and without fusion. Results, complications, and long-term follow-up. *Spine* 19:2343-2347, 1994.

29. Wilson DH, Campbell DD: Anterior cervical discectomy without bone graft. Report of 71 cases. *J Neurosurg* 47:551-555, 1977.

# Ventral Cervical Discectomy and Fusion with Allograft and Plating

## Maxwell Boakye and Regis W. Haid, Jr.

Ventral cervical discectomy for the treatment of cervical disc disease was introduced in the 1950s by Robinson and Smith[11,13] and Cloward.[5] Ventral cervical approaches remain today one of the most popular and successful operative approaches to treat cervical spinal disorders. Because of the simplicity and elegance of the procedure, and its overall versatility and success in treating ventral cervical pathologies, every general neurosurgeon and spine surgeon should be comfortable with the surgical anatomy and operative techniques of ventral cervical discectomy and fusion.

The widespread performance of these procedures has engendered several debates in the literature, including whether or not to fuse the spine after a discectomy. Although there have not been any randomized studies proving superior clinical outcome after fusion, there appears to be a decreased incidence of kyphotic deformity and pain in patients who undergo fusion.[1] If a decision is made to fuse the spine following discectomy, the surgeon must choose between using autograft bone and allograft bone. Ideally, anterior cervical fusion should be performed with autograft bone because only autograft bone is osteoinductive.[3] However, there are several problems that accompany using autograft, including graft site complications and persistent donor site problems.[10,17,19] Using allograft avoids all graft site complications associated with taking autograft. Although fusion rates are lower with allograft,[4,6,8,18,20] several recent studies suggest that fusion rates may be significantly augmented with addition of a cervical plating system following graft placement.[7,9,12,14-16] This chapter provides a description of operative techniques for ventral cervical discectomy with allograft fusion and plating.

## Preoperative Decision-Making

The surgeon should determine the above graft type before surgery. This decision depends on patient preference, nature of the pathology, patient compliance, and risk factors for pseudarthrosis. Radiographs should be examined to confirm the level of pathology, the extent of spinal cord compression, the presence or absence of kyphosis, bone quality, presence of spondylolisthesis, or instability. The surgeon should preoperatively select the most appropriate bone graft and plating system for the patient. There are a variety of plating systems currently available. Most implant systems are user friendly and there does not appear to be significant differences in single-level fusion rates between the older plating systems and the newer dynamic systems.[9] For single-level fusions, rigid or hybrid screw/plate systems suffice for most purposes.

## Operative Technique

Patients are brought into the operating room and placed supine on the table. After induction of general anesthesia, an IV bag wrapped in a surgical towel is placed under the neck to restore lordosis (Figure 168.2). The head may be placed on a doughnut. Esophageal stethoscopes and nasogastric tubes are avoided, since they can aggravate esophageal injury by retracting against rigid objects. The ventral neck region is prepped and draped in the usual sterile fashion. Prior to prepping and draping, various anatomic landmarks may be palpated in order to estimate the level of the disc space. The hyoid bone is generally at C3, the thyroid cartilage is at C5, and the cricoid cartilage is at C6. The carotid tubercle, the most reliable landmark, can be palpated at C6. In the absence of reliable anatomic landmarks, a preoperative lateral cervical radiograph may occasionally be used to determine location of the incision.

The incision for a single- or two-level discectomy generally follows one of the neck creases. The incision should extend from midline to the medial border of the SCM (Figure 168.3). Oblique incisions along the medial border of the SCM may be used if access to three or more levels is desired. The right side is generally preferred for a right-handed surgeon. There is not an increased incidence of RLN palsy with right-sided approach compared with left.[2]

After making the incision with a no. 10 blade, Bovie cautery or Metzenbaum scissors can be used to traverse the subcutaneous tissues to access the platysma muscle. Undermining the platysma muscle is critical to aid in retraction. The platysma muscle is divided and the medial border of the SCM is identified. This plane is gently developed using superficial sharp dissection. The carotid sheath is identified and its contents retracted laterally as the spine is bluntly palpated. The omohyoid muscle at C5-6 may be divided if necessary to improve access and exposure. The prevertebral fascia is divided in the middle of the vertebral body and swept off the spine using a Kittner (Sheavor). A localizing radiograph is obtained to confirm the operative disc space level by placement of a spinal needle in the disc space. The surgeon also may place an initial vertebral distraction pin into a body to aid with screw length determination. Once the level is determined, optimal exposure is obtained by cauterizing the edges of the longus colli muscle to gain access to the uncovertebral joints (Figure 168.4). This also aids in the identification of midline.

The longus colli muscle can be released with the Bovie or bipolar cautery. Bovie cautery should be used judiciously below C6 to avoid inadvertent thermal injury to the RLN. No attempt during the exposure is made to visualize the RLN. Self-retaining retractors are placed, with small teeth under the medial longus colli muscle (Figure 168.5). Larger toothed retractors can be used, but care should be taken to ensure that the teeth insert well under the longus colli. If further exposure is desired, longitudinal blunt self-retaining retractors can be placed in a rostrocaudal fashion as already shown in Figure 168.4.

A Cushing rongeur and a ¼-inch key elevator can be used to remove ventral osteophytes and to "garden" the vertebral bodies of interest (Figures 168.6 and 168.7). Vertebral body gardening further exposes the ventral disc and prepares the vertebrae for future plating. Next, the intervertebral body distractors are placed. This allows the graft to be placed under distraction. The distractors may be angled to reduce a kyphosis (Figure 168.8). If radiographs are taken, the length of the distraction pins can be used as a guide to select the appropriate screw length. A no. 15 or no. 11 blade is used to incise the annulus and anterior disc (Figure 168.9).

The disc is then removed to the level of the PLL using curettes. The spine is released by applying clicks of distraction across the disc space as the disc is removed (Figure 168.10). The PLL and disc space are usually obscured by ventral and dorsal osteophytes (Figure 168.11). The ventral lip of the superior vertebral body

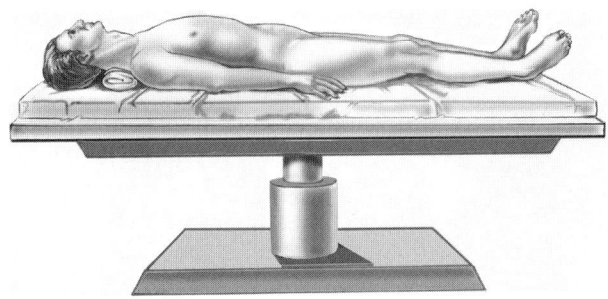

**Figure 168.2** Patient Positioning. The patient is positioned supine. A roll is placed under the neck to restore cervical lordosis.

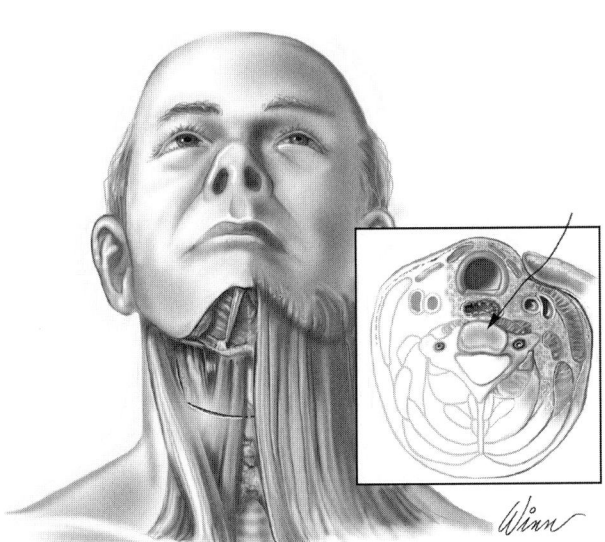

**Figure 168.3** Typical Incision for a Single- or Two-Level Discectomy. The thyroid cartilage can be palpated at C5, the cricoid cartilage at C6. The most reliable anatomic landmark is the carotid tubercle, which can be palpated at C6.

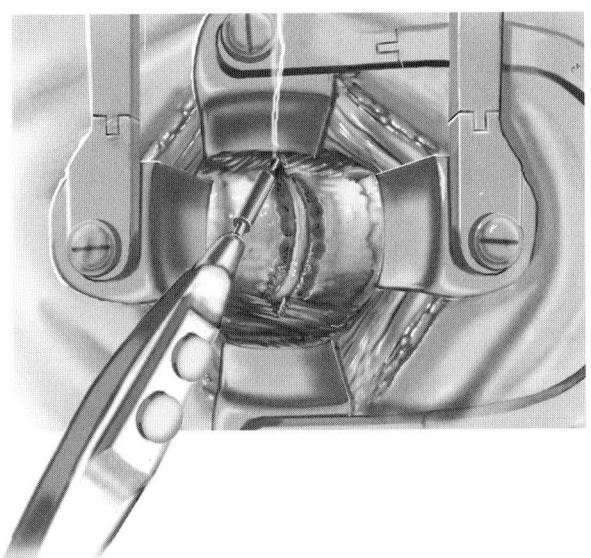

**Figure 168.4** Cauterizing the edges of the longus colli muscle to gain access to uncovertebral joints. Clear identification of the uncovertebral joints allows midline identification and facilitates foraminal decompression.

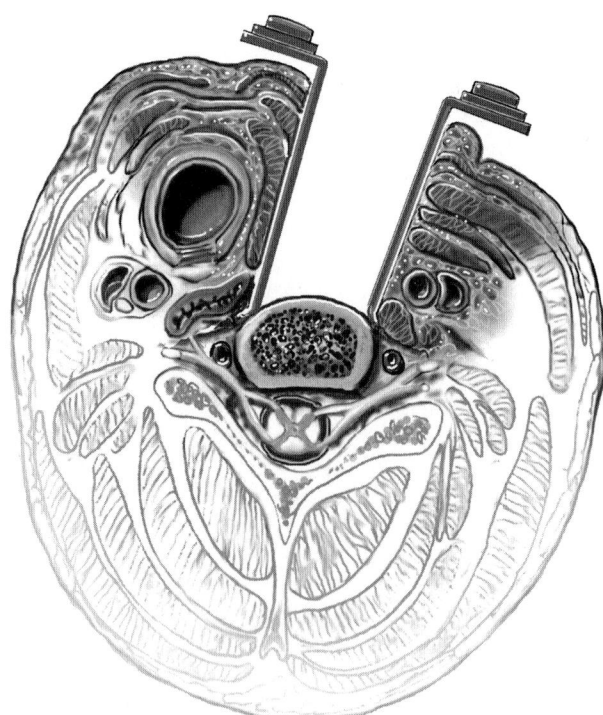

**Figure 168.5** Position of Retractor Blades under Longus Colli Muscles. Longus colli muscles are undermined and released to allow adequate retractor purchase.

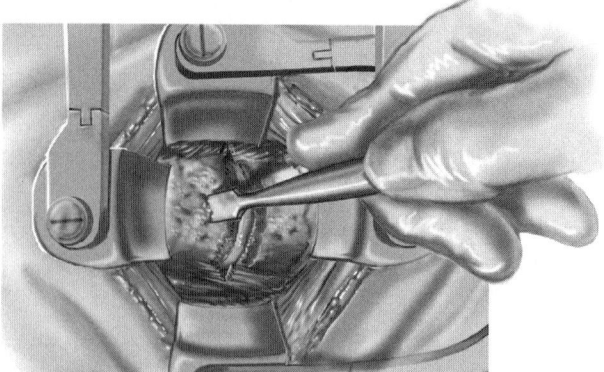

**Figure 168.7** "Gardening" with ¼-Inch Key Elevator to Expose Bone. Note that the edges of the longus colli muscle were cauterized to allow access to uncovertebral joints and lateral disc staying away from adjacent disc joints.

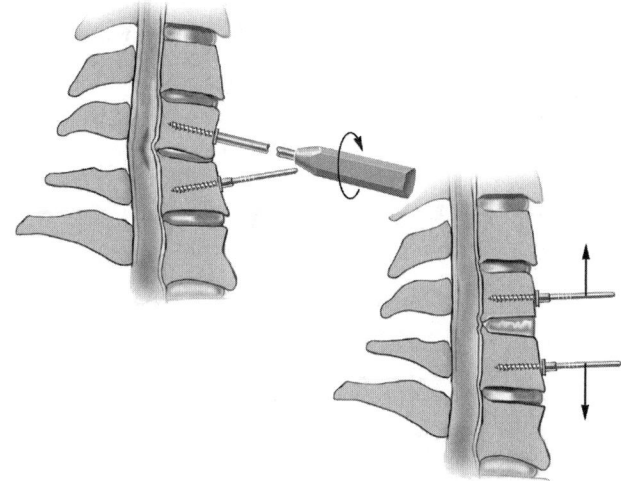

**Figure 168.8** Placement of Distraction Pins. Pins are placed in midline of the vertebral bodies and may be angled to reduce a kyphosis. Distracting the pins allows access to interspace, allows graft to be placed under distraction. In addition if a radiographic or fluoroscopy image is obtained, the pin length can be used as guide for the depth of vertebral body to choose anterior screw length.

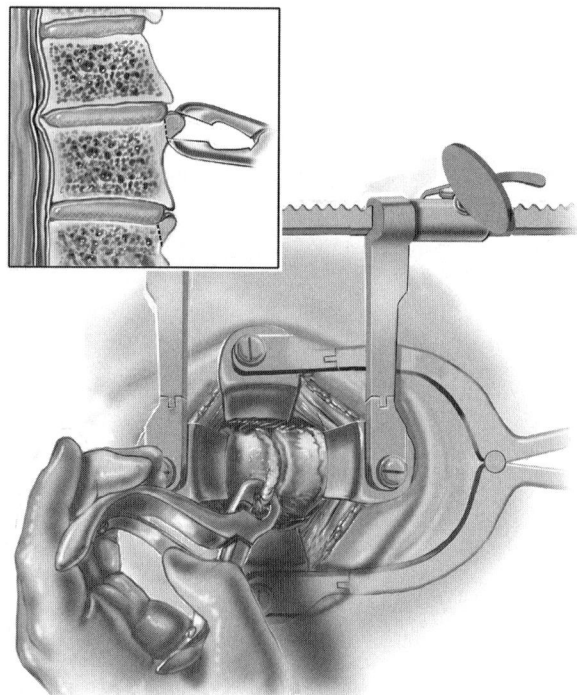

**Figure 168.6** "Gardening" the Spine with Cushing Rongeur. Soft tissue, lateral, and midline osteophytes are removed from the adjacent vertebral bodies. This prepares access to disc space.

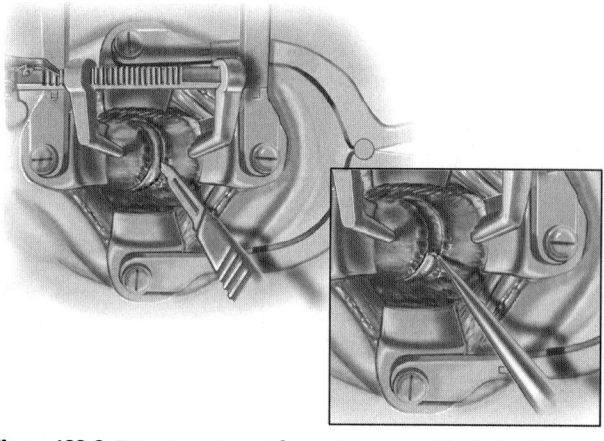

**Figure 168.9** Disc Incision with no. 11 or no. 15 Blade. Note wide disc excision and removal. Note use of large curette to remove disc from end plate.

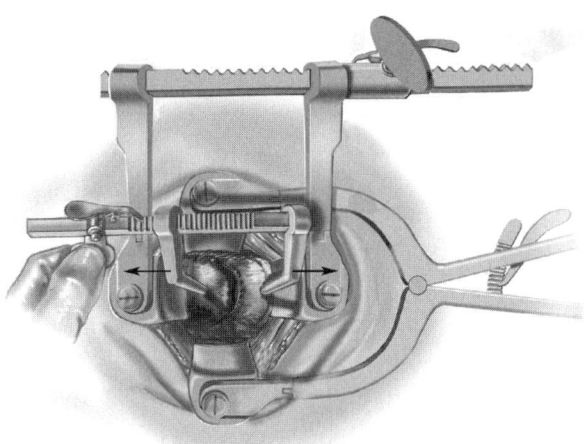

**Figure 168.10** Release of the Spine by Simultaneous Distraction and Disc Removal. This opens up the disc space and facilitates disc curettage. A few clicks of distraction are applied after each stage of disc curettage and the process is continued until the disc space is sufficiently widened.

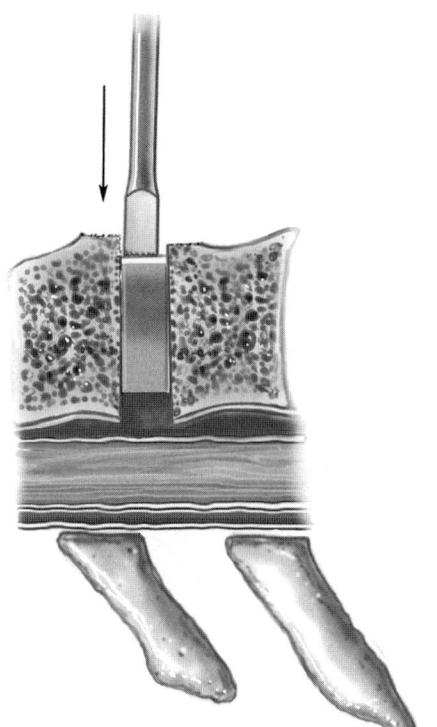

**Figure 168.11** Ventral and Dorsal Osteophyte Removal.

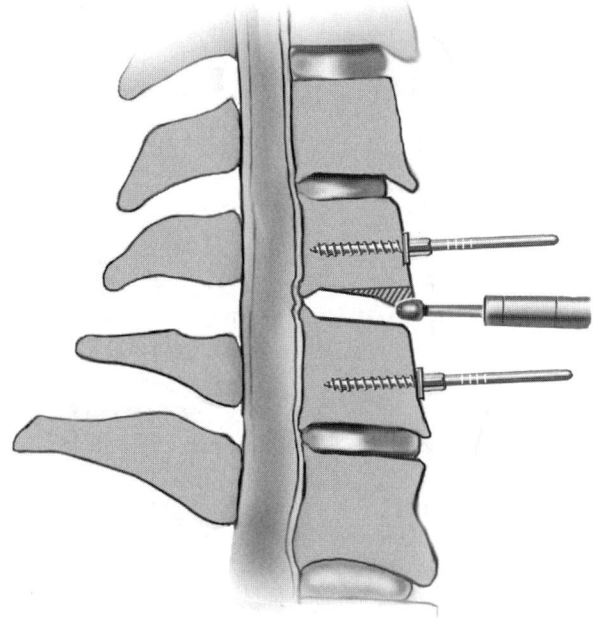

**Figure 168.12** Drilling the Ventral Lip of the Rostral Vertebral Body. The ventral lip of the rostral vertebral body is drilled to gain access to the disc space. This helps create parallel end plates, improves visualization, and prepares for graft insertion.

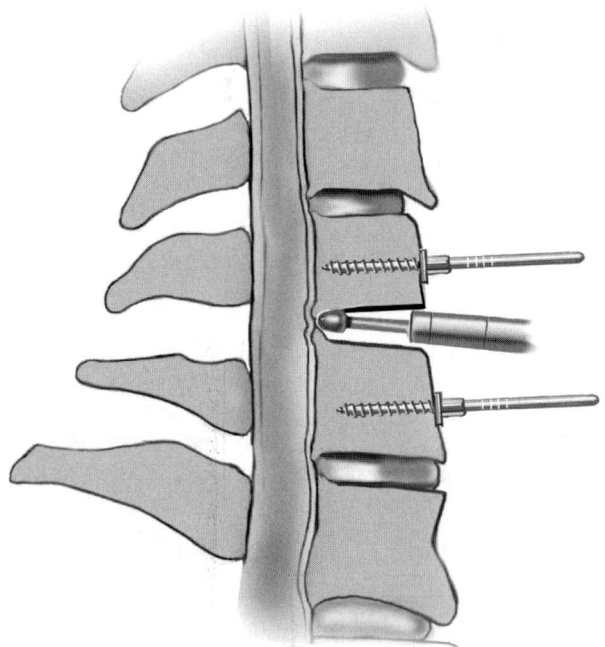

**Figure 168.13** Drilling Dorsal Osteophytes. Drilling dorsal osteophytes facilitates access to the PLL.

should be drilled to improve visualization of the disc space and prepare for graft insertion (Figure 168.12). Dorsal osteophytes and end plates should be drilled to access the PLL (Figure 168.13). The drilling of the end plates widens the disc space and increases access to the PLL (Figure 168.14). Further drilling of the dorsal vertebral body of the caudal vertebra and undercutting with 3mm thin-lipped cervical Kerrison rongeurs may be performed to

remove osteophytes and further widen the interspace (Figures 168.15 and 168.16).

Forward- and back-angled curettes may be used to cut the PLL from bone. The PLL is thinner laterally and may be easier to open laterally (Figure 168.17). The PLL is carefully removed to avoid cerebrospinal fluid leak.

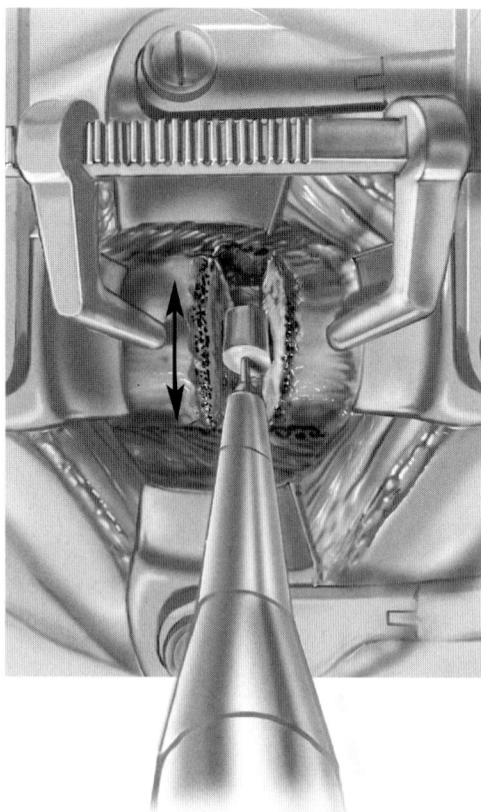

**Figure 168.14** Preparing End Plates to Gain Access to the PLL. It is important to go wide and expose the uncovertebral joints. Drilling the end plates widens the disc space and increases access to the PLL.

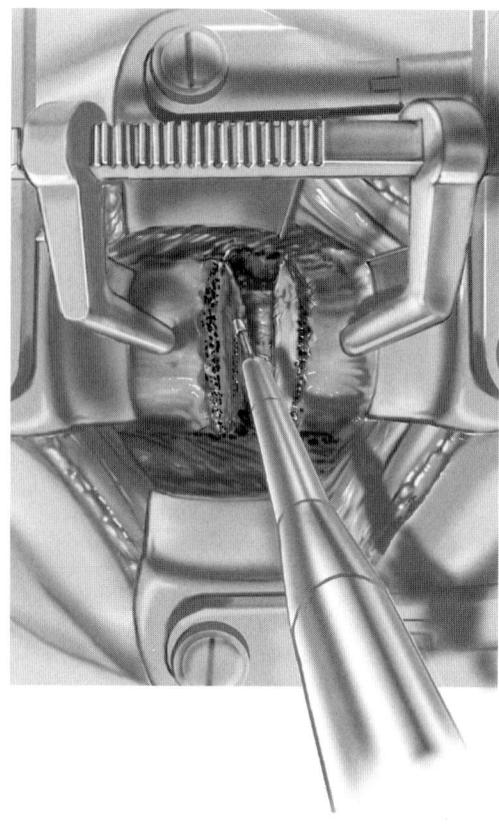

**Figure 168.15** Drilling the Dorsal Caudal Vertebral Body. This widens the interspace and removes osteophytes.

A small burr may be used to drill the lateral inferior uncovertebral joint (see Figure 168.17). This permits identification of the pedicle and the nerve root, which is rostral to the pedicle. Foraminotomies are performed as needed using a 2mm Kerrison rongeur (Figure 168.18). It is important to stay on bone to avoid epidural veins. Decompression should extend laterally until direct visualization of the medial aspect of the nerve root is achieved. Following decompression of the disc space and neural elements, the end plates are prepared for graft insertion. This may be accomplished using the cornerstone-SR cutter, which will decorticate the end plates with minimal bone removal while producing a posterior lip of bone to prevent or resist posterior graft migration. The cutter length matches the AP depth of the desired premachined allograft. The cutter is inserted until the proximal cutter face is aligned with the ventral cortex (Figure 168.19A). The cutter is then pulled medially, beginning contralaterally. The remaining thin dorsal lips may be removed with a burr to produce a final result as shown in Figure 168.19B.

Alternatively, a free-hand technique using only the burr can be used to prepare the graft site. The goal of graft site preparation when using the free-hand technique is to create a combination of cancellous and cortical bone by drilling the ventral caudal edge of the rostral vertebra and dorsal rostral edge of the caudal vertebral body (see Figure

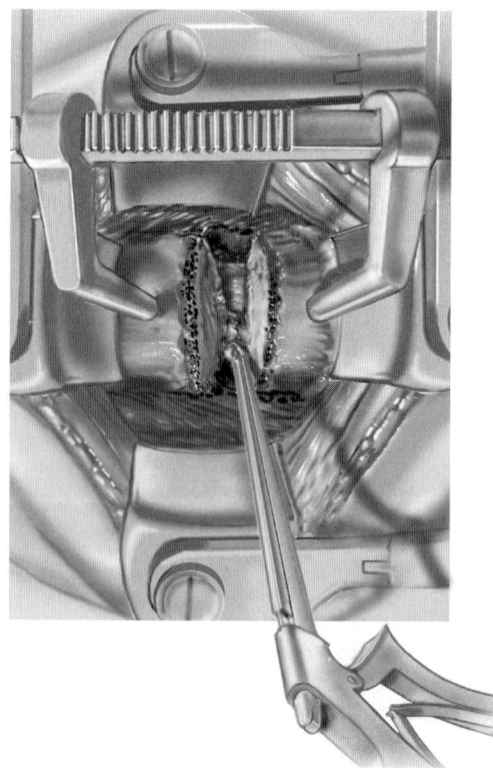

**Figure 168.16** Undercutting rostral and caudal vertebral bodies with 3mm thin-lipped cervical Kerrison rongeur.

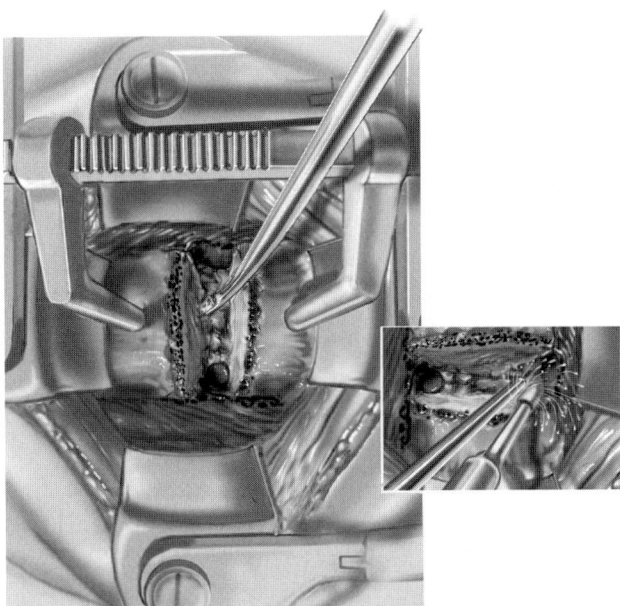

**Figure 168.17** Forward- and back-angled Karlin curettes can be used to undercut PLL from bone. A burr may be used to drill caudal inferior vertebral body uncovertebral joint. The nerve root is superior to pedicle *(inset)*.

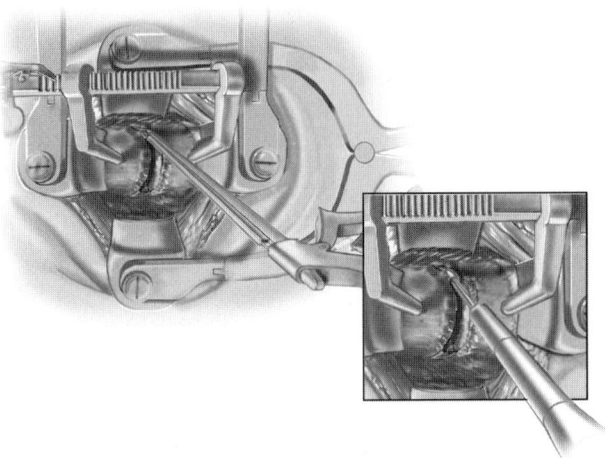

**Figure 168.18** Lateral Foraminotomy with 2mm Cervical Kerrison Rongeur. It is important to stay on bone to avoid epidural veins. Wide foraminotomy is performed. Lateral decompression is accomplished after visualization of medial aspect of nerve root.

168.19*C*). Cortical bone subverts graft subsidence while the configuration of cancellous bone enhances fusion.

## Placement of Bone Graft

Following removal of the PLL and complete decompression, the dimension of the disc space is determined and an appropriately sized strut is selected for placement (Figure 168.20). Graft options include tricortical iliac crest autograft, fibula, tibia allograft, and premachined grafts.

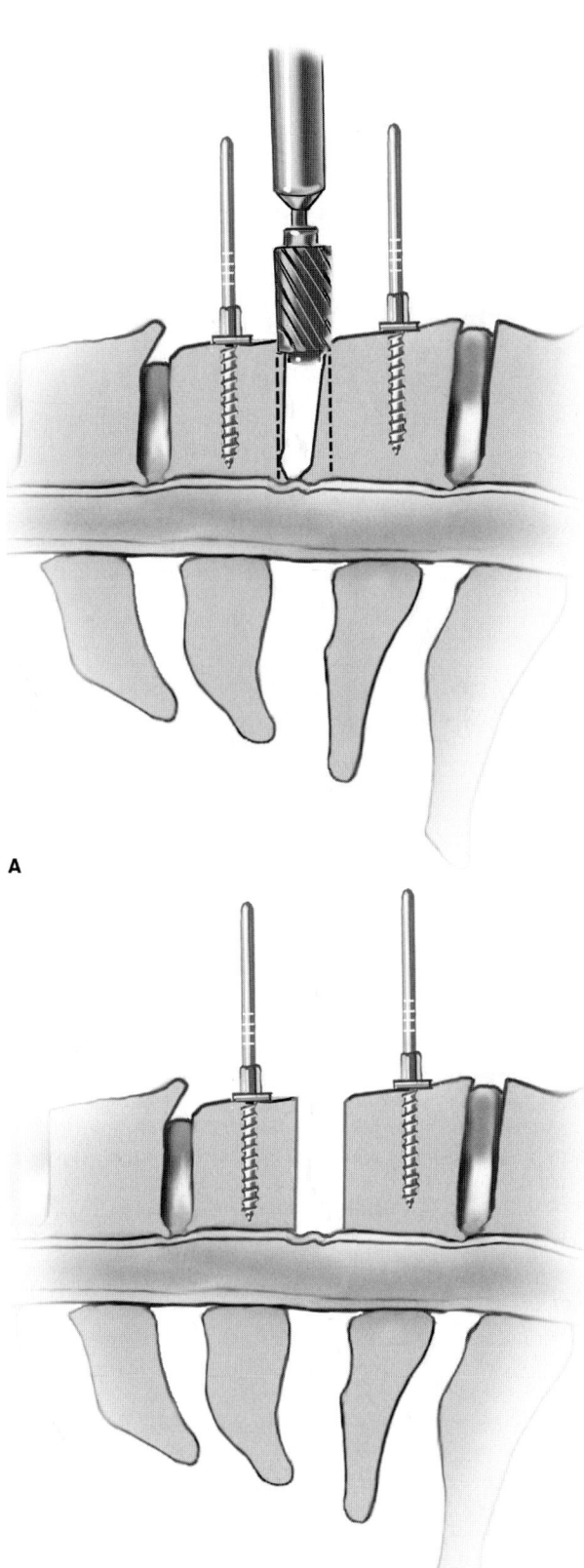

**Figure 168.19** Graft Site Preparation. (**A**) The cutter is inserted until the proximal cutter face is aligned with the ventral cortex. (**B**) After insertion in the disc space, the cutter is pulled medially starting contralaterally to produce a result as shown.

*Continued*

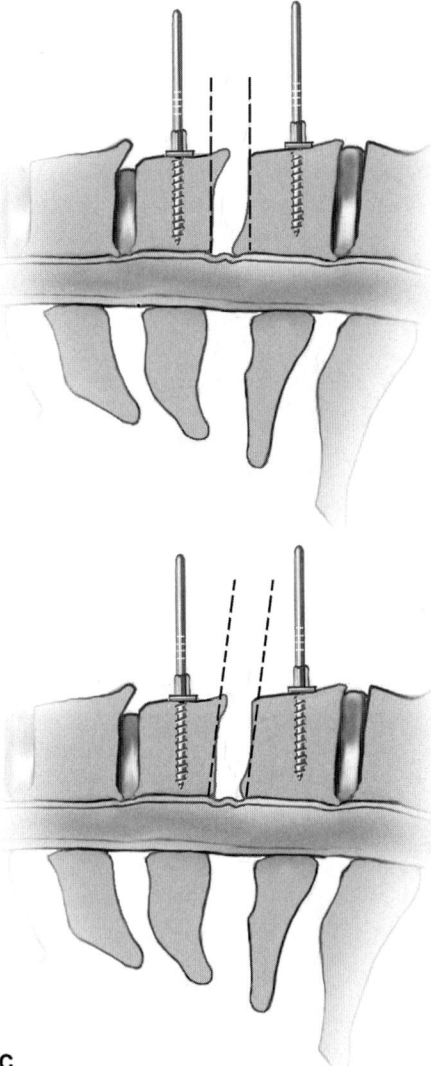

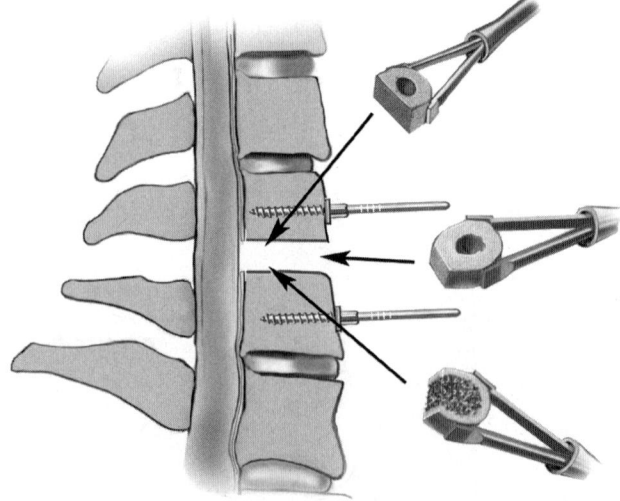

**Figure 168.20** Types of Grafts. Graft options include tricortical iliac crest, fibula or tibia allograft, and premade allografts.

**C**

**Figure 168.19** *cont'd* (**C**) Free-hand technique graft site preparation. The goal of graft site preparation when using the free-hand technique is to create a combination of cancellous and cortical bone by drilling the ventral caudal edge of the rostral vertebral bone and dorsal rostral edge of the caudal vertebral body. Cortical bone subverts graft subsidence while the configuration of cancellous bone enhances fusion.

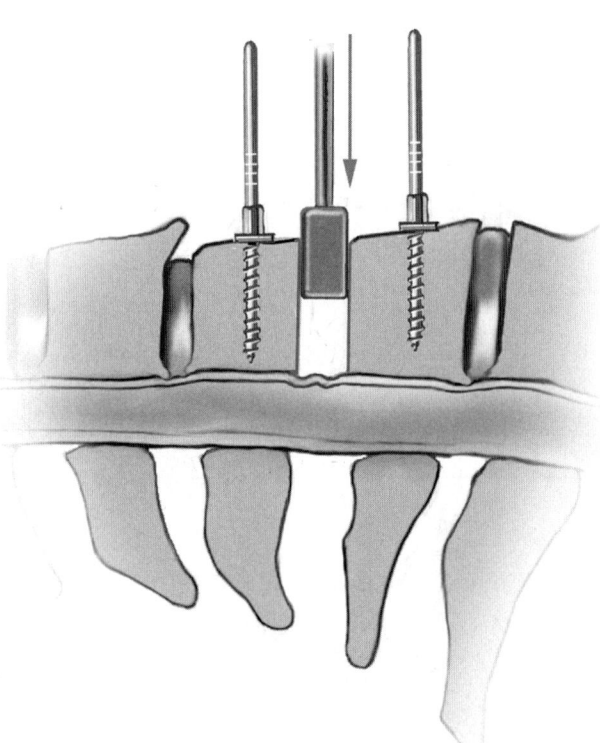

**Figure 168.21** The trial should fit flush and produce a tight fit in the disc space. If this is not possible, a larger trial should be attempted and/or the end plates should be more adequately prepared.

Successful trial selection confirms parallel end plate preparation. The trial should fit flush and produce a tight fit in the disc space (Figure 168.21). If this is not possible, a larger trial should be attempted and/or the end plates should be more adequately prepared. Thus, the trials not only help the surgeon to choose the appropriately sized graft, but they also help to determine the adequacy of end plate preparation.

Choosing a trial that is too large may produce distraction and cause the distraction pins to break out. The strut that corresponds to the final trial is chosen and gently placed into the disc space using the graft holder (Figure 168.22). The graft is tapped into the disc space using the tamp and mallet. The center of hollow implants may be filled with cancellous bone dust from the end plate drilling or with the surgeon's choice of osteoinductive material. Depending on

the bone quality, the graft may be "preloaded" by applying force on the intervertebral body pins. This permits graft compression when the distraction pins are released. Struts are typically countersunk 2 to 3mm below vertebral body surface. Tension is released on the distractors to ensure a tight fit and the distraction pins are removed (Figure

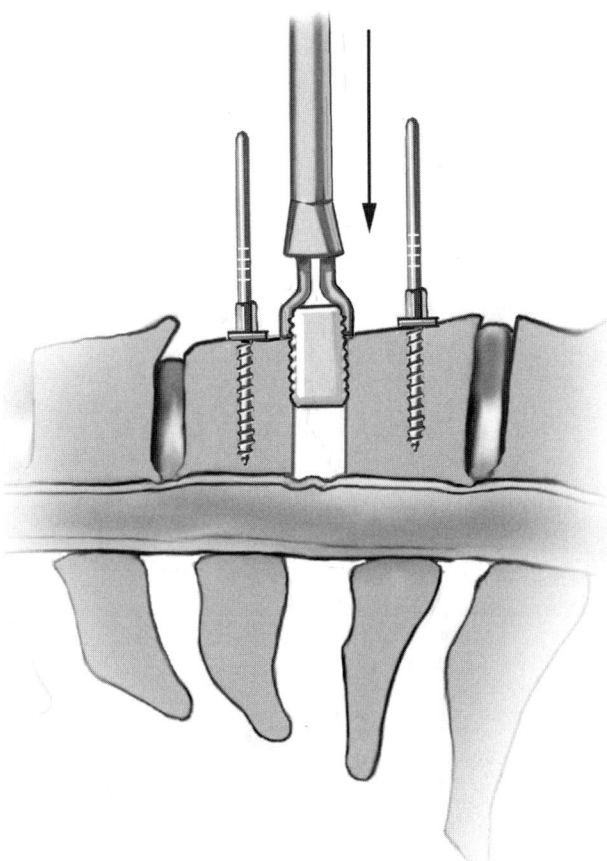

**Figure 168.22** The graft that corresponds to the final trial is chosen and gently placed into the disc space using the graft holder.

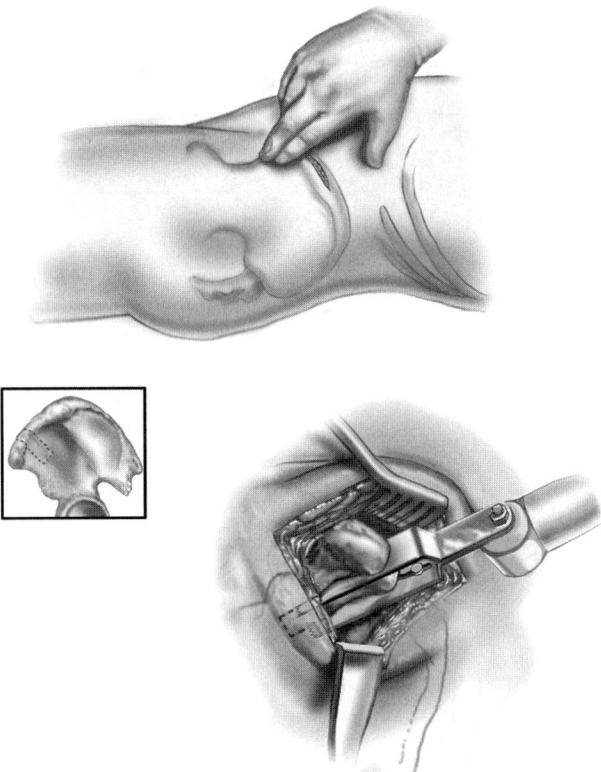

**Figure 168.24** Obtaining Iliac Crest Autograft. A double oscillating saw set to a width measured from the cornerstone template is used to make parallel cuts in the anterior iliac crest staying approximately two fingerbreadths lateral to the anterior superior iliac spine.

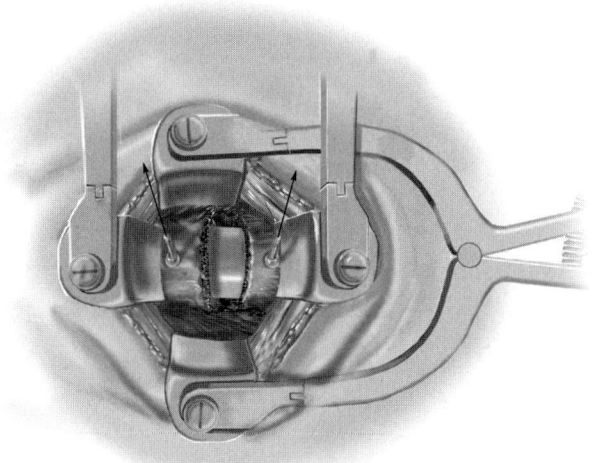

**Figure 168.23** Strut Placement. The graft is typically countersunk 2 to 3mm below vertebral body surface. Tension is released on the distractors to ensure a tight fit and the distraction pins are removed.

168.23). To check the stability of the newly placed graft, an angled curette can be used to attempt to pull the graft out of the interspace. The angled curette also may be used to palpate the posterior aspect of the graft to ensure that the graft does not compress the spinal cord.

A double oscillating saw set to a width measured from the disc interspace is used to make parallel cuts in the ventral iliac crest, remaining approximately 2 fingerbreadths lateral to the anterior superior iliac spine (Figure 168.24). After parallel cuts are completed, an osteotome bone cutter may be used to complete graft removal (Figure 168.25). Autograft is then placed in the cervical disc space in the same manner as described for allograft above.

## Anterior Cervical Plating

The vertebral bodies are then prepared for the instrumentation system. Soft tissue and ventral osteophytes should have been adequately removed in order to allow the plate to sit evenly on the spine. The Atlantis hybrid plate (Medtronic Sofamor Danek, Memphis) is described here, although any of the plating systems on the market can be used. Using the Atlantis plate, the authors typically place fixed screws caudally, and use variable screws rostrally. An appropriately sized plate is selected (Figure 168.26). The edge of the plate should not involve the adjacent unfused disc spaces.

The uncovertebral joints and the longus colli muscle are visualized in order to center the plate on the spine. Screw length is determined from the length of the distraction pin from the intraoperative radiographs or from preoperative CT, MRI, or fluoroscopy. A plate-holding pin or

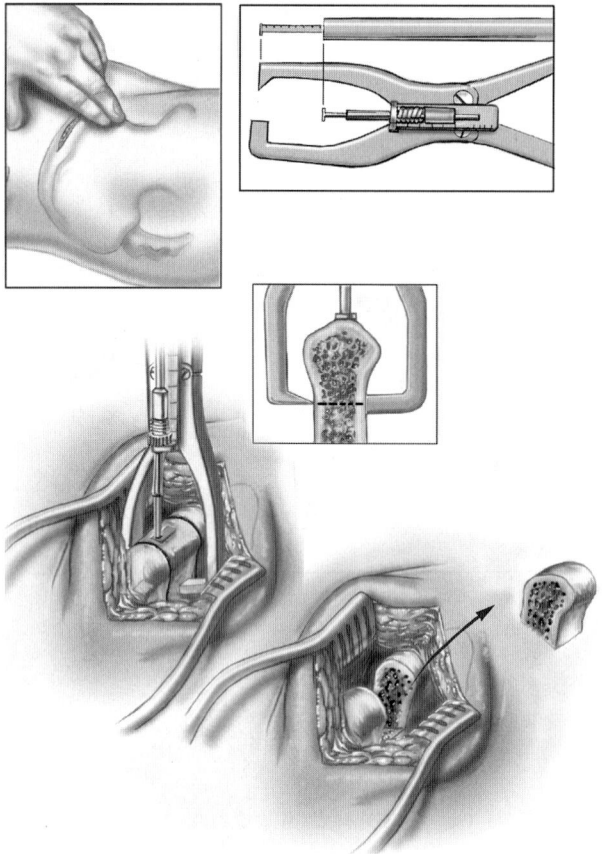

**Figure 168.25** After parallel cuts are completed with the double oscillating saw, an osteotome or bone cutter may be used to complete graft removal.

plate holder may be placed in any of the rostral or caudal screw holes to permit temporary fixation while drilling and placing screws. Alternatively, a Frazier suction device can be placed in a bone screw hole and used to hold the plate while drilling. The fixed drill guide is then seated in the caudal bone screw hole in the plate. This allows screws to be inserted at a predetermined angle of 12 degrees caudal and 6 degrees medial convergent angles.

Figure 168.27 illustrates different angles achievable with hardware allowing variable screw placement. Once the drill guide is seated, the screw hole is drilled using either a 13mm drill bit or an adjustable drill bit with an adjustable drill stop. Unless clinically indicated, the authors routinely place unicortical screws. The drilled hole is tapped at the same angle. In most cases, only the outer cortex requires tapping. If the screw length is not known at this point, a depth gage may be used to verify or select appropriate screw length. A second screw is placed diagonally from the first screw on the opposite side of the plate.

After placement of the first two screws, the plate-holding pin is removed and the remaining bone screws are placed after drilling and tapping. Final tightening is performed sequentially until the plate evenly and firmly abuts the surface of the spine. The medial angulation also enhances screw/plate stability. Problems with plating can arise if the graft is not fully seated, gardening is suboptimal, or the plate is too long (Figure 168.28).

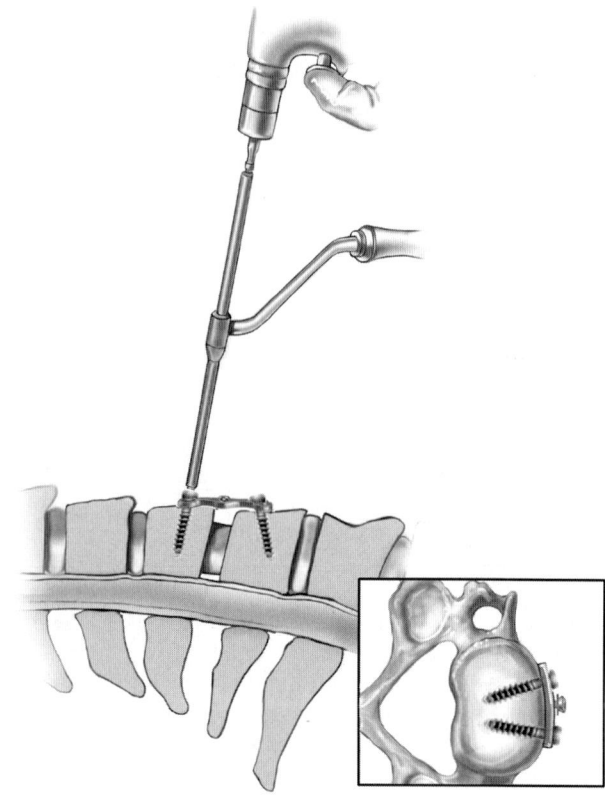

**Figure 168.26** Plate Placement. The shortest plate is selected. This allows for either placement of fixed angle screws or variable angle crews adjacent to strong subchondral bone. The edge of the plate should not involve the adjacent unfused disc spaces. The uncovertebral joints and the medial /lateral longus colli muscle are visualized in order to center the plate on the spine. The screw length is determined from the length of the distraction pin from the intraoperative radiograph or from preoperative CT, MRI, lateral radiograph, or fluoroscopy.

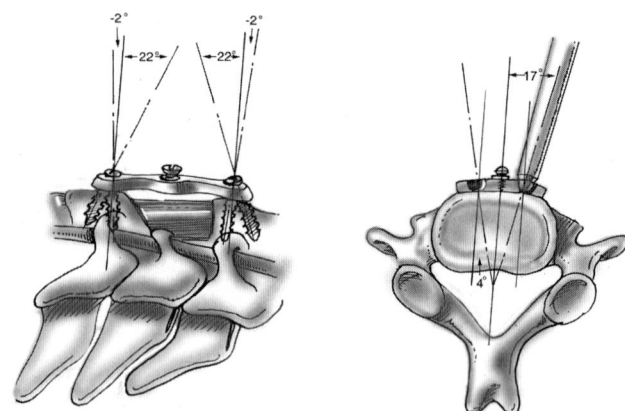

**Figure 168.27** Variable screw placement allows the surgeon to place 4.0 screws within a 22-degree distal/–2-degree proximal and 17-degree medial/4-degree lateral divergent angle.

A cross-table lateral radiograph is obtained at this point. Bleeding from epidural vessels generally responds to Gelfoam and slight pressure. A drain may be placed and the platysmal layer is approximated with 3.0 Vicryl suture. Skin closure can be performed using a subcuticular 4.0 Vicryl.

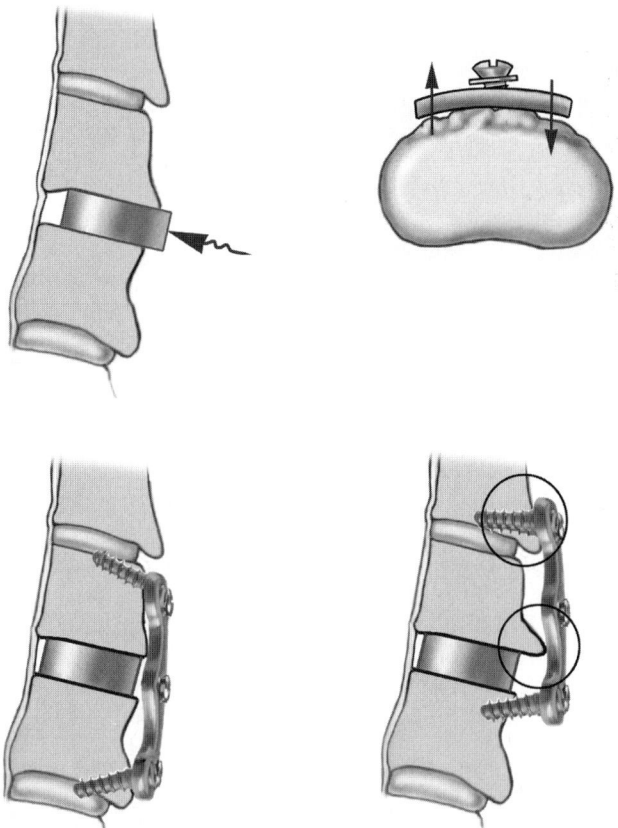

**Figure 168.28** Problems with Plating: **(A)** Graft is not fully seated. **(B)** Plate wobbles due to poor gardening. **(C)** Plate is too long. **(D)** Combination of long plate and poor gardening.

## Conclusion

This chapter presents a basic description of the ventral cervical discectomy with allograft fusion techniques. Work reported by Kaiser et al.[9] has demonstrated that fusion and excellent clinical results can be achieved using the techniques describe herein. The reader is referred to the manual from individual companies for instructions on using specific plating systems.

## REFERENCES

1. Alvarez JA, Hardy RW Jr: Anterior cervical discectomy for one- and two-level cervical disc disease: the controversy surrounding the question of whether to fuse, plate, or both. *Crit Rev Neurosurg* 9:234-251, 1999.
2. Beutler WJ, Sweeney CA, Connolly PJ: Recurrent laryngeal nerve injury with anterior cervical spine surgery risk with laterality of surgical approach. *Spine* 26:1337-1342, 2001.
3. Boden SD, Schimandle JH: Biologic enhancement of spinal fusion. *Spine* 20:113S-123S, 1995.
4. Brown MD, Malinin TI, Davis PB: A roentgenographic evaluation of frozen allografts versus autografts in anterior cervical spine fusions. *Clin Orthop* 119:231-236, 1976.
5. Cloward RB: The anterior approach for the removal of ruptured cervical discs. *J Neurosurg* 15:602-615, 1958.
6. Cloward RB: Gas-sterilized cadaver bone grafts for spinal fusion operations. A simplified bone bank. *Spine* 5:4-10, 1980.
7. Connolly PJ, Esses SI, Kostuik JP: Anterior cervical fusion: outcome analysis of patients fused with and without anterior cervical plates. *J Spinal Disord* 9:202-206, 1996.
8. Grossman W, Peppelman WC, Baum JA, et al: The use of freeze-dried fibular allograft in anterior cervical fusion. *Spine* 17:565-569, 1992.
9. Kaiser MG, Haid RW, Jr., Subach BR, et al: Anterior cervical plating enhances arthrodesis after discectomy and fusion with cortical allograft. *Neurosurgery* 50:229-236, 2002.
10. Laurie SW, Kaban LB, Mulliken JB, et al: Donor-site morbidity after harvesting rib and iliac bone. *Plast Reconstr Surg* 73:933-938, 1984.
11. Robinson R, Smith G: Anterior lateral disc removal and interbody fusion for cervical disc syndrome. *Bull Johns Hopkins Hosp* 69:223-224, 1955.
12. Schneeberger AG, Boos N, Schwarzenbach O, et al: Anterior cervical interbody fusion with plate fixation for chronic spondylotic radiculopathy: a 2- to 8-year follow-up. *J Spinal Disord* 12:215-220, 1999.
13. Smith G, Robinson R: The treatment of cervical spine disorders by anterior removal of the intervertebral disc and interbody fusion. *J Bone Joint Surg Am* 40:607-624, 1958.
14. Wang JC, McDonough PW, Endow K, et al: The effect of cervical plating on single-level anterior cervical discectomy and fusion. *J Spinal Disord* 12:467-471, 1999.
15. Wang JC, McDonough PW, Endow KK, et al: Increased fusion rates with cervical plating for two-level anterior cervical discectomy and fusion. *Spine* 25:41-45, 2000.
16. Wang JC, McDonough PW, Kanim LE, et al: Increased fusion rates with cervical plating for three-level anterior cervical discectomy and fusion. *Spine* 26:643-646, 2001.
17. Whitecloud T: Complications of anterior cervical fusion. *Instr Course Lect* 27:223-227, 1976.
18. Young WF, Rosenwasser RH: An early comparative analysis of the use of fibular allograft versus autologous iliac crest graft for interbody fusion after anterior cervical discectomy. *Spine* 18:1123-1124, 1993.
19. Younger EM, Chapman MW: Morbidity at bone graft donor sites. *J Orthop Trauma* 3:192-195, 1989.
20. Zdeblick TA, Ducker TB: The use of freeze-dried allograft bone for anterior cervical fusions. *Spine* 16:726-729, 1991.

# Ventral Cervical Discectomy and Fusion with Autograft and without Plating

Gordon R. Bell

Degeneration of the cervical spine is a common, age-related condition that may be either asymptomatic or associated with clinical symptoms. From a clinical standpoint, symptomatic degenerative cervical disc disease may produce neck pain, referred pain, radicular arm pain, or clinical myelopathy.

From a purely surgical perspective, axial neck pain, unless associated with significant or symptomatic instability, is rarely a surgically correctable condition because of the difficulty in accurately localizing the anatomic source of neck pain. Nonaxial pain may be either referred or radicular. Referred pain may be felt either interscapularly, into the shoulder or down the arm in a nondermatomal pattern. The anatomic basis for this pain is based on the embryonic location and migration of the cervical sclerotomes during embryonic development. Radicular arm pain is the most common indication for surgical intervention and, when due to neurogenic compression, can usually be successfully treated with surgery. Cervical myelopathy is commonly due to cervical spinal cord compression, and is often associated with either a congenital or acquired spinal canal narrowing. It generally portends a poorer outcome than cervical radiculopathy, may result in a permanent and significant neurologic deficit, and mandates surgical decompression. Because of inherent physiologic and anatomic differences between the nerve root and the spinal cord, recovery of spinal cord function, even after successful surgical decompression, is not assured.

This chapter focuses on indications for ventral cervical surgery, relevant surgical anatomy, the technique of ventral surgery, and complications. Attention focuses on anterior cervical discectomy and fusion (ACDF) using autogenous bone graft without the use of supplemental spinal fixation.

## Indications for Ventral Surgery

Although cervical fusion may successfully relieve neck pain, its success is limited by the inability to accurately identify the source of pain. The source of axial pain may be more accurately inferred when the pain is associated with readily identifiable instability associated with a traumatic event. Discography is a provocative test that attempts to localize the source of such pain, but it has not been universally accepted as a useful tool in determining surgical outcome. To date, there have been no good prospective studies relating the outcome of ventral cervical fusion for neck pain with the results of preoperative discography. Until such a study is done, the ultimate role of discography and cervical surgery for the diagnosis and treatment of neck pain remains controversial. The most precise and reliable role of surgery is, therefore, for dermatomal arm pain (cervical radiculopathy) or for symptomatic spinal cord compression (cervical myelopathy).

### Cervical Radiculopathy

Cervical radiculopathy is a term that refers to cervical nerve root compression in a dermatomal pattern that results in a spectrum of symptoms and signs. It may also result in paresthesia, subjective weakness, or both. Clinical signs include reflex changes, objective weakness, or sensory abnormalities. Such symptoms and signs are commonly due to nerve root compression that, when accompanied by pain, also suggests the presence of associated nerve root inflammation. The presence of compression can be identified by myelography, CT, or MRI. There

must be a precise correlation between the patient's symptoms, objective clinical findings, and imaging findings in order to demonstrate a cause-and-effect relationship between clinical and radiographic findings. Although the cervical MRI is the preferred initial imaging test, it may not show subtle degrees of nerve root compression, particularly foraminal disease, and additional imaging by postcontrast (postmyelogram) CT may be required.

The most common indication for surgery is persistent and intractable arm pain that is unresponsive to conservative measures. Other indications include the presence of a progressive neurologic deficit or a significant nonprogressive deficit that is associated with persistent arm pain. Although surgery may not restore lost strength, it can arrest further progression of the weakness.

Nerve root compression may be due to either a soft disc herniation or to bony canal or foraminal narrowing. The most common cause of unilateral nerve root compression is dorsolateral disc herniation. Other causes include foraminal bony narrowing from facet joint hypertrophy or prominent uncovertebral joints (joints of Luschka). Although a large central disc herniation may cause bilateral arm symptoms, it more commonly results in myelopathy or myeloradiculopathy. Bilateral arm symptoms suggest foraminal nerve compression.

### Cervical Myelopathy

Cervical myelopathy is a pathologic condition of the cervical spinal cord that is commonly due to spinal cord compression from a large central herniation, cervical spondylosis, or ossification of the posterior longitudinal ligament (OPLL). Pathologically, this condition is characterized by both gray and white matter destruction and by demyelinization above and below the level of compression.[23] Clinically, it is characterized by a constellation of symptoms and signs, the manifestation of which depends on the level and nature of the anatomic structures compressed. The clinical picture may be so unusual that diagnostic confusion may ensue, and the patient may be mislabeled with any one of a host of other diagnoses, including motor neuron disease, multiple sclerosis, Guillain-Barré syndrome, peripheral neuropathy, or intracranial causes. On the one hand, the patient may present with very nondescript symptoms such as a subtle gait disturbance or mild hand numbness. At the other extreme, the patient may be floridly myelopathic and present as wheelchair-bound with loss of fine motor control of the hands.

Clinical examination often reveals classical long-tract findings consisting of spasticity, hyperreflexia, clonus, plantar extensor (Babinski) response, and a Hoffman sign. Typically, the patient is neurologically normal above the level of compression, but exhibits upper motor neuron signs below the level of compression. At the level of the spinal cord compression, the patient typically exhibits a lower motor neuron dysfunction picture, characterized by hyporeflexia or areflexia and muscle weakness.

The diagnosis of cervical myelopathy is confirmed radiographically by the presence of spinal cord compression. MRI has replaced CT/myelography as the preferred imaging modality, although the latter remains a useful imaging modality because it distinguishes bone from other compressive pathology better than MRI does, and it often shows subtle degrees of foraminal pathology better than MRI does.[5] Whenever doubt exists, the clinician should have a low threshold for obtaining a myelogram and post-contrast CT scan. Radiographic findings of cervical spinal cord compression include absence of the subarachnoid space at the site of compression and compression or frank distortion with deformation of the spinal cord itself. Such findings are often associated with a narrowed spinal canal, either on a congenital or acquired basis. Such narrowing diminishes the "functional reserve" of the spinal canal, thereby permitting spinal cord compression by a comparatively smaller extradural lesion than would otherwise be required to cause symptomatic spinal cord compression. Occasionally, spinal cord signal changes may exist at sites of extreme compression, suggesting myelomalacia.

## Axial Neck Pain

Surgery for axial neck pain is subject to the same limitations as is surgery for axial low back pain: namely, the difficulty in accurately identifying the source of the pain. Unless the etiology of the pain can be precisely identified, it is probable that the pain will not be relieved by surgery. Discography for neck pain, as for back pain, is the only available provocative test for pain, but remains a controversial and unproven diagnostic entity. Therefore, most discriminating surgeons reserve cervical surgery for radicular arm pain or myelopathy rather than axial neck pain.

Surgery for axial pain, as distinguished from that for radicular pain, does not carry the imperative of neural decompression, since the goal of surgery is stabilization. Some fusion techniques for neck pain, such as the Keystone graft technique, therefore involve only partial discectomy without nerve root decompression.[28]

## Surgical Technique

### Preoperative Considerations

Meticulous preoperative preparations are essential to maximize success of surgery and to minimize complications. Precise correlation between the patient's symptoms, objective neurologic signs, and radiographic imaging findings is mandatory to optimize surgical outcome. Patients who have had prior ventral cervical spine surgery require a preoperative otolaryngology evaluation to assess vocal cord function. If normal vocal cord function is present, the surgical approach should be performed from the unoperated side of the neck, in order to permit a safer exposure by avoiding scarring associated with the prior surgery. If abnormal vocal cord function is observed, the surgical approach should be performed on the same side as the previous surgery in order to eliminate the possibility of contralateral damage to the vocal cords.

### Intraoperative Considerations
#### Positioning

General endotracheal anesthesia is administered with the endotracheal tube placed on the side opposite the intended surgical approach. For patients with cervical myelopathy or significant cervical instability, fiberoptic awake intubation should be considered. The patient is positioned supine on the operating table with a small rolled-up towel placed longitudinally between the scapulae. This allows the shoulders and clavicles to gently fall backwards and out of the way, thereby facilitating the surgical exposure. The patient's head should be supported with a foam donut and the head turned to the side opposite the intended exposure. The head is placed in slight extension in order to mimic the natural cervical lordosis and to facilitate dissection. If an autogenous iliac graft is to be harvested, a small bolster, such as a blanket, should be placed under the buttocks to facilitate the approach to the ventral iliac crest. The arms are secured at the patient's side, and Kerlix straps are looped around the patient's wrists and secured to the operating table caudally. This technique permits an unscrubbed assistant to gently pull on the arms to depress the shoulders when obtaining an intraoperative localizing radiograph, in order to better visualize the mid and lower cervical spine. The maneuver is particularly useful for patients with short, stout necks.

Antiembolic stockings or sequential compression stockings are recommended to reduce the risk of intraoperative deep venous thrombosis (DVT). If intraoperative monitoring is to be used, the recording electrodes are placed at this time. A grounding pad is secured to the patient's leg.

### Incision

The decision regarding the side of surgical approach is based on anatomic considerations related to the recurrent laryngeal nerve (RLN) and the thoracic duct. The RLN is located in the tracheoesophageal groove and is more constant in location on the left side than on the right. This has prompted some surgeons to recommend a left-sided surgical approach in order to minimize the risk of vocal cord paralysis from damage to the RLN. On the other hand, a left-handed approach is, arguably, more difficult for a right-handed surgeon than a left-sided approach. However, the greater theoretical risk of injury to the RLN from a right-sided surgical approach has not been proven clinically. A recent retrospective review of 328 ventral cervical spine fusions revealed 9 cases (2.7%) of RLN symptoms.[7] Although there was a significant difference in the incidence of RLN injury between primary and redo anterior procedures (2.3% vs. 9.5%, respectively), there was no association between side of approach and incidence of RLN symptoms.

The thoracic duct ascends from the thorax, lateral to the esophagus and loops over the subclavian artery at the level of the T1 vertebral body, approximately 3cm to 4cm above the clavicle. The risk of injury to the thoracic duct is greater with a left-sided approach to the lower cervical spine. For approaches to the lower cervical spine, either the thoracic duct should be protected or a right-sided approach should be considered.

Knowledge regarding the characteristics and location of anatomic landmarks is essential in order to place accurately the skin incision.[33] The angle of the jaw is just above the C1-2 level. The hyoid bone is generally at the level of C3, the thyroid cartilage at C4-5, and the cricoid cartilage at C6. The C7-T1 level is located approximately one fingerbreadth above the sternal notch. A common mistake is to place the skin incision too caudally. This is more likely to occur if the incision is planned with the patient's neck in extension. For exposures at C4-5 and above, the incision should be placed approximately three fingerbreadths above the clavicle. For exposures below C5, the incision should be about two fingerbreadths above the clavicle.

For one- or two-level discectomies without instrumentation or a single-level discectomy with instrumentation, a transverse incision is preferred. For more extensive surgeries, an oblique longitudinal incision along the ventral border of the SCM is usually necessary.

## Approach

The key to the surgical approach to the ventral cervical spine is understanding the fascial layers in the neck. The cervical fascia consists of one superficial and four deep layers.[16] The superficial fascia surrounds the subcutaneous tissue of the neck, including the platysma. The deep fascia consists of four components:

- The superficial layer surrounds the neck and splits to envelop the SCM and trapezius muscles.
- The middle layer is subdivided into three parts, the third portion of which is the visceral fascia that surrounds the trachea, esophagus, and thyroid gland, and fuses in the midline with the underlying alar fascia.
- The alar fascia lies dorsal to the esophagus and spreads laterally to surround the carotid sheath. It ultimately fuses with the prevertebral fascia laterally over the transverse processes.
- The prevertebral fascia surrounds the vertebral bodies and adjacent paravertebral musculature.

The clinical significance of the fascial layers lies in their ability to contain and prevent the spread of infection. Because the alar and prevertebral fasciae are fused laterally over the transverse processes, an infection involving the vertebral body is contained in the midline. On the other hand, the visceral and alar fasciae are fused in the midline so that a pharyngeal abscess is contained laterally and is prevented from spreading across the midline. The surgical significance of the fascial layers lies in the natural cleavage planes that exist between the fascial layers, which provide safe avenues for dissection.

The superficial fascia, with its enclosed platysma muscle, is divided, and the superficial layer of the deep cervical fascia surrounding the SCM and trapezius muscles is incised. The platysma muscle may either be split longitudinally or divided in the direction of the skin incision. For a one-level discectomy, the platysma muscle is generally split longitudinally. For two or more levels, it is preferable to divide the muscle. The fascial plane between the alar fascia, with its enclosed carotid sheath, and the visceral fascia, which surrounds the trachea and esophagus, is developed bluntly such that the carotid sheath is retracted laterally and the trachea and esophagus are retracted medially. By respecting the visceral fascia plane, inadvertent injury to the RLN, which is located in the tracheoesophageal groove, is minimized. Blunt dissection is continued in order to expose the prevertebral fascia and the underlying vertebral bodies. For distal exposures, the

omohyoid muscle may be divided in order to provide better visualization. It is generally not repaired during the closure.

A large-bore spinal needle is then inserted into a disc space, and a confirmatory lateral radiograph is taken to accurately localize the pathologic level. It is recommended that the needle be prebent in order to minimize the risk of inadvertently placing the needle too deeply into the disc space. It may be necessary to have an unscrubbed assistant retract the patient's arms caudally, using the previously placed Kerlix straps. This facilitates the visualization of the lower cervical spine.

After the appropriate level is exposed and the midline clearly delineated, the longus colli muscles are carefully elevated from the vertebral bodies to facilitate the placement of retractors. Care must be taken to avoid excessive stripping of the longus colli muscles in order to minimize the risk of injury to the sympathetic chain that lies over the longus colli and the longus capitus muscles. Injury to the sympathetic trunk can result in Horner's syndrome, which is characterized by ptosis, meiosis, and anhydrosis. The use of blunt, rather than sharp, self-retaining retractor blades to retract the longus colli muscles minimizes the risk of inadvertent puncture of the esophagus. The amount of retraction should be minimized in order to reduce the risk of dysphagia from esophageal injury.

It has been demonstrated that during retraction of the longus colli muscles, the larynx may be displaced against the shaft of the endotracheal tube (ET), thereby allowing impingement on the intralaryngeal portion of the RLN.[4] This can result in injury to the RLN with resulting hoarseness, vocal cord fatigue, weak cough, and/or risk of aspiration. In a clinical study involving 900 consecutive ventral cervical surgeries with plating, it was found that the risk of RLN injury could be significantly reduced by monitoring the ET cuff pressure, deflating the cuff after retractor placement, and subsequently reinflating the cuff to 15mmHg.[4] This data, and a concomitant laboratory experiment by the same authors, supported the hypothesis that injury to the RLN occurred from ET-mediated compression during retraction. Furthermore, releasing the cuff pressure could reduce the risk of vocal cord paralysis.

## Discectomy

Ventral cervical fusion for cervical spondylosis was first described by Robinson and Smith in 1955.[25,30] The original technique employed a piece of tricortical iliac graft for the fusion, a method that remains the gold standard. This method of arthrodesis restores disc space height and thereby enlarges the neural foramen, thus indirectly decompressing the nerve root. The nerve root is therefore decompressed both directly, by removal of disc material or osteophyte, and indirectly, by disc space distraction with bone graft. A successful fusion also provides stability to the level fused and therefore minimizes the risk of future segmental instability.

Cervical discectomy can be facilitated by the use of disc space distraction. This can be accomplished by the use of either Gardner-Wells tongs or Holter traction, or by the use of distractor instrumentation (Caspar; Aesculap Instrument Corp., Bethlehem, PA). The use of the latter is particularly useful, since it not only provides disc space distraction, but also permits longitudinal soft tissue retraction. Magnification and illumination is provided by either the use of magnifying loupes and headlight or the operating microscope. The microscope has several advantages, including its ability to permit superior visualization by both the surgeon and the assistant and its ability to be angled to visualize rostrally, caudally, and laterally.

The disc is incised sharply and a rectangular piece of the ALL and the ventral annulus fibrosus are excised. Disc material is removed with small straight and angled curettes and with micropituitary rongeurs. The dissection is carried down to the PLL. If a sequestered disc fragment is suspected, the PLL should be excised and the fragment identified and removed. If the disc is contained by the PLL, the ligament may be left intact. There is no particular advantage to preserving the PLL if ventral cervical plating is used, since the plate and screws provide stability. If, on the other hand, a noninstrumented fusion is planned, preservation of the PLL provides an effective tension band and adds additional stability.

The cartilaginous surfaces of the rostral and caudal end plates are removed with curettes until the underlying subchondral bone is exposed. Many authors feel that this supporting structure should be kept intact, particularly if a noninstrumented fusion is planned. The rate of pseudarthrosis can be reduced, however, by burring the end plates to expose subchondral bone.[10] Although this technique results in mild settling and a slight increase in kyphosis, clinical outcome was unchanged from that with the standard technique of preserving the end plates.[10]

There is debate about whether or not a large posterior osteophyte causing spinal cord compression should be removed, even in the presence of clinical myelopathy. Some authors feel that it may be left intact, since there seems to be no difference in clinical outcome regardless of the osteophyte, and the osteophyte frequently remodels and resorbs following successful arthrodesis.[6,19,35] Other authors have reported that spontaneous remodeling of the osteophyte may not occur, even in the presence of a solid arthrodesis.[31] The nerve root should be checked within its neural foramen and, if compressed, a foraminotomy should be performed.

If multiple discectomies are planned, the identical procedure is repeated for each of the other levels. Distraction pins for the longitudinal spreader (Caspar; Aesculap Instrument Corp., Bethlehem, PA) are placed at each vertebral body level and are left in place to serve as effective longitudinal soft tissue retractors. For a two-level discectomy, a total of three pins, therefore, will be required; for a three-level discectomy, four pins are needed. The distraction device is inserted over adjacent pins at each disc space to facilitate the discectomy at each level.

## Bone Graft Considerations

The basic principle of ventral cervical discectomy and fusion is nerve root or spinal cord decompression and spinal stabilization. In addition to neural decompression, ventral fusion provides stability, maintenance of lordosis, restoration of load sharing, and indirect foraminal decompression. Autogenous iliac crest bone graft (ICBG) is still considered

the "gold standard" material for ventral cervical discectomy and fusion. In addition to providing good structural support, it provides better osteoconductive and osteoinductive capabilities than allograft and has lower risks of disease transmission and other adverse reactions. Many surgeons still feel that the use of tricortical autogenous bone graft provides superior rates of fusion than does allograft.

The technical details of bone graft harvesting are important in order to minimize bone graft donor site morbidity and to maximize fusion. Placing a small roll under the buttocks facilitates harvest of the graft by profiling the anterior iliac crest profile and making it prominent and more easily accessible. This is particularly helpful in obese patients with a large panniculus. The incision should be placed at least 2cm lateral to the anterior superior iliac spine (ASIS) in order to minimize risk of injury to the lateral femoral cutaneous nerve. Although nerve passes anterior to the ASIS in 90% of patients, it may be injured if its course is aberrant and dorsal to the ASIS. In addition, hematoma from the graft site may cause compression of a nerve in close proximity.

The skin incision should be made parallel to, and either just below or above, the iliac crest. It should begin approximately 3cm posterior to the ASIS in order to avoid injury to the lateral femoral cutaneous nerve and to minimize the risk of fracture of the ASIS. The iliac crest is exposed, and the periosteum is incised. A periosteal elevator is used to obtain subperiosteal exposure of both the external and internal surfaces of the iliac crest, and a sponge is packed between the periosteum and the bone in order to facilitate exposure and hemostasis. Retraction of the periosteum may be achieved by utilizing two Cobb periosteal elevators, one anterior and one posterior to the crest.

The graft should be harvested with an oscillating saw, rather than an osteotome, in order to minimize the risk of producing microfractures of the weight-bearing surfaces of the bone, which could lead to graft failure and eventual collapse.[1] The graft can easily be harvested with a double oscillating saw blade that is manufactured in varying widths. The optimal thickness of a tricortical graft depends on the preoperative baseline disc height. For a preoperative disc height of 3.5 to 6.0mm, an interbody graft of 2mm above baseline thickness was found to be most appropriate.[1] In general, the graft should be at least 5mm thick in order to minimize the risk of collapse. The deep surface of the graft may be completed with a curved osteotome.

Closure of the bone graft site should be meticulous in order to minimize postoperative pain. Bleeding from the three cut surfaces of the ilium should be controlled with bone wax. If there is additional bleeding from muscle or other soft tissue, a suction drain may be inserted. The periosteum is closed with interrupted sutures. The subcutaneous tissue is closed with interrupted suture, and the skin is closed with either staples, nonabsorbable interrupted skin sutures, or an absorbable subcuticular skin closure.

## Complications
### Hoarseness

Hoarseness is a relatively common complaint in the initial postoperative period.[2,15] Usually it is due to edema from retraction and will subside within a few days. Although persistent hoarseness may indicate injury to either the superior laryngeal nerve or RLN, a more likely explanation is an endolaryngeal mechanism related to the ET. Indeed, postoperative vocal cord paralysis has been described in many noncervical spine surgeries. A series of 564 patients reported that RLN injury was caused by the ET in 11.2% of cases.[34]

Potential neurogenic causes of postoperative hoarseness include direct injury to the RLN by surgical trauma or indirect injury to it by stretching or pressure. Although injury to the superior laryngeal nerve may also cause hoarseness, it more commonly results in laryngeal fatigue. The superior laryngeal nerve is a branch of the inferior ganglion of the vagus nerve that courses with the superior thyroid artery to innervate the cricothyroid muscle.

Injury to the RLN was the most frequent neurologic complication reported by Flynn in his review of more than 36,000 anterior cervical surgery cases.[13] This nerve is more constant in location on the left side of the neck where it arises at the level of the aortic arch and passes beneath the arch to ascend between the trachea and esophagus within the visceral fascia. Injury to the RLN may result in temporary or permanent hoarseness. A left-sided surgical approach, therefore, is theoretically less risky to the nerve than a right-sided approach. However, a recent retrospective review of 187 patients undergoing anterior cervical surgery found no difference in RLN symptoms based on side of surgical approach.[7] This study was retrospective, nonrandom and relied only on voice changes (hoarseness) or subjective swallowing symptoms as evidence of potential RLN injury. Mild, asymptomatic abnormalities were not included. It is therefore possible that the incidence of nerve injury was underestimated.

## Neurologic Complications

Although uncommon, neurologic injury is the most feared complication of anterior cervical surgery. One widely quoted article surveyed 1358 neurosurgeons in 1974 to determine the frequency and severity of neurologic complications following ACDF.[13] Responses to the mailed questionnaire were received from 704 surgeons (52% response rate), involving 82,114 cases. No neurologic complications were reported in 71% of the replies (45,457 cases). There were a total of 311 neurologic complications in the remaining 36,657 cases. The single most common neurologic complication was injury to the RLN (52 cases; 16.7% of all complications). Postoperative myelopathy occurred in 78 cases. Of the 70 cases that had sufficient information for analysis, there was no apparent cause in 24 (34% of cases) and 38 (54%) were thought to be due to intraoperative trauma. The author concluded that the risk of major neurologic complication was 1 in 355 cases.

Neurologic complications following surgery for cervical myelopathy were reviewed in a series of 384 patients.[36] Two hundred four of the patients had anterior surgery, including 134 with anterior interbody fusions. Overall, 21 patients (5.5% of total) sustained neurologic deterioration related to their surgery, including 3% involving the C5 root. Deterioration involved either spinal cord function or nerve root function. Causes of spinal cord dysfunction included intraoperative spinal cord injury, malalignment of the spine associated with graft complication, and

epidural hematoma. Paralysis of the deltoid and biceps brachii muscles was related to C5 nerve root deterioration. Causes of this paralysis included direct injury to the nerve, spinal malalignment related to graft complications, and tethering or distraction of the nerve root from shifting of the spinal cord after decompression. The C5 root is short and is commonly the most ventral of the roots, since it typically lies at the point of maximal cervical lordosis. These factors make it susceptible to a traction type of injury following decompression, particularly posterior decompression. In addition, the deltoid muscle commonly has a single root innervation from C5, making an injury to this root more clinically apparent.

Less common neurologic involvement included phrenic nerve injury. Bilateral phrenic nerve palsy has been described following anterior decompression and fusion for cervical OPLL.[14] The diagnosis of bilateral phrenic nerve palsy was suspected when the patient unexpectedly failed to wean from the ventilator after surgery, and it was diagnosed radiographically by postoperative chest radiograph that showed bilateral elevation of the diaphragm. The etiology of this complication was thought to be possible bilateral C4 nerve root stretching, although a central cord etiology could not be excluded.

Neurologic injuries may also occur during positioning or intubation of the patient. In patients with myelopathy or a very stenotic canal, it is important that neck hyperextension be avoided to minimize the risk of additional canal compromise. This risk may be minimized by either placing the patient in a halo device preoperatively or by doing a fiberoptic awake intubation. Neurologic injury may also occur during the surgical approach, from decompression, during graft insertion or from epidural hematoma.

In cases of cervical myelopathy or spinal cord injury, it is imperative to maintain intraoperative blood pressure, since hypotension can exacerbate the tenuous blood supply to the spinal cord. In addition, intraoperative spinal cord monitoring, particularly with motor evoked potentials, is helpful in cases where instrumentation and alterations of spinal alignment are anticipated.

### Horner's Syndrome

Horner's syndrome is an unusual complication of ventral cervical surgery resulting from injury to the cervical sympathetic chain, which lies on the anterior surface of the longus coli muscle. Excessive dissection, retraction or electrocoagulation of the longus coli may result in injury to the sympathetics. It is characterized by ptosis, meiosis, and anhydrosis and may initially be unrecognized. The estimated incidence is 2%, with less than 1% being permanent.[13,26] Risk to the cervical sympathetics may be minimized by identifying the midline of the cervical vertebrae and by beginning the subperiosteal dissection of the longus coli at that point and avoiding excessive lateral exposure of the muscle. Caution should be exercised with using electrocautery laterally within the muscle.

### Vascular Complications

Arterial injuries during ventral cervical surgery may involve the vertebral artery, the carotid artery, or the superior and inferior thyroid arteries. The significance of injuries to the latter lies in their potential for hematoma that could cause airway obstruction. Injury to the carotid artery is rare but potentially could occur during exposure of the anterior cervical spine. The ventral approach to the cervical spine is between the alar and visceral fascia, the former surrounding the carotid sheath and the latter enveloping the trachea and esophagus. Excessive retraction of the carotid sheath could result in ischemia or stroke, and it is advisable to have the anesthesiologist check for the temporal artery pulse after placement of the retractor.

The major vascular concern in anterior cervical surgery is injury to the vertebral artery. This complication is serious both because of its potential neurologic sequelae and because of the difficulty in controlling hemorrhage. Vertebral artery injury is more likely to occur during vertebral corpectomy than with simple discectomy. In a retrospective review of 10 patients who sustained iatrogenic vertebral artery injury during cervical decompression, all injuries were associated with corpectomy, and all occurred as a result of an air drill.[29] Neurologic deficits were noted in half of the patients, although most resolved. The estimated incidence of this injury was 0.5%.

Vertebral artery injury can occur as a result of excessive lateral bone or disc removal, from distorted anatomy from tumor or infection, or if the dissection is inadvertently off the midline as a result of surgeon disorientation. The risk of arterial injury can be minimized by limiting the lateral exposure to the medial border of the longus coli muscles.[29] Abnormal course of the vertebral artery can predispose to arterial injury. An angiographic, CT and MRI review of 23 patients who underwent anterior cervical fusion revealed mild vertebral artery tortuosity in 10 patients and loop formation as a result of spondylotic changes in 3 patients.[22] Narrowing of the disc space results in a relative elongation and redundancy of the vertebral artery, which can develop a tortuous course between its fixed position in the foramen transversarium proximally and distally. During anterior decompression, the looped vertebral artery is in jeopardy by an excessively wide resection of the bone or disc. In extreme cases of vertebral artery tortuosity even routine cervical decompression can injure a looped vertebral artery.

Control of hemorrhage from vertebral artery injury can be extremely difficult. Control can be achieved by tamponade, by direct exposure with subsequent arterial repair, or by hemostasis with suture, electrocoagulation or hemostatic clip.[29] Ligation of one vertebral artery is usually not associated with any neurologic consequence unless there is arterial dominance. In this situation, one artery (usually the left vertebral artery) is dominant and supplies a greater portion of the blood supply to the hindbrain. If this situation is present, and the dominant artery is injured and ligated, cerebellar or brainstem infarction can occur. Nerve root injury can result from blind placement of a suture to control bleeding.

## Esophageal Injury

Esophageal injury following anterior cervical surgery can range from mild dysphagia to perforation.[2] Fortunately, dysphagia, although common, is usually mild and transient. Although the decompression and fusion are performed anteriorly, the surgical approach is lateral, necessitating some element of retraction of the esophagus and other tissues. Edema is felt to be a major cause of swallowing difficulties, although other causes exist. These include mechanical etiologies such as postoperative hematoma, abscess, or mechanical compression from prominent hardware or bone graft. Denervation may also play a contributing role.

Esophageal perforation is one of the most feared complications of anterior cervical surgery. The incidence of this complication is difficult to determine, but estimates range from 0.2% to 0.94%.[8,21,32] A survey of members of the Cervical Spine Research Society identified 22 cases of esophageal perforations following anterior cervical spine surgery.[21] Six were identified at the time of surgery, 6 were identified within the first postoperative week, and 10 were identified late (weeks to years later). There was one fatality due to sepsis. All of the immediately recognized cases were due to either a sharp or motorized instrument. Hardware was a contributing factor in 40% of the late cases and a prominence of either bone or polymethylmethacrylate contributed in another 40%. Diagnosis was confirmed by esophagraphy or by reexploration. Recommended treatment consisted of immediate repair, drainage, and parenteral antibiotics, although two cases were successfully treated by parenteral feeding tubes and antibiotics alone. The combination of cervical fracture with the use of hardware was thought to be a risk factor for this complication. A high index of clinical suspicion is of paramount importance in promptly and accurately diagnosing this complication. Drainage and parenteral antibiotics are the recommended and preferred treatment.

## Airway Obstruction

Upper airway obstruction following ventral cervical spine surgery is a potentially life-threatening complication that demands emergent reintubation. Etiologies include laryngospasm, hematoma, vocal cord paralysis, allergic reaction, and edema.[11] It is imperative not only that airway obstruction be promptly diagnosed, but that it be prevented. It is more common following lengthy cervical procedures and is therefore more common following corpectomy than single-level discectomy and fusion. A retrospective review of seven patients with upper airway obstruction following anterior cervical corpectomy and fusion for myelopathy spine surgery requiring immediate reintubation reported two deaths.[11] The etiology of the obstruction was hypopharyngeal edema. This review identified several common risk factors for this complication, including moderate or severe myelopathy, multilevel corpectomy, lengthy procedure (average length 5 hours), preexisting pulmonary disease, and a heavy smoking history. The risk of this complication can be reduced by maintaining the ET for 24 to 72 hours and then monitoring the patient in an intensive care unit.

## Chylothorax

The thoracic duct ascends from the chest, where it lies on the prevertebral fascia. It crosses the subclavian artery and enters the subclavian vein at the level of T1. Injury to the thoracic duct may occur during a left-sided C7-T1 approach. For anterior surgery at the C7-T1 or T1-2 levels, therefore, a right-sided approach is preferred. When identified, the thoracic duct should be double ligated.[2] If injury to the thoracic duct occurs and is unrecognized, a chylothorax may occur.

## Bone Graft Complications

Although autogenous iliac crest is still considered by most surgeons to be the gold standard graft material for anterior cervical fusion, its use is associated with donor morbidity. Donor site complication rates as high as 10% have been reported.[3,9,20] A recent retrospective review of 187 patients undergoing single-level ACDF obtained questionnaire follow-up of 134 patients (71.6% response).[27] Functional assessment and visual analogue pain scale (VAS) were evaluated. Acute symptoms (less than 3 months postoperatively) of difficulty ambulating were reported by 50.7% of patients. Chronic symptoms (greater than 3 months postoperatively) of pain at the donor site were reported by 26.1% of patients, with a mean VAS pain score of 3.8. Work and professional activity restrictions were present in 9.7% of patients. Therefore, patients need to be informed of the adverse effects, as well as the benefits, of autogenous ICBG.

The harvest of autogenous anterior iliac crest graft may be associated with injury to neural structures. Potential injury to four nerves may occur with anterior iliac bone grafting: the lateral femoral cutaneous nerve, the ilioinguinal nerve, the iliohypogastric nerve, and the femoral nerve. Injury to the lateral femoral cutaneous nerve can result in meralgia paresthetica, which produces paresthesias or pain along the lateral aspect of the thigh. The lateral femoral cutaneous nerve usually passes beneath the sartorius muscle and the inguinal ligament, both of which attach to the ASIS. The nerve therefore usually passes medial to the ASIS and is protected by staying lateral to it. In 10% of cases, however, it may be located up to 2cm lateral to the ASIS, where it is at risk for injury during anterior bone harvesting. The ilioinguinal and iliohypogastric nerves enter the inguinal canal and may be injured by traction on the nerves during harvesting of bone from the inner wall of the ilium. The ilioinguinal nerve supplies sensation to an area of skin beneath the medial half of the inguinal ligament, along the proximal and medial thigh, to the penis and portions of the scrotum. The iliohypogastric nerve provides sensation to the anterior two thirds of the iliac crest. Injury to these two nerves may result in either pain or paresthesias in the involved areas. Injury to the femoral nerve is uncommon, but the nerve is theoretically vulnerable to injury during bone harvesting from the inner table of the ilium.

## Pseudarthrosis

To a large extent, clinical outcome is proportional to fusion rate.[24] Patients with pseudarthrosis are more likely to be symptomatic than patients with solid arthrodesis. In one study of 48 patients with radiographic pseudarthrosis following ACDF, one third had symptoms at an average of 5 years follow-up.[24]

The incidence of pseudarthrosis is directly proportional to the number of levels fused.[17] For one-level noninstrumented ACDF the incidence of pseudarthrosis is approximately 5% to 10%. For ACDF at three or more levels, the nonunion rate may exceed 30%.[12,17] In most cases, the caudal-most level is the level most likely to develop a pseudarthrosis.[24] The pseudarthrosis rate can be reduced by the use of anterior cervical plating. When a symptomatic pseudarthrosis develops, the preferred method of treatment is posterior fusion. This eliminates the risk associated with having to reoperate through an area of scarring.

Some authors advocate corpectomy for multilevel anterior decompression, rather than multilevel discectomy with fusion. A higher fusion rate can be achieved by corpectomy with strut grafting than with multilevel discectomy and interbody grafting without plate fixation.[18] Whether or not the pseudarthrosis rate is less with corpectomy than with multilevel discectomy and fusion with plate fixation is unknown.

## Summary

ACDF is a reliable procedure with a low complication rate for the treatment of radicular arm pain due to neural compression. It is also indicated for cervical myelopathy from spinal cord compression. Its indication as a surgical treatment for axial neck pain is limited by the inability to identify reliably and predictably the source of neck pain. The procedure has a half century of experience and is well accepted as a gold standard for surgical treatment of anterior neural compression. Complications are well known and can be minimized by attention to detail. The use of anterior plate instrumentation is beneficial for multilevel fusion in order to reduce the pseudarthrosis rate. For single-level disease, noninstrumented fusion yields excellent results, although anterior plate fixation can accelerate fusion, thereby reducing the immobilization time in a cervical collar. Evolving technologies in the surgical treatment of axial and radicular neck pain include bone grafting alternatives and disc arthroplasty. Their ultimate role in the treatment of cervical disorders is unknown, but it is likely that they will replace, to a significant degree, current treatment methods by fusion with autogenous bone grafting.

## REFERENCES

1. An HS, Evanich CJ, Nowicki BH, *et al:* Ideal Thickness of Smith-Robinson Graft for anterior cervical fusion. A cadaveric study with computed tomographic correlation. *Spine* 18:2043-47, 1993.
2. Andreshak TG, An HS: Complications of cervical spine surgery. In An HS, Simpson JM (eds): *Surgery of the Cervical Spine.* Baltimore, Williams & Wilkins, 1994, pp 401-426.
3. Arrington ED, Smith WJ, Chambers HG, *et al:* Complications of iliac bone graft harvesting. *Clin Orthop* 329:300-309, 1996.
4. Apfelbaum RI, Kriskovich MD, Haller JR: On the incidence, cause, and prevention of recurrent laryngeal

nerve palsies during anterior cervical spine surgery. *Spine* 25:2906-2912, 2000.

5. Bell GR, Ross JS: Diagnosis of nerve root compression, myelography, computed tomography, and MRI. *Orthop Clin North Am* 23:405-419, 1992.

6. Bohlman HH: Cervical spondylosis with moderate to severe myelopathy. A report of 17 cases treated by Robinson anterior cervical discectomy and fusion. *Spine* 2:151-162, 1977.

7. Buetler WJ, Sweeney C, Connolly PJ: Recurrent laryngeal nerve injury with anterior cervical spine surgery, risk with laterality of surgical approach. *Spine* 26:1337-1342, 2001.

8. Capen DA, Garland DE, Waters RL: Surgical stabilization of the cervical spine: a comparative analysis of anterior and posterior spine fusions. *Clin Orthop* 196:229-239, 1985.

9. Ebraheim NA, Hossein E, Rongming X: Bone-graft harvesting from iliac and fibular donor sites: techniques and complications. *J Am Acad Orthop Surg* 9:210-218, 2001.

10. Emery SE, Bolesta MJ, Banks MA: Robinson anterior cervical fusion. Comparison of the standard and modified techniques. *Spine* 19:660-663, 1994.

11. Emery SE, Smith MD, Bohlman HH: Upper-airway obstruction after multilevel cervical corpectomy for myelopathy. *J Bone Joint Surg Am* 73:544-551, 1991.

12. Emery SE, Fisher JR, Bohlman HH: Three-level anterior cervical discectomy and fusion: radiographic and clinical results. *Spine* 22:2622-2624, 1997.

13. Flynn TB: Neurologic complications of anterior cervical interbody fusion. *Spine* 7:536-538, 1982.

14. Fujibayashi S, Shikata J, Yoshitomi H, et al: Bilateral phrenic nerve palsy as a complication of anterior decompression and fusion for cervical ossification of the posterior longitudinal ligament. *Spine* 26:E281, 2001.

15. Graham JJ: Complications of cervical spine surgery. In Sherk HH, Dunn EJ, Eismont FJ, et al. (eds): *The Cervical Spine*, ed 2. Philadelphia, Lippincott, 1989, pp 831-837.

16. Grodinsky M, Holyoke EA: Fasciae and fascial spaces of head, neck and adjacent regions. *Am J Anat* 63: 367-408, 1938.

17. Herkowitz, HN: A comparison of anterior cervical fusion, cervical laminectomy, and cervical laminoplasty for the surgical management of multiple level spondylotic radiculopathy. *Spine* 13:774-780, 1988.

18. Hilibrand AS, Fye MA, Emery SE, et al: Increased rate of arthrodesis with strut grafting after multilevel anterior cervical decompression. *Spine* 27:146-151, 2002.

19. Kadoya S, Nakamura T, Kwak R: A microsurgical anterior osteophytectomy for cervical spondylotic myelopathy. *Spine* 9:437-441, 1984.

20. Keene JS, McKinley NE: Iliac crest versus spinous process grafts in posttraumatic spinal fusion. *Spine* 17:790-794, 1992.

21. Newhouse KE, Lindsey RW, Clark CR, et al: Esophageal perforation following anterior cervical spine surgery. *Spine* 14:1051-1053, 1989.

22. Oga M, Yuge I, Terada K, et al: Tortuosity of the vertebral artery in patients with cervical spondylotic myelopathy: risk factor for the vertebral artery injury during anterior cervical decompression. *Spine* 21:1085-1089, 1996.

23. Ono K, Ota H, Tada K, et al: Ossified posterior longitudinal ligament: a clinicopathologic study. *Spine* 2:126-138, 1977.

24. Phillips FM, Carlson G, Emery SE, et al: Anterior cervical pseudarthrosis. Natural history and treatment. *Spine* 22:1585-1589, 1997.

25. Robinson RA, Smith GW: Anterolateral cervical disc removal and interbody fusion for cervical disc syndrome. *Bull Johns Hopkins Hosp* 96:223-224, 1955.

26. Saunders RL: Complications of corpectomy. In Tarlov EC (ed): *Complications of Spinal Surgery. Neurological Topics*. Rolling Meadows, IL, American Association of Neurological Surgeons, 1991, pp 105-113.

27. Silber JS, Anderson G, Daffner SD, et al: Donor site morbidity after anterior iliac crest bone harvest for single-level anterior cervical discectomy and fusion. *Spine* 28:134-139, 2003.

28. Simmons EH, Bhalla SK: Anterior cervical discectomy and fusion (keystone technique). *J Bone Joint Surg Br* 51: 225-237, 1969.

29. Smith MD, Emery SE, Dudley A, et al: Vertebral artery injury during anterior decompression of the cervical spine: a retrospective review of ten patients. *J Bone Joint Surg Br* 75:410-415, 1992.

30. Smith GW, Robinson RA: The treatment of cervical spine disorders by the anterior removal of the intervertebral disc and interbody fusion. *J Bone Joint Surg Am* 40:607-624, 1958.

31. Stevens JM, Clifton AG, Whitear P: Appearances of posterior osteophytes after sound anterior interbody fusion in the cervical spine: a high-definition computed myelographic study. *Neuroradiology* 35:227-228, 1993.

32. Tew JM, Mayfield FH: Complications of surgery of the anterior cervical spine. *Clin Neurosurg* 23:424-434, 1976.

33. Watkins RG: Cervical, thoracic, and lumbar complications—anterior approach. In Garfin SR (ed): *Complications of Spine Surgery*. Baltimore, Williams & Wilkins, 1989, pp 211-247.

34. Yamada M, Hirano, M, Ohkubo K: Recurrent laryngeal nerve paralysis: a ten year review of 564 patients. *Auris Nasus Larynx* 10 (suppl):1-15, 1983.

35. Yang KC, Lu XS, Cai QL, et al: Cervical spondylotic myelopathy treated by anterior multilevel decompression and fusion. follow-up report of 214 cases. *Clinic Orthop Rel Res* 161-164, 1987.

36. Yonenobu K, Hosono N, Iwasaki M, et al: Neurologic complications of surgery for cervical compression myelopathy. *Spine* 16:1277-1282, 1991.

# Ventral Cervical Discectomy with Artificial Disc

**Jan Goffin**

When considering treating a cervical disc herniation by a surgical intervention, three major strategies currently come into discussion: ACDF using autograft or allograft, ventral or dorsal foraminotomy, and, recently, ventral discectomy with placement of a disc prosthesis. In the majority of cases, the option of discectomy without fusion can be categorized in the ACDF group since about 70% of such patients spontaneously develop osseous interbody fusion in a more or less kyphotic position at the operated level during the long-term postoperative course. Incidentally, ACDF may also be performed using a cage.

At initial consideration, ventral[17] and dorsal[1,13] foraminotomy seem to be valuable therapeutic alternatives in cases were the herniation is located laterally or far laterally. However, in most cases of foraminotomy, the removal of the disc herniation is not followed by a true discectomy, which implies that the recurrence rate may be higher than expected. Furthermore, the long-term biomechanical consequences of the removal of the medial one third of the facet joint have not been studied carefully. So, even in cases of laterally located disc herniations, other therapeutic options may be desirable.

For all centrally located and for the great majority of mediolaterally located disc herniations, ACDF has been the gold standard for a number of decades. However, although natural progression of disc degeneration is known to occur over time, and has been documented even in initially asymptomatic people who were not operated on,[11] the concept of accelerated degeneration at adjacent levels after an ACDF has been widely postulated for a number of years.[3-5,8] On the contrary, it has remained controversial, until recently, whether this accelerated adjacent level degeneration is due to natural progression of the disease[14,15] <Arch Orthop Trauma Surg 1983/ 101/ 283-286> or to altered biomechanics secondary to the surgical fusion itself, resulting from increased mobility,[5,6,22] <Arch Orthop Trauma Surg 1985/ 104/ 247-250> increased longitudinal or shear strain,[18] or increased intradiscal pressure.[20] Perhaps both factors (i.e., natural progression of degeneration and altered biomechanics secondary to the fusion) contribute simultaneously.[16] If the increased motion stress at the adjacent level is the most important contributing factor, the use of an artificial intervertebral disc, which could preserve the mobility as well as the elasticity of the motion segment, might be taken into consideration.

Theoretically, the cervical spine appears to be a far better site to place an artificial disc than the lumbar area. Forces exerted on the functional spinal unit in the cervical spine are considerably less, although the range of motion in everyday life is probably greater.[7] However, given the excellent short-tem clinical results of ACDF and the low operative risks of this intervention, cervical disc prostheses will have high standards to meet. A cervical disc prosthesis will thus need to be simple and safe to implant, without a substantially increased operating time, while providing immediate clinical results comparable with those of arthrodesis.[19]

In order to assess the frequency and severity of degenerative radiographic findings at adjacent levels after anterior cervical interbody fusion and their clinical impact, as well as to contribute to the insights about their pathogenesis, 180 patients who were treated at the Department of Neurosurgery of University Hospital of the Catholic University of Leuven, Belgium by ventral cervical interbody fusion with or without additional plating and who had a follow-up of at least 60 months were clinically and radiologically examined. The long-term clinical situation

was compared to the clinical result at 6 weeks postoperatively. The same was done for the degree of degeneration at the adjacent disc levels. The results of this study were presented at the annual meeting of the Cervical Spine Research Society in Charleston, South Carolina, in November 2000[9] and have also been submitted for publication. The interval between operation and last follow-up visit ranged from 5 to more than 15 years with a mean follow-up of more than 8 years. A number of patients were treated for trauma and others for nontraumatic pathologies (mostly degenerative disc disease, causing radiculopathy and/or myelopathy, or both).

Clinically, two thirds of the patients remained the same at long-term follow-up, whereas one third presented a more or less pronounced deterioration. It was interesting that no statistically significant correlation was found between this clinical deterioration and the age of the patients at the time of surgery or the type of pathology.

At radiologic examination, only 8% of the patients demonstrated no progression in disc degeneration at both the rostral and caudal adjacent levels, whereas 92% had a more or less pronounced progression of disc degeneration at either the rostral or the caudal level, or both, at long-term follow-up. Once again this progression of disc degeneration did not correlate with the age of the patients at the moment of surgery nor with the type of pathology. However, there was a statistically significant correlation between progression of disc degeneration at adjacent levels and time interval since the operation. A suggestive trend for correlation was also found between the long-term increase in adjacent level degeneration and the clinical deterioration at a $p$-value of .06.

The similarity of progression to degeneration at adjacent levels between younger trauma cases without preexisting degenerative disc disease (mean age of 31.6 years) and older nontrauma cases (mean age of 48.8 years), as noticed in this study, suggests that interbody fusion was the most important triggering factor, and less so the natural progression of preexisting disc disease. Although, at first sight, the absence of a real matched nonsurgical control group of patients seems to be a weak point in the study, the young trauma patients might be considered as the control group (Figure 168.29), according to the suggestion by Braunstein et al.[4]

Reoperations due to adjacent level disease have been described to be performed in 7.3% to 10 % of the cases after ACDF.[2,9,12,14,21] As a consequence, the findings of accelerated disc degeneration at adjacent levels and the concepts about their pathogenesis may represent an argument in favor of replacing ACDF by an artificial disc in a great number of disc herniations, at least when the mechanics of such disc prosthesis (mobility, elasticity) would be highly comparable to the biomechanical behavior of a normal human disc. Other conditions, such as safety, immediate postoperative stability, and so on should, of course, also be fulfilled (see Chapter 125).

When considering what has been presented up to now, there are only two options: the Bristol prosthesis (also termed the Frenchay or Cummins prosthesis) and the Bryan total cervical disc prosthesis.

The Bristol prosthesis allows motion; however, its elasticity is not at all comparable to that of a normal disc.

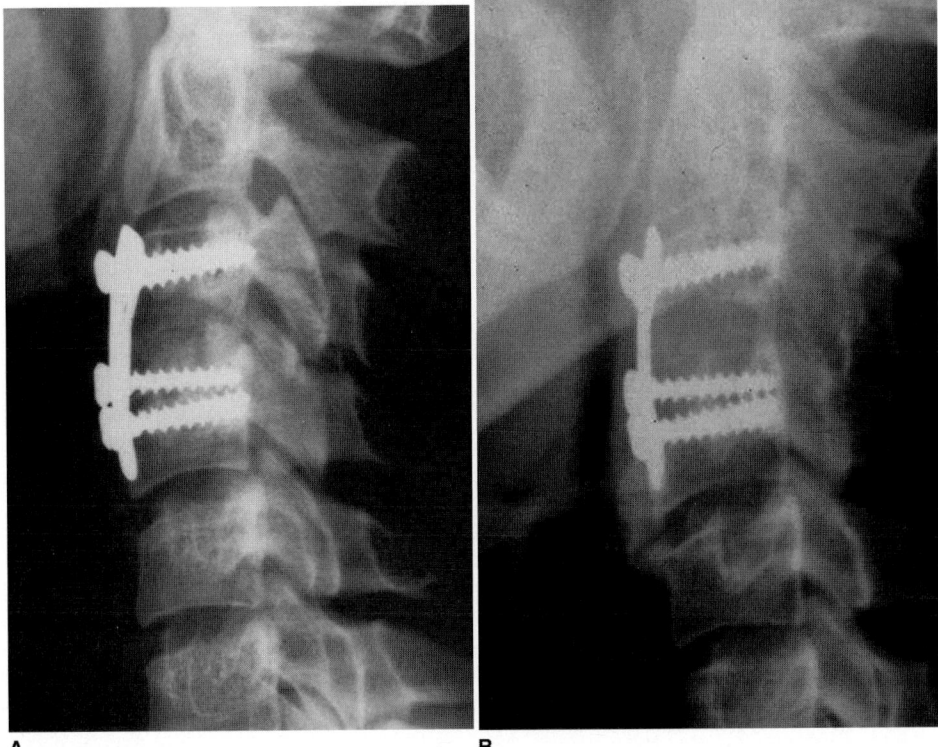

**Figure 168.29** A 32-year-old man who was treated by ventral interbody fusion and plating (Caspar plate) for a traumatic anterior subluxation at C3-4. **(A)** 3-month postoperative radiograph in lateral projection. **(B)** 8-year postoperative radiograph in lateral projection, showing ventral osteophytosis at C4-5.

Furthermore, this prosthesis has a quite large profile on a lateral radiograph film, leading in a number of cases to dysphagia[7] and extends almost up or down to the level of rostral or caudal adjacent disc. Using a Bristol prosthesis in bilevel cases seems therefore to be impossible. Because of its basic concept, as well as the satisfactory results of mechanical and animal testing, the Bryan disc prosthesis seems to be, at this point in time, the better option. Preliminary clinical experience with the Bryan disc prosthesis in a first European multicenter study has been very satisfactory, even exceeding the results obtained with ACDF-procedures.[10] However, long-term follow-up will be necessary, not only to prove continuous motion of the prosthesis at the operated level in the long run, but, most of all to assess the protective influence of the prosthesis on adjacent level disc degeneration seen in fusion cases.

## REFERENCES

1. Adamson T: Microendoscopic posterior cervical laminoforaminotomy for unilateral radiculopathy: results of a new technique in 100 cases. *J Neurosurg (Spine)* 95: 51-57, 2001.
2. Bohlman H, Emery S, Goodfellow D, Jones P: Robinson anterior cervical discectomy and arthrodesis for cervical radiculopathy. Long-term follow-up of one hundred and twenty-two patients. *J Bone Joint Surg Am* 75:1298-1307, 1993.
3. Boni M, Denaro V: [Traitement chirurgical des cervicarthroses. Révision à distance (2-13 ans) des 100 premiers cas opérés par voie antérieure]. *Rev Chir Orthop* 68:269-280, 1982. [Article in French]
4. Braunstein E, Hunter L, Bailey R: Long-term radiographic changes following anterior cervical fusion. *Clin Radiology* 31:201-203, 1980.
5. Cherubino P, Benazzo F, Borromeo U, Perle S: Degenerative arthritis of adjacent spinal joints following anterior cervical spinal fusion: clinicoradiologic and statistical correlations. *It J Orthop Traum* 16:533-543, 1990.
6. Clements D, O'Leary P: Anterior cervical discectomy and fusion. *Spine* 15:1023-1025, 1990.
7. Cummins B, Robertson J, Gill S. Surgical experience with an implanted cervical joint. *J Neurosurg* 88:943-948, 1998.
8. DePalma A, Rothman R, Lewinnek G, Canale S: Anterior interbody fusion for severe cervical disc degeneration. *Surg Gynecol Obstet* 134:755-758, 1972.
9. Goffin J, Geusens E, Vantomme N, *et al:* Long-term follow-up after interbody fusion of the cervical spine. *Proc Cervical Spine Research Society* 28:20-22, 2000 (abstract).
10. Goffin J, Kehr P, Lind B, *et al:* Early clinical experience with the Bryan cervical disc prosthesis in single-level patients. *Proc Cerv Spine Res Soc* 29: 22-23, 2001 (abstract).
11. Gore D: Roentgenographic findings of the cervical spine in asymptomatic people, a 10-year follow-up. *Spine* 26: 2463-2466, 2001.

12. Gore D, Sepic S: Anterior cervical fusion for degenerated or protruded discs. A review of one hundred forty-six patients. *Spine* 9:667-671, 1984.

13. Henderson C, Hennessy R, Shuey H, Shackelford G: Posterior-lateral foraminotomy as an exclusive operative technique for cervical radiculopathy: a review of 846 consecutively operated cases. *Neurosurgery* 13:504-512, 1983.

14. Hillibrand A, Carlson G, Palumbo M, *et al:* Radiculopathy and myelopathy at segments adjacent to the site of a previous anterior cervical arthrodesis. *J Bone Joint Surg Am* 81:519-528, 1999.

15. Hillibrand A, Yoo J, Carlson G, Bohlman H: The success of anterior cervical arthrodesis adjacent to a previous fusion. *Spine* 22:1574-1579, 1997.

16. Hunter L, Braunstein E, Bailey R: Radiographic changes following anterior cervical fusion. *Spine* 5:399-401, 1980.

17. Jho H-D: Anterior microforaminotomy for cervical radiculopathy: a disc preservation technique. *Neurosurg Operative Atlas* 7:43-52, 1998.

18. Matsunaga S, Kabayama S, Yamamoto T, *et al:* Strain on intervertebral discs after anterior cervical decompression and fusion. *Spine* 24:670-675, 1999.

19. Pointillart V: Cervical disc prosthesis in humans: first failure. *Spine* 26:E90-E92, 2001.

20. Pospiech J, Stolke D, Wilke H, Claes L: Intradiscal pressure recordings in the cervical spine. *Neurosurgery* 44:379-385, 1999.

21. Watters III W, Levinthal R: Anterior cervical discectomy with and without fusion. Results, complications, and long-term follow-up. *Spine* 19:2343-2347, 1994.

22. Woesner M, Mitts M: The evaluation of cervical spine motion below C2: a comparison of cineroentgenographic and conventional roentgenographic methods. *Am J Roentgenol* 115:148-154, 1972.

# Ethical and Medicolegal Aspects of Spine Surgery

## Andrea L. Halliday and John A. Anson

The ethical and legal principles that shape current medical practice are evolving. The principle that has increasingly gained wide acceptance in the United States is individual autonomy, or respecting the individual's right to determine his or her own destiny. Closely related to this is the principle of disclosure, or enabling a competent patient to make a rational decision by providing adequate relevant information. These principles take precedence in most circumstances over the principle of beneficence, or acting to benefit patients by promoting health, sustaining life, treating illness, and relieving pain. A fourth ethical principle that enters into medical decision making is the principle of justice, or providing for an equitable distribution of the burdens and benefits of medical treatment and research. In this chapter, three of the many possible situations to which these ethical principles could be applied are discussed: (1) the practice of withdrawing life support from a quadriplegic patient, (2) the extent of the physician's obligation to inform the patient about issues concerning the use of pedicle screws, and (3) the ability to carry out emergency research.

## Withdrawal of Life Support and the Spinal Cord Injury Patient

### Case Summary

B.L. was a white male, 37 years of age, who sustained a C2 fracture with C1-2 instability from a motorcycle accident. On examination, the physician noted that the patient was a complete quadriplegic with no movement or sensation below the neck. The patient required mechanical ventilation and blood pressure support with vasopressors. The patient was able to communicate with movements of his head, eye blinks, and the mouthing of words. The day after the patient was admitted, the physician informed the patient that (1) he had a severe spinal cord injury (SCI) and an unstable fracture of his cervical spine; (2) he would need surgery to stabilize his cervical spine, but the surgery would not restore any neurologic function; and (3) if he did not recover any neurologic function below the level of his neck over the next few days, his prognosis for neurologic recovery was very poor. The patient was able to ask if this meant that he would not walk again. The physician told him that if he did not recover significant neurologic function, he would remain quadriplegic and would be unable to breathe without the ventilator.

The patient initially stated that he wanted to think about his options and to discuss the situation with his family. On the following day, with his family's support, the patient decided not to proceed with surgery. He expressed the desire to be removed from the ventilator and to be allowed to die. The family also stated that the patient had expressed in the past that he would not want to live as a quadriplegic. On several subsequent interviews the patient consistently expressed the desire to be removed from life support. A psychiatric consult was obtained to help determine if depression or any psychiatric condition was impairing the patient's capacity to make that decision.

Repeated physical examinations documented no neurologic function below the neck. The psychiatric examination determined that the patient had the capacity to make medical decisions. The patient was asked to reconsider his decision. He was also told that he could choose to have life support withdrawn at any time. The potential for rehabilitation at the Veterans Administration Hospital near his home and other care options were discussed with the patient and the family. The patient refused the option of talking with a quadriplegic peer counselor. The patient stated that he knew two people who were quadriplegic.

The Hospital Bioethics Committee was asked to consult. Given all of the above, the Bioethics Committee supported the patient's decision. The family also continued to support the patient's decision to be removed from the ventilator. Both the patient and the family expressed concern that the patient not suffer. They were assured that the patient would be given enough intravenous medication upon his removal from the ventilator (if he chose this option) to keep him comfortable, even if this hastened his death. Four days after the patient was admitted to the hospital, the ventilator was discontinued at his request. He was given intravenous sedation and analgesia. He died with his family and the hospital chaplain at his bedside.

This case raises important ethical issues regarding the patient's decisional capacity in the acute intensive care unit setting, the duty of the physician to inform the patient, the patient's right to autonomy, the patient's right to die with dignity and comfort, and the duty of the physician to the dying patient.

### Presumption of Capacity

The Uniform Health-Care Decision Act recognizes the right of adults with decisional capacity to make their own health care decisions. *Decisional capacity* is defined as the ability to understand and appreciate the nature and consequences of proposed health care, including its significant benefits, risks, and alternatives to proposed health care, and to make and communicate an informed health care decision.[19] The presumption is that the patient has this capacity. The determination otherwise requires the opinion of two qualified health care professionals—the primary physician and a person with expertise in the assessment of functional impairment—if mental illness or developmental disability is thought to be the cause of incapacity. More than 40 states have adopted similar statutes.[16]

As with all seriously ill patients, there may be circumstances that impair the SCI patient's decision-making capacity. The assessment of the patient's capacity can be made by the primary physician after one or more interviews with the patient. If there is any doubt about the patient's ability to understand the risks and benefits or if there is some difficulty communicating with the patient, as with the intubated or sedated patient, the decision may require several interviews with the patient. If there is any concern regarding a psychiatric or emotional impediment to the patient's decision-making capacity, another physician with expertise in this area can be asked to evaluate the patient, as occurred in the B.L. case. Counseling of the patient can be timed and medication adjusted to avoid periods when the patient's decision-making capacity is impaired by medication. Because temporary factors may cloud a patient's decision-making capacity, important health care decisions should be made after several discussions with the patient. This affords the patient the opportunity to absorb the information presented and the physician the opportunity to assess the patient's ability to understand the information presented.

## Right To Be Informed

The primary physician has the duty to determine and communicate the goals of management. Treatment goals fall into one of three categories: (1) to cure the basic disease process, (2) to maintain the current state of health when the underlying disease process cannot be reversed, or (3) to maximize comfort when the patient is terminally ill. The primary physician must first determine the patient's treatment goal, communicate this with the patient and the family, and discuss the treatment options compatible with this goal. In the case of a complete-SCI patient, the treatment goal is generally stabilization of the spine, support of the patient with mechanical ventilation and vasopressors, and treatment of any resulting conditions, such as pneumonia, without reversal of the underlying SCI. Thus, the treatment goal falls under category 2. However, at some point in the critical care phase of the quadriplegic patient, the patient and family may wish to consider the withdrawal of life support, thus altering the treatment goal to category 3. The Uniform Rights of the Terminally Ill Act defines a patient as terminally ill if the medical condition is incurable and irreversible—that is, without administering life-sustaining therapy, the condition will, in the opinion of the attending physician, result in death in a relatively short period of time.[16]

At this point the primary physician's responsibility is to present the patient with the likely prognosis of the patient's medical condition, with and without treatment. In the case of high-level SCI patients, this discussion should include the effect of the injury on the chance of being ventilator-dependent, on patient mobility, bowel and bladder function, sexual activity, and reproduction. These patients should be allowed the time to assimilate the information, to discuss the treatment options with family, and to have ample opportunity to ask questions. These discussions are best conducted by a physician with expertise in the care of SCI patients, so that the quadriplegic patients can assess the potential for rehabilitation,

as well as their own ratings as they pertain to quality of life. The opportunity to meet with a patient with a similar deficit who has undergone the rehabilitation process should be offered.

## The Principle of Patient Autonomy

The supremacy of patient autonomy in medical ethics and the law has evolved over the last 20 years, beginning with the Karen Ann Quinlan case.[22] The New Jersey Supreme Court authorized her removal from the ventilator at the request of her parents on the basis of Quinlan's constitutional right to privacy.[2] In the first case heard by the United States Supreme Court involving the right to refuse life-sustaining treatment (*Cruzan v. Director, Missouri Department of Health*), the Court recognized a constitutional right of competent adults, even those not terminally ill or facing imminent death, to refuse any medical therapy, including life-sustaining and artificially provided hydration and nutrition.[2] This constitutional right is based not on the right to privacy but on the liberty interest protected by the Fourteenth Amendment to the U.S. Constitution.[2] "The principle that a competent person has a constitutionally protected liberty interest in refusing unwanted medical treatment may be inferred from our prior decisions."[8] As Justice O'Connor explained in her concurring opinion in *Cruzan v. Director, Missouri Department of Health*, the question in right-to-die cases is whether intrusion by the government into a person's right to "liberty, dignity, and freedom" is justified by the relevant state's interests.[8] In response to the *Cruzan* decision, which allowed the state of Missouri to restrict the exercise of the right to refuse treatment by surrogate decision makers, the Uniform Health Care Decisions Act was developed.[16] The Uniform Health Care Decisions Act provides for an individual's right to make health care decisions, provides for surrogate decision making when the patient lacks decisional capacity, and provides guidelines for advanced health care directives. It is illegal under this Act to continue or institute medical therapy refused by a competent patient. A professional duty to respect patient autonomy in decisions to withhold or withdraw life-sustaining therapy is supported by the ethical codes of national physician organizations and consensus statements of health care professionals.[7,14] This duty is also law in the majority of states, as a result of their adoption of a statute similar to the Uniform Health Care Decisions Act.[16]

The principle of patient autonomy has superseded another important principle in medical ethics, that of beneficence or acting to benefit patients by sustaining life, treating illness, and relieving pain.[5] With the patient's decision to withhold or withdraw medical care, the principle of autonomy overrides the principle of beneficence.[8] The options in this situation include forcing treatment on the patient, withdrawing or withholding treatment as requested by the patient, attempting to persuade the patient to accept the recommended treatment, and determining whether the patient is competent to make the decision given the stress the patient is under and the patient's risk for depression.[11] The determination of the patient's competence was the course chosen in the B.L. case, and in the psychiatrist's opinion the patient was competent to make medical decisions. The patient understood that he would die without the support of the ventilator. He also understood that with surgery to stabilize his cervical spine and rehabilitation he could sit up and achieve some degree of independence in a wheelchair. The patient consistently chose to be removed from the ventilator during discussions over the course of several days. He was also clear about his decision with his family, and they supported his decision. In this situation, to not abide by the patient's decision would have been unethical and illegal. If the attending physician is unable to comply with the patient's wishes because of his or her own personal beliefs, that physician has a duty to transfer the care of the patient to a physician who will comply.

## Patient Autonomy and the Right to Die

As a matter of law, the decision to withhold or withdraw nutrition and hydration is not treated differently from the withholding or withdrawal of other medical interventions by the United States Supreme Court's ruling in the *Cruzan* case.[15] However, a distinction is made legally, and on the part of official medical organizations, between withdrawing and withholding life-sustaining therapy and physician-assisted suicide and voluntary euthanasia.[1,23] This distinction is made even when palliative sedation or analgesia is instituted to relieve the pain and suffering that might arise from the withdrawal or withholding of life-sustaining therapy, even though the known effect is to hasten the patient's death.[1] This distinction was called into question by the decisions of two courts of appeals that overturned the New York and Washington state laws prohibiting physician-assisted suicide. In *Quill v. Vacco* the United States Court of Appeals for the Second Circuit ruled on the basis that the prohibition against physician assisted-suicide denies some patients equal protection of the law.[21] In *Compassion in Dying v. State of Washington* the United States Court of Appeals for the Ninth Circuit ruled on the basis that a person who is terminally ill has a constitutionally protected liberty interest in hastening death.[6]

The official statement of the American Thoracic Society (ATS) on withdrawing and withholding life-sustaining therapy indicates that the physician has an obligation to offer to relieve the pain and suffering that might arise from implementing the decision to withhold or withdraw life support. The patient, or surrogate, must be informed about the use of this palliative therapy and agree with it. It is acknowledged that the palliative therapy may "unintentionally contribute to the patient's death."[1] The official ATS statement then goes on to state, "Physician involvement in assisted suicide and active euthanasia, even if requested by the patient, is not endorsed by the ATS."[1]

Palliative therapy, which is routinely used (usually in the form of a morphine drip) when removing patients from the ventilator and as was used in the B.L. case, is acceptable under current medical practice and ethics. This palliative therapy is generally accepted to have a double effect: "The intent of the treatment is to relieve pain and suffering, not to end the patient's life, but the patient's death is a foreseeable potential effect of the treatment."[7] To state that this is an unintended result of the medication is to ignore the reality of what is common practice among physicians when removing a patient from the ventilator, that is, to administer enough sedation and analgesia to ensure that the patient will not experience any respiratory distress and that the patient's inevitable demise will not be prolonged, thus sparing both the patient and the family needless suffering. This is done with the full knowledge of the patient and the family (such as in the B.L. case) when the death of the patient is the acknowledged intended result of removal from the ventilator. To acknowledge this commonly accepted practice of life-ending medical conduct is, as stated in the United States Court of Appeals for the Ninth Circuit in *Compassion in Dying v. State of Washington*, "'another bridge crossed' in the journey to vindicate the liberty interests of the terminally ill."[6] Whether one terms this practice euthanasia or not, it is clearly an example of physicians assisting a patient to die. As stated in the United States Court of Appeals for the Second Circuit, "Withdrawal of life support requires physicians or those acting at their direction to remove equipment and, often, to administer palliative drugs which may themselves contribute to death. The ending of life by these means is nothing more nor less than assisted suicide. It simply cannot be said that terminally-ill persons who seek to hasten death but whose treatment does not include life support are treated equally."[21] Decisions by these two United States Courts of Appeals stress that the important distinction in these cases is that the decision to hasten one's death is a voluntary one on the part of a fully informed, competent patient. The court stated "the key factor in both dual effect and physician-assisted suicide cases is that it is the terminally ill patient's voluntary and informed wish that the doctor assist him to die through medical treatment. . . . We consider it less important who administers the medication than who determines whether the terminally ill person's life shall end."[6] The U.S. Supreme Court has agreed to review the challenges to the New York and Washington state laws banning physician-assisted suicide.

To assist a patient to die a dignified death is argued by some to compromise the integrity of the medical profession. The concern as expressed by the Council on Ethical and Judicial Affairs of the American Medical Association is that because of difficulty defining appropriate criteria for when assisting a patient to die is ethically appropriate, the "potential exists for a gradual distortion of the role of medicine into something that starkly contrasts with the current vision of a profession dedicated to healing and comforting."[7] This depends on one's view of the role of the physician. This role has been and is evolving. It is becoming increasingly accepted that one of medicine's most important purposes is to allow the terminally ill to die with as much autonomy, dignity, and comfort as possible.[16,20] An increasing number of physicians are recognizing aid in dying as not only compatible with the role of the physician but also as a *duty* of the physician. As stated by Dr. Francis Moore, "It is my credo that assisting people to leave the dwelling place of their body when it is no longer habitable is becoming an obligation of the medical profession."[18]

Assisting patients to die requires strong clinical judgment and experience to avoid its misuse, as Dr. Moore points out in his article "Prolonging Life, Permitting Life to End."[18] It may often be appropriate to inform the patient and family that the decision to withdraw care is premature or inappropriate based on the clinical situation. However, just because it is a practice that can be misused, it does not imply that it is a practice to be avoided.

A greater danger to the integrity of the medical profession lies in not openly acknowledging the practice of intentionally hastening a patient's death, by euphemistically claiming that the effect of depressing respirations by the morphine drip, thereby hastening the patient's death, is the unintended effect of the drug. There is more risk to the integrity of the medical profession and to vulnerable patients in hidden practices than there are in thoughtful, carefully defined practices. Furthermore, the uncomfortable position physicians are placed in by not being able to openly acknowledge the practice of helping terminally ill patients to hasten their death interferes with the open and honest discussion of this practice that would lead to safeguards preventing its abuse.

## Pedicle Screws and Informed Consent: The Physician's Obligation

The same respect for individual autonomy that underlies issues of the right to die also forms the basis of the ethics of informed consent. The ethics of informed consent, as with other decisions regarding medical treatment, is based on the ethical principle of respect for persons and regards patients as autonomous agents with a right to self-determination in matters of health.[4] The essential elements of informed consent include competency, voluntariness, disclosure of information, and the ability to understand the information. The Nuremberg Code, Helsinki IV, and the Council of International Organizations of Medical Sciences ethical guidelines "focus on the need for full disclosure to enable individuals to make free and informed decisions."[9] Informed consent implies that a physician has informed a competent patient of the risks and benefits of the proposed treatment and any alternative treatments, including not having the procedure or treatment, and that the patient understands this information and voluntarily decides whether or not to undergo the proposed treatment.[17] The responsibility of the physician is to disclose the information that the patient needs to make a rational decision based on the patient's own values.

The legal doctrine of informed consent has also developed out of an emphasis on individual autonomy, reflecting the right of an individual to be free from nonconsensual interference with his or her person and the moral principle that it is wrong to force another to act against his or her will.[12] Battery is the antecedent of the current legal doctrine of informed consent.[24] Initially, the physician's obligation in obtaining consent was met by a description of the procedure proposed. In the latter half of the century, the courts extended the physician's duty to obtain consent to include disclosure of information. The term *informed consent* was first used in 1957.[24] In most states, when no consent is obtained or when the procedure performed differed from the one consented to by the patient, the physician may be liable for battery. When consent is obtained but the patient is not adequately informed, the physician may be liable for negligence.[24]

The exact scope of disclosure legally required by the physician is not clear.[12,24] Some courts have adopted a standard of full disclosure.[12] A literal interpretation of full disclosure is obviously unrealistic because the physician cannot discuss with his or her patient every risk of the proposed treatment, no matter how small or remote. Furthermore, this literal type of full disclosure may not be helpful to the patient's decision-making process. Therefore, one must consider that even cases in which the term *full disclosure* is used, something less than total disclosure leaves unanswered the question of what is the physician legally and morally obligated to tell the patient about the proposed procedure.

Two standards have been most frequently applied by the courts to define the physician's duty to disclose information. The first standard, the professional standard, requires the physician to provide information that any reasonable medical practitioner in the community would provide under the same circumstances.[12,24] At the same time, some courts have argued that it is the patient's right to autonomy in medical decision making that determines the scope of the physician's duty to inform.[12,24] This second standard of disclosure requires the physician to disclose all information that a reasonable person in the patient's position would consider material to his or her decision making. Whether a risk is material to a patient's decision is a function of its frequency and severity.[24] The standard of informed consent applied by the courts differs from state to state, but most states have enacted standards adopting the professional standard.[12,24]

Recent litigation involving pedicle screws alleges a violation of informed consent on the part of physicians implanting these devices. The issue concerns whether or not the doctrine of informed consent requires physicians to inform their patients of the regulatory status, or label, assigned to a particular medical device by the Food and Drug Administration (FDA). Judge Bechtle, the presiding judge of the United States Third District Court and the judge responsible for handling all of the federal cases pertaining to bone screw litigation, invoked the legal standard of informed consent of what a reasonable patient would consider material. The judge ruled that requiring physicians to inform patients which regulatory or administrative labels have been placed on a given device by the FDA distorts the informed consent doctrine because it is not a risk of a medical procedure.[3] Furthermore, the FDA does not regulate the practice of medicine. Therefore, a physician may use a medical device for an off-label purpose if medical judgment dictates that the device will benefit the patient. The physician can be held liable for malpractice for the exercise of that judgment. However, the physician cannot be held liable under the doctrine of informed consent as long as the patient has been advised of the risks, benefits, and alternatives directly related to the use of pedicle screws. Although these risks may have led to the FDA classification of the device, the FDA regulatory status of pedicle screws is not a medical "risk."[3]

## Exceptions to Informed Consent and Emergency Research

Individual autonomy has formed the basis of ethical and legal standards of the issues regarding the right to die and informed consent. As discussed in the Belmont Report,[4] the three basic ethical principles involved in research are the principles of respect for persons, beneficence, and justice. The principle of respect for persons contains two parts: (1) respect for the individual autonomy of the competent person, which is the foundation of the ethics of the right to die and of informed consent and (2) additional protection for persons whose autonomy is absent or diminished. This generally implies obtaining informed consent for the research from the patient's next of kin or power of attorney for health care. However, an exception to the requirement for informed consent was recently granted by the FDA in the situation of emergency research where the human subject is in a life-threatening situation, available treatments are unproven or unsatisfactory, and obtaining informed consent from the patient or the family before the intervention is not feasible because of the medical condition of the patient and the narrow therapeutic window of the intervention.[10]

What is the ethical basis for enrolling patients without their, or their legal representative's, consent? To understand the ethical principles involved, we must appeal to ethical principles other than the respect for individual autonomy. To formulate the rule providing for a narrow exception to the requirement for obtaining informed consent, the FDA relied on the ethical principles outlined in the Belmont Report. They are the basis of the legal and ethical foundation of human experimentation in the United States.[4]

Most therapeutic interventions in acute care and emergency research, such as agents designed to prevent secondary injury in head trauma and SCI, must be initiated within a restricted time frame to have any chance of being effective. In these situations, it is often not feasible to obtain consent for enrollment of a patient into a protocol involving emergency research. When the expected outcome of standard therapy is poor and a promising intervention is available, the principles of beneficence and justice may take precedence over the principle of autonomy.

The principle of beneficence requires the physician to act in the patient's best interest. The principle of beneficence supports research that "makes it possible to avoid the harm that may result from the application of previously accepted routine practices, that on closer investigation, turn out to be dangerous."[4] The principle of beneficence maximizes possible benefits and minimizes possible harms. This requires that the risks associated with a research activity are outweighed by the expected benefits and that the research design is such that the possible benefits are maximized and the possible risks minimized. Harms are also minimized by careful monitoring of the study by an independent data and safety monitoring board that has preestablished rules for stopping the study should the research intervention be shown to be clearly harmful. The principle of beneficence is also the basis for society's interest in the promotion of health. One way that health is promoted is by well-designed studies that examine the possible benefits to patients of new interventions compared with established interventions, particularly when the established interventions have only been marginally efficacious. Society has an ethical obligation to conduct research that might potentially improve the outcome from head and spinal cord injury.

The principle of justice also underlies the ethical justification for the waiver of consent in emergency research. By this principle, patients should not be deprived of the opportunity to receive potentially beneficial treatment for their medical condition. If research in emergency situations is restricted to circumstances in which one can obtain informed consent, those patients who are unable to give informed consent or who do not have surrogates to give consent for them are discriminated against. It is also an ethical obligation, under the principle of justice, that the burden of research not fall on one particular class of patients, such as the poor, racial or ethnic minorities, or persons confined to institutions. Patients must be selected for reasons directly related to the problem being studied.[4]

## Summary

The primary ethical principle guiding the current practice of medical decision making is the principle of respect for patient autonomy, and two related ethical obligations include providing additional protections for patients whose autonomy may be absent or diminished and providing information necessary for the patient to make an informed rational decision that is free from coercion. However, the principles of beneficence and justice still sometimes take precedence over patient autonomy.

## REFERENCES

1. American Thoracic Society Medical Section of the American Lung Association: Withholding and withdrawing life-sustaining therapy, *Am Rev Respir Dis* 144:726-731, 1991.
2. Annas GJ: Sounding board: Nancy Cruzan and the right to die, *N Engl J Med* 323:670-672, 1990.
3. Bechtle J, Moss J: In United States District Court for the Eastern District of Pennsylvania and in the Court of Common Pleas of Philadelphia County. In re: Orthopedic Bone Screw Liability Litigation. MOL Docket No. 1014, March 8, 1996.
4. *Belmont Report*, 44 FR 23, 192 at 23, 194 (1979).
5. Bone RC, Luce JM: Concepts in emergency and critical care medicine: ethical principles in critical care, *JAMA* 263:696-700, 1990.
6. Compassion in Dying vs. State of Washington. 96 CDOS 1507, 9th Cir, 1994.
7. Council on Ethics and Judicial Affairs, American Medical Association: Council report: decisions near the end of life, *JAMA* 267:2229-2233, 1992.
8. Cruzan v. Director, Missouri Department of Health, 110 S Ct 284, 497 US at 287, 289, 1990.
9. Editorial, *JAMA* 274:844-845, 1995.
10. *Federal Register*, Vol. 61, 1996.
11. Fleetwood J: Solving bioethical dilemmas: a practical approach, *Nursing*: 63-64, 1989.
12. Furrow BR, Johnson SJ, Jost TS, Schwortzke: Liability and quality issues in health care. In: *Informed Consent: The Physician's Obligation*, pp 322-379.

13. Grin ODW: Patient education: protecting the surgeon-patient relationship through the strategy of patient education, *Spinal Instru Chap* 16:275-279.

14. Guidelines on the vegetative state: commentary on the American Academy of Neurology on certain aspects of the care and management of the persistent vegetative state, *Neurology* 39:123-126, 1989.

15. Letter to the editor. Occasional notes bioethicists' statement on the U.S. Supreme Court's Cruzan decision, *N Engl J Med* 686-687, 1990.

16. Meisel A: Nature and sources of the right to die. In *The Right to Die*, ed 2, New York, 1989, John Wiley & Sons, pp 37-42.

17. Meisel A: What we do and do not know about informed consent, *JAMA*, 246:2473, 1981.

18. Moore FD: Prolonging life, permitting life to end, *Harvard Mag* Jul-Aug:46-51, 1995.

19. New Mexico State Code. Relating to Health: Enacting the Uniform Health-Care Decision Act: Providing for an Individual's Right to Make Health-Care Decisions. House Bill 483, as amended. Chap. 182, Sec. 1, 1995.

20. Quill TE, Cassel CK, Meier DE: Sounding board: care of the hopelessly ill: proposed clinical criteria for physician assisted suicide, *N Engl J Med* 327:1380-1388, 1992.

21. Quill vs. Vacco, 60 2nd Cir, 1995: S.D. New York, 1996.

22. Quinlan, 70 NE 10, 355 A2d 647, cert denied 429 US 922, 1976.

23. Singer PA: Sounding board: euthanasia—a critique, *N Engl J Med* 322:1881-1883, 1989.

24. Sprung CL, Wintuc JB: Informed consent in theory and practice: legal and medical practices on the informed consent doctrine and a proposed reconceptualization, *Crit Care Med* 17:1346-1354, 1989.

# CHAPTER 170

# Economics and Practice Management

**Stanley Pelofsky, James R. Bean, Kevin Blaylock, Edward C. Benzel, and Christopher B. Shields**

The practice of spine surgery is not just the evaluation of spinal problems and the application of surgical techniques to solve them. Prior to surgery, even prior to seeing the first patient and after all the spinal work is done, a practice needs an infrastructure, a business organization that ensures not just financial solvency but also efficient operations, innovative management, and effective marketing. To enjoy a spinal practice, a spine surgeon needs a sound business strategy and reliable administrative support.

Surgery, and medicine in general, is practiced in an economic landscape, which changes chameleon-like from year to year. Although medical practice is relatively resistant to the fluctuating health of the general economy, with its cyclical swings from bull to bear market, medical practice remains subject to many of the same considerations that drive other businesses, such as potential for growth, competition, overhead costs of doing business, demand for and financing of innovation, interest rates, labor market conditions, economies of scale, and strategic planning.

The health care landscape has seen substantial change over the past decade, some of it predictable, some of it unexpected. The only certain lesson learned from the past 10 years is that medical practice and health care in general is mutable and is in the midst of a transformation that has yet to see an end. To thrive or even to survive future change, a spinal practice must recognize change as it occurs and adapt to it effectively. This requires an awareness of conditions in the general business and health care economies that affect the way a practice is run (macroeconomics), as well as sound decision making in managing the practice for current stability and future innovation and solvency (microeconomics).

## The Changing Economic Environment

The economic environment of health care has experienced substantial stress over the past decade, due to health care cost increases in the preceding decades.

In the 1980s the inflation rate in health care services was 10% to 12% per year, exceeding the growth in the general economy by more than 7% per year.[5] The doubling time for medical costs at this rate is 5 to 7 years, eroding the funds available for other public or private purposes, such as capital investment, business growth, personal amenities, or savings. Employee health benefits, as percentage of corporate profit, rose from 8% in 1960, to 29% in 1980, to more than 70% in 1990.[11] The need to bring health care costs under control was seen not as an option but rather as a business and government necessity.

## Factors Leading to the Unrestrained Rise in Medical Costs

To understand the response to costs, one must know the factors that payers believe have led to unrestrained rise in medical costs: (1) fee-for-service reimbursement, (2) traditional indemnity insurance, and (3) a technical complexity basis of quality medical care.

### Fee-for-Service Reimbursement

Fee for service (FFS) rewards physicians for work on a per-item basis. It provides a strong motivation to work productively, but not necessarily cost-efficiently. It is strongly favored by physicians but is viewed by payers as an incentive for physicians to overuse medical services, or at least to remove inhibitions from recommending services.

### Indemnity Insurance

Indemnity insurance covers expenses for the medical benefits defined in its plan. It allows payment for necessary, often large, and sometimes unexpected medical expenses. It insulates the patient from the true expense of treatment, lowers price sensitivity, and creates a tendency to overuse services. Physicians may order more tests and services because of defensive medicine or because payment is ensured; and patients accept more, because no personal financial consequence is perceived.

### Technical Complexity Basis of Quality

Technical complexity is the *sine qua non* of surgery. Greater benefit is perceived to be associated with instruments and techniques of greater intricacy. Greater perceived benefit is equated with higher quality, and thus, greater value. From the payer's perspective, however, greater technical complexity translates simply into greater expense, but often without better value, as measured by functional outcome.

## Methods Used to Control Costs

In response to these factors, payers have attempted to restrain financial exposure. These restraints are the instruments of managed care and, in their most basic form, are price and utilization controls. The simplest price control is a fee discount, and the simplest utilization control is approval of services for reimbursement before the service is performed (preauthorization). These managed care techniques are superimposed on the traditional indemnified FFS mode to balance the cost of recommended medical services by restrictions in permitting them.

Another form of cost control is to shift a portion of the financial risk for cost increase from third-party payers to physicians by withholding a portion of fees to pay for cost overruns (fee withhold), or by paying for expected services in advance (capitation). Financial risk sharing is perceived as an incentive for physicians to share a reluctance with the payer for creating unnecessary or excessive expense.

For the payer to control expenses, a binding agreement must be made between the payer and the patient, and between the payer and the physician. Under traditional indemnity coverage, the insurer contracted only with the patient to cover incurred expenses. Under managed care contracts, the payer agrees to pay for expenses in exchange for a patient's agreement to accept restrictions in choice of service, location of service, and physician. The payer and physician must reach contract agreement on price and acceptance of utilization restrictions. The contract between the physician and payment plan represents a fundamental shift in decision-making authority from the physician-patient relationship to the payment plan. Contract medicine has shifted economic power from the physician to payment plans, granting payers decision-making control for the allocation of resources.

## Backlash Against Managed Care

Managed care and medical service contracting have been the triggers for a profound and unexpected consumer backlash against health plan restrictions and even physicians who accept contract conditions that create an incentive to restrict patient access to services.

Within 2 years after the failure of the federal Health Security Act proposed by the Clinton administration in 1994, public denouncements of managed care tactics became widespread. Numerous state legislatures proposed, and a large number passed, "patient protection" statues restricting health plan management methods. A consistent provision, common among state proposals and included in all federal proposals, is access to specialty care, which seeks to overcome the utilization denials and gatekeeper obstructions that are built into most managed care plans and intended to reduce the higher costs attributed to specialty referrals.

In addition to federal and state legislative proposals to limit managed care restrictions, the backlash took market and judicial forms. The primary care gatekeeper health maintenance organization (HMO) products, which grew with such rapidity prior to 1995 and were projected to become the dominant form of health care plan by 2000, lost popularity and momentum as enrollment shifted back to less restrictive preferred provider organization (PPO) plans between 1997 and 2001. Capitation payment to physicians lost ground in a return to traditional fee for service. By 2000, large national health plans, such as United Healthcare, began reducing preauthorization restrictions, after finding little savings in medical expenses compared with the administrative cost to conduct preauthorization and after loss of enrollment from enrollees angered by obstructions to medical services. Additionally, several multimillion-dollar jury awards to plaintiffs against managed health care plans for injuries caused by denials of care revealed a public sentiment to retaliate against managed care restrictions with heavy punitive damages.

As managed care restrictions lessened at the end of the 1990s, the rate of rise in health care costs, which had dipped to under 2% by 1994, began to rise again, and by 2001 had again reached 11%, with the prospect of faster increase in the coming years. The change in rate of growth in costs was due almost purely to a rapid growth in the "volume and intensity" of services, meaning particularly the number of specialty services and drugs prescribed, rather than an increase in the fees paid for individual services, which have been fixed or reduced by provider contracts.

The conflict between the cost of care and the demand for care continues to be and will be the source of more economic pressure on physician practices in the future as the cycle of cost growth in health care again reaches unsustainable highs. Caught between payer budgets and patient needs in this struggle, physicians, including spine surgeons, will have to find new ways to improve the outcome of care without unacceptably expanding the cost of care. More importantly, the lesson for physicians from the managed care "revolution" is, paradoxically, a recall of traditional physician ethics: always keep patient interest and welfare foremost in mind.

# Practice Organization

Surgeons choose or join a form of practice organization according to personal preference and practice goals. Larger organizations lend the power of collective group influence to negotiations for payer contracts. As a principle, the form of organization chosen should conform to the demand in the market. Larger groups also allow for subspecialization within the practice, which improves the technical expertise of the entire practice and the reputation and marketability of the practice as a whole to the benefit of each of its members.

*Any organization is a trade-off. What the organization member gains in collective power is lost in personal autonomy.* For physicians accustomed to independent judgment, self-reliance, and personal professional accountability, the exchange may be difficult. What seems to be lost is individual control of practice conditions, professional decisions, and sometimes, personal income. What is gained, however, is the security of business economies of scale, cross-fertilization of professional knowledge and experience, division of labor, sharing of administrative expenses, and collective bargaining power in negotiations.

## Single Specialty Group

The simplest form of organization is the single specialty group practice. The advantages of this form—shared office expenses to reduce overhead, shared service call to increase free time, and shared case information to enlarge on personal experience—make professional life more efficient and productive. Beyond simple office sharing, however, lies a quantum leap in business control opportunity through corporate organization. Corporate integration allows sharing of records, production pools, owned business assets, financial risk, policies, planning, and reputation. More importantly, corporate integration, such as a professional service corporation (PSC) or limited liability corporation (LLC), allows group decisions about fees, contract participation, services offered, and extent of geographic coverage. In short, it allows, within legal antitrust limitations of group size and market monopoly, the control of price and participation conditions in the market unavailable to single practitioners.

The advantages of single specialty group practice persist into more complex arrangements, such as multispecialty network or multispecialty group arrangements. The organizational potentials of practice should be considered as multiple tiers of organization, with the larger arrangements dependent on the sound structure and function of the smaller units. The basic unit is the individual, with thorough training, reliable practice habits, and cooperative group behavior. The next level is the foundational organization: the single specialty corporate unit, with the specialty expertise on which each large unit builds and capitalizes. The last level is multispecialty affiliation, such as the independent practice association (IPA) contracting networks, which serve as the common contractor (similar to the general contractor in construction) for its individually autonomous functional specialty units. An alternative to loose affiliation is the higher integrative level of incorporated multispecialty medical groups, with central governance and shared financial risk, yet still dependent on the competence and effective functioning of its component single specialty units.

The key to single specialty groups is the efficient use of individual resources. Internal competition should be minimized, and differences in individual interests and experience should be exploited and individual strengths maximized. To do so, effort and production should be fairly rewarded (however the group collectively defines *fairly*).

The tendency toward subspecialty differentiation within specialty groups can be expected to grow. The 1995 Comprehensive Neurosurgical Practice Survey found that 23% of respondents had completed a fellowship, but only 11% listed the spine as the area of special training. Of the 16% who practiced only a subspecialty, over one third were spine surgeons.[8] About two thirds of neurosurgical practice involves spine work, traditionally, by neurosurgeons in a general neurosurgical practice.[7] As the size of neurosurgical groups grows, an increase in subspecialization may be expected, with a larger number of neurosurgeons limiting practice exclusively to spinal disorders.

Subspecialization creates higher levels of efficiency for three reasons: (1) it allows concentration of experience in a few individuals, which improves technical ability, tends to reduce both operative time and complications, and creates local expertise; (2) it allows concentration of interest, particularly for learning, researching, and designing innovative techniques; and (3) it improves marketability of the practice in a competitive market, where expertise, especially if cost-efficient, holds a high premium.

## Contracting Network

An intermediate form of integration of independent practices is the IPA, which is an affiliation of otherwise independent physicians or groups organized for the purpose of entering into contracts for medical service with one or more payers.

The IPA is a corporate entity whose physician members have signed a participation agreement with the IPA. The IPA members remain independent and enter individual participation contracts negotiated by the IPA with insurers. An IPA may be a single specialty network, but more often includes a complete multispecialty panel, which conforms to the contracting need of the health plan. Depending upon the IPA's agreement with its members, the IPA may either include all its physician members in any medical services contract it negotiates and signs or reserve the right of each physician group to accept or reject each payer contract. The former arrangement, IPA single-signature contracting authority, gives the IPA greater negotiating power and generally the potential for better contract terms. However, physician groups often balk at giving blanket contracting authority to an IPA, and sometimes prefer to reserve the right to refuse, despite the weakened bargaining position created for the IPA.

The advantage of an IPA to the physician is the opportunity to participate in contracts attracted by the organized physician panel and benefit from what negotiating clout the network may have. The disadvantage is the network's inability to collectively set fees or refuse to deal with an insurer, because antitrust restrictions limit the concerted action of independent physicians affiliated in a network. The advantage of an IPA to an insurer is the simplicity of network building, particularly when entering a new market. The disadvantage to an insurer is the possible cost-inefficiency and incoordination of a loosely affiliated physician network and the weakened control the insurer has over contract conditions with individual physicians.

For physicians outside of multispecialty group practice, where the administrative arm of the group serves as the negotiating agent for its member physicians, the IPA provides access to group-contract negotiating power, while preserving an independent practice. It does not provide all the available practice for its members but serves as a useful supplemental source of managed care contracts.

## Multispecialty Group

The most integrated medical practice organization is a multispecialty group practice. Its organizational features are similar to single specialty groups except that many or all specialties are represented. Independence is traded for group financial and practice security. Individual autonomy is traded for group market power. Practice freedoms are traded for practice stability. The defining features of an integrated multispecialty group are a single corporate billing identity and shared financial business risk.

Several advantages accrue to a multispecialty group, compared with networks. The group has greater latitude to set fees and deal collectively with managed care payers and to collectively refuse unfavorable terms. It can pool capital resources for business investment. It can share overhead expenses, information systems, management, and marketing. It can plan collectively and wield significant influence over local market conditions by group price and participation decisions.

Several disadvantages must be borne by multispecialty groups. Income from higher paid specialties may be shifted to lower paid primary care physicians to attract a needed primary care base. Personal control of practice hours, time off, and vacation time is reduced or lost. Influence over management decisions is diminished in proportion to the size and variety of the group.

The advantage of a multispecialty group to a spine surgeon depends on the local market. Academic practices are generally large multispecialty groups, although commonly with departmental autonomy, so a desire for academic practice usually implies the choice of a multispecialty group. Outside of academic practice, the choice of multispecialty group practice is commonly determined by financial factors, such as ease in start-up, and practice factors, such as ensured referrals. Two considerations make multispecialty group practice attractive. The first is the power of group influence in medical service contract negotiation. The second is shared overhead expenses, which increase under managed care conditions and require heightened efficiency and access to pooled resources.

## Reimbursement

From 1964 to 1994, payment sources, technical applications, and health care costs all grew exponentially. With managed care came both fee reductions and alternative forms of payment to shift financial risk for the cost of care to physicians. Both changes create challenges for spinal practice. The management strategies for the practice depend highly on the forms and levels of payment.

### Fee-for-Service

The traditional form of reimbursement for medical and surgical services has been an FFS system. The concept is simple, but the problems are legion. As an incentive system, it has worked only too well. It satisfies the physician's desire for compensation for the amount of work done. However, it is a major contributing factor to cost increases and is subject to assault and modification in the market.

One must understand the economic quandary in FFS to understand the changes offered in reimbursement from payer sources: (1) FFS is a cost-based additive unit pricing system without a budget, which encourages the addition of more units, thus increasing the total charge; (2) FFS discourages the bundling of unit charges into package prices and, in fact, encourages the *unbundling* of previously packaged prices, such as global surgical charges; (3) FFS developed as individual pricing strategies without a rational or consistent basis for the charges, related either to overhead (production) costs or to other physicians (competition) in the market; and (4) the lack of competitive market restraint on fees gave rise to the odd economic response wherein the buyer (insurer) established market fee limits (usual, customary, and reasonable [UCR]) rather than relying on seller (physician) competition.

The payer response to the FFS quandary has been to either modify fee pricing among physicians by contracting with physicians for modified fees or offer alternative payment schedules, such as financial risk sharing or salary. The successive modifications to fee pricing levels in FFS reimbursement have been (1) comparative community average rates (e.g., UCR), (2) discounted fee levels (e.g., 80% of charges), (3) private relative value fee schedules (e.g., California relative value scale [RVS], McGraw-Hill RVS), and (4) a public resource-based RVS (e.g., resource-based RVS [RBRVS], Medicare Fee Schedule [MFS]).

### Resource-Based Relative Value Scale

The trend in market pricing has been movement from modification #1 (UCR) to modification #4 (RBRVS). One of the goals of the Medicare RBRVS development was to establish a fee schedule that could be adopted throughout the health care system by both public and private payers in order to establish uniformity and rationality in the system's reimbursement methodology.[2] By paying on the basis of the *resources* (time, effort, practice expenses) used to provide a service, a rational basis for relating one service to another was introduced. By using a common basic RVS, the variability among different payers is reduced to a simple difference in conversion factor. Many, if not most, PPO and HMO fee schedules currently use the MFS as a benchmark for their own pricing, setting fees as a percentage of Medicare. Depending on the region, the private payer conversion factor may be higher or lower than Medicare's annually adjusted conversion factor.

Two changes in specialists' practice accounting can be made to convert from payer reimbursement to the Medicare RBRVS. The first and more radical change is the conversion of current fees to the Medicare RVS. A benchmark code, such as 63030 (lumbar disc excision), is used to establish the conversion factor equating current fees to the Medicare RVS values. This conversion factor is then applied to all other CPT code relative values, and a new RVS fee is derived for each CPT code. The new fee is compared with the practice's older fee, noting the degree of disparity. The problem for physicians is that the disparity between existing practice fees and fees derived from MFS relative values using a single conversion factor may be quite large, throwing the practice's billing temporarily into disequilibrium. The effect of disparities between current charges and RVS charges can be softened by converting current charges to the RVS incrementally over time, similar to the 4-year transition period adopted by Medicare in converting to the MFS between 1992 and 1996. The value of such a transition may be quickly realized as the relative weighting of CPT code values becomes the same in the practice's billing system as in payers' fee schedules. For spinal procedures with multiple CPT codes per procedure, this means an ability to consistently prioritize the order of the CPT codes submitted, to be sure the primary code, or base code, is the higher valued code.

The other, less radical option is to continue to use current fees, but determine the conversion factor for each fee that would equate it to the Medicare relative value. The result is a confusing array of different conversion factors for each individual CPT code that may range from $35 or less at the low end to over $75 at the high end. This calculation can be useful in equating current fees to a proposed conversion factor using the Medicare RVS and estimating the effect the offered or negotiated conversion factor would have on current fees for individual codes. To simplify the process, the 20 most commonly billed codes should be selected and analyzed to examine the bulk of revenue-producing services without getting lost in detail.

### Bundled Service (Per Episode of Care)

A variant of FFS is a bundled service for a fixed fee. There is an element of risk sharing, because the fee for the bundle is fixed in advance and any extra unexpected services are included as part of the package. There is a long tradition in surgery of charging a global surgeon's fee that includes the procedure as well as the hospital visits and postoperative outpatient visits. This is a bundled service but is risk-limited by charging FFS for any additional required surgical procedures and limiting the postoperative outpatient visits to a fixed period, such as 3 months.

Another form of bundled service is a compromise between unit pricing FFS and fixed payment over time, or capitation. This form of bundled service offers a fixed price for a bundled service that includes *all* charges anticipated for an average episode of care, including all professional fees, technical costs, and facility charges. For this bundled price, the surgeon's fee, anesthesia fee, radiology fee, operating room charge, and all inpatient hospital, pharmacy, and related outpatient charges are included in a single prospective charge to the payer. Charge calculation requires an accurate database of average utilization and FFS reimbursement for all elements of the bundled team. Profitability emerges from heightening efficiencies to reduce expenses while the bundled fee remains the same. Business efficiencies arise from standardized protocols for care, lower complication rates, better coordination among participants, and selection of more economical pharmaceuticals and technical devices.

Bundled services are a marketing tool for specialty services in a competitive market. The hope of the entrepreneur offering the package is that known reputation can be combined with reduced financial exposure to the payer to draw business for that particular procedure away from competitors. It offers specialists a niche in a competitive market where they can increase the referral base beyond usual physician sources and local health plans. The key is to select procedures that are technically complex and expensive, offering payers significant opportunity for savings by concentrating referrals to one physician group or institution. The strategy works best for high-frequency procedures, where the level of efficiency can be measurably improved and cost lowered compared with competitors; for low-frequency conditions the area of draw simply has to be widened to convert low local frequency to high regional frequency.

For spine surgery the concept of bundled service has a natural appeal because all the features coexist that lend themselves to successful bundling: (1) a competitive, oversupplied market, (2) technical complexity, (3) coordination of multiple service components, (4) high expense, (5) high variability in cost and outcome, and (6) payer control of referral.

The drawback for physicians using bundled case rates, or per-episode-of-care rates, is the risk of loss to physicians if their payment is combined with a facility payment. Any time the physician fee is included in a facility payment, the physician risks reduced reimbursement, particularly if excess facility costs are taken out of the fixed-rate payment, reducing funds available for the physician's reimbursement.

## Capitation

Capitated reimbursement is a practical means for managed care organizations (MCOs) to shift financial risk for medical care from insurers to medical providers. Two principles are involved. First, the payer's annual budget is relatively fixed by contract with providers, who become responsible for a share in cost overruns. Second, the incentive to increase services, under an FFS mode, is reversed, so that provider profit increases as service volume is reduced. Capitation usually begins with primary care physicians (gatekeepers), who are expected to control utilization of specialty referrals, hospitalization, and surgical services. Specialty capitation may follow thereafter, mandating that spine surgeons be educated about this form of reimbursement. Some plans have even reversed the order, capitating specialists and hospital services, where the highest utilization costs exist, while maintaining FFS to primary care physicians.

A specialist's association with capitation comes in several forms. In its simplest form the primary care physician is capitated, while specialists continue to receive a modified FFS reimbursement for referrals that pass the capitated gatekeeper. The model is simple for accounting purposes, but it creates conflicting incentives within the plan between primary care and specialist physicians, with a tendency to retain high specialty utilization and costs once the gatekeeper barrier has been breached.

At the next level, the specialist agrees to share risk but without fully capitating. The simplest risk sharing is a percentage withhold of fees, such as 10% to 20%, which is returned at the end of the period of risk (e.g., 1 year) if specialty-generated expenses have not exceeded budget. The more complex risk-sharing arrangement is capitation modified by risk limits. The risk limit is set in one of two ways. The first is stop-loss insurance, such that any expense above a fixed percentage of capitated risk, such as 10%, is covered by an insurance policy. The second is a window or corridor of risk negotiated with the payer. Under this arrangement the capitation rate is set based on an expected utilization. If utilization exceeds a limit, such as 110% of what was anticipated, the plan provides the physician additional reimbursement, commonly on a discounted FFS. On the other hand, cost savings for utilization less than anticipated may be shared by both plan and physician when less than a threshold amount, such as 90% of expected cost, occurs.

The highest level of risk is full capitation. For a specialist, this means receiving a periodic payment, generally once a month, for all anticipated specialty services for a defined population of plan enrollees. The advantage to the plan is that financial risk for that service is fixed in advance, and the person with most control over the generation of expenses (the specialist physician) pays the financial consequence for overuse. The advantage to the specialist is the chance to profit by careful restriction of services or a more efficient use of services. The risk, of course, is a failure to do so, resulting in the specialist's financial loss. The ultimate risk is financial insolvency, if miscalculation is profound.

Several conditions must exist before a specialty physician can safely accept a capitation reimbursement, even on a partial risk-sharing basis. They include an understanding of the change in incentives the capitation payment creates, a belief that it can work, and a determination to react responsibly by controlling unnecessary utilization without jeopardizing patient welfare. However, good intention is not enough; only data analysis can allow a practice to safely accept a capitation payment.

The calculation necessary to negotiate a capitation rate for a practice is complex and will likely require actuarial help. The first requirement is access to organized, reliable data on the physician's practice as well as data on the patient base in the plan. The two data sources are necessary to show two things: (1) how the revenue from the capitation payment will likely compare with revenue under current FFS reimbursement, and (2) what the expected utilization and, thus, the practice expenses will be. The difficult task in negotiation is to reach an equivalency between the reimbursement under FFS and the lump capitation fee, then use practice efficiency measures to reduce nonessential high-cost service utilization and convert practice expenses to profit.

Data in a practice should be collected in advance of the necessity for negotiating a capitated contract. The minimum necessary information from the practice is (1) a frequency list of CPT codes billed in the practice over 1 year; (2) the average treatment plan for the top 20 diagnoses (ICD-9-CM) or CPT codes. The treatment plan is the list of services by code that the practice provides, on average, for a particular problem, such as lumbar disc herniation. This includes (1) preoperative visits, diagnostic services, operative procedure charges, in-hospital visits, and postdischarge visits; (2) average charge per CPT code (the practice's listed charge to FFS payers); (3) average allowable per CPT code (the average amount received from all payers [note that the average practice discount equals average charge minus average allowable]); and (4) utilization rate for individual CPT codes in the practice (how often a given CPT code is used for all patient encounters, and how often for particular ICD-9-CM diagnoses).[3] These data provide a window into the volume, composition, and revenue generation of billable practice activity under FFS.

The next information needed comes from the plan itself. Demographic data (e.g., age, gender, and possibly occupation) of the plan's enrollees under FFS reimbursement for a minimum period of at least 1 year, and preferably 2 or 3 years, reinforces the accuracy of the actuarially expected utilization by the insured population. The information must be specific for the services to be covered by the capitated contract and must include all those services for all plan members, including those by other providers, which may shift to the capitated specialist under a capitation contract. The most important demographic distinction is Medicare risk versus commercial risk, where the capitation rate for Medicare may be several times greater than general commercial rates.[9]

Finally, the terms of the proposed contract must be examined in order to know exactly what services are included and what the surgeon's obligation is under the agreement. Terms such as *all necessary neurosurgery services* or *all spine surgery services* are too vague. The contract should detail the specific capitated services by CPT code. Some services that are high-expense, that are rarely done, or that the provider simply does not do may be excluded and provided either as a carveout by another provider or simply on a modified FFS basis. At the same time, it is important to know whether patients from other specialists will be shifted to the capitated provider, necessitating a higher capitation rate to cover the increased volume. Along the same vein, it is important to ensure that inappropriate patient referral, sometimes known as *dumping*, does not occur in a flood once the capitation rate ensures no increased financial risk to primary care physicians for early referral to ease their own office burden. This risk is reduced by retaining external health plan utilization controls, developing referral guidelines, using telephone consultations prior to referrals, or conducting informal or formal primary care physician education. Early referral for specialty management may be appropriate, ultimately providing cost saving, but must be covered by the capitation rate.

The actual base per member per month (PMPM) rate is calculated as a sum of individual rates for each CPT code used by the practice. To make this calculation, an actuarially determined annual utilization table is required, either from national data, such as the Medical Group Management Association data, or from local plan data. The utilization rate for each code is a fraction reflecting the expected frequency of the procedure among the defined population in 1 year (e.g., 0.000900 = the per member per year [1] [PMPY] utilization rate for CPT code 63030). The average allowable charge in the practice for each code is multiplied by the actuarially determined utilization factor to arrive at a PMPY rate that matches current average practice reimbursement. Additional services are added that compose the average treatment plan for the code, also multiplied by the actuarial utilization rate. The total (procedure plus additional services) PMPY rates for all CPT codes to be included in the capitation rate are added together and divided by 12, arriving at the PMPM rate that would allow that practice to maintain a FFS level reimbursement. This figure is used as a benchmark in negotiating a capitation rate. At this point the practice negotiator must understand that the practice expense data for the capitation rate offered by the plan is likely to be lower than the FFS equivalency rate calculated above. Only knowledge of the practice expense can reveal what the actual profit margin will be for a compromise cap rate and whether the practice is willing to accept the rate, negotiate the rate, or refuse the offer.

It is important that the number of covered lives in the contract be large enough to prevent unexpected outliers (high-expense cases) from devouring all profitability. Small populations of covered lives make this fluctuation more likely, and the chance of loss relatively high. A specialist capitated for fewer than 15,000 lives is taking a high risk. However, it may be prudent for a practice to enter capitation arrangements gradually, initially with a small proportion of the practice volume, thereby limiting the effect of errors in calculation early in the capitation experience, which later might overwhelm the practice with unanticipated expenses.

Once a practice enters a capitation contract, it becomes more important than ever to continuously track cost and utilization data, particularly with regard to the capitated population. It must be remembered that the penalty for an error in calculation or loose utilization control can quickly become catastrophic. Under FFS, unit reimbursement may be increased to cover expenses for any excess utilization. Under capitation, reimbursement is fixed in advance, based on an estimate of expenses. If utilization is higher than calculated, the only side of the ledger that goes up is expense to the business, which diminishes the profit side. Accurate and frequent analysis of practice cost and utilization data allows the practice to learn quickly whether profitability is maintained and what adjustments in utilization are necessary.

## Capitation Carveouts

A capitation carveout is a contract for a particular specialty service directed to a single provider group. A capitated plan seeks a specialty carveout either when the service is not available within its panel of capitated physicians and facilities or when it contracts with independent specialty groups and wishes to concentrate care in exchange for capitation-rate negotiation with one group. The capitation rate for the carveout services is not included in the capitation rate of any other provider under contract. A specialty group seeks a carveout when it is competing with other groups in a region and wants to lock in referral within a capitated plan. It is an unnecessary strategy when the specialty offers a full range of services and is part of a large capitated group or network without internal competitors.

Carveout services, such as all spinal specialty referrals, or designated subcategories of service, such as all spine surgeries, can be negotiated by spine surgeons. The difference between a carveout service and a bundled service is that the carveout is a capitation variant, with a fixed fee per covered member per month, whereas the bundled service is an FFS variant, with a fee per episode of care. The degree of provider financial risk is greater with the carveout because the calculation requires not just the estimated expenses per episode of care but also the estimated occurrence of need for the episode of care in the covered population.

The calculation necessary to negotiate a reasonable carveout capitation rate may combine the calculations necessary for a full capitation and for a bundled service. If a carveout capitation rate includes only the professional component, the calculation is identical to the full capitation calculation, except that the number of CPT codes analyzed is more limited (those included in the carveout). If the capitation rate includes all charges for the carveout service, including professional, technical, and facility charges, the calculation must include all the average needed services combined with an actuarial estimate of the population need for the service over a fixed period of time.

# Practice Costs, Management, Productivity, and Profitability

The amounts and types of cost incurred in operating a medical business determine, in part, how profitable the enterprise will be. Productivity is the measure of the value of output relative to the costs of input to the process. Many input costs are incurred when operating a spine surgery business, the most valuable of which are obviously the efforts of the surgeon. The strategy, therefore, is to find the optimum type and amount of cost expenditures that facilitate maximal surgery productivity. Practice manage-

ment must then endeavor to obtain fair reimbursement for the spine surgeon's production in order to ensure the desired profitability.

## Practice Cost Categories

A spine surgeon's operating costs are numerous. They include the following categories: nonprovider salaries, nonprovider benefit expense, information services expense, occupancy expense, administrative and medical supplies expense, insurance premiums, and capital expenditures such as for furniture and equipment.

The most significant operating costs are personnel costs. Nonsurgeon employees perform tasks that are more economically done by support medical personnel, such as nurses, physician assistants, and nonprofessional medical assistants. Administrative employees perform administrative functions such as billing and collection, patient registration and reception, appointment scheduling, surgery scheduling and precertification, data processing, transcription, accounting, and personnel management.

Nonprovider benefit expenses include medical, life, or disability insurance; vacation and sick pay; and retirement plans. Advantageous tax treatment is afforded these types of expenses for both physician and nonphysician employees. In order to attract and retain quality clinic employees, it is necessary to provide attractive benefits. Because employee benefits are very expensive, one must maintain flexibility with benefit plan–funding requirements and mandate at least some employee contribution toward payment of plan costs.

Information services are of ever-increasing cost and importance, perhaps, especially for spine surgeons. Most of the costs associated with information services are capital expenditures. However, also included would be hardware and software maintenance costs and service bureau fees.

Generally, occupancy costs are office space lease payments or depreciation, mortgage principal and interest, property taxes, and maintenance costs. The fluctuating conditions of the health care industry favor renting over ownership. The accompanying responsibilities of real estate ownership can be a counterproductive distraction to the physician. Changes in the practice and market conditions require flexibility in office space, either expansion or contraction; property ownership or multiyear leases often obstruct rapid adjustment to changing practice space needs. Expensively appointed accommodations could possibly be offensive to patients and payers. Medical offices should be comfortable, spacious, distinguished, and attractive, but also modest.

Insurance premiums include employee benefit insurance, general property and liability insurance, professional liability insurance, and perhaps, key-person life or business continuation insurance. Professional liability insurance is very expensive. However, because the risks involved in spine surgery are relatively high, one should usually purchase the most complete coverage reasonably available. Only if a group rating is unavailable due to previous litigation should one undertake asset protection strategies instead of appropriate insurance coverage. Also, if a surgery practice is incorporated, total liability coverage can sometimes be increased economically by purchasing separate coverage for the corporation in addition to coverage for the individual surgeons. The advisability of key-person life or business continuation insurance depends on the configuration of the practice organization and the number of practicing surgeons. This type of insurance is generally useful for covering a contractual buyout obligation between the physician and the corporation.

The final cost category is capital expenditures for fixed assets, such as furniture and equipment. Most spine surgery procedures are performed in hospitals; therefore, medical equipment is not usually required in the office. The most significant capital expenditures both in terms of cost and value are for management information and communications technologies. Computer hardware and software, network, telephone, facsimile, and transcription and reproduction systems cost tens of thousands of dollars. However, these expenditures are imperative for the successful operation of a surgical practice in the twenty-first century.

A common measure of practice expenses is the percentage contribution of each cost component to the total practice revenue. Average percentages for a neurosurgery spinal practice, for example, are less than 2% for information services, about 5% for occupancy costs, 1% for administrative supplies and services, 4% for professional liability insurance, about 13% for nonprovider salaries, and approximately 4% for nonprovider benefit expenses. Total nonphysician expenses would average about 35%. Furthermore, the average neurosurgical practice would employ 3.6 nonprovider support personnel per surgeon.[4]

## Practice Costs Behavior

All of the significant components of the total operating costs of the typical private spine surgery practice are virtually fixed over a wide range of business activities. Those expense components that vary with changes in the activity rate tend to do so in discrete increments rather than in a continuous proportional manner. For example, personnel costs generally constitute by far the largest single component of total operating costs. Usually, a private spine surgery practice employs a large number of full-time support personnel. This configuration remains constant over a wide range of practice activity. If, however, business increases or decreases beyond certain points, employment will increase or decrease in single full-time employee increments (Figure 170.1).

Some spine surgery practices are attempting to create cost structures that are more variable and flexible. These efforts generally involve greater use of hourly or part-time employees for peak activity periods, keeping full-time employment to a minimum. One option is to contract out certain administrative functions such as billing and collecting, bookkeeping, and even appointment scheduling to service bureaus, which charge based on the level of activity, thus converting relatively fixed costs to variable costs. Some personnel, such as nurses, can be leased from third parties to provide maximum flexibility.

## Cost Accounting

Cost accounting is the determination of costs of doing business, or overhead costs. The importance of performing cost accounting arises in the current market when reimbursement levels for services may be so reduced that reimbursement for those services fails to meet or exceed costs. In the past, fees could simply be raised when overhead costs cut into profitability. In contract medicine, this can no longer be done. Business efficiencies must be invoked to prevent income loss when fees are fixed or reduced by contract. One form of business efficiency is to

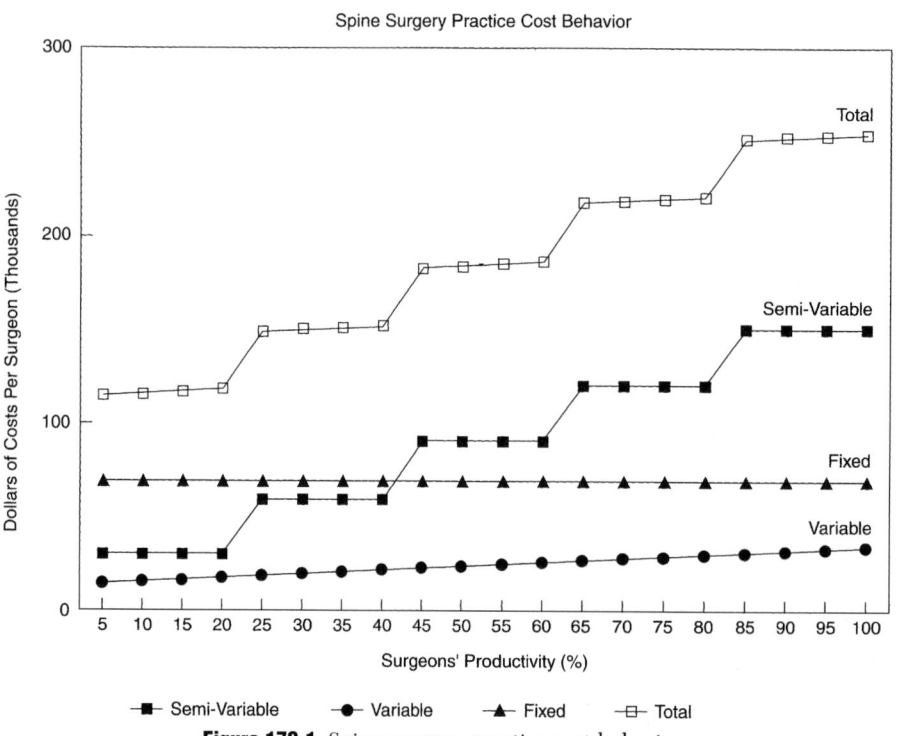

**Figure 170.1** Spine surgery–practice cost behavior.

learn which services have a narrow, or even negative, margin of profitability, and decide whether to offer those services.

Cost accounting is greatly simplified when using a fee schedule where each CPT code fee is logically related to all other fees by an RVS. A simplified method to determine costs is as follows:

1. The total expenses of the practice (E) are calculated for a year. Excluded is any discretionary physician distribution made after necessary expenses are paid. Discretionary distributions are physician salaries, bonuses, fringe benefits, and retirement funding.
2. The total number of relative value units (total RVUs) billed during the year is calculated by finding the sum of all CPT codes billed multiplied by the number of times each code was billed multiplied by the RVUs for each code.
3. An assumption is made that each CPT code participates equally in the proportion of expenses (e.g., if the practice expense ratio is 40%, then 40% of each code RVUs equals practice expense).
4. The RVU is calculated by dividing E by the total RVUs. For instance, a practice expense of $20/RVU might be calculated. Therefore, at a negotiated conversion factor of $35, the profit would be $15/RVU, or expressed differently, an expense ratio of 20/35 = 57% and a profit ratio of 15/35 = 43%.

If the practice has adopted an RBRVS fee scale, the comparison to a managed care contracted fee schedule based on the Medicare RBRVS becomes quite simple:

1. The practice's conversion factor (CF) is calculated by dividing annual net revenue (NR) by total RVUs: CF = NR/total RVUs.
2. The practice's conversion factor is compared with the managed care plan negotiated conversion factor to determine what the overhead ratio will be for that contract and whether the margin of profitability is sufficient to warrant agreement to the terms. For example, the practice CF is 50, with an expense factor of 20, for a 40% expense ratio. If a plan offers a CF of 40, the expense ratio for that business will be 20/40 = 50%.

When both plan and practice follow the same RVS, the practice expense ratio for every procedure is known as soon as the conversion factor is revealed, simplifying the mental calculation to determine whether the reimbursement offer is acceptable.

This form of cost accounting can be used for practice fees that are not on an RBRVS scale. It remains useful to determine whether negotiated fee schedules offer a sufficient margin of profit compared with calculated expenses to warrant acceptance. For instance, if the practice fee for a myelogram were $300, the calculated practice expense (40%) is $120. If a plan offered $150 reimbursement, the overhead cost for the myelogram service would be 80% (120/150 = 0.8). This allows a margin of profit of 20%, which in this case is $30. This type of calculation must be applied separately to individual codes when the fee schedule is not constructed on a relative value basis. The calculation can be used for each individual code when deciding which to accept and which to negotiate. On a practical basis the 20 most frequently billed CPT codes in the practice can be analyzed by this method to decide whether the large majority of the fees offer an acceptable margin of profit.

## Productivity

Managing operating costs is essential to a profitable practice, but it is not the only significant factor. The most valuable component of spine surgery care is the surgeon's time and efforts. The amount of the spine surgeon's available time is finite; therefore careful management of that time is the most important factor for business efficiency and productivity. Minimal operating costs are clearly not optimal if efficient use of the spine surgeon's time is compromised.

Surveys indicate that the average neurosurgeon, in 1 week, spends 16 hours evaluating patients in the office, 9 hours making hospital rounds, 19 hours performing surgery, 6 hours on other patient care activities, and 5 hours on administration.[8] Obviously, the time spent in surgery is by far the most financially productive. Therefore, increased operating costs can be offset many times by added revenue, if those costs can increase the portion of the surgeon's time spent in surgery.

Only 9% of neurosurgeons would prefer to see more patients in their office. Nearly 32%, in contrast, feel that they have time for a greater surgical volume. The volume of surgery tends to be a function of the number of office visits. The solution is to increase the number of patients that can be seen in the office without increasing the amount of surgeon time devoted to that activity. The best way to do this may be the use of physician extenders (i.e., physician assistants or clinical nurse specialists). For fee-for-service practice, the new patient or consultation visit is the most productive office time, for that is where new surgical cases are found. An optimal allocation of office visit time is increasing time for new referrals by assigning routine follow-up visits to physician extenders.

As with most personal service businesses, in a spine surgery practice the revenue producer (the surgeon) is also the owner and manager. The management of any business is usually very time-consuming. Therefore, professional managers can minimize the amount of time the surgeon must spend on business affairs and can be cost-effective. With qualified professional managers being somewhat expensive, their employment may be an option only available to a group practice, which can spread the cost among several producers.

## Profitability

Careful management of practice costs can enhance the spine surgeon's productivity and contribute greatly to the practice's profitability. Careful management of the types of patients seen by the spine surgeon and those patients' source of payment can equally determine profitability. Three payment sources of a unique character are Medicare, worker's compensation claims, and third-party liability for personal injury claims.

Medicare patients (except Social Security increment [SSI]) are older than 64 years of age. Their age may make their medical treatment more complicated and time-consuming. Medicare reimbursement rates are usually the lowest in most markets, with the only exceptions involving Medicaid patients, welfare patients, and patients with no insurance (self-pay). Workers' compensation and liability reimbursement rates are generally greater than Medicare and commercial managed care, but sometimes less than commercial indemnity FFS rates. Workers' compensation and liability patients may have their legal claims as a secondary concern to their medical well-being and can complicate their treatment; therefore, these patients may consume more of the spine surgeon's time. Because reimbursement is procedure-based and surgical procedures are reimbursed at much higher rates than evaluation and management office charges, patients who require less of the surgeon's office time, relative to surgery time, are economically preferable. When evaluating the economic profit potential of patient populations categorized according to payment source, one should consider the rate of reimbursement relative to the total surgeon time consumption implicit in the characteristics of each population subset.

Likewise, one should attempt to maximize the yield of spine surgery cases derived from the total number of patients seen in the office. This can be achieved by tracking the surgery-to-patient ratio in different groups and then favoring the groups with the higher yield. For example, if workers' compensation patients tend to have a lower than average yield, their office visits might be restricted unless the fee reimbursement rate is relatively high enough to offset the lower yield. Likewise, it might be profitable to accept a managed care plan's lower rate of reimbursement if the surgery-to-patient ratio is relatively high. However, with many spine surgery reimbursement rates either negotiated with managed care plans or imposed by government, general pricing strategies are less relevant than before.

Finally, collecting as much as possible and collecting as soon as possible is critical to profitability. Conscientious, industrious, and resourceful billing and collection personnel can be one of the most important factors in maintaining profitability. For a mature spine surgery practice, gross accounts receivable should be less than 30% of annual gross billings, and average days in accounts receivable should be kept between 30 and 45 days. Bad debts should average no more than 6% to 7%. Collection-to-charges ratios formerly ranged between 70% and 80%. However, with deep managed care discounting, the collection-to-charge ratio may be as low as 40%, reflecting the widening difference between former standard charge levels as contrasted with more recent contractual fee levels. If the charges are reduced arbitrarily to conform to typical managed care fees, the charges may be lower than other commercial payers allow, leaving "money on the table." Therefore, in order to capture less common—but available—higher fees, it is better to maintain charges at prior levels and accept the large gap between collections and charges and the higher accounts receivable.

## Data Need

Office information systems have, of necessity, become increasingly complex, as claims information requirements have grown. The growth in information requirements has paralleled the growth in cost-control managed care techniques among payers (e.g., documentation of services, prior approval, utilization review, second surgical opinion, and retrospective review). The effect has been an adaptive increase in the sophistication of administrative and financial information collection and handling, without a parallel refinement of clinical information systems. Whereas computerization of financial and demographic information has become a practical necessity for conduct of daily business, the remainder of the clinical record has remained for most practitioners a more primitive written record.

Under changing market conditions, information requirements reward new information management schemes. The market demands a more corporate form of structure in the medical community in order to adapt to payer needs. This implies that generated data must be consistent, relevant, standardized, and rapidly transmissible. The specific elements of a data system necessary to meet these requirements are (1) a fully computerized office record, including electronic medical record, (2) standardized historical, process, and outcome data sets, (3) routine analysis of data sets related to CPT codes and ICD-9-CM codes, (4) composite practice and individual utilization and outcome profiles, (5) a monthly expense analysis, including variations among individual practitioners, and (6) telecommunication capability among all participants in the health care process, including physician office, hospital, pharmacy, diagnostic facility, ancillary provider, and payer.

Particular mention must be made of the necessity for correctly coding Evaluation and Management (E&M) services according to the level of service provided and the documentation recorded in the medical record. Medicare began enforcement in 1997 of documentation guidelines first published in 1995, and revised in 1997, 1999, and 2000. The guidelines have been surrounded by controversy, particularly (1) the problem that specialties have with guidelines designed for a general practice and (2) the use of "bullets," or items required in the dictation to qualify for a level of service regardless of the type of medical problem. Nevertheless, practices have been audited for compliance with the guidelines and severely penalized by the Office of Inspector General and the Department of Justice with fines, restitution, and Medicare program exclusion for noncompliance. It is vital to the practice that office records support the levels of E&M service coded and billed, both to Medicare and to private payers, most of whom adopt the same documentation requirements.

The selection of a specific information system depends on cost and system capability. Numerous commercial systems are available, with information about them assessable from trade associations and journals, such as the Medical Group Management Association (MGMA) and American Group Practice Association (AGPA).

A database designed for a clinical spinal practice is a need yet to be satisfactorily filled. The requirements are relatively simple: (1) demographic information, (2) coded diagnostic information, (3) coded procedural information, and (4) outcome information in coded format. Demographic information acquisition is the easiest, yet the most pivotal, to acquire. Diagnostic information parallels standard diagnostic codes, such as ICD-9-CM codes. Its simplicity can obscure relevant clinical subtleties that may affect treatment and outcome (e.g., with respect to disc herniation, the severity of sciatica versus the extent of low back pain, the presence or absence of reflexes, the degree of positivity of straight leg raise testing, and the factor of time). Procedure coding is straightforward (i.e., the use of CPT codes). The problem in designing a database lies in outcome data acquisition. No standard data format is accepted industry-wide, although a number of health status questionnaire databases are currently in use. Outcome assessment tools, such as the short form health survey (SF-36) for general health assessment[10] and the more detailed Health Status Questionnaire, with a condition-specific (back pain) module,[6] are available for commercial use. It remains to be determined if these functional outcome assessments are sufficiently sensitive and accurate to lead to meaningful decisions about the value of care, particularly spine surgery.

## Marketing

Marketing is more than advertising or selling. Physicians in practice have always used marketing techniques, albeit generally unacknowledged, in building and maintaining a practice. Personal telephone calls with referral-source physicians about referred cases, local educational talks or seminars, and contacts in professional societies are all marketing strategies geared toward the referring physician. The strength of the practice is based on the breadth, stability, and reliability of the network of physician contacts. This form of marketing conforms with the traditional medical ethic that proscribed public advertising as breaching professional dignity and restraint. In fact, it fits an economic system based on a variety of factors, including (1) informal market relationships among vendors (physicians) and between suppliers and purchasers, (2) demand defined by reliance on professional judgment to determine market need, (3) supply restriction of competition by licensing and institutional privileging requirements, (4) a distribution system characterized by initial public contact via primary care physicians, (5) decision-making authority in purchasing choices accorded to consumer agents (physicians), and (6) pricing based on FFS reimbursement supported by nonrestrictive indemnity insurance.

The economic market in which medicine is practiced is changing, and in response, marketing strategies are evolving. The changes involve the aforementioned factors: (1) informal relationships are becoming formal contract relationships among physician, patient, and payer, (2) demand is defined both by patient and payer health plan needs (which often conflict), (3) supply restriction of competition by licensing and institutional privileging requirements, (4) a distribution system is structured by payer plans in contracted provider panels, (5) purchasing decisions and micromanagement authority are assumed by payers through contract agreement, and (6) pricing is shifted to market competitive payer fee schedules or to prepayment within a fixed budget (capitation). Each of these economic factors indicates a change in strategies

observed in the market and new strategies that physicians must consider.

Marketing begins with identifying customer (patient/payer) need. Next, the service or product is designed or redesigned to meet the expressed need or demand. The consumer is informed of the availability and advantages of the product or service by communication strategies. Feedback must be gathered from customers about the satisfaction with the product. This feedback must be used to improve the product and the distribution system. Finally, the market must be regularly reexamined in order to find new needs and successful competing product lines.

In a monopoly market, such as medicine was in the past, price is relatively fixed, service amenities are often neglected, quality is often judged informally and anecdotally, efficiency is deemphasized, and innovation is discouraged. However, medicine is exiting the monopoly market of professional domination and entering the competitive market of corporate business. The successful marketing strategy in this market is the identification and exploitation of a *competitive differential advantage*. This strategy mandates the identification of the strengths of the practice, as well as the building on these strengths or the identification of a market niche or unmet market demand that the practice can grow to fill. Important concepts are flexibility, sensitivity, and appropriate responses to market demands.

The standard competitive elements on which a business chooses to compete in the market are price, quality, and amenities. Price competition is usually characteristic of a commodity market with large volumes, offset by narrow profit margins per item. Price is commonly the predominant element of competition in plans offering large blocks of enrollees.

Quality is difficult to define in a medical market where common training, licensing, and accreditation standards create a presumption of quality. Current standard measurements used to estimate quality of medical care are crude (e.g., mortality, morbidity, and complication rates) and are not generally regarded as significant in purchaser decisions. However, as quality becomes defined as best value, or equivalent outcome for lower price, cost-effectiveness measures, such as length of stay and utilization rates, may become significant competitive elements when contracting with managed care plans.

Finally, the practice may compete on the basis of consumer amenities, which often implies a higher price for more convenience or a pleasing environment. Amenities refer to factors such as evening or weekend appointment times, minimal delays in appointment scheduling, short office waiting time, follow-up office calls to check on progress, pleasant office waiting areas, courteous office staff, and printed disease information and patient instruction materials. Amenities also include conveniences germane to the physician-patient relationship, including personal contact, prompt responses, courtesy, and reliability. The choice of competitive elements should be deliberate, particularly regarding price and volume versus amenities.

Service design or redesign that conforms to market research indicators may involve maneuvers as significant as adding or deleting services, or as minimal as a name change to improve public understanding and name recognition. A commonly perceived problem is the lack of public recognition of the neurosurgeon as the spine surgeon. Spine surgery is, indeed, the majority of the neurosurgeon's clinical practice. Name changes, such as *neurospinal surgery, cranial and spinal surgery,* or simply *spine surgery,* are all tactics that emphasize public recognition of what is involved with a general neurosurgery practice.

Service redesign can apply to single procedures or the integration of multiple service components. Consideration of public preference for less invasive procedures may lead to the offering of minimally invasive spinal techniques, such as endoscopic surgery for lumbar disc herniation with refractory radiculopathy. Similarly, capitated reimbursement may favor minimally invasive outpatient surgery on a cost-effectiveness basis. Discussions with employers may assist in the design of treatment protocols that conform to occupational needs and improve the referral opportunity.

Feedback is required to determine if the service and marketing strategy is effective and how each should be altered to respond to consumer perceptions. Patient satisfaction surveys, physician surveys and direct contacts, and employer or payer direct contacts complete the cycle of marketing and bring the business, once again, around to redesigning or refining the product or service.

Use of an Internet site is becoming a more common means for marketing a medical practice. It allows the practice to publicize those services it wishes to emphasize in building a competitive differential advantage. It also allows patients to become acquainted with the physicians in the practice and the patient information needs and billing requirements of the practice. A Web site also provides a means for access to postoperative instructions and answers to commonly asked questions without a phone call to the office. A Web site can include links to commercial medical information sites the practice finds would help patients better understand the conditions and surgical procedures the practice deals with most commonly.

Marketing is necessary in a competitive market. It is as much information gathering as it is information dissemination. It has a cyclical character, must be pursued continuously, and above all, must be sensitive and responsive to consumer needs.

## The Future

As tight reimbursement and rising operating costs have made it challenging to prosper solely on a spine surgeon's professional services, some are beginning to supplement their income by competing for the facility and ancillary components of health care spending. A growing number of spine surgeons have found profit opportunities by investing in diagnostic imaging, physical therapy, and even ambulatory surgery centers (ASCs). However, federal legislation commonly known as *Stark Laws* essentially prohibits referral of Medicare and Medicaid patients to diagnostic imaging and physical therapy facilities in which the physician has ownership interests.[1] Restrictions arising from Stark Laws generally do not apply to a surgeon's investment in an ASC. But, since ASCs by definition do not allow for overnight stays, a spine surgeon's ability to utilize ASCs is severely limited.

Recently, some spine surgeons have begun investing in surgical hospitals and even hospitals that specialize in treating disorders of the spine. Like the ASC, surgeon ownership of hospitals is generally exempt from Stark Laws. The shear magnitude of the investment required to develop a surgical hospital is daunting and necessitates the contribution of many surgeon and/or nonsurgeon partners. However, the profit potential is also significant. Finally, ownership of a hospital empowers the surgeon to ensure quality patient care and achieve greater professional productivity by establishing operational efficiency in the hospital.[12]

## Summary

The economics of medical and surgical practice are in transition. No longer can surgeons function independently or passively accept practice inefficiencies and cost-ineffective procedures tolerated in the past. No longer can all facilities afford to support all specialty services or the equipment and supply overhead costs of specialty, particularly spinal surgical, care. Cost cannot be ignored. No longer can data be primitive and routine treatment outcomes ignored. Practice solvency cannot be assumed based simply on technical training or past success.

Medicine faces an identity crisis: service profession versus corporate business. The pattern for the future is uncertain, but the broad general features are becoming clearer with each year. As the environmental forces and structures become defined, necessary professional and business adaptations can be more easily made. However, regardless of the changes in the landscape, several principles should guide the course of a practice:

1. Training and experience remain a surgeon's most valuable asset. Whatever the business arrangements, attend first to attaining and preserving unassailable professional competence.
2. Compassion is a fundamental requirement. Never forget who the system is intended to benefit. With the patient's interests foremost, success will follow.
3. Flexibility is vital. Know the environment and change with it. Avoid fixed ideas and responses.
4. Be proactive in learning and changing. In a highly competitive environment in transition, security lies not only in perseverance but also in foresight, innovation, and action.
5. Adopt changes incrementally, preferably in advance of absolute necessity. By this means, errors remain small learning experiences, rather than practice-disrupting disasters.

The economics of spine surgery is the engine that drives the train of the clinical and surgical practice. Attention to detail is essential. Analysis, evaluation, and education concerning market forces and changes are critical to the well-being and survival of the spine surgeon's practice.

Residents entering a practice should learn about the business of spine surgery with the same intensity devoted to acquiring knowledge of new medical technology. The practicing spine surgeon should analyze and learn about the business aspects of medicine.

# REFERENCES

1. 42 U.S.C. § 1395 nn, et seq.
2. *Annual report to Congress,* Washington, D.C., 1993, Physician Payment Review Commission, pp 135-144.
3. Beard PL: *How to negotiate capitation without losing your head,* Shawnee Mission, KA, 1994, ProStat Resource Group.
4. *Cost survey: 2001 report based on 2000 data,* Englewood, CO, 2001, Medical Group Management Association.
5. Eddy D: Health system reform: will controlling costs require rationing services? *JAMA* 272:324-328, 1994.
6. *Health status questionnaire (HSQ).* Velocity Healthcare Informatics, Minnetonka, MN.
7. Heary RF, Kaufman BA, Harbaugh RE, Warnick RE: *Annual procedural data of United States neurological surgeons: report of the 1999 AANS survey,* Park Ridge, IL, 1999, American Association of Neurological Surgeons.
8. Pevehouse BC, Gary Siegel Corporation: *1995 comprehensive neurosurgical practice survey,* Park Ridge, IL, 1996, American Association of Neurological Surgeons.
9. *Physician network insider,* Rockville, MD, 1994, United Communications Group.
10. *SF-36 health status survey,* East Greenwich, RI, Response Technologies.
11. Sokolov JJ: *Richard C. Schneider lecture,* San Diego, CA, 1994, American Association of Neurological Surgeons.
12. Tibbs RE Jr, Pelofsky S, Friedman ES, Blaylock KL: *Physician ownership of specialty spine hospitals: neurosurgical focus,* Charlottesville, VA, 2002.

# CHAPTER 171

# The Rationale for Practice Hygiene: Coding, Reimbursement, and Nomenclature

**Thomas Faciszewski and Gregory J. Przybylski**

Although the practice of spine surgery can be extremely complex, the evolving business requirements often outpace the demands of the clinical practice. The growing expanse of knowledge required to effectively manage a practice is, in part, a consequence of the highly regulated practice of medicine in the United States. In fact, surgeons must master many topics that they were likely not exposed to during their residencies and fellowships. Some of these topics include diagnostic and procedural coding, fraud and abuse legislation, and compliance programs. These once obscure matters have become among the most commonly discussed, debated, and controversial topics facing spinal care physicians.

The spectrum of importance of these coding-related topics is wide and heavily laden with political, social, and scientific issues. Why have nomenclature and coding become so important in the practice of medicine? First of all, physicians must be able to accurately describe diagnoses, treatments, and outcomes in order to discover and reliably provide the most effective advice and treatment for their patients. The diagnosis, which refers to our understanding of a given condition, must be defined accurately because it implies both the extent and limits of our knowledge regarding the etiology, pathogenesis, and prognosis of the disease. Physicians must define our diagnostic nomenclature in order to accurately describe the specific clinical facets of patients' experiences, which is the basis for offering a prognosis and for predicting responses to treatment for the diagnosed condition. Without accurately defined terms, meaningful clinical research cannot be conducted. Secondly, nomenclature and coding have become very important for economic reasons. Both reimbursement requirements as well as fraud and abuse concerns have escalated the demand for correct coding. In the United States, changes in the federal law associated with increasing civil and criminal penalties have caused a quantum shift in the importance of coding.

Consequently, it is imperative that every spine surgeon becomes familiar with coding and reimbursement methods as well as the potential consequences of inaccurately describing physician services. In order to provide the basis for understanding these systems, the historical development of diagnostic and procedural coding methods is reviewed in this chapter. Then the development of the relative value system is examined. Finally, the impact of legislative efforts upon the application of coding and reimbursement methods is highlighted with a few recent examples.

## Development of Diagnosis Coding

The basis of our current diagnostic coding system originates from a method of tracking mortality devised by John Graunt in seventeenth century England. Although others subsequently attempted to classify diseases systematically during the following century, William Farr, the first medical statistician of the General Register Office of England and Wales, is credited with the creation of a uniform classification system that permitted changes associated with advances in medicine.

The Farr classification system was evaluated annually until the first International Statistical Congress asked Farr and colleague Marc d'Espine to develop an international classification in 1853. Although the compromise method adopted by the Congress was never universally accepted, the system proposed by Farr served as the basis for the International List of Causes of Death. Subsequently, the International Statistical Institute asked a committee chaired by Jacques Bertillon to develop a classification system that represented a combination of English, German, and Swiss classification schemes, based upon the organization recommended previously by Farr. The system, entitled the *Bertillon Classification of Causes of Death,* was adopted by the Institute, along with a plan to revise the classification each decade.

However, it was not until the sixth revision during the International Health Conference in 1946 that a classification of causes of morbidity was also included. This conference is credited with the development of international cooperation in health statistics, linking national statistical institutions with the World Health Organization. The current classification, entitled the *International Classification of Diseases—ninth revision—Clinical Modification* (ICD-9-CM), represents the efforts of the World Health Organization (WHO) in 1975.[17] Modifications included the creation of fifth digits to allow two additional levels of subclassification to the previous three-digit system, as well as an independent four-digit system to classify the histopathology of neoplasms. This internationally used classification scheme provides a uniform method for tracking morbidity data and preparing claims for reimbursement.

Although primarily used for diagnostic coding, ICD-9-CM also contains codes assigned to procedures and complications.[23] Over 8000 diagnostic codes, covering the entire scope of clinical diseases, represent the most commonly used subset by physicians. The first section, including codes from 001.0 to 999.9, is divided into 17 classifications of diseases and injuries including infectious and parasitic diseases; neoplasms; diseases defined by body systems; congenital anomalies; symptoms, signs, and

2186

ill-defined conditions; and injuries and poisonings. The second section, consisting of codes from V01.0 to V82.9, describes the reasons for a patient visit other than disease or injury. V codes may be used when reporting preventive medical treatments, physical examination, postoperative follow-up examinations, physical therapy, radiographs, and laboratory tests.

Guidelines implemented by the Centers for Medicare and Medicaid Services (CMS), which was formerly called the Health Care Finance Administration (HCFA), require association of each service provided with an ICD-9-CM code, starting with the primary diagnosis.[23] The chosen diagnostic code should be of the highest degree of specificity, utilizing fourth and fifth digits when applicable. Additional secondary and tertiary diagnoses should also be included if relevant to the service provided. Although coexisting conditions affecting the patient's treatment should also be included, diagnoses that are no longer applicable (as the patient's circumstances change) should be eliminated. Services provided for reasons other than disease or injury, such as well-baby office visits, should be identified with the appropriate V code.

Since the diagnostic codes are linked to the physician service, a system exists to track the costs of managing illnesses. Third-party insurance companies, particularly managed care organizations, have utilized this association to monitor the costs attributable to individual physicians in treating patients for specific diseases. In order to maintain control of expenditures, some insurance companies have utilized this information to determine whether or not to renew contracts with physicians whose costs exceed those of the average practitioner. Consequently, the accurate and careful use of diagnostic coding has become essential to the successful physician's practice.

However, there are limitations associated with the application of ICD-9-CM. Although used to form databases for research and to guide public policy, diagnostic coding was never designed for billing purposes. In addition, ICD-9-CM offers no capacity to designate sidedness (e.g., is the intervertebral disk displacement left-sided or right-sided?) and no manner to designate acuity or severity (e.g., life threatening versus minimally symptomatic spinal cord compression). Despite its many deficiencies, ICD-9-CM is in use because it was available at a crucial time in the organization of health care and its acceptance is sufficiently universal to guarantee its perpetuation. In fact, ICD-9-CM diagnosis coding has become increasingly important as it signifies the reason a service was rendered, a test was ordered, or a procedure was performed.

The WHO planned to replace ICD-9-CM with ICD-10-CM by 1998.[24] However, although ICD-10-CM has been drafted, application has been delayed. Unlike ICD-9-CM, ICD-10-CM contains only diagnosis and no procedural codes. Some of the differences include a vastly increased number of categories of codes (2033 as compared to 855 in ICD-9-CM); a different format—a six-digit alphanumeric system with the letter at the beginning and the decimal point in the middle (e.g., C50.333); and more specificity of some codes, sometimes including severity rating and/or sidedness. Costs associated with the retooling of computers and educating staff about this new system have delayed its implementation. The potential for

a greater degree of specificity places an additional burden on documentation, which must be examined to ensure that it is comprehensive enough to assign a code.

Because ICD-10-CM contains no procedural codes, CMS has contracted with Minnesota Mining and Manufacturing to develop a system of procedural coding to be titled *International Classification of Diseases—tenth revision—Procedure Coding System* (ICD-10-PCS). This seven-character alphanumeric code system bears no resemblance to the Current Procedural Terminology (CPT) system used by the American Medical Association (AMA) (and described in the next paragraph). In addition, the two are distinctly different, and the software used to run ICD-10-CM will not interface with ICD-10-PCS. A specific date for the implementation of this system has not been determined. However, the existence of this system worries some physicians because of the potential for CMS to implement the system without physician involvement.

## Development of Procedure and Supply Coding

In order to standardize the description of physician services as well as to develop a method for compiling actuarial data, the AMA developed a list of descriptive terms and associated numerical codes for reporting medical services, which was published in 1966 as *Current Procedural Terminology*. This first edition predominantly described surgical procedures with only limited reference to medical or radiologic procedures. The second edition was published 4 years later and included an expanded description of medical services, as well as a five-digit coding system.

Two additional revisions to CPT were compiled later that decade. The fourth edition was completed in 1977 and contained substantial revisions to include improvements in medical technology. Although one of the intended applications of CPT was to facilitate communication between physicians and insurance agencies, CMS did not adopt CPT as part of their Common Procedure Coding System (HCPCS Level I) until 1983. Subsequently, CMS mandated use of this system to report services for payment under Part B of the Medicare program. Three years later, CMS also required Medicaid agencies to use the method. Given the growing interest in greater specificity of both diagnostic and procedural coding, the AMA has been working extensively on developing a significant revision to the current edition,[3] whose framework has been in place for 25 years. Efforts have included improving granularity by eliminating codes that include "and/or" and "with/without" language so that physicians can more precisely code the work that was done. The fifth edition is the current edition.

The CPT system undergoes annual revision under the direction of the CPT Editorial Panel. A 16-member physician panel meets quarterly and is comprised predominantly of 11 physicians appointed by the AMA. The 11 AMA panelists serve 4-year terms. Four of the seats rotate among specialists to allow a multidisciplinary influence. The other members of the panel include the co-chairman of the Health Care Professionals Advisory Committee (HCPAC), a representative from CMS, and appointees from the Blue Cross and Blue Shield Association, the

Health Insurance Association of America, and the American Hospital Association. AMA staff assists the CPT Editorial Panel with input from the CPT Advisory Committee, which is comprised predominantly of physicians selected by national medical specialty societies. The HCPAC was created by the Editorial Panel to facilitate participation of allied health professionals and limited license practitioners to participate in the process.

Currently, two main groupings of Category I codes are contained within CPT. For inclusion as a Category I code, the CPT Editorial Panel requires that the service or procedure is performed in multiple locations by many health care providers and has approval of the Food and Drug Administration, when required. The first group is the Evaluation and Management (E&M) codes, which describe services performed in broad subcategories, which are then further divided into two or more types of E&M service. For example, there are two types of office visits—new patient and established patient visits—and two types of hospital visits—initial patient and subsequent patient visits. The second main category is Surgical Procedures, which is subclassified according to organ system so that, generally, the five-digit codes associated with a given organ system are in the same numbering sequences. In reference to spine surgery, the majority of the arthrodesis and instrumentation codes are in the 22000 series of codes, and the decompressive procedures such as laminectomy and discectomy are in the 63000 series. In addition, there is a listing of Category III codes, which contain temporary codes for emerging technology that does not satisfy the CPT Editorial Panel requirements for Category I designation.

Although codes contained in CPT describe the procedures and services provided by physicians to patients, another national coding system was developed to describe nonphysician services, as well as supplies.[19] For example, ambulance transportation and dental services, as well as various durable medical equipment and prosthetic devices, are described by this system. These represent Level II HCPCS codes and are published and maintained by CMS. In contrast to the five-digit numeric codes of CPT, these are alphanumeric codes containing an initial letter (between A and V but excluding S) followed by four numbers. Moreover, modifiers can also append these codes, but are comprised of either two letters (-AA to -VP) or alphanumeric symbols.

Finally, a third level of codes exists which is maintained by local Medicare carriers. These Level III codes describe new procedures and supplies not accounted for by the two sets of national codes. In similarity to the Level II codes, these are also alphanumeric codes containing an initial letter (from W to Z as well as S) followed by four numbers. Although local Medicare carriers create these codes, prior approval by CMS is required before implementation is permitted. Occasionally, one may encounter service or supply descriptions in two or all three coding levels.

While these diagnostic and procedural coding systems provide a method for describing the encounter between the patient and the physician, this information must be communicated to the insurer in order for the physician to receive payment for the services provided. An understanding of information flow is necessary prior to applying coding rules to reimbursement. The process of describing physician work involves a continuous flow of information, beginning with the patient-physician encounter and ending with the submission of a bill to the patient or insurance carrier.

The patient-physician encounter is the period during which data is gathered regarding the patient's clinical condition and a diagnosis and/or treatment is rendered. It is important to note that unless the data gathered during this encounter is documented in written form, it is considered by the legal authorities and insurance carriers not to have been done. This requirement for written documentation is critical, as deficient documentation is the most common reason for later assignment of a code which overrepresented the amount of work performed (i.e., upcoding), as well as the most common reason for denied claims.

This documented encounter is then coded based upon the type and amount of physician work performed. This may reflect work related to seeing patients in the outpatient setting or work performed in the operating room. These service codes are then linked to the specific diagnostic codes that prompted the service. A billing sheet is then constructed with the diagnostic and procedural codes along with the physician charges and is mailed or sent electronically to the insurance carrier. In the case of Medicare or Medicaid patients, this claim is submitted on a HCFA 1500 form.

## Development of the Resource-Based Relative Value System

Once the insurer receives the documentation of services, the payer must determine the reimbursement to the physician for the services provided. A fee-for-service payment method based on customary, prevailing, and reasonable (CPR) charges was the cornerstone of third-party reimbursement until the 1980s. Since physician payment schedules were the basis for determining reimbursement, there was little motivation to understanding the coding systems used to track services. However, the alarming growth of health care expenditures attracted attention from both government and private insurers.

During the mid-1980s, total health care expenditures had reached $540 billion, representing an 11% share of the gross national product. In fact, proportional spending had more than doubled from the 5.6% share paid in 1965.[18] Moreover, reimbursement for physician services by Medicare grew at a 15% compound rate between 1975 and 1987, nearly twice the 7.9% growth rate of the gross national product.[28] Finally, observations of utilization of physician services suggested that excessive and unnecessary procedures further contributed to escalating costs.[2,11]

The impetus to revise the Medicare payment system arose from the rapidly increasing expenditures for payment of physician and hospital services by CMS. Efforts to control costs of physician services followed implementation in 1983 of a prospective pricing system (PPS) for hospital services reflected in Medicare Part A. Since hospital services accounted for more than two thirds of Medicare expenditures, cost-containment efforts were naturally directed at hospitals first. A diagnosis-related group

(DRG) payment was developed for approximately 500 diseases based upon the national average cost of hospital care for that particular illness. This method assumed that, over time, the cost for providing care for patients with a range of illness severity would equal the calculated DRG payment. Additional payments were also authorized to account for unusually severe illnesses requiring prolonged hospital stays. Since the payment was identical regardless of the hospital cost, the PPS provided a strong incentive for hospitals to improve cost-efficiency. As a result, the annual growth of Medicare expenditures was reduced by more than half between 1975 and 1990.

Several factors, including dissatisfaction with the original payment scheme, growing Part B Medicare expenditures, and a reasonable proposal for a new method, influenced the decision to develop an alternative method of physician payment. The original method for determining the physician payment schedule was based on CPR charges. This resembled the usual, customary, and reasonable (UCR) charge system utilized by private insurers to pay for physicians' services based upon their actual fees. However, the wide variation in the amount Medicare paid for physician services both among physician specialties as well as among geographic regions caused dissatisfaction within the medical profession.[1] Additional dissatisfaction grew among physicians because of increasing disparity between the lower valuation of patient evaluation services and procedural services.

Consideration was given toward developing a DRG system similar to that developed for hospital payments under Medicare Part A.[25] Another option was to create a managed care or capitation model of payment. Finally, a proposal was offered for replacing the CPR method with a payment schedule based on a relative value scale (RVS). Only the CPR and the payment schedule represented fee-for-service methods. Many physicians voiced concern that a DRG or capitated system would threaten clinical judgment in patient-care decisions. Moreover, the AMA opposed policies that precluded physicians from charging patients the difference between their fee and the Medicare payment (i.e., balance billing). Since the courts supported Congressional legislation to limit physicians' fees, development of an RVS seemed to provide the best alternative to the CPR method.

The concept of an RVS was not new. In fact, the California Medical Association developed an RVS in 1956 that was regularly updated for nearly 2 decades. However, it was based on a median of charges reported by California Blue Shield in 1969, thereby still representing a CPR charge methodology. Yet, physicians used this method to determine fee schedules, and government and private insurers alike used the system to establish payment rates. Subsequently, concerns raised by the Federal Trade Commission regarding the possibility of antitrust violations led the California Medical Association to discontinue updating the charge data collected.

Rather than continuing pursuit of a charge-based RVS as supported by most surgical subspecialty societies, a resource-based RVS (RBRVS) was considered in which physician services were ranked based upon the relative costs incurred in providing them. Most nonprocedural specialty societies believed that wide variations among fees for services and geographic variations failed to adequately reflect costs incurred to provide the services. As a result, the AMA chose to support an RVS based on resource costs, provided that the payment system reflected geographic variations in practice costs and did not prevent physicians from balance billing. Although the AMA submitted a proposal to CMS for development of a new RVS, continued antitrust concerns precluded direct physician involvement in their development. Consequently, the AMA accepted a proposal submitted by the Harvard University School of Public Health to perform a national study of RBRVSs for physician services.

On July 1, 1986, the Consolidated Omnibus Budget Reconciliation Act mandated that the Department of Health and Human Services develop a RBRVS to be submitted to Congress. In addition, the law created the Physician Payment Review Commission (PPRC) to study a variety of additional options for Medicare payment reform including changing CPR, capitation, and physician DRG.[26] The PPRC recommended development of a payment schedule linked to a RBRVS.[27]

Concurrently, the Harvard study commenced in December of 1985 with funding from CMS. The principal investigators, William Hsiao, Ph.D., and Peter Braun, M.D., had previously encountered limited success in a 1979 pilot study that attempted to rank 27 physician services from 5 specialties.[16] Five years later, a follow-up study demonstrated more consistent results after estimates of work alone without the addition of complexity were considered. The first phase of the national study supported by CMS developed a RBRVS for twelve physician specialties. In addition, independent funding was obtained for study of six additional specialties. Not only were specialty-specific scales developed, but also a method for creating cross-specialty links allowed integration of a single cross-specialty RBRVS. The Omnibus Budget Reconciliation Act of 1986 provided a 2-year extension for submission of RBRVS to Congress and mandated inclusion of 15 additional specialties during the second phase of the study.[12-15]

Although the AMA adopted in principle the results of the Harvard study, they also recommended that the new Medicare payment system include geographic differences in practice costs and professional liability, as well as a transition period to prevent disruptive changes between the CPR and RBRVS systems. The PPRC likewise endorsed the study and supported the AMA recommendations. However, the commission diverged from the AMA on two recommendations. Despite opposition to balance billing, the commission recommended placing limits on balance billing. In addition, expenditure targets for Medicare spending were also recommended. Since RBRVS was still a variation of a fee-for-service payment system, PPRC believed that cost containment could only be achieved with expenditure targets.

In December of 1989, Congress enacted the Omnibus Budget Reconciliation Act (OBRA 89), which mandated a Medicare payment schedule based on the RBRVS from the Harvard study with inclusion of physician work, practice expense, and professional liability costs. Geographic adjustments to all three components were included in a method for the calculation of the relative value unit (RVU) of a physician's service under the RBRVS system (Equation 1):

$$MFS = [(RVUw \times GPCIw) + (RVUpe \times GPCIpe) + RVUm \times GPCIm)] \times CF \qquad (1)$$

where MFS = Medicare Fee Schedule; RVU = relative value unit; GPCI = geographic practice cost index; w = work; pe = practice expense; m = malpractice; and CF = conversion factor.

The conversion factor for the calculated RVU was based on keeping the overall Medicare expenditure the same as the cost using the CPR system. A process was created to annually adjust the conversion factor, maintaining a "budget-neutral" value, which limited increases in expenditures to $20 million annually. Additional reductions in limits on balance billing were included.

A 5-year transition to the RBRVS Medicare payment system was to begin on January 1, 1992. Despite more than 7 years of investigation in the Harvard study, RVUs had not been assigned to all services listed in CPT by this date. At the direction of CMS, regional carrier medical directors assigned RVUs to the remaining codes until the third phase of the study was completed. The final comprehensive RBRVS for physician services was published in the November 25, 1992 *Federal Register*.

After implementation of the RBRVS fee schedule by CMS for payments by Medicare, additional health insurers have gradually implemented an RVS as well. Although RBRVS is the method most commonly used, an alternative RVS called *St. Anthony's* is also used in certain regions. This privately maintained system, formerly known as *McGraw-Hill*, utilizes relative value units based upon the time, risk, and complexity of the physician service. In contrast, the RBRVS uses physician work, practice expense, and malpractice expense as the components for determining the relative value of a particular physician service. The physician work component comprises approximately 54% of the total relative value of the service, whereas practice expense comprises 41%. In addition, a geographic practice cost index is incorporated to adjust for geographic differences. Consequently, conversion factors between RBRVS and St. Anthony's RVS are different.

In order to coordinate changes in CPT with assignment of RVU by CMS, the AMA/Specialty Relative Value Update Committee (RUC) was created in 1991.[22] Twenty-three of the twenty-eight members are appointed by major national medical specialty societies. The other five panelists include the RUC chair, the co-chair of HCPAC, and members of the AMA, American Osteopathic Association, and the CPT Editorial Panel. An RUC Advisory Committee composed of members appointed by 94 specialty societies develop and suggest RVU for new codes to the RUC. Specialty society representatives are responsible for compiling physician survey data to determine the time spent in performing the medical service and ranking the service relative to existing services. In general, procedures are valued by determining, from survey information (RUC survey), the sum of the component time, the intensity, and the risk of performing the procedure. Physician work value is added to the practice expense and to malpractice expense to form the total relative value for the specific procedure. Only the physician work value (wRVU) is pre-sented to CMS for approval. For the most part, CMS has been supportive of the RUC valuations for procedures, but CMS has authority to disapprove RUC recommendations. During the 5-year period ending in 1998, nearly 2300 relative value recommendations were made to CMS with a recent acceptance rate of more than 90%.

However, the Balanced Budget Act requires a budget neutrality adjustment. Since the development of new CPT codes requires subsequent valuation, the new RVU assigned must come from previously valued codes to maintain budget neutrality. Typically, values are maintained within a family of codes such as the musculoskeletal or neurosurgical sections of the CPT manual. Consequently, there is some disincentive to making significant changes in codes. Some allowance for new technology exists to account for innovations in medical care, thereby creating an opportunity for growth within a family of codes. The methods of maintaining budget neutrality have included reductions in practice expense as well as changes in the conversion factor. CMS decided that, beginning in 1996, annual budget neutrality adjustments would be made to the physician fee schedule conversion factor (Figure 171.1).

Although work valuations were resource-based, practice expense was based upon the AMA's Socioeconomic Monitoring System 1989 Core Survey (SMS) of a representative sample of 4000 physicians in 34 specialties. However, practice costs, including office rent, wages of nonphysician personnel, equipment, and supplies, were measured overall rather than specific to a given service. Moreover, practice expenses varied among specialties, representing 52.2% of family physicians' practice costs but only 38.9% of neurosurgeons' costs. The method enacted by OBRA 89 involved multiplying the specialty-specific practice expense factor by the average Medicare payment of the service in 1991. Similarly, professional liability was calculated based upon the proportion of cost multiplied by the Medicare payment. The average neurosurgical professional liability component of practice cost was 7.6%, compared with a 3.9% proportion for the family physician. If the service was provided by more than one specialty, a weighted average of surveyed costs was utilized.

The Omnibus Budget Reconciliation Act of 1993 mandated reductions in the practice expense of "over-valued" services. Over a 3-year period the practice expense was reduced annually by 25% of the amount that the value exceeded the physician work RVU until it was no greater than 128% of the work component. However, concerns over the nonresource-based OBRA 89 method of calculating practice expense as well as a 1994 Social Security Act amendment mandating resource-based practice expense calculations prompted CMS to contract with Abt Associates, Inc., to perform a national study of physician's practice expense. Fifteen Clinical Practice Expert Panels (CPEPs) were formed from nominations by medical associations to develop a list of direct cost components of a selected group of reference codes. In addition, a national mail survey of 5000 practices was performed to obtain a sample of practice costs and service mix to validate the CPEP estimates. However, poor response rates from physicians led CMS to abandon efforts at obtaining actual survey data. In order to meet the deadline of January 1998 set by Congress, CMS planned to implement new practice

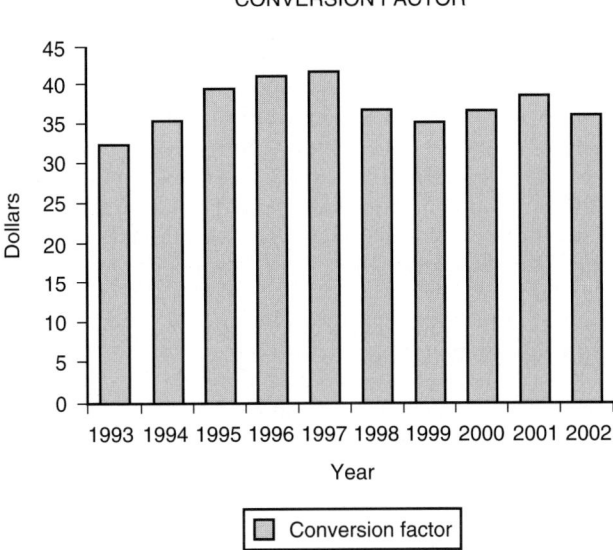

CONVERSION FACTOR

**Figure 171.1** Variation in Medicare's surgical conversion factor over the past decade.

expense values based on CPEP data. Lack of validation of the CPEP data with actual practice expense information, as well as failures to account for actual differences in practice cost among all specialties prompted the AMA to urge Congress to extend the deadline for implementation of new practice expense values. As a result, Congress not only delayed implementation until 1999, but also directed the General Accounting Office (GAO) to review HCFA's methodology and make recommendations for a valid resource-based model. The GAO report supported the concerns raised by the AMA.

Beginning in January 1999, CMS initiated a transition to a resource-based practice expense valuation that differs based on the site of the service. If a medical service can be performed either in an office or a hospital, then both a nonfacility and facility practice expense value were assigned. Whereas locations assigned nonfacility practice expense include physician offices and independent imaging or laboratory centers, facility practice expense is attributed to hospitals, surgical centers, and nursing homes. The method for estimating practice costs is based upon the AMA's SMS data. Since the SMS data came from small sample sizes with sufficient variability to introduce sampling bias, there continues to be concern regarding this methodology.

## Additional Impact of Legislative Changes Upon Coding and Reimbursement

Two recent acts of the United States Congress—the Kennedy-Kassebaum Health Insurance Portability and Accountability Act of 1996 (HIPAA) and the Balanced Budget Act of 1997 (BBA)—have created major changes in the practice of U.S. physicians. HIPPA changed the U.S. government's fraud and abuse regulations by increasing civil monetary damages from $2000 to $10,000, by

applying fraud and abuse laws to the private as well as the public sector, by permitting confiscation of personal property for health care fraud convictions, and by changing health care frauds from misdemeanors to federal felonies with mandatory prison sentences. Surgeons are liable for fraud and abuse violations in the documentation, coding, and billing tasks of their practice. Compliance plans and programs are aimed at satisfying the Office of the Inspector General's (OIG's) requirements for the constant surveillance of these responsibilities.

The overall purpose of the Balanced Budget Act was to erase the federal budget deficit, but as a part of the Act, federal regulators were enabled to more aggressively attack health care fraud and abuse, especially as it relates to the Anti-Kickback Statute. Prior to the BBA, the OIG had to pursue anti-kickback cases through the Department of Justice, as these cases were considered criminal matters. The BBA allowed the OIG to pursue anti-kickback violations for civil monetary penalties, thereby lowering the standard of proof and obviating the need to go through the Department of Justice. In addition, the BBA requires CMS to account for health care expenditures and to reimburse health care providers based upon documented physician work. CMS is now required to reimburse physicians for in-office practice expenses based upon actual, rather than "assumed," office expenses. In a brief time, these legislative acts served to change the face of the practice of medicine in the United States and pushed to the forefront the demand for precise coding and documentation by physicians and other health care providers.

Some methods for preventing fraudulent billing of services have been automated by CMS. Despite the growing number of codes to describe medical services, the work included in many codes overlapped. The process of unbundling, which involves description of a larger procedure with several codes that contain overlapping work, resulted in significant increases in health care expenditures. On January 1, 1996, Medicare initiated the Correct Coding Initiative (CCI) to reduce unbundling and inappropriate reporting of CPT codes.[21] CMS contracted with Administer Federal, an Indiana Medicare carrier, to create and maintain a computer program to be used nationally. Despite the $700,000 development cost, Medicare reported savings in excess of $700 million since the program's inception. In Version 5.1 of the CCI released on April 1, 1999, there were an estimated 120,000 coding edits.[16] Most of the edits represented payment policies in which a comprehensive code would be paid while the component code would be disallowed, whereas a small percentage of edits identified mutually exclusive codes which would not be performed concurrently.

## Nomenclature

Coding requires translation of diagnostic and procedural terms to a system that can be classified and manipulated more easily than standard language. Therefore, coding can be no more accurate than the terms being translated. An international committee of anatomists, the Federative Committee on Anatomic Terminology, has undertaken the arduous task of updating an exhaustive list of anatomic terms.[9] Although this provides standards for acceptable terms and their spelling, it does not provide definitions or include pathology.

In the field of spine care, it has been well documented that some of the most basic diagnostic terms (e.g., *herniated disc*) are not precisely defined and are commonly misunderstood in communications among physicians, patients, insurers, and those who may influence public policy on matters important to spine care. A task force of the North American Spine Society (NASS) recommended preferred terminology for disc pathology and definitions of terms related to disc disorders.[7] These efforts were expanded by a joint task force of NASS, the American Society of Neuroradiologists, and American Society of Spinal Radiologists.[8] Their work does not include attention to disorders of the vertebral canals (i.e., stenosis), disorders of the posterior elements, or procedures.

## Research Applications

For physicians trying to do meaningful clinical research, especially when relying upon methods that require retrospective retrieval of information or analysis of previously published findings on a subject, the potential for errors introduced by nonstandardized nomenclature and faulty or incomplete coding systems is obvious. The problems may be compounded further, but become less obvious, when the separation of those applying the data from those who collected the data increases, such as when data are pooled to guide social policy or administrative decisions.

Information based on the hospital or outpatient patient experience may be abstracted from patients' medical records to form "administrative databases," which have been used in attempts to describe many aspects of the delivery and utilization of health care.[4] A variety of conclusions have been drawn from the research performed using administrative databases. These conclusions can have significant and important implications for patients, providers, and society at large, to the extent that such data inform participants in current health care policy debates.[20]

Although ICD-9-CM data can be used for creating outpatient databases, the most common use of ICD-9-CM is for the coding of in-patient hospital admissions. The processing of the in-patient medical record information into ICD-9-CM–coded language follows a typical sequence. First, hospital medical records personnel abstract clinical information in the hospital medical record and discharge summary. The data identified includes diagnoses, procedures, and complication data. This information is then converted into ICD-9-CM code form. Also abstracted are patient demographic data such as age, gender, length of stay, and discharge status. With this patient demographic data and ICD-9-CM codes, a discharge abstract is constructed. Pooling of discharge abstracts has been referred to as the formation of administrative databases. Administrative databases contain regional discharge abstracts. At the state level, discharge abstracts are received from every hospital within the state. At the federal level, CMS receives nationwide discharge abstracts relating to Medicare patients.[10] These data are then available for analysis and research questions.

Several studies have been performed in order to evaluate the accuracy of the information contained within these databases, as their usefulness relates directly to the quality of the data contained within them.[5,6] The limitations of these databases are many, including nonstandardized nomenclature for labeling diagnoses and procedures, inherent deficiencies of the ICD-9-CM system, limitations of the coders assigning the codes, institutional differences in coding practices, incomplete data, and inaccurate data.

## Practice Essentials

A comprehensive description of the nuances of required coding practices and rules is beyond the scope of this chapter. However, it should be clear based upon the foregoing discussion that the practicing physician/surgeon has a comprehensive understanding of fraud and abuse legislation, anti-kickback legislation, AMA CPT coding rules, and compliance plans and programs. Legislative issues and rules change on a regular basis, so the process of maintaining competence requires at least yearly updates. The easiest and most efficient way to stay informed is via specialty society coding education courses. NASS and AANS are two societies that offer on a regular basis coding courses that are relevant to the spine surgeon's practice. Both society courses offer detailed lectures on coding, reimbursement, and compliance issues.

## REFERENCES

1. Burney IL, Schreiber GJ, Blaxall MO, Gabel JR: Geographic variation in physician's fees, *JAMA* 240: 1368-1371, 1978.
2. Chassin MR, Kosecoff J, Park RE, *et al*: Does inappropriate use explain geographic variations in the use of health care services? A study of three procedures, *JAMA* 258: 2533-2537, 1987.
3. *Current Procedural Terminology: CPT 2002*, Chicago, 2001, American Medical Association.
4. Faciszewski T: Spine update: administrative databases in spine research, *Spine* 22:1269-1275, 1997.
5. Faciszewski T, Broste S, Fardon D: Quality of data regarding the diagnosis of spinal disorders in administrative databases: a multicenter study, *J Bone Joint Surg Am* 79:1481-1488, 1997.
6. Faciszewski T, Johnson L, Noren C, Smith M: Administrative database complication coding in anterior spinal fusion procedures: what does it mean? *Spine* 20:1783-1788, 1995.
7. Fardon DF, Herzog RJ, Mink JH, *et al*: Nomenclature of lumbar disc disorders. In Garfin SR, Vaccaro AR, editors: *Orthopaedic Knowledge Update—Spine* (pp A3-A14), Rosemont, 1997, American Academy of Orthopaedic Surgeons.
8. Fardon DF, Milette PM, *et. al*: personal communication, (publication data pending).
9. *Federative Committee on Anatomical Terminology:* Terminologia Anatomica, New York, 1998, Georg Thieme Verlag.

10. Fisher ES, Whaley FS, Krushat WM, *et al:* The accuracy of Medicare's hospital claims data (progress has been made, but problems remain), *Am J Public Health* 82: 243-248, 1992.

11. Greenspan AM, Kay HR, Berger BC, *et al:* Incidence of unwarranted implantation of permanent cardiac pacemakers in a large medical population, *N Engl J Med* 318:158-163, 1988.

12. Hsiao WC, Braun P, Becker ER, Thomas SR: The resource-based relative value scale, *JAMA* 258:799-802, 1987.

13. Hsiao WC, Braun P, Dunn D, Becker ER: Resource-based relative values: an overview, *JAMA* 260:2347-2353, 1988.

14. Hsiao WC, Braun P, Dunn D, Becker ER: Results and policy implications of the resource-based relative value study, *N Engl J Med* 319:881-888, 1988.

15. Hsiao WC, Braun P, Yntema D, Becker ER: Estimating physicians' work for a resource-based relative value scale, *N Engl J Med,* 319:835-841, 1988.

16. Hsiao WC, Stason WB: Toward developing a relative value scale for medical and surgical services, *Health Care Financ Rev* 1:23-29, 1979.

17. *International Classification of Diseases*, Geneva, 1977, World Health Organization, pp 7-33.

18. Jacobs P: Behavior of supply. In *The Economics of Health and Medical Care,* ed 3, Gaithersburg, MD, 1991, Aspen, pp 168-174.

19. Jones-Burns MK: *St. Anthony's HCPCS Level II Code Book,* Reston, 1997, St. Anthony's, pp 1-3.

20. Kassirer JP: The quality of care and the quality of measuring it, *N Engl J Med,* 329:1263-1264, 1993.

21. Kirschner CG, Reyes D: *An update on Medicare's correct coding initiative, in CPT Assistant*, Chicago, 1999, American Medical Association, pp 7-9.

22. Gallagher PE (ed): *Medicare RBRVS: the Physician's Guide 2002,* Chicago, 2002, American Medical Association, pp 2-48.

23. Hart AC, Hopkins CA (eds): *Medicode ICD-9-CM professional for physicians, International Classification of Diseases, 9th revision, clinical modification,* ed 6, Reston, 2001, St Anthony's.

24. *Medicode ICD-10 Made Easy,* Reston, 2000, St Anthony's.

25. Mitchell JB: Physician DRG's, *N Engl J Med,* 13:670-675, 1985.

26. Physician Payment Review Commission: Medicare physician payment: an agenda for reform. In *Annual Report to Congress No. 68-227,* Washington, DC, 1987, U.S. Government Printing Office.

27. Physician Payment Review Commission: Medicare physician payment. In *Annual Report to Congress,* Washington, DC, 1988, U.S. Government Printing Office.

28. Roper WL: Statement before Subcommittee on Health of the Committee on Ways and Means, U.S. House of Representatives, 1988, U.S. Department of Health and Human Services, Health Care Finance Administration.

# CHAPTER 172

# Intraoperative Crisis Management in Spine Surgery: What To Do When Things Go Bad

**Michael P. Steinmetz, Jared H. Miller, and Edward C. Benzel**

In spite of all attempts to avoid complications, they occasionally "raise their ugly head." The previous chapters have addressed prevention and management. What has not been addressed is the management of catastrophic/cataclysmic complications—usually intraoperative. This, the final chapter, fills this void.

There have been many reported complications related to spine surgery. Most, however, are not crises. When a crisis occurs, swift and decisive action by the health care team is required. For the purpose of this discussion, this action is necessary either during the operative procedure or during the immediate postoperative period. Not all complications require immediate action and therefore are not discussed. For example, nerve root avulsion is a major complication but does not require immediate action. Crisis management can be divided into four sections: (1) anesthesia-related crises, (2) surgical crises, (3) monitoring issues, and (4) neurologic injuries.

## Anesthetic Crises
### Prone Cardiopulmonary Arrest

The prone position is the position of choice for most spinal operations. However, it is associated with some difficulties for the anesthesiologist. It may interfere with monitoring techniques, alter respiratory function, and limit airway and vascular access.[19] With modern anesthetic technique, cardiopulmonary resuscitation (CPR) is rarely required in the operating room (OR). Nevertheless, in some instances it becomes necessary. The prone position substantially complicates cardiopulmonary arrest management because of many factors. First, the time to acquire a stretcher and turn the patient to the supine position in order to initiate CPR may significantly delay therapy. Furthermore, the wound must be closed quickly, risking infection and costing precious time. Second, the spine may be left iatrogenically unstable, risking further injury. In addition, spinal implants may not be completely attached or they may be protruding from the wound.

Turning the patient in some situations may not be feasible because of the risk of neurologic injury. In these situations, the majority of the responsibility for patient management resides with the anesthesiologist; but the surgeon must initiate CPR. There are two options available in these circumstances. Closed CPR in the prone position has been described[17,19] and is usually used first. If sternal support is present, both hands may be placed on either side of the incision at the midthoracic level with the palms over the scapulae (Figure 172-1).[19] Compression is then initiated. One should observe the arterial wave form, blood pressure, and end-tidal $CO_2$ to monitor cardiac output and the adequacy of the resuscitation. If there is no sternal support (e.g., when the patient is placed on chest rolls), one of the surgeon's hands may be placed under the patient's chest over the lower third of the sternum clinched in a fist[17] (Figure 172-2) requiring a break in sterility. The surgeon's other hand then compresses at the midthoracic level. An associate may assist with this process.

If the aforementioned is not feasible or is unsuccessful because of a lack of adequate cardiac output or spine instability, the surgeon has the option of left dorsal thoracotomy.[17] A thoracotomy may be performed rapidly with the patient in the prone position. This procedure provides direct access to the heart. Following exposure, open internal cardiac massage or defibrillation may be performed (Figure 172.3).

## Air Embolism

Intraoperative venous air embolism (VAE) most commonly occurs with patients in the sitting position. Some surgeons avoid this position specifically to avoid air emboli. Depending on the sensitivity of the monitoring technique used, the overall occurrence of air embolism is as high as 30% in the sitting position.[23] In one report in which transesophageal echocardiography was used, 100% of patients in the sitting position exhibited venous air embolism.[13] Although the occurrence of VAE is high, the incidence of sequelae is low, as long as appropriate measures to treat the embolism are instituted rapidly. Therefore, in high-risk cases, such as surgery in the sitting position, appropriate monitoring techniques should be used. These include ECG, arterial catheter, right atrial or pulmonary artery catheter, end-tidal $CO_2$ monitor, and a precordial Doppler (the most sensitive and practical monitor for VAE).

These monitoring devices allow treatment of VAE before paradoxical air embolism or cardiopulmonary embarrassment occurs. Most often, the initial indication of the presence of VAE is via the precordial Doppler. If the VAE is significant, audible Doppler indicators may be accompanied by a decrease in end-tidal $CO_2$, ventricular arrhythmias, hypotension, and/or an increase in pulmonary artery pressure. With the first sign of VAE, the surgeon should flood the operative field with saline, wax all bleeding bone edges, and occlude any visual sources of venous bleeding. Bilateral jugular compression by the anesthesiologist increases the CVP and may help in identifying the venous source. Simultaneously, the anesthesiologist should discontinue nitrous oxide infusion, discontinue PEEP (positive end expiratory pressure [PEEP]), and aspirate air from the right atrial catheter. These steps often lead to resolution of the symptoms related to the VAE. The patient may also be placed in a head-down position with the patient's right side up, although this is rarely required.[7]

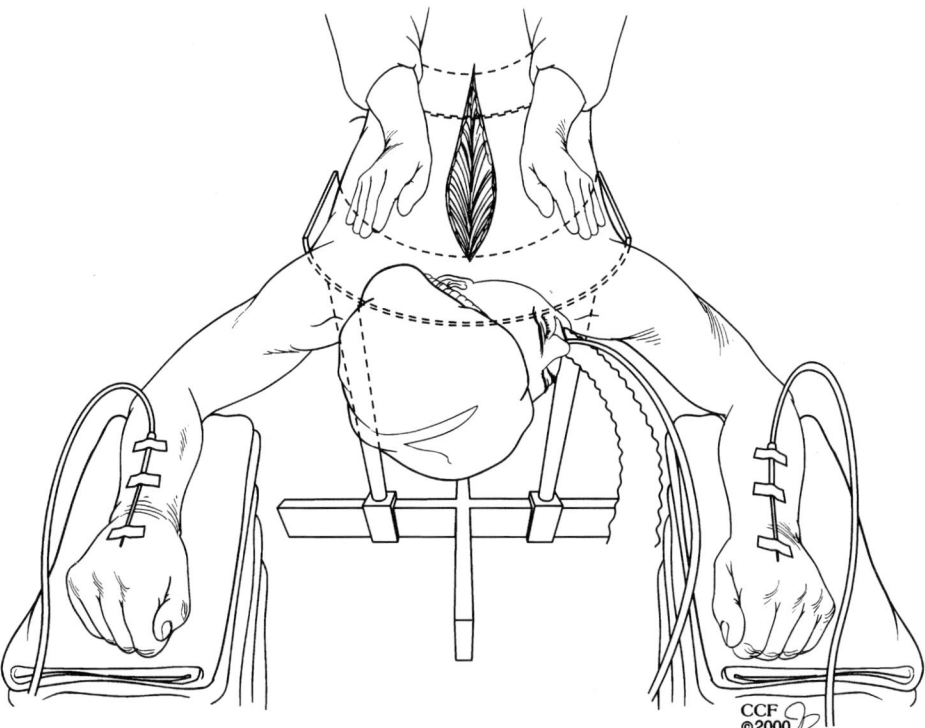

**Figure 172.1** When sternal support is available, the surgeon may place his or her hands on either side of the spine at the midthoracic level for compressions during CPR.

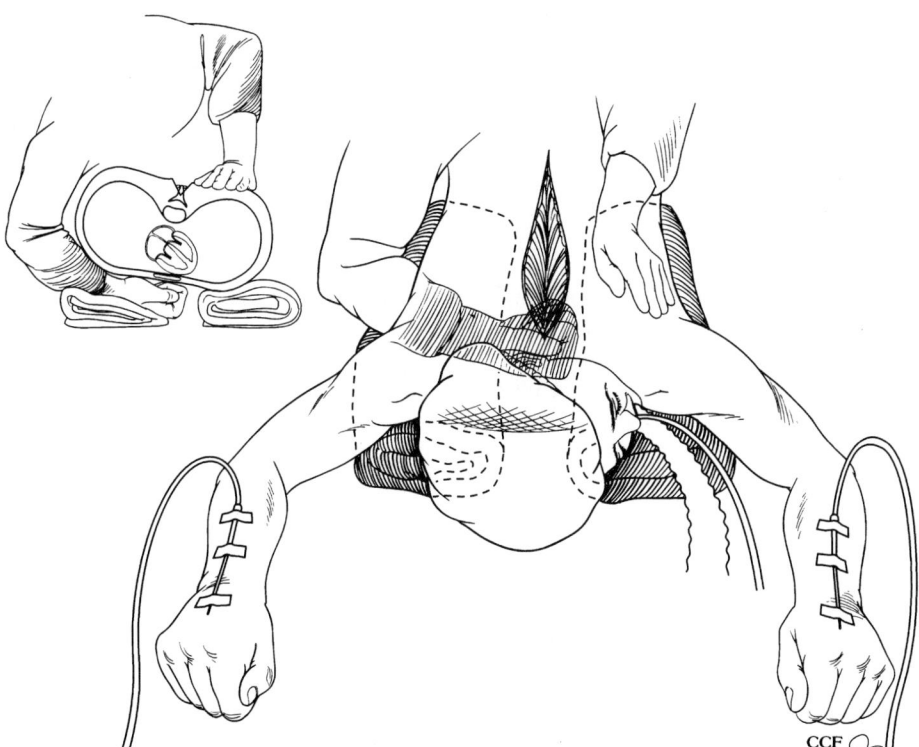

**Figure 172.2** When there is a lack of sternal support, the surgeon (or assistant) may place a clenched fist on the lower sternum and the other hand may then compress at the midthoracic level during CPR.

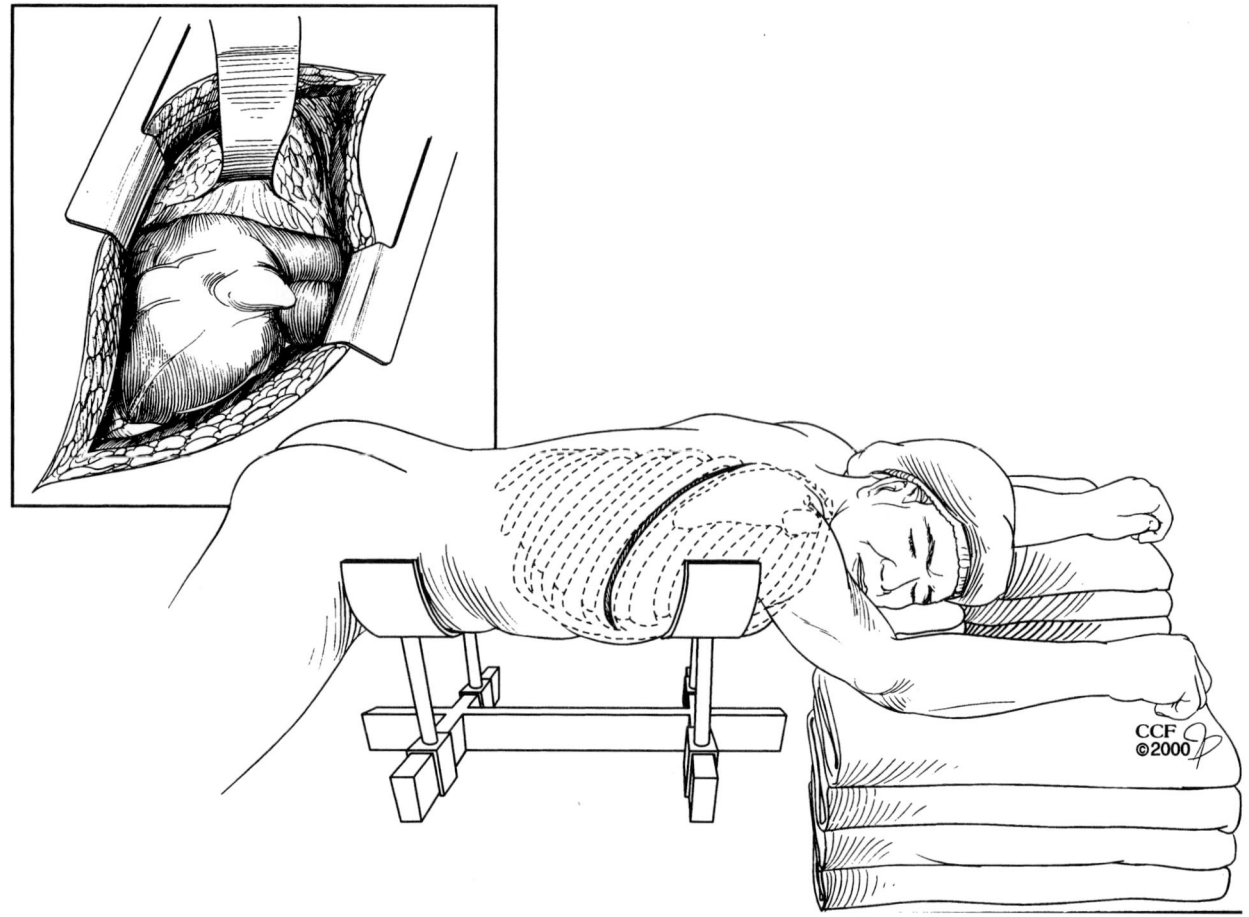

**Figure 172.3** Left dorsal thoracotomy. An incision is made between the ribs. The dissection is taken down to and through the intercostal muscles. The parietal plura is incised. The heart may now be visualized and internal cardiac massage may be undertaken.

This may aid in aspiration of the bolus of air. Nitrous oxide should be discontinued for the remainder of the case, because it is known to enlarge the gas volume of air-containing cavities.[14] PEEP should also be discontinued, because PEEP may alter right to left atrial pressure gradients and facilitate the passage of air across an existing patent foramen ovale.[2]

If the symptoms completely resolve with the aforementioned maneuvers, the procedure may be completed as planned. If the VAE is severe (does not respond to standard therapy) or continues to progress, the procedure should be terminated. The surgery may be completed at a later date with the patient in a prone position.

## Surgical Crises
### Vascular Injuries
#### Cervical Approaches

Vascular injuries occasionally occur during cervical spine surgery. However, their true incidence is unknown. During ventral approaches the carotid and vertebral arteries are at risk. The carotid artery is fully visualized during ventral exposure of the spine and is therefore rarely injured. Moreover, injury is usually readily identified and controlled with direct pressure, with or without primary vascular repair. Temporary clamping of the carotid artery may be performed while a primary or patch repair of the artery is performed.

Both ventral and dorsal cervical approaches place the vertebral artery at risk for injury. Injury may occur ventrally during lateral dissection of the vertebral body (e.g., during subperiostial elevation of the longus colli muscles or lateral drilling of the uncinate processes). Injury may occur dorsally during far lateral dissection of the lateral masses, C2 or transarticular screw placement, or aggressive foraminotomy. Because the vertebral artery is hidden as it travels through the foramen transversarium, the arterial injury is not readily visualized and is heralded by brisk arterial bleeding. Vertebral artery injury should be suspected in this situation. The first corrective maneuver should be manual pressure and the use of hemostatic agents at the site of suspected injury. Once control of the bleeding has been attained, the anesthesiologist has time to "catch up" with regard to volume replacement and, if appropriate, blood transfusion. Proximal and distal control of the artery should be sought. From either a ventral or dorsal approach, the transverse process should be dissected to expose the artery one level above and below the injury. A high-speed drill with a diamond tip burr may be used to open the foramen transversarium and expose the artery. An aneurysm clip can be placed for temporary

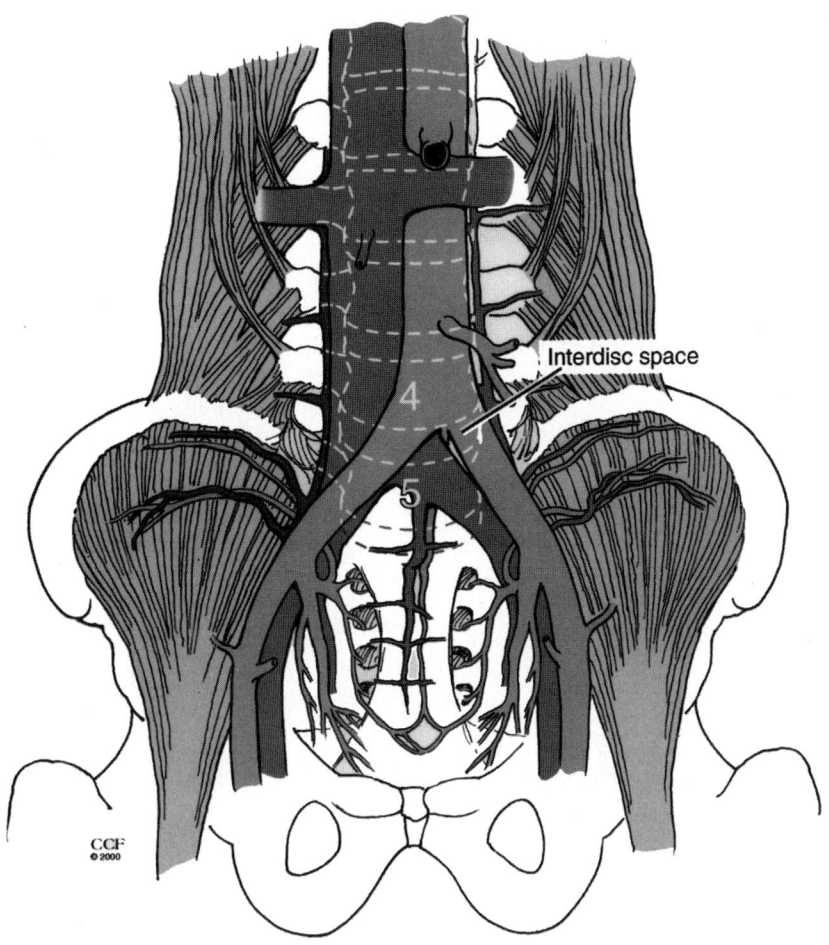

**Figure 172.4** Anatomically, the left common iliac artery ventral to the fourth lumbar disc space. This makes it the most vulnerable artery to injury during lumbar discectomy.

control of bleeding during injury repair.[8] Primary repair of the artery should be considered. If the artery cannot be reconstructed, it should be ligated proximally and distally. Alternatively, once primary control of the bleeding is attained, the patient may be taken to the endovascular suite and the vertebral artery stented or occluded.

As previously mentioned, vertebral artery injury may also occur during C2 or transarticular screw placement. Brisk arterial bleeding is usually noted during drilling or K-wire placement. Hemorrhage control can be attained by placing the transarticular screw into the drill hole, or the hole may be packed with bone wax. The former option is preferred because it plugs the hole and provides stability. Of importance, the opposite screw should not be drilled or placed because of the high risk of catastrophic sequelae associated with bilateral vertebral artery injury.

### Dorsal Thoracic and Lumbar Approaches

Vascular injury during dorsal thoracic procedures is rare. Therefore, this discussion is limited to dorsal lumbar approaches. Lumbar disc surgery is one of the most commonly performed spine operations. Vascular complications of this procedure are rare but do occur. The true incidence is unknown but is approximately 0.05% to 1.0%.[18]

The most commonly injured vessel is the left common iliac artery. This is due to its anatomical location ventral to the fourth lumbar disc interspace (Figure 172.4).[10] Other vessels potentially injured include the left common iliac vein, right common iliac artery, median sacral artery, aorta, and inferior vena cava.

Vascular injury is usually caused by a pituitary rongeur, with penetration of the ventral annulus fibrosus and a tearing of the vessel.[16] Neither the experience of the surgeon[18] nor the amount of the disc material removed[16] affects the incidence of this injury. The injury is usually not immediately evident to the surgeon because brisk bleeding from the disc interspace is only observed in 25% of such injuries.[16] Moreover, when brisk bleeding is observed, it may be from extradural veins and not an arterial injury.[18]

The injury is usually recognized in the recovery room. The patient most often is hypotensive, tachycardic, and with abdominal distension and pain. Pallor with a diminished pulse is also usually present. The patient should immediately be taken back to the operating room for laparotomy. Cross clamping the aorta allows for resuscitation.[16] All vessels should be inspected carefully. A tear in a vein may be primarily repaired with suture. The iliac artery may be divided to gain access to an injured vein. It must then be re-anastomosed. An arterial injury may be repaired primarily or with an interposition graft. If an internal iliac vessel (artery or vein) has been damaged, it may be simply ligated[16] if repair is not possible.

### Ventral Thoracic and Lumbar Approaches

Ventral approaches to the lumbar spine have increased the incidence of vascular crises. These vascular injuries usually occur during the exposure. The chance of injury is heightened if preoperative radiation therapy was used or osteomyelitis is present. Potentially injured vessels include the left iliac vein, the iliolumbar vein, the middle sacral vessels, and an arterial injury such as the left iliac artery. During ventral exposure and dissection, the middle sacral vessels (Figure 172.5A) and iliolumbar vein (Figure 172.5B) should be identified and ligated. If sudden hemorrhage occurs, direct pressure is applied to the vena cava and identification of the injured vessel is attempted. A torn lumbar or iliolumbar vein may be clamped and ligated. If an iliac vein injury is suspected, direct pressure should be applied and proximal and distal control of the vein gained. The perforation can then be repaired primarily.[22] If an artery is injured, proximal and distal control must be attained and the injury repaired, either primarily or with an interposition graft.

The aorta is rarely injured in the upper lumbar and thoracic region. This injury should be treated with immediate thoracotomy and/or laparotomy to repair the vessel. If suspected in the recovery room and the patient is stable, angiography should first be performed to identify the injury[7] prior to repair.

### Iliac Crest Graft Harvest

The superior gluteal artery is rarely injured during dorsal iliac crest bone graft harvesting. The incidence of this injury is not known. The artery is usually injured during exposure of the iliac crest. This occurs during the inadvertent placement of a sharp self-retaining retractor into the sciatic notch.[11] If encountered and the vessel is easily identified, it should be ligated. Because of vessel retraction, this is usually not possible. If it is not easily identified, the operative site should be packed and the patient taken to the angiography suite for embolization. The primary operation may be finished the next day. Direct surgical exploration and ligation is possible but requires a ventral retroperitoneal approach because the vessel usually retracts to an intrapelvic location.[12] This extensive procedure is rarely indicated in the modern era of endovascular therapy.

### Visceral Injuries

The majority of visceral injuries are not considered to be a crisis to the spine surgeon. These injuries include intestinal and ureteral injury. They are usually discovered after the operation and are dealt with postoperatively. One exception is esophageal injury. The incidence of this type of injury is unknown and rare. As previously noted, many of these injuries are discovered weeks or months after an operation. Nevertheless, one may be presented with an esophageal injury during the procedure. It is most com-

monly caused by retraction. If noted during surgery, the tear may be primarily repaired with interrupted resorbable sutures in a single layer. A nasogastric tube should be placed, and broad-spectrum antibiotics started and continued for at least 3 days. An esophagram should be obtained around day 7 and, if normal, oral feeding may be started.

Esophageal perforation may be noted in the recovery room by the observation of significant subcutaneous emphysema. The patient should be taken back to the operating room immediately for exploration. Any esophageal perforation should be repaired as previously described. Because of contamination, the wound may be left open. Consideration must be given to placing a tissue layer between the fresh suture line and the bone graft. The sternal head of the sternocleidomastoid muscle may be reflected and sutured to the contralateral paravertebral muscles to accomplish this.[20] The surgeon should strongly consider the removal of the ventral spinal implant, if placed.

### Durotomy

A durotomy can certainly be a crisis during spine surgery. Durotomies are often readily repaired (e.g., small dorsal tears that requires one simple stitch). However, a ventral tear may require a dorsal durotomy to repair the ventral defect. A dural tear is one of the most common complications of spinal surgery. It occurs in approximately 1% to 17% of cases.[6,21] Its management has been somewhat controversial. Opinions differ as to whether or not there is a place for a subfascial drain or number of days of bed rest that are optimal postoperatively in order to facilitate adequate healing of the defect. Despite the controversy, most agree that durotomies should be repaired primarily, if possible. Of significant note is that unintended durotomies have been found to result in no substantial difference in final clinical outcome of operative procedures on the lumbar spine.[21]

Dural tears, if observed, should usually be repaired primarily. The type of suture and suture technique is the surgeon's choice. The authors favor 4-0 Neurolon (Ethicon, Sumerville, NJ) suture, using a running locking technique. Adequate exposure of the tear must be achieved before suturing. Proper illumination and often magnification (loupe/microscope) are optimal. After exposure, a surgical patty is used over the tear and a smaller sucker tip is used. If the surgeon believes that primary closure may lead to excessive tension on the nerve roots, a patch may be used. There are many patch varieties available, including synthetic, cadaveric, and autologous (the authors prefer autologous tissue). If there is a small defect, the lumbar fascia may be used, which is secured to the dura mater with interrupted sutures. If a larger defect is encountered, fascia lata may be used. With very large dural defects requiring patch placement, fibrin glue may be considered.

Once the repair has been accomplished, a Valsalva maneuver should be performed to check for leak. If any is present, it should be over-sewn. A dry piece of Gelfoam may be placed over the suture line. Next, the more superficial tissues should be tightly and meticulously closed in layers. A few muscle sutures are placed using non-absorbable O-gauge braided suture. The fascia is then closed with the

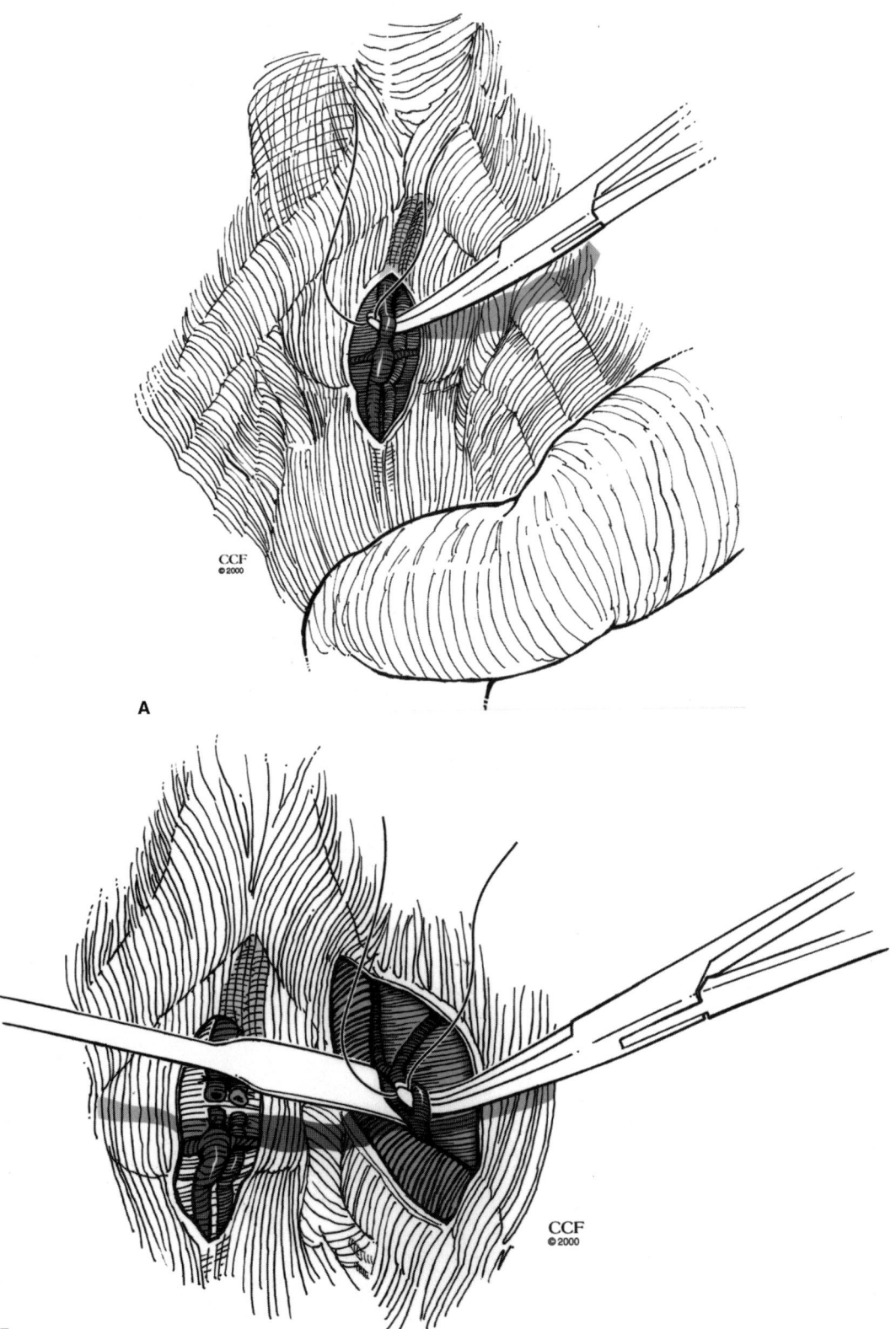

**Figure 172.5** During dissection for a ventral lumbar approach, the middle sacral vessels (**A**) and iliolumbar vein (**B**) should be identified and ligated.

same suture in a watertight manner. Next, 2-0 absorbable suture may be used to close as many layers as possible, including Scarpa's fascia and dermis. The skin should be carefully closed, usually with sutures. Interrupted vertical mattress closure should be considered because of its excel-

lent skin approximation characteristics. There is controversy regarding the use of a subfascial drain. A relatively recent paper by Wang et al.[21] demonstrated no increased incidence of myelocutaneous fistula with such drains. One can conclude that subfascial drains may be used with relative safety. One may also consider the placement of a subarachnoid drain during surgery. However, there is no conclusive evidence regarding efficacy in this regard.

## Facet Reduction

Unilateral or bilateral cervical facet dislocation often presents as a crisis to the spine surgeon. Traditionally, this problem has been addressed by closed reduction followed by dorsal arthrodesis and/or external orthosis. These procedures have stood the test of time but are not without risk. Catastrophic neurologic injury has been reported after performing closed reduction for cervical facet dislocation.[5] Until this report, little attention was given to the possibility of traumatic disc herniation associated with facet dislocation. A ventral approach to this problem allows decompression, reduction, and stabilization, and it avoids the risk of catastrophic neurologic sequela from open dorsal or closed reduction[15]

A patient with suspected unilateral or bilateral cervical facet dislocation should be considered for undergoing plain radiography, CT, and MRI. This confirms the dislocation and presence or absence of traumatic disc herniation.

For a ventral reduction and stabilization approach, the patient is positioned in the supine position and a standard approach for anterior cervical discectomy is performed. Once the discectomy is complete, vertebral body posts are placed at 10- to 20-degree diverging angles to each other (Figure 172.6,*A*). Distraction is applied, which disengages the locked facets (Figure 172.6,*B*). A dorsally directed force is then applied to the rostral body by manual pressure (Figure 172.6,*C*) or curette (Figure 172.6,*D*); this facilitates reduction. Interbody disc spreaders placed at an angle and then rotated rostrally may also be used for the reduction (Figure 172.7). After this maneuver, a plain radiograph is performed to acknowledge the reduction. If there is lack of reduction, the procedure is performed again. If reduction cannot be achieved, perhaps related to comminuted facet fractures, the patient should then undergo dorsal reduction and arthrodesis followed by ventral arthrodesis. Once adequate reduction is obtained, standard iliac crest bone harvesting and strut placement is performed. A ventral cervical fixation device is then placed.

## Level Identification

Locating the appropriate spinal level intraoperatively may be challenging at times. Identifying the correct level during all spine surgery cases is paramount. Usually, this is accomplished by performing a lateral intraoperative radiograph with a marker in place. In the lumbar spine, an Alice clamp may be placed on the presumed most appropriate spinous process, along with a Penfield no. 4 under the same lamina, both directed perpendicular to the spine.

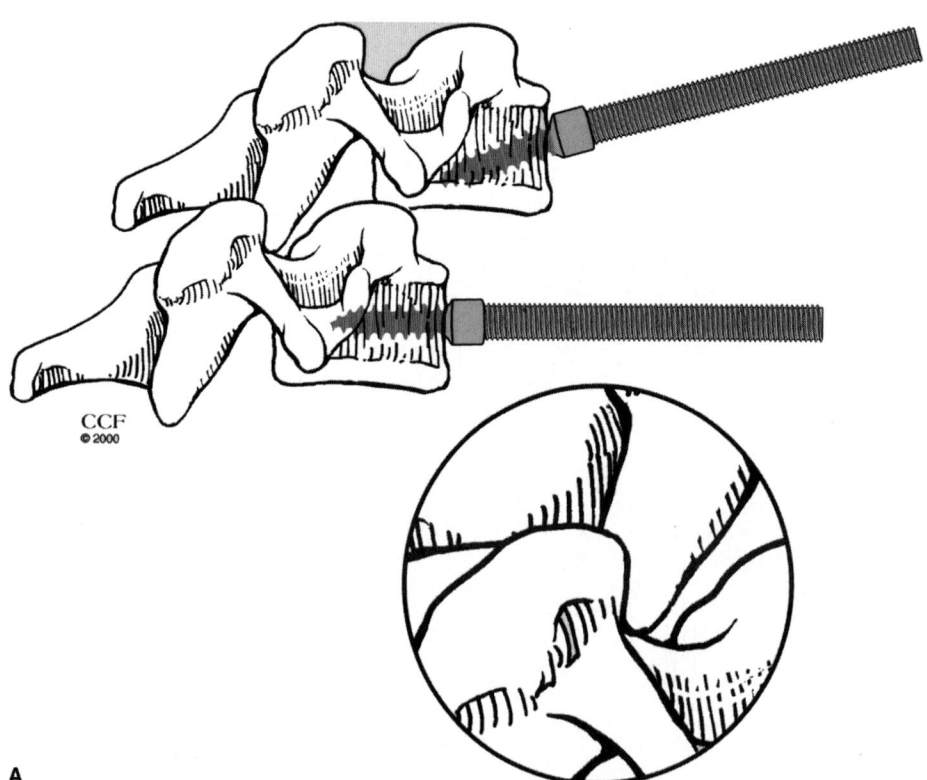

**A**

**Figure 172.6** Cervical facet dislocation management via the ventral approach. (**A**) The vertebral posts may be placed at 10- to 20-degree diverging angles to each other. When distraction is applied this will allow disengagement of the facets.

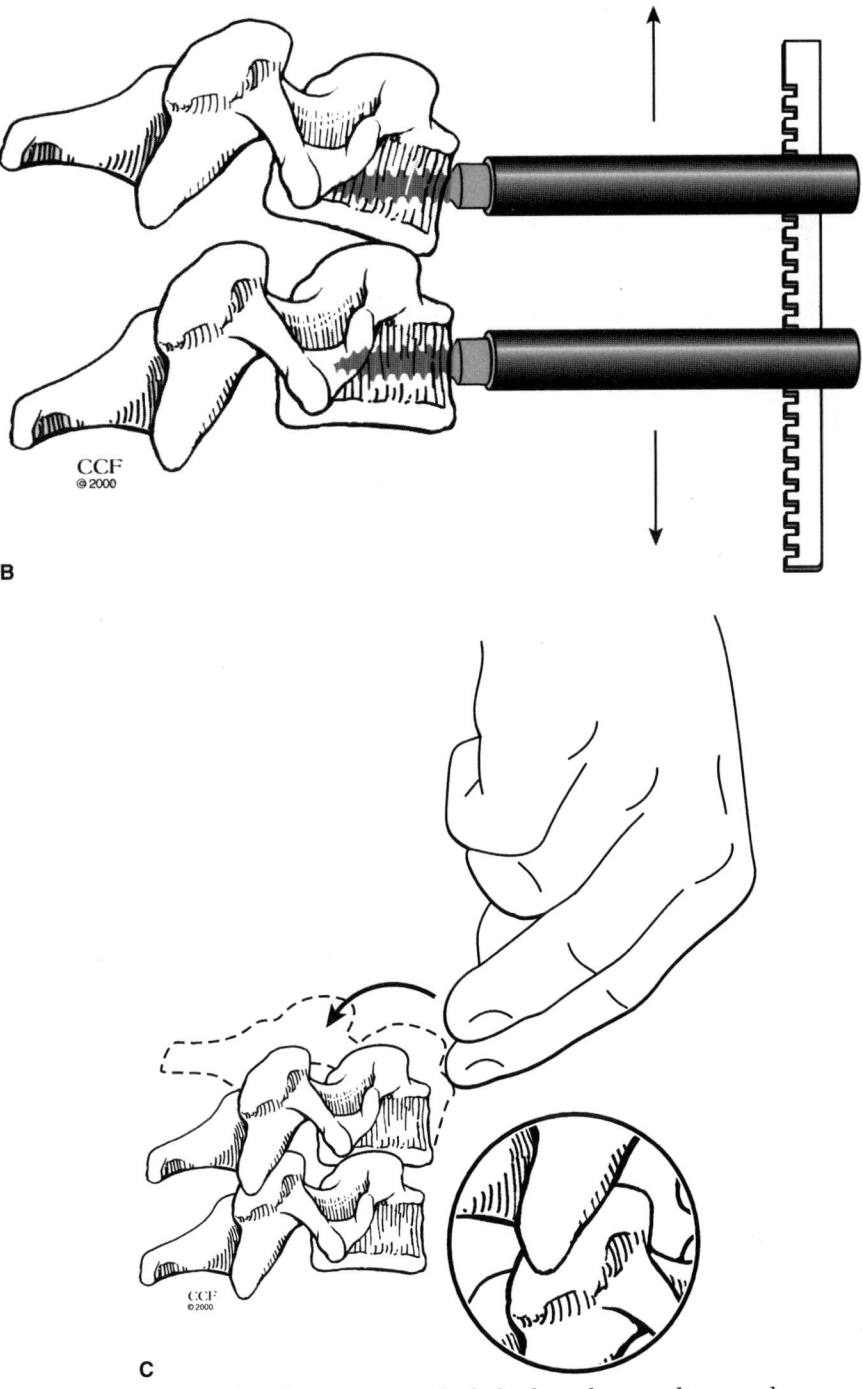

**Figure 172.6** *cont'd* (**B**) When distraction is applied, the facets become disengaged. (**C**) The rostral body may be reduced by manual pressure.

*Continued*

A lateral radiograph is obtained. Counting is performed from the sacrum to the "marked" level. Localization in the cervical spine is also accomplished in the same fashion but by counting down from the occiput.

Localization in the thoracic spine tends to be more difficult. Often an anterior posterior radiograph is obtained and ribs counted to the desired level. In the authors' opinion, this is often misleading. Localization with lateral radiographs may be used as in the lumbar or cervical spine. Marking may be performed as in the lumbar spine, but care must be taken in placing an instrument under the lamina because of the narrow spinal canal dimensions at this level. A marker may also be placed on the transverse process. A large plate radiograph is then performed, which includes the sacrum or the occiput. Counting is performed from either the occiput or the sacrum to the marker. At times there is inadequate visualization using this technique. In these circumstances, a marker (Alice clamp) may be placed at the most rostral or caudal level (spinous or transverse process) exposed. A lateral cervical or lumbar radiograph is then obtained, which

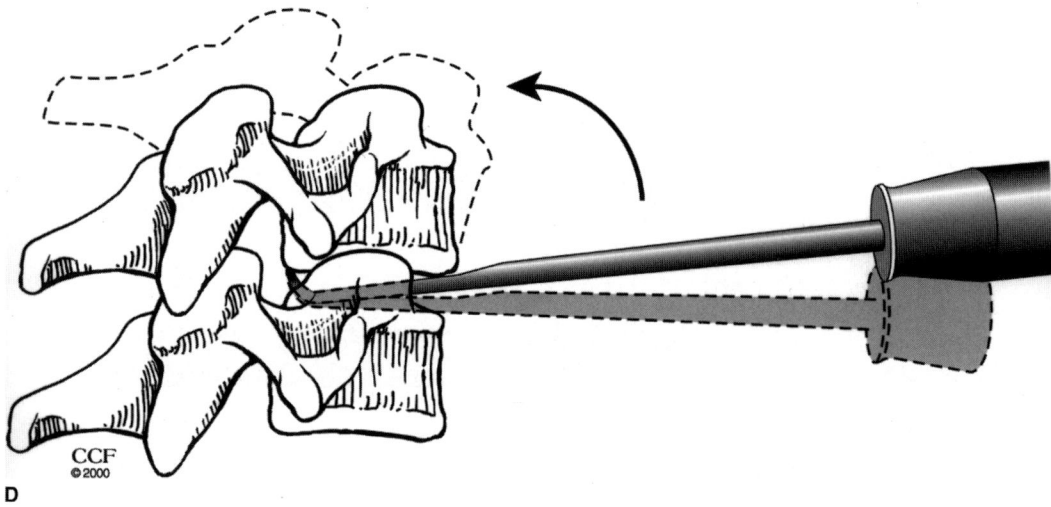

**Figure 172.6** *cont'd* (**D**) The rostral body may be reduced by placing a curette into the disc space and rotating it rostrally.

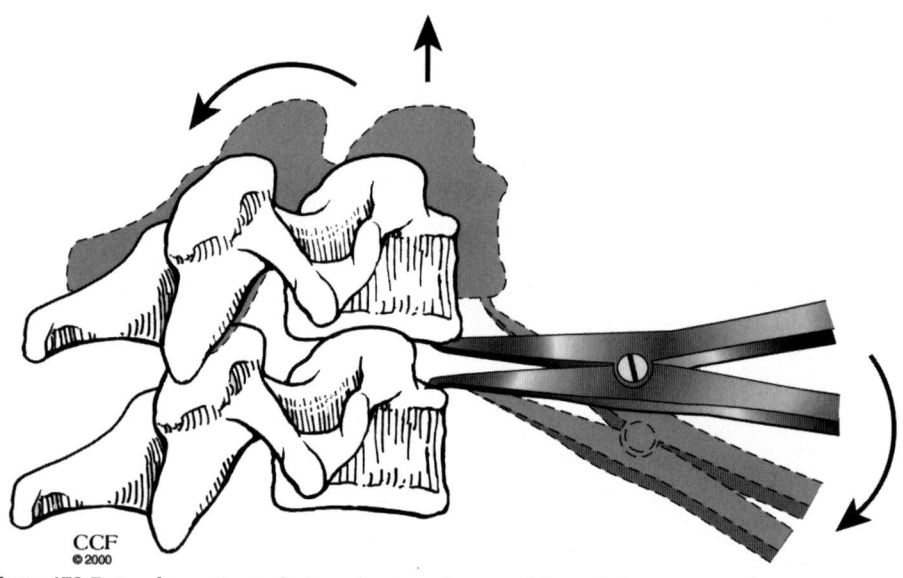

**Figure 172.7** An alternative technique for ventral cervical facet dislocation management. Disc interspace spreaders may be placed into the disc space once the facets are disengaged. Rotating the spreaders rostrally facilitates reduction.

includes the occiput or sacrum respectively, and levels are counted to this marker. A lateral radiograph of the thoracic spine is then performed, and levels are counted from the prior marked level to the pathology (which also has been marked with an Alice clamp).

Care must also be taken when marking the pathological level once it is identified. Some surgeons mark the lamina and interspinous ligament with a marking pen. However, this mark may be washed off by blood or irrigation. The level may also be marked with a small bite off the spinous process with a rongeur, or a suture may be placed through the spinous process.

If the expected pathology is not observed at the expected level, the appropriate location should be confirmed with a repeat radiograph. Lateral radiographs should continue to be performed with different marking techniques until the surgeon is satisfied that he or she is operating at the correct level.

Although radiographs can help identify pathological levels, they are only helpful if the radiographs can be correlated with preoperatively acquired images that identified the pathology. Myelography can occasionally be helpful in the thoracic spine by providing a radiographic correlate that "relates anatomically" to the pathology. Ribs can then be used with confidence as markers. This eliminates errors related to discrepancies between radiographs and MRI. Wide AP myelographic views should be obtained so that the ribs can be visualized (particularly the lowest rib) and counted.

Trajectory of beams should be considered when interpreting intraoperative radiographs. The effect of "beam trajectory error" can be minimized by placing the marker as close to the pathology in the sagittal plane as possible (Figure 172.8).

## Electrophysiological Spinal Cord Monitoring

Spinal cord monitoring has become popular, especially for deformity correction, to ensure that neural element injury has not secondarily occurred because of deformity correction maneuvers. Many monitoring techniques are available, and each is measured against the gold standard of the wake-up test (this test consists of lessening the level of anesthesia until the patient is able to follow commands, thus assessing gross motor function). Available monitoring techniques include somatosensory evoked potential (SSEP), motor evoked potential (MEP), spinal evoked potential (SpEP), and electromyographic monitoring (EMG). SSEP and SpEP monitor dorsal column integrity, whereas MEP monitors ventral column integrity. EMG monitors nerve root integrity and may be used continuously[9] or be stimulus evoked.[3] In modern spine surgery, multimodality monitoring may be used. This includes the interrogation of the ventral and dorsal spinal cord as well as the nerve roots.

The efficacies of the aforementioned monitoring techniques have been called into question. False-positive and false-negative test findings for each technique have been documented. The main reasons for a false-negative results include failure to detect minor injury, the temporal difference between the actual injury and the observed change on the monitor, and the discrepancy between the area of the spinal cord injured and the region assessed by the monitoring technique used.[3] Of even greater concern is that there is no recognized standard for the assessment of injury during electrophysiologic monitoring.[3]

Nevertheless, if electrophysiological monitoring is used, the surgeon must have a plan (strategy) for dealing with intraoperative electrophysiological abnormalities. SSEPs are commonly used most. Therefore, there is a substantial experience in treating SSEP changes. If a change is observed (e.g., a 10% change in latency or 50% change in amplitude), it is prudent to alter parameters that could be causing the change. The patient's blood pressure should be elevated (if low) and the temperature of the patient and the room should be increased. Infused blood or IV solution should be warmed. The electrodes should be checked to ensure that there are no technical problems. Inhaled anesthetic agents should be discontinued and barbiturates and opioids used. The oxygen saturation of the patient should be increased (if low). The placement of hydrogen peroxide in the wound may increase local oxygen saturation. If the aforementioned does not return the tracing to baseline, mechanical factors should be considered next. Sublaminar wires or hooks perhaps should be removed, or their position aggressively assessed. A bone graft placed in proximity in time with the SSEP change should be removed and remeasured or reassessed. Distraction forces should be relaxed. Consideration should next be given to performing a wake-up test.

Time should be given for observation of the tracing to return to baseline. The period of observation may be up to 60 minutes. A reformed bone graft should be replaced (if removed), and forces reapplied to the construct (but not in

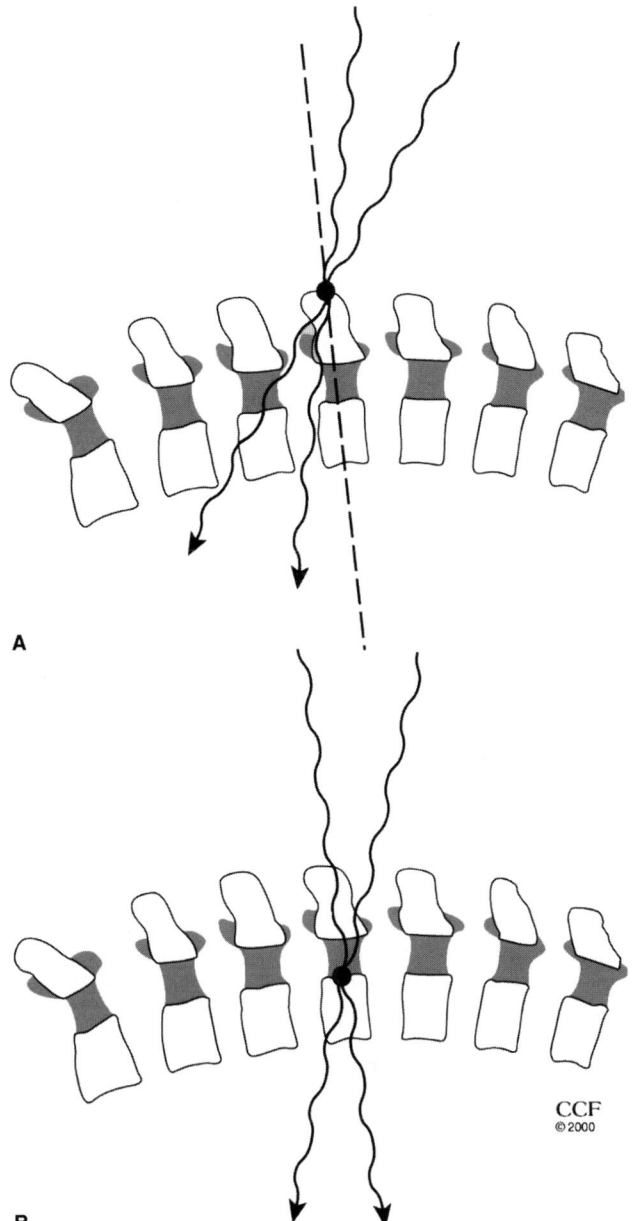

**Figure 172.8** **(A)** With the marker placed on the spinous process *(black dot)*, an alteration in the x-ray beam trajectory may misinterpret the spinal level. The dotted line is the ideal x-ray beam trajectory. Altering the beam angle in a more rostral direction *(wavy lines)* will lead to misinterpretation. In this case a level or two below the marked level will be interpreted as the marked level. **(B)** When the marker is placed near the vertebral body, altering the beam trajectory will not be nearly as misleading. Note: The wavy lines (representing different x-ray trajectories) both pass through the marked level.

excess). If evoked potentials do not return to baseline, only enough force should be placed on the implant to maintain its position. Postoperatively, serial neurologic examinations are in order. Repeat radiography and/or myelography should be considered to document the position of the construct. Aberrantly placed implants should be reexplored in the operating room.

## Neurologic Injuries

Neurologic deficits that are new and unexpected following surgery are indeed a crisis. They are most commonly observed in the recovery room immediately following the emergence from anesthesia. Early diagnosis may be imperative in many cases.

In others, an irreversible neural element injury may have already occurred. When the surgeon cannot honestly rule out an intraoperative event that might have caused such a deficit, an aggressive approach to diagnosis should be considered immediately. Bone graft misplacement, instrumentation encroachment on neural elements, and postoperative hemorrhage should be ruled out. Emergent imaging is often indicated and may include radiography, CT, and/or MRI. If an abnormality is found, it should be surgically rectified immediately, if appropriate. If there is a profound or progressive neurologic deficit, imaging is often not performed and the patient is taken back to the operating room immediately for exploration of the previous site of surgery. The "offending culprit" (e.g., epidural hematoma) is most often evident and removed and/or repaired. If no hematoma is found, the construct should be inspected. As previously described, the graft should be removed and hooks, wires, screws, and rods should be addressed. If encroachment on neural elements is identified, the construct, including the bone graft, may be removed, resized, and replaced. If there is no apparent abnormality demonstrated at the time of surgical exploration, the patient should be taken for emergent MRI. The MRI should include the region of the spine rostral and caudal to the surgical site. This may disclose a distant epidural hematoma.

Ischemia caused by radicular artery injury can only be diagnosed on an exclusionary basis. An anterior spinal cord syndrome, which is often preceded by a surgical obliteration of the contents of a neuroforaminal that includes a radicular artery such as the artery of Adamkiewicz, may be untreatable. Angiography is usually not helpful because of the variable presence of vital radicular arteries in the normal situation. Treatment of such cases should consist of the maintenance of normotension (or slight hypertension), the establishment and maintenance of a euvolemic state, and the elimination of external neural element compression.

Complete pharmacological reversal of anesthesia in situations where a new neurological deficit is suspect is imperative. Naloxone should be administered in sufficient doses to ensure reversal of opioids given during surgery. As an aside, narcotic antagonists have been shown to reverse ischemic neurological deficits.[1,4] Therefore, the administration of naloxone should perhaps be considered more liberally under such circumstances.

## Summary

Crises in spine surgery are not common, but when they occur, one must have the knowledge to effectively deal with them. Many spine "emergencies" are not identified in the operating room, but rather in the recovery room. The period for crisis management then extends beyond the operating room and into the perioperative period, requiring continued vigilance by the surgeon. These issues should be dealt with in an expedient and thorough manner to prevent further complications.

## REFERENCES

1. Baskin DS, Hosobuchi Y: Naloxone reversal of ischemic neurologic deficits in man. *Lancet* 2:272-275, 1981.
2. Bedford RF, Perkins-Pearson NAK: PEEP for treatment of venous air embolism. *Anesthesiology* 57:A379, 1982(abstr).
3. Ben-David B: Spinal cord monitoring. *Orthop Clin North Am* 19:427-448, 1988.
4. Benzel EC, Khare V, Fowler MR: Effects of naloxone and nalmefene in rat spinal cord injury induced by the ventral compression technique. *J Spinal Disord* 5:75-77, 1992.
5. Eismont FJ, Arena MJ, Green BA: Extrusion of an intervertebral disc associated with Traumatic subluxation or dislocation of cervical facets. Case report. *J Bone Joint Surg (Am)* 73:1555-1560, 1991.
6. Eismont FJ, Wiesel SW, Rothman RH: Treatment of dural tears associated with spinal surgery. *J Bone Joint Surg* 63-A:1132-1136, 1981.
7. Frost EAM: Some inquiries in neuroanesthesia and neurological supportive care. *J Neurosurg* 60:673-686, 1984.
8. Golfinos JG, Dickman CA, Zabramski JM, *et al:* Repair of vertebral artery injury during anterior cervical decompression. *Spine* 19:2552-2556, 1994.
9. Holland NR, Kostuik JP: Continuous electromyographic monitoring to detect nerve root injury during thoracolumbar scoliosis surgery. *Spine* 22:2547-2550, 1997.
10. Jarstfer BS, Rich NM: The challenge of arteriovenous fistula formation following disc surgery: a collective review. *J Trauma* 16:726-733, 1976.
11. Kahn B: Superior gluteal artery laceration, a complication of iliac bone graft surgery. *Clin Orthop* 140: 204-207, 1979.
12. Lim EVA, Lavadia WT, Roberts JM: Superior gluteal artery injury during iliac bone grafting for spinal fusion. *Spine* 21:2376-2378, 1996.
13. Mammoto T, Hayashi Y, Ohnishi Y, Kuro M: Incidence of venous and paradoxical air embolism in neurosurgical patients in the sitting position: Detection by transesophogeal echocardiography. *Acta Anaesthesiol Scand* 42:643-647, 1998.
14. Munson E: Transfer of nitrous oxide into body air cavities. *Br J Anaesth* 27:202-209, 1974.
15. Ordonez BJ, Benzel EC, Naderi S, Weller SJ: Cervical facet dislocation: techniques for ventral reduction and stabilization. *J Neurosurg (Spine 1)* 92:18-23, 2000.
16. Raptis S, Quigley F, Barker S: Vascular complications of elective lower lumbar disc surgery. *Aust N Z J Surg* 64:216-219, 1994.
17. Sun WZ, Huan FY, Kung KL, *et al:* Successful cardiopulmonary resuscitation of two patients in the prone position using reversed precordial compression. *Anesthesiology* 77:202-204, 1992.
18. Szolar DH, Preidler KW, Steiner H, *et al:* Vascular complications in lumbar disk surgery: report of four cases. *Neuroradiology* 38:521-525, 1996.

19. Tobias JD, Mencio GA, Atwood R, Gurwitz GS: Intraoperative cardiopulmonary resuscitation in the prone position. *J Pediatr Surg* 29:1537-1538, 1994.

20. van Berge Henegouwen DP, Roukema JA, de Nie JC, vd Werken C: Esophageal perforation during surgery on the cervical spine. *Neurosurgery* 29:766-768, 1991.

21. Wang JC, Bohlman HH, Riew KD: Dural tears secondary to operations on the lumbar spine. *J Bone Joint Surg* 80-A:1728-1731, 1998.

22. Watkins R: Anterior lumbar interbody fusion surgical complications. *Clin Orthop* 284:47-53, 1992.

23. Young ML, Smith DS, Murtagh F, *et al:* Comparison of surgical and anesthetic complications in neurosurgical patients experiencing venous air embolism in the sitting position. *Neurosurgery* 18:157-161, 1986.

# Index

Note: Page numbers followed by the letter b refer to boxes; those followed by the letter f refer to figures, those followed by the letter t refer to tables.